a LANGE medical book

CURRENT
EMERGENCY
Diagnosis & Treatment
fifth edition

Edited by

C. Keith Stone, MD
Professor and Chairman
Department of Emergency Medicine
Texas A&M University Health Science Center
Scott & White Memorial Hospital
Temple, Texas

Roger Humphries, MD
Assistant Professor and Residency Director
Department of Emergency Medicine
University of Kentucky College of Medicine
Lexington, Kentucky

Lange Medical Books/McGraw-Hill
Medical Publishing Division

New York   Chicago   San Francisco   Lisbon   London   Madrid   Mexico City   Milan   New Delhi   San Juan   Seoul
Singapore   Sydney   Toronto

Current Emergency Diagnosis & Treatment, 5th Edition

3 4 5 6 7 8 9 0 DOC/DOC 0 9 8 7 6 5 4

ISBN: 0-8385-1450-2

ISSN: 084-2293

Notice

Medicine is an ever-changing science. As new research and clinical experience broaden our knowledge, changes in treatment and drug therapy are required. The editors and the publisher of this work have checked with sources believed to be reliable in their efforts to provide information that is complete and generally in accord with the standards accepted at the time of publication. However, in view of the possibility of human error or changes in medical sciences, neither the editors nor the publisher nor any other party who has been involved in the preparation or publication of this work warrants that the information contained herein is in every respect accurate or complete, and they disclaim all responsibility for any errors or omissions or for the results obtained from use of the information contained in this work. Readers are encouraged to confirm the information contained herein with other sources. For example and in particular, readers are advised to check the product information sheet included in the package of each drug they plan to administer to be certain that the information contained in this work is accurate and that changes have not been made in the recommended dose or in the contraindications for administration. This recommendation is of particular importance in connection with new or infrequently used drugs.

This book was set in Adobe Garamond by Pine Tree Composition, Inc.
The editors were Shelley Reinhardt, Harriet Lebowitz, and Nicky Fernando.
The production supervisor was Philip Galea.
The book designer was Eve Siegel.
The cover designer was Mary McKeon.
The index was prepared by Coughlin Indexing Services, Inc.
RR Donnelley was the printer and binder.

This book is printed on acid-free paper.

INTERNATIONAL EDITION ISBN 0-07-121975-7
Copyright © 2004. Exclusive rights by The McGraw-Hill Companies, Inc., for manufacture and export. This book cannot be reexported from the country to which it is consigned by McGraw-Hill. The International Edition is not available in North America.

Contents

Pharmacotherapy in Advanced Cardiac Life Support . . . . Inside Front Cover

Authors vii

Preface xiii

SECTION I. SPECIAL ASPECTS OF EMERGENCY MEDICINE 1

Chapter 1. Approach to the Emergency Department Patient. 1
Mary Nan S. Mallory, MD, RDMS & Robert Perry Pringle Jr. MD

Chapter 2. Prehospital Emergency Medical Services 6
Eric M. Sergienko, MD, & Thomas N. Bottoni, MD

Chapter 3. Nuclear, Biologic, & Chemical Agents; Weapons of Mass Destruction 20
Michael W. Stava, MD, & Joachim Franklin, MD

Chapter 4. Multicasualty Incidents & Disasters 42
Louis J. Kroot, MD, & Robert B. Gray, MD

Chapter 5. Legal Aspects of Emergency Care. 60
Charles A. Eckerline, Jr., MD, FACEP, & Steven D. Rothert, MD, JD

Chapter 6. Emergency Procedures. 73
William Randall Partin, MD

SECTION II. MANAGEMENT OF COMMON EMERGENCY PROBLEMS 145

Chapter 7. Basic & Advanced Cardiac Life Support 145
Eric M. Sergienko, MD, & Thomas N. Bottoni, MD

Chapter 8. Compromised Airway 167
Harriet L. Boozer, MD, & Melissa M. Cheeseman, MD

Chapter 9. Shock. 191
Peter W. Greenwald, MD

Chapter 10. The Multiply Injured Patient. 208
Julia Martin, MD, & Michael McClurg, MD

Chapter 11. Dyspnea, Respiratory Distress, & Respiratory Failure 222
Sabina A. Braithwaite, MD, & Debra G. Perina, MD

Chapter 12. Chest Pain 240
Sean P. Barbabella, DO & William R. Dennis, Jr., MD

Chapter 13. Abdominal Pain 257
  Roger Humphries, MD, & Jon Andrew Russell, MD

Chapter 14. Gastrointestinal Bleeding 283
  Charles W. Erdman, MD, & James J. Mensching, DO, FACEP

Chapter 15. Diarrhea & Vomiting 296
  Phillip A. Clement, MD, & Jason A. Gardiner, MD

Chapter 16. Coma 311
  Steven D. Kelley, MD, & Adam Saperston, MD, MS

Chapter 17. Syncope, Seizures, & Other Causes of Episodic Loss of Consciousness 332
  Adam Saperston, MD, MS

Chapter 18. Weakness & Stroke 348
  Heidi P. Cordi, MD, MS

Chapter 19. Headache 379
  C. Keith Stone, MD, & Nancy J. Antonacci, MD

Chapter 20. Delirium & Acute Confusional States 391
  Eric W. Flach, MD, Timothy A. Coakley, MD, & James J. Mensching, MD, DO, FACEP

Chapter 21. Arthritis & Back Pain 404
  Roger L. Humphries, MD, & David O'Keefe, MD

SECTION III. TRAUMA EMERGENCIES 421

Chapter 22. Head Injuries 421
  Stephen C. Ausband, MD, FACEP, & Ritu Sahni, MD, MPH

Chapter 23. Maxillofacial & Neck Trauma 435
  Fermin S. Godinez, DO, & Susan J. Letterle, MD

Chapter 24. Chest Trauma 454
  James Svenson, MD, MS, & Désirée La Charité, MD

Chapter 25. Abdominal Trauma 467
  Luis E. Rodriguez, MD, & John E. Gough, MD, FACEP

Chapter 26. Genitourinary Trauma 477
  Geoffrey A. Wiss, MD, Claudia Whitaker, MD, & Robert B. Dunne, MD, FACEP

Chapter 27. Vertebral Column & Spinal Cord Trauma 493
  Robert Casey Wilson, MD, & Louis J. Kroot, MD

Chapter 28. Orthopedic Emergencies 510
  Luis E. Rodriguez, MD, & John E. Gough, MD, FACEP

Chapter 29. Hand Trauma 548
  Adam Saperston, MD, MS

Chapter 30. Wound Care 573
  Louis J. Kroot, MD, & David Hurst, MD

SECTION IV. NONTRAUMA EMERGENCIES 599

Chapter 31. Eye Emergencies 599
  William R. Dennis, Jr., MD, & Alia M. Dennis, MD

Chapter 32. ENT Emergencies: Disorders of the Ear, Nose, Sinuses, Oropharynx, & Mouth 626
  David C. Van, MD, MS

Chapter 33. Pulmonary Emergencies 653
  Christopher R. Pund, MD, & C. Keith Stone, MD

Chapter 34. Cardiac Emergencies 675
  Roger L. Humphries, MD, & C. Keith Stone, MD

Chapter 35. Cardiac Arrhythmias 694
  David A. Wald, DO

Chapter 36. Obstetric & Gynecologic Emergencies & Rape 725
  Melissa Platt, MD, & Mary Nan Mallory, MD, RDMS

Chapter 37. Genitourinary Emergencies 750
  Susan J. Letterle, MD

Chapter 38. Vascular Emergencies 766
  Scott W. Hines, MD, & James J. Mensching, MD, DO, FACEP

Chapter 39. Hematologic Emergencies 788
  J. Stephan Stapczynski, MD, & Geoffrey A. Martin, MD

Chapter 40. Infectious Disease Emergencies 824
  Brian Hawkins, MD, & Daniel F. Danzl, MD

Chapter 41. Metabolic & Endocrine Emergencies 867
  Micheal D. Rush, MD, & Wason W.S. Louie, MD

Chapter 42. Fluid, Electrolyte, & Acid-Base Emergencies 890
  Michael E. Chansky, MD, FACEP, Andrew Nyce, MD, & Jason Friedman, MD

Chapter 43. Burns & Smoke Inhalation 917
  Melissa M. Cheeseman, MD, & Harriet L. Boozer, MD

Chapter 44. Disorders Due to Physical & Environmental Agents 930
  D. Shannon Waters, MD, & Rebecca C. Bowers, MD

Chapter 45. Poisoning. 963
    D. Shannon Waters, MD, Darren K. Waters, MD, & Travis Sewalls, MD

Chapter 46. Dermatologic Emergencies. 1012
    Joseph A. Salomone III, MD, FAAEM, & Martha Ann Pratt, MD

Chapter 47. Psychiatric Emergencies. 1026
    Gregory Hall, MD, & Denis J. Fitzgerald, MD

Chapter 48. Pediatric Emergencies 1039
    Roger L. Humphries, MD, Keith D. Bricking, MD, & Thomas M. Huhn, MD

Index 1103

Pharmacotherapy in Advanced Cardiac Life Support (continued) . . . . Inside Back Cover

Authors

Nancy J. Antonacci, MD
President, E=mc^2, Lexington, Kentucky
Headache

Stephen C. Ausband, MD, FACEP
Assistant Professor, Department of Emergency
    Medicine, The Brody School of Medicine, East
    Carolina University, Greenville, North Carolina
ausbands@mail.ecu.edu
Head Injuries

Sean P. Barbabella, DO
Chief Resident, Naval Medical Center Portsmouth,
    Portsmouth, Virginia
spbarbabella@mar.med.navy.mil
Chest Pain

Harriet L. Boozer, MD
Emergency Medicine Staff Physician, Carolina Care,
    PA, Columbia, South Carolina
hboozer@hotmail.com
Compromised Airway; Burns & Smoke Inhalation

Thomas N. Bottoni, MD
Attending Staff Emergency Physician, Sentara
    Careplex Hampton, Hampton, Virginia
*Prehospital Emergency Medical Services; Basic &
Advanced Cardiac Life Support*

Rebecca C. Bowers, MD
Resident Physician, Department of Emergency
    Medicine, University of Kentucky Medical
    Center, Lexington
Disorders Due to Physical & Environmental Agents

Sabina A. Braithwaite, MD
Assistant Professor, Department of Emergency
    Medicine, University of Virginia School of
    Medicine, Charlottesville
sabina@virginia.edu
Dyspnea, Respiratory Distress, & Respiratory Failure

Keith D. Bricking, MD
Resident Physician, Department of Emergency
    Medicine, Indiana University School of Medicine,
    Indianapolis, Indiana
kbrickin@iupui.edu
Pediatric Emergencies

Michael E. Chansky, MD, FACEP
Chairman and Associate Professor of Emergency
    Medicine and Internal Medicine, Robert Wood
    Johnson Medical School, Camden, New Jersey;
    Cooper University Hospital, Camden, New Jersey
chansky-michael@cooperhealth.edu
Fluid, Electrolyte, & Acid-Base Emergencies

Melissa M. Cheeseman, MD
Assistant Professor and Emergency Medicine
    Physician, Department of Emergency Medicine,
    University of Kentucky College of Medicine,
    Lexington
Compromised Airway; Burns & Smoke Inhalation

Phillip A. Clement, MD
Assistant Clinical Professor and Director of Under-
    graduate Education, Department of Emergency
    Medicine, The Brody School of Medicine, East
    Carolina University, Greenville, North Carolina
clementp@mail.ecu.edu
Diarrhea & Vomiting

Timothy A. Coakley, MD
Chief Resident, Naval Medical Center Portsmouth,
    Portsmouth, Virginia
Delirium & Acute Confusional States

Heidi P. Cordi, MD, MS
Assistant Clinical Professor of Medicine, Columbia
    University College of Physicians and Surgeons;
    Assistant Attending Physician, The New York
    Presbyterian Hospital, New York, New York
hcordimd@usa.net
Weakness & Stroke

Daniel F. Danzl, MD
Professor and Chair, Department of Emergency
  Medicine, University of Louisville School of
  Medicine, Louisville, Kentucky
dandanzl@pol.net
Infectious Disease Emergencies

Alia M. Dennis, MD
Pediatric Chief Resident, Childrens Hospital of the
  Kings Daughters, Norfolk, Virginia
dennisa120@cox.net
Eye Emergencies

William R. Dennis, Jr., MD
Attending Staff Physician and Instructor, Department
  of Emergency Medicine, Naval Medical Center
  Portsmouth, Portsmouth, Virginia
dennisw120@cox.net
Chest Pain; Eye Emergencies

Robert K. Dunne, MD, FACEP
Assistant Professor, Department of Emergency
  Medicine, Wayne State University School of
  Medicine, Detroit, Michigan; Attending
  Physician, Department of Emergency Medicine,
  Sinai-Grace Hospital, Detroit, Michigan
rkdunne@sprintmail.com
Genitourinary Trauma

Charles A. Eckerline, Jr., MD, FACEP
Associate Professor, Department of Emergency
  Medicine, University of Kentucky College of
  Medicine, Lexington
caecke1@uky.edu
Legal Aspects of Emergency Care

Charles W. Erdman, MD
Resident, Department of Emergency Medicine,
  Naval Medical Center Portsmouth, Portsmouth,
  Virginia
cwerdman@mar.med.navy.mil
Gastrointestinal Bleeding

Denis J. Fitzgerald, MD
Assistant Professor, Department of Military and
  Emergency Medicine, Uniformed Services
  University of the Health Sciences, Bethesda,
  Maryland; Adjunct Assistant Professor,
  Department of Emergency Medicine,
  University of Cincinnati College of Medicine,
  Cincinnati, Ohio
Psychiatric Emergencies

Eric W. Flach, MD
Intern, Department of Emergency Medicine, Naval
  Medical Center Portsmouth, Portsmouth,
  Virginia
flache@bellsouth.net
Delirium & Acute Confusional States

Joachim Franklin, MD
Resident, Department of Emergency Medicine,
  University of Kentucky College of Medicine,
  Lexington
*Nuclear, Biologic, & Chemical Agents; Weapons of
Mass Destruction*

Jason A. Gardiner, MD
Senior Resident, Department of Emergency
  Medicine, The Brody School of Medicine,
  East Carolina University, Greenville, North
  Carolina
gardinerj@mail.ecu.edu
Diarrhea & Vomiting

Fermin S. Godinez, DO
Chief Resident, Department of Emergency
  Medicine, Naval Medical Center Portsmouth,
  Portsmouth, Virginia
Maxillofacial & Neck Trauma

John E. Gough, MD, FACEP
Associate Professor and Physician, Department of
  Emergency Medicine, East Carolina University,
  Greenville, North Carolina
goughj@mail.ecu.edu
Abdominal Pain; Orthopedic Emergencies

Robert B. Gray, MD
Resident, Department of Emergency Medicine,
  University of Kentucky Medical Center,
  Lexington
rgraydoc@hotmail.com
Multicasualty Incidents & Disasters

Peter W. Greenwald, MD
Instructor in Clinical Medicine, Columbia College
  of Physicians and Surgeons; Attending Physician,
  Columbia Presbyterian Hospital, New York
pg2014@columbia.edu
Shock

Gregory Hall, MD
Resident, Department of Emergency Medicine, University of Cincinnati College of Medicine, Cincinnati, Ohio
Psychiatric Emergencies

Brian Hawkins, MD
Resident Physician, Department of Emergency Medicine, University of Louisville Hospital, Louisville, Kentucky
bhaw481674@cs.com
Infectious Disease Emergencies

Scott W. Hines, MD
Physician, Department of Emergency Medicine, Naval Medical Center Portsmouth, Portsmouth, Virginia
Vascular Emergencies

Thomas M. Huhn, MD
Resident Physician, Department of Emergency Medicine, University of Kentucky College of Medicine, Lexington
tmhuhn0@uky.edu
Pediatric Emergencies

Roger Humphries, MD
Assistant Professor and Residency Director, Department of Emergency Medicine, University of Kentucky College of Medicine, Lexington
rlhump0@uky.edu
Abdominal Pain; Arthritis & Back Pain; Cardiac Emergencies; Pediatric Emergencies; Inside Front Cover: Drugs Commonly Used Intravenously in Emergencies; Inside Back Cover: Quick Reference Table for Pediatric Resuscitation Equipment by Weight and Age

David Hurst, MD
Resident, Department of Emergency Medicine, University of Kentucky College of Medicine, Lexington
davidghurst@hotmail.com
Wound Care

Steven D. Kelley, MD
Resident, Department of Emergency Medicine, Naval Medical Center Portsmouth, Portsmouth, Virginia
sdkelley@mar.med.navy.mil
Coma

Louis J. Kroot, MD
Associate Professor, Department of Emergency Medicine, University of Kentucky College of Medicine, Lexington
Multicasualty Incidents & Disasters; Vertebral Column & Spinal Cord Trauma; Wound Care

Désirée La Charité, MD
Assistant Professor, Section of Emergency Medicine, Department of Medicine, University of Wisconsin Medical School, Madison
ddl@medicine.wisc.edu
Chest Trauma

Susan J. Letterle, MD
Staff Physician, Department of Emergency Medicine, Naval Medical Center Portsmouth, Portsmouth, Virginia
Maxillofacial & Neck Trauma; Genitourinary Emergencies

Wason W.S. Louie, MD
Physician, Department of Emergency Medicine, Truman Medical Center, Kansas City, Missouri
Metabolic & Endocrine Emergencies

Mary Nan S. Mallory, MD, RDMS
Associate Professor, Department of Emergency Medicine, University of Louisville School of Medicine, Louisville, Kentucky
marynanmd@pol.net
Approach to the Emergency Department Patient; Obstetric & Gynecologic Emergencies & Rape

Geoffrey A. Martin, MD
Professor, Department of Emergency Medicine, University of Kentucky College of Medicine, Lexington
Hematologic Emergencies

Julia Martin, MD
Associate Professor, Department of Emergency Medicine, University of Kentucky College of Medicine; Medical Director, University of Kentucky Air Medical Services, Lexington, Kentucky
jemart2@uky.edu
The Multiply Injured Patient

Michael McClurg, MD
Resident Physician, Department of Emergency
Medicine, University of Kentucky College of
Medicine, Lexington
The Multiply Injured Patient

James J. Mensching, MD, DO, FACEP
Physician, Department of Emergency Medicine,
Good Samaritan Medical Center, Brockton,
Massachusetts; Physician, Department of
Emergency Medicine, St. Elizabeth's Medical
Center, Boston, Massachusetts
j.j.mensching.do@attbi.com
*Gastrointestinal Bleeding; Delirium & Acute
Confusional States; Vascular Emergencies*

Andrew Nyce, MD
Assistant Professor, Department of Emergency
Medicine, Robert Wood Johnson Medical School,
University of Medicine and Dentistry of New
Jersey, Newark, New Jersey; Attending Physician,
Department of Emergency Medicine, Cooper
University Medical Center, Camden, New Jersey
nyce-drew@cooperhealth.edu
Fluid, Electrolyte, & Acid-Base Emergencies

David O'Keefe, MD
Resident, Department of Emergency Medicine,
University of Kentucky College of Medicine,
Lexington
dlokeefe@hotmail.com
Arthritis & Back Pain

William Randall Partin, MD
Assistant Clinical Professor, University of Louisville
School of Medicine, Louisville, Kentucky; Attend-
ing Physician, Floyd Emergency Medicine Associ-
ates, Floyd Memorial Hospital, New Albany,
Indiana
randypartin@insightbb.com
Emergency Procedures

Debra G. Perina, MD
Associate Professor, University of Virginia School of
Medicine, Charlottesville; Director, Prehospital
Care Division, University of Virginia Health
Systems, Charlottesville
Dyspnea, Respiratory Distress, & Respiratory Failure

Melissa Platt, MD
Physician, Department of Emergency Medicine,
University of Louisville Hospital, Louisville,
Kentucky
maproc01@hotmail.com
Obstetric & Gynecologic Emergencies & Rape

Martha Ann Pratt, MD
Resident Physician and Clinical Instructor,
Department of Emergency Medicine, University
of Missouri-Kansas City School of Medicine,
Kansas City, Missouri
Dermatologic Emergencies

Robert Perry Pringle, Jr., MD
Resident, Department of Emergency Medicine
University of Louisville School of Medicine,
Lousiville, Kentucky
Approach to the Emergency Patient

Christopher R. Pund, MD
Resident, Department of Emergency medicine,
University of Kentucky, College of Medicine,
Lexington
chrispund@hotmail.com
Pulmonary Emergencies

Luis E. Rodriguez, MD
Director of Emergency Medicine, Roanoke Chowan
Hospital, Ahoskie, North Carolina; Clinical
Assistant Professor, Department of Emergency
Medicine, The Brody School of Medicine, East
Carolina University, Greenville, North Carolina
lourod2000@yahoo.com
Abdominal Trauma; Orthopedic Emergencies

Steven D. Rothert, MD, JD
Resident, Department of Emergency Medicine,
University of Kentucky College of Medicine,
Lexington
srothert@insightbb.com
Legal Aspects of Emergency Care

Micheal D. Rush, MD
Assistant Professor, Department of Emergency
Medicine, Truman Medical Center, University
of Missouri-Kansas City School of Medicine,
Kansas City, Missouri
micheal.rush@tmcmed.org
Metabolic & Endocrine Emergencies

Jon Andrew Russell, MD
Chief Resident, Department of Emergency Medicine, University of Kentucky College of Medicine, Lexington
jandrewrussell@hotmail.com
Abdominal Pain

Ritu Sahni, MD, MPH
Assistant Professor, Deaprtment of Emergency Medicine, Oregon Health and Science University School of Medicine, Portland; Medical Director, Life Flight Network, Portland, Oregon
sahnir@ohsu.edu
Head Injuries

Joseph A. Salome III, MD, FAAEM
Emergency Physician, Truman Medical Center; Associate Professor, Department of Emergency Medicine, University of Missouri-Kansas City School of Medicine, Kansas City, Missouri
joseph.salomone@tmcmed.org
Dermatologic Emergencies

Adam Saperston, MD, MS
Staff Physician, Peninsula Emergency Physicians, Inc., Hampton Careplex Hospital, Hampton, Virginia
dradam@worldnet.att.net
Coma; Syncope, Seizures, & Other Causes of Episodic Loss of Consciousness; Hand Trauma

Eric M. Sergienko, MD
Staff Physician, Naval Hospital, Guam; Medical Director, Naval EMS Guam, Agana, Guam
docz@ite.net
Prehospital Emergency Medical Services; Basic & Advanced Cardiac Life Support

Travis Sewalls, MD
Resident Physician, Department of Emergency Medicine, University of Kentucky Medical Center, Lexington
Poisoning

J. Stephan Stapczynski, MD
Professor, Department of Emergency Medicine, University of Kentucky College of Medicine, Lexington
jsstap01@uky.edu
Hematologic Emergencies

Michael W. Stava, MD
Assistant Professor, Department of Emergency Medicine, University of Kentucky College of Medicine, Lexington
Nuclear, Biologic, & Chemical Agents; Weapons of Mass Destruction

C. Keith Stone, MD
Professor and Chairman, Department of Emergency Medicine, Texas A&M University Health Science Center College of Medicine, Scott & White Memorial Hospital, Temple, Texas
kestone@swmail.sw.org
Headache; Pulmonary Emergencies; Cardiac Emergencies

James Svenson, MD, MS
Associate Professor, Section of Emergency Medicine, Department of Medicine, University of Wisconsin Medical School, Madison
jes@medicine.wisc.edu
Chest Trauma

David C. Van, MD, MS
Assistant Clinical Professor of Medicine, Department of Emergency Medicine, Columbia University College of Physicians and Surgeons, New York
Emergencies: Disorders of the Ear, Nose, Sinuses, Oropharynx, & Mouth

David A. Wald, DO
Assistant Professor, Department of Emergency Medicine, Temple University School of Medicine and Emergency Medicine Clerkship Director, Temple University Hospital, Philadelphia, Pennsylvania
waldda@tuhs.temple.edu
Cardiac Arrhythmias

Darren K. Waters, MD
Chief Resident, Department of Emergency Medicine, University of Kentucky College of Medicine, Lexington
dwa1972@hotmail.com
Poisoning

D. Shannon Waters, MD
Assistant Professor and Physician, Department of Emergency Medicine, University of Kentucky College of Medicine, Lexington
dswaters@comcast.net
Disorders Due to Physical & Environmental Agents; Poisoning

Claudia Whitaker, MD
Physician, Wayne State University School of
    Medicine; Resident Physician, Sinai-Grace
    Hospital, Detroit, Michigan
whitakermd@aol.com
Genitourinary Trauma

Robert Casey Wilson, MD
Physician, Department of Emergency Medicine,
    University of Kentucky College of Medicine,
    Lexington
rcwilsonmd@msn.com
Vertebral Column & Spinal Cord Trauma

Geoffrey A. Wiss, MD
Attending Physician, Department of Emergency
    Medicine, Sinai-Grace Hospital and Research
    Fellow, Emergency Medicine Basic Science
    Laboratory, Wayne State University School
    of Medicine, Detroit, Michigan
gwiss@yahoo.com
Genitourinary Trauma

Preface

Current Emergency Diagnosis & Treatment, fifth edition is designed to present concise, easy-to-read, practical information on the diagnosis and treatment of a wide spectrum of conditions that present to the emergency department. The chapters emphasize the immediate management of life threatening problems then present the evaluation and treatment of specific disorders. We trust that this text will aid all practitioners of emergency medicine in providing care to their patients.

OUTSTANDING FEATURES

In keeping with the tradition of the *Current* series, *CEDT* strives to provide the reader with a broad-based text written in a clear and succinct manner. Our goal is to provide practicing emergency physicians quick access to accurate and useful information that will aid in their everyday practice of emergency medicine.

Because this text focuses on the practical aspects of emergency care, there is little discussion of the basic science or pathophysiology of disease processes. In addition, discussion of management restricts the material presented to treatments routinely provided in the ED.

INTENDED AUDIENCE

CEDT will be useful to all practitioners of emergency medicine, including physicians, residents, medical students as well as physician extenders. It will also provide valuable information for emergency nurses and prehospital care providers.

ORGANIZATION

The fifth edition of *CEDT* has undergone some reorganization. A new initial section entitled "Special Aspects of Emergency Medicine" has been created. This section brings together two new chapters, on the approach to the emergency department patient and on nuclear, biologic and chemical agents and weapons of mass destruction, with chapters previously included in the section on non-trauma emergencies.

This edition retains the priority-based and problem-oriented organization of previous editions. Chapters in Section II, "Management of Common Emergency Problems," are presented in a problem-based format. Life-threatening disorders are discussed first followed by a presentation of specific disorders. This chapter format is carried out in the remainder of the book in the sections dealing with traumatic emergencies and non-trauma emergencies.

SPECIAL TO THIS EDITION

- A new chapter on the approach to the emergency patient
- A new chapter on nuclear, biological and chemical terrorism
- Updates of all chapters
- New radiographic images throughout
- Updated and color-enhanced illustrations

ACKNOWLEDGMENTS

We would like to thank the editorial staff at McGraw-Hill, especially Shelley Reinhardt, Nicky Fernando, and Christie Naglieri for their guidance, patience, and support throughout this project. In addition, we would like to thank our wives, Gail and Kris, and our children, Chase, Jack, and Maddie, for their love, understanding, and support for the time needed to dedicate to this endeavor.

C. Keith Stone, MD
Roger L. Humphries, MD
September 2003

SECTION I
Special Aspects of Emergency Medicine

Approach to the Emergency Department Patient

1

Mary Nan S. Mallory, MD, RDMS & Robert Perry Pringle, Jr., MD

What Is Emergency Medicine?
Birth & Growth of Emergency Medicine
Scope of Practice

Principles of Emergency Medicine
Conclusion

WHAT IS EMERGENCY MEDICINE?

An emergency is commonly defined as any condition perceived by the prudent layperson—or someone on his or her behalf—as requiring immediate medical or surgical evaluation and treatment. Based on that definition, the American College of Emergency Physicians (ACEP) states that the practice of emergency medicine has the primary mission of evaluating, managing, and providing treatment to these patients with unexpected injury and illness.

So what does an emergency physician do? This specialist routinely provides care and makes medical treatment decisions based on real-time evaluation of a patient's history; physical findings; and many diagnostic studies, including multiple imaging modalities, laboratory tests, and electrocardiograms. The emergency physician needs an amalgam of skills to treat a wide variety of injuries and illnesses—ranging from the diagnosis of an upper respiratory infection or dermatologic condition to resuscitation and stabilization of the multiple trauma patient. Furthermore, these physicians must be able to practice emergency medicine on patients of all ages and not just in urban tertiary-care facil-

ities. Clinical emergency medicine may be practiced in emergency departments, both rural and urban; urgent care clinics; and other settings such as at mass gathering incidents, through emergency medical services (EMS), and in hazardous material and bioterrorism situations.

Emergency medicine serves as the United States's health care safety net. It provides valuable clinical and administrative services to the health care delivery system, including care for the indigent and others who lack access to health care, and has evolved as the most visible and vital component of a patchwork of health care providers and facilities. These emergency departments have become the routine, and often the only, source of care for many of the uninsured, thereby acting as a critical safety net for our fragmented health care delivery system.

Finally, emergency departments are the only element of the health care system whose function has been delineated by federal law. Initially authorized in 1986, the Emergency Medical Treatment and Active Labor Act mandates that all emergency departments provide screening, stabilization, and appropriate transfer to *all* patients with *any* medical condition. Emergency medicine is often the last resort for many patients and frequently the access point for competent, comprehensive, and efficient medical care.

BIRTH & GROWTH OF EMERGENCY MEDICINE

By current popular opinion based on reality and dramatic television productions, emergency medicine appears to be at the forefront of medicine, providing compassionate and competent care by residency-trained emergency physicians. Unfortunately, this has not always been the case. The profession of emergency medicine is still quite young and continues to grow and mature. A brief timeline of emergency medicine growth is shown in Table 1–1. Since the first emergency medicine residency program began in 1970, the number of approved residency programs has increased dramatically (Table 1–2). Despite the rapid growth in emergency medicine residencies, a significant number of practitioners of emergency medicine are not residency trained or board certified (Table 1–3).

Table 1–1. Timeline of emergency medicine growth.

1968: Formation of American College of Emergency Physicians.
1970: University of Cincinnati established nation's first emergency medicine residency program.
1974: Emergency Medical Services Act (The White Paper) authorized the establishment and expansion of emergency medical services system and research.
1975: The American Medical Association (AMA) House of Delegates approved Section of Emergency Medicine and standards for emergency medicine residencies were established. Total number of emergency medicine residencies: 18.
1979: The AMA and the American Board of Medical Specialties recognizes emergency medicine as the 23 medical specialty.
1980: Emergency medicine specialty certification examinations begin. Total number of emergency medicine residencies: 43.
1982: Accreditation Council for Graduate Medical Education approves requirements for emergency medicine residency programs.
1985: Total number of emergency medicine residencies: 63.
1989: American Board of Medical Specialties grants emergency medicine primary board status.
1990: Total number of emergency medicine residencies: 81.
1995: Total number of emergency medicine residencies: 108.
2000: Total number of emergency medicine residencies: 122.
2001: Total number of emergency medicine residencies: 124.

Table 1–2. Emergency medicine residency statistics.

Emergency medicine residencies approved by the Residency Review Committee/Emergency Medicine (2001)	124
Total active emergency medicine residents and fellows	3,676
Average number of residents and fellows per program	29.6
Average percentage female residents	28.2%
Average percentage international medical graduate	3.4%
Average number of full-time physician faculty	20.6
Average number of part-time physician faculty	3.7
Average percentage full-time female physician faculty	24.2%
Average full-time physician faculty-to-resident ratio	0.7

SCOPE OF PRACTICE

Emergency medicine physicians are faced with an ever-growing patient volume, decreasing inpatient bed availability, decreasing reimbursement, and increased litigation. However, these same physicians have the unique responsibility for being prudent stewards of a finite amount of health care resources. Based on that responsibility, the ACEP in 2002 endorsed the following:

- The best medical interest of the patient should be foremost in any clinical decision making process.
  Criteria for appropriate use of finite resources should include:
  1. Urgency of the patient's medical condition
  2. Likelihood, magnitude, and duration of medical benefit to the patient
  3. Burdens and cost of care to the patient
  4. Cost to society

Table 1–3. Emergency physician personnel statistics.

Emergency physicians (in clinical practice in 2000)	32,020
Emergency physicians certified by the American Board of Emergency Medicine (as of December 2001)	17,300
Emergency physicians certified by the American Osteopathic Board of Emergency Medicine (as of July 2001)	1,078
Members of the American College of Emergency Physicians	21,000

- Emergency physicians should not allocate health care resources on the basis of a patient's ability to pay, contribution to society, past use of resources, or responsibility for their medical condition.

In 2001, the ACEP Core Content Task Force II published its *Model of Clinical Practice of Emergency Medicine.* In this publication, the scope of practice of an emergency physician is well defined and yet quite expansive, to include care from the prehospital environment to prevention and education. Listed below are the tasks of the emergency physician as agreed upon by the task force.

Prehospital Care

Participate actively in prehospital care and education, provide direct patient care or on-line or off-line medical direction or interact with prehospital medical providers, and assimilate information from prehospital care into patient assessment and management.

Emergency Stabilization

Conduct primary assessment, and take appropriate steps to stabilize and provide treatment to patients.

Performance of Focused History & Physical Examination

Communicate effectively to interpret and evaluate the patient's symptoms and history; identify pertinent risk factors in the patient's history; provide a focused evaluation; interpret the patient's appearance, vital signs, and condition; recognize pertinent physical findings; and perform techniques required for conducting the exam.

Modifying Factors

Recognize age, gender, ethnicity, barriers to communication, socioeconomic status, underlying disease, and other factors that may affect patient management.

Professional & Legal Issues

Understand and apply principles of professionalism, ethics, and legal concepts pertinent to patient management.

Diagnostic Studies

Select and perform the most appropriate diagnostic studies, and interpret the results.

Diagnosis

Develop a differential diagnosis and establish the most likely diagnoses in light of the history, physical examination, interventions, and test results.

Therapeutic Interventions

Perform procedures and nonpharmacologic therapies, and counsel patients.

Pharmacotherapy

Select appropriate pharmacotherapy, recognize pharmacokinetic properties, and anticipate drug interactions and adverse effects.

Observation & Reassessment

Evaluate and reevaluate the effectiveness of a patient's treatment or therapy, including addressing complications and potential errors; and monitor, observe, manage, and maintain the stability of one or more patients who are at different stages in their workups.

Consultation & Disposition

Collaborate with physicians and other professionals to evaluate and provide treatment to patients; arrange appropriate placement and transfer if necessary; formulate a follow-up plan; and communicate effectively with patients, family, and involved health care members.

Prevention & Education

Apply epidemiologic information to patients at risk; conduct patient education; and select appropriate disease and injury prevention techniques.

Documentation

Communicate patient care information in a concise manner that facilitates quality care and coding.

Multitasking & Team Management

Prioritize multiple patients in the emergency department in order to provide optimal patient care; interact, coordinate, educate, and supervise all members of the patient management team; utilize appropriate hospital resources; and have familiarity with disaster management procedures.

Other "Tasks"

Emergency medicine has evolved to include much more than the above-mentioned "tasks." For the profession of emergency medicine to continue to progress, physicians must embrace the following responsibilities:

- Basic and clinical research
- Multidisciplinary and continuous medical education
- Injury prevention
- Disaster management and mass-gathering medicine
- Toxicology and regional Poison Control Center direction
- Hazardous material and bioterrorism management
- Hospital and EMS systems administration

PRINCIPLES OF EMERGENCY MEDICINE

It is often said that emergency department patients "don't read the textbook," meaning that their presentations do not fit nicely into specific textbook diagnoses or classical presentations of illness. However, a cornerstone of an emergency physician's practice is the recognition of patterns in a patient's presentation; therefore, the prudent physician must be a detective and scientist to muddle through the muck of vague signs and symptoms to find the pattern.

The principles of emergency medicine are simply questions that must be answered to provide effective care to patients who have entrusted emergency physicians with their care. The questions are not to be used as a cookbook approach to the management of these often complex medical and psychosocial issues but are a simple method to guide the prudent emergency physician through the quagmire of clinical emergency medicine.

A. Is the Patient About to Die?

Obviously, this is the first and most important question to answer. Every patient's presentation is quickly prioritized to one of the following acuities:

1. Critical—Patient has symptoms consistent with a life-threatening illness or injury with a high probability of death if immediate intervention is not begun.

2. Emergent—Patient has symptoms of illness or injury that may progress in severity if treatment is not begun quickly.

3. Nonurgent—Patient has symptoms that have a low probability of progression to a more serious condition.

Look for *symptoms* of a life-threatening emergency, not a specific disease entity. Anticipate impending life-threatening emergencies in the apparently stable patient.

B. What Steps Must Be Undertaken to Stabilize the Patient?

Act quickly to stabilize the critically ill or injured patient. Focus on the primary survey (airway, breathing, circulation, and neurologic deficits), and make necessary interventions as each issue is identified. Do not delay necessary primary interventions while awaiting completion of ancillary testing.

C. What Are the Most Potentially Serious Causes of the Patient's Presentation?

Thinking of the worst-case scenario, develop a mental list of the most deadly causes of the patient's presentation by asking, "What will kill my patient the fastest?" Once the list has been developed, the vital signs, history, physical examination, and ancillary assessments should identify or confirm those causes highest on the list.

D. Could There Be Multiple Causes of the Patient's Presentation?

In addition to constant reevaluation and reprioritization of the differential diagnosis, continually ask, "Is this all there is?" For example, is the new-onset seizure and hypoglycemia in an older diabetic patient from intentional or accidental medication overdose or perhaps worsening renal insufficiency? Is the near-syncope and abdominal pain in an apparently intoxicated college coed from a ruptured ectopic pregnancy or perhaps a ruptured spleen secondary to undisclosed physical abuse by her boyfriend? Frequent reassessment and thoughtful inquiry as to the multiple possibilities responsible for each patient's condition are imperative.

E. Can a Treatment Assist in the Diagnosis in an Otherwise Undifferentiated Illness?

Often in emergency medicine, treatment response foretells a diagnosis. A case in point is the unconscious patient with no available collateral history. The patient's response to empiric administration of naloxone will include or exclude narcotic overdose as a contributor to the obtundation. Referred to as the "diagnostic-therapeutic" concept, it underscores the emergency medicine philosophy that an established diagnosis is not a prerequisite to initiating appropriate treatment. Pitfalls can exist. For example, sublingual nitroglycerin and so-called GI cocktails can relieve symptoms of chest pain resulting from the same cause.

F. Is a Diagnosis Mandatory or Even Possible?

After emergent issues have been addressed, the patient and emergency physician are often left with an undifferentiated symptom complex. This frequently elicits an uncomfortable response by non-emergency-medicine-trained physicians. Become accustomed to and comfortable with the notion of determining the disposition for a nonemergent patient—having treated their symptoms and excluding emergency conditions–without a specific diagnosis.

G. Does This Patient Need To Be Admitted to the Hospital?

Having appropriately answered the preceding questions, make the bottom-line disposition decision. Once assessments and treatments are under way, decide whether an emergent condition exists. Consider other subtleties. Does the patient have timely, accessible follow-up? How far away from a medical facility does the patient live? Are unresolved abuse or self-care issues involved? Are you, as the emergency physician, comfortable discharging the patient?

H. If the Patient Is Not Being Admitted, Is the Disposition Safe and Adequate for the Patient?

More frequently than not, patients are discharged home from the emergency department. However, many patients do not receive a specific diagnosis, and some symptoms may persist. Recommend appropriate follow-up, and provide written discharge instructions. Invite the patient back. Instruct the patient when to return for further evaluation should symptoms change or worsen. Provide the patient with information regarding treatment and diagnosis as well.

CONCLUSION

Since 1970, emergency medicine has seen a tremendous growth and increase in awareness of the unique aspects of the profession. It remains a challenging and fulfilling experience for many physicians and an appealing choice of specialties for medical students. As emergency medicine matures as a specialty, its importance as the United States's health care safety net and its integral status as front-line medicine will continue to expand and grow.

American College of Emergency Physicians: Definition of emergency medicine, as approved by the ACEP Board of Directors, April 2001. http://www.acep.org/3,411,0.html

American College of Emergency Physicians: Emergency medicine training, competency and professional practice principles position statement, as approved by the ACEP Board of Directors, November 2001. http://www.acep.org/3,5141,0.html

American College of Emergency Physicians: Emergency physician stewardship of finite resources, as approved by the ACEP Board of Directors, January 1997. http://www.acep.org/3,4245,0.html

American College of Emergency Physicians Core Content Task Force II: *The Model of the Clinical Practice of Emergency Medicine.* American College of Emergency Physicians, 2001.

Asplin BR, Sosnow PL, Yeh CS: *"The Safety Net and Current Federal Health Care Policy." Defending America's Safety Net.* American College of Emergency Physicians, 1999.

Prehospital Emergency Medical Services

Eric M. Sergienko, MD, & Thomas N. Bottoni, MD[1]

Components of the Emergency Medical Services System

Prehospital Skills & Techniques

The delivery of effective, organized, prehospital emergency medical services (EMS) is a development that dates to the 1960s in the United States. Although there were ambulance providers and even some local systems, there was no national approach to prehospital care until publication of the 1966 White Paper entitled "Accidental Death and Disability—The Neglected Disease of Modern Society" (National Academy of Sciences, National Research Council).

When medical emergencies are reported, trained medical personnel arrive on the scene to provide emergency care within 6–10 minutes. The skills of these personnel range from basic first aid techniques and cardiopulmonary resuscitation (CPR) to advanced life support (ALS) techniques, including defibrillation, endotracheal intubation, and the use of emergency medications. Radio communications permit ongoing discussion of patient status and treatment between emergency medical personnel at the scene and the supervising physician at the base hospital. Air ambulances (fixed-wing aircraft or helicopters staffed with medically trained flight crews) can rapidly evacuate and transport patients from a remote emergency scene to a regional medical center.

COMPONENTS OF THE EMERGENCY MEDICAL SERVICES SYSTEM

Modern EMS systems consist of several major components: (1) professional field personnel trained to provide specific levels or types of care, (2) a comprehensive emergency communications network, (3) hospital emergency department physicians and nurses who su-

pervise the treatment provided by EMS field personnel, (4) hospitals categorized according to their relationship with EMS field personnel and according to the level of care they can provide, and (5) EMS administrative officials who manage and coordinate the elements of the system.

Professional EMS Field Personnel

The health professionals and first responders who provide prehospital care are trained to carry out specific levels of care, ranging from basic first aid and CPR provided by first responders, through basic life support (BLS) given by emergency medical technicians (EMTs), to the ALS provided by advanced EMTs (paramedics). These personnel provide care only as extensions or agents of physicians and are not independently licensed to provide medical care. The care they deliver is authorized by standing orders (written authorization to administer certain treatments without prior attempt at base contact by radio) or protocols from physician directors or by orders transmitted by radio from supervisory physicians at the base hospital to EMS personnel at the scene. A critical element in the development of EMS since 1970 has been the recognition that personnel without prior medical training can be prepared through relatively short courses to provide effective prehospital care. The designations, levels of training, and skills of EMS personnel are now largely standardized according to United States Department of Transportation (DOT) curriculum and formal categories established in 1983 by the National Registry of Emergency Medical Technicians. The curriculum is regularly reviewed and updated to reflect changes in medicine and in the prehospital environment. The latest iteration released by the DOT was in 1998, with some modifications in 2000. Types of EMS field per-

[1]This chapter is a revision of the chapter by Charles E. Saunders, MD, FACEP, & Thomas Hearne, PhD, from the 4th edition.

Table 2–1. Training and procedures for emergency medical personnel.

Emergency Personnel Type	Hours of Training	Curriculum[1]	Skills and Procedures

First Responder	–40	Patient assessment
		Basic life support
		  Cardiopulmonary resuscitation
		  Bleeding and shock
		Wounds and fractures
		Medical emergencies
		  Poisoning, drug and alcohol emergencies,
		  heart attack, stroke, epilepsy, asthma,
		  emergency childbirth
		Environmental emergencies
		  Burns
		Psychiatric emergencies
		Stabilization and transfer
			Patient assessment
			Cardiopulmonary resuscitation
			Control of bleeding
			Bandaging and limited splinting
			Limited extrication

EMT-A (Basic)	81–140	Orientation and legal responsibilities
		Patient assessment
		Cardiopulmonary resuscitation
		Bleeding and shock
		Injuries
		Medical emergencies
		  Heart disease, stroke, substance abuse,
		    pediatric emergencies
		Childbirth
		Environmental emergencies
		  Burns, hazardous materials, water hazards
		Psychologic aspects of emergency care
		Patient handling and extrication
		Ambulance operations and vehicle maintenance
		  Emergency driving, communications, report
		    writing
		Optional skills
		  Intravenous therapy, advanced airway
		    management, defibrillation by EMTs
			Patient assessment
			Airway management and oxygen therapy
			Control of bleeding
			Management of shock (including Military
			    Anti-shock Trousers [MAST])
			Dressing and bandaging wounds
			Splinting (including traction splints)
			Spinal immobilization
			Extrication and triage

EMT-I (Intermediate)	110–1000	All EMT-A skills plus various advanced life
		  support skills
			All EMT-A skills plus specialized training in
			  one or more life support skills, usually
			  including:
			  Manual or automatic defibrillation
			  Intravenous therapy
			  Selected emergency medications
			  Advanced airway management

(continued)

sonnel and their training are described below and summarized in Table 2–1.

A. First Responders

First responders may include law enforcement officers, rescue squad members, firefighters, or volunteer EMS personnel. First-responder courses usually consist of about 40 hours of classroom instruction and clinical training in basic first aid and CPR. First responders are equipped with basic emergency care equipment (eg, bandages, dressings, tape, blanket and pillow, upper and lower extremity splint sets). Oxygen equipment and a self-refilling bag-valve-mask combination (eg, Ambu bag) are optional. First responders also carry basic tools to help them reach and extricate trapped individuals. Increasingly, first responders are being trained

Table 2–1. Training and procedures for emergency medical personnel. (*Continued*)

Emergency Personnel Type	Hours of Training	Curriculum[1]	Skills and Procedures
EMT-P (Advanced or Paramedic)	>1000	Role of the paramedic Human systems and patient assessment Fluids and shock General pharmacology Respiratory system Cardiovascular system Central nervous system Soft tissue injuries Musculoskeletal system Medical emergencies Obstetric and gynecologic emergencies Pediatric emergencies Management of the emotionally disturbed Communications and telemetry Multiple injuries, multiple causalities, and triage	All EMT-A skills plus specialized training in advanced life support skills, including[2] Intravenous cannulation Invasive airway management including endotracheal intubation Cardiac dysrhythmia recognition Defibrillation Emergency medications

[1]First responder curriculum adapted and reproduced, with permission, from Karen KJ, Hafen BQ: *First Responder: A Skills Approach,* 2nd ed. Morton, 1986. EMT-P curriculum from *Emergency Medical Technician Paramedic National Standard Curriculum.* U.S. Department of Transportation, National Highway Traffic Safety Administration, 1999.
[2]Advanced procedures vary widely among communities and may include procedure not listed here.

and equipped to perform defibrillation using automated external defibrillators (AEDs).

B. EMERGENCY MEDICAL TECHNICIANS (EMTs)

The National Registry of Emergency Medical Technicians currently recognizes 3 formal grades of EMTs according to the typical number of hours of training given, the breadth of skills covered, and the range of procedures authorized: EMT-A (basic), EMT-I (intermediate), and EMT-P (advanced, paramedic). Designations and levels of training may vary from state to state. Emergency physicians should be familiar with regional variations and deviations from the National Registry guidelines.

1. EMT-A—Basic EMTs constitute the essential workforce of EMS systems throughout the United States. Most state laws require at least one certified EMT on board ambulance vehicles that transport patients.

The basic EMT course requires at least 81 hours of training standardized by the DOT. Basic classes frequently exceed this minimum by up to 140 hours. Students learn basic principles of patient care, how to identify signs and symptoms central to patient assessment and diagnosis, and how to provide treatment in specific emergencies. The use of AEDs is now standard curriculum for EMTs in most regions. Optional modules for EMTs include advanced airway management, intravenous access, and assisting patients with self-administration of medications. Additionally, some states allow administration of medications, including epinephrine in anaphylaxis and aspirin in suspected cardiac chest pain.

2. EMT-I—The intermediate EMT is trained to provide a level of advanced care in areas that are underserved by paramedics. The scope of practice has evolved since 1990 to incorporate many advanced cardiac life support procedures, including cardiac monitoring, treatment of arrhythmias, defibrillation, and advanced airway management with either endotracheal intubation or an alternative airway.

3. EMT-P—Advanced EMTs (paramedics) receive over 1000 hours of training in ALS techniques. Their skills include the basic EMT procedures as well as intravenous cannulation, invasive airway management (including endotracheal intubation), recognition of cardiac dysrhythmias, defibrillation, and the use of specific emergency medications. In addition to extensive classroom training, EMT-P personnel also complete clinical training and a field internship with experienced paramedic teams.

Paramedics operate under standing orders and treatment protocols developed by a physician medical director that are usually broader and more advanced than those guiding basic EMTs. These protocols determine the type and level of care administered at the emergency site. Physicians who provide on-line medical supervision of paramedics (by radio and telemetry) from base hospitals may permit paramedics to deviate from established protocols or to provide treatment not specifically covered in standing orders.

Special Qualifications

Additional training is available at all levels of providers for specific care settings. At the first responder level, a Winter Emergency Care course has been developed for the National Ski Patrol to address special situations that occur in ski areas. Similarly there are Wilderness modules at all levels of training that provide additional training for care provided in a remote setting with anticipated long evacuations and transportation. EMT-Tactical courses train EMTs and paramedics to function in a tactical law enforcement situation in which they may support or be part of a police special tactics teams. Finally, Paramedic–Critical Care training enables the advanced provider to provide care to critically injured or ill patients who are being transferred from one facility to another.

Types of EMS Systems

EMS systems can be delivered in various ways. There are 2 basic forms of EMS response: a single-response system and a layered-response (or tiered-response) system. In a single-response system, there is only one grade of EMS unit, and the closest available unit is dispatched to any nearby emergency. In a layered-response system, 2 or more grades of EMS personnel respond hierarchically (eg, first responder, then EMT-A, then EMT-P) as needed. Layered-response systems usually provide for an EMT-A response for all less severe reported medical emergencies, reserving an EMT-P response for severe or life-threatening incidents (Table 2–2).

Communications Network

The communications network is important in tying together the components of an EMS system. A dispatcher at a communications center receives a telephone request from a caller at the site of the emergency and dispatches mobile EMS personnel via the radio network. Dispatchers may use a call triaging system (eg, Priority Medical Dispatching) to assign resources to a call. In many areas of the United States, an easily remembered emergency telephone number (9-1-1) provides the public with rapid access to the communications center. Many systems offer an "enhanced 9-1-1" service that provides immediate callback and location information to the dispatcher.

Communications between the EMS unit and medical facilities varies from region to region. For many BLS transports, contact with the base station or receiving facility is not required. In the event of an ALS transport, contact must be made with a medical facility. In some areas, the facility is called a base station hospital, which provides on-line direction and supervision for an entire EMS region. Information called into the base station hospital is then relayed to the receiving facility. In other areas, the receiving facility is called directly.

Hospital Facilities & Staffing

EMS systems typically include hospitals with a variety of treatment capabilities, ranging from local community hospitals with a limited emergency department staffing to large teaching hospitals in urban areas with emergency physicians, surgeons, anesthesiologists, and surgical teams available 24 hours a day. Hospital facilities are frequently classified according to their relationship to EMS mobile units and their ability to provide definitive care.

A. BASE STATION HOSPITALS

Physicians or specially trained nurses with physician backup in the emergency department of the base station hospital provide EMS units with on-line medical supervision during treatment. EMS units may be

Table 2–2. Alternative EMS system designs.[1]

System Type	Response		Transport	
	Emergency	Nonemergency	Emergency	Nonemergency
Single-tier basic life support (BLS)	BLS		BLS	
Single-tier advanced life support (ALS)	ALS		ALS	
Single-tier ALS with first responder	First responder + ALS	ALS	ALS	
Multitier (transport) with first responder	First responder + ALS	ALS	ALS	BLS
Multitier (response and transport) with first responder	First responder + ALS	BLS	ALS	BLS

[1]BLS = EMT-A ambulance; ALS = EMT-P ambulance; first responder = first aid or semiautomated defibrillation.

housed at the base station hospital, but this may not be necessary or feasible because the units are usually strategically deployed in the hospital's service area. In many EMS systems, the base station hospital may also be the one most capable of providing definitive follow-up care.

B. RECEIVING HOSPITALS

Receiving hospitals are facilities to which patients may be transported. For each patient, the receiving hospital is selected according to its proximity; its capability to provide definitive care; and the preference of the patient, family members, or family physician, as long as transport to the hospital does not draw the EMS unit away from its primary service area.

C. HOSPITALS CATEGORIZED BY CAPABILITY

Hospitals may be categorized by their ability to provide acute care as determined by the availability of physicians, nurse, allied health personnel, and other hospital resources (eg, operating rooms, laboratory, blood bank). Many categorization schemes exist. The Joint Commission on Accreditation of Healthcare Organizations has established 4 levels of emergency service:

1. Level I—This service offers emergency care 24 hours a day with at least one physician experienced in emergency care on duty in the emergency care area. In addition, there must be in-house physician coverage by residents at the senior level or higher for the medical, surgical, orthopedic, obstetric-gynecologic, pediatric, and anesthesiologic services.

2. Level II—This service offers emergency care 24 hours a day with at least one physician experienced in emergency care on duty in the emergency care area. Specialty consultation should be available within 30 minutes.

3. Level III—This service offers emergency care 24 hours a day with at least one physician on duty in the emergency care area available within 30 minutes through a medical staff call roster.

4. Level IV—This service is capable of performing a triage function and can administer life-saving first aid until transportation to the nearest appropriate facility is available.

D. HOSPITALS CATEGORIZED BY AREAS OF CARE

Hospitals can also be categorized by special areas of care (eg, trauma, burns, neonatal intensive care), especially where regionalization of services in these areas is practiced. The American College of Surgeons, for example,

has established the following categorization of trauma facilities:

1. Level I—This designates a full-service trauma center that can provide optimal care of the trauma patient. One or more experienced emergency physicians, a general surgeon, anesthesiology services, laboratory, blood bank, and an operating room team must be available in-house 24 hours a day. All surgical subspecialty services should be immediately available on call. A commitment to education and research in trauma must also be demonstrated.

2. Level II—This trauma center is similar to a level I center but does not necessarily include a commitment to education or research. Occasionally patients with the most severe injuries or those needing highly specialized care may be transferred from a level II center to a level I center.

3. Level III—This trauma center does not have all of the resources available at a level I or level II center but may represent the highest level available in a given community. Usually, initial stabilization and life-saving procedures are performed and the patient is then transferred to a level I or level II center.

EMS Administration

EMS systems may be administered through a variety of organizations, including local health departments, public safety agencies such as police or fire departments, hospitals, or privately owned provider agencies. Often several of these agencies operate EMS systems in the same area, and these agencies are coordinated through an EMS regional council, which interacts with hospitals, public safety agencies, and physician medical directors; sets operational standards; and monitors performance (quality assurance).

Operation of the EMS System

One way to visualize the interplay between various components of the EMS system is to review the sequence of events surrounding a typical emergency medical incident. There are 4 major phases: (1) report of the emergency and activation of the EMS system, (2) dispatch of appropriate prehospital units, (3) medical evaluation and field treatment by EMS personnel, and (4) transport of the patient to the appropriate hospital.

A. REPORT OF THE EMERGENCY

In many areas of the United States, a single, easily remembered telephone number (9-1-1) can now be used to request emergency help from the police and fire departments and to activate the EMS system.

B. DISPATCH

Dispatchers receive the emergency call, interview the caller to determine the type and severity of the emergency, and dispatch the appropriate type of emergency medical response. In systems with heavy call volumes, calls may be priority ranked and then dispatched in order of urgency of need and resource availability. In some systems, dispatchers offer advice to callers to assist patients pending the arrival of emergency units (prearrival instructions). Algorithms may be employed to guide the dispatcher in decision making (Figure 2–1). Dispatchers in layered-response emergency medical systems frequently follow specific protocols in determining which type of EMS unit to dispatch (ie, ALS, BLS,

first responder; see Table 2–2). Dispatchers may also be trained to provide CPR instructions by telephone to callers. Dispatch centers may also monitor hospital availability, manage the status and geographic deployment of EMS vehicles, and through computer-aided dispatch perform EMS management information and quality assurance functions.

C. MEDICAL EVALUATION AND TREATMENT

Most EMS systems in urban and suburban areas are capable of responding within a few minutes of receiving an emergency call. First responders can frequently arrive at the scene within 3–6 minutes, and paramedics within 5–10 minutes of receiving the call. Survival fol-

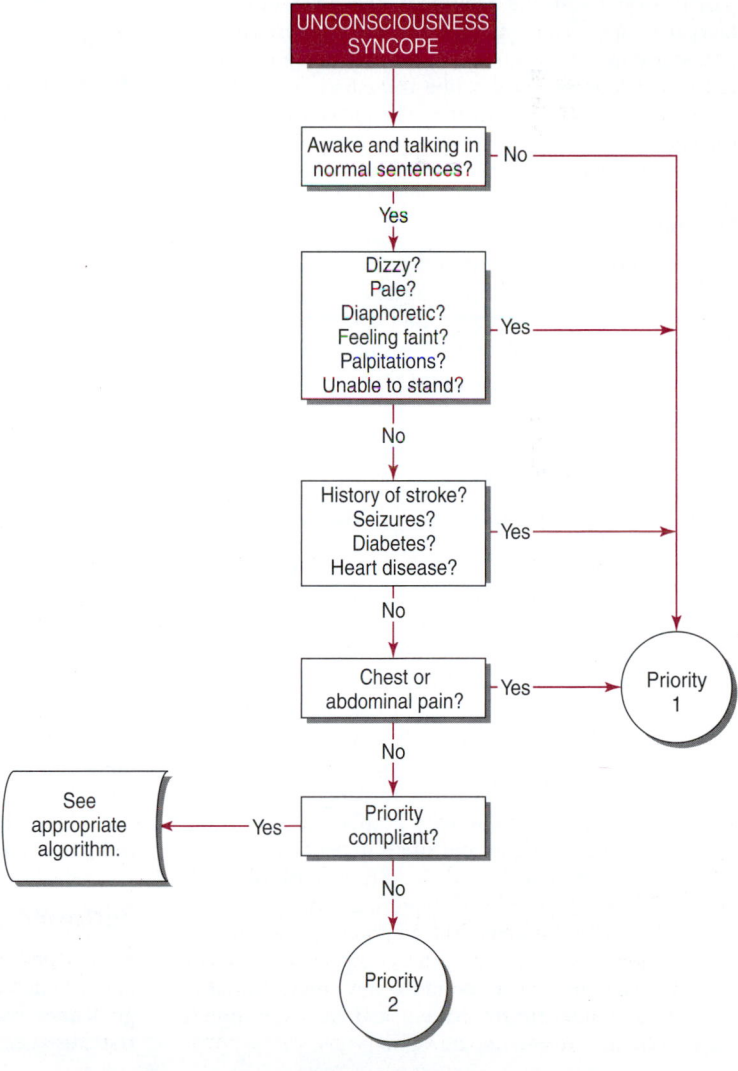

Figure 2–1. Sample algorithm to guide medical dispatchers when the patient's principal complaint or problem is unconsciousness or syncope.

lowing time-sensitive medical emergencies such as cardiac arrest is closely correlated with unit response time, especially when basic EMTs have been trained in defibrillation. In layered-response systems, paramedics are held in reserve for such critical or life-threatening incidents, where their advanced skills may provide definitive or stabilizing care to patients. Many systems have advanced-level first responders, such as engine companies manned with paramedics. These responders can provide the same interventions as ambulance-based paramedics but lack the means to transport patients. These assets can be additional resources in the single complex patient or in the multiple-patient incident.

Upon arrival at the emergency scene, EMS personnel undertake patient assessment and examination. EMT-paramedics in most cases are authorized by standing orders to proceed with patient care. Following patient evaluation and treatment, the EMS unit contacts the supervising emergency medical physician (or, in some states, a nurse) at the base station hospital by radio or telephone to describe the patient's condition and any treatment undertaken. The physician may give specific instructions for further treatment at the scene or request transport to the hospital for care.

D. TRANSPORT

The mode of transport (ground or air, with or without sirens or lights) depends on availability, stability of the patient's condition, transport time and distance, risks, and the like. Hospital destination decisions are often guided by local protocols, with critically ill patients directed to the closest, most appropriate facility. For example, a community hospital may be bypassed in favor of the nearest designated trauma center in the case of a severely injured patient. Noncritical cases may be transported to the hospital of the patient's choice.

1. Ground transport—Most patients are transported in surface ambulances. These vehicles vary slightly from state to state in their configuration and on-board equipment, but all follow guidelines set by the DOT. Emergency vehicle operators usually are allowed by local and state laws to violate certain traffic laws while responding to an emergency or carrying a patient in a life-threatening emergency. In the vast majority of cases, however, the patient's life is not in danger and posted speeds and traffic laws should be obeyed. The time gained in using red lights and sirens to get to the hospital is often outweighed by the additional risk of death and disability associated with rapid transport.

In most EMS systems, the responding unit is also the transporting unit. In others, especially layered-response systems, the responding unit may primarily evaluate and stabilize the patient and may summon a lower-level unit to provide transport.

2. Air transport—Some EMS systems and regional trauma hospitals, particularly those serving large outlying rural areas, use helicopters or fixed-wing aircraft with trained medical teams on board as additional resources for prehospital care and transportation. The majority of these aircraft are hospital based, but some are operated by municipal or state governmental agencies. Where these services are unavailable, or when search-and-rescue missions are required, aircraft equipped for medical evacuation may be sent from local military bases, operating within the Military Assistance to Safety and Traffic program.

Air ambulances are usually integrated into the EMS system and are activated according to certain locally established criteria. The decision to transport a patient by air requires careful consideration of the risks and benefits of air versus ground transport (see below).

Medical Supervision

A. ON-LINE MEDICAL DIRECTION

On-line medical direction is the direction given by radio to EMS personnel at the scene while care is being provided. It is usually given by emergency physicians or nurses at the base station hospital or receiving hospital. In most systems, the use of standing orders is allowed (Figure 2–2). This approach allows treatment to begin as soon as possible. Systems that have changed over from on-line medical control to standing orders have not shown a decrement in medical care but have shown an increase in EMS provider morale.

Even in systems that operate nearly exclusively by standing orders, some exceptions may require on-line direction. These may include cessation of CPR in a nonviable patient or the administration of restricted medications such as narcotics or paralytics. Systems that employ standing orders require effective monitoring, training, and quality assurance mechanisms.

B. OFF-LINE MEDICAL DIRECTION

Off-line medical direction is the overall direction of the activities of EMS personnel. It includes establishing protocols and standing orders, ensuring adequate training and skills, reviewing patient care records and voice tapes retrospectively, and reviewing performance and outcome data. Off-line medical direction is usually provided by a physician experienced in emergency services or by an agency in which physicians play an active role.

Performance Evaluation

System performance evaluation has many aspects, including the evaluation of input resources and operating guidelines (eg, protocol validation, personnel review, training assessment), evaluation of the process of deliv-

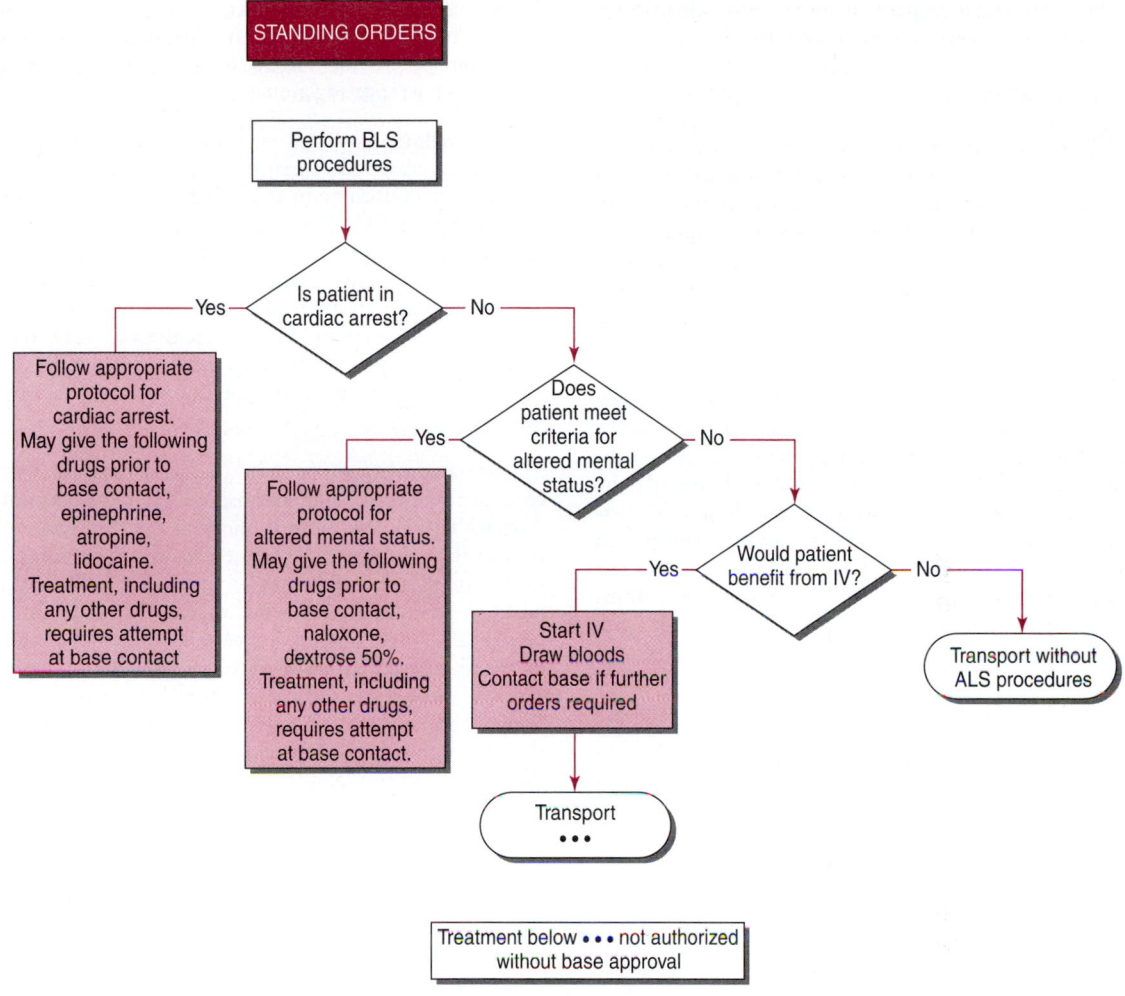

Figure 2–2. Standing orders for treatments and procedures that may be performed without prior attempt at base station contact by radio. ALS = EMT-P ambulance; BLS = EMT-A ambulance.

ering care in the field (eg, response times, service volume, treatment audits for adherence to protocols), and evaluation of the outcome of prehospital care (eg, complications, complaints, success in the performance of procedures, and patient survival). Outcome data are the most difficult to obtain.

PREHOSPITAL SKILLS & TECHNIQUES

Field Assessment

EMTs responding to a call usually have certain dispatch information, including the location, the nature of the complaint, and the number of patients. Upon arrival, they must quickly determine the presence of hazards to themselves and the patient, ascertain the probable mechanism of injury, and identify other patients, if any. Support can be summoned for hazard suppression or additional medical assistance. Patients who are conscious and in minimal distress may be able to provide historical information. Information may also be obtained from witnesses or family members.

Patients who are very ill may require that interventions be performed simultaneously with assessment. Interventions aimed at stabilizing airway, breathing, or circulation (the ABCs) will take precedence over secondary assessment. The receiving physician should expect that, if the patient is seriously ill or injured, only life-saving measures may be performed prior to arrival.

In the more stable patient, a more thorough primary and secondary survey should be performed.

Field Treatment

A. AIRWAY CONTROL

Methods of airway control depend on the EMT's level of skill and certification. Initial steps to provide an airway include positioning the jaw and suctioning secretions (taking care in the trauma victim not to hyperextend the neck). Should this fail to achieve and maintain airway patency, the basic EMT can insert an oral or nasal airway. Ventilation may be assisted by a bag-valve-mask.

EMTs and paramedics may establish alternative airways, depending on local protocol. The Combitube, a dual lumen tube designed to be placed blindly, can be used to ventilate the patient regardless of whether the tube is placed in the esophagus or the trachea. The laryngeal mask airway (LMA) is designed to be placed without laryngoscopy. It has an inflatable cuff that sits over the glottis. This allows for ventilation while minimizing gastric insufflation and aspiration. It is not as secure an airway as the endotracheal tube. An improvement on the original LMA is the LMA-Fastrach, which allows for an endotracheal tube to be passed through the LMA. Both the Combitube and the LMA have been implemented successfully in the prehospital setting.

Endotracheal intubation is the preferred method of airway control in patients with inadequate ventilation. Typically the success rate for prehospital intubation is greater than 90%. However, two recent papers have questioned the value of intubation in the field. A randomized trial involving pediatric intubation found that patients did as well with bag-valve-mask ventilation as they did with intubation. Another study found that over 25% of adult intubations in the prehospital setting were misplaced. When intubation is performed in the field it is suggested that end-tidal CO_2 detection and an esophageal detector device be used in addition to more conventional means of confirming location. After the tube is confirmed in the correct location, the risk of dislodgement should be minimized by using a commercial endotracheal tube holder and by securing the patient in a cervical collar and to a long spinal board.

B. EMERGENCY CARDIAC CARE

1. Cardiopulmonary resuscitation—The probability of survival for victims of sudden cardiac arrest is inversely related to the elapsed time before an effective cardiac rhythm is reestablished. CPR is a temporizing measure that, when initiated within 4–6 minutes, increases the chances of survival. In most systems, a paramedic unit cannot routinely reach the scene within this period. Many systems provide first responders with AEDs. AEDs have been successfully deployed with police and fire first responders. In addition, public access defibrillators provide AEDs to the public at busy venues such as sporting arenas and airports.

2. Defibrillation—Ventricular fibrillation is the initial rhythm encountered in many victims of sudden death. The sooner defibrillation is performed, the higher the survival rate. AEDs (Laerdal Heartstart 2000, others) can recognize ventricular fibrillation (or tachycardia) and deliver a countershock. The rescuer need not be able to recognize dysrhythmias but must be able to recognize cardiac arrest and operate the device. AEDs have enabled nonparamedic first responders to provide rapid defibrillation and have consequently improved survival rates.

3. Electrocardiography—In the treatment of acute coronary syndromes, the prehospital 12-lead electrocardiogram (ECG) significantly shortens the time from arrival in the emergency department to administration of thrombolytic therapy ("door to drug time"). Prehospital fibrinolytic therapy has had mixed results. In European trials, where prehospital care is typically provided by physician-staffed ambulances, 6-month and 1-year survival rates have increased. However, trials in the United States with paramedic-staffed units has not shown a significant improvement over 12-lead ECG in the field with hospital-administered fibrinolytics.

C. INVASIVE PROCEDURES

1. Venous catheterization—(See Chapter 6.) The use of intravenous techniques by EMS field personnel is usually limited to cannulation of peripheral veins of the upper extremities. In most EMS systems, the procedure can be initiated under standing order by intermediate or paramedic EMTs. Basic EMTs who have had special training in intravenous techniques and fluid therapy may also initiate intravenous lines. Studies have demonstrated that skilled paramedics in the field are able to start an intravenous line in approximately 3 minutes and achieve a success rate greater than 90%. However, when transport times are short (ie, 10 minutes or less), venous catheterization is usually unnecessary because the volume of fluid infused or the medications administered during such a short period are unlikely to be life saving. Further, in penetrating trauma to the thorax, fluid boluses may be detrimental by disrupting the clotting process. In addition, field placement of intravenous lines may increase the chances of infection. Needlestick injuries, which may occur during venous cannulation under adverse circumstances, such as in the back of a moving ambulance, are an increasing concern. Intraosseous needles may be placed by paramedics in the event that vascular access cannot be obtained in the pediatric patient.

2. Needle thoracostomy—Chest decompression for suspected tension pneumothorax may occasionally be life saving and is performed by paramedics in some systems. A 14- or 16-gauge catheter-clad needle is inserted into the second intercostal space along the midclavicular line immediately above the subjacent rib using sterile technique. The catheter is sealed with a Heimlich valve or a latex glove with the fingertip removed. (The open fingertip of the glove is secured around the catheter, allowing air to escape but preventing its reentry.)

3. Cricothyrotomy—(See Chapter 6.) Emergency entry to the airway may be life saving in cases of supraglottic airway obstruction or laryngeal trauma. Cricothyrotomy may be performed by paramedics in some EMS systems, usually after approval by the base physician via radio. Cricothyrotomy may be performed using a surgical, needle, or Seldinger technique. Because the procedure can be unexpectedly difficult, it should be performed as a last resort and only by properly trained personnel.

D. MEDICATIONS

Medications are a contentious area in the prehospital realm. Because of the lack of clinical trials, it is difficult to state what interventions are of benefit. The emergency physician should know what medications are available to their EMS providers and under what indications they may be used.

1. Advanced cardiac life support—Most drugs for advanced cardiac life support are stocked on most ALS ambulances. Consistently, epinephrine, atropine, lidocaine, sodium bicarbonate, and adenosine are stocked. In addition, nitroglycerin, aspirin, and morphine are available for treatment of acute coronary syndromes. Amiodarone often is not used because of the ongoing debate about its effectiveness and because of cost issues. Some systems do not stock diltiazem because patients with a tachydysrhythmia that requires rate control are relatively stable. Fibrinolytics are rarely used because of their cost, the staffing needed to administer and monitor them, and the minimal benefit shown in prehospital use. Other medications such as labetalol, magnesium, procainamide, and calcium chloride are typically stocked at the discretion of the agency's medical director.

2. Pulmonary—Albuterol should be available to all ALS EMS agencies. Ipratropium has been shown to be beneficial to patients with moderate to severe asthma and to those with chronic obstructive pulmonary disease. In addition to sublingual nitroglycerin, furosemide is typically stocked for treatment of pulmonary edema.

3. Other drugs—Benzodiazepines are typically stocked for treatment of seizures, anxiolysis, and sedation. The use of prehospital benzodiazepines is beneficial to patients presenting with recurrent seizures. Agents stocked include diazepam, lorazepam, and midazolam.

Glucose, in the form of 50% dextrose in water ($D_{50}W$) and oral glucose solution (occasionally $D_{25}W$ or $D_{10}W$ for pediatric patients), is stocked for treating hypoglycemia.

E. EXTRICATION

Extrication is the process of removing a patient from a condition of entrapment, usually from a motor vehicle. It requires considerable skill and experience. Often, special tools are necessary, such as heavy bolt and metal cutters or large, powered spreading devices (eg, Jaws of Life, Hurst Tool). In most EMS systems, when there is a report of a trapped victim, a fire rescue team is dispatched in addition to the EMS unit to clear fire hazards, wash away spilled gasoline, and provide additional heavy equipment and personnel.

As soon as the patient is accessible with minimal risk to emergency workers, the primary survey should be initiated while further efforts to free the patient continue. Once the patient is immobilized in place, emergency resuscitation can begin.

F. IMMOBILIZATION AND SPLINTING

1. Immobilization—Victims of trauma may have injuries to the spine or extremities, which, if manipulated, can lead to spinal cord or limb damage. Upon reaching a trauma victim, the rescue team must stabilize the patient's cervical spine. Manual stabilization is maintained throughout extrication. A cervical collar is applied as soon as practicable. Spine boards are sometimes difficult to maneuver in closed spaces, but alternative devices are available, such as the Kendrick Extrication Device (KED). In a hemodynamically unstable patient, rapid extrication onto a long spine board can be accomplished by multiple rescuers manually supporting the spine without the aid of a KED. Immobilization is not considered complete until the patient is secured to the spine board with straps, the patient's head is secured to the spine board with tape across the forehead and beneath the chin, and a cervical collar and lateral neck rolls or head immobilization device are in place.

If endotracheal control intubation is necessary, the cervical spine should remain immobilized while the procedure is performed. Should vomiting occur, the patient may be logrolled to face sideways while one rescuer maintains cervical spine traction.

2. Splinting—(See Chapters 28 and 29.) In general, extremities should be placed in an anatomic position, especially if pulses cannot be felt below a suspected fracture. If the patient protests or if resistance is felt, extremities should remain in a position of comfort. Reduction of fracture dislocations at a joint should be attempted only if vascular compromise is impending, the duration of transport is long, and the rescuer is experienced in the technique. This usually requires the base physician's approval.

A pillow, rolled-up blanket, or other material may often serve as a simple splint. Specific splinting devices include cardboard splints, inflatable air splints, the MAST (military antishock trousers) garment, and traction splints. If inflatable devices are used, care must be taken to monitor distal perfusion, because a compartment syndrome may occur with swelling of the extremity or changes in atmospheric pressure (eg, during air transport). Traction splints are used primarily with fractures of the femur.

G. PROTOCOLS AND STANDING ORDERS

Protocols are guidelines designed to assist the EMT in performing tasks in a complete and orderly fashion (Figure 2–3). Because situations vary widely and protocols cannot anticipate every variable, they are not meant to be absolute and must be accompanied by training, judgment, and experience. Each EMS system tailors its protocol to the training and skill of its EMTs and the needs of the local medical community.

Standing orders are express authorizations for the performance of a specific task or procedure. Under the standing order, an EMT may be authorized to perform a task or procedure without first obtaining verbal authorization by radio. Standing orders are useful when radio contact is impractical or would delay life-saving intervention (eg, CPR, defibrillation). Standing orders usually contain a clear list of circumstances under which the authorization applies (indications) and detailed instructions on the manner in which the procedure should be performed. They are signed by the physician medical director, who shares legal responsibility for the outcome.

H. COMMUNICATIONS

1. Equipment and frequencies—EMS units communicate with receiving hospitals by various methods. Three main radio systems exist: the HEAR network (in the 150-MHz range), the COR system (400 MHz), and the 800-MHz truncated system. The HEAR system is the oldest and has largely been replaced in urban areas by 800-MHz systems, which provide multiple frequencies for providers. In addition, cellular phones and landline telephones are used frequently for communications. Communication is simplex. Signals pass in only one direction at a time, and neither party can simultaneously speak and be heard. In rural areas, communica-

tion may be direct, via radio, without a relay station or ground lines.

2. Communication technique—Radio communication must provide information in a concise, precise, and easily understood manner. To facilitate speed and understanding, a common format is followed, with slight variations depending on the community. However, no one should hesitate to ask for clarification, because misunderstandings may prove fatal.

a. The initial contact—The caller always names the party being called first, followed by the caller's own identification:

"Central Hospital, this is medic 19, how do you copy?"

b. The initial response—The initial response confirms the contact in the same manner:

"Medic 19, Central Hospital, receiving you loud and clear, over."

c. The report—The caller gives a concise, orderly report containing pertinent history, physical findings, destination, estimated time of arrival (ETA), and any necessary request for instructions. It should be as brief as possible:

"Central Hospital, medic 19 en route to your location, ETA 8 minutes, with a 20-year old male victim of multiple, small-caliber gunshot wounds to the left chest, right flank, and right thigh. Patient is lethargic; blood pressure 80, pulse 140, respirations 46. Breath sounds absent over the left chest, abdomen soft. We have an ET tube in place, 2 IVs with lactated Ringer's wide open, and MAST garment inflated. Requesting permission for needle decompression of the left chest."

d. The report acknowledgment—This acknowledgment is kept brief; only essential queries should be made:

"Medic 19, have you checked ET tube position?"

"That's affirmative. Withdrawn 2 centimeters without improvement."

"Okay, medic 19; needle thoracostomy, left chest, is approved. Will stand by for update."

e. The sign-off—After receiving an order, the field personnel should repeat it to demonstrate that it was received accurately before signing off:

"Central Hospital, understand needle thoracostomy, left chest, is approved. Stand by."

3. 10-Codes—"Ten codes" are phrases represented by 2 numbers, the first being 10. In many areas, these are used to ensure precise communication and to add some measure of privacy to the conversation. Unfortunately, few EMS personnel have all of the possible 120 codes memorized. The result is often more confusion rather than less. Because mistakes may be dangerous, the

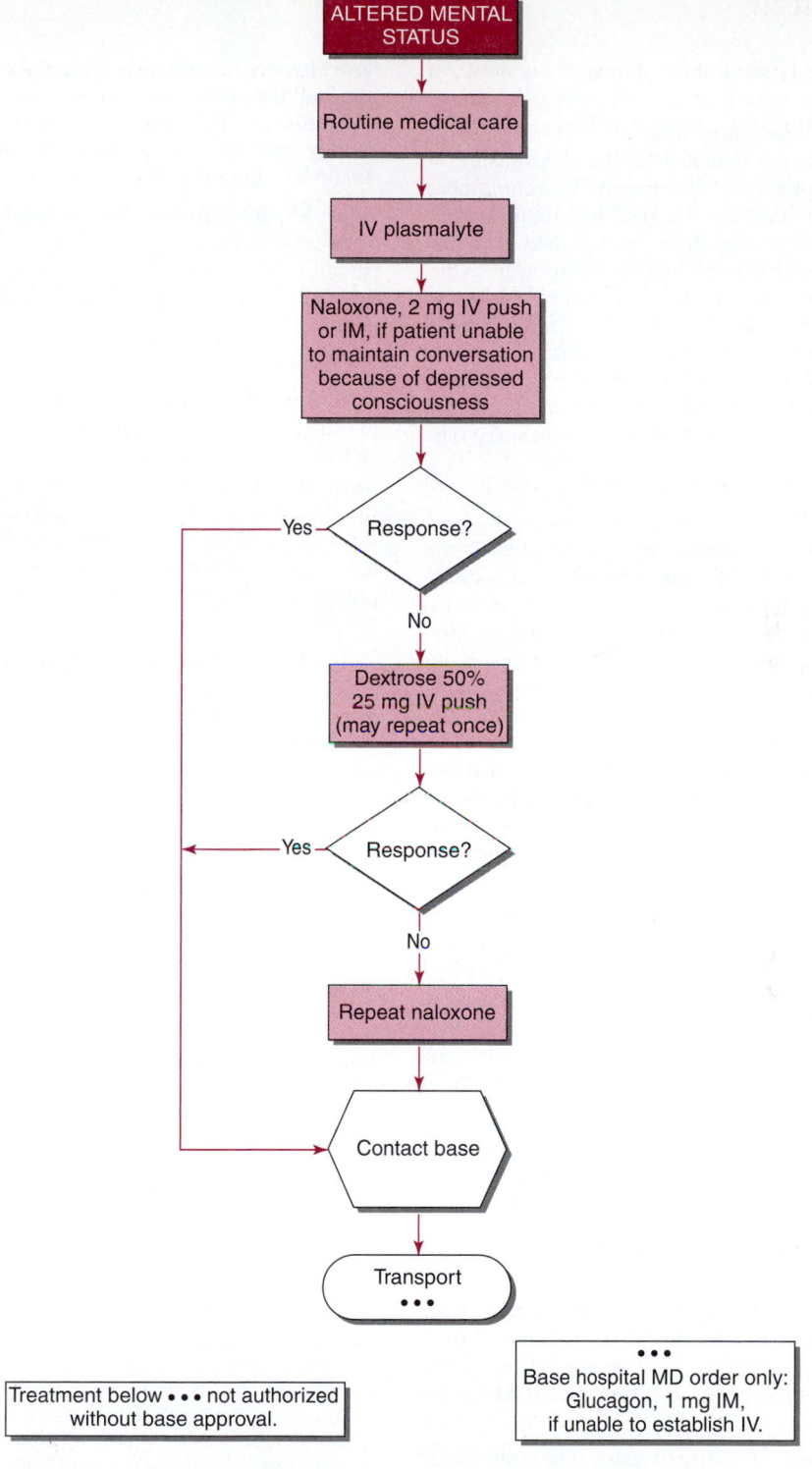

Figure 2–3. Sample protocol (in algorithmic form) for altered mental status. **Note:** The sequence for administering naloxone or glucose should be based on history and physical examination at the scene.

codes should not be used unless thoroughly understood by all parties.

4. Telemetry—Receiving hospitals and ambulances may have equipment designed for the transmission of electrocardiographic traces (telemetry). This equipment is seldom used, however, because well-trained paramedics have shown the ability to interpret unstable rhythms (eg, ventricular fibrillation, ventricular tachycardia, bradycardia, and asystole) with acceptable precision, and more complex rhythms (eg, supraventricular tachycardia) rarely require treatment that cannot be postponed until arrival at the hospital. As indicated above, the prehospital 12-lead ECG has shortened the door to drug time in patients with acute coronary syndromes.

I. Air Transport

1. Indications—As noted above, the benefits to the patient must outweigh the risks inherent in this mode of transport. Aeromedical transport is most advantageous when great distances must be covered rapidly, when ground transport is unavailable or impeded by geographic obstacles or dense traffic, or when specialized care (eg, trauma resuscitation) is needed at the scene or en route. Emergency medical helicopters serving rural areas often provide a higher level of care and more skilled procedures (eg, intubation, needle thoracostomy, cricothyrotomy) than are provided by localized services using basic EMTs. However, air transport is hazardous, and helicopters operating at night and in inclement weather have crashed.

2. Requesting service—Helicopters equipped for medical evacuation can be requested, through the EMS communications network, from an area hospital that offers such services or from a local military base that participates in the Military Assistance to Safety and Traffic program.

3. Patient preparation—Before departure, stabilize the patient on a spine board and immobilize the patient as clinically indicated. Secure airway tubes and intravenous catheters.

4. Anticipated physiologic consequences of air transport—

a. Hypoxia—Atmospheric pressure decreases with increasing altitude, as does the partial pressure of oxygen. Patients with existing heart or lung disease may suffer adverse consequences. Supplemental oxygen is required.

b. Expansion of trapped gas—The volume of trapped gas increases with decreasing barometric pressure. Thus, as altitude increases, air may expand in endotracheal tube cuffs, air splints, MAST garments, the

bowel lumen, the stomach, pneumothorax, abscess cavities, and the bottles and tubing of intravenous infusion apparatus. These compartments must be monitored frequently and vented as necessary. Intravenous flow rates should be adjusted accordingly.

c. Motion, noise, and vibration—These may cause patient discomfort. Forward acceleration with the patient's head forward may cause transient hypotension. This may be prevented by positioning the patient with feet forward.

5. Helicopter safety—

a. Site selection and lighting—A helicopter landing site should be level, approximately 100 feet square, and free of obstacles (eg, trees, wires) to approach and departure. It should also be clear of loose debris. The site should be secure from bystanders. At night, the site should be well lighted (eg, with vehicle headlights), but lights should never be directed upward toward the approaching helicopter, because they might interfere with the pilot's vision.

b. Approaching a helicopter—While the rotor blades are turning, approach the aircraft only from the front and only after prompting by the pilot. Avoid the tail rotor. Approach in a crouched position. Do not run. Never approach from uphill.

Lower tall objects such as poles associated with intravenous infusion apparatus. Secure sheets, hats, and loose clothing. Extinguish all smoking material.

Abarbanell NR, Marcotte MA: Prehospital use of intravenous diltiazem (Cardizem Lyo-Ject) in the treatment of rapid atrial fibrillation. Am J Emerg Med 1997;15:618. [PMID: 9337374]

Alspach G: Preventing prehospital delays in seeking care for acute myocardial infarction: a patient education program. Crit Care Nurs 1999;19:10. [PMID: 10808808]

Bond RJ, Kortbeek JB, Preshaw RM: Field trauma triage: combining mechanism of injury with the prehospital index for an improved trauma triage tool. J Trauma 1997;43:283. [PMID: 9291374]

Caldwell MA, Froelicher ES, Drew BJ: Prehospital delay time in acute myocardial infarction: an exploratory study on relation to hospital outcomes and cost. Am Heart J 2000;139:788. [PMID: 10783211]

Cannon CP, Sayah AJ, Walls RM: ER TIMI-19: testing the reality of prehospital thrombolysis. J Emerg Med 2000;19:21S. [PMID: 11050380] (Review.)

Canto JG et al: The prehospital electrocardiogram in acute myocardial infarction: is its full potential being realized? National Registry of Myocardial Infarction 2 Investigators. J Am Coll Cardiol 1997;29:498. [PMID: 9060884]

Collins D: The prehospital 12-lead EKG: starting outside the emergency department. J Emerg Nurs 1997;23:48. [PMID: 9128512]

Crocco TJ et al: A nationwide prehospital stroke survey. Prehosp Emerg Care 1999;3:201. [PMID: 10424856]

Deschamp C: Scene times: what is reasonable for paramedic-level prehospital care? Emerg Med Serv 2000;29:96. [PMID: 11143044]

Dickinson ET, Schneider RM, Verdile VP: The impact of prehospital physicians on out-of-hospital nonasystolic cardiac arrest. Prehosp Emerg Care 1997;1:132. [PMID: 9709354]

Doering GT: Customer care. Patient satisfaction in the prehospital setting. Emerg Med Serv 1998;27:69. [PMID: 10185418]

Fischberg BL et al: Development and use of a prehospital-oriented EMS computer bulletin board service. Prehosp Emerg Care 1999;3:243. [PMID: 10424863]

Gausche M et al: Effect of out-of-hospital pediatric endotracheal intubation on survival and neurological outcome: a controlled clinical trial. JAMA 2000;283:783. [PMID: 10683058]

Gerich TG et al: Prehospital airway management in the acutely injured patient: the role of surgical cricothyrotomy revisited. J Trauma 1998;45:312. [PMID: 9715188]

Greiff SJ: Taking it to the street: advanced monitoring and 12-lead EKGs in prehospital care. Emerg Med Serv 1998;27:47. [PMID: 10185417]

Grossman DC et al: Urban-rural differences in prehospital care of major trauma. J Trauma 1997;42:723. [PMID: 9137264]

Howes DW et al: Justification of pulse oximeter costs for paramedic prehospital providers. Prehosp Emerg Care 2000;4:151. [PMID: 10782604]

Jewkes F: Prehospital emergency care for children. Arch Dis Child 2001;84:103. [PMID: 11159280]

Jezierski M: Family violence screening: opportunities in prehospital settings. J Emerg Nurs 1999;25:201. [PMID: 10346843]

Katz SH et al: Misplaced endotracheal tubes by paramedics in an urban emergency medical services system. Ann Emerg Med 2001;37:62. [PMID: 11145768]

Loos L, Runyan L, Pelch D: Development of prehospital medical classification criteria. Air Med J 1998;17:13. [PMID: 10176557]

Ma MH et al: Compliance with prehospital triage protocols for major trauma patients. J Trauma 1999;46:168. [PMID: 9932702]

McConnel CE, Wilson RW: The demand for prehospital emergency services in an aging society. Soc Sci Med 1998;46:1027. [PMID: 9579754]

Moore L: Measuring quality and effectiveness of prehospital EMS. Prehosp Emerg Care 1999;3:325. [PMID: 10534034]

Morris DL et al: Prehospital and emergency department delays after acute stroke: the Genentech Stroke Presentation Survey. Stroke 2000;31:2585. [PMID: 11062279]

Myers RB: Prehospital management of acute myocardial infarction: electrocardiogram acquisition and interpretation, and thrombolysis by prehospital care providers. Can J Cardiol 1998;14:1231. [PMID: 9852937]

Nijs HG et al: Need for consensus development in prehospital emergency medicine: effect of an expert panel approach. Eur J Emerg Med 1998;5:329. [PMID: 9827837]

Nordlander R, Svensson L: Prehospital management of patients with acute coronary syndromes. Acta Anaesthesiol Scand Suppl 1997;110:80. [PMID: 9248542]

Ossmann EW, Bartkus EA, Olinger ML: Prehospital pearls, pitfalls, and updates. Emerg Med Clin North Am 1997;15:283. [PMID: 9183273]

Plischke M et al: Telemedical support of prehospital emergency care in mass casualty incidents. Eur J Med Res 1999;4:394. [PMID: 10477508]

Pullum JD, Sanddal ND, Obbink K: Training for rural prehospital providers: a retrospective analysis from Montana. Prehosp Emerg Care 1999;3:231. [PMID: 10424861]

Roth A et al: Potential reduction of costs and hospital emergency department visits resulting from prehospital transtelephonic triage—the Shahal experience in Israel. Clin Cardiol 2000;23:271. [PMID: 10763075]

Schou J: Duration and type of prehospital emergency therapy. Eur J Emerg Med 1999;6(3):185. [PMID: 10622381]

Seaman KG: Emergency medical service system evaluation and planning strategies for prehospital chest pain in Howard County, Maryland. MD Med J 1997;Suppl:80. [PMID: 9470352]

Shapiro SE: Outcomes of prehospital care: do we really make a difference? J Emerg Nurs 2000;26:239. [PMID: 10839853]

Spivak M: Legislating EMS. "EMS Efficiency Act of 1998" aims to improve prehospital services. Emerg Med Serv 1998;27:20. [PMID: 10185405]

Spivak M: No time to wait. An overview of recent studies and departmental programs designed to improve prehospital response to cardiac emergencies. Emerg Med Serv 1998;27:33. [PMID: 10185415]

Spivak M: Trauma care in EMS: where are we? A look at the nature, origins, controversies and future of prehospital trauma services. Emerg Med Serv 1999;28:29. [PMID: 10351460]

Stern R, Arntz HR: Prehospital thrombolysis in acute myocardial infarction. Eur J Emerg Med 1998;5:471. [PMID: 9919456]

Stiell IG et al: Improved out-of-hospital cardiac arrest survival through the inexpensive optimization of an existing defibrillation program: OPALS Study phase II. Ontario Prehospital Advanced Life Support. JAMA 1999;281:1175. [PMID: 10199426]

Streger MR: Prehospital triage. Emerg Med Serv 1998;27:21. [PMID: 10180394]

Suominen P et al: Prehospital care and survival of pediatric patients with blunt trauma. J Pediatr Surg 1998;33:1388. [PMID: 9766360]

Vaccaro AR et al: The management of acute spinal trauma: prehospital and in-hospital emergency care. Instr Course Lect 1997;46:113. [PMID: 9143955]

VanRooyen MJ, Thomas TL, Clem KJ: International emergency medical services: assessment of developing prehospital systems abroad. J Emerg Med 1999;17:691. [PMID: 10431962]

Vermeulen B et al: Prehospital stabilization of pelvic dislocations: a new strap belt to provide temporary hemodynamic stabilization. Swiss Surg 1999;5:43. [PMID: 10217975]

Warwick J: How much to do at the accident scene? Paramedic agrees with most of comments about prehospital care. BMJ 2000;320:1005. [PMID: 10753163]

Weaver J, Brinsfield KH, Dalphond D: Prehospital refusal-of-transport policies: adequate legal protection? Prehosp Emerg Care 2000;4:53. [PMID: 10634284]

Nuclear, Biologic, & Chemical Agents; Weapons of Mass Destruction

3

Michael W. Stava, MD, & Joachim Franklin, MD

Nuclear Weapons

Biologic Weapons

Bacterial Agents

1. Anthrax
2. Plague
3. Tularemia
4. Brucellosis
5. Q Fever
6. Glanders & Melioidosis

Viral Agents

1. Smallpox
2. Hemorrhagic Fever
3. Viral Encephalitis

Biologic Toxins

1. Botulinum Toxin
2. Ricin
3. T-2 Mycotoxins
4. Staphylococcal Enterotoxin B

Chemical Weapons

Nerve Agents

Pulmonary Agents

Vesicants

1. Sulfur Mustard
2. Lewisite

Cyanide Agents

Chemical Decontamination

In the past, injuries resulting from nuclear, biologic, and chemical attack were largely dealt with only in the military sector. Society as a whole, and specifically the civilian medical community, felt it unlikely that such weapons would be used against civilian populations. Recent changes in the global political environment have forced changes in this thinking. Many smaller nations, some of which are judged unstable, are attempting to develop weapons of mass destruction. Likewise, many terrorist organizations are now actively attempting to purchase or develop such weapons. In addition to the risk of an overt attack, other sources of exposure could come from accidents involving many nuclear, biologic, and chemical agents stored in facilities throughout the United States. An accident at any of these facilities could result in a large number of civilian casualties. As with most mass casualty situations, emergency physicians will be at the forefront of patient care. This chapter attempts to provide specific information regarding the management of nuclear, biologic, and chemical weapons injuries.

■ NUCLEAR WEAPONS

Several incidents in recent history, both military and civilian, have resulted in radiation injuries. The most notable, and in fact the only war-time use, involved the detonation of nuclear weapons over Hiroshima and Nagasaki, Japan. Unfortunately, many terrorist organizations have attempted to obtain nuclear weapons. A terrorist attack would most likely involve the detonation of a nuclear bomb or the detonation of a conventional explosive that also dispersed radioactive material (so-called dirty bomb).

General Considerations

Radiation-induced injury occurs when various types of ionizing radiation interact with body tissues. Radiation exposure may be external or internal. Internal contamination can occur via wound contamination or via inhalation or ingestion of contaminated particles. Four types of radioactive particles may cause damage:

1. Alpha particles—Alpha particles are large particles that are stopped by the epidermis. They cause no significant external damage. Internal contamination may cause local tissue injury.

2. Beta particles—Beta particles are small particles that can penetrate the superficial skin and cause mild burnlike injuries.

3. Gamma rays—Gamma rays are high-energy particles that can enter tissues easily and cause significant damage to multiple body systems.

4. Neutrons—Neutrons are large particles that are typically produced only during nuclear detonation. Like gamma rays, they cause significant tissue injury.

The effect that radiation will have on the body depends on the type of radiation, the amount of exposure, and the body system involved. Tissues that display higher rates of cellular mitosis, such as the gastrointestinal and hematopoietic systems, are more severely affected. At very high radiation doses, neurovascular effects will also be seen. Radiation injury may cause either abnormal cell function or cell death.

Clinical Findings

A. Symptoms and Signs

The symptoms and signs of radiation exposure occur in 3 phases: prodromal, latent, and symptomatic.

1. Prodromal phase—Patients will develop nonspecific symptoms of nausea, vomiting, weakness, and fatigue. Symptoms generally last no longer than 24–48 hours. With higher radiation exposures, symptoms will occur more rapidly and last longer.

2. Latent period—The length of the latent period depends on the dose of radiation and the body system involved (neurologic, several hours; gastrointestinal, 1–7 days; hematopoietic, 2–6 weeks).

3. Symptomatic phase—Symptoms will depend largely on the body system affected, which will depend on the radiation dose. At doses of 0.7–4 gray (Gy),[1] the hematopoietic system will begin to manifest signs and symptoms of bone marrow suppression. Because of their long life span, erythrocytes are less severely affected than are the myeloid and platelet cell lines. Neutropenia and thrombocytopenia may be significant and lead to infectious and hemorrhagic complications. At

doses of 6–8 Gy, gastrointestinal symptoms develop. Nausea, vomiting, diarrhea (bloody), and severe fluid and electrolyte imbalances will occur. The neurovascular system becomes affected at doses of 20–40 Gy. Symptoms include headache, mental status changes, hypotension, focal neurologic changes, convulsions, and coma. Exposures in this range are uniformly fatal. If an explosive device was used to disperse radioactive material, patients may also have thermal and blast injuries.

B. Laboratory and X-ray Findings

Obtain a complete blood count (CBC) with differential for all patients sustaining a radiation injury. Although symptomatic bone marrow suppression may not be evident for some weeks, a drop of the absolute lymphocyte count of 50% at 24–48 hours is indicative of significant exposure. Monitor electrolytes in patients with gastrointestinal symptoms.

Treatment

In the absence of aggressive medical therapy, the LD50 (the dose of radiation that will kill 50% of those exposed) is approximately 3.5 Gy. Aggressive medical care affords improved survival. Treat all life-threatening injuries associated with blast or thermal effects according to standard advanced trauma life support protocols. Perform surgical procedures early to avoid the electrolyte and hematopoietic effects that will occur. Clean wounds extensively and close them as soon as possible to prevent infection. Treat nausea and vomiting with standard antiemetic medications (prochlorperazine, promethazine, ondansetron). Treat fluid and electrolyte abnormalities with appropriate replacement. Anemia and thrombocytopenia can be treated with transfusion therapy. Leukopenia may be treated with hematopoietic growth factors such as sargramostim and filgrastim. In some instances bone marrow transplantation may be utilized. Follow neutropenic precautions at absolute neutrophil counts below 500. Some authors recommend prophylactic antibiotics at counts below 100. Use broad-spectrum antibiotics to treat infections. Infection is the most common cause of death in radiation patients. Despite aggressive medical care, radiation exposures above 10 Gy are usually fatal.

Decontamination

Remove all contaminated clothing. Change contaminated dressings and splints. Thoroughly clean the patient's skin with soap and water or a 0.5% hypochlorite solution. Hair should be washed and in some instances removed. Eyes may be washed with large amounts of

---

[1]The gray, a unit of measure for the dose of ionizing radiation, is equal to 1 J/kg of tissue. One gray is equal to 100 rad.

water or sterile saline. All contaminated materials should be bagged if possible and sent for proper disposal.

Disposition

Patients who have been decontaminated and have only mild transient symptoms can be safely discharged. Because of the variable and lengthy latent period involved with this disorder, early admission is not indicated. Patients should be closely monitored and admitted when warranted.

Goans RE et al: Early dose assessment in criticality accidents. Health Phys 2001;81(4):446. [PMID: 11569639] (Describes techniques for estimating the severity of radiation exposure.)

Military Medical Operations Office, Armed Forces Radiobiology Research Institute: *Medical Management of Radiological Casualties,* 1st ed. Military Medical Operations Office, Armed Forces Radiobiology Research Institute, 1999. (Produced by the U.S. Army, this text provides general information regarding all aspects of radiologic injuries.)

■ BIOLOGIC WEAPONS

Many agents can be used as biologic weapons. The most likely pathogens are presented here. Biologic agents can be classified as bacterial agents (anthrax, plague, tularemia, brucellosis, Q fever, glanders), viral agents (smallpox, hemorrhagic fever, encephalitis), and biologic toxins (botulinum, ricin, T-2 mycotoxins, staphylococcal enterotoxin B). A high index of suspicion will be required in order to identify patients who have experienced a biologic attack. A large number of patients with severe febrile illnesses will be the most likely clue. Keep in mind the attack most likely occurred several days prior to patient presentation. Aerosol release of infectious material is the most common form of biologic attack.

BACTERIAL AGENTS
(See Table 3–1.)

1. Anthrax

Bacillus anthracis is a gram-positive, sporulating rod. Anthrax infection occurs naturally after contact with contaminated animals or contaminated animal products. A biologic attack would likely involve the aerosol release of anthrax spores. The spore form of anthrax causes infection. Clinically the disease occurs in 3 forms: inhalational anthrax, gastrointestinal anthrax, and cutaneous anthrax.

Clinical Findings

A. Symptoms and Signs

1. Inhalational anthrax—Inhalation anthrax is the form of disease most likely expected after a terrorist attack. After spores are inhaled, a variable incubation period occurs, usually lasting 1–7 days. Prolonged incubation periods of up to 60 days have been observed. Initially, nonspecific symptoms of fever, cough, headache, chills, vomiting, dyspnea, chest pain, abdominal pain, and weakness occur. This stage may last from a few hours to a few days. Following these nonspecific symptoms, a transient period of improvement may be seen. When the second stage of disease is reached, high fever, diaphoresis, cyanosis, hypotension, lymphadenopathy, shock, and death will occur. Often death will occur within hours once the second stage is reached. The average time from onset of symptoms to death is 3 days. Once the initial symptoms of inhalational anthrax develop, the overall mortality rate may be as high as 95%. Early diagnosis of anthrax infection and rapid initiation of therapy may improve survival.

2. Gastrointestinal anthrax—Gastrointestinal anthrax occurs when spores are ingested into the digestive tract. Two forms of the disease occur: oropharyngeal and abdominal. Oropharyngeal disease occurs when spores are deposited in the upper gastrointestinal tract. An oral or esophageal ulcer develops followed by regional lymphadenopathy and eventual sepsis. In abdominal anthrax, the spores are deposited in the lower gastrointestinal tract. Symptoms include nausea, vomiting, diarrhea (bloody), and the development of an acute abdomen with sepsis. Mortality rates for gastrointestinal anthrax are in excess of 50%.

3. Cutaneous anthrax—Cutaneous anthrax is the most common naturally occurring form of the disease. Cutaneous anthrax occurs when spores come in contact with open skin lesions. This usually occurs on the arms, hands, and face. Following exposure, a small, often pruritic papule will develop. Eventually this papule will turn into a small ulcer (over 2 days), then progress to a small vesicle, and ultimately to a painless black eschar with surrounding edema. Then, over a period of 1–2 weeks, the eschar will dry and fall off. Regional lymphadenitis or lymphadenopathy may also occur. In some case secondary sepsis may develop. Without treatment, cutaneous anthrax has a mortality rate of 20%; however, the mortality rate drops to 1% with treatment.

4. Anthrax meningitis—Anthrax meningitis can occur as a complication of any other form of anthrax. Symptoms include headache and meningismus. Anthrax meningitis carries a mortality rate of nearly 100%.

Table 3–1. Clinical findings and treatment of bacterial biologic agent infection[1].

Agent	Syndrome	Incubation	Symptoms Early	Symptoms Late	Treatment[1] First-line	Treatment[1] Prophylaxis
Anthrax (*Bacillus anthracis*; gram-positive, sporulating)	Inhalational	1–7days	Fever, chills, nausea and vomiting, headache, cough, dyspnea, chest pain, abdominal pain.	High fever, diaphoresis, cyanosis, hypotension, lymphadenopathy, shock, death (within 3 days of late sympton onset).	Ciprofloxacin, 400 mg IV q 12 h or doxycycline, 200 mg IV, then 100 mg IV q 12 h. Without use of vaccine, treat for 60 days; with use of vaccine, treat for 30 days. As patient improves, may begin oral therapy.	Ciprofloxacin, 500 mg PO bid x 4 wk or doxycycline, 100 mg PO bid x 4 wk and begin vaccine.
	Gastrointestinal (upper)		Oral or esophageal ulcer.	Regional lymphadenopathy, sepsis.		
	Gastrointestinal (lower)		Nausea and vomiting, diarrhea (bloody).	Acute abdomen, sepsis.		
	Cutaneous	2 days	Pruritic papule → ulcer → vesicle → painless eschar.	Regional lymphadenopathy, occasional sepsis (1-2 weeks after onset).		
Plague (*Yersinia pestis*; gram-negative bacillus)	Bubonic	1–7 days	Fever, chills, malaise, lymphdenopathy.	Necrotic lymphadenitis (1-10 cm) called a bubo, possible sepsis.	Streptomycin, 30 mg/kg/d IM divided bid 10-14 d or gentamicin, 5 mg/kg IV x 10-14 d.	Doxycycline, 100 mg PO bid x 7 d or ciprofloxacin, 500 mg PO bid x 7 d.
	Septicemia (can be primary or secondary)		Fever, chills, dyspnea, hypotension, purpura.	Gangrene of nose and extremities, disseminated intravascular coagulation, death.		
	Pneumonic	1–6 days	Fever, chills, productive cough, dyspnea, hypoxia, nausea and vomiting.	Sepsis.		
Tularemia (*Francisella tularensis*; aerobic, gram-negative coccobacilli)	Ulceroglandular	Patients with any type may present with fever, chills, headache, myalgia, malaise, maculopapular rash; all types can spread hematogenously.	Papule (inoculation site) → pustule → tender ulcer (yellow exudates, black base), painful regional lymphadenopathy.		Streptomycin, 10 mg/kg/kg/d IM divided bid 10 d or gentamicin, 5 mg/kg IV x 10 d.	Doxycycline, 100 mg PO bid x 14 d or ciprofloxacin, 500 mg PO bid x 14 d.
	Glandular		Same as above except without ulcer.			

(continued)

Table 3–1. Clinical findings and treatment of bacterial biologic agent infection[1]. (*Continued*)

Agent	Syndrome	Incubation	Symptoms — Early	Symptoms — Late	Treatment[1] — First-line	Treatment[1] — Prophylaxis
	Occuloglandular			Painful conjunctivitis, lymphadenopathy, ulcerations on palpebral conjunctiva.		
	Oropharyngeal			Exudative pharyngotonsillitis, lymphadenopathy.		
	Pneumonic			Pharyngitis, bronchiolitis, hilar lymphadenopathy, pneumonia, pulmonary failure, death.		
	Typhoidal			Sepsis.		
Brucellosis (pleomorphic gram-negative coccobacilli)		1–3 weeks	Fever, chills, malaise, myalgias.	May afflict a variety of organs or organ systems.	Rifampin, 600 mg/d PO plus doxycycline, 200 mg/d PO x 6 wk.	Same as treatment course, but may be shortened to 3 weeks.
Q fever (*Coxiella burnetii*)	Can be acute or indolent in its course	5–30 days	Fever, chills, headache, malaise, myalgia, anorexia.	May afflict a variety of organs or organ systems. Endocarditis and gastrointestinal symptoms are common.	Tetracycline, 500 mg PO q 6 h x 5-7 d or doxycycline, 100 mg PO bid x 5-7 d.	Same as treatment course.
Glanders and melioidosis (*Burkholderia* spp; gram-negative bacillus)	Localized	1–2 weeks	Wound contamination, cellulitis, lymphadenopathy lymphangitis.	Sepsis can result with all modes of infection, death from sepsis occurs in 7-10 days.	Local disease: amoxicillin-clavulanate, 60 mg/kg/d divided tid x 60 d. Severe disease: ceftazidime, 120 mg/kg/d divided tid plus trimethoprim-sulfamethoxazole, 8 mg/kg/d divided qid x 2 w followed by prolonged oral therapy.	Trimethoprim-sulfamethoxazole (160 mg/800 mg) PO bid x 14 d.
	Pulmonary		Fever, chills, cough, dyspnea.			
	Septicemic		Fever, chills, malaise, abscesses, headache, pustular rash.			

[1]Alternatives to the regimens given here may be used.

B. Laboratory and X-ray Findings

Multiple laboratory studies can be used to identify anthrax. In fulminant cases, the organism may be seen on routine Gram stain. Blood cultures, wound cultures, and nasal cultures may be obtained. Given the lack of an infiltrate, sputum cultures are rarely useful. Notify laboratory personnel of a possible anthrax exposure. Often *Bacillus* spp. are thought to be the contaminant and are not pursued further. Confirmatory enzyme-linked immunoassay (ELISA) and polymerase chain reaction (PCR) tests are available at some national reference laboratories. Chest X-ray may also be useful. Patients with inhalational anthrax will display a wide mediastinum on chest x-ray. No infiltrate is typically observed.

Treatment & Prophylaxis

Because anthrax has a rapid and fulminant course, do not delay treatment while awaiting confirmatory tests. Institute empiric therapy when the diagnosis is considered. Delaying treatment for even hours may significantly increase mortality.

A. Antibiotics

Most naturally occurring strains of anthrax are sensitive to penicillin. Some strains, however, are penicillin resistant. Weapons-grade anthrax is likely to be penicillin resistant. As a result, the first-line therapy is now ciprofloxacin; doxycycline is an acceptable alternative (see Table 3–1). Treatment should continue for 60 days. If cultures were obtained, later sensitivity testing may direct antibiotic use.

B. Supportive Care

Patients may require intensive medical support such as airway management, hemodynamic support, and various measures to manage multisystem organ failure.

C. Prophylaxis

Individuals thought to be at high risk for anthrax exposure should receive treatment as though infection has occurred. Later laboratory analysis may allow discontinuation of therapy. An anthrax vaccination is available and requires injections at 0, 2, and 4 weeks, followed by injections at 6, 12, and 18 months. An annual booster is also required. If a combination of vaccination and antibiotics is used during treatment, the course of antibiotics may be shortened to 30 days.

Infection Control

No data indicate that anthrax is spread via person-to-person contact. Use standard precautions during patient care activities (Table 3–2).

Table 3–2. Levels of protection required during patient care activities.

Protection Level	Required Equipment
Standard precautions	Universal precautions; hand washing; protective gloves; gown, mask, eye protection, if splash risk exists.
Droplet precautions	Same as standard precautions, except add surgical or Hepa filter mask.
Airborne precautions	Same as standard precautions, except add negative pressure room, strict isolation; Hepa filter mask required.

2. Plague

Yersinia pestis is a nonmotile, gram-negative bacillus. Plague occurs naturally after the bite of an infected arthropod vector. Biologic attack would most likely involve the aerosolized release of *Y pestis*. Plague occurs in 3 clinical forms: bubonic plague, septicemic plague, and pneumonic plague.

Clinical Findings

A. Symptoms and Signs

1. Bubonic plague—Bubonic plague is the most common naturally occurring form of the disease. Infection begins with the bite of a contaminated flea. A latent period then occurs and may last up to 1 week, followed by fevers, chills, and weakness. Eventually the organism will migrate to the regional lymph nodes where it causes destruction and necrosis. A swollen and tender lymph node called a bubo will develop. Bubo size ranges from 1 to 10 cm. Some patients may develop secondary sepsis. Without treatment, bubonic plague has an estimated mortality rate of 50%; however, with antibiotic therapy the mortality rate falls to 10%.

2. Septicemic plague—Septicemic plague may occur either as a complication of other forms of plague or as a primary entity. Symptoms include fever, dyspnea, hypotension, and purpuric skin lesions. Gangrene of the nose and extremities may occur, hence, the name "black death." Complications of disseminated intravascular coagulation may also be evident. Without treatment, septicemic plague has an estimated mortality rate of 100%; however, with antibiotic therapy the mortality rate falls to 40%.

3. Pneumonic plague—Pneumonic plague may occur either as a complication of other forms of plague or as a primary entity. It is the most likely form of the disease to result from a terrorist attack. A latent period of 1–6 days following exposure is likely. Patients will then develop signs and symptoms of severe pulmonary infection including fever, cough, dyspnea, hypoxia, and sputum production. Gastrointestinal symptoms of nausea, vomiting, and diarrhea may also occur. Pneumonic plague has an estimated mortality rate of 100% if antibiotic therapy is not begun within 24 hours.

B. LABORATORY AND X-RAY FINDINGS

Y pestis can be identified by several different staining techniques. Routine Gram stain may reveal the organism. *Y pestis* also has a characteristic bipolar staining pattern with Wright, Giemsa, and Wayson stains. Routine blood cultures, sputum cultures, and cultures of lymph node aspirates may be useful. Specialized rapid confirmatory tests are available at some laboratories. In patients with pneumonic plague, chest x-ray will display a patchy or confluent infiltrate.

Treatment & Prophylaxis

Plague has a rapid disease progression, and any delay in treatment will cause significant increases in mortality. Institute treatment on empiric grounds, and do not delay treatment while awaiting confirmatory tests.

A. ANTIBIOTICS

Streptomycin is the drug of choice for the treatment of plague. Gentamicin may also be used and is thought to have equal efficacy (see Table 3–1). Alternative antibiotics include doxycycline, ciprofloxacin, and chloramphenicol.

B. SUPPORTIVE CARE

Patients may require intensive medical support such as airway management, hemodynamic support, and other measures to manage multisystem organ failure.

C. PROPHYLAXIS

Patients in a community experiencing a pneumonic plague epidemic should receive antibiotic therapy if they develop a cough or a fever above 38.5 °C (101.2 °F). Any person who has been in close contact with an individual with plague should receive a 7-day course of antibiotics. Antibiotic choices are the same as for treatment.

Infection Control

Pneumonic plague can be spread from person to person by aerosol droplets. Use droplet precautions, and either the patient or caregivers should wear masks (see Table 3–2). Once the patient has received 48 hours of antibiotics and has improved clinically, standard precautions may be used.

3. Tularemia

Francisella tularensis is a nonmotile, aerobic, gram-negative coccobacillus. Two strains of tularemia are known to exist. *F tularensis* biovar tularensis is considered highly virulent, whereas *F tularensis* biovar palaearctica is more benign. Tularemia occurs naturally after the bite of an infected arthropod vector or after exposure to contaminated animal products. Biologic attack would most likely involve the release of aerosolized *F tularensis*. Tularemia displays multiple clinical forms including ulceroglandular, glandular, oculoglandular, oropharyngeal, pneumonic, and typhoidal forms. The form of disease depends on the site and type of inoculation.

Clinical Findings

A. SYMPTOMS AND SIGNS

Patients with any form of tularemia may present with the abrupt onset of fever, chills, headache, malaise, and myalgias. Often a maculopapular rash is seen.

1. Ulceroglandular tularemia—Ulceroglandular tularemia usually occurs after handling infected animals or after the bite of an infected arthropod vector. At the inoculation site a papule will form that will eventually become a pustule and then a tender ulcer. The ulcer may have a yellow exudate and will slowly develop a black base. Regional lymph nodes will become swollen and painful.

2. Glandular tularemia—Glandular tularemia displays signs and symptoms similar to ulceroglandular tularemia, except that no ulcer formation is noted.

3. Oculoglandular tularemia—After ocular inoculation, a painful conjunctivitis will develop with regional lymphadenopathy. Lymphadenopathy may involve the cervical, submandibular, or preauricular chains. In some cases, ulcerations occur on the palpebral conjunctiva.

4. Oropharyngeal tularemia—After inoculation of the pharynx, an exudative pharyngotonsillitis will develop with cervical lymphadenopathy.

5. Pneumonic tularemia—Pneumonic tularemia occurs after inhalation of *F tularensis* or following secondary spread from other infectious foci. A terrorist attack will most likely cause this form of disease. The findings of pulmonary involvement are variable and include pharyngitis, bronchiolitis, hilar lymphadenitis, and pneumonia. Early in the course of disease, systemic

NUCLEAR, BIOLOGIC, & CHEMICAL AGENTS; WEAPONS OF MASS DESTRUCTION / **27**

symptoms may predominate over pulmonary symptoms. In some cases, however, pulmonary disease progresses rapidly to pneumonia, pulmonary failure, and death.

6. Typhoidal tularemia—In this form of tularemia, systemic signs and symptoms of disease are present without a clear infectious site. Signs and symptoms include fever, chills, headache, malaise, and myalgias.

Any form of tularemia may be complicated by hematogenous spread leading to pneumonia, meningitis, or sepsis. The overall mortality rates for untreated tularemia range from 10% to 30%; however, with antibiotic therapy, mortality rates drop to less than 1%.

B. LABORATORY AND X-RAY FINDINGS

F tularensis requires special growth media. Notify laboratory personnel of a possible tularemia specimen so that proper plating can be performed. Cultures may be obtained from sputum, pharyngeal, or blood specimens. Specialized ELISA and PCR confirmatory tests are also available at some reference laboratories. In the case of pneumonic tularemia, chest x-ray may demonstrate peribronchial infiltrates to bronchopneumonia. Pleural effusions are often present.

Treatment & Prophylaxis

A. ANTIBIOTICS

Streptomycin and gentamicin are considered the drugs of choice for the treatment of tularemia (see Table 3–1). Ciprofloxacin has also displayed efficacy against tularemia. Second-line agents such as tetracycline and chloramphenicol may be used, but these agents are associated with higher rates of treatment failure. A 10-day course of antibiotics should be used. For second-line agents, a 14-day course should be used.

B. SUPPORTIVE CARE

Rarely patients may require intensive medical support such as airway management, hemodynamic support, and other measures to manage multisystem organ failure.

C. PROPHYLAXIS

Some data suggest that a 14-day course of antibiotics begun during the incubation period may prevent disease. Antibiotic choices are the same as for treatment. A live attenuated vaccine for tularemia also exists and is often used for at-risk laboratory workers. Vaccination decreases the rate of inhalational tularemia but does not confer complete protection. Given tularemia's short incubation period, and the incomplete protection of the vaccine, postexposure vaccination is not recommended.

Infection Control

Significant person-to-person transmission of tularemia does not occur. Standard precautions are sufficient during patient care activities (see Table 3–2).

4. Brucellosis

Brucellae are small aerobic, gram-negative, pleomorphic coccobacilli. Many *Brucella* spp. occur naturally; however, only 4 species are infectious to humans. Each species typically infects a particular host organism, and human infection follows contact with contaminated animal material. The *Brucella* spp. that are infectious to humans are *B melitensis* (found in goats), *B suis* (found in swine), *B abortus* (found in cattle), and *B canis* (found in dogs). *B suis* has been weaponized in the past.

Clinical Findings

A. SYMPTOMS AND SIGNS

The symptoms and signs of brucellosis are similar whether infection is contracted via oral, inhalational, or percutaneous routes. The usual incubation period following infection is 1–3 weeks. Because *Brucella* spp. infection can involve multiple body systems, a wide range of clinical findings is typical. Nonspecific symptoms are common and include fever, chills, malaise, and myalgias. Osteoarticular involvement may manifest as joint infections or vertebral osteomyelitis. Respiratory symptoms include cough, dyspnea, and pleuritic chest pain. Cardiovascular complications are numerous and include endocarditis, myocarditis, pericarditis, and mycotic aneurysms. Gastrointestinal symptoms include nausea, vomiting, diarrhea, and hepatitis. Multiple types of genitourinary infections can also occur. Neurologic involvement may cause meningitis, encephalitis, cerebral abscesses, cranial nerve abnormalities, or Guillain-Barré syndrome. Patients may also develop anemia, thrombocytopenia, or neutropenia. Central nervous system and cardiac involvement, although infrequent, accounts for most fatalities. *Brucella* spp. are not known for their lethality, and infection has an estimated mortality rate of less than 2%. Its interest as a biological weapon stems from the prolonged disease course and significant morbidity.

B. LABORATORY AND X-RAY FINDINGS

Brucella spp. will grow on standard culture media. Because of their slow growth, cultures may need to be maintained for at least 6 weeks. Specialized biphasic culture techniques may improve isolation. A more common diagnostic modality is a serum tube agglutination test. ELISA and PCR studies are available at some reference laboratories. If vertebral involvement is suspected, spinal x-rays, magnetic resonance imaging, computed tomography scanning, or bone scintigraphy may be helpful.

Treatment & Prophylaxis

A. ANTIBIOTICS

Because of the high rate of treatment failure, single drug therapy is no longer recommended. A prolonged course of multiple antibiotics is now considered to be the standard of care. The most common regimen involves the use of rifampin and doxycycline given for a 6-week period (see Table 3–1). Other antibiotics that have displayed efficacy against *Brucella* spp. include gentamicin, streptomycin, trimethoprim-sulfamethoxazole, and ofloxacin. Regardless of the antibiotics chosen, combination drug therapy should be used. In patients with serious infections, a 3-drug parenteral regimen is the norm.

B. SUPPORTIVE CARE

Rarely patients may require intensive medical support such as airway management, hemodynamic support, and other measures to manage multisystem organ failure.

C. PROPHYLAXIS

No human vaccine against *Brucella* spp. currently exists. Some authors recommend a 3- to 6-week course of antibiotics following a high-risk exposure such as a biologic attack.

Infection Control

Person-to-person spread of brucellosis is thought to be uncommon. Standard precautions are sufficient during patient care activities (see Table 3–2).

5. Q Fever

Q fever is caused by a rickettsial organism known as *Coxiella burnetii. C burnetii* has a worldwide distribution and occurs naturally in many domesticated animals (dogs, cats, sheep, goats, cattle). The organism is shed in feces, urine, milk, and placental material. Much like anthrax, *C burnetii* produces a sporelike form. Humans become infected by inhaling contaminated aerosols.

Clinical Findings

A. SYMPTOMS AND SIGNS

After infection, a typical incubation period ranges from 5 to 30 days. The symptoms and signs of Q fever are nonspecific and may occur acutely or have an indolent course. Typical symptoms and signs include fever, chills, malaise, myalgias, headache, and anorexia. If

cough occurs, it tends to occur late in the disease process and may or may not be associated with pneumonia. Various cardiac manifestations may occur and include endocarditis, myocarditis, and pericarditis. Gastrointestinal findings are common and include nausea, vomiting, diarrhea, and hepatitis. A nonspecific maculopapular rash may develop. Although not as common, various neurologic symptoms may also occur.

In some patients, Q fever may become a chronic condition. Chronic Q fever is typically manifest as endocarditis and tends to affect previously diseased cardiac valves. Although Q fever can be debilitating, it is usually not fatal. Mortality rates are generally less than 2.5%.

B. LABORATORY AND X-RAY FINDINGS

C burnetii is difficult to grow in culture, and sputum analysis is equally futile. Several serologic tests are available and include indirect fluorescent antibody staining, ELISA, and complement fixation. These tests often must be conducted at specialized reference laboratories. Elevated liver enzymes are also common in *C burnetii* infection.

Treatment & Prophylaxis

A. ANTIBIOTICS

Most cases of *C burnetii* infection will resolve without antibiotic therapy. Regardless, antibiotics are recommended because treatment will lower the rate of complications. A 7-day course of either doxycycline or tetracycline is usually sufficient (see Table 3–1). Fluoroquinolones are an acceptable alternative.

B. SUPPORTIVE CARE

Rarely patients may require intensive medical support such as airway management, hemodynamic support, and other measures to manage multisystem organ failure.

C. PROPHYLAXIS

Prophylactic antibiotics should be started 8–12 days after initial exposure. Antibiotics are ineffective if started sooner. A 7-day course of either doxycycline or tetracycline is usually sufficient. Fluoroquinolones are an acceptable alternative. An investigational vaccine exists but is not yet available to the general public.

Infection Control

Person-to-person spread of the disease is unlikely. Standard precautions are sufficient while engaging in patient care activities (see Table 3–2).

6. Glanders & Melioidosis

Glanders and melioidosis are similar diseases caused by related bacteria. The causal agent of glanders is *Burkholderia mallei*; the causal agent of melioidosis is *Burkholderia pseudomallei*. Both organisms are gram-negative bacilli. Glanders and melioidosis occur naturally. Glanders is a rare disease in humans; horses and other domesticated animals are often infected. Melioidosis occurs more commonly in humans and is endemic to Southeast Asia. Infection with either organism occurs via contact with open wounds or mucous membranes or by inhalation.

Clinical Findings

A. Symptoms and Signs

Both glanders and melioidosis can cause multiple clinical syndromes.

1. Localized disease—A localized disease may be seen and typically occurs after wound contamination or mucous membrane exposure. With wound contamination, patients develop a small ulcer with associated cellulitis. Regional lymphadenopathy or lymphangitis is also common. If mucous membrane exposure occurs, patients develop a bloody purulent discharge from the infected area (eyes, nose, or mouth). If secondary systemic infection occurs, a pustular rash similar to smallpox may develop.

2. Pulmonary disease—A pulmonary form of disease may also be seen. Pulmonary disease may occur after inhalation of aerosols or after hematogenous spread. An incubation period of 1–2 weeks occurs initially. Symptoms of pulmonary disease, including fever, chills, cough, chest pain, and dyspnea, develop eventually.

3. Septicemic disease—The most severe form of infection is the septicemic form. Patients present with nonspecific symptoms and signs of fever, chills, malaise, myalgias, photophobia, rigors, diffuse body abscesses, pustular rash, and headache. This condition is usually fatal; death occurs in 7–10 days.

B. Laboratory and X-ray Findings

Both organisms can be identified by routine Gram stain and culture. Special staining with methylene blue or Wright stain may facilitate diagnosis. Growth may be enhanced by the addition of meat nutrient agar or glucose to the growth media. Specialized agglutination and complement fixation tests may also be used. If pulmonary involvement is suspected, chest x-ray may demonstrate lung abscesses, miliary nodules, or pneumonia.

Treatment & Prophylaxis

A. Antibiotics

Both glanders and melioidosis respond to various antibiotics. Appropriate antibiotic choices include amoxicillin-clavulanate, tetracycline, trimethoprim-sulfamethoxazole, rifampin, ciprofloxacin, and ceftazidime (see Table 3–1). Various combinations of antibiotics have been recommended depending on the type and severity of infection.

B. Supportive Care

Rarely patients may require intensive medical support such as airway management, hemodynamic support, and other measures to manage multisystem organ failure.

C. Prophylaxis

According to some authorities, a course of trimethoprim-sulfamethoxazole may prevent the onset of disease.

Infection Control

Person-to-person spread of the disease is uncommon but can occur with improper handling of body fluids. Standard precautions are sufficient during patient care activities (see Table 3–2).

VIRAL AGENTS

1. Smallpox

Smallpox is a disease caused by the variola virus. The variola virus is a DNA virus of the genus orthopoxvirus. It occurs in 2 strains: the more severe variola major and a milder form, variola minor. Smallpox was essentially eradicated by an aggressive treatment and vaccination campaign conducted by the World Health Organization. The last naturally occurring case was in Somalia in 1977. Two stockpiles of the virus remain, one in the Centers for Disease Control and Prevention in Atlanta, and the other in the Institute of Virus Preparations in Moscow. Concern now exists that the Russian stockpile may have been compromised.

Clinical Findings

A. Symptoms and Signs

Disease begins with inhalation of the variola virus. After an initial exposure, a 7- to 17-day incubation period begins, during which the virus replicates in the lymph nodes, bone marrow, and spleen. A secondary viremia then develops leading to high fever, malaise, headache, backache, and in some cases delirium. After approximately 2 days a characteristic rash will develop.

The rash begins on the extremities and moves to the trunk. The palms and soles are not spared. The rash follows a typical progression beginning as macules, then papules, and eventually becoming pustular. Eventually lesions will form scabs that separate, leaving small scars. Unlike chickenpox, all the lesions in smallpox will be in similar stages of development. In unvaccinated individuals, mortality rates associated with variola major are approximately 30%. Variola minor has a similar progression to variola major, but toxicity and rash are not as severe. In unvaccinated individuals, the mortality rates associated with variola minor are approximately 1%. In 10% of cases, a variant form of rash will develop. A hemorrhagic rash displaying petechiae and frank skin hemorrhage may occur. This variant of smallpox carries a mortality rate of nearly 100%. Likewise, a malignant form exists in which the pustules remain soft and velvety to the touch.

B. Laboratory and X-ray Findings

Analysis of pustular fluid will yield virus particles. All samples should be sealed in 2 airtight containers. Variola can easily be recognized via electron microscopy. The virus itself can be grown in cell cultures or on chorioallantoic egg membranes. Further characterization of strains can be accomplished via biologic assays. PCR analysis is available at some reference laboratories.

Treatment & Prophylaxis

A. Specific Therapy

Currently there is no specific therapy for smallpox. Treatment is essentially supportive care. Many investigational drugs are currently under study. Strict patient isolation, preferably in the home, should be used. Any person having close contact with infected patients should be either quarantined or monitored for signs of infection. Antibiotics may be used if secondary bacterial infection occurs.

B. Prophylaxis

Data indicate that vaccination within 4 days of smallpox exposure may lessen subsequent illness. Because of the risk of possible terrorist attack, some authorities are recommending a preemptive initiation of smallpox vaccination. This would be problematic for several reasons. First, the current supply of smallpox vaccine is inadequate to protect a large populace. Second, many complications were known to occur with smallpox vaccination. Postvaccinial encephalitis occurred in approximately 1 in 300,000 vaccinations and was fatal in 25% of patients. Immunocompromised patients may develop a condition known as progressive vaccinia. In this condition, the initial inoculation site failed to heal, be-

came necrotic, and necrosis spread to adjacent tissues. This complication was often fatal. In some patients with eczema, a condition known as eczema vaccinatum could occur. Here, vaccinial lesions would occur in areas previously involved with eczema. Fortunately, the eruption was usually self-limited. In some patients, a secondary generalized vaccinia could develop. In others, inadvertent autoinoculation of eyes, mouth, or other areas occurred. Many of these complications could be treated with vaccinia immune globulin. Unfortunately, vaccinia immune globulin is also in short supply.

Cidofovir has also displayed some efficacy in preventing smallpox infection if given within 48 hours. There is no evidence to suggest that cidofovir is more effective than vaccine. Further, cidofovir is associated with significant renal toxicity.

Individuals vaccinated prior to 1972 are likely no longer protected, given that immunity lapses over a 5- to 10-year period.

Infection Control

Smallpox is highly infectious. Infection is spread by aerosol droplets. It is generally thought that each index case will subsequently infect 10–20 secondary individuals. The period of infectivity begins with the onset of rash and ends when all scabs separate. Use airborne precautions during patient care activities (see Table 3–2). Any material in contact with patients should be either autoclaved or washed in a bleach solution.

2. Hemorrhagic Fever

Viral hemorrhagic fever represents a clinical syndrome caused by several RNA viruses. These viruses exist in 4 different families: the Arenaviridae, the Filoviridae, the Flaviviridae, and the Bunyaviridae. Numerous viruses in each family may cause slightly different forms of hemorrhagic fever. The different forms of hemorrhagic fever are often named by their geographic origin (Table 3–3). Human infection occurs after contact with infected animals or infected arthropod vectors. Many of these viruses are also highly infectious in the aerosol form. This characteristic makes them potential biological weapons.

Clinical Findings

A. Symptoms and Signs

Several clinical aspects of hemorrhagic fever are unique to the individual forms (Table 3–3). Many symptoms and signs, however, are common to all types of hemorrhagic fever. Alterations in the vascular bed and increased vascular permeability lead to the dominant features of this disease. Early symptoms and signs include

Table 3–3. Specific forms of hemorrhagic fever and typical findings seen with each form.

Disease Form	Specific Features
Arenaviridae	
Argentine hemorrhagic fever	Progression or frank hemorrhage
Bolivian hemorrhagic fever	Progression or frank hemorrhage
Venezuelan hemorrhagic fever	Progression or frank hemorrhage
Lassa fever	Severe peripheral edema, hearing loss in survivors
Bunyaviridae	
Congo-Crimean hemorrhagic fever	Hepatitis, jaundice, severe hemorrhage
Rift Valley fever	Hepatitis, jaundice, retinitis
Filoviridae	
Ebola and Marburg forms	Hepatitis, jaundice
Flaviviridae	
Dengue fever	Pulmonary involvement
Yellow fever	Hepatitis, jaundice, pulmonary involvement

fever, conjunctival injection, mild hypotension, prostration, facial flushing, vomiting, diarrhea, and petechial hemorrhages. Eventually some patients may develop shock and mucous membrane hemorrhage. In some instances, evidence of hepatic, pulmonary, and neurologic involvement will be present. Secondary bacterial infection is also common.

B. LABORATORY AND X-RAY FINDINGS

A number of nonspecific laboratory abnormalities may be seen, including leukopenia, thrombocytopenia, proteinuria, hematuria, and elevated liver enzymes. Definitive diagnosis is possible with various rapid enzyme immunoassays and with viral culture.

Treatment & Prophylaxis

A. SPECIFIC THERAPY

Ribavirin is a nucleoside analog that has been shown to improve mortality in some forms of hemorrhagic fever. Dosing is as follows: 30 mg/kg intravenously as an initial dose, followed by 16 mg/kg intravenously every 6 hours for 4 days and then 8 mg/kg intravenously every 8 hours for 6 days. Ribavirin is usually most effective if begun within 7 days. Unfortunately, ribavirin is thought

to be ineffective against the filoviruses and the flaviviruses. Convalescent plasma containing neutralizing antibodies is also effective in some cases.

B. SUPPORTIVE CARE

Intravenous lines and other invasive procedures should be limited. Use fluid resuscitation with caution. Because of increases in vascular permeability, peripheral edema and pulmonary edema are frequent complications of volume replacement. If frank disseminated intravascular coagulopathy develops, consider heparin therapy.

C. PROPHYLAXIS

A vaccine against yellow fever is currently available. Many other investigational vaccines exist but are not currently available to the general public. Protocols also exist for the use of ribavirin in high-risk exposures.

Infection Control

The causal agents of hemorrhagic fever are highly infectious. Use caution when using sharps or when coming into contact with body fluids. Some forms are spread via aerosol, and patients with significant cough should be placed under airborne precautions. All laboratory specimens should be double sealed in airtight containers.

3. Viral Encephalitis

Much like viral hemorrhagic fever, viral encephalitis represents a clinical syndrome caused by numerous viruses. Of the pathogens that cause viral encephalitis, members of the family Togaviridae are thought to have potential as biologic weapons. The family Togaviridae includes the eastern equine encephalitis (EEE) virus, western equine encephalitis (WEE) virus, and Venezuelan equine encephalitis (VEE) virus. VEE virus has been weaponized in the past. In nature, these viruses are spread by infected arthropod vectors, and they infect humans as well as equines. They are also infectious in aerosol form, hence, their utility as biologic weapons.

Clinical Findings

A. SYMPTOMS AND SIGNS

Nearly all forms of infection will cause nonspecific symptoms and signs of fever, chills, malaise, myalgias, sore throat, vomiting, and headache. A large number of associated equine deaths may lead one to suspect equine encephalitis. The degree to which encephalitis develops depends on the pathogen involved. Although nearly all cases of VEE are symptomatic, encephalitis occurs in less than 5% of cases. If encephalitis does develop, and the patient recovers, residual neurologic sequelae usually do not occur. Without encephalitis, VEE has an expected mortality rate of less than 1%. Although uncommon, if encephalitis develops, the mortality rate increases to approximately 20%. In contrast, EEE tends to progress to neurologic involvement. Encephalitis is usually severe, and residual neurologic findings are common. With EEE, mortality rates range from 50% to 75%. WEE displays an intermediate degree of severity, with an overall estimated mortality rate of approximately 10%. If encephalitis develops, confusion, obtundation, seizures, ataxia, cranial nerve palsies, and coma may occur.

B. LABORATORY AND X-RAY FINDINGS

Although nonspecific, leukopenia and lymphopenia are common. In cases of encephalitis, cerebral spinal fluid analysis will display a lymphocytic pleocytosis. A number of serologic studies such as ELISA, complement-fixation, and hemagglutination inhibition may aid diagnosis. Although time consuming, the gold standard test for VEE involves viral isolation following inoculation of cell cultures of suckling mice. Additional specialized tests may be available only at regional reference laboratories.

Treatment & Prophylaxis

A. SPECIFIC THERAPY

Unfortunately, no specific treatment for equine encephalitis exists. Supportive care is all that can be offered. Headache may be treated with typical analgesics. Seizures are treated with typical anticonvulsant medications.

B. SUPPORTIVE CARE

Patients may require intensive medical support such as airway management, hemodynamic support, and other measures to manage multisystem organ failure.

C. PROPHYLAXIS

An investigational vaccine against VEE virus exists. It does not provide protection against all strains of VEE virus, and some patients will not display an effective antibody response. In 20% of patients receiving the vaccine, fever, malaise, and myalgias may develop.

Infection Control

Infection is not spread by person-to-person contact. Standard precautions are sufficient during patient care activities. To limit the spread of disease, patient exposure to arthropod vectors should be prevented.

BIOLOGIC TOXINS (See Table 3–4.)

1. Botulinum Toxin

Botulism is caused by a protein toxin produced by *Clostridium botulinum. C botulinum* is a gram-positive, spore-forming, obligate anaerobe found naturally in the soil. Many authorities consider botulinum toxin to be among the most potent naturally occurring poisons. The toxin occurs in 7 antigenic types, designated types A through G. Once absorbed, toxin will bind to motor neurons and prevent the release of acetylcholine, causing a flaccid muscle paralysis. Natural infection occurs in 3 forms: wound botulism, foodborne botulism, and intestinal botulism. Wound botulism occurs after *C botulinum* contaminates an open wound, subsequently producing toxin. Foodborne botulism occurs after ingesting food already contaminated by the toxin. Intestinal botulism, typically seen in infants, occurs after ingesting food contaminated by *C botulinum,* which in turn produces toxin. Although not occurring naturally, botulism can also be caused by inhalation of the toxin. This is the form of botulism that will likely occur following biologic attack. Contamination of food or water supplies also represents a possible terrorist threat. Food contamination, however, is unlikely to induce the large numbers of affected persons that would be seen following aerosol exposure. Water contamination would be difficult because current purification techniques are effective in neutralizing botulinum toxin.

Clinical Findings

A. SYMPTOMS AND SIGNS

After initial exposure, an incubation period ranging from 12 to 80 hours will occur. The duration of the incubation period depends on the type and amount of exposure. After the incubation period, a flaccid symmetric muscle paralysis will affect the bulbar musculature. Patients often display ptosis, diplopia, dysphagia, dysarthria, and dysphonia. Dilated, poorly reactive pupils are common. Eventually the paralysis will extend to the lower muscle groups, leading to paralysis. Airway compromise is common, and patients may lose respiratory function.

If foodborne exposure is involved, gastrointestinal symptoms such as nausea, vomiting, and diarrhea may occur. Botulism does not cause altered sensorium, sensory changes, or fever.

B. LABORATORY AND X-RAY FINDINGS

A mouse bioassay is the definitive test for botulism. Specimens for evaluation may be obtained from suspected food, blood, gastric contents, or possibly stool. This type of diagnostic testing is not widely available,

Table 3–4. Clinical findings associated with biologic toxins.

Biologic Toxin	Latent Period	Route	Early Symptoms	Late Symptoms
Botulism (*Clostridium botulinum*)	12–80 hours	Gastrointestinal	Nausea, vomiting, diarrhea.	Both forms: lower muscle group paralysis, respiratory failure.
		Inhalational	Flaccid paralysis of bulbar musculature (ptosis, diplopic, dysphagia, dysarthria, dysphonia, mydriasis).	
Ricin (extract from castor bean)	4–8 hours	Gastrointestinal	Nausea and vomiting, hematemesis, bloody diarrhea, melena, visceral organ necrosis.	Circulatory collapse.
		Inhalational	Fever, chills, cough, chest pain, dyspnea.	Bronchitis, pneumonia, acute respiratory distress syndrome, respiratory failure.
T-2 mycotoxins (produced from fungi)		Cutaneous	Pain, erythema, blister, necrosis, ocular irritation, rhinorrhea, oral pain.	All forms: weakness, dizziness, ataxia, and bone marrow suppression.
		Gastrointestinal	Abdominal pain, nausea and vomiting, diarrhea (bloody).	
		Inhalational	Chest pain, cough, dyspnea.	
Staphylococcal entero-toxin B (staphylococcal bacteria)	4–10 hours	Ingestion	All forms: fever, chills, headache, myalgia.	Nausea and vomiting, diarrhea (bloody).
	3–12 hours	Inhalation		Chest pain, cough dyspnea, respiratory failure.

and specimens may need to be sent to specialized laboratories. In addition to laboratory studies, electromyograms may display patterns consistent with botulism.

Treatment & Prophylaxis

A. SPECIFIC THERAPY

A botulinum antitoxin can be obtained from many state health departments or from the Centers for Disease Control and Prevention. Antitoxin therapy is most effective when given early in the disease course. It acts by binding free toxin but will not restore nerve terminals that have already been compromised. The civilian antitoxin is effective in neutralizing the 3 most common types of botulinum toxin found to affect humans (types A, B, and E). If other forms of toxin are utilized, an investigational heptavalent antitoxin may be available from the military. The military antitoxin is effective against all types of toxin (types A through G). Because some patients may develop allergic reactions to the antitoxin, a test dose is recommended.

B. SUPPORTIVE CARE

Patients may require intensive medical support such as airway management and ventilator support. Parenteral or tube feedings may be required. Treat secondary bacterial infections with antibiotics. Avoid clindamycin and aminoglycoside antibiotics because they may worsen neurologic blockade.

C. PROPHYLAXIS

Some evidence suggests that initiation of antitoxin prior to the onset of symptoms may prevent disease. Unfortunately, large amounts of the antitoxin are not available. A more prudent course of action would be to institute antitoxin therapy at the first signs of illness.

Infection Control

Person-to-person transmission of botulism does not occur. Standard precautions are sufficient during patient care activities (see Table 3–2). If food is suspected of being contaminated, thorough cooking will neutralize the toxin.

2. Ricin

Ricin is a polypeptide toxin that causes cell death by inhibiting protein synthesis. Ricin occurs naturally as a component of the castor bean, from the castor plant, *Ricinus communis*. Accidental ricin toxicity has occurred following ingestion of castor beans. Although ricin is less toxic than many other potential biologic agents, it is inexpensive, easy to produce, and can be aerosolized. These characteristics make it a potential biologic weapon. Ricin may be delivered by parenteral injection, ingestion, or inhalation. Ingestion and inhalation are the likely modes of biologic attack.

Clinical Findings

A. Symptoms and Signs

The signs and symptoms of ricin intoxication depend on the type and amount of exposure. Parenteral exposure causes necrosis of local tissues and regional lymph nodes. As the toxin spreads, visceral organs become involved, manifested as a moderate to severe gastroenteritis. Parenteral exposure is an unlikely means of biologic attack. If ricin is ingested, symptoms of gastrointestinal exposure will occur and may include nausea, vomiting, hematemesis, bloody diarrhea, melena, or visceral organ necrosis. If death occurs following parenteral or gastrointestinal exposure, it is usually secondary to circulatory collapse.

The most likely means of biologic attack involve aerosol exposure. Inhalation of ricin is manifested by direct pulmonary toxicity. Between 4 and 8 hours after exposure, the patient may develop fever, cough, chest pain, and dyspnea. Findings consistent with an aerosol exposure include bronchitis, bronchiolitis, interstitial pneumonia, and acute respiratory distress syndrome. If death occurs, it is usually secondary to respiratory failure and generally will occur within 36–72 hours.

B. Laboratory and X-ray Findings

Various laboratory tests including ELISA, PCR, and immunohistochemical staining may aid in the diagnosis of ricin toxicity. In the event of pulmonary involvement, chest x-ray may display bilateral infiltrates or noncardiogenic pulmonary edema.

Treatment & Prophylaxis

The treatment of ricin toxicity depends largely on the mode of exposure.

A. Parenteral Exposure

With parenteral exposure, treatment is largely supportive.

B. Gastrointestinal Exposure

The treatment of gastrointestinal exposure primarily involves the elimination of toxin. This can be accomplished by vigorous gastric lavage and by the use of cathartics such as magnesium citrate or whole bowel irrigation. Activated charcoal may be considered. Correct electrolyte abnormalities, and maintain adequate volume status. Treat secondary bacterial infections with appropriate antibiotics.

C. Pulmonary Exposure

With pulmonary exposure, treatment involves providing adequate ventilatory support. Patients may require oxygen, intubation, and ventilator management. Treat secondary bacterial infections with appropriate antibiotics.

D. Prophylaxis

Ricin vaccines are under development.

Infection Control

Ricin intoxication is not spread by person-to-person contact. Standard precautions are sufficient during patient care activities (see Table 3–2).

3. T-2 Mycotoxins

Like penicillin, mycotoxins are a diverse group of compounds produced by fungi for environmental protection. These compounds are frequently toxic to many animal species including humans. The T-2 mycotoxins are a particular group of compounds produced by fungi in the genus *Fusarium*. Although the actions of the T-2 mycotoxins are not completely understood, they are known to inhibit DNA and protein synthesis. They are most toxic to rapidly dividing cell lines.

Many properties of these compounds make them attractive as biologic weapons. Specifically, they are resistant to destruction by ultraviolet radiation and are heat stabile. T-2 mycotoxins confer toxicity after ingestion, inhalation, or dermal exposure. Unlike most other biologic agents, they can be absorbed directly though the skin.

Clinical Findings

A. Symptoms and Signs

With T-2 mycotoxin exposure, contamination via dermal, gastrointestinal, and pulmonary routes may occur simultaneously. The earliest symptoms and signs may begin within minutes to hours. Dermal exposure may be manifest as skin pain, erythema, blistering, and skin necrosis. Toxin exposure to the eyes and upper airway may cause ocular pain, redness, tearing, sneezing, rhinorrhea, oral pain, blood-tinged mucus, and epistaxis. Patients with pulmonary involvement will display chest pain, cough, and dyspnea. Signs and symptoms of gastrointestinal toxicity include abdominal pain, nausea, vomiting, and a bloody diarrhea. With systemic toxicity, patients may develop weakness, dizziness, and ataxia. Similar to radiation exposure, these toxins may also cause bone marrow suppression resulting in thrombocytopenia and neutropenia.

B. Laboratory and X-ray Findings

Two primary forms of laboratory testing may be used to identify T-2 mycotoxins. First, antigen detection can be performed on urine samples. The metabolites of the T-2 mycotoxins are eliminated primarily in the urine and feces. These metabolites are detectable in the urine up to 1 month after exposure. Second, mass spectrometric evaluation can be conducted on various body fluids. Appropriate samples include nasal secretions, pulmonary secretions, urine, blood, and stomach contents.

Treatment & Prophylaxis

A. Specific Therapy

The treatment of T-2 mycotoxin poisoning is essentially supportive care. Remove all contaminated clothing, and wash the patient's skin with large amounts of soap and water. Treat dermal burns with standard therapy. Treat secondary bacterial infections with appropriate antibiotics. Ocular involvement requires irrigation with water or sterile saline. Activated charcoal may aid in gastrointestinal decontamination. Patients with pulmonary involvement may require advanced respiratory techniques such as intubation or ventilatory support.

B. Prophylaxis

Vaccines against the T-2 mycotoxins are under study. The early use of soap and water may prevent skin toxicity.

Infection Control

The T-2 mycotoxins are dispersed as an oily liquid. Contact with this liquid may cause cross contamination. Therefore, remove all contaminated clothing and wash the patient's skin with soap and water. Standard precautions are sufficient during patient care activities (see Table 3–2).

4. Staphylococcal Enterotoxin B

Staphylococcal aureus produces a number of exotoxins that produce disease in humans. One such exotoxin, staphylococcal enterotoxin B (SEB), is a causal agent of the gastrointestinal symptoms seen in staphylococcal food poisoning. It is a heat-stabile toxin that belongs to a group of compounds known as super antigens. These compounds have the ability to activate certain cells in the immune system, causing a severe inflammatory response. This response causes injury to various host tissues. Aside from injury caused by SEB in natural infections, it can be aerosolized, making it a potential biologic weapon. Biologic attack could involve deliberate contamination of foodstuffs, although a more likely scenario would involve an aerosol release.

Clinical Findings

A. Symptoms and Signs

After exposure to SEB, a variable incubation period occurs, ranging from 4 to 10 hours for gastrointestinal exposure and from 3 to 12 hours for inhalational exposure. Regardless of the type of exposure, nonspecific symptoms and signs will develop and include fever, chills, headache, malaise, and myalgias. If the exposure occurred via the gastrointestinal route, then patients will also develop nausea, vomiting, and diarrhea. Conversely, if the exposure occurred via an inhalational route, the patient will also develop chest pain, cough, and dyspnea. Death is rare but in severe cases may occur from respiratory failure. Patients generally recover from symptoms after 1–2 weeks.

B. Laboratory and X-ray Findings

The presence of SEB can be confirmed by identifying specific antigens via ELISA testing. Obtain serum and urine samples. Urine samples are more productive because toxin tends to accumulate in the urine. In the case of aerosol exposure, respiratory and nasal swabs may also demonstrate toxin if samples are obtained within 1 day of exposure. With inhalational exposure, the chest x-ray is usually normal but in severe cases may demonstrate pulmonary edema.

Treatment & Prophylaxis

A. Specific Therapy

The treatment of SEB exposure is largely supportive. Correct electrolyte abnormalities, and maintain volume status. If pulmonary edema develops, patients may benefit from diuretic therapy and in some cases may require intubation and ventilatory support. Steroids may be given to lessen the inflammatory response, but this approach is controversial. Treat secondary bacterial infections with appropriate antibiotics.

B. PROPHYLAXIS

Vaccines against SEB are under study.

Infection Control

Person-to-person transmission of toxin is not a hazard. Standard precautions are sufficient during patient care activities (see Table 3–2).

Arnon SS et al: Botulinum toxin as a biological weapon: medical and public health management. JAMA 2001;285(8):1059. [PMID: 11209178] (Review article discussing all aspects of botulism use as a biologic weapon).

Dennis DT et al: Tularemia as a biological weapon: medical and public health management. JAMA 2001;285(21):2763. [PMID: 11386933] (Review article discussing all aspects of tularemia use as a biologic weapon.)

Franz DR et al: Clinical recognition and management of patients exposed to biological warfare agents. JAMA 1997;278(5):399. [PMID: 9244332] (Review article discussing issues related to common biologic warfare agents.)

Henderson DA et al: Smallpox as a biological weapon: medical and public health management. JAMA 1999;281(22):2127. [PMID: 10367824] (Review article that discusses all aspects of smallpox use as a biological weapon.)

Inglesby TV et al: Anthrax as a biological weapon: medical and public health management. JAMA 1999;281(18):1735. [PMID: 10328075] (Review article discussing all aspects of anthrax use as a biological weapon.)

Inglesby TV et al: Plague as a biological weapon: medical and public health management. JAMA 2000;283(17):2281. [PMID: 10807389] (Review article discussing all aspects of plague use as a biological weapon.)

USAMRIID Medical Management of Biological Casualties Handbook, 4th ed. U.S. Army Medical Research Institute of Infectious Diseases, 2001. (Produced by the U.S. Army, this general text provides general information regarding the most probable biologic agents.)

■ CHEMICAL WEAPONS (See Table 3–5.)

Like radiation and biologic agents, many chemicals can be developed into weapons of mass destruction. Chemical weapons are particularly attractive to rogue governments and terrorist organizations because of their low cost, stability, and ease of production. In fact, chemical

Table 3–5. Clinical findings associated with chemical agents.

Chemical Agents	Latent Period	Early Findings	Late Findings
Nerve agents	Vapor: None Liquid: Up to 18 hours	Rhinorrhea, salivation, sweating, increased pulmonary secretions, fasciculations, mood swings, difficulty concentrating.	Weakness, paralysis, vomiting, diarrhea, increased urination, seizures, coma, apnea.
Lung agents (phosgene)	0–24 hours	Mucous membrane irritation, rhinorrhea, cough, dyspnea, chest pain.	Pulmonary edema, hypotension, laryngeal spasm.
Vesicants Sulfur mustard	2–48 hours	Ocular pain, conjunctivitis, photophobia, blepharospasm, erythema, burning blister formation, mucous membrane damage, cough, nausea, vomiting, diarrhea.	Corneal clouding, dyspnea, mental status changes, seizures, pulmonary edema, respiratory failure, bone marrow suppression.
Lewisite	No latency	Similar to sulfur agents, but it also directly affects vascular premeability and causes third spacing and more systemic effects.	
Cyanide	None	Tachycardia, hypertension, tachypnea, anxiety, mental status changes.	"Cherry red" appearance to skin, coma, seizures, cardiac arrest.

agents have already been used by terrorist organizations. The terrorist group Aum Shinrikyo released sarin gas in a Japan subway in 1995. Chemical agents can be delivered as liquids, vapors, or as components of explosive devices. Chemical agents are generally categorized as nerve agents, pulmonary agents, vesicants, and cyanide agents.

NERVE AGENTS

The nerve agents are a diverse group of compounds that were developed by the Germans prior to World War II. An agent known as GA (tabun) was the first nerve agent produced, followed by several others including GB (sarin), GD (soman), GF, and VX. Each of these agents has different physical characteristics, of which volatility is the most critical. The G agents are more volatile than VX; as a result, the G agents form a vapor more readily.

These agents are classified as organophosphates and induce toxicity by binding to and inhibiting various forms of the acetylcholine esterase enzyme. This causes increased levels of acetylcholine, leading to hyperstimulation of both central and peripheral muscarinic and nicotinic receptors. The stimulation of these receptors causes the clinical syndromes consistent with nerve agent toxicity. Toxicity can occur either from skin contact or from vapor exposure. Given their increased volatility, the G agents are more prone to cause vapor exposure.

Clinical Findings

A. SYMPTOMS AND SIGNS

1. Latent period—When nerve agent exposure occurs as a vapor, there is generally no significant latent period and symptoms will develop within minutes. Likewise, the clinical effects of vapor exposure do not tend to progress over time. In contrast, liquid contamination may have a significant latent period depending on the amount of skin exposure. With small exposures, latent periods of up to 18 hours may be seen. Further, with liquid contact, symptoms and signs may progress over a period of time.

2. Clinical syndromes—The findings that will develop following nerve agent poisoning depend on the amount and type of exposure. As the degree of exposure increases, so does the severity of symptoms. The general clinical syndromes of nerve agent toxicity are as follows:

a. Central nervous system—The effects on the central nervous system may range from mild to severe depending on the degree of exposure. Mild symptoms

and signs include mood swings, difficulty concentrating, poor judgment, and sleep disturbances. With more significant exposures, coma, convulsions, and apnea may occur.

b. Peripheral nicotinic stimulation—The symptoms and signs of peripheral nicotinic receptor stimulation are manifest primarily as alterations in skeletal muscle functioning. The degree of involvement depends on the degree of exposure. Initially muscle fasciculations or weakness will occur and may eventually progress to paralysis.

c. Peripheral muscarinic stimulation—The symptoms and signs of peripheral muscarinic receptor stimulation are manifest primarily as increased exocrine gland and smooth muscle activity. Typical symptoms and signs of exocrine gland stimulation include rhinorrhea, salivation, sweating, increased gastrointestinal secretions, and increased pulmonary secretions. Increased pulmonary secretions may be severe enough to compromise the patient's airway. Increased smooth muscle activity will cause vomiting, diarrhea, increased urination, and abdominal pain.

B. LABORATORY AND X-RAY FINDINGS

Acetylcholine esterase exists in various tissues within the body. Two important subpopulations of acetylcholine esterase are the plasma cholinesterase and the erythrocyte cholinesterase. Decreased activity within either population may indicate nerve agent exposure. Of the two forms, the erythrocyte cholinesterase is the more sensitive indicator of exposure.

Treatment

A. SPECIFIC THERAPY

The treatment of nerve agent toxicity involves the use of 3 primary medications. The first, atropine, is an anticholinergic medication used to counteract the hyperstimulation of peripheral muscarinic receptors. Atropine (1–2 mg intravenously; if no effect, double dose every 5 minutes until secretions dry) should generally be given until secretions begin to dry. Atropine will not prevent central nervous system or nicotinic toxicity. In contrast, pralidoxime chloride (2-PAM), 1–2 g intravenously given over 15–30 minutes, ameliorates nicotinic toxicity by breaking the bond formed between the nerve agent and the esterase enzyme. The nerve agent–esterase bond may be broken as long as the compound has not aged, a process by which the bond becomes irreversible. For most of the nerve agents, the aging process is not clinically significant. One notable exception is GD (soman), which ages after only 2 minutes and is refractory to 2-PAM therapy. Finally, a common complication of severe intoxication is seizure activity. Seizures may be treated with benzodiazepines.

B. SUPPORTIVE CARE

Patients may require intensive medical support such as airway management and ventilatory support. Frequent suctioning of secretions may also be required.

Decontamination

For more specific information on decontamination, see Chemical Decontamination, below.

PULMONARY AGENTS

Many different chemicals can be classified as pulmonary or lung agents. All have a similar mechanism of toxicity, producing delayed onset of pulmonary edema. Of these agents, carbonyl chloride (phosgene) has been the most studied. Because phosgene is the prototypical lung agent, most of the discussion here relates to phosgene; however, the principles of management can be applied to all lung agents. As a military agent, phosgene was first used during World War I and today can be found in numerous industrial applications. Because of its high volatility, phosgene forms a gas readily, often with the faint scent of freshly cut hay. It is not absorbed through the skin, but when inhaled, it causes toxicity. After inhalation, phosgene is deposited in the peripheral airways, where it undergoes acetylation reactions. Subsequent damage to the alveolar-capillary membrane will occur, resulting in pulmonary edema. Phosgene may also interact with mucous membranes, causing local irritation.

Clinical Findings

A. SYMPTOMS AND SIGNS

As noted previously, the primary effect of phosgene involves lung toxicity, although with some exposures, patients may have transient irritation to the eyes, nose, and mouth. In some cases, rhinorrhea and oral secretions may be significant. Patients may also complain of mild chest discomfort and cough secondary to bronchial irritation. In significant exposures, early death may occur secondary to laryngeal spasm. Despite these early effects, most of the toxicity of phosgene exposure is delayed. After inhalation, a variable latent period of up to 24 hours will ensue. The length of the latent period depends on the dose of phosgene delivered and will be shorter with higher exposures. Eventually the patient may develop symptoms and signs consistent with pulmonary edema, including dyspnea, hypoxia, chest pain, and cough. In some cases, pulmonary edema may be severe enough to cause hypotension. The degree to which each patient is affected depends on the severity of exposure. In severe exposures, death may occur.

B. LABORATORY AND X-RAY FINDINGS

No clinical test exists for the diagnosis of phosgene exposure. Appropriate studies such as arterial blood gas measurements and chest x-ray should be used to manage pulmonary edema. Hemoconcentration secondary to pulmonary edema may also be evident.

Treatment

A. BED REST

Any activity, even walking, may increase the severity of pulmonary edema. As a result, discourage patients from any physical activity.

B. UPPER RESPIRATORY SYMPTOMS

In some cases, upper airway secretions may be significant. Nasal, oral, or bronchial secretions should be suctioned, if needed. If bronchospasm develops, it may be treated with intravenous steroids and inhaled bronchodilators. Treat secondary bacterial infections with appropriate antibiotics.

C. LOWER AIRWAY SYMPTOMS

If pulmonary edema develops, it should be managed with standard medical interventions including supplemental oxygen, intubation, and ventilator management. Positive end-expiratory pressure is a useful ventilator adjunct. Treat secondary bacterial infection with antibiotics.

D. HYPOTENSION

Secondary hypotension may develop in the event of severe pulmonary edema. Treatment of hypotension is problematic, given the increased permeability of the alveolar-capillary membrane. Supplemental crystalloid or colloid solutions can be used but may worsen pulmonary edema. Vasopressor agents such as dopamine may also be used.

Decontamination

No specific decontamination is required except removing the patient from the phosgene gas.

VESICANTS

Vesicants are a group of related compounds known to cause skin lesions, primarily blisters. Despite their predilection for skin involvement, multiple systemic effects are also seen. Although multiple agents may be used as vesicants, sulfur mustard and lewisite are the most common.

1. Sulfur Mustard

Sulfur mustard (mustard) was first used as a chemical weapon during World War I. Mustard is a lipophilic compound that is readily absorbed through intact skin. It causes significant dermal toxicity and after systemic absorption will affect various body systems. Exposure can occur after contact with mustard vapor or liquid. At different ambient temperatures, mustard may exist in either form. It displays a characteristic odor of garlic or mustard, hence, its name. The exact mechanism of mustard toxicity is not known but appears to involve DNA alkylation. Mustard also displays mild cholinergic activity. After systemic absorption, cell lines undergoing active mitosis are affected the most.

Clinical Findings

A. SYMPTOMS AND SIGNS

The symptoms and signs of mustard toxicity depend on the dose and mechanism of exposure. Unfortunately, initial mustard exposure is not symptomatic, and the patient may be unaware of contamination. Given the initial lack of symptoms, patients may not decontaminate, thus increasing toxicity. Depending on the dose, the latent period after exposure may range from 2 to 48 hours. In mild exposures, patients may display only mild dermal injury; in severe exposures, death may occur within hours. The specific symptoms and signs of mustard toxicity depend on the body areas exposed and the degree of systemic absorption. As noted, the skin is typically affected and will display areas of erythema, burning, and blister formation. The blisters may become large and express a clear to straw-colored fluid. The fluid does not contain mustard agent.

The eyes are one of the organs most sensitive to mustard exposure and may develop symptoms and signs first. Following ocular exposure, ocular pain, photophobia, conjunctivitis, and blepharospasm may occur. The superficial layers of the cornea may be denuded, leading to corneal clouding with visual changes.

With injury to the respiratory tree, patients may develop oronasal burning, rhinorrhea, sore throat, or epistaxis. In more severe exposures, findings of cough, dyspnea, mucous membrane necrosis, airway muscular damage, pulmonary edema, and respiratory failure may be seen. Symptoms and signs of gastrointestinal exposure may result either from the direct toxicity of mustard exposure or from mustard's cholinergic affects. Nausea, vomiting, diarrhea, and constipation are common findings.

Severe mustard exposure may also affect the central nervous system; mental status changes and seizure activity are the most common findings. Given mustard's interference with DNA activity, delayed findings of bone marrow suppression may also occur.

B. LABORATORY AND X-RAY FINDINGS

With exposure to mustard, an early leukocytosis is typical. If bone marrow suppression develops, later findings of anemia, leukopenia, and thrombocytopenia may be seen. If wound or pulmonary secretions become more purulent, a secondary bacterial infection should be suspected and Gram stain and culture obtained. Gastrointestinal symptoms may require electrolyte monitoring. The primary metabolite of mustard agent thiodiglycol may be detected in the urine in contaminated patients. Such specialized testing usually can be conducted only at reference or military laboratories. In the event of pulmonary involvement, chest x-ray may demonstrate a focal or diffuse pneumonitis and occasionally pulmonary edema.

Treatment

A. DECONTAMINATION

The most critical aspect in the treatment of mustard toxicity is removal of the chemical agent. This is problematic given the initial lack of symptoms. Even delayed decontamination, however, may lessen subsequent toxicity. Washing contaminated areas with either large amounts of soapy water or 0.5% hypochlorite solution is the preferred method of decontamination. For more specific information on decontamination, see Chemical Decontamination, below.

B. SPECIFIC THERAPY

With skin injuries, leave small blisters intact and unroof larger lesions. Clean unroofed areas frequently and cover them with antibiotic cream (Polysporin, silver sulfadiazine). Treat other irritated areas of skin with systemic analgesics or topical lotions. With ocular exposure, use topical antibiotics to prevent secondary bacterial infections. Topical anticholinergics may prevent the discomfort of ciliary spasm. With pulmonary involvement, treat associated cough with typical antitussive medications. Treat episodes of bronchospasm with systemic steroids and inhaled bronchodilators. Treat secondary bacterial infection with appropriate antibiotics. Supplemental oxygen, intubation, or ventilator management may be required in some patients. Typical gastrointestinal antispasmodics may ameliorate the symptoms of gastrointestinal exposure. Bone marrow transplant, growth factor utilization, or factor replacement are alternatives for the treatment of bone marrow suppression.

Decontamination

As noted above, toxin can be removed by washing contaminated surfaces with large amounts of soapy water or 0.5% hypochlorite solution. For more specific information on decontamination, see Chemical Decontamination, below.

2. Lewisite

Much like sulfur mustard, exposure to lewisite causes injury to contaminated body surfaces and may lead to systemic symptoms. Unlike mustard, however, lewisite exposure causes symptoms and signs without a significant latent period. Lewisite is a volatile agent with the odor of geraniums. Its exact mechanism of action is unknown, but it is thought that the arsenic component of lewisite may inhibit various enzymes.

Clinical Findings

A. SYMPTOMS AND SIGNS

As noted above, the symptoms and signs of lewisite exposure begin without a significant latent period. Even though findings of exposure begin early, it may take several hours for symptoms to fully develop. The severity of clinical findings depends on the degree and method of exposure. Shortly after skin exposure, an area of dead skin will develop that will subsequently blister. These lesions may take up to 18 hours to fully develop. Skin necrosis may also be evident. Symptoms and signs of ocular exposure are similar to those associated with mustard toxicity and include conjunctivitis, iritis, edema, ocular pain, and corneal injury. If pulmonary toxicity develops, findings of cough, dyspnea, and pulmonary edema may occur. Lewisite causes increases in vascular permeability that may lead to third spacing of fluid with subsequent hypotension. In some cases, gastrointestinal, renal, and liver involvement may be seen.

B. LABORATORY AND X-RAY FINDINGS

No specific test for lewisite exposure is currently available.

Treatment

A. DECONTAMINATION

As with mustard exposure, the cornerstone of treatment involves early decontamination. Compared with mustard exposure, decontamination is usually more successful with lewisite exposure, given the early onset of symptoms. Standard washing with soap and water or 0.5% hypochlorite solution is sufficient.

B. SUPPORTIVE CARE

Patients may require intensive medical support such as airway management, hemodynamic support, and various measures to manage multisystem organ failure.

C. SPECIFIC THERAPY

British anti-lewisite (dimercaprol), 2–3 mg/kg every 4 hours, is a compound that can be given intramuscularly to decrease the effects of lewisite exposure.

Decontamination

As noted above, the toxin can be removed by washing contaminated surfaces with large amounts of soapy water or 0.5% hypochlorite solution. For more specific information on decontamination, see Chemical Decontamination, below.

CYANIDE AGENTS

Historically, cyanide was classified as a blood agent. This classification is somewhat inappropriate because many other chemical agents exert their effects after being distributed within the vascular system. Nevertheless, this classification is still used occasionally. Once cyanide is absorbed, it distributes rapidly throughout the body. It has a high affinity for trivalent iron compounds and will bond to the cytochrome a3 complex within the mitochondria. The cytochrome a3–cyanide bond effectively blocks aerobic cellular respiration, and anaerobic metabolism ensues. Cyanide exposure most often occurs naturally after inhalation of smoke from burning synthetic materials. In a biologic attack, cyanide exposure would likely follow an aerosol release. Cyanide gas is known to exhibit the scent of bitter almonds.

Clinical Findings

A. SYMPTOMS AND SIGNS

After inhalation of cyanide gas, the cytochrome a3 enzyme is effectively blocked. Because cells can no longer utilize oxygen, they will convert to anaerobic metabolism, leading to a lactic acidosis. This inability to utilize oxygen effectively smothers the patient. Tachycardia, hypertension, and tachypnea will be seen initially. As symptoms and signs progress, anxiety, mental status changes, coma, seizures, cardiac arrest, and death will occur. Because cyanide does not alter oxygen-hemoglobin saturation, cyanosis will not develop. In fact, the inability to utilize oxygen increases the venous oxygen saturation, leading to a cherry red appearance to the skin. It generally takes 6–8 minutes for death to occur following cyanide exposure.

B. LABORATORY AND X-RAY FINDINGS

An elevated blood cyanide concentration confirms the diagnosis. Given the short time interval to death, such testing is not useful in the acute setting but may later confirm the diagnosis. Two rapid tests, an elevated venous blood oxygen saturation and an increased lactic acid level, are characteristic of cyanide poisoning.

Treatment

A. SPECIFIC THERAPY

In addition to cyanide's affinity for certain iron compounds, it also has a high affinity for sulfhydryl groups and for the methemoglobin complex. These 2 characteristics are the basis of the cyanide antidote kit. The kit contains 3 components: amyl nitrite (used if no vascular access is available), sodium nitrite, and sodium thiosulfate. First, the patient is given a nitrite compound (inhalation of an amyl nitrate ampule or sodium nitrite), which will cause the formation of methemoglobin. The dose of sodium nitrite is based on the patient's weight and hemoglobin concentration although 300 mg IV is the usual dose for non-anemic adults. Given the high affinity of methemoglobin for cyanide, it will preferentially bind the compound and help to remove it from the cytochrome a3 complex. Second, the patient is given sodium thiosulfate, (typically 12.5 g IV for an adult), which interacts with cyanide, forming thiocyanate. Thiocyanate is then excreted in the urine.

B. SUPPORTIVE MEASURES

Severe lactic acidosis may be treated with bicarbonate administration. Seizures may be treated with benzodiazepines. In many cases, patients require intubation and ventilator support.

Decontamination

The only effective mode of decontamination involves removing the patient from the cyanide gas.

CHEMICAL DECONTAMINATION

Because of the risk of cross contamination to health care workers, the need for patient decontamination should be emphasized. All patients suspected of experiencing a chemical weapons attack should be decontaminated as soon as possible. Optimally, patient decontamination should be conducted in the field. Often this is not practical, and a decontamination station should be established in a secure location adjacent to the health care facility. All persons conducting decontamination duties should be provided adequate protective clothing and should receive specialized training.

Decontamination involves physical removal of toxin and chemical deactivation of toxin. The physical removal of toxin is usually the most effective means of decontamination in the acute setting. Remove all clothing, jewelry, dressings, and splints. Wash the patient with copious amounts of soap and water. Avoid vigorous scrubbing because this may facilitate toxin absorption.

After physical removal of toxin, any remaining toxin can be chemically deactivated. This may take some time and thus is considered secondary to physical removal of toxin. The most common neutralizing solution is 0.5% hypochlorite solution, which detoxifies many chemical agents via oxidation reactions. Hypochlorite solution should not be used to decontaminate open peritoneal wounds, open chest wounds, exposed neural tissue, or ocular tissue. Irrigate these areas with copious amounts of normal saline. All contaminated materials should be bagged and sent for proper disposal.

Lee EJ: Pharmacology and toxicology of chemical warfare agents. Ann Acad Med Singapore 1997;26:104. [PMID: 8830755] (Overall review of the 4 major classes of chemical agents.)

Sidell FR: *Management of Chemical Warfare Agent Casualties: A Handbook for Emergency Medical Services.* HB Publishing, 1995. (Provides basic information regarding the treatment of chemical weapons injuries; specifically catered for emergency medical services personnel.)

Reutter S: Hazards of chemical weapons release during war: new perspectives. Environ Health Perspect 1999;107:985. [PMID: 10585902] (General review of nerve and vesicant agents.)

USAMRICD Medical Management of Chemical Casualties Handbook, 3rd ed. U.S. Army Medical Research Institute of Chemical Defense, 2000. (Published by the U.S. Army, this text is an overall handbook for the care of chemical weapons injuries.)

Multicasualty Incidents & Disasters

Louis James Kroot, MD, & Robert B. Gray, MD[1]

Epidemiology of Disasters
　　Natural Disasters
　　Nonnatural Disasters
**Prehospital Management of Multicasualty
Incidents & Disasters**

Emergency Department Disaster Management
Stress Management & Psychological Support

Multicasualty incidents and disasters share a common characteristic. Both situations suddenly and unexpectedly produce victims of sufficient number and severity that local emergency medical resources are overwhelmed and special organization and resources are required. Although exact terminology varies, the term *multicasualty incident* usually refers to an isolated, geographically focused event that produces a limited number of casualties managed within a community. The term *disaster* implies a more destructive event that damages the social and physical environment of a community or region. Management of the event requires resources and assistance from outside the community.

The American College of Emergency Physicians has suggested the following terminology to categorize such events:

Level 1—A localized multiple casualty emergency wherein local medical resources are available and adequate to provide for triage, field medical treatment, and stabilization. The patients will be transported to the appropriate local medical facility for further diagnosis and treatment.

Level 2—A multiple casualty emergency in which the large number of casualties or lack of local medical care facilities are such as to require multijurisdictional (regional) medical mutual aid.

Level 3—A mass casualty emergency wherein local and regional medical resource capabilities are exceeded or overwhelmed. Deficiencies in medical supplies and personnel are such as to require assistance from state or federal agencies.

---

[1]This chapter is a revision of the chapter by Charles E. Saunders, MD, FACEP, FACP, from the 4th edition.

■ EPIDEMIOLOGY OF DISASTERS

Specific types of disasters produce different patterns and numbers of injuries and have different effects on the social and physical environment. By understanding them and anticipating their potential effects on a community, effective mitigation and preparedness may be possible.

NATURAL DISASTERS

Natural disasters are events caused by natural forces and geographical events. With the exception of war, these are historically the most common types of large-scale events (Table 4–1).

Earthquakes

An earthquake is the most likely large-scale event in the United States. Earthquake intensity is commonly measured by the Richter scale, a logarithmic scale that measures the intensity of seismic waves. An earthquake of 2.0 magnitude is barely felt, whereas an 8.0 magnitude event is greatly destructive. There have been 6 major earthquakes greater than 8.0 on the Richter scale in U.S. history (Figure 4–1). An earthquake of a given magnitude may produce varying amounts of destruction, depending on a complex interaction of many factors, including the type of ground underlying a structure, the degree of ground failure (eg, landslide, soil failures), and the construction quality of overlying structures.

Injuries are most often due to structural collapse (ie, crush injuries), falling debris, fire, and falls. Illness also occurs as a result of disruption of existing community

Table 4–1. Sudden natural disasters causing 10,000 or more deaths, 1949–1985.[1]

Year	Event	Location	Approximate Death Toll
1949	Floods	China	57,000
1954	Floods	China	40,000
1960	Earthquake	Morocco	12,000
1962	Earthquake	Iran	12,000
1963	Tropical cyclone	Bangladesh	22,000
1965	Tropical cyclone	Bangladesh	17,000
1965	Tropical cyclone	Bangladesh	30,000
1965	Tropical cyclone	Bangladesh	10,000
1968	Earthquake	Iran	12,000
1970	Earthquake/ avalanche	Peru	70,000
1970	Tropical cyclone	Bangladesh	250,000–500,000
1971	Tropical cyclone	India	10,000–25,000
1976	Earthquake	China	225,000–650,000
1976	Earthquake	Guatemala	24,000
1977	Tropical cyclone	India	20,000
1978	Earthquake	Iran	25,000
1985	Tropical cyclone	Bangladesh	10,000
1985	Earthquake	Mexico	10,000
1985	Volcanic eruption	Colombia	22,000

[1]Reproduced, with permission, from Bernstein AB, Thompson P: The natural history of natural hazards. In: *Management of Wilderness and Environmental Emergencies.* Auerbach PS, Geehr EC (editors). Mosby, 1989.

infrastructure (eg, food supply, power, sanitation, ongoing support for persons with chronic disease). Predictably, the patterns of injury seen among casualties include lacerations, contusions, fractures, head and spinal cord injuries, burns, effects of exposure, infection, and exacerbation of chronic medical problems. The speed of rescue efforts has an important bearing on the outcome (Figure 4–2).

Tropical Cyclones (Hurricanes, Typhoons, & Tropical Cyclones)

Tropical cyclones (hurricanes in the United States and Atlantic, typhoons in the eastern Pacific, tropical cyclones elsewhere) are a circulating mass of clouds, rain, and wind around a clear central area of extreme low-barometric pressure. They occur most commonly in the late summer months.

The intensity of tropical cyclones is rated on a 5-point scale. For hurricanes approaching the United States, this information is available from the National Weather Service, which can also provide information about a storm's probable path. Damage is commonly due to high winds, which can exceed 150 mph, as well as torrential rain and high seas, which may produce flooding and soil instability (eg, landslides).

Casualties may be caused by trauma from flying debris or structural collapse; by drowning; by famine related to damaged agriculture and food distribution systems; by disease related to loss of power, water, and sanitation; and occasionally by violence related to loss of public safety. Casualties may be reduced by effective early warning systems and evacuation efforts.

Tornadoes & Severe Storms

On an annual basis, tornadoes and severe thunderstorms are the most common cause of death due to natural disasters. In the United States, approximately 100,000 severe storms (eg, involving thunder, high winds, and hail) occur each year, including 1000 tornadoes. Most commonly affected are the midwestern and southern United States, usually during the summer months, and during late afternoons. Only about 3–4% of all tornadoes produce injury, and most deaths occur in a small number of highly destructive events.

Casualties are related to trauma from structural collapse, flying debris, or being knocked to the ground or thrown. Head injuries, crush injuries, fractures, contusions, and lacerations are common. As with all disasters, secondary illness and injury may occur, although tornadoes most commonly tend to produce random, isolated groups of casualties wherever they touch down, rather than diffuse area-wide casualties and destruction to community infrastructure. Casualty mitigation through early warning and evacuation is hard to manage because tornadoes are difficult to predict and the time frame for evacuation or protective cover is brief.

Floods

Floods are typically seasonal and result from one of several causes: (1) excessive rains or snow melts that lead to rivers overflowing their banks in a floodplain area, (2) tsunamis (tidal waves) or hurricanes in low-lying coastal areas, (3) flash floods in flat areas where rainfall produces surface water that exceeds the runoff or absorptive capacity of the soil, or (4) failure of a dike or dam, usually due to heavy rains.

In the United States, the number of deaths each year from floods is small and sporadic. Property damage can

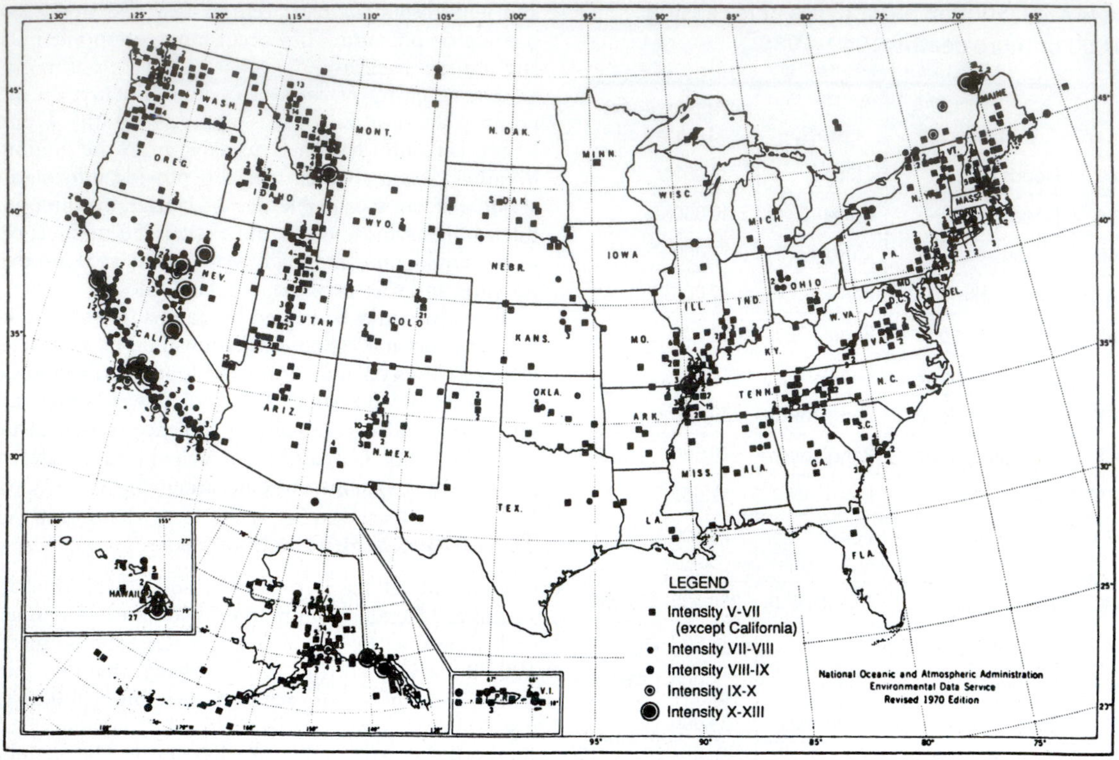

Figure 4–1. Epicenters of significant earthquakes in the United States, 1970. (Reproduced from: Centers for Disease Control: *The Public Health Consequences of Disasters.* United States Department of Health and Human Services Public Health Service, Centers for Disease Control, 1989.)

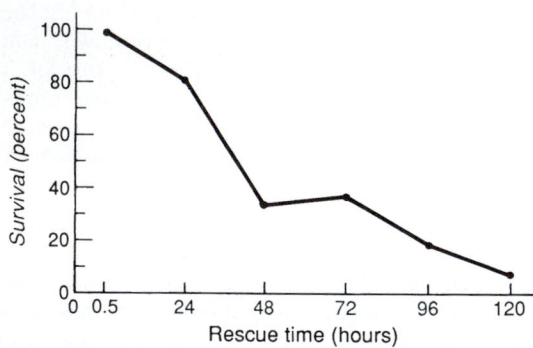

Figure 4–2. Survival rates versus rescue time for victims trapped in the Tangshan earthquake, 1976. (Adapted from Smith GS: Research issues in the epidemiology of injuries following earthquakes. In: *International Workshop on Earthquake Injury Epidemiology from Mitigation and Response.* Johns Hopkins University, 1989.)

be considerable, as are secondary effects on crops, sanitation, and vector-borne infections. When casualties occur, they are usually due to drowning.

By contrast, developing countries with poor watershed management and rapid growth of agriculture and urban development on floodplains have seen large number of casualties in isolated events. Casualties from secondary effects, such as famine, have occasionally been large (eg, in Bangladesh). Mitigation (eg, through watershed engineering projects and limiting development on floodplains) and early warning are the most effective means of reducing deaths.

Tsunamis

Tsunamis are tidal waves due to sudden geologic events occurring at sea, such as earthquakes and volcanic eruptions. A giant wave of water results that may travel from the epicenter at hundreds of miles per hour. The onset is often heralded by a sudden ebb of water that exposes the sea floor and is followed in minutes by a wall of water that may rise to 100 feet. Massive damage occurs to the shore and structures; casualties are due to drowning. Mitigation by building sea walls and locating structures on high ground and through early warning are the only effective means of reducing casualties.

Volcanoes

Volcanoes are channels of molten rock (magma) from deep in the earth that vent to the surface in one of several forms. They may cause eruptions of molten rock (lava) or spew ash and debris. Volcanoes tend to be localized to the boundaries of tectonic plates (eg, the Pacific Rim). Injury is most commonly due to falling debris, collapse of structures under the weight of ash, being buried in mudslides or lava flows, or toxic effects of gases (eg, carbon dioxide, hydrogen sulfide). Effects on agriculture and property can be extensive. In many cases, early warning, although imprecise, can allow evacuation and mitigate casualties.

Hogan DE, Askins DC, Osburn AE: The May 3, 1999 tornado in Oklahoma City. Ann Emerg Med 1999;34:225. [PMID: 104244927] (Good account of emergency room events during this disaster, outlining many of the problems encountered.)

Peleg K et al: Earthquake disasters—lessons to be learned. Isr Med Assoc J 2002;4:361. [PMID: 12040826] (A review of earthquake disasters and planning.)

NONNATURAL DISASTERS

Fires

Collectively, fires produce approximately 5000 deaths and 300,000 injuries each year in the United States, although the number has been on a steady decline since the 1950s. Under the right conditions, hot gases can produce winds that collect in a rotating cyclone (called a fire storm). Most deaths are due to asphyxiation from carbon monoxide and other toxic gases and to burns.

Transportation Accidents

Transportation accidents are the most common incidents producing multiple casualties in the United States. Airplane crashes produce a high ratio of fatalities to total injuries; highway accidents have the opposite characteristic. Railway accidents may produce significant injuries if passengers are involved and also have resulted in release of hazardous materials.

Transportation accidents are the prototypical geographically localized multicasualty events practiced in most communities' disaster drills. They are realistically apt to occur, and they lend themselves to management within the jurisdiction and structure of local emergency medical services (EMS).

The patterns of injury are well known to most emergency workers and consist of fractures, contusions, lacerations, and head and thoracoabdominal blunt injury.

Industrial Accidents

Industrial accidents that cause large-scale disasters most commonly result in the release of a hazardous material. The most notorious occurred in 1984 in Bhopal, India, where a release of methyl isocyanate killed more than 2000 and injured up to 200,000.

Injuries vary depending on the nature of the agent. Asphyxia, respiratory distress, skin and eye irritations, neurologic abnormalities, or teratogenic effects may occur.

Radiation & Nuclear Accidents

Aside from the atomic explosions in Japan in World War II, few deaths have resulted from nuclear disasters, although several significant incidents have occurred. The most deadly was the 1986 Chernobyl reactor explosion in the former Soviet Union, in which 27 people died and 135,000 were evacuated, many of whom were exposed to high radiation levels.

In nuclear accidents, injuries are due to the immediate blast effects, to exposure to toxic chemicals used at reactor sites (eg, sulfuric acid, chlorine, ammonia), and to radiation exposure.

Structural Collapse & Explosions

Structural failure of a building or man-made structure can be precipitated by natural forces (eg, earthquake) or may occur unexpectedly (eg, the Hyatt skywalk collapse in Kansas City, 1981; 113 dead, 200 injured). However, most such events in the United States have been limited in scope and have not produced many casualties. Injuries are predictable and consist of head injuries, fractures, lacerations, and blunt thoracoabdominal injuries.

Acts of Violence

Unfortunately, acts of violence do occur in the United States. Whereas casualties can be massive in armed conflicts (primarily due to explosives), in the civilian arena they are usually limited to a small number. Injuries are usually penetrating-type trauma.

Acts of Terrorism

(See Chapter 3.) Given the September 11, 2001 attack on the World Trade Center, the prior bombing there in the parking structure, the bombing of the Murrah Federal Building in Oklahoma City in 1995, the sarin gas attack in Tokyo, and the 2001 anthrax scare, it is obvious that acts of terrorism can strike close to home and affect a hospital's ability to properly care for a large influx of patients. In the World Trade Center attack and Oklahoma City bombing, a so-called second wave phenomenon occurred: The first patients arrived at the emergency department within 15 minutes of the disaster, but the highest flow occurred between 60 and 90 minutes. Patients transported by EMS have a much higher acuity and admission rate than for all other forms of transport, but in these cases EMS transported only about one third of the patients. The majority were transported by personal vehicle or other modes.

In such disasters, some experts have prepared a two-physician emergency department management scenario. The first physician would be an emergency medicine physician who is intimately familiar with the normal daily operations of the emergency department and who would be responsible for the overall medical and administrative operating of the department. The second command physician would be responsible for the delivery of trauma care, including assigning priorities for surgery and supervising the trauma teams. This role would be best filled by a trauma surgeon.

The 2001 anthrax scare in the United States, the confirmed use of biologic agents by some countries on their own citizens, and the fall of the Soviet Union and the subsequent disorganization of its biologic warfare programs have demonstrated that the threat of bioterrorism is very real. In these scenarios, the emergency department physician becomes a first responder. Without a high level of suspicion, a bioterrorism event may go unrecognized or may be dismissed as a natural epidemic until the scope of the disaster becomes catastrophic. Establishing an effective response requires hospital, local, state, and federal cooperation and training. An effective response should include four steps: (1) detection and diagnosis, (2) declaration of need, (3) defense, and (4) drug therapy.

A. DETECTION

A high level of suspicion on the part of the emergency department physician can pay off. Emergency department physicians should consider whether they have noticed multiple similar patients with similar clinical syndromes; severe illness in young and otherwise healthy people; unusual organisms identified by the lab; unusual antibiotic resistance patterns; atypical presentations of diseases; reports of sick or dead animals, birds, or plants; and the like.

B. DECLARATION OF NEED

Emergency department physicians should immediately contact the house hospital infectious disease officer,

laboratory, and local officials. They, in turn, will follow established protocols to notify state and federal authorities. The Federal Bureau of Investigations is responsible for acute crisis management, whereas the Federal Emergency Management Agency (FEMA) is responsible for consequence management. The Office of Emergency Preparedness (OEP) of the Public Health Service handles medical assistance. The OEP is currently training 120 Metropolitan Medical Response System teams. These teams would be the first to respond, along with military assistance, in the event of a large-scale biologic attack.

C. DEFENSE

Once the biologic agent is identified, each hospital should enact appropriate precautions to protect its employees and patients from further contamination (eg, isolation, barrier protection).

D. DRUG THERAPY

The determination of the biologic agent will determine drug choice and duration of therapy. Uncommon antibiotics, antivirals, vaccines, and immunoglobins may be necessary. The Centers for Disease Control are currently coordinating a regional stockpile program to augment their needs.

Brennen RJ et al: Chemical warfare agents: emergency medical and emergency public health issues. Ann Emerg Med 1999;34: 191. [PMID: 10424921] (Overview of the risks that chemical warfare agents pose to civilian populations and discussion of the emergency medical and public health issues related to preparedness and response.)

Cook L: The World Trade Center attack. The paramedic response: an insider's view. Crit Care 2001;5:301. [PMID: 11737911] (An EMS perspective on the World Trade Center attack.)

Jones J et al: Future challenges in preparing for and responding to bioterrorism events. Emerg Med Clin North Am 2002;20: 501. [PMID: 12120489] (A review of bioterrorism with an emphasis on identification and preparedness.)

Okumura T et al: The Tokyo subway sarin attack: disaster management, Part 1: community emergency response. Acad Emerg Med 1998;5:613. [PMID: 9660289] (A review of the response to the Tokyo sarin attack.)

Richards CF et al: Emergency physicians and biological terrorism. Ann Emerg Med 1999;34:183. [PMID: 10424920] (Overview of planning and response issues central to a potential bioterrorism event in light of the sarin gas attack in Tokyo, the 1993 bombing of the World Trade Center, and the 1995 bombing of the Murrah Federal Building in Oklahoma City.)

Tamber PS, Vincent JL: The World Trade Center attack. Lessons for all aspects of health care. Crit Care 2001;5:299. [PMID: 11737910] (Discussion of the implications of the World Trade Center attack on the health care system.)

■ PREHOSPITAL MANAGEMENT OF MULTICASUALTY INCIDENTS & DISASTERS

Preparation for disaster is an important responsibility of any community's public safety agencies. A community should prepare actively for those events to which the area is vulnerable based on historical, geologic, demographic, transportation, and industrial sources. Many large cities practice an airplane crash scenario each year, despite the extremely low probability of such an event occurring, in part because the local airport is mandated by the Federal Aviation Administration to conduct such drills. On occasion this has paid off. However, other realistic scenarios should not be neglected.

Organization of the Response

A. EMS VERSUS "CIVIL DEFENSE" MANAGEMENT

Most events are small level 1 events and are best managed by the local public safety or EMS jurisdiction as an extension of day-to-day operations under an organization or management system that can incorporate and coordinate outside assistance (see Incident Command System, below). At some point, large-scale events overwhelm local agencies and require the management and control to extend over a larger scale. Under the Civil Defense model, victims are collected and treated in supplementary casualty collection points or field hospitals that can stabilize them pending large-scale or distant evacuation. In many states (eg, California), plans exist for both such models, although the EMS model is most commonly employed.

B. INCIDENT COMMAND SYSTEM

The response by emergency personnel to a multicasualty event can be complex when multiple agencies are involved, jurisdictional boundaries are crossed, or the event occurs in multiple geographic locations. In order to devise a system to better coordinate events of varying size and complexity, federal, state, and local fire services joined together in 1982 in the FIRESCOPE project to devise the Incident Command System (ICS). The ICS is a management system that allows incidents of varying size and complexity to be managed effectively, regardless of the diversity of agencies and resources involved.

The ICS has several functional components coordinated within an organizational framework (Figure 4–3). At the apex is the incident commander, who directs the Operations, Planning, Logistics, and Finance sections. Within the Operations section are various functional divisions, branches, and groups that carry out the emergency response work. Various functional components or autonomous teams of individuals can maintain their group autonomy and fit into the organizational tree as a unit.

In complex incidents that have limited emergency medical needs, the EMS component may simply occupy a small division or group in the overall ICS structure. By contrast, a large, purely medical event may lead to the medical commander occupying the incident commander role.

C. MEDICAL MANAGEMENT

The organization of medical resources in response to a disaster depends on the nature and level of the event. The easiest to illustrate is the geographically focused level 1 event. An on-scene medical commander who designates functional responsibilities to individuals or teams directs the medical response: triage, treatment, transport, communications, logistics, staging, and so on. The medical commander may, in fact, be a branch of division commander within a larger ICS structure or may be the event incident commander if the event is purely medical.

In typical smaller-scale day-to-day incidents, the first-in ambulance remains out of service for the duration of the event and one paramedic assumes the role of medical commander while the other begins triage or treatment responsibilities. As additional ambulances arrive, their crews report to the medical commander, who assigns them roles or duties. Each crew then treats and transports patients in order of relative severity of injuries (as directed by a transport or loading officer).

If physicians or nurses are available, they are best used in treatment roles, because their expertise in assessing and treating patients may be considerable, whereas their experience in working with other agencies in a command role in a fast-moving prehospital environment is usually limited.

A large-scale diffuse event, such as a major earthquake, is more difficult to manage. There may be no central focus of casualties. Instead, victims may be scattered or clustered over a large area, their existence made known by many hundreds of individual telephone requests (eg, via 9-1-1), provided that telephone services remain intact. This presents a coordinating problem if a limited number of ambulances are available or radio communications with ambulances are interrupted. Such loss of communications and central coordination capability may require decentralized management: ambulance resources disperse to individual neighborhoods to organize casualty collection and treatment at that level (eg, at each fire station).

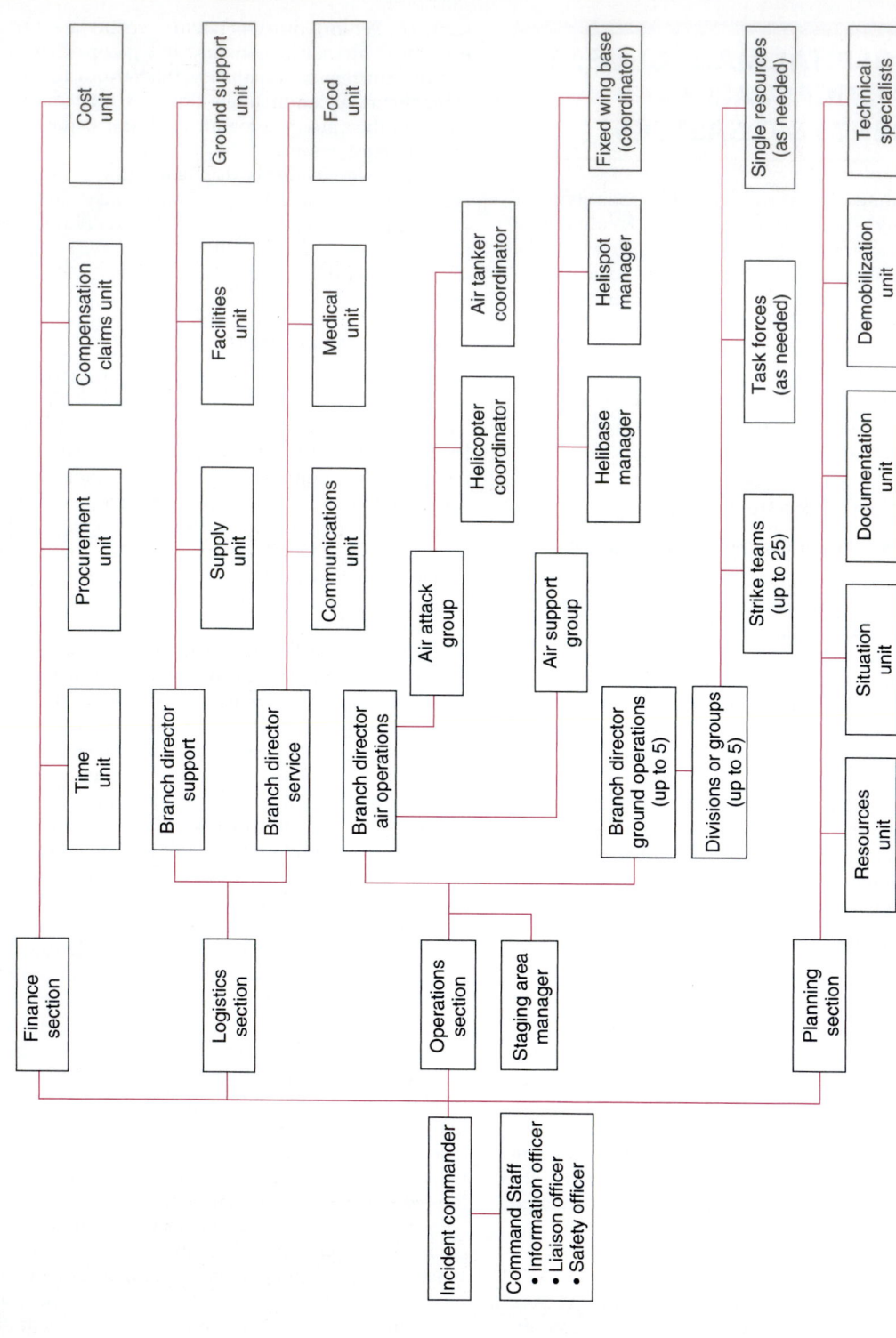

Figure 4–3. The Incident Command System (ICS) organizational diagram.

Scene Organization

Geographic factors play an important role in disaster response. In remote areas, aeromedical services may be instrumental; at sea, rescue vessels are needed; in urban areas, crowd and traffic control may be important. If a hazard is present, the area must be isolated and emergency vehicles positioned safely upwind. Figure 4–4 shows a typical ground schematic for a geographically focused multicasualty event.

Patients are most efficiently extricated and categorized (see Triage, below) if they are channeled to a single triage location and from there assigned to one of several treatment areas, depending on their level of treatment priority. From that point, patients depart the treatment areas through a single exit point. This arrangement ensures that the patients with the highest relative priority go first, no one is overlooked, and the total number of victims and their distribution are known.

Logistics

Logistics is a term applied to a support activity concerned with supplying and delivering resources to a rescue effort. Resources may be personnel, equipment, supplies, food and water, crew relief facilities, and the like. In the first few minutes of the EMS response to a

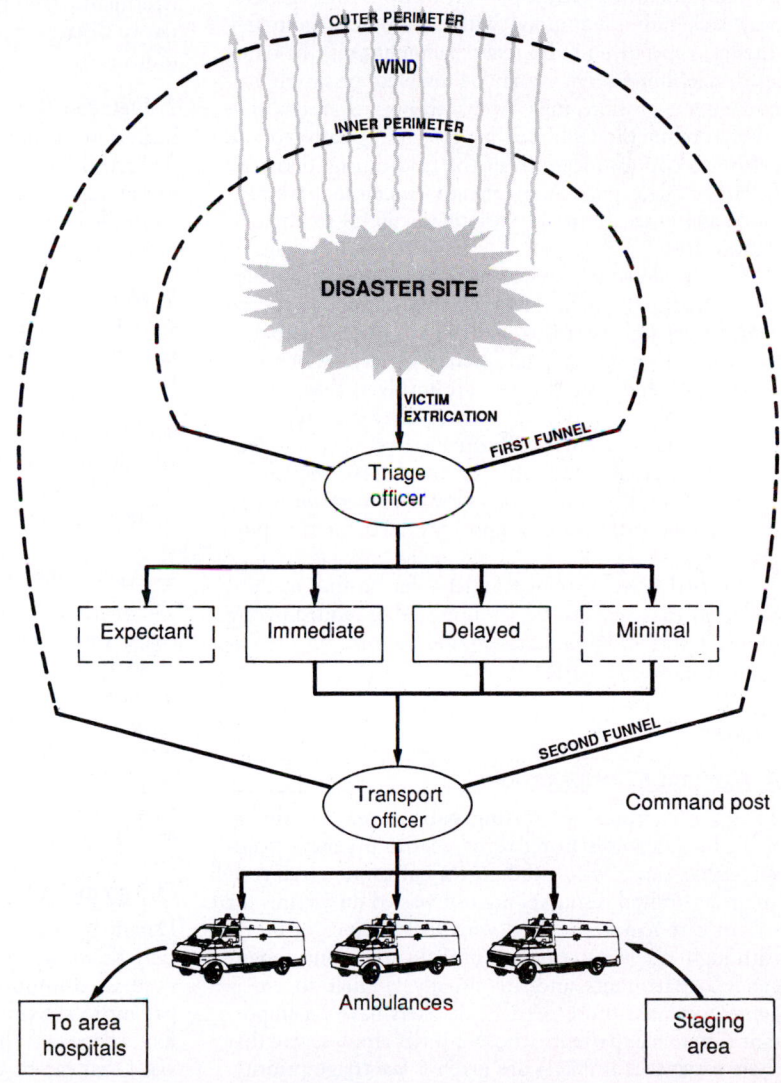

Figure 4–4. Scene diagram of a localized multicasualty incident.

typical multicasualty event, the first-in paramedic (or the medical commander) provides an initial report by radio to the dispatch or communications center, relaying information such as type of incident, estimated number of victims and severity of injuries, presence of any hazard, number and type of additional resources needed, additional agencies requested (eg, police, fire), and recommended staging location of incoming vehicles. As soon as possible, and if personnel are available, a logistics officer or team is designated by the medical commander.

Communications

Experience with modern multicasualty event management has shown communications to be the weak link in many incidents. Multiple jurisdictions and agencies may lack radios equipped with a common radio frequency, centralized radio relay equipment may be damaged, telephone services may be disabled, or simple frequency congestion may occur owing to heavy use. Lately, cellular telephones have added greatly to the ability to communicate from the field during disasters. In large-scale events, amateur radio operators have provided assistance. This is a particularly useful resource in remote areas.

In typical events, on-scene EMS units should designate a radio frequency for communications with the central dispatch center to coordinate patient distribution and requests for additional resources. When disparate ambulance companies are involved that do not usually share a common frequency, they can still communicate with a central coordinating center if the federally designated UHF Med Channels (10 frequencies set aside for communications between ambulances and receiving hospitals) are temporarily used for this purpose.

Normal base hospital telemetry for on-line medical direction may need to be temporarily suspended owing to heavy traffic. Paramedics should then act on predesignated standing orders.

Triage

A. General Considerations

Triage is a process of sorting patients and classifying them by categories in terms of relative urgency. It ensures that those who need treatment sooner receive it and that limited resources are not wasted on victims for whom care can be delayed with little chance of harm. Although triage systems are used in most busy emergency departments and are usually familiar to emergency workers, those used in disasters have an important difference: patients whose injuries are so severe that their survival is unlikely are given a *low* triage priority.

This situation can be difficult for many emergency workers to accept, but it is important because diversion of precious limited resources to moribund victims makes them unavailable to others who could be saved. The objective in disaster triage is to categorize patients in a way that will do the most good for the largest number and to ensure that limited resources are efficiently utilized.

B. Triage Categories

The most effective triage systems are simple and require no complex scoring methodology. A 4-level system is commonly used in the United States:

1. Immediate (I)—Patients have life-threatening injuries that probably are survivable with immediate treatment. Examples are tension pneumothorax, respiratory distress, major internal hemorrhage, and airway injuries.

2. Delayed (II)—Patients require definitive treatment, but no immediate threat to life exists. Patients can wait for treatment without jeopardy. Examples include minor extremity fractures, laceration with hemorrhage controlled, and burns over less than 25% of body surface area.

3. Minimal (III)—Patients have minimal injuries, are ambulatory, and can self-treat or seek alternative medical attention independently. Examples include minor lacerations, contusions, and abrasions.

4. Expectant (0)—Patients have lethal injuries and will die despite treatment. Examples include devastating head injuries, major third-degree burns over most of the body, and destruction of vital organs.

C. Assessment Methods

The method for rapidly assessing patients and deriving triage categories is based on evaluations that can be made quickly, easily, and by individuals with limited medical training. One such system employed in California is termed START (simple triage and rapid treatment; see Figure 4–5). Whatever system is used, the person with the greatest amount of experience, medical knowledge, and good judgment should be assigned the role of assigning triage categories.

D. Triage Tags

Detailed patient assessment information cannot practically be recorded in the field during a disaster, yet the need to communicate medical information about the patient to subsequent rescue workers still exists. Therefore, triage tags that are simple and visual have been devised that can be attached to the patient (Figure 4–6).

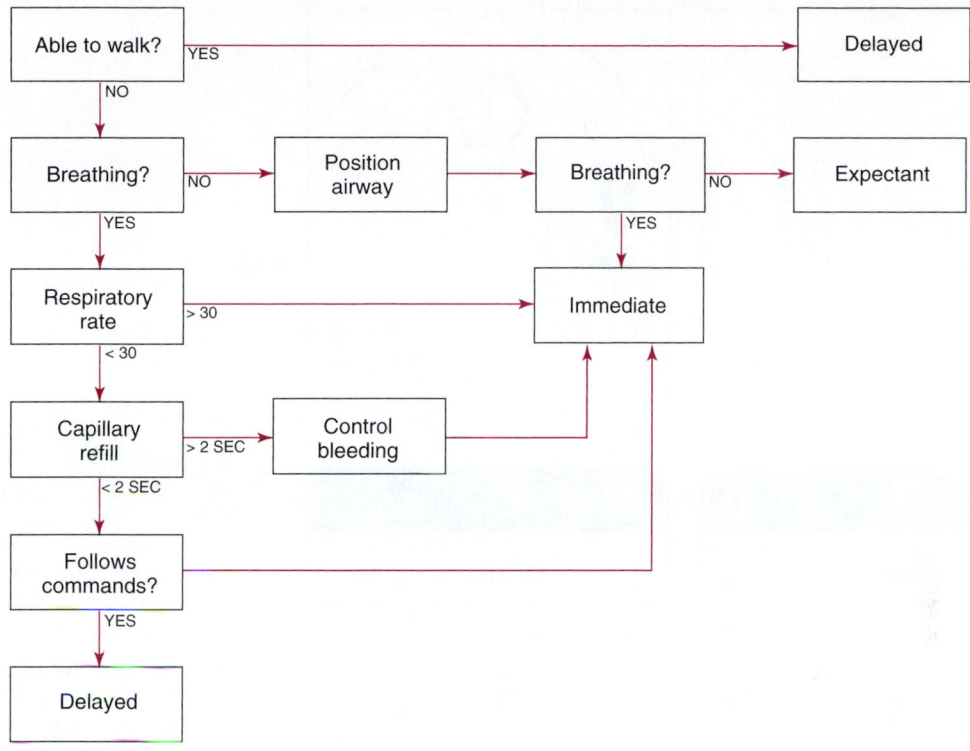

Figure 4–5. START triage algorithm.

Treatment

In a disaster or multicasualty event, personnel and equipment may be in short supply. Hence, initially, treatment is limited to *austere* medical care, that is, only essential and urgently necessary treatments, such as endotracheal intubation, pressure dressings, and intravenous lines for volume or essential drug administration. Prophylactic intravenous lines, for example, are omitted. Simplified triage using the ability to follow commands, as in the Glasgow Coma Scale, has been shown to have excellent predictive power in identifying patients who require urgent trauma care. The military has adopted the concept of "minimal acceptable care," but this has never been adopted by civilian hospitals. Indeed, surgeons of the International Committee of the Red Cross have used this approach in handling civilian casualties of military conflicts wherein 70% of the patients survived for as long as a week without definitive medical care.

Generally, a casualty collection point is designated in a convenient, safe, and sheltered location near the disaster site. The area is subdivided into sections for each triage category (ie, immediate, delayed, minimal, expectant), identifiable by colored tarps, tapes and cones,

tents, or the like. The areas should have controlled access and egress points to prevent violation of the triage and loading priority organization. Arriving EMS personnel and ancillary health care workers should be assigned by the medical commander to each area as needed. Victims, once directed to a treatment area by the triage officer, should be reassessed and treated according to need and the limitations of austere medical care. At any point, if a victim's condition changes, the victim may be moved to another area.

Victims in the expectant category are segregated and made comfortable. The dead are often not immediately extricated from the disaster site but are left for the medical examiner to remove at the conclusion of the event, unless public health reasons or security considerations require them to be moved to a temporary morgue.

Transport & Distribution of Patients

Ambulances or other transport vehicles (eg, bus or van) are directed to a specified loading location at a controlled egress point near the treatment areas. A transport officer (sometimes called loading officer) continually surveys the number of victims in each area and,

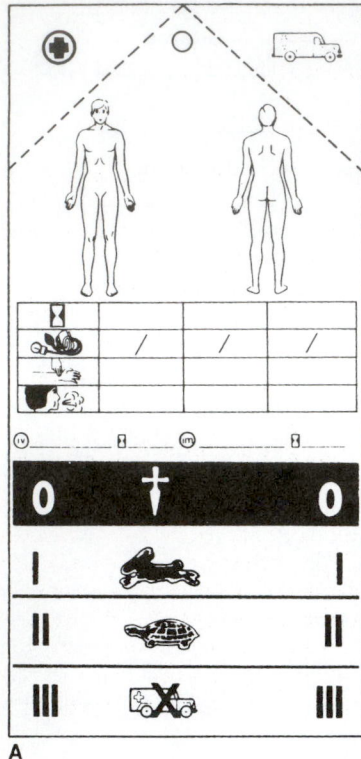
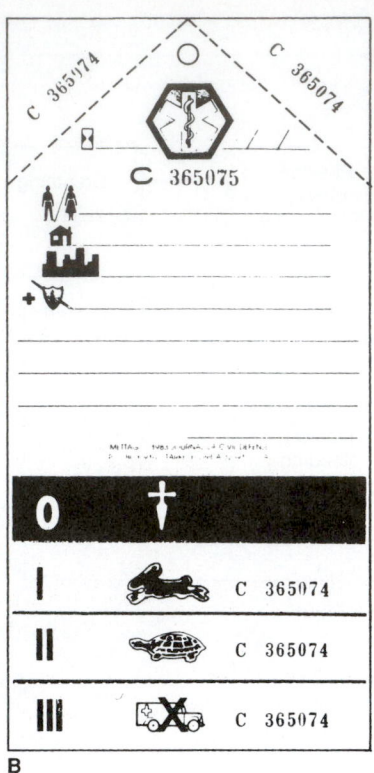

A

B

Figure 4–6. Example of triage tag, front and back. (Shown, with permission, from the *Journal of Civil Defense.*)

when ambulances arrive, assigns victims for transport in order of relative priority based on the urgency of their condition. Generally, a typical ambulance can transport more than one victim (eg, one immediate plus one or two delayed victims) depending on the stretcher and seating capacity of the ambulance and the level of attention required by the victims en route.

The distribution of victims to area hospitals differs significantly during a disaster compared with normal operations. Normally, destination may be determined by protocol factors, such as nature of problem, proximity to a given facility, or patient preference. Multicasualty events require victims to be *distributed* to area hospitals on a rotation protocol or according to each facility's capability to receive victims. This prevents the closest hospital from being inundated with large numbers of victims while more distant facilities remain idle.

Distribution can be accomplished by centrally coordinating destination assignments through the central dispatcher (if communications remain intact) or through the transport officer, who maintains a log of each departing ambulance's destination. The advantage of central coordination is that individual hospital capacity information can be solicited by dispatch personnel more easily than by on-scene rescue workers. If

feedback information is unavailable, a simple rotation protocol may be used.

Public Safety

Public safety involves protecting the public from hazards at the scene and allowing the rescue effort to unfold unimpeded by interference from the crowd. Most urban multicasualty events managed by EMS underutilize public safety personnel (ie, police and firefighters). Although firefighters have a prominent role when a hazard is present (eg, fire, explosion, collapse), an event that is predominantly medical presents a less clear role for them unless they are used to providing EMS care or to participating actively in the medical response.

Most commonly, non-EMS firefighters may be employed for hazard suppression, victim extrication and movement, and to the extent their training allows, initial triage. They should set up an inviolate perimeter barrier around the hazard area; position equipment and personnel in a safe, upwind position; and observe scene organization.

Similarly, police should enforce secure boundaries established by firefighters and EMS and maintain the crowd at a safe distance. Their assistance with traffic control and street closure may be necessary for the efficient ingress and egress of emergency vehicles.

Media Involvement

In some states, the press may have statutory right of access to a disaster site and cannot be denied access unless they interfere with ongoing rescue efforts, even if they jeopardize their own safety in the process (eg, California Penal Code, Section 409). The objectives of rescue workers and members of the press may sometimes seem at odds and lead to conflict during a disaster. However, it is usually in the broadest public interest to communicate timely, accurate information to the press.

As a general rule, the following points are worth observing:

1. Allow the press access to the disaster site, but advise them about areas and activities that are dangerous to them or that may interfere with ongoing rescue efforts or victims' treatment.

2. Actively provide the press with information that is as timely and as accurate as possible, and do so frequently. Appointing a press liaison or public relations officer is helpful.

3. Important information almost always involves the nature of the incident, number of victims, relative seriousness of injuries (eg, number of deaths), and location where the victims were taken. A source of information (eg, telephone hotline) for relatives of victims to call is an important public service.

4. Do not speculate about facts that are not known to you.

Air Medical Resources

Many communities and rural areas have access to air medical resources both for transport and for delivery of personnel and supplies. In remote areas, this may be the only form of disaster assistance. EMS helicopters may be utilized by designating a helicopter landing zone in a safe location upwind from the event. It should be distant enough that rotor noise and debris do not interfere with rescue activities, and it should be free of obstacles to landing and departing. In general, a relatively flat field (minimum of 100 feet square) with an unobstructed approach and departure path (into the wind) is ideal. An aircraft staging officer should be appointed who can coordinate arriving helicopters on a mutual radio frequency.

However, not all disasters are amenable to air medical assistance, and at times, helicopters can be a nuisance. During the Loma Prieta earthquake in 1989, many structures in the San Francisco marina area were thought to be unstable and susceptible to collapse from helicopter rotor vibrations. As a result, access to the overlying airspace was restricted.

Local Accessory Resources

Accessory resources may be needed in certain circumstances. For example, structural collapse may require heavy equipment such as bulldozers provided and operated by the city's department of public works; utility loss or live power wires may require the assistance of the local power company. The ICS is a useful organizational structure for managing these resources.

Mutual Aid

Mutual aid refers to assistance provided by local EMS and public safety agencies from neighboring counties or towns. It is intended to provide mutual back-up resources for common events that temporarily overwhelm local capabilities. Ideally, prearranged operating agreements are helpful, as is the installation of a common radio frequency for mutual communications. Requests for mutual aid are usually made rapidly at the dispatch center, although in some cases they may require authorization from a local authority, especially if an obligation for reimbursement occurs.

Special Considerations

A. HAZARDOUS MATERIALS

An incident involving a hazardous material (hazmat) requires specialty management because a threat to the rescue workers exists that may create additional casualties from among the rescuers or because contamination may spread to other areas in the community.

1. Priorities—The priorities in hazmat management are as follows:

- Identify, isolate, and contain the hazard to prevent spread of the contamination.
- Decontaminate victims.
- Protect rescue workers and EMS personnel, who should not approach or receive victims unless they are properly decontaminated, or the rescuers have appropriate protective gear, or the contamination is "contained" in a protective wrap around the victim.
- Provide advance warning to receiving hospitals so that appropriate protective measures may be taken.

2. Special training and equipment—Hazmat incidents are best managed by a specially trained team of rescue workers who wear special protective clothing and, when necessary, a respirator or self-contained breathing apparatus (Table 4–2). The appropriate training can be obtained from a variety of sources, for example, the 200-hour course provided by FEMA's National Fire Academy. Hazmat team individuals are familiar with methods of identifying hazardous substances, the nature of the substances and their effects, methods of hazard scene management, methods of hazard suppression, methods of decontamination, and operation of protective gear.

3. Specialty scene organization—The hazmat scene differs from the typical multicasualty event scene in that the immediate hazard area (the hot zone) is isolated from entry by unprotected non-hazmat personnel (Figure 4–7). Hazmat team members in protective gear enter the hot zone and extricate the victims to an intermediate zone or area where victim decontamination occurs, performed by hazmat team members also in protective gear. Hazmat team members should use triage principles to identify victims with the most immediate medical problems and the heaviest amounts of contamination. Decontamination often can be accomplished by removing the victim's clothing and dowsing the victim with copious quantities of water or another irrigant solution, taking care to prevent hypothermia and contain the effluent. Once decontaminated, victims are then transferred to awaiting EMS personnel, who perform triage and treatment as in a traditional multicasualty event.

Occasionally, victims with critical injuries require immediate lifesaving treatment before they can be decontaminated. As a result, it is helpful to include individuals in the hazmat team who have medical training (eg, paramedics), who are capable of performing triage of victims as they are extricated, and who can perform limited lifesaving care before or during decontamination efforts. If decontamination is impossible, then the contamination should be contained in an occlusive wrap and the patient transferred to EMS personnel with adequate notification of the remaining contamination hazard.

Table 4–2. Hazard exposure protective equipment.[1]

Level	Description
D	Work uniform, safety shoes, hard hat, gloves, eye protection
C	Add chemical-resistant suit, respirator
B	Add self-contained breathing apparatus (SCBA)
A	Total encapsulation with SCBA

[1]Source: Environmental Protection Agency.

B. DIFFUSELY DISTRIBUTED VICTIMS

Multicasualty events or disasters that produce victims dispersed over a large geographic area, rather than a localized event, pose a special challenge. The method of response differs in approach and method of coordination and depends on the extent to which central command, coordination, and communications remain functional.

1. The dispatch center is intact and operational—If radio and telephone communications are functioning (eg, in a moderate earthquake or natural disaster), the number of incoming 9-1-1 calls may be markedly increased with patients distributed diffusely throughout the area. Steps in managing such an event are as follows:

a. Obtain and deploy additional ambulance resources through reserve units, back-up arrangement, mutual aid, and the like.

b. Increase capacity for tracking deployed units by assigning additional dispatchers, reassigning radio frequencies, and the like. It may be necessary to suspend telemetry transmission to decongest the airwaves and free the dispatchers from nonessential duties.

c. Priority-rank incoming calls and notify callers of anticipated delays. It may be necessary to temporarily suspend response to routine service requests.

2. The dispatch center or other elements of command and communications have been rendered ineffective—In this case, there is no effective means of tracking resources, tracking incoming calls, or dispatching ambulances, and again, a large number of victims are diffusely distributed in the area. This may occur with a major natural disaster and is the most difficult situation to manage. Steps in managing such an event are as follows:

a. With loss of communications (or by declaration), centralized dispatch ceases and ambulances should disperse to predesignated station assignments in each neighborhood or area (eg, fire stations, hospitals, schools) that are natural locations for victims to self-report or around which neighborhood-level rescue efforts would be centered. Preestablished cache supplies at these sites should be utilized.

b. EMS ambulance crews should assist the local neighborhoods in organizing casualty collection, triage, and treatment areas to the extent possible. It may not be practical for EMS crews to transport victims if they are the sole resource in a

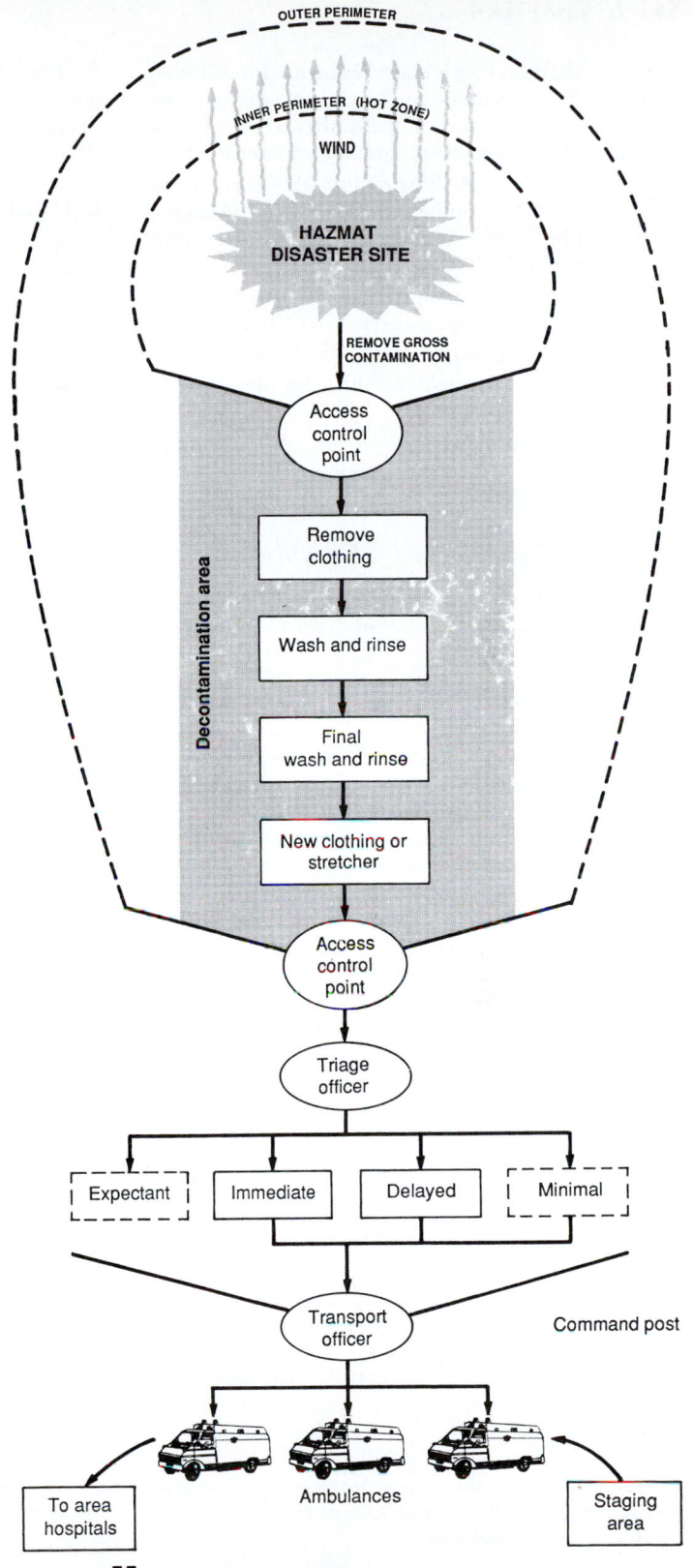

Figure 4–7. Hazmat scene organization diagram.

55

neighborhood with many casualties. Instead, they should concentrate on casualty collection and triage; use nonmedical transport, such as vans and buses, if available; and summon additional aid.

c. The numbers of casualties at each location and need for additional resources should be communicated by handheld radio or by runner to a central command post for the area.

d. Efforts to reestablish radio communications should proceed immediately.

e. Additional resources should be allocated to each area as they become available, and idle resources should be relocated.

f. Outside aid should be requested, and victim evacuation from casualty collection points should proceed if needed.

Disaster Organizations & Assistance

In addition to local mutual aid from neighboring communities, several other sources of disaster assistance are available.

A. MILITARY ASSISTANCE TO SAFETY AND TRAFFIC (MAST)

This program provides assistance from nearby military bases having a military medical mission in the form of aeromedical resources and medical support personnel in remote or rural areas. MAST can be requested directly by local public safety agencies. Usually, the response, which may consist of one or more aeromedical helicopter units, ranges from 30 to 90 minutes and consists of direct patient care and transport.

B. NATIONAL DISASTER MEDICAL SYSTEM (NDMS)

FEMA and the Department of Defense established the NDMS in 1984 as a cooperative program involving the Veteran's Administration hospital system and civilian hospitals. Its role is to provide for the distribution and care of large numbers of casualties from a major disaster or armed conflict in the United States. The principal component of the system is the network of civilian and Veteran's Administration hospitals spread throughout the United States that have pledged to provide a designated number of beds for disaster victims. The military would coordinate the collection, triage, and distribution of victims from the disaster site to these hospitals, using military airlift resources.

A second important component involves the on-scene management of casualties with disaster medical assistance teams, which consist of volunteer health care and rescue workers who are willing to be deployed to a disaster area within the United States and serve a medical clearing and staging function or serve as part of a mobile Army surgical unit.

The NDMS system can be activated by request from a governor in the event of a major disaster, with presidential approval, or by order of the secretary of defense during a military conflict.

C. OTHER MILITARY RESOURCES

Other agencies, such as the National Guard, and local military bases may be available to respond with personnel, equipment, and medical resources upon request from local, regional, or state officials.

D. DISASTER RELIEF ORGANIZATIONS

Various organizations, such as the American National or International Red Cross, Goodwill Industries, the Salvation Army, and various religious groups, are private or nonprofit organizations that provide assistance in the form of shelter, food, clothing, and services to victims of disasters. Internationally, the World Health Organization (WHO), while not directly participating in on-site disaster management, provides technical advice and assists with resources and finance. The United Nations Disaster Relief Office acts as a direct coordinator for disaster relief. Other assistance may be provided by organizations such as the Organization of American States and the regional arm of WHO, the Pan American Health Organization.

E. VOLUNTEERISM

Volunteerism by both health care and lay individuals is common during a disaster. However well-intentioned, volunteerism sometimes has drawbacks. Many volunteers are not familiar with local policies, laws, equipment, or practices; the expertise and certification of volunteers is difficult for rescue workers to verify; and volunteers may place an additional burden on the local system by their own need for food, water, and medical assistance if they are injured during rescue activities. Volunteers who have traveled to foreign countries to lend assistance during disasters have occasionally found themselves without many basic necessities, including food, shelter, and transportation home. Emergency health care workers who contemplate lending such assistance should consider these factors.

Asaeda G: The day the START triage system came to a stop: observations from the World Trade Center disaster. Acad Emerg Med 2002;9:255. [PMID: 11874794] (A case report of the World Trade Center attack.)

Auf der Heide E: Disaster planning, part 2. Disaster problems, issues, and challenges identified in the research literature. Emerg Med Clin North Am 1996;14:453. [PMID: 8635419] (A review of disaster challenges and planning principles and resources.)

Bissell RA et al: Health care personnel in disaster response. Reversible roles or territorial imperatives? Emerg Med Clin

North Am 1996;14:267. [PMID: 8635408] (A review of disaster medical response and the roles of health care providers.)

Coupland RM: Epidemiological approach to surgical management of the casualties of war. Br Med J 1994;308:1693. [PMID: 8025468] (Classic article in dealing with large numbers of wounded.)

Dormes B et al: Ethics and triage. Prehospital Disaster Medicine 2001;16:53. [PMID: 11367943] (A review of the ethics involved in mass casualty triage.)

Kennedy K et al: Triage: techniques and applications in decision-making. Ann Emerg Med 1996;28:136. [PMID: 8759576] (A review of the triage process.)

Levitin HW et al: Hazardous materials. Disaster medical planning and response. Emerg Med Clin North Am 1996;14:327. [PMID: 8635411] (A comprehensive review of hazmat procedures and planning.)

Maningas PA et al: The EMS response to the Oklahoma City bombing. Prehospital Disaster Med 1997;12:80. [PMID: 10187007] (A descriptive study of the EMS response to the Oklahoma City bombing.)

Moles TM: Emergency medical services systems and hazmat major incidents. Resuscitation 1999;42:103. [PMID: 10617329] (A review of hazmat major incidents.)

Roth PB et al: The federal response plan and disaster medical assistance teams in domestic disasters. Emerg Med Clin North Am 1996;14:371. [PMID: 8635413] (A review of national disaster response plans and resources.)

Yeskey KS et al: Operational medicine in disasters. Emerg Med Clin North Am 1996;14:429. [PMID: 8635417] (A review of medical support in military operations.)

EMERGENCY DEPARTMENT DISASTER MANAGEMENT

The term *disaster* may have a slightly different meaning to a hospital than to the prehospital community. Although a community multicasualty incident may overwhelm local EMS resources and require the activation of a community disaster plan, much of the response and resource requirement may relate to public safety needs, victim rescue, or hazard suppression, with relatively few casualties requiring hospitalization. In addition, the distribution of victims among several area hospitals may lessen the impact on a single institution, as will the existence of special destination criteria (eg, burns, trauma, pediatrics). However, internal problems at a hospital, such as utility failure, minor fires, and broken sewer lines, may require the evacuation of the hospital or shut down critical services (eg, x-ray, laboratory), causing bottlenecks or patient-flow problems. Even unexpected staffing problems coupled with a higher-than-normal emergency department census can be a minor "disaster" within a facility from time to time.

As a result, hospitals should have well-tested plans, worked out in advance, to provide special organization and management during such times.

Planning & Drilling

Community disasters large enough to require activation of a hospital's disaster plan are rare. Therefore, it is usually only through disaster drills that health care workers can gain experience with in-hospital disaster management. This is usually a committee or task force effort, and it should prominently involve input from emergency physicians and nurses in the hospital as well as from representatives of administration, plant services, security, and the like. The Joint Commission on Accreditation of Healthcare Organizations mandates that member hospitals have a disaster plan and conduct regular drills.

Disaster plans may be classified quantitatively in terms of the number of victims expected (eg, level 1, up to 20 victims; level 2, 20–50; level 3, over 50) or qualitatively in terms of the type of incident (eg, external trauma, radiation, fire, utility failure).

Mobilization of Disaster Resources

A. PERSONNEL

Additional personnel resources, such as doctors, nurses, orderlies, and registration clerks, should be quickly mobilized and sent to the emergency department where incoming patients may soon arrive. Special support areas, such as radiology, the blood bank, clinical laboratories, operating and recovery rooms, and central supply, may also need additional staff.

B. SUPPLIES

Disaster cache medical supplies, registration packets, stretchers, blood products, and the like should be delivered immediately to the emergency department.

C. SPACE

The emergency department should be surveyed quickly, and patients with non-life-threatening complaints should be moved to another area to open up treatment rooms for incoming victims. The operating and recovery rooms should be placed on standby and elective cases postponed. The intensive care units should review existing patients to identify those who can be moved to the wards. Opening a separate clinic area for minor complaints may be helpful.

Triage for Incoming Victims

An experienced physician or nurse should perform triage for arriving casualties at the door and direct them to resuscitation (or operating) areas, treatment rooms, or waiting areas, using principles similar to those outlined earlier (ie, immediate, delayed, minimal, expectant levels). Use of the triage tags applied by field paramedics is important, not only to learn about the victim's prehospital course but also to add information until a chart can be established.

Provision of Treatment

After emergency lifesaving treatment, such as airway control, has been provided, the emphasis is on providing definitive treatment rapidly for those who need it immediately and are likely to survive as a result. (Do the most good for the most people.) Unlike in the field, care need not be austere, but priority ranking is important and minor treatments may be delayed. Surgical resuscitation may be best handled in the operating room, because it tends to tie up personnel, space, and equipment in the emergency department.

Command & Communications Organization

It is important to establish early an administrative command center capable of communicating with each of the departments, coordinating logistics, and assessing resource and capacity needs. A link to the local EMS dispatch center is crucial to provide capacity information that will help the dispatchers equitably distribute patients to area hospitals.

Security Provisions

Enforcement of designated areas in the hospital and limitation of foot traffic by security personnel minimizes the stress and disorder accompanying any multicasualty event and makes the entire effort more effective.

Media Relations

A press area should be set aside and a media liaison and hospital spokesperson designated to keep the public informed of events. Accurate victim counts as well as names of victims are of intense interest to concerned relatives.

Plant Services

An assessment of the structural integrity of the facility is critical in a damaging natural disaster. Problems should be communicated to the local ambulance dispatch center so that additional victims may be diverted elsewhere.

Specialty Management of Hazardous Materials & Radiation

Variations in the basic plan are required for different types of incidents and disasters. An important variation occurs when a hazardous or radioactive substance is involved. Although sizable casualties of this type are rare in the United States, they may occur, particularly along transportation routes.

A. Notify Team

Once it is known that there are incoming contaminated victims, the hospital's radiation safety or hazmat team should be notified immediately (if one exists). Immediate information about the nature of the agent (if its identity is known), its effects, and precautions can often be obtained from the local fire department hazmat team or from a regional poison center.

B. Designate Restricted Areas

Restricted areas in the emergency department should be designated and demarcated by a strictly enforced hazard boundary line (hot zone). The area should include an intake pathway from the ambulance loading bay up to a separate decontamination area. It should also include one or more treatment or resuscitation rooms in the event that immediate resuscitation is needed before adequate decontamination is possible. Equipment, air intake vents, and floors should be covered with paper or plastic depending on the nature of the contaminant.

C. Apply Protective Clothing

Emergency personnel who will be involved in the evaluation and treatment of the victims should wear protective gear. Usually, a special hazmat suit, respirator, and self-contained breathing apparatus are not necessary. A surgical gown, scrubs, face shield, gloves, and shoe and head covering are usually adequate (the shoe covering should be removed when leaving the restricted area to prevent tracking of contamination to other areas).

D. Decontaminate the Victim

The patient should receive a triage examination away from the emergency department treatment area. Unless already decontaminated in the field, the victim should be dowsed with water or other appropriate decontamination solution and, if necessary, scrubbed with soap and water (do not abrade the skin; pay attention to hair and nails) before entry into the treatment area. Rarely, if lifesaving care cannot be delayed for decontamination, then the victim should be contained in a plastic wrap and treated by individuals protected as described above until stabilized sufficiently for decontamination.

Care should be taken to avoid washing cutaneous contamination into an open wound, where systemic absorption will be more rapid. All clothing, dressings, and tissue specimens should be collected.

E. Monitor Contamination

In the case of ionizing radiation, a monitoring device should be used to assess contamination levels of the victim and of exposed areas within the emergency department.

F. Treat

Treatment varies considerably depending on the agent involved. In some cases, specific treatments are required, such as atropine for organophosphate toxicity and sodium nitrite for cyanide toxicity. In most cases, however, treatment consists of providing airway and circulatory support and removing the offending agent.

G. Clean Up

The isolated area in the emergency department should be decontaminated thoroughly before access is granted. Depending on the agent involved, clean-up efforts should be directed by the hospital hazmat expert or radiation physicist.

Burgess JL et al: Emergency department hazardous materials protocol for contaminated patients. Ann Emerg Med 1999;34:205. [PMID: 10424922] (A review of hazmat protocols.)

Frykberg ER: Medical management of disasters and mass casualties from terrorist bombings: How can we cope? J Trauma 2002;53:201. [PMID: 12169923] (A review of the challenge, history, patterns of injury, triage, planning, and management of mass-casualty bombings.)

Hirshburg A, Holcomb JB, Mattox KL: Hospital trauma care in multiple-casualty incidents: a critical view. Ann Emerg Med 2001;37:647. [PMID: 11385336] (Review of key issues relating to trauma care during multicasualty incidents including possible redefinition of the standard of care during these events. Also discusses computer simulations and tabletop wargame-type training exercises versus mass-casualty drills to prepare for these disasters.)

Lewis CP et al: Disaster planning, part 1. Overview of hospital and emergency department planning for internal and external disasters. Emerg Med Clin North Am 1996;14:439. [PMID: 8635418] (A review of disaster planning.)

■ STRESS MANAGEMENT & PSYCHOLOGICAL SUPPORT

Multicasualty incidents and disasters are not only stressful and fatiguing to emergency workers, but they may also produce extreme psychological reactions to witnessed trauma. These reactions may be immediate or delayed, and may be manifested as anxiety, fatigue, depression, guilt, sleep disorders, and nightmares. Emergency workers who are used to working with life-and-death situations sometimes appear outwardly calm and unaffected, owing to defense mechanisms, denial, and peer effects.

In addition to an operational debriefing or so-called post-mortem event analysis, a critical incident stress team consisting of a psychologist or psychiatrist and others outside of the organization should perform a mandatory psychological debriefing. In this session, individuals should be encouraged to express their feelings and emotions related to the event and to realize that such feelings are normal, that the individuals are not alone in feeling them, and that support is available if needed.

Katz CL et al: Research on psychiatric outcomes and interventions subsequent to disasters: a review of the literature. Psychiatry Res 2002;110:201. [PMID: 12127471] (A review of the literature on postdisaster psychiatric outcomes.)

Oster NS et al: Psychiatric emergencies. Critical incident stress and challenges for the emergency workplace. Emerg Med Clin North Am 2000;18:339. [PMID: 10767889] (A review of critical incident stress debriefing.)

Legal Aspects of Emergency Care

5

Charles A. Eckerline, Jr, MD, FACEP, & Steven D. Rothert, MD, JD

General Legal Principles
  Criminal versus Civil Law
  Negligence
  Statute of Limitations
  Res Ipsa Loquitur
  Liability for the Acts of Others (Vicarious Liability)
  Duty to Provide Emergency Care
  Good Samaritan Laws
Common Legal Problems in the Emergency Department
  Consent

Psychiatric Emergencies
Abandonment
Reportable Events
The Medical Record
Emergency Physician & Medical Staff Interaction
Expert Witness
National Practitioner Data Bank
Harvesting of Organs for Transplantation

Medical malpractice lawsuits and medicolegal issues are a major concern for physicians and health care institutions. Most physicians expect to become involved in some manner in litigation alleging physician negligence. The physician may not always be a target defendant. In some circumstances, physicians who have provided treatment to a patient suing another physician may be subpoenaed to testify in court. Physicians may also become involved in litigation by agreeing to present medical opinion.

The filing of a malpractice action may generate a great deal of emotional stress for the defendant physician. This chapter discusses medicolegal problem areas in the emergency department and suggests ways in which the emergency medicine physician can avoid malpractice litigation.

The true extent of the emergency department malpractice problem is unknown, partly because emergency departments and emergency physicians are insured by many different insurance companies that have not pooled their claim information, and partly because many claims involve events that occurred not only in the emergency department but also in other parts of the hospital. It is clear, however, that disputes have increased attention to risk management, the number of emergency department malpractice claims and the size of malpractice judgments are increasing, and a malpractice insurance crisis may be brewing.

The net effect of malpractice suits has been to make emergency physicians, like physicians in general, practice so-called defensive medicine. Modern emergency departments provide mainly episodic care in a high-pressure environment that affords little time for leisurely contemplation and consultation when the diagnosis or best course of treatment is in doubt. In addition, prompt follow-up or consultation is often impossible to provide. These conditions mandate obtaining more supportive laboratory or radiographic studies than might be obtained otherwise. Whether physicians like it or not, the public demands that defensive medicine be the standard of care.

This chapter is intended to provide the practitioner with an overview of relevant medicolegal aspects of emergency medicine. The outcome of a particular malpractice case depends on its particular facts. Furthermore, both statutory and case law may vary considerably in different jurisdictions. For all these reasons, this chapter is not offered as legal advice.

■ GENERAL LEGAL PRINCIPLES

CRIMINAL VERSUS CIVIL LAW

There are 2 major types of law in the United States: criminal and civil. In a criminal lawsuit, the state or federal government sues an individual for actions considered to be against public interest, such as theft, murder, or rape. Such suits are intended to protect the public by apprehending and punishing the offender in a particular case and by deterring others from similar harmful conduct. Punishments range from fines to incarceration or even death in some jurisdictions. Given the relative severity of the punishment, the prosecution must prove its case beyond a reasonable doubt, a heavier evidentiary burden than in civil cases.

Civil cases typically involve a dispute between 2 or more persons or parties, in which the suing party (the plaintiff) seeks redress or compensation for an injury arising from the alleged wrongdoing of the defendant. Such cases may involve contract disputes, property disputes, or torts. A civil suit seeks to resolve the dispute and, if necessary, compensate the plaintiff, usually with money damages. Civil cases are concerned less with punishment than with compensation to the injured party. The suing party must prove his or her case by a preponderance of the evidence. Medical malpractice is a civil cause of action, a subset of tort law known as professional negligence.

NEGLIGENCE

Negligence, broadly defined, is the failure to do something that a reasonable person similarly situated would do, or doing something that a reasonable person similarly situated would not do. Negligence is a basic concept of tort law, and courts have long used it to remedy damages caused by such imprudent behavior. It is also the predominant (but not sole) theory of liability in medical malpractice actions. To recover against a negligent physician, a plaintiff-patient must prove each of these four elements: (1) a duty of care, (2) a breach of that duty, (3) proximate cause, and (4) damages. Thus, succinctly stated, negligence in the medical malpractice setting is the breach of a duty of care proximately causing damages.

Duty of Care

The duty of care is a physician's obligation to provide treatment according to an accepted standard of care. This obligation usually exists in the context of a physician-patient relationship but can extend beyond it in some circumstances. The physician-patient relationship clearly arises when a patient requests treatment and the physician agrees to provide it. However, creation of this relationship does not necessarily require mutual assent. An unconscious patient presenting to the emergency department is presumed to request care, and the physician assessing such a patient is bound by a duty of care. The Emergency Medical Treatment and Active Labor Act (EMTALA) requires emergency department physicians to assess and stabilize patients coming to the emergency department before transferring or discharging them. Such an assessment presumably creates the requisite physician-patient relationship. As intimated above, courts often extend this duty of care outside the immediate physician-patient relationship to include foreseeable third parties at risk for foreseeable harm.

Breach of Duty

When caring for a patient, a physician is obligated to provide treatment with the knowledge, skill, and care ordinarily used by reasonably well-qualified physicians practicing in similar circumstances. In some jurisdictions, these similar circumstances include the peculiarities of the locality in which the physician practices. This locality rule was developed to protect the rural practitioner who was sometimes deemed to have less access to the amenities of urban practices or education centers. However, the locality rule is being replaced by a national standard of care in recognition of improved information exchange, ease of transportation, and the more widespread use of sophisticated equipment and technology.

Establishing the standard of care in a given case requires the testimony of medical experts in most circumstances, unless the breach alleged is sufficiently egregious to be self-evident to the lay jury member—for example, amputating the wrong limb or leaving surgical implements in the operative field. A physician specializing in a given field will be held to the standard of other specialists in the same field, rather than to the standard of nonspecialists.

Proximate Cause

In order to recover in a malpractice lawsuit, the plaintiff must prove that the defendant's negligence more likely than not caused the injury sustained. The connection between the negligent act or omission and the injury must be reasonably foreseeable and probable in a natural course of events rather than speculative or merely possible. Courts have approached the concept of proximate cause in a number ways. The "but for" rule states that the defendant's conduct is a cause of the event if the event would not have occurred without it; that is, the event would not have occurred but for the defendant's conduct. For example, but for the physician negligently transfusing an Rh-negative woman with Rh-positive blood, the woman's unborn child would not have suffered hemolytic disease of the newborn and its complications. When it is foreseeable that 2 or more causes could result in the event, such as when a negligent act aggravates an underlying disease process, proximate cause may be found when the act in question is a substantial factor in bringing about the event.

This brief discussion of proximate cause only hints at the complexity of the issue, which is often much easier to state than to apply. The jury is charged with the responsibility of determining whether proximate cause exists and, as a practical matter, will find proximate cause if the conduct is of such closeness and significance to the event that imposition of legal liability is warranted.

Damages

Damages are awarded as compensation for loss or injury suffered as a proximate result of negligent conduct. A plaintiff may recover compensatory damages for disability or disfigurement, pain and suffering, the expense of past and future medical treatment and services, lost earnings, the loss of the services of a spouse, funeral expenses, and other expenses. In some states, punitive damages may also be awarded if the defendant acted with malicious intent or with reckless disregard for the consequences of his or her actions, that is, with willful or wanton misconduct. The jury determines the amount of damages awarded. This determination is afforded great weight by reviewing courts and will be amended only if it is clear from the evidence that the jury was moved by sympathy or prejudice in reaching its decision.

STATUTE OF LIMITATIONS

The statute of limitations is a law that specifies the time within which a lawsuit must be initiated. In other words, any person who feels that he or she may have a claim against another person must file that claim before the time period specified in the statute of limitations runs out. Failure to do so forever bars the claim. Despite its appearance, this law is not intended to shield the wrongdoer. Rather, its purpose is to promote timely filing of claims and thus to allow the defendant to prepare an adequate defense while memories are fresh, witnesses are available, and material facts are accessible.

The length of time varies for different causes of action, but the time frame for negligence actions (and, hence, most medical malpractice actions) is 2 years in most states. The time period typically begins to run once the aggrieved person knows or reasonably should know that a claim exists, not simply once the offense has occurred. However, most limitations statutes also include a longer, maximum time measured from the occurrence of the offense, known as the statute of repose. Both time periods will be extended if the offending party fraudulently conceals the negligent conduct or intentionally misleads the aggrieved party. Finally, of special note, most statutes of limitations do not begin to run against a minor until he or she reaches the age of majority. The age of majority varies from 18 to 21 years of age.

RES IPSA LOQUITUR

The plaintiff in a medical malpractice case has the burden of proving each of the elements of the cause of action and, in order to carry that burden, normally must present direct factual evidence showing that the defendant acted negligently. However, in those instances where the injury would not have occurred in the absence of negligence, such as when a patient emerges from an abdominal surgery with a shoulder injury, the plaintiff may invoke the doctrine of *res ipsa loquitur,* which translated literally means "the thing speaks for itself."

Under this doctrine, which arose in response to medical professionals' notorious unwillingness to testify against one another, the defendant's negligence may be inferred from circumstantial evidence alone when direct evidence of the cause of injury is primarily within the knowledge or control of the defendant. To invoke this doctrine, the plaintiff must demonstrate that (1) the injury is of the kind that ordinarily does not occur in the absence of negligence, (2) the injury was caused by an agency or instrumentality within the exclusive control of the defendant, and (3) the patient did nothing to contribute to the injury. The legal effect of successfully invoking this doctrine is to create an inference of a breach of the standard of care, and to shift to the defendant the burden of proving that no breach occurred. In essence, it makes the defendant speak when he or she would prefer to remain silent and about things it would be extremely difficult or impossible for the plaintiff to discover. The burden of proof shifts to the defendant only with relation to the breach of the standard of care. The plaintiff still retains the burden of proof with relation to the other elements of the cause of action. Although this doctrine is typically mentioned as a way to avoid the use of expert testimony to establish negligence, as a practical matter expert testimony is still usually required to show that the injury would not have occurred in the absence of negligence.

LIABILITY FOR THE ACTS OF OTHERS (Vicarious Liability)

Normally, a person is liable only for his or her own negligent conduct. However, according to the principles of vicarious liability, a physician or hospital may be liable for the negligent conduct of employees or agents. This doctrine was developed in the realm of employment, and a number of justifications for its use have been offered. The employer, it is deemed, has general control over the employment situation and must bear the responsibility for this supervisory control. The employer selects and trains his or her employees and should therefore pay for their negligence just as he or she profits from their efforts. The employer is better able to absorb losses and to distribute them to the public through increased prices, rates, or insurance. Essentially, these justifications describe a public policy to deliberately allocate risk. The losses caused by the torts of employees that are sure to occur in the conduct of the employer's enterprise are placed upon the enterprise itself, as a required cost of doing business.

Within the employment relationship, *respondeat superior* (Latin for "let the master answer") confers legal liability on the employer for the actions of the employee. A hospital or a physician may therefore be found liable for the negligence of an employed office worker, physician's assistant, or nurse. Similarly, a medical partnership may be held liable for the negligent acts of one of its partners, each of whom is an agent of the partnership. Liability is conferred, however, only if the agent or employee committed the negligent act within the scope of his or her employment. An employer will not be held liable for the intentionally wrongful acts of employees, such as sexual assault while at work, because such acts are not considered to be in furtherance of the business enterprise.

Traditionally, hospitals were not held liable for the negligence of physicians working in the hospital as independent contractors, such as physicians with admitting privileges. In this instance, the hospital was not deemed to have sufficient control over the actions of the physician to justify application of vicarious liability principles. In recent years, however, there has been an emerging trend to hold the hospital liable for the actions of independent contractor physicians who provide hospital-based services integral to the business enterprise of the hospital. The negligence of independent contractor physicians working in fields such as emergency medicine, radiology, and anesthesiology has been attributed to the hospitals where they work under the doctrine of apparent agency. Courts have reasoned that if the hospital holds itself out to the public as providing a given service and enters into a contractual relationship with physicians to provide this service, and the public looks to the hospital for this service without regard to the identity of the particular physician providing care, the hospital should be vicariously liable as an employer.

DUTY TO PROVIDE EMERGENCY CARE

At one time, U.S. common law did not require a physician or hospital to provide medical treatment to all who sought it. Thus private, and some public, hospitals could refuse emergency care to a patient if the treatment would result in no compensation to the hospital.

A series of abuses of the privilege not to provide emergency care and the transfers of patients to hospitals that would accept those persons unable to pay, caused mounting concern over the practice of so-called patient dumping. This concern resulted in landmark legislation that has had a huge impact on the practice of emergency medicine.

Congress enacted EMTALA as part of the Consolidated Omnibus Reconciliation Act of 1985 (COBRA). EMTALA applies to emergency care provided to all patients presenting to hospitals that have a Medicare contract and receive third-party payment from Medicare or Medicaid. EMTALA requires that anyone presenting to an emergency department requesting an examination be provided with an appropriate medical screening exam, sufficient to determine whether an emergency medical condition exists. This includes the use of appropriate ancillary services.

If no emergency medical condition is found, the duty to patients under EMTALA ends, although any alleged failure to provide appropriate care could still result in a malpractice claim. If an emergency medical condition is discovered, EMTALA requires stabilizing treatment for any emergency medical condition or labor. EMTALA restricts the transfer of patients with emergency medical conditions or women in active labor until the condition has been stabilized unless the benefits of transfer outweigh the risks.

A receiving hospital may not refuse an appropriate transfer. Hospitals that receive inappropriate transfers are required to report suspected EMTALA violations within 72 hours. The law provides for civil monetary penalties and revocation of a hospital's Medicare certification for violations. Physicians can also be subjected to fines and termination from the Medicare program. These penalties also apply to physicians who are on call and fail to appear within a reasonable time. In addition, civil suits may be filed in state or federal court, bypassing any peer review or arbitration system established in some states as part of tort reform.

EMTALA began as well-intentioned effort to address the problem of patient dumping. It has expanded far beyond its original intent to apply to inpatients, psychiatric patients, and even patients who have not yet arrived in the emergency department. This has placed an additional burden on emergency physicians as well as hospitals that transfer or receive transferred patients.

Hospitals have an interest in educating their medical staffs about EMTALA. Emergency physicians are often most knowledgeable about these issues and are looked to for leadership. The responsibilities of emergency care are so important that any hospital that does not have a qualified emergency physician on duty might find itself unable to discharge its full legal duty to the public under the law.

GOOD SAMARITAN LAWS

Good Samaritan laws are statutes enacted in each state to protect from civil liability health care professionals who render aid at the scene of an emergency. These statutes are intended to encourage assistance in emergency situations by providing an affirmative defense to suits arising from the event. Statutes vary somewhat in terms of whom they protect, ranging from physicians to all individuals. The statutes generally require that the person rendering aid act reasonably, in good faith, without compensation, and without gross negligence or harmful intent.

Good Samaritan statutes have provided protection to physicians who were not officially on call but who responded to an emergency department case. Several jurisdictions have applied Good Samaritan statutes to staff physicians called to an emergency in a hospital room. Good Samaritan protection does not apply to emergency medicine physicians seeing patients in the emergency department or to emergency medical services personnel in the field in the course of their employment. Good Samaritan statutes also do not create an affirmative duty to render aid.

■ COMMON LEGAL PROBLEMS IN THE EMERGENCY DEPARTMENT

CONSENT

General Principles Relating to Consent

Consent, as a legal doctrine, arose out of cases alleging battery by a physician. In these cases, a surgeon performing a surgery for which consent had not been obtained was likened to nonconsensual touching, which is the definition of the tort of battery. Thus it was immaterial that the patient needed the surgery, that the surgeon had performed the surgery well, or even that the patient would have consented if he or she had been asked. Infringing on the patient's right to decide what would be done with his or her body was the essential wrongdoing. The right to be free from nonconsensual touching is fundamental in U.S. civil and criminal law, in that battery is actionable in both arenas. These cases established that right in medical contexts as well.

Subsequent case law has extended this doctrine from simple consent, agreeing to a procedure despite no discussion of risks or alternative treatments, to the modern concept of informed consent, which requires physicians to give patients adequate information about proposed treatments.

Doctrine of Informed Consent

Under the modern doctrine of informed consent, a physician should discuss with the patient the following elements: the patient's diagnosis, the nature and purpose of the proposed treatment, the risks and expected outcomes of the proposed treatment, alternative treatments and their risks, and the consequences of no treatment.

In order to successfully sue for lack of informed consent, a plaintiff must prove that (1) the physician failed to obtain full and informed consent and (2) this failure proximately caused the injury, that is, that the patient would not have consented to the procedure had the material risks been disclosed. Regarding the first element, most jurisdictions follow a physician-oriented standard of disclosure. Under this standard, a physician is required to disclose what a reasonable medical practitioner of the same school in the same or similar circumstances would disclose. However, a number of jurisdictions, including New Jersey and Pennsylvania, follow a patient-oriented standard of disclosure. Under this standard, a physician is required to disclose the information that a reasonable person in the patient's situation would consider important in choosing a course of treatment. Reasonable people can disagree about which standard is more appropriate. The physician-oriented standard is sometimes derided as allowing the medical community to specify its own scope of disclosure, which may be out of touch with the needs of the individual patient. By contrast, detractors of the patient-oriented standard point out that it is too prone to misuse by sympathetic juries in cases where inevitably the undisclosed, unusual complication has occurred.

In order to prove the causation element, most jurisdictions require that the plaintiff prove that a reasonable person in the patient's situation would not have consented to the proposed treatment had adequate information been given.

Exceptions to Consent Requirements

Several exceptions to informed consent disclosure requirements have been consistently recognized throughout the United States. In medical emergencies, when the patient is unconscious or unable to communicate, or when there is no time to obtain informed consent, the physician may provide treatment under the theory of implied consent. In this circumstance, the law presumes that the compelling need for treatment outweighs the need to obtain informed consent. When a patient receives recurrent medical care and thus has prior knowledge of the nature of the ongoing treatment, as well as the material risks and alternatives, then the physician generally need not make duplicative disclosures in order to obtain informed consent. However, if the patient's condition or other circumstances change, the physician should apprise the patient of this change and renew the consent previously obtained.

A patient may expressly waive the right to informed consent by stating that he or she does not wish to be informed about certain information pertaining to the course of treatment. When this occurs, the physician should inquire why the patient does not wish to be informed and should document these reasons in the medical record. If the patient knowingly and intelligently waives this right, and has reasonable justifications for doing so, then nondisclosure will be defensible in court.

The final exception to consent requirements is known as the doctrine of therapeutic privilege. It arises in situations in which the patient is so anxious or fragile that full disclosure might cause serious emotional or physical harm. Circumstances justifying use of this doctrine are exceptionally rare, and physicians asserting this privilege must carefully document their decision making in the medical record. A physician's concern that the patient might forego recommended treatment if adequately apprised of its risks is not a sufficient reason to invoke this doctrine.

Authority to Give Consent

Informed consent obtained after adequate disclosure by the treating physician will be meaningful only if the patient has the authority to give consent. Under U.S. law, all adults are presumed to be competent to make decisions about their treatment and thus to have the authority to give or withhold consent. However, a physician should question this presumption of competence when the patient's mental capacity is altered due to physical or mental illness, intoxication, or diminished consciousness due to injury or other causes.

Competence, broadly defined, is the ability to make decisions. A competent patient is able to understand his or her medical condition and the proposed treatments in a general way and can appreciate the consequences of accepting or refusing the proposed treatment. If a patient lacks the requisite mental capacity to make informed decisions, the physician should seek consent from a qualified surrogate decision-maker. If the patient has previously been determined to be incompetent, he or she will likely have an appointed guardian with the responsibility to make medical decisions. If the patient has an advance directive such as a durable power of attorney or a living will, this document will identify the surrogate decision-maker. If no such documentation exists, most states have enacted statutes that identify a hierarchy of family members who can give or withhold consent for a patient who becomes incompetent acutely. Given the circumstances in most emergency departments, a physician should always involve an incompetent patient's closest family members in the decision-making process. Further, a physician should document in the medical record evidence justifying the determination of incompetence and his or her attempts to obtain consent from a qualified surrogate decision-maker.

Intoxicated Patients

Intoxicated patients are frequent emergency room patients and present a special risk to emergency room physicians. Their altered mental status may mask serious injuries that are too easily attributed to their intoxication, and the treating physician must exercise a heightened suspicion while evaluating such patients for injuries. Their intoxication may render them incompetent to consent to or refuse treatment, which requires that consent be obtained from a qualified surrogate decision-maker, as discussed above. In general, the emergency physician should assume that an intoxicated patient does not have the capacity to consent and that the patient may have a serious injury or illness, and should therefore perform a complete medical screening evaluation. A liberal restraint policy may be necessary to allow for proper evaluation. However, once the patient demonstrates mental competence and there is no apparent life threat, the physician has no legal right to detain the patient any longer, regardless of whether the patient's blood alcohol level is at or below the state legal limit for intoxication.

Police Custody

Patients who have been arrested and are on their way to jail, or persons already in jail, are often brought to the emergency department for treatment. Impending or actual incarceration does not alter their rights concerning consent for treatment. Sufficient consent for examination and treatment must be obtained.

Minors

In general, a minor does not have legal competence, and the consent of a minor's parent or legal guardian must be obtained before treatment can be rendered. Of course, several exceptions exist. In a medical emergency, consent will be implied by law. Most states allow an emancipated minor to consent to his or her medical care. An emancipated minor is a minor who is or has been married, who lives alone and is financially independent, or who has children of his or her own. Most states also allow minors to give consent for treatment of specific conditions such as pregnancy, sexually transmitted diseases, or chemical dependency. Consent laws vary considerably from state to state, and emergency physicians should become familiar with their own states' consent laws.

Patient Refusal to Consent

Any competent adult patient may refuse to consent to a proposed treatment, even if that treatment is necessary to save the patient's life. The guiding principle being observed is patient autonomy: all competent patients have the right to decide what will be done with their bodies.

If a patient decides to leave the emergency department without treatment and against medical advice, the risks of doing so should be explained and the patient should be asked to sign a form releasing the hospital and emergency department staff from liability. If the patient refuses to sign this form, this fact and the circumstances of the patient's departure should be documented in the medical record.

If a patient is incompetent, he or she does not have the right to refuse treatment because such a patient is not deemed to have the capacity to make an informed decision. In this circumstance, the physician has an obligation to protect the patient, restrain the patient if necessary, and render appropriate care. This delicate balancing of patient autonomy and physician authority requires a sort of cost-benefit analysis on the physician's part in each case. An intoxicated patient refusing to consent to suturing of a small laceration might be afforded greater autonomy than a previously healthy person who refuses treatment of an acute myocardial infarction. Although a physician faced with the second scenario cannot simply override a competent patient's wishes, the physician should investigate more fully the patient's understanding of his or her condition, the proposed treatment, and the likely consequences of the decision.

With these principles in mind, a few special cases should be noted. A psychiatric patient should be evaluated to determine if he or she is a threat to self or others. If so, the patient should be restrained for further psychiatric evaluation and therapy. However, the psychotic state itself does not necessarily render the patient incompetent. A psychiatric patient's right to refuse psychotropic medications has generally been upheld by the courts. The safest alternative for the emergency physician is to consult a psychiatrist to conduct this evaluation.

Narcotics users who present to the emergency department in respiratory arrest and receive naloxone may become intensely uncomfortable due to the effects of narcotic reversal and acute withdrawal. They may desire to leave the emergency department to seek more narcotics. However, naloxone has a shorter half-life than heroin and other narcotics, and the patient remains at significant risk for recurrent respiratory arrest. At a minimum, such patients should be held in the emergency department for at least one half-life of naloxone.

Emergency department personnel should use reasonable therapeutic restraint to evaluate and provide treatment to violent patients, because there is a correlation between violence and acute organic brain syndrome. If restraining such a patient places the staff at risk of harm, the patient should be allowed to "escape," and the police should be notified that the patient may be a threat to self or others. Circumstances of the incident should be carefully documented in the medical record.

The right of Jehovah's Witness patients to refuse receiving blood products is a troublesome area for physicians. Courts have generally upheld this right for competent adults, but a number of exceptions exist, depending on whether the state can demonstrate a compelling or overriding interest for authorizing the transfusion. Transfusions have been authorized when the patient has dependents or is pregnant, or when there is a reasonable doubt about the strength of the patient's convictions. Courts typically do not allow a Jehovah's Witness parent to refuse treatment for a minor. The safest course of action for a physician facing this dilemma is to contact hospital staff or legal counsel for guidance.

Finally, although parents' decisions about their child's care are typically respected, they should not be allowed to place the child at risk of serious harm. Courts have repeatedly held, under the doctrine of *parens patriae* (the state's paternalistic interest in children), that a parent does not have the right to refuse life-saving treatment for a child, even on religious grounds. If faced with such a situation, the physician should contact hospital counsel and take temporary protective custody of the child based on child neglect. The physician may be hesitant to take custody of the child, but it should not be for fear of liability; the physician is protected from civil and criminal liability under child abuse and neglect statutes. In the past 30 years, no case has been reported in which a parent has successfully sued a physician for providing nonnegligent care to a child without parental consent.

Consent for Blood Alcohol Samples

Many states have enacted statutes regarding driving under the influence; these statutes define intoxication on the basis of blood alcohol concentration. They typically specify that a person arrested under the statute is deemed to have consented to blood tests for the purpose of determining the blood alcohol level. If the patient does not allow medical personnel to obtain the sample, such refusal may result in summary suspension of the patient's driver's license. These statutes usually provide physicians with civil liability protection for use of the results of these samples in legal proceedings. In some states, this implied consent extends only to the testing of urine and breath samples but not to blood samples. The provisions of these statutes vary from state to state, and emergency physicians should become familiar with the laws of the states in which they practice.

PSYCHIATRIC EMERGENCIES
(See also Chapter 47.)

Patients with psychiatric disorders or altered mental status for other reasons (ie, drugs, alcohol, organic dysfunction) are often unable to test and evaluate external reality and may experience delusions, hallucinations, and personality disintegration. Such patients present special legal hazards with regard to the legal principles of assault and battery as well as false imprisonment. The key questions in deciding when and to what degree physical restraint can be used on a patient with mental illness is whether the patient is likely to cause self-harm or harm others. The emergency department staff may use appropriate and reasonable efforts, including the use of restraints, to protect the patient from self-harm and from harming others. If the staff fails to use necessary, reasonable restraints, it risks incurring liability to innocent third parties injured by the patient and may incur liability to the patient if the patient causes self-harm. By contrast, unnecessary or excessive force may result in liability for injuries sustained by the patient. What constitutes excessive force depends on the circumstances of each case.

Hospitals are required to have specific restraint policies and forms. Emergency department staff must be familiar with these policies and document their compliance on the appropriate forms. The emergency department record should contain an objective and thorough documentation of the patient's behavior and mental status, the physician's reason for restraints, and the method and duration of restraint.

The problem may be complicated when an alert and apparently competent patient protests against being held in the emergency department for further assessment and demands to leave before his or her evaluation is complete. The emergency department staff may be held liable for false imprisonment if such a patient is later determined not to be a danger to self or others. Actions for false imprisonment may arise when a person is unlawfully deprived of personal liberty by another person without giving consent and is aware of such deprivation, and when no defense of privilege applies. Although the potential for liability exists in such cases, the incidence of claims is low.

Conversely, emergency department staff may face liability for failure to hold and further assess a mentally unstable person if the patient is released and then causes self-harm or harms others. Physicians who discharged psychiatric patients who subsequently committed suicide have been found liable for wrongful death of these patients in lawsuits brought by the patients' survivors, if the juries concluded that the decisions to discharge their patients were made in a negligent manner. This scenario exposes the emergency department staff to a greater risk of litigation than the risk of false imprisonment.

Maintaining the patient in the emergency department for a reasonable period of time for examination and evaluation by a psychiatric health professional may be the most prudent course of action. If a psychiatrist or other mental health professional is not available, the emergency department physician must decide whether to discharge the patient or start procedures for involuntary commitment to a psychiatric faculty. Laws vary greatly with regard to emergency involuntary commitments. The emergency department staff should be familiar with the laws in their local jurisdiction. As a general principle, the decision to restrain a mentally ill patient for a thorough evaluation is more easily defended than the decision to allow a potentially dangerous patient to be discharged. The key is thorough documentation.

ABANDONMENT

Abandonment is the unilateral termination of the physician-patient relationship by the physician without the patient's consent and without giving the patient sufficient opportunity to secure the services of another competent physician. Although much emergency department care is episodic in nature and does not involve follow-up treatment, the emergency department physician and staff still have a responsibility to provide appropriate discharge instructions.

Emergency department physicians may be liable for negligent disposition of the patient if they do not give follow-up care instructions appropriate for the patient's condition. This principle also requires the translation of follow-up instructions for patients who do not read English, if the emergency department is in an area where it would be reasonable to require the presence of translating personnel in the emergency department. The area of follow-up instructions is also one of concern to the Joint Commission on Accreditation of Healthcare Organizations (JCAHO). When frequently required in an emergency care area, a means of communications should be available in the language of the predominant population groups served by the emergency department.

Follow-up Care

Emergency departments are designed to provide episodic care for emergency problems. Patients discharged from the emergency department frequently require referral for follow-up care. Due to a shortage of primary care physicians and certain specialists, and frequently a lack of financial resources by emergency department patients, arranging appropriate follow-up care can be difficult. Generally, the emergency department physician should refer the discharged patient to a physician available from the on-call list. When follow-up becomes unavailable for whatever reason, the patient should be instructed to return to the emergency department.

Instruction Sheets

Discharge instruction sheets should be provided to every emergency department patient and should be signed by the patient or guardian. The instruction sheets should be as specific as possible and appropriate for the discharge diagnosis. The patient's signatures on the instruction sheet should certify that he or she has received the form and has been given oral instructions as indicated on the sheet. A copy of the signed instruction sheet should be retained in the patient's medical record.

Telephone Consultation

Patients may also allege abandonment or negligence via telephone consultation. An example is the patient who is discharged from the emergency department, experiences a reoccurrence of symptoms, calls the emergency department, and is told not to worry about it until morning. If the patient's condition worsens, or if the patient receives any advice subsequently deemed to be inappropriate, the emergency department staff may be liable for negligence and abandonment. As a general rule, although it is reasonable to answer basic questions, the emergency department staff should not provide diagnoses or treatment to patients over the telephone.

REPORTABLE EVENTS

All governments have statutes and administrative regulations that require reporting of certain events by emergency department physicians and staff. Reportable events include child or elder abuse, rape, gunshot and stab wounds, assaults, or other suspicious injuries; certain communicable disease including most sexually transmitted diseases, hepatitis, tuberculosis, and HIV infection; animal bites; and the receipt of patients who are dead on arrival. Emergency physicians and staff should know which events are reportable and the procedure for reporting them in the area in which they practice, because these rules vary by state and county.

Child Abuse

All U.S. jurisdictions and many other countries have regulations or statutes requiring the reporting of actual or suspected child abuse. Some of the statutes allow the reporter to exercise discretion in deciding whether to report, whereas others require reporting of all cases under penalty of fine or imprisonment.

Many states' reporting statutes grant immunity from civil liability (eg, immunity from charges of slander) to the reporting party. These immunity provisions were intended to make the public (including physicians and nurses) more inclined to report suspected child abuse cases by eliminating the fear of being sued by the parents. In some states, immunity for reporting and for participating in subsequent judicial proceedings is provided without any express qualification. Other states provide immunity for actions taken "in good faith" or "without malice." Generally, no immunity provision will protect emergency department staff members who broadcast to third parties with no official status or right to know that the parents are child abusers.

In states lacking statutes granting immunity, the emergency physician and, more important, the child victim will be better off if suspicion of child abuse is reported to the appropriate agency. Failure to report a reasonably suspected case of child abuse may result in criminal penalties for failure to report according to state law and may also result in civil liability for negligence in failing to report.

Sexual Assault

All states have procedures for handling sexual assault investigations. Emergency department staff must recognize that rape is a legal conclusion and not a medical diagnosis.

Protocols for management of rape victims are given in Chapter 36.

Gunshot & Stab Wounds

Most jurisdictions require that injuries from acts of violence, such as gunshot and stab wounds, or any alleged assaults be reported to the appropriate reporting agency. Reports of violent wounds of any sort should generally be reported to the local police.

Communicable Diseases

Public health laws generally require the reporting of certain communicable diseases, including sexually transmittal infections, HIV infection, infectious encephalitis, food poisoning, hepatitis, meningococcal infections, plague, bioterrorism, anthrax, and many others. Both documented and suspected cases should be reported. Lists of reportable diseases vary by locale and should be reviewed by the emergency physician.

In general, although all medical personnel who are aware of the patient's diagnosis (including the attending physician, nurses, and laboratory personnel) are obligated to report cases of communicable disease, the hospital should develop a specific mechanism to ensure compliance with local laws. Reporting in the United States is generally accomplished by means of a short written form (the Confidential Morbidity Reporting card). With certain virulent diseases (eg, plague, botulism, anthrax), reporting by telephone or e-mail may be required for obvious reasons. In most states, failure to report is a misdemeanor punishable by fines or brief imprisonment. The physician who fails to notify the health department when he or she diagnoses a reportable event faces a risk of license revocation or civil suit if secondary cases or other damages result from the failure to report. The need of the health department to know of these conditions transcends the absolute confidentiality of the physician-patient relationship. The physician should discuss with the patient the need for reporting to preserve their therapeutic relationship.

Individuals other than the health department may be notified of the patient's diagnosis directly by the physician if there is an immediate risk to the patient's health. This notification may also be made by the health department. However, individuals not at immediate risk of contracting infection from the patient (this usually includes employers, fellow employees, landlords, and casual acquaintances) should not be informed of the patient's diagnosis by the physician. To do so could leave the physician at risk of civil liability for breach of confidentiality. The patient about whom such information is disclosed may bring a lawsuit alleging wrongful disclosure of private information. Also, the physician risks liability for defamation, which is defined broadly as that which tends to injure the plaintiff's reputation or to diminish the esteem or respect in which the plaintiff is held.

Animal Bites

Reporting laws in the United States usually require that the emergency physician and staff report an animal bite to the appropriate local health official within a specified number of hours after the bite has occurred. Such reporting is an obvious safeguard to protect the public from vicious animals and from the spread of animal-borne infections, especially rabies.

See Chapter 30 for management of bites.

Epilepsy

Epilepsy and other neurologic impairments, especially those resulting in episodic loss of consciousness, are reportable to the agency responsible for motor vehicle licensing in many states. The time period after a seizure during which a patient may not drive varies widely among the states. It is also important to provide appropriate discharge instructions to patients so that they will avoid potentially dangerous activities.

Dead on Arrival (DOA)

All states in the United States require that receipt of a body dead on arrival at the emergency department be reported to the coroner or medical examiner for possible investigation and for assessment of the need for postmortem examination. In such cases, the emergency physician and staff should do nothing to the corpse that would interfere with the gathering of evidence by the coroner or medical examiner. For example, the emergency department staff should not attempt to obtain blood and tissue for laboratory studies; all specimens in such cases should be obtained by the coroner or medical examiner. Similarly, the corpse should not be used to practice cardiopulmonary resuscitation, endotracheal intubation, or other procedures.

THE MEDICAL RECORD

The importance of medical records cannot be overstated. The medical record is both a legal document and a means of recording the cause of a patient's illness. It is subject to review by hospital administration, the medical staff including consulting or subsequent treating physicians, third-party payers, state and national accreditation agencies, patients, and occasionally attorneys.

Medical records serve many purposes, including the following:

- Recording information important to patient care now and in the future
- Delineating level of care for billing
- Providing medicolegal documentation to support compliance with the standard of care

When crucial facts such as vital signs or the results of specific examinations were not recorded in the patient's medical records, courts and juries may conclude that they were not done. Although the medical record is a summary of the patient's visit rather than a verbatim account of everything that transpired, it behooves the emergency physician and staff to document carefully with specific attention to pertinent negatives and positives for the particular presenting complaint. Invariably, should an unfavorable outcome or litigation occur, the physician would wish he or she had provided better documentation of care.

JCAHO requires that a medical record be established and maintained for every emergency department patient. The record must contain the following elements:

- Patient identification
- Time and means of arrival
- Appropriate vital signs
- Documentation of pertinent history and physical findings
- Emergency care given prior to patient arrival
- Diagnostic and therapeutic orders
- Clinical observations, including the results of treatment
- Reports of procedures, tests, and results
- Conclusions reached on completion of examination and treatment
- Diagnostic impression
- Final disposition
- Patient condition on discharge or transfer
- Documentation of discharge instructions

Other important items include the following:

- List of allergies
- Current medication
- Possibility of pregnancy, if germane
- Tetanus immunization history, if germane
- Name of patient's private physician
- Documentation of prescriptions given to the patient
- Patient's signature acknowledging receipt and understanding of discharge instructions
- Documentation of a medical screening examination
- Documentation of leaving against medical advice

The information contained in the patient's medical record is confidential and should not be disclosed to the police, press, or other parties without the patient's written consent. Exceptions arise when the patient's medical record is sought by a valid subpoena or court order. The emergency physician can be forced to release confidential information by a court order requiring such release.

Medical records of patients seen in the emergency department because of drug or alcohol abuse must be handled with particular attention to confidentially to avoid litigation for defamation. All descriptions of the patient's clinical condition must be stated in an objective manner. Extraneous subjective remarks betraying the physician's or nurse's attitudes about the patient have no place in the medical record.

EMERGENCY PHYSICIAN & MEDICAL STAFF INTERACTION

The practice of hospital-based emergency medicine involves constant interaction with many members of the medical staff as well as the hospital administration and governing body. The emergency physicians practice in something of a fish bowl, where his or her clinical skills are under constant prospective and retrospective scrutiny by the entire medical staff. As a result, emergency physicians and other staff must work in a highly charged professional environment.

A potential problem for the emergency department is created when a patient is instructed by a medical staff physician to go to the emergency department for treatment, and the physician then either fails to meet the patient and keep the appointment or fails to notify the emergency department staff of the patient's imminent arrival. The emergency physician must decide whether to exercise clinical control over the patient and institute diagnosis and treatment. If the patient is a nonemergency patient and wishes to be seen only by the private physician, there is no difficulty for the emergency department staff. However, when the patient's clinical problem requires immediate attention, the emergency physician may be sued for negligence if necessary emergency care is not given despite the wishes of the private physician. As a general rule, when in doubt, it is better to err on the side of treatment, assuming that the patient has consented to treatment in the first place. An effort should be made to contact the private physician under these circumstances, but administrative considerations should never interfere with appropriate patient care.

Another difficulty for the emergency physician is dealing with medical staff physicians' requests that the emergency physician write admission orders for patients admitted through the emergency department. The responsibility for writing admission orders should rest with the medical staff physician to whose service the patient has been admitted. Having the emergency physician write admission orders as a convenience for the medical staff still occurs at many hospitals, but it is a policy that should be discouraged. It blurs the transfer-of-care responsibility, exposes the emergency physician to unnecessary liability, and may delay prompt examination by the admitting physician.

Once a patient has been admitted through the emergency department, hospital bylaws usually specify how soon the patient must be seen by the admitting physician. If the patient's condition is serious, the patient should be seen as soon as possible after admission. All admitted patients should be seen within a reasonable time depending on their clinical condition. To ensure that this happens, the emergency physician should accurately convey the patient's clinical condition to the admitting physician. If uncertainty exists, the admitting physician should be asked to examine the patient.

Another area of potential conflict between the hospital staff and the emergency physician is the area of on-call specialty consultation. EMTALA requires hospitals to provide a list of on-call physicians who will respond to requests from emergency physicians for specialty consults and follow-up care. If emergency specialty consultation is requested and the on-call specialist fails to respond, the emergency physician may transfer the patient by certifying that the benefit of transfer outweighs the risks. Care must be taken to document requests for on-call consultation in a timely, accurate, and objective manner.

Problems such as these involving the emergency department and medical staff are of a delicate political nature. The emergency department and medical staff must keep lines of communication open so that these difficult areas can be discussed dispassionately. If this open communication does not exist, the inevitable result is strained personal and professional relations, which can cause a lowered standard of patient care and create a climate of confusion that engenders litigation.

EXPERT WITNESS

Emergency medicine physicians may be asked to provide expert witness testimony in medical malpractice cases. Regardless of how one feels about the current legal process for resolving malpractice suits, fair, accurate, and impartial opinions by emergency physicians familiar with the standard of care are essential. Serving as an expert witness can be an intimidating experience. If opposing counsel is unable to rebut the opposing expert's opinions, they often attempt to discredit the expert.

The American College of Emergency Physicians has issued expert witness guidelines for the specialty of emergency medicine (policy stated September 1995), as stated below:

> Expert witnesses are called on to assess the standard of care for emergency physicians in matters of alleged medical malpractice and peer review. Expert witnesses in the specialty of emergency medicine should meet the following criteria:
> * Be certified by a recognized certifying body in emergency medicine;

* Be in the active clinical practice of emergency medicine for three years immediately before the date of the incident;
* Be currently licensed in a state, territory, or area constituting legal jurisdiction of the United States as a doctor of medicine or osteopathic medicine;
* Abide by the following guidelines for an expert witness:
  — The expert witness should possess current experience and ongoing knowledge in the area in which he or she is asked to testify.
  — The expert witness should be willing to submit the transcripts of depositions and testimony to peer review.
  — Pursuant to Opinion 9.07 of the Current Opinions of the American Medical Association's Council on Ethical and Judicial Affairs, the expert witness should not testify on a contingency-fee basis or offer expert witness services on a contingency-fee basis through an agent, representative, or other third party.
  — The expert witness should not provide expert medical testimony that is false or without medical foundation. The key to this process is a thorough review of available and appropriate medical records and literature concerning the case being examined. The expert's opinion after this process is completed should reflect the state of medical knowledge at the time of the incident.
  — The expert witness should review the medical facts in a thorough, fair, and impartial manner and should not exclude any relevant information to create a view favoring the plaintiff or the defendant.
  — Expert witnesses are chosen on the basis of their experience in the area in which they are providing testimony and not solely on the basis of offices or positions held in medical specialty societies, unless such positions are material to the witness' expertise. Emergency physicians should not engage in advertising or solicit employment as expert witness where such advertising or solicitation contains representations about the physician's qualifications, experience, or background that are false or deceptive.

NATIONAL PRACTITIONER DATA BANK

The Health Care Quality Improvement Act (HCQIA) was passed by Congress in 1986 and called for the establishment of the National Practitioner Data Bank for Advice Information on Physicians and Other Health

Care Providers (NPDB). Its purpose is to collect data on medical malpractice payments.

All medical malpractice payments must be reported to the NPDP. What effect HCQIA and the NPDB will have on health care and the availability of insurance is yet to be determined.

HARVESTING OF ORGANS FOR TRANSPLANTATION

Emergency physicians can be expected to be confronted with the issue of organ or tissue donation. Hospitals should have specific policies in place that address the issue, and emergency staff should be familiar with them. Most states have statutes that require notification of the organ donation association in the event of any death that meets criteria for possible organ or tissue donation.

American College of Emergency Physicians Policy Statement: *Expert Witness Guidelines for the Specialty of Emergency Medicine.* American College of Emergency Physicians, 1995.

Bitterman RA: Medicolegal and risk management. In: Marx JA et al., eds. *Rosen's Emergency Medicine Concepts and Clinical Practice,* 5th ed. Mosby, 2002.

Freedman DL: National Practitioner Data Bank. ED Legal Letter 1999;10(8).

Henry GL, Sullivan DJ: *Emergency Medicine Risk Management,* 2nd ed. American College of Emergency Physicians, 1997.

Huber JR: Foresight American College of Emergency Physicians, *EMTALA—New Developments in the Regulatory Guidelines and an Update of Recent Court Opinions.* Issue 48, June 2000.

Keeton WP: *Prosser and Keeton on Torts,* 5th ed. West, 1999.

LeBlang TR, Basanta WE, Kane RJ: *The Law of Medical Practice in Illinois,* 2nd ed. Lawyers Cooperative Publishing, 1997.

Emergency Procedures

6

William Randall Partin, MD[1]

General Instructions for Skin Preparation & Sterile Technique

Upper Extremity Venipuncture

Emergency Antecubital Fossa Venous Cutdown

Peripheral Venous Catheterization with a Catheter-Clad Needle

Peripheral Venous Catheterization with a Scalp Vein (Butterfly) Needle

External Jugular Vein Catheterization

Internal Jugular Vein Catheterization

Subclavian Vein Catheterization

Femoral Vein Phlebotomy or Catheterization

Saphenous Vein Cutdown

Intraosseous Infusion

Radial Artery Puncture (For Blood Gas & pH Analysis)

Direct Laryngoscopy, Orotracheal Intubation, & Nasotracheal Intubation

Nasogastric Intubation (For Gastric Evacuation or Lavage)

Insertion of Sengstaken-Blakemore or Minnesota Tube

Cricothyrotomy

Transtracheal Jet Ventilation

Thoracentesis

Tube Thoracostomy (Insertion of a Chest Tube)

Emergency Thoracotomy

Pericardiocentesis

Focused Assessment with Sonography for Trauma

Abdominal Paracentesis

Peritoneal Catheter Insertion & Peritoneal Lavage

Insertion of Indwelling (Foley) Urinary Catheter

Percutaneous Suprapubic Cystostomy

Lumbar Puncture

Anterior & Posterior Nasal Packing for Control of Epistaxis

Arthrocentesis (Knee, Shoulder, Elbow, Ankle, Wrist, Hand, & Foot Joints)

Incision & Drainage of Superficial Abscess

Transcutaneous Cardiac Pacing

Specialized Techniques Covered in Other Chapters of This Text:

Cardiopulmonary Resuscitation (Chapter 7)

Splinting Techniques (Chapter 28)

Ophthalmologic Techniques (Chapter 31)

Dorsal Slit of the Foreskin (Chapter 37)

Wound Care & Local Anesthesia (Chapter 30)

GENERAL INSTRUCTIONS FOR SKIN PREPARATION & STERILE TECHNIQUE

Skin Preparation

There are 2 types of skin preparation: skin cleansing and skin sterilization.

A. Skin Cleansing

Cleansing of the skin is sufficient for routine injections (subcutaneous, intramuscular, intravenous) and for simple venipuncture but not for venipuncture per-formed to draw blood for culture or to permit insertion of an indwelling device.

Skin cleansing is generally performed by swabbing the skin for a few seconds with a swab saturated with alcohol (70%) or organic iodine (eg, povidone-iodine or equivalent). To reduce the pain of venipuncture, the disinfectant should be allowed to dry on the skin before the skin is punctured. *Note:* This procedure merely cleans the skin; it does not sterilize it.

B. Skin Sterilization

Skin sterilization should be performed before all procedures that involve puncturing or cutting the skin, with

---

[1]This chapter is a revision of the chapter by David Knighton, MD, FACS, Richard M. Locksley, MD, & John Mills, MD, from the 4th edition.

the exception of routine venipuncture and simple injections. This procedure eliminates superficial skin bacterial, leaving only a few organisms deep in hair follicles or sweat glands. Skin sterilization may be omitted if the delay involved would jeopardize the patients' life (eg, thoracostomy for tension pneumothorax).

A variety of techniques can be used to achieve skin sterilization:

1. Scrub the skin vigorously with copious amounts of 70% alcohol for 2 minutes. Or,

2. Using a sterile 10- × 10-cm (4- × 4-in) gauze pad, apply 2% iodine tincture to the area and allow the iodine to dry. Then remove it, using 70% alcohol on a sterile pad, because iodine may cause skin burns. Or,

3. Apply an organic iodine disinfectant (eg, povidone-iodine or poloxamer-iodine) twice, allowing each application to dry. These particular disinfectants need not be removed before the procedure is started.

The following guidelines should be observed in all cases:

- Sterilize a much larger area of skin than is required for the procedure.
- Apply the disinfectant starting at the site of the procedure and extending outward in concentrically larger circles.
- Use sterile gloves to apply the disinfectant.

Sterile Technique

It is virtually impossible to achieve sterile technique at the bedside in the emergency department comparable to that obtainable in an operating room; however, following the guidelines outlined below decreases the risk of infection. Good lighting is helpful for maintaining sterile technique and is essential for performing procedures successfully.

1. Wash hands thoroughly, preferably with antiseptic soap, before performing any procedure.

2. Have all necessary equipment assembled and opened at the bedside, so that once sterile gloves have been donned, only sterile instruments and equipment will be touched. Alternatively, an assistant can open packaged sterile supplies.

3. Don sterile gloves.

4. Sterilize the skin, as described above.

5. Enlarge the sterile field by surrounding the sterile skin with sterile drapes made of cloth or paper. These may come with a window in them that is used to isolate the area of sterile skin selected for the procedure.

6. Make sure that catheters, needles, stopcocks, and the like cannot roll off the drape onto the floor, perhaps at a critical moment.

7. When performing complicated procedures that require stricter sterile conditions (eg, insertion of a catheter for total parenteral nutrition), wear a surgical cap, mask, and gown in addition to the sterile gloves.

UPPER EXTREMITY VENIPUNCTURE

Indications

Venipuncture is performed to obtain a sample of venous blood for laboratory testing.

Contraindications

Contraindications to venipuncture are as follows:

- Cellulitis over the proposed site.
- Phlebitis.
- Venous obstruction.
- Lymphangitis of the extremity.
- Administration of intravenous fluid distal to the proposed site.

Personnel Required

One person can perform venipuncture unaided.

Equipment & Supplies Required

- Materials for skin cleansing (or skin sterilization, if blood culture is to be performed).
- Syringe of adequate size (10–50 mL) for the amount of blood needed, or Vacutainer tubes and appropriate Vacutainer syringe hub (Vacutainer equipment consists of a needle with a point at each end, evacuated glass tubes with rubber stoppers, and a plastic barrel. Blood is forced into the evacuated tube when the needle connects the tube with the vein).
- Needle (21-gauge) for the syringe, or a Vacutainer needle with an automatic valve or rubber cuff to stop blood flow while tubes are being changed. If a large amount of blood is to be drawn, it is advisable to use an 18-gauge needle. Use smaller-gauge needles or scalp vein needles for infants and children.
- Tourniquet.

- Receptacle tubes for blood for the desired laboratory tests.
- Gauze squares, 5 × 5 cm (2 × 2 in).
- Adhesive dressing.

Positioning of the Patient

The upper extremity is the site most commonly used to draw venous blood. The patient should be in a comfortable position, with the upper extremity resting on a solid object. If the patient is in bed, the supine position is best, with the arm resting on the mattress close to the patient's side. The ambulatory patient should be sitting with the arm on a table or support at a comfortable height for the operator.

Procedure

1. Assemble all necessary equipment, and position as described above.
2. Apply the tourniquet above the antecubital fossa in a manner that will allow quick removal with one hand. The tourniquet should be tight enough to occlude venous return but not so tight as to cause arterial obstruction or patient discomfort. It should be removed before the extremity turns purple.
3. Locate an appropriate vein. Have the patient open and close the fist of the selected arm to help pump blood from the muscle compartment of the arm into the superficial venous circulation.
   a. *Antecubital veins.* The superficial basilic and cephalic veins course just under the skin on the volar side of the forearm. They run along the medial and lateral edge of the antecubital fossa at the elbow crease. In slender or muscular people, these veins often stand out and are easy to enter. If one of these veins is accessible, use it. In obese people, those who have had multiple venipunctures, and intravenous drug abusers, finding a patent antecubital vein (or any other vein) may be difficult.
      Palpate the antecubital fossa with the tip of the index finger, and feel for the buoyant resilience of a distended vein. Be careful to differentiate the firm cord of a thrombosed vein from the resiliency of a patent vessel. When the veins are not visible, they must be located by feel. Even a small vein deep in the subcutaneous tissue may be detected on the basis of its resilient feel.
   b. *Arm veins.* If a patient's antecubital vein cannot be found, examine the forearm on both the volar and the dorsal surfaces. Look for the faint bluish color of a vein under the skin, or better yet, feel for a vein with the tip of the index finger.
   c. *Hand veins.* If no vein is found on the forearm, proceed to the dorsal surface of the hand, and use one of the superficial veins on the hand. These veins are small, collapse easily, and are usually inadequate for drawing a large amount of blood. If large amounts of blood are needed, it is often better to go to another anatomic site such as the femoral vein than to persist in trying to draw large quantities of blood from a small hand vein. By the time an adequate amount has been obtained, it usually clots in the syringe, and another venipuncture then becomes necessary.
      Do not give up after one examination of the arm. Carefully palpate the arm 2 or 3 times if necessary. A vein suitable for venipuncture may be obscured (eg, by hair) and may therefore be missed on initial examination. Occasionally, slapping repeatedly over the vein with the pads of the first and second fingers will help to distend a faint vein, or the patient can dangle the arm over the side of the bed to achieve the same result. Do not thrust blindly at a bluish mark on the patient's arm without first palpating the area to confirm that a patent vein is underneath.
4. Prepare the skin. Skin cleansing is adequate unless blood is being obtained for culture, in which case the skin must be sterilized (see Skin Preparation, above).
5. Grasp the syringe or Vacutainer in the dominant hand while palpating the vein with the index finger of the other hand. Exert traction on the vein by pulling distally (toward the operator) on the skin next to the puncture site. Align the needle with the course of the vein, and make sure that the bevel is facing up. With a quick but smooth motion, push the needle through the skin at an angle of about 10–20 degrees (Figure 6–1). Then carefully advance the needle into the lumen of the vein with a smooth motion.
6. When the vein has been properly penetrated, blood will flow back into the needle when the plunger is pulled away from the needle or when the Vacutainer tube is pushed onto the needle.
7. If venous blood is not obtained on the first attempt, reassess the course of the vein. Try palpating the vein proximal to the needle site. Withdraw the needle to just below the skin, and attempt a second venipuncture.
8. Once the needle is in the lumen of the vein, withdraw the required amount of blood with a steady,

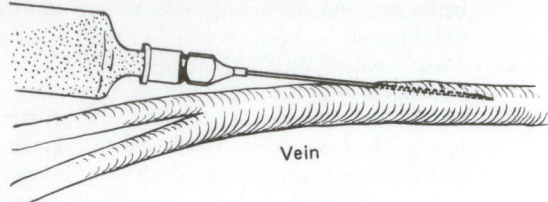

Figure 6–1. Technique of percutaneous venipuncture. The needle should be inserted into the lumen of the vein at an angle of about 10–20 degrees, and the bevel should be facing up. (Reproduced, with permission, from Krupp MA et al: *Physician's Handbook,* 21st ed. Lange, 1985.)

even pull on the plunger of the syringe. If too much force is applied and blood flow in the vein is less than the amount being drawn into the syringe, the vein will collapse, occluding the lumen of the needle. If this occurs, stop and allow the vein to fill, and then resume at a slower pace. If a

large volume of blood is required, it may be necessary to select another, larger vein.

If a Vacutainer system is being used, simply fill all of the tubes required.

9. Draw enough blood to give accurate laboratory test results; clotted or hemolyzed specimens will give misleading information.

10. When enough blood has been obtained, remove the tourniquet, and then withdraw the needle quickly and smoothly. Have the patient immediately apply firm direct pressure on a 5- × 5-cm (2- × 2-in) piece of gauze over the site for 3–5 minutes. If the site is antecubital, flex the arm to stop the bleeding. Elevating the arm will speed hemostasis.

11. Quickly fill the blood receptacle tubes with the appropriate amount of blood, and mix each tube thoroughly if anticoagulation or preservative is present in the tube. Label the tubes with the patient's name, date of birth, and date of sample, and place any specimens on ice as required.

12. It is often helpful to put an adhesive dressing on the venipuncture site to absorb any blood that might ooze out.

EMERGENCY ANTECUBITAL FOSSA VENOUS CUTDOWN

Antecubital fossa cutdown provides a secure large-bore conduit for fluid resuscitation and central venous pressure measurement without the risks associated with placement of a subclavian or internal jugular vein catheter.

Indications

Emergency antecubital fossa cutdown is performed to gain immediate large-bore access to central veins for resuscitation and venous pressure measurements.

Contraindications

Contraindications to emergency antecubital fossa cutdown are as follows:

- Previous antecubital fossa cutdown at the proposed insertion site (use the other arm or another site).
- Trauma to the extremity proximal to the proposed cutdown site.
- Known or suspected major vascular injury to the axillary or subclavian arterial or venous system on the side of the proposed cutdown.

Personnel Required

The operator may require an assistant to provide exposure and assist in insertion of the catheter.

Equipment & Supplies Required

A. Materials

- Materials for skin sterilization.
- Lidocaine, 1%, with 10-mL syringe and 25-gauge needle.
- Tourniquet.
- Topical antibacterial ointment.
- Expanded gauze roll and tape.
- Padded armboard that fits under the mattress of the patient's gurney and extends (parallel to the floor) about 15 cm (6 in) beyond the patient's outstretched arm.
- Tape to secure the patient's arm to the armboard.
- Intravenous fluid in a container with a Y-type blood infusion set and an in-line blood pump. The equipment should be flushed and fully assembled, ready for use.

B. Prepackaged Sterile Cutdown Trays

Prepackaged sterile cutdown trays are commercially available. The following items are required:

- Drapes.
- Gauze sponges (10 × 10 cm [4 × 4 in]).
- Silk ligatures (size 3-0) (2).
- Nylon or polypropylene skin suture (size 4-0) on a cutting needle.
- Needle holder.
- No. 15 and No. 11 scalpel blades, both mounted.
- Curved Kelly clamps (3).
- Mosquito clamps (2) (useful for small patients).
- Tissue dissection scissors and straight suture scissors.
- Self-retaining retractor or 2 right-angle retractors.
- Pediatric feeding tubes, sizes 5F and 10F (1 each). (Use the largest one that fits the vein.)
- Toothed and smooth forceps.
- Plastic-coated absorbent pad to place beneath the patient's arm.

Positioning of the Patient

The patient should be supine, with the arm selected for cutdown insertion extended on an armboard that has been wrapped in an absorbent pad. Tape the arm in place at the wrist.

Anatomy Review

The deep basilic vein is found medial to the brachial artery beneath the superficial fascia. Accurate identification of the basilic vein is crucial. It is usually thin-walled when compared to the brachial artery, and it has a bluish tinge. The median nerve is fibrous and relatively avascular. However, the vein may be thick-walled in an elderly person or an intravenous drug abuser, or the artery may carry desaturated blood, which may also give it a bluish tinge.

Procedure

1. Apply the tourniquet proximal to the antecubital fossa.
2. Sterilize a wide area of skin around the antecubital fossa.
3. Drape the arm.
4. Measure the catheter (pediatric feeding tube), and cut it to the required length as follows: Place the hub end of the feeding tube at the antecubital fossa of the patient's outstretched arm, and extend the catheter to the suprasternal notch. This length ensures that the catheter will be long enough to reach the central venous system (superior vena cava) without entering the right ventricle of the heart (which can cause serious ventricular arrhythmias). Cut the catheter at an angle, and trim off the sharp tip to avoid puncturing the vein distal to the insertion site.

5. Using the 1% lidocaine with the 10-mL syringe and 25-gauge needle, anesthetize the antecubital fossa over the medial aspect of the forearm at the level of the elbow crease, taking care not to puncture a superficial basilic vein. Omit this step if the patient is comatose.

6. With the No. 15 scalpel blade, make a 2.5- to 4-cm (1- to 1½-in) traverse incision on the median half of the antecubital fossa at the elbow crease. The incision should be at a right angle to the long axis of the arm and should extend down to the subcutaneous tissue. It may be helpful to palpate the brachial artery as a landmark, because the basilic vein lies medial to it. Be careful not to lacerate any large superficial veins that lie just under the skin.

7. If the patient has a large superficial basilic vein, proceed with isolation and cannulation, as described in steps 8–11. If no superficial vein is present, continue to dissect deep to isolate the basilic vein (step 8). Be sure to differentiate the vein from the brachial artery and the median nerve. (See Anatomy Review, above.)

8. Using a curved Kelly clamp with the points aimed downward, dissect the subcutaneous tissue parallel to the long axis of the arm to isolate the basilic vein. Dissect the tissue on either side and then on top of the vein. Pass the clamp under the vein and dissect the tissue there. This maneuver should separate the vein from the surrounding structures and connective tissues. Small veins may be encountered in the subcutaneous tissue. Do not attempt to cannulate these veins. They have many valves and will not allow central passage of the catheter. Use the retractors to maintain exposure of the vein.

9. Leave the Kelly clamp in the open position under the vein for support. Using the smooth forceps as a clamp, pass the 2 silk ties under the vein, one proximal and one distal to the intended venotomy site. Ligate or loosely tie the distal portion of the vein while exerting traction on the distal silk tie. Perform a venotomy with the No. 11 scalpel blade (Figure 6–2): Hold the scalpel parallel to the long axis of the vein with the blade in a hori-

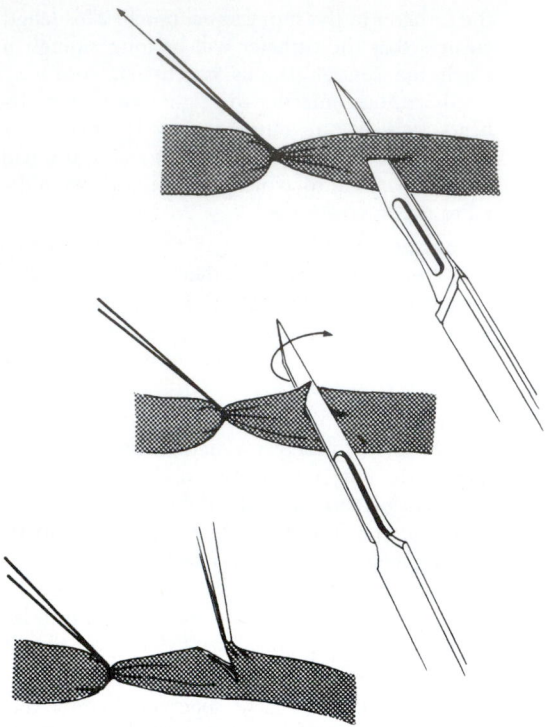

Figure 6–2. Venotomy technique. Exerting distal traction on the distal vein ligature, insert a No. 11 scalpel blade through the vein, and cut laterally. Open the venotomy incision with a mosquito clamp. (Reproduced, with permission, from Dunphy JE, Way LW [editors]: *Current Surgical Diagnosis & Treatment,* 5th ed. Lange, 1981.)

zontal position, and pass it through the midportion of the superficial (or anterior) wall of the vein. Then turn the cutting edge of the blade upward, and open the top of the vein. Be careful not to transect the vein or puncture its outer wall.

10. Insert a closed mosquito clamp into the venotomy, and gently spread the clamp to dilate the vein.

11. With the bevel up, gently insert the catheter into the vein, and advance it until the hub reaches the incision. Remove the mosquito clamp.

12. Occasionally, the catheter fails to traverse the axilla and pass into the intrathoracic venous system. In this situation, abduct the arm, and slowly advance the catheter. This maneuver straightens the course of the vein and usually facilitates passage. If the catheter meets an obstruction at a valve, move the catheter gently backward and forward while rotating it, or attempt to open the valve by infusing fluid through the catheter. If the catheter does not pass easily into the central venous system, stop. Do not push so vigorously that the vein is perforated.

   The most common problem is that the catheter has not entered the basilic vein. Withdraw the catheter, and tie off the proximal portion of the vein. Continue dissection, looking for the basilic vein. Occasionally, a basilic system vein of adequate diameter is not present, in which case an alternative method of central venous access must be found.

13. Allow blood to fill the catheter, and then remove the tourniquet. Insert the intravenous tubing in the catheter, and start the intravenous fluid drip. Ligate the distal portion of the vein with the distal silk tie, and using the same tie, secure the catheter to the ligated distal vein. Secure the catheter in the vein with a strong tie proximal to the venotomy site. Make sure that the ligatures are not so tight that they occlude the catheter (Figure 6–3).

14. Close the skin with a simple running skin stitch using the nylon or polypropylene skin suture.

15. Secure the catheter to the skin with a stitch, and tape all connections.

16. Dress the incision with the antibacterial ointment and a 10- × 10-cm (4- × 4-in) gauze sponge, and wrap the incision site with an expanded gauze roll.

17. Obtain a chest x-ray immediately to check the position of the catheter.

PERIPHERAL VENOUS CATHETERIZATION WITH A CATHETER-CLAD NEEDLE

Catheter-clad needles (eg, Angiocath) are generally preferred over needle-clad catheters (eg, Intracath) for peripheral intravenous access because they provide the largest-diameter catheter lumen possible for a given size of venipuncture. Their flexibility gives them an advantage over rigid needles for long-term use.

Indications

Peripheral venous catheterization with a catheter-clad needle is performed to gain peripheral venous access.

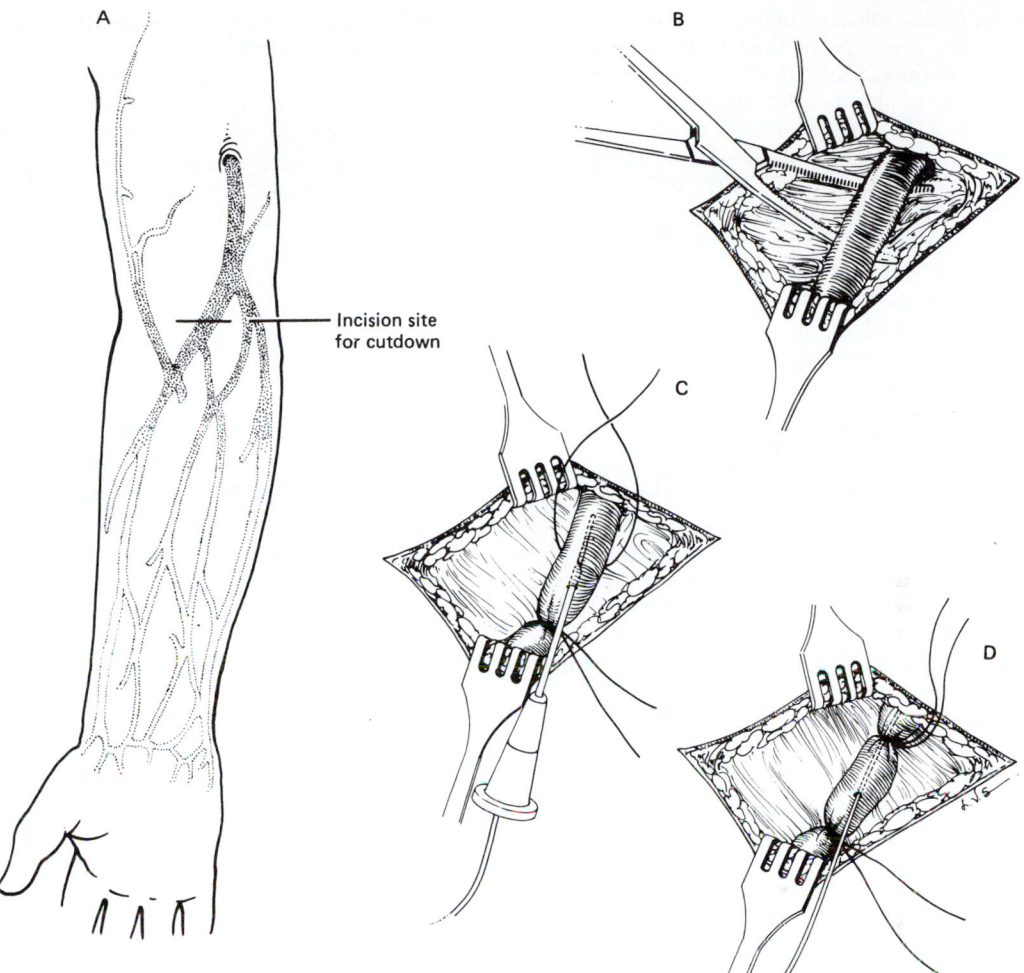

Incision site
for cutdown

Figure 6–3. Technique of cutdown insertion. After exposing the vein and making the venotomy incisions (see Figure 6–2), elevate and stabilize the vein with a straight clamp while inserting the tip of the catheter in the venotomy incision. As soon as the tip of the catheter is within the lumen of the vein, remove the clamp, slide the catheter the required distance up the vein, and tie the vein proximally and distally.

Contraindications

Contraindications to peripheral venous catheterization with a catheter-clad needle are as follows:

- Phlebitis of the extremity.
- Cellulitis over the projected site of insertion.
- Potential or existing lymphedema or venous occlusive edema of the extremity.
- Traumatic injury proximal to insertion site (eg, fracture).

Personnel Required

One person can insert a catheter-clad needle unaided.

Equipment & Supplies Required

- Materials for skin sterilization.
- Tourniquet.
- Precut tape to secure the catheter in place.
- Plastic-coated absorbent pad to place under the patient's arm.

- Catheter-clad needle (eg, Angiocath) of sufficient size for the rate and type of fluid to be infused, but smaller than the cannulated vein. For administration of electrolyte or glucose solutions at rates of less than 200 mL/h, a 20-gauge catheter is usually sufficient. For infusion of blood or colloid solutions or rapid infusion of electrolyte solutions (200-1000 mL/h), an 18-gauge catheter is mandatory and a 16–gauge is preferred. In patients with multiple trauma, who may require large volumes of blood and electrolyte solutions, a 14-gauge catheter is preferable.
- Container of fluid for intravenous administration, with proper connecting tubing. The equipment should be flushed and fully assembled ready for use.

Positioning of the Patient

Place peripheral intravenous catheters in the upper extremity if possible. Occasionally, a lower extremity intravenous catheter is necessary when all veins in the upper extremity are inaccessible and insertion of a central venous catheter is not practical. Intravenous catheters in the lower extremity are associated with a much higher incidence of infection and thrombosis than are those inserted in the upper extremity.

The patient should be in a comfortable supine or sitting position, with the extremity to be used resting on a firm surface.

Procedure

1. Connect the container of fluid with the tubing, fill the connecting tubing with intravenous fluid, and make sure that all air is flushed from the tubing.

2. Apply the tourniquet above the antecubital fossa, and secure it so that it can be quickly removed with one hand.

3. Have the patient open and close the fist to help distend the superficial veins with blood. If veins are difficult to identify, having the patient hang the arm below the level of the heart or wrapping the arm in a warm moist towel may be helpful.

4. Select an appropriate vein. The site at which 2 veins join is an excellent choice, because the vein is immobilized best in such a location. Possible sites include the radial aspect of the forearm most proximal to the wrist ("intern's vein"), the volar aspect of the forearm distal to the antecubital fossa on the ulnar side, and the dorsum of the hand. In slender people, these veins usually distend without difficulty; however, some individuals have deeply buried veins that can be found only by careful palpation. Remember that a vein does not have to be visualized in order to be successfully catheterized. Gently tapping over the vein may help to distend it and make identification and catheterization easier. If the vein lies deep in the subcutaneous tissue, make a mental picture of its course and branches by means of systematic palpation up and down the vein.

5. Inspect the catheter to make sure that it slides easily off the needle and that both the catheter and the needle are smooth.

6. Place the plastic-coated drape under the arm selected for insertion.

7. Sterilize the skin around the insertion site.

8. Either grasp the needle directly with the dominant hand or place a syringe on the needle and grasp the syringe. Insert the needle through the skin at an angle of about 10–20 degrees, either on top of or next to the vein (see Figure 6–1).

9. Pull the skin taut distal to the venipuncture site, and insert the needle and catheter into the vein. When the lumen of the vein is entered, blood flows back or can be withdrawn into the syringe.

10. Make sure that both the needle and the catheter are in the lumen of the vein. Blood may flow back when only the needle is in the vein and the catheter tip is against the wall of the vessel and has not actually entered the vessel lumen. In this position, the catheter cannot be advanced over the needle into the vein. To avoid this complication, advance the needle and catheter into the vein about 4–6 mm (⅛–¼ in) after blood initially returns. Check to be sure that blood continues to return when the needle and catheter are in this position.

11. Slide the catheter off the needle (Figure 6–4). Hold the needle steady by its hub in one hand at an angle of 10–20 degrees to the vein while gripping the hub of the catheter with the other hand, and gently push the catheter forward off the needle. Advance the catheter up to its hub while keeping the needle firmly in place. With practice, advancing the catheter and withdrawing the needle can be accomplished in one smooth motion. Be sure not to pull out both the catheter and needle at the same time. To avoid uncontrolled blood loss from the open catheter, occlude the vein proximal to the end of the catheter by applying direct pressure before pulling the needle out of the catheter.

12. *Note:* Occasionally, the catheter will encounter a valve in the vein that prevents complete advancement of the catheter. If this occurs, hold the catheter hub in place, remove the tourniquet, and connect the intravenous tubing to the catheter. Running intravenous fluid into the vein often opens the valve and allows complete insertion of the catheter.

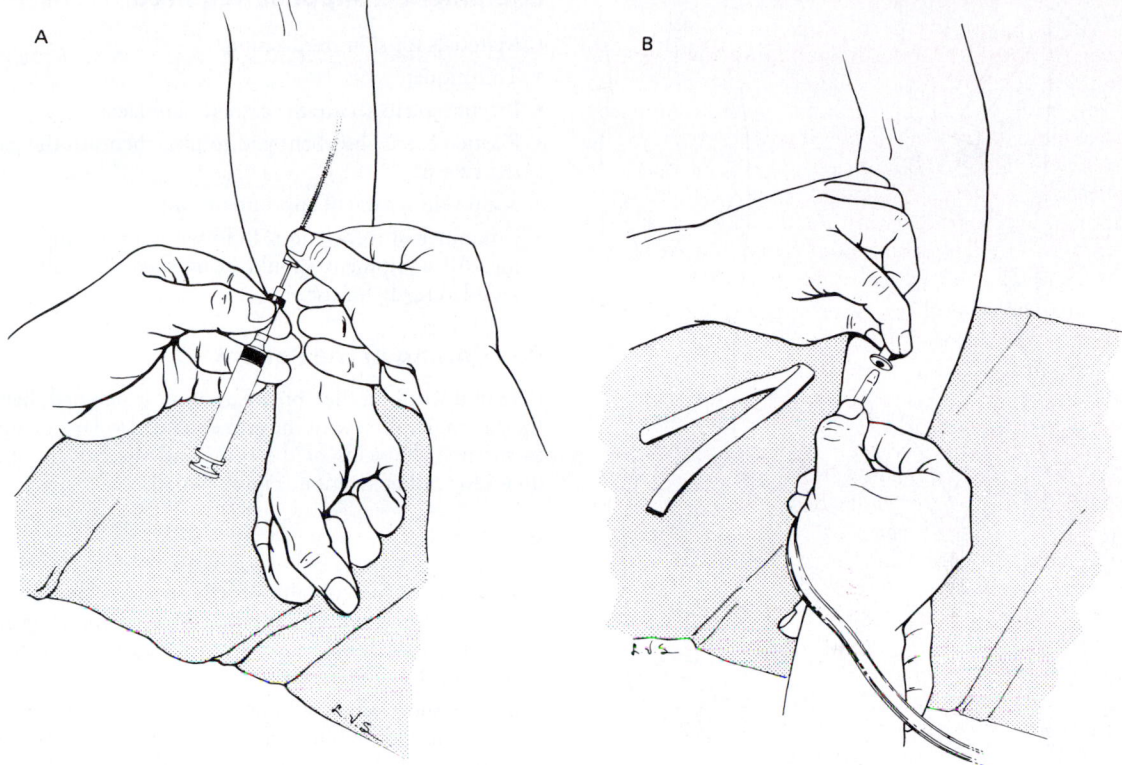

Figure 6–4. **A:** Technique of removing the needle from the catheter-clad needle. **B:** Connecting the intravenous tubing.

13. Remove the tourniquet.

14. Attach the intravenous tubing to the catheter, and check the flow. A properly located catheter should allow rapid influx of fluid. If flow is slow or there is no flow at all, withdraw the catheter a few millimeters, and watch for change in the rate of flow. Occasionally, a branch vein or valve obstructs flow, and moving the catheter will be all that is required to achieve good flow.

15. Occasionally, the catheter is pushed through the opposite wall of the vein, causing swelling and pain at the insertion site as the intravenous fluid dissects the subcutaneous tissues. In this case, withdraw the catheter and needle completely, and try a second venipuncture in another vein or in the same vein proximal to the first insertion site. (Allow enough time for the first venipuncture to clot, or leave the catheter in place to occlude the venipuncture site until the more proximal catheter is inserted, and then withdraw the unused catheter.)

16. Secure the catheter in place with tape as shown in Figure 6–5. Tape all connections. Do not apply tape completely around the arm; it can act as a tourniquet and lead to distal edema. It is helpful to write the catheter gauge and date of insertion on the tape.

PERIPHERAL VENOUS CATHETERIZATION WITH A SCALP VEIN (BUTTERFLY) NEEDLE

Scalp vein needles are useful for short-term intravenous infusions in adults and for both long- and short-term use in children. They are also useful for phlebotomy in uncooperative patients, especially children, because the flexible connecting tubing prevents dislodgment of the needle when the patient moves.

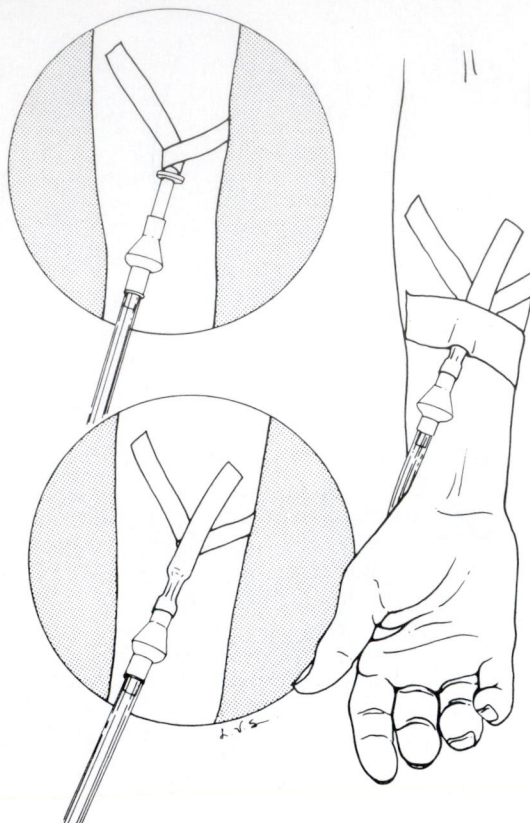

Figure 6–5. Technique of securing an intravenous catheter to the skin with tape after insertion.

Indications

Indications for peripheral venous catheterization with a scalp vein needle are as follows:

- Need to gain peripheral venous access.
- Need to perform phlebotomy in an uncooperative patient (the needle might otherwise become dislodged from the vein).

Contraindications

Contraindications to the use of scalp vein needles for peripheral venous catheterization are the same as those for catheter-clad needles.

Personnel Required

One person can perform venous catheterization with a scalp vein needle unaided if the patient is cooperative.

Equipment & Supplies Required

- Materials for skin sterilization.
- Tourniquet.
- Precut tape to secure the catheter in place.
- Plastic-coated absorbent pad to place beneath the patient's arm.
- Scalp vein needle of appropriate size.
- Container of intravenous fluid with connecting tubing. All equipment should be flushed and fully assembled ready for use.

Positioning of the Patient

If venipuncture in the upper extremity is planned, have the patient supine, with the arm extended volar side up. In infants, the veins of the scalp and the fist are also useful for catheterization (Figure 6–6A).

Procedure

1. Connect the container of intravenous fluid with the tubing, and fill the connecting tubing with intravenous fluid. Make sure that all air is flushed from the tubing.

2. The short tubing connected to the scalp vein needle should be filled with fluid before the infusion begins. This can be accomplished either by letting the blood flow back into the tubing from the vein or by filling the tubing with infusion fluid before inserting the needle. Letting blood fill the tubing can lead to clotting if the flow of intravenous fluid is not established quickly.

3. Place the plastic-coated absorbent pad under the site chosen for catheterization.

4. If an extremity is to be catheterized, apply the tourniquet above the site.

5. Sterilize the skin around the insertion site.

6. Keeping the bevel of the needle facing up, grasp the plastic wings attached to the needle between the thumb and index finger of the dominant hand, and insert the needle into the vein at a 30-degree angle (Figure 6–6B).

7. Once the needle has entered the vein (blood appears in the tubing), decrease the angle between the needle and the vein to 10–20 degrees. Then carefully thread the needle into the lumen of the vein until the entire needle is in the vein. Failure to insert the needle completely makes securing it more difficult.

8. Secure the needle to the arm with tape, as shown in Figure 6–7, and tape all connections.

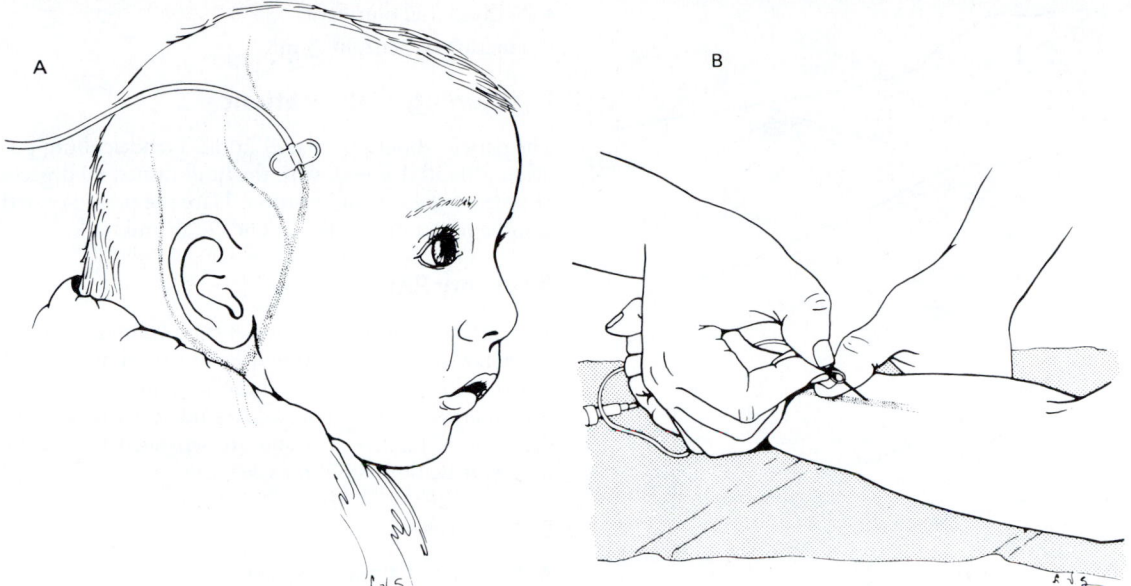

Figure 6–6. **A:** Scalp vein needle in an infant. **B:** Technique of inserting a butterfly needle. With the bevel of the needle facing up, oppose the 2 plastic "wings," and grip them between the thumb and forefinger while performing venipuncture.

EXTERNAL JUGULAR VEIN CATHETERIZATION

Indications

External jugular vein catheterization is performed to gain peripheral or central venous access when sites other than the external jugular vein (eg, internal jugular or subclavian vein) are inaccessible or if catheterization of those sites is contraindicated (eg, coagulopathy).

Contraindications

Contraindications to external jugular vein catheterization are as follows:

- Agitated, uncooperative patient (relative contraindication).
- Cellulitis at the insertion site.
- Previous neck surgery (the position of the vein may be distorted, or it may have been ligated or removed).

Personnel Required

One person can perform simple external jugular vein catheterization unaided, although an assistant is help-ful. Insertion of a central venous catheter through the external jugular vein by means of a J wire requires an assistant.

Equipment & Supplies Required

A. PERIPHERAL VENOUS ACCESS

- Materials for skin sterilization.
- Catheter-clad needle (eg, Angiocath), 16- to 18-gauge.
- Container of intravenous solution and connecting tubing.
- Precut tape for securing the catheter.
- Plastic-coated absorbent pad to place under the patient's head and neck.
- Tincture of benzoin, 5 mL.

B. CENTRAL VENOUS ACCESS

- Materials for skin sterilization.
- Materials for sterile technique (cap, mask, gloves, and gown).

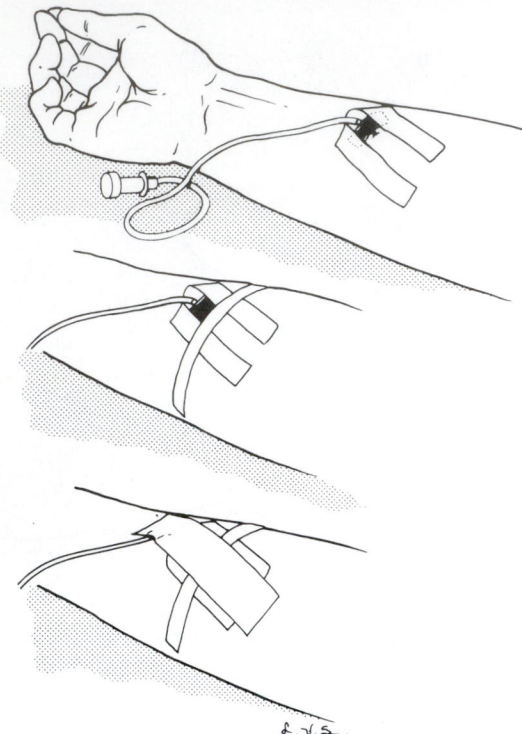

Figure 6–7. Technique of securing a butterfly needle to the skin with tape after insertion.

- Lidocaine, 1%, with 10-mL syringe and 25-gauge needle.
- Sterile medicine cup with normal saline for flushing intravenous catheters and tubing.
- Most adults will need a 16- to 18-gauge catheter-clad needle. Make sure the needles and catheters are of the proper size and construction to accept and slip over the J wire.
- J wire (flexible angiography wire) 35.5 cm (14 in) long, about 0.089 cm (½ in) in diameter, and with a curvature that has a radius of about 3 mm (⅛ in).
- Silk skin suture (size 3-0) on a cutting needle.
- Needle holder.
- Straight scissors.
- Container of intravenous fluid and connecting tubing. All equipment must be flushed and fully assembled ready for use.
- Gauze squares, 10 × 10 cm (4 × 4 in).
- Plastic-coated absorbent pad to place under the patient's head and neck.
- Sterile drapes.

- Antibacterial ointment.
- Tincture of benzoin, 5 mL.

Positioning of the Patient

The patient should be placed in the Trendelenburg position (20–30 degrees), with the head turned 90 degrees away from the side of insertion. Place the plastic-coated absorbent pad under the patient's head and neck.

Anatomy Review

The external jugular vein courses from behind the angle of the jaw across to the sternocleidomastoid muscle and superficial to it to join the subclavian vein (Figure 6–8). The internal jugular vein and carotid artery lie deep to the external jugular vein and are separated from it by the sternocleidomastoid muscle.

Procedure

A. PERIPHERAL VENOUS ACCESS

1. Assemble all necessary equipment, including the container of intravenous fluid and tubing, and make sure the tubing has been flushed to remove all air.
2. Position the patient.
3. Sterilize the skin around the area of insertion from the clavicle to the ear.

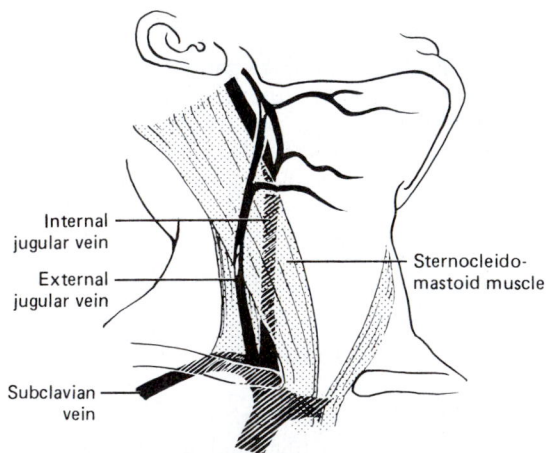

Figure 6–8. Anatomic relationships of the external jugular vein. The external jugular vein originates at the level of the angle of the mandible in the parotid gland, and it courses caudally and anteriorly across the sternocleidomastoid muscle. It enters the subclavian vein near the subclavian triangle.

4. Have the patient take a deep breath and forcibly exhale against a closed glottis (Valsalva maneuver) to increase intrathoracic pressure and distend the external jugular vein with blood. It is sometimes helpful to have the patient put a thumb in his or her mouth and blow against it. If the patient is unable to cooperate, the vein may be distended by obstructing its outflow with a finger placed on the neck above the clavicle.

5. Make a mental note of the position and size of the vein.

6. Have the patient resume normal breathing as soon as the size and position of the vein have been determined.

7. Insert the catheter-clad needle into the vein halfway between the angle of the jaw and the clavicle. While the patient performs the Valsalva maneuver, apply traction cephalad on the vein, and insert the catheter-clad needle into the vein lumen. Withdraw the needle, leaving the catheter in place. (See above for technique of catheterization using a catheter-clad needle.)

8. Connect the intravenous tubing to the catheter, and start the intravenous infusion. To avoid air embolism, make sure either that intrathoracic pressure is elevated (eg, by the Valsalva maneuver) or that the hub of the needle is occluded with a thumb or finger.

9. Tape the tubing in place. When taping an intravenous line to the neck, it is helpful to use tincture of benzoin on both the patient's skin and the tubing. Tape the tubing up the side of the patient's neck and face superior to the ear, securing the line in several places with tape (Figure 6–9). Tape all connections.

10. Short catheters inserted in the external jugular vein are difficult to secure because of the constant motion of the patient's neck. The catheter may become dislodged from the vein and cause infiltration of intravenous fluid into the soft tissues of the neck. Before administering blood or drugs through an external jugular catheter, check to see that there is free flow of fluid into the line, that the neck is not swollen, and that blood can reflux freely into the intravenous tube when the intravenous bag or bottle is lowered below the level of the patient.

B. CENTRAL VENOUS ACCESS

1. Assemble all necessary equipment, including the container of intravenous fluid and tubing, and make sure the tubing has been flushed to remove all air.

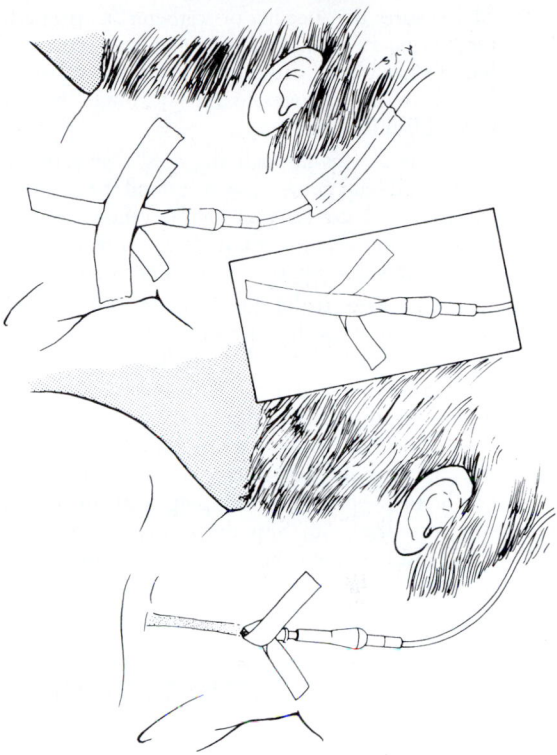

Figure 6–9. Technique of securing an external or internal jugular vein catheter to the skin with tape after insertion.

2. Position the patient.

3. Sterilize the skin around the area of insertion from the clavicle to the ear.

4. Drape the area, and observe sterile technique (don cap, mask, gloves, and gown).

5. Have the patient take a deep breath and forcibly exhale against a closed glottis (Valsalva maneuver).

6. Note the course of the vein, and then have the patient resume normal breathing.

7. Select an insertion point about 4 cm (1⅝ in) above the clavicle, and infiltrate the area with the 1% lidocaine with the 10-mL syringe and 25-gauge needle.

8. While keeping the vein distended (by Valsalva maneuver or occlusion of outflow with finger compression), insert the catheter-clad needle or the needle from a needle-clad catheter into the external jugular vein. If a catheter-clad needle is being used, remove the central needle at this point, and cover the end of the catheter hub with a thumb to prevent aspiration of air.

9. Make sure the needle or catheter is properly placed in the vein by observing the return of blood through the catheter. Inject 5 mL of sterile saline, or run intravenous fluid through the line to establish its patency.

10. Insert the J wire through the needle or catheter, curved end first; guide the wire around the bends in the course of the external jugular vein–subclavian vein junction into the intrathoracic portion of the subclavian vein–superior vena cava system.

11. Secure the wire at the skin with a clamp or a finger. Do not allow the wire to slip all the way into the vein. If a catheter-clad needle is being used, slide the catheter over the wire and into position in the intrathoracic portion of the venous system. If a needle-clad catheter is being used, remove the insertion needle, taking care to grasp the J wire firmly to keep it from slipping forward all the way into the vein. Slip the catheter over the J wire, and be careful not to let the J wire slip all the way into the vein as the catheter is being advanced.

12. Holding the catheter in place, remove the J wire, and cover the end of the catheter hub with a thumb until the setup can be tested for return of blood. Then start the intravenous infusion.

13. Secure the catheter in place with the silk suture run first through the skin and then wrapped around the catheter.

14. Take the patient out of the Trendelenburg position.

15. Obtain a portable chest x-ray immediately to confirm placement of the catheter.

16. Dress the insertion site with antibacterial ointment, cover it with a folded sterile 10- × 10-cm (4- × 4-in) gauze pad, and tape the pad in place.

17. Remember to tape all connections to prevent air embolism.

INTERNAL JUGULAR VEIN CATHETERIZATION

The internal jugular vein is used for insertion of central venous catheters. Pulmonary complications (hemothorax, pneumothorax) occur less commonly than with subclavian vein catheterization, but arterial injury (eg, to the carotid artery) is more common.

Indications

Internal jugular vein catheterization is performed to gain access to the central venous system for administration of fluids and measurement of central venous pressure.

Contraindications

Contraindications to internal jugular vein catheterization are as follows:

- Previous neck injury that might have ligated or scarred the internal jugular vein and thereby altered its anatomy.
- Superior vena cava occlusion.
- Acquired or iatrogenic bleeding disorder.
- Cellulitis over the proposed insertion site.
- Agitated, uncooperative patient (relative contraindication).
- Patient receiving cardiopulmonary resuscitation (CPR).

Personnel Required

The operator performing internal jugular vein catheterization requires an assistant to help handle sterile materials and position the patient.

Equipment & Supplies Required

A. MATERIALS

- Materials for skin sterilization.
- Materials for sterile technique (cap, mask, gloves, and gown).
- Lidocaine, 1% with 10-mL syringe and 25- and 22-gauge needles.
- Topical antibacterial ointment.
- Tincture of benzoin.
- Tape.
- Container of intravenous fluid with all necessary tubing. All equipment should be flushed and fully assembled ready for use.

B. PREPACKAGED STERILE CUTDOWN TRAYS

Prepackaged sterile cutdown trays are commercially available. The following items are required:

- Drapes.
- Gauze sponges, 10 × 10 cm (4 × 4 in).

- Nylon or silk skin suture (size 3-0 or 4-0) on a cutting needle.
- Needle holder.
- Straight scissors.
- Plastic-coated absorbent pad to place beneath the patient's arm.
- Syringe, 3-mL, with 22-gauge, 6.5-cm (2½-in) needle (for use as a probe).
- Central venous catheter and insertion set. Many kinds are commercially available; most consist of an introducing needle and radiopaque catheter, usually 30.5 cm (12 in) long.

Positioning of the Patient

Use a bed or gurney that can be placed in the Trendelenburg position and that has a removable headboard. The patient should be supine, with the head turned 90 degrees away from the side selected for insertion. Place the patient in as steep a Trendelenburg position as possible in order to fully distend the internal jugular vein and also to create increased pressure inside the vein, thus decreasing the chances of air embolism during insertion.

Anatomy Review

The internal jugular vein leaves the base of the skull and courses laterally and posteriorly to the carotid artery and the carotid sheath. It joins the subclavian vein at the thoracic outlet. The internal jugular vein runs medial to the upper portion of the sternocleidomastoid muscle, deep to the triangle formed by the 2 heads at the midportion of this muscle, and deep to its clavicular head (see Figure 6–8).

Procedure

A. MIDDLE (TRIANGLE) APPROACH

(See Figure 6–10).

1. Assemble and arrange all necessary equipment, including the container of intravenous fluid and intravenous tubing, and make sure the tubing has been flushed to remove all air.
2. Position the patient, as described above.
3. Observe sterile technique (don cap, mask, gown, and gloves). Sterilize the skin around the area of insertion from the clavicle to the ear, and drape the patient.
4. The sternocleidomastoid muscle will be clearly outlined when the patient lifts the head slightly. Make a mental picture of the triangle formed by the 2 heads of the muscle, which has its apex

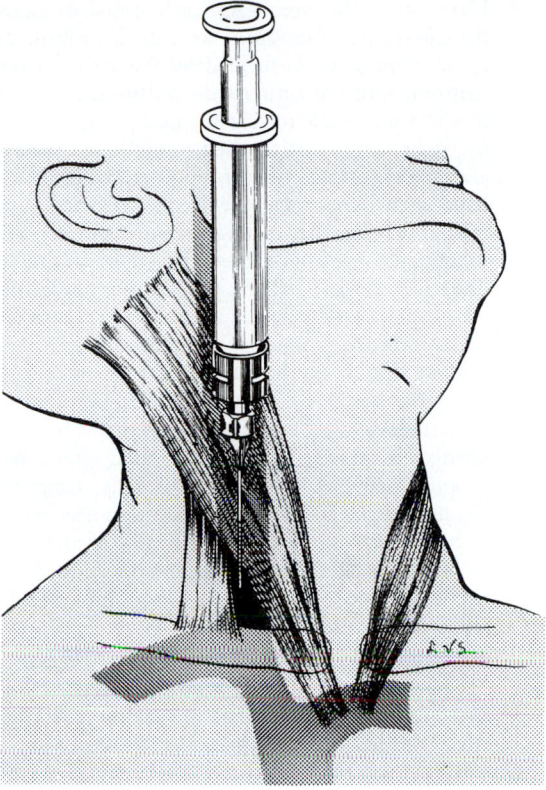

Figure 6–10. Internal jugular vein catheterization—middle approach. (Reproduced, with permission, from Dunphy JE, Way LW [editors]: *Current Surgical Diagnosis & Treatment,* 5th ed. Lange, 1981.)

pointed cephalad and its base formed by the clavicle.

5. Palpate the carotid artery, and make a mental note of the course of the internal jugular vein, which runs lateral and deep to the artery.
6. Choose a point near the apex of the triangle formed by the sternocleidomastoid, and anesthetize the skin with the 1% lidocaine with the 10-mL syringe and 25-gauge needle. Change to the 22-gauge needle, and infiltrate a path through the subcutaneous tissue toward the internal jugular vein, directing the needle downward at an angle of 45 degrees toward the ipsilateral nipple. Be careful when infiltrating the area to aspirate before injecting, so as to avoid injecting significant amounts of lidocaine into the vein. Omit this step if the patient is comatose.
7. Make a probe by placing the 22-gauge, 6.5-cm (2½-in) needle on the 3-mL syringe.

8. Use this small-gauge needle as a probe to locate the internal jugular vein. Pierce the skin near the apex of the triangle formed by the sternocleidomastoid, and direct the needle downward at a 30- to 45- degree angle toward the ipsilateral nipple. If the right hand is being used to guide the syringe and needle, palpate the carotid artery with the left hand to make sure that the needle is moving away from it. The needle should pierce the vein after advancing 2.5–4 cm (1–1½ in). If it does not, withdraw the needle until the point is just under the skin, reposition the needle in the subcutaneous tissue, and probe more medially, always keeping the left index finger on the carotid artery for reference. Once the needle has entered the internal jugular vein, dark venous blood should flow freely into the syringe. If the vein cannot be located after a few probing maneuvers, ask for assistance. *Caution:* Do not use the larger catheter insertion needle or a catheter-clad needle (eg, Angiocath) if the vein cannot be located with the probing needle. When the vein is located, withdraw the probing needle, and remove it from the syringe.

9. Place the catheter insertion needle or catheter-clad needle on the syringe, and follow the course of the probing needle to enter the internal jugular vein. Always recheck the landmarks and position of the carotid artery while inserting this large needle.

10. Maintain a slight vacuum in the attached syringe while inserting the larger needle. Once the needle has entered the vein, dark venous blood will flow freely into the syringe. While aspirating, rotate the needle 360 degrees to make sure that the bevel of the needle is completely within the vein; cessation of blood flow at any point indicates that the needle should be slowly advanced or withdrawn, because it is near one wall of the vein.

11. When it is clear that the needle is properly positioned in the lumen of the vein, disconnect the syringe, and immediately occlude the orifice of the needle to prevent air embolization during inspiration. Most central venous catheters are inserted using the Seldinger technique. This method involves the use of a flexible guide wire or J wire that is placed through the lumen of the needle. The needle is then removed while allowing the guide wire to remain in the lumen of the vein. A No. 11 scalpel blade is then used to make a small incision in the skin where the wire penetrates. Next, a semirigid dilator is advanced over the wire and into the lumen of the vein to create a tract for the more pliable catheter to follow. The dilator is removed continuing to keep the guide wire in place. Finally, the catheter is advanced over the wire and into the lumen of the vein and the guide wire is removed from the catheter leaving only the pliable catheter in place in the vein. An alternative is to place the dilator inside the catheter (most kits are designed to allow this) and then advance the dilator-catheter complex over the wire and into the vein lumen. This method permits dilation of the tract and insertion of the catheter simultaneously. After the dilator-catheter complex is advanced over the wire and into the vein lumen, the dilator and guide wire can then be removed leaving only the catheter behind in the lumen of the vein.

12. When the catheter is fully inserted, check again to be sure there is good return, attach the intravenous tubing, and start the fluid infusion. Anchor the catheter in place with the nylon or silk size 3-0 or 4-0 skin suture. Make sure that the catheter is well secured, and tape it in place, using tincture of benzoin to help secure the tape to the skin and catheter. Tape all connections. Cover the insertion site with antibacterial ointment and a sterile 10- × 10- cm (4- × 4-in) gauze pad folded in half.

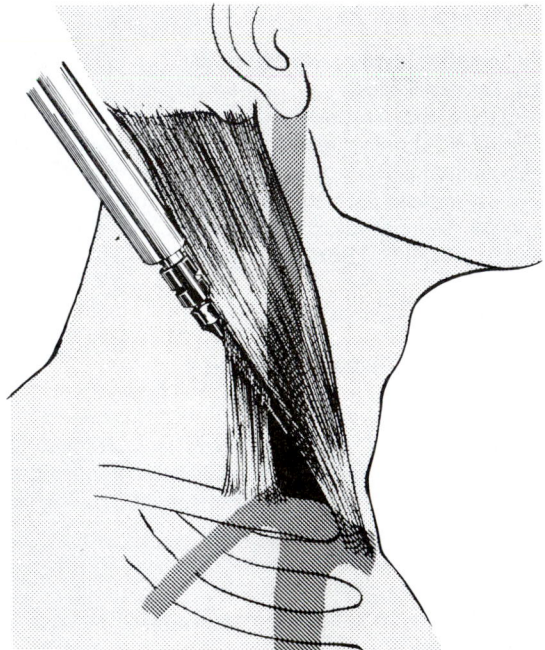

Figure 6–11. Internal jugular vein catheterization—posterior approach. (Reproduced, with permission, from Dunphy JE, Way LW [editors]: *Current Surgical Diagnosis & Treatment,* 5th ed. Lange, 1981.)

13. Take the patient out of the Trendelenburg position, and obtain a chest x-ray immediately to check placement of the catheter and to detect possible pneumothorax.

B. POSTERIOR APPROACH

(See Figure 6–11).

4. Steps 1–4 are the same as in the anterior approach.

5. Note the border where the posterior edge of the anterior belly of the sternocleidomastoid muscle meets the external jugular vein, and anesthetize with the 1% lidocaine. Use a 25-gauge needle for superficial infiltration and a 22-gauge needle for deeper anesthesia.

6. Using a 22-gauge, 6.5-cm (2½-in) needle attached to the 3-mL syringe as a probe, enter the skin just distal to the posterior edge of the sternocleidomastoid muscle about two thirds of the way down, where the external jugular vein crosses the sternocleidomastoid muscle. Enter at a 45-degree angle to the vertical axis and 20 degrees below the coronal plane. Direct the needle under the sternocleidomastoid muscle and toward the suprasternal notch. Pull back on the plunger as the needle is inserted. When the vein has been successfully entered, dark venous blood will flow back into the syringe. If the vein is not entered when the probing needle has been inserted its full length, withdraw the needle, and try again.

7. When the vein has been located with the probing needle, withdraw this needle, and insert the larger catheter insertion needle or catheter-needle combination. The needle should be attached to a syringe in which a slight vacuum is maintained.

8. When the vein has been successfully entered, dark venous blood will flow freely into the syringe.

9. Insert the catheter using the Seldinger technique, as described above.

The remaining steps are the same as in the anterior approach.

SUBCLAVIAN VEIN CATHETERIZATION

Indications

Subclavian vein catheterization is performed to gain venous access for monitoring of central venous pressure, insertion of a transvenous pacemaker, or administration of medications or intravenous fluids.

Contraindications

Contraindications to subclavian vein catheterization are as follows:

- Edema or other manifestations of superior vena cava obstruction on the proposed side of insertion.
- Previous surgery or irradiation to the subclavicular area.
- Bleeding diathesis.
- Infection or cellulitis over the proposed insertion site.
- Pneumothorax on the contralateral site.
- Uncooperative patient.
- Patient receiving CPR.

Relative Contraindications

Relative contraindications to subclavian vein catheterization are as follows:

- Assisted ventilation with high end-expiratory pressures.
- Mastectomy on the proposed side of insertion.
- Severe hypovolemia (eg, hemorrhagic shock).
- Recently discontinued subclavian line in the same area.

Personnel Required

Two people are usually required to perform percutaneous subclavian vein catheterization. The operator inserts the catheter, and an assistant opens sterile equipment and helps to position the patient.

Equipment & Supplies Required

A. MATERIALS

- Materials for skin sterilization.
- Materials for sterile technique (cap, mask, gloves, and gown).
- Lidocaine, 1%, with 10-mL syringe and 22- and 25-gauge needles.
- Topical antibacterial ointment.
- Container of intravenous fluid with connector tubing.

- Central venous catheter and insertion set. Many kinds are commercially available; most consist of an introducing needle and a radiopaque catheter, usually 30.5 cm (12 in) long.
- Tincture of benzoin.
- Tape (including precut lengths).
- Standard bath towel.

B. PREPACKAGED STERILE CUTDOWN TRAYS

Prepackaged sterile cutdown trays are commercially available. The following items are required:

- Drapes.
- Gauze sponges, 10 × 10 cm (4 × 4 in).
- Nylon or silk suture (size 3-0 or 4-0) on a cutting needle.
- Needle holder.
- Straight scissors.
- Syringe, 3-mL, with 22-gauge, 6.5-cm (2½-in) needle for use as a probe (optional).

Positioning of the Patient

Proper positioning of the patient is crucial to successful subclavian vein catheterization. Place the patient in the Trendelenburg position at an angle of 30 degrees, with the patient's head at a comfortable height for the operator. This position fully distends the subclavian vein and creates positive pressure inside the vein when the catheter is inserted, thus preventing air embolism.

Place the rolled bath towel between the patient's scapulas to allow the shoulders to fall backward and flatten the clavicles. Both arms should be at the patient's sides.

Anatomy Review

The subclavian vein courses under the clavicle near the subclavian artery and the apex of the lung (Figure 6–12). The artery is superior and deep to the vein. With a percutaneous approach, the vein is entered before the artery can be accidentally punctured. Laterally, the artery and vein drop caudally to enter the axilla.

Procedure

1. Make sure that all equipment is close at hand and ready for use. Assemble the container of intravenous fluid and tubing, and flush the tubing with fluid to remove all air.
2. Position the patient.
3. Sterilize the skin over the insertion site from the lateral aspect of the clavicle to the ear to the suprasternal notch.

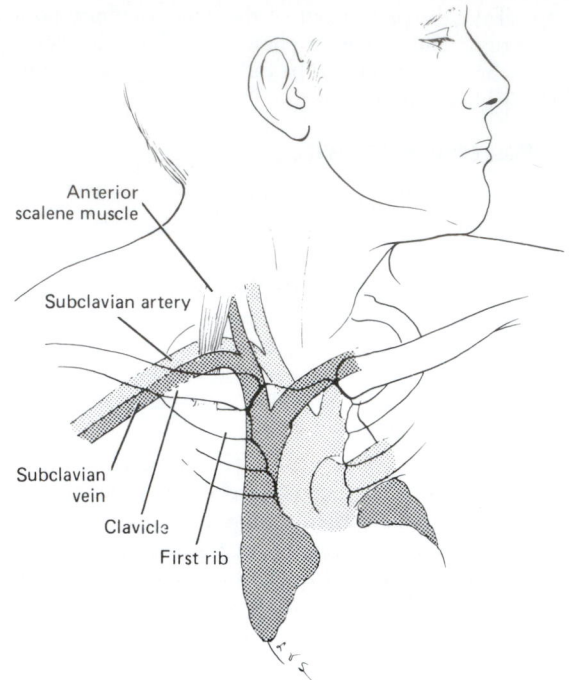

Figure 6–12. Anatomic relationships of the subclavian vein.

4. The patient's head should be rotated away from the side of insertion, with the neck twisted as far as possible.
5. Observe sterile technique (don cap, mask, gloves, and gown).
6. Assemble the introducing needle and syringe, and make sure that the catheter is close by and quickly available.
7. Drape the infraclavicular area.
8. Using the index finger, palpate inferior to the clavicle to find the costoclavicular ligament, which connects the clavicle and the first rib. This ligament lies where the clavicle bends posteriorly (about one-third the length of the clavicle from the suprasternal notch). Place the thumb between the clavicle and the first rib just lateral to this ligament, and place the index finger in the suprasternal notch. The subclavian vein traverses the imaginary line connecting these 2 fingers (Figure 6–13).
9. Anesthetize the skin with the 1% lidocaine using the 10-mL syringe and the 25-gauge needle; then use the 22-gauge needle to anesthetize the subcutaneous tissue and the periosteum of the clavicle

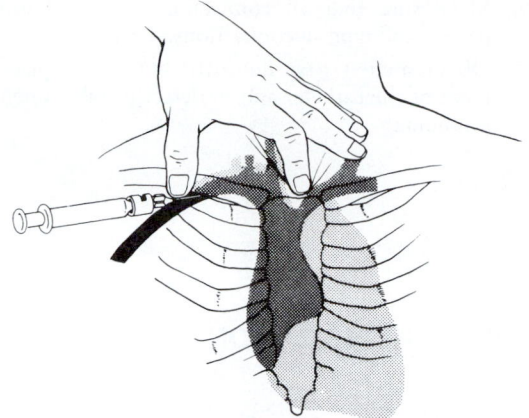

Figure 6–13. Technique of subclavian vein catheterization. With the index finger in the suprasternal notch and the thumb marking the costoclavicular ligament, insert the needle just medial to the thumb.

along the expected route of insertion (ie, the inferior border of the clavicle). When anesthetizing, make sure that the needle is not in the vein (ie, that blood does not flow back when the plunger of the syringe is gently pulled back) before injecting lidocaine.

10. Reposition the index finger in the suprasternal notch and the thumb over the costoclavicular ligament. Place the catheter insertion needle or catheter-clad needle on the 3-mL syringe, and insert the needle under the skin 3 cm (1⅛ in) caudal to the clavicle just medial to the thumb (see Figure 6–13). Insert the needle with the bevel facing up, so that its orientation can be maintained after it enters the vein. It may help to find the vein with a smaller needle (22-gauge, 6.5-cm [2½-in] needle attached to a 3-mL syringe) before using the introducing needle.

11. Advance the needle at a 10- to 20-degree angle until it contacts the clavicle. Decrease the angle of the needle until the needle shaft is parallel to the patient's back and close to the correct alignment (pointing to the finger in the suprasternal notch). Push the needle slowly inferiorly along the clavicle until it reaches the inferior surface. Always keep the tip in contact with the clavicle, and proceed slowly. When the inferior surface is reached, check the alignment of the needle with the suprasternal notch, and while pulling back on the plunger of the syringe, advance the needle toward the suprasternal notch, keeping the needle shaft parallel to the patient's back. When the needle enters the vein, venous blood will flow back into the syringe. If no blood flows out, slowly withdraw the needle while continuing to pull back on the plunger. Occasionally, blood will enter the syringe as the needle is being pulled out slowly.

12. If the first attempt fails, withdraw the needle completely, and flush it with air to clean out any tissue from the needle lumen. This maneuver is important, because a second attempt at catheterization with an obstructed needle will also fail. Occasionally, directing the needle a little cephalad or a little deeper will locate the vein, but do not make misguided attempts in all directions, because of the danger of penetrating nearby structures such as the lung or the subclavian artery. Seek assistance if 3 or 4 attempts to locate the vein fail. If assistance is not obtainable, attempt catheterization on the other side (obtain a chest x-ray first to rule out pneumothorax), or insert an internal jugular venous catheter instead.

13. After the vein has been entered, rotate the needle so that the bevel faces caudally (toward the patient's feet), and make sure that there is free flow of blood. Occasionally, if the tip of the needle lies against the wall of the vein, blood will flow if the bevel is facing cephalad but not when the bevel is rotated. If this is the case, advance or withdraw the needle a short distance, and check it again for blood flow.

14. When the needle is properly located in the lumen of the vein, hold it in place with the thumb and forefinger of one hand, remove the syringe, and immediately occlude the hub of the needle to prevent any air from entering the vein. (If a hypovolemic patient takes a deep breath just as the syringe is disconnected, air may be sucked into the vein, possibly causing air embolism.) If the needle is properly positioned, blood should flow freely from it.

15. The catheter can now be inserted using the Seldinger technique described earlier.

16. Evacuate the insertion syringe of all blood clots, attach it to the catheter hub, and withdraw some blood to make sure that the catheter is in the vein. The blood should flow freely. Remove the syringe. An assistant should then insert the intravenous tubing into the catheter hub and check for rapid flow.

17. Take the patient out of the Trendelenburg position.

18. Secure the catheter at the insertion site by placing the skin suture through the skin, tying it, and then looping it around the catheter 3 times and tying it again. Make sure that the lumen of the catheter is not constricted by the tie.

19. Position the needle and the needle guard on the patient's chest, making sure there are no kinks in the tubing or catheter. Apply a small amount of antibacterial ointment to the insertion site, cover it and the needle with a folded 10- × 10-cm (4- × 4-in) sterile gauze sponge, and tape the sponge in place after applying tincture of benzoin to the skin to help secure the tape to the skin and the catheter.

20. Make sure that all connections are tight and patent, and tape all connections.

21. Obtain a chest x-ray immediately to check placement of the catheter and to detect possible pneumothorax.

FEMORAL VEIN PHLEBOTOMY OR CATHETERIZATION

Femoral vein catheterization is an easy way to gain rapid access to the central venous system, for example, during CPR. Because infection is common at this site, the femoral vein should not be used for procedures requiring elective long-term venous access (eg, parenteral nutrition). Femoral vein phlebotomy is useful in patients in whom peripheral veins of the extremities are not palpable (eg, intravenous drug abusers). However, this route should not be used to obtain blood for culture.

Indications

Femoral vein phlebotomy is used to obtain venous blood samples in patients in whom other sites cannot be used for venipuncture. Femoral vein catheterization is performed to gain central venous access.

Contraindications

Contraindications to femoral vein phlebotomy or catheterization are as follows:

- Previous surgery in the groin.
- Prosthetic graft placement in the groin.
- Venous occlusive disease of the extremities.
- Acquired or congenital bleeding disorder.
- Cellulitis or burn over the proposed site of insertion.

Personnel Required

One operator can perform femoral vein phlebotomy or catheterization unaided if the patient is cooperative, but it is helpful to have an assistant.

Equipment & Supplies Required

A. FEMORAL VEIN PHLEBOTOMY

- Materials for skin cleansing.
- Syringe (20- to 30-mL) with 18- or 20-gauge needle.

- Gauze sponges, 5 × 5 cm (2 × 2 in).
- Specimen tubes for blood.
- Adhesive dressing.

B. FEMORAL VEIN CATHETERIZATION

- Materials for skin sterilization.
- Materials for sterile technique (cap, mask, gloves, and gown).
- Lidocaine, 1%, with 10-mL syringe and 25-gauge needle.
- Catheter-clad needle (eg, Angiocath), 16- to 18-gauge and 12.5–20.5 cm (5–8 in) long; or a central venous catheter kit.
- Container of intravenous infusion fluid with connecting tubing. All equipment should be flushed and fully assembled ready for use.
- Nylon or silk suture (size 3-0) on a cutting needle.
- Needle holder.
- Straight scissors.
- Antibacterial ointment and dressings.
- Drapes.
- Gauze sponges, 10 × 10 cm (4 × 4 in).
- Tape.

Positioning of the Patient

The patient should be supine, with the leg externally rotated on the side selected for phlebotomy or catheterization.

Anatomy Review

The femoral vein normally lies 1–2 cm (⅜–¾ in) medial to the readily palpable femoral artery (Figure 6–14). In a patient without a palpable femoral pulse, the approximate position of the vein can be determined by dividing the distance from the anterior superior iliac spine to the pubic tubercle into 3 equal segments. The artery

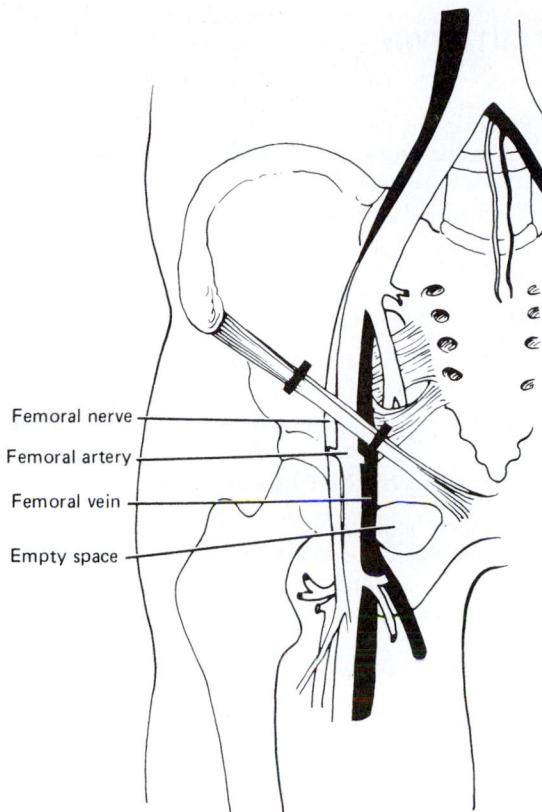

Figure 6–14. Anatomic relationships of the femoral vein at the inguinal ligament.

lies at the junction of the medial segment and the middle segment. The vein is about 1.5 cm (⅝ in) medial to this point and to the artery.

Procedure

A. FEMORAL VEIN PHLEBOTOMY

1. Cleanse the skin.
2. Locate the femoral artery with the nondominant hand.
3. Using the 20- to 30-mL syringe and the 18- or 22-gauge needle in the dominant hand, hold the needle at an angle of 90 degrees to the long axis of the vein.
4. Insert the needle under the skin about 0.5 cm (³⁄₁₆ in) medial to the artery, and pull the plunger back gently to create a slight vacuum as the needle is advanced.

5. When the needle enters the vein, dark venous blood will flow back into the syringe. The blood should flow freely.
6. After obtaining the desired amount of blood, remove the needle quickly, and apply direct pressure over the puncture site.
7. Fill the specimen tubes as described under Upper Extremity Venipuncture, above.

B. FEMORAL VEIN CATHETERIZATION

1. Assemble all equipment, and make sure that it is readily at hand.
2. If necessary, shave the side of the groin chosen for insertion.
3. Observe sterile technique (don cap, mask, gloves, and gown).
4. Sterilize the skin around the groin, and drape the area.
5. Locate the femoral artery. Infiltrate the skin 1.5 cm (⅝ in) medial to the artery with the 1% lidocaine. Omit this step if the patient is comatose.
6. Using the catheter insertion needle attached to a syringe, insert the needle just under the skin, and pull the plunger back gently to crate a slight vacuum. Then advance the needle at an angle of 45 degrees to the long axis of the vein; when the needle enters the vein, dark venous blood will flow back into the syringe. The blood should flow freely.
7. Advance the catheter into the vein. Once the catheter is in place, check to make certain that the blood flows freely. A central venous catheter could be inserted instead, using the Seldinger technique described earlier.
8. Obtain an x-ray immediately in order to check the position of the catheter.
9. If the femoral artery instead of the femoral vein is entered, brighter red blood will flow into the syringe under systemic arterial pressure. A patient in shock or cardiac arrest may have desaturated blood, with little arterial pressure, so that differentiation between arterial and venous puncture may be difficult. If the catheter is to be used solely for infusion of fluid or medication during emergency treatment (eg, CPR), temporary placement in the femoral artery is probably not harmful. If central venous access is required, withdraw the needle and catheter from the artery, maintain direct pressure over the area for 5 minutes, and then either try again on the same side or attempt catheterization on the opposite side.

Femoral nerve
Femoral artery
Femoral vein
Empty space

SAPHENOUS VEIN CUTDOWN

Indications

Saphenous vein cutdown is performed to gain emergency venous access when other sites are not available or when multiple intravenous lines are required.

Contraindications

Contraindications to saphenous vein cutdown are as follows:

- Previous use of the saphenous vein for a surgical procedure (eg, cutdown, vein stripping, coronary artery bypass surgery).
- Phlebitis.
- Evidence of severe venous obstructive disease.
- Cellulitis over the proposed site of insertion.
- Significant trauma to the legs.

Personnel Required

One person can perform saphenous vein cutdown unaided; however, an assistant is helpful.

Equipment & Supplies Required

A. Materials

- Materials for skin sterilization.
- Lidocaine, 1%, with 10-mL syringe and 25-gauge needle.
- Tourniquet.
- Topical antibacterial ointment.
- Expanded gauze roll and tape.

B. Prepackaged Sterile Cutdown Trays

Prepackaged sterile cutdown trays are commercially available. The following items are required:

- Drapes.
- Gauze sponges, 10 × 10 cm (4 × 4 in).
- Silk ligatures (size 3-0) (2).
- Nylon or polypropylene skin suture (size 3-0) on a cutting needle.
- Needle holder.
- No. 15 and No. 11 scalpel blades, both mounted.
- Kelly clamps (2).
- Mosquito clamps (2).
- Dissection tissue scissors and straight scissors.
- Self-retaining retractors or right-angle retractors (2).

- Pediatric feeding tubes, sizes 5F and 10F (1 each), cut to the proper length sufficient to extend to the knee is usually satisfactory).
- Toothed and smooth forceps.
- Plastic-coated absorbent pad to place beneath the patient's leg.

C. Other Materials

- Suitable intravenous infusion set (including blood pump and filter, if desired).
- Container of intravenous fluid with connecting tubing.

Positioning of the Patient

The patient should be supine. The foot selected for the procedure should be externally rotated to expose the medial malleolus, and the plastic-coated absorbent pad should be placed underneath the patient's leg.

Anatomy Review

The saphenous vein runs anterior to the medial malleolus, under the skin and subcutaneous tissue, but superficial to the malleolus (Figure 6–15). At this site, the vein is usually 4–5 mm (⅛–3⁄16 in) in diameter in adults.

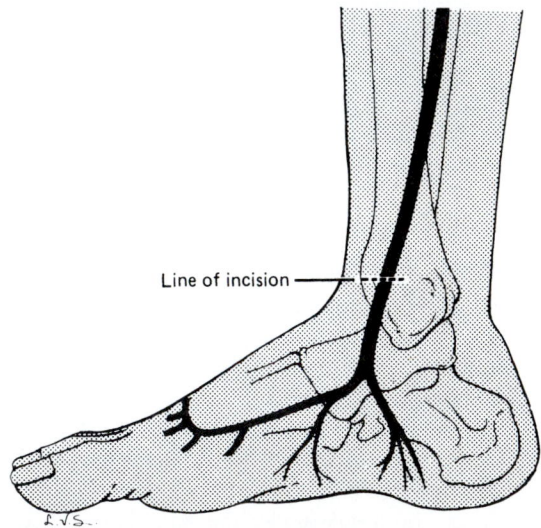

Figure 6–15. Anatomic relationships of the saphenous vein. (Reproduced, with permission, from Dunphy JE, Way LW [editors]: *Current Surgical Diagnosis & Treatment*, 5th ed. Lange, 1981.)

Procedure

1. Assemble all necessary equipment, including the container of intravenous fluid and connecting tubing, and make sure that the tubing has been flushed to remove all air.

2. Place a tourniquet around the lower extremity proximal to the venotomy site to occlude venous return and dilate the saphenous vein.

3. Sterilize the skin around the medial malleolus.

4. Drape the skin.

5. Anesthetize the area with the 1% lidocaine with the 10-mL syringe and 25-gauge needle. Omit this step if the patient is comatose.

6. With the No. 15 scalpel blade, make a 2-cm (¾-in) superficial transverse incision (the dotted line in Figure 6–15), just anterior to the medial malleolus, being careful not to cut through the vein.

7. Using a mosquito clamp, dissect the tissues in the long axis of the leg to isolate the vein. Pass the clamp under the vein and dissect the underlying tissue. Place a silk suture under the vein, and tie off the distal part of the vein. Maintain exposure with retractors.

8. Supporting the vein with an open Kelly clamp, perform a venotomy with the No. 11 scalpel blade: Hold the scalpel parallel to the long axis of the vein with the blade in a horizontal position, and pass it through the midportion of the superficial (or anterior) wall of the vein. Then turn the cutting edge of the blade upward, and open the top of the vein (see Figure 6–2). Take care not to transect the vein or puncture its outer wall.

9. Dilate the vein with the closed point of the Kelly clamp.

10. Insert the catheter (see Figure 6–3), and pass it 10–12.5 cm (4–5 in) proximally up the vein (it is unnecessary to pass it farther). Allow blood to fill the catheter, and then remove the tourniquet.

11. Connect the intravenous tubing to the catheter, and begin the infusion.

12. Now pass the second silk suture under and around the proximal portion of the vein (which now encloses the catheter). Tie this second suture around the vein and catheter proximal to the venotomy. Make it snug but not too tight, or it will cut through the vein, leaving the catheter loose.

13. Close the skin with the nylon or polypropylene suture using a simple running stitch. Secure the catheter to the skin with a skin stitch.

14. Apply antibacterial ointment to the wound, and wrap the ankle with an expanded gauze roll.

INTRAOSSEOUS INFUSION

Indications

Intraosseous infusion is a temporary means of intravenous access in children to be replaced with conventional venous access as soon as possible. It is performed when other techniques of venous cannulation have failed or would be too time-consuming (eg, in the presence of cardiac arrest, trauma, shock). Complications are infrequent (0.6%) and consist mostly of osteomyelitis and infection in adjacent tissues.

Site Selection

Several sites are suitable for infusion. In children under age 3 years, the proximal tibia or distal femur is preferred, but these sites should not be used in patients beyond age 5 years, because the red marrow is replaced by fat beyond this age. The sternum is more suitable in older children; it may be too thin and inadequately ossified in infants. The iliac crest is also acceptable.

Contraindications

Cutaneous infection or burn overlying the insertion site or major injury to the extremity proximal to the insertion site are contraindications.

Personnel Required

One person can perform the procedure. An assistant is helpful.

Equipment & Supplies Required

- Materials for skin sterilization.
- Lidocaine, 1%, with 5-mL syringe and 25-gauge needle.
- Sterile drapes.
- Sterile gloves.

- Short, large-bore bone marrow needle or 18-gauge spinal needle. (Intraosseous infusion needles are commercially available.)
- 10-mL syringe.
- Intravenous infusion set, including sterile tubing and appropriate fluids for administration.
- Gauze sponges (eg, 10 × 10 cm [4 × 4 in]).
- Adhesive tape.

Positioning of the Patient

The patient should be supine. If the proximal tibia is selected, the leg should be rotated slightly externally.

Anatomy Review

The ideal insertion site on the tibia lies 1–2 cm distal to the tibial tuberosity on the anterior medial surface. On the femur it is 2–3 cm proximal to the lateral epicondyle in the midline.

Procedure

1. Sterilize the skin.
2. Drape the area.
3. Using sterile technique, locate the desired insertion site and infiltrate the skin with 1% lidocaine over a 2- to 3-cm area. Lidocaine should also be infiltrated along the anticipated course of insertion, down to and including the periosteum.
4. Using the bone marrow needle, spinal needle, or intraosseous infusion needle, penetrate the skin perpendicularly. Advance the needle toward the bone at a 6-degree angle (directed away from the growth plate; caudal at the tibia, and rostral at the femur).
5. Use firm pressure to penetrate the cortex, employing a rotating or twisting motion. Upon entry into the marrow space, a sudden "give" will be felt. *Caution:* Errant placement of the needle can cause injury to the growth plate with resultant growth deformity.
6. Remove the trocar from the needle and attach a 10-mL syringe. Aspiration of blood and marrow contents confirms needle-tip placement in the marrow.
7. Connect a fluid-filled syringe or intravenous tubing to the needle and infuse under pressure.
8. Apply gauze 10- × 10-cm (4- × 4-in) sponges (cut midway) against the skin at the entry site, surrounding the needle. Occasionally, deep penetration of the needle through the bone cortex on the opposite side can occur, with delivery of infusion into surrounding tissue spaces. This can also occur if the needle becomes dislodged and withdrawn from its intramedullary position; tape the needle firmly in place. (Commercially available intraosseous infusion needles may have a lip to which tape can be attached or a screw mechanism, for securing the needle to the skin surface.) If a spinal needle is used, a Styrofoam cup may be placed over the needle to protect it from being bumped.

RADIAL ARTERY PUNCTURE
(For Blood Gas & pH Analysis)

Indications

Indications for radial artery punctures are as follows:

- Need to obtain arterial blood for blood gas and pH determinations.
- Need to perform phlebotomy when other sites are inaccessible.

Contraindications

Contraindications to radial artery puncture are as follows:

- Positive Allen test (see below), indicating that only one artery supplies the hand.
- Absence of palpable radial artery pulse.
- Cellulitis or other infection over the radial artery.
- Coagulation defects (relative contraindication).

Personnel Required

One person can perform radial artery puncture unaided, but it is helpful to have an assistant to maintain pressure over the puncture site while the operator prepares the sample for transport to the laboratory.

Equipment & Supplies Required

- Materials for skin cleansing.
- Lidocaine, 1%, with 5-mL syringe and 23- to 25-gauge, 1.5-cm (½-in) needle.

- Heparinized syringe, 3- to 5-mL, preferably of glass or of siliconized plastic made especially for arterial blood sampling. To heparinize the syringe, aspirate 0.5 mL of heparin (100–1000 units/mL) into the syringe, hold the syringe upright, pull the plunger all the way out to the end, and then return all of the heparin to the original container. This procedure ensures that a small amount of heparin is in the tip of the syringe and needle hub that is adequate to heparinize the arterial blood gas sample but not enough to affect the accuracy of blood gas determinations.
- Needle for arterial puncture, 23- to 25-gauge (depending on the size of the artery), 1.5-cm (½-in) long.
- Ice for transport.

Positioning of the Patient

The patient should be in a comfortable position, either supine or sitting. If respiratory difficulties require that the patient sit upright, the upper extremity selected should be extended on a stable surface such as a bedside table or on the side of the bed. The arm should be positioned with the volar side up.

Anatomy Review

The radial artery runs along the lateral aspect of the volar forearm deep to the superficial fascia. The artery runs between the styloid process of the radius and the flexor carpi radialis tendon. The point of maximum pulsation of the radial artery can usually be palpated just proximal to the wrist.

Allen Test

The Allen test should be performed to confirm the patency of the ulnar artery before any attempt is made to obtain a blood sample from the radial artery.

While the patient is elevating the arm and making a tight fist, occlude both radial and ulnar arterial flow with firm pressure over both the radial and the ulnar aspects of the volar forearm just proximal to the wrist. Allow a few minutes for the blood to drain from the hand, and then lower the arm to waist level and have the patient open the hand. Release the pressure on the ulnar artery while keeping the radial artery occluded. Normal skin color should return to the ulnar side of the palm in 1–2 seconds, followed by quick restoration of normal color to the entire palm. A hand that remains white indicates either absence or occlusion of the ulnar artery, in which case radial artery puncture is contraindicated. Failure to perform this test may result in a gangrenous finger or loss of the hand from a spasm or clotting of the radial artery where there is no collateral flow through the ulnar artery.

Procedure

1. Palpate the radial artery just proximal to the wrist, and determine where the pulse is most prominent.
2. Locate the approximate position of the artery under the pad of the index finger by slowly rolling the finger from side to side. This maneuver causes the pulse to become alternately stronger and weaker and further helps to locate the relatively small artery.
3. Cleanse the skin over the proposed site of puncture.
4. Anesthetize the skin over the proposed site of puncture with 1% lidocaine using the 3- to 5-mL syringe and 23- to 25-gauge needle.
5. Using the index and middle fingers of the nondominant hand, identify again the point of maximal pulsation of the radial artery (Figure 6–16).

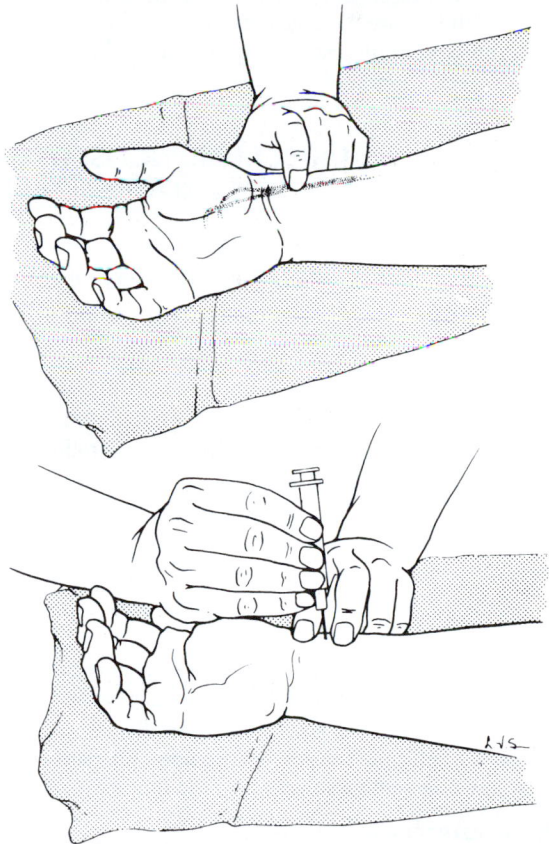

Figure 6–16. Technique of radial artery puncture. The index and middle fingers are used to identify the point of maximum pulsation.

6. Attach the 23- to 25-gauge needle to the heparinized syringe, and holding the needle perpendicular to the arm, insert the needle into the skin in the anesthetized area. The smaller the needle, the less the risk of injury to the artery and the less painful the procedure to the patient.

7. Guide the needle toward the point of maximum pulsation, and watch for a sudden gush of arterial blood into the hub of the needle or the lower part of the syringe. Once the needle has entered the lumen of the radial artery, the force of arterial pulsation should fill the syringe if it is specially designed for arterial puncture (glass or siliconized plastic). If an ordinary plastic syringe is used, a small amount of suction may be required to obtain an adequate blood sample (only 1–2 mL of blood is required for blood gas and pH analysis).

8. If no blood is obtained with these maneuvers, it is possible that the needle has completely passed through the radial artery. Advance the needle until it meets the periosteum of the radius. Slowly withdraw the syringe and needle, and look for the gush of arterial blood into the hub of the needle.

9. If this attempt is still unsuccessful, withdraw the needle to a position just under the skin, move it 1 mm (⅟₁₆ in) to ether side of the previous attempt, and try again. Make at least 3 attempts before giving up and trying another site or seeking assistance.

10. Remove the needle from the artery with a smooth, swift motion, and apply immediate direct pressure over the puncture site for 10 minutes. An assistant is helpful to apply pressure on the artery.

11. Evacuate all air bubbles from the sample by holding the syringe upright and allowing the bubbles to collect near the needle hub. Gently tapping the syringe with the end of a finger will help dislodge bubbles from the walls of the syringe. Once all of the air has been confined to the tip of the syringe, evacuate it by pushing on the plunger. Then, cap the needle with a rubber stopper, label the tube with the patient's name and number, and place the sample on ice for transport to the laboratory.

12. Return in 15 minutes, and check for adequate perfusion of the hand and for possible hematoma formation in the patient's wrist.

DIRECT LARYNGOSCOPY, OROTRACHEAL INTUBATION, & NASOTRACHEAL INTUBATION

Please see Chapter 8 for a complete discussion of airway management.

Indications

A. OROTRACHEAL INTUBATION

Indications for orotracheal intubation area as follows:

- Inadequate oxygenation (eg, decreased arterial PO_2) that is not corrected by supplemental oxygen supplied by mask or nasal cannula.
- Inadequate ventilation (increased arterial PCO_2).
- Need to control and remove pulmonary secretions (bronchial toilet).
- Need to provide airway protection in an obtunded patient or a patient with a depressed gag reflex.
- Need to perform urgent or emergent diagnostic studies in a multiply injured or intoxicated patient or in an uncooperative patient with head injury.

B. NASOTRACHEAL INTUBATION

Nasotracheal intubation is used for long-term intubation because it is more comfortable for the patient than orotracheal intubation. It is also used when access to the trachea through the oropharynx is difficult and emergency cricothyrotomy is not indicated. The advantages of nasotracheal intubation are greater comfort for the patient and greater ease in communicating with the intubated patient through lip reading. Disadvantages include need for a smaller airway, which results in increased airway resistance; need for a more skilled operator, because the tube is usually inserted without direct vision; possible bleeding caused by passage of the nasotracheal tube through the nasopharynx; and sinusitis that may result owing to obstruction of the ostia of the sinuses.

Contraindications

The following are only relative contraindications to tracheal intubation:

- Severe airway trauma or obstruction that does not permit safe passage of an endotracheal tube. Emergency cricothyrotomy is indicated in such cases.
- Cervical spine injury is no longer considered a contraindication to intubation. Rapid sequence induction followed by orotracheal intubation optimizes intubating conditions and with careful maintenance of

in-line cervical immobilization has not been shown to lead to iatrogenic cervical spinal cord injury.

- Nasotracheal intubation is still performed by those with significant experience with the technique but is contraindicated in the apneic patient.

Personnel Required

One person can perform direct laryngoscopy or tracheal intubation unaided in nontrauma patients. An assistant is required to maintain cervical spine immobilization for any patient with a history of trauma who requires intubation.

Equipment & Supplies Required

- Self-refilling bag-valve-mask combination (eg, Ambu bag) or bag-valve unit (Ayres bag), connector, tubing, end-tidal CO_2 ($ETCO_2$) detector, and oxygen source. Assemble all items before attempting intubation.
- Laryngoscope with curved and straight blades of a size appropriate for the patient.
- Endotracheal tubes of several different sizes (Table 6–1). Low-pressure, high-flow cuffed balloons are preferred. Tracheal tubes used in nasotracheal intubation should be smaller than those used for orotracheal intubation (see Table 6–1).
- Oral and nasal airways.
- Tincture of benzoin and precut tape.
- Introducer (stylets or Magill forceps).
- Suction apparatus (tonsil tip and catheter suction).
- Syringe, 10-mL, to inflate the cuff.
- Mucosal anesthetics and astringents (eg, 1% lidocaine jelly and phenylephrine nasal spray).
- Water-soluble sterile lubricant.

Table 6–1. Guidelines for endotracheal tube selection.

Age	Orotracheal Tube[1]	Nasotracheal Tube
Premature	2.0	Not applicable
Term	2.5	Not applicable
3–18 months	3–4	Not applicable
1 ½–3 years	4–5	Not applicable
3–5 years	5–6	5
5–7 years	6–6.5	5–6
8–14 years	7–8	6–7
Over 14 years		
Female	7–8	7
Male	7–9	7–8

[1]Inside diameter in millimeters.

Positioning of the Patient

Unless contraindicated as in the trauma patient, the sniffing position—patient supine, with the neck extended, the occiput elevated, and the head tilted backward—permits visualization of the glottis and vocal cords and allows passage of the endotracheal tube. A towel rolled under the head usually makes it easier for the patient to maintain this position.

In infants under age 1 month, the head and neck should be in a neutral position.

Procedure

A. MASK VENTILATION

Oxygen is delivered with a face mask at a rate of 10–15 L/min.

1. Select the proper-sized mask; it should cover the mouth and nose and fit snugly against the cheeks.
2. Place the nontrauma patient in the sniffing position.
3. Place the mask over the patient's mouth and nose with the right hand.
4. With the left hand, place the small and ring fingers under the patient's mandible, and lift up to open the airway. Grasp the mask with the thumb and index finger, and press it to the patient's face while lifting the mandible with the ring and small fingers.
5. Compress the bag with the right hand.
6. The chest should rise with each breath, and airflow should be unimpeded. If not, reposition the mask, and try again. Occasionally, insertion of an oral or nasal airway facilitates ventilation by mask. Because of the lack of support for the lips, elderly edentulous patients may be especially hard to ventilate using a mask.

B. TOPICAL ANESTHESIA

Anesthetize the mucosa of the nose, oropharynx, and upper airway with cocaine, 4%, or lidocaine, 2%, if time permits and the patient is awake.

C. DIRECT LARYNGOSCOPY

1. Place the patient in the sniffing position.
2. Check the laryngoscope and blade for proper fit, and make sure that the light works.
3. Make sure that all materials are assembled and close at hand.
4. Curved blade technique: (a) Open the patient's mouth with the right hand, and remove any dentures. (b) Grasp the laryngoscope in the left hand (Figure 6–17). (c) Spread the patient's lips, and

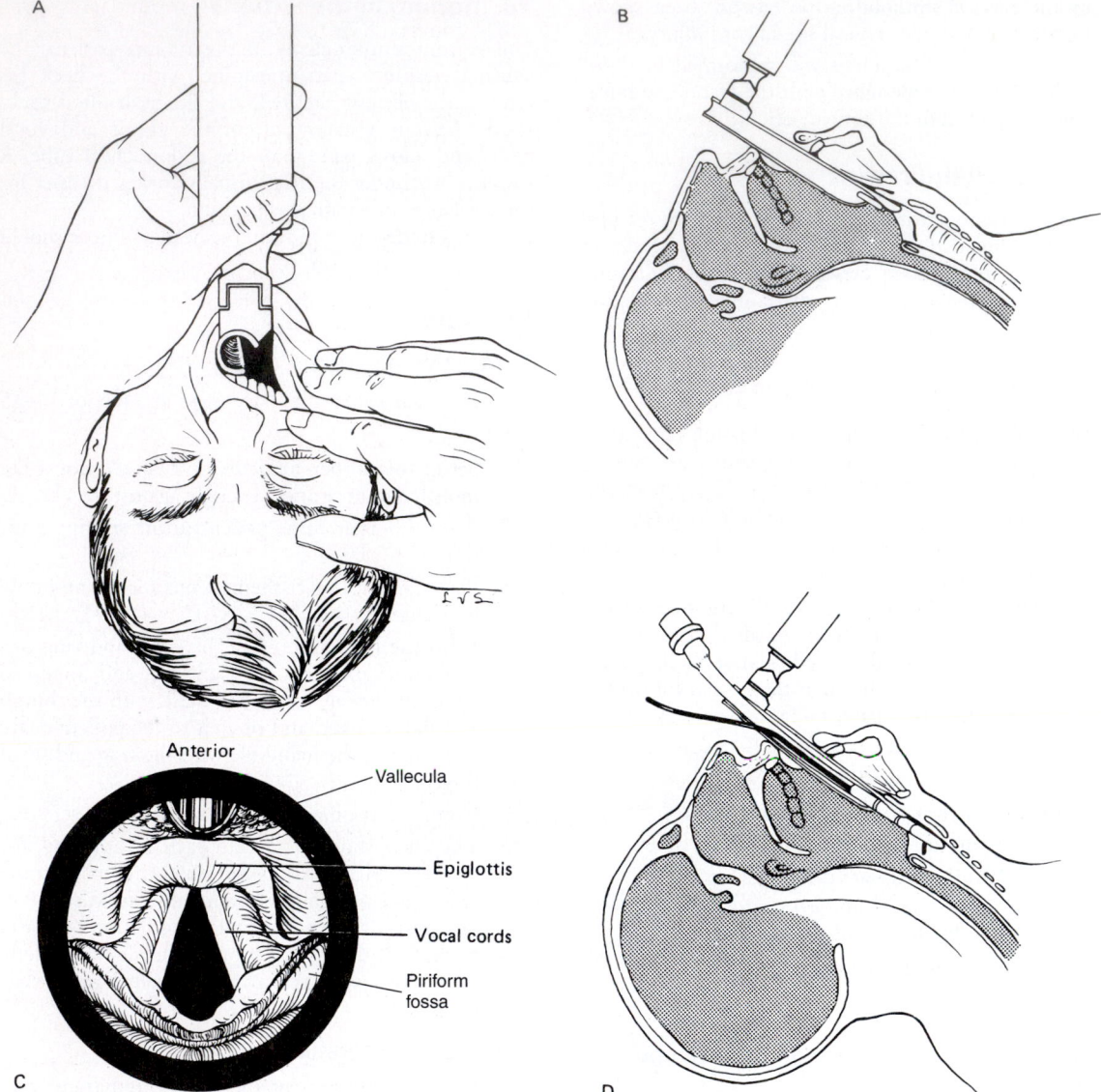

Figure 6–17. Technique of direct laryngoscopy and orotracheal intubation. **A:** The straight laryngoscope blade is passed behind the tongue and deep to the tip of the epiglottis. **B:** Lateral view showing straight laryngoscope blade deep to the tip of the epiglottis exposing glottic opening. **C:** View of glottis as seen through a laryngoscope with a curved blade. **D:** Insertion of endotracheal tube. (Parts A, B, and D reproduced, with permission, from Way LW [editor]: *Current Surgical Diagnosis & Treatment,* 3rd ed. Lange, 1977. Part C reproduced, with permission, from Kempe CH, Silver HK, O'Brien D [editors]: *Current Pediatric Diagnosis & Treatment,* 4th ed. Lange, 1976.)

insert the blade between the teeth, being careful not to break a tooth. (d) Pass the blade to the right of the tongue and advance the blade into the hypopharynx, pushing the tongue to the left and placing the tip of the blade into the vallecula. (e) Lift the laryngoscope upward and forward, without changing the angle of the blade, to expose the vocal cords.

5. Straight blade technique: Follow the steps outlined for curved blade technique, but advance the blade down the hypopharynx, and lift the epiglottis with the tip of the blade to expose the vocal cords. The tip of the laryngoscope blade fits below the epiglottis, which is no longer visible with the blade in position.

D. Orotracheal Intubation

1. Select the proper-sized tube (see Table 6–1). Most adult men take an endotracheal tube that has an inside diameter of 8–9 mm. Most adult women take an endotracheal tube that is 7–8 mm internal diameter. For children, a general rule is that the external diameter of the tube is equal to the diameter of the child's fifth digit fingernail.

2. With the 10-mL syringe, inflate the balloon with 5–8 mL of air. Make sure that the balloon is functional and intact.

3. Lubricate the end of the tube (optional).

4. Insert the stylet, and bend the tube and stylet gently into a crescent shape so that the tip of the stylet is at least 1 cm (⅜ in) proximal to the end of the orotracheal tube.

5. Be sure that the syringe and the bag-valve combination are within easy reach.

6. Ventilate the patient with the bag-valve combination for 1–2 minutes with 100% oxygen.

7. Open the patient's mouth, remove dentures, and suction secretions or vomitus from the mouth.

8. Visualize the glottis and vocal cords and, by direct laryngoscopy, gently pass the tube through the vocal cords into the trachea. Occasionally, having an assistant press posteriorly on the anterior neck at the level of the cricoid cartilage will help to bring an anteriorly placed larynx into view and facilitate intubation. This is known as the Sellick maneuver; it also helps reduce reflux of gastric contents into the hypopharynx.

9. Gently pass the tube next to the laryngoscope blade, through the vocal cords, and far enough so that the balloon is just beyond the cords.

10. Withdraw the stylet, and inflate the cuff.

11. Connect the bag-valve combination and $ETCO_2$ detector, and begin ventilation with 100% oxygen.

12. Confirm the tube is properly positioned by several methods. $ETCO_2$-detector color change confirms endotracheal intubation in the patient with spontaneous circulation but the color may not change in patients who have had cardiac arrest. Next, it is important to use auscultation to confirm appropriate placement. First, listen over the stomach with a stethoscope while ventilating the patient. If sounds of airflow are heard or if distention of the stomach occurs, the tube is in the esophagus. If the esophagus has been intubated instead of the trachea, remove the tube, ventilate the patient with a mask, and try again.

Next, listen to each side of the chest, including the axilla, to be sure that the breath sounds are equal. If the left chest has more distant breath sounds than the right chest, try withdrawing the tube 1–2 cm (⅜–¾ in) and ventilating again. This maneuver helps to correct intubation of the right main-stem bronchus as a cause of unequal ventilation. Airway anatomy makes intubation of the right main-stem bronchus more likely than intubation of the left. When breath sounds are equal on both sides and the thorax rises equally on both sides with each inspiration, note the position of the tube (eg, mark the tube at the patient's mouth).

13. Secure the tube in place with tracheostomy ribbon or tape.

14. Obtain a chest x-ray immediately to check tube placement.

15. Obtain arterial blood gas measurements to assess the adequacy of ventilation.

E. Nasotracheal Intubation

6. Steps 1–6 are the same as those for orotracheal intubation, except no stylet is needed. The tube must be checked and lubricated, and all materials must be readily at hand.

7. Examine the patient's nose, and determine if one nasal passage is larger than the other. Insert the lubricated nasotracheal tube in the external naris, and pass it directly posteriorly until it meets the floor of the nasopharynx. The technique is similar to that used to pass a nasogastric tube (see Nasogastric Intubation, below).

8. Make sure that the natural bend in the tube (without the stylet in place) corresponds to the direction of passage, and with gentle, steady pressure, continue to advance the nasotracheal tube into the posterior pharynx. At this point, the tube may meet with obstruction. If the tube fails to pass into the posterior pharynx under gentle, steady pressure, withdraw the tube, and attempt insertion in the opposite nostril.

9. Once the nasotracheal tube is in the pharynx, the patient's head may be flexed by lifting the occiput if no concern for cervical spine injury exists. This helps to guide the tube through the vocal cords anteriorly into the larynx. The patient may start to cough when the tube passes through the vocal cords.

10. If the patient is breathing spontaneously, listen at the external end of the tube. If the tube is properly positioned over the larynx, air should be heard coming in and out of the tube. If no air is heard, the tube has slipped posteriorly and is in the esophagus. Place the index finger and thumb on each side of the larynx. This allows for external palpation of the endotracheal tube if it deviates to either piriform fossa. Using the digits flanking the trachea, manually deviate the trachea toward the intubated nares to facilitate better alignment and allow for easier intubation.

11. When ventilation is heard, steady the patient's head in that position, and when inspiration begins, advance the tube into the trachea.

12. Once the tube is in the trachea, inflate the balloon and listen again to make sure that air is coming from the nasotracheal tube, and look at the tube to see the condensation of water vapor with exhalation.

13. Have an assistant steady the nasotracheal tube. Connect an air reservoir bag (eg, Ayers or Ambu bag) and $ETCO_2$ detector to the tube, ventilate the patient, and check for elevation of both sides of the chest on inspiration and the presence of breath sounds at each axilla in addition to color change on the $ETCO_2$ detector. As with orotracheal intubation, inadvertent intubation of the right main-stem bronchus (with poor ventilation of the left lung) occurs more commonly than intubation of the left bronchus.

14. When proper positioning of the tube in the trachea has been achieved, secure the tube in place with tracheostomy ribbon or tape. Make sure that there is no pressure on the external naris that might cause necrosis.

F. REMOVAL OF THE ENDOTRACHEAL TUBE

1. Ventilate the patient with a bag-valve combination for 1–2 minutes with 100% oxygen.

2. Suction the patient's trachea, mouth, and hypopharynx before removing the tube.

3. Deflate the cuff by withdrawing all air with the 10-mL syringe.

4. Have the patient take a deep breath, and remove the tube at the midpoint of expiration.

5. Suction the patient's mouth a second time to remove any remaining secretions.

6. Begin oxygen, 5 L/min, by mask. Obtain a sample of arterial blood to assess respiratory function.

NASOGASTRIC INTUBATION
(For Gastric Evacuation or Lavage)

Indications

Indications for nasogastric intubation are as follows:
- Need to suppress vomiting caused by gastric distention or paralytic ileus.
- Need to perform gastric lavage (therapeutic or diagnostic).
- Need to perform gastric decompression.
- Need to perform gastric evacuation.

Contraindications

Important contraindications to nasogastric intubation are as follows:
- Choanal atresia.
- Massive facial trauma or basilar skull fracture.
- Esophageal atresia or stricture.
- Ingestion of a caustic substance (eg, acid, lye)-unless nasogastric intubation can be performed under direct vision.

Relative contraindications to nasogastric intubation are as follows:

- Recent gastric or esophageal surgery.
- Recent oropharyngeal or nasal surgery.
- Esophageal stricture.
- Esophageal burn.
- Zenker diverticulum.

Personnel Required

One person can perform nasogastric intubation unaided, but an assistant is helpful.

Equipment & Supplies Required

- Nasogastric tube of the proper diameter. There are 2 main types of tubes: straight suction tubes and sump suction tubes (with 2 lumens). The sump tube is less likely to be sucked against the stomach wall and become plugged. The only disadvantage is that because of the second air-inlet port, it has a slightly smaller lumen for suction than a similarly sized straight suction tube. Most adults require a 16–18F sump tube. The limiting factor is the size of the naris. Children usually require a 10F nasogastric tube and infants an 8F tube. (Nasogastric size can be estimated by multiplying endotracheal tube size by 2.)
- Lubricant.
- Suction syringe with catheter tip.
- Connector (usually supplied with the nasogastric tube).
- Suction tube and suction device (wall suction, intermittent wall suction, or portable intermittent suction).
- Phenylephrine nasal spray, 0.5%, and benzocaine-tetracaine spray.
- Tincture of benzoin.
- Tape.

Positioning of the Patient

The patient should be in a comfortable, supported sitting position. Unconscious patients should either be supine and flat or supine with the head slightly elevated. Children or unusually overreactive adults may be asked to sit on their hands as a reminder to keep them away from the nose and the tube as it is being passed into the stomach.

Procedure

1. Explain exactly what the steps of the procedure will be, and explain the need for the patient's help at certain points.
2. Determine the length of tubing necessary by measuring the distance between the ear and the umbilicus.
3. Lubricate the end of the tube with lubricant.
4. Apply 0.5% phenylephrine nasal spray to both nostrils to prevent epistaxis. If intractable gagging is a problem, Benzocaine-tetracaine spray applied to the pharynx will help.
5. Insert the tube into the nostril at a 60- to 90-degree angle to the plane of the face, and advance it straight back until it meets resistance (the patient usually signs when this happens).

6. Using the gentle pressure and pushing posteriorly and perpendicularly to the long axis of the head, advance the tip of the tube inferiorly and into the nasopharynx (Figure 6–18).
7. Have the patient take a small sip of water through the straw and hold it in the mouth without swallowing. Then have the patient swallow, and advance the tube into the esophagus simultaneously. If this maneuver is successful, the patient will gag. If it fails and the tube slips into the trachea, violent coughing will usually ensue. Withdraw the tube into the oropharynx, and try again. The most important step is timing the advancement of the tube to coincide with the swallow. Patients with an altered sensorium sometimes tolerate tracheal intubation without any reflex coughing. The tube is improperly positioned if air exchange is heard.
8. When the tube is in the esophagus, advance it into the stomach. In adults, the tube is usually in the stomach when it is advanced to the next-to-the-last mark on the sump tube.
9. Once the nasogastric tube is in the stomach, withdraw some gastric juice, and with a suction syringe inject air down the tube while listening over

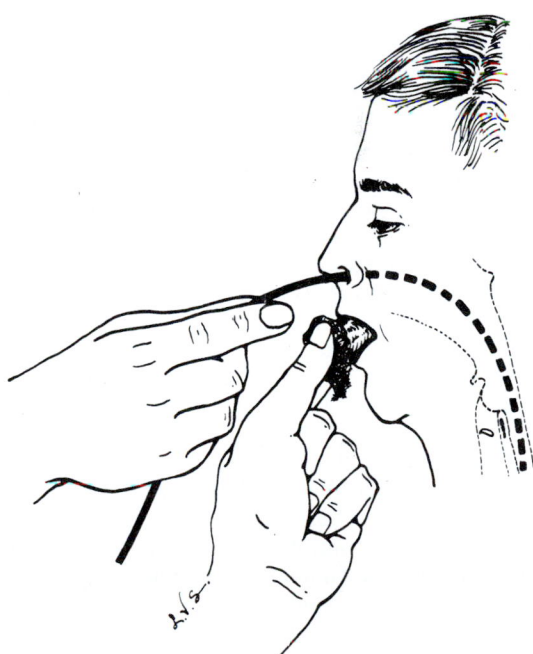

Figure 6–18. Technique of nasogastric intubation.

the left upper quadrant for the sound of air leaving the tube and bubbling in the stomach. If no sound is heard, reposition the tube, and inject more air. If several attempts fail, check to make sure that the tube is not in the trachea or curled in the patient's mouth. Obtain a chest x-ray to check the position of the tube. Injecting a small amount of water-soluble contrast medium down the tube and visualizing its position with fluoroscopy or standard x-ray is the definitive confirmatory procedure. Never assume that the tube is in the correct position without performing some confirming maneuver. Nasogastric tubes have been left in the peripheral lung, cranial vault, extraesophageal mediastinum, and peritoneal cavity.

10. Apply tincture of benzoin to the nose before securing the tube to the nose with tape, and make sure that the tube does not exert pressure on the external naris, which can result in pressure necrosis and sloughing of the naris.

Special Problems

A. INTUBATED PATIENTS

Inserting a nasogastric tube in an intubated patient can be difficult. Follow the steps outlined above, and remember to deflate the cuff of the endotracheal tube if the nasogastric tube becomes stuck in the upper esophagus. In an unresponsive intubated patient, it may occasionally be necessary to use Magill forceps and a laryngoscope to advance the tube into the esophagus under direct vision.

B. COMATOSE PATIENTS

A comatose or obtunded patient cannot swallow at the right time to facilitate passage of the tube. The natural bend of the tube as it passes into the pharynx from the naris is anterior; the tube therefore tends to enter the trachea. Any one of the following maneuvers may be helpful (they should be performed in the order given here):

1. Flex the patient's head when passing the tube. Make sure the patient does not have a cervical spine injury if this is attempted in the emergency department.

2. After the tube passes into the hypopharynx, rotate the tube to direct the natural curve posteriorly and continue to advance it.

3. Pass the tube through the nostril and into the nasopharynx, and insert a finger into the patient's mouth to manually guide the tube posteriorly into the esophagus.

4. Use a laryngoscope and Magill forceps to pass the tube into the esophagus under direct vision.

INSERTION OF SENGSTAKEN-BLAKEMORE OR MINNESOTA TUBE

Minnesota and Sengstaken-Blakemore tubes (Figure 6–19) are used to control hemorrhage from esophageal varices and the esophagogastric junction. The Sengstaken-Blakemore tube is a triple-lumen rubber tube with 2 balloons: one that is inflated in the lumen of the stomach and pressed against the esophagogastric junction, and one that is inflated in the lumen of the esophagus to press directly against the varices. Two of the lumens are used to inflate the balloons; the third opens into a port on the distal tip of the tube and is used to irrigate and drain the stomach.

The Minnesota tube is currently preferable to the other tubes that are available. This tube has 4 lumens: 2 for filling the balloons, one that permits aspiration of gastric contents, and a fourth to aspirate the esophagus above the balloon. If a tube without an esophageal port is used (eg, a Sengstaken-Blakemore tube), a nasogastric tube must be tied to the Sengstaken-Blakemore tube just above the esophageal balloon in order to remove secretions collecting there.

Effective use of the Sengstaken-Blakemore or Minnesota tube requires close attention to the pressure in each balloon and monitoring for continued bleeding from the esophagogastric varices (blood aspirated through the gastric aspiration port of the Sengstaken-Blakemore tube or above the esophageal balloon through a nasogastric tube or the esophageal port of the Minnesota tube). Proper insertion will also ensure that the gastric balloon is not inflated in the esophagus, which may lead to esophageal rupture.

With either tube, patients may require orotracheal or nasotracheal intubation first to protect the airway before balloon tamponade is attempted. Intubation must always be done in comatose patients.

Indications

Indications for insertion of a Sengstaken-Blakemore tube are as follows:

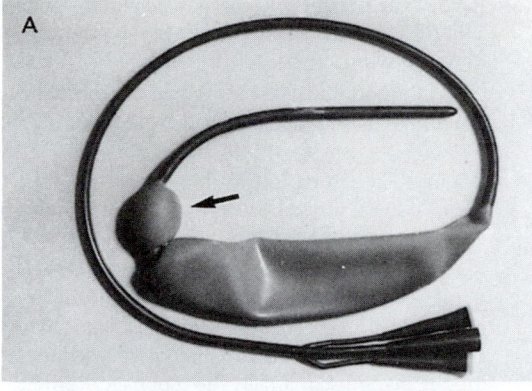

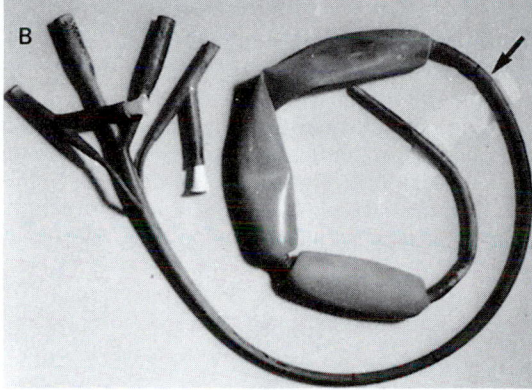

Figure 6–19. Balloon tamponade for bleeding varices. **A:** The Sengstaken-Blakemore tube has a small gastric balloon (arrow) that can be inflated to 250 mL with air. **B:** The 4-lumen Minnesota tube has a much larger gastric balloon that inflates to 450 mL and a series of aspirating ports (arrow) for removing secretions above the esophageal balloon.

- Need to control massive upper gastrointestinal tract hemorrhage presumed to be from esophageal varices in a patient with hypovolemic shock.
- Need to control documented esophagovariceal hemorrhage in a patient with or without hemodynamic compromise.

Contraindications

Insertion of a Sengstaken-Blakemore tube is contraindicated in patients who have undergone previous gastroesophageal surgery.

Personnel Required

The operator will require an assistant.

Equipment & Supplies Required

- Sengstaken-Blakemore tube or Minnesota tube.
- No. 18 Salem sump tube if Sengstaken-Blakemore tube is used.
- Constant or intermittent wall or portable suction device.
- Mercury manometer or aneroid pressure gauge.
- Y connector.
- Rubber-clad clamps (3).
- Water-soluble lubricating jelly.
- Cocaine spray, 4%.
- Glass of water and a straw.
- Manometer-grade rubber tubing, 0.6–1 m (2–3 ft).
- Irrigating syringe, 50-mL; water, basin.
- Football helmet with a face mask, if available.
- Sponge rubber to act as cuff around the tube.

Positioning of the Patient

The patient should be supine, with the head of the bed elevated 30–45 degrees if possible. It is difficult to insert the tube with the patient in the Trendelenburg position.

Anatomy Review

Esophageal varices result form portal hypertension. When the distal esophageal veins become distended, they become susceptible to erosion, and the overlying mucosa becomes thinner. Mechanical or chemical (reflux of gastric acid) irritation may rupture the varices, causing hemorrhage.

Procedure

1. Protect the airway. In stuporous patients or those with a diminished gag reflex, endotracheal intubation should be performed before passage of a Minnesota or Sengstaken-Blakemore tube.
2. Inflate the balloons to test for air leaks, and lubricate the distal end of the tube and balloons.
3. Make sure that all necessary equipment is readily at hand.
4. Deflate the balloons completely.
5. Anesthetize the patient's nasal passages, pharynx, and hypopharynx with the 4% cocaine spray or benzocaine-tetracaine spray and wait 2–3 minutes.
6. Pass the tube through one nostril with steady pressure until the tip of the tube is in the posterior pharynx.

7. Advance the tube into the esophagus as the patient swallows.

8. Advance the tube to at least the 50-cm mark. (In the typical adult, the tube should be in the stomach at this point.)

9. Fill the irrigating syringe with air, and listen over the patient's stomach with a stethoscope while injecting air through the gastric aspiration port. If the tube is properly positioned, a gurgling sound will be heard in the stomach as air escapes from the tube. If no air is heard, withdraw the tube, and insert it again. Do not inflate either balloon until the tube is known to be in the stomach.

10. When proper placement of the tube in the stomach has been confirmed, inflate the gastric balloon with air (250–275 mL for the Sengstaken-Blakemore tube; 450–500 mL for the Minnesota tube), and clamp the gastric balloon port with a rubber-clad clamp. If the patient develops substernal pain while the gastric balloon is being inflated, the balloon may be in the esophagus. Stop immediately, deflate the balloon, and push the tube farther into the stomach before attempting reinflation of the gastric balloon.

11. Pull back on the tube until resistance is felt, showing that tamponade of the gastroesophageal junction has been achieved. Secure the tube with a minimum of tension (about 0.45 kg [1 lb]) by taping a cuff of sponge rubber to the tube just distal to the patient's nostril.

12. Construct a pressure-reading mechanism by connecting the esophageal balloon port to a Y connector. Use part of the manometer-grade rubber tubing if needed. Connect the manometer or aneroid pressure gauge to one port of the Y connector and an inflating bulb of the 50-mL syringe to the other.

13. If inflation of the gastric balloon fails to stop the bleeding, inflate the esophageal balloon to 35–50 mm Hg of pressure, using manometer control. Use the lowest pressure possible that will control hemorrhage.

14. Aspirate through the gastric port of the tube, and evacuate the stomach of all blood and water. Irrigate and aspirate the stomach, if necessary, to completely evacuate all contents.

15. Continue gastric lavage for 30 minutes, and check for bright red blood. If bleeding continues, increase the esophageal balloon pressure by 5-mm Hg increments. Continue lavage to determine the exact pressure at which bleeding stops. Occlude the esophageal and gastric ports with a rubber-clad clamp proximal to the Y connector.

16. Record the pressures in the gastric and esophageal balloons, and transport the patient to an intensive care unit with one-on-one nursing.

17. Obtain a portable chest x-ray and abdominal film immediately to check for proper placement of the tube.

18. If a football helmet is available, secure the tube to the face mask instead of using pressure against the nostril to hold the tube in place.

19. If a Sengstaken-Blakemore tube is being used, pass a standard nasogastric Salem sump tube through the other nostril to evacuate all secretions that accumulate above the esophageal balloon. If a Minnesota tube is being used, attach the esophageal port to a suction device set to intermittent high suction.

20. If the patient is comatose and the tube cannot be passed through the nose, insert it through the mouth, and guide it into the esophagus with a finger. An alternative is to use direct laryngoscopy and Magill forceps to guide the tube into the esophagus. Be careful not to puncture the balloon with the forceps.

21. Secure the tube as shown in Figure 6–20.

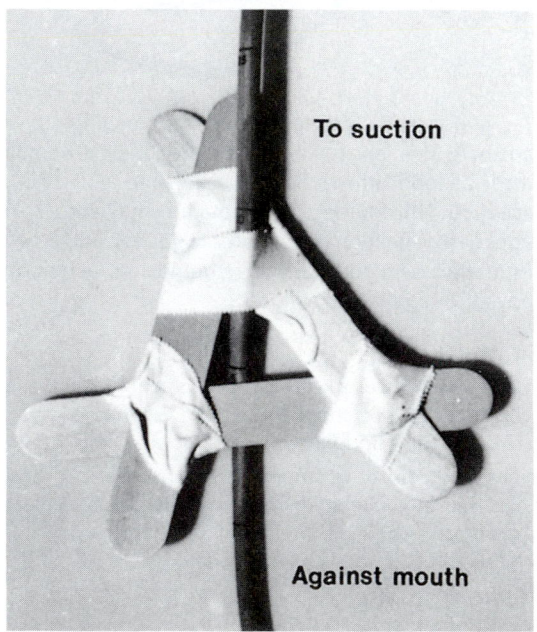

Figure 6–20. Securing tamponade tube using crossed tongue blades. The insertion tube is secured to the corner of the mouth as shown. Foam or gauze may be placed between the triangle and the patient's mouth to prevent damage to gingival mucosa.

22. The pressure in both balloons should be checked every 30 minutes by releasing the rubber-clad clamps on the tube proximal to the Y connector while the tube used for inflation is occluded. This connects the balloon to the manometer for pressure measurement, and air leaks in the balloon can be quickly detected before bleeding recurs. Periodically irrigate and aspirate through the gastric port and through the esophageal port (Minnesota tube) or Salem sump tube (Sengstaken-Blakemore tube) to make sure that no gastric or esophageal bleeding goes undetected.

CRICOTHYROTOMY

Indications

Cricothyrotomy is performed when the airway must be secured or maintained and when attempts at orotracheal or nasotracheal intubation have failed. Transection or fracture of the trachea, larynx, or cricoid cartilage are contraindications. The procedure should not be performed in children younger than age 12 years. Transtracheal jet ventilation (also known as needle cricothyrotomy) is the preferred method for this age group.

Contraindications

Cricothyrotomy is contraindicated when any other less radical means of securing an airway is feasible.

Personnel Required

One person can perform cricothyrotomy unaided, but an assistant is helpful.

Equipment & Supplies Required

Because cricothyrotomy is almost always performed when speed is essential to save the patient's life, presterilized kits containing the required materials should be available in all hospital emergency departments. The following items are required:

- Materials for skin sterilization.
- Materials for sterile technique (cap, mask, gloves, and gown).
- Lidocaine, 1%, with 10-mL syringe and 25-gauge needle.
- Sponges, 10 × 10 cm (4 × 4 in).
- Drapes and rolled bath towel.
- No. 11 scalpel blade, mounted.
- Mosquito clamps (2).
- Kelly clamps (2).
- Self-retaining skin retractors.
- Low-pressure, high-flow orotracheal tube sized to the patient (usually a small [4- to 6-mm] tube is used to fit the small opening) or, if available, low-pressure cuffed tracheostomy tubes of various sizes.
- Syringe, 10-mL, to inflate the balloon on the orotracheal tube.
- Self-refilling bag-valve-mask combination (eg, Ambu bag) or bag-valve unit (eg, Ayres bag), connector, tubing, and oxygen source.
- Tincture of benzoin.
- Tape.

Positioning of the Patient

The patient should be supine, with a rolled bath towel under the shoulders, and the neck hyperextended.

Anatomy Review

The cricothyroid membrane (conus elasticus and cricothyroid ligament) lies between the thyroid cartilage superiorly and the cricoid cartilage inferiorly (Figure 6–21). The membrane is a poorly vascularized ligamentous structure that lies under the subcutaneous tissue between the laterally placed cricothyroid muscles.

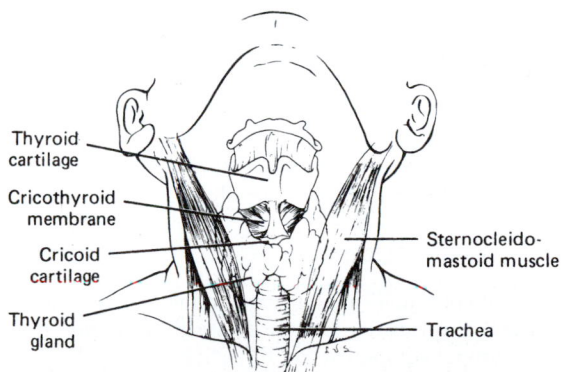

Figure 6–21. Anatomic relationships of cricothyroid membrane. (Reproduced, with permission, from Dunphy JE, Way LW [editors]: *Current Surgical Diagnosis & Treatment*, 5th ed. Lange, 1981.)

Procedure

1. Assemble all necessary equipment.
2. Position the patient.
3. Sterilize the skin of the neck from the chin to the sternal notch and laterally to the base of the neck, if time permits.
4. Observe sterile technique (don cap, mask, gloves, and gown) if time permits.
5. Check the endotracheal tube or tracheostomy tube for cuff leaks by inflating the tube with air from a syringe.
6. Identify the cricothyroid membrane. Using the 10-mL syringe with the 25-gauge needle, infiltrate the skin and underlying cricothyroid membrane with the 1% lidocaine in a line across the membrane while steadying the thyroid cartilage with the left hand. Omit this step if complete airway obstruction is present or if the patient is comatose.
7. Using the No. 11 blade, make a vertical incision in the skin overlying the cricothyroid membrane. Retract the skin with self-retaining retractors and relocate the cricothyroid membrane by palpation.
8. Make a horizontal incision through the cricothyroid membrane. Extend the incision in the cricothyroid membrane for approximately 1 cm on each side of the midline.
9. Using a mosquito or Kelly clamp in the left hand (with the point downward), insert the clamp into the incision and spread it. This maneuver alone is sufficient to provide an airway for a patient with supraglottic airway obstruction.
10. Grasp the endotracheal tube or tracheostomy tube with the right hand, and insert the tube through the incision into the trachea, directing it caudally.
11. Connect the bag-valve unit to the tube, and immediately ventilate the patient with 100% oxygen. Check for respiratory movement of the chest and the presence of bilaterally symmetric breath sounds.
12. Inflate the balloon just enough to stop any audible air leak during the inspiratory phase of positive-pressure ventilation.
13. Cut a 10- × 10-cm (4- × 4-in) gauze sponge halfway down the middle, and wrap it around the tube. If an orotracheal tube is being used, fashion a necklace of adhesive tape, apply tincture of benzoin to the tube, and tape it in place. If a tracheostomy tube is being used, secure the wings of the tube by tying the tapes around the patient's neck, leaving enough slack so that an index finger can easily slide under the tape. Tying the tape too tightly can cause erosion of the skin and venous congestion above the tie, whereas tying it too loosely invites dislodging of the tube.
14. Suction the trachea.
15. Obtain a chest x-ray immediately to check the position of the tube.

TRANSTRACHEAL JET VENTILATION

Indications

Transtracheal jet ventilation (TTJV) is an alternative to cricothyrotomy in patients who require emergency assisted ventilation when conventional methods of endotracheal intubation are not possible.

Contraindications

TTJV is contraindicated if conventional methods of endotracheal intubation can be successfully employed or if the proper equipment for TTJV is not available.

Personnel Required

One person can perform the procedure unaided, although it is helpful to have an assistant to position the patient's head and handle equipment.

Equipment & Supplies Required

- Materials for skin sterilization.
- Sterile gloves.
- Intravenous catheter, 12- or 14-gauge, or 13-gauge cannula designed specifically for TTJV that has lateral flanges to which tape may be attached.
- Bag-valve mask set.
- 50-psi Oxygen source.
- Demand valve device or Y adapter with connectors and tubing that connects to the 50-psi oxygen source.
- Adapter (eg, Luer-Lok) for connecting the demand valve outflow tubing to the catheter (Figure 6–22).
- Tape for securing catheter in place.
- Syringe, 3-mL.

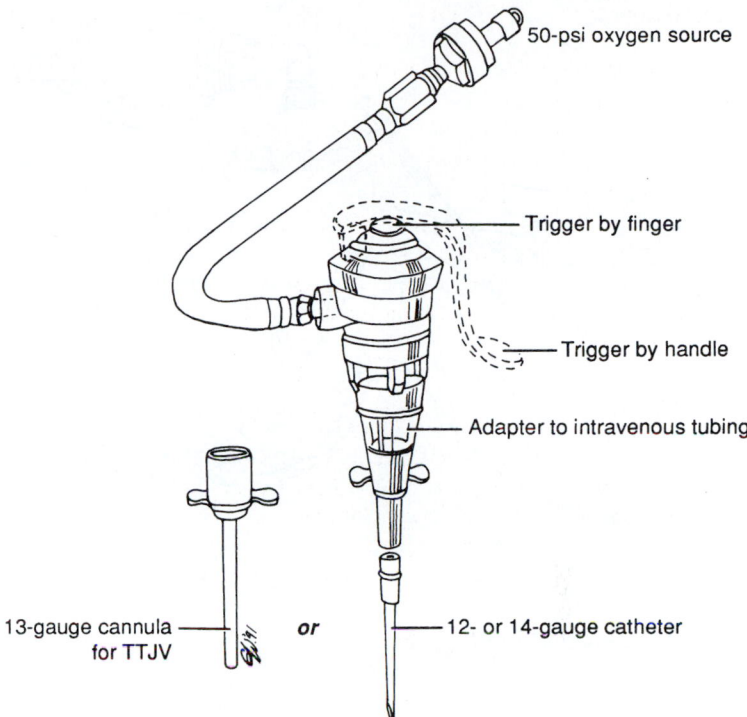

50-psi oxygen source

Trigger by finger

Trigger by handle

Adapter to intravenous tubing

13-gauge cannula for TTJV — *or* — 12- or 14-gauge catheter

Figure 6–22. 50-psi oxygen source is connected via a demand valve to the transtracheal jet ventilator.

Positioning of the Patient

The patient is positioned supine with the head in the midline. It is helpful to have the neck slightly extended unless cervical spine injury is suspected.

Anatomy Review

The cricothyroid membrane is a 1- to 1.5-cm membrane that lies inferior to the thyroid cartilage and superior to the cricoid cartilage. It can be located easily by palpating the protuberant midline portion of the thyroid cartilage ("Adams apple") and then moving the fingertip inferiorly 1.5 cm until it rests in a soft, flat depression between the thyroid cartilage and the cricoid cartilage. The examining fingertip will then be on the cricothyroid membrane.

Procedure

1. Position the head as described above. Have an assistant hold the patient's head or use the tape across the forehead to prevent unexpected motion. If the patient requires assisted ventilation, provide it by a bag-valve-mask device.

2. Prepare the anterior surface of the neck with povidone-iodine.

3. Using sterile gloves, locate the cricothyroid membrane. It may be helpful to place the thumb and index finger of the nondominant hand on either side of the cricothyroid membrane to stabilize the trachea and anchor and stretch the skin slightly.

4. Connect the catheter or cannula to the 3-mL syringe. With the catheter or cannula and syringe in the dominant hand, pierce the skin and cricothyroid membrane at a 45-degree angle, directing the catheter tip inferiorly (Figure 6–23). When the catheter tip enters the tracheal lumen, a slight "give" will be felt. The patient may also cough when the catheter stimulates the tracheal wall. Traction in the syringe plunger during the entry will confirm lumen entry when air is withdrawn freely.

5. Slide the catheter sheath forward until it is snug against the skin, and then withdraw the needle.

6. Connect the inflow tubing on the demand valve or Y adapter to the 50-psi oxygen source and the outflow tubing to the catheter via the adapter. (*Note:* 50 psi may be obtained from a step-down regulator that supplies oxygen to a demand valve or from a venturi flow regulator opened wide to deliver 15 L/min.)

7. Begin ventilation at a rate of 20 breaths per minute, by pressing the button on the demand

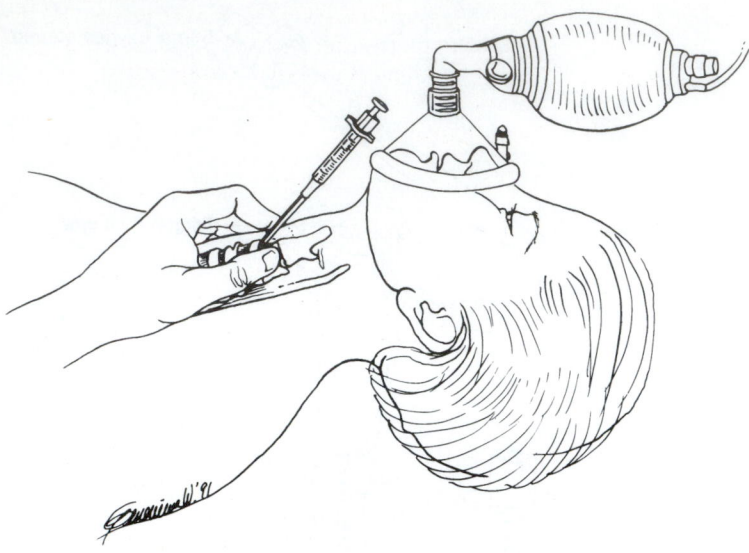

Figure 6–23. Proper orientation for introducing transtracheal catheter. The trachea is stabilized with the hand.

valve, or occluding the open port on the Y adapter, and inflating for 1 second, followed by a 2-second relaxation phase during which the patient will exhale passively through the oropharynx. Be prepared for secretions to be expelled during inflation as well as exhalation.

8. Tape the catheter firmly in place, with the hub of the catheter snug against the neck.

THORACENTESIS

Indications

Indications for thoracentesis are as follows:
- To relieve dyspnea or respiratory distress caused by accumulation of fluid in the pleural space.
- To obtain pleural fluid for diagnostic tests.

Contraindications

Contraindications to thoracentesis are as follows:

- Severe coagulopathy (should be corrected before thoracentesis, unless severe respiratory failure is present, as determined by arterial blood gas analysis).
- Agitated, uncooperative patient (relative contraindication).

Personnel Required

One person can perform thoracentesis unaided.

Equipment & Supplies Required

- Materials for skin sterilization.
- Materials for sterile technique (cap, mask, gloves, and gown).
- Lidocaine, 1%, with 5-ml syringe and 25- or 27-gauge needle.
- Sterile towels (4) or sterile paper drapes.
- Gauze sponges, 10×10 cm (4×4 in).
- Catheter-clad needle (eg, Angiocath), 16- to 18-gauge, 30.5 cm (12 in) long; and 30-mL syringe to aid in insertion.
- Three-way stopcock.
- Luer-Lok syringe, 30-mL.
- Sterile connecting tubing and empty intravenous bottle, or vacuum bottle specially designed for thoracentesis (if removal of more than a few hundred mil-

liliters of fluid is anticipated). The connecting tube should not have a drip chamber.

- Collection vessels and culture media for laboratory analysis.

Positioning of the Patient

Thoracentesis is usually performed with the operator positioned behind the seated patient. Occasionally, thoracentesis must be performed in the lateral position when the patient cannot sit.

For the posterior approach, the patient should be sitting on the edge of the bed or gurney with arms and trunk bent forward over a bedside stand and supported by the elbows or a pillow.

If the lateral approach must be used, have the patient lie at the edge of the bed on the affected side with the ipsilateral arm extended over the head. The midposterior line must be accessible for insertion of the needle. Elevating the head of the bed 30 degrees is sometimes helpful.

Anatomy Review

Access to the pleural space is gained through the intercostal spaces (Figure 6–24). Remember that nerves and blood vessels run on the underside of the rib, and that the domes of the diaphragm are highest posteriorly, occasionally as high as the 7th intercostal space.

Procedure

Position the patient, and prepare all equipment.

A. INITIAL PREPARATION

1. If removing a large volume of fluid, assemble the connecting tubing and a collection vessel.
2. Observe sterile technique (don cap, mask, gloves, and gown) if time permits.
3. Arrange all of the equipment on a sterile field on a Mayo stand or bedside table.
4. Select the thoracentesis site by localizing the level of pleural fluid either by percussion (area of dullness) or ultrasonography. Insert the needle in the intercostal space below the level of fluid in the midposterior line (posterior insertion) or the midaxillary line (lateral insertion).
5. Sterilize a wide area of skin around the proposed insertion site.

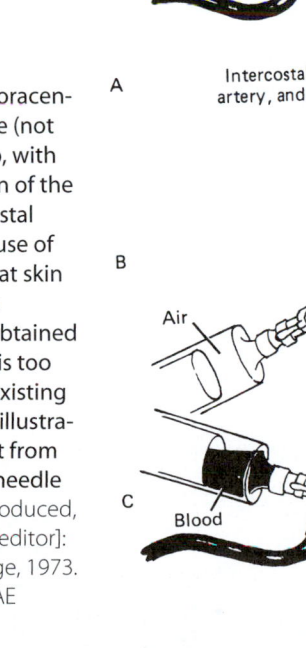
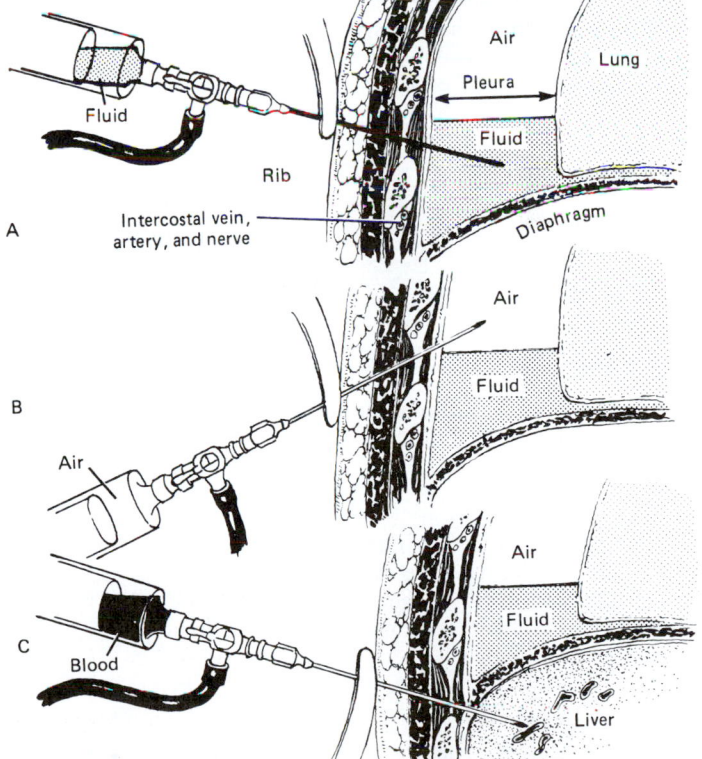

Figure 6–24. Technique of thoracentesis using a regular steel needle (not catheter-clad). **A:** Successful tap, with fluid obtained. Note the position of the needle in relation to the intercostal neurovascular bundle, and the use of the clamp to steady the needle at skin level (do not use a clamp with a catheter-clad needle). **B:** Air is obtained if the position of the needle tip is too high (lung is punctured, or preexisting pneumothorax is entered, as in illustration). **C:** A bloody tap may result from excessively low position of the needle with puncture of the liver. (Reproduced, with permission, from Wilson JL [editor]: *Handbook of Surgery*, 5th ed. Lange, 1973. Redrawn from GE Lindskog and AE Liebow.)

6. Drape the patient (this may be impossible if the patient is sitting).

7. Anesthetize the skin over the insertion site with the 1% lidocaine with the 25- or 27-gauge needle and 5-mL syringe. Then anesthetize the superior surface of the rib and the parietal pleura.

B. CATHETER-CLAD NEEDLE (EG, ANGIOCATH) INSERTION

1. Attach a 30-mL syringe to the catheter-clad needle, and insert the needle through the skin over the rib selected. Advance the needle until it hits the rib.

2. Move the tip of the needle cephalad over the edge of the rib until it encounters the superior aspect of the rib.

3. Have the patient take a deep breath and hold it against a closed glottis.

4. Advance the needle over the superior surface of the rib and through the pleura into the pleural space. Maintain constant suction on the syringe so that the pleural fluid will enter the syringe instantly when the pleural space is entered. Apply controlled, gentle, steady pressure with both hands steadied on the patient's back to keep from suddenly spearing the lung. Do not use a Kelly clamp to grip a catheter-clad needle.

5. When the catheter has entered the pleural space, angle the needle caudally, and push the catheter off the needle and into the base of the pleural space.

6. Occlude the lumen of the catheter, and have the patient exhale and breathe normally.

7. Have the patient take a deep breath again and hold it; insert the 3-way stopcock into the catheter hub. Make sure that the stopcock valve is set to occlude the catheter port. Have the patient resume normal breathing.

8. Connect the 30-mL Luer-Lok syringe to one port of the 3-way stopcock and (if needed) the intravenous tubing to the other.

9. Turn the stopcock valve to connect the syringe with the catheter, and withdraw fluid from the pleural space. Then turn the stopcock so as to connect the syringe to the intravenous tubing, and empty the syringe through the tubing into the intravenous bag or bottle. The first syringeful of fluid may be reserved for diagnostic tests.

10. Withdraw as much fluid as possible but no more than 1 L at one time. In order to completely evacuate the pleural space, the patient may have to be rocked from side to side while fluid is being withdrawn.

11. When no more fluid can be withdrawn, the patient should take a deep breath and hold it while the catheter is quickly withdrawn. Cover the insertion site with a sterile occlusive dressing.

12. Obtain an upright portable chest x-ray to check for possible pneumothorax and residual fluid.

TUBE THORACOSTOMY (Insertion of a Chest Tube)

Indications

Tube thoracostomy is performed in order to drain air or fluid from the pleural space.

Contraindications

There are no absolute contraindications to chest tube insertion. Usually, the patient is in distress, and any relative contraindication (eg, coagulopathy) is superseded by the need to reinflate a compressed lung or drain fluid from the lungs.

Personnel Required

One operator can insert a chest tube alone; however, an assistant is helpful.

Equipment & Supplies Required

Most hospitals have sterile thoracostomy trays ready for use. If a tray is not available, assemble the following instruments and materials:

- Materials for skin sterilization.
- Materials for sterile technique (cap, mask, gloves, and gown).
- Lidocaine, 1%, with 10-mL syringe and 25- and 22-gauge needles.
- Sterile towels (4) or sterile paper drapes.
- Chest tube of the appropriate size and style to suit the clinical situation (see below).
- No. 11 surgical blade, mounted.
- Mayo clamp.

- Kelly clamp.
- Surgical silk suture (size 0) with large curved cutting needle.
- Needle holder.
- Petrolatum-impregnated gauze.
- Sterile gauze sponges, 10 × 10 cm (4 × 4 in).
- Plastic adhesive tape, 5 cm (2 in) wide.
- Suction apparatus, 3-bottle, with water-seal, collection, and water-column sections (Figure 6–25). In the United States, this device is usually supplied as a unit with tall connectors and tubes included (eg, Pleur-evac).
- Sterile Y connector (if 2 chest tubes are to be connected to the same suction apparatus).

Positioning of the Patient

Tubes are usually inserted laterally when fluid, pus, or blood is drained, irrespective of whether air is also being removed. The patient should lie with the affected side up, and the ipsilateral arm extended over the head and grasping the top of the bed or the guardrail for security.

Rarely, chest tubes are inserted anteriorly to evacuate a pure pneumothorax. The patient should be supine, with the head raised about 10 degrees. Position the bed or gurney at a comfortable height to prevent back strain for the operator.

Anatomy Review

See Anatomy Review under Thoracentesis, above. Remember that the intercostal arteries and veins follow the inferior border of the rib.

Procedure

1. Prepare all necessary equipment, and arrange it on a sterile towel placed on a Mayo stand or bedside table.
2. Select the proper chest tube for insertion. In patients with trauma, insert the largest tube available (usually 36–40F). In patients without trauma, use a 26–32F chest tube, either straight or curved. In a patient with pure pneumothorax, a smaller chest tube (12–20F) is usually sufficient. A general rule is that a large tube effectively drains any substance from the pleural space and thus is preferred in emergencies, when the diagnosis may be unclear.
3. Assemble the suction apparatus according to the manufacturer's directions.
4. Connect the suction apparatus to a wall suction outlet, and adjust the suction so that a steady stream of bubbles is produced in the water column.
5. Position the patient.
6. Determine the insertion site. Most tubes are inserted in the lateral thorax at the anterior axillary line, just lateral to the nipple. This places the tube in the 4th or 5th intercostal space, ensuring that it is above the dome of the diaphragm. Palpate the nearest rib, and double-check the position; liver or spleen laceration can occur if the patient is not properly positioned.
7. Observing sterile technique, open the sterile instrument tray, arrange all necessary instruments, and make sure that everything is present.
8. Sterilize the skin over the insertion site and a wide area around it.
9. Again locate the rib for the insertion site, and anesthetize the skin over the mid to inferior aspect of the rib with the 1% lidocaine with the 10-mL syringe and 25-gauge needle. Then anesthetize the surface of the rib and the tissue superior to it with the 22-gauge needle.
10. Drape the area around the insertion site.
11. Using the No. 11 blade, make a horizontal incision through the skin along the inferior aspect of the rib. The incision should be about 1½ times as wide as the tube selected. Incise the skin down to the subcutaneous tissue.
12. Use the Mayo clamp with the tips down as a dissector. Spread the tips to open tissue planes, and create a tunnel aiming toward the superior aspect of the rib. Make sure the clamp stays next to the rib.
13. When the Mayo clamp is just over the superior edge of the rib, close the clamp, and push it with steady pressure through the parietal pleura and into the chest. This maneuver requires more pressure than might be anticipated. Use steady, even, controlled pressure to provide control of the clamp after it has perforated the pleura. A lunging motion may cause a hole in the lung, liver, or spleen.

    Once the clamp has penetrated the pleural space, air, fluid, blood, or pus may escape during expiration. Tension pneumothorax will whistle as air escapes under pressure, and the lung will collapse further during inspiration, because free air has access to the pleural space.
14. Widen the hole in the parietal pleura by spreading the Mayo clamp.
15. If a tube of large diameter is to be inserted, use the index finger to dilate the tract and hole in the pleura. This maneuver also ensures that entry has been made into the pleural space and not into a

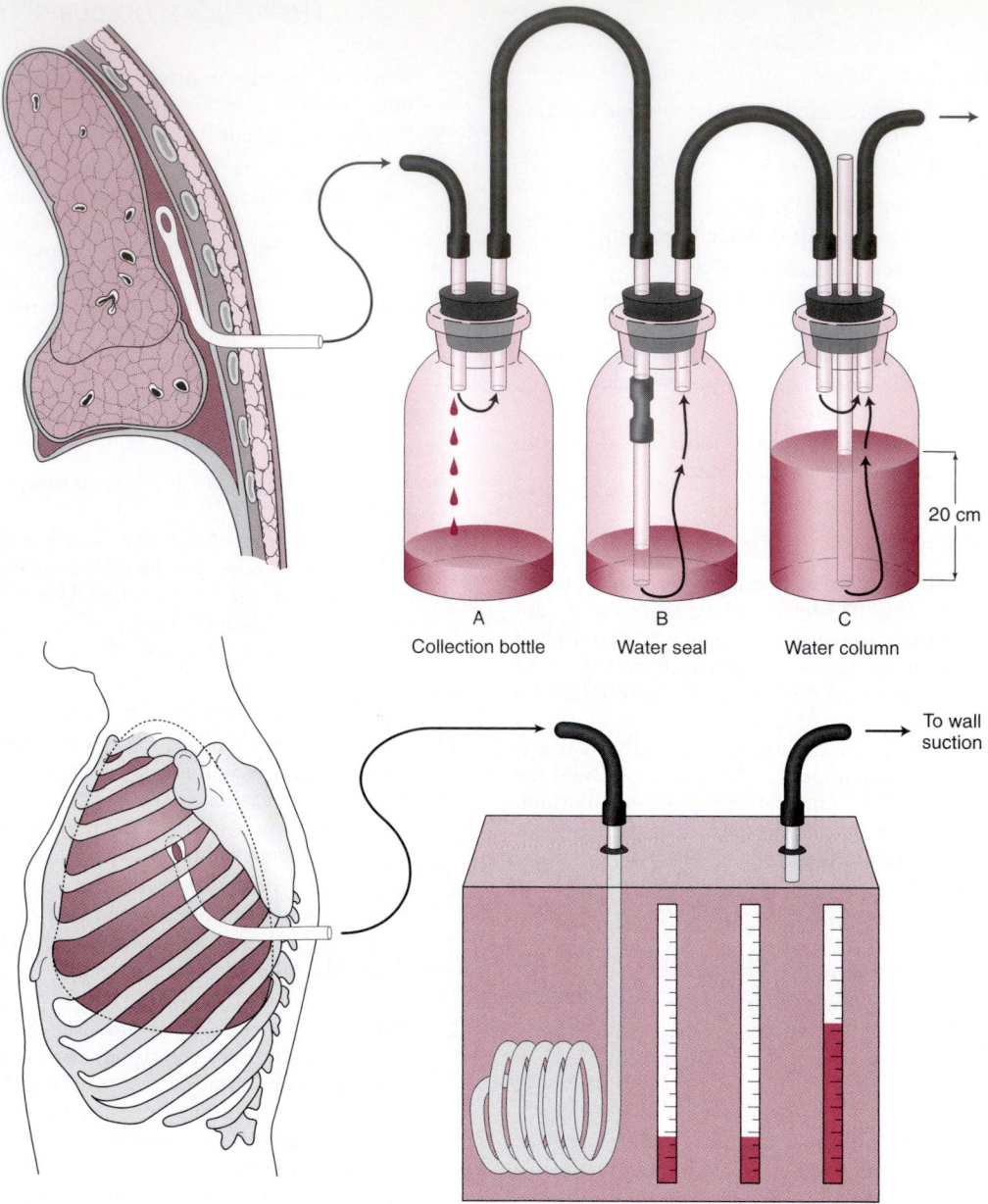

A
Collection bottle

B
Water seal

C
Water column

20 cm

To wall
suction

Commercial thorolostomy tube drainage system

Figure 6–25. Diagram of tube thoracostomy and 3-bottle suction apparatus. **Bottle A** is connected to the thoracostomy tube and collects pleural drainage for inspection and measurement of volume. **Bottle B** acts as a simple valve to prevent collapse of the lung if tubing distal to this point is opened to atmospheric pressure. Pulmonary air leak can be detected by the escape of bubbles from the submerged tube. **Bottle C** is a system for regulating the negative pressure delivered to the pleural space. Wall suction should be regulated to maintain continuous vigorous bubbling from the middle open tube in bottle C. The resulting negative pressure (in cm H_2O) is equal to the difference in the height of the fluid levels in bottles B and C. The Pleur-evac system works in a similar manner. One end is attached to the chest tube and the other end is attached to suction. Each chamber of the Pleur-Evac is filled with sterile water to the level noted in the manufacturer's instructions. (Reproduced, with permission, from Dunphy JE, Way LW [editors]: *Current Surgical Diagnosis & Treatment,* 5th ed. Lange, 1981.)

space inadvertently created between the parietal pleural and the chest wall.

16. Grasp the end of the chest tube along the index finger and guide the tube down the tract into the pleural space, making sure that the last hole in the chest tube is within the pleural space. If a curved tube is being used, direct it inferiorly so that it lies along the base of the pleural space. A straight tube may be positioned inferiorly, laterally, or superiorly, depending on the clinical situation.

17. Connect the chest tube to the suction apparatus, and make sure that the level in the water column varies with respiration. Usually, fluid, blood, or pus drains from the tube, a sign that the tube is properly positioned in the pleural space (unless the tube was inserted for pure pneumothorax). *Note:* If the tube has been inadvertently inserted between the parietal pleural and the chest wall, no fluid will drain from the tube, and the level in the water column will not vary with respiration.

18. Sew the tube to the chest wall with the silk suture. Partially close the incision with a mattress stitch, and use one throw of a square knot to close the skin around the tube. Then, wind both ends of the suture around the tube, starting at the bottom and working toward the top (as if lacing up a shoe). Tie the ends of the suture snugly around the top of the tube.

19. Wrap Xeroform or petrolatum-impregnated gauze around the tube to seal it to the skin. Cover the tube with two 10- × 10-cm (4- × 4-in) sterile gauze sponges, cut so that they fit around the tube. Tape the sponges and the tube in place. Tape connections of the chest tube to the suction tube, and tape the chest tube to the patient's side below the insertion site.

20. Obtain a portable upright chest x-ray to check the position of the tube and to make sure that the lung is expanded and that all fluid has been evacuated.

Emergency Thoracotomy (See Chapter 24.)

Emergency thoracotomy is performed to gain access to the heart and great vessels. It can occasionally be life saving, although controversy exists over the indications and the location where it should be performed. It should be performed only when the patient can be taken immediately afterward to the operating room.

Indications

1. Traumatic cardiac arrest following penetrating chest trauma with signs of life in the prehospital setting (survival rate up to 40%).

2. Traumatic cardiac arrest following penetrating or blunt trauma with signs of life in the emergency department (low survival rate for blunt trauma victims).
3. Cardiac tamponade with profound shock; patient is unresponsive to rapid volume expansion, is deteriorating, and is unlikely to survive until operation.
4. Blunt or penetrating trauma to the chest or abdomen with profound shock; patient is unresponsive to rapid volume expansion, is deteriorating, and is unlikely to survive until operation.
5. Massive chest or abdominal bleeding with profound shock; patient is unresponsive to rapid volume expansion, is deteriorating, and is unlikely to survive until operation.

Contraindications

1. Traumatic cardiac arrest with no signs of life in the prehospital setting (survival rate virtually nil).
2. Appropriate operating facilities and personnel not immediately available.
3. Patient immediately responsive to volume expansion or decompression of tension pneumothorax.

Personnel Required

One individual experienced in the technique is required to perform the procedure, another to maintain an airway and assist ventilation, and, ideally, a third to prepare and hand equipment to the operator. In most cases, patients have multiple, concomitant needs that are best met by a team.

Equipment & Supplies Required

- Materials for skin sterilization.
- Sterile drapes.
- Scalpel with No. 10 blades.
- Rib spreaders.
- Vascular clamps.
- Nonvascular clamps.
- Suture scissors.
- Metzenbaum scissors (long).
- Needle holder (long).
- Suture (2-0 silk or comparable) on cutting needle.
- 10-in DeBakey tangential occlusion clamp.
- Suction catheter.
- Tissue forceps.
- Bone rongeur.
- Rib approximator.

Positioning of the Patient

The patient should be supine. Place rolled sheet under the left scapula and lower ribs, and elevate the left arm above the head to expose the left chest and axilla. The patient should be intubated and ventilated with positive pressure (manual bag-valve method or mechanical ventilator). Advance the endotracheal tube to selectively intubate the right main-stem bronchus. This allows the left lung to be manually collapsed providing access to the heart. Remember to decrease tidal volumes by half and increase the respiratory rate to compensate for ventilation of a single lung.

Anatomy Review

The favored approach to the heart in an emergency setting is through a left thoracotomy. The incision follows the rib interspace, with care taken to avoid the intercostal vessels that run beneath each rib. The internal mammary artery runs parallel to the lateral margin of the sternum and must be ligated should hemorrhage from this vessel occur.

Procedure

1. Prepare the anterior thoracic surface generously on both sides with skin-sterilizing solution, and cover it with sterile drapes to the extent that time allows.

2. Using the No. 10 scalpel blade, make a horizontal incision in the left 4th or 5th intercostal space, extending from the sternum to the posterior axillary line. It should be deep enough to expose the intercostal muscles and should follow the superior rib margin to avoid injury to the intercostal vascular bundle beneath the rib above. In women, make the incision beneath the breast.

3. With a scalpel or scissors, make a small opening through the intercostal muscles into the pleural space. Using Metzenbaum scissors, divide the intercostal muscles the entire length of the incision, remaining close to the superior margin of the rib. Ligate the internal mammary artery above and below. Using the scalpel or heavy scissors, cut through 2 sternocostal cartilages above the interspace.

4. Insert a rib spreader and spread the ribs as widely apart as possible. If necessary (eg, in penetrating trauma to the right chest), the incision may be extended across the sternum and into the right chest to increase exposure.

5. Inspect the heart. It will appear to be bluish if cardiac tamponade is present. To relieve tamponade or perform cardiac massage, open the pericardium. Pick up the pericardium with forceps and incise it from apex to base, using Metzenbaum scissors. Be careful to avoid the phrenic nerve, which courses longitudinally along the lateral heart margin. Remove any clotted blood; suction excess blood as needed.

6. If observable cardiac contractions are inadequate, or if cardiac arrest has occurred, perform internal cardiac massage by gently compressing the heart with both hands. If ventricular fibrillation is present, a quivering motion will be observed. Perform defibrillation using the internal paddles, at an energy level of 5–50 J. If a myocardial laceration is present, it can be temporarily controlled with a fingertip or with a 3-0 polypropylene suture. Horizontal mattress sutures through Teflon pledgets will help prevent further laceration of the myocardium. Place sutures through the epicardium and myocardium only. Avoid the coronary arteries. Atrial wounds can be repaired with simple interrupted sutures.

7. Control massive bleeding from the lung or pulmonary vessels by cross-clamping the hilum of the involved lung.

8. If the patient fails to respond rapidly to volume administration, or if intra-abdominal bleeding is suspected, incise the overlying pleural and cross-clamp the aorta above the point where it enters the diaphragm. Be careful to avoid clamping the esophagus. As a temporary measure during internal cardiac massage, the aorta may be occluded with the index and long fingers placed behind the heart.

9. If resuscitation is successful, immediately transport the patient to the operating room for definitive care.

PERICARDIOCENTESIS

Blind aspiration of the pericardium was formerly the only way to detect and treat a pericardial effusion. Complications of this technique included pneumothorax, myocardial or coronary artery laceration, and iatrogenic pericardial tamponade. Many emergency departments currently utilize bedside ultrasound to detect pericardial effusion. Ultrasound is quick, noninvasive, and can even provide guidance for pericardiocentesis in the symptomatic patient with pericardial effusion. Blind pericardiocentesis should be reserved for those situations in which a critically ill patient is suspected of having tamponade and no diagnostic tests are rapidly available to assist in the diagnosis or treatment.

Indications

The following description of pericardiocentesis assumes bedside emergency ultrasound or echocardiography are not rapidly available to evaluate and treat a suspected pericardial tamponade.

Contraindications

In a patient who requires pericardiocentesis for decompensated or rapidly decompensating cardiac tamponade, there are no contraindications. In other patients, the following conditions are contraindications:

- Infection along the proposed course of pericardiocentesis.
- Bleeding diathesis (relative contraindication, especially if it can be corrected).

Personnel Required

Three people are required to perform pericardiocentesis: the operator and an assistant to monitor the electrocardiograph, and another physician besides the operator. A cardiothoracic surgeon should be available in case complications occur.

Equipment & Supplies Required

Many hospitals have prepackaged sterile pericardiocentesis trays that contain many of the required items. If these are not available, the following instruments and materials are required:

- Materials for skin sterilization.
- Materials for sterile technique (cap, mask, gloves, and gown).
- Lidocaine, 1%, with 10-mL syringe and 25-gauge needle.
- Pericardiocentesis needle: 17-gauge, 12.5-cm (5-in) thin-walled steel needle (usually a spinal needle) for aspiration. It is possible to use 16-gauge and even 14-gauge needles with plastic outer cannulas.
- Syringes: assorted sizes, including 50-mL (2), 30-mL (2), 10-mL (2), and 5-mL (1).
- No. 11 scalpel blade, mounted.
- Sterile conductive monitoring cable with alligator clamps at each end.

- Three-way stopcock.
- Silk suture (5-0) on a cutting needle.
- Straight clamp and needle holder.
- Needles: assorted sizes, including 25-gauge, 1.5-cm (⅝-in) (1); 22-gauge, 2.5-cm (1-in) (2); and 19-gauge, 4-cm (1½-in) (5), for transferring specimens.
- Drapes.
- Sterile, capped, 15-mL specimen tubes (10).
- Heparin, to lightly heparinize cytologic specimen tubes.
- Specimen tubes, 1 purple-topped and 3 red-topped.
- Clean glass microscope slides.
- Microhematocrit centrifuge tubes with occlusive sealant.
- Ice bucket to hold cytologic specimens.
- Sterile dressing for entry and exit sites.
- CPR cart and equipment and electrocardiograph.

Positioning of the Patient

The patient should be supine, and if time permits, the thorax should be elevated 30 degrees. Optimize bed height and lighting for the operator.

Procedure

A. PATIENT PREPARATION

Take the following steps, if time permits:

1. The patient should be in a bed where cardiac monitoring is available, preferably in a cardiac catheterization laboratory.
2. Position the patient, as described above.
3. Begin electrocardiographic monitoring with limb leads.
4. Gain secure intravenous access.
5. Give atropine, 0.6–1 mg intramuscularly or subcutaneously, before pericardiocentesis, because vagal responses during cardiac tamponade may be devastating.
6. Narcotics may be used as long as they do not depress consciousness or respiration.
7. Supplemental oxygen, 5-10 L/min, by mask or nasal cannula is advisable.

B. OBSERVE STERILE TECHNIQUE

1. Don cap, mask gloves, and gown.
2. Sterilize the skin in a wide area around the xiphoid process.
3. Drape the field widely with sterile towels if time permits.

C. Begin Pericardiocentesis

1. Locate the appropriate site to the right of and below the xiphoid process (Figure 6–26), and anesthetize the skin with the 1% lidocaine with the 10-mL syringe and 25-gauge needle. Switch to the 22-gauge needle, and anesthetize the tissue beneath the xiphoid process along the track of the pericardiocentesis needle. Omit this step if the patient is comatose.

2. A small incision in the skin with the No. 11 scalpel blade may facilitate entry of the pericardiocentesis needle.

3. With the help of an assistant, attach the conductive monitoring cable to the chest terminal lead of the electrocardiograph using one of the alligator clamps. Attach the other end to the hub of the pericardiocentesis needle. Operate the electrocardiograph on the V lead setting. The pericardiocentesis needle then becomes a probing electrocardiographic lead.

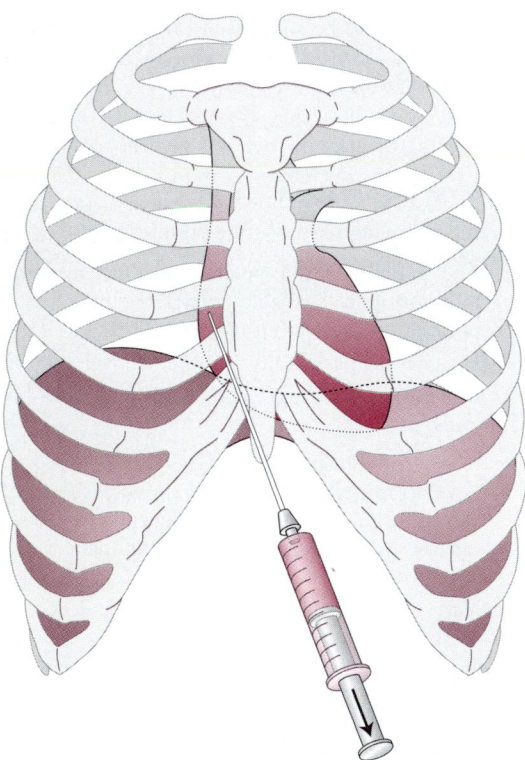

Figure 6–26. Diagram of pericardiocentesis showing position of needle and anatomic relationships. (Reproduced, with permission, from Way LW [editor]: *Current Surgical Diagnosis & Treatment,* 9th ed. Appleton & Lange, 1991.)

4. With the alligator clamp and conductive monitoring cable mounted, attach the pericardiocentesis needle to a 30-mL syringe.

5. Perform pericardiocentesis. If this procedure is being done during active CPR, make sure that everything is ready beforehand, work rapidly, and stop CPR for only as long as necessary. Enter the selected site, just caudal and to the right of the xiphoid process, and direct the needle at an angle of 30–45 degrees to the skin. Aim toward the patient's right shoulder. Advance the needle slowly, and aspirate the fluid continuously. There is usually a palpable feeling of resistance when the needle pierces the parietal pericardium.

   If the attempt to penetrate the pericardium is unsuccessful and no fluid is aspirated, bring the needle back to the subcutaneous tissue, and direct it more medially. Continue either until fluid is aspirated or until the needle hits the right side of the sternum, at which point it is safer to use fluoroscopic or echocardiographic guidance.

   Pericardial aspiration by an anterior left intercostal approach (usually the 4th left intercostal space just left of the sternum) is less satisfactory because it penetrates the pleural space and has a potential for laceration of the left anterior descending coronary artery or a branch of the internal mammary artery. This approach may be used as a last resort in a dying patient.

6. Have an assistant continuously monitoring the electrocardiograph during the procedure. When fluid is aspirated and is flowing freely, the needle can be anchored at the chest wall with a surgical clamp to keep it from penetrating any farther. A myocardial current of injury or precipitation of arrhythmias on the electrocardiograph is a sign to slowly withdraw the needle until fluid is aspirated. In cardiac tamponade due to pericardial hemorrhage, the fact that pericardial blood does not clot (whereas intracardiac blood does) may be a helpful diagnostic clue.

7. Aspirate until the pericardium is dry by slowly withdrawing fluid under constant electrocardiographic monitoring. Secure any specimens that are required for diagnostic tests. In the presence of decompensated cardiac tamponade, removal of even a small amount of pericardial fluid should result in a dramatic improvement in the patient's hemodynamic status.

8. After aspiration is completed, withdraw the needle, and gain hemostasis with pressure. A single suture may be required.

9. Cover the entry site with a sterile dressing.

FOCUSED ASSESSMENT WITH SONOGRAPHY FOR TRAUMA

Focused assessment with sonography for trauma (FAST) is a rapid, noninvasive technique for determining the presence of intra-abdominal fluid (eg, blood or urine) in the trauma victim. It does not detect retroperitoneal fluid collections or hollow viscus injury such as bowel perforation. The FAST exam is a quick screening tool and should be performed after the primary survey of the trauma victim.

Indications

- Blunt thoracoabdominal trauma.
- Penetrating thoracoabdominal trauma.
- Suspected pericardial tamponade.
- Undetermined origin of hypotension in trauma patient.

Contraindications

The FAST exam is contraindicated in the unstable trauma victim who requires immediate surgery.

Personnel Required

One operator can perform a FAST exam unaided.

Equipment & Supplies Required

- Ultrasound transmission gel (hypoallergenic).
- Ultrasound machine with 2.5- to 7.0-MHz transducer. Higher frequency allows for better resolution; however, a 3.5-MHz transducer is usually adequate for FAST exams performed on the adult trauma victim.
- An attached printer that allows images viewed to be transferred to photographic paper for documentation.

Positioning of the Patient

The patient should be supine on a level surface. Reverse-Trendelenburg position increases the sensitivity in the suprapubic view.

Anatomy Review

FAST exams evaluate fluid collections in 4 anatomic locations. In the chest, the pericardial sac is viewed. In the abdomen, the Morison pouch in the right upper quadrant, the splenorenal recess in the left upper quadrant, and the pouch of Douglas in the suprapubic area

are viewed. To optimally view the pelvis, a full bladder is required. When a Foley catheter is inserted before or during the FAST exam, remember to have the Foley drainage tubing clamped so as not to decompress the bladder. The distended bladder provides a good "acoustic window" to identify free fluid in the pelvis.

Procedure

1. Set up the ultrasound machine for FAST exams as instructed by the machine's manufacturer.
2. Enter the patient's name and medical record number using the machine's annotation keys.
3. Expose the patient's thoracoabdominal area and place ultrasound transmission gel in the following 4 locations: pericardial area, right upper quadrant, left upper quadrant, and suprapubic area (Figure 6–27).
4. Orient the transducer for sagittal sections of the body and place it in the subxiphoid region. This view identifies pericardial fluid collections.
5. Next, place the transducer on the right midaxillary region between the 4th and 5th ribs to view the Morison pouch. Keep the transducer in the intercostal space to avoid shadows created by the ribs.
6. Move the transducer, still in the sagittal plane, to the left posterior axillary line between the 9th and 11th ribs to view the splenorenal recess.
7. Finally, place the transducer, now oriented for the transverse view, about 4–5 cm superior to the pubic symphysis in the midline to view the pouch of Douglas.
8. Each view should be frozen on screen and printed. This documentation should be placed with the patient's medical record. Performing and interpreting FAST exams is not a difficult procedure, but it requires hands-on training, which should be undertaken by any emergency physician wishing to become prolific in its use.

Limitations

A FAST exam is helpful when the findings are positive; however, a negative study must be evaluated further (eg, with computed tomography [CT] scan, repeat evaluations, observation). A falsely negative FAST exam can result from several factors:

- Too little time has elapsed since the trauma for the blood to accumulate.

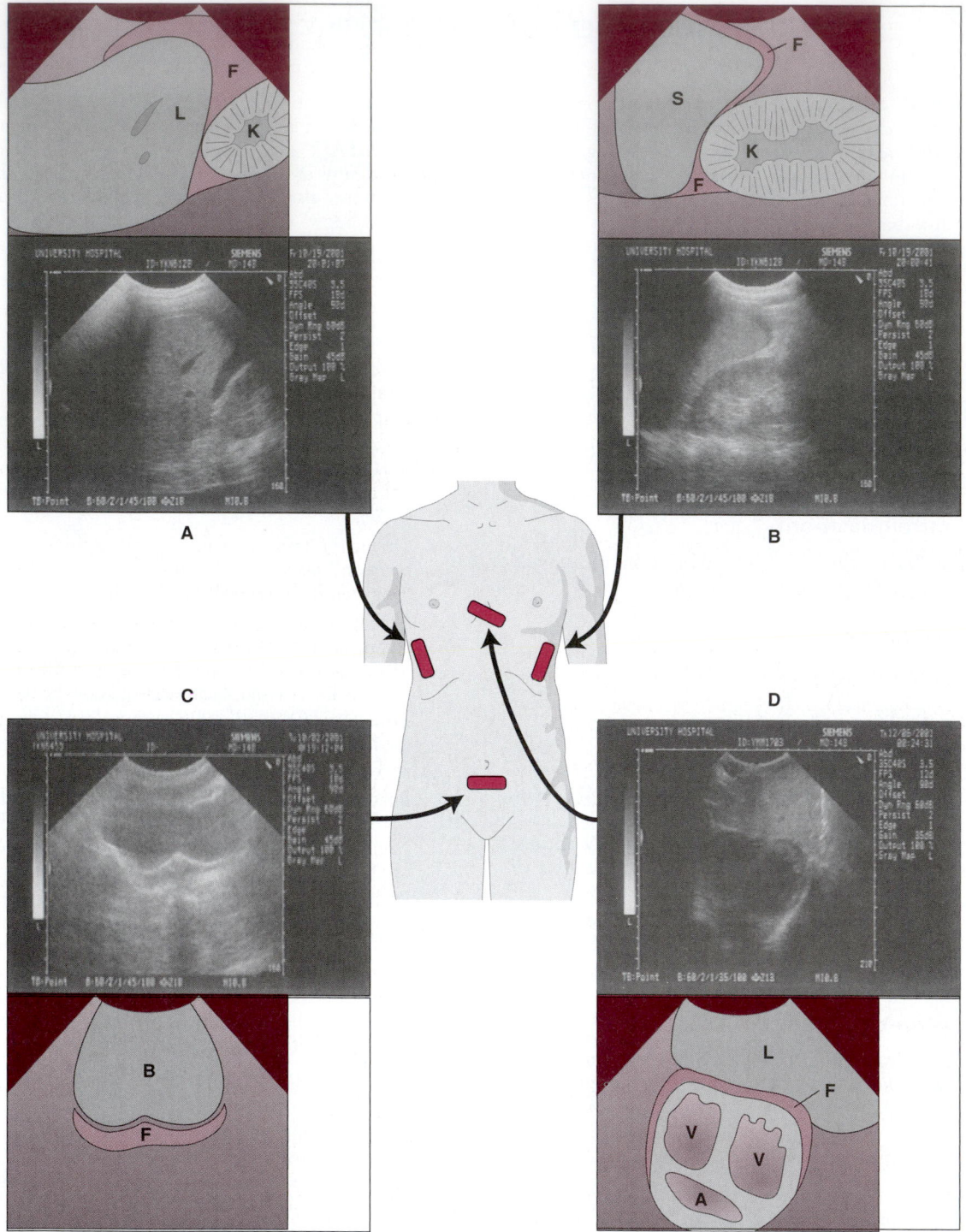

Figure 6–27. Illustration of the 4 views for the FAST exam and where fluid would be seen in each view. A = atrium; B = bladder; F = fluid; K = kidney; L = liver; S = spleen; V = ventricle.

- Bleeding may be retroperitoneal and not visible on FAST exam.
- Solid organ injury with encapsulated bleeding is present.

- Hollow viscus injury is present.
- Inadequate volume of fluid. As little as 50 cc of fluid can be detected; however, it may take up to 250 cc of fluid to create an unequivocally positive FAST exam.

ABDOMINAL PARACENTESIS

Indications

Indications for abdominal paracentesis are as follows:

- To determine the cause of ascites, including suspected intra-abdominal hemorrhage from trauma.
- To lower intra-abdominal pressure in tense ascites (rarely indicated in the emergency department).
- To obtain fluid for analysis and culture in patients with ascites who are thought to have an infection.

Contraindications

The following conditions are relative contraindications to abdominal paracentesis, and most can be corrected or circumvented if paracentesis must be performed:

- Bleeding diathesis (coagulopathy or thrombocytopenia). Correct severe bleeding diathesis before performing paracentesis. Cautious paracentesis with a 22-gauge needle may be safely performed in patients with mild to moderate bleeding tendencies.
- Previous abdominal surgery.
- Severe bowel distention (correct with nasogastric suction and a rectal tube before performing paracentesis).

Personnel Required

One person can perform paracentesis unaided if the patient is cooperative. An assistant may be helpful if the patient is obese.

Equipment & Supplies Required

- Materials for skin sterilization.
- Materials for sterile technique (cap, mask, gloves, and gown).
- Lidocaine, 1%, with 10-mL syringe and 22- and 25-gauge needles.
- Needles in various sizes, including a longer 20- or 22-gauge spinal needle and a 19-gauge catheter-clad needle (eg, Angiocath). Use a 22-gauge, 4-cm (1½-in) needle or spinal needle in patients with severe bleeding diathesis.

- Syringe, 50-mL.
- Drapes.
- Specimen tubes, both with and without anticoagulant, and a blood culture bottle.
- Ice bucket for cytology specimens.
- Gauze sponges, 10 × 10 cm (4 × 4 in).
- Topical antibacterial ointment.
- Tape and dressing material.
- Three-way stopcock, connector tubing, and 500-mL collection bottle (if therapeutic paracentesis is planned).

Positioning of the Patient

Have the patient supine at the edge of the bed nearest the operator (right side of the bed for a right-handed operator), with the trunk elevated 45 degrees. Allow 10 minutes for ascites to pool in the dependent portion of the abdomen and for air-filled bowel to float up away from the puncture site. Be sure the bladder has been emptied by voiding or catheterization.

The patient can be tipped 30 degrees to either side if paracentesis of the lower quadrants is necessary. Limited ascites can be aspirated successfully by having the patient bridge 2 beds or a bed and a chair on hands and knees. The approach in this case (a somewhat cramped one for the operator) is from below upward into the dependent abdomen.

Procedure

1. Observe sterile technique (don cap, mask, gloves, and gown).
2. Sterilize the skin between the umbilicus and symphysis pubica and both lower quadrants.
3. Drape the field widely.
4. Using the 25-gauge needle, anesthetize the skin with the 1% lidocaine in the 10-mL syringe at the selected puncture site. The preferred site is on the poorly vascularized linea alba, about halfway between the symphysis pubica and the umbilicus (Figure 6–28). Change to the 22-gauge needle,

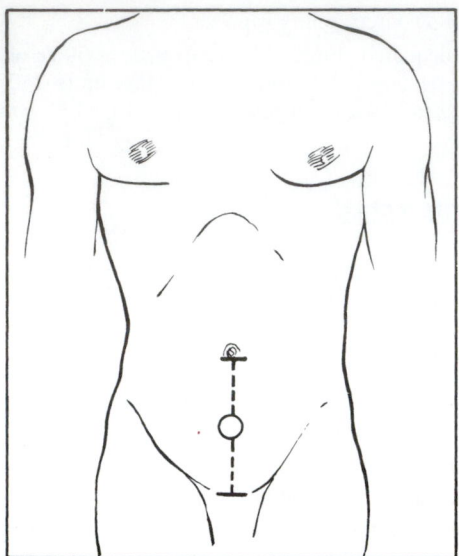

Figure 6–28. Insertion site for abdominal paracentesis. (Reproduced, with permission, from Dunphy JE, Way LW [editors]: *Current Surgical Diagnosis & Treatment*, 5th ed. Lange, 1981.)

and anesthetize down to and including the peritoneum.

5. Attach the 19-gauge catheter-clad needle to a 50-mL syringe. In patients with severe coagulopathy and thrombocytopenia, use a 22-gauge needle. In markedly obese patients, use a 20-gauge spinal needle.

6. Puncture the skin. Keeping the needle perpendicular to the abdominal wall, maintain continuous negative suction in the syringe while slowly advancing the needle. In tense ascites, it may be useful to try Z-tracking the needle to minimize persistent leaking of ascitic fluid; that is, after

penetrating the skin, move the needle and syringe 1–2 cm (⅜–¾ in) before piercing the subcutaneous tissue, but maintain the perpendicular approach. Repeat this maneuver at the level of the peritoneum, thus describing an oblique Z pattern through the various layers of tissue. In this manner, the track of the needle from the skin to the peritoneal space will not be a continuous line when the needle is removed.

7. The dense connective tissue of the peritoneum will yield a noticeable "pop" when pierced.

8. Fluid should flow freely into the syringe. To avoid bowel or visceral trauma, particularly in patients with bleeding tendencies, it is preferable to remove the steel needle, leaving the plastic catheter in place while specimens are collected. The patient can be safely moved into more dependent positions with the plastic catheter in place to facilitate draining of sufficient fluid for analysis. In most cases of diagnostic paracentesis, a single collection of 50 mL is adequate. At a minimum, fluid should be sent to the laboratory for cell count, tests for protein, cultures, and staining with Gram stain. For suspected neoplasia or for therapeutic relief of tense ascites, up to 1 L may be removed, although 750 mL is a more prudent upper limit in order to avoid adverse effects on intravascular volume. A 3-way stopcock can be used to minimize leakage while the operator is continually aspirating with a syringe. Alternatively, drainage can go directly into sterile 250- to 500-mL vacuum containers using connecting tubing.

9. After samples have been collected, remove the catheter or needle, and apply firm pressure to the site for 5 minutes.

10. Apply topical antibacterial ointment, and dress the site with a pressure dressing.

11. If leaking of ascitic fluid persists despite a pressure dressing, close the paracentesis tract with a mattress stitch.

PERITONEAL CATHETER INSERTION & PERITONEAL LAVAGE

Indications

Peritoneal lavage is performed to determine if intraperitoneal hemorrhage has occurred. With the proliferation of CT scanning and FAST exams, peritoneal lavage is used less frequently; however, it continues to have a role in evaluation of the trauma victim when the victim is too unstable to be sent for CT scan or if ultrasound is inconclusive.

Contraindications

Contraindications to peritoneal lavage are as follows:

• Previous intra-abdominal surgery of any kind.
• Pregnancy.
• Unstable patient who requires immediate surgery.

Personnel Required

One operator and an assistant are required for peritoneal lavage using the percutaneous approach. Alternatively, one operator and two assistants are required for peritoneal lavage using the operative approach.

Equipment & Supplies Required

Prepackaged trays with the necessary equipment are available commercially, or they can be made up by the hospital. The following items are required:

- Materials for skin sterilization.
- Materials for sterile technique (cap, mask, gloves, and gown).
- Sterile towels (4) or sterile paper drapes.
- Lidocaine, 1%, with 5-mL syringe and 25-gauge needle.
- No. 11 surgical blade, mounted.
- Peritoneal lavage catheter (11–18F) and introducing stylet.
- Sterile bottle containing 1 L of lactated Ringer's injection or normal saline, with intravenous connector tubing.
- Nylon suture (size 4-0) on a cutting needle (percutaneous approach); chromic catgut (size 3-0) plus silk, nylon, or polypropylene sutures (size 3-0) (operative approach).
- Needle holder and straight scissors.
- Adhesive dressing.
- For operative technique only: 2 Allis or Kocher clamps, 1 Kelly clamp, and 2 small right-angle retractors.

Positioning of the Patient

The patient should be supine on a level surface. Examine the abdomen for scars; do not perform peritoneal lavage if abdominal surgery has been performed previously. Take diagnostic abdominal x-rays before performing peritoneal lavage (the procedure may produce artifacts on the x-ray [eg, ileus or intraperitoneal air]).

Procedure

A. PREPARATORY MEASURES

1. Drain the bladder (by urination or catheterization, as required). Place nasogastric tube.
2. Position the patient, and check to see that all equipment is at hand.
3. Sterilize the skin of the anterior abdominal wall from the umbilicus to the symphysis pubica.
4. Drape the operative site.

5. Observe sterile technique (don cap, mask, gloves, and gown).
6. Using the 1% lidocaine with the 5-mL syringe and 25-gauge needle, anesthetize the skin about 2 cm (¾ in) caudal to the umbilicus in the midline. Then, directing the needle perpendicularly to the anterior abdominal wall, infiltrate the fascia (linea alba), preperitoneal space (between peritoneum and fascia), and parietal peritoneum. The needle will encounter resistance when it reaches the peritoneum.

B. PERCUTANEOUS APPROACH

1. Using the No. 11 blade, make a 0.5-cm (¼-in) transverse incision through the skin and fascia to allow easy passage of the catheter and stylet.
2. Carefully insert the catheter and stylet into the anesthetized tract with gentle, steady, controlled pressure. (*Caution:* The abdominal aorta lies in the path of the catheter.) Control is best achieved by making sure that both hands are comfortably placed on the patient's abdomen and by advancing the catheter with steady pressure applied by the thumb and forefinger. Advance the catheter through the peritoneum and into the peritoneal cavity. There will be a definite give ("pop") as the catheter penetrates the peritoneum.
3. Once the catheter has penetrated the peritoneal cavity, slide it off the stylet and into the peritoneal cavity. The catheter should slide easily. If any resistance is encountered, withdraw the catheter and stylet together, and attempt insertion again. Difficulty in advancing the catheter may indicate that the stylet has not entered the peritoneal cavity and that the catheter is being inserted into the space between the peritoneum and the fascia; alternatively, there may be adhesions in the peritoneal cavity that have fixed the intraperitoneal structures. Failure to make this important distinction may result in false-positive or false-negative findings or perforation of intraperitoneal structures.

C. OPERATIVE APPROACH

With this approach, a superficial laparotomy is performed to permit direct visualization of the peritoneum when the catheter is inserted. The advantage of this approach is that inadvertent insertion of the catheter into the preperitoneal space is unlikely to occur; however, more personnel are required to perform the procedure.

1. After the area has been anesthetized, use the No. 11 blade to make a 3-cm (1³⁄₁₆-in) vertical incision in the midline about 1 cm (¾ in) inferior to the umbilicus.

2. Using the Kelly clamp, bluntly dissect through subcutaneous tissue to the fascia of the abdominal wall. Then incise the fascia for the length of the incision. Again using a Kelly clamp, spread the preperitoneal fat, and expose the parietal peritoneum.

3. Using 2 Allis or Kocher clamps, grasp the peritoneum, and lift it up to free it from any underlying visceral structures. (Grasp a bit of peritoneum with one clamp, grasp another bit with the second clamp about 1–2 cm [⅜–¾ in] away, and release the first clamp. Repeat as needed. This method of alternately grasping and releasing the peritoneum separates it from underlying structures.)

4. Holding the peritoneum up between 2 clamps (Allis or Kocher), make a small stab wound through the peritoneum with a No. 11 scalpel blade.

5. Insert the catheter into the peritoneal cavity under direct vision.

D. RESULTS

With either approach, gross blood may return after the catheter has been placed and the stylet has been removed. This finding signifies extensive intraperitoneal hemorrhage, and the patient should be prepared for surgery.

1. If blood does not return immediately, connect the intravenous tubing to the catheter, and instill 1 L of sterile, warm Ringer's lactate or normal saline (Figure 6–29). Gently massage the abdomen to spread the fluid, and roll the patient from side to side to make sure that the lavage fluid reaches all areas of the peritoneal cavity. Lower the intravenous bottle to the floor. The fluid in the peritoneal cavity should flow out of the cavity and back into the bottle. Again, roll the patient from side to side to return as much fluid as possible to the bottle.

2. After as much of the fluid as possible has been removed from the peritoneal cavity (a reasonable return is 75–80% of the fluid instilled), remove the catheter, and close the incision. Use the size 4-0 nylon skin suture if the percutaneous approach was used, and cover it with an adhesive dressing. To close the incision made for the operative approach, close the peritoneum with chromic catgut sutures; close the anterior abdominal fascia with interrupted silk, polypropylene, or nylon sutures; approximate the subcutaneous tissue with absorbable sutures; and close the skin.

   If immediate laparotomy is necessary, leave the incision open, and cover it with a sterile dressing that has been soaked in saline.

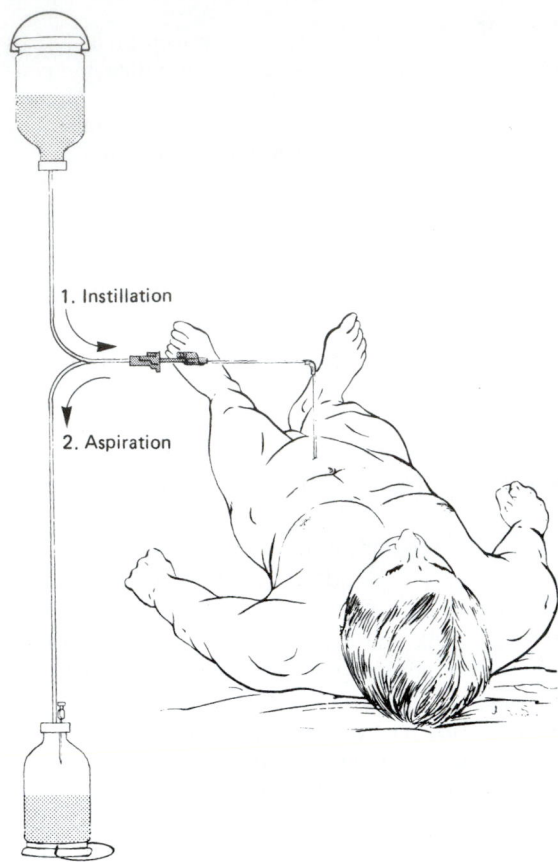

1. Instillation

2. Aspiration

Figure 6–29. Technique of peritoneal lavage. (Reproduced, with permission, from Dunphy JE, Way LW [editors]: *Current Surgical Diagnosis & Treatment,* 5th ed. Lange, 1981.)

3. Make sure to record the amount of any excess fluid left in the patient's peritoneal cavity as fluid input on the fluid intake and output computation sheet.

Interpretation

Significant intraperitoneal hemorrhage is indicated by grossly bloody lavage fluid or gross blood coming from the catheter. Lavage fluid with a hematocrit of 1% or higher also indicates significant intraperitoneal hemorrhage and suggests the need for laparotomy. Completely clear fluid indicates lack of significant intraperitoneal bleeding.

INSERTION OF INDWELLING (FOLEY) URINARY CATHETER

Indications

Indications for insertion of an indwelling urinary catheter are as follows:

- Diagnostic or therapeutic drainage of the urinary bladder.
- Need for a reliable and frequent assessment of urine output (eg, for treatment of shock).
- Need to perform retrograde cystography.

Contraindications

The following are only relative contraindications to insertion of an indwelling urinary catheter:

- Previous urethral surgery.
- Suspected or known urethra trauma (free-floating prostate, blood issuing from urethra meatus). In this case, perform a urethrogram before urethral catheterization is attempted.

Personnel Required

One person can insert an indwelling urinary catheter unaided. An assistant is helpful if the patient is uncooperative.

Equipment & Supplies Required

Note: Most hospitals have disposable Foley insertion trays that contain most of the items listed below except for the catheter. It is important to check to see that the tray contains all of the needed materials and that the catheter, if it is supplied with the set, is of the proper size and desired material and has a balloon of the proper size.

- Foley catheter of the appropriate size, material, and contour (different catheters are discussed below).
- Urinary drainage bag and connecting tube.
- Sterile lubricant.
- Antiseptic solution and sterile cotton balls to sterilize the male urethral meatus and the female perineum.
- Sterile syringe, 5- to 10-mL, filled with enough sterile water to inflate the balloon on the catheter. The size of the balloon is usually printed on the catheter (usually 5 mL).
- Sterile gloves and drapes.

Selecting a Catheter

The Foley catheter is used in almost all cases when an indwelling urinary catheter is required. It consists of a double-lumen rubber tube with a terminal retaining balloon. The larger channel is for drainage of urine, and the smaller is for inflation of the balloon. Some indwelling catheters have a third lumen, for constant bladder irrigation. Foley catheters are of standard length (46 cm [18 in]) but come in varying diameters that are numerically graded (French system), with the larger number indicating a larger diameter. Two sizes of balloon are commonly available: 5-mL balloons for routine catheterizations and 30-mL balloons for special situations. Most Foley catheters are made of rubber. Teflon or Silastic is sometimes used for long-term, indwelling catheters. (Specialized shapes and contours are not discussed here, because they should be inserted by a urologist.)

- For routine, short-term catheterization in males or females, a 14F or 18F rubber catheter with a 5-mL balloon is satisfactory. Smaller sizes are required for children.
- Men with prostatic hypertrophy may require larger catheters (eg, 20–22F).

Positioning of the Patient

A. FEMALES

The patient should be in the lithotomy position. If she is comatose or under anesthesia, flex her knees and hips, and allow the legs to abduct. If the soles of the feet are pressed together, this position can easily be held by the patient without assistance.

B. MALES

The patient should be supine.

Anatomy Review

A. FEMALES

The female urethra is short, and because there is no prostate gland, passage of a catheter is relatively easy. The only difficulty is locating the urethral meatus, which lies in the superior fornix of the vulva, above the vaginal opening and below the clitoris. It appears as a small dimple or slit in the midline.

B. MALES

The urethra leaves the bladder at the trigone, passes through the prostate, and then runs the length of the penis to exit at the meatus at the tip of the glans.

Procedure

A. CATHETERIZATION OF FEMALES

1. Assemble all necessary equipment.

2. Open the catheter tray and selected catheter, and position them on a sterile field placed on a bedside table or stand so that all required materials are readily accessible.

3. Place a generous amount of lubricant on the sterile field.

4. Put on sterile gloves, and drape the perineal area.

5. Make sure that the catheter is open and the lubricating jelly is accessible.

6. Open the antiseptic packet, and moisten the cotton swabs provided with antiseptic.

7. Be sure that the syringe is filled with enough sterile water to inflate the balloon being used.

8. Using the left hand (standing on the patient's right side), spread the labia and identify the superior fornix with the clitoris at the apex. Thoroughly cleanse the entire area with 4–5 swabs soaked in antiseptic. Clean the labia with front to back strokes with 2 successive swabs; then cleanse the urethral meatus with another 2 successive swabs.

9. The left hand continues to hold the labia spread apart from the rest of the procedure.

10. Make a loop in the Foley catheter for easier handling. Grasp the catheter with the right hand, coat the tip and proximal portion with lubricating jelly, and insert the catheter into the urethral meatus, which lies just below the clitoris. Advance the catheter until urine returns. Then advance it 4–5 cm (1⅝–2 in) farther to make sure that the balloon is well within the bladder.

11. Inflate the balloon with the appropriate amount of sterile water (usually 5 mL; the balloon volume is usually printed on the catheter), and withdraw the catheter gently until the balloon is pulled snugly against the trigone (Figure 6–30).

12. Collect a small amount of urine in a sterile container for appropriate studies (urinalysis should be obtained routinely), and then connect the catheter to the urinary drainage bag.

13. Tape the Foley catheter and the urinary drainage tube to the upper thigh, leaving enough slack so that abduction of the legs will not put tension on the catheter.

14. *Note:* The most common mistake in catheterization of the female bladder is to miss the urethral meatus and inadvertently slip the catheter into the vagina. No urine will return. Leave the catheter in place in the vagina as a marker. Obtain a new,

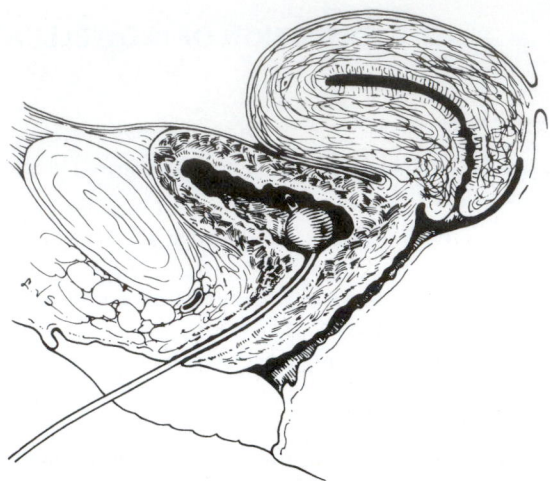

Figure 6–30. Sagittal section of female bladder showing balloon of Foley catheter fitting snugly against the trigone.

sterile catheter, and try again. Remove the other catheter.

B. CATHETERIZATION OF MALES

7. Steps 1–7 are the same as those described under Catheterization of Females, above.

8. Using the left hand (standing on the patient's right side), grasp the penis so that the shaft lies in the palm and the glans of the penis is free but secure. The penis should be held at a right angle to the abdomen. The left hand should remain in this position for the remainder of the procedure; it is no longer sterile.

9. Sterilize the glans and urethral meatus with 3–4 swabs dipped in antiseptic.

10. Put a single loop in the Foley catheter for easier handling, grasp the catheter in the right hand, and coat the tip of the catheter with lubricating jelly. It is often helpful to place some on the meatus as well.

11. Insert the catheter into the urethral meatus, and advance it down the penile urethra to the base of the penis with successive, steady movements.

12. Advance the catheter through the membranous and prostatic urethra into the bladder.

13. Advance the catheter to the hilt (even if urine is obtained earlier) to ensure that the balloon is not inflated in the urethra. As soon as the catheter has been advanced to the hilt, release the penis to free both hands for inflation of the balloon.

14. Inflate the balloon with the proper amount of sterile water for its size (usually 5 mL), and withdraw the catheter until the balloon is pulled snugly against the trigone.

15. Obtain a specimen for appropriate tests (at a minimum, routine urinalysis should be performed). Connect the urinary drainage system bag to the catheter, and tape the catheter to the upper thigh, leaving sufficient slack so that movement of the leg will not pull on the catheter.

Problem Solving

A. Males with Prostatic Enlargement or False Urethral Passages

Conventional technique usually fails in patients with significant prostatic hypertrophy or false urethral passage. Listed below are a few techniques that have proved successful in catheterizing these patients. *Caution:* Reasonable persistence in attempting catheterization is acceptable; however, there comes a time when further manipulations may rupture the urethra or create new false passages. If attempts using the guidelines outlined below are still unsuccessful, consult a urologist, or insert a suprapubic catheter instead (see below).

1. Increase the size of the catheter—Large catheters are stiffer and provide more forceful dilatation of the prostatic urethra. The larger, blunt tip tends to follow the true urethra rather than smaller false passages.

2. Lubricate the urethra—Fill a 30- to 50-mL sterile catheter-tipped syringe with the lubricating jelly and inject the jelly down the urethra with gentle pressure until no more can be injected. Then insert the catheter.

3. Inject lubricating jelly while the catheter is being passed—Fill the syringe as outlined above, insert the tip into the catheter, and fill the catheter with jelly. As the catheter is being passed, slowly inject more lubricant to ensure that the entire length of the catheter is lubricated and to help dilate the urethra just ahead of the catheter tip.

4. Use a Coudé catheter—A Coudé catheter has an upwardly deflected tip, which may navigate through a narrowed prostatic urethra more successfully than a standard Foley catheter.

B. Traumatized Patients

Most patients with major trauma have a Foley catheter inserted during resuscitation. A rectal examination must be performed before a catheter is inserted in a male patient with major blunt trauma. Feel for the prostate and make sure that it is firmly attached to the surrounding tissues. A free-floating prostate or gross blood escaping from the urethra signifies urethral rupture until proved otherwise. In either case, Foley catheterization is contraindicated, and a suprapubic catheter should be inserted instead.

PERCUTANEOUS SUPRAPUBIC CYSTOTOMY

Suprapubic bladder cystostomy is a means of bypassing the urethra to provide drainage of the urinary bladder.

Indications

Suprapubic bladder cystostomy is performed to provide bladder drainage when transurethral drainage is unsuccessful or contraindicated.

Contraindications

Contraindications to suprapubic cystostomy are as follows:

- Nondistended, nonpalpable bladder.
- Carcinoma of the bladder, because percutaneous catheterization of the bladder might lead to seeding of the cancer along the track of the catheter.
- Gross hematuria, which would require a tube of large diameter to drain clots from the bladder.

- Recent cystostomy (the percutaneous technique might disrupt suture lines).

Personnel Required

One person can perform percutaneous suprapubic cystostomy unaided, although an assistant may be helpful, particularly if the patient is uncooperative.

Equipment & Supplies Required

Many prepackaged commercial kits are available for percutaneous suprapubic cystostomy. The following items are required:

- Materials for skin sterilization.
- Materials for sterile technique (cap, mask, gloves, and gown).
- Lidocaine, 1%, with 10-mL syringe and 25-gauge, 1-cm (½-in) and 22-gauge, 4-cm (1½-in) needles.

- Sterile towels (4) or sterile paper drapes.
- Razor.
- No. 11 scalpel blade, mounted.
- Catheter-clad needle (eg, Angiocath), 14-gauge, 30-cm (12-in); or other commercially manufactured percutaneous suprapubic catheter set. A central venous catheter kit can also be used if no other equipment is available.
- Syringe, 50-mL.
- Closed urinary drainage system (sterile intravenous tubing and empty intravenous bag or bottle).
- Silk suture (size 3-0) on a curved cutting needle.
- Needle holder.
- Suture scissors.
- Antibacterial ointment.
- Sterile gauze sponges, 5 × 5 cm (2 × 2 in), and tape.
- Rolled bath towel for placement under the patient's hips.

Positioning of the Patient

The patient should be supine, with a rolled-up towel placed under the hips.

Anatomy Review

The urinary bladder lies in the midline of the lower abdomen. When it is distended, its position can be detected by palpation or percussion.

Procedure

1. Locate the distended bladder by palpation, percussion, or ultrasonography. If the bladder cannot be located, percutaneous suprapubic cystostomy should not be performed. If the bladder is not distended, it can usually be filled by oral or intravenous hydration.
2. Prepare the area just above the symphysis pubica by shaving the pubic hair and sterilizing the skin. Extend the sterile field with drapes.
3. Assemble all necessary equipment.
4. Observe sterile technique (don cap, mask, gloves, and gown).
5. Determine the insertion point by measuring cephalad 1–2 cm (⅜–¾ in) from the superior edge of the symphysis pubica in the midline (Figure 6–31).
6. Using the 1% lidocaine with the 10-mL syringe and 25-gauge needle, anesthetize the skin at the point of insertion. Then switch to the 22-gauge needle to anesthetize the subcutaneous tissue and

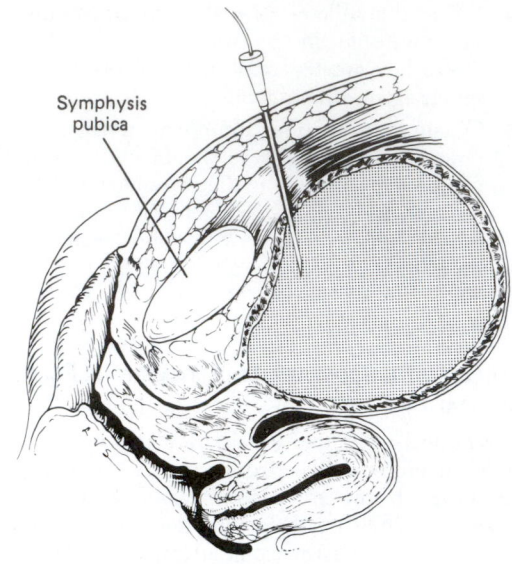

Figure 6–31. Suprapubic cystostomy. Sagittal section of distended bladder showing insertion site for catheter.

anterior wall of the bladder. If the position of the needle is correct, urine can be aspirated through the needle. Remove the needle.

7. Make a 0.5-cm (³⁄₁₆-in) transverse incision in the skin over the anesthetized area with the No. 11 scalpel blade.
8. The technique for placing the catheter depends on the type of catheter used:
   a. *Catheter-clad needle:*
   (1) Attach a 50-mL syringe to the 14-gauge, 30-cm (12-in) catheter-clad needle.
   (2) Insert the catheter unit through the skin incision.
   (3) Advance the catheter caudally at a 50- to 60-degree angle to the abdominal surface. Advance the catheter with a smooth, deliberate motion, and steady the guiding hands on the patient's abdomen as necessary. A "give" is felt as the catheter and needle penetrate each successive layer of the fascia and bladder wall. Maintaining gentle suction with the syringe will cause aspiration of urine as soon as the bladder cavity has been entered.
   (4) Once the bladder has been entered, slip the catheter tip off the needle by holding the hub of the needle in the left

hand and advancing the catheter with the right.

(5) Advance the catheter about 6–8 cm (2⅜–3⅛ in) to make sure that enough of it is within the bladder.

(6) Attach the sterile intravenous tubing to the catheter hub. If no assistant is available, reattach the 50-mL syringe to the tubing to keep the system closed. Otherwise, have an assistant attach the end of the tubing to the empty intravenous bag or bottle that is to receive the urine.

(7) Suture the catheter in place at the insertion site with the size 3-0 silk suture. Wind the ends of the suture around the catheter at least 3 times to make sure that it is secured to the abdominal wall.

(8) Apply antibacterial ointment to the insertion site, cover it with sterile 5- × 5-cm (2- × 2-in) gauze sponges, and tape the sponges in place.

(9) If not done earlier, attach the end of the tubing to the empty intravenous bag or bottle that is to receive the urine.

(10) Tape all connections.

b. *Central venous catheter kit.* Use the Seldinger technique, as previously discussed, to insert the catheter.

c. *Percutaneous suprapubic catheter.* Follow the manufacturer's instructions for use.

LUMBAR PUNCTURE

Indications

Lumbar puncture is performed to obtain cerebrospinal fluid for diagnostic tests (eg, suspected meningitis, subarachnoid hemorrhage).

Contraindications

Contraindications to lumbar puncture are as follows:

- Local infection of the lumbar area. Cervical or cisternal puncture should be performed instead.
- Suspected intracranial mass lesion (brain abscess, tumor, any posterior fossa lesion, subdural hematoma). Papilledema or focal cerebral defects (excluding ophthalmoplegia) suggest a mass lesion of the central nervous system. CT scan of the head should precede lumbar puncture in these circumstances.
- Bleeding diathesis (relative contraindication; should be corrected if time permits).
- Suspected spinal cord mass lesion (eg, epidural abscess, hematoma, or tumor). Myelography should be performed in consultation with a neurosurgeon to define the lower limit of the spinal block.

Personnel Required

One person can perform lumbar puncture unaided if the patient is cooperative. An assistant can help with positioning of the patient, lighting, handling of samples, and the like, and is essential if the patient is uncooperative.

Equipment & Supplies Required

Prepackaged sterile disposable lumbar puncture trays are commercially available. If the tray is to be assembled at the hospital, the following items are required:

- Materials for skin sterilization.
- Materials for sterile techniques (gloves and mask; cap and gown are optional).
- Spinal needles, 20- and 22-gauge (shorter, smaller-gauge needles are required for children).
- Manometer.
- Three-way stopcock.
- Cerebrospinal fluid collection tubes (5).
- Sponges, 10 × 10 cm (4 × 4 in).
- Lidocaine, 1%, with 5-mL syringe and 22- and 25-gauge needles.
- Sterile drapes.
- Adhesive dressing.
- Ice bucket for specimens that must be put on ice immediately.

Positioning of the Patient

A. LATERAL DECUBITUS

Place the patient in the lateral decubitus position lying on the edge of the bed and facing away from the operator. The patient should flex the lumbar spine as much as possible by assuming the fetal position (forehead bent toward knees and knees drawn up to abdomen). The patient's head should rest on a pillow, so that the entire craniospinal axis is parallel to the bed. Positioning is the most crucial aspect of successful lumbar puncture, and the 3 key elements of proper positioning are achieving maximal lumbar flexion (to open the intervertebral spaces), keeping the patient's spine parallel to the bed, and having the line of the patient's shoulders and pelvis be perpendicular to the bed (to facilitate orientation of the needle track). Prevent pelvic rotation by keeping the patient's knees and ankles aligned. An assistant is useful to help the patient maintain the proper position.

B. Sitting

The patient sits facing away from the operator and bends over a bedside table to maximize lumbar flexion. This position is useful when cerebrospinal fluid pressure is low (eg, dehydration) or when the patient is obese. Cerebrospinal fluid pressure can be determined by having the patient lie in the decubitus position after the needle is in place.

After the patient has been properly positioned, raise the bed until the patient's lower lumbar spine is at the mid chest level of the operator, who should be seated. Adjust the lighting for optimal effect.

Anatomy Review

Lumbar puncture should enter the subarachnoid space below the level of the conus medullaris, which extends to L1-L2 in most adults and L2–L3 in children. The L3–L4 interspace, the most commonly used site for lumbar puncture, is at the level of the posterior iliac crests (Figure 6–32). The L4–L5 interspace may be preferable, however, because a traumatic spinal tap at this level may leave cerebrospinal fluid obtained at the higher interspace uncontaminated with red blood cells (because of the caudal direction of flow of cerebrospinal fluid).

With the patient properly positioned, find the posterior iliac crest, and palpate the spine at this level for

the L3–L4 interspace. Other interspaces are counted from this landmark. The needle should enter the exact midpoint of the interspace between the spinous processes. Mark the point on the patient's skin with the end of a ballpoint pen or the indentation from a fingernail to facilitate locating the landmark after the skin has been sterilized.

It may be difficult to palpate the spinous processes in obese patients. Using the gluteal cleft to mark the midline, locate the sacral promontory, which is palpable even in obese patients. Move cephalad until the promontory ends, indicating the L5–S1 interspace; the L4–L5 interspace is then easily identified.

Procedure

1. Observe sterile technique (don mask and gloves; cap and gown are optional).

2. Prepare all equipment. Assemble the manometer and stopcock (the channel from the spinal needle to the manometer should be open), open the specimen tubes, and draw up the 1% lidocaine into the 5-mL syringe with the 25-gauge needle.

3. Sterilize the skin in a wide field around the L2–L3 to L4–L5 interspaces.

4. Place a sterile drape under the patient that extends over the edge of the bed. Contamination of gloves may be avoided by folding the edge of the drape back over the gloves, pushing the edge beneath the patient's back, and carefully removing the gloved hands.

5. Place a second sterile drape over the top side of the patient, leaving only sterilized skin between the edges of the drapes. Although a drape with a center hole is preferred by some, it obscures the rest of the spine (a valuable landmark) and makes shifting to another interspace difficult.

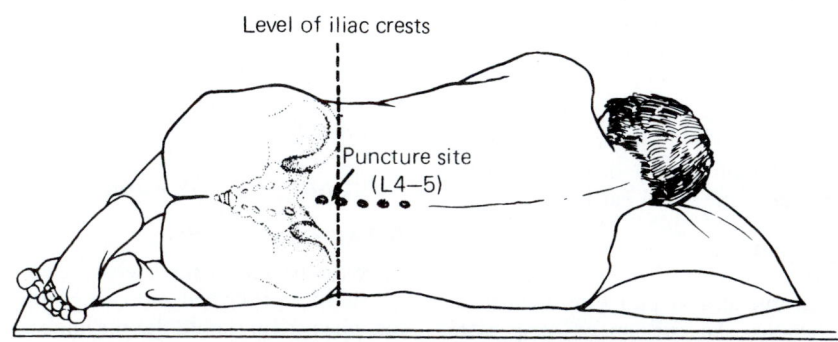

Figure 6–32. Decubitus position for lumbar puncture. (Reproduced, with permission, from Krupp MA et al: *Physician's Handbook,* 21st ed. Lange, 1985.)

6. Locate the puncture site, and anesthetize the skin using the 1% lidocaine in the 5-mL syringe with the 25-gauge needle. Change to the 22-gauge needle before anesthetizing between the spinous processes. Be sure to apply vacuum to the syringe to make sure that the needle has not entered a blood vessel (blood in the syringe).

7. Hold the spinal needle between the index and middle fingers, with the thumb over the stylet. It may be held with 2 hands, if necessary, for stability. Avoid touching the tip and shaft of the needle, because starch granules from the gloves may be introduced into the subarachnoid space and can cause sterile arachnoiditis. The 20-gauge needle is better for transmitting pressure changes in cerebrospinal fluid, but the 22-gauge needle is adequate in most cases; smaller needles should be used in children.

8. Introduce the needle in the midline perpendicular to a line connecting the iliac crests, aiming about 30 degrees rostrally toward the umbilicus. Be sure the long axis of the needle is parallel to the bed and that the plane of the patient's back is perpendicular to the bed. In infants, the entry angle is nearer to the perpendicular, whereas in elderly patients, the angle may approach 45 degrees rostrally to pass beneath the osteophytic lipping of the spinous processes. The bevel of the needle should be facing up (parallel to the spine) if the patient is in the lateral decubitus position, so that the fibers of the dura are split longitudinally.

9. Advance the needle slowly. There will be a "pop" as the needle passes through the ligamentum flavum and the spinal arachnoid membrane. Since the spinal venous plexus is anterior to the spinal canal, the chance of a traumatic spinal tap can be minimized by frequent checking of the position of the needle (withdraw the stylet).

10. If the needle hits bone deep in the penetration, withdraw to the ligamentum flavum, and redirect the tip in a more caudal direction. (The needle will follow the same course unless it is drawn back through the ligamentum flavum.) Pain radiating to the leg or buttock is an obvious indication to direct the needle toward the midline and away from the involved side.

11. When cerebrospinal fluid begins to flow from the needle, discard the first few drops. Establish free flow of cerebrospinal fluid—rotating the bevel of the needle may be helpful. Do not aspirate cerebrospinal fluid unless it cannot be obtained by other means, because a nerve root may be trapped against the needle and injured. Replace the stylet halfway in the shaft of the needle to prevent leakage. If the patient is in a seated position and if cerebrospinal fluid pressures are to be obtained, have an assistant help the patient into the decubitus position, taking care not to move the needle.

12. Remove the stylet, and attach the stopcock and the manometer to the needle.

13. If not already done, rotate the stopcock lever to open the channel between the needle and the manometer. Cerebrospinal fluid will rise into the manometer, and the opening cerebrospinal fluid pressure can be measured. Normal pressure is between 780 and 180 mm H_2O. If pressure is elevated, make sure that the patient's position is not causing jugular or abdominal compression. Have the patient slowly relax and uncurl from the fetal position (if in the lateral decubitus position) and then inhale deeply. Cerebrospinal fluid pressure falls with inspiration and rises with expiration. Check pressure changes with the patient's head first flexed and then extended. To detect mass lesions in the spinal canal, look for a block to cerebrospinal fluid that is present only on either extension or flexion. Abnormally low pressures may be caused by dehydration.

14. Remove the manometer, and begin collecting samples of cerebrospinal fluid in the specimen tubes. This is most easily achieved by removing the 3-way stopcock and using the stylet to block flow between samples by replacing the stylet halfway in the shaft of the needle. Three tubes are routinely collected: tube 1 (0.5–1 mL), tube 2 (2–3 mL), and tube 3 (2–4 mL) in adults (smaller amounts are collected in children). Frequently, however, further information is desired, and more samples are collected in the extra tubes (see section on specimen collection, below). If in doubt, collect extra fluid in additional tubes.

15. Replace the manometer, and obtain a closing pressure if spinal subarachnoid block is suspected.

16. Remove the needle, and place a small adhesive bandage over the puncture site.

17. Draw venous blood for determination of glucose concentration. The radio of blood glucose to cerebrospinal fluid glucose is helpful in the diagnosis of inflammatory disease.

18. Recommendations to have the patient lie supine after the procedure do not appear to affect the incidence of post-dural puncture headache.

Special Problems Encountered in Lumbar Puncture

A. MASSIVE OBESITY

If the patient is obese, landmarks are difficult to locate, and alternative methods for locating the L4–L5 interspace must be used (see Anatomy Review, above). Lumbar puncture with the patient sitting may be tried if attempts fail with the patient in the lateral decubitus position. The sitting position makes the midline easier to locate and increases lumbar flexion. A 12.5-cm (5-in) needle may be required. The patient must be cooperative. Cerebrospinal fluid pressures are not measured in this position, but the patient may be carefully repositioned in the lateral decubitus position after the needle is in place to record cerebrospinal fluid pressures. If lumbar puncture in the sitting position is unsuccessful, a neurosurgeon can use the cervical approach (done at the bedside), or a neuroradiologist can attempt a fluoroscopically guided approach (performed in the radiology department).

B. OSTEOARTHRITIS

As the body ages, desiccation of the nucleus pulposus of the intervertebral disk occurs, with subsequent narrowing of the disk space. This change, together with osteophytic "lipping" of the spinous process and calcification of the interspinous ligament and ligamentum flavum, combine to make lumbar puncture difficult. A larger-gauge needle (eg, 18- to 19-gauge) facilitates passage through calcified posterior ligaments. It may occasionally be necessary to resort to an oblique approach performed by a radiologist using fluoroscopy.

C. PREVIOUS LUMBAR SURGERY

Lumbosacral spine films assist in defining the extent of surgery and fusion. If all of the posterior approaches are unavailable for lumbar puncture, obtain neurologic or neurosurgical consultation.

D. INADVERTENT ARTERIAL PUNCTURE

If arterial blood is obtained during lumbar puncture, completely withdraw the needle. Obtain a fresh spinal needle for the next attempt, because clotted blood makes replacement of the stylet difficult and also contaminates the sample. If the patient has an underlying coagulopathy, it should be corrected and the patient observed for signs of compressive spinal epidural or subdural hematoma (Chapter 16).

E. HIGH OPENING PRESSURE

If high cerebrospinal pressures are unsuspected before lumbar puncture is performed, use the smallest needle possible. Collect the minimum amount of fluid necessary (usually that in the manometer is sufficient), and withdraw the needle. Watch the patient carefully for signs of impending herniation, and treat accordingly (Chapter 16). Obtain a closing cerebrospinal fluid pressure; remove only as much fluid as causes the initial pressure to drop by one-half. A rapid drop in cerebrospinal fluid pressure to low levels with removal of only a small amount of fluid may be an ominous sign

indicating impending herniation. Obtain urgent neurosurgical consultation.

F. HYPOTENSION

Cerebrospinal fluid pressure is proportionate to venous pressure and P_{CO_2}. Severe hypotension may decrease the volume of the subarachnoid space and make it difficult to penetrate. Slowly advance the needle, and each time the stylet is removed, attach a tuberculin syringe with a small air bubble in the hub, relying on the negative pressure in the epidural space to help define location (the bubble is sucked into the needle when the needle is in the epidural rather than the arachnoid space). Advancing the needle a few millimeters will place the tip within the subarachnoid space, permitting aspiration of cerebrospinal fluid.

The sitting position may be helpful in the patient with severe hypotension, provided that arterial blood pressure is sufficient to enable the patient to tolerate the upright position. The sitting position takes advantage of gravity to help raise cerebrospinal fluid pressure in the lumbar space.

G. POST–LUMBAR PUNCTURE HEADACHE

Headache following lumbar puncture is unfortunately a relatively common complication of the procedure. It does not appear to be related to the duration that a patient remains supine after the procedure. Smaller, less traumatic (pencil point) needles may reduce the incidence. Medications such as oral or intravenous caffeine may be of benefit for headaches that continue despite bed rest. For persistent headaches, an epidural blood patch is usually effective in resolving the headache.

H. BLOOD IN CEREBROSPINAL FLUID

Features that point to a traumatic spinal tap rather than to subarachnoid hemorrhage include (1) normal cerebrospinal fluid pressure, (2) absence of xanthochromia after centrifugation, (3) blood sample followed by clearer samples or bloodier samples, (4) white cell count proportionate to red cell count (700–1000 red blood cells per white blood cell; 1 mg/dL of protein per 1000 red blood cells), (5) changing red cell count in successive tubes, or (6) clot formation (rare). A repeat lumbar puncture at a higher interspace yields cerebrospinal fluid that is usually clear if the fluid was bloody owing to traumatic tap at a lower level. The presence or absence of crenated red cells is of no diagnostic value.

Specimens

At a minimum, collect 3 tubes: tube 1 (0.5–1 mL) for cell count, tube 2 (2–3 mL) for culture and Gram stain, and tube 3 for protein and glucose determinations and for chemistry studies (2–4 mL). Most authorities recommend another 0.5 mL for a VDRL study. There is

Table 6–2. Pigmentation of the cerebrospinal fluid following hemorrhage.

	Appearance	Maximum	Disappearance
Oxyhemoglo-bin (pink)	½–4 hours	24–35 hours	7–10 days
Bilirubin (yellow)	8–12 hours	2–4 days	2–3 weeks

no harm in collecting extra tubes, because a variety of other diagnostic tests may be indicated. If the specimen is bloody, perform comparison counts in tubes 1 and 3.

If subarachnoid hemorrhage is suspected, the supernatant in the tube should be examined for xanthochromia. Centrifuge 2–3 mL of cerebrospinal fluid at 1000 rpm for 5 minutes in a clinical centrifuge, and then examine the supernatant for the characteristic yellowish pigmentation of oxyhemoglobin and bilirubin. Xanthochromia does not appear until about 2–4 hours after hemorrhage, reaches a maximum around 6–48 hours, and may persist for 2–4 weeks (Table 6–2). Jaundice, hypercarotenemia, and elevated cerebrospinal fluid protein (> 150 mg/dL) may also cause xanthochromic spinal fluid. Xanthochromia does not occur in the supernatant after a traumatic spinal tap, because the bloody cerebrospinal fluid is not exposed to the enzyme in the subarachnoid space that converts hemoglobin to bilirubin.

ANTERIOR & POSTERIOR NASAL PACKING FOR CONTROL OF EPISTAXIS

Bleeding from the anterior or posterior nasal passages is a commonly encountered emergency. The patient may present with bleeding ranging from mild epistaxis that is easily controlled by local pressure to exsanguinating hemorrhage causing hemorrhagic shock.

Successful treatment of epistaxis requires careful identification of the bleeding source. To accomplish this, proper positioning of the patient, proper instruments, and a bright, hand-directed light source are a necessity.

Bleeding in the anterior nares occurs most commonly in children and can be controlled by local measures such as direct pressure or cautery. Bleeding in adults usually occurs more posteriorly in the anterior nares and often requires anterior nasal packing; epistaxis in the elderly often requires both anterior and posterior nasal packing because the site of bleeding is in the posterior nares.

Indications

Nasal packing (Figure 6–33) is performed to control hemorrhage that cannot be controlled by local measures.

Contraindications

The patient's ability or inability to cooperate during the procedure is the only limiting factor in performing nasal packing. Occasionally, direct control of the bleeding site under general anesthesia in the operating room is required.

Personnel Required

One person can perform nasal packing unaided, although it is helpful to have an assistant to position the patient and handle instruments.

Equipment & Supplies Required

A. ANTERIOR PACKING

- Cocaine solution, 4% (10 mL); benzocaine-tetracaine spray or tetracaine liquid; phenylephrine nasal spray, 0.5–1%.
- Lidocaine, 1%, with epinephrine (10 mL).
- Syringe, 5-mL, with 25-gauge needle.
- Cotton-tipped swabs.
- Silver nitrate–tipped sticks for coagulation.
- Portable electrocautery device.
- Nasal speculum.
- Headlamp, or reflective eye mirror with suitable light source.
- Continuous suction device with nasal suction tips.
- Petrolatum-impregnated gauze packing (continuous strip).
- Nasal packing forceps.
- Cotton pledgets.

B. POSTERIOR NASAL PACKING

The materials and equipment listed for anterior nasal packing are required for posterior nasal packing. The following additional items are required:

- Occluding balloon catheter (specially designed for tamponade of the bleeding site) (2).
- Absorbent cotton (4 × 5 cm [1⅝ × 2 in]), with 3 pieces of size 0 silk suture material tied around the middle (alternative to balloon catheterization).
- No. 12 or No. 14 red rubber catheter.

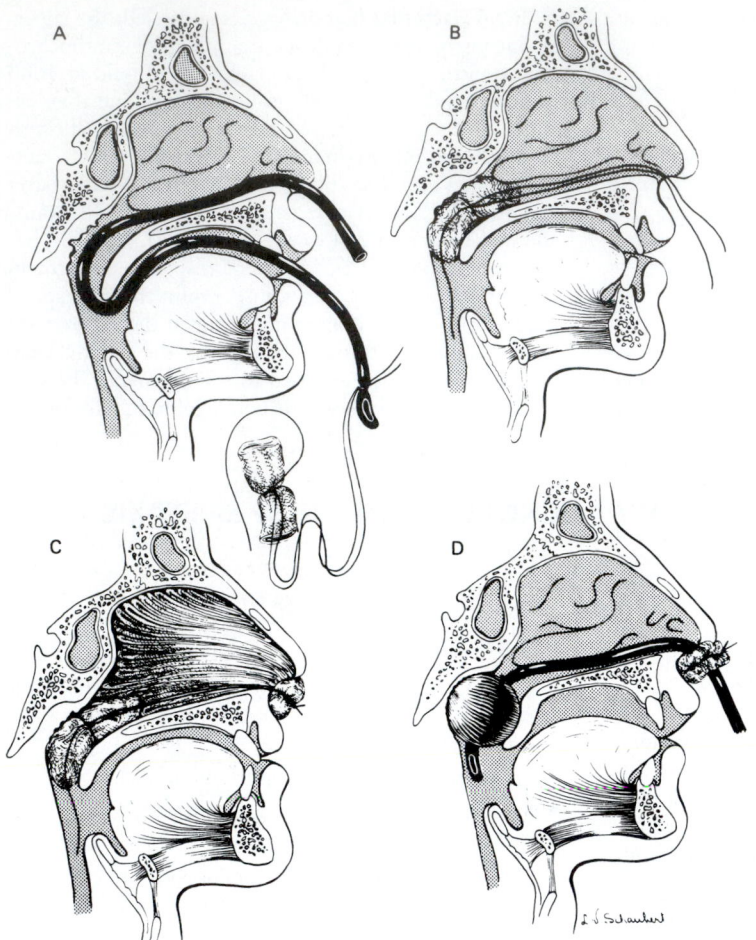

Figure 6–33. Packing to control bleeding from the posterior nose. **A:** Catheter inserted and pack attached. **B:** Pack drawn into position as catheter is removed. **C:** Strip tied over a bolster to hold pack in place with anterior pack installed "accordion pleating" style. **D:** Alternative method using balloon catheter instead of gauze pack. Anterior packing should follow placement of all posterior packs. (Reproduced, with permission, from Way LW [editor]: *Current Surgical Diagnosis & Treatment,* 9th ed. Appleton & Lange, 1991.)

- Scissors.
- Kelly clamp.

Positioning of the Patient

The patient should be either seated in an ENT chair or lying on a gurney with a back rest in the full upright position. The patient's head should also be supported.

Anatomy Review

Bleeding from the anterior nares most commonly occurs in the Kiesselbach area, located anteriorly along the nasal septum (see Figure 32–1). Bleeding that occurs more posteriorly in the anterior nares (a common occurrence in adults) may originate in the nasal turbinates. Posterior epistaxis usually occurs in elderly patients with calcified arteriosclerotic vessels, which are refractory to the normal vasospastic control mechanism in response to bleeding and which may therefore bleed briskly. These posterior vessels are not accessible in a routine nasal examination, and control of epistaxis therefore requires tamponade with a balloon or pack.

Procedure

Commercial devices such as nasal tampons and anterior nasal balloons are available and are very effective. The nasal balloons usually have a central cannula that allows for air passage.

A. Anterior Nasal Pack

1. Assemble and arrange all necessary equipment so that it is within easy reach.
2. Position the patient as described above, and make sure that the patient is comfortable but well supported and immobile.

3. Make sure that suction and adequate lighting are available.

4. While the operator is arranging equipment, an assistant can pinch the nose to stop bleeding from the septum.

5. Spread the patient's nostrils apart using the nasal speculum, and remove all blood with the suction device. Check the anterior septum for bleeding. Then examine the turbinates and the oropharynx to determine whether bleeding is occurring posteriorly.

6. If an anterior bleeding vessel is identified (eg, vessel in the Kisselbach area), bleeding can be controlled in one of 3 ways:

  a. *Local vasoconstriction.* Saturate cotton pledgets with tetracaine liquid mixed with phenylephrine nasal spray, place one in each nostril, and have an assistant or the patient firmly pinch the nostrils together for 5 minutes. The mixture will shrink the nasal mucosa and cause vasoconstriction, which, along with the pressure, often controls bleeding. An alternative method using 0.5–1% phenylephrine nasal spray and benzocaine-tetracaine spray in a similar manner is also effective.

  b. *Silver nitrate–tipped sticks.* After the bleeding site has been identified, cauterize the bleeding vessels using silver nitrate–tipped applicators. It is important to localize the site of cauterization precisely over the bleeding site. Overzealous cauterization of large areas of the nasal septum may cause septal necrosis with perforation.

  c. *Electrocautery.* A single anterior bleeding vessel may be cauterized using an electrocautery device. Exercise the same discretion required with chemical cautery.

7. Bleeding that is occurring more posteriorly in the anterior nasal passage, which cannot be controlled by local measures, requires anterior nasal packing. Using nasal forceps, pack the petrolatum-impregnated gauze in successive, tightly packed layers (accordion pleating), starting in the most posterior part of the accessible portion of the nose and working anteriorly. Insert only a small quantity of gauze at a time to ensure that the anterior naris is completely packed.

8. After the entire anterior nasal passage has been packed, check the oropharynx to see if bleeding is continuing posteriorly; if it is, insertion of a posterior pack is indicated (the anterior pack will have to be removed before this can be done). The anterior pack must then be replaced after posterior packing is completed.

B. Posterior Nasal Pack

1. Sedate the patient (for adults, diazepam, 10 mg orally; or morphine, 5–10 mg intramuscularly).

2. Anesthetize the anterior nose with cocaine-saturated cotton pledgets or benzocaine-tetracaine and phenylephrine sprays before inserting the posterior nasal pack using either of the methods outlined below.

  a. *Balloon occlusion technique:*

  (1) Balloon catheters made specifically to pack the posterior nasopharynx are available commercially. They work on the same principle as a Foley catheter, with an air inflation port to inflate the balloon.

  (2) The balloon-tipped distal end is inserted through the anterior naris into the posterior naris by guiding it directly posteriorly with gentle, steady pressure. After the catheter enters the posterior naris, inflate the balloon with the appropriate amount of air (the amount is printed on the balloon). Exert traction on the catheter to pull the balloon snugly up against the posterior nasal chamber, and secure the catheter at the external naris with gauze packing tied around the tube. Some nasal catheters have a small proximal balloon that, when inflated, will serve the same function as the gauze packing—to maintain tension on the distal intranasal balloon.

  (3) After inserting the balloon catheter, check the anterior naris for coexisting anterior bleeding and the oropharynx to determine if posterior bleeding is continuing. If bleeding is occurring from both sides, a second balloon catheter may be placed. Insert an anterior nasal pack.

  b. *Gauze technique:*

  (1) If a balloon catheter is not available, posterior packing can be accomplished using a 4- × 5-cm (1⅝- × 2-in) piece of absorbent cotton or gauze. Tie the gauze around the middle with 3 strands of size 0 silk suture material. Two of the strands will be passed through the nasal passage and tied at the anterior naris. The third strand will be cut and allowed to hang down in the throat to facilitate removal of the pack after bleeding has been controlled.

  (2) Pass the No. 12 rubber catheter through the external naris until the catheter is visible in the patient's throat.

(3) Using a Kelly clamp, grasp the end of the catheter in the throat, and bring it out through the patient's mouth (Figure 6–33A).

(4) Take the 2 ends of the size 0 silk suture material securing the gauze pack and tie them to the catheter.

(5) Pull the other end of the catheter through the patient's nose so that the sutures follow as the pack passes from the mouth to the posterior nasopharynx. This maneuver helps the pack fit snugly in the posterior nostril.

(6) Repeat the process for the other nostril. Tie the 4 silk strands (2 from each nostril) across a gauze sponge placed under the nose to prevent pressure on the nares from the septum.

(7) After the posterior packs are in place, pack the anterior nares, and check the oropharynx again to make sure that hemorrhage is controlled.

(8) In patients with preexisting cardiac or respiratory disease, draw blood for arterial blood gas determinations, because a significant drop in PO_2 may be seen.

All patients with posterior nasal packs should be hospitalized for monitoring of the airway. If the external gauze wrapping around the catheter slips, the balloon may be displaced posteriorly into the hypopharynx and may obstruct the airway. Antimicrobial prophylaxis (to prevent sinusitis) is recommended by many authorities, although its benefit is unproved. Give ampicillin, 150 mg/kg/d intravenously in 4–6 divided doses.

ARTHROCENTESIS
(Knee, Shoulder, Elbow, Ankle, Wrist, Hand, & Foot Joints)

The major peripheral joints can be aspirated safely in the emergency department. Aspiration of the hip and other joints of the axial skeleton usually requires the aid of specialists (orthopedic surgeons or rheumatologists) and the use of ancillary techniques (fluoroscopy and radionuclide scans); therefore, it is not discussed here.

Indications

Indications for arthrocentesis are as follows:

- Need to obtain synovial fluid for diagnosis.
- Drainage of hemarthrosis when conservative management is unsuccessful.
- Instillation of local analgesic and anti-inflammatory agents into a joint.

Contraindications

Contraindications to arthrocentesis are as follows:

- Soft tissue infection overlying proposed site of aspiration.
- Uncooperative patient (relative contraindication).
- Severe bleeding diathesis or anticoagulant therapy.

Personnel Required

One person can perform arthrocentesis unaided if the patient is cooperative, although an assistant is helpful for handling samples and holding young children.

Equipment & Supplies Required

- Materials for skin sterilization.
- Materials for sterile technique (mask and gloves; cap and gown are optional).
- Lidocaine, 1%, with 10-mL syringe and 22-gauge needle.
- Needles: 25-gauge, 1.5-cm (⅝-in) (2); 22-gauge, 4-cm (1½-in) (2); 20-gauge, 4-cm (1½-in) (2); 27-gauge, 1.5-cm (½-in) (1). Select a needle size appropriate to the joint to be aspirated.
- Syringes: 10-mL (2), 2-mL (2), 30-mL (1).
- Sterile gloves.
- Drapes.
- Gauze pads, 10 × 10 cm (4 × 4 in) (2); 5 × 5 cm (2 × 2 in) (2).
- Adhesive dressing.
- Sterile capped specimen tubes (2–3).
- Containers for synovial fluid: purple-topped or green-topped (EDTA or heparin anticoagulant, respectively, for cell count and differential and examination for crystals) (2); gray-topped (fluoride inhibitor for glucose) (1); red-topped (no anticoagulant) (3).
- Clean glass microscope slides and coverslips.

Positioning of the Patient

See Procedure for Specific Joints, below.

Procedure

1. Stabilize the joint to be aspirated. Identify landmarks, and mark the entry point with a scratch or indentation on the skin.

2. Sterilize the skin in a wide field around the puncture site.

3. Assemble all necessary equipment.

4. Observe sterile technique (don mask and gloves; cap and gown are optional).

5. Anesthetize the skin with the 1% lidocaine with the 10-mL syringe and 22- to 27-gauge needle; continue down to the joint capsule.

6. Select an appropriate needle (usually 20-gauge for knee, shoulder, elbow, ankle, or wrist; 25- or 27-gauge for small hand joints) and syringe (10-mL for knee, shoulder, elbow, ankle, or wrist; 2-mL for hand joints). A large-bore needle (eg, 18-gauge) may be required for aspiration of pus in larger joints. Use the 30-mL syringe for large effusions.

7. Penetrate the skin at the selected site, and cautiously advance the needle into the joint space; a "pop" will be felt when the needle passes through the synovium into the joint space. Aspirate continuously. Stop advancing the needle when joint fluid flows freely into the syringe.

8. Remove as much fluid as possible, but do not drain the joint dry if synovial biopsy is planned.

9. If joint fluid fails to flow freely, bring the needle all the way back to the subcutaneous tissue before redirecting it, in order to avoid joint trauma that might occur with deep probing.

10. After samples of fluid have been obtained, withdraw the needle, and apply firm pressure over the site for 1–2 minutes.

11. Cover the site with an adhesive dressing.

Procedure for Specific Joints

A. KNEE

The joint space of the knee may be entered either medially or laterally (Figure 6–34). In either case, the leg should be fully extended, with the patient supine. Pressure on the opposite side of the joint will make the synovium bulge more prominently and assist in directing the needle.

From the lateral aspect, the entrance site is at the intersection of lines (extended from the upper and lateral margins of the patella). A 22-gauge, 4-cm (1½-in) needle held parallel to the bed is directed medially and just deep to the patella and into the suprapatellar space.

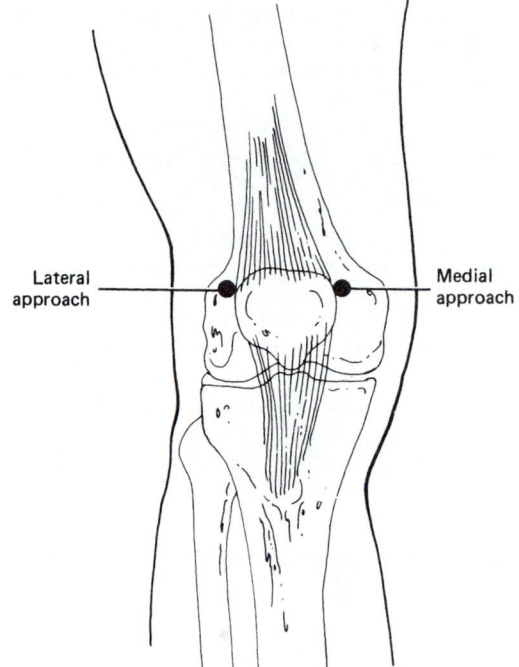

Figure 6–34. Aspiration of the knee joint.

From the medial aspect, the needle is introduced anteromedially in the space between the patella and the medial condyle. The needle (held parallel to the bed) is advanced upward (toward the undersurface of the patella) and laterally, beneath the patella and into the joint space.

B. SHOULDER

The shoulder joint can be aspirated from either an anterior or a posterior approach. The latter has the advantage of being out of the patient's line of vision.

For the posterior approach, the patient should sit in a chair and face backward (chest against the back of the chair). To open up the joint space and facilitate entry of the needle, the patient should put the arm of the site to be aspirated up against the chest and touch the opposite shoulder. This will adduct and internally rotate the arm. The head of the humerus is palpable posterolaterally. Use a 20- or 22-gauge, 4-cm (1½-in) needle, and keep it parallel to the floor. Direct it about 30 degrees medially into the joint space from a point just under the posterior inferior border of the acromion (Figure 6–35).

For the anterior approach, the patient should sit in a chair, facing forward, with the arm comfortably supported in the lap. Using a 20- or 22-gauge, 4-cm (1½-in) needle, enter the joint space at a spot medial to the head of the humerus and just below the palpable tip of

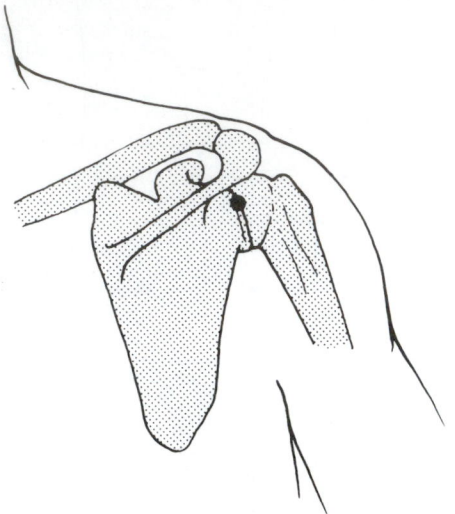

Figure 6–35. Posterior approach to shoulder joint aspiration.

the coracoid process (Figure 6–36). Direct the needle slightly laterally and superiorly into the scapulohumeral joint space.

C. Elbow

Be certain to differentiate olecranon bursitis that does not involve the elbow joint from bulging synovium.

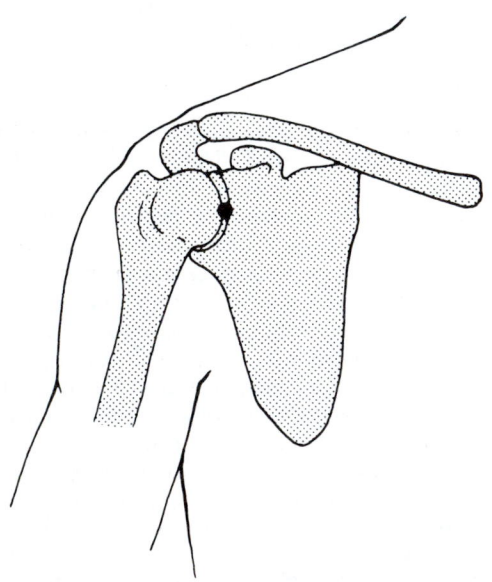

Figure 6–36. Anterior approach to shoulder joint aspiration.

Have the patient sit with the forearm supported from the elbow to the hand on a table, with the elbow joint in about 10–30 degrees of flexion. With significant effusion, the bulging synovium should be evident laterally. Introduce the needle (usually a 20- or 22-gauge, 4-cm [1½-in] needle) just below the lateral epicondyle and proximal to the olecranon process of the ulna (Figure 6–37). Advance the needle medially and slightly proximally into the joint space.

D. Ankle

Arthrocentesis of the ankle is more difficult than that of the other joints discussed here. The most common approach is anteromedial. Have the patient lie supine, with the knee extended and the foot slightly plantarflexed. Identify the extensor hallucis longus tendon by having the patient extend the great toe. Just anterior (1 cm [≅⅜ in]) and inferior (1 cm [≅⅜ in]) to the medial malleolus and lateral to the extensor tendon is a small depression. Introduce the needle in this depression, and direct it toward the tibiotalar articulation (Figure 6–38). If swelling and pain are most severe on the side of the ankle, use a similar approach but from the anterolateral aspect of the joint. When subtalar disease is suspected (eg, pain on pronation and supination of the foot), the needle is introduced more distally, at the talonavicular articulation. Although fluid is seldom obtained at the talonavicular joint, injection of anti-inflammatory agents may be readily accomplished.

E. Wrist

A bulging, inflamed joint space at the wrist can be entered dorsally at prominent areas of swelling; such areas

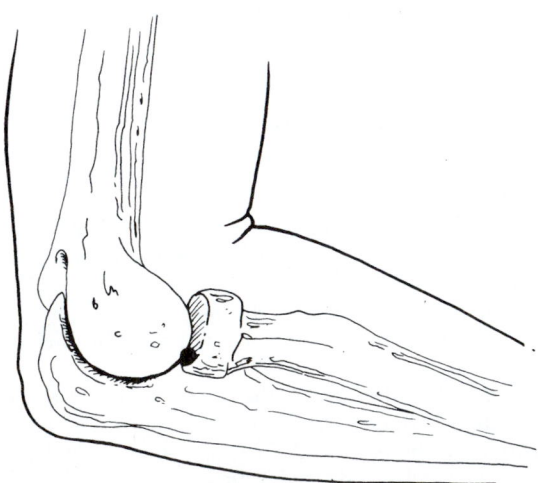

Figure 6–37. Aspiration of the elbow joint.

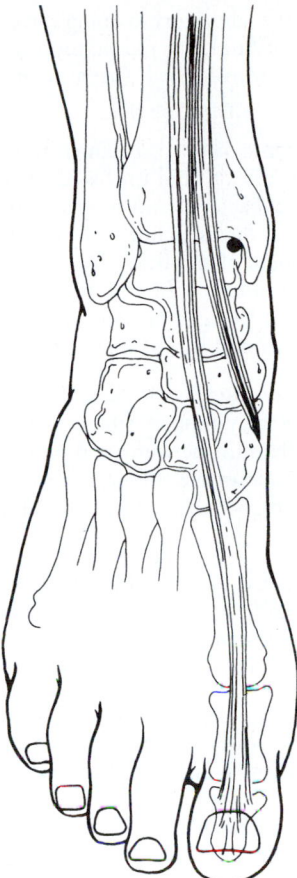

Figure 6–38. Determination of the needle entry site for ankle joint aspiration. A small depression can be palpated about 1 cm (½ in) anterior and inferior to the medial malleolus and lateral to the extensor hallucis longus.

are invariably found on the radial or ulnar aspects. Use a 20- or 22-gauge, 4-cm (1½-in) needle.

For the radial (lateral) entry, position the hand with the palmar surface down, and flex it over a rolled towel at the wrist. Aspirate the joint at the midpoint of the distal articulation of the radius, just medial to the extensor tendon of the thumb. The needle should be perpendicular to the skin during aspiration.

The ulnar, or medial, approach is made in the middle of the palpable depression between the lateral aspect of the tip of the ulna and carpus. Position the hand as for a radial approach. Direct the needle ventrally toward the palmar surface and proximally into the joint space.

To administer corticosteroids into the carpal tunnel (to treat compression of the median nerve), place the needle between flexor creases of the wrist just lateral to the palmaris longus tendon (or medial to the flexor carpi radialis), and advance it distally until resistance to injection is minimal. (See Chapter 29 for details.)

F. SMALL JOINTS OF THE HANDS AND FEET

Systemic arthritides frequently involve the proximal and distal interphalangeal joints and the first metatarsophalangeal joint. Enter the joint in the midline just lateral to the extensor tendon on the dorsolateral aspect, and gently work a 25- or 27-gauge needle into the joint space. A 2-mL syringe suffices for aspiration and is easier to handle than larger ones. Maintain a slight vacuum in the syringe, so that any trauma to digital vessels will be recognized immediately (blood will appear in the syringe). Traction on the distal portion of the phalanx helps open the joint space, allowing easier access for the needle.

Synovial Fluid Analysis

If minimal fluid is available, priorities must be established for processing the sample. If pyogenic arthritis is a diagnostic possibility, an appropriate approach would be to place one drop of fluid on a microscope slide for Gram stain, another into a hemacytometer for cell count, and the remainder of the sample for culture. If 10–20 mL or more of synovial fluid is obtained, complete synovianalysis can be performed, as outlined below; partial analysis is possible on even as little as 1 mL of fluid.

A. PHYSICAL CHARACTERISTICS

1. Determine the total volume of fluid removed.
2. Assess color and clarity of fluid (normally a crystal-clear yellowish fluid through which print can be easily read).
3. Note viscosity by allowing a drop to fall from the needle. Normal joint fluid has high viscosity and easily forms a cord several inches long.
4. Perform the mucin clot test (Ropes test) by adding 1 mL of synovial fluid to diluted acetic acid (about 5%). Normally, the mucin in the fluid congeals within minutes, forming a gel (commonly called a clot) that remains firm for hours. In the case of infection or chronic inflammation, unstable gel forms that is easily broken up by gentle agitation. Examine the gel again at 1 hour for friability; normal mucin gel should be unchanged after 1 hour.

B. LABORATORY STUDIES

The choice of studies is guided by clinical circumstances. Gram stain and culture, cell count, and examination for crystal formation should always be performed when fluid from an acutely inflamed joint is being evaluated.

1. Cell count and differential—Place 2–10 mL of synovial fluid in a purple-topped (EDTA anticoagulant) or green-topped (heparin anticoagulant) tube for laboratory examination. If fluid is scanty, use 1–2 drops counterstained with methylene blue, and perform a cell count in the emergency department with a hemacytometer. Normal synovial fluid contains fewer than 200 white cells per microliter, of which less than 25% are polymorphonuclear neutrophils.

2. Special stains—All joint fluid should be stained with Gram stain and examined by microscopy. Special stains for fungi and acid-fast bacilli should also be performed when chronic monarticular arthritis is being evaluated. These tests are specific but not sensitive for detection of fungal or mycobacterial arthritis.

3. Examination for crystals—Place a drop of synovial fluid on a clean glass microscope slide under a coverslip. Examine the specimen immediately; if this is impossible, slow the evaporation of joint fluid by sealing the edges of the coverslip with nail polish or petrolatum. Crystals can be detected using light microscopy and tentatively identified on the basis of morphologic characteristics seen at × 400 magnification. Urate crystals are needle-shaped; calcium pyrophosphate crystals are more rhomboid-shaped; and cholesterol crystals are flat, with notched corners. Polarized light microscopy demonstrates the negative birefringence of urate crystals and the positive birefringence of calcium pyrophosphate. The presence of crystals both free in fluid and within leukocytes is pathognomonic of crystal-induced arthropathy. If the laboratory is doing the examination, collect 1–2 mL of fluid in a purple-topped (EDTA anticoagulant) or green-topped (heparin anticoagulant) tube.

4. Culture—Sterile, capped specimen tubes should be filled with 1–10 mL of fluid for bacterial cultures and, if indicated, mycobacterial and fungal cultures. In suspected gonococcal disease, chocolate agar should be inoculated with some of the fluid (in the emergency department if possible). When a potentially infected prosthetic joint is being evaluated, a jar of anaerobic transport media should also be inoculated.

5. Glucose determination—Place 0.5–1 mL of synovial fluid in a gray-topped (fluoride anticoagulant) tube. The sample must be compared with a simultaneously drawn blood sample. Blood glucose that is more than 40 mg/dL higher than synovial fluid glucose suggests infection.

6. Protein—Place 0.5–1 mL of synovial joint fluid in a red-topped (no anticoagulant) tube. Determine the total serum protein of a simultaneously drawn blood sample. Normal joint protein is about one third that of serum.

7. Other studies—Less commonly indicated studies include cytology studies in possible pigmented villonodular synovitis or metastatic disease (5–10 mL in a lightly heparinized specimen tube); pH determinations (1–2 mL in a sealed heparinized syringe); complement levels; and tests for rheumatoid factor, antinuclear antibody, immunoglobulins, and various enzymes.

The presence of fat globules (often with blood) suggests intra-articular fracture.

INCISION & DRAINAGE OF SUPERFICIAL ABSCESS

Indications

A superficial abscess is incised in order to drain it.

Contraindications

There are no contraindications to incision and drainage of a superficial abscess.

Personnel Required

One person can usually incise and drain a superficial abscess unaided, although an assistant may be helpful to restrain an uncooperative patient.

Equipment & Supplies Required

Many incision and drainage kits are commercially available. The following items are required:

- Materials for skin cleansing.
- Protective gown or apron and gloves.
- No. 11 surgical blade, mounted.
- Drapes.
- Curved Kelly and mosquito clamps.
- Forceps.
- Packing material, such as gauze strip packing.
- Sterile gauze sponges, 10 × 10 cm (4 × 4 in), and tape.

- Ethyl chloride skin-freezing solution (optional).
- Lidocaine, 1%, with 25-gauge needle and 5-mL syringe.
- Culture tube and slides.
- Sterile saline for irrigation.
- Irrigating syringe and basin.
- Needle, 18-gauge, with 5-mL syringe.
- Plastic-coated absorbent pad.

Positioning of the Patient

The patient should be lying on a firm surface in a comfortable position, with the area to be drained in full view and firmly supported.

Procedure

Anesthesia is the main difficulty in incision and drainage. Superficial abscesses suitable for drainage at the bedside are painful, and the patient should be assured that pain will decrease after the pressure is relieved and the pus is drained. Incising the skin and draining the pus are painful, however, and little relief can be obtained short of general or block anesthesia, both of which require an anesthesiologist and an operating room. Spraying the area with ethyl chloride to freeze the skin will prevent some but not all pain. Infiltrating the thick layer of skin over the pointing abscess with lidocaine is impossible, and injecting lidocaine into the abscess cavity is ineffective and may create more pain from increased pressure. Narcotic analgesics (eg, morphine, 2–10 mg intramuscularly or subcutaneously) may take the edge off the pain and relieve some of the patient's anxiety, but they will not provide total relief.

If an abscess is too large to be adequately drained at the bedside or if it appears that the patient may experience too much pain to be able to cooperate effectively, incision and drainage in the operating room is always an alternative.

A. SIMPLE ABSCESS NOT INVOLVING A VITAL STRUCTURE

1. Assemble the necessary equipment, and arrange it on a table or bedside stand.

2. Position the patient. Place the plastic-coated absorbent pad under the body part with the abscess to be drained.

3. Don sterile gloves and put on a gown to protect clothing. Cleanse the skin over the area being drained. Drape the area, and have extra absorbent materials ready to catch any pus not absorbed by the drape.

4. If there is any doubt whether an abscess is actually present, take the 18-gauge needle and the 5-mL syringe, and aspirate the suspected abscess at the point of maximum fluctuance. If no pus is found, reassess the clinical situation, and proceed with incision and draining if it is deemed appropriate.

5. If ethyl chloride or lidocaine is being used, it should be given at this time.

6. Using the No. 11 blade, open the abscess at the point of maximum fluctuance, and allow the pus to drain under its own pressure. Using a quick, decisive motion minimizes the patient's discomfort. Collect the first portion of pus for Gram stain and culture and sensitivity testing.

7. After the pressure has been relieved, insert the Kelly or mosquito clamp and find the longest axis of the abscess. Point the curve of the clamp up at the farthest point from the central incision and determine the shortest possible length to be incised so that the abscess is completely drained. Incise the skin to that point, using swift upward motion of the No. 11 blade. If it is necessary to make a long incision to completely drain the abscess, infiltrate the skin in the most lateral aspect with lidocaine. Repeat the procedure in the opposite direction. Allow any further pus to drain. ***Note:*** It is important to obtain an opening in the abscess wide enough to allow complete drainage of all pus. If the abscess is not opened completely, complete drainage cannot occur, and resolution of the abscess will be delayed.

8. Using the clamp, break up any loculated pus in the cavity.

9. Irrigate the abscess with saline until all pus is removed.

10. Pack the abscess cavity with iodoform or plain gauze packing. Fill the cavity tightly enough to cause hemostasis but not so tightly that it causes pain.

11. Dress the area with the sterile 10- × 10-cm (4- × 4-in) sponge and tape. On the extremities or in areas where there is movement, consider dressing the site with an expanded bandage around the extremity.

12. Begin antimicrobial therapy, if indicated (eg, for facial abscesses, cellulitis). Dicloxacillin, 20 mg/kg/d orally in 4 divided doses, is usually satisfactory.

13. Schedule a follow-up appointment in 1–2 days.

B. INCISION AND DRAINAGE OF ABSCESSES OVER SPECIAL AREAS

1. Face, head, and neck abscesses—The clinical situation in these anatomic areas must be carefully considered before incision and drainage is performed, because the large scar left by complete incision and drainage may be cosmetically unacceptable and because of the possibility of injuring vital structures beneath the skin. In small superficial abscesses on the face, drainage can be accomplished by making a small incision at the lower part of the abscess, removing all pus, and leaving a gauze wick in the incision to keep the wound from closing. Frequent irrigation will be needed during follow-up to keep the cavity clean and promote healing. Any abscess that is large or that might involve vital structures should be drained in the operating room by personnel experienced in this procedure.

2. Abscesses around joints—Make sure that the abscess does not involve the joint space. (Consult an orthopedic surgeon if there is any doubt.) If the abscess is superficial and does not involve the joint space, proceed with incision and drainage. Remember that splinting of the joint is necessary for adequate healing.

3. Abscesses around the anus—Differentiate pilonidal abscesses from perianal abscesses caused by anal fistulas. Perianal of abscesses require surgical consultation and possibly drainage in the operating room.

4. Abscesses of the hands, wrists, ankles, and feet—The compact arrangement of many vital structures in the hand, wrist, ankle, and foot makes drainage of abscesses in these areas difficult to perform in the emergency department. It is recommended that any abscess around these structures be drained in the operating room by experienced personnel. Surgical consultation is advisable in all cases of abscesses in these areas.

TRANSCUTANEOUS CARDIAC PACING

Transcutaneous cardiac pacing is a safe, rapid, noninvasive method of temporarily treating symptomatic bradyarrhythmias and asystole. Recent advances in technology have led to the development of defibrillators that are also capable of transcutaneous pacing. With these devices, transcutaneous pacing can be initiated in the prehospital setting or in the emergency department and is the procedure of choice in the treatment of asystole and bradycardic cardiac arrest.

Indications

- Asystole.
- Symptomatic bradycardia (< 40 beats/min) unresponsive to atropine.
- Overdrive pacing for tachyarrhythmias (atrial, ventricular, torsade de pointes) unresponsive to medical and electrical cardioversion.
- Transvenous pacing is difficult or contraindicated (eg, heart block in myocardial infarction treated with thrombolytic therapy).

Complications

The main complications associated with transcutaneous pacing are pain and local skin erythema due to first-degree burns. With the newer devices, pain from cutaneous nerve and muscle stimulation is now reported as tolerable. The energy levels used for pacing have not been shown to produce any significant myocardial damage. Other persons coming into contact with the pacing impulses may experience mild tingling. The risk of inducing ventricular fibrillation during transcutaneous pacing is negligible.

Personnel Required

One person can initiate transcutaneous pacing unaided.

Equipment Required

- Transcutaneous pacing device, 2 pacing electrodes, and connecting cable.
- Optional electrodes and connecting cable for electrocardiographic monitoring are available with some models.

Procedure

1. Place one pacing electrode over the left anterior chest. Place the other electrode posteriorly in the interscapular area. Attach the connecting cables as indicated on the labels.
2. If the pacing device is equipped for electrocardiographic monitoring, attach monitor leads to both shoulders and the left upper abdomen. ***Note:*** Standard electrocardiographic monitor results are usually uninterpretable owing to the strong pacing stimulus and movement artifact.
3. Set rate at 80 beats/min; select synchronous mode for bradycardia or asynchronous mode for asystole. (Depending on the model, rate and mode may be fixed and not operator-selected.) Turn on power; turn on pacing.

4. Begin at 70–80 mA current output.

5. Check for presence of a femoral pulse. Check the monitor for evidence of electrical capture (pacer spike before each QRS complex). If no pulse is detected, gradually increase the current output until pulse appears or highest current setting is reached. *Caution:* The carotid pulse is usually difficult to detect owing to muscle contractions. A Doppler stethoscope may be needed to ascertain the presence or absence of a pulse.

6. Reduce current output to the lowest setting associated with a palpable pulse, and determine blood pressure.

7. If transcutaneous pacing is successful, interrupt pacing intermittently to check for return of spontaneous electrical activity. As soon as the patient is stable, if pacing is still needed, insert a transvenous pacemaker.

8. If transcutaneous pacing is unsuccessful and pacing is still required, attempt transvenous pacing.

SECTION II
Management of Common Emergency Problems

Basic & Advanced Cardiac Life Support

7

Eric M. Sergienko, MD, & Thomas N. Bottoni, MD

Overview of Cardiac Arrest
    Epidemiology of Cardiac Arrest
    Determinants of Cardiac Arrest Survival
    The Team Approach to Cardiac Arrest
    Family Presence During Resuscitation
Adult Basic Life Support
    The Chain of Survival
    Techniques of Basic Life Support
    Complications of Basic Life Support
    Foreign Body Airway Obstruction
    Defibrillation
Adult Advanced Life Support
    Advanced Airway Management

    Specific Rhythms
    Pharmacologic Therapy
    Postresuscitation Stabilization
    Termination of Resuscitation
Cardiopulmonary Resuscitation in Infants & Children
    Pediatric Basic Life Support
    Pediatric Advanced Life Support
Novel Approaches in Cardiac Arrest Management
    Alternative Basic Life Support Techniques
    The Scaling Exponent
    Fibrinolytic Therapy

■ OVERVIEW OF CARDIAC ARREST

EPIDEMIOLOGY OF CARDIAC ARREST

Cardiac disease is the most common cause of death in the United States. The majority of cardiac deaths occur suddenly. There are more than 300,000 cardiac arrests each year in the United States. About two thirds of these occur in the prehospital setting. Survival to discharge varies dramatically from region to region and system to system with rates ranging from 1.4% in New York City to 49% in King County, Washington. A meta-analysis of defibrillator-capable emergency medical services (EMS) showed a median survival to discharge rate of 6.4%. Of note, resuscitation within critical care areas has similar success rates. Sudden cardiac death is associated with an underlying history of coronary artery disease, but an acute thrombotic event is associated with only 20–40% of cardiac arrests. Twenty-five percent of cardiac arrests have a noncardiac origin (eg, massive pulmonary embolism, renal failure, malignancy). The most common presenting rhythm to prehospital care providers is ventricular fibrillation, which occurs in about a third of all patients. Asystole and pulseless electrical activity (PEA, formerly electromechanical dissociation) are the second and third most common rhythms, respectively, at time of first intervention.

DETERMINANTS OF CARDIAC ARREST SURVIVAL

The single most important factor for survival in the undifferentiated adult cardiac arrest victim is the elapsed time from patient collapse until the first defibrillation shock is delivered. Other factors related to a positive outcome include witnessed cardiac arrest, early bystander cardiopulmonary resuscitation (CPR), and chest pain as the presenting complaint. Early provision of advanced life support (ALS) has been shown to be of benefit, but its value in addition to defibrillation is of some debate. Factors associated with poor prognosis include dyspnea as the presenting complaint, malignancy or sepsis as the underlying cause of cardiac arrest, coexistence of pneumonia, presence of hypotension prior to cardiac arrest, and a homebound lifestyle.

A patient who is not resuscitated in the field is unlikely to be resuscitated in the emergency department. Forty-six percent of patients are deemed dead in the field, and another 16% are declared dead upon arrival in the emergency department or shortly thereafter. The risks of transporting a patient who remains in cardiac arrest after ALS procedures have been performed in the field often outweigh the likelihood of a successful resuscitation with good neurologic outcome. Medical directors should consider protocols to determine death and termination of resuscitative efforts in the field.

THE TEAM APPROACH TO CARDIAC ARREST

There are many pivotal participants in a cardiac arrest—first responder, prehospital EMS personnel, emergency department resuscitation team leader, emergency department resuscitation team members, and ancillary personnel. A successful resuscitation depends on a functional team. Roles should be identified prior to a resuscitation. Team behaviors and expectations can be established and used on a daily basis and during real-time resuscitations.

The composition of the resuscitation team is based largely on resource availability and institutional preferences. Intuitively, there must be a team leader who is responsible for the overall direction of the resuscitation.

A designated team member must manage the airway, and a second, or even third, team member can assist with airway functions, including ventilation, suctioning, and gathering and assembly of airway equipment. Multiple team members will rotate through providing chest compressions. The team leader must ensure that these providers do not become fatigued, providing for relief every 5–10 minutes. Vascular access must be obtained, and the team member performing this role can also administer medications. If a medication dispenser (eg, Pyxis) is being used, it is helpful to designate one person to manage it. Finally, it is helpful to have a recorder to record events, provide cues, track laboratory results, and communicate with areas outside of the resuscitation. The team leader must also control the number of people involved in the resuscitation. Too often the scene becomes chaotic because of those wanting to help or just take a look.

Care providers are often trained as individuals, even though they most often respond as an integrated team. Utilization of team behaviors can minimize the number of errors, duplication of efforts, and loss of information that can occur during the confusion of a resuscitation. Maintaining situational awareness is the key to being an essential team member. Reinforcing situational awareness in others (ie, cross monitoring) emphasizes the team construct. Some mechanisms to enhance cross monitoring include call outs, check backs, and hand offs. Call outs involve information that must be shared with the entire team (eg, calling out vital signs). Check backs are means to avoid order errors—the recipient of the order repeats the order verbatim, and then the orderer confirms that order verbatim. Hand offs are positive transfer of control of aspects of patient care. These techniques sustain dynamic situational awareness and allow for an organized, integrated team approach to comprehensive resuscitative care.

FAMILY PRESENCE DURING RESUSCITATION

An often vexing issue in a resuscitation is the presence of family members. The default has been to exclude the family from the resuscitation. Most surveys of family members show they would prefer to be present at resuscitations. This is true for both adult and pediatric resuscitations. Most providers who work at facilities that allow family members to be present during resuscitation feel it is beneficial. Those who work at facilities that do not allow family members to be present feel that it is not beneficial and may interfere with the resuscitation. Programs that have implemented family presence during resuscitations dedicate a staff member to be at the family's side to answer questions, provide support, and act as a liaison between the family and the resuscitation team.

Clarke JR et al: An objective analysis of process errors in trauma resuscitations. Acad Emerg Med 2000;7(11):1303. [PMID: 11073483]

Cooper S, Wakelam A: Leadership of resuscitation teams: "Lighthouse Leadership." Resuscitation 1999;42(1):27. [PMID: 10524729]

de Vreede-Swagemakers et al: Circumstances and causes of out-of-hospital cardiac arrest in sudden death survivors. Heart 1998;79(4):356. [PMID: 9616342]

Dickinson ET, Schneider RM, Verdile VP: The impact of pre-hospital physicians on out-of-hospital nonasystolic cardiac arrest. Prehosp Emerg Care 1997;1(3):132. [PMID: 9709354]

Hillman K et al: Redefining in-hospital resuscitation: the concept of the medical emergency team. Resuscitation 2001;48(2):105. [PMID: 11426471]

Soar J, Absalom A: Survival after cardiac arrest outside hospital. Heart 2000;83(1):103. [PMID: 10671071]

Soo LH et al: Resuscitation from out-of-hospital cardiac arrest: is survival dependent on who is available at the scene? Heart 1999;81(1):47. [PMID: 10220544]

Stiell IG et al: Modifiable factors associated with improved cardiac arrest survival in a multicenter basic life support/defibrillation system: OPALS Study phase I results. Ontario Prehospital Advanced Life Support. Ann Emerg Med 1999;33(1):44. [PMID: 9867885]

Tsai E: Should family members be present during cardiopulmonary resuscitation? N Engl J Med 2002;346(13):1019. [PMID: 11919313]

Weston CF, Wilson RJ, Jones SD: Predicting survival from out-of-hospital cardiac arrest: a multivariate analysis. Resuscitation 1997;34(1):27. [PMID: 9051821]

■ ADULT BASIC LIFE SUPPORT (See Figure 7–1.)

THE CHAIN OF SURVIVAL

The American Heart Association (AHA) first proposed the phrase "the chain of survival" to describe the interrelated series of interventions that must be in place to maximize functional survival from sudden cardiac death. Any failure to implement a single link in the chain will lead to a decrease in survival. As depicted by the AHA, there are 4 links in the chain of survival: early access, early basic life support (BLS), early defibrillation, and early advanced cardiac life support (ACLS). Some authors propose a total of 7 links, to include early prevention prior to the event and definitive care and rehabilitation after the event. The framework of ACLS and BLS interventions focuses on maintaining the links of this chain.

TECHNIQUES OF BASIC LIFE SUPPORT

Early Prevention

Early prevention involves both primary prevention, including lifestyle modification, and secondary prevention, including medical therapy. More pertinent, the patient and family should be taught the signs and symptoms of chest pain related to cardiac ischemia. Patients with known cardiac disease should attempt to treat the pain with sublingual nitroglycerin. If, after taking 3 doses of nitroglycerin, there is no relief, the patient should call the emergency number for his or her area. Patients without known disease should contact the emergency number if unremitting chest pain is present for more than 5 minutes. In the hospital setting, an early, organized approach to chest pain, dyspnea, and abnormal vital signs including pulse oximetry can decrease the number of cardiac arrests.

Early Access

The first responder should call the appropriate emergency number (eg, 9-1-1) after coming upon an unresponsive patient. In the adult victim, after opening the airway and confirming apnea, "phone first." In the community setting, call the emergency number (eg, 9-1-1) to initiate an organized response to the cardiac arrest. In the hospital setting, initiate the hospital's emergency response or "code" system. Early access into the system is imperative to minimize the time delay until defibrillation.

Early Basic Life Support

Upon finding an unresponsive patient, activate the EMS system and then return to the patient to provide BLS until further help arrives. Assume a position alongside the patient so that rescue breathing and chest compressions can be done without repositioning one's body. Position the patient on a hard surface to allow for efficient chest compressions. This is achieved by placing a CPR board under the patient's chest or modifying the bed to provide a firmer surface. Anticipate the arrival of a defibrillator, which is usually positioned on the left side, next to the patient's ear.

The ABCs

A. AIRWAY

Open the patient's airway using the head-tilt and chin-lift method (Figure 7–2). Place one hand firmly on the patient's forehead; apply firm downward, backward pressure to tilt the head. Hook the fingers of the other hand under the bony part of the chin, lifting up the chin. In the event of trauma, use the jaw thrust without head tilt (Figure 7–3A).

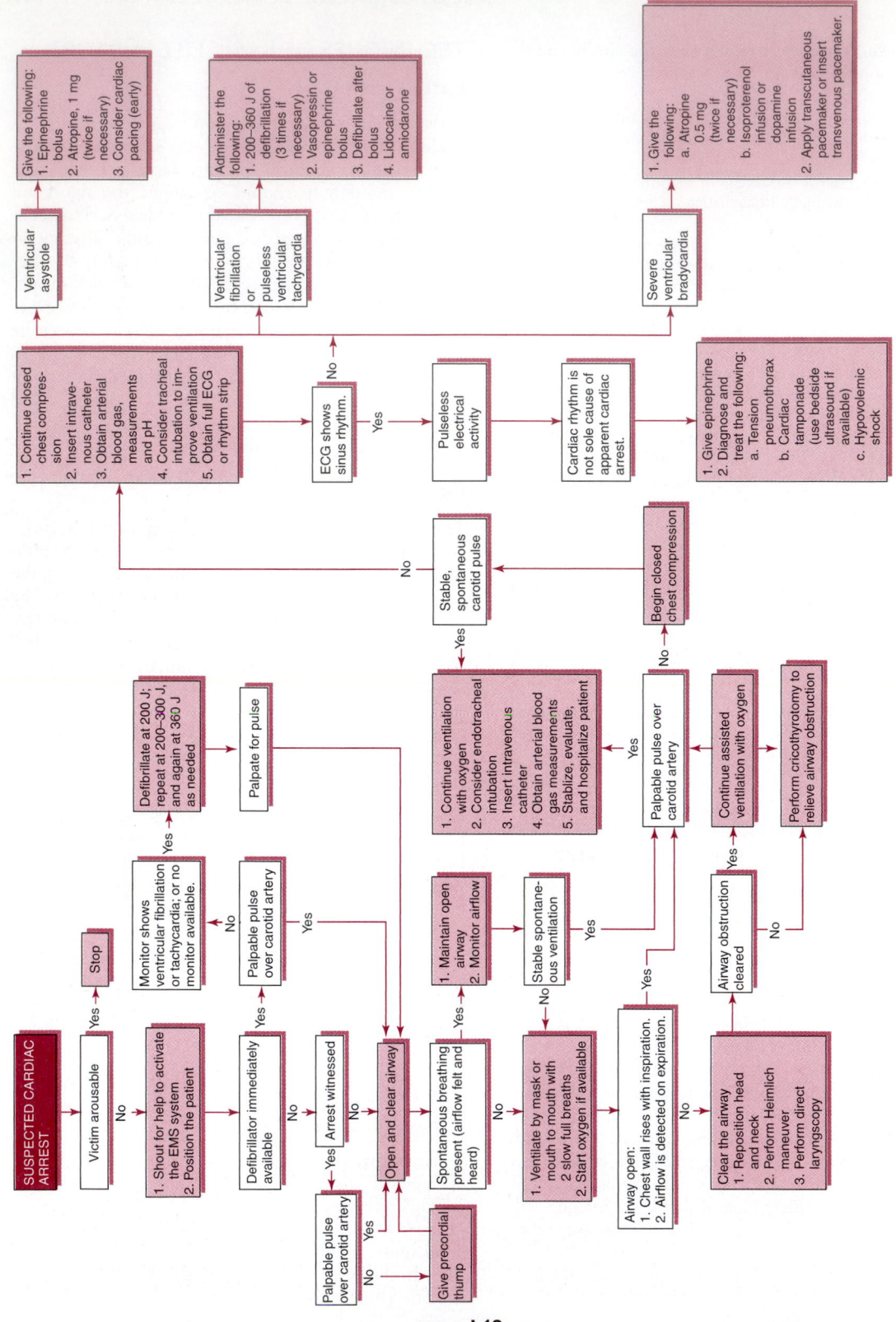

Figure 7–1. Management of suspected cardiac arrest.

148

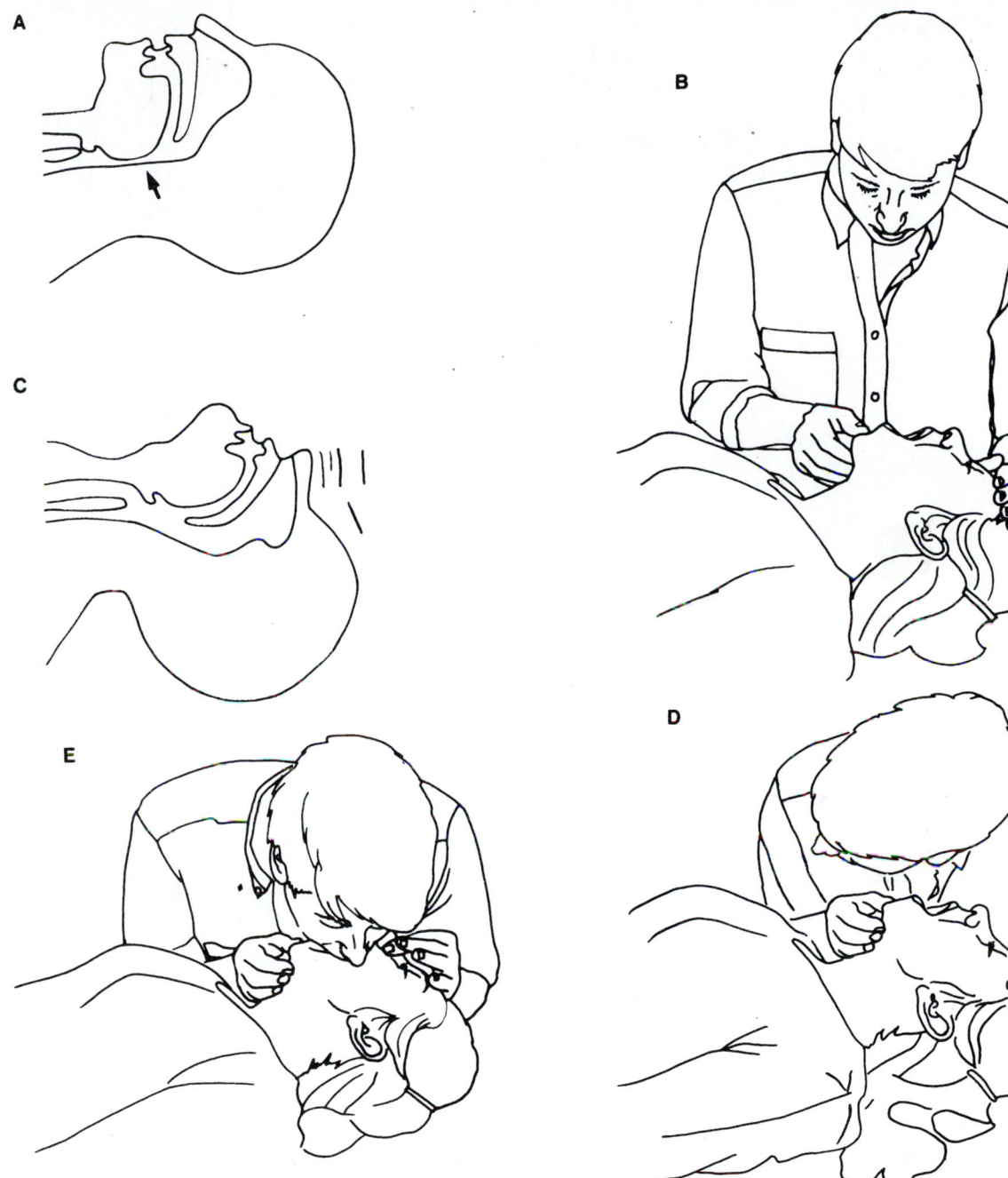

Figure 7–2. Opening the airway and providing ventilation. **A:** Obstruction of airway by posterior displacement of tongue (arrow) in resting, supine position. **B** and **C:** Relief of lingual airway obstruction in supine position by forward displacement of mandible (head-tilt and chin-lift method). **D:** Rescuer checks for spontaneous breathing by listening and feeling for exhaled air while looking for chest movement. **E:** Mouth-to-mouth ventilation. While maintaining head tilt and chin lift, the rescuer uses his or her fingers to seal the victim's nose shut; rescuer takes a deep breath, seals mouth over victim's mouth, and exhales, watching for chest movement. Look, listen, and feel for passive exhalation.

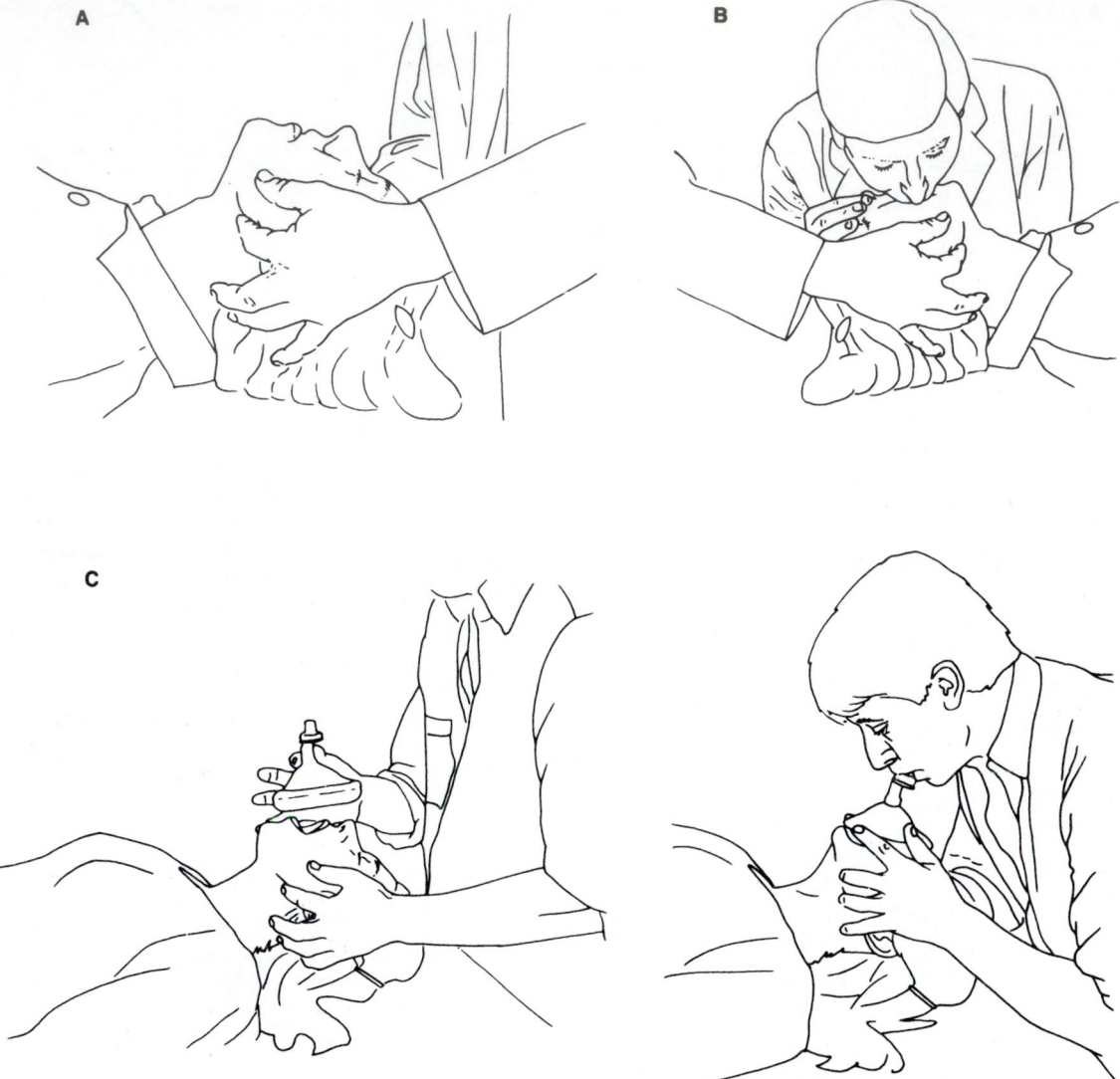

A

B

C

Figure 7–3. Jaw-thrust maneuver. **A:** If cervical spine injury is suspected, open airway by grasping and lifting angles of victim's lower jaw without tilting the head. **B** and **C:** Ventilation is best provided with the aid of a second rescuer or a pocket mask.

B. BREATHING

Assess breathing by leaning over the patient's open mouth and looking down at the chest for any rise or fall of breathing. Place an ear near the patient's mouth, listening for breathing or feeling the flow of air over the cheek (see Figure 7–2D). This should take no more than 10 seconds.

In the absence of breathing, perform mouth-to-mouth, mouth-to-mask, or bag-mask ventilation. Health

care professionals should be familiar with all of these techniques. A mask with a one-way valve should be readily available in all health care settings to minimize the risk of contamination from the patient's oral secretions. A bag-mask should be available in all critical care areas and on crash carts.

1. Mouth to mouth—The airway is maintained by using the head-tilt and chin-lift method. Pinch the patient's nose shut. Seal your lips around the patient's mouth (see Figure 7–2E). Give 2 slow breaths initially. There should be good chest rise and fall. If not, reposition the patient's airway and attempt to ventilate again. If there is still no movement of air, presume that the patient has a foreign body airway obstruction (see "Foreign Body Airway Obstruction" section, below) and attempt to clear it.

2. Mouth to mask—A clear mask with or without a one-way valve (often called a pocket mask) can be used as an adjunct to mouth-to-mouth ventilation (see Figure 7–3C). Ventilations are provided in the same way as for mouth to mouth. It is often easier and more effective for the inexperienced provider to adequately ventilate the patient with the pocket-mask than with the bag-mask. When possible the mask should be attached to supplemental oxygen. There are 2 techniques to achieve an effective seal with the mask.

a. Cephalic technique—The cephalic technique is used when there is more than 1 provider. The provider ventilating the patient is positioned at the head of the bed. The mask is applied in one of two ways, either with the thumbs and thenar eminences providing a seal, while the fingers are used to perform jaw thrust, or with the thumbs and index fingers providing a seal, while the remaining fingers provide a jaw thrust (Figure 7–4).

b. Lateral technique—When there is only 1 provider, the lateral technique must be used to allow

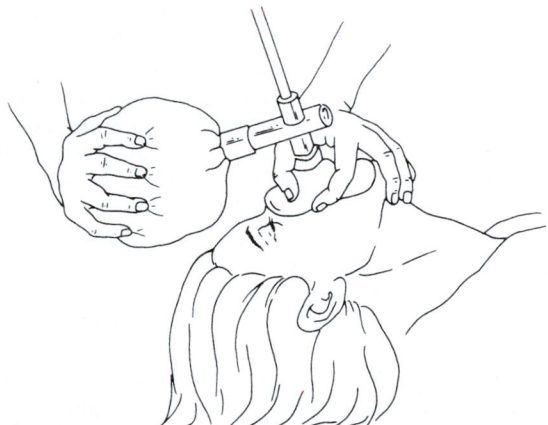

Figure 7–4. Ventilation technique using face mask and positive pressure ventilation (bag or valve). As in mouth-to-mouth ventilation, head must be tilted to keep airway open. Seal mask to face with one hand, with fingers under chin to maintain open airway. Use other hand to operate bag or valve.

the provider to perform 1-person CPR. With the provider at the patient's side, a head tilt–chin lift is applied. The hand closer to the top of the patient's head performs a head tilt while creating a seal on the upper part of the mask with index finger and thumb. The lower hand performs a chin lift with the fingers while creating a seal on the lower part of the mask with the thumb and thenar eminence.

3. Bag-mask ventilation—When ventilating a patient, use supplemental oxygen whenever possible, to provide up to a 100% concentration. The adult bag-mask is usually a 1600-mL self-inflating bag with a nonrebreathing valve attached to a face mask. There should be a reservoir for oxygen and tubing to connect to an oxygen source.

When 2 providers are available to manage the patient's airway, the mask is applied as with the cephalic technique of the pocket-mask. Ventilations are then administered by the second provider squeezing the bag over 2 seconds and then releasing for 3 seconds. If only one provider is available for airway management, he or she must provide an adequate seal with one hand, using the index finger and thumb while providing a chin lift with the other 3 fingers. The other hand is used to squeeze the bag-mask. Optimizing the head tilt by positioning towels underneath the patient's shoulders may help, especially if the patient is obese. Ventilation can be improved by squeezing the bag against the provider's body.

4. Cricoid pressure application—Cricoid pressure (Sellick maneuver) can be used to minimize gastric insufflation associated with ventilation. The cricoid cartilage is the only complete ring in the trachea. Posterior displacement of the cricoid cartilage closes off the esophagus. This should be done only in the unconscious patient. The cricoid cartilage is found by first locating the thyroid cartilage with the index finger, then moving down the neck over the cricothyroid membrane. The first cartilage ring below the membrane is the cricoid cartilage. Moderate pressure (5–10 pounds) is applied, pressing the cartilage with the thumb and index finger posteriorly toward the cervical spine.

C. CIRCULATION

Assess circulation by checking for the carotid pulse. The carotid pulse is located in the groove lateral to the trachea. Check the pulse for no more than 10 seconds. If a pulse is present, rescue breathing can continue with 1 breath every 4–5 seconds. If a pulse is absent, start chest compressions.

Chest compressions are performed on the lower half of the sternum. Identify the location by tracing the fingers of the hand nearest to the patient's feet along the costal margin to the xiphisternal junction (Figure 7–5).

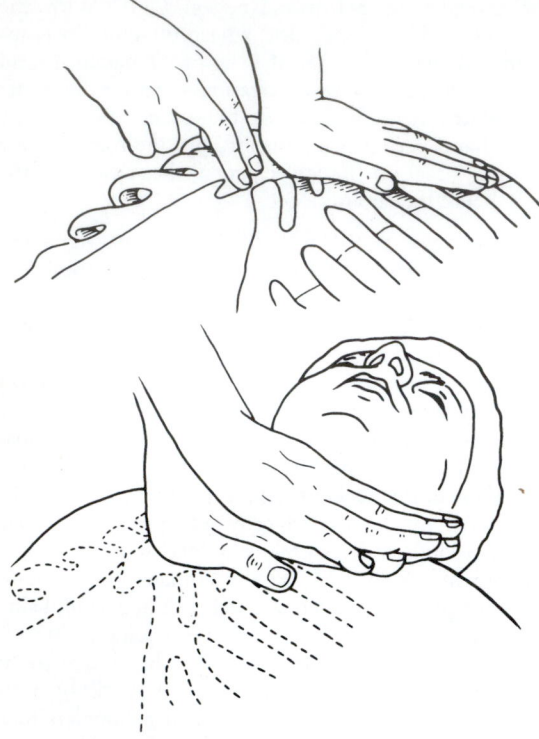

Figure 7–5. Hand placement for closed chest compression. Locate xiphoid, and place heel of one hand 2 fingerwidths cephalad to the xiphisternal notch. Only the heel of the bottom hand should touch the chest wall—not the palm or fingers.

Place the heel of the other hand on the sternum just cephalad to the fingers of the first hand. Place the first hand on top of the other hand. The long axis of the heels of both hands should be parallel to the long axis of the sternum. Fingers may be interlaced or extended but must be kept off the chest.

The provider is positioned with the knees as close to the patient as possible; the provider's shoulders, elbows, and heels of the hands are in a vertical line with the patient's sternum and chest. Provide compressions by rocking back and forth on the heels. If the patient is on a gurney, do compressions by rocking back and forth at the hips. The elbows should remain locked. Compressions should depress the sternum 1½–2 inches. Compressions should be rhythmic; the same amount of time should be spent on each phase of the cycle. The hands should not leave the chest. Give 100 compressions per minute. Until the patient is intubated, the ratio of compressions to ventilations is 15 to 2. This ratio applies to all BLS providers. It allows for greater coronary perfusion pressures than the 5:1 ratio used previously by

health care providers. Once an airway is established, ventilations and compressions can be performed asynchronously.

COMPLICATIONS OF BASIC LIFE SUPPORT

The key complication associated with ventilation is gastric insufflation. Air forced into the stomach can lead to gastric distention, which can cause regurgitation of stomach contents, diminished lung volumes, and decreased effectiveness of chest compressions. Complications occurring with chest compressions are numerous but can be minimized with correct technique. Even with correctly performed chest compressions, rib fractures can occur. Additional complications include lacerations of liver and spleen, pneumothorax, and hemothorax.

FOREIGN BODY AIRWAY OBSTRUCTION

Foreign body airway obstruction occurs in adults with ingestion of alcohol or other drugs (which result in an altered level of consciousness), in patients who have difficulty chewing or swallowing secondary to stroke or other disease process, and in denture wearers. Foreign body airway obstruction can be recognized in the conscious patient when difficulty breathing, coughing, or the universal "I'm choking" sign—clutching fingers around the throat (Figure 7–6)—is seen.

Ask the patient if he or she is choking. If the patient nods, ask if he or she can speak. If the patient has a strong cough, is not cyanotic, does not have labored breathing or retractions, and can speak, then a partial obstruction with good air exchange exists. Observe the patient, but do not intervene initially. Allow the patient to attempt to clear the obstruction by him- or herself. If the patient has a weak cough, is cyanotic, has labored breathing or stridor, or has difficulty speaking, then a partial obstruction with poor air exchange exists. Prompt intervention is indicated. If the airway is obstructed completely, the patient is unable to speak or cough and may become cyanotic. Rapid intervention is essential.

The Heimlich maneuver, or abdominal thrust, is used in the conscious choking patient (see Figure 7–6). While standing behind the patient, position the fist with the thumb facing up over the umbilicus. Roll the fist so that the thumb is against the abdominal wall. Grasp the fist with the other hand. Apply sharp upward thrusts until the foreign body is cleared or the patient collapses and becomes unconscious.

The Heimlich maneuver can be performed on a sitting patient by kneeling and reaching around the chair.

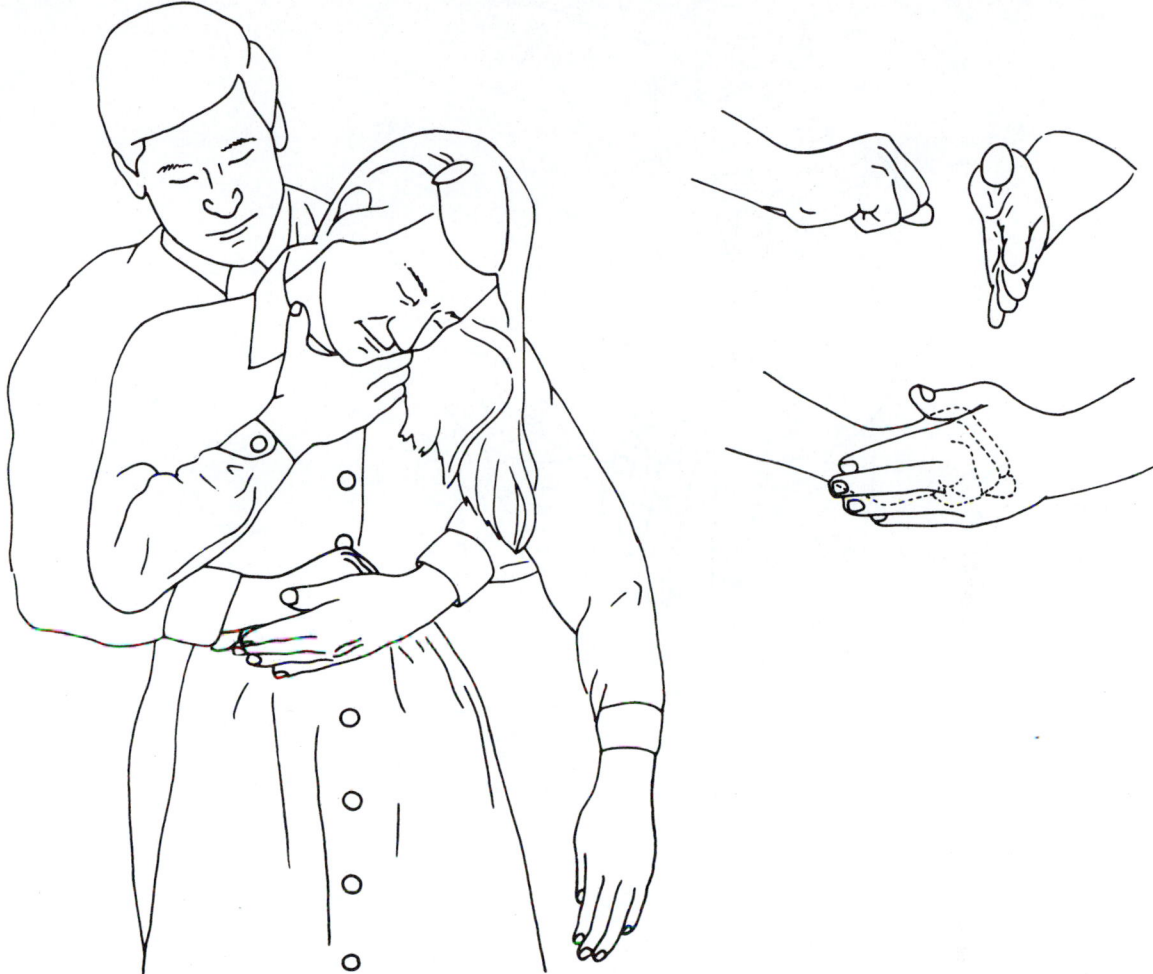

Figure 7–6. Clearing airway in conscious victim (Heimlich maneuver). Reach around the victim from the back, and deliver a sharp thrust to the epigastrium with the clenched fist, thumb-side toward the abdomen.

If the patient collapses, position him or her on the floor. Perform a tongue-jaw lift by grasping the jaw and tongue with one hand (Figure 7–7A). With the other hand, perform a blind finger sweep. Attempt to ventilate. If the first attempt does not succeed, reposition the airway and attempt to ventilate again. If the second attempt fails, perform the Heimlich maneuver by straddling the patient (Figure 7–7B and C). Place the heel of one hand in the same location as that used for the standing abdominal thrust. Place the other hand over the top of the first. Provide five sharp upward thrusts. Repeat the sequence of finger sweep, ventilation, and thrusts until the obstruction is relieved or until alternative means of clearing the airway arrive (eg, Magill forceps, surgical or needle cricothyroidotomy).

DEFIBRILLATION

Defibrillation is the intervention for the heart in ventricular fibrillation. When a critical level of energy reaches the myocardium, the ventricles become depolarized. This provides an opportunity for the sinoatrial node or another pacemaker to restore an organized perfusing rhythm. To succeed, the defibrillator must overcome the resistance, or impedance, encountered going through the chest. To minimize transthoracic impedance the provider must select the proper size paddles or self-adhesive pads; apply them in the correct position (Figure 7–8); use conductive gel, pregelled conductive pads, or saline-soaked-gauze to minimize skin resistance; and apply 25 pounds of pressure to the paddles.

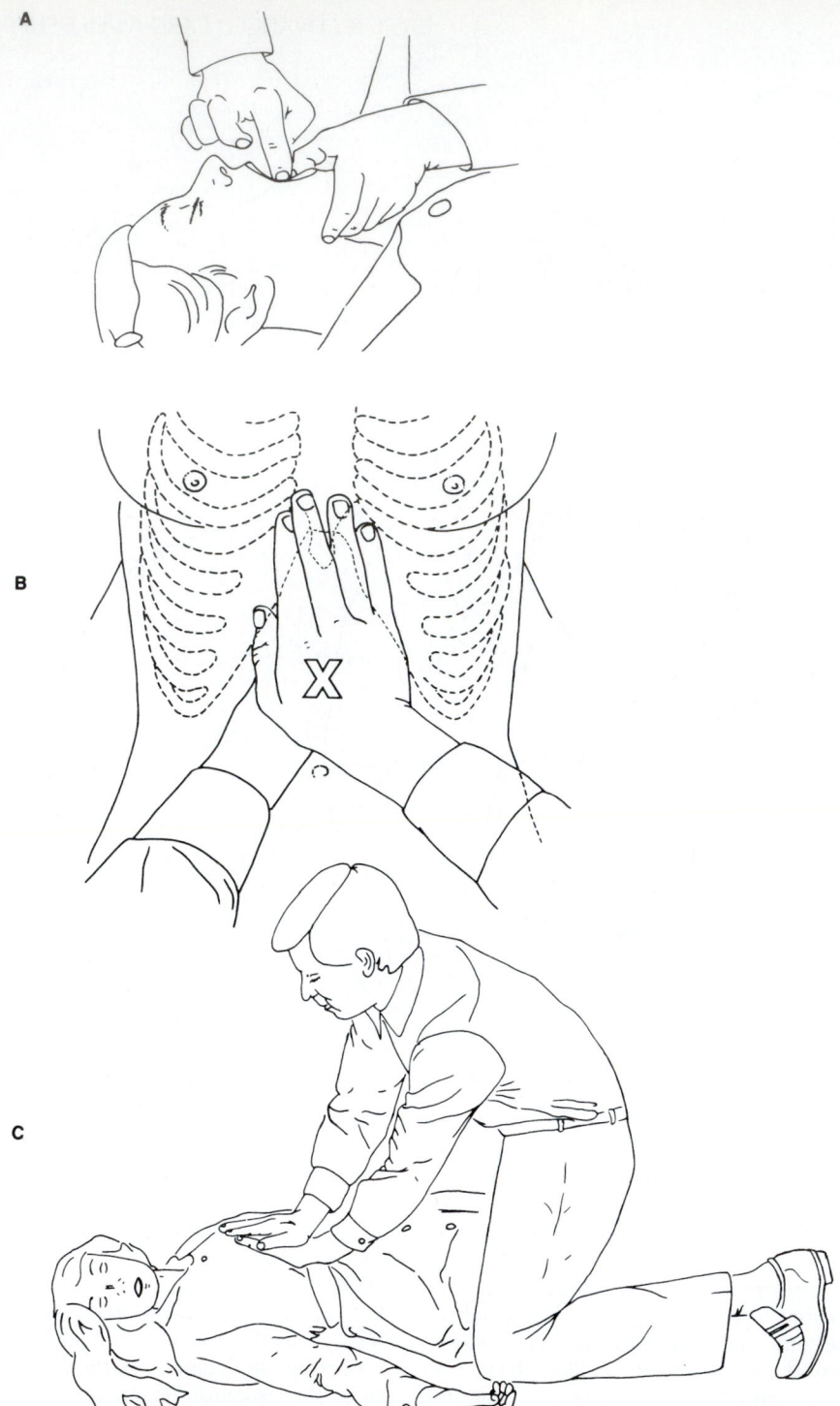

Figure 7–7. Clearing the obstructed airway. **A:** Finger sweep. Using a partially flexed index finger, sweep through far side of victim's mouth along cheek, deeply into back of the throat, and then out the near side. **B** and **C:** Supine Heimlich maneuver (subdiaphragmatic thrust). With victim level (or head down) and head turned to the side, rescuer kneels astride victim's thighs. Rescuer places heel of one hand midway between navel and xiphoid (well away from tip of xiphoid) and the other hand directly on top of the first. Deliver as many as 10 vigorous thrusts to victim's epigastrium.

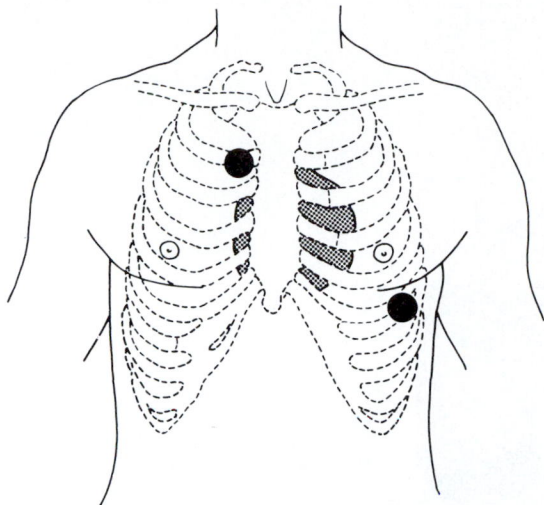

Figure 7–8. Contact points for defibrillation electrodes (solid circles). Place one paddle electrode to the right of the sternum in the second or third interspace; the other paddle should be at the cardiac apex. In children and thin adults, paddles may be placed directly over the heart in anteroposterior orientation.

Increasing the energy selected will increase the energy delivered. Repeated shocks will decrease transthoracic impedance successively.

The same techniques for defibrillation are used for synchronized cardioversion. The defibrillator must be placed in the synchronized mode. This is done by activating the "SYNCH" button on most defibrillators. This coordinates the shock so that it is not delivered during the relative refractory period (a shock during this period could result in ventricular fibrillation). Most defibrillators will revert to an unsynchronized mode after delivering a synchronized shock. This allows for rapid defibrillation if ventricular fibrillation occurs. For repeated synchronized cardioversion, the defibrillator must be resynchronized. A patient should be adequately sedated and receive analgesia prior to cardioversion, if circumstances permit.

Defibrillation Waveforms

Waveforms indicate the flow of energy between the two paddles or pads of the defibrillator. A monophasic waveform travels in one direction, whereas a biphasic waveform travels initially in one direction and then reverses flow. Old defibrillators used the monophasic

waveform. The biphasic defibrillator was first used in implanted defibrillators because it required less energy to successfully defibrillate; therefore, a smaller battery was needed. This technology was transferred to the AED (Figure 7–9), which required a small battery with a long shelf life. Compared to monophasic waveforms, biphasic waveforms have the same rate of defibrillation, with less damage to the myocardium. Theoretically the biphasic waveform should be more effective at defibrillating than the monophasic waveform, but this has not been shown in a clinical trial. Most manufacturers are making the transition to a biphasic waveform for their manual defibrillators. Although these manufacturers have differing biphasic waveforms, they all require less energy—in the range of 150–200 J per shock. Some defibrillators have escalating levels of energy, whereas others are fixed. Providers must be familiar with their defibrillator.

Automated External Defibrillation

(See Figure 7–9.) Manual defibrillation was first performed in the 1960s. With the development of waveform recognition software, it has been possible to program a defibrillator to deliver a shock in the event of ventricular fibrillation. The first defibrillators designed to deliver a shock without human interpretation of the waveform were manufactured in the late 1970s. Several trials have shown a significant increase in survival to hospital discharge with a community automated external defibrillator (AED) program. This is true regardless of what type of first responder (emergency medical technician, firefighter, or police) used the AED.

Before applying the AED, the rescuer should initiate airway management and ventilations. If the patient has no pulse, an AED should be brought to the patient's side. If two rescuers are available, one can perform CPR while the AED is sought, but obtaining the AED is the critical action. The AED requires the rescuer to power on the device, apply the self-adhesive pads to the patient's chest, press the Analyze button, and, if an electrical shock is indicated, press the Shock button. The current algorithm for AED use is shown in Figure 7–10.

The medical direction of an AED program is crucial and is discussed in Chapter 2.

Public Access Defibrillation

With the marked success of AEDs used by trained rescuers, the concept of providing public access defibrillators (PADs) evolved. PADs have a role in cardiac arrest in settings where an AED is used once in 5 years, when rescuers would take greater than 5 minutes to respond

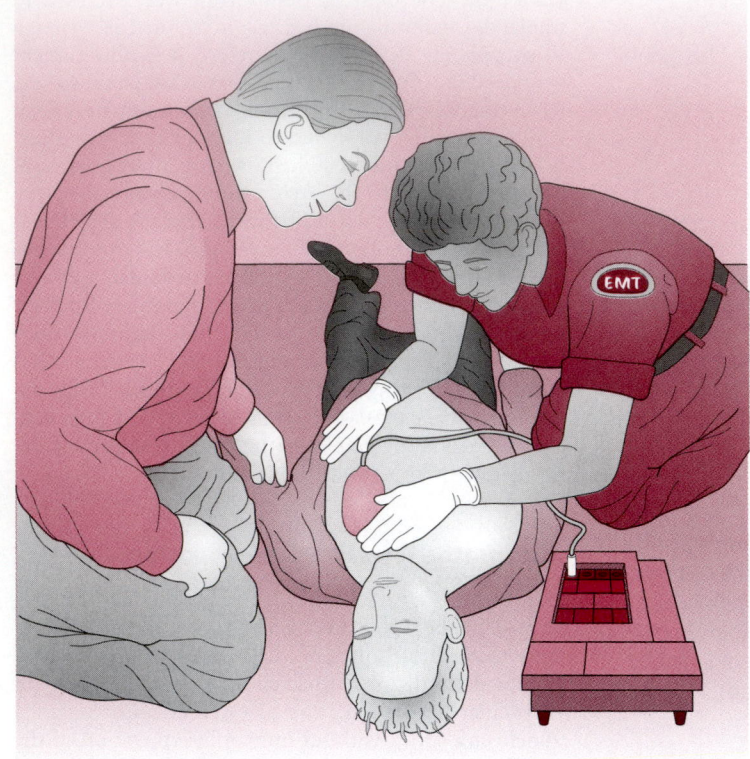

Figure 7–9. Use of the automated external defibrillator.

from time of collapse, and when it would be likely a lay rescuer could use the AED in less than 5 minutes. Suggested venues for PADs include sports arenas, shopping malls, and airports. Where PADs have been established, there have been numerous reports of positive outcomes, with no adverse outcomes related to an improperly used AED. AED malfunction is most likely to occur secondary to lack of maintenance. Many manufacturers have created AEDs that perform daily self-checks that minimize this risk. Like the AED used by first responders, the PAD requires medical direction.

Bang A, Herlitz J, Holmberg S: Possibilities of implementing dispatcher-assisted cardiopulmonary resuscitation in the community. An evaluation of 99 consecutive out-of-hospital cardiac arrests. Resuscitation 2000;44(1):19. [PMID: 10699696]

De Maio VJ et al: CPR-only survivors of out-of-hospital cardiac arrest: implications for out-of-hospital care and cardiac arrest research methodology. Ann Emerg Med 2001;37(6):602. [PMID: 11385328]

Ewy GA: Cardiopulmonary resuscitation—strengthening the links in the chain of survival. N Engl J Med 2000;342(21):1599. [PMID: 10824080]

Ginsburg W: Prepare to be shocked: the evolving standard of care in treating sudden cardiac arrest. Am J Emerg Med 1998; 16(3): 315. [PMID: 9596443]

Ho J et al: Automatic external defibrillation and its effects on neurologic outcome in cardiac arrest patients in an urban, two-tiered EMS system. Pre-hospital Disaster Medicine 1997; 12(4):284. [PMID: 10179208]

Jacobs I et al: The chain of survival. Ann Emerg Med 2001;37(4 Suppl):S5. [PMID: 11290965]

Niemann JT: Defibrillation waveforms. Ann Emerg Med 2001;37: 59. [PMID: 11145773]

White RD, Hankins DG, Bugliosi TF: Seven years' experience with early defibrillation by police and paramedics in an emergency medical services system. Resuscitation 1998;39(3):145. [PMID: 10078803]

■ ADULT ADVANCED LIFE SUPPORT

If a patient does not respond to initial CPR and defibrillation, further interventions are required. With the success of early interventions in restoring a perfusing rhythm, the patient may still require ALS (ie, airway, medications, and further evaluation) to optimize outcome.

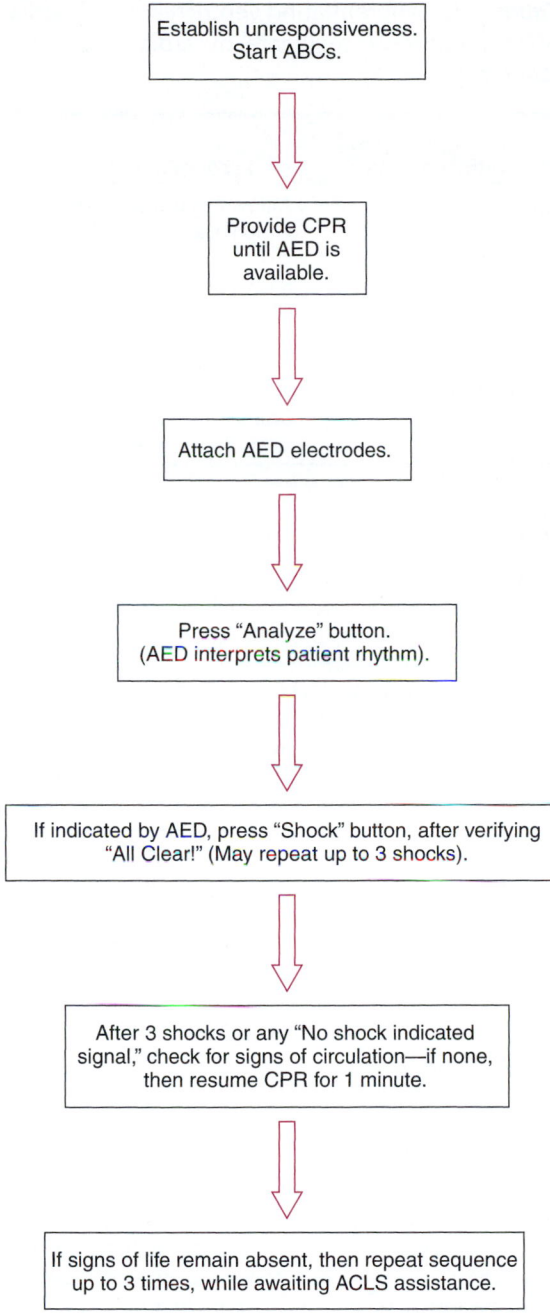

Establish unresponsiveness.
Start ABCs.

Provide CPR
until AED is
available.

Attach AED electrodes.

Press "Analyze" button.
(AED interprets patient rhythm).

If indicated by AED, press "Shock" button, after verifying
"All Clear!" (May repeat up to 3 shocks).

After 3 shocks or any "No shock indicated
signal," check for signs of circulation—if none,
then resume CPR for 1 minute.

If signs of life remain absent, then repeat sequence
up to 3 times, while awaiting ACLS assistance.

Figure 7–10. Algorithm for usage of automated external defibrillator (AED). ACLS = advanced cardiac life support.

ADVANCED AIRWAY MANAGEMENT

Advanced airway techniques include endotracheal intubation, the use of the laryngeal mask airway, or the use of a double lumen tube such as the Combitube or pharyngotracheal lumen airway.

Endotracheal intubation provides the best means of securing the airway; however, intubation should be attempted only by providers who are skilled in the procedure and who perform it at least 6–12 times per year. Placement of the tube should be confirmed by colorimetric end-tidal CO_2 detectors (although unreliable in prolonged cardiac arrest), esophageal detector devices, or capnography in addition to more traditional techniques. The details of endotracheal intubation are discussed in Chapters 6 and 8. A commercial tracheal tube holder may be more beneficial than regular tape in securing the endotracheal tube. Because of the risk of accidental and unrecognized dislodgment in the prehospital setting, it is recommended that the patient be placed in a cervical collar and on a backboard to minimize neck movement. When unable to secure an airway (either manually with advanced airway techniques or surgically) or unable to ventilate the patient using a bag-mask, the trained provider must perform a surgical or needle cricothyroidotomy.

SPECIFIC RHYTHMS
(See Figure 7–1.)

Ventricular Fibrillation or Pulseless Ventricular Tachycardia

As mentioned above, early defibrillation is the key to successful resuscitation in the patient with ventricular fibrillation. The first 3 shocks are given as stacked, sequential shocks. The paddles do not leave the chest, and the pulse is not checked between shocks. The monitor is checked between each shock. If a rhythm other than ventricular fibrillation (or ventricular tachycardia [VT] that was originally without a pulse) is noted, then a pulse check is performed. Shocks continue to be delivered between other interventions. It is acceptable to stack further shocks.

Enhancing cardiac output and blood pressure improves both coronary and cerebral perfusion. This improves the outcome of subsequent defibrillation and helps to mitigate neurologic injury. In ventricular fibrillation, vasopressin (40 units) may be used as an alternative to the first dose of epinephrine. This is a 1-time dose; epinephrine may then be used starting 10 minutes after the vasopressin (see "Pharmacologic Therapy" section, below).

Antidysrhythmics may prove beneficial in return of spontaneous circulation (ROSC). Both lidocaine and amiodarone are acceptable alternatives. Magnesium can be considered in torsade de pointes. Procainamide can be effective in recurring ventricular fibrillation.

Pulseless Electrical Activity

The key to successfully resuscitating the patient with PEA is identifying and treating the underlying cause. Assessment for these conditions can be facilitated by history, vital signs including temperature, electrocardiogram (ECG), blood gas analysis, electrolytes, and a focused physical examination. Initial interventions can be performed concurrently to address hypoxemia and hypovolemia.

Asystole

Asystole usually is a preterminal rhythm. As with PEA, the underlying causes must be addressed. Transcutaneous pacing may be considered early on, but it should be used only if the patient was witnessed entering asystole from a perfusing rhythm. If an asystolic patient does not respond to ALS interventions in the field, terminate resuscitation efforts in the field and do not consider urgent transport.

Tachydysrhythmia with a Pulse

If a patient has a tachydysrhythmia with evidence of poor perfusion (where the tachydysrhythmia is the likely source), prompt cardioversion is indicated. Chest pain, dyspnea, altered level of consciousness, hypotension, and new-onset congestive heart failure are all indications of instability. Quickly perform synchronized cardioversion. Give the patient analgesic and sedative agents if circumstances permit.

In a hemodynamically stable patient with a tachydysrhythmia, clinical evaluation is needed to determine the source of the dysrhythmia. History and ECG are the 2 key diagnostic aids. The most difficult differentiation is with the regular wide-complex tachycardias. The diagnostic dilemma is to decide whether the rhythm is supraventricular in origin with aberrant conduction or a true VT (Chapter 35). Table 7–1 indicates findings suggestive of VT versus supraventricular tachycardia (SVT). If the rhythm cannot be confirmed as SVT, the patient should be presumed to have a VT, and appropriate treatment should be rendered. Treating a VT as an SVT can have disastrous results. The use of adenosine as a diagnostic aid in distinguishing between SVT with aberrant conduction and VT is also discouraged. The conversion of VT with adenosine has been reported, most often in young, otherwise healthy patients.

Table 7–1. Differentiating ventricular tachycardia (VT) from supraventricular tachycardia (SVT) with aberrancy.

Factors Favoring SVT with Aberrancy	Factors Favoring VT
A preceding ectopic P wave	Atrioventricular dissociation
rSR' (right bundle branch block pattern) in lead V1	Fusion beats
qRS in lead V6	RS in lead V1
Response to carotid sinus massage	QRS > 0.14 s
Varying bundle branch block pattern	Age > 35 years, history of congestive heart failure, myocardial infarction, or coronary artery bypass grafting

Bradycardia

As with tachydysrhythmia, a slow rhythm with signs of inadequate perfusion needs immediate intervention, regardless of the underlying pathology. A relative bradycardia with good perfusion may be observed while preparations are made to treat the underlying cause. Atropine can be beneficial if parasympathetic tone is excessive. This is typically the case in depressed sinus node automaticity and in atrioventricular (AV) block secondary to acute myocardial infarction. Bradycardias secondary to degeneration of the conduction system (or disruption, as in a transplanted heart), or due to pharmacologic or metabolic causes, generally do not respond to atropine. Transcutaneous or transvenous pacing can be used as a bridge to a more permanent pacing mechanism.

PHARMACOLOGIC THERAPY (See Table 7–2.)

Vasoactive Agents

A. Epinephrine

Epinephrine is a mixed α and β agonist. It has been shown to increase diastolic aortic blood pressure and coronary perfusion pressure. As such, it has been the mainstay of pharmacologic therapy in the pulseless patient, regardless of the underlying rhythm. High-dose epinephrine in adults has largely been abandoned. Although it resulted in a greater rate of ROSC and admission to hospital, higher dose epinephrine did not lead to an increase in hospital discharge. Its advantageous properties are related to its α receptor stimulation, whereas its β properties may adversely lead to increased myocardial oxygen consumption. This has led researchers to seek a drug with more pure α properties.

Table 7–2. Pharmacotherapy in advanced cardiac life support.[1]

Drug Name	Adult Dose	Pediatric Dose	Indications	Frequency	Effects
Epinephrine	1 mg IV OR 2–5 mg IV via ETT	0.01 mg/kg IV or IO OR 0.1 mg/kg via ETT	Any pulseless rhythms	Every 3–5 min.	Increases perfusion to myocardium and to brain by increasing peripheral vascular resistance.
Vasopressin	40 units IV	Not indicated	VF, pulseless VT	Single dose, may be followed at 10 min by epinephrine.	Increases peripheral vascular resistance.
Amiodarone	For VF or pulseless VT: 300 mg IV push	For VF or pulseless VT: 5 mg/kg IV push	VF, pulseless VT, VT with a pulse, SVT	May use second dose of 150 mg for recurrent VF/VT. In children may be repeated in 5 mg/kg doses to a total of 15 mg/kg.	Predominately class III antiarrhythmic, but has sodium, potassium channel, and α and β receptor blockade.
Lidocaine	1.0–1.5 mg/kg IV push	Same	VF, pulseless VT, VT with a pulse	Second and subsequent doses of 0.75 mg/kg every 5 min to a total dose of 3 mg/kg.	Class IB antiarrhythmic; suppresses ventricular automaticity and electrical conduction.
Magnesium	1–2 g IV slow push	25–50 mg/kg IV slow push	Torsade de pointes, known hypomagnesemia	Single dose.	Can cause cutaneous flush, apnea, and hyporeflexia, if given too quickly.
Procainamide	17 mg/kg IV slow bolus at maximum rate of 50 mg/min	15 mg/kg IV load; 3–6 mg/kg over 5 min, not to exceed 100 mg/dose	VT with a pulse	Continue infusion (4 mg/min) until QRS widening > 50%, dysrhythmia terminated, onset of hypotension; or 17 mg/kg infused.	Decreases myocardial excitability and conduction velocity.
Atropine	Perfusing patients: 0.5 mg IV push q 5 min, to maximum of 3 mg Pulseless patients: 1.0 mg IV push q 5 min, to maximum of 3 mg	0.02 mg/kg; minimum dose of 0.1 mg	Bradycardia, asystole.	May be repeated once up to maximum dose of 3 mg.	Parasympatholytic, eliminates vagal tone.
Adenosine	6 mg rapid IV push through proximal peripheral line; central line dose is one-half	0.1 mg/kg rapid IV push; maximum dose, 6 mg	SVT	If needed, second dose of 12 mg (pediatric, double initial dose up to 12 mg); third dose of 12–18 mg.	Endogenous nucleoside causing brief asystole allowing dominant pacemaker to resume function.

(continued)

Table 7–2. Pharmacotherapy in advanced cardiac life support.[1] (*Continued*)

Drug Name	Adult Dose	Pediatric Dose	Indications	Frequency	Effects
Diltiazem	0.25 mg/kg to a maximum dose of 20 mg IV push over 2 min	Same	SVT	Second dose of 0.35 mg/kg, maximum dose of 25 mg, at 15 min; after conversion, start diltiazem drip at 5–15 mg/h.	Calcium channel blocker.
Esmolol	500 µg/kg bolus over 1 min	100–500 µg/kg bolus over 1 min	SVT	May give another bolus if desired effect is not achieved; start drip 50 µg/kg/min.	β-Blocker (short acting).
Atenolol	5 mg IV over 5 min	Not indicated	SVT, myocardial infarction	Repeat in 10 min, then give 50-mg oral load.	β-Blocker (β-1 selective).
Metoprolol	5 mg IV push	Not indicated	SVT, myocardial infarction	Repeat twice at 5-min intervals, then give 50-mg oral load.	β-Blocker (β-1 selective).
Dopamine	2–20 µg/kg/min	Same	Hypotension	Low doses are predominantly β; higher doses become predominantly α.	Inotropic agent/vasopressor (combined α and β agonists).
Dobutamine	2–20 µg/kg/min	Same	Hypotension	Titrate to effect.	Inotropic agent (β agonist).
Norepinephrine	Start at 8–12 µg/min, then titrate to 2–4 µg/min for maintenance; maximum dose of 30 µg/min if hypotension unresponsive to lower doses.	0.05–2 µg/kg/min.	Hypotension.	Titrate to effect.	Vasopressor (predominately an α agonist).
Phenylephrine	100–500 µg bolus IV.	0.1–0.5 µg/kg/min.	Hypotension.	Every 5 min until desired effect, then continuous infusion of 40–180 µg/min.	Vasopressor (pure α agonist).

ETT = endotracheal tube; IO = intraosseoulsy; IV = intravenously; SVT = supraventricular tachycardia; VF = ventricular fibrillation; VT = ventricular tachycardia.
[1]Agents are listed from most effective (and most commonly used) to least.

B. Vasopressin

Vasopressin is an endogenous hormone also known as antidiuretic hormone. It evokes more prominent vasoconstriction in the skin, skeletal muscle, and intestinal tract, while causing relatively less vasoconstriction in the coronary, cerebral, and renal vasculature. It is potentially useful as an alternative to epinephrine in ventricular fibrillation. It has been shown to have a higher rate of ROSC in the porcine model, although the results of human trials have been mixed. Vasopressin has not been shown to be useful in either asystole or PEA. Vasopressin has not been shown to be beneficial in pediatric patients.

C. Dopamine

Dopamine has mixed α, β, and dopaminergic effects that manifest in a dose-dependent fashion. At low doses of 2–4 μg/kg/min there is no inotropic effect, nor is there increased renal and splanchnic perfusion. At doses of 5–10 μg/kg/min, β-1 and β-2 inotropic effects predominate. At doses greater than 10 μg/kg/min there is a substantial predominance of α effects with a resultant decreased perfusion of the splanchnic bed. For this reason, high-dose dopamine should not be used. If hypotension remains after optimization of filling pressures, dobutamine (as an inotropic agent) or norepinephrine (as a vasopressor) should be considered.

D. Norepinephrine

Norepinephrine has predominantly α effects but has some β effects as well. Its role is in the postresuscitation management of hypotension when systolic pressures are less than 70 mm Hg.

E. Dobutamine

Dobutamine is a synthetic predominantly β-1 agonist with little β-2 or α effects. As such, it can improve myocardial contractility and increase cardiac output. It is the initial agent of choice in patients with systolic blood pressure of 70–100 mm Hg and no signs or symptoms of shock. Paradoxically it can worsen hypotension in patients with inadequate preload. Dobutamine can provoke tachyarrhythmias. It is run as an intravenous infusion of 2.5–15 μg/kg/min.

F. Phenylephrine

Phenylephrine is a pure α agonist that can be used in the postresuscitation phase to maintain diastolic blood pressure. Once blood pressure has been stabilized, an intravenous drip of 40–60 μg/min should be started and then titrated to effect.

Antidysrhythmics

A. Adenosine

Adenosine is an endogenous nucleoside that is a potent but short-lived AV nodal blocking agent. Along with vagal maneuvers, it is considered first-line therapy in paroxysmal supraventricular tachycardia (PSVT) secondary to a reentrant-type conduction defect. Adenosine should be considered only when a supraventricular rhythm is suspected. It should not be used as an aid in differentiating between PSVT with aberrant conduction and VT. It is associated with a prolonged sinus pause. The patient will often experience transient flushing, dyspnea, or chest pain.

B. Amiodarone

Amiodarone is predominantly a class III antidysrhythmic (potassium channel blocker), but it also has some properties of class I (sodium channel blockade), class II (β-blockade), and class IV (calcium channel blockade) antidysrhythmics. This wide variety of effects makes amiodarone useful in treating both supraventricular and ventricular tachydysrhythmias. There is good evidence supporting its use in PSVT for both rate control and rhythm conversion. The same dosing regimen is used for hemodynamically stable VT, but this recommendation is extrapolated from unstable VT and ventricular fibrillation studies. In ventricular fibrillation or pulseless VT, 2 prospective prehospital trials have shown a significant increase in ROSC and survival to hospital admission. This has not, however, resulted in an increase in survival to hospital discharge.

C. Atropine

Atropine is a parasympatholytic agent useful in the treatment of bradycardias due to increased parasympathetic tone (second- and third-degree AV blocks). Its use can be considered in asystole and bradycardic PEA. Dosing in the perfusing patient is 0.5 mg IV every 5 minutes up to a total of 3 mg. In the pulseless patient, the dose is 1 mg IV every 5 minutes to a total dose of 3 mg.

D. β-Blockers

β-Blockers (ie, atenolol, metoprolol, esmolol) are indicated for SVT for rate control in patients with preserved left ventricular function. Atenolol and metoprolol are β-1 (cardioselective) blocking agents available in both intravenous and oral formulations. Esmolol is a short-acting β-1 agent that must be given in a bolus and then maintained through a continuous infusion. This may be advantageous in patients who may respond negatively to β-blockade (for example, patients with chronic obstructive pulmonary disease). If an adequate response is not achieved after 5 minutes, the loading dose may be repeated and the infusion rate doubled.

E. Calcium Channel Blockers

Calcium channel blockers (ie, diltiazem and verapamil) are also indicated for rate control in SVT. They slow

AV nodal conduction and prolong the AV nodal refractory period. Calcium channel blockers are contraindicated in atrial fibrillation or atrial flutter with rapid ventricular response when an accessory pathway such as Wolf-Parkinson-White syndrome exists because it could lead to a life-threatening increase in the ventricular heart rate. Diltiazem is better tolerated in patients with impaired left ventricular function.

F. LIDOCAINE

Lidocaine is a class IB antidysrhythmic. It is the most commonly used agent for ventricular rhythms, both stable and unstable. The only large-scale observational study involving lidocaine demonstrated an increased survival to hospital admission but not to discharge. This study was confounded by the fact that the patients who were given lidocaine received treatment from ALS providers (ie, registered nurses), whereas those who were not given lidocaine received treatment from prehospital technicians. Other smaller studies have not shown a clear benefit for lidocaine.

G. MAGNESIUM

Magnesium is indicated for patients who are known or suspected to have a low magnesium level or recurrent ventricular dysrhythmias and for those with torsades de pointes. It has been used in the past for SVTs that have been unresponsive to adenosine, but no clinical trials to date support this use.

H. PROCAINAMIDE

Procainamide is a second-line agent for stable VT. It is also indicated for pulseless VT and ventricular fibrillation, but there is less support for these uses. It is a class IA antiarrhythmic that is more effective than lidocaine in converting VT, but it is hindered by the time required to administer the medication as a continuous infusion. Also, procainamide can provoke hypotension, and its use should be avoided in patients with long QT intervals or when drugs that prolong the QT interval, such as amiodarone, have already been administered.

POSTRESUSCITATION STABILIZATION

After successful ROSC, continued evaluation and management are required. Initial data gathering is needed to address the patient's history, underlying condition, and current physiologic status. Cull the patient's history from friends, family, witnesses, and prehospital care providers. Evaluate evidence of the patient's prearrest condition from the history and physical examination. Evaluate the patient's status by physical examination, laboratory and radiologic studies, and continuous hemodynamic monitoring. Routine postresuscitation studies include complete blood count, electrolytes, glucose, cardiac enzymes, arterial blood gas, and a portable chest

x-ray. Additional studies might include bedside echocardiography, pulmonary artery catheterization, heart catheterization, and computed tomography. Direct initial interventions toward maintaining stable hemodynamic parameters. The primary goal at this juncture is to restore adequate perfusion to peripheral organ systems, specifically the renal and splanchnic beds. Attach full monitoring equipment, if not done previously. Place a Foley catheter to monitor urine output. Secure intravenous lines, and replace any hastily placed lines. Provide a definitive airway if it is otherwise unsecured. If the patient requires ongoing ventilatory support, set up a mechanical ventilator.

Hyperventilation is not indicated, because this can lead to decreased cerebral perfusion. Acidemia secondary to metabolic acidosis should resolve through adequate ventilation and increased organ system perfusion.

Address postresuscitation hypotension initially with small-volume (250–500 cc) boluses of crystalloid solution. Reassess the patient and consider other causes of hypotension, such as pneumothorax and pericardial tamponade. If bolus fluid therapy fails, add vasoactive agents. The use of dopamine as a single-use agent is discouraged. Dobutamine should be used for inotropic support. Phenylephrine or norepinephrine can be used as a vasopressor.

Hyperthermia must be avoided, because this increases the cerebral metabolic rate, which creates an imbalance between delivered oxygen and demand. This can lead to anoxic cell death and can initiate a subsequent systemic inflammatory response. Hypothermia, in contrast, can be beneficial to the patient. Although studies have not shown the benefit of induced hypothermia, spontaneous mild hypothermia (34–36 °C [94–97 °F]) in the postresuscitation phase has been associated with an improved outcome.

TERMINATION OF RESUSCITATION

If there has been no response to the collective interventions in a resuscitation, the decision must be made to cease further efforts. An appropriate trial of electricity, vasoactive agents, and antidysrhythmics without any perfusing rhythm after 20–30 minutes should prompt the termination of the resuscitation. In addition, bedside echocardiography can be used to evaluate wall motion and the presence of a gel-like echo in the ventricles. Wall motion suggests the possibility that PEA has been inadequately resuscitated. A gel-like echo in the ventricle is uniformly associated with death. One exception to the standard guidelines for termination of resuscitation is hypothermic cardiac arrest, which may occur from severe exposure or cold water drowning. Because of the protective effects of hypothermia, several cases of good neurologic recovery after prolonged resuscitation from hypothermic cardiac arrest have been documented. In general, continue resuscitation efforts until the patient has been rewarmed to a core temperature of 30–32 °C (86–90 °F).

Abramson N et al: Ethics in emergency cardiac care. Ann Emerg Med 2001;37(4 Suppl):S196. [PMID: 11290981]

Cummins RO et al: In-hospital resuscitation: a statement for healthcare professionals from the American Heart Association Emergency Cardiac Care Committee and the Advanced Cardiac Life Support, Basic Life Support, Pediatric Resuscitation, and Program Administration Subcommittees. Circulation 1997;95(8):2211. [PMID: 9133536]

Glazer S, Gray WA: Futile care. What is the endpoint of unsuccessful field resuscitation? Emerg Med Serv 1995;24(7):65. [PMID: 10143873]

Herlitz J et al: Lidocaine in out-of-hospital ventricular fibrillation. Does it improve survival? Resuscitation 1997;33(3):199. [PMID: 9044490]

Jaslow D et al: Termination of nontraumatic cardiac arrest resuscitative efforts in the field: a national survey. Acad Emerg Med 1997;4(9):904. [PMID: 9305433]

Kapp MB: Evolving clinical practices and legal standards of care: softening the shock. Am J Emerg Med 1998;16(3):325. [PMID: 9596445]

Kern KB, Halperin HR, Field J: New guidelines for cardiopulmonary resuscitation and emergency cardiac care: changes in the management of cardiac arrest. JAMA 2001;285(10):1267. [PMID: 11255370]

Koster RW: Lidocaine: work still in progress. Resuscitation 1997;33(3):197. [PMID: 9044489]

Kulkarni RG, Thomas SH: Severe accidental hypothermia: the need for prolonged aggressive resuscitative efforts. Prehosp Emerg Care 1999;3(3):254. [PMID: 10424866]

Marco CA et al: Ethical issues of cardiopulmonary resuscitation: current practice among emergency physicians. Acad Emerg Med 1997;4(9):898. [PMID: 9305432]

Morris DC et al: Vasopressin can increase coronary perfusion pressure during human cardiopulmonary resuscitation. Acad Emerg Med 1997;4(9):878. [PMID: 9305429]

Nakatani K et al: Utility of colorimetric end-tidal carbon dioxide detector for monitoring during pre-hospital cardiopulmonary resuscitation. Am J Emerg Med 1999;17(2):203. [PMID: 10102328]

Part 1: Introduction to the International Guidelines 2000 for CPR and ECC: a consensus on science. Resuscitation 2000;46:3. [PMID: 10978786]

Proceedings of the Guidelines 2000 Conference for Cardiopulmonary Resuscitation and Emergency Cardiovascular Care: An international consensus on science. Ann Emerg Med 2001;37(4 Suppl):S1. [PMID: 11290963]

Sanders AB: When are resuscitation attempts futile? Acad Emerg Med 1997;4(9):852. [PMID: 9305424]

Stapleton ER: International guidelines 2000 for CPR and ECC: what do they mean for you? Emerg Med Serv 2001;30(9):45. [PMID: 11563344]

Streger MR, Kelley K: Cardiac care 2000. Field termination of cardiac arrest resuscitation. Emerg Med Serv 2000;29(9):53. [PMID: 11143036]

■ CARDIOPULMONARY RESUSCITATION IN INFANTS & CHILDREN

Epidemiologic studies of cardiac arrest in children are fraught with methodologic problems that make it difficult to ascertain the true scope of incidence. In the United States, some 16,000 children each year die of unexpected cardiopulmonary arrest. Trauma remains the leading cause of death in the pediatric population. In pediatric patients under age 1 year, sudden infant death syndrome (SIDS) is the leading nontraumatic cause of death. Lesser causes include submersion injury, pulmonary disease, asphyxia, aspiration, and primary cardiac disease.

Cardiac arrest in the pediatric population is most often secondary to respiratory arrest. Treatment prior to cardiac arrest is essential. Primary prevention has been shown to be effective in SIDS (ie, the "Back to Sleep" initiative) and with swimming pool safety education.

The pediatric patient who experiences cardiopulmonary arrest in an out-of-hospital setting uniformly has a poor outcome. A prospective study in an urban EMS system demonstrated a 2% survival rate with only 1 patient out of the 6 survivors having a good neurologic outcome. Patients not resuscitated in the field did not survive to hospital admission.

The following terms apply to the pediatric patient:

- Newborn: first 24 hours of life, wherein the patient transitions from a fetal to a neonatal circulation
- Neonate: first 28 days of life
- Infant: first year of life
- Child: ages 1–8 years

For the purposes of basic life support, an adult is someone older than age 8 years. There can be significant overlap across the age lines, in that it may be necessary to perform infant CPR on a toddler or adult chest compressions on a large child.

PEDIATRIC BASIC LIFE SUPPORT

Pediatric BLS utilizes the same basic techniques as adult BLS, but it is appropriately adapted for the size and physiology of infants and children. The first significant difference between adult and pediatric BLS is the "phone fast" rather than "phone first" rule. Because the predominant cause of pediatric cardiac arrest is respiratory arrest, in the event that help cannot be obtained simultaneously with initiating CPR (ie, the lone rescuer situation), CPR should be performed for 1 minute prior to interrupting to phone for help.

A. AIRWAY

Opening the airway in a pediatric patient is similar to the procedure followed for adults. The head-tilt and chin-lift method is used for the patient not suspected of having trauma. The jaw thrust is used when cervical spine injury secondary to trauma is a possibility. In the event of loss of consciousness secondary to foreign body airway obstruction, the rescuer may use the tongue-jaw lift to visualize the oropharynx and remove any foreign bodies.

B. BREATHING

Ventilations are provided in a manner similar to adults. In infants, the mouth–to–mouth and nose technique can be used. The rescuer's mouth is placed over the infant's mouth and nose to create an effective seal. In children, mouth-to-mouth ventilation is performed. Mouth-to-nose ventilation is an alternative when the rescuer is unable to obtain an effective seal with the preferred technique. Ventilations should be delivered over 1–1.5 seconds. Initially, 2 ventilations should be delivered. An effective ventilation occurs when there is enough force and volume provided to make the chest rise. An appropriately sized bag-mask may be used by the trained provider (250-mL bag for neonates, 500-mL bag for infants and children). Supplemental oxygen should be used with the bag-mask when available. An anesthesia bag may be used, but this requires a provider who routinely uses this with pediatric patients. In addition, the anesthesia bag requires a continual flow of oxygen. Cricoid pressure should be applied when giving a child rescue breaths prior to the insertion of an endotracheal tube. (Cuffed tubes are not recommended for infants or children.)

C. CIRCULATION

The rate of compressions should be performed faster in pediatric patients than in adults. In the infant, give at least 100 compressions per minute (newborn, 120 per minute). In the child, give 100 compressions per minute. In the infant, the preferred method for chest compressions is both hands encircling the chest with both thumbs providing compressions on the sternum (2-thumbs/encircling-hands technique). The alternative technique is using 2 fingers (either the index and middle finger or the middle and ring finger) from 1 hand to provide compressions. This technique may be more practical with a single rescuer. In children, the heel of 1 hand is used, but the technique is similar to the 2-handed method used for adults. In all patients, the depth of compression is one third to one half the depth of the chest.

Five compressions are delivered, followed by a single ventilation. This is in contrast to the adult compres-sion-to-ventilation ratio, which is 15:2 until the adult patient has been intubated.

PEDIATRIC ADVANCED LIFE SUPPORT

Pediatric ALS is directed toward the same goals of ALS in the adult: ROSC with preserved neurologic function. Hence, much of the underlying theory and algorithms are similar. Several important differences are noted below. As with adults, preparation is crucial, and in larger emergency departments, a dedicated pediatric crash cart should be assembled. Accordingly, in the prehospital arena, it may be useful to have a dedicated pediatric bag or kit on hand. These carts and kits should have age-appropriate equipment and medications. A means of estimating approximate weight, vital signs, and drug doses should be utilized. The Broselow-Luten length-based tapes are an excellent example. If these guides are unavailable, the endotracheal tube size can be estimated in children over age 1 year as follows: tube size = ¼(age) + 4. Endotracheal intubation provides another route to deliver some resuscitation medications (eg, lidocaine, epinephrine, atropine). However, in one study, endotracheal intubation in the pediatric patient in the out-of-hospital setting did not improve survival over bag-valve-mask technique.

Nonperfusing ventricular rhythms occur in up to 10% of pediatric cardiac arrests. If SIDS deaths are excluded, this rate increases to 19%. The chance of ROSC increases from about 5% in all patients to 30% in patients who present in ventricular fibrillation or pulseless VT. Appropriate paddles are 4.5 cm for infants up to age 1 year or 10 kg, and adult paddles for all others. Paddle positioning is the same as for adults. Defibrillation for ventricular fibrillation or pulseless VT is initially 2 J/kg, followed by 2–4 and then 4 J/kg. Currently, AEDs provide shocks at a fixed energy level appropriate only for adults. This energy level delivers 6–8 J/kg in the average 8 year old. This energy level would deliver too much energy to a smaller patient. Because of this, AEDs are currently not recommended for children younger than age 8 years. The other significant concern in the pediatric patient is the potential misdiagnosis of rapid sinus tachycardia as VT, leading to delivery of an inappropriate shock. Pediatric AEDs are currently in development. Any identifiably treatable causes, such as a toxic ingestion, electrolyte abnormalities, or asthmatic exacerbations, should be addressed appropriately.

Vascular access in the pediatric patient in cardiac arrest should be achieved as rapidly as possible. The most rapid means of securing such access is through the use of an intraosseous catheter. The intraosseous needle can be placed in 30–60 seconds. It can be placed in any large bone containing marrow, although the proximal tibia is most recommended. High-dose epinephrine, which had been endorsed previously in pediatric patients, has not been shown to lead to an increase in survival to discharge.

Gausche M et al: Effect of out of hospital pediatric endotracheal intubation on survival and neurological outcome: a controlled clinical trial. JAMA 2000;283:783. [PMID: 10683058]

Niermeyer S et al: International Guidelines for Neonatal Resuscitation: an excerpt from the Guidelines 2000 for Cardiopulmonary Resuscitation and Emergency Cardiovascular Care: International Consensus on Science. Pediatrics 2000;106(3): E29. [PMID: 10969113]

Sirbaugh PE et al: A prospective, population based study of the demographics, epidemiology, management, and outcome of out of hospital pediatric cardiopulmonary arrest. Ann Emerg Med 1999;33(2):174. [PMID: 9922413]

■ NOVEL APPROACHES IN CARDIAC ARREST MANAGEMENT

ALTERNATIVE BASIC LIFE SUPPORT TECHNIQUES

Several alternatives to the basic chest compression described in the "Adult Basic Life Support" section have been developed since Kouwenhoven's original proposal in 1960. Currently, 3 forms of alternative CPR remain as potential improvements over the basic chest compression.

Active Compression/Decompression CPR

Active compression/decompression (ACD) CPR requires a suction cup device, which adheres to the chest. This technique actively decompresses the chest, resulting in increased preload. This leads to greater cardiac output. Most trials of ACD have not demonstrated a significant increase in the number of patients who survive to hospital discharge. A study of 750 patients did show a significant increase in the number of patients surviving to discharge but not to 1-year survival.

Interposed Abdominal Compressions

Interposed abdominal compressions (IACs) apply positive pressure to the abdomen during the chest compressions relaxation phase. This increases the return of blood to the right ventricle, which leads to an increase in cardiac output and systemic perfusion pressure. Prospective trials have shown an increase in survival to discharge when IACs were performed in an in-hospital

cardiac arrest. These results have not been seen in prehospital trials.

"Lifestick" CPR

A combination of the other 2 techniques, referred to as "Lifestick" CPR (after the device used to perform the technique), provides improved hemodynamics over either technique alone. It has shown a significant increase in survival in the porcine model. Results of prehospital trials are pending.

THE SCALING EXPONENT

Intuitively, it was believed that the "coarser" the ventricular fibrillation, the more likely resuscitation was to be successful. Multiple studies have attempted to find a measure of this coarseness. Amplitude has a high correlation with successful defibrillation; however, patient movement, chest compressions, and other factors complicate calculation of amplitude during resuscitation. The scaling exponent is an estimate of the "roughness" or "smoothness" of the ECG waveform. It is a fractal measure that is independent of the amplitude or frequency of the waveform. Its value lies in identifying those patients who would benefit from immediate defibrillation. The calculation of the exponent is complex but can be performed in real time. Retrospective prehospital studies have identified a scaling exponent value at which CPR and pharmacologic therapy would result in a greater rate of ROSC. Animal studies have validated this value, although prospective prehospital trials are pending.

FIBRINOLYTIC THERAPY

Between 50% and 70% of patients experience sudden cardiac death secondary to intravascular thrombosis (20–40% due to an intracoronary thrombus; 20–30% related to a massive pulmonary embolus). Fibrinolytic therapy has been proposed as a means to treat these underlying causes. Multiple case reports and case series through the 1980s and 1990s showed a high rate of ROSC with a good neurologic outcome. The only prospective trial to date has supported good neurologic outcomes (Bottiger et al, 2001). Patients given tissue-type plasminogen activator had an odds ratio of 2.65 (95% CI, 1.11–6.25) for ROSC and an odds ratio of 3.11 (95% CI, 1.32–7.69) for admission to the intensive care unit. The trial was stopped early due to the significantly improved outcome of the treatment group. This study also demonstrated the safety of fibrinolytics during CPR, with no significant bleeding complications related to CPR.

The mechanism by which fibrinolysis may provide benefit in cardiac arrest is unclear. Changes in cardiac function occur within 2–12 minutes after the administration of fibrinolytics. This is not long enough to reestablish TIMI (trials in myocardial infarction) grade 3 flow. It is possible that only a small amount of flow is necessary to eliminate the insult causing the dysrhythmia or that the microvascular disease that is readily treated is the source of the insult. The neuroprotective effects of fibrinolysis are thought to be due to the reversal of an unopposed clotting cascade initiated during the cardiac arrest. Dosing of fibrinolytics is unchanged during cardiac arrest. Unfractionated heparin was administered to the patients in the largest case series and in one prospective study.

Arntz HR et al: Phased chest and abdominal compression-decompression versus conventional cardiopulmonary resuscitation in out-of-hospital cardiac arrest. Circulation 2001;104(7):768. [PMID: 11502700]

Bottiger BW et al; Efficacy and safety of thrombolytic therapy after initially unsuccessful cardiopulmonary resuscitation: a prospective clinical trial. Lancet 2001;357(9268):1583. [PMID: 11377646]

Callaway CW et al: Scaling exponent predicts defibrillation success for out of hospital ventricular fibrillation cardiac arrest. Circulation 2001;103(12):1656. [PMID: 11273993]

Dickinson ET et al: Effectiveness of mechanical versus manual chest compressions in out-of-hospital cardiac arrest resuscitation: a pilot study. Am J Emerg Med 1998;16(3):289. [PMID: 9596436]

Kern KB: Thrombolytic therapy during cardiopulmonary resuscitation. Lancet 2001;357(9268):1549. [PMID: 11377640]

Plaisance P et al: A comparison of standard cardiopulmonary resuscitation and active compression-decompression resuscitation for out-of-hospital cardiac arrest. N Engl J Med 1999;341(8):569. [PMID: 10451462]

Plaisance P et al: Benefit of active compression-decompression cardiopulmonary resuscitation as a pre-hospital advanced cardiac life support. A randomized multicenter study. Circulation 1997;18;95(4):955. [PMID: 9054757]

Skogvoll E, Wik L: Active compression-decompression cardiopulmonary resuscitation: a population-based, prospective randomized clinical trial in out-of-hospital cardiac arrest. Resuscitation 1999;42(3):163. [PMID: 10625156]

Compromised Airway

8

Harriet L. Boozer, MD, & Melissa M. Cheeseman, MD[1]

Immediate Management of the Compromised Airway	**Surgical Airways**
Principles of Intubation	**Use of Drugs to Assist in Intubation**
Nonsurgical Alternatives for Managing the Difficult Airway	**Special Cases**
	Care of the Intubated Patient
Needle Cricothyroidotomy	

■ IMMEDIATE MANAGEMENT OF THE COMPROMISED AIRWAY (See Figure 8–1.)

Securing the airway and assuring adequate ventilation are the first priorities in the resuscitation of any acutely ill or injured patient. Without a patent airway and adequate gas exchange, other resuscitative measures will usually be futile. Thus attention to the airway must precede or occur simultaneously with any other type of management. The exception is the initial defibrillation in cardiac arrest due to ventricular fibrillation, if defibrillation can be performed immediately.

Assess the Airway

Determine the patient's level of consciousness, and note the presence of any respiratory effort. In patients with known or suspected cervical spine injury, all assessments and maneuvers should be undertaken with the cervical spine immobilized in a neutral position to prevent cord injury.

A. Apneic, Unconscious Patients

Open the airway with a chin-lift or jaw-thrust maneuver. If the cervical spine is not injured, place the head in the sniffing position (Figure 8–2). Clear the airway of obstructions, using a rigid suction catheter to remove any blood, vomitus, or secretions from the oropharynx. Remove any large obstructing foreign bodies from the oropharynx manually or with Magill forceps (see Chapter 7).

If the patient remains apneic, assist ventilation using a bag-valve-mask device (eg, Ambu bag) or mouth-to-mouth breathing (see Chapter 7). If adequate personnel and equipment are available, immediately perform endotracheal intubation. Administer high-flow oxygen.

B. Patients with Respiratory Effort

Administer high-flow oxygen. Clear and position the airway as described above. Identify evidence of upper airway obstruction. Prolapse of the tongue and accumulation of secretions, blood, or vomitus are common causes of obstruction. Signs may include wheezing, sonorous respirations, stridor, cough, and dysphonia. Upper airway obstruction should be removed if present. Back blows or the Heimlich maneuver may clear the obstruction. If not, use suction or direct visualization and a Magill forceps or finger. Blind sweep is contraindicated. Obstructions that recur or persist require endotracheal intubation, either orotracheally or via cricothyroidotomy, tracheostomy, or percutaneous transtracheal jet ventilation (PTTJV) (see also Chapters 6, 7, and 48).

Evaluate the effectiveness of the patient's respiratory effort. Helpful signs include respiratory rate, tidal volume, accessory muscle use, level of consciousness, skin color, upper airway sounds, and auscultated lung sounds. Further assessment may include pulse oximetry, arterial blood gas measurement, and chest radiography.

If intubation is indicated (Table 8–1), continue high-flow oxygen and assist ventilation as needed. Assemble all items necessary for the appropriate method of intubation (Tables 8–2 and 8–3). Check for equipment malfunction. If the patient is alert, inform him or her of your plan.

---

1. This chapter is a revision of the chapter by Julia Nathan, MD, from the 4th edition.

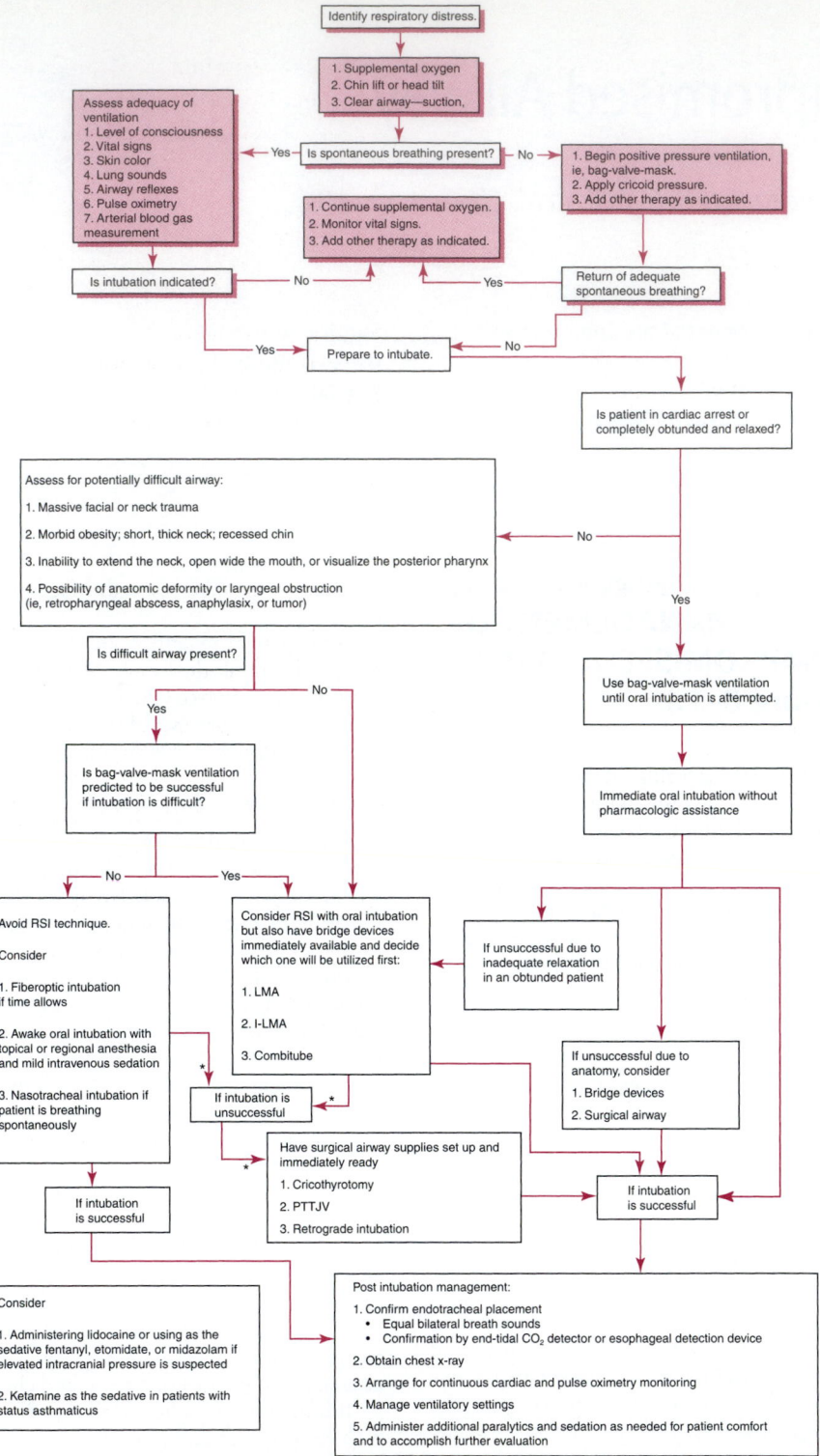

Figure 8–1. Management of the compromised airway. I-LMA = intubating laryngeal mask airway; LMA = laryngeal mask airway; PTTJV = percutaneous transtracheal jet ventilation; RSI = rapid-sequence induction.

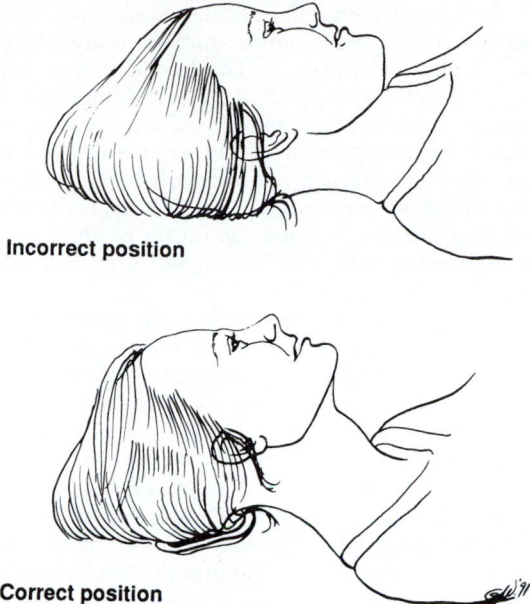

Incorrect position

Correct position

Figure 8–2. In the sniffing position, the head is slightly extended and the neck is flexed on the shoulders. This aligns the axis of the airway with the mouth and pharynx, facilitating direct visualization of the cords during intubation. It is particularly important in young children and infants, in whom the larynx is considerably more anterior. A pad beneath the occiput improves flexion of the neck. This position cannot be used when there is cervical spine injury.

Table 8–1. Indications for intubation.

Respiratory insufficiency
  Apnea
  Hypoxia
  Hypoventilation
Airway obstruction
  Foreign body
  Fixed mass
  Traumatic deformity
  Continued bleeding, secretions, or emesis
Inability to protect airway
  Altered mental status
  Loss of normal airway reflexes
Need for hyperventilation
  Head injury
  Metabolic acidosis in critically ill or injured patient
Anticipated or impending airway compromise
  Shock
  Multiple trauma
  Need for sedation or paralysis

Table 8–2. Essential airway management equipment.

Oxygen
Nasal cannula
Nonrebreathing masks of various sizes
Suction—rigid pharyngeal, flexible
Oral and nasal airways—range of sizes
Bag-value-mask units—adult and pediatric sizes
Water-soluble lubricant
Vasoconstrictive topicals
Anesthetic topicals (jelly and spray)
Laryngoscope handles
Laryngoscope blades—range of sizes (curved or straight based on operator preference)
Low-pressure cuff endoctraceal tubes of varying sizes
Stylets
Intravenous access (advised)

Prepare for Intubation

A. HIGH-FLOW OXYGEN

All patients with airway or ventilatory compromise require high-flow oxygen. Oxygen through a nasal cannula at flow rates up to 6 L/min provides a patient with 20–40% inspired oxygen concentration. A variety of masks are available that can accept oxygen flow rates of 5–15 L/min. Masks equipped with reservoirs and nonrebreathing valves can deliver oxygen concentrations close to 100% at flow rates of 10 L/min if an adequate seal can be maintained between the mask and face.

Before attempting intubation, preoxygenate the patient with 100% oxygen for 2–3 minutes. In a ventilating patient, this provides 6–7 minutes of protection against hypoxia should the patient become apneic. In an apneic patient, preoxygenation with a bag-valve-mask unit provides 2–3 minutes of protection against

Table 8–3. Optional equipment and rescue devices for difficult intubations.

Alternative laryngoscope blades and handles
Flexible-tipped stylets
Lighted stylets
Combitube cuffed oropharyngeal airway
Flexible-tipped endotracheal tubes
Fiberoptic laryngoscope or bronchoscope
Laryngeal mask airway (LMA)
Intubating laryngeal mask airway
Kit for retrograde intubation[1]
Kit for percutaneous transtracheal ventilation[1]
Kit for cricothyroidotomy[1]

[1]Either commercially available or preassembled in a sterile tray.

hypoxia. Unsuccessful attempts at intubation should be stopped at 30 seconds so that the patient may be reoxygenated.

B. Suction

A rigid-tipped suction catheter should be available at all times to keep the airway clear of blood and secretions. The suction device should be set at 120 mm Hg. After intubation, suction the tracheobronchial tree with a sterile, flexible catheter as described in the "Care of the Intubated Patient—Pulmonary Toilet" section, below.

C. Oral and Nasal Airways

When the jaw thrust or chin lift is ineffective in airway opening, a nasal or oral airway may support collapsed oropharyngeal tissues and permit adequate ventilation. A range of sizes should be readily available in all areas of the emergency department (Figure 8–3).

The oral airway is best used in an obtunded patient. It may be inserted over a tongue blade or positioned backward as it enters the mouth and rotated after the tongue is cleared. Positioned correctly, it retracts the tongue upward and anteriorly. Care must be taken not to push the tongue backward into the pharynx, worsening the obstruction. An overly long oral airway can push the epiglottis over the larynx, causing complete obstruction.

The soft, rubber, noncuffed nasopharyngeal tube tends to be better tolerated in a semiobtunded patient. Lubricate the tube with anesthetic jelly before insertion. Insert it through the least obstructed nostril, advancing it posteriorly along the floor of the nostril until it bypasses the tongue. If it is too long, it may enter the esophagus, resulting in ineffective positive-pressure ventilation and gastric distention. Epistaxis may occur during insertion, and suction should be available.

In patients with intact airway reflexes, placement of either device may cause emesis, gagging, or laryngospasm. During and after placement, head position should be maintained to optimize airway patency. Where indicated, spinal precautions must be maintained. Evaluate breath sounds after placement of either device to ensure that obstruction has not occurred. Care must be taken to avoid trauma during placement.

D. Positive-Pressure Ventilation

Following airway opening, positive-pressure ventilation may be used to preoxygenate a patient before intubation. Occasionally it may be the only form of ventilation in an apneic patient when an airway cannot be secured, or when a patient responds rapidly to other therapy. In general, however, it is not recommended for prolonged ventilation owing to gastric dilatation and technical difficulty.

The bag-valve-mask unit is the device most commonly used to provide positive-pressure ventilation in the emergency department. The bag-valve-mask unit has a self-inflating bag that accepts 15-L/min oxygen flows. A nonrebreathing valve permits reservoir air to enter through a separate port from expired air. At these flow rates, inspired air will approach 100% oxygen. The self-filling bag permits use with spontaneously breathing patients. The unit can usually be attached to an endotracheal tube after intubation for manual bag-assisted tracheal ventilation.

The procedure for using the bag-valve-mask unit is described in Chapter 6. Use of this device is difficult in the hands of a single operator because effective bag-valve-mask ventilation depends on a tight seal between the mask and face. Often this requires 2 hands and a second operator to compress the bag. Many circumstances of anatomic variation or maxillofacial trauma make a tight seal impossible. During bag-valve-mask ventilation, proper head position must be maintained to preserve airway patency. Monitor the effectiveness of ventilation closely by frequent assessments of chest wall movement, lung sounds, and gastric dilatation.

The positive pressure generated by bag-valve-mask ventilation leads to gastric dilatation and abdominal distention. This results in decreased lung compliance and significant risk of emesis and aspiration. A clear mask is recommended to reveal emesis. Suction equipment must be available. In patients with unprotected airways, cricoid pressure (the Sellick maneuver) is recommended (Figure 8–4). To perform the Sellick maneuver, apply firm, direct pressure on the circumferential cricoid cartilage. This will compress the esophagus posteriorly, decreasing gastric dilatation and reflux. If emesis occurs, release pressure on the cricoid to prevent esophageal rupture. If bag-valve-mask ventilation must be prolonged for any reason, place a nasogastric tube to reduce gastric dilatation and its consequences.

Because of operational difficulties and risks of aspiration, the bag-valve-mask is a temporizing measure under most circumstances. Patients who require bag-assisted ventilation should generally be intubated as soon as it can be accomplished safely and practically.

The mouth-to-mask technique is another method of providing positive-pressure ventilation. This method may be easier for a single operator, because both hands can be used to seat the mask. Supplemental oxygen is provided via a port in the mask or via a nasal cannula worn by the operator.

E. Esophageal Obturators and Related Devices

An esophageal obturator airway (EOA) or similar device may be placed in the prehospital setting. These tubes are designed to provide airway protection and

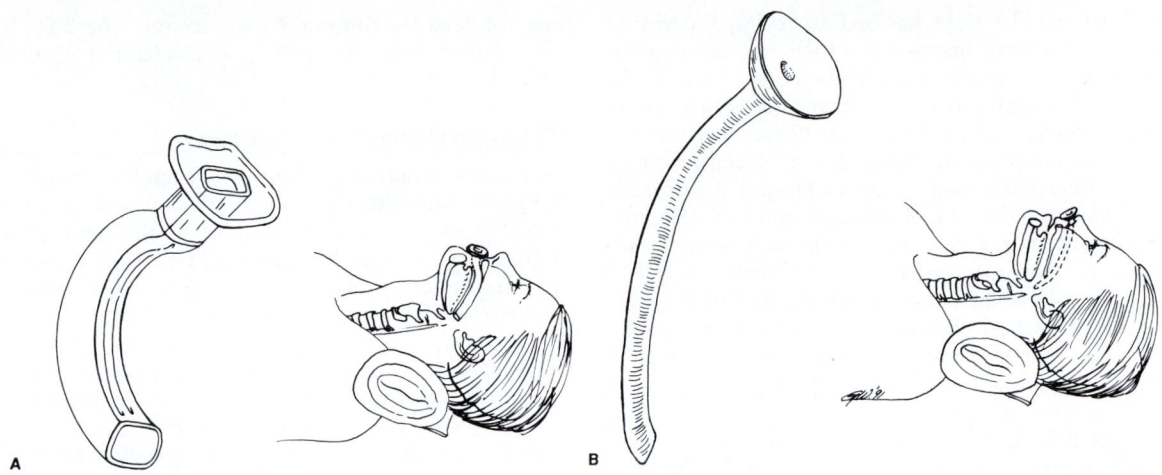

Figure 8–3. **A:** Oral airway. **B:** Nasal airway.

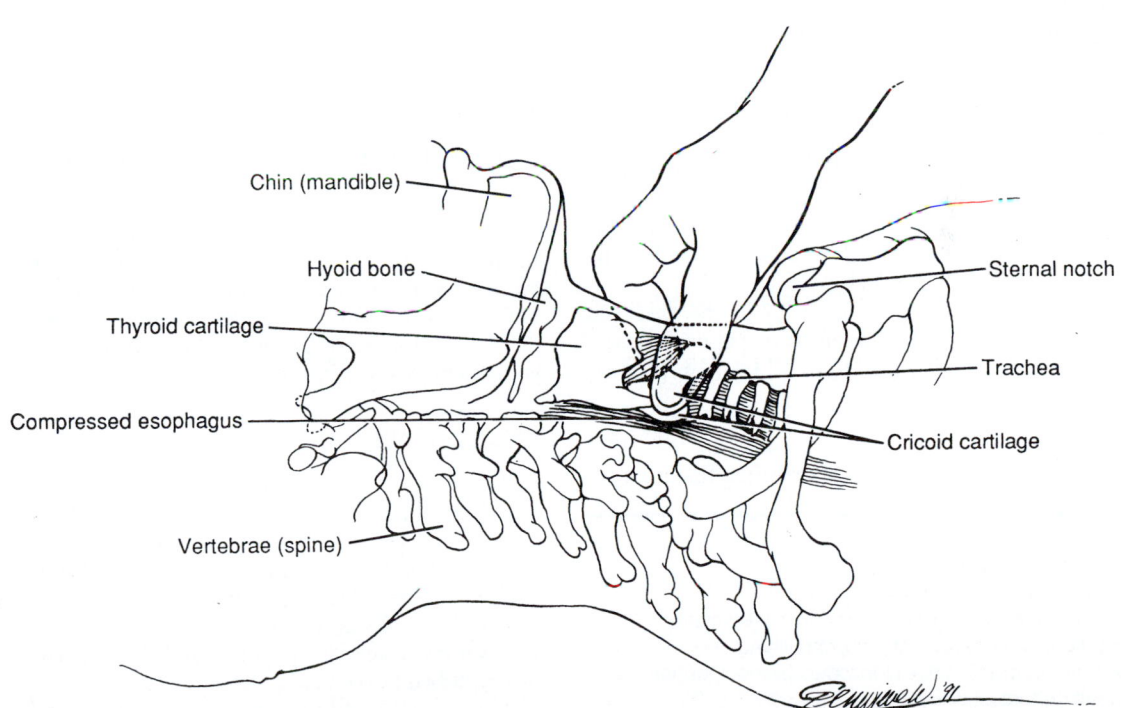

Figure 8–4. The Sellick maneuver. Firm pressure on the cricoid cartilage compresses the esophagus, preventing aspiration of gastric contents when airway reflexes are absent.

ventilation. The EOA has become mainly a device of historical interest because of a high rate of complications and uneven efficacy. The use of this device in the prehospital setting is not recommended. There are no indications for the EOA in the emergency department.

Since introduction of this device, several modifications have been made. The esophageal gastric tube (EGT) airway has a hollow esophageal tube that permits passage of a nasogastric tube for gastric decompression. The esophageal tracheal Combitube (ETC) may be used as an endotracheal tube if blind insertion results in tracheal placement. Similarly, the pharyngeal tracheal lumen airway (PTLA) may be ventilated through either a long or short tube depending on the tube position after placement.

The ETC has found favor in prehospital and emergency department settings. It comprises 2 tubes that form a single double-lumen tube. A proximal balloon isolates the hypopharynx, whereas the distal balloon occludes the esophagus or the trachea, depending on its location. The tube is inserted blindly and is fairly stiff, so that it usually enters the esophagus. Tube 1 is closed distally with side holes for ventilation. Tube 2 is open distally and gives a direct route to either the lungs or the stomach. Tube 1 is always ventilated first, when confirming placement of the tube. Advantages of the ETC include ease of placement, airway protection from aspiration, and lack of manipulation of the cervical spine in the trauma patient.

Esophageal tubes are contraindicated in awake and semiobtunded patients and in infants, children, and patients less than 120 cm in height. Do not use them when there is known esophageal injury or ingestion of caustic substances. Complications are listed in Table 8–4. Because of reports of esophageal trauma, some authors recommend Gastrografin swallow or endoscopy after use of an EOA-like device.

Patients intubated with an EOA in the field will need endotracheal intubation upon arrival in the emergency department. If an ETC or PTLA is in place, it may be used for continued resuscitation. The ETC is an effective device for prolonged mechanical ventilation.

F. Cuffed Oropharyngeal Airway

The cuffed oropharyngeal airway is a modified oropharyngeal airway with a large distal inflatable cuff. It is inserted like a traditional oral airway, and the cuff is then inflated in the supraglottic space. This device is useful in resuscitation because of its ease of insertion and the low level of skill required to place it.

Agro F et al: Associated techniques for tracheal intubation. Resuscitation 2000;47:343. [PMID: 11114469] (Review of different techniques for establishing a patent airway.)

Foley LJ et al: Managing the airway in the critically ill patient—bridges to establish an emergency airway and alternate intubating techniques. Crit Care Clin 2000;16:429. [PMID: 10941582] (Review of alternative airway management techniques.)

Levitan RM et al: Airway management and direct laryngoscopy—a review and update. Crit Care Clin 2000;16:373. [PMID: 10941579] (Review of airway management techniques.)

Orebraugh SL: Difficult airway management in the emergency department. J Emerg Med 2002;22:31. [PMID: 11809554] (Review of techniques for managing the difficult airway.)

Shuster M et al: Airway and ventilation management. Cardiol Clin 2002;20:23. [PMID: 11845543] (Review of airway management techniques.)

■ PRINCIPLES OF INTUBATION

These principles of intubation management apply to all methods of airway management described in this chapter. Airway positioning, suction, and administration of 100% oxygen must precede any attempt at advanced airway control. Keep protective gear with the airway equipment, and use it routinely.

Choice of Method

Most patients can be intubated orally by direct laryngoscopic visualization of the cords. This is the method of choice, because the best assurance of correct tube placement is seeing the tube pass through the cords into the trachea. When direct visualization is not possible (Table 8–5), airway control can be achieved using a wide variety of special equipment and alternative methods described below (Table 8–6).

Choice of a blind or surgical technique depends on the patient's condition, availability of equipment, and operator experience. Advantages, indications, and problems associated with each technique are summarized

Table 8–4. Complications of esophageal airways.

Unrecognized endotracheal intubation
Incorrect positioning in pharynx
Inadequate mask-to-face seal
Esophageal or pharyngeal trauma due to placement, cardiopulmonary resuscitation, or retching
Tracheal compression due to incorrect balloon position
Balloon rupture or leakage
Anterior displacement of larynx
Emesis on removal
Gastric rupture

Table 8–5. Relative contraindications for orotracheal intubation.

Mechanical obstruction in the hypopharynx or at the cords
Severe laryngeal/tracheal trauma
Unusual anatomic features
Presence of wiring due to jaw fracture
Greater advantage for nasotracheal intubation or tracheal airway (i.e., in patients with chronic obstructive pulmonary disease or congestive heart failure who cannot lie supine).

---

below. Most alternative procedures require some training and expertise. Become comfortable with several techniques, and be sure that the emergency department stocks the appropriate equipment.

Intubation by any method carries risks of hypoxia, aspiration, laryngospasm, unrecognized esophageal intubation, bleeding, airway trauma, spinal cord trauma, right or left main-stem intubation, arrhythmia, and death. Delayed complications include soft tissue infection, mediastinitis, tracheal stenosis, and dysphonia.

Any blind technique (nasal, digital, lighted stylet) carries increased risk of unrecognized esophageal tube placement and trauma to the hypopharynx and airway. These methods should be used only when direct visualization is dangerous or cannot be successfully completed.

Surgical and needle techniques are generally rapid but in inexperienced hands may lead to massive bleeding or trauma that makes control of the airway impossible. They share the relative contraindications of coagulopathy, goiter, overlying tumor, or overlying skin infection. There are no absolute contraindications other than the ability to obtain an airway by less invasive means. Although each invasive method of airway control has unique complications, as a group they share an increased risk of bleeding, extratracheal tube placement,

and trauma to the airway and surrounding tissues over less invasive routes. Loss of integrity of the tissues of the neck may result in barotrauma and significant soft tissue infection. Delayed complications include hoarseness and subglottic stenosis.

Universal Precautions

Airway management presents many opportunities for exposure to patient secretions. Wear adequate protective clothing, including a gown, gloves, mask, and either a face shield or goggles, any time the airway is manipulated. When the intubator's fingers are in the patient's mouth (eg, digital intubation, lighted stylet), care must be taken to prevent bite wounds. Place a bite block or dental prod before initiating intubation. Alternatively, place several layers of gauze between the intubator's hand and the patient's teeth. If the patient wears dentures, remove them before airway manipulation.

Laryngoscopy & Oral & Nasal Intubation

See Chapter 6.

Postintubation

After intubation, assess the position of the endotracheal tube by observing the chest wall for expansion. Auscultate both lung fields and the abdomen while ventilating. Inaudible lung sounds or the presence of abdominal sounds suggest esophageal placement. If breath sounds are louder on the right than the left, suspect right main-stem intubation. Withdraw the tube 1–2 cm, and auscultate again. Confirm the tube position by chest x-ray.

Levitan RM et al: Airway management and direct laryngoscopy—a review and update. Crit Care Clin 2000;16:373. [PMID: 10941579] (Review of airway management techniques.)

Table 8–6. Alternative methods of intubation.

Blind Techniques
  Nasal intubation
  Digital intubation
  Use of lighted stylet
  Laryngeal mask airway (LMA) assisted intubation
Indirect Visualization Techniques
  Fiberoptic intubating bronchoscopy
  Use of rigid fiberoptic scopes (Bullard, Shikani)
Surgical Techniques
  Retrograde intubation
  Cricothyroidotomy (percutaneous or open)
  Tracheostomy

■ NONSURGICAL ALTERNATIVES FOR MANAGING THE DIFFICULT AIRWAY

Laryngeal Mask Airway

The laryngeal mask airway (LMA) is a device that has been proved useful as an alternative for bag-valve-mask ventilation and as a rescue option in the difficult airway. The LMA is a semirigid tube with a distal inflatable mask that is inserted blindly into the hypopharynx. The mask lies over the larynx and seals around the glottic opening. The LMA does not protect against aspiration. This device has been demonstrated to be easy to insert with limited prior training. The LMA is appropriate for use in adults and pediatrics, including neonates weighing more than 2 kg. The intubating LMA (I-LMA) is a modification of the LMA that has been developed to act as a conduit to allow passage of the endotracheal tube through the glottis.

Digital Intubation

This method has been used successfully when the cords cannot be visualized because of anatomic features or copious secretions. In the hands of experienced clinicians, it is rapid and can be achieved with little movement of the cervical spine. There are no absolute contraindications to this method, but it is a blind method and should not be used when direct visualization of the cords can be safely done. Because of the risk of being bitten, use this method only in deeply comatose patients.

If necessary, one person can perform digital intubation unaided. No special equipment is necessary beyond an oxygen delivery system, suction, and an appropriately sized endotracheal tube with stylet. Lubrication may aid passage of the tube. Take precautions against the accidental or reflex bite. Place a stylet into the lubricated tube as far as the side hole, and bend the tube into a gentle hook at the end.

To perform digital intubation, stand at the patients' right shoulder. Insert the index and middle fingers into the patient's mouth, and advance along the midline of the tongue until the epiglottis is palpated. Pass the endotracheal tube along the fingers until the tip reaches the epiglottis. Move the 2 fingers posteriorly, and advance the tube past the epiglottis while exerting gentle anterior pressure to guide the tip of the tube into the trachea. Once past the cords, remove the stylet before further advancement to prevent damage to the anterior trachea. After removing the stylet, adjust the final tube position, secure the tube, and verify its placement in the usual way. Never advance the tube against resistance. Cricoid pressure may be used until the endotracheal cuff is inflated.

Complications are similar to those described for other methods of blind intubation.

Variations on Basic Equipment

Several variations on the basic equipment have been developed for managing the difficult intubation. Use of these devices may be helpful under some circumstances.

Flexible-tipped endotracheal tubes (Endotrol, others) have a built-in thread that extends from the distal tip to the proximal end, where it attaches to a plastic ring. Traction on the ring flexes the tip of the tube, directing the tube more anteriorly, simulating the function of a flexible stylet.

Specialized laryngoscope blades and handles are produced but are not widely available in most emergency departments. Several variations of the rigid fiberoptic laryngoscope also exist. These devices allow for indirect visualization of the airway through an eyepiece. The endotracheal tube is advanced off the stylet into the glottis under visualization.

Fiberoptic Techniques

A. Lighted Stylet

Lighted stylet and light wand devices have been developed to aid in blind intubation. This method can be used when blood, secretions, or vomitus fill the hypopharynx. Because laryngoscopy need not be used, lighted stylets may be advantageous when the cervical spine must remain immobilized. Blind intubation with a lighted stylet is most suitable for deeply comatose or apneic patients when there is little risk of stimulating protective reflexes or biting of the intubator's hand. Use a bite block or dental prod for protection. A lighted stylet can also be combined with direct laryngoscopy. Although there are no absolute contraindications to this technique, ambient lighting must be low to maximize its benefit. Obesity may diminish the intensity of transillumination. As for other blind techniques, avoid this method when direct laryngoscopy can be performed.

If necessary, one person can perform this technique unaided. These devices have a battery-powered light source at the top of a semiflexible stylet. A longer, floppy stylet is available for nasal intubations. The stylet is threaded into an endotracheal tube. Aside from the lighted stylet, no special equipment is required.

Form the assembly of stylet and endotracheal tube into a hook of slightly greater than 90 degrees. The patient may be approached from the head if laryngoscopy is used. Otherwise, approach the patient from the right shoulder. While placing gentle traction on the tongue, pass the assembly into the mouth. When the epiglottis is reached, use a scooping or ladling motion to place the tip into the glottis. The appearance of transillumination at the neck indicates the position of the tube. Tracheal placement results in a bright, well-circumscribed area of transillumination at the cricothyroid membrane. The endotracheal tube can then be advanced over the stylet into the trachea. Transillumination lateral to the midline indicates piriform sinus placement and need for repositioning. Esophageal placement causes little or no transillumination. The procedure is essentially the same for nasal intubation with a lighted stylet.

This procedure shares the same complications as other blind techniques: inadvertent malpositioning of the tube, hypoxia, and tissue damage.

B. Fiberoptic Bronchoscope

Fiberoptic bronchoscopes may be used to locate the opening of the glottis when direct laryngoscopy cannot be used or is unsuccessful. The endotracheal tube can then be advanced over the endoscope into the trachea. Although this procedure can be carried out without movement of the cervical spine, it requires skill and practice. It may be time consuming when the hypopharynx is filled with blood or secretions. In addition, the equipment is expensive and easily damaged.

Foley LJ et al: Managing the airway in the critically ill patient—bridges to establish an emergency airway and alternate intubating techniques. Crit Care Clin 2000;16:429. [PMID: 10941582] (Review of alternative airway management techniques.)

Levitan RM et al: Devices for difficult airway management in academic emergency departments—results of a national survey. Ann Emerg Med 1999;33:694. [PMID: 10339685] (National survey of emergency medicine residency program directors and their use of alternative airway devices.)

Orebraugh SL: Difficult airway management in the emergency department. J Emerg Med 2002;22:31. [PMID: 11809554] (Review of techniques for managing the difficult airway.)

Pollack CV: The laryngeal mask airway—a comprehensive review for the emergency physician. J Emerg Med 2001;20:53. [PMID: 11165839] (Review of the laryngeal mask airway indications, complications, and limitations.)

Rodricks MB et al: Emergent airway management—indications and methods in the face of confounding conditions. Crit Care Clin 2000;16:389. [PMID: 10941580] (Review of management of the difficult airway, which includes review of current medications used in rapid-sequence protocols.)

Shuster M et al: Airway and ventilation management. Cardiol Clin 2002;20:23. [PMID: 11845543] (Review of airway management techniques.)

■ NEEDLE CRICOTHYROIDOTOMY

Cricothyroidotomy is the standard approach to creating an emergent surgical airway. Two methods using needle penetration of the cricothyroid membrane are described below. They are acceptable alternatives to cricothyroidotomy in selected cases and may be easier and less invasive than emergent cricothyroidotomy for inexperienced operators.

Identification of the cricothyroid membrane is critical to performing either needle or surgical cricothyroidotomy (Figure 8–5). Palpation of the tracheal midline will identify the hyoid bone superiorly. Below this, the thyrohyoid space leads to the laryngeal prominence of the thyroid cartilage. The vocal cords lie behind the thyroid cartilage. The cricothyroid membrane is about 1.5 fingerwidths below the prominence and is bounded caudally by the cricoid cartilage. It is approximately 10 mm high and 22 mm wide. Each landmark must be clearly identified by palpation in the caudal and cephalad directions to prevent incision of the thyrohyoid space with entry into the hypopharynx, above the cords. Penetration of the cricothyroid membrane will enter the trachea about 1 cm below the vocal cords. Penetrate the cricothyroid membrane in the lower third of the membrane to avoid the superior cricothyroid vessels that run transversely across the upper third of the cricothyroid membrane. When subcutaneous air, trauma, or body habitus obscure the usual landmarks, the approximate position of the cricothyroid membrane may be determined by placing the small finger of the right hand in the sternal notch while the hand is held in neutral position. The cricothyroid membrane will lie approximately 4 fingerwidths above the sternal notch. If time allows, prepare the skin with an iodine skin disinfectant, and raise a wheal of local anesthetic over the cricothyroid membrane before inserting the needle.

Percutaneous Transtracheal Jet Ventilation

(See also Chapter 6.) PTTJV is an alternative technique for oxygenating and ventilating a patient who cannot be intubated in a more standard fashion. It is unique in that positive pressure is generated by high-pressure oxygen delivered as an intermittent jet through high-pressure tubing and a percutaneously placed large-bore tracheal catheter. No bag reservoir or nonrebreathing valve is employed. PTTJV is less invasive than cricothyroidotomy and less time consuming than retrograde intubation (see below). It is relatively easily learned. With attention to detail, there are few complications. It can be used in awake or obtunded patients. Other advantages include presumed protection of the cervical spine and possible expulsion of a pharyngeal foreign body by expired air. In the emergency department it is regarded as a temporizing measure while other methods of airway control can be established. Indications for PTTJV are the same as for cricothyroidotomy. PTTJV has been proved useful in the pediatric population.

Disadvantages include the need for either makeshift or commercially available special equipment. With prolonged use, retention of carbon dioxide may develop. Contraindications include anterior neck trauma, where high delivered pressures may lead to severe tissue disruption, and complete airway obstruction, where ex-

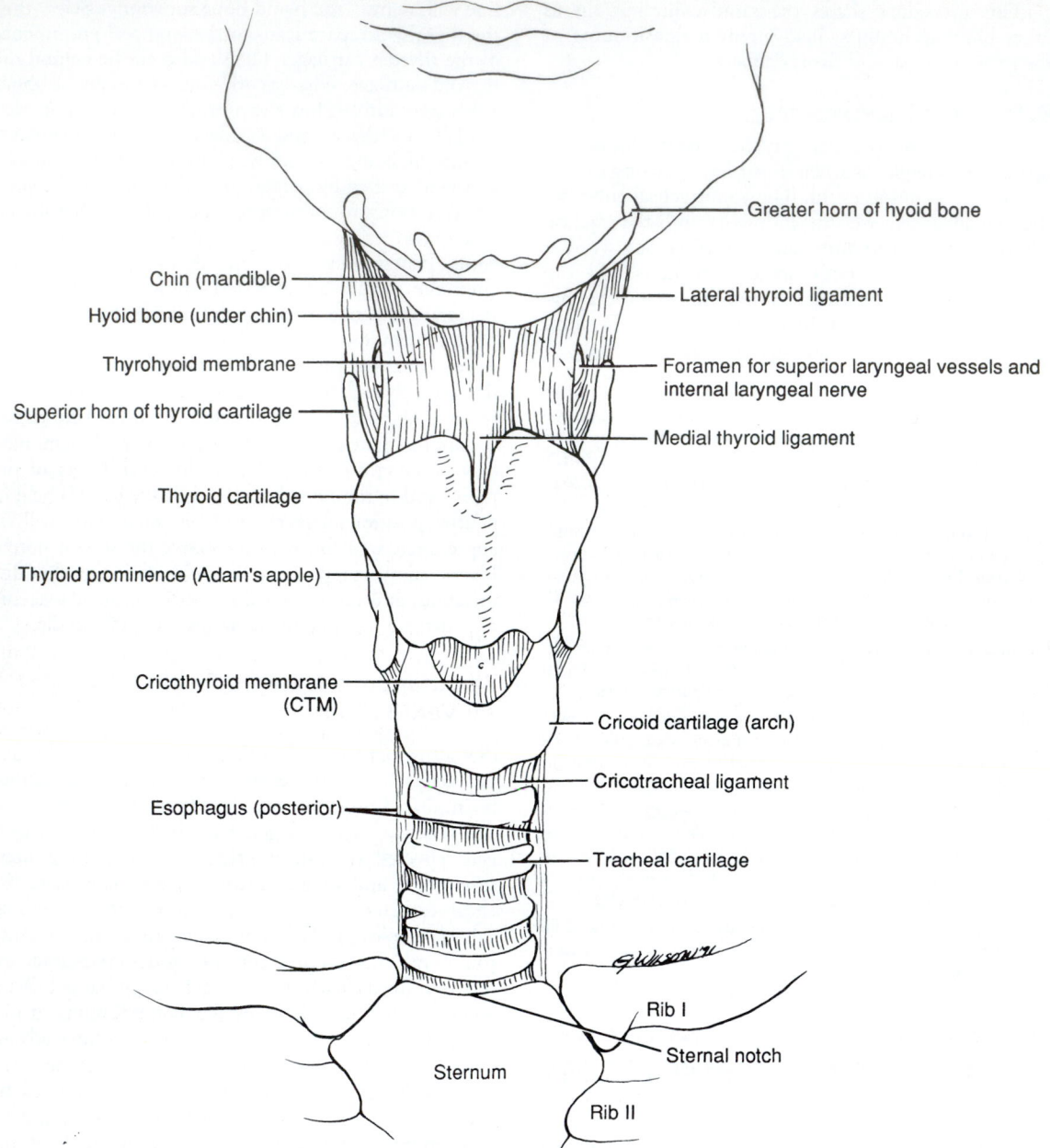

Greater horn of hyoid bone

Chin (mandible)

Lateral thyroid ligament

Hyoid bone (under chin)

Thyrohyoid membrane

Foramen for superior laryngeal vessels and internal laryngeal nerve

Superior horn of thyroid cartilage

Medial thyroid ligament

Thyroid cartilage

Thyroid prominence (Adam's apple)

Cricothyroid membrane (CTM)

Cricoid cartilage (arch)

Cricotracheal ligament

Esophagus (posterior)

Tracheal cartilage

Rib I

Sternal notch

Sternum

Rib II

Figure 8–5. Landmarks for locating the cricothyroid membrane.

pired air cannot escape through the glottis. PTTJV shares the relative contraindications mentioned above for all invasive methods of airway control. Prior unsuccessful attempts at catheter placement may lead to air leak or subcutaneous emphysema after a second, successful attempt.

The materials required for PTTJV are listed in Table 8–7. The system may be built out of items normally stocked in the emergency department and operating room. Several companies now produce specialized delivery systems and cannulas for PTTJV. The components of the system must be im-

Table 8–7. Equipment required for percutaneous transtracheal ventilation (PTTJV).

Oxygen source capable of delivering 50 psi line pressure.
Stryker valve to access high-pressure oxygen
High pressure tubing
Cut-off or interrupt valve for tubing
Luer-Lok adaptor at the catheter end of the tubing
5– to 8–cm over-the-needle, 12- to 14-g catheter
10–mL syringe for needle placement

---

mediately available to be useful in emergency department airway management.

To obtain the 50 psi of pressure necessary to generate adequate volume to expand the patient's chest, the high-pressure tubing must be attached to the oxygen tank through a step-down regulator (or demand valve). A wall oxygen outlet or the flush valve of the anesthesia machine are also potential sources of high-pressure oxygen. A bag-valve-mask unit cannot generate adequate pressure to ventilate a patient with this system.

The high-pressure tubing is fitted with an interrupt valve along its length. If an interrupt valve is not available, a Y connector or side port in the oxygen tubing can be used as an alternate port. It is then attached directly to the tracheal catheter via a Luer-Lok adapter. If necessary, an adapter can be constructed using the male end from intravenous tubing, a 3-way stopcock, or the barrel of a 3-mL syringe. All connections should be reinforced with plastic ties to prevent separation under pressure (Chapter 6).

The over-the-needle catheter must be kink-resistant and meet the specifications noted in Table 8–7. The commercially available catheters have distal side holes that diffuse the jet of air entering the trachea, preventing focal trauma. They also have a proximal flange for securing the catheter to the neck.

Significant deviations from recommended equipment may lead to inadequate ventilatory volumes, hypoxia, and hypercapnia.

To place the catheter, prepare the neck and locate the cricothyroid membrane as described above. Insert the over-the-needle catheter and needle into the lower third of the cricothyroid membrane in a caudal direction at an angle of 30–45 degrees. Aspiration of air should confirm catheter position. Advance the catheter, and remove the needle. In its final position, the tip of the catheter should be near the carina. Secure the catheter at the neck, attach the oxygen delivery system to the catheter, and begin ventilation.

When the alternate port is covered with a finger, oxygen is delivered to the patient, generating about 20 cm H_2O pressure in the airway. Much of the 50-psi pressure is lost through the glottis during oxygen delivery. When the alternate port is released, there is a period of passive exhalation while the patient's chest wall and diaphragm recoil. Recommended ventilatory rates vary from 12 to 20 cycles per minute with an inspiratory to expiratory ratio of 1:2 (eg, 1 second with the alternate port covered leading to ventilation, 2 seconds with the alternate port opened allowing passive exhalation). During ventilation, the chest wall will rise and a significant volume of oxygen will be expelled from the glottis. This produces a spray of blood and secretions through the patient's mouth and nose, creating potential for hazardous exposure. During passive exhalation, the chest wall muscles recoil, expelling (less forcefully) some of the volume, and the chest wall should fall. Monitor the rise and fall of the chest wall closely, because without chest wall recoil and passive exhalation, hypercapnia, acidosis, and barotrauma may develop quickly.

Complications include all those noted above for needle placement. Needle misplacement may cause perforation of the trachea or esophagus, leading to tissue disruption and emphysema of the deep tissues or mediastinitis owing to the high pressures of ventilation. Local subcutaneous emphysema is common. Inadequate monitoring may lead to hypoxia, hypercapnia, and acidosis as noted above. The awake patient may experience cough during the procedure. Even with good technique, prolonged ventilation using PTTJV will result in respiratory acidosis and hypoxia.

Retrograde Intubation

Retrograde intubation is indicated when oral or nasal intubation is contraindicated or technically impossible owing to anatomic, pathologic, or traumatic abnormalities. The advantages of this technique include maintenance of the cervical spine in a neutral position and the benefits of any blind technique. In addition, it requires less skill than fiberoptic intubation. Disadvantages include its time-consuming nature and the need to have the patient ventilating adequately throughout. This method is contraindicated when the airway is obstructed at or above the level of the cords. If the patient is unable to open the mouth, the retrograde wire must be passed out the nose for nasal intubation, which can be difficult and suboptimal in some settings. Contraindications include apnea and those described above, in the "Choice of Methods" section.

Retrograde intubation can be performed by one operator, although an assistant is extremely helpful. Special equipment includes a needle large enough to accept a catheter or guide wire and a wire or catheter, approximately 70 cm in length. Local anesthetic is recommended. A small clamp is useful.

The principle of retrograde intubation involves entering the trachea at the cricothyroid membrane with a guide wire that is threaded out the mouth or nose and used as a guide for blind oral or nasal intubation. After appropriate preparation of the neck, identify the cricothyroid membrane and surrounding landmarks. Pass a needle through the skin, and puncture the inferior third of the cricothyroid membrane with the needle directed about 30 degrees caudad. Aspiration of air confirms tracheal placement. Rotate the needle to about 30 degrees cephalad, and reaspirate to confirm tracheal position. Introduce the wire through the needle. As the wire is threaded through the needle, it often exits spontaneously through the mouth. Occasionally, however, it must be retrieved with fingers or forceps. When the wire is in hand at the lips or nares, the needle is removed. Fix the wire at the cricothyroid membrane with fingers or a small clamp. Thread the proximal end of the wire into the endotracheal tube through the side hole (Murphy's eye). It should pass up through the lumen of the tube, exiting at its proximal end. Advance the lubricated tube along the wire until resistance is met, indicating that the tube is in the trachea, below the cords, pulled tight against the fixed wire. Release the wire at the skin, and pull it out through the proximal end of the tube. Advance the tube to the appropriate position, and confirm placement in the usual manner.

Only a small number of cases of retrograde intubation have been described. Few serious complications have been reported.

Orebraugh SL: Difficult airway management in the emergency department. J Emerg Med 2002;22:31. [PMID: 11809554] (Review of techniques for managing the difficult airway.)

Soriano SG et al: The difficult pediatric airway—surgical airway, rigid bronchoscopy, and transtracheal jet ventilation in the pediatric patient. Anesthesiol Clin North Am 1998:16:827. (Review of alternative methods for airway control in the pediatric patient.}

SURGICAL AIRWAYS

Cricothyroidotomy

When there is complete upper airway obstruction or massive facial trauma that prohibits intubation from above, immediate access to the trachea can be obtained with cricothyroidotomy. In experienced hands, it is a rapid technique that maintains immobilization of the cervical spine. It is a radical procedure with risk of significant short- and long-term negative outcomes. It is contraindicated whenever the airway can be secured by less invasive means. In children, cricothyroidotomy becomes technically more difficult as the landmarks become smaller. Patient age less than 10 years is a relative contraindication for inexperienced practitioners. In children under age 5 years, PTTJV or a tracheostomy is preferable if possible. Other relative contraindications include preexisting laryngeal disease, coagulopathy, anatomic deformities of the neck due to trauma or other causes, and lack of familiarity with the procedure.

The equipment and technique for cricothyroidotomy are described in Chapter 6. Kits are available that use over-the-wire techniques, progressive dilatation, and trocar placement.

Early and delayed complications of cricothyroidotomy are the same as for other invasive techniques (see above).

Tracheostomy

Tracheostomy has little indication in emergency department management of the airway. Its only true indication is severe blunt trauma to the neck with fracture of the thyroid or cricoid cartilage, preventing access to the cricothyroid membrane. Tracheostomy is the preferred method of surgical airway management in the very small child when PTTJV is not possible. Because of the proximity of vascular, nerve, and visceral tissue, the risk of negative sequelae is high. A thorough knowledge of anatomy and careful surgical technique are critical to success. It should be performed only by surgeons experienced with the procedure.

Walls RM: Management of the difficult airway in the trauma patient. Emerg Med Clin North Am 1998;16:45. [PMID: 11809554] (Review of airway techniques in the trauma patient.)

USE OF DRUGS TO ASSIST IN INTUBATION

Many patients in the emergency department can be intubated without the use of pharmacologic intervention other than oxygen. However, when pharmacologic adjuncts are indicated, their use may dramatically reduce the difficulty of intubation and speed control of the airway. The patient's overall condition and the goal of intubation determine the choice of agent.

Oral or nasal intubations in awake patients are best carried out under local, topical, or regional anesthesia. Occasionally, sedation alone may be useful in preparing for intubation. For a semiobtunded or combative patient, use of neuromuscular blockade with sedation, usually in a rapid-sequence intubation (RSI) protocol, provides rapid control of the airway while protecting against aspiration of gastric contents.

Drugs that induce apnea must be used by or under the direct supervision of experienced clinicians prepared to obtain a surgical airway in the event of failed intubation. Equipment necessary for intubation and surgical airway must be prepared in advance and be available at the bedside before the patient is sedated or anesthetized.

Topical Anesthesia

A. GENERAL CONSIDERATIONS

Awake intubation presumes a patient with enough ventilatory effort to allow time to anesthetize the airway. The patient must be able to cooperate with, or at least tolerate, the noxious process of passing an endotracheal tube. Anesthesia of the airway causes loss of the normal protective airway reflexes, with concomitant risk of aspiration. Absorption of topical agents occurs more readily from tracheal tissues than from oral or nasal mucosa, increasing the risk of systemic toxicity if excessive doses are used.

B. CHOICE OF AGENT

Common choices for topical anesthesia of the airway are lidocaine and cocaine (Table 8–8). All local anesthetics have central nervous system toxicities including confusion, coma, and seizures. All local anesthetics also have cardiovascular effects including slowed conduction, myocardial depression, arrhythmogenesis, and peripheral vasodilation. Hypotension and cardiac arrest may occur.

1. Lidocaine—Topical lidocaine may be administered as a gargle of 10-mL aliquots repeated 3 times. The drug must be spat out, not swallowed, between each dose to avoid toxic systemic levels. To aerosolize, 4 mL of a 4% solution may be administered through a stan-

dard nebulizer at 8 L/min with either a mouth piece or face mask.

2. Cocaine—Topical cocaine combines anesthetic and vasoconstrictive properties. A local vasoconstrictor is unnecessary with cocaine and can be dangerous. Owing to risks associated with cocaine, its use has fallen out of favor in the emergency department. Its use is now generally limited to nasal anesthesia in the operating room (see Table 8–8).

C. TOPICAL VASOCONSTRICTORS

If nasal intubation is planned, addition of a local vasoconstrictor is necessary to decrease the risk of epistaxis (unless topical cocaine is used). The best drugs for this purpose are phenylephrine, 0.005–0.15%, or ephedrine, 1%. Topical epinephrine is ineffective.

D. TOPICAL LARYNGEAL ANESTHESIA

After nasal and oropharyngeal anesthesia is induced, the posterior pharynx and larynx may require additional local anesthesia. Gentle direct laryngoscopy will permit local anesthesia of more distal tissues with a spray. Tracheal anesthesia can also be obtained by direct injection of 2–3 mL of 1–2% lidocaine through the cricothyroid membrane.

Superior Laryngeal Nerve Block

Sensory innervation of the larynx, epiglottis, and lower pharynx is supplied by the internal branch of the superior laryngeal nerve that branches from the vagus bilaterally. It pierces the thyrohyoid membrane between the thyroid cartilage and the hyoid bone below the greater horn of the hyoid, and runs in the submucosa of the piriform fossa. It may be blocked in the sitting patient by inserting the needle laterally just above the thyroid cartilage below the greater horn and injecting 2–3 mL of 2% lidocaine. The injection is then repeated on the other side. A median approach with the needle directed

Table 8–8. Properties of local anesthetics.

	Lidocaine	Cocaine
Available concentration	2–4%	4–11%
Common routes	Gargle, spray, or atomizer	Saturated swabs or packing
Time to onset	3–5 minutes	5–10 minutes
Duration	30–45 minutes	30–90 minutes
Toxic doses	> 4–5 mg/kg or 200–250 in adults	> 3–4 mg/kg (toxicity has been reported with therapeutic doses)
Toxicities	Seizure, coma, confusion, respiratory arrest, cardiovascular depression	Tachycardia, cardiac arrhythmias, stroke, cardiac arrest, elevated blood pressure

laterally and upward toward the greater horn of the hyoid bone on either side also will be effective (Figure 8–6).

Rapid-Sequence Intubation

A. GENERAL CONSIDERATIONS

Use of sedation alone to intubate a patient in the emergency department can be difficult and risky. Titration of a narcotic or sedative to an intubating dose is time consuming. Delays in airway control can delay other care. Unwanted central nervous system or cardiovascular side effects can persist, complicating the patient's postintubation course. Hypoventilation often occurs before the patient is adequately relaxed for intubation, and prolonged bag-valve-mask ventilation may be required. Many emergency department patients present with a full stomach. These factors, combined with gastric distention due to bag-valve-mask ventilation, de-

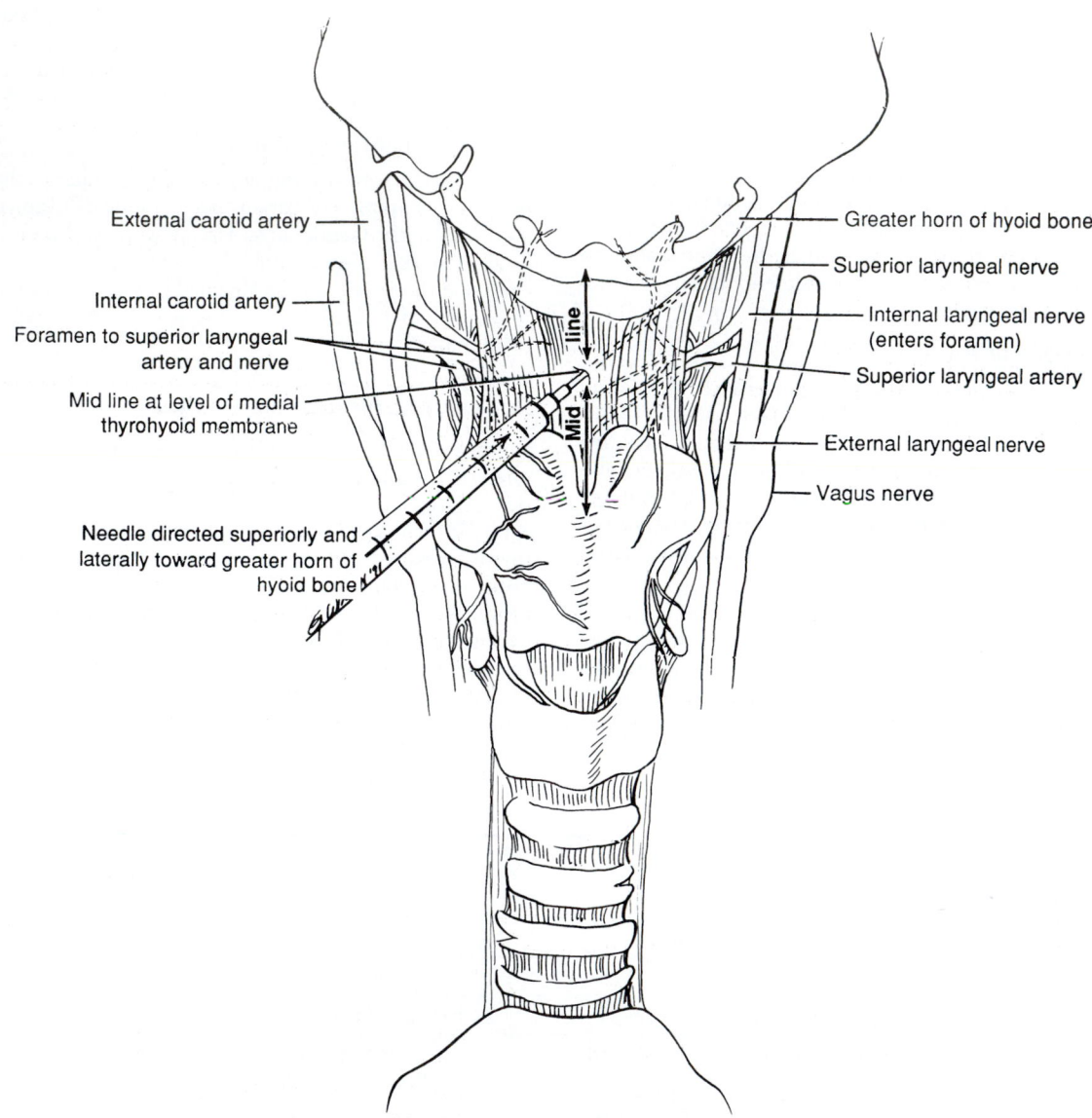

Figure 8–6. The superior laryngeal nerve block.

pressed airway reflexes, and the emetic effects of sedatives, raise the risk of aspiration.

The RSI protocol diminishes these difficulties in the awake patient who is agitated or who has altered mental status and requires oral intubation. A rapid-acting neuromuscular blocker is given to paralyze the patient. Though controversial, some protocols recommend a priming dose of a nondepolarizing neuromuscular blocker (such as vecuronium) to facilitate paralysis, reduce fasciculations, and limit elevations in intracranial pressure during laryngoscopy. Prior to administration of the paralytic, a short-acting sedative is added to decrease agitation and the noxious sensations associated with paralysis and intubation in awake or semi-conscious patients. The patient is intubated immediately after paralysis. Further sedation or paralysis may then be effected as indicated.

During the short period when the patient is paralyzed and not intubated, the airway must be protected from aspiration with cricoid pressure.

The RSI protocol is generally unnecessary in a completely obtunded, relaxed patient; however, if the patient has retained enough muscle tone to make intubation without paralytics difficult, RSI may facilitate a more rapid intubation. Contraindications include contraindications to the specific drugs that will be used. Do not induce apnea if there are contraindications to oral intubation or evidence that it is not likely to be successful and bag-valve-mask ventilation will be difficult. Because the RSI protocol will obscure the neurologic examination and physical manifestations of status epilepticus, alternative plans to follow the neurologic condition of the patient must be made before inducing paralysis.

B. EQUIPMENT AND PERSONNEL REQUIRED

At least 2 individuals must be available to safely initiate the RSI protocol. Other than the drugs, no special equipment is required to induce neuromuscular blockade. Before giving any sedative or neuromuscular blocking agent, review the checklist in Table 8–9. The choice of sedative or anesthetic and neuromuscular

Table 8–9. Checklist for initiation of RSI.

Baseline neurological exam is completed.
All materials for intubation are assembled.
Materials for surgical airways are immediately available.
Suction is working and available.
Individuals have been designated as responsible for cricoid pressure cervical spine stabilization (in the setting of trauma).
The patient is preoxygenated.

blocking agent depends on the indication for intubation, patient condition, and user familiarity.

C. PROCEDURE

Table 8–10 outlines the steps of the RSI protocol. The characteristics of the recommended drugs are mentioned in the "Drugs Used During Intubation" section, below.

D. ADDITIONAL DRUGS

Several agents may be added to the RSI protocol under specific circumstances.

1. Vecuronium—Vecuronium, 0.01 mg/kg priming dose given 3–5 minutes before succinylcholine, will abolish fasciculations. Fasciculations may cause muscle pain, increased intragastric pressure, increased intraocular pressure, and increased intracranial pressure and may displace bony fractures. Although vecuronium can attenuate these effects, many physicians use fasciculations as an indicator that paralysis is being initiated and intubate immediately upon cessation of fasciculation.

Table 8–10. Rapid-sequence induction protocol.

Preoxygenate with 100% oxygen.
  (Use bag-valve-mask ventilatory assistance only as needed.)
Give rapid intravenous injection of sedative.[1]
For trauma patients:
  Maintain in-line cervical traction from induction and until cervical collar can be replaced after the endotracheal tube has been secured.
Give rapid intravenous injection of succinylcholine,[2] 1–2 mg/kg (unless contraindicated).
Initiate cricoid pressure, and stop bag-valve-mask ventilation.
Observe for fasciculations followed by apnea.
Immediately intubate upon onset of apnea.
Begin ventilation.
Inflate endotracheal tube cuff, and release cricoid pressure.
Confirm tube position clinically (ascultate breath sounds, use end tidal CO_2 detector).
Secure tube.
Provide additional sedation and paralysis as indicated.

[1]Sedative drug choices:
  Etomidate, 0.3 mg/kg
  Methohexital, 0.5–1 mg/kg
  Midazolam, 0.1–0.3 mg/kg
  Fentanyl, 1–5 µg/kg
  Ketamine, 1–2 mg/kg
  Thiopental, 1–4 mg/kg
[2]Alternative neuromuscular blocker:
  Vecuronium, 0.1–0.25 mg/kg
  Rocuronium, 0.6 mg/kg
  (Use only when succinylcholine is contraindicated).

2. Atropine—Atropine, 0.01–0.02 mg/kg given immediately before the sedative, attenuates the vagal bradycardia associated with succinylcholine. Children, who tend to be more sensitive to the bradycardic and hypotensive effects of succinylcholine, benefit from pretreatment with atropine. Pretreat adults with bradycardia and those receiving a second dose of succinylcholine.

3. Lidocaine—Lidocaine, 1.5 mg/kg given 1 minute before intubation, may attenuate elevations in intracranial pressure associated with succinylcholine and intubation. It may have some protective effect against laryngeal spasm and ventricular arrhythmias during intubation.

4. Analgesics—If pain control is part of the management plan, a narcotic such as morphine sulfate, 0.1 mg/kg; fentanyl, 1–2 μg/kg intravenously; or other analgesic should be added after intubation, because barbiturates have little analgesic effect and neuromuscular blockers have none.

5. Anticonvulsant agents—If status epilepticus is present before intubation, load the patient with anticonvulsant medications such as phenytoin, 15 mg/kg, after intubation. The neuromuscular blockers used in the RSI protocol mask, but do not stop, central nervous system seizure activity.

Drugs Used During Intubation

A. SUCCINYLCHOLINE

Succinylcholine is a depolarizing neuromuscular blocking agent.

1. Dose—1.0–1.5 mg/kg in adults, 1.5–2.0 mg/kg in children.

2. Onset—60 seconds to complete relaxation.

3. Duration—5–10 minutes.

4. Metabolism—Degraded by pseudocholinesterase.

5. Indications and advantages—
   a. Drug of choice for the RSI protocol under most circumstances owing to rapid onset, complete muscular relaxation, and short duration.
   b. Single dose in emergency department setting usually well tolerated if appropriate precautions are taken (see below).

6. Contraindications—
   a. Risk factors for hyperkalemia (see "Adverse effects and precautions," below).
   b. Hereditary pseudocholinesterase deficiency (1 in 2800 patients).
   c. Penetrating ocular trauma or glaucoma.
   d. Known family or personal history of malignant hyperthermia.
   e. Hypersensitivity to succinylcholine.

7. Adverse effects and precautions—
   a. Cardiovascular effects include bradycardia and hypotension, ventricular arrhythmias, and tachycardia or hypertension. Use with care in setting of irritable myocardium.
   b. Fasciculations (see above for sequelae).
   c. Hyperkalemia occurs in settings of subacute burns, subacute crush injuries, upper and lower motor neuron disease, and tetanus. Levels in excess of 9 mEq/L have been reported, and cardiac arrest may occur. Use may worsen hyperkalemia in renal failure patients.
   d. Pseudocholinesterase inhibition may occur in pregnancy, in renal or hepatic insufficiency, and with a variety of drugs.
   e. Malignant hyperthermia occurs in 1 in 50,000 patients.
   f. Histamine release may cause bronchospasm or anaphylactoid reaction.
   g. Intraocular pressure is elevated during fasciculations.
   h. Intracranial pressure may increase.
   i. Intragastric pressure may increase; use cricoid pressure until endotracheal tube cuff is inflated.
   j. Always use sedation with alert patients; succinylcholine has no intrinsic analgesic or sedative effect.

B. VECURONIUM

Vecuronium is a nondepolarizing neuromuscular blocking agent (NDNMB).

1. Dose—Standard dose is 0.1 mg/kg. To achieve rapid intubating conditions, 0.25 mg/kg may be used.

2. Onset—Dose dependent; standard doses achieve paralysis in 3–5 minutes, larger doses in 1–1.5 min.

3. Duration—Dose dependent; standard doses last 20–40 minutes, and larger does may prolong paralysis 2–3 times the usual duration.

4. Metabolism—Hepatic metabolism with renal excretion. No dose changes recommended in patients with congestive heart failure or hepatic or renal insufficiency.

5. Indications and advantages—
   a. One of the NDMBDs that can be used when succinylcholine is contraindicated.
   b. Short duration allows neurologic reevaluation and provides satisfactory paralysis for procedures such as computed tomography scan in emergent setting.
   c. Minimal cardiovascular effects at usual doses.
   d. Reversible after partial recovery (evidence of head lift, respiratory effort, or muscle twitch

response) with neostigmine, 0.04 mg/kg intravenously. Atropine, 0.02 mg/kg intravenously, must also be administered to prevent muscarinic side effects.

e. Does not cause fasciculations or elevate intracranial pressure.

6. Contraindication—Know hypersensitivity to vecuronium.

7. Adverse effects and precautions—

a. Reduce dosage in patients with myasthenia gravis to avoid prolonged blockade.

b. Maintain cricoid pressure until inflation of endotracheal tube cuff.

c. Must use sedation or anesthesia in awake patients.

d. Block is prolonged by aminoglycosides, lithium, quinidine, lidocaine, and propranolol and in hypermagnesemia, hyperkalemia, dehydration, hypothermia, and respiratory acidosis.

e. Use during pregnancy only if clearly indicated.

C. ROCURONIUM

Rocuronium is a rapid onset, short-acting NDNMB.

1. Dose—0.6 mg/kg.

2. Onset—1–2 minutes.

3. Duration—30 minutes.

4. Metabolism—Minimally hepatic with excretion in stool.

5. Indications and advantages—Excellent choice for nondepolarizing neuromuscular blockade. Good alternative for use when succinylcholine is contraindicated.

6. Contraindication— Known hypersensitivity to rocuronium.

7. Adverse effects and precautions—

a. Effects potentiated by electrolyte disturbances, neuromuscular diseases, and renal or hepatic failure.

b. Use in pregnancy only if clearly indicated.

D. PANCURONIUM

Pancuronium is a longer-acting NDNMB.

1. Dose—0.05–0.2 mg/kg.

2. Onset—1–3 minutes.

3. Duration—Dose dependent, averaging 60–90 minutes.

4. Metabolism—Hepatic metabolism with renal excretion. Dosage adjustments are indicated.

5. Indications and advantages—

a. Main use is prolonged blockade after intubation is complete.

b. Does not promote bronchospasm.

c. Reversible after partial recovery (see discussion of vecuronium, above).

d. No elevated intracranial pressure or fasciculations.

6. Contraindications—

a. Known hypersensitivity to pancuronium.

b. Cardiovascular instability or history of congestive heart failure.

7. Adverse effects and precautions—

a. History of myasthenia gravis (see section on vecuronium, above).

b. Cardiovascular effects include increased heart rate, increased afterload, and ventricular arrhythmias. Use with caution in the setting of irritable myocardium.

c. Blockade is prolonged by multiple drugs (see section on vecuronium, above).

d. Onset and duration profile are not optimal for use with the RSI protocol.

e. Maintain cricoid pressure until inflation of endotracheal tube cuff.

f. Always use sedation or anesthesia in awake patients.

g. Use in pregnancy only if clearly indicated.

E. THIOPENTAL

Thiopental is a short-acting, highly lipid-soluble barbiturate sedative.

1. Dose—1–4 mg/kg.

2. Onset—60 seconds.

3. Duration—5–50 minutes.

4. Metabolism—Hepatic metabolism.

5. Indications and advantages—

a. Historically popular choice for the RSI protocol owing to rapid onset and short duration.

b. Decreases intracranial pressure and cerebral oxygen consumption.

c. Produces amnesia.

6. Contraindications—

a. Known sensitivity to barbiturates.

b. Variegate or acute intermittent porphyria.

7. Adverse effects and precautions—

a. Respiratory depression and apnea.

b. Cardiovascular effects include myocardial depression, dilation of veins, tachycardia, and hypotension. Dehydrated patients are at greatest risk for hypotension. Use with care in cardiovascular disease and shock and in hypotensive patients.

c. Cough, laryngospasm, bronchospasm, and hiccups. Consider an alternative drug for status asthmaticus.

d. Nausea and vomiting.
e. Pain on injection and local necrosis with extravasation.
f. Anaphylactoid reactions.
g. Effect prolonged or intensified by other sedatives, narcotics, probenecid, advanced age, Addison disease, renal or hepatic insufficiency, myasthenia gravis, and anemia.
h. Effect antagonized by aminophylline.
i. Consider an alternative drug in pregnancy.

F. METHOHEXITAL

Methohexital is a rapid-, ultra-short-acting barbiturate anesthetic.

1. Dose—0.5–1.5 mg/kg.

2. Onset—Less than 60 seconds.

3. Duration—5–7 minutes.

4. Metabolism—Hepatic metabolism with renal excretion.

5. Indications and advantages—
a. Slightly shorter acting alternative to thiopental in the RSI protocol.
b. See section on thiopental, above.

6. Contraindications—See section on thiopental, above.

7. Adverse effects and precautions—See section on thiopental, above.

G. ETOMIDATE

Etomidate is a short-acting sedative-hypnotic.

1. Dose—0.3 mg/kg intravenously.

2. Onset—Within 1 minute.

3. Duration—3–5 minutes.

4. Metabolism—Hepatic metabolism with delayed elimination in end-stage liver disease.

5. Indications and advantages—
a. Alternative drug for sedation in RSI.
b. Little to no cardiovascular side effects.
c. Lowers intracranial and intraocular pressures.

6. Contraindication—Known hypersensitivity to etomidate.

7. Adverse effects and precautions—
a. May cause hypotension in the hypovolemic patient.
b. May cause apnea, laryngospasm, hiccough, and cough.
c. Decreases plasma cortisol and aldosterone.
d. Local pain on injection.
e. Skeletal muscle movements such as myoclonus.

f. No recommendations for dosing in children younger than age 10 years.
g. May cause fetal malformation in pregnancy.

H. MIDAZOLAM

Midazolam is a short-acting benzodiazepine central nervous system depressant.

1. Dose—0.1–0.3 mg/kg.

2. Onset—Approximately 30 seconds, depending on rate of injection when given intravenously.

3. Duration—15–20 minutes.

4. Metabolism—Hepatic metabolism with delayed elimination in congestive heart failure, renal insufficiency, and old age.

5. Indications and advantages—
a. Alternative induction agent for sedation in the RSI protocol (may have prolonged sedative effect).
b. Minimal cardiovascular effects.
c. May produce amnesia for several hours.
d. Blunt intracranial pressure responses at high doses.

6. Contraindications—
a. Known sensitivity to midazolam or benzodiazepines.
b. Acute narrow-angle glaucoma.

7. Adverse effects and precautions—
a. Respiratory depression or arrest.
b. Cardiovascular effects usually minimal with bigeminy, premature ventricular contractions, and nodal rhythms.
c. Laryngospasm and bronchospasm, cough, and hives.
d. Local irritation at injection site.
e. Nausea and vomiting.
f. Potentiated by other central nervous system depressants; dose modifications recommended.
g. Dose modifications recommended in patients with chronic obstructive pulmonary disease or congestive heart failure, in elderly patients, and in patients with renal failure.
h. Possible increase in fetal malformations with pregnancy.

I. FENTANYL

Fentanyl is a short-acting narcotic anesthetic.

1. Dose—1–5 µg/kg intravenously.

2. Onset—60 seconds.

3. Duration—30–60 minutes.

4. Metabolism—Hepatic metabolism.

5. Indications and advantages—
   a. Alternative drug for sedation in the RSI protocol (sedation may be prolonged with thiopental).
   b. Both analgesic and sedative effects.
   c. No histamine release.
   d. Blunts intracranial pressure response to intubation.
   e. Reversible with naloxone, 1–4 mg intravenously.

6. Contraindication—Known sensitivity to fentanyl.

7. Adverse effects and precautions—
   a. Respiratory depression and apnea. Respiratory depression may persist beyond analgesic and sedative effects.
   b. Muscle rigidity, which may occur with rapid injection of high doses.
   c. Rare bradycardia or cardiovascular depression.
   d. Nausea and vomiting.
   e. Effects potentiated by other central nervous system or respiratory depressants.
   f. Dose modifications recommended in patients with chronic obstructive pulmonary disease or congestive heart failure, in elderly patients, and in patients with renal failure.
   g. Possible increase in fetal malformations. Consider alternative drugs in pregnancy.

J. KETAMINE

Ketamine is a dissociative anesthetic agent.

1. Dose—1–2 mg/kg.

2. Onset—60 seconds.

3. Duration—5–10 minutes.

4. Metabolism—Hepatic metabolism.

5. Indications and advantages—
   a. Alternative drug for sedation and analgesia during the RSI protocol, particularly in hypotension.
   b. Sedative of choice in status asthmaticus patients because it may cause bronchodilation.
   c. Airway reflexes are usually maintained. Respiratory depression is usually minimal and transient.
   d. Myocardial depression is uncommon.
   e. Prominent analgesic effects.

6. Contraindications—
   a. Hypersensitivity to ketamine.
   b. Head injury.
   c. Severe hypertension.

7. Adverse effects and precautions—
   a. Elevated blood pressure and pulse rate are the most common cardiovascular effects. Hypotension, bradycardia, and arrhythmias have been reported. Use with caution if irritable myocardium is present or when hypertension would adversely affect patient course.
   b. Respiratory stimulation and maintained airway most common, but apnea, respiratory arrest, and laryngospasm also have been reported.
   c. Dysphoric emergence reactions.
   d. Nausea and vomiting.
   e. Local irritation at injection site.
   f. Increased intracranial pressure.
   g. Intraocular pressure may be increased.
   h. Muscle rigidity or myoclonus.
   i. Increased secretions. Consider pretreatment with atropine.
   j. Possible prolonged recovery when used concurrently with narcotics or barbiturates.
   k. Consider alternative drug in pregnancy and for patients below 2 months of age.

Li J et al: Complications of emergency intubation with and without paralysis. Am J Emerg Med 1999;17:141. [PMID: 10102312] (Retrospective chart review of intubation complications with and without paralytics.)

Rodricks MB et al: Emergent airway management—indications and methods in the face of confounding conditions. Crit Care Clin 2000;16:389. [PMID: 10941580] (Review of management of the difficult airway, which includes review of current medications used in rapid-sequence protocols.)

Wadbrook PS: Advances in airway pharmacology—emerging trends and evolving controversy. Emerg Med Clin North Am 2000;18:767. [PMID: 11130938] (Review of drugs used for RSI protocol.)

■ SPECIAL CASES

Management of the Pediatric Airway

Basic principles of airway management are similar for all age groups. However, anatomic and physiologic differences affect the emergency physician's equipment needs and management decisions when confronted with a pediatric airway emergency.

A. UNIQUE FEATURES

- In infants, the head is relatively larger in proportion to the body.
- The neck is more supple owing to a greater proportion of cartilaginous support tissue.

- The airway is smaller, resulting in increased resistance and susceptibility to obstruction due to edema, blood, or secretions.
- The mucosa is looser, permitting obstruction due to positioning and greater, faster distention from blood or edema.
- The adenoidal and tonsillar lymphatic tissues are larger and more friable than those of adults.
- The larynx is more cephalad and anterior.
- The epiglottis is larger and more floppy and protrudes into the airway more prominently.
- The narrowest portion of the airway in children younger than age 5 years is the cricoid cartilage rather than the larynx, as in adults.
- The cricothyroid membrane is very small and does not lend itself to surgical manipulation.
- The carina branches symmetrically at 45 degrees.
- The chest wall is thinner, and both airway and gastric sounds radiate easily, making auscultation less reliable.
- The chest wall is more pliable, and ventilation depends significantly on diaphragmatic movement.
- Oxygen consumption is 6–8 mL/kg/min in children, whereas adults usually consume about 3–4 mL/kg/min. Hypoxemia can occur more rapidly and is tolerated less well.
- Apnea occurs suddenly during a wide range of illnesses and injuries.
- Normal vital signs vary for different age groups (Table 8–11).

B. Equipment Required

All essential equipment (oxygen delivery systems, face masks, bag-valve-mask units, oral and nasal airways, laryngoscope blades, endotracheal tubes, stylets, and suction devices) should be stocked in a variety of sizes to accommodate the anticipated population served by the facility (see Table 8–11). Oxygen should be humidified and warmed to prevent drying of secretions and subsequent airway obstruction. Endotracheal tubes for children younger than age 8 years should be noncuffed to prevent damage to the cricoid ring. Correct tube size may be obtained from a table or gauged based on one of the 3 following methods:

1. The tube size should closely approximate the size of the child's small finger at the distal interphalangeal joint.
2. The tube size should closely approximate the size of the child's nares.
3. The tube size in millimeters is equal to (16 + patient's age in years) ÷ 4.

For patients under age 4 years, a straight blade is preferred owing to the tendency of the epiglottis to protrude and cover the airway. In emergency departments where pediatric resuscitation is rare, precalculate the doses of commonly needed drugs, based on weights, and post them clearly in the resuscitation area or utilize length-based charts such as the Broselow-Luten tape.

C. Decision and Techniques

Evaluate for respiratory distress by assessing vital signs, skin signs, overall patient condition, use of accessory muscles, retractions, nasal flaring, and arterial blood gases or pulse oximetry. Supplemental oxygen must be given. Children often cannot tolerate a face mask. Adequate oxygen supplementation can frequently be achieved by directing a stream of humidified 100% oxygen across the patient's face.

Airway positioning is essential. Alert patients will often choose the position of greatest airway patency and should not be forced to lie down. Infants and obtunded patients must be placed in the sniffing position (see Figure 8–2) unless cervical spine injury is suspected or present. In this position, the neck is flexed slightly, and the head is extended on the neck. The jaw thrust or chin lift is then used to lift the soft tissues out of the airway. Obstruction should be cleared.

Table 8–11. Pediatric vital signs and airway equipment.

Age	Premature	Neonate	1 mo	6 mo	1 yr	3 yr	5 yr	7 yr	>10 yr
Weight (kg)	1	2–3	4	7	10	12–14	16–18	20–26	>30
Heart rate	145	125	120	130	125	115	100	100	75
Respiratory rate	30–40	30–40	25–35		20–30		12–25		12–18
Endotracheal tube size (inner diameter in mm)	2.5–3.0 Uncuffed	3	3.5	3.5	4	4.5	5–6	6–6.5 -------Cuffed	7
Length at teeth (cm)	8	10	12		12	16	16	18	20–22
Laryngoscope blade size	0	0–1	1		1–2	1–2	2	2–3 ------Curved	3
Suction catheter size (Fr)	5	6	6–8	6–8	8	8–10	10	10–12	12

Oral and nasal airways are less useful in children because they frequently stimulate laryngospasm or emesis when reflexes are intact. In addition, placement may traumatize the adenoidal or tonsillar soft tissues, resulting in significant bleeding, which can be difficult to control and further complicate airway management.

In obtunded or paralyzed children, cricoid pressure should be used during positive-pressure ventilation until intubation is confirmed.

Bag-valve-mask ventilation is used initially for emergent oxygenation and ventilation in children because of the ease of attaining a seal and the smaller size of the chest cavity. Adequacy of ventilation is best assessed by observing chest wall motion; auscultation is less reliable. Nasogastric tube placement should accompany bag-valve-mask ventilation when safe to decrease the risk of emesis and aspiration. Care should be taken to coordinate breaths with the bag-valve-mask unit with spontaneous ventilations, when present.

Definitive airway control involves oral endotracheal intubation. Blind nasal intubation is technically more difficult in children and is contraindicated in the emergency department. The increased adenoidal tissue is at risk for bleeding, and the anterior position of the larynx with the overlying epiglottis makes nasal tube placement more difficult.

Until age 10 years, children should be premedicated with atropine, 0.01–0.02 mg/kg, to prevent bradycardia with intubation.

Because auscultation can be unreliable, tube placement should be confirmed by a colorimetric end tidal CO_2 detector, observation of chest wall movement, skin color, and radiographs.

When a cervical fracture is suspected and immediate airway control is essential, RSI may be used with in-line traction; other options include PTTJV. PTTJV has been shown to be effective in the pediatric model. Perform needle cricothyroidotomy as described for adults. The smaller size of the airways should be taken into account. The possibility of obstruction at the cricoid cartilage must be considered, because ventilation at the level of the cricothyroid membrane would be ineffective in that situation.

Surgical airways in young children and infants are extremely difficult. They should be performed only as a last resort by surgeons with experience in pediatric head and neck surgery. There are high failure and complication rates. Most airways will be adequately managed by bag-valve-mask or oral intubation techniques.

D. Epiglottitis and Croup

These illnesses may cause severe airway edema and sudden obstruction. Diagnosis is based on clinical features and, when necessary, anteroposterior and lateral neck soft tissue views.

1. Croup—Croup progresses more slowly than epiglottitis, causes subglottic swelling and a barking cough, and is often accompanied by signs of viral upper respiratory infection. Croup rarely requires intubation. Treatment includes intravenous fluids, humidified air, steroids, and racemic epinephrine.

2. Epiglottitis—Epiglottitis progresses rapidly with a toxic-appearing, drooling child sitting in the upright position with the neck hyperextended. Abrupt, complete airway obstruction can occur with minimal stimulation of the patient. When suspicion is high for epiglottitis, supplemental oxygen should be supplied and the patient transported with minimal disturbance to the operating room, where the epiglottis can be directly visualized. More than half of patients with epiglottitis will require intubation, which is best done in the operating room by the most experienced intubator before airway obstruction occurs. If intubation fails, an emergent tracheostomy must be performed, preferably by a pediatric otorhinolaryngologist. Treatment includes antibiotics and intravenous fluids after the airway is secured (see Chapter 48).

Management of Foreign Bodies in the Airway

Management of foreign bodies in the airway is dictated by the location of the object and the patient's age and condition. Most airway obstructions due to foreign bodies occur between the ages of 1 and 5 years. More than 3000 deaths annually are due to this disorder.

Assessment begins with observation for tachypnea, air movement, stridor, retraction, agitation or lethargy, and cyanosis. Auscultation and chest x-ray may be helpful. Examination of the oropharynx may reveal the foreign body.

If the foreign body is visible, the airway may be cleared with a manual sweep. Blind sweep is not recommended. If the patient is coughing, do not interfere; the normal reflexes often clear the airway. Oxygen should be administered to all patients with foreign body aspiration.

If there is total obstruction, attempt the Heimlich maneuver in patients older than 1 year; in younger children, back blows and chest thrusts are recommended. If these methods are unsuccessful, position the airway to optimize patency. Attempt to remove the object under direct observation with a laryngoscope. If this is unsuccessful, a surgical airway is necessary. Subglottic obstructions may not be relieved by cricothyroidotomy or tracheostomy. Removal in the operating room with rigid bronchoscope may be the only option.

Management of the partially obstructed airway must be individualized. Bronchial obstructions often do not require intubation, and compromise may be subacute.

If there is air movement and the object cannot be visualized on direct observation, the safest method for removal is under general anesthesia with the rigid bronchoscope. Take care not to cause complete obstruction while inserting the laryngoscope or bronchoscope.

Management of Airway in Status Asthmaticus

The asthmatic patient requires intubation when clinical evidence of fatigue is accompanied by increasing respiratory acidosis due to carbon dioxide retention and increasing hypoxia in the face of aggressive therapy. Intubation is dangerous for asthmatic patients. These patients are susceptible to barotrauma while intubated, and intubation does not ensure bronchodilation or adequate ventilation and oxygenation. Because of the difficulties of bag-valve-mask ventilation in status asthmaticus, many practitioners prefer awake nasal intubations with topical anesthetic. The asthmatic patient's active respiratory effort helps tube placement through the cords, but agitation often complicates this procedure. If the RSI protocol is used, succinylcholine is relatively contraindicated owing to histamine-induced bronchospasm. Similarly, thiopental may worsen the condition. Better choices include vecuronium, midazolam, fentanyl, and ketamine. Unlike other choices for sedation, ketamine also has bronchodilating effects.

Management of Airway in Trauma Patients

A. Patients with Unstable Cervical Spines or Facial Injuries

When airway control must precede definitive stabilization of the spine, oral intubation with RSI and in-line maintenance of the cervical spine has been proved safe and effective. It is the method of choice in the trauma patient with suspected spinal injury. However, most large series report no bad neurologic outcomes with any technique that is carefully done. Other options for airway control include blind techniques such as nasal or digital intubation, use of lighted accessories, and transtracheal methods. The decision must be individualized based on the patient's level of consciousness and injuries, the urgency of the need for airway control, and the intubator's skill with various techniques.

Patients with severe facial and upper neck trauma present significant challenges to the emergency physician. If RSI techniques are attempted, the emergency physician should be prepared to switch immediately to a surgical airway or a bridge device to allow ventilation in the event that bag-valve-mask ventilation proves difficult or ineffective. If the airway is predicted from the beginning to be difficult, an awake intubation using topical anesthetics and intravenous sedation may be the best approach.

B. Patients with Head Trauma

Intubation of patients with severe head trauma is indicated to treat hypoventilation and hypoxia and to protect and control the airway in patients who are unstable or combative and agitated enough to require paralysis for necessary studies and procedures. Additionally, it is the only way to hyperventilate the patient to a lower PCO_2 as part of the treatment for elevated intracranial pressure. Approach to the airway must take into account other potential traumatic injuries to the mid face, cervical spine, soft tissues of the neck, and respiratory tract. Oral intubation with the RSI protocol is generally recommended. If the RSI protocol is used, lidocaine, 1.5 mg/kg intravenously, may attenuate the rise in intracranial pressure. Although succinylcholine is reported to raise intracranial pressure, it remains the recommended agent for neuromuscular blockade in the setting of head trauma because it allows for rapid control of the airway and initiation of treatment. Other sedative options available to attenuate the rise in intracranial pressure associated with laryngoscopy include fentanyl and etomidate. Vecuronium, an NDNMB, is administered at 0.01 mg/kg as a small priming dose to eliminate muscle fasciculations associated with succinylcholine use. Digital intubation or light-assisted or surgical airways may be used as indicated if oral intubation is unsuccessful.

Cummins RO et al: Guidelines 2000 for cardiopulmonary resuscitation and emergency cardiovascular care. American Heart Association Currents 2000;Fall:1. (Update of advanced cardiac life support guidelines.)

Levy RJ et al: Managing the airway in the critically ill patient—pediatric issues. Crit Care Clin 2000;16:489. [PMID: 10941587] (Review of the management of the difficult airway in the pediatric patient.)

Soriano SG et al: The difficult pediatric airway—surgical airway, rigid bronchoscopy, and transtracheal jet ventilation in the pediatric patient. Anesthesiol Clin North Am 1998;16:827. (Review of alternative methods for airway control in the pediatric patient.)

Walls RM: Management of the difficult airway in the trauma patient. Emerg Med Clin North Am 1998;16:45. [PMID: 11809554] (Review of airway techniques in the trauma patient.)

■ CARE OF THE INTUBATED PATIENT

Adjunctive Drugs

Intubated patients often require sedation to prevent coughing or "bucking" the endotracheal tube and to reduce agitation. Prolonged paralysis may be indicated during procedures or during early stages of management. In general, neuromuscular blockade should be accompanied by sedation to blunt the noxious sensation of paralysis. Paralysis may mask the manifestations of status epilepticus. Patients with ongoing status epilepticus must have full anticonvulsant loading before, during, or immediately after paralysis. If the patient remains paralyzed, control of seizures must be demonstrated with electroencephalographic recording.

Pulmonary Toilet

After the endotracheal tube position is confirmed by clinical evaluation and x-ray, it is secured by taping about the head or neck to prevent accidental extubation. All intubated patients require regular suctioning. The frequency of suctioning depends on the amount of secretion produced. Indicators of the need to suction may include visible secretions welling up in the endotracheal tube, hypoxia, agitation, and increased difficulty with bagging. In the emergency department, most patients will be manually ventilated with a bag-valve-mask unit, at least initially. If on a mechanical ventilator, a patient should be preoxygenated with several minutes of bag-valve ventilation at 100% oxygen to ensure against hypoxia during suctioning. Disposable, sterile, narrow-gauge, flexible suction catheters are available for suctioning the endotracheal tube. The diameter of the catheter should be less than half the internal diameter of the endotracheal tube. Insert the catheter with the side port open. When the catheter is in the trachea, apply suction by covering the side port. Rotate the catheter several times to suction both right and left main stems. Continue suction and rotary movement during catheter removal. The patient is then reoxygenated. No single suctioning episode should last longer than 10–15 seconds. Preoxygenate for 30–60 seconds before reinserting the catheter. Suctioning may be aided by administering 1–2 mL of sterile normal saline down the tube to moisten secretions. Complications of suctioning include hypoxia, arrhythmias, hypotension, mucosal trauma, and pulmonary collapse. There is also a surge in intracranial pressure during suctioning, which may be blunted by the use of tracheal or intravenous lidocaine. Occasionally the oropharynx must be suctioned with the rigid-tipped catheter to control oral secretions or blood.

Endotracheal Medication

Medications that are safe and probably effective when given endotracheally include epinephrine, atropine, lidocaine, diazepam, and naloxone. Because of erratic absorption, some authors recommend administering 2–10 times the normal intravenous dose for epinephrine endotracheally. Delivery is enhanced if the drugs are diluted in 10 mL of normal saline before administration and aerosolized during administration by rapid injection through a pediatric feeding tube positioned in the trachea.

Monitoring

A. Observation

Any patient intubated in the emergency department requires close observation. A respiratory technician, nurse, or physician should be present at all times. In addition to contributing critical clinical observation to the data obtained by monitoring devices, they may note complications of intubation and positive-pressure ventilation and address them before these complications compromise the patient.

Complications that may occur while a patient is intubated include barotrauma with tension pneumothorax, atelectasis, and obstructions or disconnections in the ventilatory circuit. In critically ill patients, continuous observation for changes in the patient's hemodynamic or mental status is the standard of care.

B. Pulse Oximetry

A pulse oximetry sensor can be clipped over the tip of a digit or an earlobe to detect the oxygen saturation of arterial blood. Oximetry reflects trends in oxygenation before, during, and after intubation. When the PaO_2 is greater than 60–80 mm Hg, a large change in PaO_2 may result in only a small change in oxygen saturation measured by the pulse oximeter. Oxygenation can also be maintained to some degree by hyperventilation (PCO_2 declines); however, pulse oximetry provides no information about the adequacy of ventilation. Consequently the pulse oximeter cannot substitute for arterial blood gas determinations in many clinical settings. The presence of nail polish, skin pigmentation, methemoglobin, carboxyhemoglobin, intravascular dye, hypothermia, and hypoperfusion all may reduce the accuracy of the pulse oximeter.

C. Capnography

Capnometers may be attached to the expired air circuit to monitor the end-tidal carbon dioxide tension ($P_{et}CO_2$). In healthy patients, the plateau $P_{et}CO_2$ is usually 1 mm Hg less than the PCO_2. Because the absence of $P_{et}CO_2$ indicates esophageal intubation, disposable devices are helpful to indicate successful endotracheal tube placement in patients with perfusing rhythms.

D. Esophageal Detection Device

An esophageal detection device is used to detect esophageal versus tracheal intubation. It consists of a large syringe or self-inflating bulb, which will easily aspirate air if the tube is in the trachea. Resistance to aspiration will be noted if the tube is in the esophagus. This device is useful in patients with or without perfusing rhythms. The device may be unreliable in morbidly obese, pregnant, or asthmatic patients.

E. Arterial Blood Gases

The measured pH, $PaCO_2$, and PaO_2 remain the standard for monitoring respiratory status. The method for obtaining a sample is described in Chapter 6. The main disadvantage of using the arterial blood gas measurement is the discontinuous nature of the data. Transient changes and trends may be missed. Overall, however, it remains the best indicator of gas exchange and acid-base balance.

F. Cardiac Monitoring

Most intubated patients require continuous cardiac monitoring and frequent checks of blood pressure and heart rate. Hypoxia and other complications of intubation are often reflected early in changes in vital signs.

G. Other Monitoring Methods

Several other devices may assist in monitoring an intubated patient. Some are useful only in specific settings and others when intubated patients must be held for prolonged periods in the emergency department while awaiting a bed in an intensive care unit. Transcutaneous PO_2 devices are available for neonates in whom $P_{tc}O_2$ correlates well with PaO_2. Arterial lines and pulmonary artery catheters allow intra-arterial measurement of PaO_2 and measurement of mixed venous oxygen saturation. Pulmonary functions may be monitored, particularly in patients who are likely to be extubated in the emergency department.

General Care

Paralyzed patients are unable to shift their weight from pressure points at will. Consequently, they must be turned every hour, and particular pressure points must be padded. If they are in a cool environment, they must be adequately covered. Lubricate and tape the eyes to prevent corneal ulceration.

Mechanical Ventilation

If mechanical ventilation is used in the emergency department, the choice of ventilator and ventilator settings must be individualized to the patient's condition. In many circumstances, a tidal volume of 15 mL/kg, a rate of 12, and the "assist control" mode are reasonable settings. For hyperventilation, start with a rate of 20 and check an arterial blood gas measurement for confirmation. The use of a ventilator does not obviate the need for close observation of the patient's condition by a physician or qualified nurse.

Extubation

In several circumstances, a patient may require extubation in the emergency department. Before electing to extubate, be certain that the patient has spontaneous ventilation and is able to generate a vital capacity of 15 mL/kg. The indication for intubation must be resolved, and airway reflexes should be intact. Optimally the patient should be able to follow commands and understand the planned procedure. If possible, decompress the stomach with nasogastric suction. Assemble equipment for suctioning and reintubation. Suction the oropharynx and tracheobronchial tree, manually oxygenate with 100% oxygen, release the cuff, and withdraw the tube at the end of inspiration. Ventilate with a mask, and observe for laryngospasm or respiratory insufficiency. If laryngospasm occurs, continue bag-valve-mask ventilation with 100% oxygen. Consider racemic epinephrine, 0.5 mL of 2.25% in 4 mL of normal saline via nebulizer. If these methods fail, reintubation or a surgical airway may be necessary.

Cummins RO et al: Guidelines 2000 for cardiopulmonary resuscitation and emergency cardiovascular care. American Heart Association Currents 2000;Fall;1.

Shuster M et al: Airway and ventilation management. Cardiol Clin 2002;20:23. [PMID: 11845543] (Review of airway management techniques.)

Shock

Peter W. Greenwald, MD[1]

Immediate Management of Shock
Determination of the Cause of Shock
    Approach to Shock with History of Trauma
    Approach to Shock Without History of Trauma
Emergency Treatment of Specific Causes of Shock
    Hypovolemic Shock
    Cardiogenic Shock

Obstructive Shock
    1. Cardiac Tamponade
    2. Massive Pulmonary Embolism
Distributive Shock
    1. Septic Shock
    2. Anaphylactic Shock
    3. Neurogenic Shock

■ IMMEDIATE MANAGEMENT OF SHOCK (See Figure 9–1.)

ESSENTIALS OF DIAGNOSIS

- *Early (compensated): Tachycardia, anxiety, restlessness, apprehension, delayed capillary refill, diaphoresis, widened pulse pressure.*
- *Late (decompensated): Hypotension, confusion, loss of consciousness, oliguria, acidemia.*

Shock is a state of metabolic failure. In shock, tissues do not metabolize energy properly. This may be caused either by inadequate delivery of oxygen to the tissues or by the inability of tissues to properly metabolize oxygen once it is delivered. Clinical shock is a final common pathway for a diverse group of profound physiologic disturbances. Untreated, shock leads to multiple organ system failure and death. The mortality rate among patients in shock may be as high as 70%, depending on the underlying cause. Appropriate shock management involves early recognition of the condition in addition to treatment of both the underlying causes of shock and the physiologic abnormalities associated with the shock state (Table 9–1).

Causes of Shock

Shock can be caused by qualitative defects (in which blood flow, and therefore oxygen delivery, to tissues is depleted) or quantitative defects (in which cellular oxidative metabolism is primarily affected). The goal of shock therapy, regardless of cause, is to restore homeostasis before irreversible system dysfunction develops.

On a cellular level, tissues deprived of blood flow receive insufficient oxygen and undergo a buildup of toxic metabolic byproducts. Left uncorrected, this situation leads to metabolic dysfunction severe enough that the tissue will fail to recover even if adequate oxygen flow is restored.

Cellular dysfunction plays a particularly important role in septic shock, in which a toxic stimulus (such as endotoxin) triggers an inflammatory cascade, including the release of proinflammatory monokines, cytokines, prostaglandins, leukotrienes, histamine, nitric oxide, and proteases. These chemical mediators have differing regulatory functions on a wide variety of receptors, and differing functions on the same receptors in different locations. The presence of these mediators leads to a condition known as the systemic inflammatory response syndrome. Clinically, this syndrome is defined as two or more of the following:

- Temperature > 38 °C or < 36 °C
- Pulse > 90
- Respiratory rate > 20 or $PaCO_2$ < 32 mm Hg
- White blood count > 11,000 or < 4000 or > 10% band forms

---

[1]This chapter is a revision of the chapter by Donald D. Trunkey, MD, Patricia R. Salber, MD, FACEP, FACP, & John Mills, MD, from the 4th edition.

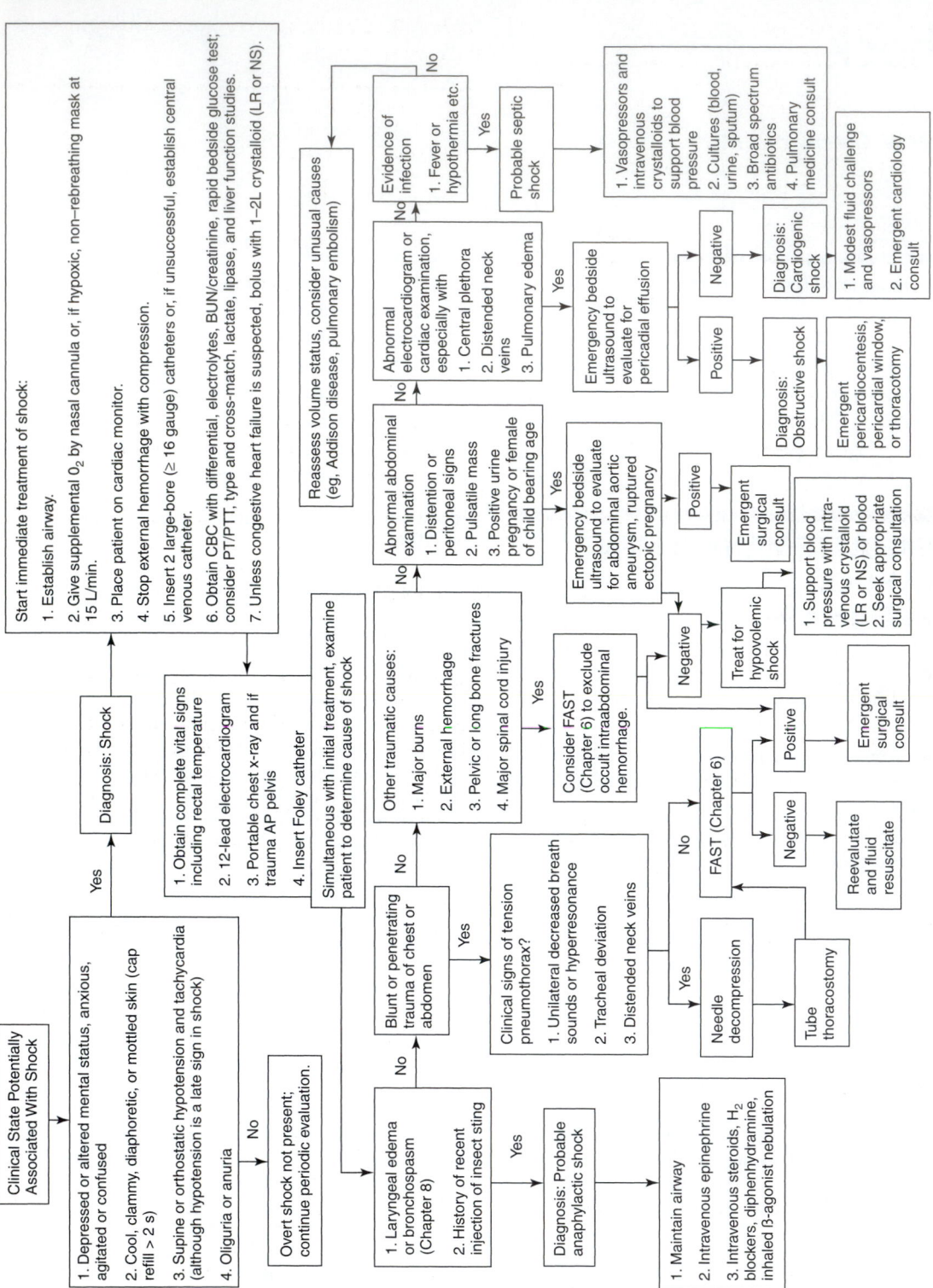

Figure 9–1. Management of a clinical state potentially associated with shock. BUN = blood urea nitrogen; FAST = focused assessment with sonography for trauma; LR = lactated Ringer's; NS = normal saline; PT = prothrombin time; PTT = partial thromboplastin time.

Table 9–1. Clinical classification of shock.[1]

	Pathophysiology	Clinical Manifestations
Mild (<20% of blood volume lost)	Decreased peripheral perfusion only of organs able to withstand prolonged ischemia (skin, fat, muscle, and bone). Arterial pH normal.	Patient complains of feeling cold. Postural hypotension and tachycardia. Cool, pale, moist skin; collapsed neck veins; concentrated urine.
Moderate (20–40% of blood lost)	Decreased central perfusion of organs able to tolerate only brief ischemia (liver, gut, kidneys). Metabolic acidosis present.	Thirst. Supine hypotension and tachycardia (variable). Oliguria or anuria.
Severe (>40% of blood volume lost)	Decreased perfusion of heart and brain. Metabolic acidosis is severe. Respiratory acidosis may also be present.	Agitation, confusion, or obtundation. Supine hypotension and tachycardia are invariably present. Rapid, deep respiration.

[1]These clinical findings are most consistently observed in hemorrhagic shock but apply to other types of shock as well.

In septic shock, the release of these mediators coincides with mitochondrial dysfunction leading to impaired oxygen utilization.

A similar impairment occurs later in the other forms of shock. As the shock state progresses, normal cellular ionic concentration gradients deteriorate due to inadequate energy production. Intracellular calcium concentrations increase, leading to further inability of mitochondria to produce adenosine triphosphate, and causing muscle to lose its ability to relax normally. Intracellular CO_2 and H^+ increase, and a generalized catabolic state, accompanied by decreased cell membrane function, leads to cellular edema by osmotic flow of water.

In shock from any cause, there comes a point at which restoration of adequate oxygenation will no longer restore tissue function and the evolution of multiple organ system dysfunction syndrome, and most likely death, will occur.

Classification of Shock

There are a variety of classification schemes for shock. Classically the causes of shock have been divided into four categories (Table 9–2).

Table 9–2. Classification of shock by mechanism and common causes.

Hypovolemic shock
  Loss of blood (hemorrhagic shock)
    External hemorrhage
      Trauma
    Internal hemorrhage
      Hematoma
      Hemothorax or hemoperitoneum
  Loss of plasma
    Burns
    Exfoliative dermatitis
  Loss of fluid and electrolytes
    External
      Vomiting
      Diarrhea
      Excessive sweating
      Hyperosmolar states (diabetic ketoacidosis, hyperosmolar nonketotic coma)
    Internal
      Pancreatitis
      Ascites
      Bowel obstruction
Cardiogenic shock
  Dysrhythmia
    Tachyarrhythmia
    Bradyarrhythmia
  "Pump failure" (secondary to myocaridal infarction or other cardiomyopathy)
  Acute valvular dysfunction (especially regurgitant lesions)
  Rupture of ventricular septum or free ventricular wall
Obstructive shock
  Tension pneumothorax
  Pericardial disease (tamponade, constriction)
  Disease of pulmonary vasculature (massive pulmonary emboli, pulmonary hypertension)
  Cardiac tumor (atrial myxoma)
  Left atrial mural thrombus
  Obstructive valvular disease (aortic or mitral stenosis)
Distributive shock
  Septic shock
  Anaphylactic shock
  Neurogenic shock
  Vasodilator drugs
  Acute adrenal insufficiency

A. Hypovolemic Shock

The chief abnormality in hypovolemic shock is decreased intravascular volume, which may occur as a result of loss of blood or plasma or of fluid and electrolytes. These losses may be exogenous (eg, gastrointestinal tract bleeding, diarrhea) or endogenous (eg, retroperitoneal hematomas or "third spacing" associated with bowel obstruction or pancreatitis).

B. CARDIOGENIC SHOCK

The chief abnormality in cardiogenic shock is abnormal cardiac function due to arrhythmia, "pump failure," myocardial depressant factors, or valvular dysfunction.

C. OBSTRUCTIVE SHOCK

The chief abnormality in obstructive shock is an impediment to filling of the right or left ventricle (decreased preload). If decreased filling is sufficiently severe, the resulting fall in cardiac output causes shock. Obstruction may occur in the systemic circulation (eg, obstruction of the vena cava) or pulmonary circulation (eg, massive pulmonary embolus) or may be due to pericardial disease (eg, cardiac tamponade) or cardiac disease (eg, atrial myxoma).

D. DISTRIBUTIVE SHOCK

The chief abnormality in distributive shock is abnormal distribution of vascular volume due to changes in vascular resistance or permeability. This can be thought of as an increase in the size of the vascular compartment. The end result is a decrease in ventricular filling that leads to inadequate cardiac output. The derangement of vascular volume characterizing distributive shock may occur as a result of sepsis, anaphylaxis, or neurogenic shock.

Physical Diagnosis of Shock

The first step in the diagnosis of shock is to suspect its presence. The most useful therapeutic interventions in shock may be those that take place in early compensated shock, when its presence may be difficult to determine.

A. SIGNS OF SHOCK

(See Table 9–1.)

1. Hypotension—Although hypotension is often mentioned first, it is a late sign of shock. Waiting for hypotension to develop before beginning treatment of shock is a potentially fatal error. Hypotension is a particularly late sign in children. In general, if a child's blood pressure is less than 2 times the child's age, plus 70, hypotension is present.

2. Tachycardia—An elevated heart rate may be one of the earliest signs that shock is present.

3. Adrenergic responses—The patient may be restless, agitated, or diaphoretic or may be cool in the extremities (due to peripheral vasoconstriction). The same mechanism may cause livedo reticularis (mottled skin) and capillary refill greater than 2 seconds.

4. Altered mental status—The patient in shock may demonstrate normal mental status but also may have restlessness, anxiety, agitation, confusion, lethargy, or more profound alterations in consciousness. These changes may be an early finding.

5. Orthostatic vital signs—The patient in early shock may evidence tachycardia or hypotension only in the standing position. If there are no contraindications to doing so, a set of vital signs taken 3 minutes after standing can be compared to a set previously taken lying down. An elevation in the heart rate, or a decrease in the blood pressure in a standing position, may indicate inadequate intravascular volume.

B. DETERMINATION OF SHOCK SEVERITY

1. Compensated shock—The body attempts to continue to perfuse vital organs as a shock state develops. Blood is preferentially shunted away from the skin, fat, skeletal muscle, and bone. As shock deepens, the liver and gut are deprived of oxygen, then the kidneys. Urine output is decreased. The body preserves blood flow to the most vital organs, the brain and heart, longest. As shock becomes severe, mental status deteriorates and arrhythmias and signs of cardiac ischemia may develop.

2. Decompensated shock—The byproducts of inadequate cellular energy metabolism eventually overwhelm the vasculature's ability to continue shunting blood to the vital organs. At this point, mental status is severely impaired, the patient is hypotensive, and the shock state is likely to lead to death even with aggressive supportive care.

Initial Treatment of Shock

There are common initial therapy points for shock of all types. These same points apply to very ill patients regardless of cause of disease. A cause of shock must be identified to provide more specific therapy. Obtain a brief history from the patient, family, friends, bystanders, police, or ambulance personnel. Use the examination to help provide clues to the cause (eg, circular erythema may indicate the prior use of "cupping" as a folk remedy to remove infectious illness).

The ABCs (and D)

A. AIRWAY

Open or maintain the airway. Is the patient speaking? If not, are sonorous respirations or stridor present, which might indicate an inadequate airway? Will suctioning or placement of a nasal airway improve the airway? If the patient tolerates an oropharyngeal airway (OPA), put it in place. A patient who tolerates an OPA has an inadequate gag reflex and will need to be intubated. Ventilate and intubate the patient if respiratory status is inadequate. For airway protection, intubate all trauma patients who have severely impaired mental status (use a Glasgow Coma Scale score of 8 or less as a guide). Avoid nasotracheal intubation if head trauma is present.

B. BREATHING

Provide supplemental oxygen at 10–15 L/min via a non-rebreathing mask. Respirations of less than 12 or greater than 30 are unlikely to be sufficient. Pulse oximetry and arterial blood gas measurements may aid in the diagnosis of respiratory insufficiency when it is not clinically apparent. Sources of respiratory insufficiency, such as pneumothorax and loss of integrity of the chest wall (flail chest), should be sought and corrected.

C. CIRCULATION

Stop obvious external hemorrhage. Obtain vascular access. Use large-bore peripheral catheters if hypovolemic shock is suspected. Administer fluids as is appropriate for the type of shock. Obtain an electrocardiogram (ECG) early if a cardiac cause is within the differential diagnosis. Patients with suspected shock should be on a cardiac monitor. If trauma is present, or if the patient is at risk for pericardial effusions (ie, history of renal failure, cancer, or pericarditis), consider bedside emergency department ultrasonography to rapidly identify correctable causes of shock such as pericardial tamponade or hemoperitoneum. Obtain a complete blood count (CBC), electrolytes, and renal function tests; and if trauma is present or hemorrhagic shock suspected, type and crossmatch blood. Cultures of blood, urine, and possibly sputum should be obtained (prior to the administration of antibiotics) if septic shock is a possibility. Foley catheter insertion is necessary to monitor urine output and response to fluid therapy in hypovolemic shock.

D. DISABILITY

If trauma is present, the above steps should take place with protection of the cervical spine using a rigid collar and long spine board. Test and document the patient's Glasgow Coma Scale response. Evaluate distal motor and sensory function. Assess pupils for evidence of cerebral herniation. Rapidly check the fingerstick blood glucose and administer thiamine and naloxone if the patient has an altered mental status.

Fink MP: Cytopathic hypoxia. Mitochondrial dysfunction as a mechanism contributing to organ dysfunction in sepsis. Crit Care Clin 2001;17(1):219. [PMID: 11219231] (A discussion of the metabolic deficits that develop with sepsis and their implications for sepsis therapy.)

■ DETERMINATION OF THE CAUSE OF SHOCK

Perform a rapid assessment of the most likely cause of shock in order to provide more specific and definitive therapy. Obtain a brief history from the patient, family, friends, bystanders, police, or ambulance attendants. Pay careful attention to clues available from the physical examination (eg, obvious trauma, melena, fever, or diarrhea).

APPROACH TO SHOCK WITH A HISTORY OF TRAUMA
(See also Chapter 10.)

Is There Obvious External Blood Loss or Penetrating Injury?

Turn the patient to examine his or her back (logroll the patient to maintain axial immobilization if cervical spine injury is suspected).

Has There Been Chest Trauma?

Chest trauma may be due to obvious penetrating injury or to blunt trauma causing hemothorax, tension pneumothorax, cardiac tamponade or rupture, or myocardial contusion. Carefully examine the patient for distended neck veins, indicating pericardial tamponade or tension pneumothorax. Tracheal deviation and unilaterally absent breath sounds are commonly noted when a tension pneumothorax is present. When tension pneumothorax is clinically suspected, needle decompression (Chapter 6) can be life saving and should not be delayed while waiting for chest x-ray confirmation. Bedside emergency department sonography enables the emergency physician to quickly assess for the presence of hemodynamically significant hemothorax or pericardial effusion.

Has There Been Abdominal Trauma?

Intra-abdominal or retroperitoneal bleeding may result from visceral or vascular injuries. **Note:** Intra-abdominal or retroperitoneal bleeding must be assumed to be present in any injured patient with severe shock, a normal chest x-ray, and no signs of significant external bleeding. Focused Assessment with Sonography for Trauma (FAST) exams (Chapter 6) can rapidly identify hemoperitoneum. In hemodynamically unstable patients with intra-abdominal free fluid, early exploratory laparotomy is required to reverse hemorrhagic shock. If emergency department sonography is not immediately available or if the results are equivocal, diagnostic peritoneal lavage should be performed to determine the patient's need for immediate laparotomy. In a more stable patient, abdominal computed tomography (CT) scan may be useful for diagnosing intra-abdominal bleeding.

Has There Been Deceleration Injury?

Deceleration injury may be associated with lacerations of the aorta, especially in the region of the isthmus. A widened mediastinum may be visible on chest x-ray, but high-resolution contrast CT, transesophageal echocardiography, or aortic angiography is required for definitive diagnosis.

Have There Been Pelvic or Thigh Injuries?

Injuries to the pelvis or thigh may be associated with a large volume of concealed blood loss. Significant pelvic injuries are suspected when anteroposterior or lateral compression of the iliac wings indicates an unstable pelvis. If pelvic instability is apparent on the primary survey, repeated testing by other physicians could exacerbate ongoing pelvic hemorrhage and should be discouraged. A portable anteroposterior radiograph of the pelvis may demonstrate pubic symphysis diastasis and widening of the sacroiliac joints. MAST trousers may be used to close the volume and stabilize the pelvis in an attempt to limit intrapelvic hemorrhage. Alternatively, a bed sheet can be tightly wrapped around the pelvis and tied in a knot to stabilize the pelvis.

Is There Evidence of Significant Spinal Cord Injury?

Neurogenic shock may occur after traumatic quadriplegia or paraplegia. However, severe shock with the patient in the supine position is usually due to other concomitant causes of shock, such as blood loss. Do not confuse neurogenic shock with spinal shock. Spinal shock is a transient dysfunction of the spinal cord associated with traumatic injury. Neurogenic shock refers to the loss of vasomotor tone leading to diffuse vasodilation and hypotension.

Did a Preexisting Medical Condition Cause Trauma?

An example of a preexisting condition that results in trauma is an acute myocardial infarction that causes a motor vehicle accident.

APPROACH TO SHOCK WITHOUT HISTORY OF TRAUMA

Is This Hemorrhagic Shock?

Blood loss may be difficult to recognize if there is preexisting anemia or if not enough time has elapsed for compensatory mechanisms to cause hemodilution. Serial hematocrit measurements are needed to rule out hemorrhagic causes of shock. Do not be reassured by the initial hematocrit being normal.

A. Seek Evidence of Gastrointestinal Tract Blood Loss

(See Chapter 14.) Ask about prior hematemesis, melena, or abdominal pain. Perform a test for occult blood on a sample of feces, and insert a nasogastric tube to search for blood loss in the gastrointestinal tract.

B. Seek Evidence of Aortic Dissection or Ruptured Abdominal Aortic Aneurysm

(See Chapter 32.) The sudden onset of severe back or abdominal pain in a patient with a history of hypertension should suggest contained aortic dissection. Hematuria, neurologic deficit, or diminished peripheral pulses may be present. Abdominal pain with a palpable abdominal mass or abdominal tenderness and distention suggests rupture of an abdominal aortic aneurysm. *Note:* Severe hemorrhagic shock in a patient without an obvious source of blood loss should be considered to be caused by a ruptured abdominal aortic aneurysm, and exploratory laparotomy should be performed immediately. Patients with aneurysms that have been repaired with aortoiliac grafts may occasionally present with massive gastrointestinal tract bleeding resulting from rupture at the suture site into the colon or duodenum.

C. Seek Evidence of Ectopic Pregnancy

Consider ruptured ectopic pregnancy in a woman of childbearing age who presents in shock, especially if there is a history of pelvic pain, vaginal bleeding, or amenorrhea. An emergency bedside ultrasound of the right upper quadrant demonstrating free fluid in the hepatorenal (Morrison) space is frequently seen in patients in shock who have ruptured ectopic pregnancies. Transvaginal ultrasound yielding no intrauterine pregnancy when the serum human chorionic gonadotropin (hCG) level is greater than 1600, or at greater than 4 weeks' gestation based on dates, should be assumed to indicate ectopic pregnancy in the setting of shock. Shock may be caused by ectopic pregnancy even when the quantified hCG is very low. Culdocentesis, blind aspiration of the rectouterine pouch, has largely been replaced by sonography. However, culdocentesis should be performed if pelvic sonography is not immediately available in the evaluation of a pregnant patient presenting in shock.

Is This Nonhemorrhagic Hypovolemic Shock?

Fluid or fluid and electrolyte loss may be the cause of hypovolemic shock in a patient with no evidence of external hemorrhage in whom serial hematocrit measurements remain stable (Table 9–2).

Is There a Cardiac Cause of Shock?

Cardiac causes of shock include arrhythmias, acute valvular dysfunction, rupture of the ventricular septum or free ventricular wall, or "pump failure" (cardiogenic shock). Pump failure can be caused by vascular obstruction, tamponade, or muscular dysfunction secondary to myocardial depressant factors. Ask about a history of hypertension, chest pain, or cardiac disease. Perform a careful physical examination, and pay special attention to the presence of distended neck veins, rales, and abnormal cardiac sounds (S_3 gallop, murmurs, rubs). An ECG may show arrhythmias or ischemic changes such as ST segment abnormalities.

Is There Evidence of Pericardial Disease?

Cardiac tamponade may occur in the patient with aortic dissection, pericarditis, uremia, or recent myocardial infarction. Occasionally patients with constrictive pericarditis present in shock. Assess the patient for pulsus paradoxus, Kussmaul sign, or distended neck veins without evidence of pump failure (clear lung fields on chest x-ray, no S_3 gallop). With bedside sonography in the emergency department, the clinician can rapidly detect significant pericardial effusions. Ultrasound can also be used to percutaneously drain pericardial effusions. If ultrasound or echocardiography is not immediately available, blind pericardiocentesis (Chapter 6) may be a life-saving procedure in patients with pericardial tamponade. If the patient is stable, obtain an echocardiogram to confirm the presence of pericardial fluid and to assist in pericardiocentesis.

Is There Evidence of Sepsis?

Fever or hypothermia, rigors, leukocytosis, or petechiae suggest septic shock. Infants, the elderly, and immunocompromised or severely leukopenic patients may lack symptoms that localize the site of infection. Consider the possibility of toxic shock syndrome in young women, especially if there is a history of tampon use or recent menses.

Does the History Suggest Anaphylactic Shock?

A history of a bee or wasp sting, recent administration of drugs, or ingestion of certain foodstuffs should raise a suspicion of anaphylactic shock. Urticaria, laryngeal edema, and bronchospasm often (but not invariably) accompany anaphylaxis. Because most cases of anaphylaxis are due to parenteral administration of medications and occur within minutes of exposure to the inciting agent, the diagnosis usually is readily apparent.

Is This Obstructive Shock?

Tension pneumothorax, an obstructive cause of shock, should be considered in a setting of chest or upper abdominal trauma when diminished breath sounds are present unilaterally with tracheal deviation. Other causes of obstructive shock, resulting from obstruction to filling of the right or left ventricle, are difficult to diagnose rapidly in the emergency department. Obstructive shock may be due to such diverse conditions as massive pulmonary embolus, mural thrombus, or atrial myxoma. (Although diseases of the pericardium such as tamponade and constriction are also obstructive disorders, symptoms and signs often permit early specific diagnosis.) Pulmonary embolus should be suspected in the patient who presents in shock with signs of right heart failure (distended neck veins, right-sided S_3 gallop), refractory hypoxemia (especially if there is evidence of decreased pulmonary compliance as manifested by difficulty in ventilating the patient with a bag-valve-mask), and an ECG that shows evidence of right heart strain (large R wave in lead V1, right axis deviation, or incomplete right bundle branch block or the classic S in lead I, Q in lead III, and T wave inversion in lead III.).

Are There Other Causes of Shock?

Unusual and infrequently encountered causes of shock include pheochromocytoma, addisonian crisis, and severe hypothyroidism (Chapter 41). Drug or toxins may also produce shock through a variety of mechanisms, including vasodilatation (eg, phenothiazines) and direct cardiac effects (eg, tricyclic antidepressants).

■ EMERGENCY TREATMENT OF SPECIFIC CAUSES OF SHOCK

HYPOVOLEMIC SHOCK

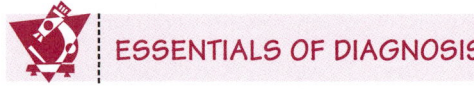 ESSENTIALS OF DIAGNOSIS

- *Shock in the setting of massive blood, fluid, or electrolyte losses (eg, from burns, vomiting and diarrhea, trauma, internal hemorrhage).*

General Considerations

Hypovolemic shock may result from loss of whole blood, plasma, or fluid and electrolytes (Table 9–2). In many patients with hypovolemic shock who are seen in the emergency department, the cause of shock will be immediately apparent (eg, obvious bleeding or history of severe diarrhea). Common causes that may not be readily apparent include ruptured abdominal aortic aneurysm, aortic dissection, splenic rupture (which may occur after seemingly inconsequential trauma), intestinal obstruction, and peritonitis.

Clinical Findings

The clinical features of shock are present. In addition, there may be signs suggesting hypovolemia as the cause, for example, obvious hemorrhage or clinical features associated with volume loss due to burns, peritonitis, bowel obstruction, or ruptured abdominal aneurysm. Central venous pressure is low, and both venous and arterial pressures improve rapidly with intravascular volume replacement.

Treatment

Perform the ABCDs as previously noted.

A. Gain Intravascular Access

The number of intravenous cannulas required depends on the severity of shock. For adults, catheters inserted should be 16 gauge or larger. During insertion of the intravenous line, blood should be obtained for CBC, electrolytes, blood urea nitrogen and creatinine, and prothrombin time. If hemorrhage is suspected, blood should be sent for blood typing and cross-matching. Arterial blood gas and lactate measurement may help in determining the severity of hypoperfusion and acidosis. Two large-bore (16-gauge or larger) peripheral catheters are sufficient for initial management. If peripheral access cannot be obtained, central access or venous cutdown might be considered.

1. Long saphenous vein—The safest site for a venous cutdown is the long saphenous vein at the ankle (Chapter 6). If shock is not severe and the vein is not collapsed, insert a 16-gauge percutaneous catheter.

2. Basilic vein—The basilic vein in the antecubital fossa is also a good site for a large-gauge percutaneous catheter or venous cutdown. It can be used to achieve central venous pressure monitoring (Chapter 6).

3. Femoral vein—A temporary percutaneous catheter inserted in the femoral vein may permit rapid access to the circulation without major complications (Chapter 6).

4. Central veins—Avoid percutaneous catheterization of the subclavian or jugular veins for treatment of hy-

povolemic shock, because the great veins are usually collapsed, and the chances of complications such as hemothorax and pneumothorax are greatly increased. (For a patient in hypovolemic shock, the additional physiologic insult of hemothorax or tension pneumothorax may be rapidly fatal.)

5. Intraosseous infusion—In infants and young children, rapid access for fluid administration can be gained through intraosseous infusion (Chapter 6).

B. Administer Intravenous Fluids

Administer intravenous fluids at once to restore adequate intravascular volume. The goal is normal cardiac output and tissue perfusion.

1. Types of fluids—Table 9–3 lists various solutions used in resuscitation of patients in shock. These solutions may be divided into 2 main types: crystalloids and colloids.

    a. Crystalloids—Crystalloid solutions include isotonic (0.9%, or normal) saline and balanced salt solutions (eg, lactated Ringer's injection, Plasma-Lyte, Isolyte). Balanced salt solutions contain varying amounts of acetate or lactate (or both) that are metabolized to bicarbonate when perfusion of the liver is adequate. Crystalloids are readily available and relatively inexpensive.

    Hypertonic sodium chloride (7.5%) has been employed experimentally for hypovolemic shock due to hemorrhage (some preparations also include 6% dextran). These fluids osmotically draw water from extravascular spaces and can quickly expand blood volume. However, their safety has not yet been established, and there is growing concern over the value of rapidly expanding intravascular volume before hemorrhage is controlled sur-

Table 9–3. Fluids used for resuscitation of the patient in shock.

Crystalloids
Isotonic sodium chloride (normal saline)
Hypertonic sodium chloride
Balanced salt solutions
Lactated Ringer's injection
Acetated Ringer's injection
Normosol, Plasma-Lyte, etc
Colloids
Blood
Low-titer O-negative (universal donor)
Type-specific
Typed and cross-matched
Washed red cells
Fresh warm blood

gically. Otherwise, hemorrhage may actually increase, accompanied by progressive hemodilution.

b. Colloids—It has been advocated that colloid (high molecular weight) solutions draw water into the pulmonary vascular space and therefore out of the interstitium. This is most likely false. There is no proven benefit to using colloids over crystalloid in the setting of shock.

c. Blood—Blood is most commonly available as packed red blood cells or whole blood. In patients in mild hemorrhagic shock, especially if blood pressure can be maintained with asanguineous fluids, typed and cross-matched packed red blood cells are preferred. Because it may take 45 minutes or longer to type and cross-match blood, patients with moderate to severe hemorrhagic shock may require type-specific, Rh-negative blood or universal donor blood (O-negative blood with low antibody titers to erythrocyte antigens) if shock persists after administration of more than 2–3 L of crystalloid solutions in adults or 20–40 mL/kg in children. Whole blood should be used as soon as possible in patients with moderate to severe hemorrhagic shock. Because hypothermia is a frequent side effect of transfusion of large amounts of blood stored at 4°C, blood should be administered through blood warmers. Critically ill patients with hematocrit less than 30% benefit from the administration of blood.

(1) Plasma or albumin solutions—Plasma or albumin solutions are effective volume expanders; however, they may be harmful if they enter the pulmonary interstitium as a result of capillary leakage.

(2) Plasma substitutes—Plasma substitutes such as dextrans have been used for initial volume replacement in hypovolemic shock, but their use is not widely accepted.

2. Choice of fluids—The choice of fluid for resuscitation depends on the type of hypovolemic shock present (hemorrhagic versus nonhemorrhagic) and on the severity of shock.

a. Mild shock—Normal saline, lactated or acetated Ringer's injection, and plasma or other blood products are equally effective in treating mild shock. Crystalloid solutions are strongly preferred because of their low cost, lack of adverse effects, and ready availability.

b. Moderate to severe shock—There has been considerable controversy regarding the correct fluid to use in patients in moderate to severe shock. Current accepted therapy is to use crystalloids as a first-line agent. Blood should be used if bleeding is extensive or ongoing. With low hematocrit and controlled bleeding, there is some debate about what constitutes an appropriate transfusion threshold. It would be prudent to

transfuse if the hematocrit is less than 30%. Assume that 3 L of crystalloid are required to achieve the same intravascular volume expansion as 1 L of blood.

E. EVALUATE THE EFFECTIVENESS OF RESUSCITATION

1. Monitor indices of resuscitation (Table 9–4)—Indicators of successful resuscitation include improved blood pressure and urine output, diminished tachycardia, improved mental status, falling lactate, and normalizing pH. Additional guidelines include improved state of consciousness and peripheral perfusion (as measured by clinical criteria, including arterial blood pH). In an intensive care setting, measurements of cardiac output are also useful.

a. Atrial filling pressure—The only estimate of atrial filling pressure available in most emergency departments is the central venous (right atrial) pressure. New, noninvasive measures of cardiac output, such as thoracic bioimpedance or real-time transnasal esophageal echocardiography, may prove useful in emergency department resuscitation management. Central venous O_2 saturation is being used by some groups as a measurement to approximate cardiac output in order to help guide emergency department fluid and pressor therapy without necessitating a pulmonary artery catheter. It is generally a good measure of intravascular volume but may be unreliable in patients with cardiac or pulmonary disease or in those who require mechanical ventilatory support. Such patients require measurement of pulmonary capillary wedge pressure.

Normal central venous pressure is 3–8 cm H_2O. As a general rule of thumb, maintaining central venous pressure at 8–12 cm H_2O when managing shock is prudent. A growing body of literature suggests that supranormal values of cardiac indices may reduce mortality in perioperative patients. This also may be true early in septic shock.

b. Urine output—Urine output is a good index of visceral blood flow (specifically, renal blood flow)

Table 9–4. Indices of successful resuscitation.

Improved blood pressure
Diminished tachycardia
Falling lactate
Normalizing pH
Increasing central venous O_2 saturation
Urine output > 0.5 mL/kg/h or improving (in children, > 1 mL/kg/h; in infants, > 2 mL/kg/h)
Level of consciousness improving
Peripheral perfusion improving
Cardiac output increasing (normal ≥ 3.5 L/min in adults)

and should be maintained at more than 0.5 mL/kg/h in adults, 1 mL/kg/h in children, and more than 2 mL/kg/h in infants. This measurement is unreliable in patients with preexisting serious renal damage or when renal damage has occurred as a result of prolonged shock (eg, acute tubular necrosis).

2. Record progress of resuscitation—Documentation, preferably entered on an emergency department critical care flow sheet, is essential both for emergency department management and for later management once the patient has been transferred to an intensive care unit or operating room. The following information should be systematically recorded:

a. Vital signs—Record blood pressure, pulse, and respiration rate every 5–15 minutes.

b. Fluids—Note the quantity and type of fluid administered.

c. Central venous pressure—If central venous access has been obtained, measure and record central venous pressure every 30–60 minutes or as dictated by the progress of resuscitation.

d. Urine output—Measure and record urine output every 30–60 minutes (use an indwelling catheter).

e. Other factors—Obtain and record serial hematocrits, arterial blood gas determinations, electrolyte measurements, and renal function tests as indicated.

F. AGGRESSIVELY SEARCH FOR THE CAUSE OF PERSISTENT SHOCK

Persistent shock or recurrence of shock in a patient who initially responded to treatment suggests ongoing, often occult hemorrhage. Obtain serial hematocrit measurements, give blood, and search for hidden sources of blood loss. Patients with severe, refractory shock may require immediate surgery (eg, left thoracotomy to cross-clamp the aorta, exploratory laparotomy). Possible sources of blood loss include the following:

1. Thorax—Each hemithorax may contain up to 2 L of blood; therefore, a quick upright or lateral decubitus chest x-ray should always be obtained before surgery is considered.

2. Abdomen—Hidden blood loss in the abdomen is common. Distention is a late and unreliable sign. Intra-abdominal hemorrhage must be assumed to be present in any patient in shock who has a normal chest x-ray and no external signs of significant bleeding. Bedside sonogram of the abdomen has become the preferred imaging modality to detect intra-abdominal free fluid, which can be assumed to be blood in the presence of trauma-induced shock. In an unstable patient, free fluid is an indication for emergent exploratory laparotomy. Diagnostic peritoneal lavage (Chapter 6) may be helpful

if gross blood is found or if a hematocrit of 2% or more is noted on the lavage sample. Absence of these signs does not exclude the possibility of intra-abdominal bleeding. A CT scan may demonstrate intraperitoneal fluid and help identify injury to specific solid organs. Its use should be restricted to patients who are relatively stable and for whom it can be obtained rapidly.

3. Retroperitoneum—Bleeding in the retroperitoneum cannot be diagnosed with routine studies. A CT scan is a helpful diagnostic tool, if the patient's condition is stable enough to permit this delay.

4. Pelvis—The pelvis may conceal a large amount of blood; hemorrhagic shock is a common sequela of pelvic fracture.

5. Thigh—The thigh may contain 3–4 L of blood after a major fracture or crush injury.

Disposition

All patients in hypovolemic shock must be hospitalized.

Felbinger TW, Suchner U, Goetz AE: Treating patients with severe sepsis. N Engl J Med 1999;341(1):56. [PMID: 10391763] (A current review of sepsis care.)

Hebert PC: Transfusion requirements in critical care (TRICC): a multicentre, randomized, controlled clinical study. Transfusion Requirements in Critical Care Investigators and the Canadian Critical Care Trials Group. Br J Anaesth 1998;81(Suppl 1):25. [PMID: 10318985] (A prospective randomized trial of transfusion in critically ill patients that shows lower mortality rates during hospitalization in a group randomized to a restrictive transfusion threshold.)

Kohli-Seth R, Oropello JM: The future of bedside monitoring. Crit Care Clin 2000;16(4):557. [PMID: 11070805] (A discussion of technology under development that may expand the information available to the bedside physician.)

Wu WC et al: Blood transfusion in elderly patients with acute myocardial infarction. N Engl J Med 2001;345(17):1230. [PMID: 11680442] (A retrospective observational study of 79,000 patients with myocardial infarction, demonstrating much higher mortality rates in patients with lower hematocrit.)

CARDIOGENIC SHOCK

 ESSENTIALS OF DIAGNOSIS

- *Shock in the setting of cardiac outflow obstruction (eg, hypertrophic subaortic stenosis) or pump failure (eg, massive myocardial infarction, severe myocardial disease, arrhythmia).*

General Considerations

Broadly defined, the term *cardiogenic shock* denotes a shock syndrome resulting from some abnormal cardiac function, such as arrhythmias, valvular disease, or pericardial disease (eg, cardiac tamponade), as well as shock resulting from severe myocardial dysfunction (pump failure). This section considers mainly pump failure. Shock due to pericardial disease or cardiac tumors is discussed in the "Obstructive Shock" section, below. Further discussion of the diagnosis and treatment of arrhythmias, valvular disease, and pericardial disease is found in Chapters 34 and 35.

Cardiogenic shock due to pump failure is often associated with acute myocardial infarction but may also result from end-stage cardiac disease of any cause, including valvular heart disease or cardiomyopathy. Cardiogenic shock is a complication of acute myocardial infarction in about 10% of patients and carries a grave prognosis (mortality rate > 50%) even with appropriate therapy. Potentially correctable myocardial— and nonmyocardial—factors may contribute to, or be the sole cause of, shock in a patient with myocardial infarction (Table 9–5). These factors must be sought and treated vigorously.

Clinical Findings

A. Symptoms and Signs

The hallmark of cardiogenic shock is hypotension (systolic blood pressure usually < 90 mm Hg, although it may be higher accompanied by clinical signs of increased peripheral vascular resistance (weak, thready pulse; cool, clammy skin) and inadequate organ perfusion (altered mental status, decreased urine output). The patient also shows signs of acute myocardial infarction or preexisting severe cardiac disease.

Table 9–5. Potential correctable causes of cardiogenic shock.

Cardiac
Mitral regurgitation from papillary muscle dysfunction or rupture; rupture of chordae tendineae
Acute aortic regurgitation
Rupture of interventricular septum
Ventricular aneurysm
Rupture of free ventricular wall
Severe valvular or infravalvular stenosis
Arrhythmias
Pericardial
Cardiac tamponade
Pericardial constriction

1. Early signs—Tachycardia and decreased pulse pressure (due to elevated systemic vascular resistance) are early signs of decreased cardiac output and should alert the physician to potential problems even if systolic blood pressure is normal. Diaphoresis or other signs of an increase in circulating catecholamines may be present. Restlessness, agitation, or confusion is an early manifestation of decreased cerebral blood flow.

2. Central venous pressure—Central venous pressure (assessed by examination of the patient's neck veins) varies in cardiogenic shock depending on intravascular volume and the degree of associated right ventricular failure. Central venous pressure is not a reliable means of diagnosing severe left ventricular failure.

B. Imaging Studies

Transthoracic echocardiography (TTE) can be a useful diagnostic modality, allowing visualization of hypodynamic myocardium. Determination of dilated right ventricle with TTE may point to a diagnosis of pulmonary embolus. TTE can also elucidate valve dysfunction.

Treatment

Initial treatment of cardiogenic shock should be started in the emergency department, definitive therapy often requires hemodynamic monitoring using pulmonary and other systemic pressure catheters.

An intra-aortic balloon pump may provide stabilization for patients in profound cardiogenic shock. If cardiogenic shock is from an acute coronary occlusion, reperfusion by percutaneous transluminal coronary angioplasty may improve survival, although overall mortality still remains high. Reperfusion by fibrinolytic therapy has not been shown to be beneficial in cardiogenic shock.

A. Airway

Using arterial blood gas measurements as guidelines, establish adequate ventilation and oxygenation. Give supplemental oxygen, 2–5 L/min, by nasal cannula, pending the results of blood gas determinations; adjust oxygen supplementation to maintain arterial P_{O_2} at 65 mm Hg or higher. Pulse oximetry may also be used to maintain oxygen saturation ($\geq$ 90%). If hypercapnia and acidosis are present, tracheal intubation may be necessary (Chapter 6).

B. Position

Place the patient supine or supine with the legs elevated if systolic blood pressure is less than 70–80 mm Hg. Conversely, a patient with pulmonary edema and a normal or low normal blood pressure should be seated upright.

C. INTRAVENOUS ACCESS

If hypotension is profound (systolic blood pressure < 70 mm Hg) and there is no evidence of pulmonary edema, gain intravenous access and infuse a crystalloid solution (normal saline or lactated Ringer's injection).

D. BLOOD WORK

Draw a sample of venous blood for CBC, electrolyte measurements, renal function test, cardiac enzymes (assays may include CK, CK-MB isoenzymes, troponin, and myoglobin). Coagulation studies (prothrombin and partial thromboplastin times and platelet count) are essential if invasive monitoring or placement of a central venous catheter is anticipated.

E. CARDIAC MONITORING

Obtain a 12-lead ECG, and begin continuous cardiac monitoring.

F. URINE OUTPUT

Monitor urine output hourly. Bladder catheterization may be necessary.

G. NONMYOCARDIAL FACTORS

Search for and treat nonmyocardial factors that may be causing or contributing to shock.

1. Acidosis—(See Chapter 42.) Respiratory acidosis (low arterial blood pH, high P_{CO_2}) in cardiogenic shock is due to hypoperfusion, with production of lactic acid. In addition to measures to improve cardiac output, sodium bicarbonate may be given if the blood pH is less than 7.1 and the acidosis is metabolic. Give 0.5–1.0 mEq/kg over 5–10 minutes, and repeat as needed, using arterial blood gas determinations as a guideline. *Caution:* Do not administer sodium bicarbonate through the same intravenous line as catecholamines.

2. Arrhythmias—(See Chapter 35.) Cardioversion is the treatment of choice for tachyarrhythmias causing hypotension. Initial treatment for bradyarrhythmias causing hypotension is atropine, 0.5 mg intravenously every 5 minutes up to a total dose of 2 mg for adults; in children, give 0.02 mg/kg, with a minimum single dose of 0.1 mg and a maximum total dose of 1 mg. A transcutaneous pacemaker should be put in place only until transvenous pacing becomes available. If the patient has responded to atropine, then the transcutaneous pacer should be left on the patient, in the "off" mode, so that it is readily available should the bradycardia reoccur or worsen.

3. Hypovolemia—In the patient with acute myocardial infarction, recent use of diuretics, excessive sweating, vomiting, or diarrhea may cause hypovolemia. In the patient without supine hypotension, measurement of orthostatic vital signs may provide a valuable clue to possible depletion of intravascular volume. Cautious administration of intravenous fluid should be attempted in patients who have no evidence of pulmonary edema. Give intravenous fluids in 50- to 100-mL increments over 5–10 minutes, and watch closely for signs of improvement (decreased heart rate, increased blood pressure) or deterioration (increased dyspnea or decreased arterial P_{O_2}).

4. Tamponade—Rupture of the free ventricular wall or pericarditis with effusion may result in cardiac tamponade and may be confused with cardiogenic shock of myocardial origin. Perform a careful physical examination, and look for evidence of cardiac tamponade (elevated neck veins with clear lung fields on chest x-ray, pulsus paradoxus, pericardial friction rub, low voltage on the ECG). As mentioned previously, bedside sonography in the emergency department can be used, if available, to rapidly identify and drain pericardial effusions causing tamponade. If ultrasound is not available, emergent blind pericardiocentesis may be life saving.

5. Acute valvular disease or ventricular septal rupture—Listen carefully for characteristic murmurs. Definitive diagnosis may require cardiac catheterization or echocardiography. Treatment with intra-aortic balloon pumping or drugs that reduce afterload may gain time to prepare the patient for life-saving surgery (Chapter 34).

H. PHARMACOLOGIC THERAPY

If the patient fails to respond to intravenous fluids, give dopamine, 200 mg in 250 mL of 5% dextrose in water (800 µg/mL) at the lowest rate that maintains adequate blood pressure (usually 4–15 µg/kg/min).

Dobutamine may be the mainstay for therapy of cardiogenic shock. This is especially true if left-sided congestive heart failure with low blood pressure is present. Dobutamine can increase cardiac contraction (positive inotropy) without raising afterload. This results in improved cardiac output. Because dobutamine has minimal α-receptor activity, it has little effect on the systemic blood pressure, making dopamine, not dobutamine, the inotropic agent of choice in profound hypotension. Norepinephrine can be considered as a second-line agent after dopamine. It will raise the blood pressure but will also cause increased infarct size and must be delivered via a central line.

Stabilization in the emergency department may require maintaining blood pressure by means of such vasoconstriction while the patient is awaiting transfer to the intensive care unit.

Digitalis glycosides have no role in the initial treatment of cardiogenic shock.

I. Intensive Care Unit

Assess the need for urgent transfer of the patient to an intensive care unit. A patient with frank pulmonary edema and hypotension is difficult to manage in the emergency department, and every effort should be made to transfer the patient as rapidly as possible to an intensive care unit for hemodynamic monitoring and drug therapy.

J. Treatment for Pulmonary Edema

If the patient's blood pressure is only slightly decreased and the major clinical findings suggest pulmonary edema (elevated neck veins, rales, and decreased oxygenation) rather than decreased tissue perfusion (hypotension, clammy skin, and the like), small doses of intravenous furosemide (adults, 20–40 mg; children, 0.5–1.0 mg/kg) or a preload reducing agent (nitroglycerin ointment, 1.5–2.0 cm under an occlusive dressing) may be tried. Pay close attention to the effect of these drugs on blood pressure and clinical signs of tissue perfusion.

Disposition

All patients in cardiogenic shock should be hospitalized in an intensive care unit.

OBSTRUCTIVE SHOCK

Obstructive shock results from impaired filling of the ventricles (decreased preload) that is severe enough to cause a significant fall in cardiac output (Table 9–2). With the exception of acute cardiac tamponade and tension pneumothorax, obstructive disorders are difficult to diagnose and even more difficult to treat in the emergency department. Knowledge of the patient's medical history can be crucial in management. Clues to the specific cause of shock are discussed below.

1. Cardiac Tamponade
(See also Chapter 34.)

A history of cancer, uremia, or infectious illness should suggest the possibility of pericardial effusion; distended neck veins without evidence of pump failure (clear lung fields on chest x-ray, absent S_3 gallop) suggest cardiac tamponade. Pulsus paradoxus, a fall in systolic blood pressure of 12 mm Hg or more during inspiration, occurs in almost every case of cardiac tamponade. A peri-

cardial friction rub may or may not be present. Distant heart sounds, an enlarged cardiac silhouette on chest x-ray, and low voltage on the ECG are additional (but insensitive) clues to the presence of pericardial effusion. Sudden onset of shock in a patient with recent myocardial infarction may be due to rupture of the free ventricular wall that causes cardiac tamponade. Bedside emergency ultrasound plays an important role in rapid identification and treatment of pericardial effusions causing cardiac tamponade. If ultrasound is unavailable, blind pericardiocentesis is required for suspected tamponade and may be a life-saving intervention. If the patient's condition permits, obtain an echocardiogram to confirm the diagnosis and to guide pericardiocentesis. In the desperately ill patient, blind pericardiocentesis (Chapter 6) may be life-saving. See Chapters 10 and 34 for a more complete discussion of the diagnosis and treatment of cardiac tamponade.

2. Massive Pulmonary Embolism
(See also Chapter 33.)

Ask about a history of thrombophlebitis, pulmonary emboli, or hypercoagulable state (use of oral contraceptives, pregnancy status, family history of thromboembolic disease, cancer). Search for evidence of lower extremity venous thrombosis or for some other predisposing factor (lower extremity injury, recent prolonged immobility). Pleuritic chest pain, dyspnea, apprehension, or cough occurs frequently in patients with massive pulmonary embolism; hemoptysis or syncope occurs less commonly. Accentuation of the pulmonary closure sound (P_2) may occur. Massive pulmonary embolism with acute pulmonary hypertension may result in signs of right ventricular overload, for example, jugular venous distention and a right-sided S_3 gallop. The ECG may show evidence of acute right heart strain, for example, R > S in lead V1, S1Q3T3 pattern (large S wave in lead I, Q wave in lead III, inverted T wave in lead III). Patients with massive pulmonary embolism typically are hypoxemic. Pulse oximetry does not improve much with the administration of O_2 (a pulmonary embolism acts physiologically like an atrioventricular shunt). Attempt to maintain blood pressure with intravenous fluids (an initial bolus of 500–1000 mL of normal saline should be infused rapidly); if the patient fails to respond, give vasopressors as described above. Administration of thrombolytic agents such as streptokinase or tissue plasminogen activator is indicated for massive pulmonary embolization. Current indications include shock, recent cardiac arrest, and severe respiratory failure; however, the prognosis in patients with massive pulmonary embolism is poor. See Chapter 33 for further discussion. Emergency surgery (eg, Trendelenburg procedure) is rarely successful.

Atrial myxoma, mitral thrombus, coarctation of the aorta, obstructive valvular disease, and pulmonary hypertension are rare causes of shock in patients presenting to the emergency department. Emergent decompression of tension pneumothorax is discussed in Chapters 12 and 24. Supportive treatment usually includes fluids, vasopressors, and oxygenation. Echocardiography and right heart catheterization may help to establish the diagnosis in obstructive shock.

DISTRIBUTIVE SHOCK

Distributive shock occurs when distribution of intravascular volume is markedly abnormal as a result of decreased vascular resistance (as occurs in fainting, when blood pools in the venous rather than the arterial portion of the circulation). Cardiac output may be increased, normal, or low in patients with this type of shock. The causes of distributive shock are diverse and include septic shock, anaphylactic shock, and neurogenic shock, which are discussed below; acute adrenal insufficiency is discussed in Chapter 41. Some drugs and toxins may produce vasodilation and may also result in distributive shock. See Chapter 45 for a discussion of drug overdose and poisoning.

1. Septic Shock
(See also Chapter 46.)

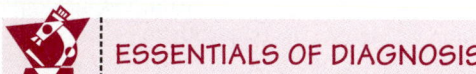 **ESSENTIALS OF DIAGNOSIS**

Systemic Inflammatory Response Syndrome (SIRS)

- *Respiratory rate greater than 20 or $PaCO_2$*
- *Temperature > 38 °C or < 36 °C.*
- *White blood cell count > 12,000 or < 4000 or > 10% band forms.*
- *Heart rate greater than 90 beats/min.*

Sepsis

- *Presence of SIRS and infection confirmed.*

Severe Sepsis

- *Sepsis associated with organ dysfunction, hypoperfusion abnormality, or sepsis-induced hypotension.*

Septic Shock

- *Sepsis-induced hypotension despite adequate fluid resuscitation.*
- *Persistence of hypoperfusion abnormalities or organ dysfunction.*

- *Includes patients needing pressor agents to maintain blood pressure.*

General Considerations

Septic shock is the number one cause of death in U.S. intensive care units. The incidence of septic shock continues to increase. Septic shock is usually caused by gram-negative bacteria that invade the bloodstream (endotoxic shock), although other bacteria and some fungi may produce a similar syndrome. Septic shock may occur without frank bacteremia if there is extensive local infection (eg, intra-abdominal abscess). Shock also occurs in toxic shock syndrome as a result of absorption of a staphylococcal toxin.

Factors predisposing to development of septic shock include trauma, diabetes, leukemia, severe granulocytopenia, disease of the genitourinary tract, radiation treatment, and treatment with corticosteroids or immunosuppressive agents. Immediate precipitating causes may include surgical or other manipulation of the urinary, biliary, or gynecologic tracts.

Hypotension results from multiple factors. There is a loss of vascular integrity, leading to third spacing of fluids. There is a loss of contractile ability of the vasculature, leading to increased size of the vascular compartment. Energy metabolism becomes impaired on the cellular level, and cardiac function is depressed by chemical mediators.

Clinical Findings

Clinical features of shock and infection are present.

A. SYSTEMIC SIGNS

Rigors, fever (hypothermia is noted in 5–10% of patients), petechiae, leukocytosis, or leukopenia with a shift to the left may be noted.

B. LOCALIZED SIGNS

Abdominal tenderness, perirectal abscess, and extensive pneumonia may be present. Localizing symptoms and signs may be absent, however, especially if the patient is immunocompromised, very young, or very old. Typical sites of occult infection include the urinary tract, biliary system, pelvis, retroperitoneum, and perirectal area.

C. OTHER SIGNS

Hyperventilation with hypocapnia is common. The presence of infection should be confirmed by microscopic examination, culture, or other definitive test. Samples of body fluids and tissues that may harbor infection should be submitted for culture, including 2 or 3 blood cultures.

In toxic shock syndrome, toxins from localized staphylococcal colonization or infection cause severe hypotension or shock associated with a diffuse red rash (which later desquamates) and other symptoms and signs (nausea and vomiting, diarrhea, thrombocytopenia). The incidence of toxic shock syndrome increased in the late 1980s due to the marketing of highly absorbent, occlusive tampons that facilitated an anaerobic vaginal environment. With the removal of these tampons from the market, the incidence of this disease has fallen.

Treatment

A. MEDICAL MEASURES

1. Pharmacologic therapy—Over a decade of pharmaceutical investigation and clinical trials of drugs designed to block various parts of the pro-inflammatory cascade of sepsis has failed to yield a drug with proven clinical benefit for septic shock. Drugs that have gone through clinical trials include antiendotoxin antibodies, anticytotoxin antibodies, interleukin therapy, and antibodies to tumor necrosis factor. One study demonstrated that early, aggressive therapy in the emergency department may confer some survival advantage.

2. Volume replacement—The amount of fluid administered follows the same guidelines governing fluid replacement in severe hypovolemic shock (see above). In general, for adults, 1–2 L given over 30–60 minutes (children, 10–20 mL/kg) will improve blood pressure and urine output; further administration of fluid depends on clinical response (ie, urine output, blood pressure, and pulse).

3. Inotropic agents—Give dopamine (with both inotropic and vasopressor properties), 3–15 µg/kg/min, if the patient fails to respond to measures that raise central venous or pulmonary capillary wedge pressure to normal levels. Norepinephrine may also be used for this purpose. Follow the dosage guidelines given in the table on the inside front cover. Vasopressin may also be useful in the setting of septic shock.

4. Antibiotic therapy—Antibiotic treatment should be specific for the causative organism, but the etiologic agent may not be known at the onset of shock. Prompt empiric treatment with antibiotics should be started. Antibiotic recommendations change frequently and vary depending on host and local resistance patterns. Therapy decisions should be based on the likely source of the infection (see Table 40–1). Because the mortality rate of septic shock is 40–70%, empiric therapy should be broad and aggressive, and later tailored to the culture results. Evidence suggests that many patients ill enough to be admitted to the intensive care unit receive inadequate antibiotic therapy and that this inappropriate therapy may contribute to mortality.

B. SURGICAL MEASURES

Antibiotics and fluid replacement are much less effective if an abscess or other localized source of infection is not drained. It is therefore critical to identify as soon as possible any source of sepsis (eg, intra-abdominal abscess, biliary obstruction with cholangitis) or any other disorder requiring surgery.

C. SPECIAL MEASURES

1. Corticosteroids—Administration of pharmacologic doses of glucocorticoids has no beneficial effect in patients with septic shock and may even be harmful. Therefore, high-dose corticosteroids should not be used as adjunctive therapy in septic shock. It is still a matter of debate whether patients will benefit from physiologic doses of steroids.

2. Heparin—Disseminated intravascular coagulation (Chapter 39) may occur in septic shock. If treatment of septic shock is successful, consumption of coagulation factors usually ceases and rapid regeneration of these factors occurs. If coagulation studies confirm the presence of persistent disseminated intravascular coagulation (prolonged prothrombin and partial thromboplastin times, decreased number of platelets, depressed fibrinogen levels, and the presence of fibrin degradation products) and if there is significant bleeding, give heparin, 100 units/kg intravenously to start, followed by 10–40 units/kg/h by continuous intravenous administration (infusion pump preferred). Response to heparin is indicated by slowing of bleeding and a rise within 12 hours of the levels of fibrinogen and factors V and VII. Platelet counts may rise at a slower rate. Discontinue heparin therapy when the cause of disseminated intravascular coagulation has been corrected and coagulation factors have been restored to hemostatic levels.

Disposition

All patients should be hospitalized, preferably in an intensive care unit.

Alia I et al: A randomized and controlled trial of the effect of treatment aimed at maximizing oxygen delivery in patients with severe sepsis or septic shock. Chest 1999;115(2):453. [PMID: 10027447] (A prospective, randomized controlled trial of maximizing cardiac performance in septic shock that did not demonstrate any benefit to patients. Interventions in the intensive care unit may be too much, too late, when it comes to septic shock.)

Fitch S, Gossage J: Optimal management of septic shock. Postgrad Med 2002;111(3):53. [PMID: 11912997] (A review summarizing the diagnosis and treatment of septic shock.)

Gossage J: Early intervention in massive pulmonary embolism. Postgrad Med 2002;111(3):27. [PMID: 11912996] (A guide to the evaluation and triage in the first hour of patients with suspected massive pulmonary embolism.)

Holmes CL et al: Physiology of vasopressin relevant to management of septic shock. Chest 2001;120(3):989. [PMID: 11555538] (Discussion of the pathophysiology and therapeutic role of vasopressin in septic shock.)

Kollef MH et al: Inadequate antimicrobial treatment of infections: a risk factor for hospital mortality among critically ill patients. Chest 1999;115(2):462. [PMID: 10027448] (A prospective surveillance study in which 9% of patients in the intensive care unit were administered inappropriate antibiotics. The mortality rate among these patients was more than double those receiving appropriate antibiotics.)

Rivers E et al: Early goal-directed therapy in the treatment of severe sepsis and septic shock. N Engl J Med 2001;345(19):1368. [PMID: 11794169] (A prospective randomized trial of algorithm-based intensive care aimed at maximizing cardiac parameters in the emergency department in the treatment of septic shock that shows significant reductions in mortality and morbidity. There may be a narrow window of opportunity to treat sepsis before irreversible deficits are established.)

2. Anaphylactic Shock

ESSENTIALS OF DIAGNOSIS

- *Shock in the presence of massive histamine release.*
- *Uticaria, soft tissue edema, wheezing secondary to bronchospasm, stridor due to laryngeal edema, hypotension due to vasodilatation.*
- *Cutaneous and extremity perfusion is maintained.*

General Considerations

Anaphylactic shock is a catastrophic and frequently fatal type of allergic reaction that occurs within minutes after parenteral (rarely oral) administration of drugs or nonhuman proteins, including foods, sera, or venoms. In cases obviously caused by injections of drugs or sera, there is seldom any reason for delayed treatment.

Clinical Findings

Symptoms and signs include marked apprehension, generalized urticaria or edema, back pain, a choking sensation, cough, bronchospasm, or laryngeal edema. In severe cases, hypotension, loss of consciousness, dilatation of the pupils, incontinence, and convulsions may be present; sudden death may occur.

Three modes of presentation of anaphylaxis (based on the most conspicuous presenting features) are recognized; however, any combination of these may occur: (1) urticaria or angioedema that may be associated with upper airway obstruction and laryngeal edema, (2) bronchospasm, or (3) vascular collapse (ie, severe hypotension).

Treatment

Begin treatment as soon as anaphylaxis is suspected. *Do not wait until it is fully developed.*

A. POSITION

Place the conscious patient in a comfortable position and ensure unimpeded ventilation. The unconscious patient should be placed supine, in a level or slightly head-down position (do this as quickly as possible).

B. AIRWAY

Keep the airway open (Chapter 8), and give supplemental oxygen by mask or nasal prongs at a rate of 5–10 L/min. If the patient is not breathing, assist ventilation with a bag-mask until endotracheal intubation can be performed (Chapters 6 and 8). If equipment for insertion of an endotracheal tube is not available or if intubation is unsuccessful because of airway obstruction by laryngeal edema, cricothyrotomy (Chapter 6) may be necessary.

C. INTRAVENOUS ACCESS

Insert an intravenous catheter and begin infusion of a balanced salt solution or normal saline (adults, 0.5–1 L over 30 minutes; children, 5-15 mL/kg), with further administration governed by blood pressure and urine output.

D. PHARMACOLOGIC THERAPY

Epinephrine administered intravenously or via an endotracheal tube is central to the initial therapy for the very ill patient with anaphylaxis.

1. Aqueous epinephrine—For anaphylaxis with mild to moderate symptoms, give epinephrine (adults, 0.3–0.5 mg [0.3–0.5 mL of 1:1000 solution] intramuscularly; children, 0.01 mL/kg/dose up to a maximum of 0.4 mL/dose). For severe anaphylaxis, epinephrine should be administered intravenously or via an endotracheal tube (1.0 mL of 1:10,000 solution). Repeat every 5–10 minutes if symptoms continue or recur. A continuous infusion may be necessary in some patients. Add 1 mg of a 1:1000 solution of epinephrine to 250 mL of 5% dextrose in water (10 μg/mL); for adults, begin the infusion at a rate of 1 μg/min (children, 0.1 μg/kg/min) and increase up to 10 μg/min as needed. Caution should be used in patients with cardiac or hypertensive histories.

2. Diphenhydramine—Give diphenhydramine (adults, 50 mg; children, 2 mg/kg) intravenously or intramuscularly, early in treatment.

3. Histamine blockers—Administer ranitidine, 50 mg, or famotidine, 20 mg, intravenously to additionally block receptors and ameliorate the histamine reaction.

4. Glucocorticoids—A soluble glucocorticoid preparation should be given as an adjunct to epinephrine. Give hydrocortisone sodium succinate, 100–250 mg intravenously; or methylprednisolone sodium succinate, 50–100 mg intravenously. Benefit from glucocorticoids will not be seen for several hours.

5. β-Agonist aerosol—If bronchospasm is present, give albuterol or another β-agonist inhalant solutions, 0.5 mL in 2.5 mL normal saline, by nebulizer every 30–60 minutes.

Prevention

Inquire carefully about any history of drug allergy before giving drugs. In drunk, unconscious, or obtunded patients, search for a card, bracelet, or necklace specifying drug allergies or medical conditions (eg, diabetes) requiring special attention. Be cautious when administering parenteral medications to patients with a history of drug allergy. If there is a history of previous reaction to the agent to be injected, use an alternative drug whenever possible. Given intravenous injections slowly, and observe individuals who have received parenteral medication for at least 30 minutes after injection. Patients with a history of anaphylactic reactions to insect venoms or other environmental agents that cannot be easily avoided should be prescribed a kit with epinephrine for self-administration and should be advised to carry it at times of high risk of exposure.

Disposition

Recurrent episodes of anaphylaxis may occur 12–24 hours after the initial episode; therefore, patients who have experienced life-threatening anaphylaxis should be hospitalized for observation and treatment. Patients who have shown only mild manifestations of anaphylaxis (eg, urticaria) that have resolved with treatment may be discharged from the emergency department after treatment (Chapter 46) and 6 hours of symptom-free observation. Follow-up is based on the principles outlined in Chapter 46.

3. Neurogenic Shock

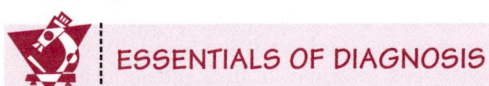

ESSENTIALS OF DIAGNOSIS

- *Hypotension in the presence of spinal cord injury.*

- *Cutaneous and extremity perfusion is maintained.*

General Considerations

Neurogenic shock is due to failure of vasomotor regulation that results in pooling of blood in dilated capacitance vessels and a subsequent fall in blood pressure. True neurogenic shock should be distinguished from vasovagal syncope (Chapter 17). Although the mechanism of hypotension is similar in both conditions—sudden failure of vasomotor regulation—the condition is not prolonged enough in vasovagal syncope to produce diffuse tissue ischemia and clinical features of shock.

Neurogenic shock is rare. It is most commonly due to traumatic quadriplegia or paraplegia (spinal shock), although a similar syndrome can be induced by high spinal anesthesia and is occasionally seen in severe Guillain-Barré syndrome and other neuropathies. In patients with traumatic spine injuries, it is important to remember that hypovolemic shock (due to associated injuries) is still the most common cause of shock and must be presumed to be present until proved otherwise.

Clinical Findings

The symptoms and signs of neurogenic shock are similar to those of hypovolemic shock. Signs of neurologic disease often associated with neurogenic shock are also present (eg, traumatic quadriplegia or paraplegia).

Treatment

Place the patient supine and give oxygen. If blood pressure and peripheral perfusion are not rapidly restored, begin other measures.

The treatment of choice is volume replacement with crystalloid solution to "fill up" the dilated capacitance vessels. For adults give 1 L (children, 10-20 mL/kg) of crystalloid solution intravenously over 20–40 minutes (depending on the severity of shock). If initial fluid therapy is insufficient to bring the mean arterial pressure to greater than 80, an intravenous vasopressor agent with α-agonist activity, such as dopamine in high doses (> 10–20 µg/kg/min) or norepinephrine (4 mg in 500 mL normal saline started at 1–1.5 cc/min) should be started.

Disposition

All patients should be hospitalized, preferably in an intensive care unit.

The Multiply Injured Patient

Julia Martin, MD, & Michael McClurg, MD

Immediate Management of Life-Threatening Problems
    Preparation
    Initial Assessment
        1. Primary Survey
        2. Initial Resuscitation
    Hemorrhagic Shock
Emergency Treatment of Specific Disorders
    Injuries to the Neck Region
        1. Cervical Spine
        2. Upper Airway
        3. Esophagus
        4. Vascular Injury

Tension Pneumothorax
Flail Chest
Pulmonary Contusion
Cardiac Tamponade
Myocardial Contusion
Traumatic Aortic Rupture
Abdominal Trauma
Head Trauma
Genitourinary Trauma
Extremity Trauma
Spinal Trauma

■ IMMEDIATE MANAGEMENT OF LIFE-THREATENING PROBLEMS (See Figure 10–1.)

The primary goal in providing care to the trauma patient is effective resuscitation while minimizing the time from injury to definitive care.

PREPARATION

Trauma care begins at the scene of the accident. It is important for hospitals to have good working relationships with local fire departments and emergency medical services (EMS) to ensure that proper care is provided early. Preparation efforts should be coordinated between the emergency departments and the local EMS systems, including prehospital protocols related to the treatment and transport of trauma patients. Transport protocols should incorporate decision-making guidelines including information regarding transporting patients to the most appropriate facility and the proper use of air medical transport. Prehospital providers should be trained to detect specific injuries and know the mechanism of forces which could predict the possibility of severe injury (Table 10–1). Prehospital personnel should provide early notification to the emergency department for all major trauma patients to allow emergency department preparedness.

Injury-scoring systems such as the Glasgow Coma Scale (GCS), Trauma Score, and Revised Trauma Score may be used to help quantify the degree of injury (Figure 10–2). Maintain a high index of suspicion with pediatric, geriatric, and obstetric patients. Their physiologic responses to major trauma differs from that of other patients, and their injuries are often missed or delayed in diagnosis. Early transfer to definitive care improves outcomes in these patient groups.

Emergency department response should include a stepwise notification system to alert local surgeons or trauma teams and ancillary services such as x-ray, computed tomography (CT) scan, laboratory, blood bank, and operating room personnel. Initial stabilization and resuscitation is done most effectively if a well-organized team approach is used. The key to an organized system is the designation of a person in charge to oversee the total care of the patient. The team leader should assign specific tasks to emergency department team members. It is important for everyone to understand their roles, know where equipment is located, adhere to universal precautions, and keep noise and extraneous conversation to a minimum. Constant reassessment of the pa-

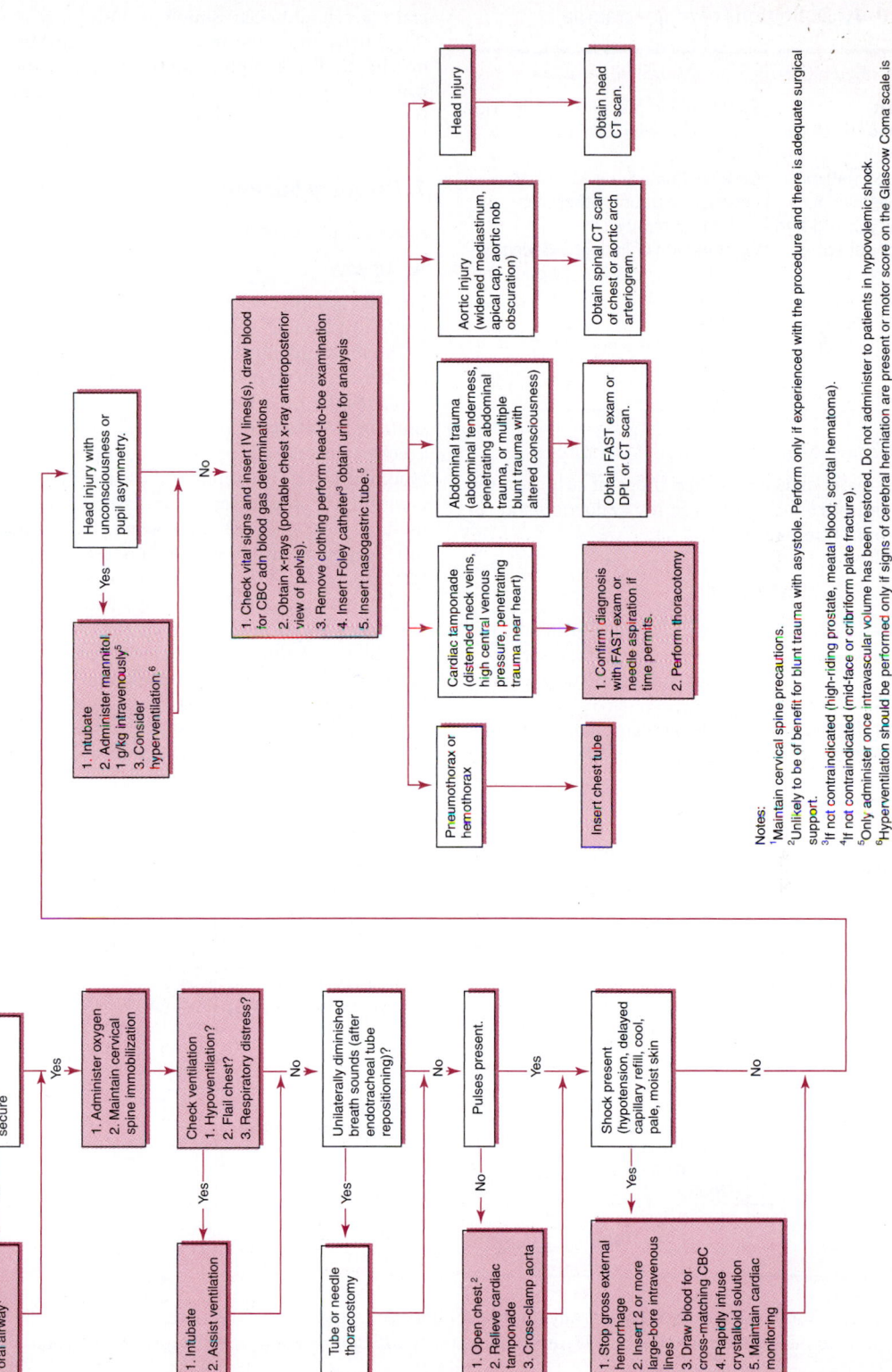

Figure 10–1. Assessment of the patient with multiple injuries. DPL = diagnostic peritoneal lavage; FAST = focused assessment with sonography for trauma.

Table 10–1. Definitions of major trauma.

Mechanism of Injury	Clinical Information
Falls > 20 ft	Systolic blood pressure < 90 mm Hg
Rollover motor vehicle collision	Respiratory rate < 10/min or > 29/min
Crash speed > 40 mph	Glasgow Coma Scale score < 10
Auto-pedestrian or auto-bicycle collision	Penetrating trauma other than distal extremity
Ejection of patient	Combination of 2nd- or 3rd- degree
Occupant fatality in same vehicle	burns over > 15% of the body and multiple trauma
Major auto deformity > 20 in Blast injury	Trauma score < 13
	Revised trauma score < 11
	Pelvic fractures
	Paralysis

tient and maintenance of a high index of suspicion for possible injuries are important in the evaluation and resuscitation of trauma patients.

INITIAL ASSESSMENT

The initial assessment consists of a rapid primary survey, initiation of resuscitative measures, followed by a secondary survey. The primary survey includes evaluation of the airway, breathing, and circulation and a brief neurologic exam. Problems identified in the primary assessment should be corrected immediately. Several tasks should occur simultaneously such as assessing the patient; initiating resuscitation; placing the patient on the cardiac monitor, pulse oximetry, and supplemental oxygen; and initiating intravenous lines. Rapid stabilization of airway, breathing, circulation, and neurologic status is paramount for patient survival.

1. Primary Survey

Assessment of ABCs

A. AIRWAY

(See also Chapter 8.) Airway management and maintenance of adequate oxygenation are extremely important in the multiply injured patient. Shock leads to an oxygen deficit, which increases the body's demands and necessitates the need for supplementary oxygen. Cervical spine immobilization is considered part of airway management in trauma patients. To open the airway, a modified jaw thrust should be used with cervical spine control. An oropharyngeal or nasopharyngeal tube is useful to help maintain an airway. The nasopharyngeal tube may be used in semiconscious patients with an intact gag reflex. The oropharyngeal airway should be used only in unconscious patients without a gag reflex; otherwise, it may induce vomiting.

Obtain a definitive airway in any patient who is not breathing, has inadequate ventilation or oxygenation, has an unprotected airway without a gag reflex, or has a decreased level of consciousness with a GCS score less than 8. Emergency department providers should be

A Glasgow Coma Scale

Eye opening	Spontaneous	4
	To verbal command	3
	To pain	2
	None	1
Verbal responsiveness	Oriented	5
	Confused	4
	Inappropriate words	3
	Incomprehensible sounds	2
	None	1
Motor response	Obeys	6
	Localizes	5
	Withdraws (pain)	4
	Flexion (pain)	3
	Extension (pain)	2
	None	1
	Total: _____	

B Revised Trauma Score

Respiratory rate (breaths/min)	10–29	4
	> 29	3
	6–9	2
	1–5	1
	0	
Systolic blood pressure (mm Hg)	> 89	4
	76–89	3
	50–75	2
	1–49	1
	No pulse	0
Glasgow conversion scale	13–15	4
	9–12	3
	6–8	2
	4–5	1
	< 4	0
	Total: _____	

Figure 10–2. Trauma scores used to quantify degree of injury. **A:** Determine total on Glasgow Coma Scale. **B:** Convert Glasgow Coma Scale total to Revised Trauma Score points and determine Revised Trauma Score total.

knowledgeable about and skilled with a variety of surgical and nonsurgical methods of securing an airway. Patients with inadequate ventilation and oxygenation require bag-mask ventilation until intubation is accomplished. Tracheal intubation may be accomplished by 2 methods: nasotracheal or orotracheal. Both methods require good cervical spine immobilization including manual stabilization of the neck. With adequate training and experience, rapid sequence intubation (RSI) offers many advantages in the multiply injured trauma patient. RSI involves the use of paralytics to rapidly achieve muscle relaxation and sedatives to render the patient unconscious and unaware of laryngoscopy and intubation. Use of paralytics helps protect against a rise in intracranial pressure associated with laryngoscopy, and with good manual cervical spine stabilization there is less risk of additional cervical spine injury. The use of paralytics and sedation requires a good working knowledge of the medications' indications, their side effects, and their contraindications, in order to minimize complications associated with the procedure. Being well trained in backup airway maneuvers such as the laryngeal mask airway, lighted stylet, fiberoptic intubation, and surgical airway options is imperative prior to initiating RSI in a patient. RSI is relatively contraindicated in patients who cannot be ventilated with a bag-valve-mask if intubation proves difficult or impossible. If orotracheal or nasotracheal intubation is unsuccessful, a surgical airway such as a cricothyrotomy should be performed.

B. BREATHING

Assess adequacy of ventilation by inspecting the chest wall for adequate expansion; looking for paradoxical rise of the chest, flail segments, and sucking wounds; and noting labored respirations or auxiliary muscle use. Auscultate the lungs for the presence of symmetrical breath sounds.

If breath sounds are unilaterally diminished and the patient is intubated, consider withdrawing the endotracheal tube 2–3 cm in case the tip is residing in a mainstem bronchus, and then recheck the breath sounds. Persistently diminished breath sounds imply pneumothorax. If the patient is hypotensive, in shock, or laboring to breathe, perform a tube thoracostomy immediately. Should a delay exist before this can occur, decompress the chest with a 14-gauge angiocatheter or other catheter-clad needle inserted in the 2nd intercostal space at the midclavicular line. A stable patient with diminished breath sounds may await a chest x-ray for confirmation prior to decompression with a needle or thoracostomy tube.

Treat a sucking chest wound by sealing the wound with an occlusive dressing (eg, petrolatum-impregnated dressing) at 3 points and then performing a tube thoracostomy (not through the chest wall defect). Adequacy of ventilation can be confirmed with arterial blood gas measurements.

C. CIRCULATION

Rapidly assess blood pressure and pulse. A narrowed pulse pressure suggests hypovolemic shock. Hypotension is evidence of severe intravascular depletion. Rapidly evaluate the abdomen because it is frequently a source of significant hemorrhage in the multiply injured patient. Severe pelvic fracture or pelvic ring disruptions can be associated with massive intrapelvic hemorrhage. Give the patient crystalloid initially and then blood, if needed, to improve perfusion.

1. Traumatic arrest—If spontaneous cardiac activity is not detected by palpation of the carotid artery, begin cardiopulmonary resuscitation immediately. If the patient has blunt trauma and has been pulseless for less than 5 minutes, or if there is penetrating chest trauma and the patient has been pulseless for less than 15 minutes, consider emergent thoracotomy. Only experienced physicians trained in emergent thoracotomy should perform this procedure. If the patient has been pulseless longer than the above time limits, thoracotomy is not indicated and has not been shown to improve survival. Initiate closed chest compressions with volume resuscitation with crystalloids and cardiac drugs per advanced cardiac life support guidelines (Chapter 7).

2. External hemorrhage—Stop obvious external hemorrhage using direct pressure with sterile dressings. Scalp wounds, even small ones, can produce significant blood loss if not controlled. Sometimes direct pressure and dressings are not sufficient. For uncontrolled scalp wound hemorrhage, the wound should be closed with sutures, staples, or, if available, Raney scalp clips, preferably using sterile technique. If a nonsterile technique is used, the wound should be inspected carefully, cleansed, and then definitively closed using sterile technique when the patient stabilizes. Bleeding vessels should not be clamped indiscriminately. Rarely will compression be insufficient to control an exsanguinating arterial hemorrhage from an extremity. A blood pressure cuff inflated proximal to the wound can serve as an effective tourniquet temporarily until surgical control of the bleeding can be achieved. Except as a last resort, avoid tourniquets. If a tourniquet is required, monitor and document the application time.

3. Shock—(See also Chapter 9.) Shock is defined as inadequate tissue perfusion and is further classified as mild, moderate, or severe, based primarily on clinical criteria. Cool, pale skin; diaphoresis; delayed capillary refill (> 2 sec); tachycardia; and mental status changes are reliable indicators of shock. Hypotension and oliguria are presumed to be due to shock until proved otherwise. Do not assume that perfusion is adequate on the basis of supine pulse and blood pressure alone, because these signs may not change until late in shock. This is particularly true in young healthy adults—who are the most common victims of multiple trauma. Patients taking β-blockers (or other medications that blunt the normal response to adrenergic stimulation) may not exhibit tachycardia despite profound shock.

Shock in the traumatized patient is due to hypovolemia from hemorrhage in the majority of the cases. Cardiac tamponade, tension pneumothorax, or spinal cord or brain injury may contribute to shock or (rarely) may cause shock without concurrent volume loss. In a trauma patient, shock should be treated as hypovolemic shock with volume infusions until other causes of shock are found.

Brief Neurologic Exam

A quick neurologic exam may be accomplished by using the GCS (see Figure 10–2). The GCS allows for quick assessment of the patient's level of responsiveness to determine if he or she is awake and alert; responds to verbal stimuli with eye opening or following of commands; responds to painful stimuli (eg, sternal rub, muscle or tendon squeeze) by appropriate movement, localization, or posturing; or is unresponsive.

Assess the patient's pupils for symmetry, size, and reactivity. An asymmetrically enlarged pupil in a unresponsive patient may imply transtentorial herniation, which should be treated with endotracheal intubation. Among the other interventions to reduce intracranial pressure is short-term hyperventilation (Chapter 22).

2. Initial Resuscitation

Evaluation and treatment must proceed rapidly and simultaneously. During the primary survey, correct any identified problems immediately. Place the patient on a cardiac monitor, including pulse oximetry with supplemental oxygen administered. Initiate intravenous lines and order initial laboratory studies. Place a Foley catheter after examination of the perineal area and rectal exam. Do not insert a urethral catheter if there is obvious injury to the external genitalia, obvious urethral bleeding, scrotal hematoma, a malpositioned or high-riding prostate on rectal examination, or difficulty in passing the catheter. Monitoring of urine output is important in evaluating the patient's response to resuscitative efforts. Urinary output below 0.5 cc/kg/h indicates significant hypovolemia.

Intravenous Access

Insert multiple large-bore (≥ 16-gauge) catheters in a patient with profound shock. Initiate at least 2 intravenous lines. Consider a central line to administer large amounts of fluids rapidly or to monitor central venous pressure in patients with poor peripheral venous access in profound shock, in the elderly, and in patients with significant comorbid disease.

Laboratory Tests

Obtain blood specimens for hematocrit or complete blood count, electrolyte measurements, renal function tests, and coagulation (prothrombin and partial thromboplastin times). Obtain a urine sample for gross blood. Obtain a pregnancy test from female patients of childbearing age. If abdominal trauma is present, request laboratory studies for liver enzymes, amylase, and lipase. If severe shock is evident or suspected, type and cross-match for 4 units of packed red blood cells, and obtain an arterial blood gas and serum lactate. Trauma patients have high rates of alcohol and drug use, and a blood alcohol level or urine drug screen may be useful in evaluating patients with altered mental status.

Fluid Resuscitation

If clinical evidence of shock is present, initiate intravenous infusion of crystalloid solution. Give up to 2 L of crystalloid solution to support intravascular volume before giving blood. Give cross-matched or type-specific blood, if available, to a patient in persistent shock unresponsive to crystalloids. If typed and cross-matched blood is not available, then give type O blood. Reserve type O-negative blood for females under age 50 years; all others should receive type O-positive.

Initial Radiographic Studies

During the acute phase of evaluation and resuscitation, the most valuable x-rays are of the chest and pelvis. These x-rays assist in the evaluation of potential injuries associated with a large amount of blood loss. Although spine x-rays are important, the spine can be protected from further injury by adhering strictly to spinal immobilization precautions during the initial evaluation and resuscitation.

Large hemorrhages can also be found in the abdominal cavity. The abdomen can be rapidly evaluated in the unstable trauma patient by using bedside emergency ultrasound and performing a FAST (Focused Assessment with Sonography for Trauma) exam to look for free fluid. The more traditional approach to the unstable patient was the use of a diagnostic peritoneal lavage (DPL), which should be performed by the surgeon caring for the patient if ultrasound is unavailable. In stable trauma patients, a contrasted CT scan of the abdomen and pelvis provides useful information regarding the extent of specific organ injuries. Because ultrasound and CT scan are poor in evaluating bowel injuries, maintain a high index of suspicion so that this type of injury is not overlooked, especially in pediatric patients.

Ongoing Evaluation & Resuscitation

Frequently reassess a multiply injured trauma patient for evidence of new or ongoing signs of shock. In the multiply injured patient, hemorrhage is the most common cause of shock. Even so, it is important to conscientiously assess the patient for other underlying causes of shock. Early surgical consult is important for any trauma patient with signs of shock. Splint fractures, administer antibiotics and tetanus toxoid when needed, and keep patients warm. Pay close attention to the prevention of further injury. Avoiding infection, hypothermia, coagulopathy, and ongoing blood loss is important for minimizing possible mortality and morbidity.

Melio FR: Priorities in the multiple trauma patient. Emerg Med Clin North Am 1998;16:29. [PMID: 9496313] (Overview of the initial approach to the multiply injured trauma patient.)

HEMORRHAGIC SHOCK

ESSENTIALS OF DIAGNOSIS

- *Evidence of external blood loss.*
- *Injuries with associated internal blood loss.*
- *Tachycardia.*
- *Decreased level of consciousness.*
- *Decreased urine output.*
- *Delayed capillary refill.*
- *Hypotension (late sign).*

General Considerations

Defined as inadequate tissue perfusion due to decreased cardiac output secondary to blood loss, hemorrhagic shock accounts for the overwhelming majority of trauma patients in shock. Clinical signs are due to compensatory mechanisms. For example, excess sympathetic nervous system stimulation causes tachycardia and peripheral vasoconstriction, whereas decreased peripheral and renal blood flow result in decreased urine

output, pallor, delayed capillary refill, and weak peripheral pulses.

Clinical Findings

A. OBVIOUS SOURCES OF BLOOD LOSS

Identify and control external hemorrhage during the primary survey. Logroll trauma patients to examine their backs. A single hematocrit may provide a baseline but is not helpful in detecting acute occult hemorrhage.

B. HIDDEN SOURCES OF INTERNAL BLOOD LOSS

Serial hematocrits over several hours are useful in determining continued blood loss, because a single initial value may be deceivingly normal. Major sources of occult blood loss are as follows:

1. Thorax—Each hemithorax may contain 1–2 L of blood, primarily as a result of a pulmonary laceration or laceration of intercostal vessels or internal mammary artery due to either penetrating or blunt trauma. Suspect hemothorax in cases of shock associated with decreased or absent breath sounds or when dullness to percussion is present on the affected side. A supine chest x-ray may only show haziness over the hemithorax.

2. Abdomen—Assume intra-abdominal hemorrhage in patients in shock with a normal chest x-ray and no external sources of bleeding. Abdominal distention is a late and unreliable sign. Kehr sign is referred left shoulder pain due to diaphragmatic irritation associated with hemoperitoneum and splenic injuries. Cullen sign (periumbilical ecchymosis) is a late finding in intra-abdominal hemorrhage. Use a FAST exam or DPL to examine unstable patients. Stable patients should undergo CT scan of the abdomen.

3. Retroperitoneum—The retroperitoneum can accumulate approximately 4 L of blood before tamponade occurs, and retroperitoneal hemorrhage may not be detected by abdominal ultrasound or DPL. Grey-Turner sign (flank ecchymosis) is a late finding on physical examination. CT scan of the abdomen and pelvis is necessary to confirm the diagnosis.

4. Pelvis—Pelvic fractures may result in extensive bleeding from the bone itself or from disruption of the presacral venous plexus. The presence of blood can be identified with FAST exam or DPL; however, identification of the definitive source of bleeding requires CT scan, angiography, or laparotomy.

5. Soft tissues (ie, thigh, upper arm, calf)—Between 1 and 4 L of blood can accumulate in the soft tissues due to long bone fractures and may not be immediately apparent on physical examination.

Treatment

A. DIRECT PRESSURE

Obvious external hemorrhage can usually be controlled with direct pressure over the bleeding site or over a proximal artery. Tourniquets are rarely indicated. Never blindly place a clamp into a wound.

B. INDIRECT PRESSURE OR PNEUMATIC ANTISHOCK GARMENT

Immediate temporary stabilization of an unstable pelvis fracture can decrease the pelvic volume and help tamponade bleeding. This can be accomplished by internally rotating the lower legs and tying them together with a sheet, followed by another sheet tied around the pelvis itself. Although they have not been shown to improve survival in patients with hemorrhagic shock, military antishock trousers (MAST) can be applied and inflated as a temporary measure to splint pelvic or femur fractures and help control hemorrhage. MAST are contraindicated in severe head or chest trauma, evisceration, diaphragmatic rupture, pulmonary edema, cardiogenic shock, or advanced pregnancy.

C. SUPPORTIVE MEASURES

Guidelines for volume resuscitation are set forth in Chapter 9.

1. Crystalloid solutions—As a general rule, administer 3 cc of crystalloids for every 1 cc of estimated blood loss. Consider administering blood products if the patient's hemodynamic response is not favorable after the first 2 L of crystalloids.

2. Blood products—The amount of blood or blood products given depends on the clinical situation and the patient's response to fluid resuscitation. Ideally the hematocrit should be kept at approximately 30% (35–40% in elderly patients and those with preexisting cardiopulmonary disease).

3. Autotransfusion—Autotransfusion is the administration of autologous blood collected from the patient's thoracic cavity. The blood is collected from chest tube drainage into containers with sodium citrate added as an anticoagulant. The blood can then be filtered and reinfused into the patient. Advantages include blood that is immediately available and already warm, with no risk of infectious disease transmission or transfusion reaction.

4. Warming of blood—Hypothermia is a common side effect of transfusion of stored blood. New combination pressure infusers and fluid warmers are ideally designed to avoid hypothermia during aggressive fluid resuscitation of trauma patients.

Disposition

Admit patients for surgery or observation as indicated.

■ EMERGENCY TREATMENT OF SPECIFIC DISORDERS

INJURIES TO THE NECK REGION (See also Chapter 23.)

 ESSENTIALS OF DIAGNOSIS

- *Immobilize to prevent further injury.*
- *Examine neck for both blunt and penetrating trauma.*
- *Evaluate neck for expanding hematoma, crepitus, subcutaneous air, external hemorrhage, trachea midline, and cervical spine tenderness or deformity.*

1. Cervical Spine

Clinical Findings

(See Chapter 23.)

Treatment

Maintain in-line axial immobilization if a cervical spine injury is suspected (Chapter 23).

Disposition

Admit all patients with injury to neck structures, other than minor blunt or superficial penetrating injuries.

2. Upper Airway

Clinical Findings

Injury to the upper airway is characterized by hoarseness or aphonia, apnea or respiratory distress, stridor, subcutaneous emphysema, or bubbling of blood during inspiration and expiration in open neck wounds.

Treatment & Disposition

Early definitive airway management using RSI or cricothyrotomy may be life-saving if indicated. If the airway is exposed, intubate directly through the wound. If subcutaneous emphysema is present, assume a tracheobronchial injury is present and attempt to pass the endotracheal tube distal to the site of injury if possible.

All patients with injuries to the upper airway require admission.

3. Esophagus

Clinical Findings

Esophageal injury is uncommon, even in penetrating trauma. Difficulty swallowing and neck pain are common, but overt clinical signs may be minimal initially. Chest x-ray may reveal pneumomediastinum, but definitive diagnosis requires esophagoscopy or contrasted swallowing studies.

Treatment & Disposition

Insert a nasogastric tube and administer broad-spectrum antibiotics (ie, penicillin). Obtain surgical consultation.

4. Vascular Injury

Clinical Findings

The neck is divided into 3 anatomic zones. Zone I is below the cricoid cartilage, zone II is between the cricoid and the angle of the mandible, and zone III is above the angle of the mandible. Clinical findings of a vascular injury are variable and may be subtle or absent initially. Traditionally, surgical exploration was advocated for all zone II injuries deep to the platysma and for others with clinical indications (expanding hematoma, active bleeding, diminished carotid pulsation, hemoptysis, crepitus, dysphonia, hematemesis, dysphagia, or Horner syndrome). Some authors advocate selective management with angiography, Gastrografin swallow, and esophagoscopy. Because of difficulties in accessing the major vascular structures in zone III and especially zone I, arteriography (Table 10–2) and the other studies mentioned above continue to be utilized for evaluation of injuries in these zones.

Table 10–2. Indications for arteriography following trauma.

Penetrating neck injuries: zones I and III and selected zone II
Suspected thoracic aortic rupture after indeterminate CT scan of the chest or transesophageal echocardiography
Pelvic fractures with massive hemorrhage
Penetrating extremity trauma associated with an abnormal pulse or Doppler pressure index such as the ankle-brachial index or wrist-brachial index
Knee dislocation

Treatment & Disposition

Treat hemorrhagic shock as indicated (Chapter 9). Prompt surgical consultation with or without arteriography is essential.

TENSION PNEUMOTHORAX
(See also Chapter 24.)

 ESSENTIALS OF DIAGNOSIS

- *Respiratory distress.*
- *Asymmetrical lung sounds.*
- *May or may not have external signs of trauma to chest wall.*
- *Tracheal shift is late sign.*
- *Distended neck veins may not be present in patients with hypovolemic shock.*

General Considerations

Tension pneumothorax interferes with venous return to the heart and thus decreases cardiac output and perfusion. Oxygenation is also impaired. A simple pneumothorax can be converted to a tension pneumothorax during positive pressure ventilation.

Clinical Findings

Tension pneumothorax is manifested by respiratory distress, distended neck veins, contralateral tracheal shift, asymmetry of breath sounds, and percussion tympany. Chest x-ray confirms the diagnosis; however, tension pneumothorax is a clinical diagnosis and treatment should not be delayed while waiting for radiographs. Profound shock and cardiac arrest may be refractory to usual treatment unless the tension is relieved. Therefore, if a tension pneumothorax is clinically suspected, and an appropriate mechanism of injury is identified, emergent needle thoracostomy should be performed.

Treatment

Tension pneumothorax may be treated initially by inserting a large-bore (ie, 14-gauge) needle into the 2nd intercostal space, in the midclavicular line on the affected side. A rush of air confirms the diagnosis. If the tension pneumothorax is due to an open pneumothorax creating a 1-way valve (ie, sucking chest wound), then application of an occlusive dressing sealed on 3 sides can prevent the development of further tension. Definitive treatment is tube thoracostomy in the fifth intercostal space, in the midaxillary line, as soon as possible (Chapters 6 and 24).

Disposition

Hospitalization is required for all patients with tension pneumothorax.

FLAIL CHEST
(See also Chapter 24.)

 ESSENTIALS OF DIAGNOSIS

- *Paradoxical chest wall motion.*
- *Respiratory distress.*
- *If signs of hypoxia or ventilatory failure are present, intubation is required.*

Clinical Findings

Flail chest is diagnosed clinically with careful inspection and palpation revealing paradoxical motion of the flail segment (inward movement with inspiration and outward movement with expiration).

Treatment

The goal is maintenance of adequate ventilation and careful fluid resuscitation, because the underlying injuries are sensitive to both inadequate resuscitation of shock and fluid overload. In some patients, flail chest can be managed without mechanical ventilation; however, intubation and mechanical ventilation may be necessary at the first sign of ventilatory failure or hypoxia. All patients with flail chest should receive supplemental oxygen.

Disposition

All patients with flail chest require hospitalization in an intensive care unit and may eventually require intubation as pulmonary contusions worsen and the increased work of breathing and pain contribute to poor respiratory function.

PULMONARY CONTUSION
(See also Chapter 24.)

 ESSENTIALS OF DIAGNOSIS

- *Respiratory distress.*
- *Worsening hypoxia with time.*

- *Radiographic findings often delayed in comparison to a rapid decline in respiratory function based on clinical examination.*
- *Diffuse pulmonary opacities on chest x-ray.*

General Considerations

Pulmonary contusion is one of the most common potentially lethal injuries to the chest, with respiratory failure developing over time. The severity of injury generally peaks between 48 and 72 hours.

Clinicial Findings

The diagnosis of pulmonary contusion is based on chest x-ray findings of diffuse opacities following traumatic chest trauma. A high index of suspicion is required, because radiographic findings may be delayed more than 24 hours. CT scan of the chest can confirm the diagnosis earlier than chest x-ray.

Treatment

Careful monitoring of oxygenation and ventilation (including oxygen saturation and arterial blood gases) is required. Administer supplemental oxygen as indicated. Any patient with significant hypoxia (PaO_2 < 65 or oxygen saturation < 90%) despite high-flow supplemental oxygen should be intubated and mechanically ventilated. Associated medical conditions (ie, chronic obstructive pulmonary disease, renal failure) increase the likelihood that a patient will require early intubation and ventilatory assistance.

Disposition

Hospitalize all patients for observation and monitoring.

CARDIAC TAMPONADE
(SEE ALSO CHAPTER 24.)

 ESSENTIALS OF DIAGNOSIS

- *Hypotension.*
- *Jugular venous distension may or may not be present.*
- *Muffled heart sounds.*
- *Electrical alternans on electrocardiogram.*
- *Positive FAST exam for pericardial fluid.*

General Considerations

Cardiac tamponade most commonly results from penetrating injuries and interferes with diastolic filling, thus leading to inadequate cardiac output and end organ perfusion.

Clinical Findings

The classic presentation consists of the Beck triad, although this is not always present. The triad includes hypotension, jugular venous distention, and muffled heart tones. However, jugular venous distention is common in supine patients without tamponade and may not be seen in hypovolemic patients with tamponade. In addition, muffled heart sounds are difficult to hear during a noisy resuscitation. Although not commonly seen, electrical alternans on electrocardiogram (ECG) (positive and negative QRS axis alternating with each beat) is pathognomonic for the condition. A FAST exam can rapidly confirm the diagnosis (Chapters 6 and 9).

A. Penetrating Injury

Suspect cardiac tamponade in any patient with penetrating trauma to one of the hemithoraces, because it has been estimated to occur in approximately 2% of patients with anterior penetrating chest injury. However, injury to the heart can occur even with remote wounds (ie, abdomen, back, and flank), and especially following gunshot injuries.

B. Blunt Trauma

Blunt anterior chest trauma occasionally causes tamponade, with blood originating from injuries to the heart itself, the great vessels, or pericardial vessels. Associated myocardial contusion is common, and the clinical findings of tamponade may be delayed.

Treatment

If cardiac tamponade is suspected before the patient is in extremis, an emergency echocardiogram can be useful in confirming the diagnosis. Studies have shown transesophageal echocardiogram (TEE) to be nearly 100% accurate in diagnosis of posttraumatic pericardial tamponade. Pericardiocentesis (Chapter 24) may be beneficial as temporary treatment; however, all patients with a positive pericardiocentesis after trauma require open thoracotomy to further evaluate the heart and great vessels.

If shock is rapidly progressive despite treatment or if cardiac arrest occurs due to tamponade, immediate emergency thoracotomy is required in order to decompress the pericardium (Chapter 24).

Disposition

Immediate hospitalization and operative thoracotomy are required.

MYOCARDIAL CONTUSION
(See also Chapter 24.)

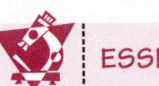 **ESSENTIALS OF DIAGNOSIS**

- *High-velocity blunt chest trauma.*
- *New conduction abnormalities on electrocardiogram.*
- *Hypotension.*
- *Wall motion abnormalities on echocardiogram.*

Clinical Findings

Suspect myocardial contusion (also known as blunt cardiac injury) in any patient who sustains high-velocity blunt chest trauma. The classic mechanism is an unrestrained driver in a head-on motor vehicle collision, in which a bent steering wheel or deformed steering column results. Clinically important sequelae include hypotension and wall motion abnormalities on 2-dimensional echocardiography, although significant conduction abnormalities may be the most potentially lethal manifestations and usually occur in the first 12 hours following injury. Unlike myocardial infarction, the contused area usually heals completely; however, a significant number of patients may have a clinically significant decrease in cardiac output. The diagnosis is established via ECG; unexplained sinus tachycardia is the most common finding. Other ECG abnormalities associated with the condition include arrhythmias (both atrial and ventricular), ST and T wave changes, and heart blocks. Echocardiogram and elevated cardiac enzymes have also been used to evaluate myocardial contusion, although they are not usually recommended as screening tools because they are unreliable and do not predict complications.

Treatment

Treat arrhythmias as indicated (Chapter 35). Obtain serial ECGs to assess for changes (including premature ventricular contractions, atrial fibrillation, bundle branch block, and ST-segment abnormalities).

Disposition

There is evidence that hemodynamically stable patients younger than age 55 years, with normal ECGs and no significant medical history, can be discharged to home. However, all other patients with significant blunt chest trauma should be considered for admission with continuous cardiac monitoring and observation for 12–24 hours.

TRAUMATIC AORTIC RUPTURE
(See also Chapter 24.)

 ESSENTIALS OF DIAGNOSIS

- *Mechanism of injury at risk for aortic rupture.*
- *X-ray findings consistent with aortic rupture.*
- *Positive definitive diagnostic study such as CT scan, aortography, or transesophageal echocardiogram.*

Clinical Findings

The diagnosis of traumatic aortic rupture requires a high index of suspicion, based on mechanism of injury (eg, deceleration injuries, pedestrian struck by a vehicle, falls > 30 feet) and radiographic findings. Making the diagnosis can be difficult because specific signs and symptoms are frequently absent and the physical examination is neither sensitive nor specific.

A. SYMPTOMS AND SIGNS

Pseudocoarctation, with blood pressure higher in the upper extremities than in the lower extremities; diminished femoral pulses; or a new harsh systolic murmur suggest the possibility of aortic injury. However, up to 50% of patients are without external evidence of chest trauma.

B. X-RAY FINDINGS

The following findings on chest x-ray indicate aortic injury:

- Widened mediastinum (> 8 cm on supine x-ray)
- Tracheal or nasogastric tube deviation to the right
- Widening of the right paratracheal stripe (> 5 mm)
- Depression of the left main-stem bronchus
- Indistinct aortic knob
- Left apical capping

C. OTHER IMAGING STUDIES

Although helical CT scanning of the chest with intravenous contrast is highly sensitive for aortic injury, aortography remains the gold standard for diagnosis. TEE has also been reported to have very high sensitivity and specificity for thoracic aortic injury. Although not widely practiced for evaluation of traumatic aortic in-

jury, TEE can be performed in the unstable patient either in the emergency department or in the operating room.

Treatment & Disposition

Patients with significant blunt chest trauma and possible aortic rupture should be hospitalized for surgical consultation, diagnostic studies, and immediate surgery if indicated. Unstable patients require immediate thoracotomy. Otherwise, support blood pressure with intravenous crystalloids and blood, and maintain hematocrit at greater than 30%. Maintain systolic blood pressure at 100–120, and use β-blockade (ie, esmolol) and afterload reduction (ie, nitroprusside) to control hypertension.

Zinck SE: Radiographic and CT findings in blunt chest trauma. J Thorac Imag 2000;15:87. [PMID: 10798627] (Review of the use of CT scan to diagnose traumatic chest injuries. Includes incidence of common injuries and diagnostic criteria.)

ABDOMINAL TRAUMA
(See also Chapter 25.)

 ESSENTIALS OF DIAGNOSIS

- *Mechanism of injury.*
- *Abdominal tenderness, distension, rigidity, or bruising.*
- *FAST exam, DPL, or CT scan is diagnostic.*
- *Laboratory studies: CBC, amylase, lactate.*

General Considerations

Significant amounts of blood may be present in the abdominal cavity without any dramatic change in appearance or abdominal dimensions. Injuries may be blunt (related to compression or crushing injury or deceleration) or penetrating. In blunt injuries, the spleen is the most commonly injured organ, and in penetrating injuries, the liver and small bowel are the most commonly injured organs.

Clinical Findings

History, including mechanism of injury, and physical examination (with involuntary muscle guarding as a reliable sign of peritoneal irritation) must be supported by further diagnostic studies, unless the patient has no history of abdominal injury, is alert and oriented, and has a completely unremarkable abdominal examination. Laboratory studies include complete blood count, electrolytes, lactate, serum alcohol, urine drug screen, and urine pregnancy test as indicated. Radiographic studies include FAST exam and CT scan of the abdomen with intravenous, oral, or occasionally rectal contrast. DPL may be required for evaluation of unstable patients when ultrasound is not available or the results are equivocal.

A. Stable Patients

Hemodynamically stable patients may be sent to the radiology suite for CT scanning of the abdomen, followed by DPL if the CT scan is negative and a strong suspicion for bowel injury remains. A negative CT scan may be followed by serial abdominal examinations or serial FAST exams.

B. Unstable Patients

Hemodynamically unstable patients should remain in the emergency department and undergo FAST examination. If the FAST exam is positive and the patient subsequently stabilizes, then CT scanning of the abdomen with intravenous or oral contrast can be performed for further diagnosis and assessment of the extent of injury. Otherwise, the unstable patient with a positive FAST exam requires laparotomy. If the initial FAST exam is negative, but a high index of suspicion for intra-abdominal injury remains, then DPL or serial FAST exams may be performed. A positive DPL is an unstable patient requires laparotomy.

Treatment & Disposition

Treatment is determined by the results of the above-noted studies and may include operative or nonoperative treatment of specific organ injuries depending on the injury severity and the patient's stability. Serial abdominal examinations or serial FAST exams are indicated for patients undergoing nonoperative treatment of intra-abdominal organ injury.

Boulanger BR, Rozycki GS, Rodriquez A: Sonographic assessment of traumatic injury. Surg Clin North Am 1999;79:6. [PMID: 10625980] (Review of the FAST examination in general, with historical perspectives and possible future applications.)

Boulanger BR et al: The routine use of sonography in penetrating torso injury is beneficial. J Trauma 2001;51:2. [PMID: 11493792] (Description of the use of the FAST exam at a level I trauma center and its benefit in early identification of intraperitoneal injury.)

Chiu WC et al: Abdominal injuries without hemoperitoneum: a potential limitation of focused abdominal sonography for trauma (FAST). J Trauma 1997;42:617. [PMID: 9137247] (Article providing evidence as to why a negative FAST exam does not definitively rule out intraperitoneal injury.)

HEAD TRAUMA
(See also Chapter 22.)

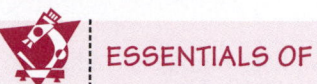

ESSENTIALS OF DIAGNOSIS

- *Evidence of external trauma.*
- *Altered mental status with or without focal neurologic findings.*
- *Hemotympanum, Battle sign, or raccoon eyes.*
- *Unequal or unreactive pupils.*
- *Decreasing Glasgow Coma Scale score.*

Clinical Findings

A. Symptoms and Signs

Suspect head injury in any trauma patient with cranial lacerations or hematomas, and in any patient with an altered mental status with or without focal neurologic findings.

Examine the scalp and cranium for evidence of lacerations, hematomas, or other structural deformities (ie, depressions). Examine the nose and ears for any clear fluid, which must be assumed to be cerebrospinal fluid.

Physical examination findings suggestive of a basilar skull fracture include hemotympanum, cerebrospinal fluid leakage from the nose or ears, a postauricular hematoma (Battle sign), bilateral periorbital ecchymosis (raccoon eyes), or 7th cranial nerve palsy.

B. Neurologic Examination

Perform a rapid and directed neurologic exam on all patients. The GCS is used to quantify neurologic findings and allows a uniformed, standardized description of head injury severity. It assesses eye opening and verbal and motor responses. This standardized format allows for rapid identification of changes in neurologic status on subsequent evaluation. In addition, the following factors should be evaluated:

- Level of consciousness: a simplified approach uses the AVPU mnemonic (**a**wake, responds to **v**erbal or **p**ainful stimuli, and **u**nresponsive).
- Pupillary response, extraocular movements, and the presence or absence of decorticate or decerebrate posturing.
- General motor function and motor response to painful stimuli.
- Deep tendon reflexes, including assessment of Babinski reflex.

Serial neurologic exams are used to identify changes in neurologic status.

C. IMAGING STUDIES

CT scan of the head without contrast should be performed on all patients suspected of having a closed head injury following trauma, especially if there is a history of more than a momentary loss of consciousness, amnesia, persistent vomiting, or severe headache.

Treatment

An initial goal is to achieve euvolemic fluid status, because fluid overload or dehydration can be detrimental. In addition, the goal is to maintain a P_{CO_2} of 35–40 mm Hg, with hyperventilation indicated only for impending uncal herniation. Even when hyperventilation is indicated, the P_{CO_2} needs to be maintained above 25 mm Hg. Mannitol may be given as an osmotic diuretic for signs of increasing intracranial pressure. Decompressive craniotomy or burr holes may be indicated for extremely rapid neurologic deterioration.

GENITOURINARY TRAUMA
(See also Chapter 26.)

 ESSENTIALS OF DIAGNOSIS

- *Evidence of pelvic injury or fracture.*
- *Blood at urinary meatus, scrotal or perineal hematoma, high-riding prostate, or vaginal lacerations.*

Clinical Findings

Injuries such as pelvic fractures are often associated with genitourinary injuries. Initial physical examination findings suggestive of genitourinary injury include blood at the urinary meatus, scrotal or perineal hematoma, or a high-riding, ballotable prostate on rectal examination in males. Patients with blood at the urinary meatus should undergo a retrograde urethrogram prior to insertion of an indwelling urinary catheter to identify injuries anterior to the urogenital diaphragm. If a catheter is placed and gross hematuria is identified, then obtain a cystogram to identify injuries posterior to the urogenital diaphragm. Renal or ureteral injuries in hemodynamically stable patients are evaluated by CT scan of the abdomen with intravenous contrast.

Treatment

Treat shock as indicated.

Disposition

Hospitalize patients as required. Obtain urologic consultation. Hematuria without identifiable genitourinary or renal structural abnormalities may be followed by a urologist on an outpatient basis.

EXTREMITY TRAUMA
(See also Chapters 28 & 29.)

 ESSENTIALS OF DIAGNOSIS

- *Deformities.*
- *Swelling, soft tissue ecchymosis.*
- *Abnormal neurovascular examination.*
- *Early splinting decreases further damage.*

General Considerations

The goal in the initial assessment and management of extremity injuries is to rapidly identify injuries that pose a threat to life or limb. Early definitive management can prevent or limit complications from extremity injuries that can lead to long-term loss of function.

Clinical Findings

During the secondary survey, examine all bones and joints, and obtain x-rays at 90-degree angles to one another of areas of suspected injury.

Crush injuries are characterized by massive swelling and soft tissue ecchymosis, and are suggested by the mechanism of injury. They place the patient at risk for developing a compartment syndrome, with immediate or delayed neurovascular compromise.

Treatment

Splinting of fractures (Chapter 28) prevents excessive fracture site motion, which helps control blood loss, reduce pain, and prevent further soft tissue or neurovascular damage. Cover open fractures with sterile saline-moistened dressings. Administer intravenous antibiotics (ie, cefazolin, 1 g ± penicillin and aminoglycoside depending on the type and severity of contamination) and tetanus prophylaxis if indicated. Obtain orthopedic consultation.

If compartment syndrome is suspected, compartment pressures should be measured (> 35 mm Hg exceeds the tissue perfusion pressure and suggests impending neurovascular compromise). Fasciotomy may be required. Evaluate patients for rhabdomyolysis via measurement of creatinine kinase and urine myoglobin. Treatment of associated myoglobinuria consists of aggressive fluid resuscitation and osmotic diuresis to maintain high renal tubular volume and urine flow. Alkalinization of the urine with sodium bicarbonate reduces the precipitation of myoglobin in the renal tubules.

Disposition

Hospitalize patients for observation or surgery as indicated.

SPINAL TRAUMA
(See also Chapter 27.)

 ESSENTIALS OF DIAGNOSIS

- *Immobilize to prevent further damage.*
- *Direct spinal tenderness on physical examination.*
- *Swelling or deformity over spine.*
- *Neurologic deficits in extremities.*
- *Sensory loss.*
- *Decreased rectal sphincter tone or perineal sensation.*

General Considerations

Proper immobilization of the entire spine with a semirigid cervical collar, head blocks, and long spine board are required until vertebral or spinal cord injuries are excluded.

Clinical Findings

Evaluation consists of logrolling the patient to examine the entire spine, including a rectal examination to evaluate rectal sphincter tone and perineal sensation. Evaluate any painful areas radiographically, and perform a detailed motor and sensory examination on all extremities. Neurologic deficits may or may not be present initially; therefore, a high index of suspicion must be maintained while in-line spinal immobilization is continued.

Treatment & Disposition

Immobilization and hospitalization are required for patients with evidence of spinal trauma, with the exception of alert and oriented patients with a thoracolumbar strain or those with a cervical strain, who may be discharged to home in a cervical collar with outpatient follow-up in 1–2 weeks for reevaluation for possible ligamentous injury. Orthopedic or neurologic consultation is indicated for fractures or neurologic deficits.

Grabber MA et al: Cervical spine radiographs in the trauma patient. Am Fam Phys 1999;59(2):331. [PMID: 9930127] (Summary of the clinical and radiographic evaluation of the cervical spine. Includes useful tables, algorithms, and x-rays with accompanying drawings.)

Dyspnea, Respiratory Distress, & Respiratory Failure

11

Sabina A. Braithwaite, MD, & Debra G. Perina, MD[1]

Immediate Management of Life-Threatening Problems
- Cardiac Arrest
- Severe Upper Airway Obstruction
- Altered Mental Status with Shallow Breathing
- Tension Pneumothorax
- Massive Aspiration
- Severe Pulmonary Edema
- Severe Asthma, Chronic Obstructive Pulmonary Disease, or Pulmonary Fibrosis

Further Diagnostic Evaluation

Emergency Treatment of Specific Disorders
- Chest Wall Defects
    1. Flail Chest
    2. Neuromuscular Diseases
- Pulmonary Collapse
    1. Pneumothorax
    2. Hydrothorax & Hemothorax (Pleural Fluid or Blood)
    3. Massive Atelectasis

Loss of Functional Lung Parenchyma
1. Pulmonary Edema
2. Pneumonia
3. Diffuse Interstitial Pulmonary Disease
4. Aspiration

Airway Disease
1. Upper Airway Obstruction
2. Asthma, Chronic Obstructive Pulmonary Disease, & Cystic Fibrosis

Pulmonary Vascular Disease
1. Acute Pulmonary Embolism
2. Chronic Pulmonary Vascular Obstruction (Repeated Small Pulmonary Emboli)

Miscellaneous Conditions
1. Pleurisy
2. Metabolic Acidosis
3. Anemia, Pregnancy, & Thyrotoxicosis
4. Neurogenic Hyperventilation
5. Psychogenic Hyperventilation & Pulmonary Neurosis

■ IMMEDIATE MANAGEMENT OF LIFE-THREATENING PROBLEMS (See Figure 11–1.)

Assess Severity & Give Immediate Necessary Care

The first step in the evaluation of the patient with suspected respiratory disease is to quickly assess the severity by noting the patient's general appearance and heart and respiratory rate. Rapidly perform a focused examination of skin color and temperature, oropharynx, neck, lungs, heart, chest, and extremities. Any patient with severe respiratory distress should receive immediate oxygen supplementation during assessment and treatment. If severe respiratory distress is present (eg, too short of breath for speech)—and especially if it has developed over a short period of time (minutes to hours) —proceed rapidly with simultaneous evaluation and therapy (see Figure 11–1). As in all life-threatening conditions, providing and maintaining an adequate airway is the first consideration.

Assess Adequacy of Oxygenation

In the patient with severe respiratory distress, assessment and management are concurrent. Clinical assessment of airway and ventilatory status drives the decision-making process. The clinical picture is augmented by immediately available data to allow rapid decisions and treatment interventions required by the critically ill patient.

---

[1]This chapter is a revision of the chapter by John Mills, MD, & John M. Luce, MD, from the 4th edition.

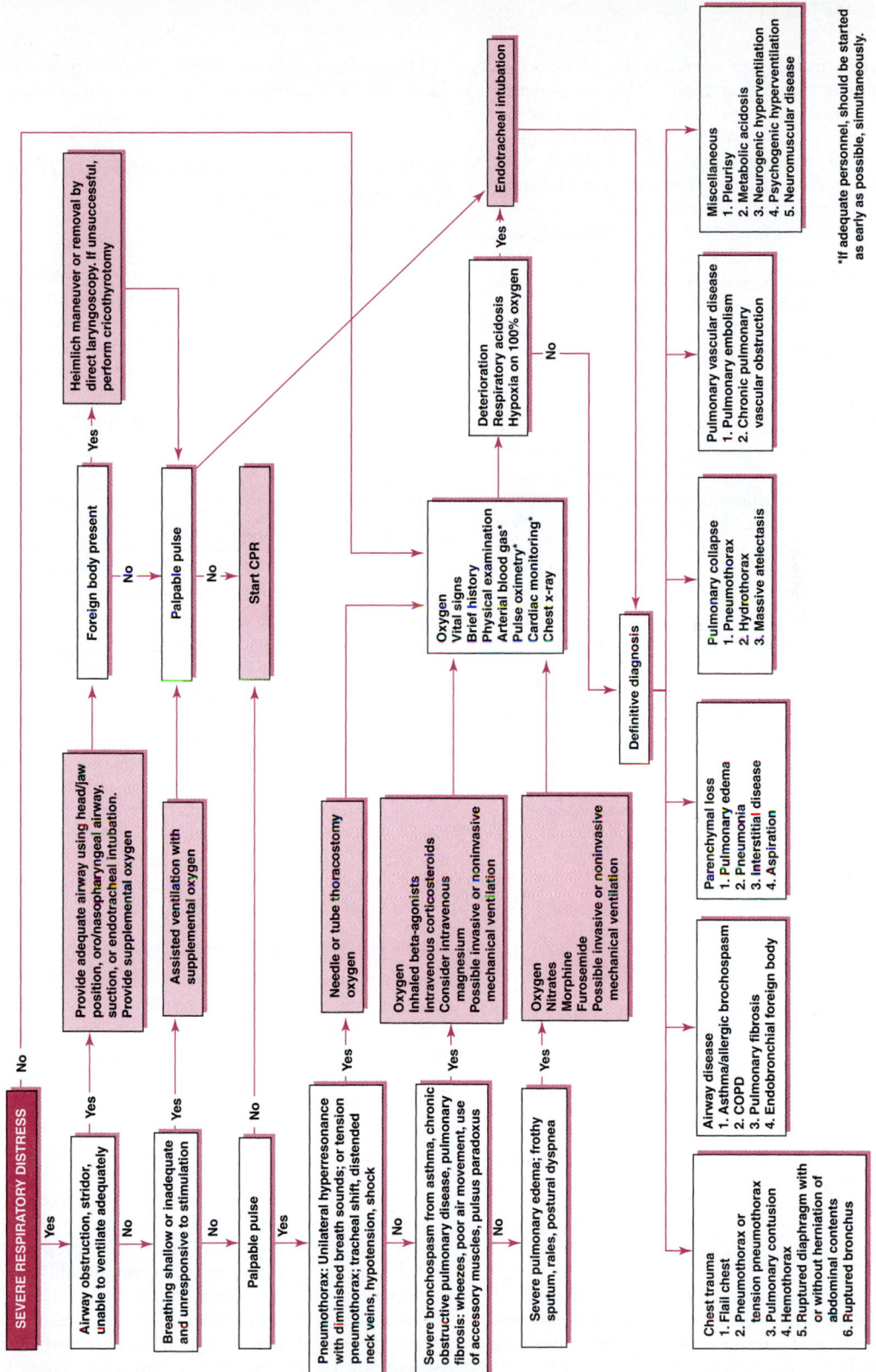

Figure 11–1. Management of severe respiratory distress.

223

Signs including inability to speak, stridor, diaphoresis, accessory muscle use, tripod position, pulsus paradox, and altered mental status may be associated with severe respiratory distress. Pulse oximetry, waveform capnography, and rapid electrolyte and pH machines offer prompt, invaluable data on oxygenation, gas exchange, and acid-base status. This information will drive treatment decisions and urgency for interventions such as noninvasive or invasive mechanical ventilation, or surgical airway. Additional modalities such as imaging, arterial blood gas sampling, and other laboratory tests that require more time are used to refine the treatment plan following initial assessment and stabilization.

Pulse oximetry measures the percent oxygen saturation of hemoglobin and provides a guide to the oxygenation of arterial blood. However, because hyperventilation can raise the PO_2, a normal saturation may be observed despite an abnormal elevated alveolar-arterial PO_2 gradient. Pulse oximetry provides no information about PCO_2 tension or adequacy of ventilation. It is inaccurate when carbon monoxide is present in the blood. Probes may not read properly in patients with hypotension, severe vasoconstriction, or severe peripheral vascular disease. Patients with severe hypoxemia (eg, saturation < 90%) or ventilatory insufficiency should also have arterial blood gas determinations. Recall that a PaO_2 of 60 mm Hg is equivalent to a saturation of 90%. However, patients on supplemental oxygen with normal ventilation should have PaO_2 of greater than 40 mm Hg and so should have a saturation of 100%. Because oximetry readings begin to change only toward the lower end of this gradient, reading less than 95% (particularly in patients receiving supplemental oxygen) should be addressed promptly, before the patient becomes hypoxic.

CARDIAC ARREST

Clinical Findings

In unresponsive patients, check for airway patency and properly position the head and jaw to open the airway (Chapter 7). Evaluate respiratory effort and assist ventilations if inadequate. Assess for presence of a carotid pulse. In cardiac arrest, terminal gasping respirations may simulate respiratory distress; conversely, conditions that produce severe respiratory distress may lead to hypoxic cardiac arrest.

Treatment & Disposition

Start cardiopulmonary resuscitation (CPR) at once if the carotid pulse is not palpable, and continue with appropriate basic and advanced life support measures (Chapter 7).

Hospitalization in an intensive care setting is mandatory for these patients if they survive initial resuscitation.

SEVERE UPPER AIRWAY OBSTRUCTION (SEE ALSO CHAPTER 8.)

Clinical Findings

Listen for inspiratory and expiratory stridor. Look for increased work of breathing, which may include suprasternal, supraclavicular, and intercostal retractions. When coupled with cyanosis, significant upper airway obstruction is present. Patients with complete upper airway obstruction are in extremis and will lose consciousness and progress to cardiac arrest quickly without definitive treatment.

Treatment

A. AWAY FROM HOSPITAL

(See also Chapter 7.) Remove possible obstructing foreign bodies by performing the Heimlich maneuver repeatedly until successful. If the victim loses consciousness, call for help to activate the Emergency Medical Services system, and perform 6–10 supine subdiaphragmatic thrusts (supine Heimlich), followed by a finger sweep and attempt to ventilate. Repeat these steps until the obstruction is cleared. If the victim is markedly obese or in the third trimester of pregnancy, use closed chest compressions instead of the Heimlich maneuver. A foreign body may be removed by trained rescue personnel under direct visualization using a laryngoscope and suction device or forceps. Rarely, cricothyrotomy may be necessary, but it should be performed by rescuers trained in the technique.

B. IN A HOSPITAL EMERGENCY DEPARTMENT

Immediate direct laryngoscopy is indicated if the obstruction cannot be removed quickly. This may be the first step in emergency department treatment. Foreign bodies may be removed under direct visualization using forceps. Obstruction caused by soft tissue swelling or local edema (as in anaphylaxis or angioedema) may be relieved by passage of an endotracheal tube. Anaphylaxis requires specific treatment (Chapter 9). Epiglottitis may cause upper airway obstruction in either children or adults; if this condition is suspected, avoid patient agitation or repositioning until prepared to provide a definitive airway (Chapter 32). A physician skilled in difficult airway management should care for these patients and may use adjuncts such as fiberoptic intubating bronchoscopy for diagnosis or securing the airway. If less invasive methods fail, immediate cricothyrotomy or tracheostomy is required (Chapter 6).

Disposition

Patients with easy, uncomplicated removal of an obstructing foreign body may be sent home following a period of observation with instructions to eat more slowly, chew more thoroughly, and swallow more carefully. Patients who lost consciousness but otherwise appear well should be examined and observed in the emergency department. Patients requiring intubation or surgery or who remain symptomatic should be hospitalized for treatment and observation.

ALTERED MENTAL STATUS WITH SHALLOW BREATHING

Clinical Findings

Altered mental status in a patient with obvious respiratory distress may be due to carbon dioxide retention or profound tissue hypoxia. However, the patient may have unlabored shallow respirations. Absence of a gag reflex (unprotected airway) or severe hypercapnia or hypoxemia on arterial blood gas studies (ie, respiratory failure) together with clinical assessment of underlying causes of altered mental status combine to support the necessity for endotracheal intubation in the emergency department.

Treatment

Ventilatory support should be given until endotracheal intubation can be accomplished. Provide high-flow (10–15 L/min) supplemental oxygen by nonrebreather mask or bag-valve-mask ventilation, as indicated.

As soon as oxygenation and carbon dioxide exchange have been partially corrected by assisted ventilation, the patient should be intubated. An endotracheal tube provides a definitive airway by preventing aspiration and facilitating effective respiratory support.

If there is doubt about the need for intubation, err on the side of intubation. Evaluation and treatment of other causes of altered mental status should follow airway management (Chapters 17, 18, and 20).

Disposition

Hospitalize these patients for further diagnosis and treatment.

TENSION PNEUMOTHORAX

Clinical Findings

Severe respiratory distress associated with tension pneumothorax usually occurs following blunt or penetrating chest trauma (including chest compressions during CPR). Rarely, it may occur spontaneously in patients with spontaneous pneumothorax. Contralateral tracheal shift, ipsilateral hyperresonant hemithorax with markedly decreased or absent breath sounds, hypotension, and distended neck veins are classical signs, although they are not invariably present. Treatment should be based on findings of acute cardiorespiratory collapse in the appropriate clinical setting.

Treatment

Give oxygen, 10–15 L/min by nonrebreather mask. Perform tube thoracostomy (Chapter 6). For immediate relief, perform needle thoracostomy in the 2nd intercostal space in the midclavicular line with a large-bore (14- to 16-gauge) needle if delay is anticipated in obtaining equipment for chest tube insertion. The risk of needle or tube thoracostomy without x-ray confirmation of tension pneumothorax must be weighed against the severity of respiratory distress or hemodynamic compromise and the likelihood of the clinical diagnosis. If the procedure is properly performed, the risks of tube thoracostomy are minimal even in a patient without pneumothorax.

Disposition

Hospitalize these patients for further treatment.

MASSIVE ASPIRATION

Clinical Findings

If the patient with severe respiratory distress has vomitus with particulate matter in the oropharynx, significant aspiration is likely.

Treatment

Clear the airway with a large-bore, hard-tipped suction device. Endotracheal intubation is often required because of depressed consciousness with hypercapnia and severe hypoxemia, or inability to protect the airway. Begin oxygen, 10–15 L/min by nonrebreather mask.

Antibiotics and corticosteroids have been suggested by some authorities because of the risk of bacterial pneumonia. However, there is evidence that antibiotics are ineffective acutely in this situation, because the initial infiltrate appearing on chest x-ray is due to a chemical pneumonitis. Corticosteroids have also not been shown to be effective in decreasing the death rate from aspiration pneumonitis. In addition, pneumonia due to gram-negative organisms is more likely to develop in patients who have received corticosteroids than in those who have not.

Disposition

Hospitalize these patients for definitive treatment.

SEVERE PULMONARY EDEMA
(See also Chapters 33 & 34.)

Clinical Findings

Patients with severe pulmonary edema are extremely dyspneic, especially in the supine position, and may cough up frothy, pink sputum. Rales (crackles) are present, and the chest x-ray usually reveals bilateral interstitial infiltrates (Figure 11–2). Fever is uncommon. In cardiogenic pulmonary edema, other manifestations of heart failure are often present: tachycardia, distended neck veins or hepatojugular reflux, peripheral edema, cardiomegaly, or a ventricular (S_3) gallop. Wheezing may also be present (so-called cardiac asthma, probably caused by reflex bronchospasm). Patients with cardiogenic pulmonary edema often give a history of heart disease and have had pulmonary edema before.

Noncardiac pulmonary edema has many causes. Drug overdose (especially from heroin and other narcotics), septic shock, pulmonary contusion, pancreatitis, and fat embolism are the most common causes.

Treatment

Aggressive early management can decrease the need for intubation as well as the length of stay in intensive care. All patients with severe pulmonary edema should receive supplemental oxygen, 10–15 L/min, by nonrebreather mask. If the patient remains hypoxic, noninvasive positive-pressure ventilation (NIPPV) via continuous positive airway pressure (CPAP) or bilevel positive airway pressure (BiPAP) may allow adequate gas exchange for hours to days until pharmacologic interventions produce improvement. Endotracheal intubation rates in congestive heart failure are significantly decreased by NIPPV use. Endotracheal intubation with mechanical ventilation may be required if the patient does not tolerate NIPPV or has refractory hypoxia and respiratory acidosis.

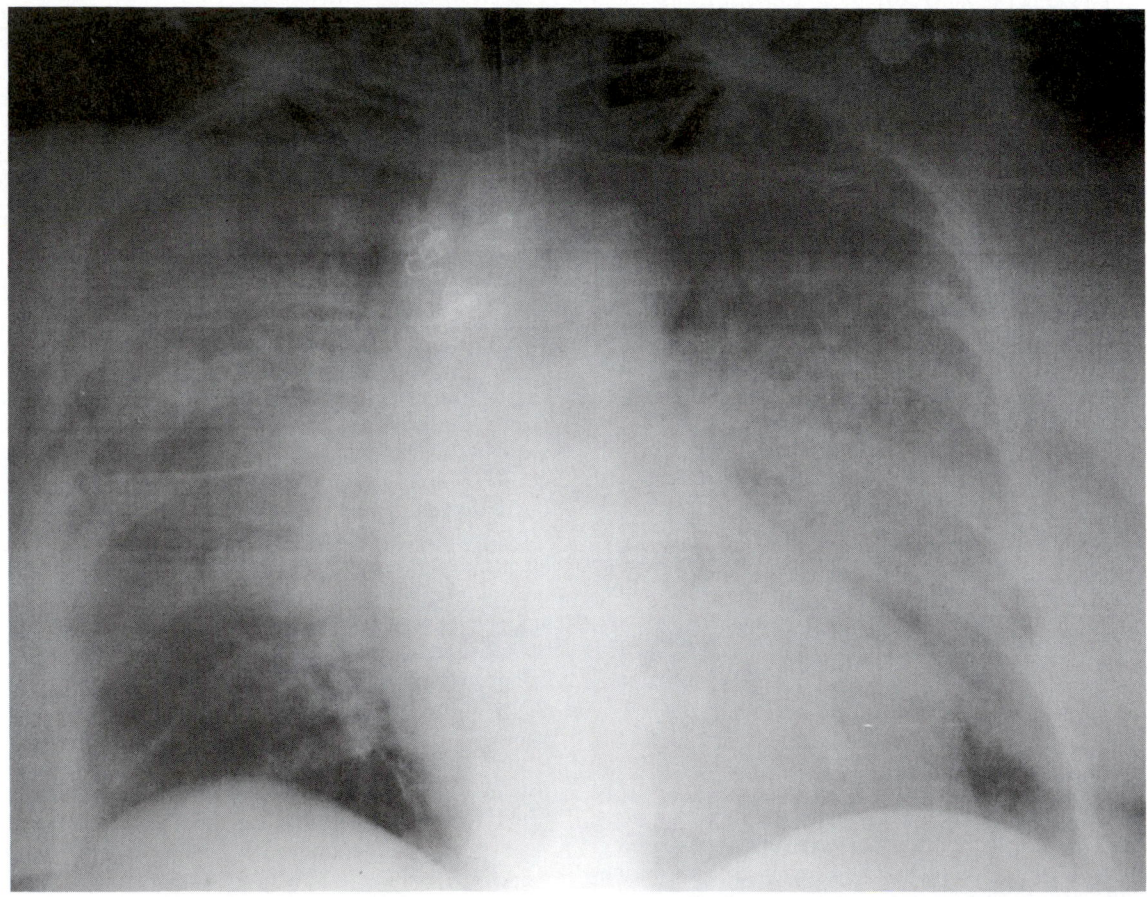

Figure 11–2. The radiographic appearance of severe pulmonary edema.

Morphine, 2–10 mg intravenously; and/or nitrates given sublingually (0.4 mg), cutaneously (1–2 inches of nitroglycerin ointment), or by intravenous infusion (begin at 5–10 μg/min, and titrate to desired effect) cause peripheral vasodilation. Diuresis using furosemide, 40–80 mg intravenously, or bumetanide, 1–2 mg intravenously, will often improve respiratory function in patients with both cardiogenic and noncardiogenic pulmonary edema. Use caution with morphine, because its use is associated with increased endotracheal intubation rates. Angiotensin-converting enzyme inhibitors (ACE-I) have the opposite effect in congestive heart failure.

Additional treatment depends on whether the edema is cardiogenic or noncardiogenic (Chapters 33 and 34). Determination of a pulmonary artery wedge pressure is essential to the differential of these conditions. This procedure is usually not performed in the emergency department. Long-term ACE-I therapy decreases readmission rates in patients with congestive heart failure.

Disposition

Hospitalize these patients for further diagnosis and treatment. Some patients with a mild exacerbation of known cardiogenic pulmonary edema referable to an easily reversible cause such as medication or dietary noncompliance may be evaluated, diuresed, and observed in the emergency department. They may be discharged home with close follow-up when they return to baseline.

SEVERE ASTHMA, CHRONIC OBSTRUCTIVE PULMONARY DISEASE, OR PULMONARY FIBROSIS (See also Chapter 33.)

Clinical Findings

Patients with asthma, chronic obstructive pulmonary disease, or pulmonary fibrosis may present with severe dyspnea and respiratory distress similar to that found in patients with pulmonary edema. However, dyspnea in the former group of patients is less likely to be postural. Cough is common to the obstructive disorders, but sputum production is variable. Most important, patients with asthma, chronic obstructive pulmonary disease, or pulmonary fibrosis usually have wheezing on auscultation of the chest, unless tidal volume is inadequate. In such patients, the principal physical findings are tachypnea, tachycardia, cyanosis, chest hyperexpansion, and globally diminished breath sounds. In severe episodes, a pulsus paradoxus may be present. The use of the sternocleidomastoid muscles during inspiration is common, and intercostal retractions, nasal flaring, and tripod position may be noted. Chest x-ray shows only hyperexpanded lung fields unless another pathologic process such as bacterial pneumonia is present. These patients frequently do not have pneumonia; rather, viral or (rarely) bacterial tracheobronchitis or exposure to an allergen has exacerbated their chronic underlying disease. Multiple objective measures can be utilized to assess response to therapy. A visual analog scale or other validated dyspnea assessment tool, as well as peak expiratory flow rate or forced expiratory volume in 1 second, may be measured in the emergency department. These measurements can be used to follow improvement, compare the degree of obstruction to a known baseline, and guide treatment and disposition for a given patient.

Treatment

Several practice guidelines are available to help direct care. Further management of patients with these disorders is discussed in Chapter 33.

A. OXYGEN

Give oxygen, 1–3 L/min to raise arterial saturation to at least 95% or PO_2 to between 60 and 80 mm Hg without causing respiratory depression and a marked increase in arterial PCO_2. Pulse oximetry is preferred, but arterial blood gas analysis may be indicated to help direct therapy. Tracheal intubation and mechanical ventilation should be avoided but may be necessary if a patient is in acute respiratory failure. Do not withhold oxygen from the acutely hypoxic patient.

B. β-ADRENERGIC SYMPATHOMIMETIC BRONCHODILATORS

In adults, β-adrenergic sympathomimetic bronchodilators should be given in aerosol form if possible; otherwise, they may be given parenterally. A typical regimen is albuterol, 0.2–0.3 mL in 3 mL normal saline, delivered by nebulizer over 5 times every 30 minutes. β-agonists may be nebulized in combination with ipratropium bromide (0.5 mg, up to 3 doses). For patients who are able to use them properly, metered-dose inhalers are as efficacious as nebulized therapy.

In general, parenteral therapy offers little benefit over nebulization, except in the most extreme cases. If used, parenteral therapy includes epinephrine, 0.2–0.3 mL (1:1000 dilution) every 20–30 minutes subcutaneously, or terbutaline, 0.25 mg subcutaneously every 2–4 hours. Parenteral therapy may have value in younger patients with severe exacerbation. However, parenteral administration of sympathomimetics can produce marked tachycardia and may induce myocardial ischemia, especially in elderly patients or those with preexisting coronary artery disease. Therefore, they should be used cautiously in this group and be withheld if chest pain or extreme tachycardia develops.

C. CORTICOSTEROIDS

Corticosteroids should be given within the first hour of treatment to patients who do not respond adequately to nebulized or parenteral β-adrenergic agents alone. The recommended regimen is methylprednisolone, 125 mg intravenously initially, or prednisone, 60 mg orally. If the patient is to be discharged from the emergency department, a short course of oral steroids is warranted.

D. MAGNESIUM SULFATE

Magnesium sulfate has a bronchodilating effect that may be of benefit in asthma. Its use should be reserved for life-threatening bronchospasm that is refractory to all other interventions. Adult dosing of magnesium sulfate is 1–2 g intravenously over 15–30 minutes; pediatric dosage is 40 mg/kg intravenously. Effects are short-lived after the infusion is discontinued. Blood pressure should be monitored and the infusion stopped if hypotension occurs. Intravenous calcium should be immediately available to counteract cardiac dysrhythmias related to magnesium. Deep tendon reflexes will be lost once serum magnesium concentration reaches 7–10 mEq/L (normal concentration is 1.5–2.0 mEq/L); the infusion should be stopped if reflexes are lost. At higher concentrations, respiratory depression and cardiac arrest may occur. However, the dose used for asthma is relatively low (approximately one-fourth the dose used in preeclampsia).

Disposition

Hospitalize patients with significant bronchospasm that does not respond promptly to treatment, or those with moderate bronchospasm that fails to improve after several hours of treatment. Discharged patients should receive short-term outpatient corticosteroid therapy such as prednisone, 40–60 mg/d with or without a taper over 6–10 days.

Barton ED: Tension pneumothorax. Curr Opin Pulm Med 1999;5:269. [PMID: 10407699] (A review of the pathophysiology, diagnosis, and treatment of tension pneumothorax.)

Emerman CL et al: Prospective multicenter study of relapse following treatment for acute asthma among adults presenting to the emergency department. Chest 1999;115:919. [PMID: 10459087] (Study of patient factors associated with relapse following acute asthma treatment in the emergency department.)

Howes DS et al: Triage and the initial evaluation of the oral facial emergency. Emerg Clin North Am 2000;18:371. [PMID: 10967730] (A review of initial evaluation of facial emergencies to include acute airway obstruction.)

Hunt SA et al: ACC/AHA Guidelines for the Evaluation and Management of Chronic Heart Failure in the Adult: Executive Summary. A Report of the American College of Cardiology/American Heart Association Task Force on Practice Guidelines (Committee to Revise the 1995 Guidelines for the Evaluation and Management of Heart Failure). Circulation 2001;104:2996. [PMID: 11739319] (Provides evidence-based recommendations for prevention and treatment of heart failure in various stages.)

Kosowsky JM et al: Continuous and bilevel positive airway pressure in the treatment of acute cardiogenic pulmonary edema. Am J Emerg Med 2000;18:91. [PMID: 10674543] (Review of literature regarding use of noninvasive ventilatory support in acute congestive heart failure.)

Lee-Chiong TL Jr: Pulmonary aspiration. Compr Ther 1997;23:371. [PMID: 9239486] (A comprehensive review of pulmonary aspiration.)

Lerner DL et al: Prevention and treatment of upper airway obstruction in infants and children. Curr Opin Pediatr 1998;10:265. [PMID: 9716888] (A review of airway obstruction causes in the pediatric population.)

■ FURTHER DIAGNOSTIC EVALUATION

Diagnostic Information

A. DATA BASE

After supplemental oxygen has been started and life-threatening problems have been corrected, proceed as follows to construct an emergency cardiopulmonary data base:

1. Obtain brief history directed toward cardiopulmonary disease and comorbidities, including potential triggers or causes, previous similar episodes, previous need for mechanical ventilation, and duration of this attack of dyspnea.

2. Obtain complete list of prescribed and unprescribed medications (current and recent past), including most recent dosage history and history of steroid use.

3. Conduct physical examination of the heart, lungs, abdomen, extremities, and other areas as indicated.

4. Obtain complete blood count, urinalysis, serum creatinine or blood urea nitrogen, serum electrolytes, and glucose, depending on the patient's history and examination findings.

5. Monitor pulse oximetry and peak expiratory flow rate, and conduct dyspnea scale assessment. Arterial blood gas may be performed based on pulse oximetry or concomitant clinical findings.

6. Order chest x-ray and electrocardiogram, if indicated.

7. Order additional indicated tests such as D-dimer or other imaging studies (ie, chest computed tomography [CT] scan, angiogram, ventilation-perfusion scan).

B. INTERPRETATION OF DIAGNOSTIC DATA

Information from this data base usually will allow the emergency physician to identify the cause of dyspnea (further discussed below and in Table 11–1). The basis of this categorization is discussed below and in greater detail in Chapter 33.

Disposition

(See also specific conditions, below.) If the emergency data base suggests a significant acute abnormality, but an exact diagnosis cannot be made that would permit specific therapy to be started, hospitalize the patient even if the clinical status would not otherwise warrant hospitalization. Sometimes more than one abnormality is present in the same patient (eg, acute exacerbation of chronic bronchitis and pneumonia).

■ EMERGENCY TREATMENT OF SPECIFIC DISORDERS

CHEST WALL DEFECTS

1. Flail Chest

Clinical Findings

Posttraumatic flail chest is usually apparent on physical examination as painful paradoxical motion of the rib cage or sternum (inward with inhalation and outward with exhalation). Crepitation or subcutaneous emphysema may be noted on examination together with decreased breath sounds on the affected side.

Treatment

Provide supplemental oxygen. Use a bag-mask to support ventilation of patients with obvious hypoventilation. Continuously monitor pulse oximetry.

Intubation for respiratory support need not be performed immediately if saturation is greater than 90% or arterial blood gas levels are satisfactory (PO_2 > 65 mm Hg, PCO_2 < 44 mm Hg). However, endotracheal intubation and positive-pressure ventilation are likely to be required, and prolonged saturations of less than 95% or hypoventilation due to pain should trigger intervention.

Provide analgesia (morphine, 1–4 mg intravenously, or fentanyl, 25–50 μg intravenously), and watch carefully for signs of respiratory depression. Do not use analgesia if respiratory failure is imminent.

Disposition

All patients with flail chest injuries require hospitalization for treatment and evaluation of this and potential associated injuries.

2. Neuromuscular Diseases

Clinical Findings

Patients with dyspnea or respiratory distress associated with progressive neuromuscular disease usually have hypoventilation (decreased pulse oximetry readings or arterial blood gases showing hypoxemia and hypercapnia) and objective weakness of other muscle groups, though the latter is not always present. Among many possible causes are Guillain-Barré syndrome, myasthenia gravis, periodic paralysis, botulism, and tick paralysis.

Treatment & Disposition

Believe the patient's complaints of dyspnea, and evaluate respiratory status using pulse oximetry, arterial blood gas analysis, and pulmonary function tests (eg, vital capacity and maximal inspiratory force). Intubation may be postponed if initial blood gas levels are satisfactory. Specific therapy should focus on the neuromuscular disease (Chapter 18). Immediate hospitalization is indicated.

PULMONARY COLLAPSE

Moderate degrees of pulmonary collapse that do not cause severe respiratory distress or obvious physical findings can be apparent on chest X-ray. Treatment depends on the specific cause as discussed below.

1. Pneumothorax

Clinical Findings

The patient often has chest pain and severe respiratory distress, with decreased breath sounds and tympany elicited by chest percussion of the affected side. The degree of dyspnea or respiratory distress depends on the amount of collapse and on the degree of pressure (ie, tension pneumothorax). Chest x-ray shows lung collapse and air in the pleural space (Figure 11–3). Small amounts of fluid may also be present in the pleural space. Tension pneumothorax presents in a similar manner, and late findings include shift of the mediastinum away from the involved side, distended neck veins, hypotension, and shock.

Treatment

Immediate thoracostomy is indicated for bilateral pneumothoraces or unilateral tension pneumothorax, even if the patient appears stable, because sudden deterioration

Table 11–1. Essentials of diagnosis of diseases causing dyspnea and respiratory distress.[1]

Disorder	Specific Condition	Onset History	Symptoms Other Than Dyspnea	Signs	Chest X-ray	Comment
Chest wall defect	Flail chest.	Trauma.	Pain with respiration.	Paradoxical motion of chest wall.	Rib fractures.	Coexistent pneumothorax common.
	Muscular weakness.	Gradual onset.	Weakness of other muscles.	Weakness of non-respiratory muscles	Normal.	Diminished inspiratory force.
Pulmonary	Pneumothorax.	Sudden onset; occasionally trauma.	Cough and chest pain common.	Tympany and decreased breath sounds; decreased blood pressure and tracheal shift if tension.	Lung collapse; mediastinal shift if tension.	
	Hydrothorax.	Gradual onset.		Dullness and decreased breath sounds.	Pleural effusion (decubitus views)	
	Atelectasis.	Variable onset.		Variable.	Signs of atelectasis.	
Loss of functional lung parenchyma	Pulmonary edema	Usually abrupt onset (hours to days).	Cough common; dyspnea on exertion, paroxysmal nocturnal dyspnea, orthopnea.	Bibasilar rales (occasional wheezing); jugular venous distention with or without peripheral edema.	Bilateral alveolar infiltrates, often symmetric.	Most common cause is cardiogenic, in which case will have associated signs of heart failure.
	Pneumonia.	Usually abrupt onset (hours to days).	Cough, pleurisy common.	Rales with or without dullness over affected areas; fever.	Patchy alveolar infiltrates, usually asymmetric.	Leukocytes and often bacteria in sputum.
	Diffuse interstitial disease.	Previous dyspnea common.	Cough.	Often dry rales.	Interstitial disease (or negative).	Patient often aware of diagnosis.
	Aspiration.	Abrupt onset; history of vomiting	Cough.	Vomitus in oropharynx, or on endotracheal suction.	Normal or infiltrate.	Usually associated with coma or obtundation, underlying disease.
Airway disease	Upper airway obstruction	Often sudden onset.	Hoarseness or aphonia.	Inspiratory stridor.	Normal.	Soft tissue x-rays of neck may be helpful.
	Asthma.	Usually previous attacks;	Wheezing.	Wheezing; hyperinflation and decreased breath sounds in status asthmaticus.	Hyperinflation	Patient usually aware of diagnosis.
	Chronic obstructive lung disease and cystic fibrosis.	Previous dyspnea common; onset variable.	Cough, wheezing.	Wheezing; hyperinflation and decreased breath sounds.	Hyperinflation; occasional pneumonitis.	Clubbing with cystic fibrosis; patient usually aware of diagnosis.

(continued)

Table 11–1. Essentials of diagnosis of diseases causing dyspnea and respiratory distress.[1] *(Continued)*

Disorder	Specific Condition	Onset History	Symptoms Other Than Dyspnea	Signs	Chest X-ray	Comment
Pulmonary vascular disease	Acute pulmonary embolism.	Abrupt onset.	Cough, pleurisy, hemoptysis.	Tachycardia; occasionally signs of acute cor pulmonale.	Usually normal; occasionally infiltrates, atelectasis, elevated hemidiaphragm. "Hampton's hump"	Ventilation-perfusion lung scan, CT angiogram, pulmonary arteriogram for diagnosis. D-dimer.
	Repeated small pulmonary emboli.	Gradual onset.	Rarely, pleurisy or chest pain.	Occasionally signs of cor pulmonale.	Rarely helpful.	May require formal pulmonary function tests for diagnosis.
Miscellaneous	Pleurisy.	Often abrupt	Pleuritic pain	Rub (about 80%).	Normal.	Rule out pulmonary embolism.
	Metabolic acidosis.	Gradual onset.	Often not dyspneic.	Hyperventilation.	Normal.	Low arterial blood pH and bicarbonate.
	Neurogenic.		Usually not dyspenic.	Signs of cardiac or neurologic disease.	Normal.	Stroke, heart failure are usual causes.
	Psychogenic.	Previous attacks common; abrupt onset with stress.	Circumoral and acral tingling.	Tetany.	Normal.	Relief obtained with rebreathing system (eg, paper bag). Low P_{CO_2}.

[1] The most helpful tests or findings are shaded.

is likely. Unilateral large (> 20% of the pleural space) simple (nontension) pneumothoraces are also best treated by thoracostomy tube in the emergency department before hospitalization. Other types of pneumothoraces may be treated with a chest tube or, if the pneumothorax is simple and uncomplicated, by catheter aspiration or by observation of the patient in the emergency department with the catheter connected to a Heimlich valve for 6 hours. If a follow-up chest x-ray demonstrates persistent lung reexpansion or unchanged pneumothorax size, the patient may be discharged with close follow-up and instructions to return if symptoms reappear.

Disposition

Hospitalization is indicated for patients who have received tube thoracostomy, including all patients who present with tension pneumothorax or bilateral pneumothoraces of any type or who fail to maintain lung reexpansion after catheter aspiration.

Patients with small to moderate-sized unilateral simple pneumothoraces of recent onset may be observed

for a few days in the hospital without a chest tube to see if the condition is stable or improving. Those with recurrent pneumothorax should be admitted and considered for surgical intervention.

Patients with first-time stable small spontaneous unilateral pneumothoraces that remain asymptomatic with stable repeat chest radiograph after 4–6 hours with no symptoms may be referred for follow-up on an outpatient basis. These patients should be seen within 1–2 days.

2. Hydrothorax & Hemothorax (Pleural Fluid or Blood)

Clinical Findings

Fluid in the pleural space results in pulmonary collapse. Small amounts of air may be present as well. The patient shows moderate dyspnea or respiratory distress and has dullness with chest percussion of the affected side. Chest x-ray is diagnostic (Figure 11–4).

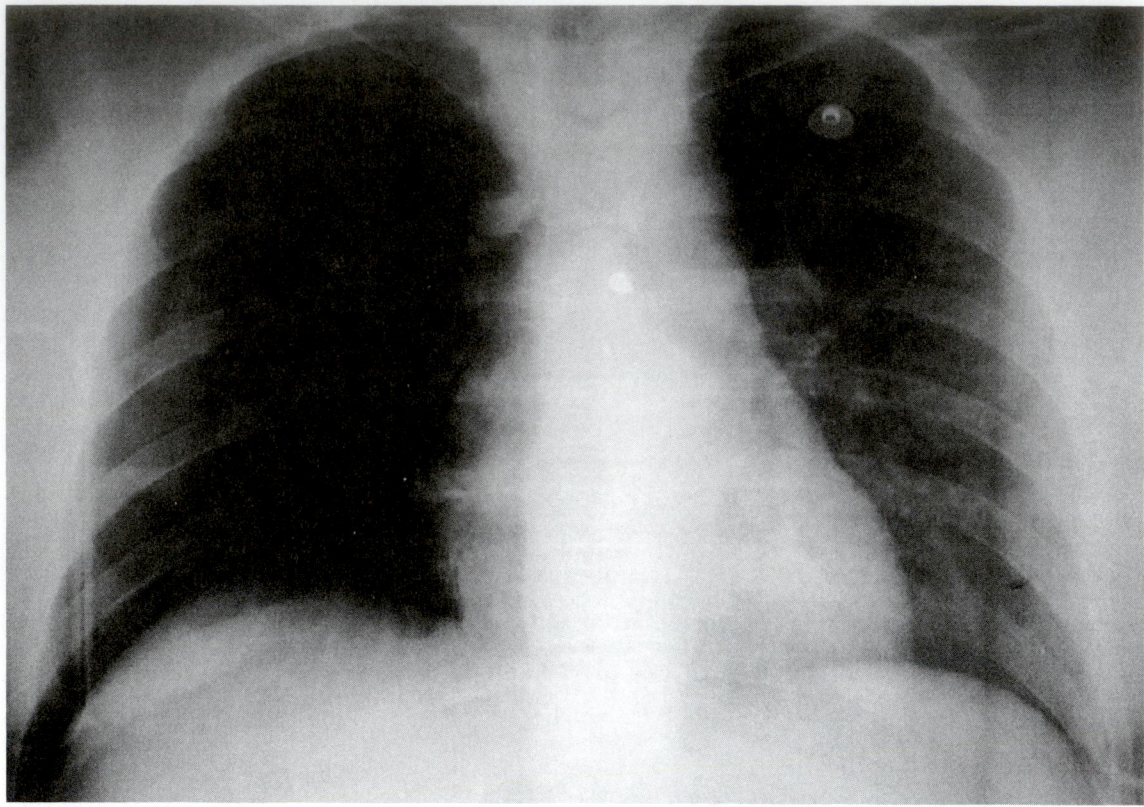

Figure 11–3. Small right-sided pneumothorax.

Treatment

A. Hydrothorax

If dyspnea of acute onset is thought to be secondary to hydrothorax, immediate drainage in the emergency department is indicated. A needle or small-gauge catheter should be used if the fluid is watery. Viscous effusions may require tube thoracostomy. No more than 1–2 L should be removed at any one time because of the risk of expansion injury to the lung. The fluid should be sent for analysis (pH, specific gravity, cell count, glucose, protein, lactate dehydrogenase, and amylase), culture (for *Mycobacterium tuberculosis* and other bacteria), and cytologic studies.

B. Hemothorax

In hemothorax due to penetrating trauma, autotransfusion may be indicated. Otherwise, thoracentesis or tube thoracostomy (or both) should be done, followed by investigation into the source of bleeding (eg, aortic angiography, exploration) as indicated (Chapter 24).

Disposition

Hospitalization is required for all patients except those with chronic recurrent pleural effusions of known cause and without significant hypoxia or respiratory impairment.

3. Massive Atelectasis

Clinical Findings

Atelectasis is alveolar collapse that is not due to pneumothorax or hydrothorax (Chapter 33). Decrease in chest motion on the affected side, dullness to percussion, and decreased to absent breath sounds are noted. Dyspnea, tachycardia, and cyanosis may be present. The disorder is evident radiologically as an increase in density of the collapsed lung, with reduced volume of the involved hemithorax (narrowed rib interspaces, elevated hemidiaphragm, and mediastinal shift to the side of involvement).

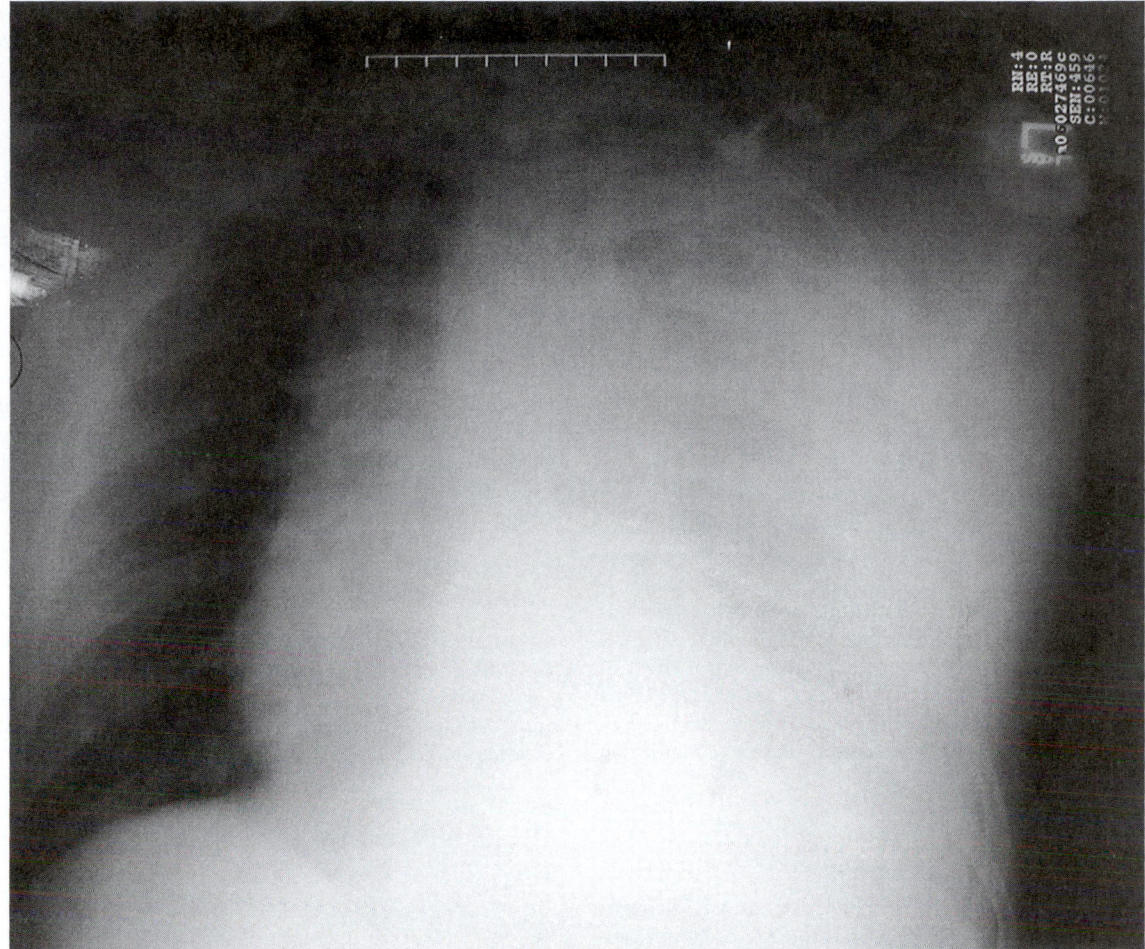

Figure 11–4. Large left-sided hemothorax.

Treatment

In general, patients with atelectasis exhibit some degree of respiratory distress, which can be quite variable. In the rare patient with respiratory failure, respiratory support (administration of oxygen and usually also assisted ventilation) should be initiated in the emergency department. Administration of oxygen is indicated for patients with hypoxia on pulse oximetry while the underlying cause is determined.

Disposition

Hospitalization is required unless the process is known to be chronic and nonprogressive.

LOSS OF FUNCTIONAL LUNG PARENCHYMA

A number of conditions can produce acute or chronic dyspnea through loss of functional pulmonary parenchyma.

The hallmarks of diseases causing loss of functional lung parenchyma are inspiratory rales (crackles) on physical examination, dullness to percussion, auscultatory pitch changes (eg, egobronchophony, bronchophony, and bronchial breath sounds), and one or more infiltrates on chest x-rays.

These disorders may be divided into those associated with (1) pulmonary edema, (2) pneumonia (including aspiration pneumonia), and (3) interstitial disease. Pulmonary contusion following blunt chest trauma is covered in Chapter 24.

In patients with dyspnea, several processes may be occurring simultaneously. For example, aspiration pneumonia may be a combination of chemical pulmonary edema and bacterial pneumonia, with varying degrees of airway obstruction; viral pneumonias are often interstitial in their early phases; and cardiogenic pulmonary edema starts as interstitial edema before progressing to the alveolar filling stage. Additionally, it may be difficult to differentiate these conditions initially in the emergency department (eg, pneumonia from pulmonary edema).

1. Pulmonary Edema

Clinical Findings

The clinical presentation of less severe pulmonary edema is similar to that associated with the more severe form discussed above. Patients generally are less dyspneic and have a history of symptoms and signs such as paroxysmal nocturnal dyspnea, gradually increasing peripheral edema, and intermittent chest pain if the pulmonary edema is cardiogenic. Noncardiogenic edema usually begins more abruptly and is more severe than the cardiogenic form. Chest x-ray shows cephalization (Figure 11–5).

Treatment

Give oxygen as needed. Additional treatment depends on whether the diagnosis is cardiogenic or noncardiogenic pulmonary edema (Chapter 33 and 34). Endotracheal intubation may be required if hypoxemia cannot be corrected with high-flow oxygen by mask.

Disposition

Many patients with dyspnea from acute pulmonary edema require hospitalization. Some patients with chronic or recurrent pulmonary edema (usually cardiogenic) can be managed on an outpatient basis.

2. Pneumonia
(See also Chapter 40.)

Clinical Findings

Patients with pneumonia generally give a history of fever and cough; dyspnea is a secondary or late symptom. Production of purulent sputum and pleuritic chest pain are common.

Physical examination usually shows a febrile patient with localized rales and dullness on percussion, often associated with signs of consolidation (egobronchophony, bronchial breath, and vocal sounds). In children, fever and cough are the only constant symptoms.

Chest x-ray (Figure 11–6) shows one or more infiltrates, except in patients with early pneumonia or concomitant dehydration, in whom observation and rehydration over 4–6 hours generally will make the infiltrates visible on x-ray. Immunosuppressed patients may also have pneumonia without infiltrates.

Patients with AIDS may develop pneumonia due to *Pneumocystis carinii*. Despite cough, fever, dyspnea, and hypoxemia (or an elevated alveolar-arterial PO_2 gradient calculated from arterial blood gas data), the clinical findings may be few and x-ray findings extremely subtle or normal. However, typical x-ray findings, if present, are a diffuse heterogeneous alveolar or interstitial infiltrate.

Treatment

Begin antibiotics promptly based on the clinical situation, likely pathogen, and the results (if available) of a Gram-stained smear of sputum. (See Chapter 40 for a more extensive discussion of evaluation and treatment of pneumonia.)

Disposition

Hospitalization is warranted for all seriously ill patients, for very young or very old patients, for patients with significant concurrent illnesses, for unreliable patients, and for patients with pneumonia of unknown cause. Patients with *Pneumocystis* pneumonia should be admitted.

Adolescents and young adults with mild viral, mycoplasmal, or pneumococcal pneumonia usually can be managed on an outpatient basis (Chapter 40). Practice guidelines for management of community-acquired pneumonia provide support for specific dispositions.

3. Diffuse Interstitial Pulmonary Disease (See also Chapter 33.)

Clinical Findings

Most patients with interstitial pulmonary disease have a history of chronic dyspnea, are aware of their diagnosis, and come to the emergency department because of recent worsening of symptoms. If the patient has not sought medical attention previously, interstitial pulmonary disease may be suspected if the physical examination shows diffuse "dry" rales, the chest x-ray shows interstitial infiltrates, and arterial PCO_2 and PO_2 are low.

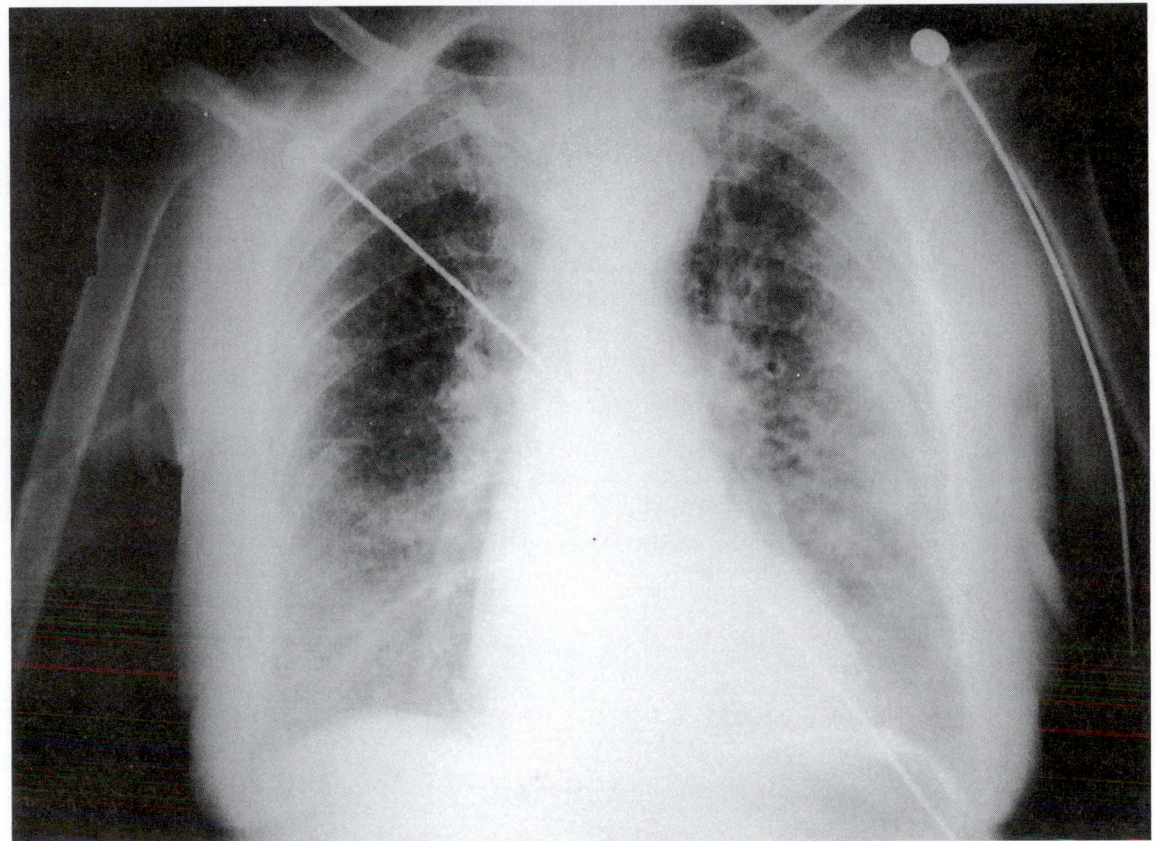

Figure 11–5. Mild to moderate pulmonary edema with cephalization of pulmonary vasculature.

Treatment

Supportive care is the only treatment recommended in the emergency department.

Disposition

Hospitalization should be considered for all newly diagnosed patients and for patients with known interstitial disease with significant recent increase in dyspnea or hypoxemia.

4. Aspiration

Clinical Findings

Aspiration may present clinically as pneumonia without obvious prior aspiration or as respiratory distress *with* obvious aspiration (vomitus in mouth and on clothing and elsewhere). This latter presentation is more common in patients with altered mental status.

Treatment

Supportive care should be given immediately in all cases. If obvious aspiration has occurred, clearing the airway is the most important emergency measure. This is best accomplished with a large-bore, hard-tipped suction device. Endotracheal intubation for better airway control and pulmonary toilet should be considered, as should emergency bronchoscopy.

Disposition

Hospitalize all patients. The patient's initial status is not a reliable guide to the need for hospitalization, because pulmonary function may worsen progressively for 24–72 hours after aspiration.

AIRWAY DISEASE

Obstruction to airflow (airway obstruction) is a principal manifestation of all types of airway disease.

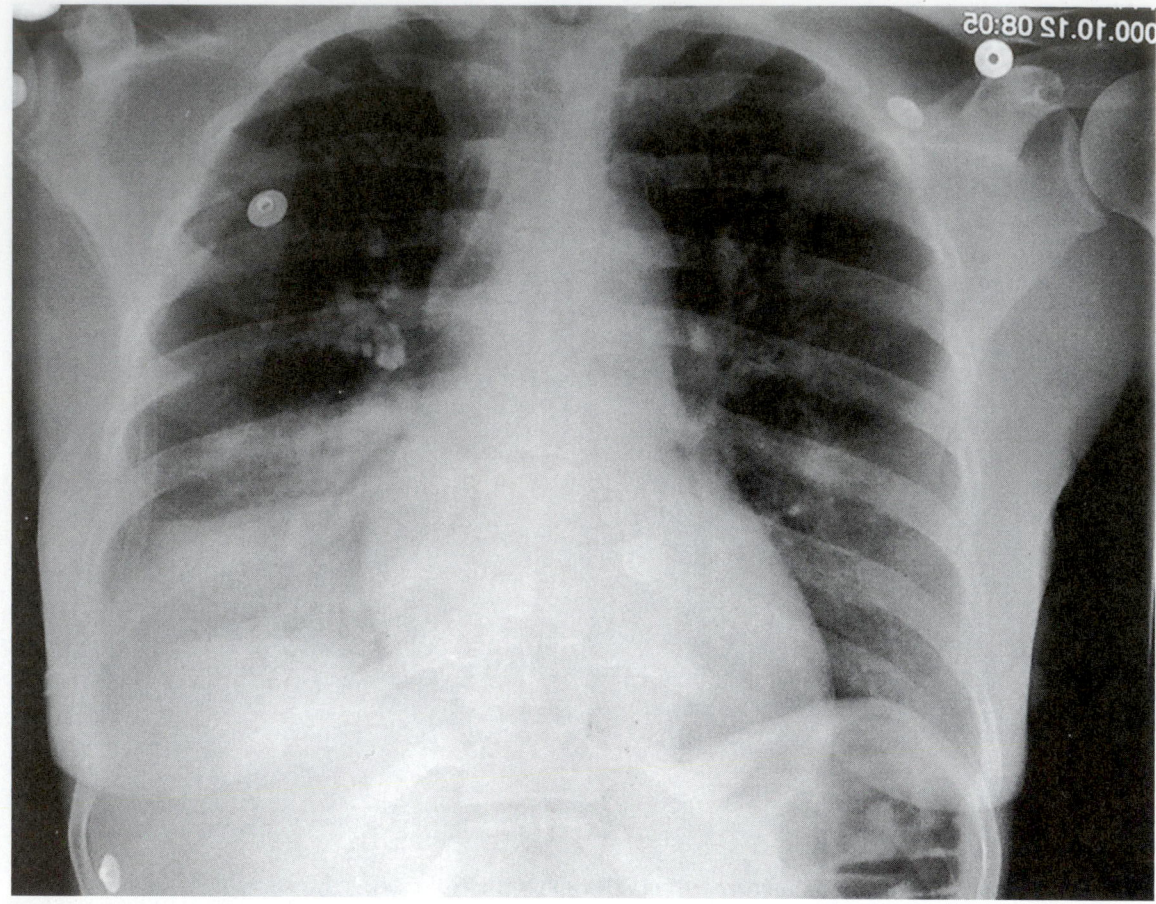

Figure 11–6. Radiographic appearance of a right lower lobe pneumonia.

1. Upper Airway Obstruction

Lesions of the oropharynx, larynx, or trachea may occlude the airway sufficiently to cause dyspnea.

Clinical Findings

Upper airway obstruction usually causes pronounced stridor (obstruction of inspiratory airflow equal to or greater than expiratory airflow), which may be accentuated by forced ventilatory efforts. The stridor may be accompanied by intercostal, suprasternal, or supraclavicular retractions or other signs of increased respiratory effort. The diagnosis can be made with lateral soft-tissue x-rays of the neck. In some cases, fiberoptic laryngoscopy is helpful.

Causes of upper airway obstruction include foreign bodies, tonsillar hypertrophy, croup, epiglottitis, anaphylaxis with laryngeal edema, retropharyngeal abscess, and tumors. If epiglottitis is suspected, obtain a lateral neck x-ray before attempting to visualize the upper airway directly (Chapter 32). Young children may aspirate small objects (eg, beads, coins, or peanuts) that lodge in the trachea or main-stem bronchus. Wheezing may be mistaken for bronchospastic disease. An expiratory chest x-ray is diagnostic, showing unilateral hyperexpansion on the affected side due to the ball-valve effect of the obstructing object (which may not be visible).

Treatment

A foreign body should be removed if present. Anaphylaxis with laryngeal edema requires immediate intramuscular injection of epinephrine, 0.5–1.0 mg (0.5–1.0 mL of 1:1000 solution). Alternatively, give 0.1–0.2 mg (1–2 mL of 1:10,000 solution) intravenously. Repeat in 3–10 minutes as needed (Chapter 9). Additionally, administration of diphenhydramine, 25–50 mg intramuscularly or intravenously, or selective histamine blockers such as famotidine, 20 mg intravenously, will block further histamine release. Discharged patients should receive diphenhydramine, 25 mg orally every 6 hours for 24–48 hours, to prevent recurrence. Surgical cricothyrotomy may be emergently required if obstruction progresses. Occasionally patients with hereditary angioedema (due to C1q esterase inhibitor deficiency) will present with signs and symptoms similar to those of allergic anaphylaxis. These patients are affected little by epinephrine and require C1q esterase inhibitor replacement (or fresh-frozen plasma if C1q esterase inhibitor is unavailable).

Children with epiglottitis (Chapter 48) should not receive direct or indirect laryngoscopy in the emergency department, because laryngeal spasm may precipitate complete obstruction. They should be carefully intubated in the operating room with surgeons present who can perform an emergency tracheostomy if needed. Adults with epiglottitis are less prone to sudden airway obstruction but should be admitted and monitored closely. Both children and adults should receive intravenous antibiotics.

Other disorders should be treated specifically to the extent possible.

Disposition

Patients with dyspnea from documented or suspected upper airway obstruction require hospitalization unless the problem is chronic, mild, and nonprogressive or is due to a foreign body that can be removed in the emergency department. Successfully treated upper airway obstruction due to anaphylaxis may recur when epinephrine wears off. Therefore, a 4- to 6-hour period of observation (or hospitalization) is advisable.

2. Asthma, Chronic Obstructive Pulmonary Disease, & Pulmonary Fibrosis (See also Chapter 33.)

In these disorders, expiratory airflow tends to be reduced proportionately more than inspiratory flow. Patients with dyspnea caused by these types of airway disease usually have a history of respiratory symptoms and are aware of their diagnosis.

Clinical Findings

Cough is commonly a feature, although sputum production is variable. Most of these patients have wheezing on auscultation, accentuated during forced expiration. Other findings are similar to those discussed earlier in this chapter.

Treatment

The therapy discussed under treatment of severe forms of these disorders is also of value in less severe presentations.

Disposition

Hospitalization is indicated for patients with severe or rapidly worsening dyspnea that does not respond to a few hours of treatment in the emergency department. Adult patients with asthma who are discharged home should receive corticosteroid therapy: oral for those with moderate symptoms, and oral or inhaled for those with minor symptoms. Children benefit from intramuscular steroids or high-dose inhaled steroids.

PULMONARY VASCULAR DISEASE

Dyspnea from pulmonary vascular disease may be one of the most difficult diagnostic problems confronting the emergency physician. The manifestations of pulmonary vascular disease are extremely varied in character and severity, and there is a significant risk of labeling patients with these illnesses as hysterical personalities or malingerers.

1. Acute Pulmonary Embolism (See also Chapter 33.)

Clinical Findings

Patients with acute pulmonary embolism and infarction usually have dyspnea, tachypnea, pleuritic chest pain, tachycardia, hypoxemia, and hypocapnia. Low-grade fever, cough, hemoptysis, and wheezing may also be present. Pulmonary infiltrates, occasionally with effusion, may be seen on x-ray.

Patients with embolization without infarction have similar manifestations but often without pulmonary infiltrates, fever, and hemoptysis.

In massive pulmonary embolization, crushing anterior chest pain, dyspnea, severe hypoxemia, syncope, shock, and cardiac arrest are common.

Patients with right-sided endocarditis and other causes of septic pulmonary embolization usually have high fever and rigors associated with symptoms of embolization; the chest x-ray often shows multiple, scattered infiltrates that frequently cavitate after several days of illness.

Progressive, noninvasive evaluation strategies that consider specific risk factors and physical findings have essentially replaced invasive methods of diagnosis. D-dimer, venous lower extremity Doppler ultrasound, spiral CT, CT angiography, and ventilation-perfusion scanning have significantly decreased the need for conventional pulmonary angiography in suspected pulmonary embolism.

Treatment

Give oxygen. Give morphine as necessary for pain. Treat shock if present. Heparin should be started (unless contraindicated) if embolization is strongly suspected. *Do not give heparin to patients with suspected septic embolization.* For adults, give a bolus of 10,000 units per hour, adjusting the rate to maintain the prothrombin time at 1.5–2 times control values. Selected patients may be appropriate for low-molecular-weight heparin therapy (enoxaparin sodium, 1 mg/kg subcutaneously every 12 hours). Thrombolytic therapy (Chapter 33) should generally be reserved for patients with moderate to severe right ventricular dysfunction.

Disposition

Patients with suspected or documented pulmonary embolization almost always require hospitalization.

2. Chronic Pulmonary Vascular Obstruction (Repeated Small Pulmonary Emboli)

A much more difficult problem is presented by patients with repeated small pulmonary emboli without infarction or with progressive pulmonary vascular occlusion from other causes (intravenous drug abuse, sickle cell anemia, vasculitis).

Clinical Findings

These patients usually complain of dyspnea yet may have no abnormal findings in the emergency cardiorespiratory data base. Although significant hypoxemia and hypocapnia are often present, blood gas values are occasionally normal at rest. Evidence of pulmonary hypertension and right ventricular overload is found infrequently and then only in patients with advanced illness. A normal perfusion lung scan virtually excludes pulmonary emboli and is evidence against other types of pulmonary vascular disease. By contrast, abnormal ventilation lung scans can be produced by practically any type of pulmonary disease: asthma, bronchitis, and emphysema are the most common offenders in patients with normal chest x-rays.

Treatment & Disposition

Obtain pulse oximetry and possibly an arterial blood gas sample for determination of PO_2, PCO_2, and pH before starting treatment. Start low-flow oxygen, 2 L/min

by nasal cannula, and adjust the flow to maintain oxygen saturation at 95% or greater.

Hospitalization is indicated for patients with respiratory failure or if symptoms are worsening rapidly. Dyspneic patients with unexplained hypoxemia should not be discharged home without arranging for home oxygen and an evaluation to exclude pulmonary vascular disease (screening pulmonary function tests with diffusing capacity, measurement of the alveolar-arterial PO_2 gradient during rest and exercise, perfusion lung scan, pulmonary arteriography, and the like). Furthermore, if a patient comes to the emergency department on 2 or 3 occasions with dyspnea, and no abnormalities are noted in the cardiopulmonary data base, referral to a pulmonologist is warranted for evaluation and complete pulmonary function testing.

MISCELLANEOUS CONDITIONS

1. Pleurisy

Clinical Findings

Pleurisy and pleuritic pain from any cause may produce a sensation of dyspnea. Even conditions such as rib fractures that produce pleuritic pain in the absence of significant underlying pulmonary parenchymal abnormalities may cause splinting and atelectasis sufficient to produce hypoxemia. When pleural fluid forms, the pain and friction rub may lessen or disappear. Pleurisy is often part of a viral syndrome (which may occasionally be accompanied by pericarditis). Fever, myalgias, headache, nasal congestion, or flulike symptoms may be present. A chest x-ray is required to exclude underlying lung disease, pleural effusion, or pneumothorax.

Treatment

Other than measures for relief of pain, therapy must be directed toward the underlying lesions.

Disposition

Hospitalization is required if the patient is severely hypoxemic (arterial $PO_2 \leq 60$ mm Hg as a new finding), if parenteral analgesia is required for pain relief, or if the underlying disease requires hospital treatment.

2. Metabolic Acidosis

Clinical Findings

Metabolic acidosis (eg, diabetic ketoacidosis, salicylate overdose) can produce secondary hyperventilation that may be taken for dyspnea or respiratory distress. Arterial blood gas analyses usually show a normal or high PO_2, marked hypocapnia (PCO_2 of 10–20 mm Hg), and metabolic acidosis (low serum bicarbonate concentration).

Treatment & Disposition

Treatment depends on the underlying condition. Patients almost always require hospitalization for management of the underlying cause of metabolic acidosis (Chapter 42).

3. Anemia, Pregnancy, & Thyrotoxicosis

These 3 conditions may at times have accompanying dyspnea, and therapy for the underlying condition is all that is required.

4. Neurologic Hyperventilation

Primary central nervous system disease can produce a variety of abnormal breathing patterns, including central hyperventilation and Cheyne-Stokes respiration, any of which could be mistaken for respiratory distress. Cheyne-Stokes respiration may also occur when the circulation is slowed, as in heart failure.

Clinical Findings

The diagnosis is based on finding obvious neurologic or cardiac disease consistent with the respiratory pattern. The arterial PO_2 is usually normal; PCO_2 may be low or high.

Treatment

No treatment of the respiratory condition is required.

Disposition

Disposition depends on the underlying disease.

5. Psychogenic Hyperventilation & Pulmonary Neurosis

Clinical Findings

Patients with psychogenic hyperventilation usually present with a history of acute dyspnea and anxiety, often precipitated by personal or environmental factors. Hyperventilation to the point of tetany is diagnostic. Lightheadedness (due to cerebral vasoconstriction) and circumoral or limb paresthesias are often present. Another helpful feature is that the dyspnea often improves with exercise. Patients can be calmed enough to speak,

whereas in organic dyspnea, patients may not be capable of speech. There are usually no abnormalities on the screening data base other than a low arterial PCO_2, normal or high arterial PO_2, and elevated pH. Most of these patients can be diagnosed in the emergency department as having neuroses, but the possibility of pulmonary vascular disease must be considered.

Treatment

There is no specific treatment. Reassurance is usually helpful. Patients with symptomatic hypocapnia (circumoral tingling, carpopedal spasm, tetany) or marked respiratory alkalosis (pH > 7.55) should breathe into an airtight bag for several minutes to relieve hypocapnia.

Disposition

The patient should be referred to a pulmonary clinic or internist for complete evaluation and reassurance.

Guthrie R: Community-acquired lower respiratory tract infections: etiology and treatment. Chest 2001;120(6):2021. [PMID: 11742937] (A review of the cause and treatment of community-acquired pneumonia.)

Jain SK et al: Spontaneous pneumothorax: determinants of surgical intervention. J Cardiovasc Surg 1998;39:107. [PMID: 9537545] (Describes success of varying levels of intervention in spontaneous pneumothorax.)

Karnik AM: Management of pneumothorax and barotraumas: current concepts. Compr Ther 2001;27:311. (A comprehensive review of all aspects of pneumothorax.)

Kline JA et al: New diagnostic tests for pulmonary embolism. Ann Emerg Med 2000;35:181. [PMID: 10650235] (Review of noninvasive methods of evaluation for pulmonary embolism with specific emphasis on emergency department assessment and management.)

Pezzella AT, Silva WE, Lancey RA: Cardiothoracic trauma. Curr Probl Surg 1998;35:647. [PMID: 9739342] (A review of cardiothoracic trauma.)

Scribano PV et al: Provider adherence to a clinical practice guideline for acute asthma in a pediatric emergency department. Acad Emerg Med 2001;8:1147. [PMID: 11733292] (Describes a practice guideline and issues relating to adherence to the guideline.)

Sivaloganathan M, Stephens R, Grocott M: Management of flail chest. Hosp Med 2000;61:811. [PMID: 11198758] (A short review of cases and treatment of flail chest.)

Smoller JE et al: State of the art: panic anxiety, dyspnea, and respiratory disease. Theoretical and clinical considerations. Am J Respir Crit Care Med 1996;154:6. [PMID: 8680700] (A review of hyperventilation and panic disorders and their relationship.)

Stollberger C et al: Multivariate analysis-based prediction rule for pulmonary embolism. Thrombosis Research 2000;97:267. [PMID: 10709901] (Offers and validates a prediction rule for pulmonary embolism based on rapidly obtainable patient-specific information.)

Chest Pain[1]

Sean P. Barbabella, DO & William R. Dennis, Jr., MD[2,3]

Immediate Management of Life-Threatening Problems
    Initial Management
    Management of the Patient with Chest Pain & Abnormal Hemodynamics
    Management of the Patient with Severe Chest Pain & Normal Hemodynamics
Further Evaluation of the Patient with Chest Pain
Management of Specific Disorders Causing Chest Pain
    Cardiovascular Disorders
        Acute Coronary Syndrome
        Myocardial Infarction
        Mitral Valve Prolapse
        Aortic Stenosis & Regurgitation
        Pericarditis
        Aortic Dissection
    Pulmonary Disorders
        Pleurisy & Pleurodynia
        Spontaneous Pneumothorax
        Traumatic Pneumothorax

Pneumomediastinum
Pulmonary Hypertension
Pulmonary Embolism
Pneumonia
Gastrointestinal Disorders
    Esophageal Disorders
    Perforated Esophagus
    Perforated Stomach or Duodenum
    Pancreatitis
    Cholecystitis
Musculoskeletal Disorders
    Costochondral Separation, Rib Fractures, & Intercostal Muscle Strain
    Disk Disease (Cervical & Thoracic)
    Tietze Syndrome (Costochondritis)
    Muscle Spasm ("Stitch")
Miscellaneous Disorders
    Intrathoracic Neoplasm
    Zoster

■ IMMEDIATE MANAGEMENT OF LIFE-THREATENING PROBLEMS (See Figure 12–1.)

INITIAL MANAGEMENT

Begin Supplemental Oxygen

Give oxygen, 4 L/min, by nasal cannula or face mask, pending further evaluation.

---

[1]Chest pain due to trauma is discussed in Chapter 24.
[2]This chapter is a revision of the chapter by Mary T. Ho, MD, MPH, & John Mills, MD, from the 4th edition.
[3]The views expressed in this article are those of the authors and do not reflect the official policy or position of the U.S. Department of the Navy, the U.S. Department of Defense, or the U.S. government.

Begin Continuous Cardiac Monitoring

Begin cardiac monitoring with pulse oximetry, and treat life-threatening arrhythmias (Chapters 7 and 35).

Look for Markedly Abnormal Hemodynamics

A. SHOCK

Look for signs of shock. Arterial hypotension and poor peripheral perfusion cause altered sensorium; pale, clammy skin; oliguria; and, frequently, respiratory distress.

B. CENTRAL VENOUS HYPERVOLEMIA

Central venous hypervolemia is manifested initially by distended superficial veins (best seen in the neck); later, pulmonary edema (causing cough, dyspnea, rales, and frothy sputum) or peripheral edema may be seen, al-

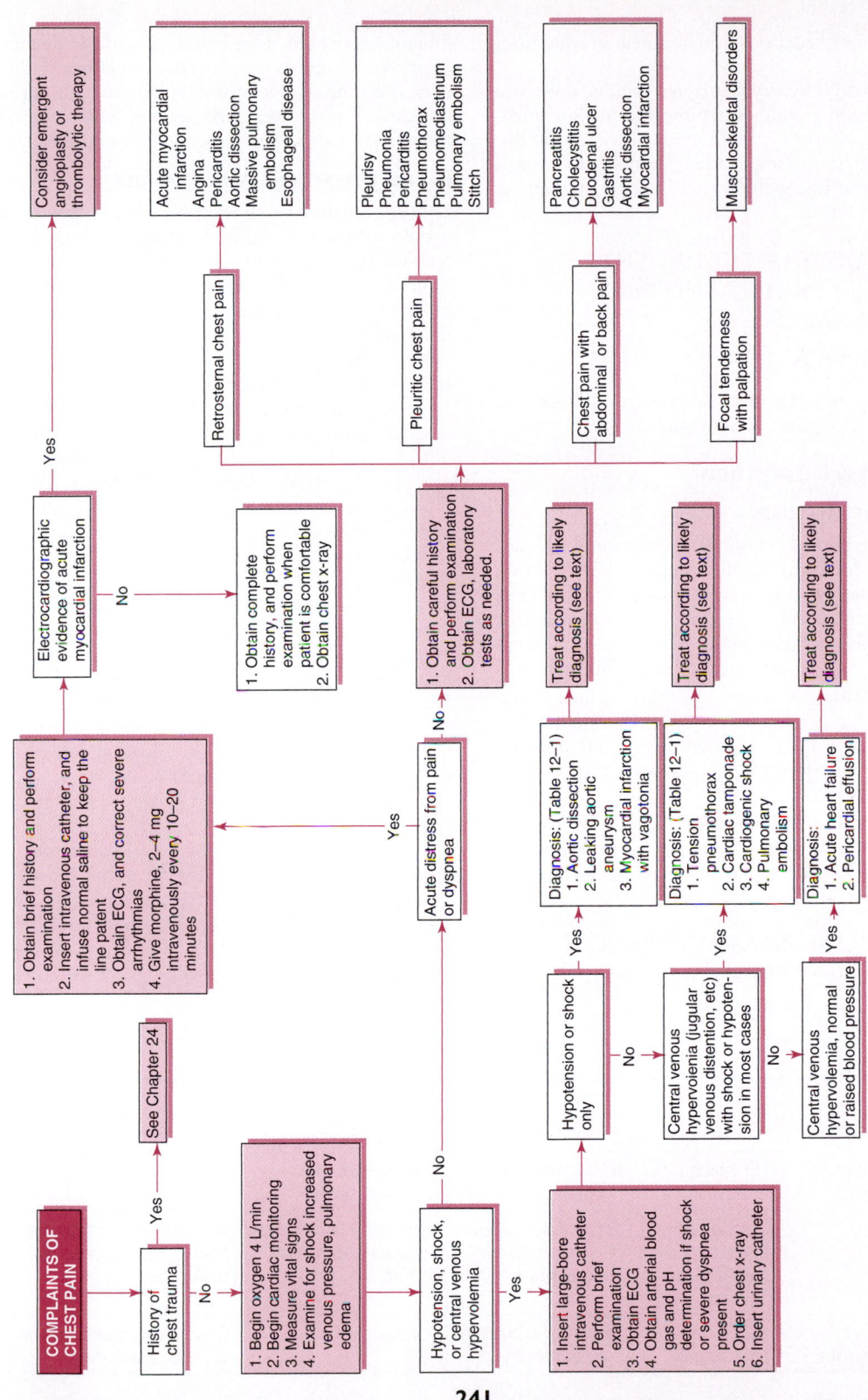

Figure 12-1. Management of complaints of chest pain.

though peripheral edema is usually absent in conditions of acute onset.

Central venous hypervolemia may be caused by conditions obstructing venous return (eg, tension pneumothorax, pulmonary embolization) or by cardiac disease (eg, infarction, tamponade). Pulmonary edema is usually not seen in conditions causing only interference with venous return.

MANAGEMENT OF THE PATIENT WITH CHEST PAIN & ABNORMAL HEMODYNAMICS

Clinical Findings

The patient is in acute distress, and signs of abnormal hemodynamics are obvious on examination.

Treatment & Disposition

A. Immediate Measures

Insert 2 large-bore (≥ 16-gauge) intravenous catheters. Draw blood for complete blood count (CBC), serum electrolyte measurements, glucose, and tests for renal function; reserve 2 tubes for other studies that may be needed. Begin administration of intravenous fluids based on estimate of intravascular fluid volume.

1. Hypotension or shock present—Infuse intravenous crystalloid solutions (eg, normal saline or lactated Ringer's), about 300–500 mL in 20 minutes. Monitor the response (blood pressure, urine output, sensorium).

2. Central venous hypervolemia (with or without shock or hypotension)—Pending more precise diagnosis, infuse normal saline to keep the intravenous catheter patent.

Briefly examine the pulmonary and cardiovascular systems, and palpate the abdomen for presence of a pulsatile mass. Obtain a 12-lead electrocardiogram (ECG).

Obtain arterial blood for blood gas and pH determinations. Avoid unnecessary arterial punctures if the patient is a candidate for thrombolytic therapy for acute myocardial infarction. Arrange for a portable chest x-ray as soon as possible. Insert a urinary catheter.

B. Life-Threatening Abnormalities

1. Hypotension or shock present—Hypovolemia is manifested by collapsed neck veins, clear lung fields on physical examination or chest x-ray, and absence of peripheral edema. The central venous and pulmonary capillary wedge pressures are low. Table 12–1 lists the differentiating features of the 3 most important conditions causing chest pain with hypotension but without central venous hypervolemia.

If the diagnosis is uncertain, treatment should be oriented primarily toward aortic dissection (Chapter 38).

Type and cross-match for 6–10 units of whole blood. Expand intravascular volume with administration of intravenous crystalloid solution. Consider inserting a central venous catheter. For severe hypovolemia with shock, up to 3 L of crystalloid solution may be given rapidly (over 30–60 minutes) to restore normal hemodynamics until cross-matched blood is available. If blood is needed immediately, type-specific or universal donor blood (O-negative, low antibody titer or erythrocyte antigens) may be used (Chapter 39). Maintain blood pressure with continued infusion of blood and crystalloid solution. Blood should be given to keep the hematocrit above 30%.

Obtain emergency vascular or thoracic surgical consultation.

Reexamine the patient for pulse deficits or an abdominal mass, and check urine for occult blood; these findings indicate aortic aneurysm or dissection. Obtain a portable chest x-ray and if the patient is stable consider computed tomography (CT) scan of the chest or abdomen and pelvis if indicated.

Table 12–1. Differentiating features of conditions causing chest pain with hypovolemia.

Diagnosis	Findings			
	History	Examination	ECG	X-Rays
Myocardial infarction with vagotonia	Crushing chest pain; nausea	Bradycardia; stable hypotension	Acute infarction pattern and bradycardia	Nonspecific.
Aortic dissection	Tearing chest pain; back pain; often history of hypertension	Tachycardia; pulse deficits; progressive hypotension	Nonspecific or may show ischemia or infarction pattern, left ventricular hypertrophy	Widened mediastinum; pleural fluid. CT scan is more sensitive than x-ray.
Leaking upper abdominal aortic aneurysm	Chest and epigastric pain	Tachycardia; pulsatile epigastric mass	Nonspecific	CT scan or ultrasound is more sensitive than x-rays.

Management of thoracic aortic dissection consists of β-blockade to maintain heart rate less than 60–80 beats/min (esmolol, loading dose 500 μg/kg/min followed by an infusion at 50 μg/kg/min to maintain desired heart rate) and vasodilators to maintain a systolic blood pressure less than 120 mm Hg (nitroprusside, 0.3–10 μg/kg/min to desired blood pressure), establishing the β-blockade first.

Hospitalize the patient in an intensive care setting immediately for further evaluation and treatment.

2. Central venous hypervolemia with hypotension or shock—Superficial veins (especially neck veins) are distended; pulmonary and peripheral edema may be present. See Table 12–2 for guidelines to differential diagnosis. Consider tension pneumothorax immediately, because this condition may be quickly and reliably differentiated from the others and is easy to treat. Look for marked respiratory distress, laterally deviated trachea away from the affected side, and a hyperresonant hemithorax with markedly decreased or absent breath sounds on the affected side. Chest x-ray confirms the diagnosis, but treatment should not be delayed to obtain a chest x-ray, because many patients require definitive treatment quickly.

Cardiac tamponade should also be diagnosed early, because treatment is reasonably effective but differs markedly from that for cardiogenic shock, heart failure, or pulmonary embolism. Look for hypotension, jugular venous distension, and muffled heart sounds (Beck triad) and for low voltage on all leads of the ECG, electrical alternans, or diffuse ST-segment elevation typical of pericarditis. A narrow pulse pressure and pulsus paradoxus may also be present. Pulmonary edema is rare. Chest x-ray is not helpful, because acute tamponade does not cause a detectable increase in heart size. Definitive diagnosis by noninvasive methods is best done by bedside emergency ultrasound or formal echocardiography, but tamponade may be confirmed (and treated) by pericardiocentesis alone in desperate cases.

a. Tension pneumothorax—(See Chapter 24.) Insert a thoracostomy tube if one is readily available (Chapter 6). Otherwise, a 14-gauge needle inserted in the 2nd intercostal space at the midclavicular line or in the 4th intercostal space at the anterior axillary line relieves tension in the chest until a thoracostomy tube can be inserted. Hospitalize the patient for further care.

b. Cardiac tamponade—(See Chapter 24.) Attempt volume expansion with intravenous administration of 500–1000 mL of crystalloid solution over 20–30 minutes if the diagnosis is confirmed (this therapy is disastrous for cardiogenic shock). If the initial trial succeeds in elevating the blood pressure, volume expansion may be repeated once in a patient whose systolic blood pressure subsequently drops to less than 90 mm Hg.

If time permits, obtain emergency cardiothoracic consultation for therapeutic pericardiocentesis, which should be performed in the operating room or under echocardiographic or fluoroscopic guidance. Otherwise, perform immediate pericardiocentesis (under ultrasound guidance if available) (Chapter 6) if rapid, progressive hypotension develops and the patient fails to respond to volume expansion. Hospitalize the patient at once in an intensive care unit.

c. Cardiogenic (arrhythmogenic) shock—See Chapter 35 for further details on the diagnosis and treatment of cardiac arrhythmias.

(1) Severe bradyarrhythmia (heart rate usually < 40 beats/min)—Give atropine, 0.5 mg intravenously; if necessary, repeat every 5–10 minutes up to a total dose of 0.04 mg/kg. An external transcutaneous pacemaker (Chapter 6) may be applied to increase the heart rate until a percutaneous transvenous pacemaker can be inserted, if indicated. Dopamine can be used to support blood pressure and increase myocardial contractility. Mix 200 mg of

Table 12–2. Distinguishing features of conditions causing chest pain, hypotension, or shock in association with distended neck veins.

Diagnosis	Helpful Distinguishing Features
Tension pneumothorax	Hyperresonant hemithorax with decreased breath sounds; chest x-rays diagnostic, trachea deviates away from affected side.
Cardiac tamponade	Faint heart sounds; ECG with diffuse low voltage or electrical alternans. Pulmonary edema rare. Echocardiography diagnostic.
Cardiogenic shock (arrhythmogenic)	ECG or cardiac monitor shows severe bradycardia (ventricular rate < 50 beats/min, usually < 40 beats/min, usually > 180 beats/min). Signs of myocardial ischemia may also be present.
Cardiogenic shock (myocardial)	Pulmonary edema almost always present. ECG almost always shows pattern diagnostic of infarction.
Pulmonary embolism (massive)	Physical examination, ECG, and chest x-ray show signs of right heart strain. Chest x-ray may show infiltrates, effusion, or truncation of pulmonary vasculature. Confirm diagnosis by ventilation-perfusion scanning, spiral CT scan of chest or pulmonary arteriography.

dopamine in 250 mL of 5% dextrose in water for a solution of 800 µg/mL. Infuse at a rate of 5–12 µg/kg/min by continuous intravenous infusion, and observe the response. The dosage may be increased as needed but should not exceed 20 µg/kg/min. If the response is inadequate with dopamine, start an epinephrine infusion. Mix 1 mg of 1:1000 epinephrine in 50 cc normal saline, begin the infusion at 2–10 µg/min, and titrate to desired effect.

Isoproterenol may be given as a last resort until a temporary pacemaker becomes available. Give 2–4 µg/min initially by continuous intravenous infusion, and increase as needed up to 20 µg/min. Isoproterenol must be used with extreme caution and only with continuous cardiac monitoring and frequent blood pressure readings, because it may cause arrhythmias. Because of the vasodilatory (β_2-adrenergic) effect of isoproterenol, blood pressure may fall if the heart rate does not increase.

Occasionally patients will present with hypotension or shock due to severe bradyarrhythmia and without central venous hypervolemia. For these patients, fluid challenge may be given as described in the section on cardiac tamponade. If the patient does not respond to the above measures or if the patient develops left heart failure with fluid challenge, insert a percutaneous transvenous pacemaker, which is the treatment of choice. Hospitalize all patients in an intensive care unit.

(2) Severe tachyarrhythmia (heart rate usually > 180 beats/min)—Immediate cardioversion is the treatment of choice. Deliver 50–100 J of synchronized direct current countershock initially, and increase the shock by 50- to 100-J increments if there is no response.

d. Cardiogenic shock (myocardial infarction)—(See also Chapter 9). In patients with no evidence of pulmonary edema, ensure adequate intravascular volume; give intravenous crystalloid solution, 300–500 mL over 30 minutes. If blood pressure improves, maintain the infusion at a rate of 100–200 mL/h.

Give dobutamine, dopamine, or a combination of both if no change in blood pressure occurs or if severe shock or pulmonary edema is present initially. Mix 500 mg (2 vials) of dobutamine in 250 mL of 5% dextrose in water for a 2 mg/mL solution, and give at a rate of 2.0–20 µg/kg/min by continuous intravenous infusion. Begin at the lower dose, and increase as needed, guided by clinical response. Dobutamine is the drug of choice for treatment of cardiogenic shock due to pump failure. *Caution:* Observe for signs of arrhythmia.

Give morphine, 2–4 mg intravenously every 5–20 minutes, until pain and dyspnea are controlled. If hypotension is a concern, then fentanyl may be used for pain. Carefully monitor the patient's respiratory status. Avoid unnecessary arterial punctures in patients who may be candidates for thrombolytic therapy.

Nitroglycerin ointment, 1.25–2.5 cm (½–1 in) applied under an occlusive dressing, can be used for addi-

tional preload reduction. If the patient's condition worsens because of the effect of the ointment, it can be discontinued by simply wiping it off.

Notify the cardiology consultant immediately if an acute infarction pattern is evident on the 12-lead ECG. Ideally, patients eligible for thrombolytic therapy (Chapter 34) should have treatment begun in the emergency department by the emergency physician, avoiding the delay necessitated by obtaining cardiologic consultation or transporting the patient to the coronary care unit. Emergency reperfusion therapy with thrombolytic agents or percutaneous transluminal coronary angioplasty has been shown to be of benefit in decreasing the mortality rate and the size of the infarct.

Hospitalize the patient immediately in a coronary care or intensive care unit, and insert a pulmonary artery (Swan-Ganz) catheter and an arterial line as soon as possible to monitor blood pressure and cardiac output.

e. Massive pulmonary embolism—(See Chapter 33.) Because massive pulmonary embolism is an uncommon diagnosis and is difficult to confirm rapidly, every attempt should be made to exclude other causes of chest pain with shock. Consider an emergent echocardiogram if available. Findings consistent with massive pulmonary embolism include right ventricular hypokinesis and dilation. Right ventricular dysfunction from pulmonary embolism predicts increased mortality.

Attempt volume expansion with administration of 300–500 mL of normal saline over 20–30 minutes to elevate systolic blood pressure. The dose may be repeated if the trial is successful and if heart failure does not develop. In the rare patient with hypotension without central venous hypervolemia, a fluid challenge should also be given, but a larger dose (500–1000 mL of normal saline instead of 300–500 mL) may be administered.

Give dopamine (see above). If clinical signs strongly suggest pulmonary embolism and thoracic dissection has been ruled out, begin heparin (unfractionated or a low-molecular-weight heparin) (see Pulmonary Embolism, below, and Chapters 33 and 34). Obtain pulmonary consultation, and consider thrombolytic therapy.

3. Central venous hypervolemia with normal or elevated blood pressure—Superficial veins (especially neck veins) are distended. Pulmonary and peripheral edema is common. Blood pressure is normal or (more commonly) elevated.

Acute congestive heart failure is the most common cause. It generally occurs as an exacerbation of preexisting disease but occasionally results from acute myocardial infarction (acute cardiogenic pulmonary edema), although acute myocarditis or pericardial effusion without frank tamponade may be present rarely.

a. Nitroglycerin—Give nitroglycerin, 0.4 mg sublingually, or use nitroglycerin ointment, 1.25–2.5 cm (½–1 in) applied under an occlusive dressing. Nitroglycerin by intravenous infusion, beginning with a rate of 10 μg/min and increasing by 5–10 μg/min every 3–5 minutes as needed, can be started in the emergency department. Monitor the blood pressure closely, and if hypotension develops, place the patient in the Trendelenburg position and decrease the infusion rate. Do not give nitrates to patients taking sildenafil (Viagra).

b. Furosemide—Give furosemide, 0.5–1.0 mg/kg by bolus intravenous injection. The initial effect of rapid preload reduction is of immediate benefit; diuresis occurs later.

c. Morphine—Give morphine, 2–4 mg intravenous, and repeat every 5–10 minutes until pain and dyspnea are relieved.

d. Aspirin—Give aspirin, 160–325 mg chewed, if not contraindicated. If the patient has an allergy to aspirin, use clopidogrel, 75 mg orally.

e. Angiotensin-converting enzyme (ACE) inhibitors—Captopril or enalapril are associated with reduced admission rates to the intensive care unit and decreased endotracheal intubation rates. Acutely, a reduction in preload and afterload has been seen. For oral or sublingual captopril, a one-time dose of 12.5 mg or 25 mg is given; enalapril is given as a 1.25 mg intravenous infusion over 5 minutes. Avoid using ACE inhibitors in patients who are hypotensive, pregnant, or hyperkalemic or in those who are allergic to ACE inhibitors.

f. Positive-pressure ventilation—If the patient continues to deteriorate, consider early noninvasive positive-pressure ventilation (BiPAP or CPAP); this approach may even prevent the need for endotracheal intubation.

g. Inotropic agents—Short-term inotropic therapy can improve hemodynamic parameters. These agents may be beneficial for patients who are unable to receive conventional therapy. Milrinone may be administered as a 50 μg/kg bolus over 10 minutes, followed by an infusion at 0.25–0.75 μg/kg/min. Another choice is dobutamine, at an infusion rate of 2.5–15.0 μg/kg/min.

h. Nesiritide—Nesiritide (human B-type natriuretic peptide) is now recommended for the treatment of severe decompensated congestive heart failure. It is administered as a bolus of 2 μg/kg over 1 minute, followed by a continuous infusion of 0.01 μg/kg/min. Hypotension is the major dose-limiting side effect. Nesiritide has been shown to improve both hemodynamic parameters such as pulmonary capillary wedge pressure and clinical variables such as dyspnea and fatigue in patients admitted with congestive heart failure.

i. Hospitalization—Hospitalize the patient immediately in an intensive care setting, and monitor hemodynamic status with a pulmonary artery catheter and arterial catheter as needed.

MANAGEMENT OF THE PATIENT WITH SEVERE CHEST PAIN & NORMAL HEMODYNAMICS

Clinical Findings

The patient is in acute distress because of chest pain but is neither hypotensive nor in shock.

Treatment

A. OXYGEN

Give oxygen, 4 L/min, by nasal cannula or mask. Begin continuous electrocardiographic monitoring.

B. VENOUS ACCESS

Insert an intravenous catheter (18-gauge is satisfactory), and begin an infusion of normal saline as slowly as necessary to keep the catheter open.

C. ELECTROCARDIOGRAM

Obtain a 12-lead ECG within 10 minutes of the patient's arrival. If the ECG reveals evidence of acute myocardial infarction, evaluate the patient for possible thrombolytic therapy (Chapter 34).

D. DRUG THERAPY

Give aspirin, 160–325 mg chewed, if not contraindicated. If the patient has an allergy to aspirin, give clopidogrel, 75 mg orally.

Give nitroglycerin, 0.4 mg sublingually. Sublingual nitroglycerin may be repeated twice with 5 minutes between doses. If pain continues despite morphine and sublingual nitroglycerin and if acute myocardial infarction is suspected, begin nitroglycerin by intravenous infusion (see above).

Give morphine, 2–4 mg slowly intravenously; morphine may be repeated every 10–20 minutes until the patient is more comfortable.

E. LABORATORY FINDINGS

Send blood samples to the laboratory for CBC; renal function tests; and serum electrolyte, glucose, lipase, and amylase determinations. Send blood samples for cardiac enzyme measurements (CK-MB isoenzymes, troponin I/T, myoglobin) if myocardial infarction is suspected and the patient is to be hospitalized.

F. TREATMENT OF ARRHYTHMIAS

Correct any significant cardiac arrhythmias (Chapter 35).

G. HISTORY AND PHYSICAL EXAMINATION

Take a thorough medical history with emphasis on the quality, radiation, severity, timing, and duration of chest pain, and perform a complete physical examination (see below).

H. CHEST X-RAY

Obtain a chest x-ray. An anteroposterior view with portable equipment is satisfactory if the patient is too sick to tolerate a better examination.

I. OTHER TESTS

Obtain additional tests as indicated on the basis of the history, physical examination, and results of laboratory tests.

Disposition

Patients with chest pain severe enough to cause objective distress should be hospitalized or admitted to an observation unit for further evaluation.

American Heart Association in collaboration with the International Liaison Committee on Resuscitation. Guidelines 2000 for cardiopulmonary resuscitation and emergency cardiovascular care. Circulation 2000;102(8 Suppl):1. [PMID: 10966667]

Antonelli M et al: A comparison of noninvasive positive-pressure ventilation and conventional mechanical ventilation in patients with acute respiratory failure. N Engl J Med 1998; 339:429. [PMID: 9700176]

Brady WJ, Harrigan RA: Evaluation and management of brady-arrhythmias in the emergency department. Emerg Med Clin North Am 1998;16(2):361. [PMID: 9621848]

Colucci WS et al: Intravenous nesiritide in the treatment of decompensated congestive heart failure: Nesiritide Study Group. N Engl J Med 2000;343:246. [PMID: 10911006]

Hollenberg, SM, Kavinsky CJ, Parillo JE: Cardiogenic shock. The pathophysiology and management. Ann Intern Med 1999; 131(1):47. [PMID: 10391815]

Jouriles NJ: Atypical chest pain. Review of aortic dissection, pulmonary embolism, and pericarditis. Emerg Med Clin North Am 1998;16(4):717. [PMID: 9889737]

Lee TH, Goldman L: Evaluation of the patient with acute chest pain. N Engl J Med 2000;342:1187. [PMID: 10770985]

Spodick DH: Pathophysiology of cardiac tamponade. Chest 1998; 113(5):1372. [PMID: 9596321]

Wiesenfarth J: Aortic dissection; the symptoms, diagnosis and treatment. eMedicine; www.emedicine.com

Wigder HN et al: Pressure support noninvasive positive pressure ventilation treatment of acute cardiogenic pulmonary edema. Am J Emerg Med 2001;19:179. [PMID: 11326339]

Zevitz ME et al: Heart failure. eMedicine; www.emedicine.com.

■ FURTHER EVALUATION OF THE PATIENT WITH CHEST PAIN

Differential Diagnosis by Location & Quality of Pain

Evaluation of patients who complain of chest pain but are not in severe distress should proceed in a systematic fashion. The single most useful means of evaluation is the carefully elicited history supplemented by examination of the heart, lungs, abdomen, and peripheral vessels in conjunction with electrocardiograhy, chest x-ray, and arterial blood gas measurements. Consider most of the diagnostic possibilities at least briefly in every patient who presents with chest pain (Table 12–3).

A. RETROSTERNAL DISCOMFORT

Retrosternal discomfort, especially if it is a tightness, pressure, or "squeezing" pain, should suggest serious underlying disease, for example, myocardial infarction, unstable angina due to atherosclerosis or valvular heart disease, pericarditis, dissection of the aorta, or pulmonary embolism. When the above diagnoses are excluded, esophageal disease (eg, spasm, esophagitis) is the most common cause of retrosternal distress (see below). Because esophageal disease is relatively benign and rarely requires hospitalization, the more serious causes of retrosternal discomfort must be excluded with a high degree of certainty before concluding that the pain is of esophageal origin.

Consider hospitalization for all adult patients with retrosternal pain for observation unless a condition not requiring hospitalization is diagnosed with certainty.

B. PLEURITIC PAIN

Pain that is markedly worse on inspiration should suggest pleurisy associated with pneumonia, pulmonary embolism, or isolated pleuritis. The pain of pneumothorax, pneumomediastinum, ruptured esophagus, and pericarditis frequently has a pleuritic component. The fleeting pain of a "stitch in the side" is often pleuritic in nature as well. Chest pain due to myocardial infarction may have a pleuritic component.

One of the most serious causes of pleuritic chest pain, pulmonary embolism, is also one of the most difficult to diagnose given the widely varied presentations of the disease with nonspecific history and physical examination findings. Because of the increased mortality associated with misdiagnosis, consider pulmonary embolism in all patients presenting with pleuritic chest pain (Chapters 33 and 34).

Table 12–3. Diagnostic clues to cause of chest pain.[1]

Cause	Previous Attacks of Similar Pain	History — Pain — Location	History — Pain — Character	History — Pain — Onset	History — Duration	Common Associated Findings	Signs	Other Abnormalities	Other Comments
Angina	Usually	Retrosternal, radiating to arms, neck, back, or epigastrium	Squeezing, dull ache	Often with stress or exercise	2–10 minutes up to 20–30 minutes	Occasionally dyspnea; dizziness and syncope rare.	Often none. S₄ occasionally.	ECG often normal between attacks.	Relieved by nitroglyerin.
Acute myocardial infarction	In some cases	Retrosternal, radiating to arms, neck, back, or epigastrium	Squeezing, dull ache, increases with time.	No precipitating factor necessary	> 30 minutes	Nausea and vomiting, diaphoresis, dyspnea	Heart failure, restlessness, shock; cardiac examination often normal.	ECG may be diagnostic or normal.	Elevated CK, CK-MB isoenzymes, and Troponin I or T. Normal isoenzymes levels on one determination do not exclude diagnosis.
Mitral valve prolapse	Usually	Variable	Variable	Variable	Variable; usually hours	Dyspnea, dizziness common; syncope in some	Midsystolic click or murmur in most cases.	ECG may show inverted T waves on leads II, III, and aVF. Echocardiogram is diagnostic.	Arrhythmia or sudden death may occur. Usually seen in young women. High-arched palate or chest or spine deformities may be present.
Aortic stenosis	May have occurred	Like angina	Like angina	Like angina	Like angina	Syncope, dyspnea	Systolic ejection murmur transmitted to carotid arteries; delayed carotid pulse.	ECG usually shows left ventricular hypertrophy. Echocardiography and angiography are diagnostic.	More common in older men.
Aortic regurgitation	May have occurred	Like angina	Like angina	Like angina	May be prolonged	Dyspnea	Diastolic murmur transmitted to carotid arteries. Water-hammer and Quincke's pulse. Wide arterial pulse pressure	ECG may be normal or may show left ventricular hypertrophy. Echocardiography and angiocardiography are diagnostic.	History of rheumatic heart disease, connective tissue disease, or syphilis.

(continued)

Table 12-3. Diagnostic clues to cause of chest pain.[1] (Continued)

Cause	History – Previous Attacks of Similar Pain	History – Pain – Location	History – Pain – Character	History – Pain – Onset	History – Pain – Duration	Common Associated Findings	Signs	Other Abnormalities	Other Comments
Pericarditis	May have occurred	Retrosternal	Variable; often pleuritic and relieved by sitting	Variable	Hours to days	Variable	Pericardial friction rub in many.	ECG may be diagnostic, nonspecific, or normal. Echocardiography often shows fluid.	Recent history of upper respiratory infection.
Aortic dissection	No	Retrosternal and back	Tearing, maximal at onset	Sudden	Variable	Myocardial infarction, stroke, limb ischemia, syncope	Stroke, absent pulses, hematuria, shock.	Chest x-ray may show widened mediastinum or be normal. ECG may show acute myocardial infarction. Pulsatile abdominal mass.	Angiography or CT scan is definitive. Hypertension or connective tissue disease may be present.
Pleurisy	In some cases	Variable; usually lateral thorax	Pleuritic	Usually sudden	Variable	Subjective dyspnea	Often none. Occasionally friction rub, low-grade fever.	Occasionally pleural effusion.	Negative lung scan, spiral chest CT scan, or pulmonary angiogram.
Pneumothorax	May have occurred	Variable	Variable often pleuritic	Usually sudden	Variable	Dyspnea and cough; shock if tension pneumothorax is present	Tachycardia, lung collapse with or without mediastinal shift	Chest x-ray is diagnostic but needs careful examination.	
Pneumomediastinum	No	Retrosternal	Variable; often pleuritic	Usually sudden	Variable	Dyspnea	Mediastinal crunch.	Chest x-ray is diagnostic. Pneumothorax common.	Consider esophageal perforation as cause.
Pulmonary hypertension	Usually	Retrosternal	Like angina	Like angina	Variable	Dyspnea, fatigue, exercise syncope	Loud P_2, right ventricular lift.	ECG shows right heart strain. Chest x-ray shows signs of pulmonary hypertension.	

248

Pulmonary embolism	May have occurred	Variable; usually lateral thorax	Usually strong pleuritic component	Usually sudden	Minutes to hours	Dyspnea, cough, and tachypnea; hemoptysis sometimes	Friction rub or splinting in some	Hypoxemia and hypocapnia. Chest x-ray usually abnormal, but findings are not specific.	Abnormal ventilation-perfusion radionuclide lung scan, spiral CT chest, or pulmonary angiogram.
Pneumonia	Rare	Over affected lobe	Pleuritic	Variable	Variable	Fever and chills, cough, dyspnea, sputum production	Fever, rales with or without consolidation, friction rub.	Infiltrates on chest x-ray; purulent sputum.	
Esophagitis Esophageal spasm Hiatal hernia	Usually	Retrosternal or epigastrium	Changes with eating	Usually gradual	Variable	Gastrointestinal symptoms	None	Positive barium swallow or endoscopy.	Relieved by antacids, H$_2$ blockers, or proton pump inhibitors.
Perforated esophagus	No	Retrosternal	Severe	Usually sudden	Variable	Variable	Subcutaneous emphysema, mediastinal crunch.	Chest x-ray usually shows pneumomediastinum, pneumothorax, or pleural effusion. Esophagogram or esophagoscopy is diagnostic.	History of severe retching or vomiting or esophageal trauma or instrumentation.
Perforated duodenal ulcer	No, or milder pain of ulcer	Retrosternal to epigastrium	Severe	Variable	Variable	Variable	Epigastric pain. May have prominent findings of peritoneal irritation	Free air in peritoneal; elevated amylase.	Rare as cause of chest pain.
Pancreatitis	May have occurred	Retrosternal to epigastrium	Variable	Variable	Hours to days	Vomiting, anorexia	Epigastric or upper quadrant tenderness.	Markedly elevated serum or serum lipase.	Rare as cause of chest pain.

(continued)

249

Table 12–3. Diagnostic clues to cause of chest pain.[1] (Continued)

Cause	Previous Attacks of Similar Pain	History Pain Location	History Pain Character	History Pain Onset	Duration	Common Associated Findings	Signs	Other Abnormalities	Other Comments
Cholecystitis	Usually	Right upper quadrant; occasionally epigastrium or retrosternal	Variable	Usually sudden	Hours to days	Vomiting, anorexia, fever	Epigastric or right upper quadrant tenderness.	Abnormal liver function tests. Sonography usually diagnostic.	Rare as cause of chest pain.
Musculoskeletal disorder (eg, Tietze syndrome, stitch), rib fracture	Variable	Costochondral junctions; retrosternal and lateral	Pleuritic ache, "sticking" sensation	Gradual to sudden	Variable; fleeting for stitch	Splinting	Tender (or, rarely, swollen), costosternal junctions, especially first and second ribs. Point tenderness over affected ribs.	None.	Relieved by lidocaine-corticosteroid injection.

[1]The shaded areas are the most helpful diagnostically.

C. BACK OR ABDOMINAL PAIN WITH CHEST PAIN

Abdominal pain that is inferior to the xiphoid process and associated with chest pain should suggest intra-abdominal disease, dissecting aortic aneurysm, or possibly myocardial ischemia. In stable patients, CT scan of the chest and abdomen with intravenous contrast can reliably exclude the diagnosis of dissecting or ruptured aortic aneurysm. Even after aortic catastrophes are excluded, patients with chest pain often require hospitalization or admission to an observation unit to rule out myocardial ischemia.

D. MUSCULOSKELETAL DISCOMFORT

Musculoskeletal disease with chest pain (Tietze syndrome, rib fracture) is usually associated with marked tenderness localized over the affected site. Patients with chest pain referred from intrathoracic structures may also have some associated tenderness of superficial structures. Most patients with chest pain from musculoskeletal disorders can receive treatment in the emergency department and be discharged for outpatient follow-up care.

■ MANAGEMENT OF SPECIFIC DISORDERS CAUSING CHEST PAIN

CARDIOVASCULAR DISORDERS

ACUTE CORONARY SYNDROME
(See Chapter 34.)

MYOCARDIAL INFARCTION
(See Chapter 34.)

MITRAL VALVE PROLAPSE

 ESSENTIALS OF DIAGNOSIS

- *Has late systolic click.*
- *Palpitations are the most frequent complaint.*

Clinical Findings

Consider mitral valve prolapse in any patient with a mitral regurgitation murmur or clicks (without other known heart disease or other cause of chest pain) who presents with recurring atypical chest pains. The ECG may show nonspecific T-wave abnormalities. Echocardiography is required for definitive diagnosis.

Treatment

No specific emergency therapy is required. Although life-threatening arrhythmias may occur, they are rare. β-blocker therapy (eg, metoprolol, 50 mg orally twice daily) may be offered to patients who are uncomfortably symptomatic.

Disposition

Refer patients to a cardiologist or primary care physician for definitive evaluation and management.

AORTIC STENOSIS & REGURGITATION

 ESSENTIALS OF DIAGNOSIS

- *Classic triad: angina, syncope, and heart failure.*
- *Crescendo-decrescendo systolic murmur is classic finding in aortic stenosis, loudest at 2nd right intercostal space.*
- *Aortic regurgitation is a high-pitched, blowing decrescendo diastolic murmur.*

Clinical Findings

Chest pain in patients with severe aortic stenosis or regurgitation is clinically similar to that of angina and is probably the result of a similar mechanism, that is, relative myocardial ischemia secondary to diminished coronary blood flow.

Anginal pain in a patient with aortic valve disease may indicate that hemodynamically significant abnormalities of the valve are present, with a higher risk of impending sudden death. Murmurs of aortic stenosis or regurgitation are present on physical examination, often with adjunctive findings indicating severe valvular disease (eg, thrill over the carotid artery, wide pulse pressure; see Table 12–3).

Treatment

Provide symptomatic treatment pending further evaluation for definitive treatment. Begin oxygen, 4 L/min, by nasal cannula, and obtain an ECG. Insert an intravenous catheter (18- to 20-gauge) and begin an infusion of normal saline to keep the catheter open. Give nitroglycerin, 0.3–0.4 mg sublingually, for pain. If nitroglycerin is not effective, give morphine, 2–4 mg intravenously. Monitor the patient closely and discontinue medication if any signs of decompensation develop.

Disposition

Hospitalization is warranted because of the imminent risk of decompensation or sudden death. Patients should be evaluated for cardiac catheterization or valve replacement with or without coronary bypass.

PERICARDITIS
(See Chapter 34.)

AORTIC DISSECTION
(See Chapter 38.)

PULMONARY DISORDERS

PLEURISY & PLEURODYNIA
(See also Chapter 33.)

 ESSENTIALS OF DIAGNOSIS

- *Coxsackievirus B is most common cause.*
- *Sudden lancinating chest pain.*
- *Associated with fever, malaise, and headaches.*

Clinical Findings

Patients with idiopathic pleurisy or pleurodynia are generally young, and the onset of illness is acute, with severe pleuritic chest pain. Apart from low-grade fever in some patients and possible friction rub, other findings on physical examination are usually normal. Chest x-ray may show a small pleural effusion, with or without a small pulmonary infiltrate. Viruses (especially enteroviruses) are the usual causative agents.

An accurate diagnosis of pleurisy is important because its symptoms are similar to those of pulmonary embolism. Pleurisy is often a diagnosis of exclusion.

Treatment

Pleurisy and pleurodynia are benign, self-limited diseases, and only symptomatic measures are necessary. Although aspirin is sufficient for most patients, indomethacin, 25–50 mg orally 3 times daily, is reported to be more effective.

Disposition

Hospitalization is rarely indicated, and then only for relief of severe pain. Refer patients to an outpatient clinic for turberculin testing and repeat chest x-ray.

SPONTANEOUS PNEUMOTHORAX
(See Chapter 33.)

TRAUMATIC PNEUMOTHORAX
(See Chapter 24.)

PNEUMOMEDIASTINUM
(See also Chapter 33.)

 ESSENTIALS OF DIAGNOSIS

- *"Crunch" of subcutaneous air is felt on exam.*
- *Chest x-ray is diagnostic.*
- *Retrosternal pain.*

Clinical Findings

Pneumomediastinum is frequently associated with pneumothorax. It is characterized by severe boring pain located retrosternally or in adjacent areas; the pain sometimes radiates to the back. Chills, fever, and shock may be present, especially if there is concurrent mediastinitis. A mediastinal "crunch" on auscultation or air in the mediastinum on chest x-ray is diagnostic.

Treatment

Give oxygen, 3–5 L/min, by nasal cannula or mask. Insert an intravenous line (≥ 16-gauge), and keep it open with normal saline. Give morphine, 2–4 mg intravenously, for pain; the dose may be repeated.

Treat pneumothorax with tube thoracostomy as indicated. Evaluate the patient thoroughly to rule out serious underlying disease, ruptured bronchus, or a ruptured esophagus. Rupture of the esophagus is invariably associated with mediastinitis.

Disposition

Hospitalize patients for observation and examination to rule out serious precipitating factors such as rupture of the trachea, bronchus, or esophagus. Refer patients with chronic or recurrent pneumomediastinum for outpatient care.

PULMONARY HYPERTENSION
(See also Chapter 34.)

 ESSENTIALS OF DIAGNOSIS

- *Dyspnea, exertional syncope, and exertional chest pain.*

- Evidence of right ventricular failure almost always present.
- Prominent P2 (pulmonic) heart sound.
- Doppler echocardiography can help make diagnosis.

Clinical Findings

Severe or sudden onset of significant pulmonary hypertension may cause an oppressive retrosternal sensation or frank angina associated with dyspnea on exertion. A history of easy fatigability, weakness, syncope on exertion, and hemoptysis may be elicited. A loud P_2 and right ventricular lift on physical examination suggest pulmonary hypertension. The ECG may reveal strain in the right side of the heart or cor pulmonale (right axis deviation; depressed ST segment and inverted T waves in leads II, III, aVF, and V1–5; and tall, peaked P waves in leads II, III, and aVF). A large right ventricle or large pulmonary vessels on chest x-ray are diagnostic.

Treatment

No specific treatment is available for pulmonary hypertension. Administer oxygen for hypoxia and treat other abnormalities (bronchopulmonary infection, recurrent pulmonary emboli, heart failure) that may be exacerbating the pulmonary hypertension.

Disposition

Hospitalization is indicated for patients with severe pain, hypoxia, or severe heart failure. Refer patients to a cardiologist for complete evaluation to rule out repairable lesions and to evaluate patients for treatment with anticoagulants or other investigational treatments.

PULMONARY EMBOLISM
(See Chapter 33.)

PNEUMONIA
(See Chapter 40.)

GASTROINTESTINAL DISORDERS

ESOPHAGEAL DISORDERS

Clinical Findings

Esophageal disorders such as esophagitis, spasm, motility disorders, and gastroesophageal reflux frequently cause retrosternal chest pain that can be difficult to differentiate from pain due to cardiac causes. When cardiac disease is excluded, esophageal disorder is the most common cause of chest pain. Characteristic features of chest pain of esophageal origin include pain that is burning in nature, often radiates along the sternum, is made worse by lying down and relieved by sitting, may be induced by swallowing, and often persists for hours after a shorter episode of more intense pain. Rest, sublingual nitroglycerin, "GI cocktails," and calcium-channel blockers can relieve pain of both cardiac and esophageal origin and should not be used as diagnostic aids. Because cardiac disease is more life threatening, cardiac causes of chest pain must be excluded with a high degree of certainty before esophageal disorder is diagnosed as the cause of pain.

Diagnostic tests include barium swallow, endoscopy, manometry, and pH monitoring. Definitive emergency diagnosis of the esophageal disorder is seldom warranted.

Treatment

General symptomatic treatment can be offered to patients who are in discomfort, because the specific esophageal disorder is not usually known at the time of the emergency visit. A trial of viscous lidocaine, 15 mL mixed with 15 mL of an antacid given orally, can be tried for acute relief. Clinicians are cautioned to avoid attributing chest pain symptoms to an esophageal cause based entirely on improvement in chest discomfort after a "GI cocktail." Other measures include eating frequent small meals, using antacids, avoiding food before sleep, and using bed blocks (10–15 cm [4–6 in] high) under the head of the bed. If gastroesophageal reflux is suspected, H_2-receptor blocker or proton-pump inhibitor therapy may be tried.

Disposition

If esophageal disorder is diagnosed as the cause of chest pain and cardiac disease or other life-threatening conditions can be excluded with confidence, refer the patient for outpatient care within 1–2 weeks.

PERFORATED ESOPHAGUS
(See also Chapter 24.)

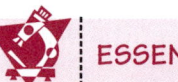 ESSENTIALS OF DIAGNOSIS

- Severe chest pain.
- Pain increased with swallowing or breathing.
- Chest x-ray may reveal air within the mediastinum, pleural cavity, pericardium, or subcutaneous tissue.

Clinical Findings

Esophageal perforation is marked by agonizing retrosternal chest pain associated with pneumomediastinum, pneumothorax, pneumonia, or purulent pleural effusion. A recent history of severe retching, vomiting, or endoscopy is often present. The diagnosis is confirmed by an esophagogram using water-soluble contrast medium or esophagoscopy.

Treatment

See Chapter 24.

Disposition

Hospitalize the patient for evaluation for possible surgery.

PERFORATED STOMACH OR DUODENUM
(See also Chapter 13.)

ESSENTIALS OF DIAGNOSIS

- *Often a history of peptic ulcer disease.*
- *Vomiting is common.*
- *Acute distress.*
- *Acute abdominal x-ray may reveal free air in the abdomen.*

Clinical Findings

Perforation distal to the esophagus is characterized by sudden onset of severe pain that is usually epigastric but may be retrosternal and may radiate to the back. A history of chronic epigastric pain or ulcer disease often is present. Epigastric tenderness and diminished or absent bowel sounds may be found. If peritonitis has supervened, rebound tenderness and a rigid abdomen are present. Air under the diaphragm may be seen on an x-ray. Serum amylase or lipase levels may be elevated as a result of posterior perforation into the pancreas. Leukocytosis with a shift to the left often is present.

Treatment

Insert a large-bore (≥ 16-gauge) intravenous catheter, and give crystalloid solutions intravenously to support blood pressure. Give morphine, 2–4 mg intravenously, for pain; the dose may be repeated.

Insert a nasogastric tube, and begin continuous suction. Obtain urgent surgical consultation. Begin prophylactic intravenous antibiotics (cefoxitin, 2 g intra-

venously, and gentamicin, 2 mg/kg intravenously; see also Table 13–1).

Disposition

Hospitalize the patient at once for emergency surgery.

PANCREATITIS
(See Chapter 13.)

CHOLECYSTITIS
(See Chapter 13.)

MUSCULOSKELETAL DISORDERS

COSTOCHONDRAL SEPARATION, RIB FRACTURES, & INTERCOSTAL MUSCLE STRAIN
(See also Chapter 24.)

ESSENTIALS OF DIAGNOSIS

- *Pain associated with movement.*
- *X-rays may reveal a fractured rib.*
- *Often a history of trauma.*

Clinical Findings

In this group of musculoskeletal disorders, pain is usually worse with movement and breathing. A history of minor trauma, strenuous exercise, or severe coughing often is present. Pain is localized and elicited by palpation. Chest x-ray may be normal or may show rib fractures if they are present.

Treatment

Oral analgesics and nonsteroidal anti-inflammatory drugs (NSAIDs) are effective for analgesia. Local heat alone may provide relief. Narcotic analgesics may be required if respiratory effort is affected because of pain. Splinting is generally not recommended for rib fractures, because it may impair respiratory function and promote atelectasis or pneumonia. For patients with rib fractures, ensure that a pneumothorax is not present on x-ray.

Disposition

Refer the patient for outpatient follow-up if pain is severe or persistent.

DISK DISEASE
(Cervical & Thoracic)

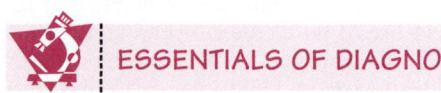 ESSENTIALS OF DIAGNOSIS

- *Pain radiates from neck or back to arms.*
- *Paresthesia in fingers.*
- *Weakness in arm with decreased reflexes.*

Clinical Findings

Disk disease may cause paroxysmal pain radiating from the back of the neck into the arms and fingers. The pain is aggravated by coughing, sneezing, and straining. Neck movement is restricted by cervical muscle spasm. The patient may have paresthesias and pain in the fingers, weakness of hand and forearm muscles, and decreased biceps and triceps reflexes. Narrowing of the vertebral interspace is seen on a plain film, and magnetic resonance imaging confirms the diagnosis.

Treatment

Treatment is symptomatic. Local heat may be of value. In mild cases, a light cervical collar during the day may be helpful.

Disposition

Hospitalization is rarely required even for patients with severe disk disease. Outpatient follow-up by a spinal surgeon is recommended. Mild cases can be treated on an outpatient basis.

TIETZE SYNDROME
(COSTOCHONDRITIS)

 ESSENTIALS OF DIAGNOSIS

- *Remember that cardiac pain also can be reproducible by palpation.*
- *Pain is localized to a specific point.*

Clinical Findings

Tietze syndrome affects the costochondral or chondrosternal junctions, with visible swelling and erythema of the overlying skin and localized tenderness.

Treatment

Pain usually is relieved by NSAIDs or other oral analgesics. Injection of lidocaine-corticosteroid preparations into the joints also relieves pain.

Disposition

Refer the patient for outpatient follow-up if pain is severe or persistent.

MUSCLE SPASM
("STITCH")

 ESSENTIALS OF DIAGNOSIS

- *History of trauma or exercise.*

Clinical Findings

The patient complains of aching pain, usually in localized areas but sometimes more generalized. Pain often increases with movement and palpation. A history of minor trauma or strenuous exercise may be present.

Treatment

Massage, heat, and other local treatments are effective. Aspirin or other NSAIDs are useful.

Disposition

Refer the patient for outpatient follow-up as needed. A search for more serious illnesses (eg, myositis, arthritis, Pancoast tumor) may be necessary in recurrent or persistent cases that have no obvious cause.

MISCELLANEOUS DISORDERS
INTRATHORACIC NEOPLASM

 ESSENTIALS OF DIAGNOSIS

- *History of fever, night sweats, and weight loss.*
- *Cough or hemoptysis.*
- *Chest x-ray may reveal a mass.*

Clinical Findings

Intrathoracic neoplasm is suggested by a mass seen on chest x-ray with no other explanation for the chest pain.

Treatment

Give analgesics and other supportive measures as required.

Disposition

Depending on their general condition, patients with intrathoracic neoplasms should be either hospitalized or referred for timely evaluation by a pulmonologist.

ZOSTER
(See also Chapter 46.)

 ESSENTIALS OF DIAGNOSIS

- *Vesicles in a dermatomal pattern.*
- *Does not cross midline.*
- *Pain may precede vesicles.*

Clinical Findings

In the preeruptive stage of zoster, pain felt on the skin surface in dermatomal distribution may occur several days before the characteristic skin lesions (clusters of clear, fluid-filled vesicles in a dermatomal distribution) appear. Pain is typically unilateral and does not cross the midline. Hypoesthesia in dermatomal distribution may also be present.

The appearance of the skin lesions confirms the diagnosis. Rarely, patients may present with pain as the only manifestation of the disease; in such patients, a rise in antibody titer is diagnostic.

Treatment

Give analgesics as necessary; narcotics may be required for relief. Acyclovir, 800 mg orally 5 times daily for 7–10 days, or famciclovir, 500 mg orally 3 times a day for 7 days, if given within 72 hours of onset may alleviate symptoms, shorten the duration of illness, and reduce the incidence of postherpetic neuralgia, a special concern in elderly patients. Local nerve block with long-acting anesthetics (eg, bupivacain [Marcaine, Sensorcaine]) is effective and obviates the need for narcotics and their associated side effects. It may also decrease the incidence and severity of postherpetic neuralgia. Prednisone, 60 mg orally daily (tapered over 2 weeks), may also decrease the incidence and severity of postherpetic neuralgia in elderly patients.

Disposition

Patients with severe cases (extensive localized disease, dissemination) may require hospitalization for pain control and possible treatment with intravenous acyclovir. Other patients may be referred for outpatient evaluation and continued treatment (analgesia).

Bonow RO et al: ACC/AHA guidelines for the management of patients with valvular heart disease. J Heart Valve Dis 1998;7: 672. [PMID: 9870202]

Bouknight DP et al: Current management of mitral valve prolapse. Am Fam Physician 2000;61:3343. [PMID: 10865929]

Brady WJ et al: Electrocardiographic diagnosis of acute myocardial infarction. Emerg Med Clin North Am 2001;19(2):295. [PMID: 11373980]

Jouriles NJ: Atypical chest pain. Review of aortic dissection, pulmonary embolism, and pericarditis. Emerg Med Clin North Am 1998;16(4):717. [PMID: 9889737]

Kontos MC: Evaluation of the emergency department chest pain patient. Cardiol Rev 2001;9(5):266. [PMID: 11520450]

Ng SM et al: Ninety-minute accelerated critical pathway for chest pain evaluation. Am J Cardiol 2001;88:611. [PMID: 11564382]

Rubin LJ: Primary pulmonary hypertension, review of the treatments. N Engl J Med 1997;336:111. [PMID: 8988890]

Stankus SJ, Dlugopolski M, Packer D: Management of herpes zoster (shingles) and postherpetic neuralgia. Am Fam Physician 2000;61:2437. [PMID: 10794584]

Zalenski RJ, Shamsa F, Pede KJ: Evaluation and risk stratification of patients with chest pain in the emergency department. Predictors of life-threatening events. Emerg Med Clin North Am 1998;16:495. [PMID: 9739772]

Abdominal Pain

13

Roger Humphries, MD, & Jon Andrew Russell, MD[1]

Immediate Management of Life-Threatening Problems

Further Evaluation of the Patient with Abdominal Pain

  History

  Physical Examination

  Laboratory Examination

  Radiologic Examination

Additional Measures for the Management of Acute Abdomen

Management of Specific Disorders Causing Abdominal Pain

  Intestinal Disorders

    1. Appendicitis

    2. Intestinal Obstruction

    3. Perforated Peptic Ulcer

    4. Perforation of the Bowel

    5. Diverticulitis

    6. Intestinal Strangulation

    7. Gastroenteritis

    8. Idiopathic Inflammatory Bowel Disease

  Hepatobiliary Disorders

    1. Biliary Colic

    2. Acute Cholecystitis

    3. Acute Suppurative Cholangitis

    4. Hepatic Abscess

    5. Hepatitis

  Vascular Disorders

    1. Ruptured Aortic Aneurysm

    2. Ischemic Colitis

    3. Mesenteric Thrombosis

    4. Rupture of the Spleen

    5. Splenic Infarct

  Urinary Disorders

    1. Renal Colic

    2. Pyelonephritis

    3. Renal Infarct

  Acute Pancreatitis

  Gynecologic Disorders

    1. Ectopic Pregnancy with Rupture

    2. Acute Salpingitis (Pelvic Inflammatory Disease)

    3. Ruptured Ovarian Follicle Cyst

    4. Ovarian Torsion

    5. Endometriosis

  Primary Peritonitis

  Retroperitoneal Hemorrhage

Conditions Causing Acute Abdominal Pain That Are Not Amenable to Surgery

■ IMMEDIATE MANAGEMENT OF LIFE-THREATENING PROBLEMS (See Figure 13–1.)

Perform Brief Examination

Record complete vital signs, including blood pressure and pulse with the patient in the sitting (or standing) position if blood pressure is normal in the supine position. Assess peripheral perfusion (alertness; skin and extremity temperature). Gently examine the abdomen to find an obvious aortic aneurysm or the presence of an "acute" abdomen, ie, boardlike (involuntary) guarding. Perform a rectal examination, and check the stool for blood. A brief history may often be obtained simultaneously. (If there has been abdominal trauma, proceed as outlined in Chapter 25.)

Caution: Patients with acute myocardial infarction, especially involving the inferior or posterior wall, may present with epigastric or upper abdominal pain. A carefully elicited history and an electrocardiogram (ECG) should be obtained, especially if no abdominal

---

[1]This chapter is a revision of the chapter by Richard A. Crass, MD, & Donald D. Trunkey, MD, from the 4th edition.

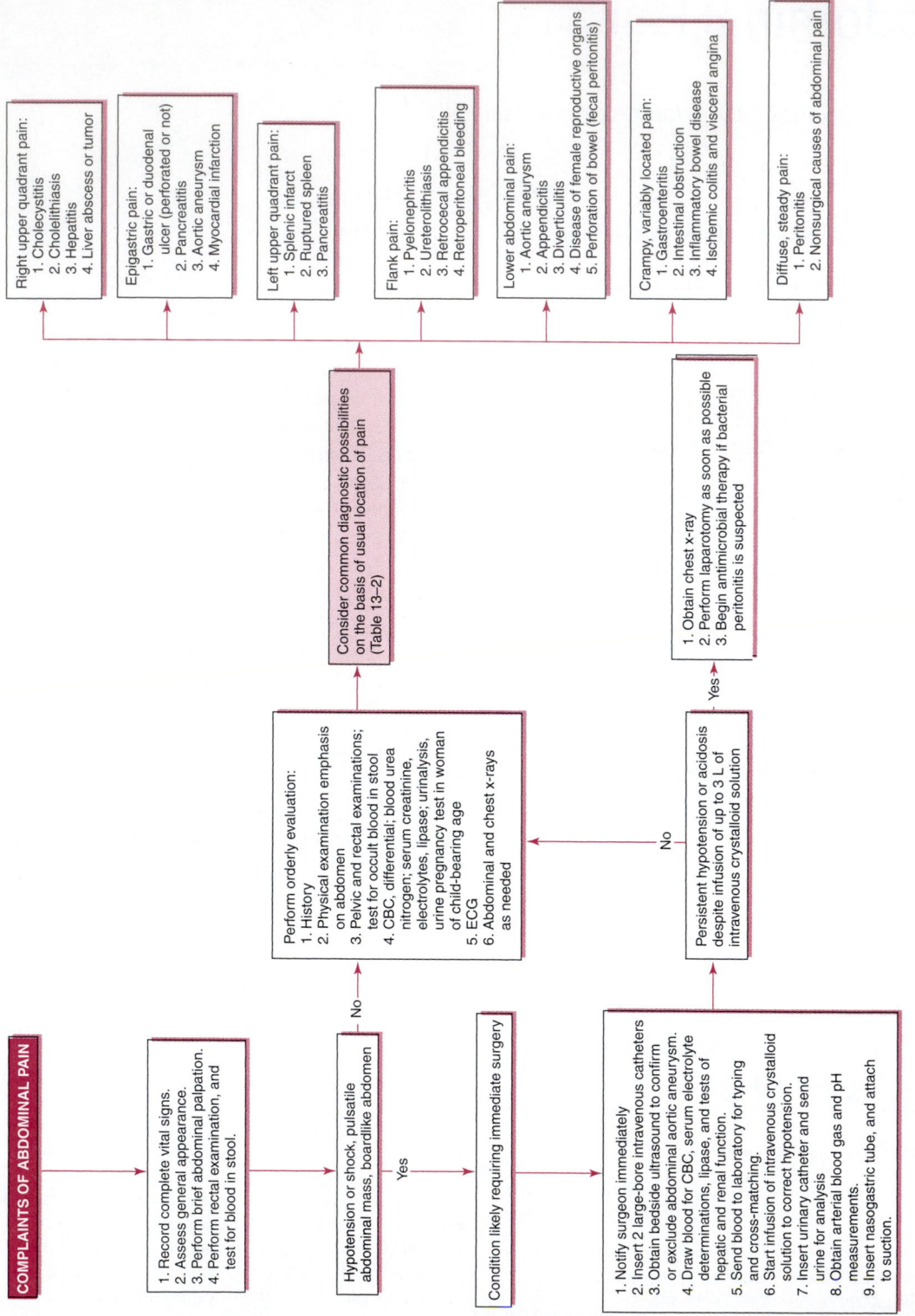

Figure 13–1. Algorithmic approach to complaints of abdominal pain.

258

disorder is clearly identified. In addition, patients with diabetic ketoacidosis may present with severe abdominal pain and vomiting.

Identify Candidates for Urgent Surgery

If hypotension (supine or postural) without gastrointestinal bleeding, an aneurysm, or a rigid abdomen is present in the patient with abdominal pain, there is a strong possibility of underlying life-threatening disease requiring early surgical correction. The on-call surgeon and operating room personnel should be notified.

Treat Shock

Note: Persistent shock despite fluid resuscitation in the patient with acute abdominal pain requires urgent laparotomy.

Treat hypotension or frank shock (Chapter 9). To reiterate—

1. Insert 2 large-bore ($\geq$ 16-gauge) intravenous catheters in an upper extremity.

2. Obtain blood for complete blood count (CBC) with differential, serum electrolyte measurements, lipase determination, renal function tests, and a rapid bedside glucose determination. Send a tube of clotted blood for typing and cross-matching.

3. Immediately begin rapid infusion of crystalloid solution (eg, a balanced salt solution). Adjust the rate of infusion based on blood pressure; initially, give 1 L over 10–20 minutes (adult dose).

4. Administer oxygen, 5–10 L/min, by nasal cannula or mask to keep oxygen saturation on pulse oximetry above 95%.

5. Insert a urinary catheter to monitor urine output, which is a sensitive indicator of visceral blood flow. Send a urine sample for analysis and for pregnancy test in women of child-bearing age.

6. Obtain arterial blood gas and pH measurements, because they are a useful guide to the patient's overall physiologic condition.

7. Insert a nasogastric tube if the patient shows evidence of peritonitis, severe ileus, intestinal obstruction, or gastrointestinal bleeding. The tube should be inserted before other diagnostic measures are undertaken.

8. Obtain a 12-lead ECG, and begin continuous cardiac monitoring.

9. If bacterial peritonitis is suspected, begin antibiotics after appropriate cultures have been obtained (Table 13–1).

Table 13–1. Antimicrobials for the acute abdomen.

Drug	Dose
Cefoxitin	150 mg/kg/d intravenously in 4–6 divided doses
Cefotetan	1–2 g every 12 hours
Ampicillin-sulbactam	1.5–3.0 g every 6–8 hours
Ticarcillin-clavulanate	3.1 g every 4–6 hours
Aztreonam	2 g every 6 hours
plus	
Clindamycin[1]	900 mg every 8 hours

[1]Metronidazole (500 mg every 6–8 hours) may be substituted for clindamycin.

Farber MS, Abrams JH: Abdominal emergencies: has anything changed? Antibiotics for the acute abdomen. Surg Clin North Am 1997;77:1396. [PMID: 9431346]

■ FURTHER EVALUATION OF THE PATIENT WITH ABDOMINAL PAIN

When vital functions have been normalized, reassess the patient as described below unless immediate surgery is required (Table 13–2).

Pain is usually present in acute intra-abdominal disorders. Diagnosis depends on meticulous history taking and physical examination. The history is usually the most important diagnostic aid, though physical examination and laboratory and x-ray studies provide important confirmation data. In general, 85–90% of diagnoses may be based on history alone, whereas laboratory examination alone or physical examination alone accounts only for an additional 5–8% of diagnoses each. The physician's time should be allocated accordingly.

Often it is impossible to diagnose abdominal pain definitively in the emergency department. If pain is significant, it is prudent to hospitalize the patient for observation and further diagnostic procedures.

HISTORY

If there is a history of abdominal trauma, the diagnostic approach differs from that for spontaneous abdominal pain and is discussed in Chapter 25. Pelvic pain in women is discussed in Chapter 36.

Table 13–2. Differential diagnosis of the common causes of acute abdominal pain.

Disease	Location of Pain and Prior Attacks	Mode of Onset and Type of Pain	Associated Gastrointestinal Symptoms	Physical Examination	Helpful Tests and Examinations
Acute appendicitis	Periumbilical or localized generally to right lower abdominal quadrant.	Insidious to acute and persistent.	Anorexia common; nausea and vomiting in some.	Low-grade fever. Epigastric tenderness initially; later, right lower quadrant.	Slight leukocytosis. CT scan of the abdomen or ultrasound of the appendix may be helpful if diagnosis is uncertain.
Intestinal obstruction	Diffuse.	Sudden onset. Crampy.	Vomiting common.	Abdominal distention; high-pitched rushes.	Dilated, fluid-filled loops of bowel on abdominal x-ray.
Perforated duodenal ulcer	Epigastric. History of ulcer in many.	Abrupt onset. Steady.	Anorexia; nausea and vomiting	Epigastric tenderness Involuntary guarding.	Upright abdominal x-ray shows air under diaphragm. CT scan.
Diverticulitis	Left lower quadrant. History of previous attacks.	Gradual onset. Steady or crampy.	Mild diarrhea common.	Fever common. Mass and tenderness in left lower quadrant.	CT scan shows inflammatory mass.
Inflammatory bowel disease	Diffuse; primarily in lower abdomen. Prior attacks common.	Gradual onset. Often crampy.	Diarrhea common, often with blood and mucus.	Fever. Diffuse abdominal tenderness.	Blood and leukocytes in stool. CT scan. Abnormal results on proctosigmoidoscopy or barium enema.
Acute cholecystitis	Epigastric or right upper quadrant; may be referred to right shoulder.	Insidious to acute.	Anorexia; nausea and vomiting.	Right upper quadrant tenderness.	Right upper quadrant sonography shows gallstones. Radionuclide scan shows nonvisualization of gallbladder.
Biliary colic	Intermittent right upper quadrant. Prior attacks common.	Often abrupt onset. Dull to sharp.	Anorexia; nausea and vomiting common.	Right upper quadrant tenderness.	Sonography shows gallstones.

Condition	Location of pain	Onset and character	Nausea, vomiting, diarrhea	Physical findings	Laboratory and imaging
Ischemic colitis	Epigastric; diffuse. Prior attacks common.	Often abrupt. Crampy.	Diarrhea, commonly bloody.	Diffuse abdominal tenderness. Vascular disease elsewhere.	Barium enema shows "thumbprinting" of mucosa. CT scan. Visceral angiography shows vascular obstruction.
Ruptured abdominal aortic aneurysm	Epigastrium and back.	Abrupt. Sharp and severe.	Variable; may be none.	Hypotension or shock. Abdominal aneurysm.	Sonography, CT scan, or angiography shows aneurysm.
Rupture of spleen	Left upper quadrant or diffuse. May be referred to left shoulder. History of trauma common.	Abrupt. Severe.	Usually none.	Hypotension or shock. Peritonitis. Left upper quadrant tenderness; fractured left ribs in some.	CT scan or liver-spleen scan shows rupture. Peritoneal lavage reveals blood.
Renal colic	Costovertebral or along course of ureter.	Sudden. Severe and sharp.	Frequently nausea and vomiting.	Flank tenderness.	Hematuria. Abnormal Noncontrast CT scan of the abdomen or excretory urogram (obstruction, hydronephrosis)
Acute pancreatitis	Epigastric penetrating to back.	Acute. Persistent, dull, severe.	Anorexia; nausea and vomiting common.	Epigastric tenderness.	Elevated serum lipase. CT scan shows pancreatic inflammation.
Acute salpingitis	Bilateral adnexal; later, may be generalized.	Gradually becomes worse.	Nausea and vomiting may be present.	Cervical motion elicits tenderness. Mass if tubo-ovarian abscess is present	Ultrasound can rule out tubo-ovarian abscess.
Ectopic pregnancy	Unilateral early; may have shoulder pain after rupture.	Sudden or intermittently vague to sharp.	Frequently none.	Adnexal mass. Tenderness.	Pelvic ultrasound reveals adnexal mass or blood. Positive urine pregnancy test.

Mode of Onset of Abdominal Pain

(See Figure 13–2 and Table 13–2.)

A. ABRUPT ONSET

If the patient was well one moment and seized with agonizing (explosive) pain the next, the most probable diagnosis is rupture of a hollow viscus or a vascular accident (eg, ruptured aortic aneurysm). In these instances, the pain is maximal or nearly maximal at time of onset.

Pain that begins abruptly, is only moderately severe at first, and worsens rapidly suggests acute pancreatitis, mesenteric thrombosis, or small bowel strangulation. If pelvic pain is present, consider a possible ruptured ectopic pregnancy or ovarian follicle cyst (Chapter 36).

B. GRADUAL ONSET

Gradual onset of slowly worsening pain is characteristic of peritoneal infection or inflammation. Patients with appendicitis or diverticulitis often report gradual onset of pain.

Character of Pain

(See Figure 13–2.)

A. SEVERE PAIN

Severe abdominal pain may be caused by several conditions including renal and biliary colic or vascular conditions such as myocardial infarction, rupture of an abdominal aortic aneurysm, or mesenteric ischemia. Other conditions associated with severe pain include acute pancreatitis, perforation of a hollow viscus, or peritonitis.

B. DULL PAIN

Pain that is dull, vague, and poorly localized and does not require analgesia is also likely to have been gradual in onset. Such findings strongly suggest an inflammatory process or a low-grade infection. Appendicitis and diverticulitis are associated with this type of pain.

C. INTERMITTENT PAIN WITH CRAMPS

The clinical picture of intermittent pain with cramps is common in gastroenteritis. However, if the pain comes in regular cycles, rises in crescendo fashion, and then subsides to a pain-free interval, the most likely diagnosis is mechanical small bowel obstruction. Occasionally, this type of pain occurs in early subacute pancreatitis or in renal colic.

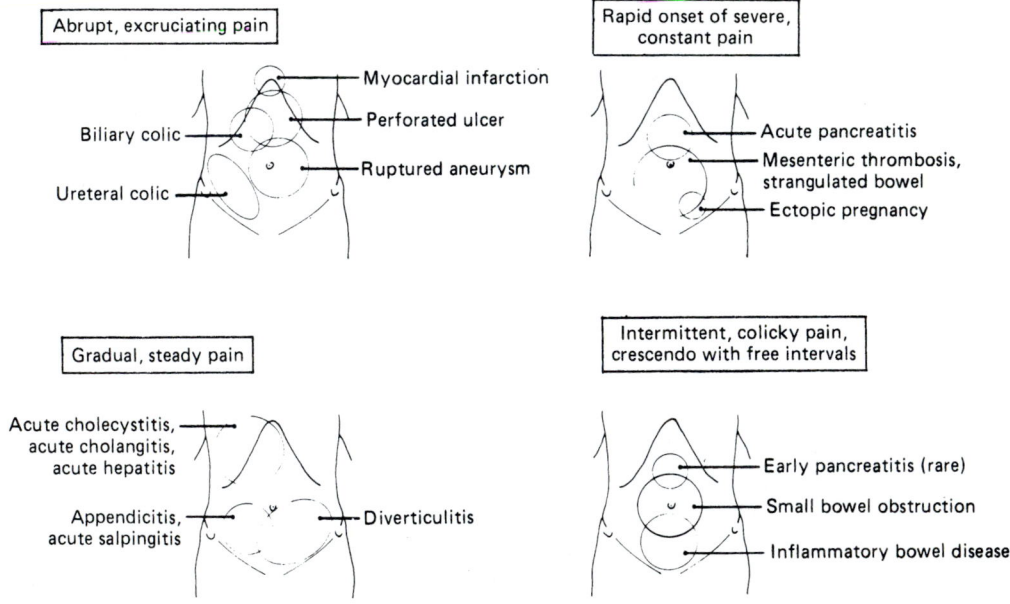

Figure 13–2. Correlation between nature of abdominal pain and underlying condition.
(Reproduced, with permission, from Way LW [editor]: *Current Surgical Diagnosis & Treatment,* 9th ed. Lange, 1991.)

D. ABSENCE OF PAIN

Occasionally, a patient presents with no abdominal pain but rather a sense of fullness and a feeling that a bowel movement would bring relief. A bowel movement, whether it is spontaneous or due to administration of cathartics or an enema, usually fails to relieve discomfort, however. This so-called gas stoppage sign is characteristic of retrocecal appendicitis but may be present when any inflammatory lesion is walled off from the free peritoneal cavity.

Location of Pain

Generally, pain fibers within the abdominal cavity are confined to the visceral peritoneum, parietal peritoneum, and blood vessels. The parietal peritoneum is innervated by somatic nerve fibers and will therefore localize pain. Pain due to visceral peritoneal involvement alone is poorly localized. In conditions that do not involve the parietal peritoneum, the most common sources of pain are distention of a hollow viscus and visceral ischemia. These general principles are a useful guide to a systematic evaluation of the cause of abdominal pain.

A. LOCALIZED ABDOMINAL PAIN

(See Table 13–2.) In general, when abdominal pain becomes localized, it does so over or near the involved viscus, for example, epigastric or right upper quadrant pain of acute cholecystitis, or right lower quadrant pain of appendicitis. However, the physician must remember anatomic variants (eg, an inflamed retrocecal appendix produces flank pain or nonlocalizing abdominal pain) and must consider all structures that might cause pain (eg, vascular disease).

B. RADIATION OF PAIN OR SHIFT IN LOCALIZATION

Radiation of pain or shift in localization of pain has particular diagnostic significance.

1. Shoulder pain—Shoulder pain may be due to ipsilateral diaphragmatic irritation from air, blood, or infection in the peritoneal cavity. For example, cholecystitis may be associated with referred right shoulder pain or even epigastric and left shoulder pain mimicking angina.

2. Diffuse periumbilical and epigastric pain—Diffuse periumbilical and epigastric pain gradually localizing to the right lower quadrant is a classic sign of appendicitis. With early appendicitis, only the visceral peritoneum surrounding the appendix is involved in the inflammatory process, and localization is therefore poor. As inflammation spreads and involves the parietal peritoneum, pain then localizes to the right lower quadrant. If the appendix is retrocecal, however, as it is in

15% of cases, the parietal peritoneum is not involved, and then pain remains poorly localized.

3. Pain radiating from the flank—Pain radiating from the flank to the groin or genitalia usually signifies ureteral colic, as seen in urolithiasis.

Anorexia; Nausea & Vomiting

Anorexia and nausea and vomiting occur more commonly in disease of the upper abdomen; however, advanced intra-abdominal disease may be present without any of these symptoms. If the peritoneum is well protected from infection or inflammation, as in retrocecal appendicitis or when the appendix is completely isolated by omentum, the patient may retain a normal appetite.

If nausea and vomiting precede the onset of pain, an acute abdominal emergency requiring operation is unlikely. The most likely diagnoses are gastroenteritis and food poisoning, acute gastritis, acute pancreatitis, and (much less frequently) common duct stone and high intestinal obstruction. In most acute surgical emergencies, nausea and vomiting are not dominant or early symptoms, although they may be present by the time the patient seeks medical attention.

Severe vomiting with retching—particularly after a dietary indiscretion or an alcoholic bout—followed by abdominal pain with or without hematemesis should immediately suggest mucosal laceration of the gastroesophageal junction (Mallory-Weiss syndrome) or an esophageal perforation (Boerhaave syndrome). Massive hematemesis or severe pain radiating into the chest and left shoulder in association with severe vomiting and retching are classic symptoms of Boerhaave syndrome. The presence of pleural fluid on chest x-ray further supports the diagnosis.

Fever & Rigors

Fever is common with most causes of acute abdominal pain. In appendicitis, the temperature is usually not high, and rigors (shaking chills) are uncommon. High fever or rigors in suspected appendicitis strongly suggest diffuse peritonitis from perforation of a viscus, pylephlebitis (septic thrombophlebitis of the portal vein), or another disorder entirely (eg, pyelonephritis). High fever with peritoneal signs in a female patient with no apparent general systemic illness is characteristic of acute salpingitis with pelvic peritonitis. Repeated shaking chills and fever are most common in infections of the biliary or urinary tract. Patients with acute cholangitis or acute pyelonephritis usually present with intermittent rigors and fever. Chills, fever, rigors, jaundice, and hypotension suggest suppurative cholangitis, which is a surgical emergency.

Diarrhea, Constipation, & Obstipation

Diarrhea, constipation, and obstipation may occur in the acute abdomen patient but are not often major symptoms in acute intra-abdominal disease requiring surgery. Colitis (vascular or some other kind) usually is associated with early and severe diarrhea. Occasionally, patients with diverticulitis, appendicitis, or salpingitis may also experience diarrhea.

PHYSICAL EXAMINATION

The basic steps of the physical examination of the acute abdomen are outlined in Table 13–3. Remember that physical findings may be subtle in elderly or immunocompromised patients.

Inspection

The physician should first inspect the abdomen and look for striking features such as the scaphoid, contracted abdomen of an early perforated viscus; the visible peristalsis and distention of mechanical obstruction; or the soft, doughy distention of early ileus.

Auscultation

A silent abdomen, with complete absence of audible peristalsis, usually signifies diffuse peritonitis; however, peristalsis may persist in the face of established peritonitis. Other manifestations of diffuse peritonitis such as rigidity and distention are usually also present. It may be necessary to listen for as long as 2–3 minutes to establish absence of peristalsis, because peristalsis diminishes if the patient has not eaten.

High-pitched, tinkling bowel sounds are suggestive of acute small bowel obstruction. There may also be intermittent peristaltic rushes that coincide with the onset of pain. These findings will usually be associated with abdominal distention.

Table 13–3. Routine for physical examination of acute abdomen.

Inspection
Auscultation
Palpation
    Examination of hernial rings and male genitalia
    Cough tenderness
    Rectus muscle spasm
    One-finger palpation
    Costovertebral angle tenderness
    Deep palpation
Percussion
Special signs (iliopsoas and obturator signs, etc)
Pelvic and rectal examinations

In gastroenteritis, dysentery, and active ulcerative colitis, there may be abnormal high-pitched peristalsis with rushes that are not synchronous with the episodes of pain.

Palpation

A. EXAMINE HERNIAL RINGS AND MALE GENITALIA

Examine the inguinal and femoral canals in both sexes and the genitalia in the male, and look for incarcerated hernias that may be causing intestinal obstruction. This must be done by asking the patient to cough but should be done gently so as to cause as little discomfort as possible.

B. ELICIT COUGH TENDERNESS

In most acute inflammatory conditions arising within the abdomen, coughing elicits pain in the involved area. Directing the patient to point one finger to the area of pain provides objective localization of the lesion. With this information, the examiner can proceed to examine the abdomen and deliberately examine last the area now known to be most tender.

C. FEEL FOR SPASM OF RECTUS ABDOMINIS MUSCLE

The next step is to establish the presence or absence of true muscle spasm by placing a hand gently over the rectus abdominis muscle and depressing it slightly and gently without causing pain. The patient is asked to take a long, slow breath. If the spasm is voluntary, the muscle will immediately relax underneath the gentle pressure of the palpating hand. If there is true spasm, however, the muscle will remain taut and rigid through the respiratory cycle. This maneuver alone may be sufficient to establish the presence of peritonitis.

Except for rare neurologic disorders, renal colic, or rectus muscle injury, only peritoneal inflammation produces abdominal muscle rigidity (for reasons not understood). In renal colic, the spasm is confined to the entire rectus muscle on the involved side. This distinction is important, because marked rigidity of the entire length of one rectus muscle with relaxation of the opposite rectus cannot occur in peritonitis, because the peritoneal cavity is not compartmentalized. It is possible to have segmental spasm of a rectus muscle involving only the upper or lower portion of one side, or to have segmental spasm of both rectus muscles in upper or lower abdominal peritonitis. In generalized peritonitis, however, both muscles are usually involved to the same degree.

D. PERFORM ONE-FINGER PALPATION

Abdominal tenderness must be assessed with one finger, because it is impossible to localize peritoneal inflammation accurately if palpation or tenderness is done with the entire hand. Careful one-finger palpation, beginning as far away as possible from the area of tenderness elicited by coughing and gradually working toward it, will usually enable the examiner to delineate the area of abdominal tenderness precisely. In early acute appendicitis, this area is often no larger than 3 cm (1 ³⁄₁₆ in) in diameter and sometimes smaller. Diffuse abdominal tenderness without associated involuntary rigidity of the muscles suggests gastroenteritis or some other inflammatory process of the intestines without peritonitis.

Do not test for peritoneal inflammation by looking for classic rebound tenderness (deep palpation of the abdomen with abrupt release). This maneuver yields no additional information and is so painful in patients with significant abdominal tenderness that further examination may be impossible.

E. Look for Costovertebral Angle Tenderness

Palpation should be followed by gentle percussion of the costovertebral angles. This will cause pain in individuals with pyelonephritis, retroperitoneal abscesses, and retrocecal appendix. Avoid excessively vigorous percussion, because it is not helpful in localizing tenderness and the pain it causes will make further examination difficult.

F. Perform Deep Palpation

Having established the presence or absence of muscular rigidity and localized the area of tenderness, the examiner now palpates more deeply for the presence of abdominal masses. Often, it is difficult to perform a reliable physical examination of the abdomen in an anxious patient. Some patients are so anxious that they begin to guard with voluntary contraction of the abdominal musculature before the examiner performs even light palpation. This barrier to palpation can occasionally be overcome by palpating with a stethoscope while auscultating bowel sounds.

Among the more common lesions identifiable by careful palpation in patients with acute abdominal pain are the distended, tender gallbladder found in acute cholecystitis; the right lower quadrant tender mass of appendicitis with early abscess formation; the left lower quadrant mass of sigmoid diverticulitis; and the midline pulsatile mass indicating a leaking abdominal aneurysm.

Percussion

In free perforation of a hollow viscus with air under the diaphragm, there may be diminished or absent liver dullness. Tympany located laterally in the midaxillary line, 5 cm (2 in) or more above the costal margin, is due to free air; tympany located anteriorly over the liver may be due to air in distended loops of bowel.

Special Signs

Several maneuvers in physical examination may help localize an acute abdominal lesion.

A. Iliopsoas Sign

(See Figure 13–3.) The patient flexes the thigh against the resistance of the examiner's hand. A painful response indicates an inflammatory process involving the psoas muscle.

B. Obturator Sign

(See Figure 13–4.) The patient's thigh is flexed to a right angle and gently rotated, first internally and then externally. If pain is elicited, an inflammatory lesion involving the obturator internus muscle (pelvic appendicitis, diverticulitis, pelvic inflammatory disease) is present.

C. Murphy's Sign (Inspiratory Arrest)

The patient is asked to take a slow, deep breath as the examiner gently palpates the right upper quadrant. With descent of the diaphragm with the liver and gallbladder, an acutely inflamed gallbladder comes in contact with the examining fingers, causing pain, and the patient stops inspiration in an attempt to avoid the pain.

Pelvic & Rectal Examination

The importance of pelvic and rectal examination cannot be overstressed. In men a rectal examination plus simultaneous lower abdominal palpation with the other hand often reveals masses or localized pain not disclosed by abdominal examination alone. Likewise, pelvic examination in women provides essential information not revealed by other maneuvers. Evaluation of

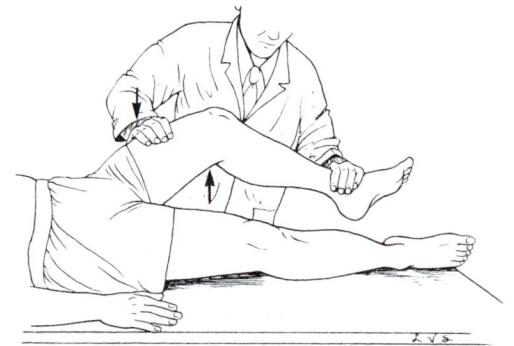

Figure 13–3. Performing the iliopsoas test.
(Reproduced, with permission, from Way LW [editor]: *Current Surgical Diagnosis & Treatment*, 6th ed. Lange, 1983.)

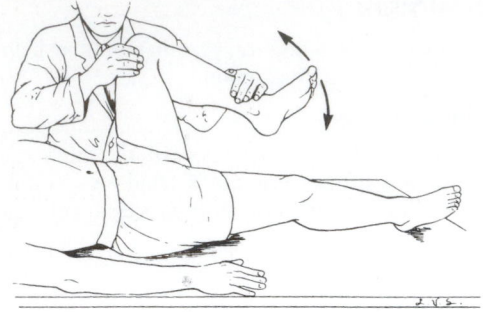

Figure 13–4. Performing the obturator test. (Reproduced, with permission, from Way LW [editor]: *Current Surgical Diagnosis & Treatment,* 6th ed. Lange, 1983.)

lower abdominal pain in women is discussed further in Chapter 36.

Examination of stool for occult blood must be performed in every patient with abdominal pain. Occult blood may result from intestinal tumors (possibly causing intestinal obstruction), inflammatory bowel disease, and ischemic bowel disease.

LABORATORY EXAMINATION

CBC with differential, lipase measurements, and urinalysis are called for in most cases. Electrolyte determinations and tests of renal function should be obtained if vomiting, diarrhea, hypotension, or shock are present or if there is a strong chance that surgery will be performed.

Blood Count

The hematocrit reflects changes both in plasma volume and in red cell volume. It is most useful diagnostically if it is markedly elevated (indicating dehydration) or depressed (indicating anemia). Additionally, the hematocrit should be corrected toward normal values (between 30% and 45% is usually satisfactory) in preparation for surgery in hemodynamically unstable patients.

The white cell count may be helpful if it is significantly elevated. However, normal or even low counts can occur in established peritonitis or sepsis (although usually with a marked shift to the left), and elevated counts may occur in gastroenteritis. A normal or low white count, particularly with lymphocytosis, may suggest viral infection. A progressively rising white count is of considerable diagnostic value and usually indicates progression of an inflammatory or septic process. A shift to the left on a blood smear may be a clue to an inflammatory reaction in the presence of a normal or only moderately elevated white count.

Serum Amylase & Lipase

Serum amylase and lipase levels require cautious evaluation. Patients with abdominal pain and elevated serum amylase or lipase usually have acute pancreatitis. However, some patients with severe hemorrhagic pancreatitis have normal or low serum amylase, and patients with persistent or chronic pancreatitis often have normal serum amylase levels. In the presence of pancreatic pseudocysts, however, serum amylase often remains elevated.

Serum amylase may be elevated in mesenteric arterial thrombosis, intestinal obstruction, or perforated duodenal ulcer and occasionally in other conditions. It is also elevated in macroamylasemia, a common benign condition in which urinary amylase clearance is markedly reduced as a result of complex formation with other serum proteins.

Lipase is a more specific marker for pancreatitis because it is found only in the pancreas. Vissers et al. (1999) have suggested using lipase as the more accurate screening test for patients with suspected pancreatitis and that there is no clinical utility to obtaining both amylase and lipase in the emergency department. In emergency department patients with abdominal pain, lipase sensitivity (100%) was better than amylase sensitivity (72%) for the diagnosis of pancreatitis. In addition, for patients with radiographically proven alcoholic pancreatitis, the sensitivity of lipase was superior to amylase (100% vs. 55%, respectively). Unfortunately, the degree to which either marker is elevated cannot predict the severity of the condition or any associated complications of pancreatitis.

Vissers RJ, Abu-Labari RB, McHugh DF: Amylase and lipase in the emergency department evaluation of acute pancreatitis. J Emerg Med 1999;17(6):1027. [PMID: 10595892] (Review.)

Hepatic Function Tests

Hepatic function testing is indicated for patients who have right upper quadrant pain or tenderness, jaundice, acholic stools, or tea-colored urine and for patients in whom hepatitis is a concern.

Urine

Urinalysis (including microscopic examination of the sediment) is critical in ruling out urinary tract infection, urolithiasis, and diabetes. Hematuria strongly suggests urolithiasis. Rarely, however, urolithiasis with complete obstruction of the ureter may be associated with normal results on urinalysis. Low urine specific gravity associated with severe vomiting may be the earliest clue to renal disease. Obtain a urine pregnancy test in all women of child-bearing age.

Serum Electrolytes & Tests of Renal Function

Serum electrolyte determinations and a test of renal function (blood urea nitrogen, serum creatinine, or both) are required to document the nature and extent of fluid losses if vomiting or diarrhea has been significant or if the illness has lasted for more than 48 hours with diminished oral intake. Abnormalities should be corrected as much as possible in preparation for surgery (Chapter 42).

Pregnancy Test

A urine pregnancy test should be obtained in all women of child-bearing age unless pregnancy is physically impossible (eg, complete hysterectomy, bilateral oophorectomy). Women with a history of pelvic infection, current intrauterine device use, prior ectopic pregnancy, and failed tubal ligation are at increased risk for ectopic pregnancy.

Electrocardiogram

A 12-lead ECG should be obtained in patients with epigastric or upper abdominal pain in whom no clear cause of the pain is identified and cardiac ischemia is a possibility.

Peritoneal Fluid

In peritoneal dialysis or chronic liver disease patients, examination of the peritoneal fluid is often warranted if abdominal pain, tenderness, or fever are present.

RADIOLOGIC EXAMINATION

Radiologic examination may provide important evidence for diagnosis of acute abdominal disease. Close cooperation between the radiologist and the physician caring for the patient is essential.

Suggested Studies

Abdominal radiographs are most helpful in the evaluation of patients with suspected bowel obstruction or hollow viscus perforation and in children or mentally handicapped adults with possible foreign body ingestion. An acute abdominal series consists of three films: an upright anteroposterior chest x-ray, a supine anteroposterior abdominal x-ray, and an upright or left lateral decubitus abdominal x-ray. To maximize the diagnostic utility and limit unnecessary abdominal x-rays, Böhner suggests limiting these studies to patients with two or more of the following findings: prior abdominal surgery, increased bowel sounds, abdominal distention, peritoneal signs, history of constipation or vomiting, and age over 50 years.

Interpretation

When the films are reviewed, the following questions should be asked: (1) Are the outlines of the liver, spleen, kidneys, and psoas muscles clearly defined? (2) Are the peritoneal fat lines identifiable? (3) Is the gas pattern in the stomach, small bowel, and colon within normal limits? (4) Is there evidence of air outside the bowel or beneath the diaphragm? (5) Is there air in the biliary ducts and ductules? (6) Are there abnormal opaque shadows such as gallstones; ureteral stones; fecaliths; or calcification in lymph nodes, pancreas, aorta, or other soft tissue masses?

On the basis of these observations, the following important pieces of evidence may be obtained:

A. PSOAS SHADOW

Obliteration of the psoas shadow may indicate a retroperitoneal hematoma or abscess (Figure 13–5).

B. GAS PATTERNS

Gas patterns are of particular importance. Dilated loops of small bowel with air-fluid levels and no gas in the

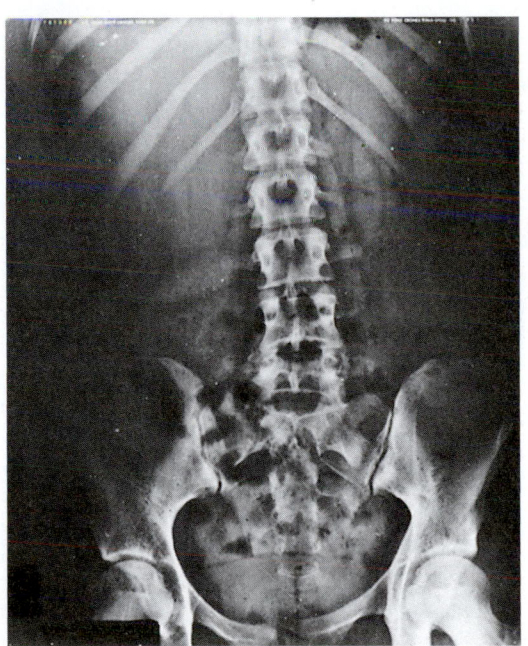

Figure 13–5. Obliteration of the psoas shadow on the right by a subhepatic abscess.
(Reproduced, with permission, from Way LW [editor]: *Current Surgical Diagnosis & Treatment*, 6th ed. Lange, 1983.)

colon are indicative of small bowel obstruction (Figure 13–6).

C. Cecum

Marked dilatation and rotation of the cecum or sigmoid are typical of volvulus.

D. Dilatations

Marked dilatation of the entire colon suggests colonic obstruction. Massive dilatation of the colon in acute colitis indicates toxic megacolon. Distention of both the small and the large bowel is characteristic of ileus, peritonitis, and pseudo-obstruction of the bowel (Figure 13–7). The differentiation between distended small and large bowel may at times be difficult. In advanced cases, the clinical signs may be more reliable than x-rays in the differentiation between intestinal obstruction and peritonitis.

E. Air in Abnormal Locations

Except following laparotomy, laparoscopy, or recent percutaneous gastrotomy tube placement, free air under the diaphragm usually indicates a perforated viscus, most

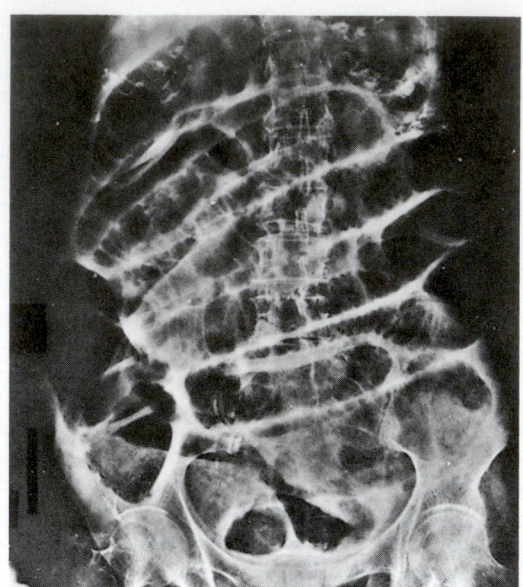

Figure 13–7. Abdominal x-ray showing dilated loops of small and large bowel without air-fluid levels, typical of diffuse peritonitis. (Reproduced, with permission, from Way LW [editor]: *Current Surgical Diagnosis & Treatment,* 6th ed. Lange, 1983.)

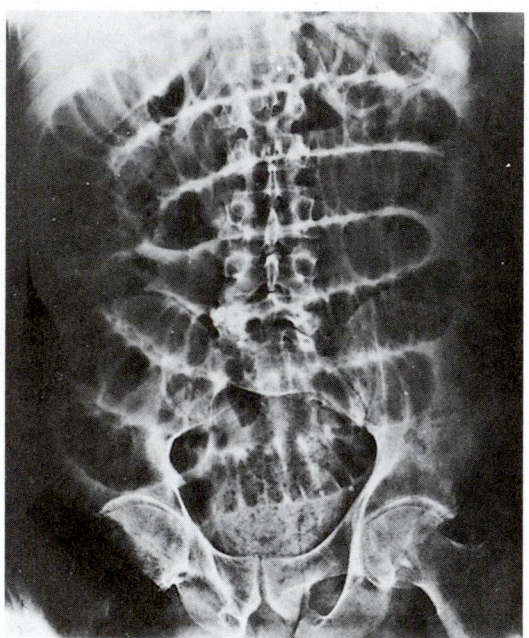

Figure 13–6. Upright abdominal x-ray showing dilated loops of small bowel with air-fluid levels and no gas in the colon. Patient had small bowel obstruction. (Reproduced, with permission, from Way LW [editor]: *Current Surgical Diagnosis & Treatment,* 9th ed. Lange, 1991.)

commonly seen in perforated duodenal or gastric ulcer (Figure 13–8). Massive amounts of air beneath the diaphragm suggest colonic perforation. An encapsulated air shadow outside the contours of small or large bowel may indicate localized perforation of the intestine. Air in the biliary tract is diagnostic of a free communication between some portion of the gastrointestinal tract and the biliary tree. If evidence of intestinal obstruction is present, this pattern is characteristic of gallstone ileus. Air in the portal venous system indicates pylephlebitis with a gas-forming organism but also occurs in pneumatosis cystoides intestinalis and has been described following the introduction of hydrogen peroxide into the rectum. Rarely, free air in the peritoneum may be seen in asymptomatic or minimally symptomatic women with no signs of apparent underlying disease. The free air has presumably entered the peritoneum from the genital tract.

F. Calcifications and Opacities

X-rays of the abdomen may establish the presence of gallstones, ureteral stones, pancreatic calcification, retroperitoneal calcification, and vascular calcification. Such findings must be carefully correlated with the history and physical examination to establish their significance.

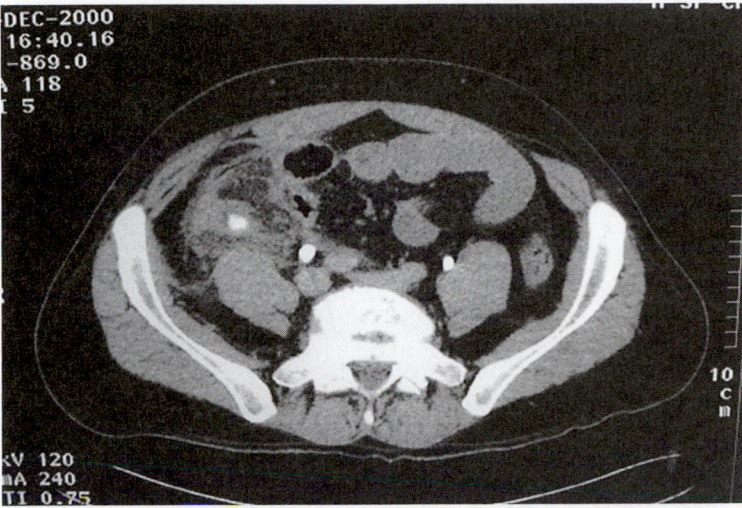

A

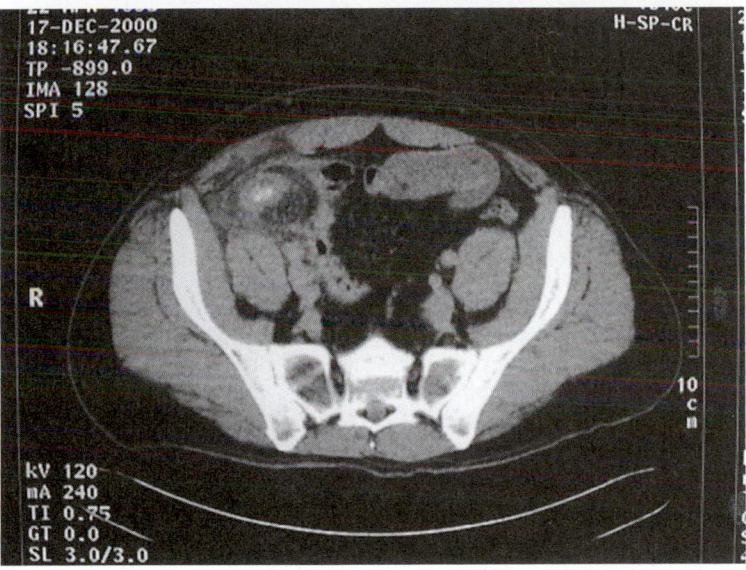

B

Figure 13–8. CT scan of the abdomen with oral and intravenous contrast in a patient with right lower quadrant pain. The study demonstrates a calcified appendolith (A and B) with associated stranding in the right lower quadrant. A dilated, fluid-filled appendix is noted (C).

Special Studies

(See Table 13–4.) Special x-ray contrast studies, ultrasonography, or computed tomography (CT) scans may be helpful.

A. Barium Enema

Avoid barium enema if possible in the presence of acute abdominal disease and peritonitis. In rare cases, a water-soluble contrast enema is necessary to establish a diagnosis of sigmoid volvulus or a low, partial colonic obstruction due to carcinoma.

B. Ultrasonography

Ultrasonography is a useful technique for evaluating the gallbladder, biliary ducts, pancreas, appendix, kidneys, and abdominal aorta. It is probably the best single diagnostic test for evaluating patients with right upper quadrant pain (see Table 13–4).

C. CT Scan

The CT scan of the abdomen with oral and intravenous contrast is frequently obtained to gain information about not only the solid organs and retroperitoneal

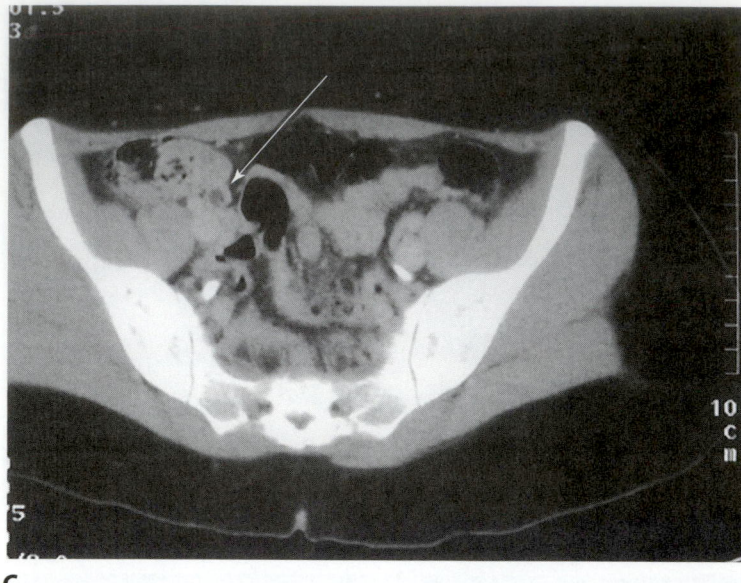

Figure 13–8. (Continued)

C

structures but also the hollow organs of the abdomen. Abdominal CT scanning has taken a prominent role in the evaluation of many patients with right lower quadrant pain and suspected appendicitis.

D. ANGIOGRAMS

Angiograms are used less frequently than before in trauma, because CT scan has been found to be more useful in cases of rupture of a solid viscus such as the spleen or kidney. Mesenteric angiography is the best way to identify the site of bleeding in massive lower gastrointestinal tract hemorrhage, although radionuclide blood pool scans are more sensitive in intermittent or less severe hemorrhage (Chapter 14).

■ ADDITIONAL MEASURES FOR THE MANAGEMENT OF ACUTE ABDOMEN

Repeated Examination

When the diagnosis is in doubt and the patient is not critically ill, a period of active observation is in order. Frequent inquiries about progression or alteration of symptoms combined with repeated, gentle examinations of the abdomen and, occasionally, repeat laboratory tests will avoid many unnecessary operations without risking dangerous delays. If the physician feels that

a diagnosis cannot be made within 6–12 hours, the patient should be hospitalized for observation. Observation in the emergency department for more than 4–6 hours is unwarranted for reasons of patient comfort, quality of care, and cost. Even in the absence of a tentative diagnosis, hospitalization is indicated for patients with severe pain and abdominal tenderness or peritoneal signs and for those with laboratory test abnormalities suggesting significant disease.

Relief of Pain

Although some surgical consultants may still oppose the administration of narcotics until a definitive diagnosis or plan for laparotomy has been established, parenteral narcotic analgesics should be given at once to relieve severe pain. Evaluation of acute abdominal disease can be performed more accurately after severe pain is relieved and the patient can cooperate. In addition, studies have demonstrated no adverse effects on the ability to diagnose acute surgical conditions when patients with an acute abdomen receive narcotics. What at first appears to be diffuse tenderness may become better localized. Abdominal masses not palpable initially often become obvious after moderate sedation and relief of pain.

Antimicrobials

Antimicrobial agents should be withheld until the diagnosis is at least tentatively established, except in the presence of obvious signs of systemic infection (high

Table 13–4. Definitive diagnosis of conditions causing acute abdominal pain.

Usual Location of Pain	Condition	Most Sensitive and Specific Signs and Diagnostic Tests
Right upper quadrant	Cholecystitis	right upper quadrant sonogram; radionuclide scan
	Biliary colic	Right upper quadrant sonogram
	Cholangitis	Right upper quandrant sonogram
	Hepatitis	Liver function tests, especially transaminases
	Liver abscess or tumor	Right upper quadrant sonogram; CT scan; radionuclide liver scan
	Right lower lobe pneumonia	Chest x-ray
Epigastrium or midline	Peritonitis	Smear and culture of peritoneal fluid; laparoscopy or laparotomy
	Pancreatitis	Serum lipase; CT scan
	Duodenal perforation	Upright or left decubitus flat plate of abdomen; CT scan with water-soluble oral contrast media
	Abdominal aortic aneurysm	Sonogram; CT scan
	Myocardial infarction	ECG; CK/troponin isoenzymes
Left upper quadrant	Rupture of spleen	Sonogram, peritoneal lavage; CT scan of abdomen
	Splenic infarct	CT scan
Flank	Pyelonephritis	Urinalysis and Gram's stain of urine; urine culture
	Renal colic	Urinalysis; noncontrast CT scan of abdomen; excretory urogram
	Renal infarct	Urinalysis; renal scan or angiography
Lower abdomen	Appendicitis	History and examination; CT scan with oral and intravenous contrast; sonogram; laparoscopy or laparotomy
	Diverticulitis	History and examination; CT scan with oral and intravenous contrast
	Ectopic pregnancy	Pelvic sonogram; laparoscopy or laparotomy; positive urine pregnancy test
	Salpingitis	History and examination; pelvic sonogram
	Ruptured ovarian follicle cyst	Pelvic sonogram
Diffuse or variable	Gastroenteritis	History and examination; stool smear and culture (Chapter 19)
	Intestinal obstruction	History and examination; supine and upright abdominal x-ray
	Volvulus and intestinal strangulation	Supine and upright abdominal x-ray
	Intestinal perforation	Supine and upright abdominal x-ray; CT scan with intravenous and water-soluble oral contrast
	Ischemic colitis	CT scan; visceral angiography; barium enema
	Idiopathic inflammatory bowel disease	CT scan with intravenous and water-soluble oral contrast
	Retroperitoneal hemorrhage	CT scan
	Mesenteric thrombosis	History and examination; visceral angiography; laparotomy; CT scan with intravenous and soluble oral water-contrast
	Porphyria	History; hirsutism; elevated urinary porphobilinogens
	Addison's disease	Low serum sodium and high serum potassium; low serum cortisol level

(continued)

Table 13–4. Definitive diagnosis of conditions causing acute abdominal pain. (Continued)

Usual Location of Pain	Condition	Most Sensitive and Specific Signs and Diagnostic Tests
Diffuse or variable	Poisoning	Toxicology screen (lead, arsenic, iron)
	Familial Mediterranean fever	History—patient and family
	Diabetic Ketoacidosis	Diabetes, previous attacks
	Tertiary syphillis	Presence of syphillis; previous attacks
	Preeruptive zoster	Unilateral dematomal distribution

fever, rigors, hypotension). In obscure cases, antibiotic therapy may mask progression of disease and lead to serious complications with increased illness (eg, appendicitis).

Surgical Consultation

Early surgical consultation is helpful for both the patient and the surgeon. Because the surgeon, like the emergency physician, must rely on repeated examinations for diagnosis, the earlier observation begins, the faster a definitive diagnosis can be made. Furthermore, delays in consultation may allow worsening of the condition, with possible disastrous sequelae.

Cook C, Campbell-Smith TA, Hopkins R: The abdominal radiograph: a pictorial review. Hosp Med 2002;63:726. [PMID: 12512199]

Thomas SH et al: Effects of morphine analgesia in diagnostic accuracy in emergency department patients with abdominal pain: a prospective, randomized trial. J Am Coll Surg 2003;196:18. [PMID: 12517545]

■ MANAGEMENT OF SPECIFIC DISORDERS CAUSING ABDOMINAL PAIN

INTESTINAL DISORDERS

1. Appendicitis

Clinical Findings

The initial symptom is poorly localized abdominal pain around the umbilicus or epigastrium, rarely in the right lower quadrant over McBurney's point. Later, the pain shifts from the periumbilical region to the right lower quadrant. Anorexia and nausea and vomiting usually accompany the illness. Localized abdominal tenderness

and guarding are noted on physical examination. Fever is low grade, and the white count may be moderately elevated. Variations from the classic clinical picture are common, especially in retrocecal appendicitis, where the pain commonly remains poorly localized. Abdominal CT with intravenous and water-soluble oral contrast has become a widely accepted tool in the evaluation of patients with possible appendicitis (see Figure 13–8). The sensitivity and specificity of abdominal CT scan in the evaluation of appendicitis are 90–100% and 91–99%, respectively. In addition, when appendicitis is not present, the CT scan demonstrates an alternative diagnosis two thirds of the time. Ultrasonography of the appendix may be helpful if the diagnosis is uncertain.

Treatment & Disposition

The patient should be hospitalized and prepared for surgery within a few hours. Administer intravenous crystalloid solution to replace any volume deficits. Antimicrobial therapy generally is not used until the decision is made to operate.

Paulson EK, Kalady MF, Pappas TN: Clinical practice. Suspected appendicitis. N Engl J Med 2003;348:236. [PMID: 12529465] (Review.)

2. Intestinal Obstruction

Clinical Findings

The patient usually complains of intermittent colicky abdominal pain of sudden onset that rises to a peak and then subsides. Bowel habits may be altered. Vomiting may occur and will be feculent if obstruction is distal and long-standing. The abdomen is distended and tender, and peristaltic rushes as well as high-pitched tinkling may be heard. Dilated loops of bowel with air-fluid levels on abdominal x-ray confirm the diagnosis (see Figure 13–6). Differentiation between small and large bowel is often based on the mucosal patterns demonstrated on the abdominal radiograph. In the small intestine, the valvulae conniventes cross the width of the lumen, and in the large intestine the haustra do not cross the entire width of the lumen. Occasionally, x-ray findings are absent, and the diagnosis is based on clinical suspicion or abdominal CT scan with contrast.

Treatment & Disposition

Nasogastric suction and intravenous hydration should be initiated and the patient hospitalized for evaluation and possible surgery. Some cases resolve without surgery.

3. Perforated Peptic Ulcer

Clinical Findings

Perforation of a duodenal ulcer usually causes sudden severe upper abdominal pain. The pain of perforation subsides when gastric contents are diluted by peritoneal secretions but reappears later, with progressive worsening. Shoulder pain may occur owing to diaphragmatic irritation. The patient is usually in severe distress, with shallow breathing and knees drawn up to the chest in an effort to minimize pain. Upper abdominal tenderness is accompanied by boardlike rigidity of the abdomen. X-ray with the patient upright may show air under the diaphragm (Figure 13–9). When abdominal radiographs are nondiagnostic and perforation is suspected, abdominal CT scan with intravenous and water-soluble oral contrast can be diagnostic.

Treatment & Disposition

Insert a nasogastric tube for drainage of gastric acid. Administer crystalloid solution intravenously to correct volume depletion. Initiate broad-spectrum intravenous antibiotics. Immediate hospitalization for surgery is necessary.

4. Perforation of the Bowel

Clinical Findings

Perforation of the bowel is accompanied by sudden or explosive onset of severe, agonizing mid or lower abdominal pain. Shock may be present and can be profound. Nausea and vomiting are common. The abdomen is rigid and tender. The temperature may be high and is accompanied by leukocytosis. A history of diverticulitis can often be elicited.

Treatment & Disposition

Treat shock with intravenous crystalloid solution. Insert a nasogastric tube for continuous gastric suction. Obtain blood and urine cultures. Begin antimicrobials (see Table 13–1). Hospitalize the patient, and prepare for surgery within 1–2 hours.

Jamieson GG: Current status of indications for surgery in peptic ulcer disease. World J Surg 2000;24:256. [PMID: 10658057] (Review.)

Svanes C: Trends in perforated peptic ulcer: incidence, etiology, treatment, and prognosis. World J Surg 2000;24:277. [PMID: 10658061] (Review.)

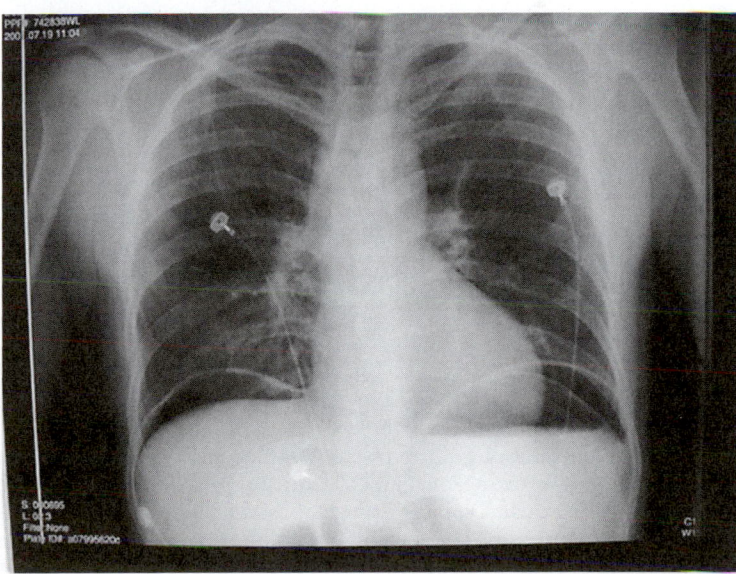

Figure 13–9. Upright anteroposterior chest x-ray demonstrating pneumoperitoneum from a perforated peptic ulcer.

5. Diverticulitis

Clinical Findings

Diverticulitis is associated with lower abdominal pain that is usually gradual in onset and localized, predominantly in the left lower quadrant, but that may be mid-abdominal or in the right lower quadrant. A history of diverticulosis may be present. Fever is low grade, accompanied by slight leukocytosis. Other findings may include abdominal tenderness, a palpable abdominal mass, and alterations in bowel function (either constipation or frequent defecation).

Treatment & Disposition

Most patients should be hospitalized for administration of intravenous fluids and antimicrobial drugs (see Table 13–1) and further observation. Patients without significant nausea or vomiting, fever, or other systemic signs of infection or any peritoneal signs may be candidates for outpatient treatment with oral antibiotics as long as the patient is reliable. Instructions should include a clear liquid diet initially and to return if vomiting, worsening pain, or fever develop.

6. Intestinal Strangulation

Clinical Findings

Intestinal strangulation occurs most frequently in volvulus or femoral hernia and occasionally in inguinal hernia. Onset of pain is usually rapid. Pain increases in severity and may be intermittent and colicky. The patient may complain of an urge to defecate. The abdomen is distended, rigid, and diffusely tender. Exquisite tenderness is present in the region of strangulation. Shock appears early. Other findings usually include nausea and vomiting, high fever, and leukocytosis. In the case of volvulus, findings on abdominal x-ray may be diagnostic.

Treatment & Disposition

The patient should be hospitalized and prepared for surgery within 1 hour.

7. Gastroenteritis
(See also Chapter 15.)

Clinical Findings

The patient complains of mild to severe cramping and pain that may have come on gradually or abruptly. There may be nausea and vomiting, retching, and diarrhea, in any combination. These symptoms usually precede the onset of pain, in contrast to conditions requiring surgery, in which pain is usually the first symptom. Abdominal examination reveals generalized discomfort. In contrast to situations requiring surgery, involuntary guarding, localized tenderness, and peritoneal signs (eg, cough tenderness) are absent. Fever is generally absent or mild, although patients with shigellosis typically have high fever and rigors. The patient may be dehydrated. Stool should be tested for blood, examined microscopically for leukocytes, and sent for culture if the patient has prolonged or severe diarrhea associated with fever.

Treatment & Disposition

Severely ill or dehydrated patients should be hospitalized. Mild to moderately ill patients can be sent home with instructions for rehydration. If symptoms persist or worsen, patients should receive follow-up evaluation. Bismuth subsalicylate (Pepto-Bismol, many others) may be used for symptomatic relief. Opiate-containing antidiarrheal agents (diphenoxylate with atropine [Lomotil, many others]) should be used, with caution, only in patients with mild diarrhea without evidence of dysentery. See Chapter 15 for details.

8. Idiopathic Inflammatory Bowel Disease

Clinical Findings

The patient complains of abdominal cramps and intermittent bloody diarrhea and usually gives a history of previous episodes of the same symptoms. A long history of colitis may be present. Weight loss, fever, and anemia may be present. Cramps may come on gradually or suddenly. The abdomen is slightly tender. Infectious causes of colitis (eg, *Shigella, Clostridium difficile, Campylobacter, Entamoeba histolytica*) should be systematically ruled out.

Treatment & Disposition

A. FOR THE SERIOUSLY ILL PATIENT OR FOR UNCERTAIN DIAGNOSIS

Treat hypotension or shock with administration of intravenous crystalloid solution. Give nothing by mouth; nasogastric suction may be helpful if the patient is vomiting. Abdominal radiographs or CT scan may provide important information about possible complications of inflammatory bowel disease such as perforation, bowel obstruction, or intraperitoneal abscess. Hospitalize the patient for definitive diagnosis and treatment. Indications for hospitalization are uncertain diagnosis, shock, fever, toxic megacolon, anemia, or gross blood in the stool.

B. For the Ambulatory Patient with Certain Diagnosis

For patients under the care of a gastroenterologist, discuss the options with the patient's physician regarding outpatient treatment with oral antibiotics, steroids, and other anti-inflammatory medications such as sulfasalazine.

Berg DF et al: Acute surgical emergencies in inflammatory bowel disease. Am J Surg 2002;184:45. [PMID: 12135718] (Review.)

Ferrell RJ, Peppercom MA: Ulcerative colitis. Lancet 2002;359:331. [PMID: 11830216] (Review.)

Marteau P: Inflammatory bowel disease. Endoscopy 2002;34:63. [PMID: 11778131] (Review.)

HEPATOBILIARY DISORDERS

1. Biliary Colic

Clinical Findings

Biliary colic is due to intermittent obstruction of the biliary tree by stones, usually at the cystic duct. The pain occurs in discrete episodes (frequently after ingestion of food), which usually begin abruptly and subside gradually. During an attack, steady upper abdominal pain extends all the way across the abdomen but is more severe on the right. Pain may be referred to the scapula. A careful history often reveals prior attacks of similar pain. Abdominal examination shows right upper quadrant tenderness and, occasionally, a palpable gallbladder. A right upper quadrant sonogram is diagnostic and shows gallstones or a dilated gallbladder and cystic duct. Dilation of the common bile duct is commonly seen with choledocholithiasis.

Treatment

In the absence of acute cholecystitis, ascending cholangitis, choledocholithiasis, or pancreatitis, no specific emergency treatment is necessary. Provide adequate analgesia.

Disposition

Refer the patient for possible elective cholecystectomy. Outpatient treatment involves controlling the symptoms with oral analgesics and possibly antiemetics.

2. Acute Cholecystitis

Clinical Findings

Acute cholecystitis is characterized by acute right upper quadrant pain and tenderness that may be referred to the right scapula. A history of similar episodes may be present. The discomfort may be moderate to severe and prostrating. Anorexia and nausea and vomiting usually occur also. Low-grade fever and leukocytosis are usually present. In some cases, the gallbladder is palpable. Elderly patients with acute cholecystitis are more likely than younger patients to have few localized right upper quadrant signs and symptoms.

Ultrasonography of the abdomen demonstrating gallstones, dilatation of the intra- or extrahepatic bile ducts or thickening of the gallbladder wall, and pericholecystic fluid (if present) confirms the diagnosis. Ultrasonography is the preferred diagnostic technique, because it is sensitive, specific, rapid, inexpensive, and without adverse effects. A sonographic Murphy's sign, specific tenderness of the gallbladder noted during the ultrasound exam, has a sensitivity of 88% and a specificity of 80% for acute cholecystitis. Nonvisualization on nuclear imaging (HIDA) of the biliary tract is also diagnostic and remains the gold standard for acute cholecystitis.

Treatment

Give analgesics intravenously or intramuscularly. Insert a nasogastric tube and attach it to continuous suction if the patient is vomiting. Give crystalloid solution (lactated Ringer's injection or equivalent) intravenously if the patient is dehydrated. Administer empiric antibiotics if the patient has systemic signs of infection such as fever. A second-generation cephalosporin such as cefuroxime, 1.5 g every 8 hours, and metronidazole, 500 mg every 8 hours, are recommended. Give nothing by mouth.

Disposition

Hospitalize patients with cholecystitis, and obtain immediate surgical consultation.

Indar AA, Beckingham IJ: Acute cholecystitis. Br Med J 2002;325:639. [PMID: 12242178] (Review.)

Trowbridge RL, Rutkowski NK, Shojania KG: Does this patient have acute cholecystitis? JAMA 2003;289:80. [PMID: 12503981] (Review.)

3. Acute Suppurative Cholangitis

Clinical Findings

Acute suppurative cholangitis is a surgical emergency commonly accompanied by bacteremia and septic shock. Symptoms are abdominal pain, jaundice, fever and chills, mental confusion, and shock. Because of the overwhelming suppurative process, the biliary obstruction may not be apparent, and the diagnosis is sometimes missed. Right upper quadrant sonography is the diagnostic procedure of choice and shows dilated, obstructed intrahepatic biliary ducts. Bile and blood cultures are often positive for aerobic organisms such as *Escherichia coli, Klebsiella,* enterococcus, *Enterobacter, Pseudomonas, Serratia,* and *Proteus* species. The most common anaerobe is *Bacteroide fragilis.*

Treatment

Treat shock with infusion of intravenous crystalloid solution. Insert a nasogastric tube and connect it to a continuous suction device if the patient is vomiting. Insert a Foley catheter to monitor urine output.

Administer antimicrobials: classical treatment of cholangitis has included an aminoglycoside, a penicillin, and metronidazole. Less nephrotoxic regimens include monotherapy with imipenem, mezlocillin, ciprofloxacin, or ampicillin-sulbactam.

In the case of acute cholecystitis complicated by choledocholithiasis, endoscopic retrograde cholangiopancreatography can retrieve obstructed stones to decompress the common bile duct.

Disposition

Hospitalize the patient, and prepare for surgery or endoscopic papillotomy within 1–2 hours.

Ahmed A, Cheung RC, Keeffe EB: Management of gallstones and their complications. Am Fam Physician 2000;61:1673. [PMID: 10750875] (Review.)

Lillemoe KD: Surgical treatment of biliary tract infections. Am Surg 2000;66:138. [PMID: 10695743] (Review.)

4. Hepatic Abscess

Clinical Findings

When liver abscess results from other intra-abdominal infections, increasing toxicity, high fever, jaundice, and a deteriorating clinical picture are seen. Right upper quadrant pain may be present. In primary liver abscess (eg, caused by Entamoeba histolytica), the onset is insidious, and it may be several weeks before the disease becomes fulminant. High fever and leukocytosis often accompany the abscess, and rigors occur in approximately one fourth of patients. The liver becomes enlarged and is often tender. Right upper quadrant sonography, CT scan, or liver scan is diagnostic. Obtain blood for culture and amebic serologic tests. Many patients with amebic liver abscesses do not have intestinal

amebiasis; hence, stool examination for parasites is not helpful.

Treatment & Disposition

Hospitalize the patient immediately for evaluation and treatment. Empiric antimicrobial therapy must be active against amebas, anaerobes, and coliform bacteria. CT-guided aspiration can assist in diagnosis. Empiric antibiotics should include an aminoglycoside, a penicillin, and metronidazole. In elderly patients or those with impaired renal function, a third-generation cephalosporin can be substituted for the aminoglycoside. Metronidazole alone (800 mg 3 times a day for 5 days) will resolve 95% of uncomplicated amebic abscesses.

Krige JE, Beckingham IJ: ABC of diseases of the liver, pancreas, and biliary system, liver abscesses and hydatid disease. Br Med J 2001;322:537. [PMID: 11230072]

5. Hepatitis

Clinical Findings

Hepatitis is manifested by anorexia, nausea and vomiting, malaise, symptoms of upper respiratory tract infection or flulike syndrome, and bilirubinuria. Fever, jaundice, and an enlarged, tender liver are usually present. The white cell count is low or normal, and liver function tests show elevated bilirubin and hepatic enzymes (AST [SGOT], ALT [SGPT], and alkaline phosphatase).

The most common causes are viral infection (hepatitis viruses, yellow fever, cytomegalovirus, Epstein-Barr virus) and alcohol. Alcoholic hepatitis can often be distinguished from viral hepatitis by the history and physical examination (evidence of alcohol abuse) and by AST and ALT levels (usually < 100 IU/L in alcoholic hepatitis). In alcoholic hepatitis, AST (SGOT) levels are the same or higher than ALT (SGPT) levels; in viral hepatitis, the situation is reversed.

Treatment & Disposition

Severely ill patients with persistent vomiting, dehydration, hypoglycemia, hepatic encephalopathy, or significant coagulopathy (prothrombin time > 15 seconds) should be hospitalized. Other patients can be referred to a primary care physician and receive treatment at home. The patient should be instructed to maintain hydration and strict hygiene and to avoid potential hepatotoxins (alcohol). Patients with viral hepatitis must avoid handling food that will be consumed by others.

Tests that help in specific diagnosis (eg, HBsAg and hepatitis A IgM antibody) can be obtained in the emergency department if the physician so chooses. Close family contacts should be advised regarding appropriate immunizations if hepatitis viruses are suspected.

Bondesson JD, Saperston AR: Hepatitis. Emerg Med Clin North Am 1996;14(4):695. [PMID: 8921765] (Review.)

VASCULAR DISORDERS

1. Ruptured Aortic Aneurysm

Clinical Findings

Rupture of an abdominal aneurysm is accompanied by severe abdominal pain of sudden onset that may radiate into the back. In some patients, pain is confined to the flank, low back, or groin. Faintness or syncope may occur as a result of blood loss. After the first hemorrhage, pain may lessen and faintness may disappear, but these symptoms recur and progress until shock finally supervenes. While dissection is occurring, a discrete pulsatile mass can be palpated in the abdomen. If rupture occurs in the retroperitoneum, a poorly defined midabdominal fullness can be felt, and shock becomes profound. Emergency department bedside ultrasound can rapidly confirm the diagnosis. Most patients with a leaking or ruptured abdominal aortic aneurysm are too unstable to be diagnosed by CT scan. A chest x-ray should also be obtained to evaluate the thoracic aorta.

Treatment

(See also Chapter 32.) Insert at least 2 large-bore ($\geq$ 16-gauge) percutaneous catheters for vascular access. Consider a central venous catheter. Draw blood for CBC, electrolytes, PT and PTT, and tests of renal function. Type and cross-match for 8 units of whole blood. Treat shock with intravenous crystalloid solution followed by whole blood as soon as available. In patients who are exsanguinating, type-specific or universal donor blood may be used until cross-matched blood is available (Chapter 39). Obtain immediate vascular or general surgical consultation. Prepare the patient for surgery as rapidly as possible.

Disposition

All patients must be hospitalized; the mortality rate is virtually 100% without surgical treatment.

Mancini MC: Abdominal aortic aneurysm. Emedicine.com; www.emedicine.com/med/topic3443.htm

2. Ischemic Colitis

Clinical Findings

Patients with ischemic colitis are usually elderly and have evidence of vascular disease elsewhere in the body. A history of similar attacks, abrupt in onset and of varying degrees of severity, is often present. The pain may be localized anywhere in the abdomen or may be diffuse. Severe colitis is usually accompanied by bloody diarrhea. Ischemic areas may progress to gangrene if the ischemia is sufficiently severe; if ischemia is milder, the areas may heal, often with strictures. Routine laboratory tests do not show specific abnormalities, although hemoconcentration and azotemia are common. Tests that confirm the diagnosis of ischemic colitis include sigmoidoscopy or colonoscopy, barium enema, and visceral angiography.

Treatment

Treat shock and hemoconcentration with intravenous crystalloid solution. Administer antimicrobials (see Table 13–1).

Disposition

All patients with suspected or documented ischemic colitis should be hospitalized for further diagnostic tests and possible surgery.

MacDonald PH: Ischaemic colitis. Best Pract Res Clin Gastroenterol 2002;16:51. [PMID: 11977928] (Review.)

3. Mesenteric Thrombosis

Clinical Findings

The patient usually complains of the sudden onset of severe, diffuse abdominal pain in the mid or lower abdomen. The pain is poorly localized and severe, often not relieved by narcotics. It is constant rather than crampy. Nausea and vomiting and diarrhea, with gross or occult blood in the stool, may be present. Physical findings are absent initially. As the condition progresses, abdominal distention and tenderness appear and shock supervenes. Marked leukocytosis, hemoconcentration, azotemia, and acidosis are commonly associated with mesenteric thrombosis.

Treatment & Disposition

Treat shock and hemoconcentration with intravenous crystalloid solutions, and administer antimicrobials (see Table 13–1). Hospitalize the patient and prepare for emergency surgery. Visceral angiography or abdominal

CT scan with oral and intravenous contrast may be used to confirm the diagnosis.

Kim AY, Ha HK: Evaluation of suspected mesenteric ischemia: efficacy of radiologic studies. Radiol Clin North Am 2003;41:327. [PMID: 12659341] (Review.)

4. Rupture of the Spleen
(See also Chapter 25.)

Clinical Findings

Rupture of the spleen is usually caused by trauma to the lower left rib cage that is often associated with rib fractures. Occasionally, the spleen may rupture after trivial or overlooked injury, usually when pathologic enlargement has occurred (eg, infectious mononucleosis, AIDS, leukemia). Actual splenic rupture may occur several days after initial injury. Blood leaking into the peritoneal cavity causes abdominal pain and tenderness that may radiate to the left side of the neck or left shoulder. Tachycardia, hypotension, and falling hematocrit are present, and shock may develop. Occasionally, patients present with syncope, hypotension, or shock without abdominal symptoms. Palpation of the left upper quadrant may reveal tenderness, mild spasm, and distention. Tenderness over the 9th and 10th ribs on the left is a diagnostic clue. Emergent bedside ultrasound, specifically the FAST exam (Chapter 25) can rapidly identify intraperitoneal fluid, which in the setting of blunt trauma must be assumed to represent blood. The spleen is intra-abdominal solid organ most commonly injured in blunt trauma. CT scan of the abdomen is useful for diagnosis of splenic rupture in stable patients.

Treatment

Insert at least 2 large-bore (≥ 16-gauge) percutaneous intravenous lines. Obtain a CBC, and type and cross-match for 6 units of whole blood. Treat shock initially with intravenous infusion of crystalloid solution. Administer whole blood as soon as available, using hematocrit, blood pressure, pulse, and urine output to gauge the effectiveness of resuscitation.

Disposition

All patients with suspected splenic rupture should be hospitalized. Hemodynamically stable patients with less severe splenic injuries may be observed nonoperatively. Patients with hypotension and shock require emergent splenectomy.

Debnath D, Valerio D: Atraumatic rupture of the spleen in adults. J R Coll Surg Edinb 2002;47:437. [PMID: 11874265] (Review.)

5. Splenic Infarct

Clinical Findings

Infarction of the spleen usually occurs in patients with abnormal spleens due to hematologic disease (eg, sickling hemoglobinopathies). Rarely, it occurs as a result of arterial embolization (eg, in patients with endocarditis). Left upper quadrant pain of variable degree, occasionally referred to the shoulder, is present. Left upper quadrant tenderness is usually present as well. CT scan is helpful in confirming the diagnosis.

Treatment

No specific treatment is necessary. Symptomatic measures (eg, relief of pain) and treatment of the underlying disease may be necessary.

Disposition

Hospitalization is advisable until the diagnosis is confirmed. Likewise, hospitalization may be required for pain relief or treatment of the underlying disease.

URINARY DISORDERS

1. Renal Colic
(See also Chapter 37.)

Clinical Findings

Sudden, severe flank pain followed by hematuria is characteristic of renal colic. A history of passage of stones may be present. Examination reveals costovertebral angle tenderness on the side of the stone, with the pain shifting anteriorly and inferiorly as the stone progresses down the ureter toward the bladder. The stone can usually be visualized on x-ray. Excretory urography confirms the diagnosis by demonstrating obstruction to urinary flow. In most centers, noncontrast CT scan of the abdomen has replaced the intravenous pyelogram as the preferred diagnostic modality for the evaluation of renal colic (Figure 13–10). Noncontrast CT scan is helpful in identifying the size and location of ureteral stones. Another benefit of noncontrast CT scan is that alternative diagnoses such as appendicitis or diverticulitis may be identified and the treatment modified appropriately. Urinary tract infection may coexist, and urinalysis should be performed in every case along with urine culture for organisms if infection is suspected.

Treatment & Disposition

A severe clinical picture requires hospitalization for administration of parenteral analgesia and maintenance of

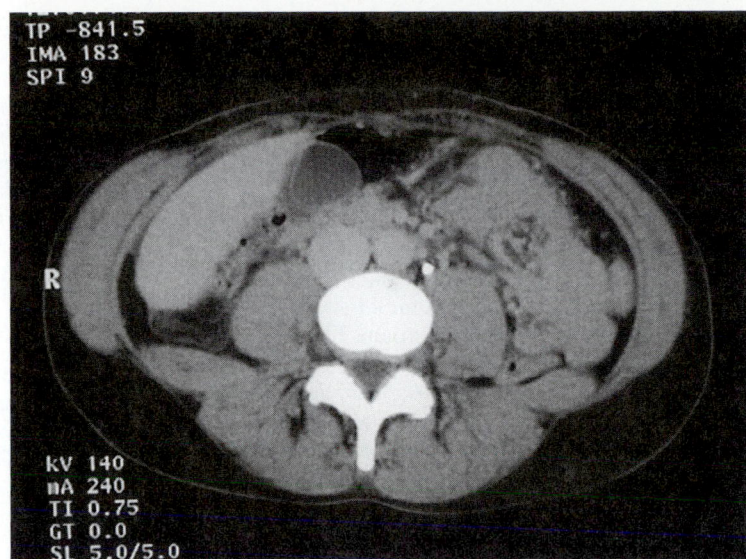

TP -841.5
IMA 183
SPI 9

R

kV 140
mA 240
TI 0.75
GT 0.0
SL 5.0/5.0

Figure 13–10. Noncontrast CT scan of the abdomen in a patient with left flank pain. Study demonstrates a dense calcification (ureterolithiasis) involving the mid portion of the left ureter, confirming the diagnosis of renal colic.

hydration. Patients with either renal insufficiency or pyelonephritis and ureterolithiasis generally require admission for possible operative intervention. Patient with small stones can receive treatment on an ambulatory basis, with appropriate oral analgesia, hydration, and follow-up care with a primary care physician or urologist.

2. Pyelonephritis (See also Chapter 40.)

Clinical Findings

Patients with pyelonephritis typically have dysuria, urinary urgency and frequency, fever, and sometimes rigors. Pain, if present, is usually over the costovertebral angle or occasionally the abdomen. The pain is dull and usually gradual in onset. Malaise and nausea and vomiting are commonly present as well. Many bacteria and leukocytes are seen on stained smears of the urinary sediment.

Treatment & Disposition

A patient who is severely ill (vomiting, high fever, rigors), pregnant, very young or very old, or immunocompromised, or who has know anatomic abnormalities of the genitourinary tract, requires hospitalization for intravenous hydration and parenteral antibiotics. Gentamicin and ampicillin or monotherapy with ceftriaxone or a fluoroquinolone provide reasonable empiric coverage for pyelonephritis. Outpatient therapy is appropriate for some patients with pyelonephritis, including those tolerating oral intake, those with telephone access, and those reliable to return if their condition worsens. Sequential therapy utilizing an initial parenteral dose of an antibiotic followed by an oral regimen as an outpatient is often recommended.

Miller O, Hemphill RR: Urinary tract infection and pyelonephritis. Emerg Med Clin North Am 2001;19:655. [PMID: 11554280] (Review.)

3. Renal Infarct

Clinical Findings

Infarction of the kidney usually occurs because of arterial embolization (eg, from endocarditis or atrial fibrillation). In addition to flank pain and tenderness, hematuria is usually present. The diagnosis may be confirmed by CT scan, renal scan, or angiography.

Treatment

No specific treatment is required for renal infarct. However, anticoagulation or other measures may be required to treat the underlying disease.

Disposition

Hospitalization is advisable for definitive diagnosis, administration of appropriate analgesia, treatment of underlying disease, and rapid anticoagulation measures if indicated.

ACUTE PANCREATITIS

Clinical Findings

Acute pancreatitis is characterized by abrupt onset of severe, unrelenting epigastric pain radiating to the back, often accompanied by vomiting and retching. In severe cases, the patient may be in shock. A predisposing condition (alcoholism, glucocorticoid administration, diabetes mellitus) may be present. Abdominal examination reveals decreased or absent bowel sounds and tenderness usually localized to the epigastrium. Rarely, an abdominal mass is palpated in the epigastrium. Elevated serum amylase and lipase levels, mild fever, and leukocytosis are often present. As discussed previously, lipase has better specificity and sensitivity for pancreatitis than amylase. If the diagnosis is uncertain, abdominal CT scan can often demonstrate changes pathognomonic of pancreatitis (although CT scan can be normal initially in 30% of patients with pancreatitis). Patients may have a history of recurrent pancreatitis; alcohol abuse is a common predisposing factor.

Treatment

Send blood for CBC; serum electrolyte, glucose, calcium, and lipase measurements; and renal and hepatic function tests. Insert an intravenous catheter ($\geq$ 18 gauge), and begin an infusion of crystalloid solution. Give morphine, 2–4 mg intravenously, for pain; the dose may be repeated. Insert a nasogastric tube attached to a suction device if the patient is vomiting or if the abdomen is distended, especially if ileus is present. Give nothing by mouth to patients who are more severely ill.

Disposition

Patients with severe pain or persistent vomiting should be hospitalized for analgesia, intravenous hydration, and correction of electrolyte abnormalities. Even if they are not acutely ill, patients with no history of pancreatitis should be hospitalized for evaluation and treatment. Patients with chronic and recurrent pancreatitis may not require hospitalization if they can take fluids by mouth and do not require parenteral analgesics. Patients with recurrent acute pancreatitis due to alcohol abuse may receive oral analgesics and hydration on an outpatient basis if they are not severely ill.

GYNECOLOGIC DISORDERS (SEE ALSO CHAPTER 36.)

1. Ectopic Pregnancy with Rupture

Clinical Findings

In ectopic pregnancy with rupture, the patient experiences sudden, severe, unilateral abdominal or pelvic pain that may be referred to the shoulder. Prior to rupture, pain may be vague or intermittent. There may be occasional nausea and vomiting but usually no fever. Irregular menses or other symptoms of pregnancy may be present as well. Postural hypotension or shock may be found on initial examination. Pelvic examination often reveals a unilateral doughy mass and tenderness on movement of the cervix. Pelvic sonography reveals free fluid and an adnexal mass. A urine pregnancy test is positive in almost all cases.

Treatment & Disposition

Treat shock or hypotension with intravenous crystalloid solution and blood if necessary. Hospitalize the patient at once for emergency surgery or for laparoscopy if the diagnosis is in doubt (Chapter 36).

Dart RG: Role of pelvic ultrasonography in evaluation of symptomatic first-trimester pregnancy. Ann Emerg Med 1999;33: 310. [PMID: 10036346]

Mateer JR et al: Outcome analysis of a protocol including bedside endovaginal sonography in patients at risk for ectopic pregnancy. Ann Emerg Med 1996;27:283. [PMID: 8599484]

2. Acute Salpingitis (Pelvic Inflammatory Disease) (See also Chapter 40.)

Clinical Findings

The patient with salpingitis experiences gradual onset of pelvic and lower abdominal pain that slowly increases in severity. There may be headache and lassitude with high fever and tachycardia. Nausea and vomiting may be present. The patient shows exquisite tenderness to vaginal examination and particularly to movement of the cervix. Adnexal fullness or mass (tubo-ovarian abscess) may be present. A pelvic sonogram is diagnostic for tubo-ovarian abscess.

Treatment & Disposition

Hospitalization of patients with pelvic inflammatory disease is recommended for the following situations: diagnosis is uncertain (eg, cannot exclude appendicitis); patient has severe symptoms such as nausea, vomiting, or high fever; patient is an adolescent or is pregnant or has failed outpatient treatment; patient is unable to follow up; or patient is immunocompromised (eg, HIV with low CD4 count). Surgery may be necessary if abdominal symptoms persist or if the patient's condition deteriorates.

Quentin R, Lansac J: Pelvic inflammatory disease: medical treatment. Eur J Obstet Gynecol Reprod Biol 2000;92:189. [PMID: 10996679]

3. Ruptured Ovarian Follicle Cyst

Clinical Findings

Patients with ruptured ovarian follicle cyst experience sudden, moderately severe pelvic or lower abdominal pain. Gastrointestinal symptoms usually are absent, and the patient is afebrile without leukocytosis. Tenderness may be elicited over the affected ovary. There should be no masses on pelvic examination, and the serum pregnancy test should be negative.

Treatment & Disposition

Keep the patient under observation in the hospital until the diagnosis is confirmed. Operation is not necessary.

4. Ovarian Torsion

Clinical Findings

Torsion of the ovary is characterized by sudden unilateral lower abdominal or pelvic pain precipitated by a change in position. The pain is often sudden onset, sharp or colicky in nature, radiating into the groin, back or flank of moderate to severe intensity. Gastrointestinal symptoms include nausea and vomiting. Patients with ovarian torsion may have a history of ovarian abnormalities such as cysts or masses.

Treatment & Disposition

The patient should be hospitalized for observation and possible surgery.

Houry D, Abbott JT: Ovarian torsion: a fifteen-year review. Ann Emerg Med 2001;38:156. [PMID: 11468611]

5. Endometriosis

Clinical Findings

Patients with endometriosis usually have a history of infertility, dysmenorrhea, and previous cyclic attacks of cramps and pains in the lower abdomen and possibly in the flank. Pain is worse with menses. Onset of symptoms may be gradual or sudden if there is associated bleeding. Painful defecation and dyspareunia are present. Aching pelvic discomfort and general tenderness on pelvic examination suggest endometriosis. Acquired secondary dysmenorrhea should be attributed to endometriosis until proved otherwise.

Treatment & Disposition

If symptoms are mild, give the patient analgesics and refer her to the obstetrics and gynecology department for follow-up. If pain is severe, the patient should be hospitalized for evaluation and possible surgery.

PRIMARY PERITONITIS

Clinical Findings

Primary peritonitis occurs almost exclusively in patients with preexisting ascites, especially those with cirrhosis or nephrotic syndrome. (Peritonitis secondary to traumatic fecal soilage is discussed in Chapter 25.) The symptoms and signs vary, but fever and abdominal pain and tenderness are common. The most helpful tests are blood culture and abdominal paracentesis for Gram-stained smear, cell count, and culture. A polymorphonuclear (PMN) cell count of greater than $250/mm^3$ is highly suspicious for spontaneous bacterial peritonitis and is an indication for initiation of empiric antibiotics. Most cases of primary bacterial peritonitis demonstrate positive blood cultures, peritoneal fluid leukocyte counts over $1000/mm^3$ (with a predominance of PMNs), and bacteria on Gram-stained smears or culture. In 40% of cases, all of these findings are present except that peritoneal fluid smears and cultures are negative. Familial Mediterranean fever produces sterile peritonitis that is difficult to distinguish from bacterial peritonitis.

Treatment

Culture blood and peritoneal fluid (include a culture for Mycobacterium tuberculosis). Treat shock, if present, with intravenous crystalloid solution. Begin parenteral antimicrobials: administer a cephalosporin in full doses (eg, cefotaxime, 2 g every 8–12 hours for 5 days). Alternatively, fluoroquinolones can be used.

Disposition

All patients with suspected or confirmed acute peritonitis should be hospitalized for diagnostic evaluation and treatment.

Rimola A et al: Diagnosis, treatment and prophylaxis of spontaneous bacterial peritonitis: a consensus document. J Hepatol 2000;32:142. [PMID: 10673079] (Review.)

RETROPERITONEAL HEMORRHAGE

Clinical Findings

Retroperitoneal hemorrhage is a rare condition that may occur secondary to minor trauma in individuals with defective clotting factors resulting from medication or disease. Back pain and abdominal pain are present, and the psoas sign is often positive. Abdominal CT scan localizes the bleeding in most cases.

Treatment

Treat shock with intravenous crystalloid solution, followed by cross-matched whole blood as soon as available. Correct coagulation defects by administering platelets or clotting factors as needed.

Disposition

Patients with copious hemorrhage, active bleeding, severe clotting abnormalities, or severe pain should be hospitalized.

■ CONDITIONS CAUSING ACUTE ABDOMINAL PAIN THAT ARE NOT AMENABLE TO SURGERY

A variety of conditions not amenable to surgery may cause abdominal pain. Aside from common conditions such as pyelonephritis, salpingitis, myocardial infarc-

tion, and lobar pneumonia, a number of these conditions are capable of mimicking abdominal disorders requiring surgery. Most of these conditions simulate acute diffuse peritonitis. Helpful differential diagnostic tests are listed in Table 13–4.

Gastrointestinal Bleeding

14

Charles W. Erdman, MD, & James J. Mensching, DO, FACEP[1]

Immediate Management of Life-Threatening Bleeding
    Assess the Rate and Volume of Bleeding
    Conduct Initial Assessment
    Determine Site of Bleeding
Further Evaluation of Gastrointestinal Bleeding
Emergency Treatment of Specific Disorders Causing Upper Gastrointestinal Bleeding
    Peptic Ulcer Disease
    Gastritis
    Mallory-Weiss Syndrome
    Esophageal Varices

    Hemobilia
    Aortic Aneurysm (Aortoenteric Fistula)
Emergency Treatment of Specific Disorders Causing Lower Gastrointestinal Bleeding
    Diverticulosis
    Angiodysplasia
    Hemorrhoids
    Colonic Polyps
    Colitis
    Crohn Disease
    Solitary Rectal Ulcer
    Meckel Diverticulum

For the majority of patients presenting with gastrointestinal (GI) bleeding, hematemesis (vomiting of blood), hematochezia (passage of bright red stools), or melena (black and tarry stools caused from the breakdown of large amounts of blood) will be the chief complaint. Occasionally patients may present with only dizziness, weakness, or syncope. If no obvious cause of shock is present, gastric lavage and a rectal examination should be performed promptly as part of the initial assessment. The severity of blood loss must be assessed quickly so that life-saving therapeutic interventions can be instituted.

■ IMMEDIATE MANAGEMENT OF LIFE-THREATENING BLEEDING (See Figure 14–1.)

ASSESS THE RATE AND VOLUME OF BLEEDING

Any patient presenting to the emergency department with ongoing hematemesis or hematochezia is at significant risk of exsanguination, and prompt volume resuscitation must begin at once. Proceed with initial stabilization procedures as described below.

CONDUCT INITIAL ASSESSMENT

Place the patient in a monitored bed and obtain temperature, pulse rate, blood pressure, respiratory rate, and oxygen saturation via pulse oximetry. If the initial systolic blood pressure is greater than 100, and the pulse is less than 100 beats/min in the supine position, consider obtaining orthostatic blood pressure and pulse rate measurements.

Recognize Risk Factors for Severe Gastrointestinal Bleeding

Signs, symptoms, or history that may indicate ongoing hemorrhage are as follows:

- Profuse hematemesis or hematochezia
- Hypotension, tachycardia, or signs of shock (see Table 9–1)
- Postural hypotension, tachycardia, or lightheadedness
- Possible aortoenteric fistula (history of abdominal aortic aneurysm repair, or palpable pulsating abdominal mass)

---

[1]This chapter is a revision of the chapter by Richard A. Crass, MD, John P. Cello, MD, & Donald D. Trunkey, MD, from the 4th edition.

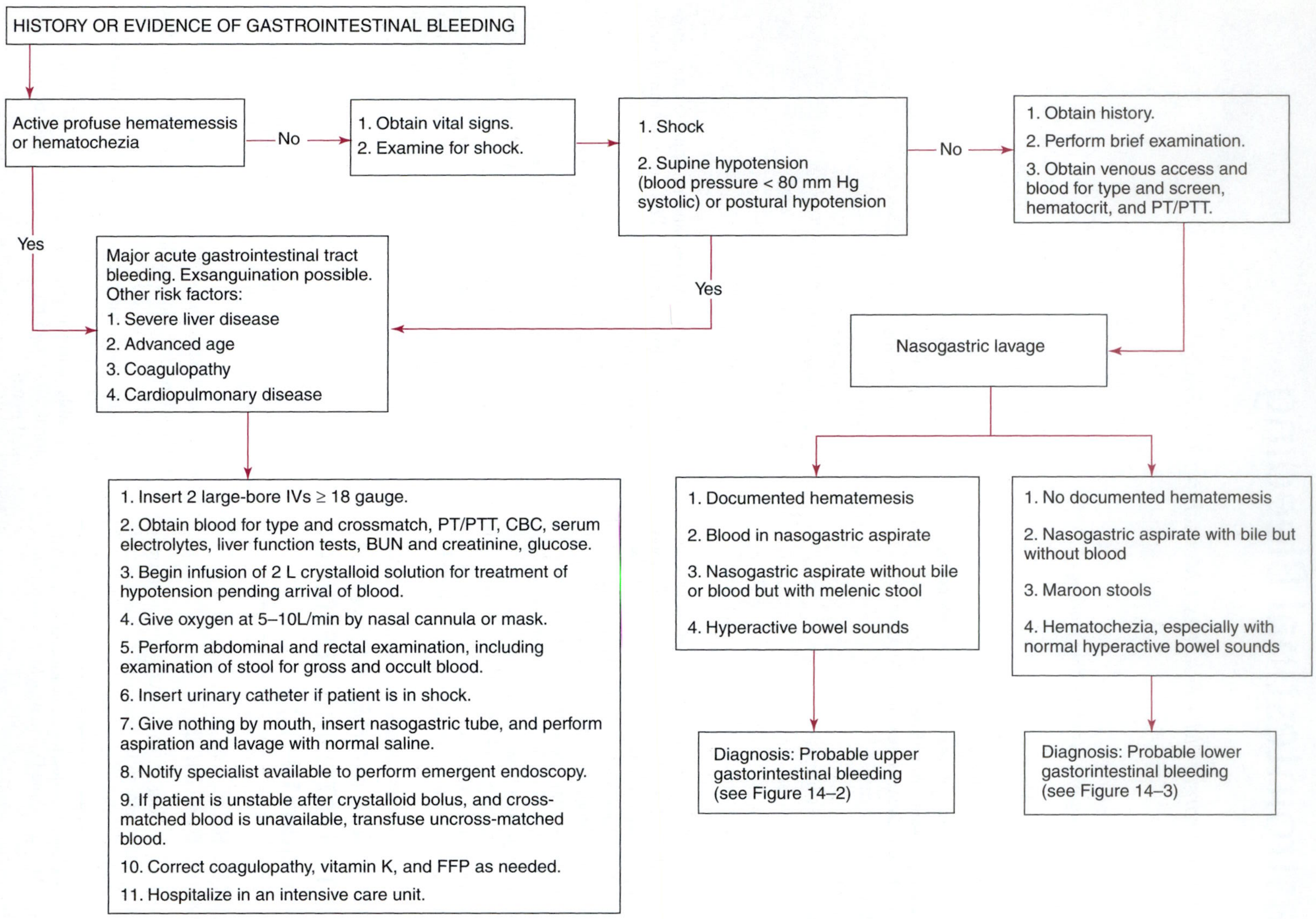
HISTORY OR EVIDENCE OF GASTROINTESTINAL BLEEDING
Active profuse hematemessis or hematochezia
No
1. Obtain vital signs.
2. Examine for shock.
1. Shock
2. Supine hypotension (blood pressure < 80 mm Hg systolic) or postural hypotension
No
1. Obtain history.
2. Perform brief examination.
3. Obtain venous access and blood for type and screen, hematocrit, and PT/PTT.
Yes
Major acute gastrointestinal tract bleeding. Exsanguination possible. Other risk factors:
1. Severe liver disease
2. Advanced age
3. Coagulopathy
4. Cardiopulmonary disease
Yes
Nasogastric lavage
1. Insert 2 large-bore IVs ≥ 18 gauge.
2. Obtain blood for type and crossmatch, PT/PTT, CBC, serum electrolytes, liver function tests, BUN and creatinine, glucose.
3. Begin infusion of 2 L crystalloid solution for treatment of hypotension pending arrival of blood.
4. Give oxygen at 5–10L/min by nasal cannula or mask.
5. Perform abdominal and rectal examination, including examination of stool for gross and occult blood.
6. Insert urinary catheter if patient is in shock.
7. Give nothing by mouth, insert nasogastric tube, and perform aspiration and lavage with normal saline.
8. Notify specialist available to perform emergent endoscopy.
9. If patient is unstable after crystalloid bolus, and cross-matched blood is unavailable, transfuse uncross-matched blood.
10. Correct coagulopathy, vitamin K, and FFP as needed.
11. Hospitalize in an intensive care unit.
1. Documented hematemesis
2. Blood in nasogastric aspirate
3. Nasogastric aspirate without bile or blood but with melenic stool
4. Hyperactive bowel sounds
1. No documented hematemesis
2. Nasogastric aspirate with bile but without blood
3. Maroon stools
4. Hematochezia, especially with normal hyperactive bowel sounds
Diagnosis: Probable upper gastorintestinal bleeding (see Figure 14–2)
Diagnosis: Probable lower gastorintestinal bleeding (see Figure 14–3)

Figure 14–1. Immediate management of life-threatening bleeding. BUN = blood urea nitrogen; FFP = fresh frozen plasma; PT = prothrombin time; PTT = partial thromboplastin time.

- Known or suspected varices
- Previous history of GI bleeding
- History of diverticulosis

Initial Stabilization Procedures

A. Obtain Venous Access

Insert 2 intravenous catheters into peripheral veins, preferably 18 gauge or larger in an adult. If peripheral access cannot be obtained, consider placement of a central venous line.

B. Assess Need for Airway Management

If the patient is having ongoing hematemesis or if signs and symptoms of shock are present, consider securing the airway with an endotracheal tube via rapid sequence intubation (Chapter 8). If immediate airway control is not needed, give oxygen via nasal cannula or face mask as needed to maintain oxygen saturation at greater than 93%.

C. Perform Laboratory Studies

Send blood for complete blood count (CBC). Type and cross-match blood for 2–6 units, depending on the extent of bleeding and the patient's status. Measure prothrombin and partial thromboplastin time to assess for any coagulopathy. Measure serum electrolytes and renal and liver functions. Blood urea nitrogen is elevated in many patients with upper GI bleeding. Venous blood gas and lactate may be helpful in assessing tissue perfusion status.

D. Begin Fluid Resuscitation

Rapidly bolus either warmed lactated Ringer's or normal saline to restore intravascular volume.

E. Assess the Need for Immediate Blood Transfusion

For persistent hypotension despite the infusion of 2 L of crystalloid, consider immediate transfusion of cross-matched blood if available. If not, then transfuse O-negative blood until cross-matched blood is available. Continue transfusion to maintain systolic blood pressure at greater than 90.

F. Perform Electrocardiogram

Obtain an electrocardiogram (ECG) for any patient over 50 years of age; for any patient with a history of ischemic heart disease or significant anemia; and for any patient with chest pain, shortness of breath, or severe hypotension. If the initial ECG demonstrates ongoing ischemia in the face of ongoing GI bleeding, then consider immediate transfusion of packed red blood cells. If a patient's initial hematocrit is less than 30% and he or she has a history of ischemic heart disease, early transfusion is probably indicated.

G: General Examination

Assess the patient's general appearance; vital signs; mental status (including restlessness); and skin signs such as pallor, moisture, telangiectasia, and petechiae. Also, perform a cardiac and pulmonary examination to assess for abnormal heart or lung sounds that indicate cardiac dysfunction.

H. Perform Abdominal Examination

Inspect the abdomen for any skin changes (ie, telangiectasia, ecchymoses, or old surgical scars). Auscultate for any bruits that may indicate an aneurysm. Palpate for tenderness, mass, or hepatosplenomegaly.

I. Perform Rectal Examination

Inspect the anus and rectum for evidence of hemorrhoids or fissure. Obtain stool for hemoccult testing.

J. Perform Bladder Catheterization

If a patient is in shock or has a history of cardiac or renal dysfunction, insert a Foley catheter into the bladder to monitor urinary output. Order a urine analysis to assess for hematuria, which may indicate an abdominal aneurysm.

K. Insert Nasogastric or Orogastric Tube

If hematemesis has not been documented, prepare the nasal passageway and posterior pharynx with topical anesthetic, place a nasogastric tube, and lavage with room temperature normal saline (cold fluids may impede normal coagulation) until aspirate is clear. Persistent bleeding during lavage indicates potential life-threatening upper GI bleeding, and immediate consultation with a gastroenterologist or surgeon should be obtained.

If persistent bleeding is noted and the endoscopist gives instructions to do so, place an Ewald orogastric tube for gastric lavage with increments of 200–300 mL of either saline or tap water because the fluid does not have to be sterile. The patient should be in the left lateral decubitus position with the bed in the Trendelenburg position. Lavage until the return is clear.

L. Withhold All Fluids and Antacids

Patients waiting for endoscopy should receive nothing by mouth. Do not administer fluids or antacids because they may impair adequate visualization during endoscopy.

M. Correct Coagulopathy

Patients taking Coumadin or who show signs of hepatic failure (eg, jaundice) may require vitamin K and fresh frozen plasma to correct coagulopathy before bleeding can be controlled.

N. Seek Early Consultation

After initial stabilization of the patient, contact the on-call general surgeon or gastroenterologist for either immediate endoscopy and therapy or further instructions. If emergent endoscopic services are unavailable at the treating facility, the emergency physician should find an accepting physician at a facility capable of providing these services and arrange rapid transport.

Disposition

Based on certain clinical criteria such as age, comorbid disease, presenting vital signs, laboratory data, and availability of next-day follow-up, a subgroup of patients with GI hemorrhage can be discharged home. This decision should be made with the gastroenterologist. Intensive care unit admission should be reserved for patients with continued bleeding, abnormal vital signs, significant comorbid disease, or need for transfusion therapy and for those at increased risk for rebleeding (ie, esophageal varices).

DETERMINE SITE OF BLEEDING

Once the patient is stabilized, attempt to determine the bleeding site if it is not already obvious. In 90% of patients presenting with GI hemorrhage, the bleeding has an upper GI source (ie, proximal to the ligament of Treitz); in only about 10% of patients is the source of bleeding distal to this proximal portion of the duodenum. In about 80–85% of patients with GI hemorrhage, the bleeding will cease prior to the patient's arrival in the emergency department.

Diagnostic Characteristics of Upper Gastrointestinal Bleeding

See Figure 14–2.

A. HEMATEMESIS

Hematemesis (excluding hemoptysis or swallowed blood from epistaxis) is observed. Blood or material in the nasogastric lavage tests positive for blood.

The aspirate will be negative in approximately 10% of patients with a duodenal source of GI hemorrhage. A duodenal source cannot be excluded unless gastric lavage contents reveal bile. Even if bile is returned, the bleeding may have resolved spontaneously prior to arrival. If a patient reports unwitnessed hematemesis and gastric lavage is inconclusive, consultation with a gastroenterologist for early endoscopy is warranted.

B. MELENA AND HEMATOCHEZIA

Melena is usually due to bleeding from an upper GI source. Hematochezia from an upper source usually indicates severe hemorrhage and corresponds with signifi-

cant increases in mortality, need for transfusion, complications, and need for surgery.

C. ABSENCE OF BLEEDING

If nasogastric lavage reveals bile and no blood, then active bleeding from an upper GI source is less likely. Between 80% and 85% of bleeding resolves spontaneously prior to the patient's arrival; therefore, in otherwise stable patients, close follow-up with an endoscopist should be arranged.

Diagnostic Characteristics of Lower Gastrointestinal Bleeding

A. HEMATOCHEZIA

An upper GI source is found for suspected lower GI bleeding in up to 15% of patients presenting with hematochezia. In these instances, consider aortoenteric fistula (in patients with abdominal aortic aneurysm repair) or duodenal ulcer. Otherwise, bleeding distal to the ligament of Treitz is usually associated with hematochezia.

B. MELENA

Melena is rarely associated with lower GI bleeding except when motility in the intestinal tract is decreased. Melena occurs more commonly as a result of an upper GI bleed.

C. BRIGHT RED BLOOD

When seen as streaks on stool or on toilet paper after wiping, bright red blood usually indicates a hemorrhoidal source of bleeding. Consider anal fissures as well if the patient complains of painful bowel movements and bright red blood on the stool.

D. ABSENCE OF BLEEDING

Spontaneous cessation of bleeding occurs in about 80–85% of cases without intervention, although cessation can be intermittent, and bleeding can restart at any time.

■ FURTHER EVALUATION OF GASTROINTESTINAL BLEEDING

The unstable patient should be rapidly resuscitated and stabilized prior to completing a detailed history and physical examination. Once the patient's hemodynamic

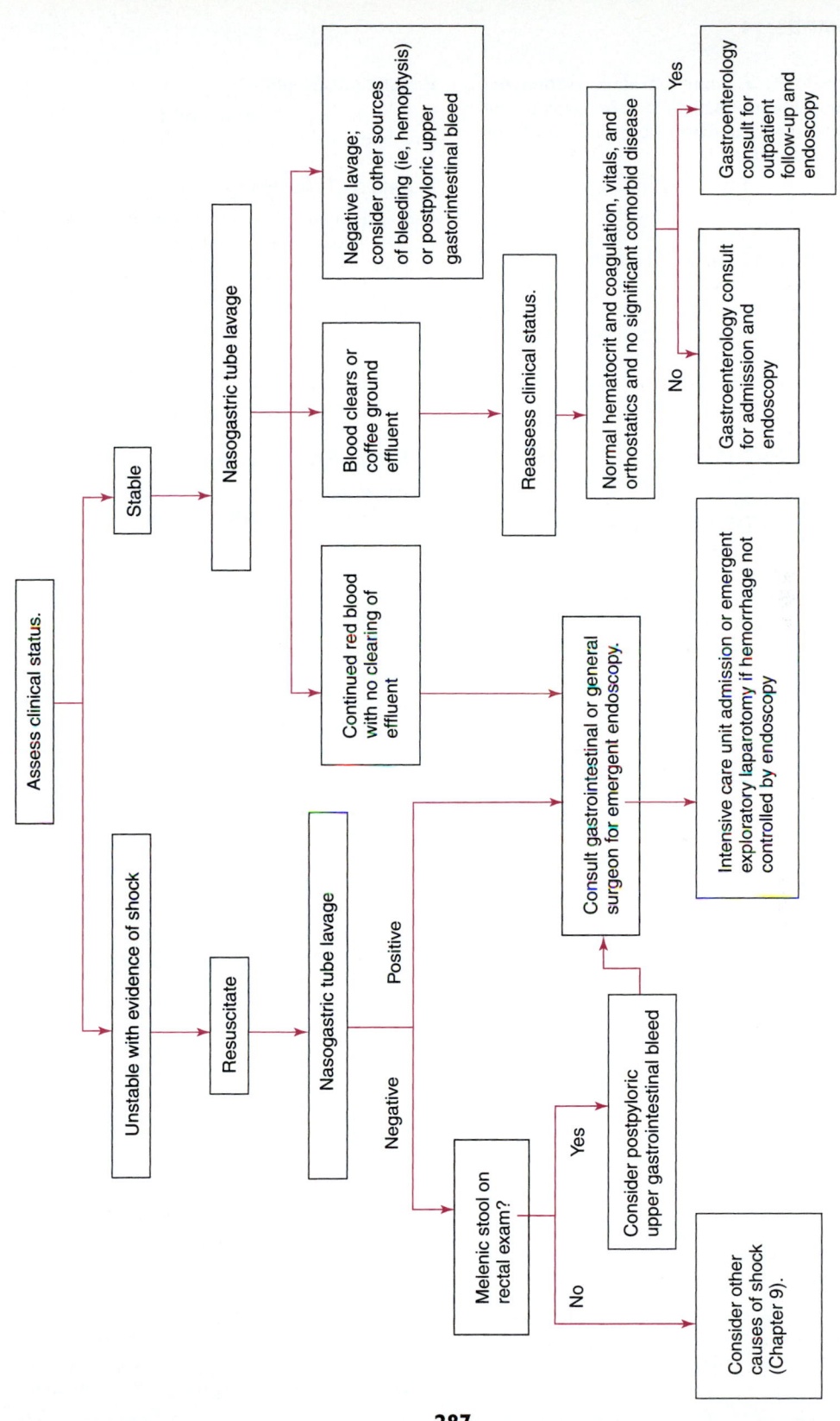

Figure 14-2. Hematemesis or suspected upper GI bleeding.

status has stabilized, a more thorough examination should be done. For the patient not in extremis and otherwise stable, this examination can performed during the initial assessment.

History

Inquire about history of GI bleeding, esophageal varices, alcohol or nonsteroidal anti-inflammatory drug (NSAID) use, oral anticoagulation, recent weight loss, change in caliber of stools, abdominal pain suggestive of ulcer or gastritis, abdominal aneurysm repair, liver disease, or abdominal surgery. Recent vigorous retching or vomiting prior to onset of hematemesis suggests the presence of Mallory-Weiss tears.

Inquire about history of hemorrhoids, anal fissures, or rectal trauma (eg, rectal intercourse, placement of foreign objects in rectum).

In patients with AIDS and in otherwise immunocompromised patients, bleeding may be related to Kaposi sarcoma, lymphoma, or cytomegalovirus ulcerations. Visceral Kaposi sarcoma is usually associated with cutaneous lesions with classical dusky violaceous nodules.

Physical Examination

A. Vital Signs

Reassess vitals signs every 15 minutes or more frequently as needed.

B. Cardiopulmonary Examination

Evaluate the patient for any evidence of cardiac dysfunction (ie, murmurs, rubs, gallops, arrhythmias). Listen to the lungs for abnormal sounds that may be suggestive of heart failure or an infectious process.

C. Liver Disease

Examine the patient for signs of chronic liver disease (eg, hepatosplenomegaly, ascites, spider angiomas, enlarged abdominal vessels, jaundice, hepatojugular reflex, asterixis, palmar erythema). Although the presence of liver disease constitutes a higher likelihood of esophageal varices, GI bleeding will be from another identifiable source in 50% of patients with varices who present with GI bleeding.

D. Osler-Weber-Rendu Disease (Hereditary Hemorrhagic Telangiectasia)

The presence of telangiectasias of the skin (particularly the digits) and lips may indicate this disease, which causes GI bleeding secondary to vascular malformations.

E. Surgical Scars

Inspect the patient for surgical scars that indicate previous abdominal surgery or possible vascular repair.

F. Pain or Tenderness

Epigastric tenderness to palpation is common with gastritis or peptic ulcer disease. Any patient who has had multiple episodes of vomiting may also have diffuse tenderness of the abdomen. A patient whose complaints of abdominal pain are out of proportion to the examination and who also has melena should be considered at risk for mesenteric ischemia. Significant tenderness or peritoneal signs may indicate perforation and warrant immediate surgical consultation.

G. Rectal Examination

Obtain a stool sample for hemoccult testing, and check for evidence of hemorrhoids or anal fissures.

Special Examinations

A. Upper Gastrointestinal Bleeding

1. Endoscopy—Endoscopy is the most accurate diagnostic tool for upper GI bleeding; it locates the source of bleeding in 75–95% of patients. If the patient is actively bleeding, endoscopy should be performed as soon as possible. If the patient is stable and has no active bleeding, endoscopy should be performed within 24 hours, according to most experts. Advances in endoscopy hemostasis techniques also make it of therapeutic benefit to the patient (sclerotherapy and banding for varices).

2. Upper gastrointestinal series—Once used for initial evaluation of the patient who is not actively bleeding, an upper GI series is no longer recommended for evaluation of upper GI bleeding. If done prior to endoscopy, the contrast material may obscure the endoscopist's view.

3. Angiography—Because endoscopy has been the mainstay for diagnosis, angiography is used in only about 1% of patients with upper GI bleeding. It may be useful if endoscopy cannot identify a bleeding source even when active bleeding is suspected.

B. Lower Gastrointestinal Bleeding

1. Anoscopy/proctosigmoidoscopy—Examination of the rectum and distal sigmoid colon should be undertaken as soon as the patient has been stabilized. If there is evidence of hemorrhoidal bleeding and no blood is noted above the rectum, the bleeding source is in the rectum. The presence of blood above the rectum reliably indicates bleeding from a more proximal site.

2. Barium enema—This radiographic study is no longer commonly used as a diagnostic study for lower GI bleeding. The barium would interfere not only with endoscopic visualization but also with visceral angiography, should that be necessary.

3. Colonoscopy—Once considered of no value in the acute evaluation of lower GI bleeding, colonoscopy is now considered by many endoscopists to be the modality of choice for diagnosis as well as for therapeutic intervention. A definitive diagnosis is made in approximately 75% of cases. Epinephrine injection can be performed if active bleeding sites are identified.

4. Mesenteric angiography—If the bleeding rate is estimated to be greater than 0.5–1 mL/min, angiography allows for selective embolization or vasopressin infusion. Complications associated with angiography include dye-induced renal failure, arterial dissection, and bowel infarction. This test should be ordered only after consultation with a general surgeon or gastroenterologist.

5. Technetium red cell scintigraphy—Technetium bleeding scans may be indicated if the bleeding rate is greater than 0.1 mL/min. A portion of the patient's red blood cells are labeled with technetium-^{99}m and reinfused, followed by scanning. The scan can be repeated periodically to help localize the bleeding site within the GI tract. This testing modality can be used prior to angiography to increase the yield and decrease the risk associated with the procedure. These exams are usually performed after consultation with the on-call endoscopist.

Monitoring for Rebleeding

A. GASTRIC LAVAGE

After placement of a nasogastric tube, continue reassessment for rebleeding by using intermittent low continuous suction. Continued bleeding or rebleeding is an indication for emergent endoscopy.

B. STOOL

Record frequency, color, and approximate amount of stool passed by the patient. Continued passage of bright red, maroon, or melenic stools may indicate need for further studies or transfusion.

C. HEMOGLOBIN AND HEMATOCRIT

Frequent checking of hemoglobin and hematocrit (every 4 hours) is essential in patients with active bleeding after they are hemodynamically stabilized. Often the initial hematocrit is normal. After fluid resuscitation and equilibration of intravascular volume, the hemoglobin and hematocrit should be rechecked.

Almela P et al: Outpatient management of upper digestive hemorrhage not associated with portal hypertension: a large prospective cohort. Am J Gastroenterol 2001;96:2341. [PMID: 11513172]

Fallah MA et al: Acute gastrointestinal bleeding. Med Clin North Am 2000;84:1183. [PMID: 11026924]

Jensen DM et al: Urgent colonoscopy for the diagnosis and treatment of severe diverticular hemorrhage. N Engl J Med 2000;342:78. [PMID: 10631275]

Kollef MH et al: BLEED: a classification tool to predict outcomes in patients with acute and lower gastrointestinal hemorrhage. Crit Care Med 1997;25:1125. [PMID: 9233736]

Lefkovitz Z: Radiology in the diagnosis and therapy of gastrointestinal bleeding. Gastroenterol Clin 2000;29:489. [PMID: 10836191]

O'Neil BB et al: Cinematic nuclear scintigraphy reliably directs surgical intervention for patients with gastrointestinal bleeding. Arch Surg 2000;135:1076. [PMID: 10982513]

Peter DJ et al: Evaluation of the patient with gastrointestinal bleeding: an evidence based approach. Emerg Med Clin North Am 1999;17:239. [PMID: 10101349]

Podila PV et al: Managing patients with acute, nonvariceal gastrointestinal hemorrhage: development of a clinical care pathway. Am J Gastroenterol 2001;96:208. [PMID: 11197254]

Shetzline MA et al: Provocative angiography in obscure gastrointestinal bleeding. South Med J 2000;93:1205. [PMID: 11142458]

Wilcox CM et al: Causes and outcomes of upper and lower gastrointestinal bleeding: The Grady Hospital. South Med J 1999;92:44. [PMID: 993282]

■ EMERGENCY TREATMENT OF SPECIFIC DISORDERS CAUSING UPPER GASTROINTESTINAL BLEEDING

 ESSENTIALS OF DIAGNOSIS

- *May present with hematemesis or melena; massive upper GI bleeding may have hematochezia.*
- *Peptic ulcer disease accounts for 50% of upper GI bleeding; consider initiating proton-pump inhibitor therapy.*
- *Endoscopy diagnostic and often therapeutic.*

Table 14–1 lists the most likely sites of upper GI bleeding. Figure 14–2 is an algorithm for identification of the bleeding site. Esophagogastroduodenoscopy (EGD) is the procedure of choice for either acute hemorrhage or in the stable patient without active bleeding. Specific conditions and their management are discussed below.

PEPTIC ULCER DISEASE

Peptic ulcer disease accounts for approximately half of all episodes of upper GI bleeding (see Table 14–1).

Clinical Findings

Patients with peptic ulcer disease usually present with epigastric pain that can be made worse or even better with food depending on the location of the ulcer. Many patients have had dyspeptic symptoms for years. Up to 40% of patients may not relate pain prior to onset of bleeding.

The severity of bleeding determines the clinical presentation:

- Acute: Sudden onset with massive hemorrhage with symptoms and signs suggestive of shock upon presentation.
- Chronic: Increased fatigue, weakness, occult blood in stool, and anemia due to slow bleeding may be the only symptoms among elderly patients with ulcer disease.

Treatment

Provide emergent management as discussed above, in the "Immediate Management of Life-threatening Bleeding" section. All patients with known peptic ulcer disease should be given a proton-pump inhibitor such as omeprazole or rabeprazole. If the patient has suspected peptic ulcer disease, consider initiating treatment with a proton-pump inhibitor in the emergency department.

Somatostatin is an endogenous peptide that reduces splanchnic blood flow and GI motility, inhibits acid secretion, and may have gastric cytoprotective effects. Octreotide is a synthetic analogue of somatostatin that, when used in the presence of upper GI hemorrhage, may reduce the risk of continued bleeding from actively bleeding peptic ulcer disease. With a very short half-life, it is typically given as an infusion of 25–50 µg/h.

Patients should be instructed not to smoke, consume alcohol, or use NSAIDS or aspirin on a regular basis. Recurrent or persistent hemorrhage requires evaluation for surgical intervention.

Disposition

Patients with active bleeding, tachycardia, hypotension, anemia, age greater than 65 years, or significant comorbid disease should be admitted for evaluation and observation. If none of the above risk factors is present, and close follow-up with a gastroenterologist can be arranged within 24-48 hours, the patient may be discharged home. All patients should be given a proton-pump inhibitor as an outpatient, if not already prescribed by their primary care physician.

GASTRITIS

Gastritis is a more frequently recognized entity with the advent of upper endoscopy as the preferred diagnostic modality in the evaluation of upper GI bleeding. Gastritis is commonly associated with alcohol ingestion as

Table 14–1. Cause and severity of upper gastrointestinal tract hemorrhage in all patients undergoing diagnostic endoscopy at the San Francisco General Hospital over 3 years.

Source of Hemorrhage	Severity of Hemorrhage (%)	
	Mild-Moderate (n = 246 patients)	Severe (n = 140 patients)
Esophagus		
Esophagitis	12	7
Ulcer	2	2
Mallory-Weiss tear	5	19
Esophageal varices	5	31
Total, esophagus	24	59
Stomach		
Gastric ulcer	15	14
Prepyloric ulcer	2	4
Pyloric channel ulcer	4	2
Gastric erosions	2	0
Gastritis	7	0
Varices	1	2
Portal-hypertensive gastropathy	2	
Gastric cancer	2	
Polyp	0	2
Dieulafoy lesion	0	
Total, stomach	35	24
Duodenum		
Ulcer	31	15
Duodenitis	8	
Aortoenteric fistula	2	
Pancreatic pseudocyst		2
Total, duodenum	41	17
	100	100

well as aspirin and NSAID use. Esophagitis and duodenitis may also coexist as findings on endoscopy. The presence of esophagitis on endoscopy indicates dysfunction of the gastroesophageal sphincter with reflux of gastric secretions.

Clinical Findings

Although gastritis is asymptomatic in many cases, patients may experience anorexia, nausea, dyspepsia, pain, and immediate postprandial emesis. The diagnosis is made by endoscopy and cannot be reliably made by an upper GI series. Gastritis rarely results in massive bleeding by itself, but it can occur in the presence of portal hypertension and coagulopathies.

Treatment

Provide therapy as directed above. Continue nasogastric lavage until brisk bleeding has resolved.

For nonbleeding, clinically suspected gastritis, a trial of an antacid with viscous lidocaine ("GI cocktail") may provide quick relief. Consider prescribing a proton-pump inhibitor or recommending any of the many over-the-counter histamine H_2 antagonists (eg, ranitidine, famotidine).

Instruct patients to avoid aspirin, NSAIDS, and alcohol until reevaluated by their primary care physician.

Disposition

Patients with active bleeding should be hospitalized and receive treatment as outlined above. For patients who meet previously mentioned criteria for discharge, ensure timely follow-up with either their doctor or a gastroenterologist.

MALLORY-WEISS SYNDROME

Tears in the esophageal mucosa and submucosa that usually occur after forceful retching and vomiting are responsible for approximately 10% of acute upper GI bleeding. The majority of cases (75%) originate in the stomach; the rest occur at the gastroesophageal junction. Bleeding usually resolves spontaneously, but 3% of deaths from upper GI bleeding have been attributed to Mallory-Weiss tears.

Clinical Findings

In addition to retching and vomiting, this disorder has been reported following chest compressions, coughing, sneezing, or even straining with bowel movement. Many cases have no discernible predisposing factor. Alcohol abuse is a significant risk factor. EGD is the diagnostic gold standard.

Treatment

Provide emergency management as outlined earlier. Nasogastric lavage until clear. For persistent bleeding, consult with the on-call endoscopist for emergent EGD with possible therapeutic epinephrine injection, coagulation, or embolization of the vessel.

Disposition

For bleeding that does not resolve spontaneously, hospitalize the patient for observation and treatment.

ESOPHAGEAL VARICES

Patients with underlying liver disease and portal hypertension are at increased risk for esophageal or gastric variceal bleeding. Approximately 40% of these patients will experience a variceal bleed. The mortality rate for these patients is 30–50%. Alcohol-induced cirrhosis is the most common cause of esophageal varices in the United States, but parasitic infestations of the liver are a frequent cause of cirrhosis in underdeveloped countries.

Clinical Findings

Upper GI bleeding secondary to varices cannot be clinically diagnosed based on signs and symptoms alone. As mentioned earlier, in approximately 50% of patients with known varices who present with GI bleeding, the bleeding is from a source other than the varices. Endoscopic verification is mandatory for accurate diagnosis and treatment.

Treatment

A. EMERGENCY MEASURES

Provide emergent resuscitative efforts as outlined above.

B. AIRWAY MANAGEMENT

If the patient has altered mental status or profuse hematemesis, protective intubation is recommended.

C. MONITOR CARDIOVASCULAR STATUS

If the patient is unstable and has significant comorbid disease, consider invasive monitoring of central venous pressure and arterial blood pressure.

D. MEDICAL THERAPY

The immediate use of octreotide has been proven effective in controlling bleeding. Octreotide decreases splanchnic and hepatic blood flow as well as transhepatic and variceal pressures. Vasopressin has fallen out of favor because of its systemic effects and risk of ischemia.

E. ENDOSCOPIC THERAPY

Sclerotherapy involves the injection of various sclerosing agents to promote thrombus formation. Band ligation uses endoscopically placed rubber bands, which block blood flow and promote thrombus formation. Both therapies work well in over 90% of patients, but band ligation is associated with fewer complications.

F. BALLOON TAMPONADE

In rare circumstances it may be necessary to insert the Sengstaken-Blakemore tube (Chapter 6) to tamponade uncontrolled hemorrhage prior to endoscopic confirmation. Patients must be intubated prior to insertion of the tube.

Disposition

Essentially all patients with variceal bleeding are admitted to an intensive care area for further observation and treatment.

HEMOBILIA

Hemobilia can occur secondary to trauma, hepatic tumors, gallstones, and parasites. It can cause bleeding into the biliary tract, resulting in upper GI bleeding.

Clinical Findings

Hemobilia presents as GI bleeding. During EGD, bleeding is noted from the ampulla of Vater. Bleeding is typically mild. Angiography can further delineate the bleeding site.

Treatment & Disposition

Patients should be hospitalized for observation and treatment. Embolization via interventional radiographic technique is the therapy of choice.

AORTIC ANEURYSM (Aortoenteric Fistula)

Clinical Findings

Upper GI bleeding in the presence of an abdominal aortic aneurysm (or graft) should be assumed to be secondary to an aortoenteric fistula until proven otherwise.

Bleeding may be moderate at first, but profuse hemorrhage will eventually occur unless proper treatment is given. If the patient has a GI bleed and a history of an abdominal aortic aneurysm or graft repair, or if the history and physical examination are suggestive of such, obtain immediate surgical consultation after performing initial resuscitation. If the patient is hemodynamically unstable, emergent surgery is indicated. Consider bedside ultrasonography followed by computed tomography scan for confirmation in the stable patient.

Treatment

Stabilize as previously outlined and obtain immediate surgical consultation.

Disposition

All patients with the above diagnosis should be placed in an intensive care setting for close monitoring.

Almela P et al: Outpatient management of upper digestive hemorrhage not associated with portal hypertension: a large prospective cohort. Am J Gastroenterol 2001;96:2341. [PMID: 11513172]

Avgerinos A et al: Early administration of somatostatin and efficacy of sclerotherapy in acute oesophageal variceal bleeds: the European Acute Bleeding Oesophageal Variceal Episodes (ABOVE) randomized trial. Lancet 1997;350:1495. [PMID: 9388396]

Fallah MA et al: Acute gastrointestinal bleeding. Med Clin North Am 2000;84:1183. [PMID: 11026924]

Imperiale TF et al: Somatostatin or octreotide compared with H2 antagonists and placebo in the management of acute nonvariceal upper gastrointestinal hemorrhage: a meta-analysis. Ann Intern Med 1997;127:1062. [PMID: 94122308]

Peter DJ et al: Evaluation of the patient with gastrointestinal bleeding: an evidence based approach. Emerg Med Clin North Am 1999;17:239. [PMID: 10101349]

Podila PV et al: Managing patients with acute, nonvariceal gastrointestinal hemorrhage: development of a clinical care pathway. Am J Gastroenterol 2001;96:208. [PMID: 11197254]

■ EMERGENCY TREATMENT OF SPECIFIC DISORDERS CAUSING LOWER GASTROINTESTINAL BLEEDING

 ESSENTIALS OF DIAGNOSIS

- *Patients present with hematochezia; 10% may be from an upper GI source.*
- *80–85% of lower GI bleeding resolves spontaneously.*
- *Sigmoidoscopy or colonoscopy can diagnose most sources of lower GI bleeding.*

General Considerations

Lower GI bleeding is most commonly a result of diverticular disease, followed by angiodysplasia, colonic ulcers, and other miscellaneous causes. The most common cause depends on the patient's age. In the adolescent or young adult, Meckel diverticulum, inflammatory bowel disease, and polyps are the most likely causes. In adults up to age 60 years, diverticula, inflammatory bowel disease, and neoplasms are the more common causes. In patients over age 60 years, angiodysplasia, diverticula, and neoplasms predominate.

In 80–85% of patients with lower GI bleeding, the bleeding resolves spontaneously, often making it difficult to locate the source of bleeding. Massive bleeding can occur from any site in the lower GI tract, although diverticular bleeding originates in the colon.

DIVERTICULOSIS

Clinical Findings

Although typically asymptomatic, patients with diverticulosis may present with cramping, lower abdominal pain, and left lower quadrant tenderness to palpation. Tenesmus, constipation, or diarrhea may be associated with diverticulosis. Massive bleeding may occur acutely without any signs or symptoms of diverticulitis.

Treatment & Disposition

(See Figure 14–3.) Perform emergency stabilization as outlined above. Colonoscopy is becoming the modality of choice for initial evaluation in many cases after bowel prep. If massive hemorrhage is present, surgery may be necessary. Selective angiography with embolization is also an option for bleeding control. Most patients should be admitted for further observation and treatment.

ANGIODYSPLASIA

Clinical Findings

Angiodysplasia is characterized by painless bleeding that may be mild or massive. Signs may range from occult blood in stools to melena to hematochezia. Most patients are elderly and have a history of cardiac or renal disease.

For bleeding rates 0.1 mL/min or greater, technetium red cell scan is fairly reliable, although the diagnostic modality of choice may vary between consultants. Colonoscopy may reveal spider angioma–like lesions.

Treatment & Disposition

Stabilize the patient as previously discussed. Electrocoagulation has shown good results for treatment of bleeding lesions visualized during colonoscopy. If bleeding is localized via radionucleotide scanning, then embolization through angiography can be curative in many cases. Angiography can also provide accurate localization of the bleeding when surgical intervention is necessary.

Hospitalize patients for further work-up and observation as directed by the consultant.

HEMORRHOIDS

Clinical Findings

Bleeding is usually the first symptom of internal hemorrhoids. There may be a history of straining on defecation, and the patient will present with frank hematochezia often mixed with well-formed, normal-appearing stools. Occasionally, recurrent bleeding can result in marked anemia. Exsanguinating hemorrhage is rare unless portal hypertension is present. The diagnosis should be confirmed by proctoscopy in the emergency department. Careful anoscopy must be done to fully visualize hemorrhoids. If a flexible fiberoptic sigmoidoscope is used, retroflexion of the insertion tube (bending the section back to examine the rectum from above) is necessary to ensure good visualization of the anorectal junction.

Treatment

A. MEDICAL MEASURES

Most early cases can be managed with high-roughage diet, local measures (sitz baths, suppositories for hemorrhoids [Anusol, many others]), and stool softeners (psyllium [Metamucil, many others], dioctyl sodium sulfosuccinate [Colace, many others]).

B. SURGICAL MEASURES

Surgery is required occasionally to arrest hemorrhage not controlled by medical measures.

Disposition

Hospitalize patients for surgery to arrest persistent brisk bleeding. It is prudent to hospitalize patients with portal hypertension as well. Otherwise, refer patients to an outpatient clinic for follow-up.

COLONIC POLYPS

Clinical Findings

Painless rectal bleeding and discovery of a polyp on sigmoidoscopy, colonoscopy, or barium enema confirm the diagnosis of colonic polyposis.

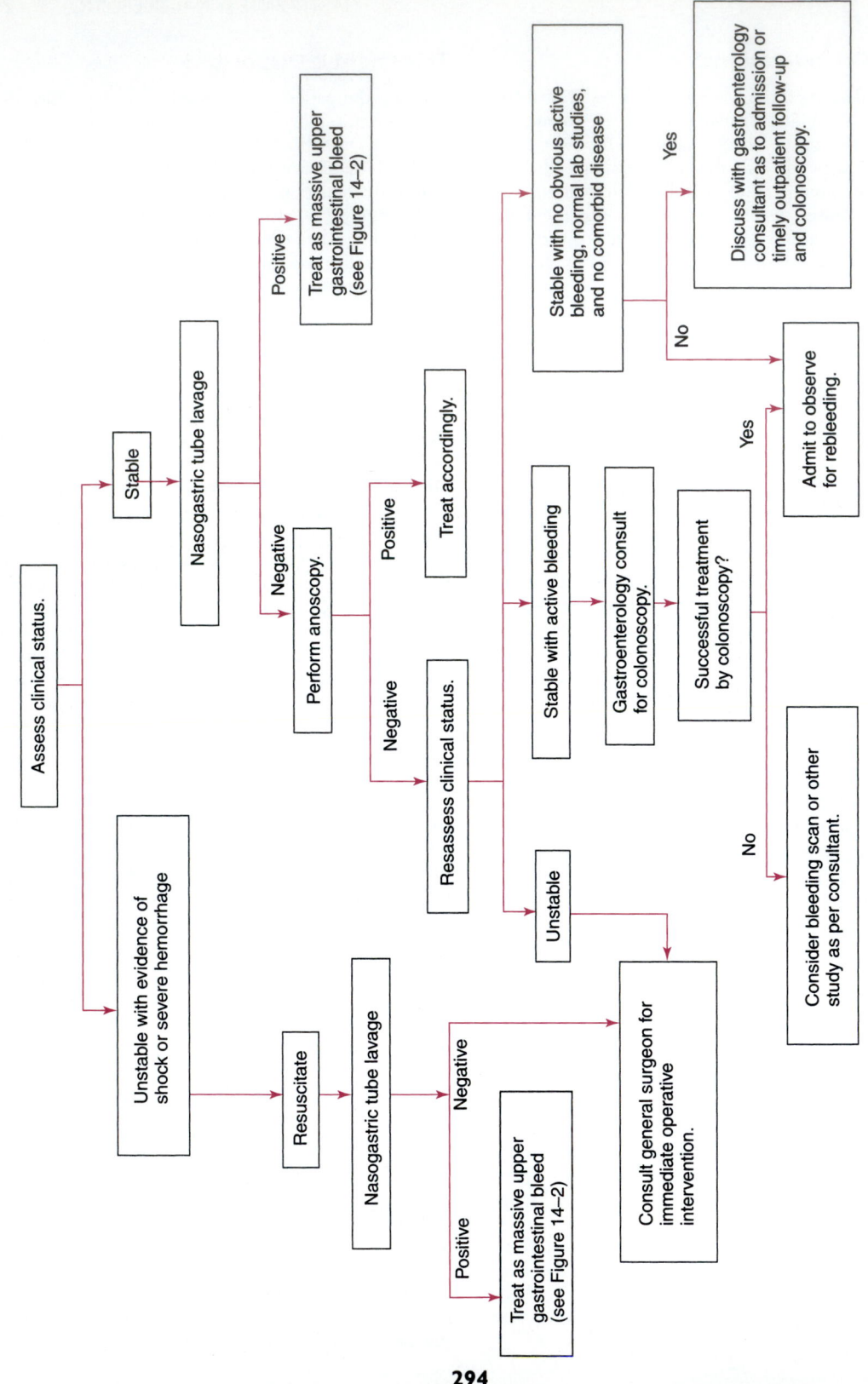

Figure 14-3. Hematochezia or suspected lower GI bleeding.

Treatment

For significant bleeding, see "Immediate Management of Life-Threatening Bleeding" section. If bleeding persists, the polyps should be removed immediately. If bleeding has stopped, patients can be referred for elective colonoscopic polypectomy.

Disposition

Hospitalization is necessary if bleeding persists; otherwise, refer patients for outpatient colonoscopic polypectomy.

COLITIS

Clinical Findings

The chief findings are abdominal cramps, diarrheal stools containing blood and mucopurulent material, fever, weight loss, and anemia. On sigmoidoscopy, the rectal mucosa is eroded and friable. Infectious causes of colitis (particularly *Shigella, Campylobacter, Entamoeba histolytica, Clostridium difficile,* and *Salmonella*) must be ruled out (Chapter 40).

Occasionally, particularly in elderly patients, ischemic colitis can occur with brisk hematochezia. Differentiation from idiopathic or infectious colitis is often possible on sigmoidoscopy. Ischemic colitis rarely, if ever, involves the rectum, whereas other forms of colitis almost always involve the rectum.

Treatment

See "Emergency Management of Life-Threatening Bleeding" section. Medical measures can usually control most symptoms in mild to moderate cases. Surgery is reserved for severe problems.

Disposition

Severe cases are medical emergencies requiring immediate hospitalization. Mild cases can be referred to the proper clinic for further evaluation and treatment after stool samples have been collected for evaluation for enteric pathogens.

CROHN DISEASE

Clinical Findings

Frank blood is seen in about one third of patients with Crohn disease, but massive bleeding is unusual. Patients have abdominal pain and tenderness; diarrhea occurs but is rarely a prominent symptom. There may be fever and sepsis.

Fistula formation, fissures, and hemorrhoids are common. However, Crohn disease may not involve the rectum or sigmoid. A normal proctosigmoidoscopic examination does not exclude Crohn disease.

Treatment

Chrohn disease should be managed medically. Surgery is indicated only rarely, when massive bleeding is not controlled by medical measures. Amebic disease must be excluded before corticosteroids are used.

Disposition

Patients with severe bleeding or systemic symptoms (eg, fever, weight loss) must be hospitalized for observation and treatment. Patients with mild Crohn disease can be referred for outpatient follow-up.

SOLITARY RECTAL ULCER

Clincial Findings

Rectal ulcer is an unusual lesion associated with rectal prolapse. It may result from straining at stool. The patient passes blood and mucus per rectum. Many patients are elderly and have chronic constipation.

Treatment & Disposition

Offer general measures to aid defecation (eg, hydration, stool softeners). Surgery should be avoided. Refer the patient to the appropriate clinic for evaluation and follow-up.

MECKEL DIVERTICULUM

Clinical Findings

About 25% of patients with Meckel diverticulum become symptomatic, and 25% of these patients have lower GI bleeding. This disorder usually occurs before age 2 years and rarely after age 10 years. Symptoms may mimic acute appendicitis. Meckel diverticulum may be diagnosed by technetium pertechnetate scintigraphy or angiography.

Treatment & Disposition

Hospitalize patients for observation, because surgery may be required for severe bleeding.

Billingham RP: The conundrum of lower gastrointestinal bleeding. Surg Clin North Am 1997;77:241. [PMID: 9092113]

Fallah MA et al: Acute gastrointestinal bleeding. Med Clin North Am 2000;84:1183. [PMID: 11026924]

Jensen DM et al: Urgent colonoscopy for the diagnosis and treatment of severe diverticular hemorrhage. N Engl J Med 2000;342:78. [PMID: 10631275]

O'Neil BB et al: Cinematic nuclear scintigraphy reliably directs surgical intervention for patients with gastrointestinal bleeding. Arch Surg 2000;135:1076. [PMID: 10982513]

Diarrhea & Vomiting

Phillip A. Clement, MD, & Jason A. Gardiner, MD

Immediate Management of Life-Threatening Problems
    Hypotension & Shock
    Acute Abdominal Emergencies
    Toxic Exposures
    Other Emergencies
Further Evaluation of the Patient with Diarrhea & Vomiting
    History & Physical Examination

Laboratory & Diagnostic Studies
Emergency Evaluation & Management of Infectious Causes of Diarrhea & Vomiting
    Viral Gastroenteritis
    Bacterial Gastroenteritis
    Parasitic Enteritis
    Empiric Management & Disposition of Patients with Infectious Gastroenteritis

Diarrhea and vomiting are common reasons for emergency department visits. Although the majority of cases are of an infectious, self-limiting nature, the differential diagnosis is broad with the potential for significant morbidity and mortality. Many pathologic processes involve gastrointestinal symptoms. Included are intracranial pathology (trauma, masses, infections), cardiac disease (myocardial infarction, angina), toxic exposures (digoxin, carbon monoxide, heavy metals), acute abdominal pathology (intestinal obstruction, mesenteric ischemia), and endocrine abnormalities (diabetic ketoacidosis, adrenal insufficiency), among others. In addition, infectious causes of diarrhea and vomiting can cause significant harm, especially in the elderly, in infants, and in immunocompromised individuals (Figure 15–1).

■ IMMEDIATE MANAGEMENT OF LIFE-THREATENING PROBLEMS

HYPOTENSION & SHOCK

ESSENTIALS OF DIAGNOSIS

- *Signs of decreased perfusion.*
- *Hypotension, tachycardia, oliguria, and orthostasis.*
- *Cool, pale skin; dry mucous membranes; and altered mentation.*

Clinical Findings

Obtain complete vital signs, including blood pressure, pulse and respiratory rate, pulse oximetry, and a rectal temperature. Look for signs of decreased perfusion (ie, cool, pale skin; altered mentation; decreased urinary output; dry mucous membranes). Hypotension (systolic pressure < 90 mm Hg), tachycardia, oliguria, and orthostasis may indicate impending hemodynamic instability. Look for evidence of sepsis, gastrointestinal bleed, cardiac pump dysfunction, surgical abdominal pathology, toxic exposures, endocrine abnormalities, or anaphylaxis.

Treatment & Disposition

Insert a large-bore intravenous catheter and draw blood for a complete blood count (CBC), electrolytes, renal and liver function, serum lipase, and a pregnancy test, if indicated. Type and cross-match if blood loss is suspected. Start supplemental oxygen, cardiac monitoring, and pulse oximetry together with normal saline volume resuscitation while the underlying cause is sought. If appropriate, initiate empiric antibiotic therapy. Hospitalize the patient for continuous monitoring, supportive treatment, and further investigation if the cause is uncertain. Initiate specific treatment once the cause is determined.

ACUTE ABDOMINAL EMERGENCIES

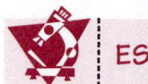 **ESSENTIALS OF DIAGNOSIS**

- *Focal abdominal pain or signs of peritoneal inflammation (rebound).*
- *Pain that precedes the vomiting or diarrhea.*
- *Pain out of proportion to the physical examination.*

Clinical Findings

Patients with acute surgical abdominal pathology may present with diarrhea and vomiting and are at risk of being mislabeled as having gastroenteritis. Inquire about the nature and location of pain, the existence of upper gastrointestinal (GI) symptoms (vomiting) and lower GI symptoms (diarrhea). Determine which symptom began first and clarify the patient's understanding of the term *diarrhea*. Signs and symptoms suggestive of an acute abdominal emergency include focal abdominal pain, an exam consistent with peritoneal inflammation, pain that precedes the vomiting and diarrhea, protracted vomiting with nonspecific abdominal pain, or pain out of proportion to the physical examination. Consider entities such as acute appendicitis, intestinal obstruction, mesenteric ischemia, ectopic pregnancy, GI bleed, intussusception, and gonadal torsion (Table 15–1). Serial abdominal exams in the emergency department may help differentiate early acute abdominal emergencies with vomiting or diarrhea from gastroenteritis. In patients with arteriovascular disease who present with pain out of proportion to the exam, mesenteric ischemia must be ruled out. Consider intussusception in infants and children with abdominal pain, vomiting, and diarrhea (often bloody).

Treatment & Disposition

Treatment ultimately depends on the cause of the symptoms. Obtain complete vital signs; gain intravenous access; and draw blood for a CBC, electrolytes, renal and liver function tests, serum lipase, pregnancy test if appropriate, and blood type and cross-match. An acute abdominal series may demonstrate a small or large bowel obstruction. A computed tomography (CT) scan or ultrasound may help identify the cause of the

Table 15–1. Conditions that may cause peritoneal inflammation (surgical abdomen) in association with vomiting and diarrhea.

Acute appendicitis
Intestinal obstruction
Mesenteric ischemia
Gastrointestinal bleed
Ectopic pregnancy
Intussusception
Gonadal torsion
Pancreatitis
Cholecystitis
Diverticulitis
Pyelonephritis
Pelvic inflammatory disease
Hepatitis
Volvulus
Inflammatory bowel disease
Tubo-ovarian abscess
Toxic megacolon
Radiation therapy
Gastrointestinal cancer
Hirschsprung disease

acute abdomen. If intussusception is suspected, an air contrast or barium enema can be both diagnostic and therapeutic. If the patient's condition is unstable, seek appropriate surgical consultation early.

TOXIC EXPOSURES

 ESSENTIALS OF DIAGNOSIS

- *Cholinergic or sympathomimetic syndromes.*
- *Ingestion of mushrooms, herbal or plant preparations, or seafood.*
- *Occupational exposures; exposure to heavy metals, pesticides, or carbon monoxide.*
- *Medications: digoxin, salicylates, or others.*

Clinical Findings

Diarrhea and vomiting are often the presenting symptoms of toxic exposures. The list of toxins is extensive (Figure 15–1). Obtain key historical information including medications, occupational exposures, use of herbal preparations, consumption of mushrooms or plant products, ingestion of seafood, exposures to heavy metals, and

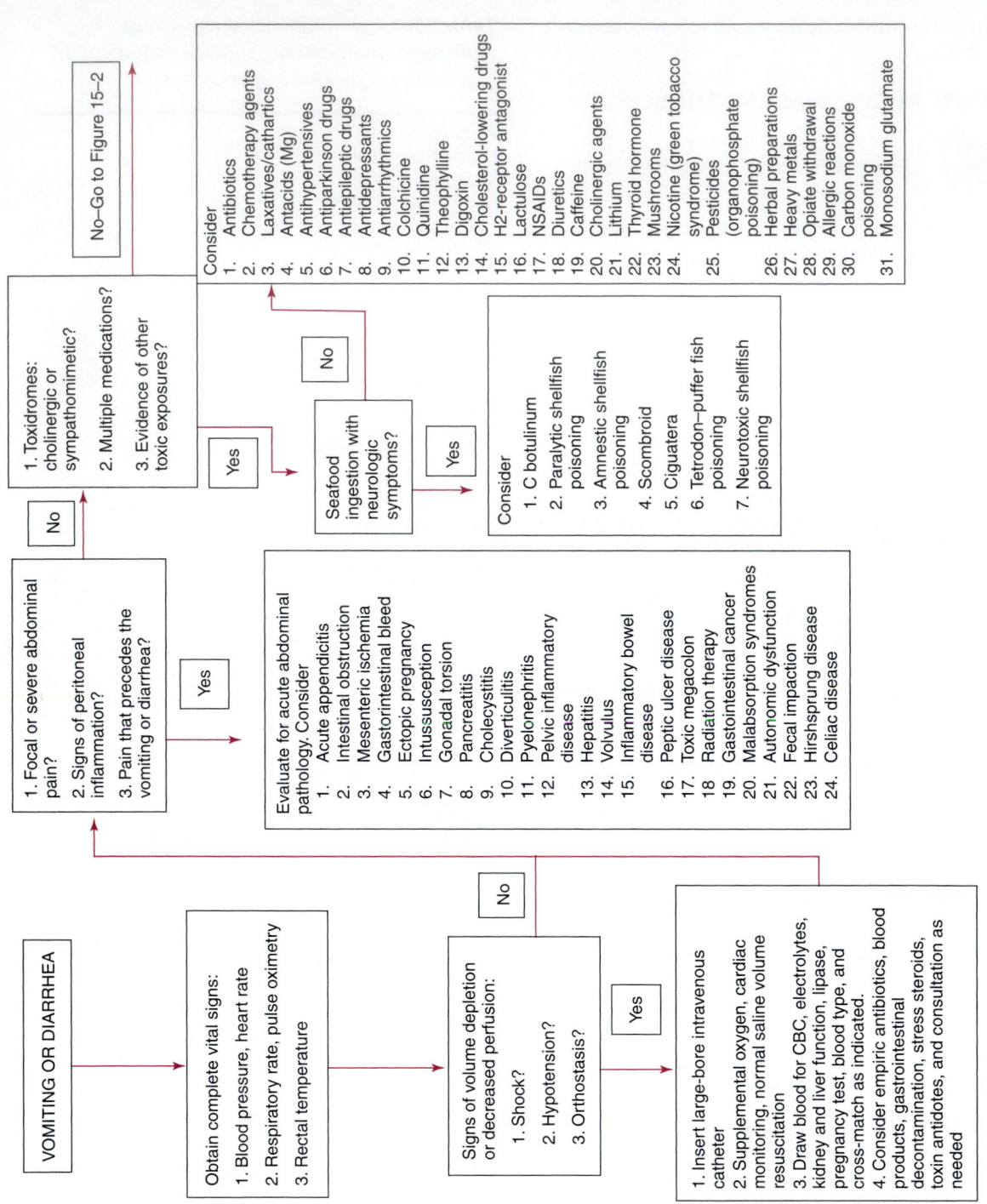

Figure 15–1. Approach to the patient with vomiting and diarrhea, part 1. NSAIDs = nonsteroidal anti-inflammatory drugs.

a history of allergic reactions. Search for specific toxin-induced syndromes such as cholinergic or sympathomimetic reactions. Consider common toxins such as digoxin, salicylates, and carbon monoxide. If neurologic symptoms exist, consider botulism or shellfish poisoning.

Treatment & Disposition

Begin treatment with the proper decontamination method. Give patients with toxic ingestions activated charcoal and a cathartic. Patients with cutaneous and inhalation exposures should be removed from the source and the contaminant diluted. Initiate supportive care and continuous monitoring. Administer specific antidotes if appropriate.

OTHER EMERGENCIES

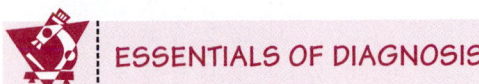

ESSENTIALS OF DIAGNOSIS

- *Chest pain, shortness of breath, diaphoresis, acute pump failure.*
- *History of cardiac, central nervous system, endocrine disease or trauma.*
- *Abnormal neurological exam, altered mentation, fevers, headache.*
- *Laboratory and physical abnormalities.*

Clinical Findings

Cardiac, central nervous system, or endocrine disorders may include vomiting or diarrhea as presenting symptoms (Figure 15–2). Evidence of a cardiac-related disorder include chest pain, shortness of breath, diaphoresis, a history of cardiac disease, or evidence of acute pump failure. Indications of central nervous system pathology include a history of trauma, an abnormal neurological exam, altered mentation, fevers, cephalgia, and evidence of other toxic or metabolic pathology affecting the central nervous system. Search for historical, physical, and laboratory evidence of endocrine dysfunction.

Treatment & Disposition

Patients with a suspected cardiac, central nervous system, or endocrine causes of vomiting or diarrhea should receive aggressive evaluation and management. This may include an electrocardiogram, continuous cardiac monitoring, intravenous access, supplemental oxygen, pulse oximetry, and a complete set of labs including clotting studies and cardiac enzymes as indicated. Obtain x-rays, CT scans, and consultations as needed.

■ FURTHER EVALUATION OF THE PATIENT WITH DIARRHEA & VOMITING

Once life-threatening conditions have been sought and treatment begun, an attempt should be made to further identify the cause of vomiting and diarrhea. Consider the following historical, physical, and laboratory investigations (Table 15–2).

History

A. Features of the Present Illness

Important features of the present illness include time of onset, the nature of symptoms, and duration of illness. Differentiate acute (less than 2 weeks) from chronic symptoms. Clarify the patient's use of the term *diarrhea*. Identify associated symptoms. Inquire about fever, abdominal pain, anorexia, diarrhea, constipation, tenesmus, myalgia, vomiting, cephalgia, and neurologic symptoms such as paresthesias, weakness, or cranial nerve palsies. Inquire about the presence of blood or mucus in the stool and about the character of the vomitus (bloody or bilious). Determine the onset and severity of diarrhea and vomiting in relation to other symptoms. Abdominal cramps after copious, watery diarrhea is consistent with gastroenteritis. However, abdominal pain followed by nausea and loose stool could represent appendicitis. The symptom complex of profuse diarrhea, fever, myalgias, and cephalgia is consistent with dysentery, whereas a symptom complex of sudden severe headache, nausea, vomiting, and loose stool could represent a process such as subarachnoid hemorrhage.

B. Medical and Surgical History

Inquire about the patient's medical and surgical history. Give special attention to immunocompetency. Inquire about a history of HIV, diabetes mellitus, GI bleed, abdominal surgeries, malignancies, and endocrine disease. Ask about recent chemotherapy or radiation therapy.

C. Medications and Antibiotic Use

Inquire about medications including prescription, over the counter, herbal preparations, and drugs of abuse. Give particular attention to recent antibiotic or laxative use.

D. Exposure Risk; Similar Illness in Others

Ask about common source exposures such as daycare or community outbreaks. Inquire about a history of hospitalization or institutionalization.

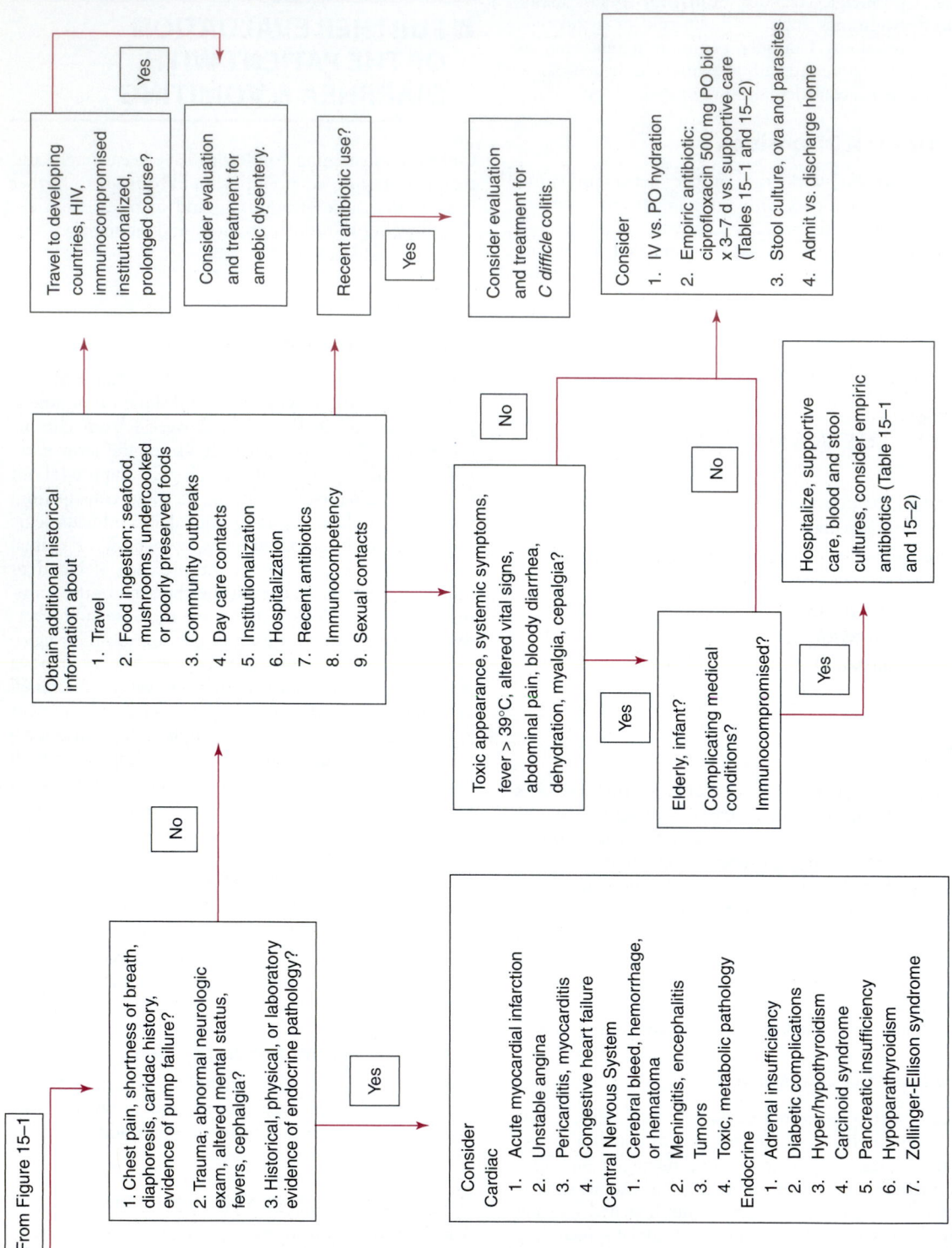

Figure 15–2. Approach to the patient with vomiting and diarrhea, part 2.

From Figure 15–1

1. Chest pain, shortness of breath, diaphoresis, caridac history, evidence of pump failure?

2. Trauma, abnormal neurologic exam, altered mental status, fevers, cephalgia?

3. Historical, physical, or laboratory evidence of endocrine pathology?

No

Yes

Consider
Cardiac
1. Acute myocardial infarction
2. Unstable angina
3. Pericarditis, myocarditis
4. Congestive heart failure
Central Nervous System
1. Cerebral bleed, hemorrhage, or hematoma
2. Meningitis, encephalitis
3. Tumors
4. Toxic, metabolic pathology
Endocrine
1. Adrenal insufficiency
2. Diabetic complications
3. Hyper/hypothyroidism
4. Carcinoid syndrome
5. Pancreatic insufficiency
6. Hypoparathyroidism
7. Zollinger-Ellison syndrome

Obtain additional historical information about
1. Travel
2. Food ingestion; seafood, mushrooms, undercooked or poorly preserved foods
3. Community outbreaks
4. Day care contacts
5. Institutionalization
6. Hospitalization
7. Recent antibiotics
8. Immunocompetency
9. Sexual contacts

Travel to developing countries, HIV, immunocompromised, institutionalized, prolonged course?

Yes

Consider evaluation and treatment for amebic dysentery.

Recent antibiotic use?

Yes

Consider evaluation and treatment for *C difficile* colitis.

Toxic appearance, systemic symptoms, fever > 39°C, altered vital signs, abdominal pain, bloody diarrhea, dehydration, myalgia, cepalgia?

No

Yes

Elderly, infant?
Complicating medical conditions?
Immunocompromised?

Yes

No

Hospitalize, supportive care, blood and stool cultures, consider empiric antibiotics (Table 15–1 and 15–2)

Consider
1. IV vs. PO hydration
2. Empiric antibiotic: ciprofloxacin 500 mg PO bid x 3–7 d vs. supportive care (Tables 15–1 and 15–2)
3. Stool culture, ova and parasites
4. Admit vs. discharge home

Table 15–2. Evaluation of acute vomiting and diarrhea.

History

Present illness: time of onset, duration and nature of symptoms, associated symptoms (fevers, abdominal pain, myalgias, cephalgia, anorexia, neurologic symptoms)

Travel: international or domestic, backpacking, new water supplies

Exposures: community outbreaks, daycare exposure, hospitalization or institutionalization

Ingestion: mushrooms, plant products, herbal preparations, seafood, 24-hour food history

Toxins: medications, recreational drugs, recent antibiotic use, exposure to heavy metals, pesticides, carbon monoxide

Radiation therapy or chemotherapy

Medical and surgical history: endocrine disorders, HIV, malignancies, gastrointestinal bleeds, abdominal surgeries

Sexual contacts

Physical examination

General appearance: patient's overall health, toxic appearance, jaundice or evidence of volume depletion

Complete set of vital signs: blood pressure, heart rate, respiratory rate, pulse oximetry, rectal temperature

Abdominal exam: focal tenderness, signs of peritoneal inflammation, pain out of proportion to the exam, distended abdomen

Rectal exam: fecal impaction, melena, hematochezia, occult blood

Laboratory and diagnostic studies

Fecal cell count: limited clinical utility because fecal erythrocytes and leucocytes are associated with dysentery and noninfectious processes

Stool cultures: in patients who appear toxic, patients who are immunocompromised, and those with chronic diarrhea

Stool for ova and parasites: in patients with chronic diarrhea, those with history of international travel, HIV-infected patients, and daycare exposures

C difficile toxin: consider if recent antibiotic use

Giardia antigen: consider in HIV-infected patients, in patients with history of travel to developing countries, in those with a history of backpacking, and in daycare exposures

Complete blood count, blood urea nitrogen, creatinine, glucose, lipase, liver function test, and blood cultures: as indicated

Urinalysis: urinalysis and a urine pregnancy test if indicated

Radiographic evaluation: consider an acute abdominal series in suspected bowel obstruction; abdominal CT scan or ultrasound as indicated

E. DIETARY HISTORY

Inquire about unusual foods, dairy products, eggs, seafood, or unpasteurized or undercooked food. Ask about the ingestion of mushrooms or other plant products.

F. TRAVEL HISTORY

Inquire about recent international travel, especially to developing countries. Ask about recent domestic travel or outdoor activities, especially backpacking or exposure to new water sources.

G. TOXIN EXPOSURES

Assess the risk of exposure to toxins, including heavy metals, carbon monoxide, salicylates, and digoxin (see Figure 15–1). Ask about occupational history as it relates to toxin exposures. In farm workers, consider pesticides (organophosphate poisoning) and nicotine (green tobacco syndrome). Inquire about a history of allergic reactions.

H. SEXUAL EXPOSURES

Inquire about sexual contacts. Amebiasis, giardiasis, campylobacteriosis, salmonellosis, and shigellosis can be transmitted by both heterosexual and homosexual contact. *Chlamydia trachomatis,* herpes simplex, and *Neisseria gonorrhoeae* are also possible causes of lower GI symptoms. HIV-positive and immunocompromised individuals are subject to infections with *Cryptosporidium,* cytomegalovirus, and *Mycobacterium avium intracellulare.*

Physical Examination

Use the physical examination to assess the patient's hydration status, evaluate for sepsis, rule out the acute abdomen, and determine the presence of blood in the stool.

A. GENERAL APPEARANCE

Assess the patient's overall health. Look for evidence of volume depletion, a toxic appearance, or jaundice.

B. FEVER

Fever is consistent with invasive bacterial or parasitic causes of gastroenteritis (ie, dysentery). Fever could also indicate a process requiring acute surgical intervention. Less commonly, fever may be associated with a viral or noninvasive bacterial gastroenteritis. Food poisoning should not be associated with fever.

C. BLOOD PRESSURE AND PULSE RATE

Hypotension and tachycardia are typical responses to volume depletion. If the volume status is not apparent, evaluate for orthostasis with the patient supine, sitting, and standing to detect more subtle degrees of volume depletion (systolic pressure drop $\geq$ 10 mm Hg and pulse rise $\geq$ 15 beats/min). Young, healthy adults may maintain normal vital signs even with significant dehydration. Look for a blunted response in patients who are taking atrioventricular nodal blockers.

D. ABDOMINAL EXAMINATION

Significant abdominal pain should prompt the search for causes other than infectious gastroenteritis. If abdominal examination elicits focal tenderness, or if signs of peritoneal inflammation are present, consider acute surgical pathology. However, subjective, diffuse, and crampy abdominal pain or tenderness may occur after extensive vomiting or diarrhea. In addition, several infectious agents, most notably *Yersinia enterocolitica* and *Campylobacter* sp., may mimic appendicitis and cause right lower quadrant pain, anorexia, low grade fever, and vomiting preceding the onset of diarrhea. Appendicitis must be ruled out in patients with this presentation.

E. RECTAL EXAMINATION

Perform rectal examination to detect fecal impaction, melena, or hematochezia.

Laboratory & Diagnostic Studies

Laboratory and diagnostic tests are of limited value in the routine evaluation of diarrhea and vomiting. Testing should be carried out, as indicated, in patients with a suspected noninfectious cause of vomiting or diarrhea, in those who are hemodynamically unstable, the very young, the elderly, and immunosuppressed individuals. In addition, testing may be necessary in patients with a prolonged course or in those not responding to conservative management.

A. FECAL CELL COUNT

Fecal erythrocytes and, to a greater degree, leukocytes have been used as a guide to determine who should receive empiric antibiotics. Both findings are associated with inflammatory diarrhea, of which bacterial dysentery is a common cause. However, there are many noninfectious causes of inflammatory diarrhea, which may also produce fecal red and white cells. These include inflammatory bowel disease, chemotherapy and radiation therapy, hypersensitivity, and autoimmune disorders.

Just as the presence of erythrocytes and leukocytes is not specific for a bacterial process, their absence by stool smear does not rule it out. Furthermore, the cell count has not been shown to be a good indicator of which patients will benefit from empiric antibiotic treatment.

B. BACTERIAL CULTURE OF STOOL

Consider bacterial culture of stool in patients experiencing a prolonged course, in infants, in the elderly, in immunocompromised patients, and in patients who appear toxic.

C. STOOL FOR OVA AND PARASITES

Consider testing for ova and parasites in patients with chronic diarrhea, those with a history of travel to developing countries, patients with HIV infection, and those with exposure to infants in daycare.

D. *CLOSTRIDIUM DIFFICILE* TOXIN

Consider testing for *C difficile* toxin if the patient reports recent antibiotic use. Diarrhea may be delayed as long as 12 weeks after antibiotic therapy. Clindamycin, penicillins, and cephalosporins are commonly implicated.

E. *ESCHERICHIA COLI* 0157:H7 TOXIN

Test patients with suspected hemolytic-uremic syndrome for *E coli* 0157:H7 toxin.

F. *GIARDIA* ANTIGEN

Consider testing for *Giardia* antigen in HIV-infected patients, in those with a history of travel to developing countries or a history of backpacking, and in those with daycare exposure.

G. CBC, BLOOD UREA NITROGEN/CREATININE, GLUCOSE, LIPASE, AND LIVER FUNCTION TESTS

Order other blood tests as indicated, especially if significant dehydration is suspected.

H. URINALYSIS

A urinalysis and a urine pregnancy test should be obtained if indicated.

I. RADIOGRAPHIC EVALUATION

Radiographic evaluation is indicated for patients thought to have a surgical abdomen. If abnormal bowel sounds, bilious vomiting, or abdominal distention are present, consider an acute abdominal series. An abdominal CT scan or an ultrasound may be appropriate as indicated.

J. REFERRAL

Referral to a gastroenterologist may be indicated in the evaluation of chronic diarrhea.

■ EMERGENCY EVALUATION & MANAGEMENT OF INFECTIOUS CAUSES OF DIARRHEA & VOMITING

The specific agent responsible for an episode of infectious gastroenteritis is difficult to identify in the acute setting. However, viral agents account for the majority of episodes, up to 70% by some estimates. Of the remaining infectious causes, bacterial agents account for approximately 24% and parasitic agents account for 6%.

VIRAL GASTROENTERITIS

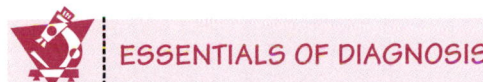

ESSENTIALS OF DIAGNOSIS

- *Mild systemic symptoms; generally no fever or abdominal pain.*
- *Fecal erythrocytes and leukocytes are uncommon.*
- *Dehydration may be mild to severe.*

Clinical Findings

Most viral agents produce a secretory diarrhea. Viral cytotoxins lead to an increased cellular permeability and result in the secretion of water and electrolytes into the intestinal lumen. Unlike invasive dysentery, viral gastroenteritis usually lacks significant systemic symptoms and is not generally associated with fever and abdominal pain. Fecal erythrocytes and leukocytes are uncommon. The most frequently identified agents are Norwalk virus and rotavirus.

Treatment & Disposition

Like other causes of nondysenteric gastroenteritis (Table 15–3), viral gastroenteritis tends to be self-limiting and to require only supportive care. However, significant dehydration can occur and lead to severe illness, especially in those at the extremes of age or those with other compromising medical conditions.

BACTERIAL GASTROENTERITIS

ESSENTIALS OF DIAGNOSIS

- *Cytotoxin-mediated bacterial gastroenteritis is clinically similar to viral gastroenteritis.*
- *Invasive bacterial enteritis produces dysentery with fever, diarrhea, abdominal cramps, and other systemic symptoms.*
- *Fecal erythrocytes and leukocytes are common in invasive disease.*

Clinical Findings

Bacterial agents may produce either an inflammatory or a secretory diarrhea. Secretory diarrhea is cytotoxin mediated and may be caused by toxins that are preformed and are therefore rapid acting, as with *Staphylococcus aureus* food poisoning, or by toxins formed after bacterial colonization, as with *Vibrio cholerae* (see Table 15–3). Inflammatory diarrhea is caused by direct bacterial invasion of the intestinal mucosa. The result is release into the intestinal lumen of water, electrolytes, blood, proteins, and mucus. The clinical presentation is dysentery and may include fever, abdominal pain, bloody diarrhea, anorexia, myalgia, cephalgia, dehydration, and weight loss. With invasive enteritis, stool smears generally contain both erythrocytes and leukocytes.

Treatment & Disposition

Among patients with gastroenteritis, those with dysentery tend to experience the greatest morbidity and mortality. Several invasive bacterial agents, most notably *Salmonella* and *Shigella,* may result in bacteremia, sepsis, and death. This is especially of concern in the elderly, infants, and the immunocompromised. However, any bacterial agent can cause significant harm in susceptible patients. Worldwide, *V cholerae* accounts for a significant number of deaths annually. Treatment depends on the causative agent; however, in the acute setting an empiric strategy is often required (see below).

PARASITIC ENTERITIS

ESSENTIALS OF DIAGNOSIS

- *Acute amebic dysentery may be clinically similar to bacterial dysentery.*

Table 15–3. Differential diagnostic features of common types of nondysenteric gastroenteritis.

Cause	Mode of Transmission	Incubation	Comments	Therapy in Adults
Staphylococcus aureus	Previously cooked proteinaceous foods (ham, shrimp, cream-filled goods, potato salad, chicken and egg salads)	1–6 hours	Nausea, severe vomiting, mild diarrhea, and abdominal cramps. Fever is rare. The source is an infected food handler. Symptoms are caused by preformed enterotoxins.	Supportive care. Intravenous versus oral rehydration. Symptomatic treatment. Antibiotics ineffective against preformed enterotoxins.
Bacillus cereus	Previously cooked meats, fried rice, vegetables, dried fruit and powdered milk	1–6 hours	Abrupt onset of nausea and vomiting, mild diarrhea. Fever is rare. Induced by preformed enterotoxins.	Self-limiting. Supportive care. Oral or intravenous rehydration and symptomatic treatment.
Clostridium perfringens	Previously cooked or poorly reheated meats, gravy, and poultry	8–24 hours	Abdominal cramps, nausea, watery diarrhea with minimal vomiting. Fever is rare. Caused by enterotoxins formed both before and after gastrointestinal colonization.	Supportive care. Self-limiting illness. Intravenous versus oral rehydration and symptomatic treatment.
Clostridium botulism	Home-canned fruits and vegetables; commercial fish products	12–36 hours	Very rare. Mild gastrointestinal symptoms, followed by weakness, malaise, fatigue, drymouth, diplopia, dysphagia, and muscle incoordination. Progressive cranial nerve palsies and muscle weakness may lead to respiratory failure.	Hospitalization, supportive care and ventilatory support as needed. Consider gastrointestinal decontamination and intravenous trivalent antitoxin administration if appropriate.
Enterotoxigenic Escherichia coli	Most outbreaks are due to contaminated water	12–72 hours	Accounts for 30–70% of traveler's diarrhea. A major cause of infantile diarrhea in the developing world. Adults are usually afebrile; infants may have a fever. Causes a cholera-like illness with profuse watery diarrhea.	Usually self-limiting. Prevention is through good hygiene. Supportive care. If severe, ciprofloxacin, 500 mg orally twice daily for 3–5 days.
Vibrio cholerae	Raw or undercooked seafood (oysters, crabs, shrimp); contaminated water or fecal-oral transmission	12–72 hours	Summer and early fall. In North America most cases are along the Gulf Coast of Texas and Louisiana. Explosive rice-water diarrhea up to 1 L/hr. Vomiting, fever, abdominal cramps, dehydration, lactic acidosis, and death if untreated. Enterotoxins are formed after bacterial colonization.	Fluid resuscitation is the essential treatment. Antibiotics may shorten the disease course. Ciprofloxacin, 1.0 g orally for 1 dose. Alternatively, tetracycline or TMP-SMZ.

	Incubation period	Clinical features	Treatment
Scombroid poisoning	Contaminated scombroid fish (tuna, bonito, mackerel); dolphin fish (mahi-mahi)	1–2 hours	Numbness and tingling of the mouth; dysphagia; headache; dizziness; diffuse flushing of the face, neck, and upper trunk. May develop palpitations, nausea, vomiting, abdominal pain, and diarrhea. Bronchospasm occurs rarely. Caused by histamine-like substance released form contaminated fish muscle.	Antihistamines: parenteral diphenhydramine, 50 mg. Histamine receptor antagonist, cimetidine, or ranitidine. Give fluid and bronchodilators as needed.
Paralytic shellfish poisoning	Bivalve shellfish (clams, oysters, mussels, scallops)	Up to 1 hour	Nausea, vomiting, diarrhea, abdominal cramps, paresthesias of face and extremities, headache, ataxia, vertigo, cranial nerve palsies, and muscle weakness; in severe ingestions, paralysis.	Gastrointestinal decontamination and supportive care. Hospitalization for 24-hour observation. May require ventilatory support.
Viral gastroenteritis	Fecal-oral, person-to-person transmission; contaminated food or water; day-care; cooler months	12–72 hours	Norwalk and rotavirus are the most common agents. Nausea, vomiting, and watery diarrhea. May have mild abdominal cramps and myalgias. Usually afebrile. Occasionally epidemics occur, especially in infants and small children.	Self-limiting. Supportive care. Oral or intravenous rehydration and symptomatic treatment.
Giardia lamblia	Contaminated food or water; fecal-oral, person-to-person transmission	1–4 weeks	Backpackers, travelers, elderly. Most common intestinal parasite in the United States. Causes bloating, crampy abdominal pain, excessive flatus, and malabsorptive diarrhea. Vomiting is rare. A common cause of chronic diarrhea.	Metronidazole, 250 mg orally three times daily for 7 days.

TMP-SMZ = trimethoprim-sulfamethoxazole.

• Consider parasitic causes in patients with chronic diarrhea, a travel history to developing countries, or a history of institutionalization or immuno-compromise.

Clinical Findings

Parasitic agents are rarely identified in the emergency department. Acute amebic dysentery, caused by *Entamoeba histolytica,* may be difficult to distinguish clinically from dysentery of a bacterial cause. Consider parasitic causes in patients with a travel history to developing countries, in institutionalized patients, or in immunocompromised patients. Also consider parasitic causes in those with a prolonged course and in those not responding to conventional treatment. Laboratory analysis of stool may be of benefit for diagnosing suspected parasitic enteritis.

Treatment & Disposition

Treatment is best determined by the results of stool analysis. In the acute setting, empiric treatment may be required (see next section).

EMPIRIC MANAGEMENT & DISPOSITION OF PATIENTS WITH INFECTIOUS GASTROENTERITIS

Supportive Care

Initial treatment consists of supportive care with special attention to the patient's hydration status. For many patients, this may be the only treatment necessary. Oral rehydration may be used for mild to moderate dehydration. In pediatric patients, oral rehydration can be accomplished by giving 50–100 ml/kg of a glucose-electrolyte solution over 4 hours.

In patients with evidence of more severe dehydration, initiate intravenous fluid resuscitation with normal saline or lactated Ringer's solution. Give pediatric patients a bolus of 20 mL/kg of normal saline, which may be repeated as needed. Because children are particularly susceptible to hypoglycemia after prolonged vomiting and poor oral intake, a rapid bedside glucose determination should be performed in ill-appearing pediatric patients.

Empiric Chemotherapy

Interruption of the fecal-oral pathway should be the initial treatment for infectious gastroenteritis and can be accomplished by adherence to strict hygiene. Viral and noninvasive bacterial gastroenteritis, as well as many cases of bacterial dysentery, tend to be self-limiting and to require only supportive therapy. Initiate empiric antibiotic treatment in patients with a suspected invasive bacterial process and severe diarrhea, systemic symptoms, fever, and abdominal pain or in those who appear toxic. Fecal cell count is of limited utility in deciding whom to treat. Admit patients with this presentation if they are immunocompromised, have complicating medical conditions, are elderly, or are infants. For these patients, base ultimate treatment on culture results. Young, healthy adults may be candidates for outpatient treatment.

Because the results of cultures are usually unavailable in the acute setting, treatment must be empiric and guided by knowledge of common causes of dysentery (Table 15–4). Ciprofloxacin, 500 mg orally twice daily for 3–5 days, has been shown to be more effective than trimethoprim-sulfamethoxazole (TMP-SMZ). Use empiric treatment with caution in pediatric patients and the elderly because of an association with hemolytic-uremic syndrome. This association has been shown with both ciprofloxacin and TMP-SMZ and is most strongly associated with treatment of enterohemorrhagic *E coli* 0157:H7. *Salmonella* and *Shigella* have also been implicated. If possible, therefore, treatment in these patients should be based on culture results.

Because no broad empiric strategy exists for the treatment of parasitic agents, drug therapy is best guided by laboratory analysis. However, if amebic dysentery is of concern, treatment with metronidazole should be considered. A second agent, such as iodoquinol, is needed after initial treatment. In patients with a history of previous antibiotic use and suspected *C difficile* colitis, *C difficile* toxin assay followed by oral vancomycin or metronidazole is appropriate therapy.

Symptomatic Treatment

A. ANTIEMETICS

Intravenous hydration helps reduce emesis and should be used as initial therapy. Often this is the only therapy needed. For patients with uncontrollable, protracted vomiting, the use of an antiemetic can be considered. However, these agents may cause somnolence and complicate evaluation in a potentially septic population. In addition, side effects are common, especially dystonic reactions with the phenothiazines (prochlorperazine or promethazine). For patients with vomiting significant enough to require antiemetics, obtain intravenous access and give an initial fluid bolus. Administer antiemetics intravenously or as a suppository. Consider the following:

Table 15–4. Differential diagnostic features of common types of dysentery.

Cause	Mode of Transmission	Incubation	Comments	Therapy in Adults
Salmonella spp.	Contaminated food or water (eggs, poultry, milk). Animals or pets (turtles, chicks, lizards). Group gatherings.	8–72 hours	Very common. Fever, abdominal pain, headache, myalgia, diarrhea with little vomiting. Risk of sepsis in the young, elderly, or the compromised (sickle cell disease, diabetes, HIV, intravenous drug abusers, the asplenic). Rare fecal RBCs; common WBCs.	Treat infection in those with severe illness or sepsis, the immunocompromised, or the hospitalized. Ciprofloxacin, 500 mg orally (400 mg intravenously) twice daily for 3–7 days. Alternative: azithromycin or ceftriaxone.
Shigella spp.	Fecal-oral, person-to-person transmission, or contaminated food. Daycare and institutions. Poor sanitation. Highly contagious.	1–3 days	Very common. Children aged 1–5 years, institutionalized patients. Fever, headache, abdominal pain, myalgia, diarrhea with little vomiting. Febrile seizures and a toxic appearance may prompt lumbar puncture. Diarrhea may begin during the procedure. Fecal RBCs common; sheets of WBCs.	Treat infection in those with severe dysentery, sepsis, or institutional outbreaks. Ciprofloxacin, 500 mg orally (400 mg intravenously) twice daily for 3–5 days. Alternative: TMP-SMZ or azithromycin.
Campylobacter spp.	Unchlorinated water, contaminated food (unprocessed milk, poultry). Animals or pets. Natural water supplies in the national parks.	1–7 days	Very common. Backpacker's diarrhea, summer months, children and young adults. Fever, headache, abdominal pain, myalgias for several days followed by diarrhea with little vomiting. May mimic appendicitis. Fecal RBCs and WBCs common.	Treat infection in those who are compromised or appear toxic. Ciprofloxacin, 500 mg orally twice daily for 5 days. Alternative: azithromycin.
Yersinia enterocolitica	Contaminated food or water (pork, milk). Fecal-oral, person-to-person transmission. Wild and domestic animals.	1–5 days	Children and young adults. Anorexia, low-grade fever, right lower quadrant abdominal pain, and vomiting may precede diarrhea and mimic appendicitis. Bacteremia is rare. Fecal RBCs and WBCs common.	Treat infection in severely ill patients. Usually self-limiting. Ciprofloxacin, 500 mg orally twice daily for 3–5 days. Alternative: TMP-SMZ.
Vibrio parahaemolyticus	Contaminated food or water. Raw or undercooked shellfish.	8–72 hours	Most common during the summer months and in adults. Common in Japan. Diarrhea, abdominal cramps, low-grade fever, headache and nausea with minimal vomiting. Bacteremia is rare. Fecal RBCs and WBCs common.	None proven. Usually self-limiting. In vitro sensitivity to fluoroquinolones or doxycycline.

(continued)

Table 15–4. Differential diagnostic features of common types of dysentery. (Continued)

Cause	Mode of Transmission	Incubation	Comments	Therapy in Adults
Enterohemorrhagic *Escherichia coli* 0157:H7	Contaminated food or water. Raw under-cooked meats, hamburger. Fecal-oral, person-to-person transmission. Institutions, daycare.	3–8 days	Children and the elderly. Fever, abdominal pain, vomiting, grossly bloody diarrhea. May mimic gastrointestinal bleed or mesenteric ischemia. Hemolytic uremic syndrome (common cause of renal failure in children) occurs in 5%, 5–20 days postinfection. Fecal RBCs and WBCs common.	Supportive care. Antibiotics are not recommended. May increase the risk of complications (hemolytic uremic syndrome).
Aeromonas hydrophilia	Contaminated water.	1–5 days	More common in the elderly or the compromised. More severe in children. Cause of 10–15% of cases of pediatric diarrhea. Diarrhea, vomiting, and abdominal cramps with or without fever. Chronic infection may mimic inflammatory bowel disease. Fecal RBCs and WBCs common.	Ciprofloxacin, 500 mg orally twice daily for 3–7 days. Alternative: TMP/SMZ or tetracycline.
Strongyloides stercoralis	Soils with fecal contamination. Warm climates, poor sanitation, institutions.	Weeks to months	Fever, abdominal pain, vomiting, diarrhea, and sepsis in the immunocompromised. The compromised may develop cutaneous, pulmonary, or central nervous system symptoms.	Thiabendazole, 25 mg/kg orally twice daily for 3–5 days.
Clostridium difficile (antibiotic associated)	Recent antibiotic use. Clindamycin, penicillins, and cephalosporins are most commonly implicated.	1–12 weeks	More common in adults. More severe in children. Fever, abdominal pain, diarrhea, rarely vomiting. May cause significant illness especially in the elderly, the compromised, or the very young. Fecal RBCs and WBCs common.	Discontinue associated antibiotics. Metronidazole, 500 mg orally three times daily for 10–14 days, or vancomycin, 125 mg orally 4 times daily for 10–14 days
Entamoeba histolytica (amebic dysentery)	Contaminated food or water. Poor sanitation, institutions. Travel to developing countries.	1–12 weeks	Patients with acute amebic dysentery present with abrupt onset of fever, abdominal pain, tenesmus, and bloody diarrhea. Vomiting is rare. Chronic dysentery causes malaise, weight loss, bloating, and blood-streaked diarrhea. May develop an hepatic abscess. Fecal RBCs and WBCs common.	Metronidazole, 750 mg orally three times daily for 10 days followed by iodoquinol, 650 mg orally 3 times daily for 20 days.

RBCs = red blood cells; TMP-SMZ = trimethoprim-sulfamethoxazole; WBCs = white blood cells.

- Prochlorperazine (Compazine): adults, 5–10 mg intravenously, or 25 mg rectally; children > 10 kg, 0.1 mg/kg rectally every 6 hours (use is contraindicated in children < 10 kg).
- Promethazine (Phenergan): adults, 12.5–25.0 mg intravenously or rectally; children, 0.25–1.0 mg/kg rectally every 4–6 hours.
- Metoclopramide (Reglan): adults, 5–10 mg intravenously; children, 0.1–0.2 mg/kg intravenously every 6–8 hours.

B. ANTIDIARRHEAL AGENTS

The literature remains divided over use of antimotility agents in treating acute enteritis. Most beneficial effects are modest with the possible introduction of adverse effects. Of concern is the association of morphine administration with *Salmonella* and *Shigella* bacteremia. An additional association has been suggested between the use of opiates, loperamide, or diphenoxylate with atropine and the precipitation of toxic megacolon in patients with ulcerative colitis or antibiotic-associated colitis. Therefore, the use of these agents should be limited in the acute setting. Commonly used agents and some associated risks are listed below:

- Loperamide (Imodium): Avoid in patients with antibiotic-associated colitis, inflammatory bowel disease, or dysentery.
- Bismuth subsalicylate suspension (Pepto-Bismol): Avoid in pediatric patients because of concern about Reye syndrome. It may cause salicylate toxicity.
- Kaolin-pectin suspension (Kaopectate): May cause constipation, bloating. Avoid if intestinal obstruction is suspected.
- Diphenoxylate with atropine (Lomotil): Avoid in pediatrics patients. May precipitate toxic megacolon in patients with inflammatory bowel disease. May cause central nervous system depression.
- Opiates: Avoid in patients with antibiotic-associated colitis, inflammatory bowel disease, or dysentery.

Disposition

Hospitalization is rarely required for vomiting or diarrhea due to food poisoning or viral gastroenteritis. Even though symptoms may be severe, the vomiting or diarrhea rarely persists long enough to require inpatient parenteral hydration. Patients with dysentery and a toxic appearance, severe dehydration, or persistent vomiting or diarrhea; those with complicating medical conditions; and the very young or elderly may require hospitalization. Hospitalization may be required in the following cases:

- Extremes of age: newborns and the very elderly tolerate fluid depletion poorly.
- Systemic toxemia, as indicated by high fever and rigors.
- Possible toxic exposures requiring further evaluation or treatment.
- Massive diarrhea or extreme dehydration.
- Severe vomiting (preventing oral replenishment) with diarrhea.
- For further evaluation of unexplained causes of vomiting or diarrhea.
- Poor home environment where required support cannot be provided.

Aranda-Michel J, Giannella RA: Acute diarrhea: a practical review. Am J Med 1999;106(6):670. [PMID: 10378626]

Besser RE et al: *Escherichia coli* O157:H7 gastroenteritis and the hemolytic uremic syndrome: an emerging infectious disease. Annu Rev Med 1999;50:355. [PMID: 10073283]

Cleary RK: *Clostridium difficile*–associated diarrhea and colitis: clinical manifestations, diagnosis, and treatment. Dis Colon Rectum 1998;41(11):1435. [PMID: 9823813]

Daniels NA et al: *Vibrio parahaemolyticus* infections in the United States, 1973–1998. J Infect Dis 2000;181(5):1661. [PMID: 10823766]

Dryden MS et al: Empirical treatment of severe acute community-acquired gastroenteritis with ciprofloxacin. Clin Infect Dis 1996;22:1019. [PMID: 8783703]

Dupont HL: Guidelines on acute infectious diarrhea in adults. Am J Gastroenterol 1997;92(11):1962. [PMID: 9362174]

Eliason BC, Lewan RB: Gastroenteritis in children: principles of diagnosis and treatment. Am Fam Physician 1998;58(8):1769. [PMID: 9835852]

Fine KD, Schiller LR: AGA technical review on the evaluation and management of chronic diarrhea. Gastroenterology 1999;116(6):1464. [PMID: 10348832]

Framm SR, Soave R: Agents of diarrhea. Med Clin North Am 1997;81(2):427. [PMID: 9093236]

Gomi H et al: In vitro antimicrobial susceptibility testing of bacterial enteropathogens causing traveler's diarrhea in four geographic regions. Antimicrob Agents Chemother 2001;45(1):212. [PMID: 11120968]

Hogan DE: The emergency department approach to diarrhea. Emerg Med Clin North Am 1996;14(4):673. [PMID: 8921764]

Kroser JA, Metz DC: Evaluation of the adult patient with diarrhea. Prim Care 1996;23(3):629. [PMID: 8888349]

MacFarlane AS et al: Morphine increases susceptibility to oral *Salmonella typhimurium* infection. J Infect Dis 2000;181(4):1350. [PMID: 10762566]

Manatsathit S et al: Guideline for the management of acute diarrhea in adults. J Gastroenterol Hepatol 2002;17(Suppl):S54. [PMID: 12000594]

Mathan VI: Diarrhoeal diseases. Brit Med Bull 1998;54(2):407. [PMID: 9830206]

McNeely WS et al: Occult blood versus fecal leukocytes in the diagnosis of bacterial diarrhea: a study of U.S. travelers to Mexico and Mexican children. Am J Trop Med Hyg 1996;55(4):430. [PMID: 8916801]

Nazarian LF: A synopsis of the American Academy of Pediatrics' practice parameter on the management of acute gastroenteritis in young children. Pediatr Rev 1997;18(7):221. [PMID: 9203830]

Oldfield EC et al: The role of antibiotics in the treatment of infectious diarrhea. Gastroenterol Clin North Am 2001;30(3):817. [PMID: 11586559]

Slutsker L et al: *Escherichia coli* 0157:H7 diarrhea in the United States: clinical and epidemiologic features. Ann Intern Med 1997;126:505. [PMID: 9092315]

Coma

16

Steven D. Kelley, MD, & Adam Saperston, MD, MS[1]

Immediate Management of Life-Threatening Problems
   Initial Evaluation & Treatment
Further Evaluation of the Comatose Patient
Emergency Treatment of Specific Disorders
  Supratentorial Mass Lesions
    1. Subdural Hematoma
    2. Hypertensive Intracerebral Hemorrhage
    3. Brain Abscess
    4. Brain Tumor
    5. Cerebral Infarction (Stroke)
  Subtentorial Mass Lesions
    1. Basilar Artery Thrombosis or Embolic Occlusion
    2. Pontine Hemorrhage
    3. Intracerebellar Hemorrhage or Infarction

    4. Subdural & Epidural Hematoma (Subtentorial)
    5. "Locked-In" Syndrome
  Postictal State
  Metabolic Encephalopathies
    1. Hypoglycemia
    2. Hypoxemia
    3. Drug Overdose
    4. Hepatic Encephalopathy
    5. Disorders of Electrolytes & Osmolality
    6. Hyperthermia & Hypothermia
    7. Meningoencephalitis
    8. Subarachnoid Hemorrhage
  Psychogenic Coma
Criteria for Brain Death

■ IMMEDIATE MANAGEMENT OF LIFE-THREATENING PROBLEMS (See Figure 16–1 and Table 16–1.)

Evaluation of the comatose patient should progress as for any patient in the emergency department. (For coma in victims of trauma, see Chapter 10 and 22.) Priorities include the initial ABCs, monitoring, venous access, and high-flow oxygen. Maintain cervical spine stabilization if trauma cannot be ruled out. The patient should be completely undressed and his or her body inspected for signs of trauma or drug use (ie, needle marks). Examine pupils for reactivity to light and evaluate movement of extremities for rapid determination of cause (ie, diffuse versus structural). The "coma cocktail" is an empiric treatment for common conditions presenting as coma. It consists of thiamine, glucose,

and naloxone and should be administered early to the comatose patient. Thiamine is an important cofactor for several enzymes, and its depletion can lead to Wernicke encephalopathy with associated mental confusion. Administer a 100-mg intravenous dose of thiamine in all cases of coma. Hypoglycemia is another common condition that may present as coma. Administer a 25-g intravenous dose of glucose (50 cc 50% dextrose) unless fingerstick testing can be done immediately at the bedside and reveals a normal glucose level. The order of thiamine and glucose is not important. Intravenous naloxone, 0.4–2.0 mg, will temporarily reverse opiate narcosis. The half-life of naloxone is shorter than that of more commonly abused opiates and will require repeated doses or continuous infusion.

Essential laboratory studies should be ordered, including complete blood count, prothrombin time, partial thromboplastin time, chemistry panel, toxicologic screen, and blood cultures. Flumazenil, a specific benzodiazepine receptor blocker that can reverse benzodiazepine-induced coma, is not included in the coma cocktail because of its ability to induce seizures and cardiac arrhythmias. It should be used only if coma is definitively caused by benzodiazepine use (ie, the iatrogenic cause of moderate sedation).

---

[1]This chapter is a revision of the chapter by Roger P. Simon, MD, from the 4th edition.

311

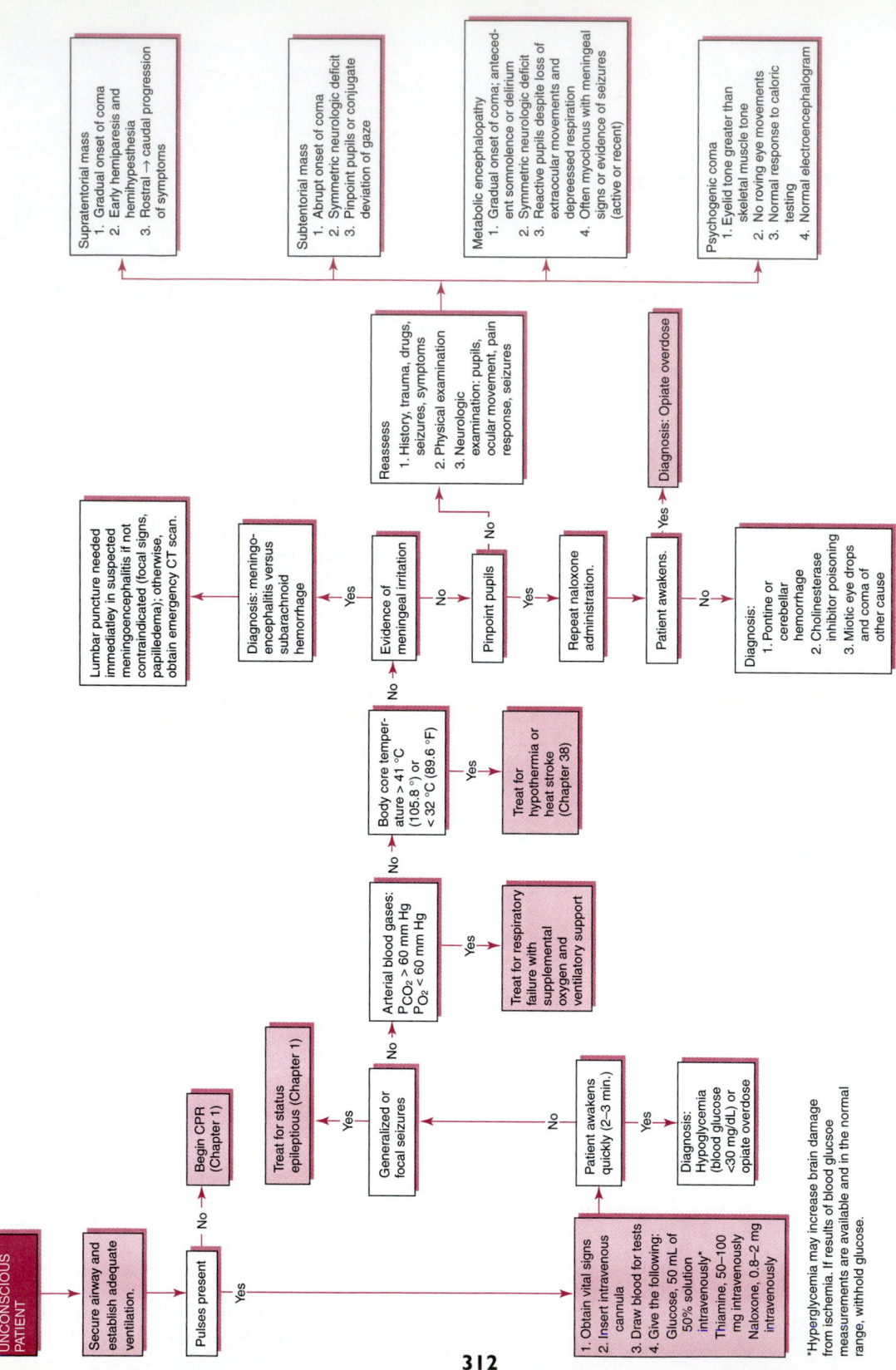

Figure 16-1. Approach to the unconscious patient.

312

Table 16–1. Assessment and management of coma.

ABCs
   Airway: Control airway with nasopharyngeal or oropharyngeal device.
   Breathing: Control oxygenation and ventilation initially with bag-valve-mask; maintain cervical spine stabilization.
   Circulation: Obtain intravenous access.
Immediate therapies (coma cocktail)
   Thiamine: 100 mg intravenously
   Dextrose 50%: 50 cc intravenously (if immediate fingerstick is normal, may hold)
   Naloxone: 0.4–2.0 mg intravenously (may repeat)
Laboratory studies
   Complete blood count
   Chemistries
   Prothrombin time/partial thromboplastin time
   Toxicologic screen
   Blood cultures
Emergent conditions and diagnostics
   Elevated intracranial pressure: Head CT scan
   Meningitis/encephalitis: Lumbar puncture, blood cultures
   Myocardial infarction: Electrocardiogram
   Hypertensive encephalopathy: Early treatment
   Status epilepticus: Electroencephalogram
   Acute stroke: Consider thrombolytics
History and physical examination
Early tests to consider:
   Head CT scan
   Lumbar puncture
   Angiogram
   Electrocardiogram
   Electroencephalogram

Monitor Cardiac & Pulse Oximetry

Place the patient on a cardiac monitor to rule out lethal arrhythmias and to monitor for change in cardiac status. Use a pulse oximeter to monitor the patient's oxygenation status.

Obtain Venous Access

Establish two large-bore (≥ 18-gauge) intravenous lines in an upper extremity. Secure them in place for later use.

Obtain Arterial Blood Gas Measurements

Arterial blood gas levels help to assess the adequacy of ventilation (by PCO_2 and PO_2), and blood pH is a useful clue to some drug intoxications (eg, salicylates) or metabolic encephalopathies.

Perform Brief Evaluation

A. Obtain History from Relatives, Friends, or Others

Obtain a description of the onset of coma and a history of any chronic illnesses, medications, allergies, or ingestions (eg, diabetes, hypertension, drug abuse, persistent headaches).

B. Obtain Complete Vital Signs

Include core body temperature in measurement of vital signs. If hypothermia is suspected, use a thermometer capable of measuring temperatures less than 33.3 °C (92 °F).

C. Perform a Rapid Physical Examination

Look for major abnormalities, especially traumatic injury (including injury of the back), cardiopulmonary disease, and meningismus.

D. Monitor Cardiac Rhythm

Rule out or treat life-threatening arrhythmias. Obtain an electrocardiogram as soon as possible.

Continue Treatment of Specific Disorders

A. Hypoglycemia

The intravenous glucose given empirically should promptly lessen hypoglycemic coma unless irreversible brain damage has occurred. ***Note:*** Beware of rebound hypoglycemia from long-acting insulin and oral hypoglycemic agents. A repeat dose of glucose or a glucose infusion may be necessary.

B. Wernicke Encephalopathy

The intravenous thiamine given empirically usually protects against Wernicke disease and will reverse the abnormalities over hours to days. Repeat daily until the patient starts a normal diet.

C. Opiate Overdose

The naloxone given empirically should reverse abnormalities related to opiate overdose. ***Note:*** Symptoms of opiate intoxication may recur, particularly if the patient has taken a long-acting drug (eg, methadone), because naloxone has a short half-life. Repeat as necessary.

D. Hypoxemia or Hypercapnia

Severe hypoxemia or hypercapnia may present as coma. Generally, PCO_2 must rise acutely to greater than 80 mm Hg and PO_2 must fall to less than 40 mm Hg before coma occurs. Give assisted ventilation with supplemental oxygen at once if blood gas abnormalities are life-threatening (PCO_2 > 60 mm Hg, PO_2 < 60 mm Hg). Marked elevation in PCO_2 levels that are chronic (ie, near-normal pH) should not be rapidly corrected. See Chapter 33 for further details.

E. STATUS EPILEPTICUS

Nonconvulsive status epilepticus can be mistaken for coma and should be considered in the differential diagnosis. Patients with prolonged convulsive status epilepticus may have decreased motor activity that may disappear altogether but continue to seize unnoticed. They may also present with nonconvulsive complex or absence status epilepticus. On physical examination, patients should be scrutinized for subtle eye and motor movements. If anticonvulsants are to be given empirically, phenytoin, fosphenytoin, lorazepam, or diazepam are good choices. The diagnosis of nonconvulsive status epilepticus must be confirmed by electroencephalogram. See Chapter 17 for detailed management of seizures.

F. HYPOTHERMIA OR HYPERTHERMIA

(See Chapter 44.) Body temperatures above 41–42 °C (105.8–107.6 °F) or below 32 °C (89.6 °F) may cause coma. *Hyperthermia in particular may cause rapid, irreversible brain injury and requires immediate corrective action.* If body temperature is 41 °C (105.8 °F) or higher, strip the patient and spray him or her with cool water while using a fan to blow air onto the patient.

Hypothermia is generally much better tolerated than hyperthermia, and the physician may start corrective measures at a more deliberate pace.

G. MENINGITIS AND ENCEPHALITIS

Antibiotics given early in the course of meningitis or encephalitis can improve patient outcome and can be accomplished early in the evaluation of a comatose patient. Any comatose patient with a fever or nuchal rigidity should be given appropriate empiric antibiotic therapy (ceftriaxone, 2 g intravenously, and ampicillin, 2 g intravenously) immediately. It is prudent to wait to perform the lumbar puncture after a computed tomography (CT) scan of the head has been obtained to rule out intracranial mass lesion or mass effect. *Early administration of antibiotics is of the utmost importance in this clinical situation.* No patient should be transferred to the CT scanner without first receiving antibiotics.

See Chapters 19 and 40 for further comments on the management of meningitis and Chapter 6 for the technique of lumbar puncture and evaluation of the cerebrospinal fluid.

Assess for Increased Intracranial Pressure

Increased intracranial pressure (ICP) should be considered if any head trauma is present or if the patient has a history of intracranial tumor or infection. Head trauma, papilledema, pupillary abnormalities, and decerebrate posturing suggestive of herniation should lead to prompt intervention in lowering ICP and obtaining a head CT scan. The most rapid method of decreasing elevated ICP is to hyperventilate the patient to a PCO_2 of 30–35 mm Hg. Mannitol, 0.75–1.0 g/kg, can also be used and will begin lowering the ICP in about 30 minutes. In the emergency setting it is not necessary to restrict fluids; the cerebral perfusion pressure (CPP) must be maintained, and intravenous fluids may be needed to maintain adequate blood pressure in response to the increase in ICP (CPP = mean arterial pressure [MAP] − ICP). Early neurosurgical consultation is recommended because more definitive surgical treatment may be required.

H. HYPERTENSIVE ENCEPHALOPATHY

Hypertension in a patient with altered mental status can result from malignant hypertension or from elevated ICP with resultant papilledema and secondary elevation of the blood pressure. Patients with malignant hypertension are young to middle aged and will usually demonstrate findings of end organ damage, especially hypertrophic cardiomyopathy and renal insufficiency. If suspected, hypertensive encephalopathy should be treated immediately with nitroprusside, labetalol, or another fast-acting intravenous antihypertensive agent.

Look for Pinpoint Pupils

A. OPIATE OVERDOSE

Repeat administration of a narcotic antagonist (naloxone, 0.4–2 mg intravenously), particularly if the history and physical examination (eg, sclerosed veins) suggest intravenous drug abuse.

B. CHOLINESTERASE INHIBITOR POISONING

Consider cholinesterase inhibitor poisoning if the patient has a history of exposure to insecticides or nerve gas and if paralysis, salivation, bronchorrhea, sweating, spontaneous defecation, or muscle fasciculations are present.

If cholinesterase inhibitor poisoning is suspected, give atropine, 1–2 mg intravenously (adult dose), at once. Repeat every 2–5 minutes until signs of atropine effect (dilated pupils, flushed face, tachycardia) occur. See Chapter 45 for further details on evaluation and treatment of poisoning.

C. FACTITIOUS PINPOINT PUPILS

Occasionally pinpoint pupils are due to miotic eye drops used by the patient, and some other condition has caused the coma. This finding can be seriously misleading unless the use of miotic eye drops is considered and excluded (primarily on the basis of history).

FURTHER EVALUATION OF THE COMATOSE PATIENT

Definitions

Coma has been defined as total or near total unresponsiveness with the inability to induce a purposeful response. Other terms used to describe decreased levels of consciousness are as follows:

- Stupor: severely impaired arousal with some response to vigorous stimuli
- Obtundation: a lesser state of decreased arousal with some response to touch or voice
- Lethargy: a state in which arousal, though diminished, is spontaneously maintained or requires only light stimulation
- Confusion: a state of impaired attention; implies adequate arousal to perform mental status tests of this ability
- Delirium: a state of confusion with periods of agitation and sometimes hypervigilance, irritability, and hallucinations typically with alternating periods of depressed level of arousal

Up to 75% of patients in a comatose state, without obvious cause, will likely have a diffuse systemic disorder. Structural lesions make up the remaining causes of coma; supratentorial lesions are more common than subtentorial lesions (Table 16–2).

History

A history may be obtained from friends and family (at the hospital or by telephone), police, or ambulance technicians. Crucial points include the following:

- Recent head trauma, even though seemingly trivial
- Drug use (including alcohol), recent or past (ask for pill containers)
- History of seizures, diabetes, hypertension, cirrhosis, or previous neurologic disease that might explain the comatose state
- Precomatose activity and behavior (eg, headache, confusion preceding coma); sudden versus gradual onset of coma

Table 16–2. Differential diagnosis of coma.

Diffuse	Focal
Hypoxia	**Supratentorial Lesions**
Hypoglycemia	Intracerebral
Hypoperfusion	hemorrhage
Thiamine deficiency	Epidural hemorrhage
Hyperammonia	Subdural hemorrhage
Uremia	Pituitary apoplexy
CO_2 narcosis	Infarction
Hyperglycemia	Thrombotic arterial
Central nervous system	occlusion
toxins	Embolic arterial
Cellular toxins	occlusion
Alcohols	Venous occlusion
Acid poisons	Tumors
Sedatives/narcotics	Abcesses
Anticonvulsants	**Subtentorial Lesions**
Psychotropics	Cerebellar hemorrhage
Isoniazid	Posterior fossa
Heavy metals	subdural/extradural
Endocrine disorders	hemorrhage
Electrolyte abnormalities	Cerebellar infarct
Hypothermia	Cerebellar tumor
Heat stroke	Cerebellar abscess
Neuroleptic malignant	Basilar aneurysm
syndrome	Pontine hemorrhage
Malignant hyperthermia	Brainstem infarct
Intracranial hypertension	Basilar migraine
Pseudotumor cerebri	demyelination
Meningitis	
Encephalitis	
Encephalopathy	
Cerebral vasculitis	
Subarachnoid hemorrhage	
Traumatic axonal shear	
injury	
Seizures/postictal state	

- Multiple patients with coma or confusion, suggesting carbon monoxide poisoning or exposure to some other common-source toxin

Physical Examination

Physical examination should include the following:

- Obtain complete vital signs and rectal temperature along with pulse oximetry. Observe the respiratory pattern.
- Search carefully for signs of head trauma. (Evidence of trauma elsewhere on the body is presumptive evidence of head trauma.)
- Examine for signs of meningeal irritation (nuchal rigidity, Brudzinski sign).

Neurologic Examination

The neurologic examination will be the most useful in determining the nature of the patient's unconsciousness. It is essential to record the results of the exam accurately, because treatment decisions will depend on whether subsequent examinations show improvement or deterioration in the patient's condition. Evaluation of the following areas assists in determining involvement of the central nervous system (CNS).

A. RESPIRATORY PATTERN

Cheyne-Stokes, hyperventilation, apneustic breathing, or Biot breathing may be present. Apneustic breathing is characterized by a prolonged pause at the end of inspiration and suggests a lesion in the mid to caudal pons. Biot breathing is characterized by a chaotic or ataxic pattern with loss of regularity and suggests a lesion in the medulla or lower pons.

B. PUPILS

Pinpoint pupils suggest opiate intoxication, cholinergic toxicity, or lesions in the pontine tegmentum. Large pupils have many causes. Adrenergic stimulation is the most common cause and can be from stimulant drug toxicity (eg, cocaine, phencyclidine) or from drug withdrawal. Pupillary asymmetry is usually caused by third nerve palsies. Loss of pupillary response, irregularly shaped pupils, and asymmetric sizes can be caused by lesions in the midbrain. Because ocular surgery has become more frequent than in the past, care must be taken not to confuse postoperative pupil abnormalities with neurologic abnormalities.

C. EYE MOVEMENTS

Observe the position of the eyes at rest. Note dysconjugate gaze and spontaneous movements. Voluntary eye movement occurs in "locked-in" syndrome. (Ask the patient to open their eyes and look at your finger. A positive reaction indicates the syndrome.)

1. Ocular bobbing—These quick downward conjugate movements are associated with a caudal pontine lesion.

2. Convergence and retraction nystagmus—These movements are associated with a midbrain lesion.

3. Ping pong gaze—This type of gaze, with pauses at extremes of horizontal gaze, is associated with vermian and bilateral hemispheric lesions.

4. See-saw nystagmus—One eye intorts and rises while the other extorts and falls; this movement is associated with a lesion in the rostral midbrain near the anterior third ventricle.

5. Dissociated nystagmus—This movement is associated with posterior fossa lesions.

6. Oculocephalic testing—Note movements in the horizontal and vertical planes. (Ensure that no cervical spine trauma is present.)

7. Oculovestibular testing—If the patient does not respond to the doll's eye maneuver (in which movement of the head in one direction produces conjugate eye movement in the opposite direction), use cold water calorics (irrigation of the contralateral ear with ice water). Horizontal movements are elicited by irrigating each ear separately. Irrigating both ears simultaneously tests vertical movements. No response suggests a lesion in the brain stem.

D. OTHER CRANIAL NERVES

Spontaneous blinking indicates intact facial nerve and nucleus. Intact blink in response to corneal stimulation indicates intact trigeminal input and facial nerve output.

E. MOTOR RESPONSES AND REFLEXES

Symmetry and spontaneous movements may give clues to side of focal lesions. Decorticate and decerebrate posturing are usually caused by hemispheric lesions. Deep tendon reflexes and plantar responses may also suggest lateralized lesion. Note any subtle repetitive motions suggestive of nonconvulsive seizures. Check for motor responses to pain both centrally (pressure on the supraorbital ridge) and peripherally (pressure on the nail beds of feet or hands).

Ancillary Studies

A. ELECTROLYTES

Electrolyte studies may show abnormalities such as hyponatremia, hypernatremia, or hypocalcemia.

B. BICARBONATE

Bicarbonate studies may indicate the presence of metabolic acidosis or acid-base disorders.

C. CREATININE AND BLOOD UREA NITROGEN

Creatinine and blood urea nitrogen studies will show worsening of renal function.

D. ARTERIAL BLOOD GAS

Arterial blood gases may show acid-base disturbances and will usually include a carboxyhemoglobin level to diagnose carbon monoxide poisoning.

E. Pulse Oximetry

Pulse oximetry provides a fast and accurate measure of oxygen saturation to rule out hypoxemia.

F. Complete Blood Count

Rarely useful, the complete blood count (CBC) may show thrombocytopenia or elevated or depressed white blood cell count.

G. Urinalysis

Urine glucose suggests hyperglycemia and hyperosmolar coma. The presence of white blood cells, nitrite, or bacteria suggests urosepsis. Calcium oxalate crystals suggest ethylene glycol poisoning. Cultures should be obtained as well.

H. Blood and Urine Toxicology Screen

These tests rarely change management but should be ordered when no obvious cause of coma is found.

I. Head CT Scan

If no metabolic cause for coma can be found, a noncontrast head CT scan should be obtained.

■ EMERGENCY TREATMENT OF SPECIFIC DISORDERS

SUPRATENTORIAL MASS LESIONS

 ESSENTIALS OF DIAGNOSIS

- Unilateral hemispheric dysfunction; progression of deficits from rostral to caudal.
- Aphasia (nondominant cerebral hemisphere); agnosia (nondominant cerebral hemisphere).
- Somnolence and coma (diencephalon).
- Unilateral pupil dilation and impaired cranial nerve III function (early midbrain).
- Marked unilateral pupillary dilatation, loss of light reactivity, and oculocephalogyric reflexes (midbrain herniation).
- Midline unresponsive, dilated pupils, no extraocular movements (pons).
- Most mass lesions will appear on noncontrast CT scan. Use angiography is CT scan or MRI is unavailable.

Clinical Findings

In supratentorial mass lesions, symptoms and signs of unilateral hemispheric dysfunction are usually present before onset of coma. These symptoms and signs persist into the early stages of coma. Neurologic deficits follow a characteristic progression from rostral to caudal (cerebral hemisphere to medulla) involvement. Results on neurologic examination are consistent with the anatomic level of involvement of the brain (Figure 16–2). The lesion can usually be demonstrated by CT scan or angiography.

A. Cerebral Hemispheres

Patients are generally alert. Hemiparesis and hemihypesthesia are commonly present. Aphasia may also be present with involvement of the dominant hemisphere, or agnosia (denial of the deficit) with nondominant involvement.

B. Diencephalon

Somnolence and eventually coma occur because of bilateral cortical involvement or diencephalic compression. Asymmetric motor and sensory abnormalities usually persist because of prior involvement of the cortex. Surgical removal of the mass when involvement does not exceed the level of the diencephalon generally results in recovery of consciousness.

C. Midbrain

1. Early stage—Herniation of the medial portion of the temporal lobe (the uncus) across the cerebellar tentorium produces midbrain signs, including unilateral pupillary dilation and impaired medial rectus muscle (oculomotor nerve) function, which may occur prior to loss of consciousness.

Results on the remainder of the neurologic examination may be normal. It is critical to recognize that these findings represent early involvement at the midbrain level and carry the same serious prognosis as the more classic midbrain state resulting from transtentorial herniation (see Figure 16–2).

2. Midbrain stage (fully developed)—Progressive uncal herniation causes loss of consciousness, and the fully developed midbrain stage appears rapidly. Marked ipsilateral pupillary dilatation and loss of reactivity to light are noted, and caloric testing fails to produce medial deviation of the eye ipsilateral to the lesion. Painful stimuli elicit decerebrate (extensor) posturing. If the patient's condition progresses to full midbrain dysfunction (absent oculocephalogyric reflexes), the chances of survival without severe neurologic impairment decrease rapidly, especially in adults.

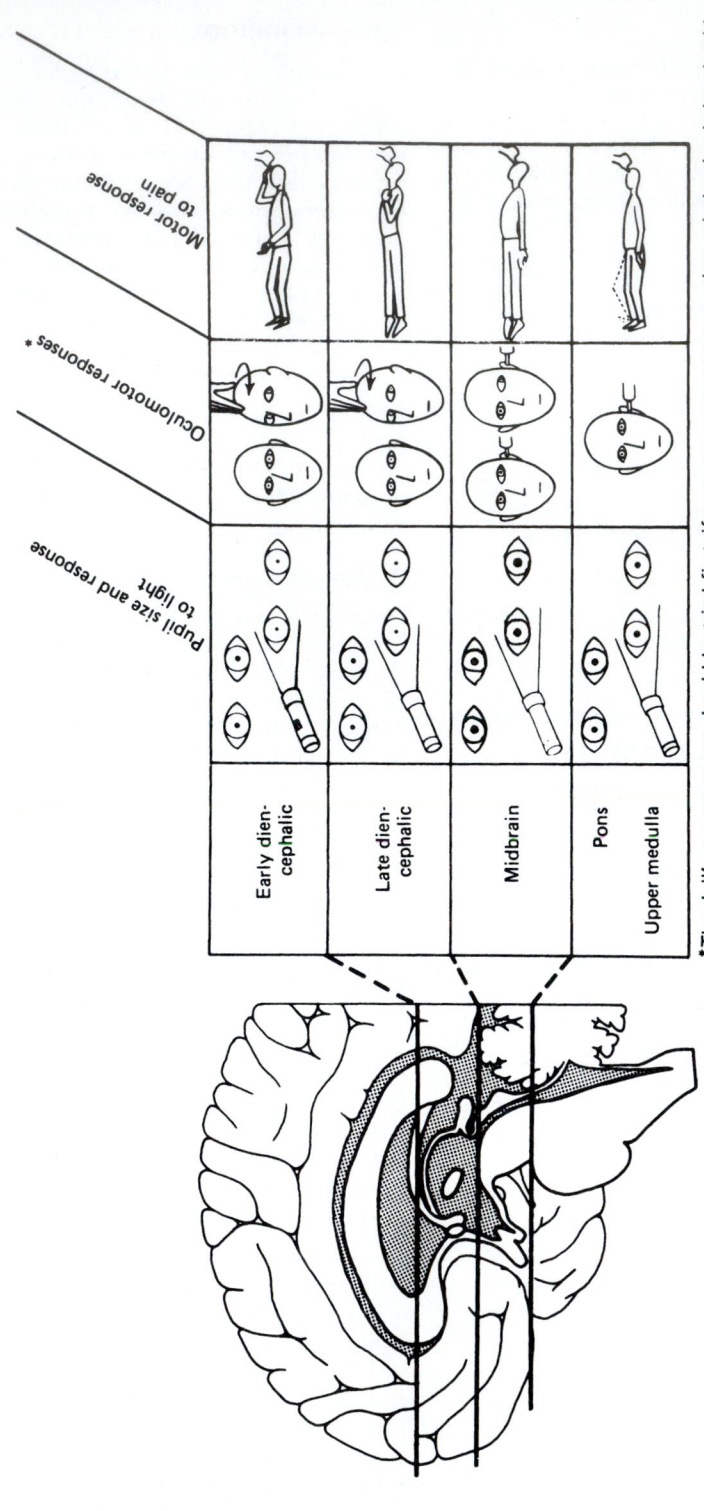

Figure 16–2. Symptoms at various levels of anatomic involvement of the brain. (Adapted and reproduced, with permission, from Plum F, Posner JB: *The Diagnosis of Stupor and Coma*, 3rd ed. Davis, 1980.)

D. PONS

Pupils remain in mid position and are unreactive to light. Extraocular movements (in response to the doll's eye maneuver and caloric testing) are absent. (Barbiturates and other drugs also abolish oculomotor reflexes.) Death is inevitable once the supratentorial mass lesion produces pontine-level dysfunction.

Focal pontine lesions (eg, pontine or cerebellar hemorrhage or infarction), as distinct from transtentorial herniation to the pontine level, produce pinpoint pupils that react to light when viewed with a magnifying glass. (Pinpoint pupils induced by opiates and pilocarpine must be excluded.) Extraocular movements are not inducible.

Treatment

A. IMMEDIATE MEASURES

If a delay in surgery is unavoidable and the patient's neurologic status is worsening, hyperventilation to an arterial P_{CO_2} of 30–35 mm Hg and administration of mannitol and the most rapidly acting intravenous glucocorticoids to reduce cerebral edema (Table 16–3) may delay progression of the neurologic deficit.

B. IMMEDIATE PALLIATIVE SURGERY

If the patient's neurologic status is worsening rapidly (eg, from cerebral hemispheric to midbrain level in less than 1 or 2 hours), immediate exploratory/decompressive craniotomy may be indicated, even if it must be done in the emergency department and even if the available personnel are not fully trained in neurosurgery.

C. DEFINITIVE SURGERY FOR REMOVAL OF MASS

If a supratentorial mass lesion is suspected, emergency neurosurgical consultation is mandatory. Hematomas, tumors, and abscesses are the most common lesions causing supratentorial compression, and all may be amenable to surgery.

If neurologic signs and symptoms are stable and the lesion is at the diencephalic level or above, a CT scan or magnetic resonance imaging (MRI) scan should be done. If the routine CT scan is normal, contrast media should be used and the scan repeated. Angiography and radionuclide brain scanning are also valuable diagnostic aids if CT scanning or MRI is unavailable.

Disposition

Immediate hospitalization is mandatory in all patients.

1. Subdural Hematoma

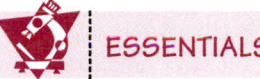 **ESSENTIALS OF DIAGNOSIS**

- *Headache, vomiting.*
- *Confusion, paresis, depressed consciousness.*

Table 16–3. Drug therapy for cerebral edema.

Drug	Dose	Route	Indications/Comments
Glucocorticoids			
Dexamethasone	Bolus 40–100 mg intravenously then 40–100 mg/d	Intravenous or oral	Dexamethasone preferred for the least mineralocorticoid effect; effective after 6–12 hours; concomitant antacid or H_2 blocker treatment probably indicated.
Prednisone	60 mg, then 25 mg 4 times a day	Oral	
Methylprednisolone	60 mg, then 25 mg 4 times a day	Intravenous or oral	
Hydrocortisone	300 mg, then 130 mg 4 times a day	Intravenous or oral	
Dehydration agents			
Mannitol	1.5–2 g/kg over 30 minutes to 1 hour	20% Intravenous solution	Effective immediately; major dehydrating effect is on normal tissue; osmotic effect is short-lived, and more than 2 intravenous doses are rarely effective; cause osmotic diuresis and electrolyte imbalance.
Urea	1–5 g/kg	Intravenous	
Glycerin (glycerol)	1.5–4 g/kg/d	Oral	Effective orally. Nausea and vomiting common.
Furosemide	40–120 mg	Intravenous	Can be used as an adjunct to mannitol to reduce fluid in the brain and decrease intracranial pressure.

- Pupil asymmetry, motor asymmetry, memory loss.
- CT scan or MRI findings.

General Considerations

The possibility of subdural hematoma must be considered in any comatose patient. Trauma is the most common cause, but in about 25% of cases, there is no history or evidence of trauma.

Clinical Findings

Symptoms and signs are notoriously nonspecific, nonlocalizing, or absent (Table 16–4) and may be either stable or rapidly progressive. The frequency of bilateral hematomas makes localization of the lesion even more difficult, as does the coexistence of associated cerebral contusion. Hemiparesis, when present, is contralateral to the lesion in approximately 60% of cases, and ipsilateral pupillary dilatation occurs in approximately 75% of cases. Seizures may occur. CT scan is the diagnostic study of choice, revealing a hyperdense extra-axial crescent-shaped collection of blood, which rarely crosses the faux or tentorium. Subacute lesions may appear as isodense, and MRI would be preferred. Skull x-rays are not helpful.

Note: Lumbar puncture is contraindicated. Cerebrospinal fluid abnormalities are nonspecific and cannot differentiate subdural hematomas from cerebral contusion without hematoma.

Treatment & Disposition

Immediate hospitalization and emergency neurosurgical consultation are mandatory in all cases. Seek radiologic confirmation of the diagnosis in stable patients and in those with slowly worsening mild neurologic dysfunction. Unstable patients with rapid worsening (minutes to hours) neurologic deficit thought to be due to an expanding subdural hematoma may require emergency exploratory craniotomy without benefit of preoperative radiologic diagnosis.

Hyperventilation, mannitol, and glucocorticoids (see Table 16–3) may be used to minimize cerebral damage while the patient is awaiting surgery.

2. Hypertensive Intracerebral Hemorrhage

Clinical Findings

Intracerebral hemorrhage nearly always begins when the patient is awake. There are no prodromal features. Obtundation is unremitting and worsens steadily over

Table 16–4. Common findings in patients with subdural hematomas.[1]

Clinical Findings	Acute[2] (82 Cases) (%)	Subacute[3] (91 Cases) (%)	Chronic[4] (216 Cases) (%)
Symptoms			
Headache	11	44	81
Confusion	12	41	37
Vomiting	24	31	30
Paresis	20	19	22
Seizures	6	3	9
Visual symptoms	0	0	12
Speech disturbance	6	8	6
Vertigo	0	4	5
Signs			
Depressed consciousness	100	88	59
Motor asymmetry	44	37	41
Pupillary inequality	57	27	20
Confusion/ memory loss	17	21	27
Papilledema	1	15	22
Drysphasia	6	12	11
Hemianopia	0	4	3
Facial weakness	0	3	3

[1]After McKissock W: Subduran hematoma: a review of 389 cases. *Lancet* 1960;1:1365.
[2]Within 3 days of trauma.
[3]Within 4–20 days of trauma.
[4]More than 20 days after trauma.

minutes to hours, most often progressing to stupor or coma. Almost all patients are hypertensive (blood pressure ≥ 170/90 mm Hg) when seen, and high blood pressure persists even into the late stages of transtentorial herniation.

The ocular fundi may show hemorrhages secondary to the acute increase in ICP. Conjugate deviation of the eyes is common, with gaze directed toward the side of the supratentorial (or away from the subtentorial) hemorrhage.

Headache occurs in 30–50% of patients and may be moderately severe; it overlies the location of the lesion. Vomiting and nuchal rigidity may also occur. Hemiplegia (contralateral to the hemorrhage) is a common early sign, because the site of hemorrhage (basal ganglia, 50% of cases; thalamus, 10%) abuts the internal capsule in most cases. Seizures are rare. CT scan provides the definitive diagnosis. The cerebrospinal fluid is grossly bloody in 90% of cases, and the pressure usually is above 200 mm H_2O and often greater than 600 mm H_2O. The total protein content is as high as 300–1200 mg/dL. The cerebrospinal fluid glucose level is normal initially but may fall later. The cerebrospinal fluid red blood cell count may be as high as 1 million/μL, and white cells are present in proportion (one white cell per thousand red cells). Peripheral blood leukocytosis (15,000–20,000/μL) is often present.

Treatment

Lowering of the blood pressure can be accomplished using labetalol, a fast-, short-acting agent, with both α and β adrenergic blocking ability. Dosing is a 10 mg bolus intravenously, followed by 10–20 mg every 10 minutes until the desired effect or maximum dose of 160 mg is achieved. Sodium nitroprusside can also be used at 2 μg/kg/min titrated to a mean arterial pressure of 100–125 mm Hg or systolic blood pressure of 140–160 mm Hg.

Methods of treatment are frustratingly limited, especially because the hemorrhage occurs over a brief period and then stops. Bleeding probably does not recur, but the patient's condition worsens because of secondary cerebral edema. Survivors of intracerebral hemorrhage may recover with minimal neurologic deficit as the clot resolves over a period of months.

Elevated intracranial pressure may respond temporarily to mannitol (see Table 16–3). Glucocorticoids are not efficacious.

For hemorrhages originating deep within the brain (eg, basal ganglia, thalamus), surgical attempts to evacuate the clot are as disappointing as supportive care alone. Surgery may be life saving, however, for patients with hemorrhage into cortical white matter (lobar hemorrhage).

Disposition

Immediate hospitalization is required, primarily for supportive care.

3. Brain Abscess

 ESSENTIALS OF DIAGNOSIS

- Stupor.
- Elevated temperature (50% of patients have normal temperature).
- Elevated white blood cell count (25% of patients have white blood cell count < 10,000/μl).
- CT scan or MRI findings.

Clinical Findings

Brain abscess accounts for only 2% of intracranial masses. Progression to stupor and coma may be rapid, occurring over days or, rarely, hours. Often the usual signs of infection are absent. The temperature is normal in half of patients, and the white blood cell count is below 10,000/μL in over one fourth of patients. Brain abscess should be considered in patients with AIDS who develop changes in mentation (may be caused by *Toxoplasma gondii*).

Lumbar puncture is contraindicated. The results are nondiagnostic, varying between normal findings and those suggestive of meningitis. CT scan, radionuclide brain scan, or MRI will demonstrate the lesions in over 90% of cases. Antibiotics should be initiated immediately without awaiting the results of a CT scan if meningitis is suspected. Begin intravenous therapy with nafcillin, 2 g every 4 hours, plus cefotaxime, 150–200 mg/kg in 4 divided doses, plus metronidazole, 30 mg/kg/d in 4 divided doses (Chapter 40).

Treatment

Neurologic and neurosurgical consultation are necessary. Hospitalize the patient for definitive diagnosis and treatment.

4. Brain Tumor

 ESSENTIALS OF DIAGNOSIS

- Headache.
- Focal weakness.
- Altered or depressed consciousness.
- Seizures.
- Papilledema.
- Chest x-ray (lung cancer metastasized to the brain), CT scan, MRI findings.

Clinical Findings

A. Symptoms and Signs

Coma is seldom the presenting symptom in primary or metastatic tumors of the CNS, although coma may result from seizures induced by the tumors. The patient typically has a history of days to weeks of headache, focal weakness, and altered or depressed consciousness. Papilledema is present in 25% of cases.

B. IMAGING STUDIES

The chest x-ray is a useful screening test for brain tumors, because lung cancer that has metastasized to the brain is the most common intracranial tumor. Other common CNS metastases often involve the lung before they affect the brain.

Treatment & Disposition

Treatment with glucocorticoids is often dramatically effective in reducing surrounding edema and improving the neurologic deficit (see Table 16–3). Hospitalize the patient for diagnosis and treatment.

5. Cerebral Infarction (Stroke) (See also Chapter 18.)

ESSENTIALS OF DIAGNOSIS

- *Hemiparesis.*
- *Hemisensory losses.*
- *Aphasia (dominant side involvement).*
- *CT scan findings.*

General Considerations

The brain swelling of cerebral edema following massive hemispheric infarction can produce contralateral hemispheric compression or transtentorial herniation that will result in coma. Such cerebral swelling becomes maximal 48–72 hours after the infarct.

Clinical Findings

The principal findings are hemiparesis or hemisensory loss (and aphasia if the dominant hemisphere is involved). Evolving transtentorial herniation progresses slowly over many hours or several days to stupor and coma. Absence of blood in the cerebrospinal fluid or on CT scan of the brain rules out cerebral hemorrhage.

Treatment

Consider the use of thrombolytics if the patient meets the criteria. See Chapter 18 for specific treatment of stroke.

Disposition

Hospitalization is indicated for all patients.

SUBTENTORIAL MASS LESIONS

ESSENTIALS OF DIAGNOSIS

- *Coma (sudden onset).*
- *Conjugate gaze toward lesion.*
- *Disconjugate eye movement with doll's eye or caloric testing.*
- *Internuclear ophthalmoplegia.*
- *CT scan findings.*

Clinical Findings

Clinical findings depend on the anatomic level of brain involvement. Generally there is coma of sudden onset without antecedent hemispheric signs (eg, hemiparesis or hemihypesthesia). With conjugate gaze deviation, the eyes are directed away from the side of the lesion and toward the hemiparesis. Disconjugate eye movements—especially internuclear ophthalmoplegia (lateral deviation of one eye on doll's eye maneuver or caloric testing without concomitant medical deviation of the contralateral eye)—strongly suggest a subtentorial lesion. Motor responses are not helpful in differentiating subtentorial from supratentorial lesions, because decerebrate or flaccid responses to painful stimulation occur with supratentorial lesions that progress to involve subtentorial structures. Respiration may be ataxic, gasping, or agonal. Differentiating a primary subtentorial process from transtentorial herniation in the late stage may be impossible except by extrapolating from the history.

In pontine or cerebellar hemorrhage or infarction, pinpoint pupils are often present. (Remember that intoxication with cholinesterase inhibitors or opiates also produces pinpoint pupils.)

Treatment

Emergency neurosurgical consultation is mandatory. If surgery must be delayed and neurologic abnormalities are progressive, use glucocorticoids, mannitol, and hyperventilation (reduce P_{CO_2} to 25–35 mm Hg) to try to control swelling of the brain (see Table 16–3).

Disposition

Immediate hospitalization is required in all cases.

1. Basilar Artery Thrombosis or Embolic Occlusion

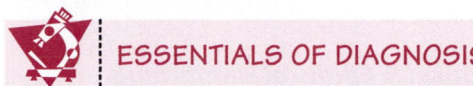

ESSENTIALS OF DIAGNOSIS

- Coma, altered mental status.
- Respiratory pattern irregular.
- Pupillary abnormalities, absent or abnormal horizontal eye movements.
- Hemiparesis, hyperreflexia, positive Babinski sign.
- CT scan findings.

General Considerations

Basilar artery thrombosis and embolic occlusion are relatively common vascular syndromes that cause coma because of direct involvement of the penetrating arteries supplying the central core of the brain stem. Patients are usually elderly and often have a history of hypertension or transient ischemic attacks or evidence of other atherosclerotic vascular disease.

Clinical Findings

Basilar artery transient ischemic attacks are characterized by (in order of frequency of occurrence) dizziness (rarely the only symptom), diplopia, weakness and ataxia, slurred speech, and visceral sensations (nausea and vomiting).

Basilar artery occlusion causes coma in half of affected patients, and almost all present with some alteration of consciousness. Focal subtentorial signs are present from the onset, and the respiratory pattern is irregular. Pupillary abnormalities vary with the site of the lesion and include poorly reactive pupils of normal size (3 mm), pupils fixed in mid position (5 mm), or pinpoint pupils. Skew deviation of the eyes is common. Horizontal eye movements are absent or asymmetric during the doll's eye maneuver or caloric testing. Conjugate eye deviation, if present, is directed away from the side of the lesion and toward the hemiparesis. Vertical eye movements in response to the doll's eye maneuver may be intact. Symmetric or asymmetric motor signs (hemiparesis, hyperreflexia, and Babinski sign) may be present. The cerebrospinal fluid is free of blood.

Treatment

Current opinion supports anticoagulation for progressive subtotal lesions, although evidence for the efficacy of this treatment is inconclusive.

Disposition

Hospitalize the patient for treatment and supportive care. The prognosis varies directly with the degree of brain stem injury.

2. Pontine Hemorrhage

ESSENTIALS OF DIAGNOSIS

- Coma.
- Ocular bobbing, pinpoint pupils, loss of lateral eye movement.
- Fever.
- Lumbar puncture or CT scan findings.

Clinical Findings

Coma of apoplectic onset is the hallmark of pontine hemorrhage. Physical examination reveals many of the findings noted in basilar artery infarction, but there is no history of transient ischemic episodes preceding pontine hemorrhage. Additional features especially suggestive of pontine involvement include ocular bobbing, pinpoint pupils, and loss of lateral eye movements. Fever greater than 39.5 °C (103 °F) may occur in patients surviving for more than several hours. The cerebrospinal fluid is grossly bloody and under increased pressure. CT scan of the brain is almost always diagnostic, demonstrating high density (blood) in the brain stem.

Treatment

There is no effective treatment, and the mortality rate is high.

Disposition

Hospitalize the patient for confirmation of the diagnosis and for supportive care.

3. Intracerebellar Hemorrhage or Infarction

ESSENTIALS OF DIAGNOSIS

- Sudden onset headache, nausea, vomiting.
- Ataxia.
- Small reactive pupils.

- *Ipsilateral facial nerve palsy, nuchal rigidity, ipsilateral cerebellar limb ataxia.*
- *Lumbar puncture or CT scan findings.*

General Considerations

Hypertension is the cause of intracerebellar hemorrhage in approximate three fourths of patients. The remaining cases result from ruptured intracerebellar arteriovenous malformations. Most affected patients are over age 50 years.

Clinical Findings

The clinical picture ranges from sudden brain stem compression progressing rapidly to death (a picture virtually indistinguishable from primary pontine hemorrhage) to a progressive syndrome developing over hours or even several days (as commonly seen with cerebellar infarction). The onset is sudden and characterized by headache and nausea and vomiting, with marked ataxia of gait that may progress to complete inability to walk or stand. ***Caution:*** Early stages of cerebellar hemorrhage are sometimes misdiagnosed as drug or alcohol intoxication.

Other features include small reactive pupils with conjugate gaze deviation away from the side of the lesion, preserved vertical eye movements, and an ipsilateral peripheral facial palsy in some cases. Nuchal rigidity is present in half of patients. Hemiparesis is rare and, if present, mild in degree. The incidence of ipsilateral cerebellar limb ataxia varies, but when this sign is present, it is of obvious value in locating the lesion. Cerebrospinal fluid becomes grossly bloody within several hours after intracerebellar hemorrhage.

Prompt diagnosis, preferably with CT scan of the brain (in which increased density seen on the scan represents blood in the cerebellar hemisphere), is crucial. Surgical decompression may be life saving.

Treatment

The only treatment for symptomatic cerebellar hemorrhage is surgical decompression, which may dramatically reduce symptoms. Pharmacologic reduction of cerebral edema may briefly delay progression of symptoms until surgery can be performed (see Table 16–3).

If appropriate treatment is given, lethargic or even stuporous patients may survive with minimal or no residual damage and with intact intellect. If the patient is in a deep coma, the chances for meaningful survival are small.

Disposition

Hospitalize the patient immediately for emergency surgical decompression.

4. *Subdural & Epidural Hematoma (Subtentorial)*

 ESSENTIALS OF DIAGNOSIS

- *Vomiting.*
- *Cerebellar signs.*
- *Ataxia, progressive obtundation, nuchal rigidity.*
- *Papilledema (chronic).*
- *CT scan findings.*

General Considerations

Subtentorial subdural and epidural hematomas are rare lesions with similar clinical pictures. Prompt and accurate diagnosis is important, because these potentially fatal disorders may be treated effectively. Occipital trauma frequently precedes the onset of brain stem involvement by hours to weeks.

Clinical Findings

Physical findings are those of extrinsic compression of the brain stem: vomiting, cerebellar signs with ataxia, and progressive obtundation. Nuchal rigidity may be present. Papilledema may occur in chronic cases.

In most patients, skull x-rays reveal a fracture line crossing the occipital venous sinuses. CT scan confirms the diagnosis.

Treatment & Disposition

Hospitalize the patient immediately for an urgent surgical decompression.

5. *"Locked-In" Syndrome*

 ESSENTIALS OF DIAGNOSIS

- *Patient is awake and alert.*
- *Patient is quadriplegic and unable to speak.*
- *Decerebrate posturing, flexor spasms.*
- *One or more voluntary movements is preserved: eye opening, vertical eye movement, convergence.*

• *Physical exam, lumbar puncture, and CT scan findings.*

General Considerations

The portion of the reticular formation responsible for consciousness lies above the level of the mid pons. Therefore, "transection" of the low brain stem by basilar artery stroke, encephalitis, demyelinating disease, or an infiltrative tumor can produce an akinetic and mute state with preserved consciousness (hence the term *locked-in*).

Clinical Findings

Patients with "locked-in" syndrome are in fact awakened and alert but appear comatose because they are quadriplegic and unable to speak. Decerebrate posturing or flexor spasms may be noted. However, one or more voluntary movements such as eye opening, vertical eye movement, or convergence are preserved. Therefore, always instruct an apparently comatose patient to "open your eyes" or "look up at my finger" at least once during the examination. *Voluntary movement of any kind is inconsistent with true coma.*

Treatment & Disposition

Hospitalize the patient for treatment and rehabilitation. Some patients will recover significant function after a month or more.

POSTICTAL STATE

ESSENTIALS OF DIAGNOSIS

- *Patient is unresponsive to pain.*
- *Nonfocal neurologic exam.*
- *Babinski sign (transient).*
- *Todd paralysis.*
- *Signs of recent seizure: tongue trauma, incontinence, rapidly clearing anion gap lactic acidosis.*
- *Study findings: electrolytes, calcium, magnesium, lumbar puncture, CT scan.*

General Considerations

Coma resulting from seizure disorders is usually not a difficult diagnostic problem, because recovery of consciousness is rapid following the end of the seizure. Pro-

longed postictal coma (several hours) followed by several days of confusion may occur after status epilepticus, in patients with brain damage (eg, multiple cerebral infarctions, head trauma, encephalitis, mental retardation), and in patients with metabolic encephalopathy that alters consciousness and induces seizures (eg, hyponatremia, hyperglycemia).

Clinical Findings

Patients may initially be unresponsive to deep pain and exhibit sonorous respirations. The neurologic examination is usually nonfocal, although Babinski sign may be transiently present. Uncommonly, there may be focal abnormalities (Todd paralysis) referable anatomically to the focus of seizure activity in the brain.

Other evidence of a recent seizure may be present, such as trauma to the tongue from biting, incontinence, or a rapidly clearing anion gap (lactic) acidosis. The rapid resolution of coma in a patient with a witnessed seizure or known seizure disorder should suggest the diagnosis of the postictal state as the cause of coma. Coma that is at first thought to be postictal but that fails to improve should prompt an investigation for underlying processes contributing to mental status depression, including metabolic encephalopathy, underlying diffuse brain damage, encephalitis, and structural lesion. Appropriate investigations should include measurements of serum electrolytes, calcium, and magnesium; CT scan; and lumbar puncture.

Treatment

Treatment depends on the underlying cause of the seizure. Be alert for metabolic causes and treat them appropriately. See Chapter 17 for details of management.

Disposition

Immediate hospitalization is required for all cases of status epilepticus and prolonged postictal coma and for seizures due to metabolic causes that are not quickly correctable. Outpatient management may be possible for stable patients.

METABOLIC ENCEPHALOPATHIES

ESSENTIALS OF DIAGNOSIS

- *Progressive somnolence.*
- *Intoxication, toxic delirium.*
- *Agitation, stupor, coma.*
- *Headache.*
- *Symmetric neurologic findings.*

- Reactive pupils.
- Hypoventilation, abnormal respiratory pattern.
- Study findings: serum glucose, CBC, arterial blood gas, alcohol level, liver function tests, serum osmolality, serum electrolytes, rectal temperature, lumbar puncture, CT scan, electroencephalogram, electrocardiogram.
- Loss of extraocular movements.

Clinical Findings

Metabolic encephalopathies are characterized by a period of progressive somnolence, intoxication, toxic delirium, or agitation, after which the patient gradually sinks into a stuporous and finally comatose state. Subarachnoid hemorrhage is an exception: loss of consciousness is rapid. Headache is not an initial symptom of metabolic encephalopathy except in the case of meningitis, subarachnoid hemorrhage, or poisoning due to organophosphate compounds or carbon monoxide.

Neurologic examination fails to reveal focal hemispheric lesions (hemiparesis, hemisensory loss, aphasia) before loss of consciousness. Neurologic findings are symmetric except in some patients with hepatic encephalopathy and hypoglycemic coma, which may be accompanied by focal signs (especially hemiparesis) that may alternate sides. Myoclonus and, during consciousness, asterixis may be present.

The hallmark of metabolic encephalopathy is reactive pupils (a midbrain function) in the presence of impaired function of the lower brain stem (eg, hypoventilation, loss of extraocular movements), an anatomically inconsistent set of abnormalities. Respiratory patterns in metabolic coma vary widely and may help establish the cause of coma (see Table 16–1).

Treatment & Disposition

Treatment depends entirely on the cause of coma. All patients require hospitalization for supportive care and specific therapy.

1. Hypoglycemia
(See also Chapter 41.)
General Considerations

Unlike other organs, the brain relies mainly on glucose to supply its energy requirements. Abrupt hypoglycemia rapidly interferes with brain metabolism and quickly produces symptoms. Insulin and oral hypoglycemic drug overdose are the most common causes of hypoglycemia.

Clinical Findings

Signs of sympathetic nervous system activity (tachycardia, sweating, and anxiety) may warn patients of impending hypoglycemia, although these signs may be masked by propranolol and other β-blockers and are absent in patients with diabetic autonomic neuropathy. Common neurologic abnormalities are delirium, seizures, focal signs that often alternate sides, stupor, and coma. Table 16–5 summarizes the symptoms and signs of insulin-induced hypoglycemic shock.

Hypoglycemic coma may be tolerated for 60–90 minutes, but once the stage of flaccidity with hyporeflexia has been reached, glucose administration within 15 minutes is mandatory to avoid irreversible damage.

Treatment & Disposition

Give glucose, 50 mL of 50% solution intravenously (adult dose). Once the diagnosis of hypoglycemia is confirmed by analysis of blood drawn before treatment, give an additional 50 mL as needed or begin an infusion of dextrose 5% in water. Patients should be observed for 1–2 hours after glucose supplementation has

Table 16–5. Signs and symptoms of hypoglycemia after insulin administration.[1]

Time After Insulin Administration	Symptoms
30 minutes	Perspiration Salivation Somnolence Excitement and restlessness Tachycardia if stimulated (bradycardia if somnolent)
2–3 hours	Loss of contact with environment Myoclonus Primitive reflexes (grasping, sucking) Reactive, dilated pupils
4–5 hours	Comatose Depressed responses to pain Roving eye movements Tonic and torsional muscular spasms Extensor plantar response
5–6 hours	Decerebrate rigidity
6–7 hours	Small pupils Bradycardia Flaccid tone Depressed reflexes

[1]Modified and reproduced, with permission, from Himwich HE: Brain Metabolism and Cerebral Disorders. Williams & Wilkins, 1951.

been discontinued to ensure that hypoglycemia does not recur before they are discharged from the hospital. In some cases, hospitalization may be necessary, especially if hypoglycemia recurs despite treatment or in the event of long-acting insulin or oral hypoglycemic agent overdose.

2. Hypoxemia

Clinical Findings

Hypoxemia produces brain damage only as a result of concomitant cerebral ischemia. Cerebral blood flow diminishes and brain ischemia occurs when the arterial PO_2 falls to 20–45 mm Hg. In cerebral anoxia due to cardiac arrest, where the duration can be timed precisely, 4–6 minutes of asystole begins to result in permanent CNS damage. Following asystole, the pupils dilate rapidly and become fixed, and tonic posturing is observed. A few seizure-like tonic-clonic movements are common.

Treatment & Disposition

Treatment of hypoxemia depends on the cause. Support cardiac output, and maintain arterial PO_2 above 60 mm Hg by supplemental oxygen or mechanical ventilation. Hospitalize all patients for diagnosis and treatment.

3. Drug Overdose

Drug overdose is one of the most common causes of coma in patients presenting to the emergency department in coma. Many drugs may be implicated, including sedative-hypnotics, opiates, tricyclic antidepressants, and antiepileptics. Details of management can be found in Chapter 45.

Alcohol Intoxication

Alcohol intoxication produces a metabolic encephalopathy similar to that produced by sedative-hypnotic drugs, although nystagmus during wakefulness and early impairment of lateral eye movements are not as common. Peripheral vasodilatation is a prominent manifestation and produces tachycardia, hypotension, and hypothermia.

In individuals who are not chronic alcoholics, stupor occurs when blood alcohol levels reach 250–300 mg/dL, and coma occurs when levels reach 300-400 mg/dL. Because alcohol has significant osmotic pressure (100 mg/dL = 22.4 mOsm), alcohol intoxication is one cause of hyperosmolality.

Management is discussed in Chapter 45. Patients should be observed until improvement has occurred (normal orientation and judgment; satisfactory coordination). Hospitalize patients who have abnormalities that would usually require hospitalization (eg, metabolic abnormalities, Wernicke encephalopathy).

Narcotic Overdose

In narcotic overdose, hypoventilation is almost always present, along with pinpoint pupillary constriction and absent extraocular movements in response to the doll's eye maneuver. Pinpoint pupils are also associated with other disorders that must be ruled out: use of miotic eye drops, pontine hemorrhage, Argyll Robertson pupils from syphilis, and organophosphate insecticide poisoning.

Narcotic intoxication is confirmed by rapid pupillary dilation and awakening after administration of a narcotic antagonist such as naloxone, 2 mg, by rapid intravenous injection. ***Note:*** Patients who have overdosed on certain narcotics (eg, propoxyphene [Darvon, many others]) may not respond to 2 mg and may require 4 mg or more. Patients intoxicated with alcohol may awaken briefly after administration of naloxone.

The duration of action of naloxone varies with the dose and route of administration. Repeat doses are frequently necessary, especially following intoxication with long-acting narcotics (eg, methadone).

Treatment of drug overdose and poisoning is outlined above and discussed more fully in Chapter 45. Hospitalization should be considered for patients who do not recover completely in the emergency department or who have taken long-acting narcotics.

γ-Hydroxybutyrate

γ-Hydroxybutyrate is a CNS depressant and can induce coma. The drug has become popular at rave parties and has also been called the "date rape drug." Detection of the drug is difficult, because most of it is eliminated through the lungs.

Treatment is primarily supportive and may involve endotracheal intubation. Some evidence indicates that physostigmine can be used as an antidote. Some patients require hospitalization for prolonged supportive care.

4. Hepatic Encephalopathy

Clinical Findings

Hepatic encephalopathy can occur in patients with severe acute or chronic liver disease. Jaundice need not be present. In the patient with preexisting liver disease, encephalopathy may develop rapidly following an acute insult such as gastrointestinal hemorrhage. Patients with surgical portacaval shunts are especially predisposed to encephalopathy.

Mental status is altered and ranges from somnolence to delirium or coma. There is increased muscle tone; hyperreflexia is common. Prominent asterixis occurs in the somnolent patient. Seizures—generalized or focal—occur infrequently. Hyperventilation with respiratory alkalosis is nearly universal and may be demonstrated by measuring arterial blood pH. Cerebrospinal fluid is normal but may appear xanthochromic in patients with serum bilirubin levels higher than 4–6 mg/dL.

Treatment & Disposition

The emergency department should provide initial supportive measures only. Hospitalization for definitive treatment is indicated for all patients.

5. Disorders of Electrolytes & Osmolality

Clinical Findings

A. HYPEROSMOLALITY AND HYPOOSMOLALITY

Coma with focal seizures is a common presentation of hyperosmolality. Consciousness is altered if serum osmolality is less than 260 mOsm/kg H_2O or greater than 330–350 mOsm/kg H_2O.

B. HYPONATREMIA

Delirium and seizures are common presenting features of hyponatremia. Hyponatremia may cause neurologic symptoms when serum sodium levels are below 120 mEq/L, and symptoms are frequent with levels below 110 mEq/L. When the serum sodium level falls rapidly, symptoms occur at higher serum sodium levels.

Treatment & Disposition

The diagnosis and treatment of these entities are discussed in Chapter 42. Hospitalization is mandatory.

6. Hyperthermia & Hypothermia

Clinical Findings

Hyperthermia and hypothermia are associated with symmetric neurologic dysfunction that may progress to coma. *All comatose patients must have rectal temperature taken with an extended-range thermometer if the standard thermometer fails to register.*

A. HYPOTHERMIA

Internal body temperatures below 26 °C (78.8 °F) uniformly cause coma; hypothermia with core temperatures above 32 °C (89.6 °F) does not cause coma. Body temperatures of 26–32 °C (78.8–89.6 °F) are associated with varying degrees of obtundation. Pupillary reaction

will be sluggish below 32 °C (89.6 °F) and lost below 26.5 °C (80 °F).

B. HYPERTHERMIA

Internal body temperatures above 41–42 °C (105.8–107.6 °F) are associated with coma and may also rapidly cause permanent brain damage. Seizures are common, especially in children.

Treatment & Disposition

If hyperthermia is present, begin to lower body temperature immediately by undressing the patient, spraying with cool water, and directing the breeze from a fan onto the patient. Further diagnostic and treatment measures are discussed in Chapter 44. Hospitalization is mandatory.

7. Meningoencephalitis

Clinical Findings

A. PRODROMAL SYMPTOMS

Prodromal symptoms such as fever, headache, malaise, or upper respiratory tract symptoms are present for hours to days; 20% of patients are in a coma when first seen by a physician.

B. HEADACHE

Headache is a common and characteristic symptom, and stuporous patients should be aroused and asked if they have a headache.

C. MENINGEAL SIGNS

Look carefully for meningeal signs so that lumbar puncture can be performed if necessary and a diagnosis made as soon as possible. Can the neck be fully flexed so that the chin touches the chest (with the mouth closed), or is movement limited? Is there knee flexion, even slight, during passive neck flexion? Does the neck or contralateral knee flex during unilateral raising of the straight leg? These signs of meningeal irritation may be absent in deep coma or at the extremes of age.

D. CEREBROSPINAL FLUID

Cerebrospinal fluid pressure may be as high as 600 mm H_2O. White cell counts can range from as few as 10 monocytes/mL in patients with viral meningoencephalitis to over 10,000 cells/mL, mainly polymorphonuclear neutrophils, in patients with purulent bacterial meningitis. Cerebrospinal fluid may be acellular on the first lumbar puncture in rare cases of viral encephalitis and in some cases of overwhelming bacterial meningitis, but in overwhelming bacterial meningitis, organisms may be seen on gram-stained slides. In patients with bacterial meningitis, cerebrospinal fluid glucose is commonly below 40 mg/dL (often in the range of 5–10 mg/dL) when blood glucose is normal; in viral encephalitis, cerebrospinal fluid glucose is almost always normal.

Treatment & Disposition

Start antibiotic therapy immediately based on clinical findings and microscopic examination of cerebrospinal fluid (see Table 40–3). Hospitalization is indicated for all patients with meningitis who present in coma.

8. Subarachnoid Hemorrhage

General Considerations

Blood may be found in the cerebrospinal fluid of a patient with intracerebral hemorrhage or head trauma; however, the term *subarachnoid hemorrhage* normally implies bleeding from a ruptured cerebral aneurysm or, less commonly, hemorrhage from a cerebral arteriovenous malformation. Aneurysmal bleeding is uncommon before age 30 years, whereas arteriovenous malformations may bleed much earlier, even in childhood. Ruptured mycotic aneurysm from subacute infective endocarditis is rare but may be seen at any age. About one half of patients die within the first month following bleeding. Coma from subarachnoid hemorrhage is the result of many factors, including the contusive force of the bleeding, communicating hydrocephalus, cerebral vasospasm, altered critical metabolic activity, and transtentorial herniation. Risk factors for subarachnoid hemorrhage are smoking, female gender, African American race, alcohol abuse, and binge drinking.

Clinical Findings

The onset of symptoms is abrupt and accompanied by headache that is unique in the patient's experience and not necessarily severe. Consciousness is often lost at the onset. Markedly elevated blood pressure (seen in 50% of patients) is a common result of the hemorrhage and is not an indication of preceding hypertension. Decerebrate posturing or, rarely, seizures may also occur early, and moderate to marked confusion is frequent if the patient is conscious. Prominent focal signs are uncommon; bilateral extensor plantar responses occur. Meningeal irritation (as shown by nuchal rigidity) may take several hours to develop and may disappear when the patient is in deep coma. Optic fundi may show acute hemorrhages secondary to suddenly increased ICP or the more classic superficial subhyaloid (preretinal) hemorrhages.

CT scan has a 92% sensitivity within 24 hours of symptoms. If the CT is negative and subarachnoid bleed is still suspected, a lumbar puncture should be performed to confirm the diagnosis. Cerebrospinal fluid pressure is usually markedly elevated, often higher than 600 mm H_2O, and the cerebrospinal fluid is grossly bloody and contains from 100,000 to more than 1 million red blood cells per microliter. In rare cases, fewer than 100,000 red cells are seen. The white blood cell to erythrocyte ratio in cerebrospinal fluid is initially the same as in the peripheral blood. The noninfectious meningitis that results from blood in the subarachnoid space may produce a pleocytosis of several thousand white blood cells during the first 48 hours. A reduction in cerebrospinal fluid glucose resulting from this "chemical" meningitis may occur between the fourth and eighth days after hemorrhage.

Useful radiologic aids include a CT scan (which shows blood in the subarachnoid space in more than 85% of patients) and cerebral angiography (which demonstrates the site of bleeding).

Treatment

Protect the airway. Establish the diagnosis by CT scan or, if CT scan is not diagnostic, by lumbar puncture. Sedate the patient with diazepam, 5–10 mg intravenously or orally, if needed. Avoid hypotension by correcting fluid imbalance with infusion of crystalloid solutions. Obtain emergency neurosurgical consultation.

Disposition

All patients require hospitalization.

PSYCHOGENIC COMA

 ESSENTIALS OF DIAGNOSIS

- *Patient is unresponsive.*
- *Normal physical examination.*
- *Flaccid symmetric decreased muscle tone.*
- *Normal and symmetric reflexes; normal Babinski sign.*
- *Ice water calorics.*
- *L Electroencephalogram findings.*

Clinical Findings

Coma is a diagnosis of exclusion that should be made only after careful documentation. The general physical examination should elicit no abnormalities; neurologic examination generally reveals flaccid, symmetrically decreased muscle tone, normal and symmetric reflexes, and the normal downward response to Babinski plantar stimulation. The pupils are normal in size (2–3 mm) or occasionally larger and respond briskly to light. Lateral eye movements elicited with the doll's eye maneuver may or may not be present, because visual fixation can suppress this reflex.

Differentiating Psychogenic Coma from Organic Coma

A. Eye Movements

The slow, conjugate roving eye movements of patients in metabolic coma cannot be imitated and, if present, are incompatible with a diagnosis of psychogenic unconsciousness.

B. Eyelid Tone

The slow, often asymmetric and incomplete eyelid closure commonly seen in organic forms of coma following passive opening of the lids cannot be mimicked. In addition, the patient with psychogenic coma usually shows some voluntary muscle tone of the eyelids during passive opening by the examiner.

C. Ice-Water Caloric Response

A helpful objective test in diagnosing psychogenic unconsciousness is the caloric test: there is no response at all or tonic deviation to the side of the irrigation in organic coma, but nystagmus occurs in psychogenic coma. Because the quick (return) phase of nystagmus requires an intact cortex, its presence is incompatible with a diagnosis of true coma.

D. Electroencephalogram

The electroencephalogram in psychogenic coma is that of a normal, awake person. In coma due to other causes, it is invariably abnormal.

Treatment & Disposition

Obtain psychiatric consultation. Hospitalization may be required. See Chapter 47 for details.

◼ CRITERIA FOR BRAIN DEATH

Brain death is defined as the irreversible loss of function of the brain, including the brain stem. Before a patient may be evaluated for the diagnosis of brain death, the patient must meet certain criteria:

- Clinical or neuroimaging evidence of catastrophic CNS event compatible with the clinical diagnosis of brain death.
- Exclusion or correction of medical conditions that may confound clinical assessment:

  – Acid-base disorders
  – Severe electrolyte disorders
  – Endocrinopathies
  – Absence of drug intoxication/poisoning
  – Patient core temperature > 32 °C (90 °F)

Once these criteria have been met, the patient can be tested for the diagnosis of brain death. If the patient meets the following criteria, the patient is observed for at least 6 hours and clinical testing is repeated. If patient testing remains unchanged, a diagnosis of brain death can be made.

- Coma (unresponsiveness): no cerebral motor response to pain
- Absence of brain stem reflexes (all of the below):
  – No pupillary response to light
  – No oculocephalic reflex (doll's eyes maneuver)
  – No response to cold water calorics
  – No corneal reflexes
  – No jaw reflex
  – No grimacing to painful stimulus
  – No gag reflex
  – No cough response to tracheal/bronchial stimulation
  – Apnea over 8 minutes with P_{CO_2} > 60 mm Hg

Confirmatory testing may be used when complicating factors are present such as severe facial trauma, preexisting pupillary abnormalities, or toxic drug levels. Confirmatory tests result in findings that are consistent with brain death and are not diagnostic. The standard confirmatory tests include cerebral angiography, transcranial Doppler ultrasonography, technetium-[99]m hexamethylpropyleneamineoxime brain scan, and somatosensory-evoked potentials. In some cases these tests may aid in the diagnosis and in others they may confuse the picture. Documentation of the diagnosis of brain death should include the cause and irreversibility of the condition, the absence of brain stem reflexes, the absence of any motor response to pain, the formal apnea test results, and the justification for and results of any confirmatory tests. The initial and repeat exams should be included. Currently most authorities feel that the same criteria above can be used for full-term infants more than 7 days old. Criteria for premature and newborns are still unclear.

American College of Emergency Physicians: Clinical policy for the initial approach to patients presenting with altered mental status. Ann Emerg Med 1999;33:251.

Bialer PA: Designer drugs in general hospital. Psychiatr Clin North Am 2002;25:231. [PMID: 11912942]

Caldicott DG, Kuhn M: Gamma-hydroxybutyrate overdose and physostigmine: teaching new tricks to an old drug. Ann Emerg Med 2001;37:99. [PMID: 11145779]

Cantrill SV: Brain death. Emerg Med Clin North Am 1997; 15:713. [PMID: 9255142]

Feske SK: Coma and confusional states: emergency diagnosis and management. Neurol Clin 1998;16:237. [PMID: 9537961]

Hoffman RS, Goldfrank LR: The poisoned patient with altered consciousness: controversies in the use of a coma cocktail. JAMA 1995;274:562. [PMID: 7629986]

McCabe JM: Uniform Determination of Death Act. Health Law Vigil 1985;8:21. [PMID: 10270263]

Plum F, Posner JB: The Diagnosis of Stupor and Coma, 3rd ed. Davis, 1980.

Qureshi AI, Suarez JI: Use of hypertonic saline solutions in treatment of cerebral edema and intracranial hypertension. Crit Care Med 2000;28:3301. [PMID: 11008996]

Riggs JE: Neurologic manifestations of electrolyte disturbances. Neurol Clin 2002;20:227. [PMID: 11754308]

Stieg PE, Kase CS: Intracranial hemorrhage: diagnosis and emergency management. Neurol Clin 1998;16:373. [PMID: 9537967]

Syncope, Seizures, & Other Causes of Episodic Loss of Consciousness

Adam Saperston, MD, MS[1]

I. Immediate Management of Life-Threatening Problems
   Status Epilepticus
II. Evaluation of the Conscious Patient with a History of Syncope
III. Emergency Treatment of Specific Disorders Causing Episodic Loss of Consciousness
  Seizures (Epilepsy)
  Vasovagal Syncope (Simple Faints)
  Cardiopulmonary Syncope
    Cardiac Arrest
    Acute Myocardial Infarction
    Cardiac Arrhythmias
    Cardiac Inflow Obstruction
    Cardiac Outflow Obstruction

    1. Aortic Stenosis
    2. Pulmonary Stenosis
    3. Hypertrophic Obstructive Cardiomyopathy
    Pulmonary Vascular Disease
  Cerebrovascular Syncope
    Basilar Artery Insufficiency
    Subclavian Steal Syndrome
    Migraine
    Carotid Sinus Syncope
  Orthostatic Hypotension
  Miscellaneous Rare Causes of States of Altered Consciousness
    Hyperventilation
    Psychiatric Causes
    Meniere Disease

■ I. IMMEDIATE MANAGEMENT OF LIFE-THREATENING PROBLEMS (See Figure 17–1.)

STATUS EPILEPTICUS

ESSENTIALS OF DIAGNOSIS

- *A prolonged seizure lasting 10–15 minutes.*
- *Continuous or multiple seizures without intervening periods of consciousness.*

Clinical Findings

A prolonged seizure (lasting more than 10–15 minutes), continuous seizures, or multiple seizure episodes without intervening periods of consciousness constitute status epilepticus.

Search carefully for seizure activity in the comatose patient. Manifestations may be subtle (eg, deviation of head or eyes; repetitive jerking of fingers, hands, or one side of the face).

Immediate Measures for Patient with Active Seizures

Perform the following in the order given here:

A. PROTECT THE AIRWAY

Roll the patient onto one side if possible. Insert a nasopharyngeal airway. Administer 100% oxygen by nasal cannula or nonrebreathing face mask and monitor with pulse oximetry. Prepare for possible endotracheal intubation in the event that anticonvulsants fail to terminate the seizure. Do not waste time trying to insert a bite block or tongue blade through clenched teeth, be-

---

[1]This chapter is a revision of the chapter by Roger P. Simon, MD, from the 4th edition.

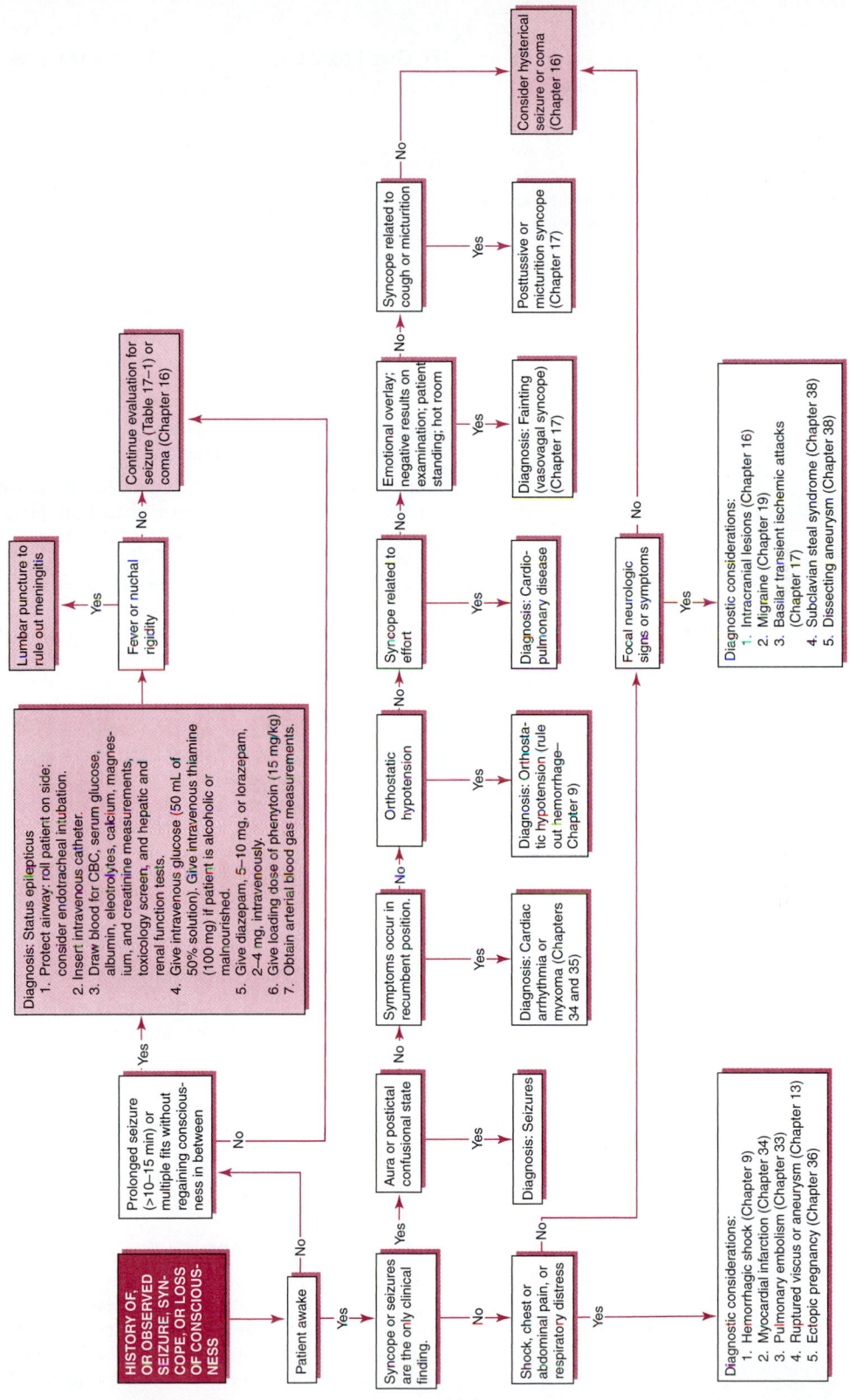

Figure 17–1. Assessment of patients with seizure, syncope, or loss of consciousness.

333

cause it does not protect the airway and may cause broken teeth.

B. INSERT AN INTRAVENOUS CATHETER

To start diagnostic evaluation (Table 17–1), obtain blood specimens for glucose, electrolytes, magnesium, and calcium determinations; hepatic and renal function tests; and complete blood count (CBC); as well as 3–4 tubes of blood for possible toxicology screen or drug levels (including anticonvulsants if patient is known or suspected to be taking them).

C. RULE OUT HYPOGLYCEMIA

Give glucose, 50 mL of 50% solution intravenously over 5 minutes. **Note:** If malnutrition is suspected, give thiamine, 100 mg intravenously, slowly prior to, or at the same time as, glucose.

Table 17–1. Emergency evaluation of the patient with seizures.

Vital signs
    Pulse: Rule out dangerous cardiac dysrhythmia, including cardiac arrest.
    Blood pressure: Rule out postural hypotension and shock.
    Body temperature: Rule out hyperthermia (> 41–42 °C [105.8–107.6 °F]).
History
    Trauma
    Previous seizures
    Drug or alcohol use
    Medications
Physical examination
    Papilledema
    Focal neurologic signs
    Evidence of systemic disease
    Heart murmur
Laboratory and special examinations
    Serum glucose: Hypoglycemia or hyperglycemia
    Arterial blood gases: Hypoxemia, hypercapnia, acidosis
    Electrocardiogram: Cardiac arrhythmia
    Serum electrolytes: Hyponatremia or hypermatremia
    Approximate serum osmolality calculation (normal range: 270–290 mOsm/L):

$$\text{Osmolality} = 2(\text{Na}^+ \text{ mEq/L}) + \frac{\text{Glucose mg/dL}}{18}$$

    Complete blood count with differential
    Serum calcium and magnesium measurements
    Hepatic and renal function studies
    Lumbar puncture (if signs of increased intracranial pressure are absent)
    Blood and urine samples for toxicologic studies (if indicated)
    Computed tomography scan (if focal signs are present)

D. GIVE LORAZEPAM OR OTHER BENZODIAZEPINE

Give lorazepam, 0.1 mg/kg intravenously at 1–2 mg/min up to 10 mg total, or diazepam, 0.2 mg/kg intravenously at 2 mg/min up to 20 mg total, as a one-time dose. These drugs have been shown to be equally effective as first-line choices. Diazepam has a faster onset than lorazepam (2 versus 3 minutes); however, lorazepam has a longer duration of action (12–24 hours) compared to diazepam (15–30 minutes). Because of this property, lorazepam is currently considered the drug of choice. If venous access cannot be obtained, diazepam can be given rectally, endotracheally, or intraosseously, or midazolam, 0.2 mg/kg, can be given intramuscularly.

E. ADMINISTER A LOADING DOSE OF PHENYTOIN OR FOSPHENYTOIN

Regardless of the effect of the benzodiazepine, a maintenance drug is required. Give phenytoin in normal saline, 15–18 mg/kg by intravenous infusion at a rate of 50 mg/min or slower. Infusion of phenytoin at more rapid rates (especially if given into centrally placed intravenous lines) can precipitate cardiac arrhythmias or hypotension. These unwanted hemodynamic and cardiac side effects can be avoided by the use of fosphenytoin, a prodrug of phenytoin. Fosphenytoin dosages are expressed as phenytoin equivalents (PE). Advantages of fosphenytoin are that it can be administered faster than phenytoin (150 PE/min) and intramuscularly if needed. The standard dose is 15–20 mg PE/kg intravenously. The disadvantage is that it is more expensive. Oral phenytoin loading is less expensive and safe and probably appropriate if the patient is awake on arrival, alert, not vomiting nor intubated, and has not had repeated seizures or status epilepticus after arrival in the emergency department.

F. MEASURE ARTERIAL BLOOD GASES AND pH

Arterial blood P_{CO_2} is a sensitive indicator of the adequacy of ventilation (hypercapnia is present in proportion to the degree of hypoventilation). Metabolic acidosis due to lactic acidosis resulting from status epilepticus is commonly present for as long as 1 hour after a seizure, depending on the duration and vigor of muscular activity. This acidosis requires no treatment. Acidosis lasting longer than 1 hour should prompt a search for other causes of acidosis (Chapter 42).

G. MAINTAIN VENTILATION

Patients in status epilepticus or those given anticonvulsant medications that are strong respiratory depressants may require endotracheal intubation to protect the airway and maintain adequate ventilation. Monitor arterial blood gas measurements to assess adequacy of ventilation ($P_{O_2} \geq 80$ mm Hg and P_{CO_2} at an appropriate level).

H. RULE OUT MENINGITIS

Perform lumbar puncture immediately to rule out meningitis if fever (body temperature > 38.5 °C [> 101.2 °F]) or nuchal rigidity is present. However, the muscle activity of status epilepticus alone produces transient fever higher than 38.5 °C (> 101.2 °F) in up to 79% of patients. Hyperthermia should be treated with passive cooling measures. Status epilepticus may also produce a mild transient cerebrospinal fluid pleocytosis(< 100 cells/μL).

I. USE ALTERNATIVE DRUGS IF NECESSARY

If a benzodiazepine and phenytoin fail to stop the convulsions, use alternative drugs (Table 17–2).

J. SEARCH FOR THE UNDERLYING CAUSE OF SEIZURE

Emergency evaluation of the patient should proceed as outlined in Table 17–1. Common causes of seizures of acute onset are listed in Table 17–3.

Prevention of Injury

Prevent injury to the patient during the seizure by padding the environment. Do not use rigid restraint (fractures may result) or insert objects into the patient's mouth during the seizure.

Treatment During Postictal State

Do not give lorazepam or diazepam if the patient has postictal stupor or coma rather than active seizures. Further evaluation of the patient in stupor or coma should proceed as described in Chapter 16.

Phenytoin or fosphenytoin, 15–18 mg/kg loading dose orally or intravenously (Table 17–4; see also Table 17–2), should be given to all patients except those who have a short-term metabolic condition known to cause seizures, such as alcohol withdrawal or hypoglycemia, which does not require or respond to phenytoin.

Alldredge BK et al: A comparison of lorazepam, diazepam, and placebo for the treatment of out-of-hospital status epilepticus. N Engl J Med 2001;345:631. [PMID: 11547716]

DeToledo JC, Ramsay RE: Fosphenytoin and phenytoin in patients with status epilepticus: improved tolerability versus increased costs. Drug Saf 2000;22:459. [PMID: 10877039]

Johnson J, Wrenn K: Inappropriate fosphenytoin use in the ED. Am J Emerg Med 2001;4:293. [PMID: 11447516]

Lowenstein DH, Alldredge BK: Status epilepticus. N Engl J Med 1998;338:970. [PMID: 9521986]

Treiman DM et al: A comparison of four treatments for generalized convulsive status epilepticus. N Engl J Med 1998;339:792. [PMID: 9738086]

■ II. EVALUATION OF THE CONSCIOUS PATIENT WITH A HISTORY OF SYNCOPE

The emergency department evaluation of the patient presenting with syncope consists of a careful history, a physical examination that includes orthostatic blood pressure measurements and a 12-lead electrocardiogram (ECG). This initial workup will provide a diagnosis approximately 50% of the time. The initial goal should be to identify life-threatening causes of syncope.

Confirm that Loss of Consciousness Is Caused by Syncope

Syncope is a symptom characterized by transient, self-limited loss of consciousness. It is associated with a loss of postural tone, usually resulting in falling. Syncope must be differentiated from other symptoms such as dizziness, presyncope, and vertigo, all of which do not result in loss of consciousness. Typically syncopal episodes are brief, lasting no longer than 20 seconds. Recovery from syncope is usually characterized by almost immediate restoration of appropriate behavior and orientation. Syncope should not be confused with other causes of loss of consciousness such as epilepsy, hypoxia, hyperventilation, hypoglycemia, cataplexy, and intoxications.

Rule Out Blood Loss

In the *awake* patient with a history of one or more episodes of loss of consciousness, rule out acute blood loss due to various causes.

A. MEASURE BLOOD PRESSURE AND PULSE

Supine hypotension (systolic blood pressure < 90 mm Hg) or severe peripheral vasoconstriction should be considered evidence of hemorrhagic shock until proven otherwise (Chapter 9).

Orthostatic vital signs should be obtained, though they may be contraindicated in patients who have supine hypotension; those in shock; and those with severe altered mental status, spinal injuries, or pelvic and lower extremity injuries. Measure blood pressure and pulse after the patient has been lying down for 3 minutes. Record blood pressure, pulse, and symptoms again after the patient has been standing for 1 minute. A positive test for orthostatic hypotension is an increase of pulse of 30 beats/min or more, or a decrease in systolic blood pressure of 20 mm Hg or a decrease in systolic blood pressure to less than 90 mm Hg. The presence of

Table 17–2. Drug treatment of status epilepticus.

Drug	Dose and Route	Advantages, Disadvantages, and Complications
First-line drug: Diazepam (Valium, others) *or* Lorazepam (Ativan, others) *or* Midazolam (Versed)	0.2–0.4 mg/kg intravenously, up to 20 mg; or 0.2–0.5 mg/kg rectal get 0.1 mg/kg intravenously over 2 minutes. 0.2 mg/kg intravenously over 2 minutes, or can be given intramuscularly.	Fast acting (lipid-soluble), short half-life intravenously (½–4 hours for diazepam; up to 16 hours for lorazepam). Respiratory depression occurs, especially if barbiturates must be added. Other complications are bradycardia and hypotension. ***Note:*** Regardless of effectiveness of diazepam, maintenance drug (phenytoin or phenobarbital) must be added to prevent recurrence of seizures.
Proceed immediately to phenytoin. Phenytoin (Dilantin, others) *or* Fosphenytoin	1000–1500 mg (15–18 mg/kg) slowly intravenously at a rate not greater than 50 mg/min, given directly into the vein (cannot be given through dextrose-containing solutions; use saline only). 15–20 PE/kg at 100–150 PE/min, either intravenously or intramuscularly	No respiratory depression. Therapeutic drug levels in the brain are achieved by the time the infusion has been completed. Effective as maintenance drug. Hypotension and cardiac arrhythmias may occur, especially in elderly patients. infusion rate of 100 mg/min is safe during active seizures.
If seizures persist following total dose of phenytoin, immediately proceed to phenobarbital. Phenobarbital (Luminal, many others)	700 mg (10 mg/kg) intravenously at a rate of 50–100 mg/min.	Respiratory depression and hypotension common with increasing doses (intubation and ventilatory support should be immediately available). Effective as maintenance drug.
If the above is ineffective, the following third-line drugs may be tried, or one can proceed immediately to general anesthesia. Paraldehyde	Rectally: 5–10 mL diluted in 2 volumes of mineral oil *or* Intramuscularly: 5–10 mL (maximum 5 mL/site) *or* Intravenously: 0.1–0.5 mL/kg (4% solution: 200 mL paraldehyde in 500 mL normal saline).	Decomposes with storage; can cause metabolic acidosis, pulmonary hemorrhage, cardiovascular depression, and proctitis (if given rectally). Use glass syringe (paraldehyde causes plastic to break down); safely administered intravenously in 4% solution. Absorption is rapid following intramuscular administration but slow with the rectal route.
Lidocaine (Xylocaine, many others)	50 mg intravenously. If effective, then 50–100 mg diluted in 250 mL of 5% dextrose and infused at a rate of 1–2 mg/min.	Higher dose may cause seizures. Minimal adverse effects on cardiac output and evaluation. Reduce dose in congestive heart failure or liver disease.
If the above is ineffective, proceed immediately to general anesthesia. Pentobarbital (Nembutal, others)	15 mg/kg slowly intravenously; then 0.5–1 mg/kg/h.	Hypotension is limiting factors; respiratory depression is routine.
Thiopental (Pentothal)	15 mg/kg slowly intravenously, followed by 5 mg/kg/h drip.	Brain half-life less than 30 minutes; hypotension is limiting factor; respiratory depression is routine.
Amobarbital (Amytal, others)	200–1000 mg slowly intravenously.	Hypotension is limiting factor; respiratory depression is routine.

PE = phenytoin equivalents.

Table 17–3. Common causes of seizures of acute onset.

Disorder	Comment
Primary central nervous system disorders	
Idiopathic epilepsy	Onset uncommon after age 25.
Head trauma	Especially acute trauma or when associated with depressed skull fracture or subdural hematoma.
Stroke	Especially hemorrhagic stroke.
Central nervous system mass lesion	Primary or metastatic tumor; brain abscess; arteriovenous malformation.
Metabolic or systemic disorders	
Cerebral hypoperfusion (hypoxia)	Cardiopulmonary arrest; cardiac dysrhythmia; severe hypotension, etc (Chapters 7, 9, 34).
Meningitis, encephalitis	Acute or chonic; bacterial, viral, fungal, parasitic, etc. (Chapter 40).
Hyponatremia	Serum sodium usually less than 120 and often less than 110 mEq/L (Chapter 42).
Hypoglycemia	Serum glucose usually less than 40 mg/dL (Chapter 41).
Hyperosmolality	Serum osmolalty usually greater than 300 mOsm/L (Chapter 42).
Hypertensive encephalopathy	Blood pressure usually greater than 250/150 mm Hg; seizures may occur at lower pressures (usually > 160/100 mm Hg) when hypertension occurs suddently (eg, in children with acute renal failure) (Chapter 34).
Uremic encephalophathy	
Hepatic encephalopathy	Respiratory alkalosis nearly always present.
Eclamptogenic toxemia	Develop and utilize a protocol for managing pregnancy-related seizures.
Acute drug overdose	Especially with tricyclic antidepressants, theophylline (aminophylline), phencyclidine (PCP), lidocaine, phenothiazines, isoniazid (Chapter 45).
Acute drug withdrawal	Anticonvulsants, ethanol, or sedative-hypnotic drugs (with habituation to daily doses of 600–800 mg secobarbital or its equivalent.
Benign febrile convulsions of childhood	Do not occur after age 5; always consider other causes.
Hyperthermia	Internal body temperature usually above 41–42 ºC (105.8–107.6 ºF); *immediate* reduction of body temperature to 39 ºC (102.2 ºF) is mandatory (Chapter 44).

symptoms such as dizziness or syncope should also be noted as a positive test. Many conditions can produce postural hypotension in the absence of hypovolemia (Table 17–5). The utility of orthostatic vital signs in children is questionable. Also, paradoxical bradycardia may occur in the presence of blood loss.

B. Gain Venous Access

Use an intravenous catheter (≥ 18 gauge), and administer a crystallized solution (eg, normal saline) as needed. If blood loss is suspected and the hematocrit or hemoglobin is normal, a repeat determination after volume repletion may confirm blood loss. Serial CBCs may be helpful in detecting active bleeding, and a dextrose test may be helpful if the history or physical examination suggests hypoglycemia. However, obtaining routine blood tests (for electrolytes, renal function, blood sugar, and hemoglobin) is not recommended, because they rarely uncover the cause of syncope.

C. Obtain Stool Sample

Check stool specimens for blood (gross and microscopic).

D. Look for Possible Gastrointestinal Tract Bleeding

Nasogastric intubation may be indicated in suspected gastrointestinal tract bleeding or in syncope with unexplained postural hypotension. *Caution:* Upper gastrointestinal tract bleeding cannot be ruled out unless the nasogastric tube aspirate contains bile. Otherwise, brisk bleeding distal to the pyloric sphincter (eg, duodenal ulcer) may be missed if the sphincter is closed (Chapter 14).

Table 17–4. Summary of anticonvulsant drug therapy.

| Drug | Dose | | Serum Half-Life (Normal Renal and Hepatic Function) | Serum Levels (μg/mL) | | Symptoms of Toxicity | Indications |
	Intravenous Loading	Oral Loading	Maintenance		Therapeutic	Toxic		
Phenytoin (Dilantin, others)	1000–1500 mg (15–18 mg/kg) directly into a large vein, not exceeding 50 mg/min. Continuous electrocardiographic monitoring is mandatory. Cannot be infused in dextrose solutions (eg, 5% dextrose in water).	1000 mg in 24 divided doses over 12–24 hours.	300–400 mg/d in a single dose or 23 divided doses.	Oral: 22 hours. Intravenous: 12 hours. (Kinetics are dose-dependent and may vary widely.)	10–20.	Above 30.	Ataxia, nystagmus, somnolence. (Nystagmus on extreme lateral gaze suggests therapeutic drug level.)	Grand mal, focal motor, and complex partial (temporal lobe) seizures.
Phenobarbital (Luminal, many others)	700 mg (10 mg/kg) over 10–20 minutes. Ventilatory support equipment must be available at bedside.	180 mg twice a day for 3 days.	90–180 mg in a single daily dose.	4 days.	10–30.	Above 40.	Ataxia, somnolence.	Grand mal, focal motor, and complex partial (temporal lobe) seizures.
Carbamazepine (Tegretol, others)	No intravenous preparation.	200 mg twice a day; increase by 200 mg daily to maintenance dose.	400 mg 2–3 times a day	15 hours.	4–8.	Above 8.	Nausea, ataxia, diplopia.	Complex partial (temporal lobe) and grand mal seizures.
Valproic acid (Depakene, Depakote, others)	10–15 mg/kg/d. Infuse over 60 minutes not to exceed 20 mg/min.	None.	750–2000 mg/d twice daily.	6–13 hours.	50–150.	Above 150 mg/dL.	Drowsiness and nausea at onset.	Myoclonic, photic-induced absence (petit mal) and refactory seizures.

Table 17–5. Causes of orthostatic hypotension.

Drug-induced
    Phenothiazines (chlorpromazine, etc)
    Tricyclic antidepressants (amitriptyline, etc)
    Antihypertensives
    Diuretics
    Nitrates (nirtoglycerine, etc)
    Levodopa
    Monoamine oxidase inhibitors
Peripheral neuropathies (see Chapter 16)
    Diabetic
    Amyloid
Hypovolemia or hemorrhage
Addison disease
Acute or chronic spinal cord injury
Degenerative diseases of the central nervous system
    Parkinsonism
    Shy-Drager syndrome (anhidrosis, sphincter dysfunction, impotence)
Posterior fossa tumors
Sequelae of surgical sympathectomy

E. CONSIDER OTHER POSSIBLE CAUSES OF BLEEDING

Consider pelvic bleeding (eg, ruptured ectopic pregnancy) or trauma, especially that which is not visually obvious, such as splenic, hepatic, retroperitoneal, or pelvic injury.

Determine Presence or Absence of Related Symptoms

A. SYNCOPE ASSOCIATED WITH CARDIAC ARRHYTHMIAS OR CONDUCTION ABNORMALITIES

Obtain an ECG. This quick, easy, noninvasive test is indicated in all cases of syncope except those with an otherwise clear cause. ECG abnormalities suggesting an arrhythmic cause of syncope are listed in Table 17–6.

B. SYNCOPE ASSOCIATED WITH PROMINENT ABDOMINAL OR PELVIC PAIN

Patients with abdominal or pelvic pain may have hypovolemic syncope secondary to gastrointestinal hemorrhage, leaking aortic aneurysm, or ruptured ectopic pregnancy. Aortic dissection and rupture of a viscus into the peritoneal cavity may also produce syncope initially by vagal stimulation or later as a result of blood loss. See Chapter 13 for further evaluation.

C. SYNCOPE ASSOCIATED WITH CHEST PAIN OR DYSPNEA

Consider myocardial infarction, pulmonary embolism, tension pneumothorax, or dissecting aortic aneurysm.

Table 17–6. Common causes of syncope due to cardiopulmonary and cerebrovascular disease.

Cardiac arrest due to any cause
Acute myocardial infarction
Cardiac dysrhythmias
    Tachyarrhythmias
        Supraventricular
            Paroxysmal atrial tachycardia
            Atrial flutter
            Atrial fibrillation
            Accelerated junctional tachycardia
        Ventricular
            Ventricular tachycardia
            Ventricular fibrillation
    Bradyarrhythmias
        Sinus bradycardia
        Sinus arrest
        Second-degree or complete (third-degree) heart block
        Implanted pacemaker failure or malfunction
    Mitral valve prolapse (click-murmur syndrome)
    Prolonged QT interval syndromes
    Sick sinus syndromes (tachycardia-bradycardia syndrome)
    Drug toxicity (especially digitalis, quinidine or procainamide, propranolol, phenothiazines, tricyclic antidepressants, potassium)
Cardiac inflow obstruction
    Left atrail myxoma or thrombus
    Constrictive pericarditis or cardiac tamponade
    Tension pneumothorax
Cardiac outflow obstruction
    Aortic stenosis
    Pulmonary stenosis
    Hypertrophic obstructive cardiomyopathy (idiopathic hypertrophic subaortic stenosis)
Severe pulmonary hypertension due to any cause
    Pulmonary hypertension
    Acute pulmonary embolus
Cerebrovascular syncope
    Basilar artery insufficiency
    Subclavian steal syndrome
    Migraine
    Takayasu disease
    Carotid sinus syncope
Orthostatic hypotension

D. SYNCOPE ASSOCIATED WITH NEUROLOGIC SYMPTOMS (EG, HEADACHE, VERTIGO, DIPLOPIA)

Obtain neurologic consultation for possible basilar artery insufficiency, migraine, and subclavian steal syndrome. Loss of consciousness as an isolated symptom is rarely if ever caused by basilar artery ischemia.

Further Evaluation of Syncope

A detailed, accurate history from the patient, family, observers, or ambulance attendants is the most important factor in making the diagnosis. A head computed tomography (CT) scan must be obtained in the emergency department if the patient has focal neurologic findings. In the fully recovered patient with a normal neurologic exam, the head CT scan can be obtained either in the emergency department or at a follow-up outpatient visit. The most helpful features are the following:

A. Epileptic Aura

History of an epileptic aura preceding the syncopal attack or a period of confusion (postictal state) upon regaining consciousness strongly suggests seizures as the diagnosis. This aura must be differentiated from symptoms of decreased cerebral blood flow (eg, those occurring before a syncopal episode or as a result of orthostatic hypotension or cardiac arrhythmia).

B. Position of the Patient at Time of Loss of Consciousness

Episodes beginning when the patient is lying down suggest seizure or cardiac arrhythmia, whereas orthostatic hypotension and vasovagal syncope occur when the patient is standing or sitting up.

C. Syncope Related to Active Physical Exertion

Syncope following active physical exertion is frequently noted in cardiac outflow obstruction (eg, aortic stenosis, hypertrophic obstructive cardiomyopathy [idiopathic hypertrophic subaortic stenosis], myxoma) and is elicited occasionally in patients with cardiac arrhythmias or pulmonary vascular disease (rare).

D. Other Causes of Syncope

Micturition and coughing are associated with distinctive syncopal syndromes. Simple fainting may occur during the first trimester of pregnancy and must be differentiated from syncope due to blood loss from ectopic pregnancy. Rare causes of syncope include glossopharyngeal neuralgia (throat or neck pain), hyperventilation, psychiatric causes, and Meniere disease (look for associated deafness and vertigo).

E. Disposition

Deciding whether to admit the patient with syncope is based on 2 different objectives: for diagnosis or for treatment. When the cause of syncope remains unknown, a risk assessment can be used for the admission decision. The following risk factors warrant consideration for hospitalization: (1) suspected or known heart disease, (2) ECG abnormalities suspicious for arrhythmic syncope, (3) syncope with onset during exercise, (4) family history of sudden death, and (5) syncope causing severe injury. Reasons for admission for patients who require treatment include the following: (1) syncope due to cardiac arrhythmia, ischemia, or structural cardiac disease, (2) cerebrovascular accident or focal neurologic deficits, and (3) severe orthostatic hypotension.

Clinical policy: critical issues in the evaluation and management of patients presenting with syncope. Ann Emerg Med 2001; 37:771. [PMID:11385356]

Kapoor WN: Primary Care, Syncope. N Engl J Med 2000; 343: 1856. [PMID: 11117979]

Meyer MD, Handler J: Evaluation of the patient with syncope: an evidence based approach. Emerg Med Clin North Am 1999;17:189. [PMID: 10101346]

■ III. EMERGENCY TREATMENT OF SPECIFIC DISORDERS CAUSING EPISODIC LOSS OF CONSCIOUSNESS

SEIZURES (Epilepsy)

General Considerations

Seizures can result from a primary central nervous system disorder or may be a manifestation of a serious underlying metabolic or systemic disorder. The distinction is critical, because therapy must be directed at the underlying disorder as well as at control of the seizure. A list of common central nervous system, metabolic, and systemic disorders that may cause seizures is given in Table 17–3.

Clinical Findings

Clinically, seizures are diagnosed by episodes of loss of consciousness (or depressed consciousness) associated with an aura preceding the seizure (50% of patients) and a period of confusion (postictal state) following it. The most common type of seizure is grand mal epilepsy (generalized major motor convulsions). Firm diagnosis of subtler types of seizure (partial seizures, eg, complex partial or temporal lobe attacks) may require an electroencephalogram. For alcohol and drug withdrawal seizures, see Chapter 20.

Seizures, especially those of status epilepticus, are accompanied by the following clinical abnormalities:

A. FEVER

Internal body temperatures as high as 42 °C (107.6 °F) may develop because of intense muscular activity. Temperatures higher than 40 °C (104 °F) should be corrected (Chapter 38).

B. LEUKOCYTOSIS

The peripheral leukocyte count may reach 60,000/μL, perhaps as a result of demargination of leukocytes secondary to catecholamine release; band cells, however, are rare.

C. ACIDOSIS

Lactic acidosis is universal after a single major motor seizure, owing to maximal muscle exertion; arterial blood pH may reach 6.8–7.1. Lactic acidosis due to seizures is transient (< 1 hour) and benign and need not be corrected. It is not associated with shifts in potassium or hyperkalemia. Acidosis does not follow psychogenic seizures.

D. TRAUMA

Trauma, especially tongue and cheek bites, occurs commonly during seizures. Fractures and joint dislocations may occur.

E. CEREBROSPINAL FLUID ABNORMALITIES

Elevation of the cerebrospinal fluid leukocyte count (usually less than 50/μL, and predominantly polymorphonuclear neutrophils) may follow severe seizures. Infection must be ruled out by cultures.

Treatment

For treatment of status epilepticus, see preceding discussion and Table 17–2. Pharmacologic characteristics of the most commonly used anticonvulsant drugs are listed in Table 17–4.

Disposition

Patients with abnormal head CT scans or persistent focal abnormalities should be hospitalized so that diagnostic studies can be performed and the patient observed. Patients with established seizure disorders may be sent home several hours after the seizures have ceased if no acute abnormalities are found. They should be referred to their regular source of medical care within a few days. Patients with alcohol withdrawal may have seizures for 6–12 hours following the first occurrence; 95% of any additional seizures occur during this period. No antiepileptic drugs have been shown to be effective in this syndrome. Phenytoin is clearly ineffective; phenobarbital and lorazepam, while useful in theory, have not demonstrated efficacy in controlled studies. Chronic anticonvulsant administration is not necessary for alcohol withdrawal seizures alone. Hospitalization for alcohol withdrawal seizures is usually not needed if the patient can be reliably observed (eg, at a detoxification center or by family or friends) and the seizures treated with benzodiazepines.

VASOVAGAL SYNCOPE (Simple Faints)

ESSENTIALS OF DIAGNOSIS

- *Usually occurs when patient is standing or sitting.*
- *Lasts 10 seconds to a few minutes.*
- *Associated with lightheadedness, nausea, pallor, sweating, and blurred vision.*
- *No postictal period.*

General Considerations

Vasovagal disorders account for most episodes of syncope. Examples of vasovagal syncope include situational syncope (eg, micturition, cough, or defecation), emotional fainting, and carotid-sinus massage. Common precipitating factors are shown in Table 17–7.

Physiologic decreases in both arterial pressure and heart rate mediated by the vagus nerve combine to produce central nervous system hypoperfusion and subsequent syncope. Prolonged cerebral hypoxia with resultant tonic-clonic movements is more likely to occur if the patient remains upright.

Table 17–7. Common factors precipitating vasovagal syncope (fainting).

Emotional upset
Sight of blood
Sudden exposure to cold
Prolonged motionless standing
Medical or surgical procedures
Injury
Pain
Blood loss
Cough
Micturition
Migraine
Early pregnancy

Clinical Findings

Vasovagal episodes begin in a standing or sitting position and only rarely in a supine position.

A. PRODROME

The prodrome lasts from 10 seconds to a few minutes and includes weakness, lightheadedness, nausea, pallor, sweating, salivation, blurred vision, and tachycardia.

B. SYNCOPE

Brain hypoperfusion causes dimming of vision; the patient then loses consciousness and sinks to the ground. Examination reveals an unconscious individual who is pale and sweating and who has dilated pupils and a slow, weak pulse. With loss of consciousness, bradycardia replaces tachycardia.

C. ASSOCIATED SYMPTOMS

Abnormal movements may be noted during the period of unconsciousness. These are mainly tonic or opisthotonic, but tonic-clonic activity is occasionally manifested. Urinary incontinence may occur, but tongue biting is rare.

D. POSTSYNCOPAL FINDINGS

The patient is lucid and awake seconds to less than a minute after sinking to a recumbent position; a postictal confusional state is absent unless a convulsion has occurred. However, nervousness, dizziness, headache, nausea and vomiting, pallor, perspiration, and an urge to defecate may persist for hours.

E. RECURRENCE

Syncope may recur, especially if the patient stands up within 30 minutes after the attack. Syncope due to a specific precipitating factor (eg, cough) can be reproduced in the emergency department.

Treatment

Reassurance and a recommendation to avoid precipitating factors are usually all that is necessary. Cough suppression and sitting down to urinate are helpful in posttussive and micturitional syncope. Adequate nutrition and hydration should be encouraged.

Disposition

Refer the patient to an outpatient clinic or primary care physician after a period of observation and confirmation of the diagnosis in the emergency department.

CARDIOPULMONARY SYNCOPE

General Considerations

A cardiovascular origin for syncope is suggested when it occurs during recumbency, during or following physical exertion, or in a patient with known heart disease. Loss of consciousness in cardiac disease is most often due to an abrupt decrease in cardiac output, with subsequent cerebral hypoperfusion producing symptoms identical to those of fainting. Such cardiac dysfunction may result from rhythm disturbances (bradyarrhythmias or tachyarrhythmias), cardiac inflow or outflow obstruction, acute myocardial infarction, intracardiac right-to-left shunts, leaking or dissecting aortic aneurysms, or acute pulmonary embolus. Table 17–6 lists some of the more common cardiopulmonary causes of syncope.

CARDIAC ARREST (SEE ALSO CHAPTER 7.)

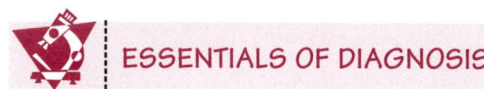 ESSENTIALS OF DIAGNOSIS

- *Suspect cardiac arrest and arrhythmias as possible causes in syncope.*

Clinical Findings

Loss of consciousness due to cardiac arrest (ventricular fibrillation or asystole) from any cause occurs in 3–5 seconds if the patient is standing or within 15 seconds if the patient is recumbent. The patient usually rapidly regains consciousness if adequate cardiac output is restored promptly; most patients who regain consciousness within 12 hours will recover without neurologic sequelae.

Seizures are uncommon but are more likely to occur the longer the cerebral hypoperfusion lasts. A postictal confusional state occurs in patients who have convulsed.

Treatment & Disposition

Initiate cardiopulmonary resuscitation; see Chapter 7 for further details. Immediate hospitalization in an intensive care unit for evaluation and treatment is required.

ACUTE MYOCARDIAL INFARCTION (SEE ALSO CHAPTER 34.)

Rarely, myocardial infarction is manifested by syncope without chest pain. Hospitalization is required in every case.

CARDIAC ARRHYTHMIAS
(See also Chapter 35.)

Clinical Findings

See Table 17–6 for arrhythmias associated with syncope. Palpitations, fatigue, dyspnea, or chest pain may precede loss of consciousness. Atypical chest pain (mainly nonexertional, left precordial, sharp, and of variable duration) suggests mitral valve prolapse.

Rapid (≥ 160 beats/min), slow (≤ 50 beats/min), or irregular pulse must be carefully investigated. Tachycardia of 180–200 beats/min will produce syncope in half of healthy persons. In patients with underlying heart disease or atherosclerosis, tachycardia as slow as 135 beats/min or bradycardia as fast as 60 beats/min may result in loss of consciousness.

Chest auscultation with the patient in various positions (eg, sitting, left lateral decubitus, squatting) may disclose abnormal murmurs and clicks in the case of mitral valve prolapse.

The ECG may confirm the diagnosis of arrhythmia, heart block, sick sinus, or prolonged QT interval. However, a single ECG, obtained when the patient is asymptomatic, is frequently normal or nondiagnostic of a rhythm abnormality responsible for the syncope. A diagnosis can be firmly established only by demonstrating arrhythmias during symptomatic periods.

Treatment & Disposition

Patients with syncopal attacks thought to be due to structural cardiac disease or an arrhythmia should be hospitalized for further evaluation.

CARDIAC INFLOW OBSTRUCTION
(SEE ALSO CHAPTER 34.)

 ESSENTIALS OF DIAGNOSIS

- Suspect with syncope due to change in position.
- Look for physical exam findings: cardiac findings, engorged neck veins, weak pulse, or hypotension.

Clinical Findings

Patients with atrial or ventricular myxomas and atrial thrombi usually present with embolization but may also have sudden loss of cardiac output and syncope; syncope occurring with change in position is classic but uncommon. Left atrial myxoma often mimics mitral stenosis but is occasionally manifested by mitral regurgitation murmur. Mitral valve prolapse may also cause syncope.

Constrictive pericarditis or cardiac tamponade causes reduced cardiac output and may result in syncope. Any maneuver or drug that decreases heart rate or venous return will further impair cardiac output. The diagnosis is suggested by the presence of engorged neck veins, clear lung fields on chest x-ray, weak pulse, and hypotension (Chapter 34).

Tension pneumothorax reduces cardiac output by decreasing venous return and may produce syncope. There is usually a history of chest trauma or chronic pulmonary disease with bullae. Chest x-ray and physical examination confirm the diagnosis. See Chapter 24 for details.

Treatment & Disposition

Patients with syncope thought to be due to cardiac inflow obstruction require immediate treatment and hospitalization.

CARDIAC OUTFLOW OBSTRUCTION

 ESSENTIALS OF DIAGNOSIS

- Consider with syncope related to exertion.
- Look for cardiac physical findings.

1. Aortic Stenosis

Loss of consciousness secondary to congenital or acquired severe stenosis may occur in all age groups. Exertional syncope occurs as a result of cerebral hypoperfusion due to exercise-induced vasodilation in the presence of a fixed cardiac output. Two other pathophysiologic events are recognized: (1) acute transient left ventricular failure with normal sinus rhythm and (2) transient arrhythmia or cardiac stand-still, causing an acute drop in cardiac output. Sudden death may result. Autonomic insufficiency also has been reported in these patients. Reflex peripheral vascular vasodilation (presumably due to left ventricular baroreceptor activity) has been demonstrated in the absence of cardiac arrhythmia.

Clinical Findings

Syncope usually follows exercise and is often associated with dyspnea, anginal chest pain, and sweating. Physical findings that occur with hemodynamically severe aortic stenosis include the following:

- Characteristic midsystolic ejection murmur (often associated with a palpable thrill)
- Sustained and prolonged left ventricular lift
- Paradoxically split second sound
- Delayed upstroke and reduced amplitude (pulsus parvus et tardus) on the carotid pulse

Treatment & Disposition

Promptly hospitalize all patients with symptomatic aortic stenosis (angina, congestive heart failure, or syncope) to evaluate them for possible valve replacement. Median survival time following the initial episode of syncope due to aortic stenosis in the patient who does not receive a prosthesis is 1.5–3 years.

2. Pulmonary Stenosis

Clinical Findings

Severe pulmonary stenosis may produce syncope, especially following exertion. A hemodynamic process similar to that of aortic stenosis is responsible. Physical findings include right parasternal lift, systolic ejection murmur at the upper left sternal border, a prominent S_4, and a conspicuous a wave in the jugular venous pulse.

Treatment & Disposition

Immediate hospitalization is required, because the pathophysiology and prognosis of this condition are similar to those of aortic stenosis.

3. Hypertrophic Obstructive Cardiomyopathy[2]

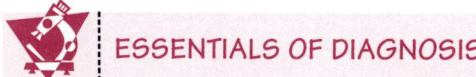 ESSENTIALS OF DIAGNOSIS

- *Syncope with exercise, dyspnea on exertion, and chest pain.*
- *Cardiac findings including systolic ejection murmur, S_4 and perhaps a thrill.*

Clinical Findings

Symptoms include syncope with exercise, dyspnea on exertion, and chest pain. Physical findings include a prominent fourth heart sound, ventricular lift, transient arrhythmias, and systolic ejection murmur and perhaps

[2]Hypertrophic obstructive cardiomyopathy is also known as asymmetric septal hypertrophy or idiopathic hypertrophic subaortic stenosis.

a thrill, both of which increase with exertion and with decreased left ventricular chamber size (eg, as produced during the Valsalva maneuver). Echocardiography confirms the diagnosis.

Treatment & Disposition

Hospitalize the patient for further evaluation and treatment.

PULMONARY VASCULAR DISEASE (See also Chapter 27.)

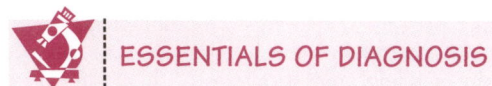 ESSENTIALS OF DIAGNOSIS

Pulmonary Embolism

- *Suspect pulmonary embolism as a cause of syncope.*
- *Complaints of dyspnea and pleuritic chest pain when awake.*
- *Look for tachypnea and tachycardia.*

Clinical Findings

A. PULMONARY HYPERTENSION

Syncope, often exertional, can be the presenting symptom of pulmonary hypertension. A history of dyspnea is invariably obtained as well. Signs of right ventricular failure (parasternal lift, increased pulmonary second sound, right-sided S_4, and murmurs of pulmonary and tricuspid valvular insufficiency), electrocardiographic evidence of right ventricular hypertrophy, and tachypnea are often found.

B. MASSIVE PULMONARY EMBOLISM

Syncope is the presenting symptom in approximately 20% of patients experiencing massive pulmonary embolism. When the patient regains consciousness after syncope, pleuritic chest pain, dyspnea, and apprehension are present. Hypotension, tachycardia, tachypnea, and significant hypoxemia frequently accompany large embolism, and death may occur. Syncope or sudden altered mental status was noted (retrospectively) as a prodrome in 60% of cadavers diagnosed with massive pulmonary embolism at autopsy.

Treatment & Disposition

Provide supplemental oxygen (10 L/min) and assisted ventilation where necessary. See Chapter 27 for further evaluation and treatment. Hospitalization is usually required.

CEREBROVASCULAR SYNCOPE

Although syncope resulting from cerebrovascular disease is often diagnosed, such an association is in fact uncommon, because consciousness is lost only when the function of both cerebral hemispheres or the brainstem reticular formation is compromised (see Table 17–6 and Chapter 16).

BASILAR ARTERY INSUFFICIENCY
(See also Chapter 18.)

Clinical Findings

Basilar artery transient ischemic attacks (TIAs) usually occur after age 65 years. Loss of consciousness is a rare manifestation.

Diplopia, vertigo, dysphagia, dysarthria, lateralized sensory or motor symptoms, and sudden bilateral leg weakness suggest brain-stem ischemia. Syncope is rarely if ever the initial or isolated symptom.

TIAs typically are of sudden onset and brief duration (seconds to minutes), but when loss of consciousness has occurred, recovery is frequently prolonged (30–60 minutes or longer).

Treatment & Disposition

Accurate diagnosis of basilar artery insufficiency is often difficult, and neurologic referral is recommended. Hospitalization is indicated, especially when syncope has occurred. Treatment with aspirin should be started; the specific effective dose has not yet been clarified.

SUBCLAVIAN STEAL SYNDROME

Clinical Findings

Patients with subclavian steal syndrome present with symptoms of vertebrobasilar artery insufficiency combined with symptoms of ipsilateral upper extremity ischemia.

The diagnosis is confirmed by the episodic signs and symptoms of basilar artery ischemia, syncope, vertigo, diplopia, limb paresis, paresthesias, and ataxia. Brainstem infarction (stroke) has not been reported to result from subclavian steal syndrome alone.

Blood pressures measured in the upper extremities are nearly always unequal. The average difference is a 45–mm Hg decrease in systolic pressure in the arm supplied by the stenotic vessel.

Treatment & Disposition

If subclavian steal syndrome is suspected, elective hospitalization for arteriography and perhaps surgical correction is indicated.

MIGRAINE
(See also Chapter 19.)

Syncope occurs in 10% of patient with migraine when they stand up suddenly. The timing of attacks suggests that loss of consciousness is due to orthostatic hypotension.

CAROTID SINUS SYNCOPE

Clinical Findings

Carotid sinus syncope classically results from pressure on an abnormally sensitive carotid sinus by a tight collar, neck mass, enlarged cervical nodes, or tumor. This pressure causes vagal stimulation that slows the sinoatrial and atrioventricular nodes and inhibits sympathetic vascular tone. The resulting bradycardia and systemic hypotension may then produce syncope. Bradycardia or hypotension may also occur without syncope. The syndrome may be reproduced in the emergency department by pressure on the carotid sinus for 5–10 seconds while the patient is both supine and erect; cardiac monitoring or ECG documents the induced bradyarrhythmia. Such pressure may also produce syncope resulting from cerebral ischemia if the examiner compresses the artery contralateral to an occluded carotid artery. Syncope is then due to cerebral hypoperfusion secondary to cerebrovascular disease and not to hypersensitivity of the carotid sinus.

Treatment

The patient with syncope should be placed supine and pressure on the carotid sinus relieved (eg, by loosening a tight collar). Further therapy is seldom required. Unusually severe or persistent bradycardia can be abolished in some cases by administration of atropine, 0.5 mg intravenously.

Disposition

Refer the patient to an outpatient clinic or primary care physician for evaluation. The patient should be told to avoid possible causes of the attacks (eg, tight collars).

ORTHOSTATIC HYPOTENSION

Orthostatic hypotension occurs more often in men than in women and is most common in the sixth and seventh decades, although it may occur even in teenagers. Orthostatic hypotension may result from multiple disorders; the more common causes are listed in Table 17–5.

Clinical Findings

Syncope often occurs following rapid change in the upright position, that is, from lying to sitting or from sitting to standing. Prolonged motionless standing, especially after exercise, or standing after prolonged bed rest, may also cause syncope. Patients usually describe lightheadedness, dimming of vision, weakness, and a fainting sensation. True vertigo does not occur.

Blood pressure that is significantly lower (> 20 mm Hg systolic difference) when the patient is standing than when he or she is supine is diagnostic. Orthostatic tachycardia may be present as well.

A stool sample should be evaluated for the presence of blood. CBC may reveal anemia or hemoconcentration due to blood loss or dehydration, respectively. Electrolyte determinations should be made to detect abnormalities produced by dehydration or drugs. Serum drug levels should be obtained as indicated.

Treatment

Discontinue any offending medication. Encourage oral fluid intake, or administer intravenous fluids to maintain hydration. Replace blood if acute blood loss is significant, and locate the source of bleeding. Instruct patients to stand up gradually, elevate the head of the bed on blocks, and use elasticized support stockings.

Disposition

Hospitalize the patient (1) if postural hypotension is currently producing symptoms and cannot be corrected easily in the emergency department, or (2) if an acute underlying cause of hypotension persists (eg, vomiting, diarrhea) or warrants hospitalization in any case (eg, gastrointestinal bleeding). Otherwise, refer the patient to an outpatient clinic or primary care physician.

MISCELLANEOUS RARE CAUSES OF STATES OF ALTERED CONSCIOUSNESS

HYPERVENTILATION

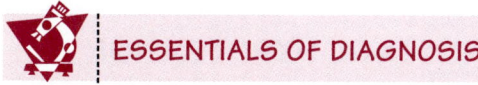

ESSENTIALS OF DIAGNOSIS

- *Diagnosis of exclusion.*
- *Numbness and tingling (especially circumoral).*
- *Muscle twitching and carpal pedal spasm.*

General Considerations

Psychogenic hyperventilation is a frequent cause of altered consciousness (eg, faintness, lightheadedness) but rarely culminates in syncope. Acute anxiety is the usual cause. The disorder is usually benign, but serious cardiopulmonary causes of hyperventilation or subjective dyspnea must be ruled out (Chapter 11).

Clinical Findings

Common symptoms include lightheadedness, shortness of breath, numbness and tingling (especially circumoral or acral), muscular twitching, and in severe cases, carpal pedal spasm. Positive Chvostek and Trousseau tests are noted during the acute stage. Respiratory alkalosis without other abnormalities (eg, metabolic acidosis) is noted on arterial blood gas analysis. Symptoms are reproduced by hyperventilating in a controlled setting (eg, emergency department).

Treatment & Disposition

Reassure the patient, and alleviate underlying anxiety. If the patient is acutely hyperventilating, ask the patient to count to 3 slowly between breaths. Patients experiencing a panic attack may benefit from alprazolam, 0.25–0.5 mg orally. Rebreathing from a paper bag is no longer recommended because of the potential risk of hypoxia.

PSYCHIATRIC CAUSES

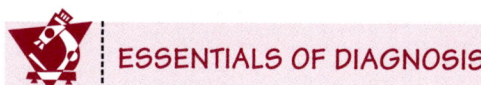

ESSENTIALS OF DIAGNOSIS

- *Diagnosis can be made only after careful exclusion of other causes.*
- *Presence of bizarre postures or movements.*

General Considerations

Psychiatric causes of syncope include major depression, general anxiety disorder, and panic disorder. Fainting is a known manifestation of somatization disorder. Alcohol or drug abuse can lead to syncopal episodes. Malingering may be a factor; patients may use the episodes of feigned unconsciousness to manipulate other people for secondary gain. Patients with factitious disorder also may fake unconsciousness, but they do so for psychological reasons.

Clinical Findings

Features that suggest psychiatric causes of syncope are lack of any prodrome, presence of bizarre postures or movements, lack of pallor, and prolonged unconsciousness. Most patients are young and have a well-documented history of psychiatric responses to stress; without such a history, a psychogenic cause in a patient over 30 years of age can be made only after thorough evaluation has excluded other causes of syncope.

While the patient is unconscious, caloric testing may be used to distinguish coma due to psychiatric causes from coma due to structural lesions or metabolic causes. In coma of organic cause, when ice water is directed against the tympanic membrane, the eyes will remain in mid position or will tonically deviate to the side of the irrigation. In psychogenic coma, the caloric test induces brisk nystagmus, or the patient awakens because of discomfort (Chapter 16).

Treatment & Disposition

Refer the patient to an outpatient clinic or primary care physician for follow-up.

MENIERE DISEASE
(See also Chapter 32.)

 ESSENTIALS OF DIAGNOSIS

- *Recurrent attacks of vertigo.*
- *Associated with tinnitus.*
- *Progressive hearing loss.*

Clinical Findings

Recurrent attacks of severe vertigo persisting for several hours associated with tinnitus and progressive hearing loss are diagnostic of Meniere disease. A few patients experience loss of consciousness for a few seconds at the onset of an attack.

Treatment & Disposition

Meclizine, 50 mg orally once or twice daily, is often helpful. Refer the patient to an otolaryngologist. See Chapter 32 for details.

Basilico FC: Cardiovascular disease in athletes. Am J Sports Med 1999;27:108. [PMID: 9934429]

Bloomfield DM: Strategy for the management of vasovagal syncope. Drugs Aging 2002;19:179. [PMID: 12027777]

Fedderly RT: Left ventricular outflow obstruction. Pediatr Clin North Am 1999;46:369. [PMID: 10218081]

Fenton AM et al: Vasovagal syncope. Ann Intern Med 2000; 133:714. [PMID: 11074905]

Grubb BP et al: Syncope resulting from autonomic insufficiency syndromes associated with orthostatic intolerance. Med Clin North Am 2001;85:457. [PMID: 11233955]

Kenny RA: Neurally mediated syncope. Clin Geriatr Med 2002; 18:191. [PMID: 12180243]

Mack G, Silberbach M: Aortic and pulmonary stenosis. Pediatr Rev 2000;21:79. [PMID: 10702320]

Martin PJ: Vertebrobasilar ischaemia. QJM 1998;91:799. [PMID: 10024945]

Martinon-Torres F et al: The relation between hyperventilation and pediatric syncope. J Pediatr 2001;138:894. [PMID: 11391335]

Roth HL et al: Seizures. Neurol Clin 1998;16:257. [PMID: 9537962]

Schnipper JL, Kapoor WN: Diagnostic evaluation and management of patients with syncope. Med Clin North Am 2001; 85:423. [PMID: 11233954]

Taylor CL et al: Steal affecting the central nervous system. Neurosurgery 2002;50:679. [PMID: 11904017]

Wood KE: Major pulmonary embolism: review of a pathophysiologic approach to the golden hour of hemodynamically significant pulmonary embolism. Chest 2002;121:877. [PMID: 11888976]

Weakness & Stroke

18

Heidi P. Cordi, MD, MS[1]

I. Immediate Management of Life-Threatening Problems Associated with Weakness

II. Further Evaluation of the Patient with Weakness

Spinal Cord Disease

Anterior Horn Cell Involvement (Poliomyelitis)

Neuromuscular Blockade

Peripheral Neuropathy

Muscle Disease (Acute Myopathy)

Hysteria

III. Emergency Management of Specific Weakness Disorders

Disorders of the Spinal Cord

Metastatic Tumor

Transverse Myelitis

Spinal Epidural Abscess

Disease of Anterior Horn Cells

Poliomyelitis

Postpoliomyelitis Syndrome

Peripheral Neuropathies

Mononeuropathies

1. Bell Palsy (Facial Weakness)

2. Compressive Mononeuropathies

Polyneuropathies

1. Guillain-Barré Syndrome (Infectious Polyneuritis)

2. Arsenical Neuropathy

3. Acute Intermittent Porphyria

4. Tick Paralysis

5. Diphtheritic Polyneuritis

6. Paralytic Seafood Poisoning

Diseases of the Neuromuscular Junction

Botulism

Organophosphate Poisoning

Myasthenia Gravis

Primary Acute Myopathies

Hypokalemic Periodic Paralysis

Acute Electrolyte Abnormalities

Rhabdomyolysis

IV. Immediate Management of Life-Threatening Problems Associated with Stroke

V. Further Evaluation of the Patient with Stroke

VI. Management of Specific Stroke Syndromes

Hemorrhagic Stroke

Subarachnoid Hemorrhage

Intracerebral Hemorrhage

Ischemic Stroke

Lacunar Stroke

Arterial Dissection

Transient Ischemic Attacks

The term *weakness* is broad and encompasses a diverse spectrum of disease processes. There is a great deal of overlap in the various clinical manifestations of muscle weakness. It can range from a primary muscular disorder to a neurologic dysfunction. Disorders characterized by rapid onset of loss of motor function are discussed in this chapter. With the exception of some stroke syndromes, consciousness is not impaired by the primary disease process, although secondary respiratory insufficiency may cause hypercapnia leading to obtundation.

Caution: The major error to be avoided in dealing with patients presenting with acute weakness is misinterpreting the symptoms as psychogenic or hysterical. These patients usually are awake and alert and may not appear critically ill. They may be able to walk. *Complaints of weakness of recent onset require careful evalua-*

---

[1]This chapter is a revision of the chapter by Roger P. Simon, MD, & Mary T. Ho, MD, MPH, from the 4th edition.

tion before judgments are made about the cause of symptoms.

I. IMMEDIATE MANAGEMENT OF LIFE-THREATENING PROBLEMS ASSOCIATED WITH WEAKNESS (See Figure 18–1.)

Stabilize Ventilation

Treat dyspnea or objective respiratory distress in a patient with weakness as a potential life-threatening emergency. Respiratory muscles may be affected even though strength in the extremities is relatively unimpaired.

A. OXYGEN

Give oxygen, 5 L/min by mask or nasal cannula, if breathing is labored, if there is obvious hypoventilation (patient is barely able to speak), or if there is evidence of hypoxemia (eg, cyanosis of digits). Distal extremity paresthesias and increased respiratory effort associated with the basic disease process (eg, Guillain-Barré syndrome) may support the impression of psychogenic hyperventilation.

B. LABORATORY TESTS

Arterial blood gases, vital capacity, and maximum inspiratory force should be measured immediately. Measurements of vital capacity and maximum inspiratory force will be abnormal even before alterations in arterial blood gases occur.

C. SUPPORTED VENTILATION

Frank hypoventilation (P_{CO_2} > 50 mm Hg) is an indication for emergency supported ventilation (eg, bag-valve-mask), followed as quickly as possible by endotracheal intubation and mechanical ventilation.

Even if arterial blood gas measurements are normal or nearly normal, a markedly diminished vital capacity (<10 mL/kg) and in particular a diminished maximum inspiratory force (<15 cm H_2O) in a patient with progressive weakness are indications for intubation and supported ventilation. In these cases, a delay of 1–2 hours is permissible to allow intubation under optimal conditions, as long as the patient is under close observation.

D. HOSPITALIZATION

Hospitalize all patients who complain of dyspnea and weakness unless the vital capacity, maximum inspiratory force, and arterial blood gases remain normal during the period of observation.

Rule Out Spinal Cord Compression

Quickly assess the possibility of a mass compressing the spinal cord, because emergency operation or radiation therapy may be needed to prevent permanent paraplegia or quadriplegia.

A. LOCATE LEVEL OF LESION

Acute spinal cord compression is associated with weakness and sensory loss caudad to the level of involvement. Cord-mediated functions cephalad to this level and cranial nerve examination will be normal.

1. Cervical level—Both upper and lower extremity weakness are present, but cranial nerve function is normal. Respiratory insufficiency is especially likely with high cervical cord lesions.

2. Thoracic level—Lower extremity weakness is present, but the upper extremities and cranial nerves are spared. Because spinal cord compression involves sensory and motor pathways, a sensory level should be carefully sought by eliciting reactions to pinprick or a cold object placed against the skin.

3. Lower spinal cord, or cauda equina, involvement—Signs and symptoms include bladder or bowel incontinence, sensory loss in sacral (saddle) distribution, and lower extremity weakness.

4. Vertebral body involvement—If spinal cord compression is due to a process that also involves the vertebral bodies (eg, metastatic tumor, epidural abscess), focal tenderness during vertebral percussion will be noted. Radiologic evidence of bony erosion or collapse of the vertebral column at the spinal cord level responsible for the abnormal neurologic findings virtually establishes the diagnosis.

B. PERFORM EMERGENCY IMAGING AND SURGERY

Patients with suspected spinal cord compression due to any cause require emergency neurosurgical consultation and imaging (preferably magnetic resonance imaging [MRI], if available).

Caution: In case of suspected spinal cord compression, do not perform lumbar puncture in the emergency department, because it may worsen symptoms and make more difficult subsequent attempts to enter the subarachnoid space (eg, for myelography).

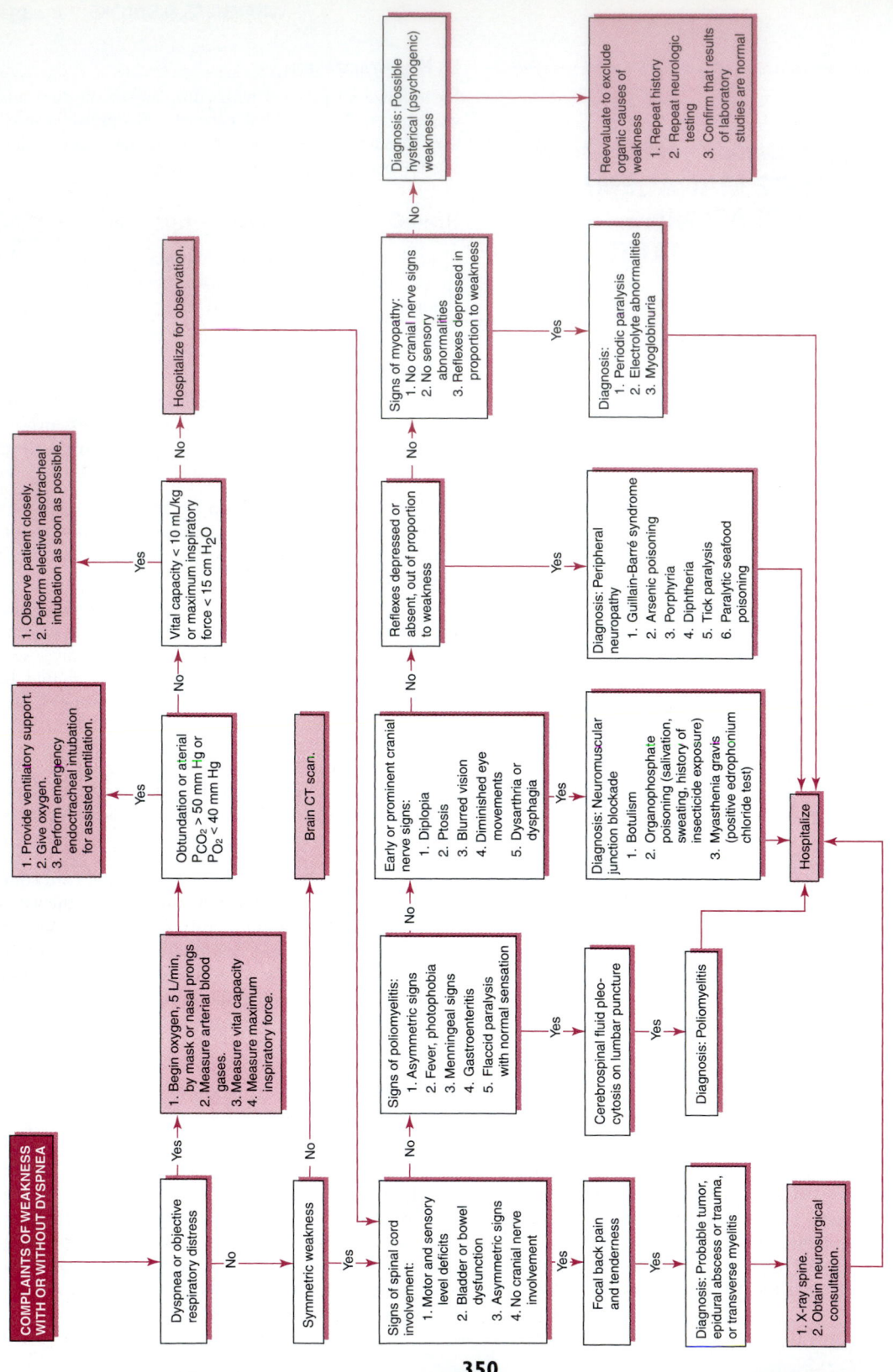

COMPLAINTS OF WEAKNESS WITH OR WITHOUT DYSPNEA

Dyspnea or objective respiratory distress

Yes →

1. Begin oxygen, 5 L/min, by mask or nasal prongs
2. Measure arterial blood gases.
3. Measure vital capacity
4. Measure maximum inspiratory force.

Obtundation or arterial $P_{CO_2} > 50$ mm Hg or $P_{O_2} < 40$ mm Hg

Yes →

1. Provide ventilatory support.
2. Give oxygen.
3. Perform emergency endotracheal intubation for assisted ventilation.

No →

Vital capacity < 10 mL/kg or maximum inspiratory force < 15 cm H_2O

Yes →

1. Observe patient closely.
2. Perform elective nasotracheal intubation as soon as possible.

No →

Hospitalize for observation.

No →

Signs of myopathy:
1. No cranial nerve signs
2. No sensory abnormalities
3. Reflexes depressed in proportion to weakness

No →

Diagnosis: Possible hysterical (psychogenic) weakness

Reevaluate to exclude organic causes of weakness
1. Repeat history
2. Repeat neurologic testing
3. Confirm that results of laboratory studies are normal

Yes →

Diagnosis:
1. Periodic paralysis
2. Electrolyte abnormalities
3. Myoglobinuria

Reflexes depressed or absent, out of proportion to weakness

Yes →

Diagnosis: Peripheral neuropathy
1. Guillain-Barré syndrome
2. Arsenic poisoning
3. Porphyria
4. Diphtheria
5. Tick paralysis
6. Paralytic seafood poisoning

No →

Early or prominent cranial nerve signs:
1. Diplopia
2. Ptosis
3. Blurred vision
4. Diminished eye movements
5. Dysarthria or dysphagia

Yes →

Diagnosis: Neuromuscular junction blockade
1. Botulism
2. Organophosphate poisoning (salivation, sweating, history of insecticide exposure)
3. Myasthenia gravis (positive edrophonium chloride test)

No →

Symmetric weakness

No →

Brain CT scan.

Yes →

Signs of spinal cord involvement:
1. Motor and sensory level deficits
2. Bladder or bowel dysfunction
3. Asymmetric signs
4. No cranial nerve involvement

No →

Signs of poliomyelitis:
1. Asymmetric signs
2. Fever, photophobia
3. Meningeal signs
4. Gastroenteritis
5. Flaccid paralysis with normal sensation

Yes →

Cerebrospinal fluid pleocytosis on lumbar puncture

Yes →

Diagnosis: Poliomyelitis

Yes →

Focal back pain and tenderness

Yes →

Diagnosis: Probable tumor, epidural abscess or trauma, or transverse myelitis

1. X-ray spine.
2. Obtain neurosurgical consultation.

Hospitalize

Figure 18–1. Assessment of complaints of weakness with or without dyspnea.

350

■ II. FURTHER EVALUATION OF THE PATIENT WITH WEAKNESS

After the immediate measures described above have been taken, further evaluation should proceed so as to localize the anatomic site of weakness into one of the following categories (see Table 18–1 and detailed discussions of specific disorders).

SPINAL CORD DISEASE

 ESSENTIALS OF DIAGNOSIS

- *Traumatic causes: concussion, incomplete cord (anterior cord, Brown-Séquard syndrome, central cord, conus medullaris, cauda equina), complete cord.*
- *Nontraumatic (infectious) causes: epidural abscess, meningitis, subdural abscess, intramedullary abscess.*

Clinical Findings

Spinal cord disease should be suspected if weakness and sensory loss are found caudad to a horizontal plane in the body. Cranial nerve examination should be normal. The most common disorders producing rapidly progressive weakness or involvement of the nervous system at the spinal cord level are essentially confined to 4 processes: (1) disk protrusion (Chapter 21), (2) spinal epidural metastases, (3) transverse myelitis, and (4) spinal epidural abscess. Other causes such as radiation myelitis and ruptured arteriovenous malformations are rare. A diagnosis of suspected spinal cord compression by abscess or tumor demands immediate confirmation by MRI or myelography and prompt surgical decompression and antibiotics for abscess and emergency radiation therapy or surgical decompression for tumor. In transverse myelitis, no such mechanical compression of the spinal cord exists, and surgery only increases the morbidity.

A. IMAGING

MRI is the study of choice; if it is unavailable, myelography is done. Obtain cerebrospinal fluid only at the time of myelography, because the subarachnoid space may be difficult to enter a second time. Remove only a small amount of cerebrospinal fluid for study, and use small volumes of contrast media (<2 mL), because spinal cord herniation may follow removal or instilla-

tion of larger amounts below a complete block. If a complete block to cerebrospinal fluid flow is anticipated, enter the subarachnoid space above the lesion via a lateral C1-C2 puncture, if possible.

B. OTHER DIAGNOSTIC MEASURES

Table 18–2 lists features helpful in differentiating the other entities causing spinal cord dysfunction.

Treatment & Disposition

Hospitalize the patient, and seek immediate neurologic or neurosurgical consultation.

ANTERIOR HORN CELL INVOLVEMENT (Poliomyelitis)

Clinical Findings

A. SYMPTOMS AND SIGNS

Poliomyelitis should be suspected if several of the following are present with weakness:

- Asymmetric weakness with intact sensation. This asymmetry of motor involvement is virtually unique to poliomyelitis in patients who have not been vaccinated or in immunocompromised patients.
- Gastrointestinal signs or symptoms.
- Fever, headache, photophobia.
- Meningeal signs.

B. IMAGING

MRI scan may show localized inflammation to the anterior horn cells.

C. LUMBAR PUNCTURE

Perform lumbar puncture if poliomyelitis is suspected. Spinal cord compression (abscess), transverse myelitis, and poliomyelitis are the only conditions commonly producing acute weakness associated with cerebrospinal fluid pleocytosis.

D. DIFFERENTIAL DIAGNOSIS

Spinal cord compression and myelitis will produce a sensory deficit. Peripheral neuropathies may spare sensory nerves; motor involvement is usually symmetric.

Treatment & Disposition

Treatment is primarily supportive. The prognosis is poor in the bulbar form of the disease, with a mortality rate of approximately 50%. Hospitalize all patients who have a clinical diagnosis of poliomyelitis. If bulbar involvement has produced respiratory failure, support respiration with supplemental oxygen and assisted ventilation (bag-valve-mask or endotracheal intubation).

Table 18–1. Differential diagnosis of acute weakness by anatomic localization.

Location	Disease State	Location of Weakness	Cranial Nerve Involvement	Sensory Abnormalities	Meningeal Signs	Reflexes	Bladder Paralysis	Cerebrospinal Fluid
Cerebral hemispheres	Stroke.	Unilateral (ie, hemiplegia or hemiparesis).	Unilateral facial weakness.	Hemihypesthesia.	Rare.	Asymmetric; decreased acutely; then increased, with upgoing toes (Babinski sign).	Rare.	Variable. Usually normal in thrombosis, bloody with hemorrhage.
Spinal cord	Compression by tumor or abscess; protruding disk or transverse myelitis.	Paraplegia or quadriplegia (may have a unilateral predominance).	None.	Depressed below level of lesion.	Present in one third to one half of patients	Decreased acutely; then increased, with upgoing toes (Babinski sign).	Prominent.	Highly variable: from normal to markedly increased in cells and protein. Myelographic block very common with mass lesions.
Anterior horn cell	Poliomyelitis, other enterovirus infection.	Scattered, focal, asymmetric.	10–20% of cases.	None.	Common.	Depressed in involved limbs.	Uncommon, transient.	Increased white blood cells (25–500/μL) early. Increased protein later. Glucose normal.
Peripheral nerve	Guillain-Barré syndrome, arsenical neuropathy, diphtheritic neuropathy, porphyria, tick paralysis.	Proximal or distal; usually symmetric.	Common in Guillain-Barré syndrome, especially facial muscles (seventh nerve).	Distal (stocking-glove distribution).	Rare.	Decreased or absent early and out of proportion to muscle weakness.	None.	Increased protein but may be normal acutely. Few or absent cells (albumino-cytologic dissociation).
Neuromuscular junction	Botulism, organophosphate poisoning, myasthenia gravis, aminoglycoside toxicity.	Proximal, symmetric.	Prominent and early involvement, especially eye movements. Pupils may be unreactive to light.	None.	None.	Decreased in relation to degree of muscle weakness.	None.	Normal.
Muscle	Hypokalemia, hyperkalemia, periodic paralysis, myoglobinuria, hypophosphatemia, hypermagnesemia.	Proximal, symmetric. Upper and lower extremities equally involved.	None.	None.	None.	Decreased in relation to degree of muscle weakness.	None.	Normal.

Table 18–2. Differential diagnosis of acute weakness at the spinal cord level.[1]

	Epidural Abscess	Epidural Tumor	Transverse Myelitis
Age (years)	11–77	Rare in childhood	1–65
Back pain	100%	90%	36%
Vertebral tenderness	100%	90%	58%
Fever	86%	0%	51%
White count > 10,000/μL	62%	0%	32%
Cerebrospinal fluid cells (cells/μL)	2–720	Normal	0–8800
Cerebrospinal fluid protein (mg/dL)	36–2000	82–822	18–216
Cerebrospinal fluid glucose (mg/dL)	Normal	Normal	Normal
Duration (from onset to maximum deficit)	Days to months	Hours to months	Minutes to weeks
Complete block to cerebrospinal fluid flow on myelogram	86%	81%	7%
Bony erosion or osteomyelitis (on spinal x-ray)	30–83%	85%	0%

[1]Based on 105 cases of spinal metastases, 65 cases of transverse myelopathy, and 65 cases of abscess selected from the literature.

NEUROMUSCULAR BLOCKAGE

Clinical Findings

A. SYMPTOMS AND SIGNS

Diseases affecting the neuromuscular junction are marked by early and prominent involvement of cranial nerves, causing difficulty in speaking and swallowing, facial weakness, blurred vision, diplopia, and ptosis. Involvement of respiratory and extremity muscles follows. There are no sensory abnormalities, and reflexes are preserved, though responses may be depressed in proportion to the degree of weakness.

B. CAUSES

Diseases causing neuromuscular blockage include organophosphate (insecticide or nerve gas) poisoning, botulism, myasthenia gravis, and envenomations. Certain antibiotics (eg, aminoglycosides) may rarely cause neuromuscular blockade, but this occurs only in hospitalized patients with contributory conditions (eg, myasthenia gravis).

Differential Diagnosis

It is important to make a rapid diagnosis, because both botulism and organophosphate poisoning require immediate specific therapy.

A. ORGANOPHOSPHATE POISONING

Poisoning with organophosphates causes marked miosis and prominent glandular hypersecretion (sweating, salivation, lacrimation, and bronchorrhea). Most patients have been recently exposed to insecticide spraying, a fact easily elicited by questioning.

B. BOTULISM

Botulism affects the neuromuscular junction and causes nausea and vomiting followed by paralysis of muscles of accommodation, respiratory muscles, extraocular muscles, extremity muscles, and the lower bulbar muscles. Glandular secretion is not affected.

C. MYASTHENIA GRAVIS

Patients with myasthenia gravis usually know their diagnosis. The rare patient with undiagnosed acute myasthenia gravis should improve in response to edrophonium (Tensilon, others). Give 2 mg intravenously over 15–30 seconds; if no reaction occurs within 1 minute, give 8 mg more. Edrophonium has a rapid onset but brief duration of action, both of which permit quick assessment of cranial nerve weakness. Testing of limb muscles may require use of the longer-acting cholinesterase inhibitor neostigmine (1.5 mg intramuscularly, together with atropine, 0.5 mg intramuscularly). Edrophonium and neostigmine will not affect symptoms due to botulinum toxin or organophosphate poisoning.

D. VENOMOUS ANIMAL INJURIES

(See also Chapter 44.) Certain bites can also produce acute symptoms, including weakness.

1. Snakes—Compounds can be found in a poisonous snake's venom that can cause a variety of reactions depending on the species involved. For example, the bite of the pit viper (the most common poisonous snake in the United States) can cause many systemic symptoms, including weakness, tingling, muscle fasciculations, and metallic taste. Coral snake venom contains compounds that block neuromuscular transmission at the acetylcholine receptor site, thereby inhibiting cardiac and skeletal muscle. The first appreciated sign is ptosis of the eyes; other signs include proximal muscle weakness, slurred speech, and dysphagia.

2. Gila monsters—Gila monster bites are associated with weakness, pain, and edema. They are rarely fatal.

3. Black widow spider—Black widow spider neurotoxin depletes acetylcholine from presynaptic nerve channels, thereby destabilizing the membranes. The patient complains of weakness, ptosis, difficulty speaking, and muscle cramps.

4. Brown recluse spider—Bites from this spider can produce weakness, nausea, and vomiting.

5. Scorpions—Toxicity varies within the species. The more dangerous type will have the more toxic effect. Systemic reactions include muscle spasms, hemiplegia, blurred vision, pseudoseizures, cardiac dysrhythmias, and respiratory arrest.

Disposition

Hospitalization is mandatory for all patients with suspected neuromuscular blockade.

PERIPHERAL NEUROPATHY

Clinical Findings

Disorders involving the peripheral nerves can produce sensory or motor symptoms or (most often) both.

A. SYMPTOMS AND SIGNS

Weakness may preferentially involve either the distal or, rarely, the proximal musculature. Sensory loss is usually restricted to a distal (ie, stocking-glove) distribution. Weakness owing to cranial nerve involvement may occur but is not a common presenting feature.

Reflexes are markedly depressed or absent early; this is helpful in identifying peripheral nerve impairment even before objective weakness can be documented.

B. LABORATORY FINDINGS

Cerebrospinal fluid protein is commonly elevated, but this may not occur until days after onset. The cell count is usually normal.

Treatment

Provide supportive care (eg, respiratory support as required). None of the illnesses causing peripheral neuropathy are relieved by specific emergency therapy except for tick paralysis, which responds to the removal of the tick (usually found in the hair).

Disposition

Hospitalization may be necessary for further evaluation and treatment.

MUSCLE DISEASE
(Acute Myopathy)

 ESSENTIALS OF DIAGNOSIS

- *Causes vary.*
- *Malaise, fatigue, and symmetric proximal weakness.*
- *Atrophy, hyporeflexia.*
- *Dark urine.*
- *No sensory complaints.*

Clinical Findings

Prompt diagnosis of primary muscle disease is important, because effective specific therapy is available for some of the conditions causing muscular weakness.

A. SYMPTOMS AND SIGNS

Weakness is characteristically more proximal than distal, and lower extremity weakness is often greater than that in the upper extremities. Cranial nerve and respiratory abnormalities occur in severe cases; eye movements are spared. Objective sensory loss does not occur. Deep tendon reflexes are depressed in proportion to the muscle weakness.

B. LABORATORY FINDINGS

Collect urine for myoglobin testing (positive test for hemoglobin on dipstick in the absence of erythrocytes on microscopy; confirm by chemical assay) and blood for determination of muscle enzymes (CK, AST [SGOT]) and potassium in serum.

Treatment & Disposition

Hospitalization is generally required, although mild attacks of recurrent familial hypo- or hyperkalemic paralysis may be treated adequately in the emergency department. If hypokalemia is present, give potassium chloride, 1–2 mEq/kg (equivalent to 5–10 g of potassium chloride) orally, and repeat once or twice at hourly intervals until strength is regained. Treat hyperkalemia associated with muscular weakness by infusing glucose and insulin (Chapter 42).

HYSTERIA

 ## ESSENTIALS OF DIAGNOSIS

- *Conversion disorder can suggest a neurologic disease, but no explanation can be found despite physical and diagnostic testing.*
- *Complete and comprehensive psychosocial history is important.*

Hysteria as a cause of weakness can be diagnosed only after all other causes have been eliminated. A history of hysteria or psychosomatic illnesses may be helpful, but one must also search for and eliminate other causes of weakness, because organic causes of weakness are frequently misdiagnosed initially as hysteria. Psychiatric evaluation should be obtained.

Arce D et al: Recognizing spinal cord emergencies. Am Fam Physician 2001;64:631. [PMID: 11529262] (A review of spinal cord emergencies.)

Della-Giustina DA: Emergency department evaluation and treatment of back pain. Emerg Med Clin North Am 1999;17:877. [PMID: 10584107] (A review of emergency diagnosis and management of back pain.)

■ III. EMERGENCY MANAGEMENT OF SPECIFIC WEAKNESS DISORDERS

DISORDERS OF THE SPINAL CORD

METASTATIC TUMOR

 ## ESSENTIALS OF DIAGNOSIS

- *Slowly progressive.*
- *Stuttering neurologic deficit.*

Clinical Findings

The most common primary malignant neoplasms producing epidural metastases and spinal cord compression are breast cancer (20%), lung cancer (10%), Hodgkin disease (10%), and prostate cancer (7%).

A. SYMPTOMS AND SIGNS

Local vertebral column pain at the level of the spinal cord lesion is the presenting symptom in the vast majority of patients. This symptom usually precedes neurologic deterioration by weeks to months, but occasionally it may be present for only a few hours.

Onset of radicular radiation of the pain (involvement of the territory of a nerve root) heralds progression. Radiation of the pain may be bilateral, especially when the thoracic spine is involved. This is followed by weakness, paresthesias, and sensory impairment (especially to vibration) of the distal lower extremity. Bladder and bowel dysfunction occurs with rapid progression of symptoms over hours to days. Sensory and motor impairment soon ascends to a spinal cord level just below the site of the lesion.

B. IMAGING

X-rays of the spine will usually reveal bony destruction by the tumor at the involved vertebral level. Demonstrate the extent of the lesion by MRI. If a myelogram is necessary, access to the subarachnoid space above the lesion is most easily obtained via a lateral C1-C2 puncture.

Treatment & Disposition

Patients with this diagnosis should be given corticosteroids immediately to reduce peritumoral edema (eg, dexamethasone, 10 mg intravenously, followed by 4 mg every 6 hours intravenously or orally). Obtain emergency neurosurgical and neurologic consultation.

Hospitalization is required for decompression by laminectomy or local radiotherapy. The latter is as effective as surgery (regardless of the tumor type) and is associated with fewer side effects.

TRANSVERSE MYELITIS

 ## ESSENTIALS OF DIAGNOSIS

- *Rapid onset of motor and sensory loss.*
- *Sphincter disturbances.*

General Considerations

Transverse myelitis is a poorly defined entity that is usually idiopathic but may be a manifestation of a known systemic disease (eg, multiple sclerosis, systemic lupus erythematosus, vitamin B_{12} deficiency). It may also result from acute hyperextension injury of the cervical spine (central cord syndrome).

Clinical Findings

A. Symptoms and Signs

The presenting symptoms are equally divided between motor weakness, sensory loss or paresthesia, and back and radicular pain. Symptoms and signs of transverse (bilateral) cord involvement may progress to a maximum level within hours. Vertebral tenderness to percussion is noted in about half of cases.

B. Imaging

An MRI or myelogram is *required* to exclude a compressive lesion; myelography will almost always demonstrate free flow of contrast material.

Treatment & Disposition

Treatment is supportive only. Partial to full recovery may occur over a period of weeks to months. Hospitalization is recommended for diagnosis and supportive care. Steroid treatment is frequently used, but its benefit is uncertain.

SPINAL EPIDURAL ABSCESS

 ESSENTIALS OF DIAGNOSIS

- *Majority located along spinal neuraxis.*
- *Hematogenous spread with seeding of epidural space (eg, intravenous drug use, infected indwelling catheters, urinary tract infection, abdominal infection).*
- *Extension of adjacent vertebral osteomyelitis, penetrating trauma, or recent neurosurgery.*
- *Fever, localized back pain; maybe subtle, radiating pain (along nerve root); sensory disturbances.*
- *Tenderness to percussion or palpation.*
- *Reflexes may be hypoactive, absent, brisk, or spastic.*

- *Immediate imaging: MRI (procedure of choice), CT scan myelography, conventional myelography.*
- *Lumbar puncture relatively contraindicated.*

Spinal epidural abscess is one eighth as common as transverse myelitis, but it may be associated with remarkably similar signs and symptoms.

Clinical Findings

The most common predisposing conditions include local staphylococcal infections of the skin and surgical wounds (including intravenous sites), bacteremia, vertebral osteomyelitis, and intravenous drug abuse.

A. Symptoms and Signs

Patients are usually febrile and appear acutely ill on presentation. Focal pain and localized tenderness over the abscess are nearly consistent findings. Classically, symptoms progress over a few days from local vertebral column pain to radiating radicular pain. Cord compression with weakness and sensory loss below the level of the lesion follows.

B. Imaging

Plain x-rays of the spine reveal osteomyelitic lesions in about 85% of cases, especially in patients with symptoms of long duration (weeks). MRI or myelography will show a complete block of cerebrospinal fluid flow in over 80% of cases.

C. Laboratory Findings

Lumbar puncture (*only* at the time of myelography) should be done with great care; the operator should aspirate frequently to make certain that the needle is not advanced through the abscess, allowing pus to enter the subarachnoid space. Culture of cerebrospinal fluid is usually negative, but Gram-stained smears and cultures of pus from the abscess reveal the causative organism in almost all cases. The cerebrospinal fluid cell count, glucose, and protein content are listed in Table 18–2.

Treatment & Disposition

Hospitalization is required for emergency surgical decompression by laminectomy, abscess drainage, and intravenous antimicrobial therapy. Selected patients without significant weakness can be managed with antibiotics alone.

DISEASE OF ANTERIOR HORN CELLS

POLIOMYELITIS

 **ESSENTIALS OF DIAGNOSIS**

Nonparalytic

- *Headache, fever, sore throat, nausea, vomiting, muscle aches.*

Paralytic

- *Severe muscle pain, spasms, weakness.*
- *Asymmetric: lower limbs affected more than upper limbs.*
- *Flaccid muscle tone.*
- *Brisk to absent reflexes.*
- *Patient complains of paresthesias but with no sensory loss.*

Bulbar Form

- *Involves spinal cord.*
- *Dysphagia, dysphasia.*
- *Shallow respirations, hiccups.*
- *Diaphragm paralysis.*
- *Autonomic dysfunction.*

General Considerations

Although now uncommon in the western world, poliomyelitis continues to occur in single cases or isolated epidemics in unimmunized populations. Other enteroviruses and attenuated (vaccine) strains of poliovirus may cause a similar syndrome.

Clinical Findings

A. Symptoms and Signs

Poliomyelitis begins as a viral syndrome with fever, myalgias, headache, and upper respiratory or gastrointestinal symptoms. Nuchal rigidity and photophobia are common. Neurologic involvement follows this prodrome in about 1% of cases, with rapid onset of weakness that progresses over 3–5 days. Flaccid paralysis then occurs, is usually asymmetric or even unilateral, and more commonly involves the legs than the arms.

Sensation is unimpaired. Cranial nerves are involved in 10–20% of cases (bulbar poliomyelitis); the most common manifestations are facial and pharyngeal weakness, which can be unilateral. Diaphragmatic and intercostal muscle involvement may lead to respiratory failure.

B. Laboratory Findings

Lumbar puncture will show a cerebrospinal fluid cell count of 25–500 cells/μL. Neutrophils predominate early, and lymphocytes predominate later. Cerebrospinal fluid protein and glucose are normal early. The diagnosis can be confirmed by recovery of virus (from stool, cerebrospinal fluid, or throat washings) or by demonstration of a 4-fold rise in antibody titer against the virus.

Treatment & Disposition

Hospitalization is mandatory, and public health associates should be notified promptly (by telephone, fax machine, or e-mail). No specific therapy is available.

POSTPOLIOMYELITIS SYNDROME

Clinical Findings

Postpoliomyelitis syndrome is characterized by the onset of new, slowly progressive weakness, fatigue, and pain in patients with a history of paralytic poliomyelitis years previously. Symptoms are the result of ongoing denervation of muscles involved in the prior attack that had subsequently reinnervated. Electromyography and muscle biopsy confirm active denervation.

Treatment & Disposition

Hospitalization is rarely needed, because progression of dysfunction is slow. No specific treatment is available, but physical therapy may be beneficial.

PERIPHERAL NEUROPATHIES

MONONEUROPATHIES

1. Bell Palsy (Facial Weakness) (See also Chapter 32.)

 ESSENTIALS OF DIAGNOSIS

- *Cranial nerve VII paralysis.*
- *Abrupt, isolated, unilateral, peripheral facial paralysis.*

- *Diagnosis of exclusion; unknown cause.*
- *Entire face is involved on affected side (unlike in cortical stroke, where upper third of face is spared).*
- *Clinical findings determine tests to be ordered.*

General Considerations

Bell palsy is a common condition of unknown cause (although some authorities suggest a link with herpes simplex infection). Although manifestations of the disorder are dramatic, recovery usually begins within 1 month, and complete resolution of symptoms occurs in 70–85% of patients. All patients with initial subtotal facial paralysis will make a cosmetically complete functional recovery.

Clinical Findings

Diagnostic features include the following:

- Development of symptoms over less than 24–48 hours
- Unilateral involvement of the facial nerve
- No signs of other nervous system involvement
- Postauricular pain (not required for diagnosis)

Differential Diagnosis

The major differential diagnostic possibilities—and those of most concern to patients—are stroke and tumor. Tumors in the region of the facial nerve rarely cause sudden onset of symptoms and usually produce abnormalities of other facial nerves, resulting in nystagmus, decreased hearing, and ataxia. Facial numbness may suggest involvement of the trigeminal nerve, but patients with Bell palsy often describe pure facial weakness in sensory terms (eg, "My face is numb.").

Stroke with facial weakness is associated with weakness of the ipsilateral arm and probably the ipsilateral leg also (most easily detectable in the extensors of the arm and the flexors of the leg). Stroke produces an upper motor neuron lesion, thereby sparing the muscles of the forehead. Bell palsy, however, involves the facial nerve itself and produces unilateral weakness of all facial muscles (those of the forehead, those responsible for eye closure, and those around the mouth). Other facial nerve functions may be involved, such as unilateral decrease of lacrimation and taste and increase in apparent intensity of sounds (eg, when talking on the telephone).

Laboratory Tests & Other Examinations

When the diagnosis is clear on clinical grounds, no further evaluation or radiographic studies (CT scans or MRI) are indicated.

Treatment & Disposition

Although Bell palsy is cosmetically disfiguring during the acute phase, the more serious concern is the risk for eye injury owing to inability to close the eyelid completely. Artificial tears should be instilled frequently during waking hours, and the lid should be taped closed (under careful instruction) when the patient is asleep to prevent corneal abrasions and ulcers. Corticosteroids may affect the ultimate recovery of motor function; corticosteroids such as prednisone, 40–60 mg/d orally for 10 days, decrease the postauricular pain often associated with acute Bell palsy. Acyclovir, 400 mg 5 times daily for 10 days with steroids, has been shown to provide a faster recovery. All patients should be referred to a neurologist, otolaryngologist, or primary care physician within a few days, regardless of whether corticosteroids have been given. Hospitalization is not required.

2. Compressive Mononeuropathies

General Considerations

Compressive mononeuropathies usually occur because prolonged compression of a superficial peripheral nerve interrupts blood flow, producing ischemic injury. This may result from sleep in an unusual position or from prolonged fixed position of a limb due to drug intoxication or general anesthesia.

Radial Nerve Palsy

Paralysis of the radial nerve produces complete but isolated wrist and finger drop (inability to extend the wrist or fingers) with inconsistent sensory loss over the radial portion of the dorsum of the hand. Such injuries occur from compression of the nerve against the humerus in patients sedated with alcohol or other drugs (Saturday night palsy) or during sleep with a partner (bridegroom's palsy). If the radial nerve is compressed in the axilla, as occurs in crutch palsy, the triceps muscle is affected as well, resulting in the additional finding of weakness of extension at the elbow.

Complete recovery over weeks to months is the rule. Immediate treatment measures include splinting of the wrist or application of a sling and referral to a primary care physician, hand specialist, or neurologist.

Ulnar Palsy

Acute injury of the ulnar nerve occurs at the elbow following fracture or dislocation. Delayed ("tardy") ulnar nerve palsies result from repeated trauma, such as resting of upper body weight on the elbows. Wasting and weakness of the hands ultimately produce a claw posture (hyperextension at the metacarpophalangeal joint and flexion at the interphalangeal joints that are maximal in the fourth and fifth digits). Sensory loss occurs in the ulnar border of the dorsal and palmar aspects of the hand below the wrist, extending to involve the fourth and fifth fingers. Injury to the ulnar nerve in the palm (eg, cycle-racing palsy) spares the sensory fibers.

Initial management consists of padding of the elbow and referral to a primary care physician, hand specialist, or neurologist.

Peroneal Nerve Palsy

Nerve compression occurs at the head of the fibula as a result of acute trauma (eg, fibular fracture, or sleeping or sitting with the legs crossed). The resulting footdrop produces a high-stepping gait in the involved limb, with inability to dorsiflex or evert the foot on examination. Some sensory loss may be found over the dorsum of the foot and the lateral aspects of the leg.

Lesions at the root of L5 (eg, disk disease) also produce footdrop but involve other muscles innervated by L5 as well (eg, foot invertors and knee flexors).

Immediate management in the emergency department or upon referral to an orthopedist, primary care physician, neurologist, or physical medicine specialist consists of splinting the foot at a right angle (cock-up splint) to normalize the gait.

POLYNEUROPATHIES

1. Guillain-Barré Syndrome (Infectious Polyneuritis)

ESSENTIALS OF DIAGNOSIS

- *Most common acute neuromuscular paralytic syndrome in the United States.*
- *Acute ascending progressive neuropathy starting in lower extremities; weakness is symmetric.*
- *Paresthesias, hyporeflexia.*
- *Muscle weakness may lead to respiratory failure (25% of cases).*
- *Labile autonomic dysfunction (labile vital signs).*
- *Pain in low back, buttocks, thighs, shoulders.*

- *Facial weakness, dysphasia, or dysarthria may be present.*
- *Anhidrosis, paralytic ileus, urinary hesitancy.*
- *Decreased to absent reflexes.*
- *History of gastrointestinal or respiratory infection (approximately 1–3 weeks prior to onset of weakness).*

General Considerations

Guillain-Barré syndrome is a common disease of uncertain cause involving the peripheral nerves and occurring in both sexes and all age groups, although the disease seems milder in children.

In one half to two thirds of cases, a mild upper respiratory infection or gastroenteritis precedes the onset of the neurologic disease by 1–3 weeks. Well-documented cases have also been recorded following surgery, other viral infections, immunization (eg, influenza vaccine), and acute glomerulonephritis or as an acute seroconversion reaction to HIV infection. Marked hypophosphatemia can produce a nearly identical syndrome.

Clinical Findings

A. SYMPTOMS AND SIGNS

Symmetric weakness is the major symptom. It may be either proximal or distal at onset and usually begins in the lower extremities. The weakness classically progresses in an ascending manner, involving first the lower and then the upper extremities and finally the cranial nerves within 1–3 days of symptom onset. The weakness does not ascend in all cases, however.

Subjective and objective sensory disturbances (numbness or paresthesias) of brief duration are common initially and may be the presenting complaint. These dysesthesias most commonly occur in a distal (stocking-glove) distribution. Muscle pain or tenderness is also an early symptom in about half of cases.

Absence of the deep tendon reflexes (or, rarely, only distal areflexia with definite hyporeflexia of biceps and knee jerks) almost always occurs by the time of presentation to a physician. **Note:** This loss of reflexes is the most important clue to diagnosis and is found even in muscles that cannot yet be shown to be weak by objective testing.

Cranial nerve (CN) involvement is common; involvement of every nerve except CNs I and II (olfactory and optic) has been described. The nerve most commonly affected is CN VII (facial); facial weakness (usually bilateral) occurs in half of cases. Cranial nerve palsies may be the most prominent feature of the illness, as in the Guillain-Barré variant of ophthalmoplegia, ataxia, and areflexia.

Peripheral autonomic nervous system involvement also occurs and may be manifested by hypertension, tachycardia, facial flushing, postural hypotension, and electrocardiographic changes. Respiratory musculature weakness requiring assisted ventilation occurs in 25% of cases.

B. LABORATORY FINDINGS

Increased spinal fluid pressure is seen only in severe cases. The cerebrospinal fluid cell count is normal initially in most patients; less than 10% of patients have more than 10 leukocytes per microliter. The classic elevation in cerebrospinal fluid protein to levels as high as 100–400 mg/dL in the absence of significant pleocytosis (so-called albuminocytologic dissociation) may not be seen until several days after the onset of symptoms. These cerebrospinal fluid findings support the diagnosis of Guillain-Barré syndrome, but they are not specific and may be seen occasionally in any acute or chronic polyneuritis.

Treatment & Disposition

Endotracheal intubation and ventilatory support should be considered in the emergency department for patients in respiratory failure. Plasmapheresis begun within 10 days of the first symptoms in the severely affected patient may shorten the need for mechanical ventilation. Corticosteroids are ineffective and may prolong the disease in elderly patients. All patients should be hospitalized.

2. Arsenical Neuropathy

ESSENTIALS OF DIAGNOSIS

- *Arsenic is found in certain water supplies and seafood; used in production of glass and semiconductors (industrial exposure).*
- *Painful peripheral neuropathy.*
- *Acute poisoning: vomiting and severe diarrhea leading to dehydration and shock.*
- *Chronic poisoning: classical dermatitis, peripheral neuropathy, chronic renal and hepatic damage.*
- *Arsenic gas: acute hemolytic anemia and chills, hemoglobinuria (black urine).*

General Considerations

The neuropathy of arsenic poisoning is a rapidly progressive sensorimotor polyneuropathy that in many ways mimics Guillain-Barré syndrome. Common sources of arsenic include rat and ant poison and the copper acetoarsenite contained in insecticides (eg, Paris green). Fowler's solution, once used for psoriasis, also contains arsenic. Patients with chronic symptoms may represent attempted murder.

Clinical Findings

A. SYMPTOMS AND SIGNS

Abdominal pain, nausea and vomiting, and diarrhea occur minutes to hours following ingestion. A rapidly progressive polyneuropathy ensues 7–14 days later. Symmetric ascending paresthesias, initially distal, begin in the lower extremities and progress to overt sensory loss.

Diffuse muscle aches and tenderness are common, as is a burning pain on the soles of the feet that is markedly aggravated by touching the skin. Deep tendon reflexes are depressed early and in the same distribution as the sensory loss.

Symmetric motor impairment follows as the neuropathy progresses over days to a few weeks and is typically more severe distally and in the lower extremities and can lead to flaccid paralysis. The cranial nerves, rectal sphincter, and respiratory muscles are unaffected.

Cutaneous stigmata of arsenical poisoning include increased skin pigmentation and marked exfoliation (especially of the hands and feet). Mees's lines (transverse white, nonpalpable lines on the nails) are especially suggestive of arsenic poisoning but do not appear until 40–60 days after ingestion because of the slow rate of nail growth.

B. LABORATORY FINDINGS

Cerebrospinal fluid findings are similar to those seen with Guillain-Barré syndrome: glucose and cell counts are normal, and protein is elevated, although usually less than 100 mg/dL.

The diagnosis is established by documenting elevated concentrations of arsenic in urine (upper limits of normal: 0.1 mg/24 h) or hair protected from external contamination, most commonly pubic hair (upper limits of normal: 0.1 mg/100 g of hair).

C. IMAGING

If continued ingestion of arsenic is suspected, abdominal x-ray may be helpful, because arsenic is radiopaque.

Treatment

(See also Chapter 45.) Symptomatic patients should be given a chelating agent to facilitate excretion of arsenic.

Treatment must be started within 24 hours after ingestion to influence the course of the neuropathy. Give dimercaprol, 3–4 mg/kg/dose intramuscularly every 4 hours for 48 hours, then 3 mg/kg every 12 hours for a total of 10 days; or penicillamine, 100 mg/kg/d orally (maximum: 1 g/d) divided into 4 doses for 5 days. Either course may be repeated if the patient is still symptomatic. Follow urine arsenic levels, because hair and nail levels do not reflect acute changes.

Disposition

If arsenic poisoning is diagnosed or suspected, hospitalization is indicated for evaluation and treatment.

3. Acute Intermittent Porphyria

 ESSENTIALS OF DIAGNOSIS

- *More common in 18- to 40-year-old age group.*
- *Autonomic neuropathy: constipation, colicky abdominal pain, vomiting, hypertension.*
- *Peripheral neuropathy.*
- *Seizure, delirium, coma.*
- *Depression.*
- *Areflexia.*
- *Any nerve can be involved.*

General Considerations

Acute intermittent porphyria (the most common form) is recognized as an autosomal dominant with variable penetrance disorder. It involves porphyrin metabolism producing episodic clinical symptoms, most commonly in the third to sixth decades. Women are affected much more frequently than men. Attacks are often precipitated by drugs that affect porphyrin metabolism (especially barbiturates and sulfonamides; see Table 18–3), infection, or fasting.

Clinical Findings

A. SYMPTOMS AND SIGNS

Abdominal pain is the most common manifestation of porphyria (85% of cases). The abdominal pain is severe, often colicky, and may be generalized or localized. Onset of pain may precede development of other signs or symptoms by several weeks. Vomiting, constipation, and abdominal distention often lead to exploratory laparotomy, even though these signs are manifestations of an autonomic peripheral neuropathy.

Table 18–3. Contraindicated and accepted drugs in treatment of acute intermittent porphyria.

Contraindicated drugs
Barbiturates (including thiopental anesthesia)
Sulfonamids
Griseofulvin
Chlordiazepoxide
Meprobamate
Phenytoin
Glutethimide
Imipramine
Ergot preparations
Methyprylon
Methsuximide
Tolbutamide
Amidopyrine-containing compounds (antipyrine)
Oral contraceptive agents
Drugs that may be safely used
Meperidine
Chlorpromazine and most other phenothiazines
Aspirin
Penicillins
Tetracyclines
Digoxin
Diazepam
Diphenhydramine

Weakness due to a predominantly motor polyneuropathy is the major neurologic manifestation. It is usually symmetric, beginning in the upper or lower extremities and most often proximally rather than distally. The neuropathy usually progresses slowly over days to weeks and is believed to result from axonal degeneration. Occasionally, completed flaccid quadriparesis with associated respiratory paralysis requiring mechanical ventilation occurs over a few days.

Cranial nerve involvement is common, especially CN VII, the vagus nerve (CN X), and the nerves to the extraocular muscles. Deep tendon reflexes are depressed or absent, except for a curious preservation of the ankle jerks in some patients. Signs of sensory or autonomic neurologic involvement are usually less prominent.

Seizures, acute psychosis, hypotension, oliguria, and hyponatremia also occur. Tachycardia (> 100 beats/min) is nearly always present because of catecholamine release during acute attacks.

B. LABORATORY FINDINGS

Cerebrospinal fluid pressure and glucose concentration are normal; protein concentration is slightly elevated (not over 100 mg/dL), and there may be a modest pleocytosis (<10 leukocytes per microliter). The diagnosis is established by measurement of excess urinary porphobilinogen, for which rapid qualitative determination is available with the Watson-Schwartz test.

Treatment & Disposition

Hospitalization is indicated for initiation of high-carbohydrate therapy (eg, intravenous glucose) and management of pain. Opiates, phenothiazines, and benzodiazepines (eg, diazepam) may be used safely for relief of pain and anxiety. Barbiturates are contraindicated. The autonomic manifestations associated with the attack can be treated with propranolol. The neuropathy and abdominal pain may be relieved by protoporphyrin IX (Hematin), 3–4 mg/kg/d for 4 days. Cimetidine has been used for Hematin-resistant cases. Maintain electrolyte balance.

4. Tick Paralysis

General Considerations

Tick paralysis is a rapidly ascending motor paralysis caused by an injected neurotoxin from the female *Dermacentor andersoni* (wood tick) and *Dermacentor variabilis* (dog tick). Symptoms begin after the ticks have been attached to the patient for 5–7 days. The disease is endemic in the southeastern and northwestern United States and in western Canada.

Clinical Findings

A. Symptoms and Signs

Most cases occur in children. Neurologic symptoms begin with ataxia and lower extremity weakness, the latter progressing over 24–48 hours to involve the upper extremities and cranial nerves. Reflexes are diminished or absent early. Respiratory depression occurs and may be fatal. Distal extremity paresthesias are common, but objective sensory loss is rare.

B. Laboratory Findings

Cerebrospinal fluid and peripheral blood examinations are normal.

Treatment

The tick may be attached to any portion of the body but is most commonly hidden in long hair about the head and neck. Removal of the entire tick by application of ether, gasoline, or petroleum is followed by symptomatic improvement within hours. Complete re-

solution of symptoms occurs within a few days to a week.

Disposition

Patients in the acute phase must be hospitalized for supportive management.

5. Diphtheritic Polyneuritis

 ESSENTIALS OF DIAGNOSIS

- Patients may present with nonspecific symptoms (fever, malaise, hoarseness, nausea and vomiting).
- Neurologic exam includes cranial nerve and peripheral nerve palsies in lower extremities.
- Progressive proximal to distal weakness.

Clinical Findings

A. Symptoms and Signs

In diphtheritic polyneuritis, the cranial and peripheral nerves are affected 2–3 weeks following infection—the cranial nerves first, especially the palate and the muscles of ocular accommodation. The patient complains of inability to focus secondary to impaired visual accommodation paresis of the ocular muscles. Although this disease is rare in the United States, it is still seen elsewhere. Involvement of the nerve supply to the pharynx, larynx, face, extraocular muscles, and extremities occurs as the illness progresses over days to weeks. Reflexes are lost early. Sensory signs are not prominent, although distal paresthesias may be noted.

Symptoms are usually maximal within 1–2 weeks. Gradual (usually complete) improvement then follows over months, although associated myocarditis may produce a significant number of deaths.

B. Laboratory Findings

Cerebrospinal fluid protein is elevated to 100–400 mg/dL. Recovery of the organisms from the pharynx or wound confirms the diagnosis, although such cultures may be negative by the time neuropathy is manifested.

Treatment & Disposition

There is no specific treatment. Administration of diphtheria antitoxin will not abort the neuropathy once symptoms have appeared. Patients must be hospitalized for supportive care.

6. Paralytic Seafood Poisoning
(See also Chapter 44.)

ESSENTIALS OF DIAGNOSIS

- *One of four distinct shellfish poisonings.*
- *Paresthesias of lips, tongue, gums within 30 minutes of ingestion.*
- *Muscle weakness, paralysis, cranial nerve dysfunction.*
- *Nausea, vomiting, diarrhea.*
- *Airway support required.*

Clinical Findings

Saxitoxin may be present in Atlantic and Pacific shellfish, especially between May and October, and can produce a fulminating sensorimotor polyneuropathy. Numbness and tingling of the fingers, toes, and perioral region are associated with a rapidly ascending motor paralysis that can begin within minutes following ingestion. Bizarre dysesthesias (eg, sensation that teeth are loose in their sockets; reversal of hot and cold sensation) are common and specific to saxitoxin or ciguatoxin poisoning. Ingestion of puffer fish containing tetrodotoxin may produce the same symptoms.

Treatment & Disposition

There is no available antitoxin. Supportive care (including mechanical ventilation if indicated) is followed by complete recovery. Hospitalization is indicated for infants and elderly victims and for patients with respiratory insufficiency or objective weakness.

DISEASES OF THE NEUROMUSCULAR JUNCTION
BOTULISM

ESSENTIALS OF DIAGNOSIS

- *Afebrile (unless other infection is present).*
- *Symmetric neurologic symptomatology.*
- *Patient remains responsive.*
- *Heart rate is normal or bradycardic; hypotension is absent.*

- *Progressive, symmetric, descending weakness, first in muscles innervated by cranial nerves, then neck, arms, and legs.*
- *Dry mouth, diplopia, dysarthria, generalized weakness.*

General Considerations

Clostridium botulinum toxin attacks the neuromuscular junction by impairing the release of acetylcholine at all peripheral synapses. Paralysis occurs mainly following the ingestion of foods contaminated with the toxin and only rarely from infected wounds. In infants, cases have resulted from colonization of the gastrointestinal tract by *C botulinum* (originating, in some cases, from ingested honey). Although commercially canned foods have caused epidemics, most cases have been due to improperly home-canned vegetables, fruits, meat, and fish. Ingestion of even a few drops of contaminated food may cause botulism. The distribution of the toxin in the contaminated vehicle may not be uniform. Fruits or vegetables contaminated with type A or B toxin will taste spoiled; other foods may not. Contaminated foods must be boiled for over 10 minutes in order for the toxin to be reliably inactivated.

Clinical Findings

A. SYMPTOMS AND SIGNS

Symptoms usually begin 12–48 hours following toxin ingestion and may progress over hours to days (Table 18–4). The shorter the interval between ingestion and the appearance of symptoms, the more severe the disease. The nervous system is involved in descending

Table 18–4. Symptoms and signs of botulism in approximate order of frequency.

Symptoms	Signs
Nausea and vomiting	Extraocular muscle weakness
Generalized weakness	Ptosis
Blurred vision	Bilateally dilated and unreactive pupils
Diplopia	Dry mucous membranes
Dysphagia	Limb weakness
Dyspnea	Respiratory impairment
Dry mouth	Postural hypotension
Dizziness (especially postural)	
Constipation	
Abdominal fullness	

fashion, beginning with the muscles innervated by the cranial nerves. This contrasts with Guillain-Barré syndrome, in which there is usually ascending involvement.

Nausea and vomiting are the initial symptoms in one third of cases (prominent with type E toxin). Blurring of vision (due to paralysis of muscles of accommodation) is the most common initial neurologic symptom. Diplopia, dysphagia, and dysphonia come on in sequence as lower bulbar muscles become involved. Weakness of respiratory and extremity muscles follows as the paralysis descends. Ptosis, extraocular muscle paralysis, and pupillary dilatation and fixation follow, and then weakness of jaw and palate function. Some deep tendon reflex activity remains until muscle paralysis is complete.

Dryness of mucous membranes and orthostatic hypotension have been prominent features in some patients. Sweating, salivation, and bronchorrhea (seen in cholinesterase inhibitor poisoning) do not occur. There are no sensory abnormalities.

Infant botulism is characterized by poor feeding, poor muscle tone, episodes of aspiration, and constipation.

B. Laboratory Findings

Examination of cerebrospinal fluid and peripheral blood smears is not helpful unless a superimposed condition develops (eg, aspiration pneumonia). Specimens of blood or contaminated food should be saved for laboratory assay for botulinum toxins (available through local public health departments). Blood samples should consist of 30 mL of clotted, nonheparinized blood, which need not be centrifuged or separated but must be collected before the antitoxin is started. In infants, save a sample of stool for culture for *C botulinum* (consult the local public health department for details).

C. Electrocardiographic Findings

T wave inversions, conduction abnormalities, and ventricular arrhythmias may occur.

Treatment

A. Antitoxin

Bivalent or trivalent antitoxin should be given as soon as possible after diagnosis. Skin testing should be performed before administration of antitoxin because of the risk of anaphylaxis. The current recommended dose of licensed botulinum antitoxin is a single 10 mL vial (per patient), diluted 1:10 in a 0.9% saline solution and given in a slow intravenous infusion. Antitoxin and consultation may be obtained in the United States by telephoning the Centers for Disease Control in Atlanta: (404) 639-2206 (days) or (404) 639-2888 (nights, week-

ends, and holidays). The local health department should be notified immediately as well (by any telecommunications method). Although the mortality rate has been reported to be as high as 60–70%, rapid diagnosis and adequate respiratory support should improve the outlook. Recovery of neurologic function occurs over weeks to months; complete recovery is common.

Serum sickness may develop as a result of administration of antitoxin. Neostigmine and other drugs effective in treating myasthenia gravis are not helpful in botulism.

B. Antibiotics

The treatment of wound botulism is debridement and penicillin, 300,000 units/kg/d intravenously, in addition to other measures described above. Clindamycin, 30 mg/kg/d intravenously, or chloramphenicol, 50 mg/kg/d intravenously, may be used in penicillin-allergic patients. Aminoglycosides may worsen neuromuscular blockade and should be avoided.

C. Additional Measures

Careful monitoring of vital capacity, maximum inspiratory force, and arterial blood gases is mandatory, because respiratory insufficiency may develop rapidly. Cathartics and enemas must be given early to remove any toxin remaining in the bowel. Emesis or gastric lavage is indicated if the contaminated food was ingested less than 6–8 hours before arrival at the emergency department. All other persons who have also eaten the suspected food should be given antitoxin, emetics, and cathartics even if they are asymptomatic.

Disposition

The patient must be hospitalized for observation and treatment.

ORGANOPHOSPHATE POISONING (See also Chapter 45.)

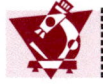

ESSENTIALS OF DIAGNOSIS

- *DUMBELS: **d**iarrhea, **u**rination, **m**iosis, **b**ronchospasm, **e**mesis, **l**acrimation, **s**alivation.*
- *Organophosphates can be absorbed through lungs, skin, gastrointestinal tract, mucous membranes.*
- *Symptoms appear within hours of exposure (but immediately with large doses).*
- *Respiratory paresis.*

General Considerations

Organophosphates exert their toxic effect by inhibiting acetylcholinesterase, producing stimulation and then inhibition at the myoneural junction by the uncatabolized acetylcholine. Poisoning is most commonly due to insecticides (eg, parathion, malathion) and occurs during spraying or dusting of crops. Certain poison gases used in war have a similar action.

Clinical Findings

Rapidity of onset and severity of symptoms vary with the dose and route of administration; symptoms of poisoning may occur within 5 minutes to 12 hours after exposure.

A. SYMPTOMS AND SIGNS

(See Table 18–5.) Initial symptoms are fatigue, headache, dizziness, nausea and vomiting, and increased salivary and sweat production. Weakness of skeletal and bulbar muscles with marked fasciculations follows, and finally loss of consciousness occurs.

Examination often reveals the characteristic garlic odor of the organophosphate compound. Lacrimation is common, and pupils are pinpoint and may be unreactive to light. Muscle fasciculations and complete motor paralysis may be present.

B. LABORATORY FINDINGS

Hyperglycemia with prominent glycosuria may occur. Polymorphonuclear leukocytosis is common. Laboratory demonstration of depressed plasma and erythrocyte cholinesterase activity confirms the clinical diagnosis.

Treatment

See also Chapter 39.

A. DECONTAMINATION

Maintain airway and respiratory function, and remove residual organophosphate by washing the skin and removing exposed clothing. Ingested organophosphates should be removed by lavage and catharsis. Induction of emesis is usually contraindicated because of the early onset of drowsiness and risk of aspiration. In this case, protect the airway and perform gastric lavage.

B. SPECIFIC MEASURES

Atropine, a specific antidote, is the treatment of choice; however, it does not reverse paralytic symptoms. Large doses may be required. Start with 2 mg intravenously (children, 0.5 mg), followed by repeated doses of 2–4 mg every 5–10 minutes (children < age 12 years, 0.05–0.10 mg/kg every 15 minutes, repeated as needed

Table 18–5. Manifestations of organophosphate poisoning.[1,2]

Symptoms and Signs	Severity of Poisoning		
	Severe (%)	Moderate (%)	Mild (%)
Weakness	100	100	100
Headache	100	100	95
Hyperhidrosis	100	91	91
Nausea and vomiting	100	100	77
Salivation and lacrimation	93	73	45
Miotic pupils	100	55	23
Dyspnea	100	55	14
Difficulty in walking	100	73	0
Diarrhea	64	36	36
Muscle fasciculation	100	55	0
Disturbance in speech	100	55	0
Disturbance in consciousness	100	55	0
Abdominal pain	36	36	27
Fever	64	55	0
Bronchopharyngeal secretions	71	36	0
Increase in blood pressure	71	18	0
Loss in pupillary reflex	71	0	0
Muscle cramps	64	0	0
Cyanosis	57	0	0

[1]Based on 47 cases of parathion poisoning; presented as percentage of total cases.
[2]Modified and reproduced, with permission, from Namba T et al: Poisoning due to organophosphate insecticides. *Am J Med* 1971;50:475.

for symptom control) until signs of atropinization occur: flushing, mydriasis, drying of secretions, and tachycardia. The use of up to 50 mg in 24 hours is not unusual.

Pralidoxime (Protopam, 2-Pam) releases organophosphates from acetylcholinesterase and should be given to all patients with significant poisoning. It should not be used for carbamate poisoning, because carbamates are not irreversibly bound to acetylcholinesterase. The dose is 20–40 mg/kg in saline intravenously over 20–30 minutes. The dose may be repeated in 1–2 hours. Adequate renal function is a prerequisite for use of pralidoxime, because it is excreted in the urine.

Benzodiazepines may be used for seizure control.

Disposition

All patients except for the very mildly ill with stable or improving symptoms require hospitalization. The earlier treatment is instituted, the lower the mortality rate.

MYASTHENIA GRAVIS

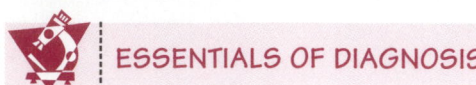

ESSENTIALS OF DIAGNOSIS

- *Rare, autoimmune disorder.*
- *Bulbar muscles most common and severe (ptosis, diplopia, blurred vision, difficulty swallowing, dysarthria).*
- *Muscle weakness provoked by repetitive use of muscles involved (eg, climbing stairs) with recovery during rest.*
- *Decreased ability to clear secretions or generate adequate respirations.*

Clinical Findings

Musculature innervated by the cranial nerves is commonly the earliest and most severely involved in myasthenia gravis, as manifested by ptosis and by impaired eye movements, facial expressions, chewing, swallowing, and speaking. Pupillary responsiveness is preserved. There is increasing weakness on repetitive muscle use ("fatigability"). Sensory abnormalities are absent. The diagnosis in previously untreated myasthenia gravis is confirmed by objective and unequivocal improvement following anticholinesterase drugs, for example, edrophonium (Tensilon, others) (for dosage, see differential diagnosis in "Neuromuscular Blockade" section, above) or the longer-acting neostigmine (Prostigmin) (1–1.5 mg intramuscularly; effect in 45-

90 minutes). Stable patients with myasthenia gravis will be following one of the drug regimens listed in Table 18–6.

The acute occurrence of respiratory insufficiency or the inability to handle oropharyngeal secretions in a previously stable myasthenic patient constitutes a myasthenic crisis. Crises may be precipitated by intercurrent infection or surgery or may have no obvious cause. The subjective complaint of dyspnea in such patients demands immediate and careful evaluation.

The difference between myasthenic and cholinergic crisis is of little practical importance; the latter, however, appears to be uncommon.

Treatment

Immediately evaluate the need for respiratory assistance and endotracheal intubation, as described above. Temporizing with drug therapy may have disastrous consequences, because the patient may worsen within minutes. Discontinue anticholinesterase therapy in the intubated patient. Treat precipitating causes if present (eg, infection), but avoid aminoglycoside antibiotics because they may worsen myasthenia gravis. Plasmapheresis may temporarily reduce symptoms or help the patient to get over the crisis. Intravenous immunoglobulin appears to have a role in acute treatment intervention when other modalities have failed.

Disposition

All patients in myasthenic crisis require immediate hospitalization. Stable patients without any respiratory symptoms (not in crisis) may receive medical treatment (Table 18–6) and be referred for outpatient care. Patients newly diagnosed as having myasthenia gravis may be hospitalized for evaluation and treatment or started on a medical regimen (Table 18–6) and referred to a clinic or private medical care.

Table 18–6. Drug therapy of stable myasthenia gravis.

Drug	Preparation	Dose	Duration of Action
Pyridostigmine (Mestinon)	60-mg tablets	1–4 tablets orally every 3–6 hours.	3–5 hours
Pyridostigmine (Mestinon)	180-mg sustained release capsules	1–3 capsules orally at bedtime.	6–12 hours
Neostigmine bromide (Prostigmin)	15-mg tablets	1–4 tablets orally every 36 hours.	2–4 hours
Neostigmine methylsulfate (Prostigmin, others)	Solution for injection; 1:1000, 1:2000, 1:4000	1 mg (2 mL of 1:2000) intramuscularly or subcutaneously.	2–4 hours

PRIMARY ACUTE MYOPATHIES

HYPOKALEMIC PERIODIC PARALYSIS

 ESSENTIALS OF DIAGNOSIS

- *May occur up to age 30 years, rare after age 50 years.*
- *Severe symmetric complete weakness.*
- *Symptoms can last up to 1 week.*
- *Exacerbated by high carbohydrate meals, cold temperatures.*
- *Potassium may be decreased but is not necessarily below normal.*
- *Increased urinary sodium, potassium, chloride.*
- *Decreased serum phosphorous.*

General Considerations

Hypokalemic periodic paralysis is characterized by episodes of profound weakness that may occur at intervals ranging from a day to years. Episodes are often precipitated by a large carbohydrate meal or a period of strenuous exercise, especially when followed by rest or sleep.

Clinical Findings

A. SYMPTOMS AND SIGNS

An attack of weakness usually lasts 2–24 hours. The weakness is painless and generalized, often beginning in the lower extremities and becoming more severe proximally. Paralysis of cranial and respiratory musculature is rare, and for this reason fatal episodes are uncommon. Extremity musculature is hypotonic during attacks. Reflexes are reduced in proportion to the muscle weakness. Sensory examination is normal.

B. LABORATORY FINDINGS

A markedly reduced serum potassium level (usually 2–3 mEq/L) during the attack, with normal potassium levels and physical examination between episodes, confirms the diagnosis.

Treatment

Give potassium chloride, about 1 mEq/kg orally at hourly intervals, until improvement occurs (usually within 3–4 hours). Many patients will require intravenous potassium chloride, with the rate of administration not exceeding 20 mEq/h. The frequency and severity of attacks can be reduced with acetazolamide, 250 mg orally 2 or 3 times a day.

Disposition

Patients having acute attacks can usually receive treatment in the emergency department and be sent home.

ACUTE ELECTROLYTE ABNORMALITIES

Profound magnesium and phosphate depletion can cause acute muscle weakness and in particular must be considered in alcoholic patients. However, the vast majority of acute clinical syndromes of muscle weakness are due to high or low serum potassium concentrations (Table 18–7). Although the onset of weakness is not well correlated with serum potassium levels, values below 3 mEq/L or above 7.5 mEq/L are most commonly associated with symptoms. Specific therapy is dictated by the cause, but the potential for life-threatening cardiac arrhythmias from severe hypokalemia or hyperkalemia demands immediate therapy (see Chapter 42).

Table 18–7. Disorders of serum potassium causing acute muscle weakness.

Hyperkalemia
  Potassium administration, orally or intravenously
  Renal insufficiency
  Potassium-retaining drug therapy: triamterene or
    spironolactone
  Acute tissue necrosis secondary to trauma or chemotherapy
  Addison disease
  Myoglobinuria
  Rhabdomyolysis
  Hypoaldosteronism
Hypokalemia
  Gastrointestinal postassium wastage
    Chronic vomiting or nasogastric suction
    Chronic diarrhea or laxative abuse
    Villous adenoma
    Draining gastrointestinal fistulas or ureteroileostomy
  Renal potassium wastage
    Drugs (diuretics, amphotericin B)
    Hyperaldosteronism
    Cushing disease or corticosteroid therapy
    Renal tubular acidosis
    Licorice (glycyrrhizic acid) intoxication

RHABDOMYOLYSIS

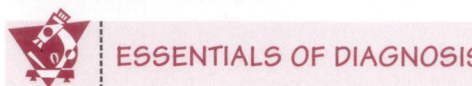

ESSENTIALS OF DIAGNOSIS

- *Myalgias and muscle weakness.*
- *Dark urine.*
- *Tenderness, decreased muscle strength, swelling, soft extremities (vs. compartment syndrome) may be present.*
- *May be secondary to infection.*

General Considerations

Release of myoglobin from the body musculature may be due to many causes (Table 18–8). Weakness presumably results from loss of this contractile protein from muscle cells. Important consequences of rhabdomyolysis with myoglobinuria are acute renal failure and marked elevations of serum potassium.

Clinical Findings

A. SYMPTOMS AND SIGNS

Pain and swelling of the involved muscles and weakness of the limbs occur, especially in proximal distribution. Reflexes are depressed in proportion to muscle weakness. Sensory examination is normal.

B. LABORATORY FINDINGS

The urine is red-tinged and turns dark brown on standing. Myoglobinuria may be suggested by a heme-positive (dipstick) test in erythrocyte-free urine and confirmed by specific chemical testing. Muscle enzymes (CK) are massively elevated in most cases.

Treatment

Treatment consists of hydration to ensure high urine volumes and prevent precipitation of myoglobin in renal tubules. If anuria is present, fluids should be administered cautiously. A recommended regimen is normal saline at a rate of 1.5 L/h. Maintain urine output at 300 mL/h. Consider mannitol and sodium bicarbonate to alkalinize the urine. Neither, however, has been shown to be superior to saline alone. Monitor urine output closely.

Disposition

Hospitalization is mandatory. Serum potassium levels should be followed closely. The prognosis of this disorder is good even with profound muscle necrosis and renal failure.

Arnon SS et al: Botulinum toxin as a biological weapon: Medical and public health management. JAMA 2001;285:1059. [PMID: 11209178]. (A review on how to recognize, diagnose and treat botulinum.)

Bella I et al: Neuromuscular disorders and acute respiratory failure. Neurol Clin 1998;16:391. [PMID: 9537968] (A review of neuromuscular disorders.)

Chao D et al: Spinal epidural abscess: A diagnostic challenge. Am Fam Physician 2002;65:1341. [PMID: 11996416] (A review on all aspects of epidural abscess.)

Dellon AL: Management of peripheral nerve problems in the upper and lower extremity using quantitative sensory testing. Hand Clin 1999;15:697. [PMID: 10563271] (A review of management of peripheral nerve problems.)

Greenstein P: Tick paralysis. Med Clin North Am 2002;86(2):441. [PMID: 11982312] (A compressive review of tick paralysis.)

Gutmann L: Periodic paralyses. Neurol Clin 2000;18:195. [PMID: 10658175] (A review of metabolic myopathies.)

Howard JF et al: Intravenous immunoglobulin for the treatment of acquired myasthenia gravis. Neurology 1998;51:S30. [PMID: 9851728] (Consensus of an expert panel on acute treatment interventions in the rapidly progressive weakness or as chronic maintenance therapy for myasthenia gravis.)

Hu H: Exposure to metals. Prim Care 2000;27:983. [PMID: 11072295] (A review of the diagnosis and treatment of heavy metal poisoning.)

Jackson CG et al: The facial nerve. Current trends in diagnosis, treatment, and rehabilitation. Med Clin North Am 1999;83: 179. [PMID: 9927969] (A comprehensive review of the diagnosis and treatment of facial nerve disorders including Bell palsy.)

Mines D et al: Poisonings: food, fish, shellfish. Emerg Med Clin North Am 1997;15:157. [PMID: 9056574] (A review of seafood-associated poisoning.)

Posner MA: Compressive ulnar neuropathies at the elbow: I. Etiology and diagnosis. J Am Acad Orthop Surg 1998;6:282. [PMID: 9753755] (A review of the diagnosis of ulnar neuropathies.)

Proposed diagnostic criteria and nosology of acute transverse myelitis. Neurology 2002;59:499. [PMID: 12236201] (A review of transverse myelitis.)

Reid RL: Radial nerve palsy. Hand Clin 1988;4:179. [PMID: 3294243] (A review article on radial nerve palsy.)

Ross MA: Acquired motor neuron disorders. Neurol Clin 1997;15:481. [PMID: 9227949] (A review article discussing acquired motor disease including poliomyelitis.)

Table 18–8. Common causes of rhabdomyolysis.

Muscle compression and necrosis secondary to prolonged coma (alcoholism, drug overdose, stroke)
Vigorous exercise, especially with poor conditioning and high environmental temperature
Status epilepticus
Delirium tremens
Chronic potassium depletion
Influenza or other acute viral infections

Sauret JM et al: Rhabdomyolysis. Am Fam Physician 2002;65:907. [PMID: 11898964] (A comprehensive review on the diagnosis and treatment of rhabdomyolysis.)

Simpson et al: Recognition and management of acute pesticide poisoning. Am Fam Physician 2002;65:1599. [PMID: 11998835] (A review of pesticide poisoning management.)

Suarez JI et al: Acute intermittent porphyria: Clinicopathologic correlation. Report of a case and review of the literature. Neurology 1997;48:1678. [PMID: 9191786] (A review of intermittent porphyria.)

Wetzel FT et al: Management of metastatic disease of the spine. Orthop Clin North Am 2000;31:611. [PMID: 11043100] (A review of the management of metastatic diseases of the spine.)

■ IV. IMMEDIATE MANAGEMENT OF LIFE-THREATENING PROBLEMS ASSOCIATED WITH STROKE

Stroke is a cerebrovascular disorder resulting from impairment of cerebral blood supply by occlusion (eg, by thrombi or emboli) or hemorrhage. It is characterized by the abrupt onset of focal neurologic deficits. The clinical manifestation depends on the area of the brain served by the involved blood vessel. Stroke is the most common serious neurologic disorder in adults and occurs most frequently after age 60 years. The mortality rate is 40% within the first month, and 50% of patients who survive will require long-term special care.

Stabilize Ventilation

A. ESTABLISH AIRWAY

Assess adequacy of airway and ventilation in all stroke patients, especially in the presence of depressed level of consciousness, absent gag reflex, respiratory difficulty, or difficulty managing secretions.

B. CONSIDER INTUBATION

Patients with inadequate ventilation (respiratory acidosis) or difficulty managing secretions will require intubation.

Search for Head Trauma

Stroke patients may sustain head injury due to incoordination or weakness. Conversely, patients with focal neurologic findings due to head trauma may be mistakenly diagnosed as suffering from stroke. If head injury is suspected from the history or clinical findings, immobilize the cervical spine. Refer to Chapter 22 for management.

Treat Cerebral Edema

Deterioration of neurologic deficits or the presence of brainstem involvement (depressed sensorium, pupillary or extraocular movement abnormality, decorticate or decerebrate posturing) suggests significant cerebral edema and impending herniation. With the exception of temporizing measures prior to surgical decompression in cerebellar or superficial lobar hemorrhage, medical therapy for cerebral edema (see Table 16–3) associated with ischemic stroke does not alter the outcome.

Treat Seizures

(See Chapter 17 for management of seizures.) Consider prophylaxis for acute seizure in patients with embolic stroke or subarachnoid hemorrhage. Give intravenous phenytoin, 15–18 mg/kg at a rate not greater than 50 mg/min, or fosphenytoin, 15—20 mg/kg PE (phenytoin equivalents) intravenously.

Treat Hypoglycemia

Occasionally patients with hypoglycemia may have focal neurologic deficits that may mimic a stroke. Confirm the presence of hypoglycemia using a glucometer or reagent strips before giving 50 mL of 50% dextrose solution. Stroke patients with elevated serum glucose may have a worsened outcome.

Obtain Emergency CT Scan

Emergency CT scan of the head should be obtained early. This is the most readily available method for reliably detecting the presence of hemorrhage and focal cerebral edema. MRI, especially diffusion weighted, has enhanced the diagnosis of ischemic stroke.

■ V. FURTHER EVALUATION OF THE PATIENT WITH STROKE

Accurate diagnosis and identification of the underlying cause of the stroke are important for appropriate evaluation and treatment. Conditions that predispose to strokes should be sought and corrected. A systematic approach to the evaluation of the patient with stroke is detailed below and can be modified depending on the urgency of the patient's condition.

History

A. DETERMINE TIME COURSE OF DEFICITS

Transient ischemic attacks (TIAs) and deficits progressive in a stepwise pattern over hours to days suggest thrombotic vascular occlusion. Abrupt onset of full neurologic deficit is characteristic of embolic stroke. Abrupt onset and rapid evolution of deficits are associated with intracerebral hemorrhage. Rapid response to stroke can result in little apparent damage. Contrarily, a stroke left undiagnosed or untreated for too long can result in neurologic damage or even death. The goal is to determine the exact time of onset of symptoms because the current recommended window of opportunity for thrombolytic therapy is 3 hours.

B. IDENTIFY RISK FACTORS

Hypertension, diabetes mellitus, TIAs, hyperlipidemia, smoking, family history, and use of oral contraceptives predispose to atherosclerotic disease. Cardiac disorders such as changing cardiac rhythms (especially atrial fibrillation), dyskinetic myocardium, and valvular heart disease are associated with increased risk for embolic strokes (Table 18–9). Bleeding dyscrasias, hypercoagulable states, blood disorders (especially sickle cell disease), and vascular disorders are also associated with a risk for stroke. Carotid artery bruits in patients with

Table 18–9. Sources of emboli.

Cardiac
  Changing rhythms, especially atrial fibrillation
  Valvular disease
    Rheumatic heart disease
    Valve prosthesis
    Bacterial and fungal endocarditis
    Myxomatous vegetation
    Congenital heart disease
    Mitral valve prolapse
  Atrial tumor
  Myocardial dysfunction
    Myocardial infarction
    Ventricular aneurysm
Noncardiac
  Foreign body
  Air, nitrogen, or other gases
  Fat
  Tumor
  Atheromatous material
  Thrombus

TIAs or stroke suggest the possibility of emboli derived from atheromatous plaques. Acute stroke syndromes, especially intracerebral hemorrhages, have been associated with cocaine and, less commonly, amphetamine use.

C. IDENTIFY OTHER ASSOCIATED SYMPTOMS

Severe headache and vomiting often accompany intracerebral hemorrhage. Patients with migraine headaches rarely may suffer strokes due to vascular spasm.

Physical Examination

A. GENERAL

A thorough examination may reveal the underlying cause for the stroke and direct treatment.

1. Vital signs—Record the body temperature. Hypertension is a risk factor for stroke, and systolic pressure above 200 mm Hg may require treatment.

2. Head—Arteriovenous malformations may be detected by auscultation of the head for bruits. Palpate the temporal arteries for tenderness, nodularity, or absence of pulse suggestive of giant cell arteritis. Search for any evidence of trauma.

3. Eyes—Examination of the retina may reveal visible emboli in the retinal vessels. Subhyaloid hemorrhage is diagnostic for subarachnoid hemorrhage.

4. Neck—The carotid arteries should be examined (one at a time) for presence of bruits and reduction of pulsation. Although these findings are not specific for carotid disease, further carotid studies may be warranted to evaluate for possible carotid endarterectomy.

5. Heart—Changing cardiac rhythms and murmurs or valvular disease are associated with increased risk of embolization from the heart.

6. Skin—Ecchymosis and petechiae may suggest blood disorders or vasculitis as causative factors. Presence of recent needle tracks or subungual splinter hemorrhages suggest the possibility of septic emboli derived from infected heart values.

7. Lung sounds—Ausculate for possible aspiration pneumonia or pulmonary edema.

B. NEUROLOGIC EXAMINATION

A rapid neurologic examination should be performed in the emergency department and should focus on (1) localizing the anatomic site of deficit as an aid in determining the specific stroke syndrome (which dictates treatment) and (2) assessing the degree of neurologic impairment, from which improvement or worsening can be assessed.

1. Level of alertness—Reduced mental alertness can be a sign of extensive injury from hemorrhage, brainstem infarction or herniation, or metabolic changes.

2. Cognitive—Assess response to commands and fluency of speech. Aphasia and apraxia are associated with involvement of the cerebral cortex and anterior (carotid) circulation; lacunar infarction or disturbance of posterior (vertebrobasilar) circulation is unlikely.

3. Cranial nerves—Visual field abnormalities exclude lacunar infarction. Abnormal pupillary reflexes and ocular palsies are brain-stem findings and are associated with disturbance of posterior circulation or impending brain herniation.

4. Motor—Hemiparesis can be associated with disturbance of the anterior or posterior circulation. Generally, in anterior circulation strokes, the face, hand, and arm are affected more than the leg. In lacunar infarction and posterior circulation strokes, this pattern is less common. Hemiparesis involving one side of the face and the other side of the body is due to disturbance of posterior circulation.

5. Sensory—Hemisensory deficits without associated motor involvement are usually due to lacunar infarcts. Astereognosis (inability to identify objects by touch) and agraphesthesia (inability to recognize figures traced on the skin) are cortical sensory deficits and are due to disturbance of anterior circulation.

6. Cerebellar—Hemiataxia suggests involvement of the cerebellum or the brain stem, or lacunar infarction deep in white matter.

Laboratory Tests

A. Blood Tests

The following blood tests should be obtained in most patients with focal neurologic deficits:

- Complete blood count and platelet count (to detect blood dyscrasias), and prothrombin time and partial thromboplastin time for coagulation disorders
- Glucose level, because both hyperglycemia and hypoglycemia may cause focal neurologic findings that can mimic stroke
- Erythrocyte sedimentation rate to detect vasculitis or arteritis

- Serologic test for syphilis
- Toxicologic screen if drug use is suspected

B. Electrocardiogram

An electrocardiogram may reveal new arrhythmias or reversion to a normal rhythm, both of which are associated with increased risk for emboli. Presence of myocardial infarction or persistent changes suggestive of a ventricular aneurysm also increase the risk for stroke.

C. CT or MRI Scan

These studies are essential for localizing the lesion; distinguishing hemorrhagic from occlusive stroke; and identifying other intracranial disease, such as tumor or abscess, that can be confused with strokes. A CT or MRI scan should be obtained in any suspected stroke patient.

D. Lumbar Puncture

Occasionally, in patients suspected of having subarachnoid hemorrhage but whose CT scan is negative or equivocal, a lumbar puncture may be diagnostic (the cerebrospinal fluid is bloody or the supernatant is xanthochromic [yellow]). Lumbar puncture is often useful in patients with meningoencephalitis and vasculitis.

Caution: In patients with focal neurologic findings, a CT or MRI scan should be performed prior to lumbar puncture.

E. Vascular Studies

Cerebral angiography may be indicated in patients suspected of having a surgically correctable condition such as cerebral aneurysm, arteriovenous malformation, and carotid atherosclerosis or stenosis. Noninvasive vascular studies such as ophthalmodynamometry, Doppler sonography, thermography, and ultrasonic studies may be useful to identify patients with suspected carotid atherosclerotic disease who may need angiography.

Bella I et al: Neuromuscular disorders and acute respiratory failure. Neurol Clin 1998;16:391. [PMID: 9537968] (A review of neuromuscular disorders.)

Chalk CH: Acquired peripheral neuropathy. Neurol Clin 1997;15:501. [PMID: 9227950] (A review of acquired peripheral neuropathies.)

Ross MA: Acquired motor neuron disorders. Neurol Clin 1997; 15:481. [PMID: 9227949] (A review article discussing acquired motor disease including poliomyelitis.)

Simpson et al: Recognition and management of acute pesticide poisoning. Am Fam Physician 2002;65:1599. [PMID: 11998835] (A review of pesticide poisoning management.)

Walter FG et al: Envenomations. Crit Care Clin 1999;15:353. [PMID: 10331133] (A review article on management of envenomations.)

Younger DS et al: Diagnosis in neuromuscular diseases. Neurol Clin 1996;14:135. [PMID: 8676841] (A review of acute myopathies.)

◼ VI. MANAGEMENT OF SPECIFIC STROKE SYNDROMES

HEMORRHAGIC STROKE

SUBARACHNOID HEMORRHAGE
(See also Chapter 16.)

ESSENTIALS OF DIAGNOSIS

- *Sudden onset of severe headache.*
- *Sentinel headache may be warning for aneurysmal subarachnoid hemorrhage.*
- *Nausea and vomiting, low back pain, bilateral leg pain.*
- *Photophobia, visual changes.*
- *Loss of consciousness.*

General Considerations

Subarachnoid hemorrhage occurs secondary to bleeding in the subarachnoid space. It is a medical emergency. Approximately 80% are due to saccular or berry aneurysms. The rest may be due to

- Trauma
- Arteriovenous malformation (which usually bleeds earlier than aneurysms, often becoming symptomatic in childhood or before age 30 years)
- Sickle cell disease
- Coagulopathies
- Central nervous system vasculitis
- Cocaine use
- Amphetamine use
- Moyamoya disease
- Intracranial neoplasm or metastatic disease

Clinical Findings

Patients usually complain of "the worst headache of my life" or "thunderclap" headache. Commonly associated symptoms include nausea and vomiting, neck stiffness, photophobia, back pain, and leg pain. Patients who present with stupor (localizing to pain) or coma are at high risk for mortality.

A high index of suspicion must be raised in patients presenting with early warning signs of a sentinel leak, because they are frequently missed in the diagnosis of subarachnoid hemorrhage, and early diagnosis can be life saving. Grading of subarachnoid bleeds is based on the patient's condition on presentation. The grading scale is as follows:

Grade	Neurologic Status
I	Asymptomatic
II	Severe headache or meningismus, cranial nerve palsy
III	Drowsy; confused, minimal neurologic deficits
IV	Stuporous; moderate to severe hemiparesis
V	Deep coma; decerebrate posturing; no motor response

A CT scan should be performed as the first diagnostic study (Figure 18–2). CT scan is up to 95% accurate within the first 24 hours; sensitivity decreases to 80% after 3 days and to 50% after 1 week. Selective catheter cerebral angiography aids in diagnosing cerebral aneurysms as the cause of subarachnoid hemorrhage. Lumbar puncture should be performed if the CT scan

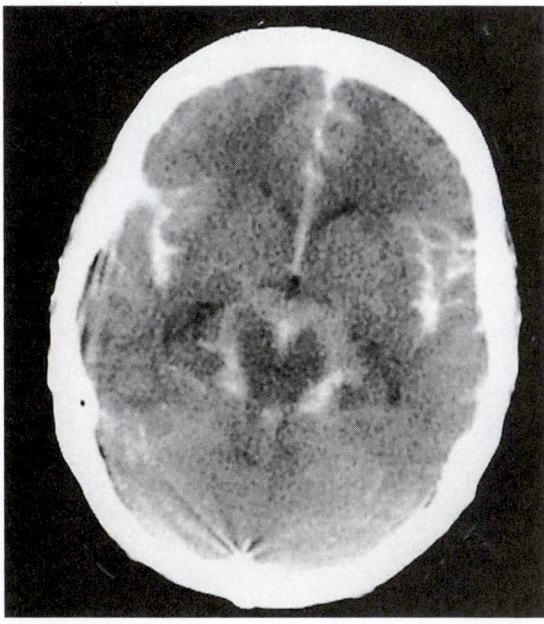

Figure 18–2. A noncontrast head CT scan demonstrating diffuse subarachnoid blood.

does not demonstrate blood but the suspicion for subarachnoid hemorrhage remains high. Lumbar puncture may demonstrate xanthochromic fluid or may even be bloody.

Complications & Treatment

The American Heart Association Special Writing Group of the Stroke Council has made various recommendations for subarachnoid hemorrhage:

A. ANEURYSMAL REBLEEDING

Aneurysmal rebleeding may be secondary to uncontrolled hypertension or aneurysmal clot fibrinolysis. Surgical clipping is strongly recommended to reduce the rate of rebleeding.

B. SEIZURE

Because seizures increase the risk of rebleeding after a subarachnoid hemorrhage, prophylactic use of an anticonvulsant for example, intravenous fosphenytoin or phenytoin, 15–20 mg/kg, is recommended.

C. HYPOVOLEMIA AND HYPONATREMIA

Hypovolemia and hyponatremia can occur secondary to the syndrome of inappropriate secretion of antidiuretic hormone. Treatment involves intravenous hydration with isotonic crystalloid. A central intravenous monitor is desirable.

D. HYDROCEPHALUS

1. Acute obstructive hydrocephalus—This form of hydrocephalus occurs in about 20% of patients after subarachnoid hemorrhage. Ventriculostomy is recommended, although it may increase the risk of rebleeding or infection.

2. Chronic communicating hydrocephalus—This form of hydrocephalus is a frequent occurrence after subarachnoid hemorrhage. A temporary or permanent cerebrospinal fluid diversion is recommended in symptomatic patients.

E. VASOSPASM

Vasospasm, or delayed cerebral ischemia, remains a frequent complication with high morbidity and mortality rates. Nimodipine, 60 mg orally every 4 hours, is strongly recommended.

F. NEUROSURGICAL CONSULTATION

Seek neurosurgical consultation for definitive management.

INTRACEREBRAL HEMORRHAGE
(See also Chapter 16.)

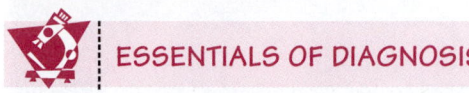 ESSENTIALS OF DIAGNOSIS

- *No specific signs or symptoms reliably distinguish between intracerebral hemorrhage and ischemic stroke.*
- *Symptoms vary depending on affected area and extent of bleeding.*
- *Patients are more likely to exhibit signs of increased intracranial pressure; seizures more common.*
- *Headache often severe and sudden.*
- *Nausea and vomiting, hypertension, altered sensorium.*

General Considerations

Intracerebral hemorrhage is twice as common as subarachnoid hemorrhage and even more likely to result in a major disability or death. Bleeding occurs primarily in the brain parenchyma, although blood appears in the cerebrospinal fluid in the majority of patients. Symptoms are due to mass effect of the hematoma with displacement and compression of adjacent brain tissue. The most common cause is advancing age and damage of intracerebral arterioles by long-standing systemic hypertension. Other causes include anticoagulation, drug and alcohol abuse, thrombolytic therapy, bleeding diathesis, neoplasms, cerebral amyloid angiopathy, infections, and arteriovenous malformations.

Clinical Findings

Clinical findings depend on the site of the hemorrhage but occur abruptly and progress within minutes to a few hours. Headache and vomiting are frequent symptoms. Focal neurologic deficits are prominent, because most bleeding sites abut the basal ganglia, thalamus, and internal capsule. Abrupt onset of coma and prominent brain-stem findings (pinpoint pupils, absent extraocular movements) are characteristic of pontine hemorrhage. A CT scan is diagnostic and is the imaging study of choice. MRI and magnetic resonance angiography are useful in detecting structural abnormalities such as malformations and aneurysms (Figure 18–3).

Ataxia and cerebellar abnormalities, with absent or mild hemiparesis, are characteristic of cerebellar hemorrhage. It is particularly important to diagnose hypertensive intracerebellar hemorrhage rapidly, because fatal brain-stem compression may occur rapidly; emergency

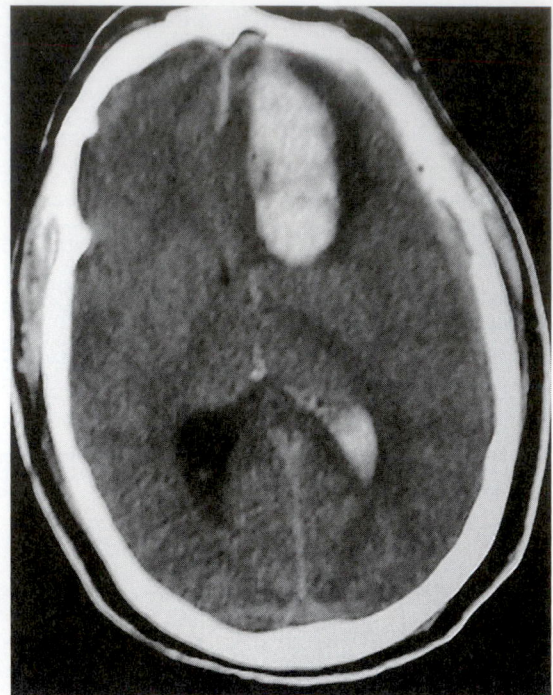

Figure 18–3. A noncontrast head CT scan demonstrating a large frontal intercerebral hemorrhage.

surgical decompression can be life saving. Because the clinical differentiation from acute vestibular dysfunction may be difficult, patients with sudden onset of disequilibrium and vomiting may need a CT scan of the brain to exclude cerebellar hemorrhage.

Treatment & Disposition

As with all other emergencies, initial management of a patient with intracerebral hemorrhage is directed toward airway, breathing, and circulation. A directed history and physical examination are essential to assess for underlying clues and deficits. If the patient exhibits need for airway protection, orotracheal intubation should be performed.

Blood pressure management is based on a theoretical rationale: lower the blood pressure and decrease the risk of ongoing bleeding from ruptured small arterioles. The converse theory therefore holds that aggressive treatment of blood pressure may decrease cerebral perfusion pressure and worsen brain injury. The American Heart Association Special Writing Group of the Stroke Council recommends that blood pressure levels be maintained below a mean arterial pressure of 130 mm Hg in persons with a history of hypertension.

Neurosurgical consultation should be obtained. The decision about whether and when to operate remains controversial.

ISCHEMIC STROKE

 ESSENTIALS OF DIAGNOSIS

- *Secondary to thrombosis or embolism.*
- *Consider in acute neurologic deficit (focal or global) or altered level of consciousness.*
- *No historical feature distinguishes ischemic from intracerebral stroke, although headache, nausea and vomiting, and altered level of consciousness are more common in intracerebral stroke.*
- *Abrupt onset of hemiparesis, monoparesis, or quadriparesis; dysarthria, ataxia, vertigo; monocular or binocular visual loss, visual field deficits, diplopia.*
- *Symptoms occur alone or in combination.*
- *Establish time of onset.*
- *Beware of stroke mimics.*

General Considerations

Stroke is the third leading cause of death in the United States. It is also the leading cause of severe neurologic disability. Many significant advances in medical and surgical technologies for patients with TIAs and acute ischemic strokes have occurred, and research is ongoing.

Ischemic strokes, comprising thrombotic, embolic, and lacunar occlusions, account for over 75% of all strokes and result in cerebral ischemia or infarction. A variety of disorders of blood, blood vessels, and heart can cause occlusive strokes, but the most common by far are atherosclerotic disease (especially of the carotid and vertebrobasilar arteries) and cardiac abnormalities. Risk factors for atherosclerosis are listed in Table 18–10.

Clinical Findings

Occurrence of TIAs preceding the stroke is the hallmark of stroke. The neurologic deficits may evolve over minutes to hours or days and are typical for a specific vascular distribution. Motor and sensory pathways are impaired. Headache and vomiting are rare. The diagnosis is made on the basis of the clinical findings and ex-

Table 18–10. Risk factors for atherosclerosis

Nonmodifiable	
Age	
Race	
Gender	
Modifiable	
Hypertensin	Smoking
Cardiac disease	Heavy alcohol use
Atrial fibrillation	Obesity
Prior transient ischemic	Physical inactivity
attack or stroke	Oral contraceptive use
Diabetes	
Hyperlipidemia	

clusion of hemorrhage by CT scan. MRI and repeat CT scan at 48–72 hours will often confirm the diagnosis when the initial study is normal.

Treatment & Disposition

In 1996, the U.S. Food and Drug Administration approved the use of thrombolytic therapy for acute ischemic stroke, and the American Heart Association and the American Academy of Neurology published guidelines for its use. Management of acute ischemic stroke is handled on a case-by-case basis. Intravenous tissue plasminogen activator (t-PA) can be used if the following criteria are met:

- The time of onset of the stroke is clearly defined, and treatment is started within 3 hours after the onset of symptoms.
- A noncontrast CT scan has excluded hemorrhage prior to treatment.
- Systolic blood pressure is less than 185 mm Hg, and diastolic blood pressure is less than 110 mm Hg.
- The patient has no history of intracranial hemorrhage, head injury in the preceding 3 months, or gastrointestinal or urinary tract hemorrhage in the past 3 weeks.

  Dosage and administration of t-PA:

- Give 0.9 mg/kg body weight of intravenous t-PA up to a maximum of 90 mg.
- Give 10% of the dose as a bolus and then administer the rest of the dose as a continuous infusion over 1 hour.
- Do not give anticoagulants or antiplatelet drugs for 24 hours after treatment.

  Acute stroke patients should be admitted to stroke units (which have demonstrated improved outcomes).

LACUNAR STROKE

 ESSENTIALS OF DIAGNOSIS

- *Most frequent in basal ganglia and internal capsule.*
- *Five classical lacunar syndromes:*

Pure Motor Stroke/Hemiparesis

- *Most common syndrome.*
- *Affects face, arm, leg equally.*
- *Dysarthria, dysphagia.*
- *Transient sensory symptoms (but not signs) may be present.*

Ataxic Hemiparesis

- *Second most common syndrome.*
- *Weakness and clumsiness on one side of body; legs affected more commonly than arms (homolateral ataxia and crural paresis).*
- *Onset over hours to days.*

Dysarthria/Clumsy Hand

- *Variant of ataxic hemiparesis.*

Pure Sensory Stroke (Thalamus)

- *Persistent numbness or tingling on one side of the body (face, arm, leg, trunk).*
- *Unpleasant sensation.*

Mixed Sensorimotor Stroke

- *Hemiparesis or hemiplegia noted.*
- *Ipsilateral sensory impairment.*

Clinical Findings

Lacunar stroke results from occlusion of the small penetrating arteries of the brain by lipohyalinotic deposits, which are a product of long-standing hypertension. The areas of infarction are generally small, and multiple old infarct sites may also be identified on CT scan. The clinical findings are distinct and may range from pure motor or pure sensory deficits to incoordination and clumsiness of the hand or ataxia of the arm or leg. CT scan is often normal or may show small lucencies in the affected areas, usually in the internal capsule, pons, cerebellum, or subcortical white matter.

Treatment & Disposition

Treatment is supportive and consists mainly of blood pressure control. The prognosis is generally good. Patients should usually be hospitalized for observation.

ARTERIAL DISSECTION

 ESSENTIALS OF DIAGNOSIS

- *Nonspecific presenting signs and symptoms, neurologic deficits.*
- *Headache, facial pain, neck swelling, amaurosis fugax, pulsatile tinnitus.*
- *More common in young adults.*
- *May follow traumatic event or simple manipulation of the neck, or may be spontaneous.*
- *Horner syndrome/bruit.*

Clinical Findings

An acute progressive syndrome of carotid or vertebral artery ischemia almost invariably associated with anterior or posterior neck pain suggests carotid or vertebral artery dissection, respectively. A history of recent neck trauma is frequent and may be relatively trivial, such as chiropractic manipulation. Angiography is diagnostic and shows the markedly reduced intravascular lumen caused by dissection of the intimal layer, producing the characteristic "string sign."

Treatment & Disposition

Surgical intervention is not indicated. Vessels recanalize spontaneously over months. Current opinion favors anticoagulation acutely and for several months thereafter to reduce the potential for distal embolization of platelet aggregates formed on the damaged vessel wall.

TRANSIENT ISCHEMIC ATTACKS

 ESSENTIALS OF DIAGNOSIS

- *Rapid onset.*
- *Manifestations are variable, lasting 2–15 minutes and rarely up to 24 hours.*
- *Review history and medications.*

Clinical Findings

Neurologic deficits occur suddenly and persist from minutes to hours but resolve completely within 24 hours. The National Stroke Association estimates that 40% of patients who had a TIA are likely to have a major stroke at some point in the future. A TIA should therefore be promptly evaluated to institute therapy to decrease the risk of stroke. These episodes are caused by small platelet, fibrin, or atheromatous emboli originating in extracranial vessels or the heart. Clinical findings depend on the area of the brain affected. Transient monocular blindness due to embolus in the retinal artery (amaurosis fugax) usually signifies ipsilateral carotid artery disease, but unlike hemispheric TIA, amaurosis fugax is associated with less risk for subsequent carotid stroke.

Treatment

Treatment is directed at identifying and correcting the underlying cause (eg, treat hypertension, evaluate for carotid endarterectomy). Antiplatelet agents are typically the treatment of choice for prevention of future strokes in patients who have experienced a TIA of presumed atherosclerotic origin. The selection of a specific agent is typically based on interpretation of the results of randomized trials that have tested these agents in populations of patients who have had a recent TIA or stroke.

Four different antiplatelet agents have shown efficacy in preventing stroke or other vascular events in patients with cerebrovascular disease:

A. ASPIRIN

Aspirin is the most economical and frequently chosen (except in intolerant patients) antiplatelet regimen in patients with TIA. The U.S. Food and Drug Administration advocates the use of aspirin in doses of 50–325 mg/d for the prevention of stroke.

B. TICLOPIDINE

Ticlopidine prevents platelet aggregation induced by adenosine diphosphate. Its use has been approved in the United States for prevention of stroke in patients with TIA or minor stroke. Typically used in patients who are intolerant to aspirin or who have had an ischemic event despite taking aspirin, its usefulness is limited by its side effects. The recommended dosage is 250 mg 2 times a day.

C. CLOPIDOGREL

Clopidogrel works by inhibiting platelet aggregation by adenosine diphosphate. It offers another alternative to patients intolerant to aspirin or who have had an ischemic event despite taking aspirin. It has a good safety profile. The recommended dosage is 75 mg/d.

D. DIPYRIDAMOLE AND ASPIRIN

A combination of a cyclic nucleotide phosphodiesterase inhibitor and a cyclooxygenase inhibitor has been found to be effective. This medication contains 200 mg extended-release dipyridamole and 25 mg aspirin. The recommended dose is 1 capsule 2 times a day.

E. ANTICOAGULATION

Oral anticoagulation with warfarin continues to be the therapy of choice for stroke prevention in atrial fibrillation in patients who have had a TIA and in primary prevention of stroke in patients with atrial fibrillation. In patients in whom oral anticoagulation is contraindicated, aspirin is recommended. Current recommendations suggest a target range international normalized ratio of 2.0–3.0 for most indications for oral anticoagulation.

F. SURGICAL INTERVENTIONS

1. Carotid endarterectomy—This intervention is used to remove atherosclerotic plaque from a carotid artery when the vessel is blocked. It has proved beneficial in preventing future strokes in certain patients with minor strokes or TIAs. The procedure is indicated when the vessel has a 70–99% blockage. When the vessel is 50–69% blocked, carotid endarterectomy is recommended; and when the vessel is less than 50% stenosed, there is no benefit from the procedure and medical management is recommended.

2. Stereotactic microsurgery of arteriovenous malformations and aneurysms—This technique involves the use of computer technology and geometric principles to pinpoint the precise location of the arteriovenous malformation, allowing neurosurgeons to use microscope-enhanced methods and delicate instruments without affecting normal brain tissue.

3. Stereotactic radiosurgery for arteriovenous malformations—This technique uses the same basic principle as microsurgery. Once located, the arteriovenous malformation can be obliterated by focusing a beam of radiation that causes it to clot and then disappear.

4. Revascularization of the blood supply—This technique is used to treat aneurysms or blocked cerebral arteries. It provides a new route of blood to the brain by grafting another vessel to a cerebral artery or providing a new source of blood to the brain.

5. Carotid angioplasty and stent placement—This method has had a high degree of technical success, and low complication rates have been reported.

6. Decompressive hemicraniectomy—This technique is performed in patients with massive nondominant infarcts, who would otherwise succumb to herniation.

Disposition

Most patients with TIAs should be hospitalized. Patients who have had recent thorough evaluation for TIAs or who are not candidates for therapy may be referred to their primary care physician for outpatient follow-up.

Adams HP et al: Guidelines for thrombolytic therapy for acute stroke: A supplement to the guidelines for the management of patients with acute ischemic stroke: A statement for healthcare professionals from a special writing group of the Stroke Council, American Heart Association. Circulation 1996;94:1167. [PMID: 8790069] (Provides updated recommendations for use of thrombolytic therapy in clinical practice as approved by the American Heart Association Science Advisory and Coordinating Committee.)

Albers GW et al: Supplement to the guidelines for the management of transient ischemic attacks. A statement from the Ad Hoc Committee on Guidelines for the Management of Transient Ischemic Attacks, Stroke Council, American Heart Association. Stroke 1999;30:2502. [PMID: 10548693] (Provides updated advances in medical and surgical therapies for patients with TIAs along with new data regarding underlying risk factors, as approved by the American Heart Association Science Advisory and Coordinating Committee.)

Broderick JP et al: Guidelines for the management of spontaneous intracerebral hemorrhage. A statement for healthcare professionals from a special writing group of the Stroke Council, American Heart Association. Stroke 1999;30:905. [PMID: 10187901] (Addresses this common stroke subtype and stresses the fact that there are a limited number of randomized controlled studies for treatment of intracerebral hemorrhage.)

Culebras A et al: Practice guidelines for the use of imaging in transient ischemic attacks and acute stroke. A report of the Stroke Council, American Heart Association. Stroke 1997;28(7):1480. [PMID: 9227705] (Provides useful recommendations regarding various diagnostic imaging studies for cerebrovascular disease.)

Gorelick P et al: Prevention of first stroke. A review of guidelines and a multidisciplinary consensus statement from the National Stroke Association. JAMA 1999;281(12):1112. [PMID: 10188663] (A panel of experts convened to provide this consensus report to identify and modify cardiovascular and cerebrovascular risk factors to help prevent first stroke.)

Hinton RC: Thrombosis and cerebrovascular disease. Med Clin North Am 1998;82(3):523. [PMID: 9646778] (A review on acute thrombotic disease.)

Lewandowski C et al: Treatment of acute ischemic stroke. Ann Emerg Med 2001;37:202. [PMID: 11174240] (A state-of-the-art article on all aspects of treatment of acute ischemic stroke in the emergency department.)

Moonis M et al: Considering the role of heparin and low-molecular-weight heparins in acute ischemic stroke. Stroke 2002;33:1927. [PMID: 12105378] (A review on the use of heparin in acute ischemic stroke.)

Rabb CH et al: Surgical treatment strategies in ischemic stroke. Neuroimaging Clin N Am 1999;9:527. [PMID: 10433643] (Addresses current indications and techniques for the surgical treatment of ischemic stroke.)

Stahmer SA, Raps EC, Mines DI: Carotid and vertebral artery dissections. Emerg Med Clin North Am 1997;15:677. [PMID: 9255140] (A review of management of carotid and vertebral dissections.)

Stieg PE et al: Intracranial hemorrhage: Diagnosis and emergency management. Neurol Clin 1998;16:373. [PMID: 9537967]

(A review of emergency management of intracranial hemorrhage.)

Tuhrim S: Management of hemorrhagic stroke. Curr Cardiol Rep 2002;4:158. [PMID: 11827640]

Wolf PA et al: Preventing ischemic stroke in patients with prior stroke and transient ischemic attack. A statement for healthcare professionals from the Stroke Council of the American Heart Association. Stroke 1999;30:1991. [PMID: 10471455] (A review of factors placing patients at higher risk of developing stroke recurrence.)

Headache

19

C. Keith Stone, MD, & Nancy J. Antonacci, MD[1]

Immediate Evaluation & Management of Headache Caused by Life-Threatening Conditions
Approach to the Diagnosis of Headache
Management of Specific Disorders Causing Acute Headache
    Subarachnoid Hemorrhage
    Cerebrovascular Accident (Stroke)
    Meningitis & Meningoencephalitis
    Postural (Post–Lumbar Puncture) Headache
Management of Specific Disorders Causing Subacute Headache
    Posttraumatic Headache

Trigeminal Neuralgia
Intracranial Mass (Brain Tumor)
Pseudotumor Cerebri (Idiopathic Intracranial Hypertension)
Temporal Arteritis (Giant Cell Arteritis)
Management of Specific Disorders Causing Chronic Headache
    Tension Headache
    Migraine
    Cluster Headache
    Headache Due to Hypertension

■ IMMEDIATE EVALUATION & MANAGEMENT OF HEADACHE CAUSED BY LIFE-THREATENING CONDITIONS
(See Figure 19–1.)

Has Head Trauma Occurred?

If recent head trauma has occurred, evaluation of this problem takes precedence (Chapter 22).

Have Seizures Occurred?

Patients may have headache following one or more grand mal seizures. However, because the seizures may themselves be due to serious underlying disease (eg, subdural hematoma), evaluation of this problem takes precedence (Chapter 17).

Are There Focal Neurologic Abnormalities?

The presence of new focal neurologic abnormalities with headache, especially if papilledema is present as well, is strongly suggestive of a mass lesion (tumor, hematoma, abscess). Computed tomography (CT) scan or magnetic resonance imaging (MRI) should be done as soon as practical to make the diagnosis. Further evaluation is discussed in Chapter 18.

Is Headache New or of Recent Origin?

The single most important item of information to obtain from a patient with headache is whether the headache is new. A new headache is one occurring in a patient without a history of headaches, or a novel pattern or quality of pain in a patient with a history of headaches. New headaches demand immediate careful evaluation.

Is the Complaint Consistent with Meningitis or Meningeal Irritation?

If the headache is acute (sudden) or subacute (hours to days) in onset, subarachnoid hemorrhage (with resultant irritative [chemical] meningitis) or meningitis must be suspected. The usual manifestations are signs of meningeal irritation (stiff neck; positive Kernig and Brudzinski signs) and fever (usually absent in subarachnoid hemorrhage). These findings may be minimal or even absent in very young or very old patients. Seizures, confusion, or coma may be present as well. Subarachnoid hemorrhage should be strongly suspected in a patient with abrupt onset of headache that is unique to

[1]This chapter is a revision of the chapter by Roger P. Simon, MD, from the 4th edition.

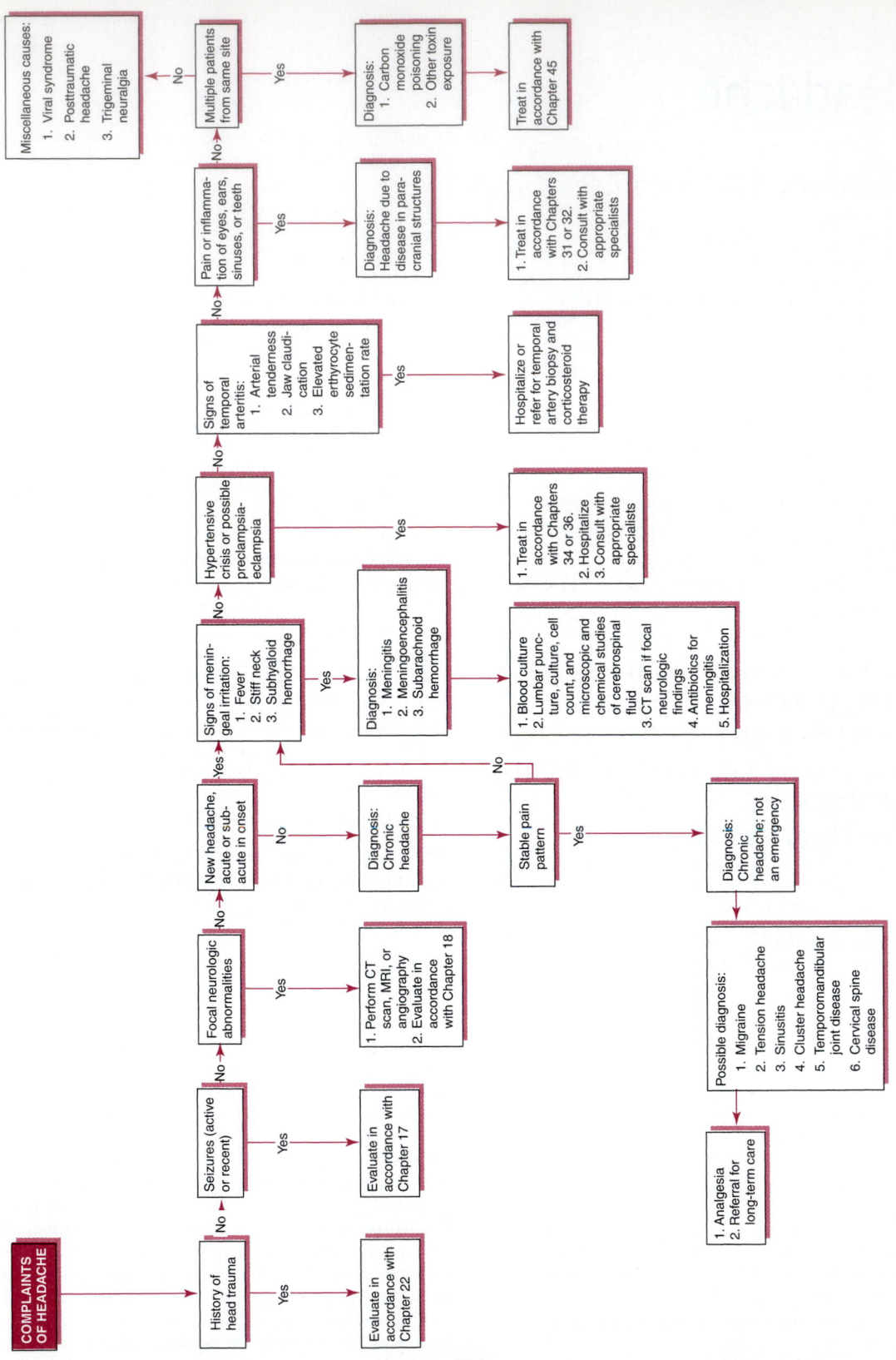

Figure 19–1. Management of complaints of headache.

the patient's experience, especially if meningeal irritation or focal neurologic findings are present. An emergency CT scan is required; if the diagnosis is still unclear, lumbar puncture should be performed. If meningitis is also a possibility, antibiotic therapy should be started as soon as possible (based on microorganisms most common for each age group) and before the CT scan is obtained (Chapter 40).

Meningitis should be strongly suspected in a patient who presents with headache accompanied by fever, especially if signs of meningeal irritation are present. A lumbar puncture should be performed immediately and antibiotics begun as soon as possible (Chapter 40).

If there are signs of altered mental status or if there are focal neurologic findings in a patient with fever, a brain abscess should be suspected. Lumbar puncture should be delayed until a CT scan is performed.

Is Headache Due to Hypertensive Encephalopathy or Preeclampsia-Eclampsia?

Moderate elevations of blood pressure alone seldom cause headache; however, severe hypertension as seen in hypertensive crises and eclampsia is associated with headache. If hypertension is present and the patient is pregnant or has signs of cerebral dysfunction (confusion, obtundation, or coma) or other end-organ damage (retinitis; nephritis with proteinuria), a life-threatening emergency exists. *Note:* In pregnancy, a slight increase in blood pressure may be more significant than in the nonpregnant patient. See Chapter 34 (hypertensive crisis) or Chapter 36 (eclampsia).

Is This Temporal Arteritis?

Temporal arteritis is a rare but treatable disease with serious sequelae that must be considered in every elderly patient with new headache. The principal manifestations are headache with temporal artery tenderness (not found in every case) and a markedly elevated erythrocyte sedimentation rate. Sudden monocular blindness may occur. If this condition is suspected, hospitalization is warranted to confirm the diagnosis by means of temporal artery biopsy and to begin therapy. For details of diagnosis and management, see later in this chapter.

Is Headache Due to Disease in Paracranial Structures?

New or acute headaches are often caused by disease in the eyes, ears, sinuses, or teeth. Look carefully for iritis or acute glaucoma (Chapter 31) or for sinusitis, otitis media, or dental caries or abscess (Chapter 32). Treatment should be focused on the primary condition.

Are There Multiple Patients from the Same Vicinity?

Multiple patients from the same vicinity with complaint of headache suggest carbon monoxide poisoning or other toxin exposure. Patients should be questioned specifically about heating sources (eg, gas heat or oven), burning materials (eg, charcoal) in poorly ventilated areas, use of household cleaners, or other chemical exposure. Specific treatment of carbon monoxide poisoning and other toxin exposure is discussed in Chapter 45.

Disposition

Even after careful initial history and physical examination, the diagnosis may not be apparent in the patient with new headache. Patients with recent onset of new headache should be hospitalized if there is any suspicion of a life-threatening process. Increasing severity of subacute headache over days or weeks, even without focal signs, suggests serious intracranial disease, and the patient should undergo appropriate diagnostic procedures. Subacute headaches without progressive symptoms and chronic headaches may be evaluated on a nonemergency basis.

Godwin SA, Villa J: Acute headache in the ED: Evidence-based evaluation and treatment options. Emergency Medicine Practice 2001;3:1. (A comprehensive review article on the diagnosis and management of acute headaches in the emergency department.)

■ APPROACH TO THE DIAGNOSIS OF HEADACHE

Pain-Sensitive Structures & Their Projections

Headache is caused by traction, displacement, inflammation, or distention of pain-sensitive structures in the head or neck. Disorders of the scalp, teeth, eyes, and ears and of the mucous membranes of the nose, sinuses, and oropharynx can produce pain. Pain-sensitive structures about the calvarium include the scalp and its blood vessels, the neck muscles, and the upper cervical nerves. The skull, brain, and most of the dura are not pain-sensitive. In general, discrete intracranial lesions above the cerebellar tentorium produce pain in trigeminal distribution (anterior to ears), whereas lesions in the posterior fossa project pain to the second and third cervical dermatomes (posterior to ears).

History

A. Time of Onset

Chronic headache (duration of months or more) is usually not due to a serious disorder, but headache of acute onset or of a changing pain pattern demands prompt evaluation in the emergency department. If the patient has a chronic headache disorder, determine whether the present headache differs from or is identical to the patient's chronic problem.

Although the sudden onset of pain or "the worst headache I ever had in my life" typifies subarachnoid hemorrhage, the associated headache will be unique but *need not be severe.*

B. Precipitating Factors

1. Tension headache—Tension, emotional stress, and fatigue.

2. Migraine—Hunger, nitrite-containing foods (hot dogs, salami, sausage), chocolate, aged cheeses, bright lights, menses, alcohol, caffeine, monosodium glutamate, aspartame, and insomnia.

3. Cluster variant of migraine—Alcohol.

4. Trigeminal neuralgia and the jaw claudication of temporal arteritis—Chewing and eating.

C. Location of Pain

1. Migraine or the cluster variant—Hemicranial or retroocular pain.

2. Tension headache—Commonly diffuse, occipital, or bandlike pain.

3. Mass lesion headache—Often focal ("right here").

4. Trigeminal neuralgia—Stabbing pain localized to the second or third division of the trigeminal nerve.

D. Quality of Pain

1. Migraine or the cluster variant—Commonly described as throbbing and often preceded by prodromal symptoms or auras, for example, scintillating scotomas or other visual changes.

2. Tension headache and mass lesion headache—Usually steady pain.

3. Trigeminal neuralgia—A shooting or stabbing character.

E. Timing

1. Mass lesion headache—Commonly maximal on awakening.

2. Cluster variant of migraine—Frequently awaken patients from sleep and often recur at the same time of day or night.

3. Tension headache—May develop at regular intervals, especially with recurrent stressful situations.

F. Factors Influencing Severity

1. Migraine or the cluster variant—Frequently relieved by pressure on the ipsilateral temporal or carotid artery; by darkness, sleep, or vomiting; or during pregnancy.

2. Mass lesion headache—Often exacerbated by events such as coughing and sneezing that transiently raise intracranial pressure.

G. Associated Symptoms

Nausea or vomiting is common with migraine and posttraumatic headache syndromes and may be seen late in the course of mass lesions. Photophobia is prominent with migraine headache but occurs also with meningitis, especially viral (aseptic) meningitis. Myalgias of pericranial muscles (eg, posterior neck muscles) often accompany tension headaches and viral syndromes. Rhinorrhea and lacrimation during headache typify the cluster variant of migraine and are ipsilateral to the pain.

Physical Examination

A. Vital Signs

1. Fever—The presence of fever supports a diagnosis of meningitis, encephalitis, or headache associated with viral infection. A low-grade fever may also occur in temporal arteritis.

2. Blood pressure—Hypertension per se rarely causes headache, but chronic hypertension is the major risk factor for stroke, especially intracerebral hemorrhage, and stroke may be associated with acute headache. Blood pressure may be markedly elevated during hypertensive encephalopathy or as a result of preeclampsia-eclampsia, subarachnoid hemorrhage, or brain-stem stroke.

B. Skin

Neurofibromas or café au lait spots of Recklinghausen disease may be associated with benign or malignant intracranial tumors.

Cutaneous angiomas sometimes accompany arteriovenous malformations of the central nervous system; rupture results in subarachnoid hemorrhage and acute headache.

C. Scalp and Head

1. Temporal arteries—Note nodularity or tenderness compatible with temporal arteritis.

2. Sinuses—Note tenderness, erythema of overlying skin, or nasal discharge.

3. Temporomandibular joints—Look for tenderness or limitation of motion.

4. Orbits—A bruit heard when the stethoscope is placed on the eyeball over closed eyelids may suggest intracranial arteriovenous malformation.

D. NECK AND BACK

1. Muscle spasm—Cervical muscle spasm may be a sign of tension or may occur with migraine.

2. Meningeal signs—Can the patient touch chin to sternum? If not, is the limitation of motion mainly in the anteroposterior direction, suggesting meningeal irritation, or in all directions, as is common with cervical spine disorders? Is there any discomfort, neck flexion, or contralateral knee flexion during straight leg raising (Kernig sign)? Most important, is there even slight flexion of the knee (Brudzinski sign) during passive neck flexion?

a. Lumbar puncture—Any evidence of meningeal irritation in a patient with acute headache demands lumbar puncture to rule out meningitis and subarachnoid hemorrhage. The only exception to this rule is the presence of obvious lateralizing findings suggesting a mass lesion (brain abscess, tumor), in which case confirmatory studies (CT scan or MRI) should be done first. If there will be a delay (>1 hour) in obtaining the CT scan, begin antimicrobials (see Table 40–3).

b. Absence of meningeal signs—Meningeal signs may be absent or difficult to demonstrate in the early stages of subacute meningitis (eg, tuberculous meningitis), several hours may elapse before evidence of meningeal irritation develops after subarachnoid hemorrhage, and these signs disappear if the patient lapses into deep coma. Meningeal signs may also be minimal in the very young or very old.

E. NEUROLOGIC EXAMINATION

Unilateral cranial nerve, cerebellar, motor, or reflex abnormalities suggest a diagnosis of intracranial mass lesion.

F. MISCELLANEOUS PHYSICAL FINDINGS

Papilledema, the hallmark of increased intracranial pressure, should always be sought.

Acute confusion or altered consciousness is common after subarachnoid hemorrhage and with purulent meningitis.

G. SPECIAL SIGNS

It is helpful to observe the patient for diagnostic signs during a headache. Ipsilateral conjunctival injection, lacrimation, and rhinorrhea support a diagnosis of cluster headache. Scalp tenderness is characteristic of migraine headache, subdural hematoma, and temporal arteritis.

Clinch CR: Evaluation of acute headaches in adults. Am Fam Phys 2001;63:685. [PMID 11237083] (A review article on the evaluation of headaches in adults.)

Headaches: Treatments vary with the type. Mayo Clin Health Lett 2001;19:1. [PMID: 11547602] (Review on the diagnosis and treatment of tension, migraine, and cluster headaches.)

■ MANAGEMENT OF SPECIFIC DISORDERS CAUSING ACUTE HEADACHE

SUBARACHNOID HEMORRHAGE

Subarachnoid hemorrhage is a life-threatening cause of acute headache. Patients typically present with a sudden onset of severe headache and most will go on to have focal neurologic signs. Diagnosis is best made with CT scan or MRI. Lumbar puncture is recommended for patients with negative neuroimaging. A detailed discussion of subarachnoid hemorrhage is found in Chapters 16 and 18.

van Gijn J, Rinkel GJ: Subarachnoid haemorrhage: Diagnosis, causes and management. Brain 2001;124:249. [PMID: 11157554] (A comprehensive review article on the diagnosis, cause, and treatment of subarachnoid hemorrhage.)

CEREBROVASCULAR ACCIDENT (STROKE)
(See also Chapter 18.)

 ESSENTIALS OF DIAGNOSIS

- *Sudden-onset focal neurologic deficit.*
- *Symptoms related to vasculature involved.*

Clinical Findings

Thrombotic or embolic strokes may be associated with mild to moderate nonthrobbing headaches that are mainly contralateral to the paralysis. The headache may precede or accompany the stroke.

Treatment & Disposition

Treat stroke as described in Chapter 18. Hospitalize the patient for evaluation and treatment.

Godwin SA, Villa J: Acute headache in the ED: Evidence-based evaluation and treatment options. Emergency Medicine Practice 2001;3:1. (A comprehensive review article on the diagnosis and management of acute headaches in the emergency department.)

MENINGITIS & MENINGOENCEPHALITIS
(See also Chapter 40.)

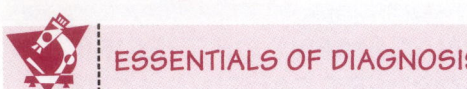

ESSENTIALS OF DIAGNOSIS

- *Headache, fever.*
- *Nuchal rigidity.*

Clinical Findings

Headache, confusion, and nuchal rigidity developing over hours to days are classic features of meningitis (infectious, carcinomatous, or irritative [chemical]). However, in rapidly progressive pyogenic meningitis, fever and altered consciousness are the most prominent presenting signs. In patients with subacute meningitis (eg, cryptococcosis, tuberculosis), headache is an early symptom that may precede nuchal rigidity and other meningeal signs. The headache of meningitis is continuous and throbbing and, although generalized, usually most prominent over the occiput. The pain is increased by head shaking, jugular vein compression, or any other maneuver that increases intracranial pressure (eg, coughing, sneezing, straining at stool). Pain is not relieved by changes in posture. Neck stiffness and other signs of meningeal irritation must be sought with care, because they may not be obvious early.

If meningitis or meningoencephalitis is suspected, perform lumbar puncture (Chapter 6) and obtain blood for culture. Relative contraindications to lumbar puncture are (1) papilledema and (2) prominent focal neurologic findings, suggesting mass lesion.

Treatment

A. ANTIMICROBIALS

Begin antibiotics immediately after taking samples of blood and cerebrospinal fluid for culture if bacterial meningitis is suspected. If lumbar puncture must be delayed for anatomic studies (CT scan), obtain 2 blood culture samples, and begin antimicrobials; perform lumbar puncture and culture cerebrospinal fluid as soon as possible. The choice of drug depends on the clinical circumstances and the results of Gram stain and culture of cerebrospinal fluid (see Table 40–3).

B. SUPPORTIVE CARE

General supportive care should be initiated in the emergency department. Protect the patient's airway, and provide padded bed rails or restraints for agitated or delirious patients. If seizures have occurred, start anticonvulsant therapy (Chapter 17). Concomitant corticosteroid treatment in purulent meningitis has been shown in children to decrease the incidence of residual hearing impairment.

Disposition

Immediate hospitalization is warranted except perhaps in the case of a patient with aseptic (viral) meningitis who appears well and can be observed at home by a third party and has close follow-up within 24 hours for reexamination.

Williams AJ, Nadel S: Bacterial meningitis: Current controversies in approaches to treatment. CNS Drugs 2001;15:909. [PMID: 11735611] (A comprehensive review article on the treatment of bacterial meningitis.)

POSTURAL (POST–LUMBAR PUNCTURE) HEADACHE

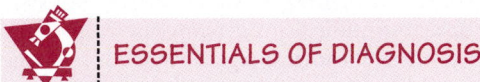

ESSENTIALS OF DIAGNOSIS

- *Follows lumbar puncture.*
- *Headache exacerbated by the upright position.*
- *Headache relieved by recumbency.*

Clinical Findings

Postural headache may follow lumbar puncture, especially if a large needle is used. This type of headache is worse in the upright position and nearly absent in recumbency. The onset of headache is usually within the first 24–48 hours and rarely occurs later. The site of the headache may be bifrontal, occipital, or in the neck and upper shoulders.

Treatment & Disposition

Recumbency for 18–24 hours, good hydration, and analgesics are usually sufficient management. For more persistent cases, refer the patient to an anesthesiologist for an epidural blood patch at the site of the puncture (epidural injection of autologous blood at the site of the puncture will clot to seal the dural opening and prevent further leakage of cerebrospinal fluid).

Chordas C: Post-dural puncture headache and other complications after lumbar puncture. J Pediatr Oncol Nurs 2001;18:244. [PMID: 11719905] (A review article on the pathophysiology, diagnosis, treatment, and prevention of post–lumbar puncture complications.)

■ MANAGEMENT OF SPECIFIC DISORDERS CAUSING SUBACUTE HEADACHE

POSTTRAUMATIC HEADACHE

ESSENTIALS OF DIAGNOSIS

• *History of head trauma.*
• *May have associated dizziness, vertigo, insomnia.*

Clinical Findings

Headache caused by head injury may begin immediately or within weeks after trauma. Chronic posttraumatic headache is defined as a headache that continues for greater than 8 weeks after the trauma occurs. The symptoms are not necessarily proportionate to the severity of the traumatic event. Persistent worsening of headache, particularly after trauma, suggests subdural hematoma (Chapter 22). Associated dizziness, vertigo, insomnia, depression, and personality change may occur. This constellation of symptoms is referred to as posttraumatic syndrome. Posttraumatic headache usually presents no special diagnostic or distinguishing features, although it may be suggestive of tension headache or migraine. Pain usually remits after days to weeks but occasionally persists for years.

Treatment & Disposition

The character of the headache dictates the treatment of posttraumatic headache. The pharmacologic treatments used for migraine and tension headache are appropriate for posttraumatic headache and should be chosen by the constellation of the patient's symptoms. Hospitalization is not indicated for posttraumatic headache, although referral for prophylactic therapy is indicated if symptoms persist.

Solomon S: Posttraumatic headache. Med Clin North Am 2001;85:987. [PMID: 11480269] (A review of the classification, clinical features, pathophysiology, diagnosis, and management of posttraumatic headache.)

TRIGEMINAL NEURALGIA

ESSENTIALS OF DIAGNOSIS

• *Excruciating, stabbing, facial pain.*
• *Pain in the distribution of the trigeminal nerve.*

Clinical Findings

In trigeminal neuralgia, lightninglike stabs of excruciating pain characteristically recur over seconds to minutes and spontaneously abate. Occurrence during sleep is rare. Sensory stimulation (eg, touch, cold, wind, talking, chewing) of trigger zones about the cheek, nose, or mouth precipitates paroxysms of pain.

Trigeminal neuralgia usually develops after the fourth decade. Pain-free intervals may last minutes to weeks, but permanent spontaneous remission is rare. Pain is confined mainly to areas supplied by the second or third divisions of the trigeminal nerve (maxillary and mandibular areas of the face). Physical examination must show no abnormalities of trigeminal nerve function (facial sensation, muscles of mastication, corneal reflex) that would support a diagnosis of posterior fossa lesions. Involvement of the first division of the trigeminal nerve (the forehead) or bilateral disease occurs in less than 5% of cases.

Treatment

Phenytoin, 250 mg intravenously over 5–10 minutes, may abort an acute attack. Remission of symptoms with carbamazepine (Tegretol, others) occurs in so many patients that it has been used as a diagnostic test. Begin with 100 mg orally twice daily, and increase by 100 mg every other day until the patient is pain-free or side effects develop.

Baclofen (Lioresal, others) is also beneficial and has synergistic effects when used with carbamazepine or phenytoin. Begin with 5 mg orally 3 times daily, and increase by 5 mg every other day until the patient is pain-free or side effects (eg, dizziness, gastrointestinal upset) occur. Abrupt cessation of baclofen can cause seizures or hallucinations; the dosage should be decreased gradually. Lamotrigine (Lamictal) has also been shown to be useful in the treatment of trigeminal neuralgia, with a starting dose of 25 mg daily with an increase of 25 mg each week until a maintenance dose is reached.

Disposition

Neurologic referral for evaluation and treatment is appropriate. Hospitalization is not usually indicated.

Sindrup SH, Jensen TS: Pharmacotherapy of trigeminal neuralgia. Clin J Pain 2002;18:22. [PMID: 11803299] (An evidence-based review of the pharmacologic treatment of trigeminal neuralgia.)

Zakrzewska JM: Diagnosis and differential diagnosis of trigeminal neuralgia. Clin J Pain 2002;18:14. [PMID: 11803298] (A review article on the diagnosis and differential diagnosis of trigeminal neuralgia.)

INTRACRANIAL MASS
(Brain Tumor)

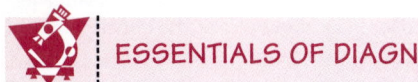

ESSENTIALS OF DIAGNOSIS

- *Mild to moderate headache increasing in frequency or duration.*
- *Becomes associated with a focal neurologic deficit.*

Clinical Findings

Headache due to primary or metastatic intracranial tumor is usually mild to moderate in severity and described as deep, aching, and initially intermittent. Pain is maximal on awakening and during episodes of increased intracranial pressure (eg, coughing, sneezing, or straining at stool). Headaches increase in frequency and duration over weeks to months and become associated with focal neurologic signs. One third to one half of patients with brain tumor present with this classic history. A CT scan obtained with intravenous contrast will usually confirm the diagnosis. MRI, which is more sensitive, may be used as well.

Treatment & Disposition

If an intracranial mass lesion is found to be the cause of headache, urgent neurologic or neurosurgical consultation is indicated. Hospitalization may be required for initiation of treatment. The distinction between primary and metastatic tumor is essential, because treatment differs.

Macarthur DC, Buxton N: The management of brain tumours. J R Coll Surg Edinb 2001;46:341. [PMID: 11768575] (A review of the presentation, diagnosis, and surgical management of brain tumors.)

PSEUDOTUMOR CEREBRI
(Idiopathic Intracranial Hypertension)

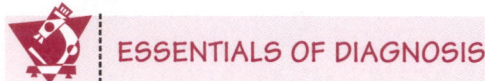

ESSENTIALS OF DIAGNOSIS

- *Papilledema.*
- *Increased intracranial pressure with normal cerebrospinal fluid.*
- *Normal brain imaging study.*

Clinical Findings

Pseuotumor cerebri is a syndrome characterized by papilledema, increased intracranial pressure (with normal cerebrospinal fluid), and a normal brain imaging study demonstrating normal or small-sized ventricles. Women are affected much more commonly than men; the peak incidence occurs in the third decade. Diffuse headache is almost invariably a presenting symptom. Complaints of diplopia and blurred vision or transient visual obscuration occur in greater than 60% of cases. Moderate to severe papilledema is seen in over 40% of affected persons. The course in idiopathic cases is generally self-limited over several months, but visual loss may occur. Differentiation from space-occupying intracerebral mass lesions is critical and can be achieved by CT scan.

Treatment & Disposition

Hospitalization is necessary for evaluation and treatment in patients with newly diagnosed pseudotumor cerebri in the emergency department. Appropriate treatments include repetitive lumbar punctures, carbonic anhydrate inhibitors (acetazolamide), thiazide diuretics, and corticosteroids. Surgical maneuvers, including shunt or optic nerve sheath decompression, may be required. Patients who present to the emergency department with a known diagnosis of pseudotumor cerebri should receive treatment in consultation with the patient's neurologist, neurosurgeon, or ophthalmologist.

Kosmorsky G: Pseudotumor cerebri. Neurosurg Clin North Am 2001;12:775. [PMID: 11524298] (An exhaustive review of the physiology, pathogenesis, epidemiology, clinical manifestations, and treatment of pseudotumor cerebri.)

TEMPORAL ARTERITIS
(Giant Cell Arteritis)

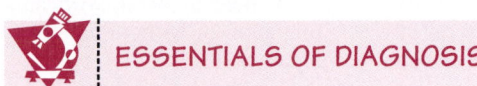

ESSENTIALS OF DIAGNOSIS

- *Age greater than 50 years.*
- *Unilateral headache.*
- *Usually tender over the temporal artery.*
- *Elevated erythrocyte sedimentation rate.*
- *Unilateral vision loss if treatment is delayed.*

Clinical Findings

Temporal arteritis, although uncommon in the general population, is the most common form of systemic vasculitis. The disease preferentially involves large- to medium-sized arteries. It affects women twice as often as men and is rarely seen before the age of 50 years. Nonspecific signs and symptoms are typical: malaise, myalgia, weight loss, arthralgia, and fever. The headache is classically of rapid onset, unremitting, and located over the temporal arteries. It is often unilateral. Associated scalp tenderness may be a prominent complaint, especially when patients lie with their head on a pillow or brush their hair. Pain during chewing (jaw claudication) is strongly suggestive of temporal arteritis. Permanent unilateral blindness, usually sudden in onset, occurs in about half of patients if treatment is delayed; half of patients so affected go on to develop bilateral blindness.

The temporal arteries may be normal on examination, although focal tenderness, thickening, nodularity, or decreased pulsation may be found. The diagnosis should be suspected if the erythrocyte sedimentation rate is greater than 50 mm/h.

The diagnosis can be established by demonstration of vasculitis in biopsy specimens of an affected artery. The biopsy specimens must be carefully examined (multiple sections) because involvement is segmental.

Treatment

Temporal arteritis responds dramatically to corticosteroid treatment. Begin prednisone, 40–60 mg/d orally, as soon as the diagnosis is suspected. Biopsy should be obtained within 2–3 days after beginning corticosteroids. Patients presenting with visual loss warrant immediate ophthalmology consult and should receive intravenous steroids in the emergency department.

Disposition

For patients with severe symptoms or visual loss, hospital admission is urgently indicated for evaluation and treatment with intravenous steroids. Patients with minimal symptoms may be discharged with oral prednisone but should make arrangements for close follow-up and biopsy within 3 days.

Levine SM, Hillmann DB: Giant cell arteritis. Curr Opin Rheumatol 2002;14:3. [PMID: 11790989] (A comprehensive review of the epidemiology, pathophysiology, diagnosis, and treatment of temporal arteritis.)

Smetana GW, Shmerling RH: Does this patient have temporal arthritis? JAMA 2002;287:92. [PMID: 11754714] (A literature review to assess accuracy of clinical signs and symptoms in the diagnosis of temporal arteritis.)

■ MANAGEMENT OF SPECIFIC DISORDERS CAUSING CHRONIC HEADACHE

TENSION HEADACHE

ESSENTIALS OF DIAGNOSIS

- *Gradual onset.*
- *Band or pressure pain about the head.*
- *Constant, nonthrobbing-type pain.*

Clinical Findings

Tension headache, although the most prevalent form of headache, is not the most severe. However, it has significant societal impact with lost workdays and reduced effectiveness when at work. Women are affected three times as commonly as men, and the age at onset is usually between the third and fifth decades. Headaches are often associated with emotional stress and have no prodrome. The pain typically comes on gradually; is bilateral, occipital, or frontal in location; and is described as a tight band or pressure about the head. The pain is constant and nonthrobbing and persists for hours or for the entire day. Nausea and photophobia are frequent accompanying symptoms but are milder than with migraine. Muscle spasm or tension, especially nuchal-occipital, is usually present. About half of patients have headaches 10–30 times a month, and about one fifth are never completely free of headache. Results on neurologic examination are normal.

Treatment

The treatment approach for tension headaches in the emergency department is pharmacotherapy. Nonsteroidal anti-inflammatory drugs remain the therapy of choice in abortive treatment of tension headache. Combination medications that contain caffeine, analgesics, and sedatives have been found to be effective. Muscle relaxants (cyclobenzaprine, methocarbamol) may also be appropriate when muscle tension appears to play a strong role. Referral for prophylactic treatment with antidepressants (amitriptyline) and incorporation of a "wellness" component is appropriate for patients expressing depression or anxiety as precipitants to their headaches.

Disposition

If simple measures are not successful, neurologic referral may be necessary. Hospitalization is not indicated.

Schulman EA: Overview of tension-type headache. Curr Pain Headache Rep 2001;5:454. [PMID: 11560811] (A review of classification, causes, and treatment of tension headaches.)

MIGRAINE

ESSENTIALS OF DIAGNOSIS

- *Throbbing-type pain.*
- *Associated nausea, vomiting, and photophobia are common.*
- *May have associated neurologic symptoms.*

General Considerations

Migraine headache is a primary brain disorder in which neural events result in vasodilation of blood vessels that causes pain and further nerve activation. Most cases occur in women, there is an inherited predisposition, and onset may be as early as the first decade. Recurrent vomiting during childhood may be the earliest manifestation of migraine. A family history of migraine is commonly present.

Clinical Findings

Migraine headaches are classified as being with aura (formerly called classic migraine) or without aura (formerly called common migraine).

Migraine with aura is preceded by transient neurologic symptoms (the aura). The most common auras are visual disturbances: hemianopic field defects, scotomas, and scintillations that enlarge and spread peripherally. As the aura fades, vasodilatation occurs, producing the headache; however, aura can occur without headache. Migraine is said to be hemicranial, but half of migraine headaches are bilateral, and some are occipital. Migraine without aura lacks the classic aura and is bilateral in over half of cases.

The pain is throbbing in most cases. Associated symptoms include nausea and vomiting, photophobia, and, less often, fluid retention, diarrhea, lightheadedness, and fainting. Continuing pain may cause cervical muscle contraction, leading to an erroneous diagnosis of tension headaches. Scalp tenderness may occur.

Attacks may be precipitated by certain foods such as tyramine-containing cheeses, wine, meats with nitrite preservatives, chocolate containing phenylethylamine, and monosodium glutamate (a flavor enhancer). Fasting, emotion, menses, drugs (especially oral contraceptive agents and vasodilators such as nitroglycerin), and bright lights may also trigger attacks. Over half of patients experience no more than one attack a week lasting less than a day. Remissions are common during pregnancy and after menopause.

Treatment

A. ANALGESICS AND ANALGESIC COMBINATIONS

These drugs remain appropriate first-line therapy for acute migraine attacks. Commonly patient will have tried at least one or several analgesics prior to presentation to the emergency department. Appropriate analgesics include aspirin, nonsteroidal anti-inflammatory drugs and combination medications that contain caffeine, analgesics, and sedatives. Opiates should be avoided because they can exacerbate gastrointestinal symptoms and have a high abuse potential.

B. DOPAMINE ANTAGONISTS (ANTIEMETICS)

Several dopamine antagonist have been shown to be effective in aborting acute migraine headaches. Prochlorperazine and metoclopramide are most widely used. Prochlorperazine dosing is 10 mg intravenously. Side effects included hypotension and akathisia. Metoclopramide is also effective in doses of 10 mg intravenously.

C. TRIPTANS

The triptans have an advantage of being selective pharmacologic agents for the treatment of migraine headaches. These compounds are serotonin 5-HT receptor agonists. All of these drugs have been shown to be effective in aborting acute migraine headaches. However, they have significant side effects and cannot be used in patients with a history of cardiovascular disease. The following triptans can be used in the treatment of migraines in the emergency department:

- Sumatriptan, 6 mg subcutaneously, which may be repeated after 1 hour; or 25–100 mg orally, which may be repeated after 2 hours
- Naratriptan, 1–2.5 mg orally, which may be repeated after 4 hours
- Almotriptan, 6.25–12.5 mg orally, which may be repeated after 2 hours
- Rizatriptan, 5–10 mg orally, which may be repeated after 2 hours
- Zolmitriptan, 1.25–2.5 mg orally, which may be repeated after 2 hours

D. ERGOT DERIVATIVES

Ergot preparations have been used widely in the past for the acute treatment of migraine headaches. These drugs have complex pharmacology, and there is little evidence to support their use. With the effectiveness of dopamine agonists and triptans, ergot preparations should be abandoned for abortive therapy in the emergency department.

E. PROPHYLACTIC DRUGS

Prophylatic therapy may be useful in preventing migraine headaches, but it should not be initiated in the emergency department. Patients should be referred to a neurologist for evaluation for preventive treatment.

Disposition

Referral to a neurologist or primary care physician is indicated. Hospitalization (other than a brief stay in the emergency department for parenteral medication) is rarely needed.

Ducharme G: Canadian Association of Emergency Physicians guidelines for the acute management of migraine headache. J Emerg Med 1999;17:137. [PMID: 96650404] (A review of emergency department treatment of acute migraine headaches.)

Elrington G: Modern management of migraine. Hosp Med 2001;62:687. [PMID: 11762100] (Examines diagnostic as well as therapeutic and prevention strategies for migraine headaches.)

Goadsby PJ, Lipton RB, Ferrari MD: Migraine—current understanding and treatment. N Engl J Med 2002;346:257. [PMID: 11807151] (Review of current understanding of the epidemiology, pathophysiology, and treatment of migraine.)

CLUSTER HEADACHE

 ESSENTIALS OF DIAGNOSIS

- *Clusters of daily attacks separated by week to months of pain-free intervals.*
- *Attacks consist of severe unilateral headache.*
- *Associated cranial autonomic symptoms include lacrimation, miosis, conjunctival injection, nasal congestion, and rhinorrhea.*

Clinical Findings

Cluster headache is a syndrome of distinct attacks of severe, unilateral headache with ipsilateral cranial autonomic symptoms. The autonomic symptoms may include ptosis, lacrimation, miosis, conjunctival injection, nasal congestion, and rhinorrhea. It is more common in men than in women and begins later in life than migraine headaches. There is often no family history of similar headaches.

Pain occurs in distribution of the trigeminal nerve and most commonly in the ocular, frontal, and temporal areas. Each attack builds in intensity over 10–15 minutes and may last up to 3 hours. Attacks recur 1–3 times daily, often at nearly the same time for periods of weeks to 2–3 months that may be separated by headache-free interval remission periods that usually last for months or years. A subset of patients experience chronic cluster headaches without remission. These patients have attacks for greater than 1 year without remission or with remissions lasting less than 14 days.

Episodes may be precipitated by alcohol or vasodilator-type drugs. Nitroglycerin challenge can be diagnostic, producing a typical headache in 30–60 minutes.

Treatment

Standard treatment for acute attacks is oxygen (7 L/min for 15 min) delivered by face mask; this treatment has a reported 70% response rate. Sumatriptan, 6 mg subcutaneously, although contraindicated in patients with known cardiovascular disease, has proved effective: 80% of patients experience complete or near complete relief. Less effective agents such as dihydroergotamine and ergotamine are also commonly used. Lidocaine, 20–60 mg given intranasally, provides some relief within 10 minutes in most patients, but complete relief is rare.

Due to the severity, reoccurrence, and chronicity of attacks, prophylaxis should follow treatment for the acute headache. Prophylactic treatment should be initiated at the first sign of an attack and continued for 2 weeks past the last attack. Prophylactic agents include verapamil, ergotamine, lithium, methylsergide, and steroids. Verapamil is considered the agent of choice at dosages of 240–480 mg/d. Higher dosages (up to 1200 mg/day) may be given to patients with chronic cluster headache. Surgical intervention has been recommended for intractable chronic cluster headaches that have become resistant to medical management.

Disposition

Neurologic referral is indicated.

Ekbom K, Hardebo JE: Cluster headache: aetiology, diagnosis and management. Drugs 2002;62:61. [PMID: 11790156] (Review of the pathophysiology, diagnosis, and management of cluster headaches.)

Newman LC, Goadsby P, Lipton RB: Cluster and related headaches. Med Clin North Am 2001;85:997. [PMID: 11480270] (Review of the etiology, diagnosis, and treatment of cluster headaches with emphasis on differentiation between cluster headaches and related disorders.)

Zakrzewska JM: Cluster headache: review of the literature. Br J Oral Maxillofac Surg 2001;39:103. [PMID: 11286443] (Literature review of papers on cluster headaches using the Cochrane systematic review guidelines; treatment and guidelines proposed based on evidence of this review.)

HEADACHE DUE TO HYPERTENSION

Headache is not a prominent feature of chronic hypertension. Research has shown that patients with hypertension and complaints of headache did not have blood pressure levels different than those during their headache-free periods. In addition, blood pressures preceding the headache pain were not significantly different than those measured at the onset of pain, and the majority of patients had their maximal blood pressures during headache-free periods.

The acute onset of headache and severe blood pressure elevation are components of hypertensive crisis (Chapter 34) and also are commonly present following subarachnoid hemorrhage. As a result, patients presenting with headache and a history of hypertension should undergo a full evaluation, and the headache should not be presumed due to elevation of blood pressure.

Kruszewski P et al: Headache in patients with mild to moderate hypertension is generally not associated with simultaneous blood pressure elevation. J Hypertens 2000;18:437. [PMID: 10779095] (A study looking at the correlation of headaches and blood pressure in patients with mild to moderate hypertension.)

Delirium & Acute Confusional States 20

Eric W. Flach, MD, Timothy A. Coakley, MD, & James J. Mensching, MD, DO, FACEP[1,2]

Immediate Management of Life-Threatening Problems

Emergency Management of Specific Disorders

Seizure Disorders
1. Postictal Confusion
2. Interictal & Postictal Psychosis

Metabolic Encephalopathies
1. Systemic Metabolic Disorders
2. Drug Withdrawal Syndromes (Ethanol & Other Sedative-Hypnotic Drugs)
3. Wernicke Encephalopathy (Acute Thiamine Deficiency)
4. Drug Intoxication

Reye Syndrome

Amnestic Syndromes
1. Amnestic Episodes
2. Transient Global Amnesia

Acute Strokes (Cerebrovascular Accidents)
1. Fluent Aphasia
2. Agitated Confusion

Confusion Associated with Psychiatric Disease
1. Psychotic Confusional States
2. Hysteria

Confusional States of Uncertain Cause

■ IMMEDIATE MANAGEMENT OF LIFE-THREATENING PROBLEMS (See Figure 20–1.)

Delirium and acute confusional states are among the most difficult problems confronting the emergency physician. The patient's mental status can be assessed quickly using a classification scheme. Such schemes classify patients according to whether or not they are alert, their ability to attend, and their memory capability, allowing the physician to differentiate among coma, delirium, and dementia. These are the 3 main categorizations of a patient with an acutely altered mental status. This chapter focuses on delirium and acute confusional states.

Confused patients are often uncooperative or combative, making evaluation difficult. Signs and symptoms may be manifestations of a life-threatening underlying condition demanding prompt diagnosis and treatment to prevent irreversible brain damage (Table 20–1). Although evaluation may be difficult, every patient with an acutely altered state of consciousness must be examined and a history taken so that the cause can be established, if possible, in the emergency department. If the diagnosis cannot be established with certainty, the patient should be hospitalized.

Immediate Measures

A. Maintain Airway

Clear secretions as needed. Begin oxygen, if necessary, 5–10 L/min, by mask or nasal cannula. Restrain the patient only if necessary.

B. Gain Intravenous Access

Insert a large-bore (≥ 18-gauge) intravenous catheter. Draw blood for complete blood count (CBC); serum glucose, electrolyte, calcium, and magnesium determinations; and hepatic and renal function tests. Obtain urine for urinalysis and toxicology screen.

Administer the following intravenously: (1) thiamine, 100 mg by slow bolus injection; (2) 50% dextrose in water, 50 mL over 3–5 minutes, if the patient is hypoglycemic by bedside fingerstick glucose testing; and (3) naloxone (Narcan, others), 2 mg by bolus injection. **Caution:** Administration of glucose may worsen

---

[1]This chapter is a revision of the chapter by Roger P. Simon, MD, from the 4th edition.

[2]The views expressed in this chapter are those of the authors and do not reflect the official policy or position of the Department of the Navy, Department of Defense, or the U.S. government.

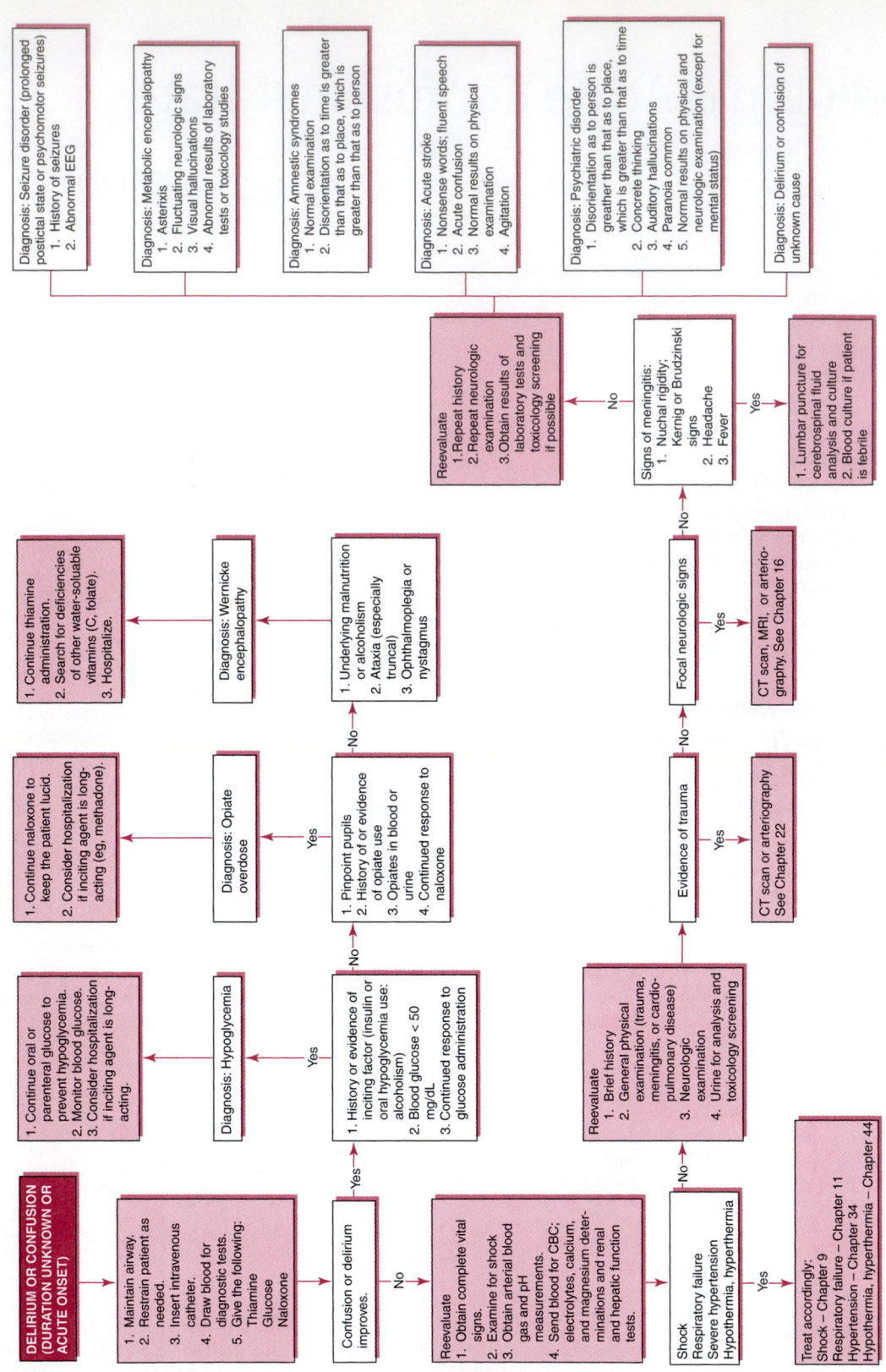

Figure 20–1. Assessment of delirium or confusional states.

392

Table 20–1. Conditions associated with acute confusion or delirium that may cause rapid cerebral damage.

Hypoglycemia
Wernicke encephalopathy
Hypotension and shock
Respiratory failure (hypercapnia or hypoxemia)
Hyperthermia or hypothermia
Meningitis or encephalitis
Stroke
Mass lesions (including intracranial bleeding)
Poisoning (methanol, ethylene glycol, carbon monoxide)

---

brain injury by increasing lactate in ischemic areas. Do not give glucose to patients during the acute phases of stroke or after cardiac arrest if serum glucose is normal.

C. TREAT SHOCK

Hypotension and shock with associated peripheral hypoperfusion may be associated with delirium or confusion. Treat shock with immediate intravenous administration of crystalloid solutions unless the patient is in cardiogenic shock, and follow with more specific measures (Chapter 9).

D. CORRECT RESPIRATORY FAILURE

Hypoxemia or hypercapnia that develops abruptly may be associated with delirium. Assess ventilatory status by means of arterial blood gases, and correct hypoxemia or hypercapnia by administration of oxygen, assisted ventilation, or both, as needed (Chapter 11).

E. TREAT HYPERTHERMIA OR HYPOTHERMIA

Markedly elevated body temperatures (40.6 °C [105 °F]) may be associated with delirium or acute confusional states. Hypothermia is likely to produce confusion at body temperatures below 32.2 °C (90 °F) and unconsciousness at temperatures below 26.6 °C (80 °F). Treat by lowering or raising core temperature, as needed (Chapter 44).

F. TREAT SEVERE HYPERTENSION

Severe hypertension (when associated with papilledema and encephalopathy) is a medical emergency requiring rapid reduction of diastolic pressure toward 100 mm Hg (Chapter 34). The diagnosis of hypertensive encephalopathy must be firmly established before antihypertensive therapy is started, however, because reduction of blood pressure when cerebral ischemia is present can severely exacerbate ischemic brain injury.

Initial Evaluation

1. Obtain complete vital signs, including temperature.
2. Assess for shock (peripheral hypoperfusion).
3. Obtain results of arterial blood gas and pH determinations.
4. Does the delirium lighten after administration of intravenous glucose, thiamine, and naloxone? If so, consider the following possibilities:
   - Hypoglycemia (diagnosis is confirmed by finding of low serum glucose)
   - Wernicke encephalopathy (look for associated alcoholism, malnutrition, ataxia, ophthalmoplegia, and peripheral neuropathy)
   - Opiate overdose (diagnosis is confirmed by positive response to naloxone and toxicology screen)

Further Evaluation

See Table 20–2.

A. EXAMINATION AND DIAGNOSTIC TESTS

1. History—Obtain a brief history from the patient, family, friends, neighbors, ambulance attendants, or bystanders. Ask in particular about prior episodes of confusion or delirium, duration and other features of the present episode, drug usage, and previous illness.

2. Physical and neurologic examination—Perform a general physical examination, and look especially for signs of trauma, meningeal irritation, and cardiac disease. Complete a basic neurologic examination, including tests of orientation and memory.

3. Laboratory studies—Send blood to the laboratory for CBC; serum electrolyte, glucose, calcium, and magnesium determinations; renal and liver function tests; carboxyhemoglobin level; and toxicology studies. Obtain urine for urinalysis and toxicology studies.

4. Electrocardiogram—Obtain an electrocardiogram in order to seek any abnormalities that might suggest a cardiac cause of the confusional state (eg, myocardial infarction, cardiac arrhythmias, prolonged intervals). T-wave changes, however, are nonspecific and may be seen with acute intracranial events.

5. Special studies—Special studies may be indicated based on the results of history and physical examination (eg, lumbar puncture for cerebrospinal fluid in the patient with confusion and fever or signs of meningeal irritation).

6. Gastric contents evaluation—Administer an activated charcoal slurry (50-100 mg of activated charcoal

Table 20–2. Differential diagnosis of conditions causing delirium or confusion.

Etiologic Category	Clinical Findings
Central nervous system mass lesion (subdural hematoma, cerebral infarction, brain tumor)	Somnolence; neurologic examination shows focal or asymmetric abnormality. Posterior nondominant parietal lobe strokes present with an agitated delirium, without hemiparesis.

Meningitis or meningoencephalitis
    Infectious, carcinomatous, or chemical meningitis
      secondary to subarachnoid hemorrhage
	Headache, fever, meningeal signs, cerebrospinal fluid pleocytosis.

Seizure disorders
    Confusional states following seizures (postictal states)
    Psychomotor status epilepticus
	History or evidence of seizures, especially seen in seizure patients with superimposed metabolic abnormality, encephalitis, or diffuse cerebral damage, in whom postictal state may be prolonged.

Amnestic states	Findings confined to recent memory loss.
Fluent aphasias	Sudden onset; patient alert; mild right hemiparesis (may be absent). Excessive speech with frequent word substitutions and nonsense phrases.
Psychiatric disease (thought disorders and hysteria)	Paranoia prominent; auditory hallucinations common; disorientation as to person, which is greater than that as to place, which is greater than that as to time. Recent memory preserved.
Head trauma (acute posttraumatic delirium, post-concussion syndrome)	Recent history or evidence of head trauma.
Metabolic encephalopathy; drug intoxication or withdrawal	Fluctuations in mental status (lucid intervals); asterixis; myoclonus; tremor; visual hallucinations; disorientation as to time, which is greater than that as to place, which is greater than that as to person; nystagmus.

admixed with water or sorbitol) and consider gastric lavage if ingestion or overdose of a toxin is a diagnostic possibility.

B. Trauma

If there is evidence of trauma—even if the head itself appears uninjured—consider the possibility of traumatic brain damage (eg, subdural or epidural hematomas). Computed tomography (CT) scan may be indicated (Chapter 22). Hospitalization is required even if no specific abnormality is found.

C. Meningeal Irritation

Look first for signs of meningitis due to infection or subarachnoid hemorrhage. Headache is common and may not be severe. Fever is common in infectious meningitis but is absent in the initial stage of subarachnoid hemorrhage. Signs of meningeal irritation (meningismus: stiff neck, positive Kernig and Brudzinski signs) are almost invariably present in meningitis or subarachnoid hemorrhage except in very young or very old patients. The most helpful diagnostic maneuver is passive flexion of the patient's neck, which elicits reflex knee flexion (usually unilateral) if meningeal irritation

is present (positive Brudzinski sign). Perform lumbar puncture immediately in patients with meningismus in the absence of signs of increased intracranial pressure (papilledema, focal neurologic findings) for evaluation of cerebrospinal fluid (Chapter 19). Bacterial meningitis requires urgent treatment (Chapter 40).

D. Focal Neurologic Findings

(See Table 20–2.) Although focal signs may be found in metabolic brain disease (notably the fluctuating hemiparesis that may occur with hypoglycemia and hepatic encephalopathy), such asymmetric findings should be assumed to reflect a structural brain lesion until proved otherwise; appropriate neurologic or neurosurgical consultation should be obtained.

The principal differential diagnostic considerations are cerebrovascular accidents (thrombotic or embolic) and mass lesions. Lumbar puncture is contraindicated, and the patient should be evaluated with CT scan.

In patients with fever and focal neurologic findings, a brain abscess must be considered along with meningitis and encephalitis. A lumbar puncture is contraindicated until a CT scan has eliminated the possibility of a mass lesion. To avoid delay of needed treatment for possible meningitis while awaiting the results of the CT scan, obtain blood cultures, and begin antibiotics immediately (Chapter 40).

E. OTHER CAUSES OF DELIRIUM OR CONFUSION

Once life-threatening conditions have been ruled out, a more specific diagnosis can be attempted. Main causes are shown in Table 20–2 and described below. Delirium or confusion occurring in patients with AIDS is discussed in Chapter 40.

Johnson J: Identifying and recognizing delirium. Dement Geriatr Cogn Disord 1999;10:353. [PMID: 10473939]

Liptzin B: What criteria should be used for the diagnosis of delirium? Dement Geriatr Cogn Disord 1999;10:364. [PMID: 1047394]

■ EMERGENCY MANAGEMENT OF SPECIFIC DISORDERS

SEIZURE DISORDERS
(See Chapter 17.)

ESSENTIALS OF DIAGNOSIS

- *Present in patients who have known seizure or have an underlying seizure disorder.*
- *Mental status abnormalities and focal neurologic symptoms are usually present.*
- *May be associated with psychiatric symptoms.*
- *Administer appropriate anticonvulsant treatment as necessary.*

1. Postictal Confusion
Clinical Findings

Postictal confusion is a fairly common phenomenon with seizures. It is usually diagnosed after a witnessed seizure in a patient who has an underlying seizure disorder. This confusion may be associated with psychiatric symptoms such as delusions, hallucinations, and behavioral changes. Although the psychiatric symptoms are usually brief, the patient may remain in a confusional state for some time.

Treatment & Disposition

Hospitalize the patient and give appropriate treatment if the cause of the psychiatric and confusional symptoms is not identified or the symptoms fail to resolve.

2. Interictal & Postictal Psychosis
Clinical Findings

Interictal psychosis is the presence of confusion and psychiatric symptoms (eg, apathy and diminished affect) in seizure patients that are unrelated to their seizures. Because these symptoms are not related to the seizure episode, this is a difficult diagnosis and should be considered in the delirious or confused patient who has an underlying seizure disorder.

Postictal psychosis occurs predominately after a repeated number of seizures. Patients present with mood changes and psychiatric symptoms, mainly paranoid delusions. Hallucinations occur less frequently.

Treatment & Disposition

Hospitalize the patient, administer the necessary anticonvulsant therapy, and monitor appropriately.

Bostwick JM: The many faces of confusion. Timing and collateral history often hold the key to diagnosis. Postgrad Med 2000; 108:60. [PMID: 11098259]

Kaplan PW: Assessing the outcomes in patients with nonconvulsive status epilepticus: nonconvulsive status epilepticus is underdiagnosed potentially overtreated, and confounded by comorbidity. J Clin Neurophysiol 1999;16:341. [PMID: 10478707]

Lancman M: Psychosis and peri-ictal confusional states. Neurology 1999;53:S33. [PMID: 9139290]

Murphy BA: Delirium. Emerg Med Clin North Am 2000;18:243. [PMID: 10767881]

METABOLIC ENCEPHALOPATHIES

ESSENTIALS OF DIAGNOSIS

- *Will see changes in patient's mental status with lucid intervals and no focal abnormalities.*
- *Patient tends to remain oriented to person but not place or time.*
- *Similar withdrawal profile is seen with alcohol, barbiturates, and other sedative-hypnotic drugs.*
- *Delirium tremens is life threatening and must be treated promptly.*

• Patients with Wernicke encephalopathy present with ophthalmoplegia, ataxia, and confusion. Wernicke encephalopathy is a medical emergency and should be treated promptly with thiamine.

1. Systemic Metabolic Disorders

Systemic metabolic disease, acute drug intoxication, or sedative-hypnotic drug withdrawal can produce an altered mental status ranging from florid, agitated delirium to lethargy or coma.

Clinical Findings

Marked fluctuation in the patient's mental state with intermittent periods of lucidity, without focal abnormalities, is characteristic of metabolic encephalopathy. A history of systemic illness (Table 20–3) or drug ingestion should be sought in every patient with a confusional state. Helpful clinical findings include the following:

• Symmetric nystagmus is found in sedative-hypnotic drug and phencyclidine ingestion.

• Asterixis is most commonly associated with hepatic or renal insufficiency.

• Hallucinations occur in metabolic disorders and are typically visual, as exemplified by delirium tremens.

• Orientation as to time is lost early in metabolic encephalopathy and is followed later by loss of orientation as to place, but orientation as to person is almost invariably preserved. This characteristic pattern of metabolic brain disease contrasts with that of psychiatric disorders, in which patients may know the correct day and date but are uncertain who or where they are.

• Arterial blood gas and pH measurements may suggest a metabolic cause for acute confusional states and are useful in distinguishing the metabolic causes of coma.

Treatment & Disposition

Seek and correct the cause of the metabolic disorder. Hospitalize the patient for treatment and diagnosis as indicated.

2. Drug Withdrawal Syndromes (Ethanol & Other Sedative-Hypnotic Drugs)

General Considerations

Several well-recognized syndromes are associated with acute withdrawal from alcohol, barbiturates, or other sedative-hypnotic drugs (Table 20–4). Manifestations of acute alcohol withdrawal are as follows:

• Acute alcoholic tremulousness

• Acute intoxication (inebriation, stupor, or combative states)

• Alcohol withdrawal seizures

• Tremor and transitory hallucinations

• Typical delirium tremens

• Atypical delirious-hallucinatory states

• Acute auditory hallucinations

• Other miscellaneous manifestations, including Wernicke-Korsakoff syndrome

Acute tremulous and hallucinatory states that are distinct from delirium tremens are more common and less serious than delirium tremens and are seen within

Table 20–3. Systemic illnesses associated with confusion due to metabolic encephalopathy.

Renal	Respiratory
Renal failure with azotemia	Hypercapnia
Electrolyte	Hypoxemia
Hypernatremia	**Cardiac**
Hyponatremia	Heart failure
Dehydration	Endocarditis
Hypercalcemia	**Other**
Hypocalcemia	Sepsis
Hyperglycemia	Shock
Hypoglycemia	Drug ingestion
Hypermagnesemia	Thiamine deficiency
Hypomagnesemia	(eg, Wernicke-Korsakoff syndrome)
Hepatic	
Hepatic failure	Hyperthyroidism
Lactic acidosis	Hypothyroidism

Table 20–4. Sedative drugs reportedly followed by clinical abstinence syndromes after withdrawal from excessive dosage.

Barbiturates (phenobarbital, many others)
Alcohol
Meprobamate (Equanil, Miltown, others)
Glutethimide (Doriden, others)
Methyprylon (Noludar)
Ethinamate (Valmid)
Ethchlorvynol (Placidyl)
Benzodiazepines

the first 6–36 hours following relative or absolute abstinence from alcohol, whereas classic delirium tremens syndrome typically appears after 3–4 days of abstinence (range: 24 hours to 5 days or more).

Clinical Findings

A. Delirium Tremens

Note: Delirium tremens is an uncommon but life-threatening illness that requires prompt recognition and treatment for the best outcome. Symptoms and signs include the following:

- Profoundly delirious state associated with tremulousness and agitation.
- Excessive motor activity (most notable as a tremor that affects the face, tongue, and extremities but that may also involve speech) and purposeless activity such as picking at the bedclothes.
- Hallucinations, classically visual rather than auditory, are a prominent feature, especially if patients are specifically asked, "What do you see? What's over there? Is there anything frightening you?" These patients may be quite suggestible and may be persuaded to light an imaginary cigarette or identify the color of a nonexistent piece of string.
- Autonomic nervous system hyperactivity: tachycardia, dilated pupils, fever, and hyperhidrosis.
- Loss of orientation as to time and place. Such patients are often oblivious to the most obvious features of the surrounding environment (eg, they do not know whether they are in bed or on a chair or wearing a suit or pajamas).

Duration of delirium tremens is less than 24 hours in 15% of cases and less than 3 days in over 80%.

B. Withdrawal Seizures

Withdrawal seizures, a syndrome distinct from delirium tremens, may result from abrupt decrease or cessation of alcohol consumption. About 90% of such convulsions occur 6–48 hours after abstinence.

Because delirium tremens requires a longer period of abstinence than withdrawal seizures, pure withdrawal seizures (ie, those occurring only during periods of withdrawal) always occur before delirium tremens. Therefore, any seizures occurring after delirium tremens must be assumed to be due to some cause other than alcohol withdrawal, and further evaluation is required.

C. Sedative-Hypnotic Drug Withdrawal

A syndrome nearly identical to delirium tremens but somewhat more protracted may follow withdrawal from short-acting barbiturates or other sedative-hypnotic drugs (Table 20–4) in habituated patients. These drug-induced withdrawal reactions occur only when the patient has become habituated to large doses of the drug.

D. γ-Hydroxybutyrate

Since the early 1990s, a prolonged withdrawal syndrome has emerged with chronic frequent use of γ-hydroxybutyrate (GHB). GHB is an increasingly popular drug of abuse owing to its euphoric effects. It has been used in the past as an anesthetic agent, bodybuilding supplement, or sexual enhancer or to incapacitate victims for assault. Its precursor is readily available for purchase on the Internet.

The onset of symptoms is typically between 1–6 hours after the last use of GHB, and symptoms can last from 5 to 15 days. Initially patients experience anxiety, insomnia, and tremor. These symptoms progress rapidly to severe delirium with psychosis and agitation, and patients may require physical restraint and sedation. Autonomic instability and death can occur.

Treatment

A. Delirium Tremens

Note temperature, pulse, and blood pressure, and record results twice hourly to monitor for hyperpyrexia and hypotension. Consider lumbar puncture to rule out meningitis if fever or meningismus is present.

1. Fluids—Fluid requirements on the first day of treatment may be as high as 4–10 L because of profound dehydration. Intravenous fluid should contain glucose to prevent hypoglycemia.

2. Thiamine—Thiamine, 100 mg/d, prevents Wernicke encephalopathy. Other water-soluble vitamins (B complex and C) should also be given.

3. Sedatives—Judicious use of sedative drugs does not eliminate established delirium but does protect the patient against self-induced trauma and permit continued treatment. Sedatives (eg, benzodiazepines) may also prevent patients with impending delirium tremens from developing a full-blown case.

    a. Initial dose—A suggested regimen is diazepam (Valium, others), 10 mg intravenously given over at least 2 minutes, followed by 5 mg intravenously every 5 minutes until the patient is calm. The total dose required to calm a patient may be as high as 200 mg (rarely, even 700 mg or more). Drug-induced hypotension and respiratory depression during administration of diazepam for delirium tremens are uncommon if adequate hydration is maintained and overzealous treatment avoided. After delirium tremens has been controlled, the patient may sleep without interruption for up to 36 hours but can nonetheless be easily aroused.

b. Maintenance doses—Administer diazepam, 5–10 mg, intravenously or orally as needed. Avoid intramuscular administration, because absorption by this route is erratic. Sedation is achieved within a few minutes following intravenous injection but may be delayed for 3 hours or longer following intramuscular injection if associated obesity, hyperpyrexia, or complicating illness (eg, pneumonia) is present.

4. ACTH or corticosteroids—Do not administer ACTH or corticosteroids for delirium tremens; they are ineffective and potentially harmful.

5. Phenothiazines—Phenothiazines have been used and may promptly control hallucinatory symptoms; however, these drugs are not recommended, because they may cause hypotension or precipitate seizures.

6. β-Blockers—The concomitant administration of β-blocking drugs decreases the associated autonomic hyperactivity.

B. Withdrawal Seizures

Pure withdrawal seizures are self-limited and usually do not require anticonvulsant therapy. Observation is necessary, because about 60% of patients will have more than one seizure, 95% of which will occur within 12 hours after the initial seizure and 80% within 6 hours. Repetitive alcohol withdrawal seizures can be controlled pharmacologically with a single loading dose of phenobarbital (750 mg, intravenously slowly); phenytoin is ineffective. Patients with withdrawal seizures, unless previously investigated, should receive outpatient follow-up. Most should be investigated at least once for structural causes. Hospitalization is rarely required.

C. Sedative-Hypnotic Drug Withdrawal

Supportive care is usually all that is necessary for sedative-hypnotic withdrawal syndromes. This may entail short-term airway protection (about 8 hours) via endotracheal intubation. Associated delirium requires benzodiazepine treatment as outlined above in treatment of delirium tremens.

Treatment

The most important therapeutic aspect of care is attention to management of the airway. Effort should also be given to protecting the patient from harming him- or herself. Specific side effects from withdrawal are treated accordingly, as described above.

Disposition

Hospitalization is indicated for all patients with sedative-hypnotic drug withdrawal who have active delir-

ium tremens or possible impending delirium tremens (tremor, tachycardia, and agitation). Patients with more benign withdrawal states (tremulousness alone, hallucinatory states other than delirium tremens, withdrawal seizures) may be sent home after 6–12 hours of observation and treatment in the emergency department.

3. Wernicke Encephalopathy (Acute Thiamine Deficiency)

Clinical Findings

Wernicke encephalopathy is a medical emergency characterized by ophthalmoplegia, ataxia, and confusion. Most cases are associated with alcoholism, malnutrition, or both. Failure to initiate prompt thiamine therapy in a patient with any of these features may result either in death or in permanent neuropathy or loss of cognitive function.

A. Ocular Abnormalities

Nystagmus (horizontal alone or horizontal and vertical) may occur. Isolated vertical nystagmus is rare. Bilateral lateral rectus muscle (sixth cranial nerve) palsies and conjugate gaze palsies may be present. Other types of ophthalmoplegia may occur. The response to irrigation of the external ear canal with ice water (caloric test) is invariably abnormal and reveals unilateral or bilateral absence of ocular movement.

B. Ataxia

Ataxia is similar to that associated with alcoholic cerebellar degeneration. Truncal ataxia is most common, with a wide-based, unsteady gait as the major finding. Limb ataxia is less common than ataxia of gait and affects the lower extremities much more than the upper extremities.

C. Confusion

Frank delirium occurs in about 20% of cases. Blatant apathy, manifested as inattention, drowsiness, and decreased spontaneous speech, is present in most cases. In the recovery phase, Korsakoff psychosis may become more prominent, with marked impairment of recent memory and inability to retain new information. Confabulation is common.

D. Cardiovascular Abnormalities

Tachycardia, exertional dyspnea, minor electrocardiographic abnormalities, and orthostatic hypotension are common. Overt beriberi heart disease with heart failure is rare.

E. Neuropathy

Peripheral neuropathy is associated with Wernicke encephalopathy in approximately 80% of cases.

Treatment

A. VITAMINS

Give thiamine, 100 mg intravenously, immediately upon diagnosis of Wernicke encephalopathy. Patients should be hospitalized and thiamine continued in doses of 50 mg/d intravenously until adequate diet and bowel function are reestablished. Other water-soluble vitamins (B complex and C) should be given, because multiple deficiencies are common in these patients. The need for folate or vitamin B$_{12}$ should be assessed based on the CBC (presence of hypersegmented polymorphonuclear leukocytes, and macrocytosis). Deficiencies of fat-soluble vitamins (A, D, and E) are rare.

Magnesium deficiency is common in alcohol withdrawal states, and magnesium should be replaced based on blood levels (Chapter 42).

B. BED REST

Bed rest is necessary because of the patient's fragile cardiovascular status (deaths have been reported following trivial physical exertion).

C. OUTCOME

With thiamine therapy, oculomotor abnormalities may begin to improve within minutes to hours, and complete recovery will occur within 1–4 weeks, except for persistent lateral gaze nystagmus. Global confusional state, ataxia, peripheral neuropathies, and Korsakoff psychosis in particular clear much less quickly, and permanent disability is common.

Disposition

All patients with thiamine deficiency syndromes should be hospitalized for supportive care and continued administration of thiamine.

4. Drug Intoxication

Centrally Acting Anticholinergic Drugs

Intoxication with a wide variety of anticholinergic medications that penetrate the central nervous system may produce agitated and confusional states. Table 20–5 lists representative prescription and over-the-counter medications.

Delirium, psychosis, anxiety, hallucinations, breathlessness, hyperactivity, disorientation, seizures, and coma are typically associated with signs of peripheral cholinergic blockade: tachycardia, mydriasis, hyperpyrexia, urinary retention, decreased bowel motility, decreased sweating, and decreased bronchial, pharyngeal, and salivary secretions. The patient is hot, dry, red, and "mad as a hatter."

Table 20–5. Drugs that may cause a central anticholinergic syndrome.[1]

Anticholinergics
Atropine (eg, belladonna, Donnatal)
Scopolamine (also found in Jimsonweed [*Datura* sp])

Tricyclic antidepressants
Amitriptyline (Elavil, many others)
Doxepin (Adapin, Sinequan, others)
Imipramine (Tofranil, many others)

Phenothiazines
Chlorpromazine (Thorazine, many others)
Trifluoperazine (Stelazine, many others)
Thioridazine (Mellaril, many others)

Antihistamines
Chlorpheniramine (Omade, Teldrin, many others)
Diphenhydramine (Benadryl, many others)
Promethazine (Phenergan, many others)

Ophthalmic preparations
Atropine, 1% ophthalmic solution
Cyclopentolate (AK-Pentolate, Cyclogyl, others)
Tropicamide (Mydriacyl, others)

Antispasmodics
Methantheline (Banthine)
Propantheline (Pro-Banthine, others)

Antiparkinsonism agents
Benztropine (Cogentin, many others)
Biperide (Akineton)
Trihexyphenidyl (Artane, others)

Over-the-counter drugs (hypnotics, analgesics)
Sominex (diphenhydramine)
Sleep-Eze (diphenhydramine)
Contac (chlorpheniramine)
Dristan (chlorpheniramine)

[1]Only selected representatives from each group are listed.

Treatment is discussed in Chapter 45. Hospitalization is required for supportive care.

Stimulants & Hallucinogenic Drugs

Some commonly abused drugs, for example, cocaine, amphetamine, LSD (lysergic acid ethylamide), jimsonweed, and PCP (phencyclidine), can cause an agitated confusional state. Cocaine is currently the most frequent culprit and can produce agitation, anxiety, depression, psychosis, paranoia, suicidal ideation, or any combination of these conditions. Symptoms are independent of the route of drug administration. Treatment is discussed in Chapter 45. Short-term psychiatric admission often is required.

Beaver TM et al: Treatment of acute anticholinergic poisoning with physostigmine. Am J Emerg Med 1998;16:505. [PMID: 9725967]

Brown TM: Drug-induced delirium. Semin Clin Neuropsychiatry 2000;5(2):113. PMID: 10837100

Dyer JE: Gamma-hydroxybutyrate withdrawal syndrome. Ann Emerg Med 2001;37:147. [PMID: 11174231]

Myrick H et al: New developments in the pharmacotherapy of alcohol dependence. Am J Addict 2001;10:3. [PMID: 11268820]

Olmedo R et al: Withdrawal syndromes. Emerg Med Clin North Am 2000;18:273. [PMID: 10767884]

Talbot-Stern JK et al: Psychiatric manifestations of systemic illness. Emerg Med Clin North Am 2000;199. [PMID: 10767878]

REYE'S SYNDROME

 ESSENTIALS OF DIAGNOSIS

- *Associated with fatty degeneration of the liver.*
- *A link exists between viruses, specifically chicken-pox and influenza, and salicylates.*
- *Extremely rare in individuals over age 20 years.*

General Considerations

Reye syndrome, an encephalopathy associated with fatty degeneration of the liver, is a major cause of delirium progressing to coma in infants and children. The degree of central nervous system impairment does not correlate well with the degree of hepatic dysfunction. The disease is extremely rare in individuals over age 20 years. Seasonal occurrence from November to April with a peak incidence in February has been noted. There may be a history of a preceding viral illness. Epidemiologic evidence has firmly linked Reye syndrome with chickenpox and influenza virus infections. An association between Reye syndrome and the use of salicylates during an antecedent illness has been demonstrated.

The number of cases has dropped dramatically since the 1980s. Several authors have noted a correlation between the decrease in reported cases to almost zero and the discovery of many new metabolic disorders that have a common pathophysiology. New diagnostic techniques to identify these inborn errors of metabolism have revealed that many cases of Reye syndrome mimicked these disorders. It is now recommended that any infant or child suspected of having Reye syndrome undergo extensive testing to rule out the treatable inborn metabolic disorders.

Clinical Findings

Illness begins with protracted vomiting and delirium that progresses to coma within 2 days. Seizures are common but are usually self-limited. Decerebrate posturing is common, but focal neurologic signs are rare once coma is established. Sustained hyperventilation and hepatomegaly are usually noted. Cerebrospinal fluid examination reveals normal protein and cell count. Blood glucose is frequently reduced because of hepatic failure and may be reflected in low levels of cerebrospinal fluid glucose. Serum transaminase and blood ammonia levels are characteristically elevated. Prothrombin time is prolonged. Serum bilirubin is normal, so that icterus makes the diagnosis of Reye syndrome doubtful.

Treatment & Disposition

Hospitalization is invariably required for control of intracranial pressure and supportive care. Early placement of an intracranial pressure monitor and measures to lower intracranial pressure may be helpful. There is no specific treatment.

Orlowski JP: What ever happened to Reye's syndrome? Did it ever really exist? Crit Care Med 1999;27:1674. [PMID: 10470768]

AMNESTIC SYNDROMES

 ESSENTIALS OF DIAGNOSIS

- *Recall must be specifically tested for the identification of memory loss.*
- *Amnestic syndromes are identified by their onset and duration; then a specific cause can be found.*

1. Amnestic Episodes

Clinical Findings

The neurologic abnormality of memory loss is easily missed unless recall is specifically tested. Confused patients may present with only memory loss and no alteration of consciousness; the general physical examination may be entirely normal. Such patients have markedly abnormal recent memory (eg, they cannot remember 3 objects after 60 seconds or even 30 seconds). Other cognitive functions and past memory are relatively intact. Such patients are confused about where they are and what they are doing.

Table 20–6. Causes of amnestic syndromes.[1]

Amnesia of sudden onset with gradual but incomplete recovery
  Bilateral hippocampal or thalamic infarction
  Diencephalic or bilateral temporal lobe injury following subarachnoid hemorrhage
  Brain injury due to hypoxemia
Slowly progressive amnestic states
  Third ventricular tumors
  Alzheimer disease and other degenerative disorders
Amnesia of sudden onset and transient duration
  Temporal lobe seizures
  Postconcussive states
  Transient global amnesia
  Hysteria
Amnesia of subacute onset with variable recovery
  Wernicke-Korsakoff syndrome
  Herpes simplex encephalitis
  Granulomatous meningitis (tuberculosis, sarcoidosis, etc)

---

[1]Modified and reproduced, with permission, from Victor M: The amnesic syndrome and its anatomical basis. *Can Med Assoc J* 1969;100:1115.

The causes and differential diagnosis of the amnestic syndromes are presented in Table 20–6. The history, cerebrospinal fluid examination, CT or magnetic resonance imaging (MRI) scan, clinical course, or associated findings establish the cause in most cases.

Treatment & Disposition

Administer thiamine, 100 mg intravenously, because Wernicke syndrome is a diagnostic possibility. All patients with new onset of memory loss should be hospitalized for evaluation.

2. Transient Global Amnesia

Clinical Findings

Transient global amnesia occurs suddenly in previously normal middle-aged or elderly patients. Men are affected more frequently than women. Episodes of amnesia occur without warning and without associated headache or findings suggesting epilepsy. Cerebrovascular disease affecting thalamic or temporal lobe structures is the most likely cause. The results of laboratory studies are completely normal.

During an attack, agitation is not a feature. Patients' responses to the illness are variable: some may be unaware of their deficit, but most realize that something is wrong; a few may recognize that their memory is impaired. During these episodes, patients may repeatedly ask the same questions regarding their current condition.

The period of retrograde amnesia varies from a day to a few months or even years. Recovery usually occurs within hours, but amnesia for the entire episode is total and permanent.

Treatment & Disposition

No specific treatment is available. Hospitalization is indicated, in part to prevent injury.

Lewis SL: Aetiology of transient global amnesia. Lancet 1998;352: 397. [PMID: 9717945]

ACUTE STROKES (Cerebrovascular Accidents)

 ESSENTIALS OF DIAGNOSIS

- *When the possibility of stroke is present, the appropriate cerebrovascular accident protocol should be followed (Chapter 18).*
- *Sudden onset, seen most commonly in the elderly and in those with valvular or ischemic disease.*
- *These patients tend to have acute onset of confusion with an associated fluent aphasia.*

1. Fluent Aphasia

General Considerations

Lesions of the dominant posterior frontal lobe may produce a nonfluent (expressive) aphasia and prominent tight hemiparesis. Lesions in a more posterior location may partially or completely spare motor function but produce a fluent (receptive) aphasia easily mistaken for confusion or delirium. Such lesions occur suddenly and are usually caused by embolic strokes in patients at risk of stroke (eg, the elderly or those with valvular or ischemic heart disease predisposing to embolization).

Clinical Findings

Patients talk volubly. Their speech is well-articulated and grammatically correct but has little content. Sentences are characterized by word substitutions (eg, *glass* instead of *clock*), replacement of real words by nonsense words (eg, *dreislen* for *finger*), and substitution of explanatory phrases for words that cannot be recalled (eg, "the thing you write with" for *pen*).

Deficits of comprehension are evident. Patients are unable, for example, to carry out the command, "Put your left hand on your right ear," or to repeat the simple phrase, "No ands, ifs, or buts."

The isolated inability to name objects (anomia) without deficits of comprehension and repetition may represent a form of fluent aphasia due to a structural lesion but most commonly occurs with metabolic encephalopathies of any cause.

Treatment & Disposition

Hospitalization is indicated for new cases to provide supportive care and determine the cause of the aphasia. A CT scan should be obtained. Emboli with an origin in the heart are a common cause and require short-term treatment with anticoagulants. Chronic cases do not require hospitalization.

2. Agitated Confusion

Clinical Findings

The acute onset of an agitated confusional state may occur with infarctions of the inferior division of the right middle cerebral artery. Such strokes spare motor cortex, so that localizing signs (eg, hemiparesis) are mild or absent. A homonymous hemianopia may be present on examination. The diagnosis is suggested by the abrupt onset of agitated confusion and is confirmed by CT or MRI scan. Embolus with an origin in the heart is common.

Treatment & Disposition

Hospitalize the patient for treatment and observation. Evaluation for the source of the embolus and treatment with anticoagulants may be indicated.

Hankey GJ: Management of the first-time transient ischemic attack. Emerg Med 2001;13:70. [PMID: 11476418]

Lewandowski C et al: Treatment of acute ischemic stroke. Ann Emerg Med 2001;37:202. [PMID: 11174240]

CONFUSION ASSOCIATED WITH PSYCHIATRIC DISEASE

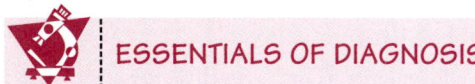 ESSENTIALS OF DIAGNOSIS

- All forms of organic causes must be evaluated and ruled out prior to considering the possibility of psychiatric disease.
- Patients tend to be fully oriented to place and time, and disorientation tends to be to person.
- Short-term memory is preserved, and hallucinations are auditory in nature.

General Considerations

Differentiation between organic and psychiatric causes of confusion (psychosis or hysteria) may be difficult. If careful evaluation (described below) is performed, few patients with metabolic diseases will be improperly diagnosed as having psychiatric illness. Additional useful differential features are outlined in Table 20–7.

1. Psychotic Confusional States

Clinical Findings

The presentation of patients with psychotic confusional states differs from that of patients with confusional states due to organic causes. The classic psychotic state is schizophrenia. Psychiatric causes of confusion have varying characteristics from organic as demonstrated below:

- Psychotic patients may be fully oriented or, if disoriented, exhibit disorientation as to person that is at least as great as or greater than their disorientation to time and place. In organic brain disease, by contrast, disorientation as to time and place is invariably greater than to person.
- Psychotic patients usually retain recent memory and are able to perform simple calculations and other cognitive tasks adequately. In contrast, these functions are rarely preserved in organic confusional states.
- Auditory hallucinations are the mainstay with psychotic states, as opposed to the visual hallucinations seen in organic confusional states.

Treatment & Disposition

Obtain psychiatric consultation. Hospitalization in a secure ward is required for patients with acute psychosis or abrupt worsening of chronic psychosis. Parenteral antipsychotics, for example, haloperidol (Haldol, others), 5–10 mg intramuscularly every 30 minutes to 1 hour, should be given until the patient shows improvement. Chlorpromazine (Thorazine, many others), 25–50 mg intramuscularly, is equally effective but is less commonly used because of side effects of sedation and postural hypotension.

2. Hysteria

Clinical Findings

Hysteria is a diagnosis of exclusion and should be made only after all other possibilities have been ruled out. The differential features listed in Table 20–7 are helpful, but few guidelines are absolute. It is useful to remember that amnesia is probably the most common

Table 20–7. Differentiating features of organic and psychiatric disorders of mentation.

Features	Organic	Psychiatric (Hysteria or Psychosis)
Age	Any; older more susceptible.	Younger; puberty to mid 30s.
Premorbid personality	Any.	Previous functional illness common.
Onset	Often acute.	Usually gradual and insidious.
Weakness, fatigue	Rare.	Common.
Level of awareness	Fluctuates between confusion and lucidity.	Usually consistent.
Hallucinations	Common; predominantly visual, tactile, and olfactory.	Common; predominantly auditory.
Orientation	Impaired: disorientation as to time is greater than that as to place, which in turn is greater than that as to person.	Impaired: disorientation to person is greater than that as to place, which is greater than that as to time; may be unimpaired, however.
Memory	Usually affected; recent memory more affected than remote memory.	Total amnesia, including self-identity; or memory may be completely unimpaired.
Other evidence of organic central nervous system disease	Present.	Usually absent.
Electroencephalogram	Frequently abnormal, usually slow.	Usually normal.
Asterixis and multifocal myoclonus	Diagnostic if present.	Never seen.

hysterical disturbance of mental function. Hysterical amnesia usually includes the inability both to form new memories and especially to recall any past experience with certainty. For example, such patients often deny knowledge of their own name, a finding that in an awake and alert person is essentially restricted to the hysterical personality. The disparity between alleged mental incapacity and the ability to function in the immediate surroundings is often quite striking.

The most helpful differentiating features on physical examination are asterixis and myoclonus, which, when present, point to a metabolic cause of the symptoms. Asterixis and myoclonus do not occur as features of psychiatric or hysterical illness.

An electroencephalogram is often helpful in diagnosis, because it is nearly always normal in psychiatric disease and is frequently abnormal (usually slowed) in organic or metabolic disease. The presence of very fast β-wave activity on the tracing may be seen with sedative-hypnotic drug intoxication and provides a helpful clue to proper diagnosis.

Treatment & Disposition

Refer the patient for psychiatric consultation. Anxiolytics, for example, diazepam (Valium, others), 5–10 mg orally, may be helpful. Hospitalization may be required if a protected home environment is not available.

CONFUSIONAL STATES OF UNCERTAIN CAUSE

Even after all the above diagnoses have been considered, for many patients in confusional states, no clear diagnosis can be established in the emergency department. These patients, especially the elderly, are often found to have subclinical mild metabolic or drug-induced abnormalities or infection, and correction of the underlying disorder may restore patients to their customary normal state. Hyperthyroidism or hypothyroidism must be considered, especially in elderly patients.

Hospitalization is indicated for further evaluation of all patients with confusional states of uncertain cause.

Fisher CM: Hysteria: a delusional state. Med Hypotheses 1999; 53:152. [PMID: 10532711]

Marsh CM: Psychiatric presentations of medical illness. Psychiatr Clin North Am 1997;20:181. [PMID: 9139290]

Arthritis & Back Pain

21

Roger L. Humphries, MD, & David O'Keefe, MD[1]

I. Evaluation of the Patient with Acute Arthritis

II. Emergency Treatment of Specific Conditions Causing Acute Arthritis

   Monarthritis or Oligoarthritis

      Traumatic Arthritis

      Acute Gouty Arthritis

      Acute Pseudogout

      Septic Arthritis

   Oligoarthritis or Polyarthritis

      Osteoarthritis (Degenerative Joint Disease)

      Rheumatic Fever & Poststreptococcal Reactive Arthritis

   Polyarthritis

      Rheumatoid Arthritis

      Spondyloarthropathies

         1. Psoriatic Arthritis & Intestinal Arthritis

         2. Reiter Syndrome

         3. Ankylosing Spondylitis

      Viral Arthritis

      Systemic Lupus Erythematosus

   Nonarticular Rheumatism

      Tendonitis

      Bursitis

III. Evaluation of the Patient with Acute Back Pain

IV. Emergency Treatment of Specific Conditions Causing Back Pain

      Traumatic Back Pain

      Acute Lumbosacral Strain & Chronic Degenerative Disk Disease

      Sciatica

      Epidural Compression Syndrome

      Facet Syndrome

      Spinal Infections

      Ankylosing Spondylitis

      Neoplasm

      Zoster

■ I. EVALUATION OF THE PATIENT WITH ACUTE ARTHRITIS (See Figure 21–1.)

Is the Patient Systemically Ill?

Whenever a patient with acute joint pain also presents with fever, rigors, systemic symptoms, or signs of involvement of additional organ systems, careful evaluation is necessary to rule out potentially life-threatening processes such as infection or diffuse vasculitis.

Hospitalization and consultation for evaluation of rheumatic or infectious disease are usually required for patients with arthritis and systemic symptoms. Obtain blood cultures, and perform the evaluation outlined below.

Is This Disseminated Gonococcal Infection?

In young adults, hematogenous gonococcal infection is one of the most common causes of acute arthritis. Arthritis may be the sole manifestation of disseminated gonococcal infection. Skin lesions are few and are found on the extremities, frequently around a joint, and are pustular or hemorrhagic, rarely bullous. Gram-stained smears of material contained in the pustules may reveal gram-negative diplococci within polymorphonuclear neutrophils. Tenosynovitis classically involves tendons of the hand or foot. The primary (mucosal) site of gonococcal infection is often asymptomatic. If disseminated gonococcal infection is suspected, culture of blood and secretions from the pharynx, rectum, and urethra or cervix should be obtained.

---

[1]This chapter is a revision of the chapter by Peter G. Trafton, MD, from the 4th edition.

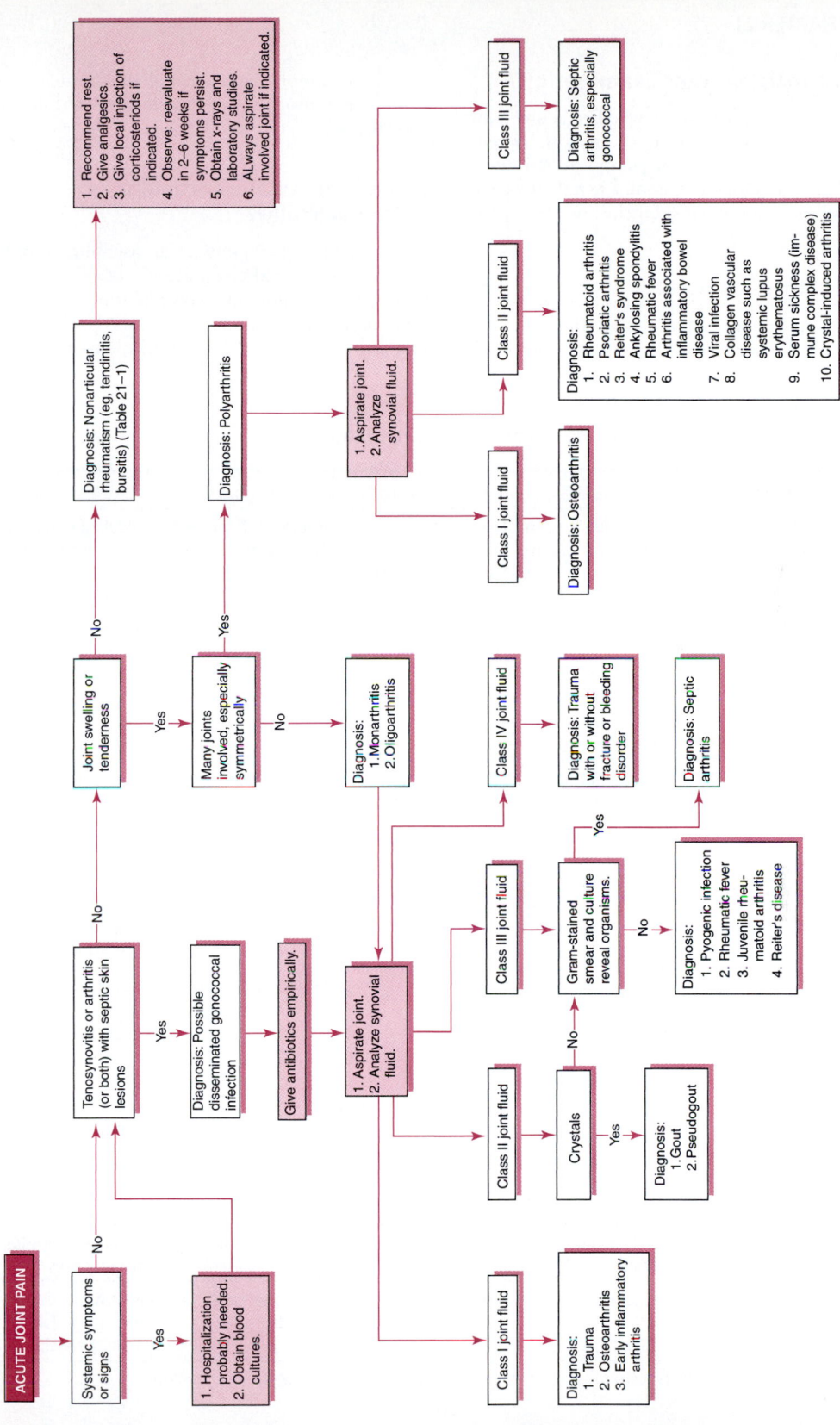

Figure 21–1. Assessment of patients with acute joint pain.

Is There Arthritis on Joint Examination?

Ascertain by careful examination whether acute joint pain is due to an intra-articular process. Is there redness, diffuse warmth, effusion, or painful limitation of active and passive motion? If the joint is not involved, consider cellulitis, tenosynovitis, bursitis, or other periarticular lesions.

If It Is Not Arthritis, What Is It?

The shoulders and upper extremities are frequent sites of acute painful extra-articular processes. Table 21–1

lists the common syndromes of nonarticular rheumatism. These disorders are described more fully later in this chapter.

Is the Process Oligoarticular or Polyarticular?

Involvement of 1–3 joints in an asymmetric pattern is generally considered characteristic of oligoarthritis, although this asymmetric involvement may occur early in some polyarticular conditions such as juvenile rheumatoid arthritis. Common causes of oligoarthritis include

Table 21–1. Some common syndromes of nonarticular rheumatism.

	History	Findings	X-Rays	Diagnosis	Treatment[1]
Shoulder	Severe pain, subacromial with or without midarm pain, worse with abduction.	Point tenderness in rotator cuff. Painful abduction.	Negative, or calcific deposit overlying greater tuberosity	Rotator cuff tendinitis (subacromial bursitis)	Local infiltration of corticosteroid. Physical therapy to preserve motion.
	Overuse. Pain and decreased motion of shoulder.	Resistance to elbow flexion and extension reproduces pain. Point tenderness over bicipital groove.	Negative, or calcium in bicipital tendon	Bicipital tendinitis	Anti-inflammatory drugs. Rest. Local infiltration of corticosteroid.
Elbow	Sharp lateral pain radiating posteriorly to wrist with lifting and twisting.	Point tenderness over lateral epicondyle or radial head.	Negative; rarely shows calcium	Tennis elbow (lateral epicondylitis)	As above. Eliminate or modify activity causing pain.
	Overuse. Trauma, often seemingly trivial. Swelling and pain over olecranon. Male.	Swollen, hot, tender olecranon bursa. Aspirate reveals purulent material.	Negative	Olecranon bursitis (infection, trauma, gout)	Needle drainage. Hospitalization. Specific therapy (for staphylococcal infection, gout).
Wrist	Moderate pain with use of thumb and grip on radial side of wrist.	Positive Finkelstein test. Tender swelling over extensor digitorum brevis and abductor pollicis longus tendon sheath.	Negative	De Quervain stenosing tenosynovitis	Usually responds to local corticosteroid injection. Splint early; then mobilize.
Hip	Pain over hip and thigh.	Swelling and tenderness over greater trochanter.	Negative	Trochanteric bursitis	Rest. Local corticosteroid infiltration.
Knee	Swollen knee; pain occasionally.	Swelling and slight tenderness over prepatellar bursa.	Negative	Prepatellar or infrapatellar bursitis	Rest. Local injection of corticosteroids for resistant cases.
	Tender patella; swelling variable.	Tenderness of patella.	Negative	Patellofemoral chondromalacia	Rest, anti-inflammatory drugs. Eliminate activity causing pain.

[1]Nonsteroidal anti-inflammatory agents such as ibuprofen or naproxen may be useful in any of these conditions.

infection, crystal deposition (eg, gout), and trauma. The polyarthritis syndromes involve many joints, usually in a symmetric fashion.

Perform Arthrocentesis

If one of the affected joints is acrally located (eg, wrist, elbow, knee, ankle), arthrocentesis should be attempted in the emergency department, using local anesthesia (Chapter 6). Arthrocentesis of shoulders and hips is best done by a specialist. The joint fluid should be analyzed and the results used to classify the arthritis according to the scheme in Table 21–2.

Classification of Arthritis

See Table 21–2.

A. Noninflammatory (Class I)

Acute arthritis in the presence of normal joint fluid usually indicates trauma, or osteoarthritis. Rarely, early joint aspiration in inflammatory arthritis produces a similar result.

B. Inflammatory (Class II)

Inflammatory arthritis may be present in acute gout, pseudogout, Reiter syndrome, rheumatoid arthritis, and rheumatic fever. Gram stain and culture of synovial fluid should be done to rule out early infectious arthritis.

C. Septic (Class III)

Purulent joint fluid (class III) is seen almost exclusively in bacterial and fungal infections. Gram stain of joint fluid may help to identify the causative organism before cultures become positive.

D. Hemorrhagic (Class IV)

Hemorrhagic joint fluid is seen in trauma with or without fracture; the presence of fat globules suggests fracture. A tear in the anterior cruciate ligament is the most common cause of hemarthrosis in the knee when no fracture is present. Also frequent are peripheral meniscus tears and patellar dislocations (with medial retinaculum tears). Hemorrhagic effusion is more likely to be associated with acute pain than is the noninflammatory effusion that can occur with minor joint trauma, because blood within the joint space generally causes an inflammatory reaction. Hemorrhagic fluid is also seen in hemophilia and in synovial neoplasms.

Table 21–2. Classification of abnormal synovial fluid.

Type of Joint Fluid	Viscosity	Clarity	Color	Leukocyte Count (per µL)	Gram Stain and Culture	Other Findings
Normal	High	Clear	Light yellow	< 200	Negative	. . .
Noninflammatory (class I)	High	Clear	Light yellow	< 4000	Negative	. . .
Inflammatory (class II)	Low	Cloudy	Dark yellow	> 2000–< 50,000	Negative	Crystals are diagnostic of gout or pseudogout (differentiate with polarizing microscopy); usually seen with class II joint fluid.
Septic (class III)	Low	Cloudy	Dark yellow	Usually > 50,000	Usually positive[1]	Bacteria on culture or Gram-stained smear. Usually seen with class III joint fluid but may be seen with class II; rarely, class I.
Hemorrhagic (class IV)	Variable	Cloudy	Pink-red	Usually > 2000[2]	Negative	Fat globules strongly suggest intra-articular fracture and are usually seen with class IV joint fluid.

[1]Most common exception is gonococcal infection (only about 25% of cases have positive culture or Gram stain).
[2]Many red cells also found.

■ II. EMERGENCY TREATMENT OF SPECIFIC CONDITIONS CAUSING ACUTE ARTHRITIS

MONARTHRITIS OR OLIGOARTHRITIS

TRAUMATIC ARTHRITIS

 ESSENTIALS OF DIAGNOSIS

- *Effusions often develop immediately after trauma.*
- *Fever or other systemic signs or symptoms are not present.*

Clinical Findings

Severe joint pain associated with trauma is usually related temporally to an obvious injury. Mild pain may occur some time after the injury. Fever and other systemic signs usually are not present. The presence of noninflammatory or hemorrhagic synovial fluid confirms the diagnosis. Because patients with septic arthritis may also give a history of recent trauma, Gram stain and culture of fluid should be performed.

The presence of many small fat globules in hemorrhagic joint fluid strongly suggests intra-articular fracture; x-rays should be carefully scrutinized to locate occult fractures. Well-localized tenderness over a bone is an important sign of fracture (Chapter 28). Scaphoid fractures are particularly difficult to locate and require careful correlation with clinical findings (eg, localized tenderness in the anatomic snuffbox). X-rays that show only joint effusion or periarticular soft tissue swelling are consistent with occult fractures or other joint injuries such as spontaneously reduced dislocations, ligamentous injuries, meniscus tears, avulsion fractures, and osteochondral fractures.

Joint effusions that accumulate immediately following trauma are uniformly hemorrhagic and usually do not require arthrocentesis for diagnostic purposes.

Treatment & Disposition

Splinting, protection from weight bearing, and follow-up care are essential. Analgesia may be needed. See Chapter 28 for more specific details and guidelines for treatment and disposition.

ACUTE GOUTY ARTHRITIS

 ESSENTIALS OF DIAGNOSIS

- *Presence of negative birefringent urate crystals in joint fluid and a negative Gram stain and culture.*
- *Uric acid level is not helpful for diagnosis in an acute attack.*

Clinical Findings

Patients with acute gouty arthritis have monarthritis or oligoarthritis with class II or class III joint fluid, urate crystals in the synovial fluid, and a negative synovial culture.

A. SYMPTOMS AND SIGNS

There is sudden onset of warmth, hyperemia, induration, and extreme pain in a joint, most commonly the metatarsophalangeal joint of the great toe. The next most commonly involved joint is the knee. Although most patients present with only one painful joint, several joints may be involved.

B. LABORATORY FINDINGS

Elevated serum uric acid concentration is supporting evidence of gouty arthritis, although during an acute attack the serum urate level may be normal. Therefore, a uric acid level should not be ordered. Definitive diagnosis requires use of a polarizing microscope to demonstrate characteristic negative birefringence of urate crystals in the synovial fluid.

Treatment

A. NONSTEROIDAL ANTI-INFLAMMATORY DRUGS

Indomethacin or other nonsteroidal anti-inflammatory drugs (NSAIDs) may be indicated if a diagnosis of gout is well established. Aspirin is contraindicated, because small doses may cause hyperuricemia.

1. Indomethacin—Give 50 mg orally every 8 hours for 2 days. Then reduce the dosage to 25 mg 3–4 times daily for 3 days. Peptic ulcer disease is a contraindication to indomethacin.

2. Other drugs—Ibuprofen, 600 mg orally every 6 hours, or naproxen, 500 mg orally every 12 hours, may be used. Other NSAIDs in appropriate doses can be effective in acute gout.

B. COLCHICINE

Oral or intravenous colchicine, if administered within 24 hours of acute arthritis, can provide dramatic relief. Colchicine should not be used in patients with renal or hepatic dysfunction. Response to colchicine also strongly supports a diagnosis of gout.

1. Oral treatment—Give colchicine, 0.6 mg every hour until pain has resolved, a maximum dose of 4–6 mg is reached, or side effects of nausea and diarrhea cannot be tolerated.

2. Intravenous treatment—Gastrointestinal toxicity can be reduced by giving colchicine, 1–2 mg intravenously in 50 mL of normal saline over 20 minutes; repeat this dose every 6 hours until the patient is asymptomatic or to a total dose of 4 mg. After a full course of colchicine, no further doses should be administered for 1 week.

C. CORTICOSTEROIDS

Corticosteroids are useful in patients who cannot take NSAIDs or colchicine. Prednisone, 40 mg daily for 1–3 days followed by a slow taper over 1–2 weeks, is recommended. Alternatively, a single dose of adrenocorticotropic hormone (ACTH) or corticotrophin, 40 units intramuscularly, boosts the patient's endogenous steroid production and can provide relief from a gouty flare-up.

Disposition

Hospitalization is rarely necessary. The patient should receive follow-up evaluation in a few days.

ACUTE PSEUDOGOUT

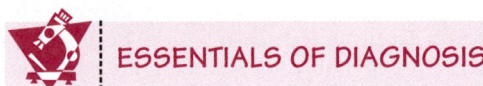

ESSENTIALS OF DIAGNOSIS

- *Calcium pyrophosphate crystals in the joint.*

Clinical Findings

Patients with acute pseudogout have acute oligoarthritis with class II joint fluid and calcium pyrophosphate crystals in the synovial fluid. Pseudogout simulates gout in middle-aged or elderly patients. It differs from gout in that the knee is the most commonly involved joint.

Serum uric acid levels are usually normal. Chondrocalcinosis may be present although not necessarily in the acutely involved joint. The presence of chondrocalcinosis, however, regardless of location, is not diagnostic. Definitive diagnosis depends on the presence of calcium dihydrate (pyrophosphate) crystals in synovial fluid.

Treatment

Aspiration of the joint is often adequate for relief of symptoms. NSAIDs may be helpful (see Acute Gouty Arthritis, above). Unlike patients with gouty arthritis, patients with acute pseudogout do not respond as well to colchicine.

Disposition

Hospitalization is rarely necessary. Refer the patient to a primary care physician.

SEPTIC ARTHRITIS

ESSENTIALS OF DIAGNOSIS

- *Joint is painful, erythematous, and tender.*
- *Systemic symptoms: fever and chills are common.*
- *Definitive diagnosis by aspiration of the joint. Fluid may demonstrate the infecting organism by Gram stain or culture.*

General Considerations

Septic arthritis is one of the more common causes of oligoarthritis, but often only one joint is affected. The most frequent pathogen in septic oligoarthritis is the gonococcus, which, although difficult to demonstrate in joint fluid, often produces typical pustular skin lesions or tenosynovitis. The most common pathogen in monarticular septic arthritis is *Staphylococcus aureus.* Another common pathogen is *Streptococcus* spp. In intravenous drug users and immunocompromised hosts, gram-negative and anaerobic organisms may be seen.

Clinical Findings

Patients with septic arthritis show evidence of infection in the joint (bacteria on Gram-stained smear or culture, or rapid response to antimicrobial therapy). Class III joint fluid is usually present.

A. SYMPTOMS AND SIGNS

Patients with septic arthritis usually present with a severe monarticular process characterized by marked pain, erythema, and tenderness. The onset of septic arthritis is usually less precipitous than that of gout. A few patients with staphylococcal or gonococcal arthritis may present with 2 or more involved joints. Acute migratory oligoarthritis followed in 1–2 days by acute arthritis localized to 1 or 2 joints is especially suggestive of gonococcal arthritis. If multiple joints are involved in septic arthritis, the distribution is usually asymmetric. Systemic symptoms and signs of infection (eg, fever, chills, leukocytosis) are common.

B. LABORATORY FINDINGS

A definitive diagnosis is established by demonstrating the infecting organism in synovial tissue or joint fluid. Joint fluid shows high leukocyte counts, usually over 50,000/μL. The higher the white blood cell count in joint fluid, the greater the likelihood of bacterial or fungal arthritis. The glucose content of synovial fluid is usually reduced. If no antimicrobial therapy has been given, smears and cultures of joint fluid usually reveal organisms.

In gonococcal arthritis, however, Gram-stained smears and even cultures of joint fluid are frequently negative, although in most cases, cultures of exudate from the cervix, urethra, pharynx, or rectum demonstrate gonococci. In gonococcal arthritis, the diagnosis may also be confirmed by prompt response to antimicrobial therapy (Chapter 40).

Treatment

A. JOINT ASPIRATION

Aspiration of the joint is essential. Obtain cultures of blood and joint fluid. If gonococcal arthritis is suspected, cervical, urethral, and possibly pharyngeal and rectal cultures should be obtained. If sepsis is considered likely, as much fluid as possible should be removed from the joint.

B. ANTIBIOTICS

Begin an antibiotic deemed appropriate based on clinical findings and Gram-stained smears. Narrow the antibiotic coverage once results of Gram stain, culture, and sensitivities are reported. The treatment of gonococcal arthritis is discussed in more detail in Chapter 40.

Disposition

Hospitalize all patients with suspected or documented septic arthritis and start them on intravenous antibiotics. Consult an orthopedic surgeon for possible incision and drainage of the infected joint. Patients with mild gonococcal arthritis often can be discharged early and given antibiotics to be taken orally, provided that they are reliable patients and careful follow-up can be ensured.

Brusch JL: Septic arthritis. eMedicine; http://www.emedicine.com/med/topic3394.htm

OLIGOARTHRITIS OR POLYARTHRITIS

OSTEOARTHRITIS (Degenerative Joint Disease)

 ESSENTIALS OF DIAGNOSIS

- Usually polyarticular involvement. Most commonly involves hips, knees, spine, and distal and proximal interphalangeal joints.
- Systemic signs and symptoms (fever and chills) should be absent.
- Radiographs usually demonstrate cartilage changes with osteophytes.

Clinical Findings

Osteoarthritis is a chronic, progressive disease in which the smooth hyaline cartilage develops irregularities due to mechanical and cellular alterations. The adjacent bone then develops irregularities and osteophytes. Diagnosis is made by the clinical features of pain, decreased movement, and muscle wasting combined with radiographic findings of joint space narrowing, osteophytes, irregular joint surfaces, and bony sclerosis. Osteoarthritis is usually polyarticular but can be monarticular. The most commonly infected joints are knee, hip, cervical and lumbar spine, and distal and proximal interphalangeal joints.

Treatment & Disposition

In the emergency department, newly diagnosed osteoarthritis must be carefully distinguished from the septic joint. Once osteoarthritis is diagnosed, patients should be discharged with medication and exercise instructions. First-line treatment is acetaminophen, 4000 mg every 24 hours in divided doses. Acetaminophen is as effective for osteoarthritis as NSAIDs and has fewer side effects. If NSAIDs are prescribed, select ibuprofen, 600 mg every 6 hours, as initial therapy.

If patients are at high risk for gastrointestinal bleeding, select a COX-2 inhibitor instead of NSAIDs. Aerobic exercise, walking, and range of motion exercises have all shown benefits in knee and hip osteoarthritis. Patients should follow-up with their primary care physician within 1 week.

RHEUMATIC FEVER & POSTSTREPTOCOCCAL REACTIVE ARTHRITIS

 ESSENTIALS OF DIAGNOSIS

- *Evidence of recent strep infection.*
- *Constitutional symptoms: fever, malaise.*
- *Often oligoarthritis with associated cardiac involvement, subcutaneous nodules, and erythema marginatum.*

Rheumatic fever or poststreptococcal reactive arthritis may present early as acute monarticular joint pain. Acute rheumatic fever is diagnosed using the Jones criteria found in Table 21–3. Poststreptococcal reactive arthritis will have only some of the Jones criteria and is usually oligoarticular. Carditis is rare, and the arthritis tends to be severe. Patients should be hospitalized if rheumatic fever is suspected. Initial treatment is penicillin and salicylates.

Table 21–3. Revised Jones criteria for diagnosis of rheumatic fever.[1]

Major criteria
Pericarditis, myocarditis, or endocarditis
Chorea
Subcutaneous nodules
Erythema marginatum
Polyarthritis
Minor criteria
Fever
Arthralgias
Laboratory findings: elevated sedimentation rate, evidence of preceding streptococcal infection (increased titer of antistreptolysn O), increased C-reactive protein
History of rheumatic fever or rheumatic heart disease; increased PR interval on ECG

[1]The presence of 2 major or 1 major and 2 minor criteria with supporting evidence of recent infection with group A streptococcus indicates a high probability of rheumatic fever.

Jansen TL et al: Acute rheumatic fever or post-streptococcal reactive arthritis: a clinical problem revisited, Br J Rheumatol 1998;37:335. [PMID: 9566678]

POLYARTHRITIS

RHEUMATOID ARTHRITIS

 ESSENTIALS OF DIAGNOSIS

- *Often subacute joint pain.*
- *Usually symmetric polyarthritis.*
- *Radiographs demonstrate juxta-articular osteoporosis and later cartilage erosions.*

Clinical Findings

Rheumatoid arthritis generally presents as a symmetric, chronic polyarthritis with prominent involvement of proximal interphalangeal and metacarpophalangeal joints, often with ulnar deviation. Distal interphalangeal joints are not involved.

A. SYMPTOMS AND SIGNS

Rheumatoid arthritis is a common cause of subacute joint pain involving multiple joints in adults. Although symmetric involvement is classic, the disease may begin with asymmetric involvement. In a typical acute presentation, joints may only be warm, tender, or swollen.

B. LABORATORY FINDINGS

Rheumatoid factor is positive in 85% of patients; therefore, a negative test does not rule out rheumatoid arthritis. Elevated erythrocyte sedimentation rate and C-reactive protein are also common but nonspecific findings.

C. X-RAY FINDINGS

Early x-ray examination generally reveals soft tissue swelling and juxta-articular osteoporosis. Erosions are seen later.

Treatment

Aspirin and other NSAIDs have proven effective for the initial treatment of rheumatoid arthritis. However, the simultaneous administration of other drug classes in addition to NSAIDs is now common. For example, steroids, gold, penicillamine, methotrexate, cyclosporine, and sulfasalazine are being used. Initial management in the emergency department should consist of aspirin or NSAIDs in appropriate doses with urgent rheumatologist follow-up or consultation for additional prescriptions if indicated.

Disposition

The patient should be referred early to a rheumatologist or primary care physician. Consider admission for patients with severe systemic involvement (eg, disabling polyarthritis, fever, or weight loss) or vasculitis.

SPONDYLOARTHROPATHIES

Spondyloarthropathies are a cluster of chronic inflammatory rheumatic diseases that include psoriatic and intestinal arthritis, Reiter syndrome, and ankylosing spondylitis. They are not associated with rheumatoid factor but have a strong association with HLA-B27. Anatomic sites include the following: the entheses (sites of ligament and tendon insertion into bone), the sacroiliac joints, limb joints, and nonarticular sites (eg, gut, skin, and eye).

1. Psoriatic Arthritis & Intestinal Arthritis

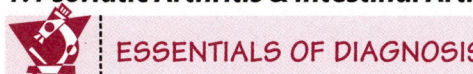 ESSENTIALS OF DIAGNOSIS

- *Common in patients with psoriasis or inflammatory bowel disease.*

Clinical Findings

Psoriatic arthritis is an inflammatory arthritis seen in 10% of patients with psoriasis. Nail involvement (pitting, dystrophy, or onycholysis) is a clue to the diagnosis. The arthritis occurs before psoriasis is seen in 15% of patients.

Intestinal arthritis is an inflammatory arthritis seen in patients with ulcerative colitis or Crohn disease. In one study, this form of arthritis occurred in approximately 40% of these patients. The arthritis can be in the limb joints or the sacroiliac.

Treatment & Disposition

Initial treatment is with NSAIDs. Sulfasalazine should be added if the patient cannot take or does not respond to NSAIDs.

2. Reiter Syndrome

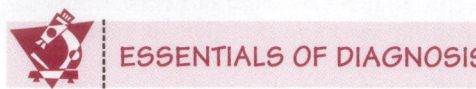 ESSENTIALS OF DIAGNOSIS

- *Usually affects young males.*
- *Arthritis, conjunctivitis, and urethritis.*
- *Arthritis is polyarticular and asymmetric, developing after chlamydial or bacterial gastroenteritis.*

Clinical Findings

Reiter syndrome is a reactive arthritis with the classic triad of arthritis, conjunctivitis, and urethritis. It is most commonly seen in men aged 15–35 years. The arthritis affects primarily the weight-bearing joints of the lower extremities.

Reactive arthritis occurs within 1 month of a genitourinary (*Chlamydia trachomatis*) or enteral (*Shigella, Salmonella, Yersinia, Campylobacter*) infection. It is asymmetric and polyarticular. Arthrocentesis reveals a class II inflammatory joint fluid.

Treatment & Disposition

NSAIDs are the mainstay of treatment. Tetracycline improves recovery time for reactive arthritis due to *Chlamydia* but not for enteral causes. The typical reactive arthritis lasts 4–5 months, but patients can develop chronic or recurrent arthritis.

3. Ankylosing Spondylitis

 ESSENTIALS OF DIAGNOSIS

- *Patients under age 40 years.*
- *Back pain of gradual onset.*
- *Stiffness worse in morning.*
- *X-rays show sacroiliitis.*

Clinical Findings

Ankylosing spondylitis is the most common spondyloarthropathy. Its classic findings include the following: gradual onset, age less than 40 years, back pain and morning stiffness worse with inactivity and made better with exercise, at least 3 months' duration, and radiographic evidence of sacroiliitis. Often a history of uveitis can be elicited.

An asymmetrical arthritis is manifested in peripheral joints because areas of enthesitis (Achilles and plantar fascia) are commonly involved. Arthrocentesis reveals a class II inflammatory joint fluid. Some patients will have constitutional complaints of malaise, decreased appetite, and fever.

Treatment & Disposition

NSAIDs and strengthening exercises are used for treatment. Follow-up with a rheumatologist should be arranged.

VIRAL ARTHRITIS

General Considerations

Viral arthritis is acute, symmetric, and polyarticular. The two most common viruses causing secondary arthritis are rubella and hepatitis B. Mumps, adenoviruses, enteroviruses, and Epstein-Barr viruses have also been implicated. The arthritis is caused by deposition of immune complexes that cause an inflammatory reaction.

Clinical Findings

Diagnosis is made by history. Recent viral infection or vaccination aid in diagnosis. The most frequently affected joints are the proximal interphalangeal joints, metacarpophalangeal joints, knee, and ankle. The symptoms are usually self-limiting after several weeks but can last years.

Treatment & Disposition

Treatment is symptomatic and includes NSAIDs. Refer patients to their primary care physician.

SYSTEMIC LUPUS ERYTHEMATOSUS

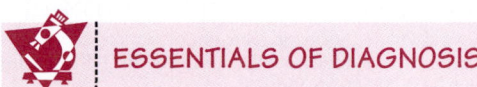

ESSENTIALS OF DIAGNOSIS

- *Arthritis associated with other systemic symptoms: rash, fever.*

- *Positive anti-double-stranded DNA or positive antinuclear antibody test.*

Clinical Findings

Almost all patients with systemic lupus erythematosus will have arthritis. Patients usually also have fever, rash, or other features of the disease. Diagnosis in patients who present only with arthritis requires demonstration of a positive antinuclear antibody test or anti-double-stranded DNA along with other criteria set forth by the American Rheumatism Association.

Treatment & Disposition

The acute arthritis of systemic lupus erythematosus is treated with NSAIDs. Patients should be referred to a rheumatologist for diagnostic evaluation and appropriate care.

NONARTICULAR RHEUMATISM

In the emergency evaluation of joint pain, it is important to distinguish between true articular (arthritis) and extraarticular (tendonitis and bursitis) causes. The clinical features of the common tendonitis and bursitis syndromes are set forth in Table 21–1.

TENDONITIS

ESSENTIALS OF DIAGNOSIS

- *Pain and tenderness more localized to the tendon.*
- *Although rare, always consider infectious causes of inflammation.*

Clinical Findings

In contrast to diffuse pain, warmth, and tenderness across an arthritic joint, tendonitis generally produces more localized pain that is reproduced with stretching of the affected tendon. Tendonitis is thought to be caused by repetitive overuse resulting in damage and inflammation to the tendon and surrounding structures. If the history reveals a puncture or laceration over a tendon with erythema, pain along the tendon, fever, and severe pain on minimal passive tendon motion, an infectious process must be ruled out.

Treatment

A. ADJUNCTIVE MEASURES

Relative rest from exacerbating activities, effective splinting, and ice as needed are the mainstays of treatment. NSAIDs and an exercise program to maintain joint motion and build muscle strength are helpful.

B. LOCAL INJECTION

Local injection of anesthetic and depot glucocorticoid preparations may be appropriate for some patients (see Bursitis, below). However, this procedure should be performed only by an individual skilled in the procedure, because complications (eg, local atrophy and rupture of the tendon) can result if corticosteroids are errantly injected into a weight-bearing tendon.

C. ANTIMICROBIALS

Suspicion of an infectious tendonitis requires orthopedic consultation for possible incision and debridement and hospital admission for appropriate intravenous antibiotics to cover presumptive staphylococcal and streptococcal species.

Disposition

Most patients with tendonitis can receive treatment on an outpatient basis, with referral to an orthopedist if necessary.

BURSITIS

ESSENTIALS OF DIAGNOSIS

- *Inflammation localized to the bursa, not the entire joint.*
- *Common sites involved are elbow and prepatellar area.*
- *Consider infection as cause of inflammation, especially if systemic symptoms such as fever and chills are present.*

Clinical Findings

A bursa is a sac normally containing a thin film of synovial fluid that cushions the interface between bone with ligaments and the overlying skin. Bursitis is inflammation of the bursa. Like tendonitis, bursitis may be due to trauma or infection (most commonly found in the olecranon and prepatellar bursa) or may be idiopathic. Clinical findings are pain, tenderness, and swelling of the involved bursa.

Treatment

A. ASPIRATION

The olecranon and prepatellar bursa should be aspirated for diagnosis and treatment if fluctuance and infectious signs are present.

B. ANTIBIOTICS

Septic bursitis is usually due to *S aureus* and, pending results of culture and susceptibility testing, should be treated with a penicillinase-resistant, β-lactamase-resistant antimicrobial (eg, nafcillin, 150 mg/kg/d intravenously in 4–6 divided doses; or cefazolin, 60 mg/kg/d intramuscularly or intravenously in 3 divided doses).

C. ANTI-INFLAMMATORY AGENTS

NSAIDs, combined with rest, are most effective.

D. CORTICOSTEROID INJECTION

Locally injected corticosteroids are useful in treatment of aseptic bursitis. However, injections should be given only by physicians skilled in the procedure because complications can include infection.

E. SURGERY

Septic bursitis rarely requires incision and debridement.

Disposition

Patients with septic bursitis require intravenous antibiotics either via home parenteral therapy or in the hospital. Patients with aseptic bursitis may be discharged with primary care follow-up within 1 week.

Almekinders LC, Temple JD: Etiology, diagnosis, and treatment of tendonitis: an analysis of the literature. Medicine and Science in Sports and Exercise 1998;30:1183. [PMID: 9710855]

Barth WF, Kinim S: Reactive arthritis (Reiter's syndrome). Am Fam Physician 1999;60:499. [PMID: 10465225]

Brent LH: Ankylosing spondylitis and undifferentiated spondyloarthropathy. eMedicine; http://www.emedicine.com/med/topic2700.htm

Easton BT: Evaluation and treatment of the patient with osteoarthritis. J Fam Pract 2001;50:791. [PMID: 11674913]

Jansen TL et al: Acute rheumatic fever or post-streptococcal reactive arthritis: a clinical problem revisited. Br J Rheumatol 1998;37:335. [PMID: 9566678]

Kaplan J: Gout and pseudogout. eMedicine; http://www.emedicine.com/emerg/topic221.htm

Khan MA: Update on spondyloarthropathies. Ann Intern Med 2002;136:896. [PMID: 12069564]

Laupland KB, Davies HD: Olecranon septic bursitis managed in an ambulatory setting. The Calgary Home Parenteral Therapy Program Study Group. Clin Invest Med 2001;24:171. [PMID: 11558851]

Meader RJ: Acute rheumatic fever. eMedicine; http://www.emedicine.com/med/topic2922.htm

Sack K: Monoarthritis: differential diagnosis. Am J Med 1997; 102(Suppl 1A):30S. [PMID: 9217557]

Smith HR: Rheumatoid arthritis. eMedicine; emedicine.com/med/topic2024.htm

■ III. EVALUATION OF THE PATIENT WITH ACUTE BACK PAIN (See Figure 21–2.)

Perform Baseline Evaluation

An established routine for evaluating patients with acute back pain will ensure that life-threatening disease is not missed. Patients who do not fit into the categories below have acute back pain due to a nonemergent cause (eg, disk disease, facet syndrome, strains, and sprains) without underlying disease.

A. History

1. Is trauma present or did a precipitating event occur?—Often the patient reports trauma or a precipitating event causing acute back pain. In patients with chronic back problems, even minor trauma such as a cough can cause acute back pain.

2. Is visceral disease present?—The emergency physician's first goal should be to identify emergent causes of back pain and to exclude nonorthopedic causes (Table 21–4). Evaluation and treatment should focus then on the organ thought to be involved.

3. Are red flags present?—Red flags in the history will help the emergency physician recognize associated life threats. In patients younger than age 18 years, consider spondylolysis, spondylolisthesis, infection, tumor, and developmental disorders. In patients older than age 50 years consider aortic abdominal aneurysm, fracture, and malignancy first. A history of trauma or chronic steroid use increases the possibility that back pain is related to a vertebral fracture. If bowel or bladder incontinence, saddle anesthesia, or bilateral neurologic defect is reported, then an epidural compression syndrome (ie, spinal cord compression, cauda equina, or conus medullaris syndrome) is likely and must be investigated

emergently. Weight loss, night pain, fever, chills, history of cancer, or intravenous drug use is concerning for malignant or infectious causes of back pain.

4. Is associated arthritis present?—When back pain is associated with arthritis (oligoarthritis or polyarthritis), both disorders are usually due to the same cause. For example, ankylosing spondylitis commonly causes peripheral and vertebral arthritis concurrently. Evaluate these patients and provide treatment as if they had acute arthritis.

5. Is a neurologic deficit present?—A new neurologic deficit in association with back pain, saddle anesthesia, or decreased rectal tone may indicate an epidural compression syndrome due to infection, tumor, or disk disease and calls for emergent management. Seek consultation with a neurosurgeon immediately, and consider magnetic resonance imaging (MRI). These patients may require hospitalization for diagnosis and treatment.

6. Does the pain have a radicular distribution?—Unilateral back pain in a nerve root distribution suggests preeruptive zoster or nerve root compression. Refer the patient for follow-up care after providing appropriate analgesics.

B. Examination

Examine the back for deformity, tenderness, and range of motion; test for limitation of straight-leg raising and evaluate gait. Examine the heart, peripheral pulses, lungs, and abdomen. Perform a neurologic evaluation that includes reflexes, muscle strength, sensory examination of the legs and perineum, and assessment of rectal sphincter strength. Pay particular attention to vital signs because fever, tachycardia, or hypotension suggest a serious or possibly life-threatening cause of back pain. A rectal examination does not have to be performed in every patient with back pain, but it must be performed in all patients who have neurologic complaints or deficits. Red flags in the physical examination include decreased rectal tone, saddle anesthesia, motor weakness, and absent reflexes. These findings indicate possible epidural compression syndrome. A herniated disc is strongly suggested in the setting of diminished reflexes and positive straight-leg and crossed straight-leg raise tests.

C. X-ray and Laboratory Findings

Obtain plain x-rays of the spine for patients with trauma and spinal tenderness, for children or adolescents with atraumatic back pain, and when red flags for infection or malignancy are present. MRI may be indicated to rule out an epidural compression syndrome. Laboratory studies such as complete blood count (CBC) with differential, erythrocyte sedimentation rate,

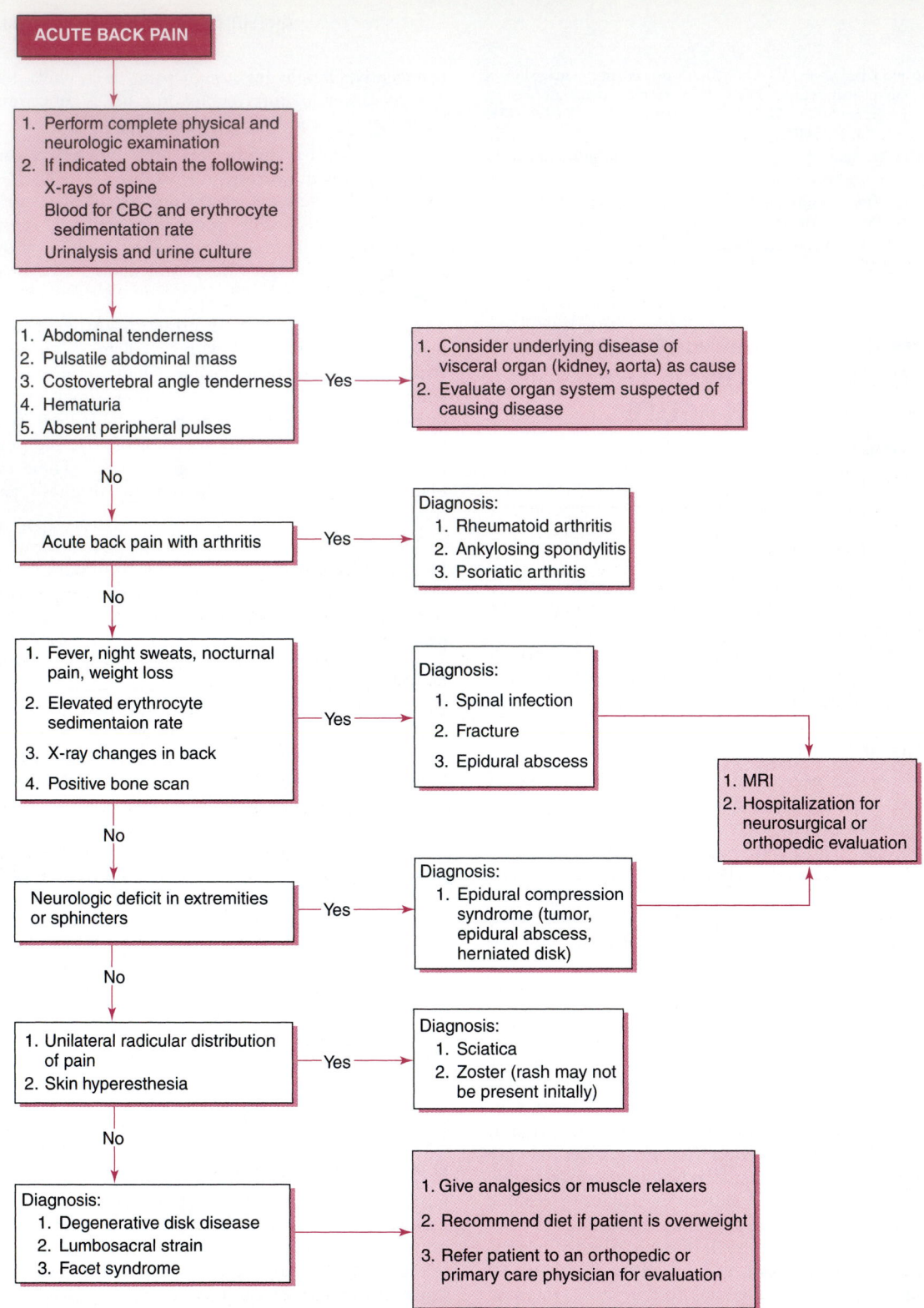

Figure 21–2. Assessment of patients with acute back pain.

Table 21–4. Nonorthopedic (visceral) causes of acute back pain.

Diagnosis	Common Clinical Findings
Pyelonephritis	Flank pain, fever, pyuria, dysuria
Nephrolithiasis	Flank pain, hematuria
Abdominal aortic aneurysm	Hypotension, pulsatile mass, abnormal emergency bedside ultrasound or CT, scan
Aortic dissection	Absent pulses, hematuria, abnormal chest x-ray
Pancreatitis	Elevated serum amylase; tender abdomen, pancreatic calcification
Ruptured abdominal viscus	Tender abdomen, air under diaphragm

and urinalysis should be performed if red flags are present. Patients with uncomplicated acute lumbosacral strains of less than 1 month's duration usually do not require imaging or laboratory testing.

D. DISPOSITION

See below under specific conditions.

◼ IV. EMERGENCY TREATMENT OF SPECIFIC CONDITIONS CAUSING BACK PAIN

TRAUMATIC BACK PAIN

Back pain associated with trauma may imply a fracture or dislocation of the thoracic or lumbar spine. The patient should remain flat on his or her back and be moved only by logroll. Perform a careful examination for other injuries. After the examination is completed, logroll the patient, maintaining in-line spinal immobilization. If a spine board is present, remove it at this time to avoid soft tissue injury. With the patient on his or her side, carefully palpate the thoracic and lumbar spine for tenderness and deformity, and perform a rectal exam. Roll the patient back to a supine position, and obtain a careful neurologic exam. Order thoracic and lumbar spine x-rays if appropriate. Other evaluation and treatment should proceed as indicated depending on the injuries present (Chapters 10 and 27).

ACUTE LUMBOSACRAL STRAIN & CHRONIC DEGENERATIVE DISK DISEASE

 ESSENTIALS OF DIAGNOSIS

- *Often pain develops after lifting or twisting.*
- *No associated constitutional symptoms (such as fever or weight loss).*
- *Normal neurologic examination.*
- *X-rays may show evidence of chronic degenerative disk disease.*

Clinical Findings

A. SYMPTOMS AND SIGNS

Acute lumbosacral strain and chronic degenerative disk disease differ only in their chronicity. The pain is typically a deep steady pain in the mid or low back that may be episodic. It is commonly unilateral and may radiate into the buttocks and posterior thigh. Pain is relieved by bed rest and aggravated by activity. There should be no red flags in the history or physical exam.

B. PHYSICAL EXAMINATION

The physical examination may show normal results or may disclose one or more of the following: increased lumbar lordosis, scoliosis, limited back motion, asymmetric lateral bending, local deep tenderness, or tight hamstring muscles. Red flags, including positive stretch tests, are not present.

C. LABORATORY FINDINGS

CBC, urinalysis, and erythrocyte sedimentation rate are not indicated. If obtained, they are normal.

D. X-RAY FINDINGS

X-rays are not indicated. If obtained, they may be normal or may show one or more of the following signs of degenerative disk disease: disk space narrowing, horizontal anterior osteophytes, spondylolisthesis, posterior facet subluxation, sclerosis, or spurs.

Treatment

A. ANALGESICS

Give drugs (NSAIDs or acetaminophen). Consider the COX-2 inhibitors or muscle relaxers for patients who cannot tolerate NSAIDS. If opioids are required, limit duration to less than 1 week and arrange close follow-up. If adequate pain control is not possible in the emergency department, consider hospitalization.

B. BED REST

Bed rest is no longer indicated. Patients should resume normal activities as tolerated by pain. Research indicates that back exercises are not beneficial in the acute setting, and patients who perform activities as tolerated recover more quickly than those who are on bed rest.

C. MUSCLE RELAXERS

If spasm of the lumbar musculature is present, muscle relaxers for the first several days may be helpful. These agents may cause sedation.

D. DIET

Weight loss is important if obesity is a causative factor in acute lumbosacral strain.

Disposition

Hospitalization is rarely required. Refer the patient to a primary care physician or orthopedist if symptoms do not improve within 2 weeks. Patients must have instructions to return to the emergency department or their physician if any of the following red flags develop: new neurologic symptoms, bowel or bladder incontinence, worsening pain, fever, or night pain.

SCIATICA

 ESSENTIALS OF DIAGNOSIS

- *Often acute on chronic flare-ups of pain.*
- *Radiation of pain in radicular fashion along the distribution of the sciatic nerve.*

- *Positive straight- and crossed-leg raise tests.*

Sciatica usually represents an acute episode in a chronic degenerative process. Patients may have a history of chronic episodic low back pain.

Clinical Findings

Pain usually begins abruptly, often with trivial trauma such as sneezing. The pain is often described as stabbing or shooting; is worse with coughing, Valsalva maneuver, or sitting; and is often incapacitating. Radiation in the distribution of the sciatic nerve is common. The main distinguishing feature of sciatica is radicular pain that extends below the knee. It affects 2% of patients with acute low back pain. In most cases it is caused by herniation of the nucleus pulposus, known most commonly as a herniated disc, that compresses a nerve root. Sciatica is 88% specific for a herniated disc. Other causes include intraspinal tumor or infection, foraminal stenosis, piriformis syndrome, and lumbar spinal stenosis.

The radicular pain is usually only in one leg and may be characterized by paresthesias, loss of sensation, or motor weakness (Table 21–5); 95% of herniated discs occur at the L4–L5 or L5–S1 levels. The most common pathologic findings of the L5 nerve root are foot drop, loss of dorsiflexion of the great toe, and pain in the great toe. Findings in S1 include heel pain, decreased plantar flexion of the great toe, and decreased ankle jerk.

The difference between lumbosacral strain and sciatica is the presence of abnormal neurologic findings, pain below the knee, and positive straight-leg and crossed straight-leg raise tests in the latter case. Plain x-rays and laboratory evaluation are not indicated for sciatica unless associated red flags for fracture, malignancy, infection, or epidural compression syndrome are present.

Table 21–5. Neurologic findings in herniated lumbosacral disk.

Disk	Root	Motor Findings	Sensory Findings	Reflexes	Sciatic Stretch Tests
L5–S1	S1	Weak foot evertors and plantar flexors	Decreased response on lateral side of foot and leg	Achilles jerk depressed or absent	Strongly positive
L4–5	L5	Weak extensor hallucis longus	Decreased response on mid dorsum of foot	No changes	Moderately positive
L3–4	L4	Weak knee extension	Decreased response on medial foot and anteromedial leg	Knee jerk depressed or absent	May be negative

Treatment & Disposition

Treatment is nearly the same as that for lumbosacral strain, including instructions for activity as limited only by pain. Opioids may need to be used more frequently in the short term. The only treatment difference is that selected patients with sciatica may need epidural steroid injections. Systemic steroids have no proven benefit.

Approximately 80% of patients with a herniated disc improve without surgery. Only 5–10% will require surgery. More than 50% will improve within 6 weeks with conservative therapy. Therefore, patients meeting the criteria for sciatica alone may be safely discharged to follow up with their primary physician in 2 weeks and return to the emergency department for the same reasons as listed under lumbosacral strain.

Back Pain in Children

A child who presents with back pain should be evaluated carefully. Red flags include decreased activity secondary to pain, fever, and nocturnal pain. These are possible indicators of tumor or infection. If the child has recently been involved in strenuous sports or exercise programs, consider spondylolysis and spondylolisthesis. Bacteremia increases the risk of spinal infections. Therefore, a history of recent febrile illness is important. Spine x-rays should be taken of virtually every child who presents with back pain. Consider obtaining CBC, urinalysis, and erythrocyte sedimentation rate if any red flags are raised. Consider admission for further workup and observation.

EPIDURAL COMPRESSION SYNDROME

 ESSENTIALS OF DIAGNOSIS

- *Bowel or bladder incontinence.*
- *Saddle anesthesia, decreased or absent rectal sphincter tone, lower extremity deficits.*

Clinical Findings

Epidural compression syndrome is a true emergency. Consider this possibility in every patient who presents with back pain. Red flags in the history and physical examination are used to screen for this syndrome. The hallmark symptoms include urinary retention marked by overflow incontinence, saddle anesthesia, decreased rectal tone, and bilateral motor and sensory deficits. If any of these red flags is present, obtain a urinary postvoid residual. If the postvoid residual is less than 50–100 mL, then cauda equina syndrome can usually be ruled out (negative predictive value is 99.99%). However, if a patient has other significant red flags, pursue an epidural compression syndrome with imaging regardless of a normal postvoid residual. Causes include a large central disc herniation, tumors, trauma, epidural abscess, and hematomas.

Treatment & Disposition

If an epidural compression syndrome is likely, start steroid therapy immediately before waiting for confirmatory MRI results. Dexamethasone is usually given in doses ranging between 10 mg and 100 mg intravenously depending on severity and rapidity of presentation and progression. The next step is to consult a neurosurgeon while ordering an emergent MRI. If unable to obtain an MRI scan, order a CT (computed tomography) scan with myelography.

FACET SYNDROME

Excessive overriding of lumbar or thoracic facets usually occurs as a consequence of disk space narrowing associated with degenerative disk disease. Facet syndrome is unusual and episodic and is characterized by the onset of acute scoliosis after asymmetric lifting. The diagnosis is usually made by exclusion. Patients should be instructed in the fundamentals of proper back care.

SPINAL INFECTIONS
(See also Chapter 40.)

 ESSENTIALS OF DIAGNOSIS

- *Usually occurs in patients with predisposition for infections: diabetic patients, intravenous drug users, transplant patients, cancer patients.*
- *Fever and back pain are the hallmarks.*
- *MRI or CT scan of the spine is essential.*

General Considerations

Disk space infections today are most commonly seen in intravenous drug users, diabetics, transplant patients, and cancer patients. Vertebral osteomyelitis should be suspected in patients who have recently undergone spinal surgery and present with red flags for infection. Epidural abscess and vertebral osteomyelitis are the most common spinal infections. The organism most commonly implicated is *S aureus*.

Clinical Findings

Red flags for disk space infections are night pain, cough pain, night sweats, fever, and an elevated erythrocyte sedimentation rate. Be alert for the rare low-grade presentations of tuberculous and fungal diskitis. Systemic evidence of infection is usually present.

The typical x-ray changes of disk space narrowing with adjacent vertebral end-plate destruction do not appear until 10–14 days after onset of symptoms. Bone scans are usually positive early in the illness before x-ray changes appear. Epidural or paraspinous abscess may appear as an ill-defined mass on x-ray. If a spinal infection is suspected, an MRI scan (gold standard) or CT scan must be ordered. Blood and urine cultures should also be collected.

Treatment & Disposition

Spinal infections require hospitalization and orthopedic consultation, needle aspiration for bacteriologic diagnosis, and appropriate antibiotics. Occasionally surgical drainage is required.

A neurologic deficit in association with signs of spinal infection often means that an epidural or paraspinous abscess is present. This is a major emergency demanding immediate MRI or CT myelography, consultation, hospitalization, and possibly emergent decompression.

ANKYLOSING SPONDYLITIS

See above for details of diagnosis, treatment, and disposition.

NEOPLASM

Metastatic tumor is the most common neoplastic process causing back pain. Bone marrow tumors such as multiple myeloma are second in frequency. Primary tumors of the spinal column or spinal cord are rare.

Fifty percent of bone must be lost before a lesion is evident on plain x-rays. Multiple lesions are common. Bone scan is more sensitive for early diagnosis.

Red flags are weight loss; night pain in the absence of day pain; and a history of insidious and progressive pain that has not responded to conservative measures, especially in elderly patients. Laboratory findings may include an elevated erythrocyte sedimentation rate, significant anemia, proteinemia, and findings in other organ systems that suggest neoplasm.

ZOSTER

Preeruptive zoster may mimic degenerative disk disease. The pain of zoster is burning and dysesthetic, with striking unilateral radicular distribution that does not cross the midline. Skin hyperesthesia over the painful area is the earliest physical finding. See Chapter 46 for details.

Aree D et al: Recognizing spinal cord emergencies. Am Fam Physician 2001;64:631. [PMID: 11529262]

Della-Giustina D et al: Back pain: cost-effective strategies for distinguishing between benign and life-threatening causes. Emergency Medicine Practice 2000;2(2):1.

Della-Giustina DA: Emergency department evaluation and treatment of back pain. Emerg Med Clin North Am 1999;17:877. [PMID: 10584107]

SECTION III
Trauma Emergencies

<table>
<tr><td>

Head Injuries

</td><td>

22

</td></tr>
</table>

Stephen C. Ausband, MD, FACEP, & Ritu Sahni, MD, MPH

Immediate Management of Life-Threatening Problems
Management of Other Symptoms
Emergency Treatment of Specific Head Injuries
  Soft Tissue Injuries
   1. Scalp Lacerations
   2. Hematoma
  Skull Fractures
   1. Closed Skull Fractures
   2. Open Skull Fractures
   3. Depressed Skull Fractures
   4. Basilar Skull Fractures

Intracranial Injury
   1. Epidural Hematoma
   2. Subdural Hematoma
   3. Cerebral Contusion
   4. Traumatic Subarachnoid Hemorrhage
   5. Diffuse Axonal Injury
Minor Head Injuries
Special Considerations for Pediatrics
Indications for Hospitalization
Discharge Instructions
Intoxicated Patients

■ IMMEDIATE MANAGEMENT OF LIFE-THREATENING PROBLEMS

Cervical Spine Immobilization

Any patient with blunt force injury to the head should be suspected of having cervical spine injury until proven otherwise. Penetrating injuries to the torso and extremities not associated with blunt force are rarely associated with cervical spine injury. Cervical spine injury is associated with 5% of all blunt force injuries to the head; the greater the force, the greater the incidence of associated cervical spine injury. Immobilization of the cervical spine must include an appropriately sized and fitted cervical collar; head blocks; and a long, rigid spine board to which the patient is secured. Immobilize the cervical spine during evaluation by manual stabilization and logrolling the patient. Do not apply traction to the cervical spine.

Airway

Hypoxia is associated with increased morbidity and mortality in trauma patients. Hypoxia must be avoided or corrected immediately. All patients with traumatic head injury should receive 100% oxygen by high-flow nonrebreathing mask as initial therapy. Keep the airway clear by suctioning of blood and secretions as needed. Remove foreign bodies, avulsed teeth, and dental appliances. Loss of gag reflex, inability to adequately clear secretions, or GCS score of 8 or less are all indications to secure the airway with an endotracheal tube. Use clini-

421

cal judgment to determine if a patient needs to be intubated in other situations, with priority on maintaining the airway during resuscitation, evaluation, and transport. Ventilate apneic or hypoventilating patients with an Ambu bag and 100% oxygen until intubation can be accomplished. Avoid using a bag to provide positive-pressure ventilation to an actively breathing patient because this induces gastric distention.

Perform intubation while maintaining manual in-line cervical immobilization without applying traction. Rapid sequence intubation should be strongly considered for all patients. Once sedatives and paralytics have taken effect, remove the cervical collar and maintain manual stabilization. After intubation, replace the cervical collar.

Orotracheal intubation is preferred because of the technical difficulty of nasotracheal intubation as well as the complications of bleeding, elevated intracranial pressure, and possible passage of the endotracheal tube through a fractured cribiform plate into the cranium. If orotracheal intubation is not successful, intubate the patient using a retrograde Seldinger technique, fiberoptic-guided intubation, or cricothyroidotomy depending on the equipment available immediately and the procedures with which the physician is most skilled. In addition, consider a temporizing device, such as a laryngeal mask airway, in the patient who is difficult to intubate. After intubation, confirm endotracheal tube position by auscultation over the lung fields and epigastrium. Additional devices, such as color capnometers and aspiration devices may be used to confirm tube placement. Data show that any single test of endotracheal tube position is substantially less accurate than using 2 tests of position. Immediate portable chest X-ray must also be used to visualize endotracheal tube position. After successful intubation, place an orogastric tube. Avoid nasogastric tubes in patients with head trauma for the same reasons that nasotracheal intubation is to be avoided.

Any change in the patient's condition or oxygen saturation and any substantial movement of the patient, such as to or from a computed tomography (CT) gantry, necessitates reevaluation of the endotracheal tube position by auscultation.

The emergency physician must be familiar with advanced airway techniques to be able to perform rapid sequence intubation and guarantee definitive airway access in any patient.

Breathing

Once the airway is secured by intubation, assess the patient's respiratory status with an arterial blood gas. Use serial arterial blood gases or end-tidal carbon dioxide monitoring to maintain arterial P_{CO_2} level in the normal physiologic range. Hypercapnia is associated with increased morbidity and mortality. Hypocapnia is associated with decreased cerebral blood flow and decreased cerebral oxygen perfusion. Patients should not be hyperventilated in order to decrease P_{CO_2} levels, and P_{CO_2} should be maintained at 35 mm Hg or more. Frequently reassess the respiratory status of patients who do not require intubation. All patients with head trauma should be monitored with transcutaneous pulse oximetry during evaluation.

Circulation

Hypotension is associated with increased morbidity and mortality in trauma patients. Care should be taken to maintain an adequate blood pressure, defined as a mean arterial pressure greater than 90 mm Hg. Treat shock aggressively with warmed intravenous lactated Ringer's or normal saline and blood products as needed. Avoid hypotonic fluids. Avoid glucose-containing fluids because of the risk of hyperglycemia, which is deleterious to the injured brain. Do not attribute hypotension to head injury alone. Elevated blood pressure associated with bradycardia is a sign of increased intracranial pressure.

Disability

Establish a Glasgow Coma Scale (GCS) for any patient with a head injury. Repeat the GCS periodically during reassessment. In addition, measure pupillary response and symmetry and also consider doll's eye (oculocephalic) movements and caloric stimulation (oculovestibular) tests, if needed, to gauge the patient's level of cortical and brain-stem functioning. Note any asymmetry in neurologic examination or focal neurologic findings. In an unresponsive patient, motor response may be elicited by nailbed pressure. If motor responses are asymmetric, the best response is a more accurate predictor of outcome and should be used for calculating the GCS. Document initial neurologic examination findings prior to administering sedative or paralytic agents, if possible.

As for any patient with altered mental status, the clinician is advised to check for and treat any easily reversible causes of decreased level of consciousness, including hypoglycemia (bedside fingerstick blood glucose); hypoxemia (pulse oximetry); narcotic overdose (naloxone administration); and, in malnourished or alcoholic patients, Wernicke encephalopathy (thiamine administration).

Exposure

As with all trauma patients, the patient should be completely undressed and the entire body examined, including the back. Once initial examination is complete, cover the patient with warm blankets. Take care to avoid hypothermia by warming the examination room and using warm blankets and warm fluids. Rewarm the patient if he or she is already hypothermic.

■ MANAGEMENT OF OTHER SYMPTOMS

Seizures

Seizure prophylaxis should be considered in patients with an initial GCS of 8 or less and in those with cerebral contusion, depressed skull fracture, intracranial hematoma, or penetrating head wound. In adults, phenytoin, phosphenytoin, or carbamazepine are the prophylactic drugs of choice. In children, phenobarbital has been used prophylactically. Treat any acute post-traumatic seizure rapidly with lorazepam, phenytoin, phosphenytoin, or phenobarbital to prevent worsening hypoxemia associated with the seizure and to limit secondary brain injury.

Combativeness

Evaluate a combative patient first for hypoxia, hypotension, hypoglycemia, and pain. Avoid physical restraints if possible, or, if needed, use them only long enough to allow for proper sedation and analgesic administration. Patients should never be allowed to struggle against restraints. Occasionally, patients who cannot be controlled with sedation and analgesia alone will require paralysis and endotracheal intubation for protection of the spine and to accomplish diagnostic studies.

Pain Control

After initial evaluation, do not withhold sedatives and analgesics. Narcotics and benzodiazepines are safe and effective medications for sedation and analgesia and should be used in doses high enough to be effective. Care must be taken to ensure that patients who are paralyzed and intubated have sufficient analgesic and sedative medications.

Systemic Hypertension

If blood pressures are elevated, evaluate the patient for adequate sedation and analgesia. Hypertension associated with bradycardia is a sign of elevated intracranial pressures. Isolated systemic hypertension that is high enough to constitute a hypertensive urgency or emergency is rare. If present, systemic hypertension should be treated with caution to avoid rapid decrease in blood pressure or decrease in blood pressure below 10% of initial values.

Intracranial Hypertension

Elevations of intracranial pressure are heralded by bradycardia and hypertension, signs of transtentorial herniation, or progressive neurologic deterioration without other attributable cause. Mannitol is the drug of choice for treating elevated intracranial pressure. It is vitally important to maintain serum osmolality below 320 mOsm and to maintain euvolemia with intravenous fluid replacement during mannitol administration. Elevation of serum osmolality above 320 mOsm can lead to a reversal of the osmotic gradient with subsequent increase in cerebral edema. Mannitol administration should be initiated in consultation with a neurosurgeon, if possible.

Gruen P, Liu C: Current trends in the management of head injury. Emerg Med Clin North Am 1998;16:63. [PMID: 9496315]

■ EMERGENCY TREATMENT OF SPECIFIC HEAD INJURIES

SOFT TISSUE INJURIES

Although often dramatic in nature, soft tissue injuries of the head cause little long-term sequelae and most can be easily managed in the emergency department. However, soft tissue injuries of the head can be an indicator of possible significant intracranial injury. For example, one study found that any sign of trauma above the clavicles is an independent predicator of possible intracranial abnormality on CT scan.

1. Scalp Lacerations

 ESSENTIALS OF DIAGNOSIS

- *Diagnosed through thorough inspection and palpation.*
- *May be significant source of blood loss.*
- *Evaluate for underlying skull fracture.*

Clinical Findings

Scalp lacerations are primarily diagnosed by palpation and a visual inspection of the patient's scalp. A complete and thorough examination of the scalp must be performed to find any evidence of laceration or hematoma. Once a laceration is located, palpate the area thoroughly to determine if any signs of skull fracture are present. Because the scalp has tremendous vascularity, scalp lacerations can be a source of significant blood loss.

Treatment

Most scalp lacerations can be easily closed with either staples or simple interrupted sutures. Clipping of the hair may facilitate easier closure. Alternatively, water-soluble lubricating jelly (eg, Surgilube) may be used to keep hair out of the laceration during closure. Shaving of the scalp may lead to increased risk of infection. The scalp is highly vascular and may be closed up to 12 hours after initial injury. Any patient with a scalp laceration and significant traumatic mechanism or alteration of consciousness should undergo CT scanning prior to closure of the scalp laceration. The wound should be copiously irrigated with normal saline before closure. Occasionally, layered closure with absorbent sutures may be required (Chapter 30).

Disposition

Patients with scalp lacerations and no other complications may be discharged safely to home. Follow-up should occur in 3–5 days for recheck; the staples or sutures may be removed in 10–14 days.

2. Hematoma

 ESSENTIALS OF DIAGNOSIS

- Diagnosed by inspection and palpation.
- Strongly consider CT scan.

Clinical Findings

Scalp hematoma is diagnosed by palpation and visual inspection. A hematoma has little long-term significance on its own but may be an indicator of more serious intracranial abnormality. Patients with scalp hematoma and significant mechanism of injury or alteration in level of consciousness should undergo CT scanning.

Treatment

A scalp hematoma is treated primarily like a hematoma or contusion in any other part of the body. Ice, elevation, and nonsteroidal anti-inflammatory drugs should

be the mainstay of treatment. Aspiration of a scalp hematoma has little, if any, benefit and should rarely be attempted.

Disposition

Patients with only a scalp hematoma may be safely discharged home and referred for standard follow-up.

SKULL FRACTURES

Skull fracture is strongly associated with other more serious intracranial abnormalities. Studies have shown that 40–100% of all intracranial abnormalities are associated with skull fracture. The skull fracture itself, however, is typically of little clinical consequence to the patient.

1. Closed Skull Fractures

 ESSENTIALS OF DIAGNOSIS

- Use CT scan for diagnosis because CT shows fractures and other associated injuries.
- Admit for observation.

Clinical Findings

Closed fractures of the skull are detected primarily on noncontrast CT scan. Because these fractures are often associated with more serious injury, it is prudent to evaluate the injury with CT scan rather than plain skull x-rays.

Treatment

There is no specific treatment for linear skull fractures. Close observation is recommended to detect the development of an epidural hematoma after an initially negative CT scan.

Disposition

Patients with isolated closed skull fractures with no evidence of brain injury require admission to the hospital for a minimum of 24 hours of observation.

2. Open Skull Fractures

 ESSENTIALS OF DIAGNOSIS

- Use CT scan for diagnosis because CT shows fractures and other associated injuries.

- *Underlie scalp lacerations.*
- *High risk of infection.*

Clinical Findings

Open fractures underlie scalp lacerations and are often palpated during evaluation of the scalp laceration. These fractures have a serious risk of infection. Definitive diagnosis is made with noncontrast CT scan, and more serious intracranial abnormality should be ruled out. Open skull fracture is likely if pneumocephalus is noted on CT scan (Figure 22–1).

Treatment

Initiate intravenous antibiotics such as cefazolin, and refer the patient to the appropriate surgical subspecialty for possible operative debridement.

Disposition

Hospitalize all patients with open skull fracture.

3. Depressed Skull Fractures

ESSENTIALS OF DIAGNOSIS

- *Often found with inspection or palpation.*
- *Use CT scan for diagnosis because CT shows fractures and other associated injuries.*

Clinical Findings

Depressed skull fractures are often palpable or visible during examination. However, swelling around the area of the injury can mask a depressed skull fracture and make it appear to be a simple hematoma. Like all skull fractures, depressed skull fractures are often associated with more serious intracranial injury, and patients need to be evaluated accordingly. Noncontrast CT scan is the test of choice to determine whether the patient has intracranial injury or depressed skull fracture (Figure 22–2).

Treatment

Depressed skull fractures without intracranial injury represent a cosmetic situation. Open depressed skull fractures are at high risk of infection, similar to open nondepressed skull fractures.

Disposition

Patients should be admitted to the hospital for observation and referred to the appropriate surgical subspecialist for possible elevation of the depression and debridement if the fracture is open.

4. Basilar Skull Fractures

ESSENTIALS OF DIAGNOSIS

- *Use CT scan for diagnosis because CT shows fractures and other associated injuries; may be missed on CT.*
- *Associated with hemotympanum, Battle sign, raccoon's eyes, cerebrospinal fluid leaking from ear or nose, or hearing loss.*

Clinical Findings

Basilar skull fractures are skull fractures at the base of the skull, typically at the petrous portion of the temporal bone. Clinical signs include hemotympanum, Battle sign (ecchymosis along the mastoid area of the skull), raccoon's eyes (periorbital ecchymosis), cerebrospinal fluid leak from the nose or ear, or hearing loss. Patients with any of these signs should undergo noncontrast CT evaluation for possible basilar skull fracture and to rule out more serious intracranial abnormality.

Treatment

Initiate intravenous antibiotics such as cefazolin.

Disposition

Patients with documented basilar skull fracture or significant signs of a basilar skull fracture should be admitted for observation. If a more serious intracranial abnormality is present, obtain neurosurgical consultation.

INTRACRANIAL INJURY

The primary goal in evaluating patients with potential head injury is to determine if an intracranial abnormality is present and then to determine if that injury requires surgical intervention. There has long been controversy as to which patients require CT scanning. Of patients presenting to the emergency department with head injury and a GCS of 15, 6–8% have an intracranial abnormality. The vast majority of these injuries are

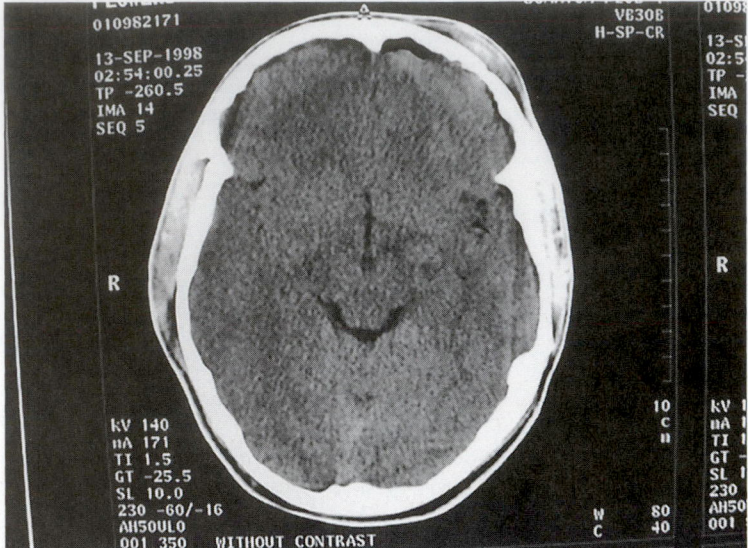

A

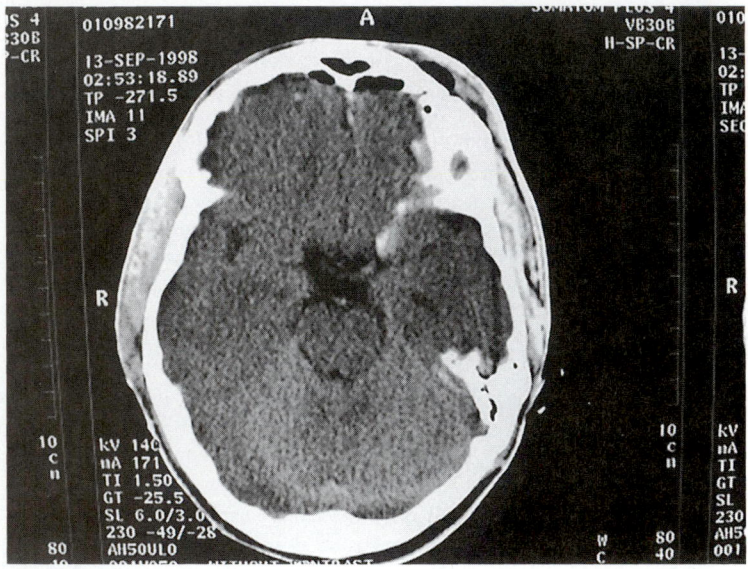

B

Figure 22–1. Depressed right temporal and nondepressed left frontal skull fractures not well visualized on typical brain windows (**A** and **B**) but clearly seen on bone windows. Also note the associated frontal pneumocephalus.

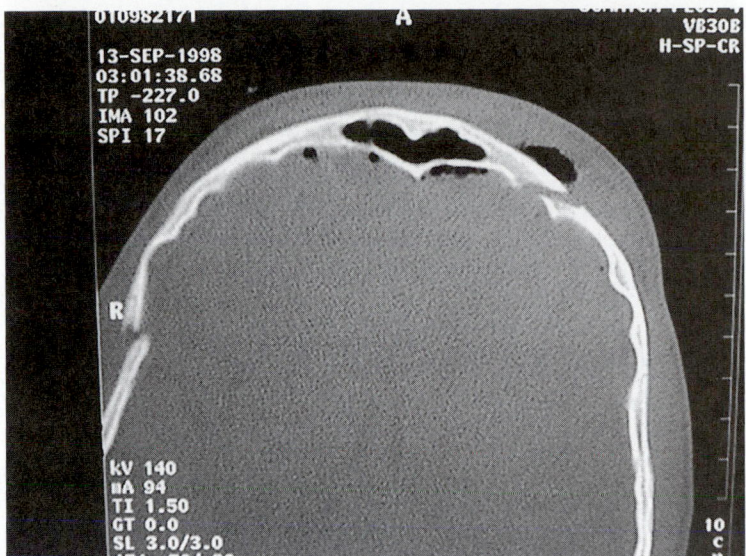

C

Figure 22–1. (continued) Depressed right temporal and nondepressed left frontal skull fractures not well visualized on typical brain windows but clearly seen on bone windows (**C**). Also note the associated frontal pneumocephalus.

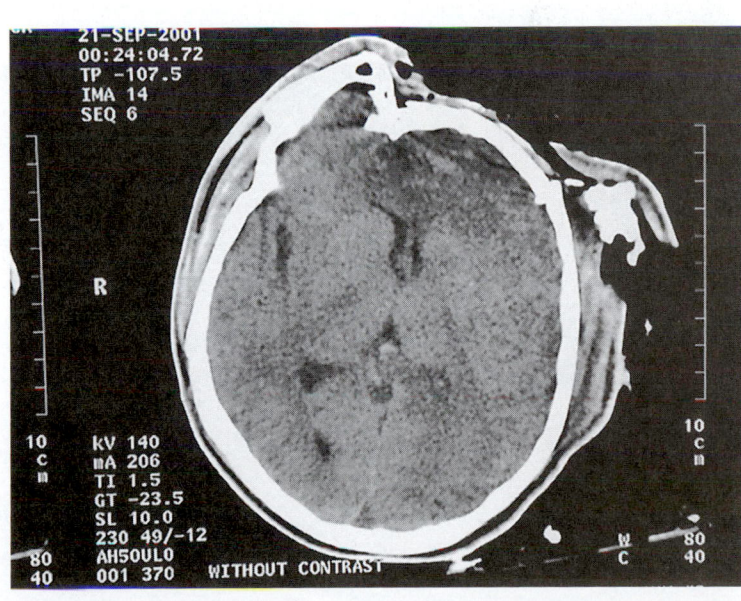

Figure 22–2. Severely depressed frontal skull fracture with significant impingement on the frontal lobes.

nonsurgical, but they may have long-term cognitive implications for the patient. There are currently few recommendations as to when a patient requires CT scanning. The emerging practice is to obtain a CT scan whenever a patient has had an alteration in the level of consciousness at any time or amnesia to the event of injury. There have been some prospective validations of criteria that may allow CT scan to be safely foregone in a small percentage of these patients. However, it is difficult to determine which patients with a GCS of 15 will have intracranial abnormalities.

1. Epidural Hematoma

 ## ESSENTIALS OF DIAGNOSIS

- *Brief loss of consciousness followed by transient lucid interval.*
- *Arterial bleeding source.*
- *Diagnosis made by CT scan, which shows a biconvex hematoma.*
- *Requires rapid neurologic evaluation for decompression.*

An epidural hematoma is a collection of blood and clot between the dura mater and the bones of the skull. Sources of bleeding from epidural hematoma include the meningeal arteries (often the middle meningeal artery) or occasionally the dural venous sinuses. These bleeds generally have a lenticular (biconvex) shape. Patients with epidural hematoma may have an initial, brief loss of consciousness followed by a lucid interval during which they may be neurologically intact. This interval is then followed by rapid clinical deterioration. All patients with epidural hematoma typically require rapid intervention by a neurosurgical specialist. An epidural hematoma represents a space-occupying lesion to the brain, often from a high-pressure arterial source. Therefore, rapid expansion of this hematoma can lead to herniation of brain contents. Patient outcome is related directly to the patient's level of consciousness on presentation and to the time until decompression of potential space-occupying lesions (Figure 22–3).

2. Subdural Hematoma

 ## ESSENTIALS OF DIAGNOSIS

- *Venous bleeding source.*
- *Diagnosis made by CT scan, which shows concave hematoma.*
- *May be chronic, acute, or acute on chronic.*
- *Admit for neurosurgical evaluation.*

A subdural hematoma also represents a space-occupying lesion. This lesion, however, lies in the space between

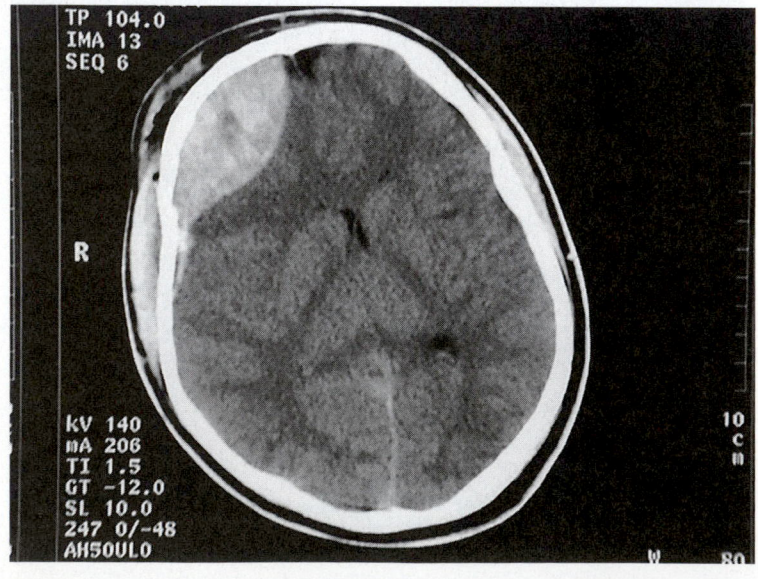

Figure 22–3. Large acute right frontal epidural hematoma with associated mass effect on the frontal lobes and slight midline shift.

the dura mater and the arachnoid mater and usually conforms to the convexity of underlying cerebral cortex (Figure 22–4). The source of bleeding is often the bridging veins, which are more likely to tear in patients with significant brain atrophy (eg, elderly or alcoholic patients). These patients can develop large chronic subdural hematomas with minimal neurologic deficit. A subdural hematoma may or may not require surgical drainage. Acute bleeds can develop in areas of chronic subdural hematoma (often from new trauma) and cause neurologic deterioration (Figure 22–5). All patients with subdural hematoma should receive prompt neurosurgical evaluation.

3. Cerebral Contusion

ESSENTIALS OF DIAGNOSIS

- *Diagnosis made by CT scan.*
- *Associated edema may require intervention.*

Cerebral contusion represents a non-space-occupying discrete lesion within the brain matter itself. These lesions are less likely to lead to herniation than are other types of intracranial lesions. Significant edema can occur around areas of cerebral contusion, which can lead to increased intracranial pressure and midline shift. Typically no surgical intervention is required for cerebral contusion. However, if the contusion is large enough and significant shift occurs, then intracranial pressure monitoring may be instituted by the neurosurgical specialist.

4. Traumatic Subarachnoid Hemorrhage

ESSENTIALS OF DIAGNOSIS

- *Diagnosis made by CT scan.*
- *Can lead to elevated intracranial pressure owing to cerebrospinal fluid obstruction.*

It was once thought that subarachnoid hemorrhage was relatively rare and had a poor outcome. However, it appears now that subarachnoid hemorrhage in a traumatic setting is much more common than previously believed. Traumatic subarachnoid hemorrhage is not a space-occupying lesion but can lead to increasing intracranial pressure, primarily by blocking the outflow of cerebrospinal fluid from the 3rd and 4th ventricles in the brain. Patients with asymptomatic subarachnoid hemorrhage may be admitted for observation and no further intervention. Patients with altered level of consciousness or other neurologic findings may require intracranial pressure monitoring in the critical care unit setting (Figure 22–6).

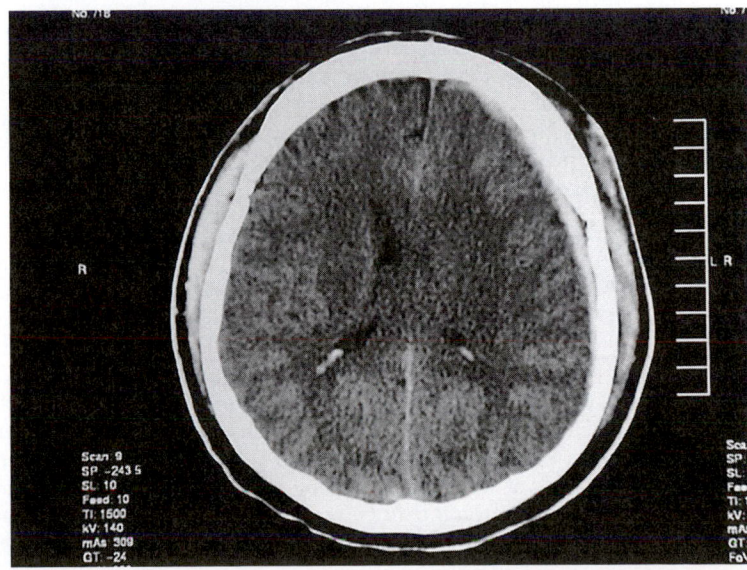

Figure 22–4. Small left subdural hematoma with effacement of the left lateral ventricle.

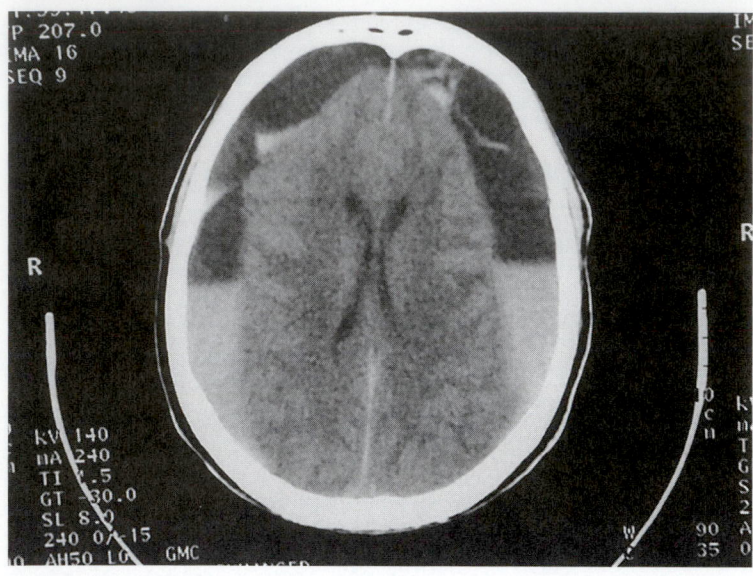

Figure 22–5. Bilateral acute on chronic subdural hematoma with significant mass effect compressing both cerebral hemispheres. Note the acute component of the hematoma layering posteriorly (dependent position).

5. Diffuse Axonal Injury

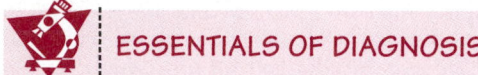

ESSENTIALS OF DIAGNOSIS

- *Diagnosis made by burring of gray- to white-matter margin, punctate cerebral hemorrhages, or cerebral edema.*
- *Associated with posttraumatic coma.*

Shearing forces from sudden deceleration during blunt trauma can cause severe intracranial injury. Diffuse axonal injury is a frequent cause of posttraumatic coma. This injury is typically manifested on noncontrast CT by a blurring of the margin between the gray and white matter, punctate hemorrhages often in the internal capsule, and cerebral edema (Figure 22–7).

■ MINOR HEAD INJURIES

The vast majority of patients with head injury who present to the emergency department have minor head injuries. One study found no significant intracranial injuries in the absence of all of the following findings: headache, vomiting, age greater than 60 years, intoxication, deficits in short-term memory (anterograde amnesia), physical evidence of trauma above the clavicles, and seizure. The negative predictive value of the absence of these clinical variables was 100%.

The first goal in caring for a patient with a head injury is to determine if a significant or serious intracranial mass lesion is present. Once serious injury is ruled out by examination, history, or CT scan, the patient falls into the category of minor head injury. Remember that any patient with amnesia to the event or any history of alteration of level of consciousness or loss of consciousness should undergo CT scanning. Patients who present with minor head injury complaints and have a negative CT scan and are neurologically completely normal may be discharged to home, especially if in the care of a responsible adult.

A significant question often arises regarding whether the injury is a concussion and what type of postconcussion restrictions are needed. Concussion is often wrongly thought of as transient loss of consciousness if CT findings are negative. Most current precaution guidelines, of which there are many, consider concussion to be a trauma-induced alteration in mental status that may or may not include loss of consciousness. The primary hallmarks of concussion are confusion and amnesia. Concussion is of significant importance because long-term neuropsychiatric testing on athletes who have sustained frequent concussions has shown that multiple concussions over a lifetime can lead to cognitive impairment. As a result, guidelines have been developed that grade concussion and recommend activity level by an athlete who undergoes concussion. Although these guidelines have not been fully used with

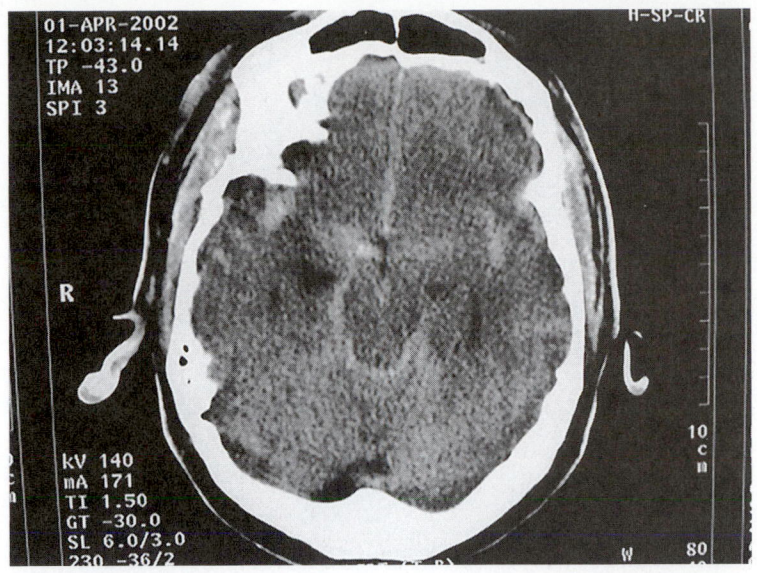

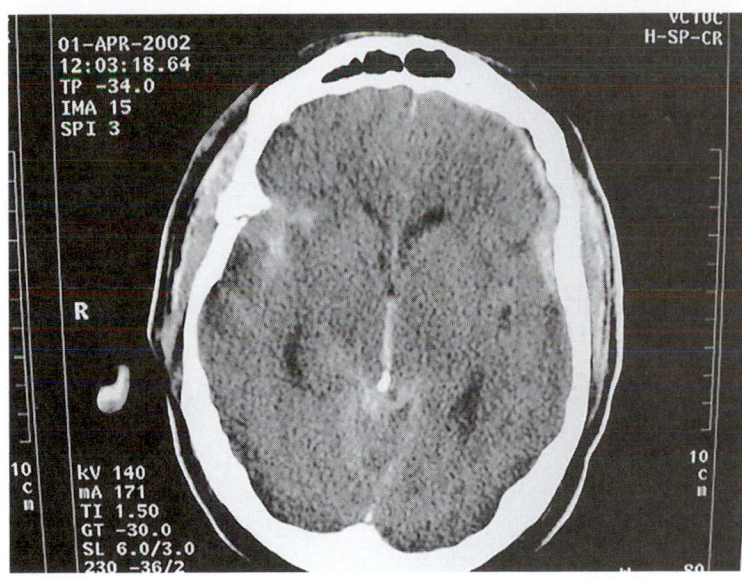

Figure 22–6. Right temporal subarachnoid hemorrhage (**A–D**) with extension into basal cistern (**A**), third ventricle (**B**) and lateral ventricles (**C** and **D**). Also note the moderate sized left frontotemporal subdural prominently seen on B–D.

non-athlete patients, some of these guidelines can be used to guide the outcome of non-athlete patients. Current guidelines have divided concussions into three grades (Table 22–1). The length of time the athlete or patient should refrain from strenuous activity is based on both the grade of the concussion and the history of prior concussions. Patients with a history of prior concussions have longer restrictions. Current recommenda-

tions for immediate treatment and restrictions are also available.

Postconcussion syndrome is characterized by headache, dizziness, and cognitive impairment (memory) and occurs acutely in 50% of patients experiencing a mild traumatic brain injury. These symptoms can occur singly or with other symptoms, and they generally resolve over the initial weeks to months after a concussion.

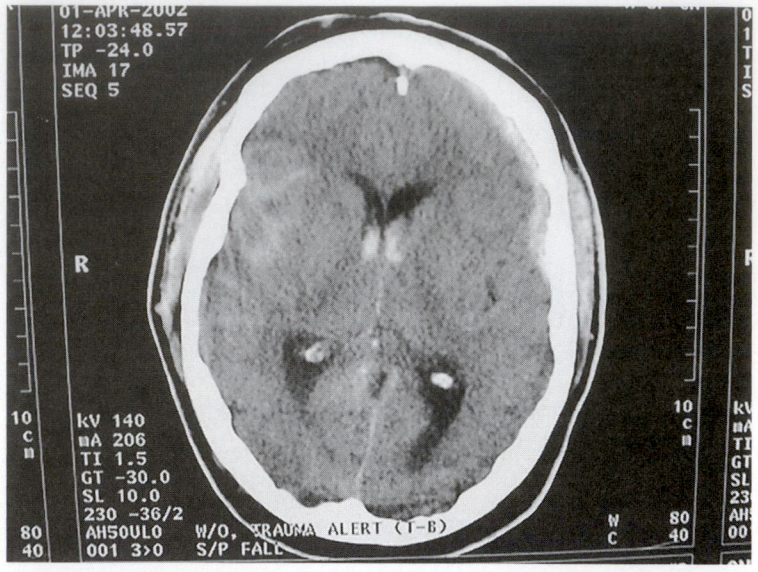

C

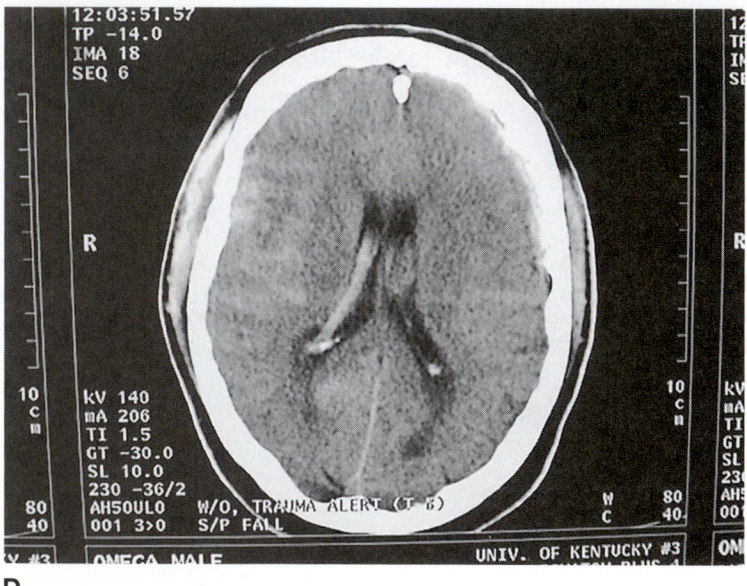

D

Figure 22–6. (continued) Right temporal subarachnoid hemorrhage (**A–D**) with extension into basal cistern (**A**), third ventricle (**B**) and lateral ventricles (**C** and **D**). Also note the moderate sized left frontotemporal subdural prominently seen on B–D.

■ SPECIAL CONSIDERATIONS FOR PEDIATRICS

Although it is difficult to determine when adult patients need further workup, the question is even more difficult to resolve for pediatric patients. Smaller children (younger than age 2 years) are even more difficult

to evaluate for possible loss of consciousness, transient confusion, and amnesia. Some conservative guidelines favor obtaining noncontrast CT scan on any child under age 2 years with any sign of trauma to the head, including minor hematomas and scratches. A more traditional approach has been to obtain imaging studies only for children with a history of loss of consciousness, altered mental status, vomiting, seizures, or focal neurologic deficits after a traumatic event.

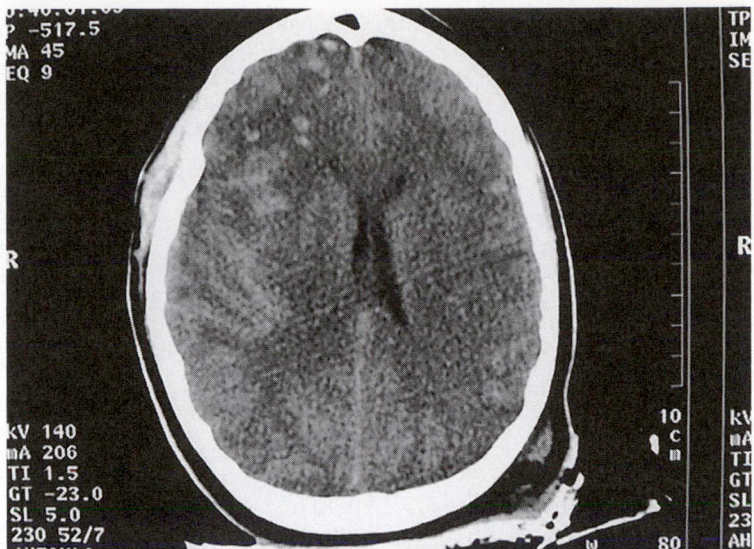

Figure 22–7. Diffuse axonal injury with punctate hemorrhages (mainly right frontal), changes of generalized edema with poor gray-white matter discrimination in the right hemisphere, and mass effect on the right lateral ventricle.

■ INDICATIONS FOR HOSPITALIZATION

In general, patients with minor head injury who have no clinical history findings that suggest neurologic injury, no neurologic abnormality on examination, and a normal CT scan can be discharged to home. Patients who have persistent amnesia, persistent alteration in level of consciousness, or any abnormality on CT scan should be admitted for observation. Patients with significant mass or space-occupying lesions should receive immediate neurosurgical consultation.

■ DISCHARGE INSTRUCTIONS

Various methods have been proposed for ongoing evaluation after discharge of patients with minor head injury. These methods have ranged from having the patient's caregiver evaluate the patient every 30 minutes to once per night. None of these discharge instructions has been validated in any prospective manner. Currently, with relatively liberal use of CT scan, the possibility of return for worsening head injury is unlikely. It is not unusual, however, for patients to present with postconcussive symptoms days or weeks after a minor head injury. Dis-

Table 22–1. Concussion grading and outcomes for a first concussion (American Academy of Neurology).

	Grade		
	1	2	3
Symptoms	Transient confusion; no loss of consciousness; concussion symptoms last less than 15 minutes.	Transient confusion; no loss of consciousness; concussion symptoms last more than 15 minutes.	Any loss of consciousness.
Immediate treatment	Removal from contest.	Removal from contest without return that day.	Removal from contest and transport to nearest emergency department.
Projected return	Same day after symptom-free for 15 minutes.	After 1 full asymptomatic week.	After 1 full asymptomatic week if loss of consciousness is brief (seconds). After 2 full asymptomatic weeks if loss of consciousness is prolonged (1 minute).

charge instructions for these patients should include being aware of any nausea or vomiting, alteration in level of consciousness, and any seizure activity.

The interval at which patients should be reevaluated is unclear. Patients with minimal clinical findings or negative CT scan and a history not suggestive of or not including loss of consciousness or amnesia are unlikely to have a significant space-occupying lesion. The exception may be the patient with an epidural hematoma during the lucid interval. Therefore, patients with minor head injury should be observed for some period of time in the emergency department before discharge home.

■ INTOXICATED PATIENTS

Intoxicated patients frequently present to the emergency department after being found unresponsive or with a decreased level of consciousness. Alcoholic patients are at increased risk of obtaining a head injury secondary to ataxia, frequent falls, and other types of trauma. A detailed examination looking for signs of head trauma, pupillary abnormalities, or other lateralizing neurologic deficits is critical in early identification of head injuries in intoxicated patients. Frequent reexamination is also important to ensure that an intoxicated patient's level of consciousness is improving over time. Any deterioration in the level of consciousness or the development of new deficits should prompt an emergent noncontrast CT scan for further evaluation.

American Academy of Neurology: Practice parameter: the management of concussion in sports (summary statement). Neurology 1997;48:581. [PMID: 9065530]

Committee on Quality Improvement, American Academy of Pediatrics. Commission on Clinical Policies and Research, American Academy of Family Physicians: The management of minor closed head injury in children. Pediatrics 1999;104:1407. [PMID: 10585999]

Coombs JB, Davis RL: A synopsis of the American Academy of Pediatrics' practice parameter on the management of minor closed head injury in children. Pediatr Rev 2000;21:413. [PMID: 11121498]

Haydel MJ et al: Indications for computed tomography in patients with minor head injury. N Engl J Med 2000;343:100. [PMID: 10891517]

Jogoda AS et al: Clinical policy: neuroimaging and decision-making in adult mild traumatic brain injury in the acute setting. Ann Emerg Med 2002;40:231. [PMID: 12140504]

Kelly JP, Rosenberg JH: The development of guidelines for the management of concussion in sports. J Head Trauma Rehabil 1998;13:53. [PMID: 9575257]

Preboth M: AAFP and AAP issue a practice parameter on the management of minor closed head injury in children. Am Fam Physician 1999;60:2698. [PMID: 10606000]

Schutzman SA et al: Evaluation and management of children younger than two years old with apparently minor head trauma: proposed guidelines. Pediatrics 2001;107:983. [PMID: 11331675]

Servadel F et al: Defining acute mild head injury in adults: a proposal based on prognostic factors, diagnosis and management. J Neurotrauma 2001;18:657. [PMID: 11497092]

Simon B et al: Pediatric minor head trauma: indications for computed tomographic scanning revisited. J Trauma 2001;51:231. [PMID: 11493779]

Smally AJ: Management of minor closed head injury in children. Pediatrics 2001;107:1231. [PMID: 11388318]

Woodcock RJ, Davis PC, Hopkins KL: Imaging of head trauma in infancy and childhood. Semin Ultrasound CT MR 2001;22:162. [PMID: 11327530]

Maxillofacial & Neck Trauma

23

Fermin S. Godinez, DO, & Susan J. Letterle, MD[1]

I. Immediate Management of Life-Threatening Problems
Ensure Airway
Stop Bleeding
Stabilize Cervical Spine
II. Further Diagnosis & Evaluation
Neck Trauma
Facial Trauma
III. Emergency Management of Specific Injuries
Facial Fractures
Mandibular Fractures
Maxillary (Le Fort) Fractures
1. Le Fort I Fracture
2. Le Fort II Fracture
3. Le Fort III Fracture (Craniofacial Dysjunction)
Zygomaticomaxillary Complex (ZMC) Fractures
Orbital Floor ("Blowout") Fractures
Nasal Fractures
Frontal Sinus Fractures

Temporal Bone Fractures (Basilar Skull Fracture)
1. Tympanic Bone Fractures
2. Longitudinal Fractures
3. Transverse Fractures
Tooth Injuries
Avulsion of Teeth
Subluxation of Teeth
Tooth Fractures
External Ear Trauma
Otohematoma
Lacerations of the Auricle
Middle & Inner Ear Disorders Following Head Trauma
Cerebrospinal Fluid Otorrhea
Facial Nerve Paralysis
Conductive Hearing Loss
Sensorineural Hearing Loss
Vertigo
Care of Facial Lacerations

■ I. IMMEDIATE MANAGEMENT OF LIFE-THREATENING PROBLEMS

Emergency management of life-threatening associated conditions is described in Chapter 10.

ENSURE AIRWAY

Evaluate the pharyngeal, laryngeal, and tracheal components of the airway in patients with head and neck trauma. Stabilize the head and axial spine with a cervical collar and full spine board immobilization until cervical spine injury can be excluded.

Caution: Any patient with injury to the neck should be managed and monitored conservatively in anticipation of rapid airway obstruction. If acute airway obstruction is a reasonable expectation (eg, in the presence of expanding hematoma, edema, hoarseness, subcutaneous emphysema, or persistent laryngeal pain), serious consideration should be given to rapid sequence intubation (RSI). At times controversial, RSI by a skilled laryngoscopist with in-line cervical stabilization in a patient with a cervical spine injury has a high degree of success. Emergency physicians should be cautioned to avoid RSI techniques in patients with airway injuries that would preclude bag-valve-mask ventilation should intubation prove unsuccessful.

In some circumstances, intubation while the patient is awake, using topical anesthetic and intravenous sedation, may be a better approach. If time permits, fiber optic bronchoscopy–assisted intubation can be an excellent alternative. A surgical airway should be immediately available at bedside and should be the next intervention if attempts at oral intubation are unsuccessful.

---

[1]This chapter is a revision of the chapter by Roger L. Crumley, MD, from the 4th edition.

Patients with an altered level of consciousness and no evidence of craniofacial injury, should have a nasogastric tube inserted after intubation to empty stomach contents. In patients with contraindications to nasogastric tube insertion, orogastric placement is recommended.

Pharyngeal Airway Injury

Massive injuries of the tongue or mandible may compromise or obliterate the pharyngeal airway. Because of this distorted anatomy, intubation may be difficult. The base of the tongue may be used as a landmark to help locate the epiglottis and secure the airway.

If there is no air exchange, immediately perform a jaw thrust and clear the oral cavity and pharynx of blood and loose teeth while preparing a laryngoscope for emergency intubation (Chapter 6).

Laryngeal Airway Injury

If there is evidence of injury below the level of the hyoid bone with compromise of the airway, assume that laryngeal fracture or laryngotracheal crush injury is present.

Cricothyrotomy (Chapter 6) should be performed to secure the airway in patients with pharyngeal or laryngeal airway obstruction when laryngoscopy is difficult, delayed, or contraindicated. After a small-bore endotracheal tube is inserted through the cricothyrotomy, a standard tracheotomy should be performed.

Tracheal Airway Injury

If there is injury below the cricothyroid membrane, a standard tracheotomy will be necessary to bypass the obstructive lesion.

In patients with no air exchange, it is permissible to attempt orotracheal intubation for 60 seconds, but preparations for cricothyrotomy or tracheotomy must be initiated simultaneously.

Intubation of the Trachea Through a Traumatic Opening

Occasionally, patients will come to the emergency department with impending asphyxia and with a gaping wound of the lower anterior neck. In some of these patients, removal of dressings and clots in the wound exposes a traumatic defect of the trachea that can be intubated. Patients with dashboard injuries or "clothes-line-fence" snowmobile or motorcycle injuries often present with laryngotracheal separation immediately above or below the cricoid cartilage. If there is no open wound, immediate tracheotomy is the preferred method of airway management. Oral intubation or paralysis may

precipitate airway obstruction and cause death. Direct intubation of the trachea is sometimes possible through an open wound on the anterior neck.

STOP BLEEDING

Control Hemorrhage

Patients with neck trauma (penetrating or blunt) may have rapidly expanding cervical hematomas from arterial or venous bleeding. Hematomas may cause airway obstruction and death if not recognized and treated. Facial and neck wounds may also be associated with external arterial or venous bleeding. Do not remove penetrating objects from the wound; they may be tamponading vessels at the site of injury.

A. PRESSURE

If venous oozing occurs, apply a pressure dressing in the emergency department. Do not wrap the neck with a circumferential dressing because it may increase intracranial pressure and act as a noose if edema or a cervical hematoma worsens.

B. PRESSURE AND CLAMPING

If major arterial bleeding occurs in an open wound, try applying pressure first. If that fails—and only then—hemostats may be applied carefully under direct vision. Clamping of large amounts of soft tissue without good visualization is contraindicated, because the vagus nerve or phrenic nerve may be included in the clamp (Figure 23–1). A firm pressure dressing is the safest hemostatic agent.

C. TRACHEOTOMY

Exsanguinating oral hemorrhage after penetrating trauma may be controlled by endotracheal intubation through a cricothyrotomy or tracheotomy (with immediate inflation of the cuff to prevent aspiration), followed by pharyngeal packing.

Treat Shock

If hypovolemic shock is present as a result of bleeding from face or neck injuries, it is managed with infusion of intravenous crystalloid solution or blood as described in Chapter 9. Management of shock may be described briefly as follows:

Insert 2 or more large-bore (≥ 16-gauge) intravenous catheters. Draw blood for a complete blood count, electrolytes, renal function tests, serum glucose, prothrombin and partial thromboplastin times, and blood clot for typing and cross-matching blood products. If the patient is hemodynamically unstable after initial crystalloid bolus of 1–2 liters, 2 units of packed red blood cells (cross-matched if available) should be infused.

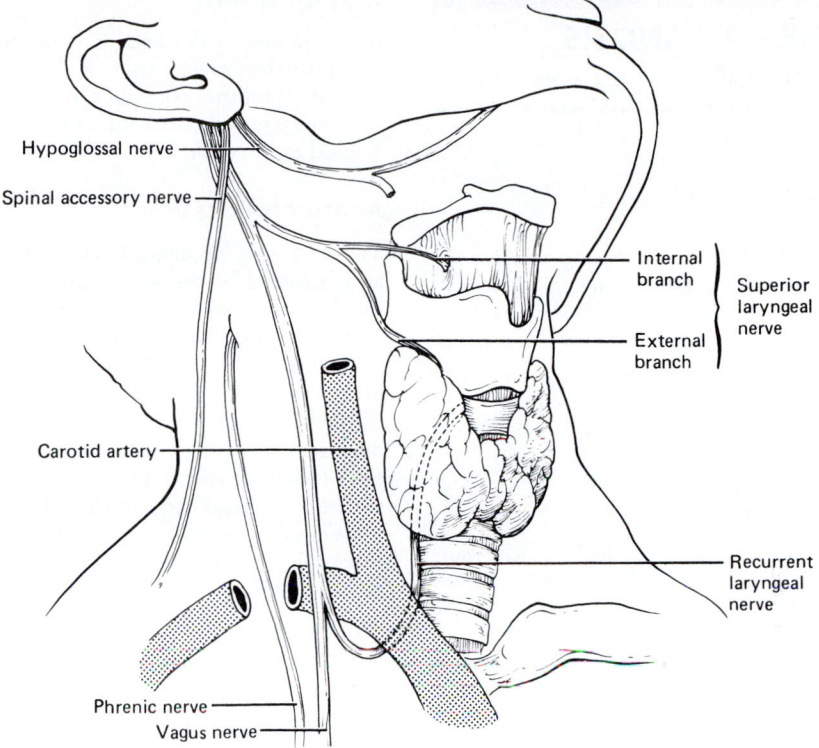

Figure 23–1. Location of nerves passing through the anterior neck that are susceptible to injury from penetrating trauma.

Infuse crystalloid solution (up to 2–3 L in 30–60 minutes) to support blood pressure and urine output. Insert a urinary catheter to monitor urine output if no urethral injury exists.

STABILIZE CERVICAL SPINE

While the airway and bleeding are being managed, the emergency physician should be thinking about the cervical spine. Unless the physician is certain that the cervical spine is intact, the patient's head should not be moved. The head, axial spine, and lower extremities should be routinely immobilized until a reliable clinical exam, cervical spine radiographs, or computed tomography (CT) scan have excluded obvious injury. In-line cervical immobilization must be maintained by an assistant during intubation attempts. If unable to obtain a definitive airway with RSI, then a surgical airway is required. Once the airway is established and the patient is hemodynamically stable, anteroposterior, lateral, and odontoid cervical spine films or CT scans should be obtained whenever blunt head or neck trauma are present or if uncertainty exists due to the influence of drugs or alcohol. See Chapter 27 for further evaluation and management.

Mandavia DP et al: Emergency airway management in penetrating neck injury. Ann Emerg Med 2000;35(3):221. [PMID: 10692187] (A retrospective study examining the approach to penetrating neck trauma, initial airway management, and their relative effectiveness from an urban level-1 trauma center and emergency medicine training program.)

Desjardins G et al: Airway management for penetrating neck injuries: the Miami experience. Resuscitation 2001;48(1):71. [PMID: 11162884] (Review.)

Tayal VS et al: Rapid-sequence intubation at an emergency medicine residency: success rate and adverse events during a two-year period. Acad Emerg Med 1999;6(1):31. [PMID: 9928974] (An observational study of a large cohort of RSI patients at an urban level-1 trauma center and emergency medicine training program.)

Walls RM: Management of the difficult airway in the trauma patient. Emerg Med Clin North Am 1998;16(1):45. [PMID: 9496314] (Review of management of the difficult airway in the trauma patient, available devices for management, and rescue maneuvers.)

■ II. FURTHER DIAGNOSIS & EVALUATION

NECK TRAUMA

Type of Trauma

A. PENETRATING INJURY

1. Knife wounds—If the penetrating instrument is still in situ, *leave it there* and obtain posteroanterior and lateral neck films or CT scan to determine its exact location (Figure 23–2). Even if the weapon or object causing the injury has been removed, it is still useful to know the length and shape of the penetrating object, as well as the direction of entry. Knowing the direction and depth of the injury provides information about what structures may have been injured.

2. Bullet wounds—Trauma from high-velocity missiles cannot be accurately assessed externally. Bullets frequently do not travel in a straight line. They may be deflected or fragmented as they pass through various tissues or strike bone. Bullets with high kinetic energy cause cavitation and tissue injury remote from the missile track. High-velocity missile injuries may require surgical intervention after evaluation by CT scan, angiography, 2-dimensional Doppler, or esophagoscopy.

B. BLUNT TRAUMA

Blunt trauma to the neck is associated primarily with injury to the cervical spine and airway. Vascular and esophageal injuries are rare. Thus, careful assessment in the emergency department can identify the need for surgical exploration.

Anatomic Location

The neck may be divided into 3 zones: Zone I is the area bordered by the suprasternal notch, clavicles, and inferior aspect of the cricoid cartilage. Zone II is the area between the inferior cricoid cartilage and the angle of the mandible. Zone III is the area between the angle of the mandible and the base of the skull. The anatomical division of the neck into zones is relevant to the management of neck injuries because of the difficulty establishing proximal and distal control of vascular structures surgically in zones I and III.

Wounds that penetrate the platysma should not be probed in the emergency department; they should be explored in the operating room.

Airway Injury

Airway injury may be manifested by an air leak, subcutaneous or mediastinal emphysema, or pneumothorax, indicating frank airway laceration. Stridor, hoarseness, painful phonation, and hemoptysis and hemothorax

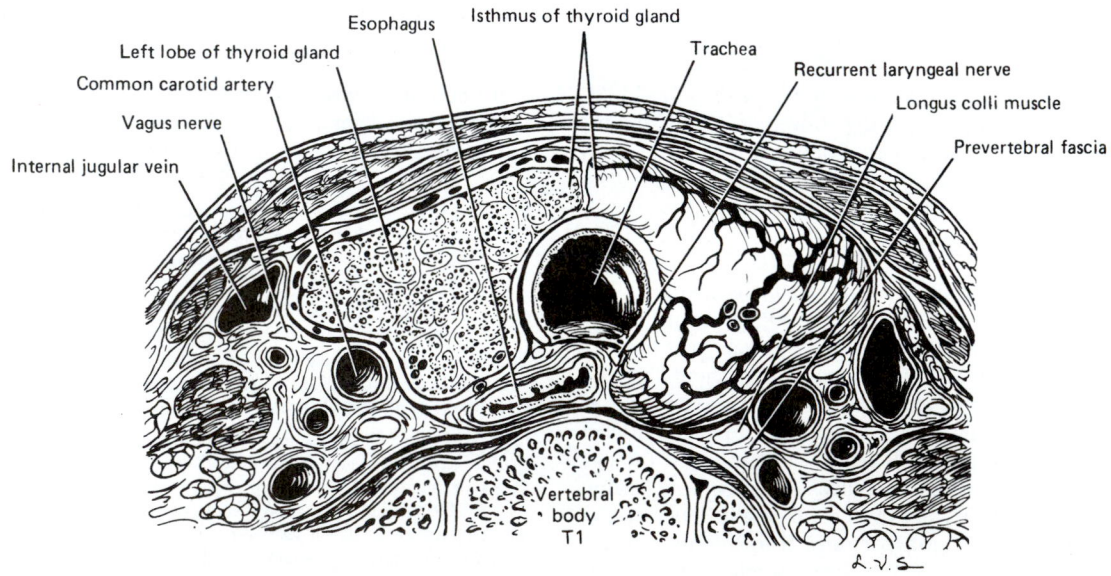

Internal jugular vein
Vagus nerve
Common carotid artery
Left lobe of thyroid gland
Esophagus
Isthmus of thyroid gland
Trachea
Recurrent laryngeal nerve
Longus colli muscle
Prevertebral fascia
Vertebral body T1

Figure 23–2. Cross section of the anterior neck at the level of C6, looking down from above, showing structures that may be injured.

may also indicate airway injury (pharynx, larynx, or trachea). Posteroanterior and lateral neck and chest x-rays or CT scans should be considered during evaluation of neck injury. Direct or indirect laryngoscopy must be performed before surgery to determine the exact nature of the airway injury.

Esophageal Injury

Injuries to the upper esophagus are associated with soft tissue crepitus, dysphagia, odynophagia, and drooling. An esophagogram with water-soluble contrast may demonstrate dye extravasation indicating perforation. However, esophagoscopy is virtually always necessary if the esophagram does not demonstrate an injury.

Vascular Injury

(See also Chapter 38.) Vascular injury may be immediately apparent if there is external bleeding, a bruit or thrill, or a cervical hematoma, or it may be hidden if bleeding occurs into the pleural space. Neurologic deficit may indicate intracranial vascular insufficiency.

Suspected vascular injuries may be managed operatively once specific injuries are identified by 2-dimensional Doppler, angiography, esophagoscopy, or dynamic CT scan (Chapter 38). Injuries occurring in zone I or zone III usually require angiography. Zone I injuries may require thoracotomy to control hemorrhage.

Nerve Injury

(See Figure 23–1.) Assess the nerves in the neck that are susceptible to injury.

A. Vagus, Recurrent Laryngeal

Record the character of the patient's voice, and examine the vocal cords via indirect (mirror) or fiberoptic laryngoscopy.

B. Spinal Accessory

Test for function of the sternocleidomastoid and trapezius muscles.

C. Hypoglossal

Test for deviation of the protruded tongue to the side of the injury.

D. Phrenic

Assess movement of the diaphragm on chest examination or by x-ray.

Disposition

Patients with penetrating trauma of the neck should be hospitalized unless local exploration of the wound shows it to be superficial to the platysma. Patients with blunt trauma with no evidence of significant injury (by physical examination and x-rays of the neck and chest) may be safely discharged.

FACIAL TRAUMA

Type of Injury

Most facial injuries consist of blunt trauma or cutting injury of the superficial soft tissue (eg, lacerations). High-velocity missile injuries of the face usually involve the central nervous system, and such injuries take priority for management (Chapter 22).

Airway Injury

Severe trauma to the lower face may compromise the airway. If obvious measures such as suction or pulling the tongue forward do not correct the problem, diverting the airway around the injury by performing endotracheal intubation, cricothyrotomy, or tracheotomy is preferred.

Vascular Injury

Bleeding from facial injuries typically is profuse but rarely causes hypovolemia or shock. *Control bleeding by direct pressure only;* hemostatic clamping may injure important nonvascular structures.

Nerve Injury

Blunt or penetrating trauma may injure branches of the trigeminal, facial, auditory, lingual, or hypoglossal nerves. The best chance to diagnose such injuries is often in the emergency department before edema and pain worsen. A careful assessment of both motor and sensory function of these nerves, especially the facial nerve, is imperative.

A. Facial Nerve

Branches of the facial nerve can be tested by these maneuvers:

1. Temporal branch (to the frontalis muscle)—Ask patient to wrinkle forehead.

2. Zygomatic branch (to the orbicularis oculi muscles)—Ask patient to squeeze eyes shut tightly.

3. Buccal branch (to the smile muscles)—Ask patient to wrinkle nose, elevate upper lip, smile, and "show your teeth."

4. Marginal mandibular branch (to the lower lip depressors)—Ask patient to pucker or whistle.

5. Cervical branch—Ask patient to wrinkle the neck.

B. TRIGEMINAL NERVE

Test for sensation over the entire face and upper neck.

C. AUDITORY NERVE

Test hearing in both ears.

D. LINGUAL NERVE

Test for sensation on both sides of the anterior tongue.

E. HYPOGLOSSAL NERVE

Test for ability to protrude tongue in midline and to both sides.

Parotid Gland Injury

An irregular quadrilateral area connecting the tragus, the angle of the mandible, the lateral commissure of the mouth, and the lateral canthus of the eye bounds an area where lacerations are most apt to injure Stensen's duct or branches of the facial nerve (Figure 23–3). Stensen's (parotid) duct courses anteriorly from the

parotid gland in the preauricular area through the cheek to enter the buccal mucosa near the maxillary (upper) molar teeth. The initial evaluation of Stensen's duct requires only gentle probing with lacrimal probes, entering through the buccal surface. If the end of the probe appears in the cheek lacerations, Stensen's duct has been disrupted and requires surgical repair. If lacerated and unrepaired, the duct will spill saliva into the cheek or externally, creating a troublesome salivary fistula. This complication is easy to prevent but difficult to treat.

Mouth Injuries

Test for pain on jaw movement or biting, feel for crepitus on movement of upper or lower teeth, and look for obvious malocclusion indicating fracture of the mandible or maxilla. Look for loose or fractured teeth. Inspect the buccal mucosa, tongue, floor of mouth, teeth, palate, and pharynx for evidence of injury. Grasp the upper alveolar bone, and check for movement that suggests a maxillary fracture. Carefully palpate the remainder of the face to determine if other areas are potentially fractured. Obtain x-rays, a mandibular Panorex, or CT scan of the face to determine the extent of injury.

Eye Injury

(See also Chapter 31.) Look for obvious injury to the globe. Either enophthalmos or complaints of diplopia should arouse suspicion of orbital bone fracture.

Bilateral periorbital hematomas ("raccoon eyes") are a sign of anterior basilar skull or ethmoid bone fracture, and a search for cerebrospinal fluid rhinorrhea should be made. Cerebrospinal fluid rhinorrhea may accompany closed head or maxillofacial injury. It should be suspected whenever clear fluid or watery bloodstained fluid drains from the nose. If cerebrospinal fluid rhinorrhea is suspected, a CT scan followed by otolaryngologic and neurosurgical consultation is indicated. There is no reliable method available in the emergency department for distinguishing cerebrospinal fluid from nasal mucus.

Nasal Injury

Inspect the nose for obvious deformity or septal hematoma. Palpate for the presence of nondisplaced fracture. If active epistaxis is present, use packing or cautery to control the bleeding. Look for cerebrospinal fluid rhinorrhea (see above), which, if present, would require a CT scan of the brain and face with otolaryngologic or neurosurgical consultation.

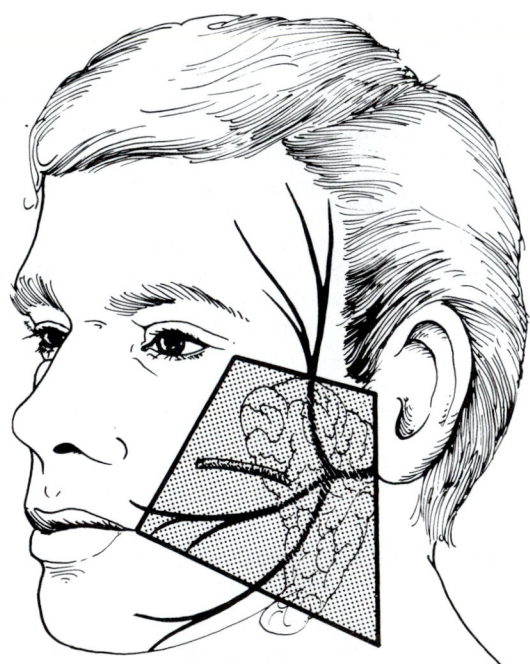

Figure 23–3. Area of the face where facial lacerations may injure the parotid gland, Stensen's duct, or facial nerve branches.

Ear Injury

Inspect the external ear, ear canal, and tympanic membrane. Test hearing if possible. A direct blow to the external ear may produce otohematoma, auricular laceration, ossicular disruption, or perforated tympanic membrane (conductive hearing loss). Blunt head trauma may fracture the temporal bone (basilar skull fracture; Chapter 22), which is associated with hemotympanum, blood in the external canal, postauricular hematoma (Battle sign), cerebrospinal fluid otorrhea, facial nerve palsies, or sensorineural hearing loss.

Disposition

Most patients with extensive or open fractures or with serious injuries of the eye, ear, or salivary gland should be hospitalized. Uncomplicated fractures of the mandible, maxilla, and nasal bone—as well as contusions or lacerations of the skin—may be managed without hospitalization. (See discussion of specific injuries for details.)

Hernandez JJ et al: Penetrating neck trauma. E-medicine Journal 2001;2(9). http://www.emedicine.com/med/topic2802.htm (Review of the relevant anatomy of the neck, image modalities for evaluation of neck injuries, and future and current controversies in the management of penetrating neck trauma.)

Kendall JL et al: Penetrating neck trauma. Emerg Med Clin North Am 1998;16(1):85. [PMID: 9496316] (Review of the anatomy of the neck, methods for obtaining airway control, and management issues related to penetrating neck trauma.)

Kim MK et al: Penetrating neck trauma in children: an urban hospital's experience. Otolaryngol Head Neck Surg 2000;123(4):439. [PMID: 11020182]. (Chart review of the selective management of head and neck trauma in children.)

▪ III. EMERGENCY MANAGEMENT OF SPECIFIC INJURIES

FACIAL FRACTURES

MANDIBULAR FRACTURES

 ESSENTIALS OF DIAGNOSIS

- Note any obvious facial swelling or asymmetry.
- Ask the awake and alert patient some simple questions: (1) "Do your teeth feel normal?" (2) "Does your bite feel normal?" (3) "Do you have any pain in your mouth, jaw, or ears? Point to where it hurts."

General Considerations

With the exception of the nasal bones, the mandible is by far the most frequently fractured facial bone. Initial evaluation of the patient with mandibular fracture should be thorough and include a detailed evaluation of sensory and motor function of the oral cavity. The oral cavity must be cleaned and suctioned of foreign bodies and debris, and a patent airway ensured. Laryngeal, cervical spine, and intracranial injuries must be sought first and treated. Failure to recognize a mandibular fracture may result in serious sequelae such as osteomyelitis, permanent malocclusion, or nonunion.

Clinical Findings

A. SYMPTOMS AND SIGNS

Mandibular fractures may be detected simply by the presence of gross facial asymmetry on inspection or by malocclusion. If the patient has a sensation of dental malocclusion, mandibular or maxillary fractures should be strongly suspected. The body, condyles, and angle of the mandible and symphysis are common sites for fracture. In some studies, multiple fractures were present in almost half of patients with mandibular fractures.

Pain is always present following mandibular fracture and may be so severe that the patient will refuse to open or close the jaw. The patient will usually point to the fracture site when asked to localize pain associated with mandibular movement. The "tongue blade test" is performed for each side of the mouth by having the patient bite down on a tongue blade between the molars. If the patient can stabilize the tongue blade between the molars on each side of the mouth while the examiner twists the stick until it breaks, the patient is unlikely to have a mandibular fracture. The sensitivity of this test is 95%.

Tenderness is best ascertained by bidigital examination with the examiner's thumbs in the mouth on the teeth or dental alveoli (in edentulous patients). The fingers then palpate externally along the lower border of the mandible. By "rocking" the mandible from side to side, the physician can sense mobility in the midline area.

B. IMAGING

X-ray evaluation for mandibular fracture should include a Panorex examination (Figure 23–4), which gives a panoramic view of the entire mandible on one film and will usually show all fractures present. If Panorex technology is unavailable (or if patients with

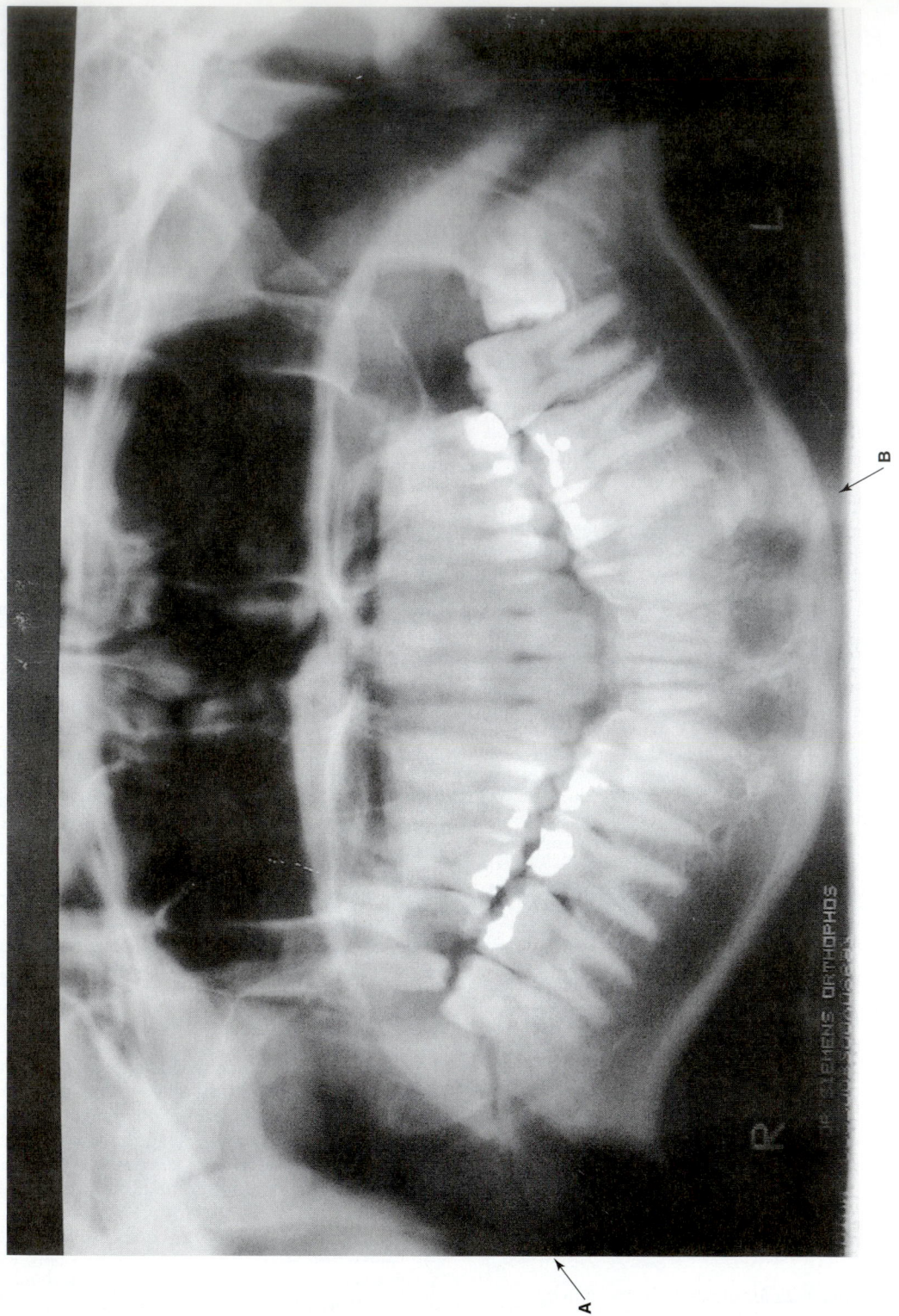

Figure 23–4. Panorex of the mandible, demonstrating a right ramus fracture (**A**) and a left para-symphyseal fracture (**B**).

multiple injuries cannot be positioned properly), a coronal facial CT scan will be a more useful imaging study and offer better visualization of the condylar processes.

Treatment

Once the diagnosis of mandibular fracture has been established, the following measures should be carried out:

A. Tetanus Prophylaxis

Give tetanus toxoid or tetanus-diphtheria toxoid as needed (Chapter 30).

B. Antibiotics

Choice of antibiotic should provide adequate coverage for oral aerobes and anaerobes. Penicillin G intravenously or penicillin VK orally will be sufficient. Clindamycin should be used in penicillin-allergic patients.

C. Barton Bandage

To provide comfort and initial stabilization of the fracture, a Barton bandage should be applied. This is simply a wrap-around gauze or Kerlix dressing that passes under the mandible and over the top of the head so as to close the mandible. Care must be taken, however, to maintain airway patency.

Disposition

Ideally, patients with mandibular fractures should be treated definitively in the emergency department before discharge. If necessary, however, patients with simple mandibular fractures may be discharged and referred to an otolaryngologist, plastic surgeon, or oral surgeon within a few days for definitive treatment. Provide adequate analgesics and antibiotics, and instruct the patient to drink plenty of liquids through a straw.

Patients with open or severely displaced mandibular fractures should be seen by the maxillofacial consultant and hospitalized for treatment.

MAXILLARY (LE FORT) FRACTURES

General Considerations

René Le Fort, a French surgeon, identified and described patterns of injuries and fractures of the midface. The maxilla and associated structures of the middle third of the face are injured more often as a result of blunt trauma. Although this classification system is beneficial, it does not include unilateral Le Fort injuries, combinations of Le Fort types, or more extensive fractures and intracranial injuries. However, this system is still useful in providing the examiner with potential sites and patterns of injury. Using this knowledge the clinician can pay particular attention during physical examination and determine the necessity and utility of diagnostic imaging.

Clinical Findings

The most helpful clinical findings are malocclusion, local tenderness, and maxillary mobility. The latter finding is elicited by grasping and rocking the anterior portion of the maxilla intraorally with one hand while stabilizing the head with the other hand. Motion is elicited in bilateral maxillary fractures if they are not seriously impacted. Diagnosis is confirmed by a facial CT scan. Le Fort fractures can be classified into 3 types (Figure 23–5).

1. Le Fort I Fracture

Clinical Findings

Le Fort I is a fracture parallel to the alveolar process and hard palate of the maxilla. The fracture extends posteriorly behind the maxillary molars, and across the lateral wall of the maxillary sinus anterior to the piriform aperture (Figure 23–5A). This fracture essentially separates the maxillary teeth and alveolar bone from the rest of the maxilla and face. There are usually no airway complications associated with such a fracture.

Treatment

After completion of a careful evaluation and reasonable exclusion of any other serious injuries, no specific emergency treatment is indicated. Provide the patient with adequate pain control.

Disposition

Patients with uncomplicated Le Fort I type injuries may be managed as outpatients after maxillofacial consultation (otolaryngologist, plastic surgeon, or oral and maxillofacial surgeon). Patients with more complex or open fractures should be hospitalized.

2. Le Fort II Fracture

Clinical Findings

Le Fort II fracture is a pyramidal fracture involving the bony nasal skeleton and the middle third of the face, and it includes the fracture lines of Le Fort I injury (Figure 23–5B). Displacement of the maxillary dentition due to fracture may cause malocclusion. Examination usually reveals ecchymosis of the nasal dorsum, the lower eyelids, and the maxillary gingival buccal sulcus. This injury pattern includes the infraorbital nerve canal, potentially causing nerve injury and a sensory

Anterior views

Lateral views

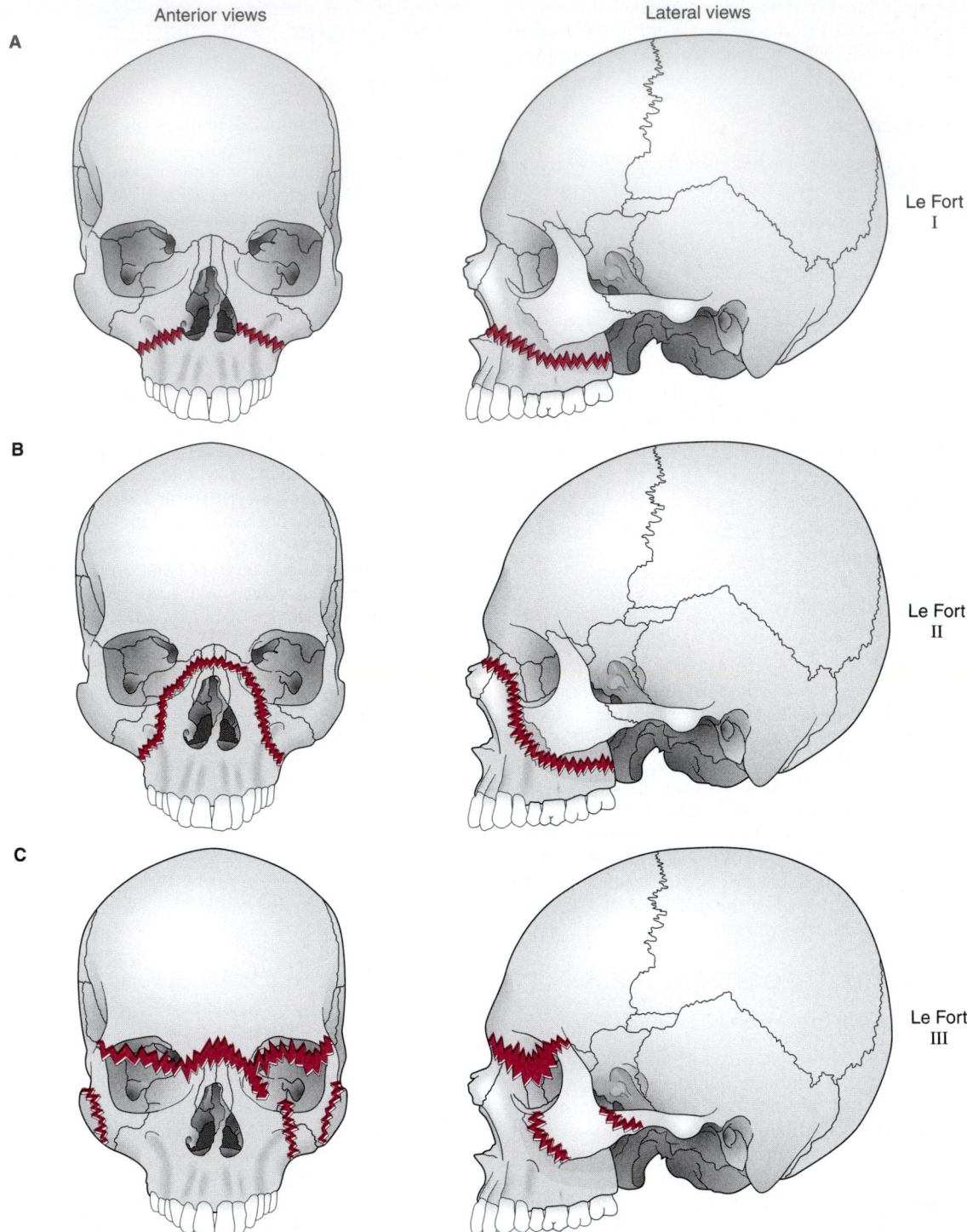

A

Le Fort
I

B

Le Fort
II

C

Le Fort
III

Figure 23–5. Anterior (*left*) and lateral (*right*) views of Le Fort maxillary fracture sites. **A:** Le Fort I. **B:** Le Fort II. **C:** Le Fort III.

deficit inferior to the involved lower eyelid. The face may appear elongated, and the anterior portion of the mid face will be mobile relative to the forehead. A CT scan of the face is the preferred imaging modality. If CT is not immediately available, a Waters view x-ray may demonstrate these fractures.

Treatment

No specific immediate treatment is necessary. Provide adequate analgesics.

Disposition

Consultation with a maxillofacial consultant (otolaryngologist, plastic surgeon, or oral and maxillofacial surgeon) should be obtained in the emergency department. The consultant should determine the final disposition based on the extent of the patient's injuries and the timing of any planned operative intervention.

3. Le Fort III Fracture (Cranial Dysjunction)

Clinical Findings

A LeFort III fracture, or craniofacial dysjunction, involves separation of all the facial bones (including the zygoma, maxilla, and nasal bones) from the cranial base. The Le Fort III injury pattern includes fracture lines extending through the ethmoid bones and orbits and into the sphenopalatine fossa. The lines then pass medially across the glabellar region (bridge of nose). In some patients, the zygoma may become completely separated by fracture lines (Figure 23–5C, left side). Patients with Le Fort III fracture tend to have massive facial edema and ecchymosis and occasionally airway obstruction secondary to dissection of hematoma into the palate, pharyngeal walls, or tonsillar pillars. Patients frequently have associated mandibular fractures with posterior prolapse of the tongue and hematoma formation.

Treatment

If airway obstruction is present or impending, secure a definitive airway with orotracheal intubation. If orotracheal intubation is unsuccessful, cricothyrotomy is indicated for impending rapid airway obstruction. Nasotracheal intubation is contraindicated due to the possibility of intracranial passage of the endotracheal tube. Provide adequate analgesics.

Disposition

In virtually all cases, a maxillofacial consultant should examine the patient in the emergency department to determine the need for hospitalization.

ZYGOMATICOMAXILLARY COMPLEX (ZMC) FRACTURES

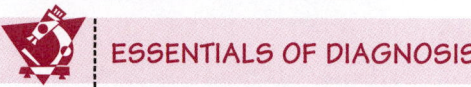 **ESSENTIALS OF DIAGNOSIS**

- *Lower eyelid swelling and ecchymoses.*
- *Flattened arch and decreased sensation of intra-orbital nerve distribution.*
- *Double vision with upward gaze.*
- *Trismus.*

General Considerations

Malar (zygomaticomaxillary complex) fracture most commonly results from lateral-to-medial blunt force applied to the face. Three fracture lines are associated with ZMC fractures (Figure 23–6). The lateral orbital rim is fractured at the zygomaticofrontal suture. The orbital floor is disrupted, with the anterior end of the fracture line passing across through the zygomaticomaxillary suture line or the infraorbital foramen. The third fracture is through the zygomaticotemporal suture. When associated with ZMC fracture, the orbital

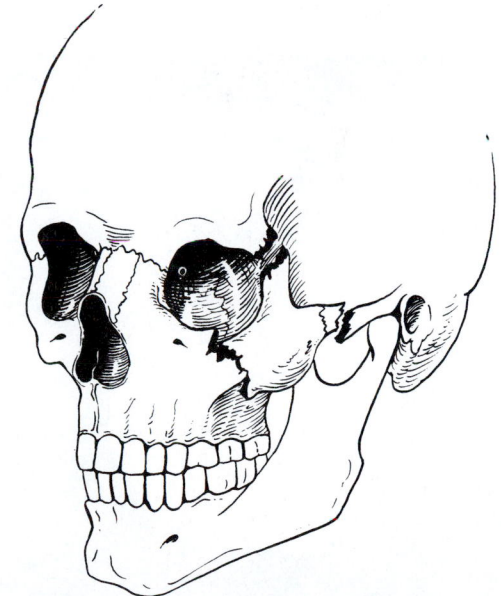

Figure 23–6. Diagram of a zygomaticomaxillary complex (ZMC) fracture. Note disruption of both the lateral orbital rim and the orbital floor, as well as the zygomatic arch.

floor fracture line is not a blowout fracture and should not be confused with one.

Clinical Findings

Epistaxis occurs, because the bony floor of the orbit is also the roof of the maxillary sinus. Periorbital edema and ecchymosis are present. Examination and palpation show flattening of the normal malar prominence and depression or separation of the lateral or inferior orbital rim.

Facial paresthesias or hypesthesias of the upper lip and cheek occur if the infraorbital nerve is damaged at the infraorbital foramen or more posteriorly in the orbital floor. Diplopia may be present as a result of orbital hematoma or slight displacement of the eyeball. Herniation of orbital contents into the antrum (maxillary sinus) is less common in ZMC fracture than in orbital blowout fracture. Subcutaneous emphysema of the face indicates that the fracture has extended into the paranasal sinuses. Make sure there is no evidence of retrobulbar hematoma or a tense globe requiring immediate intervention.

X-ray confirmation is readily obtained with a facial CT scan. Three-dimensional CT scanning provides a much more detailed view of the displacement of fracture fragments (Figure 23–7).

Treatment

Control epistaxis with nasal packing or cautery, and provide adequate analgesics. Administer antimicrobials if the fracture extends into the sinuses. Penicillin or amoxicillin may be used. Fluoroquinolones, doxycycline, or clindamycin may be other alternatives for penicillin-allergic patients, if antibiotic therapy is indicated.

Disposition

Before being discharged from the emergency department, the patient should be examined by a maxillofacial consultant to determine the need for hospitalization. Ophthalmologic consultation is also recommended.

In general, simple closed fractures of the zygomatic arch alone do not require further specific treatment or hospitalization. True ZMC fractures—especially those that are open or displaced, or with displacement of orbital contents—require open reduction under general anesthesia. Final disposition after the patient has been examined by a maxillofacial consultant should be determined based on the extent of injuries in addition to the method and timing of any planned surgical interventions.

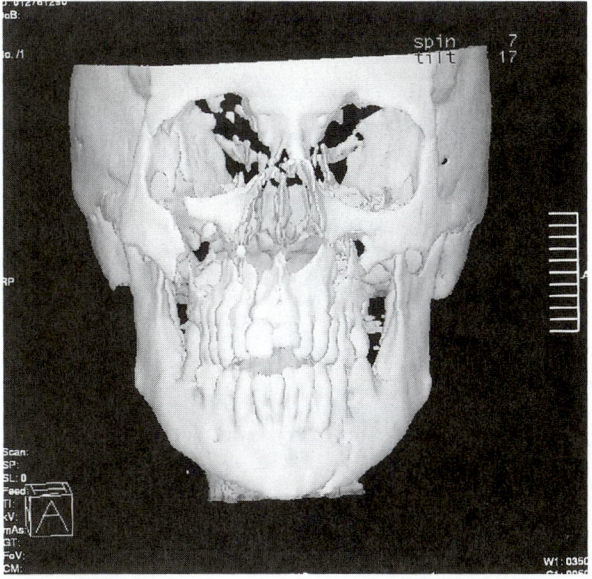
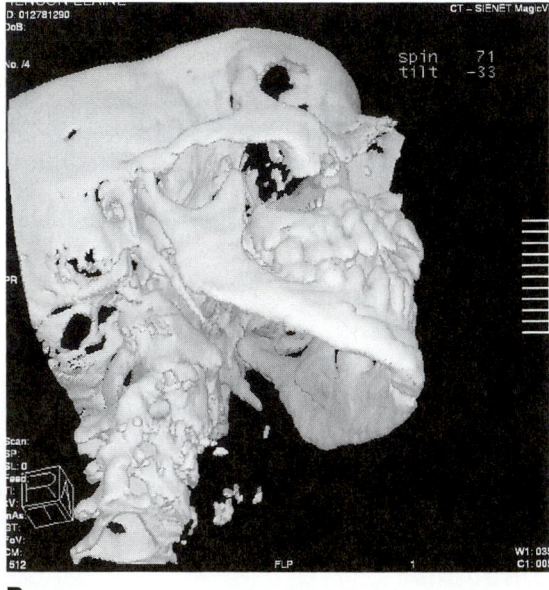

A

B

Figure 23–7. Three-dimensionally reconstructed facial CT scan. **A.** Left parasymphyseal mandibular fracture. **B.** Right zygomaticomaxillary complex (ZMC) fracture with inferior and lateral displacement of the ZMC.

ORBITAL FLOOR ("BLOWOUT") FRACTURES

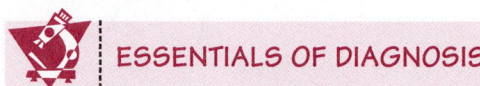

ESSENTIALS OF DIAGNOSIS

- Decreased eye movement.
- Limitation of eye movement.
- Decreased sensation of the infraorbital nerve distribution.
- Enophthalmos.
- Double vision, especially with upward gaze.

General Considerations

A. PURE BLOWOUT FRACTURE

Pure blowout fracture results from blunt anteroposterior force directed against the eyeball. Intraocular pressure rises markedly and is exerted in all directions. The orbital floor gives way because it is the weakest component of the orbital skeleton. Orbital fat, bone from the orbital floor, and occasionally extraocular muscles may be forced into the maxillary antrum. For this reason, ocular injuries and complications are more extensive with this fracture than with any other fracture. Because the infraorbital rim is not involved, tenderness may not be palpable on the face, and the diagnosis may be missed if the physician is not aware of the fracture and its mechanism. Unrepaired blowout fractures may result in permanent diplopia or disfiguring enophthalmos.

B. IMPURE BLOWOUT FRACTURE

Impure blowout fracture results from anteroposterior blunt force similar to that causing pure blowout fracture, but in this instance the force is also exerted against the infraorbital rim, producing a fracture. Impure blowout fracture is more common than pure blowout fracture. Because the force is dissipated by the rim fracture, the globe usually sustains less trauma, resulting in fewer ocular complications (eg, hyphema, retinal detachment, commotion retinae, lens dislocation) than in pure blowout fractures.

Clinical Findings

Suspect blowout fracture in any patient who has sustained blunt ocular or periorbital trauma. Diplopia and restricted upward gaze may confirm ocular muscle entrapment as a result of the fracture. Infraorbital nerve injury with infraorbital hypesthesia is common in both pure and impure blowout fractures. Epistaxis may be

present from laceration of the mucosa of the roof of the maxillary sinus.

Ocular injuries are usually associated with pure blowout fractures. Palpable fracture of the infraorbital rim occurs with impure blowout fractures and is absent in pure blowout fractures.

Coronal CT scans of the orbital floor are often helpful in delineating the extent of the fracture (Figure 23–8).

Treatment & Disposition

Consult with an otolaryngologist and ophthalmologist before discharging the patient from the emergency department.

Patients with blowout fractures and orbital entrapment (ie, diplopia or limitation of ocular mobility) should be hospitalized for exploration of the orbital floor, under general anesthesia. Reduction and internal fixation of associated facial fractures may have to be performed simultaneously.

Patients with orbital floor or rim fractures with no limitation of ocular mobility and without associated injury of the globe (Chapter 31) may be discharged from the emergency department and referred to an otolaryngologist to be seen within a few days.

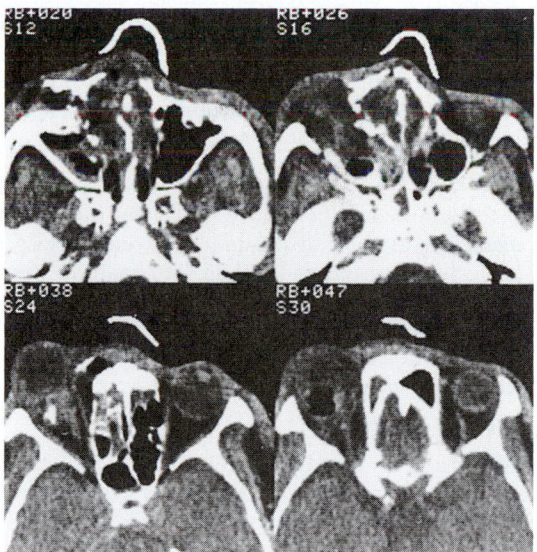

Figure 23–8. Orbital blowout fracture (impure type) on CT scan. Sequential horizontal cuts through the mid skull show blowout fracture of the right orbit, with rupture of the orbital contents into the maxillary sinus (*upper left frame*). Edema of the orbital contents is causing protrusion of the right eyeball (*lower left frame*).

NASAL FRACTURES

General Considerations

The nasal bones are sometimes fractured laterally in one fragment, but more commonly there is impaction of the nasal skeleton into the piriform aperture (bony nasal vault), requiring that the septum and nasal bones be disimpacted anteriorly before they can be reduced laterally. Open nasal fractures are rare.

Clinical Findings

There is a history of a blow to the nose, often associated with epistaxis. Tenderness, crepitation, or movement of nasal bones on palpation is present. Septal hematoma may be found on examination.

X-rays of the nasal bones seldom provide additional information and are not recommended for routine use.

Treatment

Nasal fractures without deformity or septal hematoma may be treated with analgesics. If airflow obstruction develops in nasal passages or if obvious deformity is revealed when the swelling subsides, the patient should be referred to an otolaryngologist. Ideally, nasal fractures with deformity but no associated soft tissue swelling should be reduced immediately before swelling develops. If swelling develops, reduction should be delayed until the swelling subsides. Reduction should occur after consultation with an otolaryngologist. Instruct the patient on preventing reinjury. Provide adequate analgesics and a nasal decongestant spray for the first 3 days to provide some symptomatic relief.

A. Provide Anesthesia

Most fractures can be reduced following topical intranasal anesthesia with cocaine. Roll cotton pledgets into a cylindric shape, and soak in 4% cocaine solution. Insert with nasal forceps into the upper and lower nasal cavities, and leave in place for about 15 minutes. Occasionally, topical anesthesia must be supplemented by injected local anesthetic.

B. Reduce Fracture

Simple, laterally displaced fractures may be reduced by exerting thumb pressure on the nose in the direction opposite to the initial fracture force.

Comminuted fractures must be manipulated anteriorly and laterally. This is most easily done with a Kelly clamp or Asch septal forceps inserted in the nose up the fracture site (Figure 23–9). If the nose then has normal external configuration, reduction is successful and should be maintained by applying tape over the nose, perhaps supplemented by an anterior nasal pack of petrolatum-impregnated gauze.

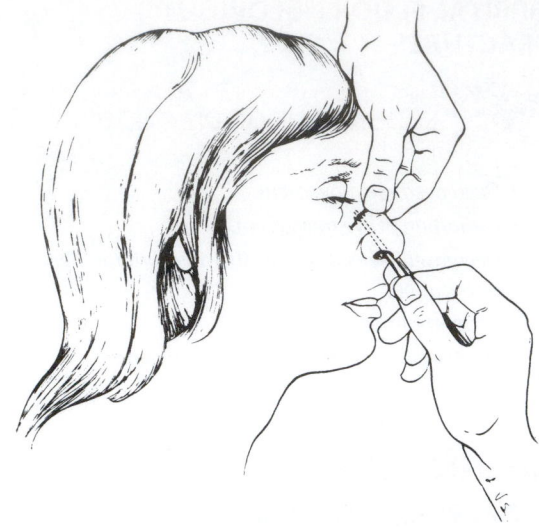

Figure 23–9. Reduction of nasal fracture by anterior traction with forceps. (Redrawn and reproduced, with permission, from Wang MK, Macomber WB: Maxillofacial injuries. Chapter 14 in: Echert C [editor]: *Emergency Room Care,* 4th ed. Little, Brown, 1981.)

If the fracture has been reduced or if it was nondisplaced, arrange for otolaryngologic consultation. If the emergency physician cannot achieve adequate reduction of a nasal fracture, an otolaryngologist should be consulted immediately. Simple lacerations without associated septal dislocation should be copiously irrigated and closed primarily. Antimicrobial prophylaxis (see below) should be given. Deep or complex lacerations or those associated with septal deviation, nasal deformity, or dislocated cartilage should not be repaired until the otolaryngologist or plastic surgeon has examined the patient.

C. Drain Hematomas

Septal hematomas should be drained by incision through the anterior nasal mucosa at the time of fracture reduction. If septal hematoma is allowed to persist and results in abscess formation, the entire septal cartilage may be lost, resulting in a disfiguring "saddle" deformity of the nose. Give antimicrobial prophylaxis (eg, amoxicillin or erythromycin).

Disposition

Hospitalization is rarely required for nasal fractures. Patients should be told that the nasal air passages may become narrowed on one side or the other, thereby requiring septorhinoplasty at a later date.

FRONTAL SINUS FRACTURES

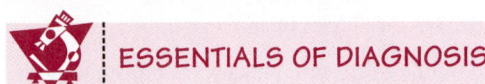

ESSENTIALS OF DIAGNOSIS

- *Facial trauma; think about the mechanism of injury.*
- *Rare in children; unlikely in early teens.*
- *Consider intracranial injury.*

General Considerations

Frontal sinus fractures most commonly result from motor vehicle trauma in which the patient's head strikes the dashboard. Patients with frontal sinus fractures require thorough head, neck, and neurologic examination, including ophthalmologic consultation. If there are variations in the level of consciousness, neurosurgical consultation should be obtained immediately. Fractures of the posterior wall of the frontal sinus may cause dural tears or brain injury, whereas fractures of the floor of the sinus often injure the nasofrontal duct.

Clinical Findings

There will usually be a history as well as evidence of trauma to the forehead. Cerebrospinal fluid rhinorrhea is common following fractures of the posterior wall of the frontal sinus, and a specific note about its presence or absence should be entered in the emergency department record. Epistaxis may represent associated direct nasal trauma or frontal sinus hemorrhage.

Axial and coronal CT scan of the face and CT scan of the head will provide the most important information on the extent of injury and potential for further intervention.

Associated injuries frequently include other facial fractures, depressed skull fractures, and orbital fractures.

Treatment

When brisk hemorrhage from the nasal cavity accompanies these fractures, it is acceptable to pack the anterior nasal vault tightly with 1.25-cm (1/2-in) iodoform gauze. Elevation of the head will reduce venous pressure and bleeding while the patient's condition stabilizes or arrangements are made for surgery. Obtain urgent otolaryngologic and neurosurgical consultation.

If the fracture is open, the wound should be covered with saline-soaked gauze. Avoid manipulation of bony fragments in the emergency department, because this may produce further dural injury.

Antibiotics are needed because the fracture lines cross the contaminated mucosal surfaces of the nose and sinus. Prior to surgical intervention by the neurosurgeon or otolaryngologist, vancomycin or a third-generation cephalosporin may be used.

Surgery is indicated for cerebrospinal fluid rhinorrhea, open fractures, markedly displaced fractures, and fractures involving the posterior wall or floor of the sinus.

Disposition

All patients with frontal sinus fractures should be hospitalized.

TEMPORAL BONE FRACTURES (Basilar Skull Fracture)

General Considerations

Most basilar skull fractures include temporal bone fractures. The temporal bone is shaped like a pyramid with its base directed laterally and its apex medially. Because it houses the cochlea, vestibule, facial nerve canal, jugular vein, and internal carotid artery, fractures through the temporal bone may have serious sequelae.

Diagnosis is based on the history of trauma and the presence of bleeding; ecchymosis of the external ear, mastoid tip (Battle sign), or ear canal; bilateral, periorbital ecchymoses ("raccoon eyes"); hemotympanum; hearing loss (conductive or sensorineural); or anosmia.

Clinical features depend on the type of fracture. Because basilar skull fractures may be associated with intracranial bleeding, brain injury, or subsequent meningitis, neurosurgical consultation, in addition to otolaryngologic consultation, should be obtained for all patients with suspected temporal bone fracture.

1. Tympanic Bone Fractures

Clinical Findings

The anterior face of the tympanic bone is the glenoid fossa of the temporomandibular joint. Hence, the mandibular condyle may be driven posteriorly into the middle ear or the external auditory canal. Patients with facial trauma who have ecchymosis, bleeding, or lacerations of the anterior external auditory canal often have such a fracture. A CT scan confirms the diagnosis.

Treatment

The ear canal is anesthetized by injection of a local anesthetic, and tympanic bone displacement is reduced by means of a metal speculum in the ear canal. This procedure is usually performed by an otolaryngologist.

Disposition

Hospitalization is not usually necessary unless associated injuries are present.

2. Longitudinal Fractures

Clinical Findings

Longitudinal fractures are so named because the fracture line parallels the long axis of the temporal bone (petrous pyramid). These fractures account for 80% of all fractures of the temporal bone. The tympanic membrane is frequently torn, and a step-off may be seen in the roof of the external auditory canal. Ossicular chain dislocation with conductive hearing loss is frequent. The hearing loss in longitudinal fractures is usually conductive rather than sensorineural, because the fracture line does not traverse the cochlea. When facial nerve paralysis is present, it is usually delayed. Delayed facial paralysis implies a better prognosis than does immediate paralysis, which indicates lacerations or other disruption of the nerve trunk and thus requires surgical exploration of the bony nerve canal as soon as the patient's condition permits.

Treatment & Disposition

Obtain immediate otolaryngologic consultation. All patients with this injury require hospitalization.

3. Transverse Fractures

Clinical Findings

Although less frequent than longitudinal fractures, the transverse fracture causes more severe injuries to the contents of the temporal bone. It usually starts near the internal auditory canal and runs a course perpendicular to the longitudinal axis of the temporal bone. Consequently, these fractures frequently traverse the cochlea, resulting in complete sensorineural hearing loss. Facial nerve injuries occur in over half of patients, and paralysis is commonly immediate, requiring exploration of the facial nerve canal.

Treatment & Disposition

Patients with suspected transverse temporal bone fractures require hospitalization for evaluation and surgery. Immediate otolaryngologic consultation should be obtained.

TOOTH INJURIES

AVULSION OF TEETH

Stop gingival bleeding with pressure. While holding the tooth by the crown so as not to damage the periodontal ligaments, wash it with saline and replace it immediately in the tooth socket. Obtain emergency oral surgical consultation, because avulsed teeth can be successfully reimplanted in some cases. For this reason, an attempt should be made to retrieve avulsed teeth from the scene of the accident.

SUBLUXATION OF TEETH

Gently manipulate the tooth back into its proper position. Obtain oral surgical consultation, because the loose tooth will have to be immobilized with a splint until it has reattached to periodontal and gingival tissues.

TOOTH FRACTURES

Exposure of the pulp or dentin is exquisitely painful, and a dentist should cover the tooth with a temporary plastic crown affixed with zinc oxide–eugenol paste. Follow-up care should be provided by the patient's regular dentist within a few days.

EXTERNAL EAR TRAUMA

OTOHEMATOMA

Clinical Findings

Bleeding between the auricular cartilage and the perichondrium frequently follows contusions or other injuries to the auricle. Such injuries are frequent in boxers and wrestlers. If untreated, they will result in cauliflower ear deformity, because blood under the perichondrium results in proliferative scarring and new cartilage formation.

Treatment

Treatment consists of aspiration or incision and drainage of hematomas, followed by application of saline-soaked cotton balls that conform to the auricular formation. A firm compression dressing should be wrapped around the head to prevent further hematoma formation.

Disposition

The patient should be seen by an otolaryngologist within 1–2 days. No specific instructions need be given. Hospitalization is not required.

LACERATIONS OF THE AURICLE

Treatment

Lacerations of the auricle result in deformity if they are not meticulously repaired. Debridement of devitalized tissue is important. Approximation of lacerated cartilage and perichondrium should be performed with a single layer of synthetic absorbable sutures. This layer is followed by 6-0 nylon skin sutures or skin tapes. Apply a petrolatum gauze dressing under slight pressure.

Disposition

Patients with extensive lacerations of the auricle should be hospitalized for surgical repair. Smaller lacerations repaired in the emergency department should be inspected by an otolaryngologist or plastic surgeon in 1–2 days.

MIDDLE & INNER EAR DISORDERS FOLLOWING HEAD TRAUMA

CEREBROSPINAL FLUID OTORRHEA

Clinical Findings

Cerebrospinal fluid otorrhea often results from minimal head injuries. Small cracks in the tegmen tympani (roof of the middle ear) provide a route for leakage of cerebrospinal fluid into the middle ear cavity. If the eardrum has a chronic perforation or has been torn at the time of injury, such leaks will result in cerebrospinal fluid otorrhea. This flow is best demonstrated in the head-down position. If the eardrum is intact, however, the fluid may pass through the auditory tube and produce cerebrospinal fluid rhinorrhea. In either case, meningitis is a potential complication. A CT scan will help diagnose the injury and eliminate the possibility of associated intracranial bleeding or brain injury.

Treatment & Disposition

Hospitalization and neurosurgical consultation are indicated for all patients with suspected leakage of cerebrospinal fluid. Prophylactic antibiotics have not been shown to be of benefit and are not recommended.

FACIAL NERVE PARALYSIS

Clinical Findings

Facial nerve paralysis may result from a small temporal bone fracture. The facial nerve passes through the middle ear cavity, where it is exposed to risk of injury from fractures and from foreign bodies introduced through the ear canal. Complete assessment of facial nerve integrity should be performed. Lost or decreased movements of the face, decreased tear production, or altered taste sensation on the affected side may indicate facial nerve paralysis or injury. An otolaryngologist should be consulted to evaluate the patient.

Treatment & Disposition

Patients with temporal bone fractures and immediate facial paralysis should be hospitalized and otolaryngologic consultation obtained immediately.

CONDUCTIVE HEARING LOSS

Clinical Findings

Disarticulation of the ossicular chain may result from head injuries with or without temporal bone fracture. One or more of the tiny ossicles may be jarred free from attachments and prevent normal function of the middle ear conduction mechanism. Patients with such injuries complain of acute hearing loss. Evidence of temporal bone fracture may or may not be present. If a step-off is seen at 12 o'clock at the medial end of the ear canal, it is further evidence of such an injury. Bone conduction is greater than air conduction in tuning fork tests. Audiometric examination reveals whether a coexisting sensorineural hearing loss is present.

Treatment & Disposition

Patients should be referred to an otolaryngologist within a few days for surgical reconstruction of the ossicular chain in the middle ear. Immediate hospitalization is not required.

SENSORINEURAL HEARING LOSS

Clinical Findings

More severe temporal bone fractures may produce sensorineural hearing loss. Such hearing losses are often total, and patients have severe vertigo during the first few days following injury.

Treatment & Disposition

Intravenous diazepam, 2–5 mg over 5–10 minutes, is an effective labyrinthine suppressant for control of vertigo. Patients should be hospitalized for evaluation and urgent otolaryngologic consultation.

VERTIGO

Clinical Findings

Some patients with head injuries complain of vertigo even though a CT scan of the head shows the temporal bone to be intact. These symptoms are thought to result from jarring of the delicate membranous inner ear structures within the bony labyrinth. In most instances, the vertigo is described as difficulty in walking or as a floating sensation. Occasionally, vertigo is so severe as to be associated with nystagmus.

Treatment & Disposition

Symptoms diminish over time. Reassurance and sedation with diazepam, 2–5 mg orally 2–4 times daily, or meclizine, 25 mg orally 3–4 times daily, are usually all that is required. Hospitalization is rarely necessary. The patient may be referred to an otolaryngologist for follow-up.

CARE OF FACIAL LACERATIONS (See also Chapter 30.)

Closure of Lacerations

Facial laceration repair requires attention to detail. Excellent wound preparation and precise tissue edge approximation with fine suture material are needed for the best possible restoration of anatomic structures and lines. If complex or extensive facial wounds are present, request assistance from the most appropriate consultant (eg, otolaryngologist, ophthalmologist, oral and maxillofacial, or plastic surgeon).

Injuries to the upper and lower lip are extremely common and likewise require precise repair. A soaking wet gauze sponge should be used to clean the lip of all blood and foreign debris. The vermilion border can be seen most easily if left wet. Closure of lacerations of this area should begin with placement of a small "sentinel" suture to align this border. The repair then progresses in either direction from it.

Replacement of Avulsed Tissue

Debridement of devitalized pieces of tissue should be done with caution and conservatism. Likewise, small avulsed pieces of external ear, nose, or facial soft tissue with skin may be cleaned, debrided, and replaced with a reasonable chance for survival. Larger pieces, as in total or subtotal avulsion of the external ear or scalp, are best reattached by microvascular techniques in the operating room. The physician should ask the patient with an avulsion injury if a friend or relative can return to the scene of the accident to retrieve lost fragments of tissue.

Delay in Closing Lacerations

In general, lacerations of the eyelids, lateral orbital region, nasal dorsum, and mandibular region should not be closed until x-rays of the facial bones have been taken. The otolaryngologist or maxillofacial consultant may prefer reduction and fixation of the fracture fragments through these lacerations.

Because of the rich blood supply of the area, it is acceptable to close facial lacerations as much as 12–24 hours after injury when necessary. When delayed closure is necessary, the wound should be packed open with saline sponges. Antibiotics (eg, dicloxacillin, cephalexin, or erythromycin for penicillin-allergic patients) may be considered for delayed closure. Pressure dressings can be used to control hemorrhage, or hemostats may be applied if bleeding vessels can be identified.

Repair Technique

Once more extensive injuries have been excluded (ie, facial nerve or parotid duct transections), local anesthetic can be infiltrated in the wound edges, or a regional block (supraorbital, infraorbital, or mental) should be employed. After the wound has been irrigated completely and conservatively debrided, the laceration should be further explored to remove any foreign debris and wound closure may proceed. Careful approximation with a fine suture material will provide the best result. The extent of the injury, number of layers or structures involved, and experience with repair of facial wounds will dictate choice of suture. Synthetic absorbable suture (eg, polyglycolic acid, polydioxanone, polyglactic acid, polytrimethylene carbonate, or polyglecaprone) may be used to close subcutaneous structures. These sutures have various periods of complete absorption, good tensile strength, and minimal inflammatory response compared to natural products.

Subcutaneous tissue should be sutured using a "buried knot" (see Figure 30–9). Synthetic nonabsorbable monofilament sutures (eg, polypropylene, polybutester, or nylon) are a good choice for skin closure; they have high tensile strength and minimal inflammatory response but require attention to securing knots. During repair, care should be taken to avoid injury of nerves or vessels. The superficial passage of the needle should be very close to the skin edge, so that after this layer is complete, the skin is already approximated and the skin sutures serve only to ensure accuracy of repair.

Facial skin should be sutured with 6-0 nylon or polypropylene on a nontraumatic reverse cutting needle. An important aspect of plastic closure of such lacerations is the angle of entry of the needle into the skin and the eversion produced by each suture (see Figure 30–10). Because the subcuticular layer has already approximated the skin, the skin sutures need not be tied tightly. A surgeon's knot (2 loops) should be tied and pulled down loosely so that the skin edges just touch. The next loop of suture should be tied with the opposite twist, so that a square knot results. If this second loop is not tied down tightly, a small loop results between the first (surgeon's) knot and the second loop; this is thought to reduce tissue strangulation when wound edema causes the skin edges to swell against the sutures. At least 2 additional knot loops should be tied on top of this second knot.

For linear lacerations, a running (uninterrupted) suture is acceptable. The same important principles of an everting needle angle and gentle tension will give the most cosmetic repair. Cyanoacrylate tissue adhesive provides a liquid alternative for 5-0 suture or smaller for selective wound closures. Avoid mucous membranes and the eyes during application. Do not use it in areas of high tension and where hair is present. Prior to application, if no local anesthetic is used, warn the patient that this liquid may cause increased pain or an intense burning sensation.

Facial skin sutures should be removed not later than the fourth day. An ophthalmic suture scissor or a No. 11 Bard-Parker blade is best for removing these fine sutures. After suture removal, both sides of the laceration should be painted with tincture of benzoin and the wound closed with adhesive dressings (eg, Steri-Strips) so that the opposing edges of the wound are pulled together. This will eliminate any tension on the closure and minimize widening and hypertrophy of the scar. The patient should be told that facial scars mature for 12 months and that facial scar revision may be done after that time.

Bruns TB et al: Using tissue adhesive for wound repair: a practical guide to Dermabond. Am Fam Physician 2000;61:1383 [PMID: 10735344] (Provides practical information regarding the use of cyanoacrylate for wound repair.)

Dale RA: Dentoalveolar trauma. Emerg Med Clin North Am 2000;18(3):521. [PMID: 10967737] (This review provides the emergency physician with an understanding of the initial evaluation and treatment of dentoalveolar trauma.)

Druelinger L et al: Radiographic evaluation of the facial complex. Emerg Med Clin North Am 2000;18(3):393. [PMID: 10967732] (A review of imaging modalities of use in the clinical assessment of maxillofacial trauma.)

Ellis E III et al: Assessment of patients with facial fractures. Emerg Med Clin North Am 2000;18(3):411. [PMID: 10967733] (This review provides emergency physicians with a fundamental understanding of the evaluation and treatment of a variety of facial fractures.)

Hollander JE et al: Laceration management. Ann Emerg Med 1999;34(3):356. [PMID: 10459093] (This review presents current management and treatment options available for the repair of lacerations seen in the emergency department.)

Laskin DM et al: Current trends in the treatment of maxillofacial injuries in the United States. J Oral Maxillofac Surg 2000;58(2):207. [PMID: 10670601] (This article presents the results of a survey questionnaire of oral and maxillofacial surgeons to assess regional and national trends in the management of maxillofacial trauma.)

Parsa T et al: Initial evaluation and management of maxillofacial injuries. eMedicine Journal 2001;2(11). http://www.emedicine.com/med/topic3222.htm (This article discusses the clinical presentation, classifications, and approach to patients with maxillofacial trauma.)

Schwab RA, Genners K, Robinson W: Clinical predictors of mandibular fractures. Am J Emerg Med 1998;16(3):304. [PMID: 9596439] (Prospective study in an urban emergency department of 119 patients presenting with mandibular trauma.)

Segal Z et al: Facial trauma, zygomatic complex fractures. eMedicine Journal 2002;3(1). http://www.emedicine.com/plastic/topic531.htm (This article presents historical, anatomic, and biomechanical information related to the evaluation and treatment of ZMC fractures.)

Chest Trauma

James Svenson, MD, MS, & Désirée LaCharité, MD

24

Immediate Management of Life-Threatening Problems
Establish ABCs
Emergency Department Thoracotomy
Pain Control
Immediately Life-Threatening Thoracic Injuries Identified on Primary Survey
Tension Pneumothorax
Open Pneumothorax
Massive Hemothorax
Cardiac Tamponade
Flail Chest
Potentially Life-Threatening Injuries Identified on Secondary Survey
Pulmonary Contusion

Myocardial Contusion
Diaphragmatic Hernia
Esophageal Disruption
Aortic Disruption
Tracheobronchial Injury
Other Injuries
Rib Fractures
Sternal Fracture
Systemic Air Embolism
Traumatic Asphyxia
Penetrating Trauma

Up to half of all trauma patients sustain some degree of thoracic injury. Between 20% and 25% of all trauma deaths are directly attributable to chest trauma. Thoracic trauma is a contributing factor in another 25% of trauma deaths.

IMMEDIATE MANAGEMENT OF LIFE-THREATENING PROBLEMS

ESTABLISH ABCS

Address the ABCs as previously outlined in Chapters 9 and 10. Specific issues must be considered in evaluating the ABCs in the patient with blunt or penetrating chest trauma. The airway can be obstructed at any level from the pharynx to the trachea. Abnormalities in breathing can be caused by several mechanisms: (1) impairments in the chest wall or musculature, for example, secondary to pain or because chest wall motion is not coordinated, (2) impairments in gas exchange secondary to atelectasis, contusion, or disruption of the respiratory tract, or (3) central nervous system (CNS) impairments secondary to drugs or head trauma. Hypoxia is the most important feature of chest injury. Early interven-

tions should attempt to ensure that an adequate amount of oxygen is delivered to the portions of the lung capable of normal ventilation and perfusion. Abnormalities in circulation can be caused by blood loss, increased intrapleural pressure, blood in the pericardial sac, vascular disruption, or myocardial dysfunction. Because shock will most often be caused by blood loss, the first step is to ensure adequate fluid resuscitation.

EMERGENCY DEPARTMENT THORACOTOMY

The role of emergency department thoracotomy is controversial. Indications for thoracotomy are (1) penetrating thoracic wound with agonal state or recent loss of vital signs, deterioration or cardiac arrest after care has been initiated, or uncontrolled hemorrhage from the thoracic inlet or out of a chest tube, (2) need for open cardiac massage or occlusion of the descending thoracic aorta before laparotomy, or (3) suspected subclavian vessel injury with intrapleural exsanguination. Contraindications to thoracotomy include penetrating trauma with no signs of life in the field or blunt trauma with no signs of life on arrival in the emergency department. Perform thoracotomy only if immediate surgical backup is available.

Aihara R et al: Emergency room thoracotomy for penetrating chest injury: effect of an institutional protocol. J Trauma 2001; 50(6):1027. [PMID: 11426116]

Feliciano DV, Rozycki GS: Advances in the diagnosis and treatment of thoracic trauma. Surg Clin North Am 1999;79 (6):1417. [PMID: 10625986] (Review.)

PAIN CONTROL

Pain may impair chest wall expansion and impede oxygenation. Pain should be relieved with small, frequent doses of narcotic medications (eg, 1–5 mg morphine, or 50–100 µg fentanyl, every 5–10 minutes). Reassess the patient's pain level constantly to ensure adequate analgesia.

■ IMMEDIATELY LIFE-THREATENING THORACIC INJURIES IDENTIFIED ON PRIMARY SURVEY

Several injuries need to be considered in the patient with chest trauma. These entities can cause severe hypoxia or shock. The diagnoses are made clinically and need to be addressed without waiting for any diagnostic testing. Patients presenting with any one of these entities should receive treatment as outlined below and be admitted to the hospital for further care.

TENSION PNEUMOTHORAX

 ESSENTIALS OF DIAGNOSIS

- *Absent or decreased breath sounds.*
- *Hyperresonance to chest wall percussion on the affected side.*
- *Tracheal deviation away from the pneumothorax in the setting of respiratory distress and hypotension.*

General Considerations

Tension pneumothorax develops when a one-way valve air leak occurs from either the lung or the chest wall. Air enters the pleural space but cannot escape, leading to increased intrapleural pressure, collapse of the lung, and shift of the mediastinal contents to the opposite side. Tension pneumothorax can result from blunt chest injury with resultant parenchymal lung injury but can also be secondary to positive pressure ventilation. Occasionally a small penetrating wound can cause a valve-like effect that allows air to enter the pleural space on inspiration but not exit on expiration. The collapse of the lung leads to right-to-left pulmonary shunting and resultant hypoxia. In addition, increased intrathoracic pressure and pressure on the vena cava can reduce venous return to the heart and lead to decreased cardiac output and shock.

Clinical Findings

Pneumothorax is characterized by respiratory distress, tachypnea, and hypoxia. There will be hyperresonance to percussion and decreased or absent breath sounds on the affected side. With tension pneumothorax, the trachea will be deviated away from the affected side. Neck veins may be distended, but this sign may be absent if the patient is hypovolemic. The diagnosis of tension pneumothorax is made clinically. Patients with a tension pneumothorax need immediate treatment and should not wait for x-ray. Figure 24–1 is a chest x-ray of a patient whose physical exam findings should have led the physician to perform a needle decompression instead of an x-ray. For stable patients, in whom a

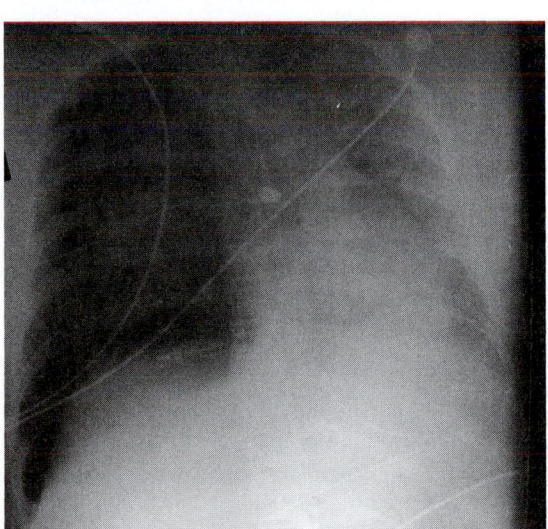

Figure 24–1. An ill-advised chest x-ray demonstrating tension pneumothorax. Clinical signs alone should be sufficient to diagnose this condition and avoid the life-threatening delay involved in obtaining an x-ray.

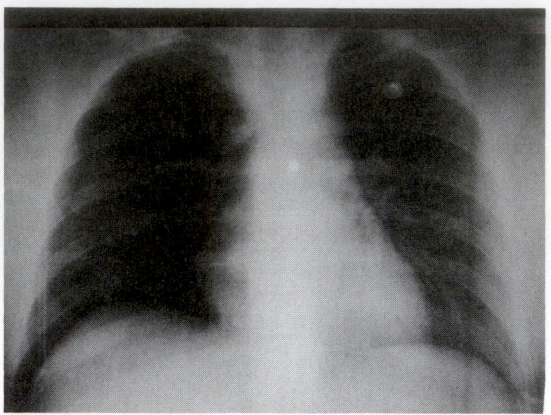

Figure 24–2. The chest x-ray demonstrates a large right pneumothorax with widening and deepening of the right costophrenic angle, also known as the deep sulcus sign. Occasionally this sign is the only radiographic indication of a pneumothorax in a supine patient.

pneumothorax is suspected, diagnosis is confirmed with chest x-ray (Figure 24–2).

Treatment

Treatment for a tension pneumothorax is immediate tube thoracostomy (Chapter 6). If a chest tube is not immediately available, needle thoracostomy with a large-bore ($\leq$ 16-gauge) needle in the second intercostal space in the midclavicular line will convert the tension pneumothorax into a simple pneumothorax until a tube can be placed. In this instance, leave the needle in until a definitive chest tube can be placed. Opening the wound further with a gloved finger or a clamp can relieve a tension pneumothorax associated with a penetrating injury. For patients with simple pneumothoraces secondary to trauma, traditional teaching has been to drain the pneumothorax through a tube thoracostomy and admit the patient for observation. However, it has been shown that patients with small pneumothoraces detected on computed tomography (CT) scan appear at low risk for complications and may not require drainage. In addition, serial observations or simple aspiration have been shown to be safe in patients presenting later or with small simple pneumothoraces.

Di Bartolomeo S et al: A population-based study on pneumothorax in severely traumatized patients. J Trauma 2001;51(4):677. [PMID: 11586158]

Miller A: Management of pneumothorax. Practitioner 2002;246 (1631):108. [PMID: 11852618] (Review.)

OPEN PNEUMOTHORAX

General Considerations

Large penetrating wounds of the thorax result in an immediate pneumothorax. Because there is equilibration between intrathoracic and atmospheric pressure, negative intrathoracic pressure cannot be generated. Effective ventilation is thus impaired because air goes through the chest wall rather than into the lung, resulting in severe hypoxia. The diagnosis is obvious, and therapy should be instituted immediately.

Treatment

Cover the chest wound with an occlusive dressing (eg, petrolatum gauze) taped on three sides. This temporarily seals the wound and prevents development of a tension pneumothorax. More definitive treatment involves placing a large-bore chest tube on the affected side and closing the wound.

MASSIVE HEMOTHORAX

 ESSENTIALS OF DIAGNOSIS

- *Decreased breath sounds and dullness to chest wall percussion on the affected side.*
- *Respiratory distress and hypotension.*

General Considerations

Injury to the chest wall, great vessels, or lung can result in intrapleural bleeding or hemothorax. Most commonly these are secondary to penetrating injury disrupting pulmonary or systemic blood vessels. In hemothorax associated with great vessel injury, 50% of patients die immediately, 25% live 5–10 minutes, and 25% live 30 minutes or longer. Respiratory insufficiency depends on how much blood is lost. In massive injury, the affected lung is collapsed, producing a right-to-left shunt. The loss of blood also leads to circulatory compromise.

Clinical Findings

A. Symptoms and Signs

Respiratory distress, tachypnea, and a variable degree of hypoxia are present. There is dullness to percussion and decreased breath sounds on the affected side. Depending on the degree of blood loss, hypotension and flat neck veins may be present. Pulse pressure is narrow. Small hemothoraces may be difficult to detect in supine patients.

B. IMAGING

Diagnosis is confirmed by chest x-ray (Figure 24–3). Small hemothoraces (<350 mL) are usually visible only as a small effusion on an upright chest x-ray. Moderate effusions (350–1500 mL) are seen as diffuse increased opacity on the affected side. Large effusions (> 1500 mL) have a ground-glass appearance on the supine film.

Treatment

For massive hemothorax, perform tube thoracostomy immediately without waiting for diagnostic tests. For smaller hemothoraces, diagnosis can be confirmed before instituting therapy. Tube thoracostomy using one or two large-bore chest tubes allows for accurate assessment of current and ongoing blood loss. Consider autotransfusion for patients with large bleeds (> 1 L). Initial blood loss of more than 1–1.5 L or ongoing continuing loss of more than 250 mL/h requires surgery.

McGhee A, Swinton S, Watt M: Use of autologous transfusion in the management of acute traumatic haemothorax in the accident and emergency department. J Accid Emerg Med 1999;16(6):451. [PMID: 10572824]

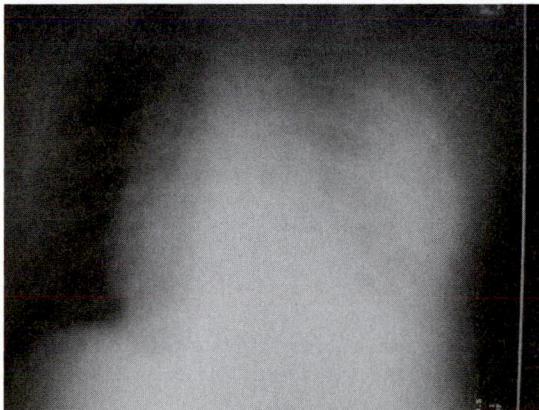

Figure 24–3. Blunt trauma patient with left hemothorax.

CARDIAC TAMPONADE

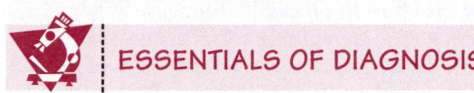

ESSENTIALS OF DIAGNOSIS

- *Signs and symptoms include dyspnea, narrow pulse pressure, hypotension, and tachycardia.*
- *Bedside focused assessment with sonography for trauma (FAST) exams can be diagnostic.*

General Considerations

Cardiac tamponade occurs when arterial, ventricular, or atrial injury causes blood to leak into the pericardium. True tamponade is rare and is most often associated with penetrating injuries. The pericardium is acutely not very distensible, and tamponade can occur even with a small amount (200 mL) of blood. The increased intrapericardial pressure compresses the heart and decreases cardiac output. In addition, venous return and cardiac filling decrease. Increased pressure may also lead to a decrease in myocardial perfusion. These factors lead to a decrease in cardiac output. Hypotension and shock then can result.

Clinical Findings

A. SYMPTOMS AND SIGNS

Symptoms and signs of tamponade are nonspecific. Tachycardia and narrow pulse pressure are usually present. Beck's triad of hypotension, muffled heart tones, and distended neck veins is present in a minority of patients with tamponade from blunt trauma. Jugular venous distension may be absent because of coexisting hypovolemia.

B. IMAGING

No specific findings on chest x-ray will confirm the diagnosis. Because tamponade can occur with a small effusion, heart size may not be significantly increased. Bedside focused assessment with sonography for trauma (FAST) exams (Chapters 6 and 25) are performed in many emergency departments to quickly identify pericardial effusions in patients with blunt or penetrating trauma. FAST exams allow rapid detection of pericardial fluid, with high sensitivity and specificity. An emergent thoracotomy can be life saving in an unstable patient with a pericardial effusion. In a stable patient, the diagnosis of pericardial effusion can be confirmed with transthoracic or transesophageal echocardiogram.

Echocardiography can also define the hemodynamic impact of the effusion on cardiac function. When ultrasound or echocardiography is not available, for the stable patient, CT scan is sensitive for detection of pericardial fluid. However, CT scan does not allow assessment of cardiac dynamics.

Treatment

Pericardiocentesis has been advocated in the past as both a diagnostic and a therapeutic modality. However, there are serious limitations. Pericardiocentesis has been reported to result in up to 80% false negatives and 35% false positives. In acute injury a large part of the pericardial blood may be clotted and so will not be aspirated through even a large-bore needle. Pericardiocentesis may injure the heart or other organs and may cause delays in definitive care. With these caveats, in a stable patient, ultrasound-guided pericardiocentesis has been shown to be safe and reliable. In patients who are unstable or in severe shock with signs and symptoms consistent with cardiac tamponade, immediate thoracotomy allows relief of the tamponade and control of myocardial injury.

Exadaktylos AK et al: Do we really need routine computed tomographic scanning in the primary evaluation of blunt chest trauma in patients with "normal" chest radiograph? J Trauma 2001;51(6):1173. [PMID: 11740271]

Salem K, Mulji A, Lonn E: Echocardiographically guided pericardiocentesis—the gold standard for the management of pericardial effusion and cardiac tamponade. Can J Cardiol 1999;15(11):1251. [PMID: 10579740]

Tsang TS et al: Diagnostic value of echocardiography in cardiac tamponade. Herz 2000;25(8):734. [PMID: 11200121]

FLAIL CHEST

Flail chest occurs when a segment of the chest does not have bony contiguity with the rest of the thoracic cage. When negative intrathoracic pressure is generated on inspiration, the flail segment moves inward, thus reducing tidal volume. Usually a significant blunt force is required (eg, motor vehicle collision or a fall from a height). The major complication is respiratory failure due to the underlying pulmonary injury.

Clinical Findings

The two major symptoms of flail chest are pain and respiratory distress. Tachypnea with shallow respirations secondary to pain will be seen. Paradoxical chest wall movement may not occur in a conscious patient due to splinting of the chest wall. Crepitus is often present. Even with marked flail chest, the patient may be able to compensate initially for the reduced tidal volume by hyperventilating. When fatigue or underlying pulmonary injury develops, frank respiratory failure may supervene.

Treatment

Supplemental oxygen is the first-line treatment. Pain control with intravenous morphine or fentanyl should be instituted early. Epidural or intercostal nerve blocks have also been used but usually not in the immediate management of these injuries. Consider early intubation and mechanical ventilation. Approximately 50% of patients will need immediate intubation. Indications for early ventilation include marked hypoxia or inadequate breathing. External chest wall supports (taping, sandbags) reduce pain with movement of the flail segment, but they also reduce vital capacity and may worsen respiratory function; therefore, they are not indicated.

Albaugh G et al: Age-adjusted outcomes in traumatic flail chest injuries in the elderly. Am Surg 2000;66(10):978. [PMID: 11261629]

Sivaloganathan M, Stephens R, Grocott M: Management of flail chest. Hosp Med 2000;61(11):811. [PMID: 11198758] (Review.)

■ POTENTIALLY LIFE-THREATENING INJURIES IDENTIFIED ON SECONDARY SURVEY

A careful and thorough secondary survey will identify multiple non-life-threatening chest injuries. Their prompt recognition and treatment may lead to an overall reduction in morbidity and mortality.

PULMONARY CONTUSION

 ESSENTIALS OF DIAGNOSIS

- *Signs and symptoms include dyspnea, hemoptysis, tachycardia, palpable rib fractures, chest wall bruising, decreased breath sounds, or crackles on pulmonary auscultation.*
- *Initially a pulmonary contusion may not be well visualized by chest radiograph.*

General Considerations

Pulmonary contusions are injuries of the lung parenchyma with hemorrhage and edema without associated laceration. They are the most frequent intrathoracic injuries in nonpenetrating chest trauma. They occur in approximately 30–75% of patients with significant blunt chest trauma. Pulmonary contusions typically occur at the site of impact and are often associated with other thoracic injuries such as rib fractures and flail chest, although they may occur alone. Pneumonia is the most common complication of pulmonary contusions, but their presence is a risk factor for the development of acute respiratory distress syndrome and long-term disability.

Clinical Findings

A. Symptoms and Signs

Pulmonary contusion is often silent during the initial trauma evaluation. Significant trauma as well as the presence of other associated thoracic and extrathoracic injuries should raise the clinician's suspicion that pulmonary contusion is present. The most important sign of pulmonary contusion is hypoxia. The degree of hypoxemia correlates directly with the size of the contusion. Large contusions lead to significant respiratory distress. Other clinical findings suggestive of pulmonary contusion include dyspnea, hemoptysis, tachycardia, and other evidence of chest injury such as palpable rib fractures, chest wall bruising, decreased breath sounds, or crackles on pulmonary auscultation.

B. Imaging

Chest x-ray findings may range from patchy interstitial infiltrates to complete lobar opacification. Chest x-ray will initially miss a substantial number of pulmonary contusions, but as a result of ongoing hemorrhage and edema, radiographic evidence of contusion is usually apparent within 6 hours of injury. Because the size of the contusion may help predict the clinical course, a thoracic CT scan may provide additional useful information. Animal studies suggest that CT scans will identify contusions in 100% of those with experimentally induced pulmonary injury. Therefore, chest x-ray should be followed by CT scan when the likelihood of undetected injury is high and identification of the injury will alter its management.

Treatment

Early recognition and treatment of pulmonary contusion is essential to prevent long-term complications. The mainstay of treatment is supportive care and consists of the careful use of intravenous fluids to ensure euvolemia, supplemental oxygen, chest physiotherapy, and if severe, the use of mechanical ventilation with positive end-expiratory pressure (PEEP).

Disposition

All patients with radiographic evidence of pulmonary contusion or clinical findings suggestive of pulmonary contusion should be admitted for monitoring and respiratory support.

Greenberg MD, Rosen CL: Evaluation of the patient with blunt chest trauma: an evidence based approach. Emerg Med Clin North Am 1999;17(1):41. [PMID: 10101340] (Review.)

Miller PR et al: ARDS after pulmonary contusion: accurate measurement of contusion volume identifies high-risk patients. J Trauma 2001;51(2):223; discussion, 229. [PMID: 11493778]

Moomey CB Jr et al: Cardiopulmonary function after pulmonary contusion and partial liquid ventilation. J Trauma 1998;45 (2):283. [PMID: 9715185]

MYOCARDIAL CONTUSION

Between 15% and 20% of patients sustaining significant thoracic trauma have some degree of cardiac involvement. Myocardial contusions are distinct areas of hemorrhage that are typically subendocardial but may extend transmurally. The right ventricle is most commonly involved due to its proximity to the sternum. Contusions of the myocardium typically produce wall motion abnormalities that may lead to conduction defects, dysrhythmias, or a decrease in cardiac output leading to cardiogenic shock.

Clinical Findings

The clinical presentation of myocardial contusion is nonspecific. Patients are often asymptomatic but may complain of chest pain, have subtle electrocardiographic changes, or present with hypotension secondary to cardiac dysmotility. Specific standardized criteria for the diagnosis of myocardial contusion do not exist. Studies that have been used to make the diagnosis include the following:

A. Electrocardiogram

A normal electrocardiogram (ECG) does not exclude the possibility of myocardial contusion, but it is the best screening tool. Obtain an ECG whenever significant thoracic trauma is present, particularly if concomitant injuries such as flail chest, rib fractures, or pulmonary contusion are present. Similarly, obtain an ECG for trauma patients complaining of chest pain, for those with unexplained hypotension, and for those with a history of coronary artery disease. The most common finding by ECG in myocardial contusion is sinus tachycardia followed by nonspecific ST and T wave changes.

A range of dysrhythmias and conduction disturbances may be evident, however, including ST elevation, atrial fibrillation, atrial flutter, premature ventricular contractions, ventricular tachycardia, ventricular fibrillation, first-degree heart block, and right bundle branch block. Although a normal ECG cannot exclude the presence of a myocardial contusion, the literature suggests that very few patients with normal ECGs develop complications.

B. BIOCHEMICAL MARKERS

There is much debate in the literature regarding the value of obtaining cardiac enzymes in the evaluation of the patient with potential myocardial contusion. Although troponin and CK-MB are specific markers for myocardial injury in myocardial infarction, they should not be obtained routinely in the evaluation of these patients. Cardiac enzymes have not been shown to diagnose clinically significant contusions or predict the development of complications or need for hospital admission.

C. ECHOCARDIOGRAPHY

Transthoracic and transesophageal echocardiography should not be used as screening tools for myocardial contusion. They are best used in the evaluation of patients with unexplained hypotension or persistent electrocardiographic abnormalities to exclude other potential cardiac injuries such as pericardial tamponade and ventricular rupture. Although both studies will identify wall motion abnormalities consistent with myocardial contusion, they have not been shown to predict or prevent clinical complications.

Treatment

There is no particular treatment for myocardial contusion other than to treat the potential complications as they arise. Monitor patients at all times. Treat dysrhythmias as discussed in Chapter 35. There is no role for the administration of prophylactic antidysrhythmics. Patients who subsequently develop myocardial infarction should receive appropriate treatment, but thrombolytics should not be given to trauma patients.

Disposition

Asymptomatic stable patients with normal ECGs and no evidence of other thoracic injury may be safely discharged from the emergency department. Elderly patients and those with a history of coronary artery disease, significant blunt thoracic trauma, ECG changes, or hypotension should be admitted for monitoring.

Bertinchant JP et al: Evaluation of incidence, clinical significance, and prognostic value of circulating cardiac troponin I and T elevation in hemodynamically stable patients with suspected myocardial contusion after blunt chest trauma. J Trauma 2000;48(5):924. [PMID: 10823538]

Feliciano DV, Rozycki GS: Advances in the diagnosis and treatment of thoracic trauma. Surg Clin North Am 1999:79 (6):1417-29. [PMID: 10625986] (Review.)

Greenberg MD, Rosen CL: Evaluation of the patient with blunt chest trauma: an evidence based approach. Emerg Med Clin North Am 1999;17(1):41. [PMID: 10101340] (Review.)

DIAPHRAGMATIC HERNIA

 **ESSENTIALS OF DIAGNOSIS**

- *Delayed presentation is common.*
- *A chest radiograph demonstrating a nasogastric tube above the diaphragm is diagnostic.*

General Considerations

Diaphragmatic hernias have been reported in 1–5% of patients sustaining blunt chest or abdominal trauma. They result either from direct violation of the diaphragm or from significant intra-abdominal or intrathoracic pressure applied to the diaphragm resulting in its rupture. The right side is affected up to three times less often than the left because it is relatively well protected by the liver. Up to 50% of these injuries are missed on the initial trauma evaluation, and their delayed presentation may not be clinically significant until herniation of abdominal contents through the diaphragm results in obstruction, incarceration, strangulation, perforation, or even death. Once a tear in the diaphragm occurs, it will not heal spontaneously, allowing for the herniation of abdominal contents into the chest cavity. Delayed presentations of patients with blunt diaphragmatic rupture have been reported up to 50 years after the primary traumatic event.

Clinical Findings

A. SYMPTOMS AND SIGNS

Patients with diaphragmatic hernias may be asymptomatic, particularly in the acute phase, or may present with symptoms of bowel obstruction. Delayed presentation is common with nonspecific respiratory or bowel complaints, given that early diagnosis is difficult to establish and often missed.

B. IMAGING

The chest x-ray is a valuable screening tool in detecting blunt diaphragmatic rupture. The initial x-ray is interpreted as normal in up to 50% of acute cases but will be abnormal in almost 100% of delayed presentations. Findings on an upright chest x-ray suggestive of diaphragmatic rupture include elevation or irregularity of the diaphragmatic border, unilateral pleural thickening, obvious herniation of abdominal contents into the chest cavity, and the presence of a nasogastric tube in the chest cavity (Figure 24–4). CT scans are often used preoperatively in the hemodynamically stable patients but have had less than satisfactory results in reporting isolated diaphragmatic injuries. Right-sided lesions are often missed because the contour of the right diaphragm is difficult to discern from the contour of the liver.

Treatment

Surgical reduction of the hernia and repair of the diaphragm is mandatory in all patients with diaphragmatic rupture. Care should be taken to avoid abdominal injury when placing a chest tube in patients with concomitant hemothorax or pneumothorax.

Nursal TZ et al: Traumatic diaphragmatic hernias: a report of 26 cases. Hernia 2001;5(1):25. [PMID: 11387719]

Shanmuganathan K, and Mirvis SE: Imaging diagnosis of nonaortic thoracic injury. Radiol Clin North Am 1999;37(3)533. [PMID: 10361545] (Review.)

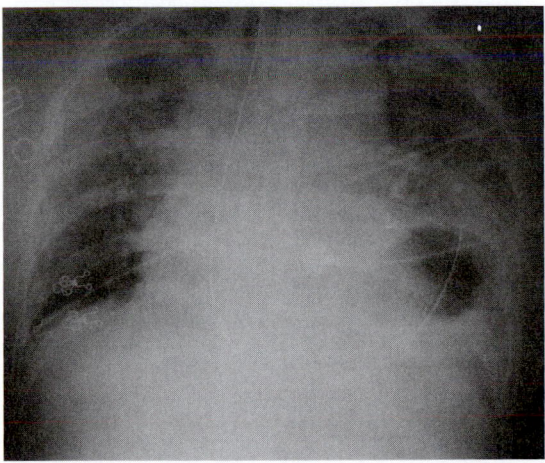

Figure 24–4. Adult female with blunt thoracoabdominal trauma from a motor vehicle collision. Chest x-ray demonstrates the nasogastric tube in the chest indicative of a ruptured left hemidiaphragm.

Singh S et al: Diaphragmatic rupture presenting 50 years after the traumatic event. J Trauma 2000;49(1):156. [PMID: 10912874] (Review.)

ESOPHAGEAL DISRUPTION

Esophageal disruption or perforation is an infrequent injury sustained secondary to blunt trauma. The mechanism of injury is unclear, but most occur during high-speed motor vehicle collisions and are typically associated with other serious thoracic injuries. Although their occurrence is rare, the reported mortality is more than 20% because of resultant complications of mediastinitis, which include pericarditis, pneumonitis, empyema, and even aortic erosion.

Clinical Findings

A. SYMPTOMS AND SIGNS

Esophageal injuries are difficult to diagnose. The symptoms and signs are often nonspecific and masked by other serious injuries. It should always be suspected in the patient with evidence of serious neck, thoracic, back, or abdominal injury. Patients may complain of throat pain, dysphagia, odynophagia, hoarseness, choking, chest pain, hematemesis, dyspnea, or continued neck pain despite appropriate treatment and immobilization. Neck redness, swelling, unexplained tachycardia, subcutaneous emphysema of the neck or chest, and bloody nasogastric tube contents may be found on physical exam.

B. IMAGING

Chest x-ray findings suggestive of esophageal injury include pneumomediastinum, widened mediastinum, and left pleural effusion. Gastrografin followed by barium swallow and esophagoscopy are probably the best diagnostic tools available for the detection of esophageal perforation; however, detailed exploratory surgery may be necessary for definitive diagnosis.

Treatment

Treatment of esophageal perforations depends on the location and the extent of the injury. Nonoperative management with drainage, antibiotics, and nutritional support may be appropriate for some injuries, but most require aggressive surgical management to prevent extensive spread of infection to the mediastinal and pleural cavities.

Monzon JR, Ryan B: Thoracic esophageal perforation secondary to blunt trauma. J Trauma 2000;49(6):1129. [PMID: 11843720]

Nakai S et al: Esophageal injury secondary to thoracic spinal trauma: the need for early diagnosis and aggressive surgical treatment. J Trauma 1998;44(6):1086. [PMID: 9637167]

Shanmuganathan K, Mirvis SE: Imaging diagnosis of nonaortic thoracic injury. Radiol Clin North Am 1999;37(3)533. [PMID: 10361545] (Review.)

AORTIC DISRUPTION

ESSENTIALS OF DIAGNOSIS

- Consider the diagnosis in all patients with rapid deceleration injuries.
- Signs and symptoms include chest pain, back pain, dyspnea, intrascapular murmur, and extremity pain caused by ischemia.

General Considerations

Traumatic aortic rupture is a common cause of death in blunt trauma. Injury is typically caused by rapid deceleration and shearing forces sustained in motor vehicle collisions, falls, and crush injuries and most commonly involves the descending segment of the aorta just past the origin of the left subclavian artery. More than 80% of patients die at the scene. Another 10–20% of patients with aortic disruption will die within the first hour. Rapid diagnosis and treatment are essential to limit the mortality associated with these injuries.

Clinical Findings

A. SYMPTOMS AND SIGNS

Consider aortic injury in all patients involved in rapid deceleration accidents. Clinical signs and symptoms suggestive of aortic injury include chest pain, back pain, dyspnea, intrascapular murmur, and extremity pain caused by ischemia. Patients may be hypertensive or hypotensive or may present with pseudocoarctation in which the upper extremities are hypertensive and the lower extremities have minimal blood pressure and pulse deficits. Fewer than 50% of patients have external signs of trauma.

B. IMAGING

Chest x-ray is an excellent screening tool for blunt aortic injury and is commonly used to determine the need for further studies. Mediastinal widening greater than 8 cm is the chest x-ray abnormality that most com-

monly leads to further workup. Other findings suggestive of aortic injury include indistinct aortic knob, left mainstem bronchus depression, tracheal deviation to the right, nasogastric tube deviation, widening of the right paratracheal stripe (> 5 mm), apical capping, and obliteration of the space between the pulmonary artery and the aorta (Figure 24–5). Despite its use as a screening tool, chest x-rays are normal in 2–7% of patients with aortic injury.

Angiography remains the gold standard for diagnosis of aortic injury. Angiography is expensive, time consuming, invasive, and requires a large dye load. Because the clinical indicators for blunt aortic injury are often nonspecific, a large number of aortograms have been performed in patients with normal aortas.

More recently, CT scan of the chest has been utilized in the evaluation of aortic injury and angiography is saved for those patients with abnormal findings by CT. CT is less expensive than angiography and can be performed much more quickly. With the newer-generation scanners and the use of intravenous contrast and consistent protocols, the sensitivity and specificity for aortic injury approaches 100%, particularly when criteria for positive scans include periaortic hematoma along with direct signs of aortic injury.

Treatment

Treatment of blunt aortic injury includes pharmacologic management of blood pressure and prompt surgical repair.

Dyer DS et al: Thoracic aortic injury: how predictive is mechanism and is chest computed tomography a reliable screening tool? A prospective study of 1,561 patients. J Trauma 2000;48 (4):673. [PMID: 10780601]

Feliciano DV, Rozycki GS: Advances in the diagnosis and treatment of thoracic trauma. Surg Clin North Am 1999;79(6): 1417. [PMID: 10625986] (Review.)

Greenberg MD, Rosen CL: Evaluation of the patient with blunt chest trauma: an evidence based approach. Emerg Med Clin North Am 1999;17(1):41. [PMID: 10101340] (Review.)

Nagy K et al: Guidelines for the diagnosis and management of blunt aortic injury: an EAST Practice Management Guidelines Work Group. J Trauma 2000;48(6):1128. [PMID: 10866262]

TRACHEOBRONCHIAL INJURY

ESSENTIALS OF DIAGNOSIS

- Signs and symptoms include dyspnea, subcutaneous emphysema of the neck or upper thoracic region, hemoptysis, and hypoxia.

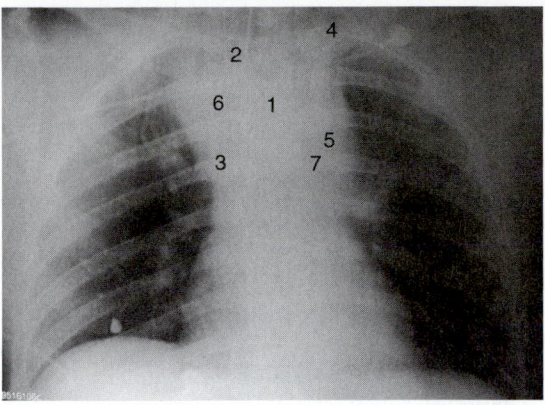

A

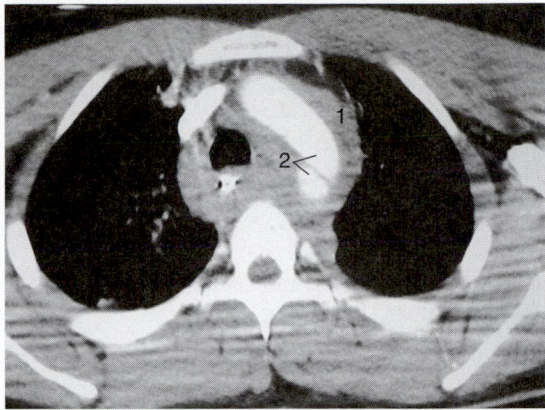

B

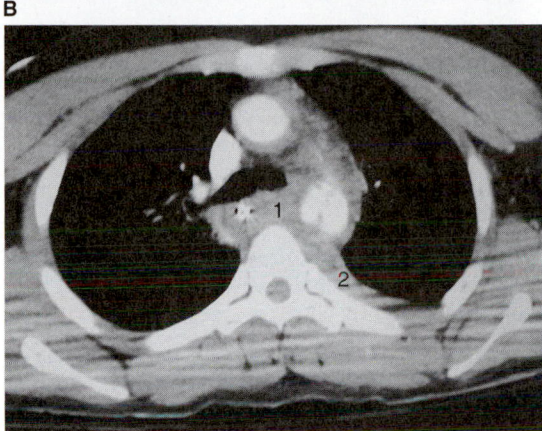

C

Figure 24–5. **A:** Chest x-ray of hypotensive adult male injured in a high-speed motor vehicle collision. Findings: (1) widened mediastinum, (2) deviation of the trachea to the right, (3) widening of the right paratracheal stripe, (4) left apical cap, (5) blurring of the aortic knob, (6) deviation of the nasogastric tube to the right, and (7) obliteration of the aorto-pulmonary window. **B:** Computed tomography (CT) scan of the chest demonstrates (1) periaortic hematoma and (2) a true and false aortic lumen; widening of the right paratracheal stripe is also noted. **C:** (1) Periaortic hematoma is present with (2) a small left hemothorax.

- *Suspect tracheobronchial injury if pneumothorax persists despite appropriate tube thoracostomy.*

General Considerations

Injury to the trachea or bronchus as a result of blunt trauma is relatively uncommon but can be quite severe. Approximately 80% of patients with tracheobronchial injuries die before reaching a hospital. Tracheobronchial injuries are usually the result of motor vehicle collisions and crush injuries. Right-sided bronchial injuries occur more commonly and are typically more severe; almost 80% occur within 2 cm of the carina. The diagnosis of tracheobronchial injury is missed in at least 25% of patients during the initial trauma evaluation.

Clinical Findings

A. Symptoms and Signs

Patients may be comfortable on room air or may present in acute respiratory distress. The most common

clinical symptoms and signs suggestive of injury to the trachea or bronchus are dyspnea and subcutaneous emphysema of the neck or upper thoracic region but may also include hoarseness, hemoptysis, hypoxia, and persistent pneumothorax despite appropriate tube thoracostomy.

B. Imaging

Chest x-ray findings indicative of tracheobronchial injury include subcutaneous emphysema, pneumomediastinum, pneumothorax, and peribronchial air.

Treatment

Patients in respiratory distress with suspected tracheobronchial injury should be endotracheally intubated, preferably over a bronchoscope if time allows. Blind intubation is discouraged because it may result in the complete disruption of small tracheal lacerations. Stable patients with suspected trauma to the trachea or bronchi should undergo immediate bronchoscopy for definitive evaluation and localization of the injury followed by operative repair.

Cassada DC et al: Acute injuries of the trachea and major bronchi: importance of early diagnosis. Ann Thorac Surg 2000;69(5): 1563. [PMID: 10881842] (Review.)

Kiser AC et al: Blunt tracheobronchial injuries: treatment and outcomes. Ann Thoracic Surg 2001;71(6):2059. [PMID: 11426809] (Review.)

Shanmuganathan K, Mirvis SE: Imaging diagnosis of nonaortic thoracic injury. Radiol Clin North Am 1999;37(3)533. [PMID: 10361545] (Review.)

■ OTHER INJURIES

RIB FRACTURES

Rib fractures are the most common injury sustained in blunt thoracic trauma. They are usually sustained in motor vehicle collisions. Fractures of the first rib usually indicate severe trauma because of the force necessary to produce such an injury. Fractures may cause localized pain, crepitus, pain with inspiration, and dyspnea and may even cause pneumothorax or hemothorax. Mortality increases with the number of ribs involved. The pain associated with rib fractures may lead to hypoventilation, atelectasis, retained secretions, and finally pneumonia.

Clinical Findings

Chest x-ray is the screening tool of choice for the detection of rib fractures, although up to 50% of rib fractures cannot be detected on chest x-ray. They may also be identified by specific rib x-rays and CT scan.

Treatment

Rapid mobilization, respiratory support, and pain management are the mainstays of treatment for multiple rib fractures. Continuous body positioning and oscillation therapy prevent hypoventilation and atelectasis by promoting redistribution of ventilation and perfusion to various lung segments. Mechanical ventilation allows for healing of the ribs and prevention of complications in the patient with respiratory failure. Incentive spirometry is excellent supportive therapy in stable patients. Pain control is paramount in facilitating adequate ventilation. Epidural anesthesia with bupivacaine controls pain without causing sedation and impairing the cough reflex.

Disposition

Treatment of isolated rib fractures in young, healthy patients without evidence of other serious underlying injury involves pain medications and deep breathing exercises with incentive spirometry. These patients do not require routine admittance or serial radiographic studies. Consider admitting elderly or other patients with serious underlying lung disease and isolated rib fractures. These patients have a higher complication rate due to a higher prevalence of hypoventilation, atelectasis, and pneumonia.

Easter A: Management of patients with multiple rib fractures. Am J Crit Care 2001;10(5):320. [PMID: 11548565] (Review.)

STERNAL FRACTURE

Most sternal fractures are associated with blunt trauma (eg, motor vehicle collisions). They are most common in postmenopausal females.

Clinical Findings

Pleuritic midline chest pain with focal tenderness over the sternum. There may be some pain with respiration, but there should be no pulmonary compromise. Because sternal fractures can be associated with myocardial contusions, evaluate patients for any evidence of myocardial injury as outlined previously.

Treatment

In the absence of complications, therapy for sternal fractures is mainly symptomatic. Give adequate analgesia with narcotics as necessary.

Disposition

Patients who have isolated sternal fractures and no evidence of other injuries can be safely sent home. Admit patients who have cardiovascular complications. Consider admission for patients who require more than standard doses of narcotics for analgesia or for patients who have limited social support.

Sadaba JR, Oswal D, Munsch CM: Management of isolated sternal fractures: determining the risk of blunt cardiac injury. Ann R Coll Surg Engl 2000;82(3):162. [PMID: 10858676] (Review.)

SYSTEMIC AIR EMBOLISM

Lung trauma in which air passages, lung parenchyma, or blood vessels are lacerated may result in a direct communication between these structures. Air can enter the pulmonary venous system as a result of a gradient caused by low pulmonary venous pressure (hypovolemia) or increased airway pressure (positive pressure ventilation, tension pneumothorax). Pulmonary venous air embolizes systemically, including coronary and cerebral circulation. Air embolization occurs most commonly after penetrating trauma.

Clinical Findings

Hemoptysis, circulatory, and CNS dysfunction immediately after initiation of positive pressure ventilation suggest air embolism. Focal neurologic abnormalities in the absence of head injury are common. Circulatory arrest after the initiation of mechanical ventilation suggests air embolism. Funduscopic examination may reveal air in the retinal vessels. Air in arterial blood gases (not due to froth) is diagnostic. Transesophageal echocardiography has been suggested as a diagnostic tool.

Treatment

Oxygenation is the first-line treatment. Selective lung ventilation has been advocated as a means of isolating the affected lung and stopping or minimizing the flow of gas into the circulation. Alternatively, high-frequency ventilation has been shown to be effective by allowing decreased ventilatory volumes and pressures. For moribund patients, thoracotomy and clamping of the hilum of the affected lung has been advocated. Cerebral air embolism has been treated with hyperbaric oxygen therapy, but other priorities may preclude or delay its use.

Ho AM, Ling E: Systemic air embolism after lung trauma. Anesthesiology 1999;90(2):564. [PMID: 9952165] (Review.)

TRAUMATIC ASPHYXIA

Severe crush injury of the thorax or abdomen can cause retrograde flow of blood from the right heart into the great veins of the head and neck.

Clinical Findings

The face and neck are a purplish-bluish color. Subconjunctival and retinal hemorrhages are common. Intracerebral bleeds are uncommon, but loss of consciousness or neurologic abnormalities can be caused by cerebral hypoxia. Traumatic asphyxia can indicate the possibility of other intrathoracic injuries associated with the severe crushing force.

Treatment & Disposition

There is no specific therapy except oxygenation. Treat other injuries appropriately. Hospitalize patients for observation.

COMMOTIO CORDIS

Commotio cordis is the condition of sudden cardiac death or near sudden cardiac death after blunt, low-impact chest wall trauma in the absence of structural cardiac abnormality. Ventricular fibrillation is the most commonly reported arrhythmia induced in commotio cordis. Young male athletes aged 5–18 years are particularly at risk for this catastrophe. It has been described after blows to the chest from baseballs, softballs, hockey pucks, and other objects. Death is usually instantaneous, and successful resuscitation is uncommon.

Link MS et al: What is commotio cordis? Cardiol Rev 1999;7 (5):265. [PMID: 11208236] (Review.)

■ PENETRATING TRAUMA

Penetrating trauma to the chest is usually inflicted by stabbing or gunshot but can include other foreign bodies or impalement injuries. Stab wounds commonly injure the ascending aorta, whereas gunshot wounds more typically injure the descending thoracic aorta, although laceration of the pericardium and any of the thoracic great vessels may occur.

Diagnosis

Information regarding the type of weapon, length or caliber of weapon, distance from the weapon, and amount of hemorrhage at the scene can be helpful when evaluating the patient with penetrating thoracic trauma. Most patients are hemodynamically unstable, and a rapid but thorough examination is essential. Address the ABCs first.

Clinical Findings

During the secondary survey, evaluate patients for signs of vascular injury including unequal blood pressures of the extremities, new vascular bruits, and the classic signs of pericardial tamponade: distended neck veins, muffled heart sounds, and hypotension. Obtain a chest x-ray immediately to identify pneumothorax, hemothorax, or foreign body. Placing radioopaque markers at the sites of wound entry and exit can be helpful in the interpretation of the chest x-ray. Bedside emergency FAST exams for the evaluation of pericardial tamponade can be extremely helpful in identifying the need for thoracotomy in the penetrating trauma patient with signs of shock. The same life-threatening and potentially life-threatening injuries described in blunt trauma can occur with penetrating trauma to the chest and should be managed as discussed in those sections.

Treatment

Address significant shock immediately with intravenous fluid boluses and blood transfusion, although some data suggest that aggressive fluid resuscitation may increase the amount of uncontrolled hemorrhage and subsequent mortality. Patients with pericardial tamponade require emergent pericardial window or thoracotomy. Perform tube thoracostomy in patients with evidence of pneumothorax or hemothorax. Autotransfusion is indicated in patients with large hemothoraces. Patients with initial chest tube blood loss exceeding 1500 mL, significant ongoing hemorrhage of more than 250 mL/h, or persistent hypotension should be taken directly to the operating room.

Never remove impaled objects in the emergency department because they may provide tamponade to surrounding vascular structures. The patient should be stabilized and the object removed in the operating room. Angiography is the gold standard for the evaluation of hemodynamically stable patients at high risk for great vessel injury based on the trajectory of the wound, although CT angiography has increasingly demonstrated reliability.

Disposition

Asymptomatic patients sustaining low-risk peripheral wounds with normal physical examinations and negative initial chest x-rays may be safely discharged to home after a 3-hour observation and repeat negative chest x-ray. Patients who develop delayed pneumothorax during this observation period require tube thoracostomy and admission.

Role of Emergency Department Thoracotomy in Penetrating Injuries

Emergency department thoracotomy is best utilized in patients sustaining penetrating thoracic injuries who have a witnessed cardiopulmonary arrest in the emergency department or lose signs of life during a short transport to the emergency department. Survival rates for cardiac injuries and stab wounds are typically better than noncardiac injuries and gunshot wounds. Thoracotomy for penetrating injuries yields an overall survival rate of approximately 11%.

Practice management guidelines for emergency department thoracotomy. Working Group, Ad Hoc Subcommittee on Outcomes, American College of Surgeons-Committee on Trauma. J Am Coll Surg 2001;193(3):303. [PMID: 11548801]

Shatz DV et al: Efficacy of follow-up evaluation in penetrating thoracic injuries: 3- v. 6-hour radiographs of the chest. J Emerg Med 2001;20(3):281. [PMID: 11267818]

Stern SA: Low-volume fluid resuscitation for presumed hemorrhagic shock: helpful or harmful? Curr Opin Crit Care 2001; 7(6):422. [PMID: 11805545]

Wall MJ Jr et al: Thoracic aortic and thoracic vascular injuries. Surg Clin North Am 2001;81(6):1375. [PMID: 11766181] (Review.)

Abdominal Trauma

25

Luis E. Rodriguez, MD, & John E. Gough, MD, FACEP

Immediate Management of Life-Threatening Injuries
Emergency Treatment of Specific Injuries
  Splenic Injuries
  Diaphragmatic Injuries
  Liver Injuries

Pancreatic Injuries
Renal Injuries
Bladder Injuries
Intestinal Injuries
Flank Injuries

IMMEDIATE MANAGEMENT OF LIFE-THREATENING INJURIES

Abdominal injuries may be life threatening and should be approached cautiously. After trauma, the abdomen may be a sanctuary for occult bleeding that, if not discovered and corrected expeditiously, may lead to deleterious consequences. Traditionally these injuries are classified as either blunt trauma, the majority of which are from motor vehicle collisions, and penetrating injuries, which are predominantly secondary to gunshot or stab wounds. Rapid assessment, stabilization, and early surgical consultation are recommended.

Assessment

Initial management of patients with abdominal trauma is the same as for all other trauma patients. Begin the assessment with a rapid primary survey, including evaluation of the airway, breathing, circulation, disability, and exposure.

A. AIRWAY

Administer high-flow oxygen, and intubate the patient if necessary. Maintain cervical spine immobilization until potential injury is ruled out.

B. BREATHING

Auscultate for breath sounds. Inspect for asymmetry of chest wall movement, open wounds, or flail segments. Pulse oximetry and capnography may be useful. Perform needle decompression or tube thoracostomy if tension pneumothorax is suspected.

C. CIRCULATION

Stop gross external hemorrhage with direct pressure. Assess pulses, capillary refill, and blood pressure. Obtain intravenous access with at least 2 large-bore (≥ 16-gauge) catheters. If peripheral intravenous access is inadequate, place a central venous catheter. Fluid resuscitation is an area of controversy (see below).

D. DISABILITY

Complete a brief, focused neurologic examination to document the patient's baseline. The examination should include an assessment of pupillary size and reactivity, a determination of the patient's Glasgow Coma Scale score, and notation of any focal neurologic deficits such as unilateral weakness or poor muscle tone. Ideally, perform the examination before administering pain medications, sedatives, or paralytics.

E. EXPOSURE

Completely undress the patient. Begin a more thorough secondary survey, including logrolling the patient and examining all skin folds, the back, and axillas for occult penetrating injuries. Identify any puncture wounds and document their location. To help identify the trajectory of bullets, place a radiopaque marker (eg, paper clip) at the wound site prior to obtaining x-rays. Do not remove impaled foreign bodies because they may be providing hemostasis from a vascular injury. Foreign body removal should be performed with surgical consultation in a more controlled setting. Avoid using terms such as entrance or exit wound on initial presentation, because it is often difficult to correctly make this assessment visually. These determinations are best left to a forensic pathologist.

Any penetrating injury below the level of the nipple line warrants evaluation for intra-abdominal injury. In patients in motor vehicle collisions, look for ecchymosis or erythema in the area of the clavicles or across the abdomen. The classic "seatbelt sign" may indicate intra-abdominal trauma.

Examine the abdomen for any tenderness, rigidity, or guarding. It is often difficult to assess bowel sounds at this stage of the exam. Evaluate the pelvis for antero-posterior or lateral instability with gentle pressure; this does not require much force. Examine the genitalia and look for blood at the urethral meatus, especially in males. Perform digital rectal examination in any patient with abdominal trauma. Look for gross blood, assess sphincter tone, and note any other evidence of trauma. There is no role for occult blood testing acutely in a trauma. If blood at the urethral meatus or a high-riding prostate is present, placement of a urinary catheter is contraindicated and a retrograde urethrogram is required to evaluate for potential urethral injury.

Treatment

A. Fluid Resuscitation

The concept of acute fluid resuscitation has evolved and may represent an area of some controversy. Animal and human studies have demonstrated deleterious effects of aggressive fluid resuscitation, particularly if penetrating trauma is present. Rapid infusion of large amounts of crystalloids may disrupt the formation of the soft clot and dilute the clotting factors, leading to increased bleeding. The results are less clear in the setting of blunt trauma. Also, blood pressure alone is not the best indicator of the level of shock. Attempts to make the patient normotensive are not recommended. A more reasonable goal may be to obtain systolic blood pressure of 80–90 mm Hg or a mean arterial pressure of 70 mm Hg. Crystalloids remain first-line fluids, followed by infusions of packed red blood cells. Other blood products may be indicated on an individual basis. Synthetic hemoglobin preparations are under evaluation.

B. Indications for Emergency Laparotomy

Patients with gunshot wounds that have an intra-abdominal trajectory require exploratory laparotomy. Most other patients with penetrating abdominal injuries will also require laparotomy given the high incidence of intra-abdominal injury once the fascia has been violated. Hemodynamically unstable patients sustaining blunt or penetrating trauma with a positive screening test (such as focused assessment with sonography for trauma [FAST] exam or diagnostic peritoneal lavage [DPL]) require laparotomy to control hemorrhage and evaluate for intra-abdominal injuries. Patients with obvious diaphragmatic injury noted on chest x-ray require emergent laparotomy.

C. Surgical Consultation

Seek surgical consultation early in the management of patients with abdominal trauma, especially if the patient is hemodynamically unstable.

Pepe PE, Mosesso VN, Falk JL: Prehospital fluid resuscitation of the patient with major trauma. Prehosp Emerg Care 2002; 6:81. [PMID: 11789657]

Velmahos GC, Tatevossian R, Demetriades D: The "seat belt" sign: a call for increased vigilance among physicians treating victims of motor vehicle accidents. Am Surg 1999;65:181. [PMID: 9926756]

Wotherspoon S, Chu K, Brown AF: Abdominal injury and the seat-belt sign. Emerg Med 2001;13:61. [PMID: 11476415]

Diagnostic Testing

A. Laboratory Evaluation

Initial laboratory evaluation should include hemoglobin and hematocrit to establish a baseline, and a blood-type and screen in case transfusion of packed red cells is needed. A lactate level may be obtained and, if elevated, is an excellent indicator of shock. Base deficit is another indicator of shock. The role of amylase in abdominal trauma is uncertain. Examination of the urine may reveal gross hematuria, which suggests significant injury to the urogenital tract (Chapter 26).

B. Other Diagnostic Modalities

1. Plain radiography—Almost all major trauma patients require plain x-rays of the chest, pelvis, and cervical spine. Although rarely utilized today, a one-shot intravenous pyelogram may be useful in patients with flank wounds or gross hematuria who are unable to undergo further diagnostic testing prior to operative intervention. Plain radiography of the abdomen is generally not helpful.

2. Diagnostic peritoneal lavage—Although DPL is still used occasionally, concern has been raised that DPL is overly sensitive, leading to nontherapeutic laparotomies. Recent literature has advocated the use of DPL in conjunction with computed tomography (CT) scanning or laparoscopy, particularly in low-velocity penetrating trauma (ie, stab wounds), to decrease the number of negative or nontherapeutic laparotomies. If DPL is considered, it should be performed only after consultation with the trauma surgeon, who should perform this diagnostic study in most cases.

3. CT scanning—In the hemodynamically stable patient, CT scanning is an excellent diagnostic modality that is easy to perform. If significant intra-abdominal injury is suspected and the hospital is not equipped to manage such patients, it is unwise to delay transfer in order to obtain a CT scan, assuming a reasonably expeditious transfer is possible.

4. Ultrasonography—Emergency ultrasonography has been studied extensively and is accurate. Also, it is safe in special patient populations (eg, pediatrics, obstetrics). FAST exam (see Chapter 6) is a bedside test that has demonstrated good accuracy with minimal experience (at least 30 examinations). The FAST exam consists of an initial subxiphoid view of the pericardium, followed by examination of the right upper quadrant looking for the Morison pouch (hepatorenal space). The Morison pouch is one of the most dependent parts of the abdomen and often shows the first signs of intraperitoneal fluid collection (blood). Subsequently the splenorenal interface in the left upper quadrant (Figure 25–1) is evaluated, followed by the pelvis. Unlike CT, a FAST exam is rapid, can be performed bedside in the emergency department, and is easily repeatable.

5. Laparoscopy—The use of laparoscopy, with or without CT scanning or DPL, is being studied. It is less invasive than traditional laparotomies and may shorten hospital stays and decrease patient costs, although it requires surgical consultation. The role of laparoscopy is not well defined at this time.

DeMaria EJ et al: Complementary roles of laparoscopic abdominal exploration and diagnostic peritoneal lavage for evaluating abdominal stab wounds: a prospective study. J Lapraroendosc Adv Surg Tech A 2000;10:131. [PMID: 10883989]

Gonzales RP et al: Abdominal stab wounds: diagnostic peritoneal lavage criteria for emergency room discharge. J Trauma 2001;51:939. [PMID: 11706344]

Gonzales RP, Ickler J, Gachassin P: Complementary roles of diagnostic peritoneal lavage and computed tomography in the evaluation of blunt trauma patients. J Trauma 2001;51:1134. [PMID: 11740265]

Goodwin H, Holmes JF, Wisner DH: Abdominal ultrasound examination in pregnant blunt trauma patients. J Trauma 2001;50:689. [PMID: 11303166]

Gracias VH et al: Defining the learning for the focused abdominal sonogram for trauma (FAST) examination: implications for credentialing. Am Surg 2001;67:364. [PMID: 11308006]

Nagy KK, Roberts RR, Joseph KT: Experience with over 2500 diagnostic peritoneal lavages. Injury 2000;31:479. [PMID: 10908739]

Patel JC, Tepas JJ: The efficacy of focused abdominal sonography for trauma (FAST) as a screening tool in the assessment of injured children. J Pediatr Surg 1999;34:44. [PMID: 10022141]

Taner AS et al: Diagnostic laparoscopy decreases the rate of unnecessary laparotomies and reduces hospital costs in trauma patients. J Laparoendosc Adv Surg Tech A 2001;11:207. [PMID: 11569509]

Types of Injury

A. BLUNT ABDOMINAL INJURY

Blunt injury occurs most frequently with motor vehicle collisions. Injuries occur secondary to shearing, tearing, or direct impact forces. The presence of a seatbelt sign is indicative of intra-abdominal injury in at least 25% of cases. Ascertain if only a lap belt was used, especially

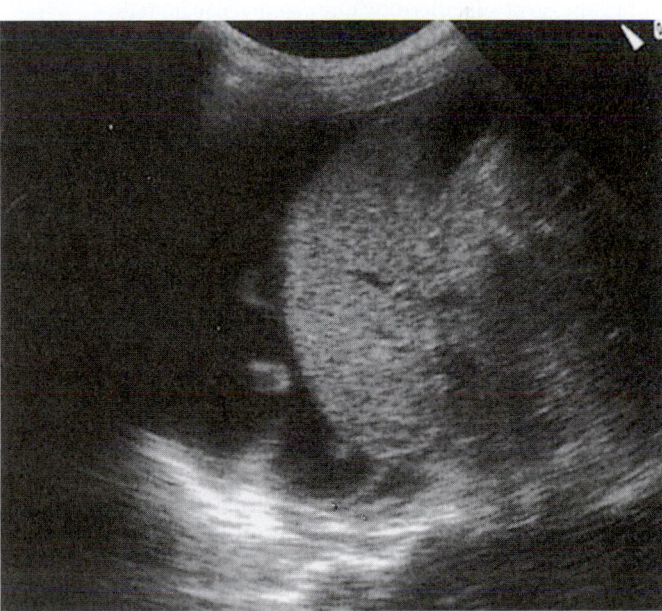

Figure 25–1. Positive FAST exam demonstrating a large amount of fluid surrounding the spleen.

in children. Lap-only restraints in children predispose them to intra-abdominal injuries such as intestinal perforations. These injuries may be associated with transverse lumbar spine fractures (Chance fractures).

B. Penetrating Injuries

Any wound inferior to a line drawn transversely between the nipples should be treated as having the potential for intra-abdominal trajectory. As noted earlier, intravenous fluids should be used judiciously in the prehospital setting. Before arrival at the emergency department, patients may be given enough fluids to maintain a systolic blood pressure of 90 mm Hg, rather than a multiliter resuscitation. If penetrating injuries are present, initiate antibiotic therapy and administer a tetanus booster early in treatment.

1. Gunshot wounds—All gunshot wounds with an intra-abdominal trajectory require exploratory laparotomy. Patients presenting with hypotension despite crystalloid resuscitation will need immediate exploratory laparotomy, antibiotics to cover abdominal flora, and a tetanus booster. Once intraperitoneal invasion has been ruled out, conservative management of wounds that are superficial and tangential to the abdomen may be used. Seek surgical consultation in all cases of abdominal gunshot wounds.

2. Stab wounds—Patients with stab wounds require resuscitation as well as tetanus booster and antibiotics if intraperitoneal violation is suspected. Stab wounds differ from gunshot wounds in that the former may be locally explored to determine if the peritoneum has been violated. A surgeon should conduct this procedure for all but the most superficial wounds, and adequate staff and lighting are required. DPL, CT scanning, and laparoscopy may be utilized. If peritoneal violation has been ruled out, patients may be safely discharged with local wound care instructions. If the peritoneum has been violated, exploratory laparotomy is required.

■ EMERGENCY TREATMENT OF SPECIFIC INJURIES

SPLENIC INJURIES

ESSENTIALS OF DIAGNOSIS

- *Most common in blunt trauma.*
- *Left upper quadrant pain and tenderness, often with radiation to left shoulder.*
- *May cause significant hemodynamic instability.*
- *CT scan is noninvasive and sensitive in stable patients; use FAST exam or laparotomy for unstable patients.*
- *Delayed rupture may occur.*

Clinical Findings

Splenic injuries commonly occur secondary to blunt injury. Patients may present with small hematomas, lacerations, devascularization, or complete rupture (Figure 25–2). There are numerous classifications of splenic injury. Most classifications range from simple lacerations to complete rupture.

Treatment & Disposition

Management of splenic injury has evolved. Not all injuries require splenectomy. Hemodynamically stable patients with low-grade lesions may be observed. Children are excellent candidates for conservative therapy. Elderly patients are poor candidates, particularly if they have high-grade injuries or if CT scan demonstrates free fluid. If hypotension unresponsive to 2 L of intravenous crystalloid infusion is present, blood transfusion should be given and the patient prepared for surgery. All splenic injuries require consultation with a trauma surgeon. Consider admission for patients with any splenic injury.

DIAPHRAGMATIC INJURIES (See also Chapter 24)

ESSENTIALS OF DIAGNOSIS

- *May be secondary to blunt or penetrating forces.*
- *Rupture occurs predominantly on left side.*
- *Often difficult to visualize on initial chest x-ray (nasogastric tube may enhance diagnosis).*
- *CT scan or laparoscopy more sensitive.*
- *Delays in diagnosis lead to increased morbidity and mortality.*

Diaphragmatic injuries are frequently difficult to detect initially. The presence of abdominal contents in the thorax may not be obvious on initial chest x-ray. Insertion of a nasogastric tube may facilitate the diagnosis

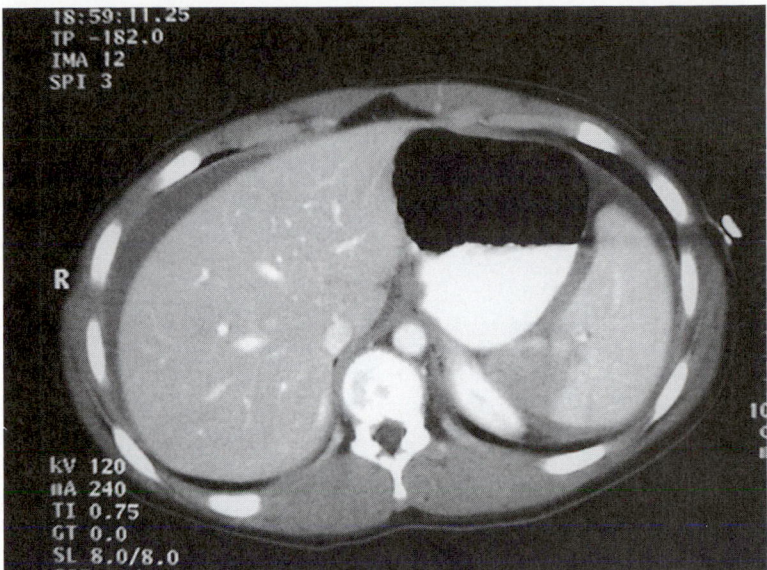

A

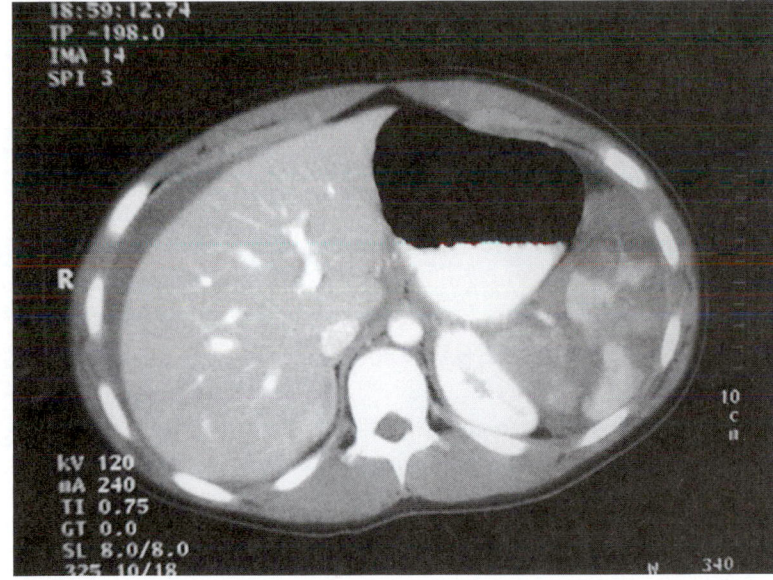

B

Figure 25–2. Adult male blunt trauma patient with splenic injury. Multiple large lacerations of the spleen are noted with associated perisplenic hematoma. Perihepatic free fluid is also noted. Images **A** and **B** were obtained shortly after the initial bolus of intravenous contrast. Note the compression of the left kidney by the perisplenic hematoma.

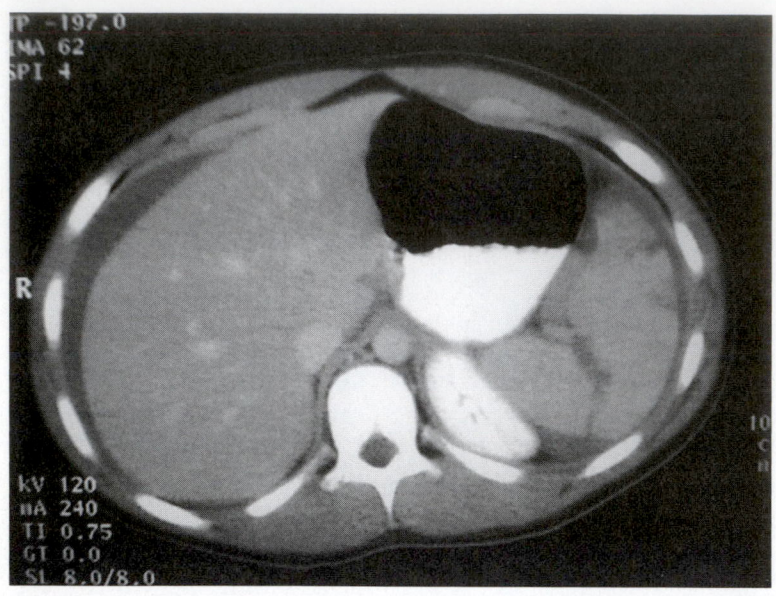

C

Figure 25–2. (Continued) Adult male blunt trauma patient with splenic injury. Image C was obtained after the initial bolus of intravenous had cleared the spleen. A large laceration on the posterior surface of the spleen is more clearly visualized extending anteriorly to the hilum.

(Figure 25–3). However, diaphragmatic ruptures may be missed even on initial CT scan. If abdominal viscera are seen in the thoracic cavity, then the diagnosis is made easy. Undiagnosed diaphragmatic injuries are a significant cause of morbidity and mortality.

LIVER INJURIES

 ESSENTIALS OF DIAGNOSIS

* Most common in blunt trauma.
* Right upper quadrant pain and tenderness, often with radiation to right shoulder.
* May cause significant hemodynamic instability.
* CT scan is noninvasive and sensitive in stable patients; use FAST exam or laparotomy for unstable patients.

Most liver injuries are managed with observation and conservative management. Liver injuries include lacerations, hematomas, or rupture (Figure 25–4). Because of the significant blood supply from the hepatic artery and portal vein, large defects are technically difficult to manage and may result in exsanguination and death.

PANCREATIC INJURIES

 ESSENTIALS OF DIAGNOSIS

* Uncommon, usually seen after blunt trauma.
* Patients may present with epigastric or back pain.
* Serum pancreatic enzyme levels are not sensitive or specific for injury.
* CT scan is noninvasive and sensitive.

Pancreatic injuries are rare and often difficult to diagnose. The pancreas may be lacerated or contused. Amylase levels are not specific and often are not helpful, particularly early in the evaluation of the patient. CT scan or radiologist-performed ultrasound may be helpful. Patients with pancreatic injuries should be admitted.

RENAL INJURIES
(See also Chapter 26)

 ESSENTIALS OF DIAGNOSIS

* Hematuria should raise suspicion for injury.
* CT scan is noninvasive and sensitive in stable patients; one-shot intravenous pyelogram may be

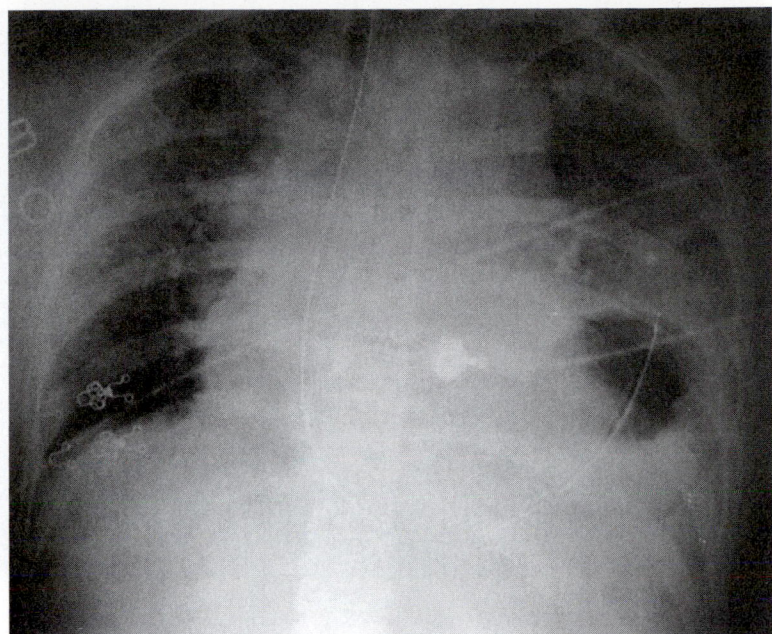

Figure 25–3. Adult female blunt trauma patient with blurring of the left hemidiaphragm and an abnormal nasogastric tube and stomach bubble location, representing a left diaphragmatic injury.

used in unstable patients, but it has limited sensitivity.

The kidney may sustain lacerations, contusions, shattering, or devascularization injuries. After a urinary catheter is inserted during the initial assessment, determine whether gross hematuria is present. Microscopic analysis is not needed in adults. In children, the presence of at least 5 red blood cells per high-power field on microscopic examination indicates possible urinary tract injury. These findings warrant urologic consultation in the emergency department (see Figure 26–5).

BLADDER INJURIES
(See also Chapter 26)

 ESSENTIALS OF DIAGNOSIS

- *Most commonly seen with pelvic fractures.*
- *Hematuria should raise suspicion for injury.*
- *Retrograde cystogram may identify injury (as well as associated urethral injury).*
- *CT scan may also be utilized with cystogram.*

Bladder injuries may be either intraperitoneal or extraperitoneal. The diagnosis is suspected in a patient with abdominal pain and hematuria and is confirmed with a retrograde cystogram. Patients with intraperitoneal rupture require immediate surgery (see Figures 26–6 and 26–7).

INTESTINAL INJURIES

 ESSENTIALS OF DIAGNOSIS

- *May occur with blunt and penetrating injuries.*
- *Peritoneal signs may be delayed.*
- *May be missed on initial plain x-rays and CT scans.*
- *May have delayed presentation (eg, duodenal hematomas).*

Both penetrating and blunt injuries can cause intestinal perforations. These perforations may be subtle initially and may be missed on CT scan (Figure 25–5). Such injury may be present even if the patient can tolerate a trial of fluids by mouth in the emergency department. The emergency physician should be cautious if this diagnosis is suspected. Give patients who are to be discharged thorough instructions, including for follow-up

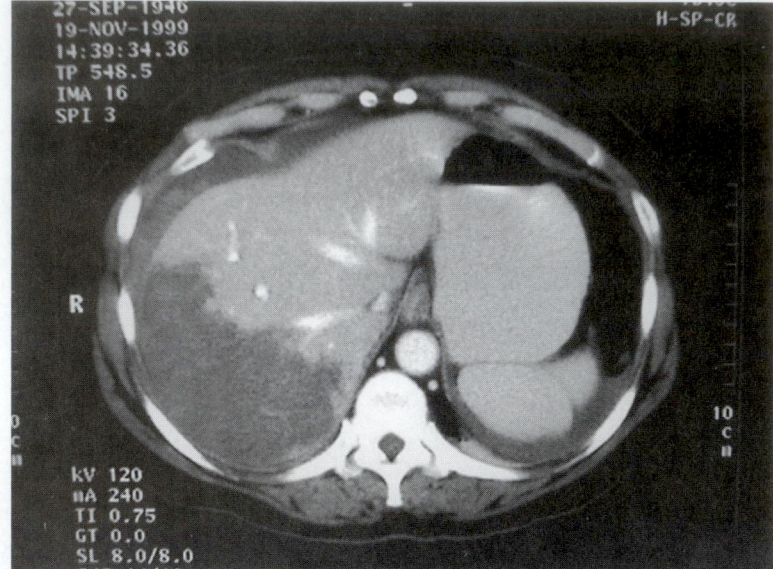

A

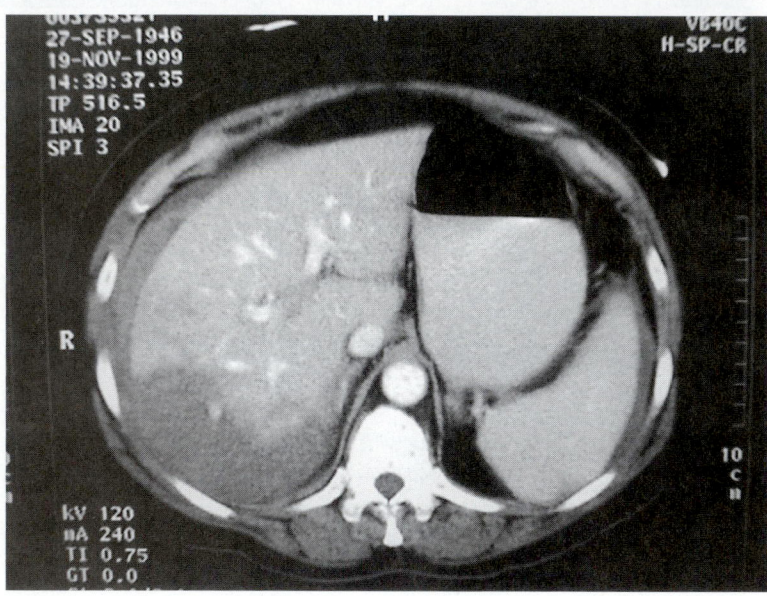

B

Figure 25–4. Adult male blunt trauma patient with a large posterior hepatic contusion with associated perihepatic and perisplenic hemorrhage.

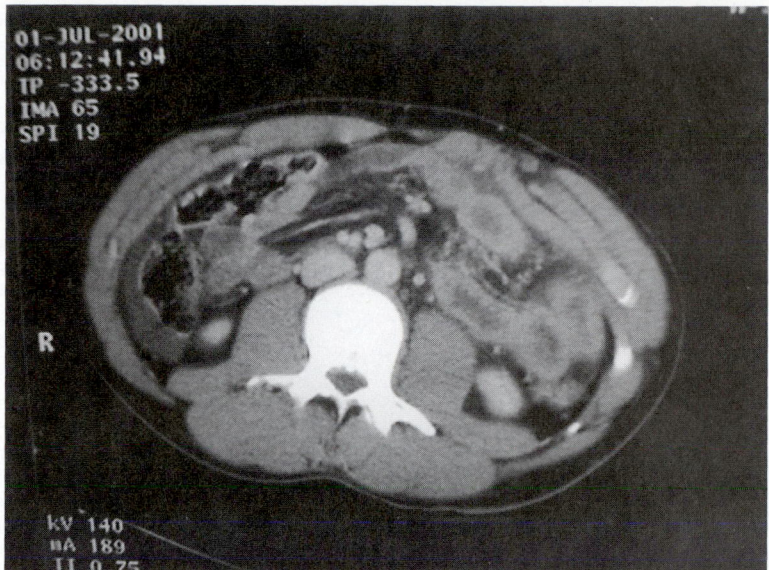

A

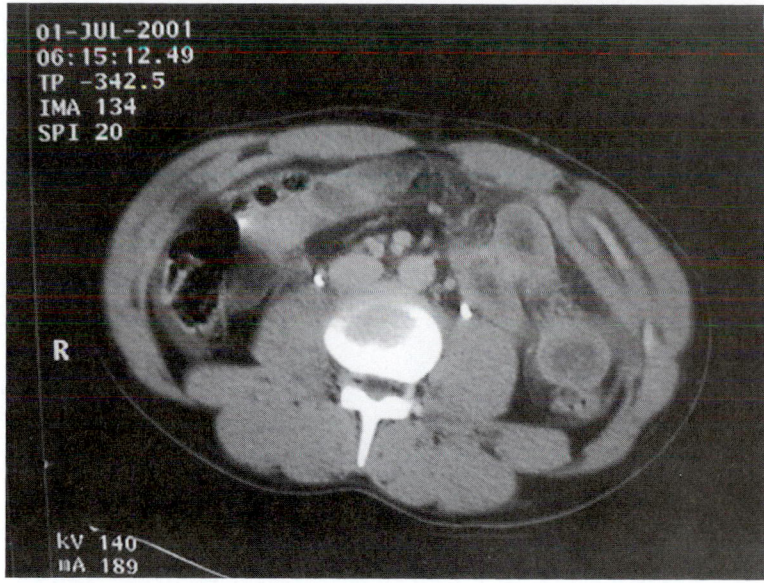

Figure 25–5. Adult male blunt trauma patient with left-sided intra-abdominal free fluid, small bowel wall thickening, and stranding in the mesenteric fat planes. Patient underwent exploratory laparotomy and was found to have a mesenteric tear with perforated and devascularized jejunum.

B

care. Patients have been able to walk out of the emergency department only to return later with fever and a rigid abdomen. Rare cases of traumatic appendicitis have been reported in the literature. If injuries involving impact, or "spearing," with bicycle handlebars are present, consider evaluating the patient for a duodenal hematoma, which can be managed conservatively.

FLANK INJURIES

 ESSENTIALS OF DIAGNOSIS

- *May be associated with renal injuries.*
- *Retroperitoneal hematoma may be false positive on diagnostic peritoneal lavage or ultrasound.*
- *CT scan is noninvasive and sensitive in stable patients.*

Flank injuries are more difficult to manage than other types of injuries because differentiating intraperitoneal from retroperitoneal involvement can be difficult. An abdominal CT scan or one-shot intravenous pyelogram may be beneficial to diagnose ureteral or retroperitoneal injury. These studies should be performed in consultation with the trauma surgeon.

Albrecht RM, Schermer CR, Morris A: Nonoperative management of blunt splenic injuries: factors influencing success in age > 55 years. Am Surg 2002;68:227. [PMID: 11893099]

Carlin AM et al: Factors affecting the outcome of patients with splenic trauma. Am Surg 2002;68:232. [PMID: 11893100]

Livingston DH et al: Admission or observation is not necessary after negative abdominal computed tomographic scan in patients with suspected blunt abdominal trauma: results of a prospective, multi-institutional trial. J Trauma 1998;44:273. [PMID: 9498497]

Nagy KK et al: Routine preoperative "one-shot" intravenous pyelography is not indicated in all patients with penetrating abdominal trauma. J Am Coll Surg 1997;185:530. [PMID: 9404875]

Genitourinary Trauma

26

Geoffrey A. Wiss, MD, Claudia Whitaker, MD, & Robert K. Dunne, MD, FACEP

Immediate Management of Life-Threatening Injuries
Emergency Treatment of Specific Injuries
   Renal Injuries
   Ureteral Injuries
   Bladder Injuries
   Urethral Injuries
     1. Posterior Urethra
     2. Anterior Urethra

External Genital Injuries
   1. Penile Rupture
   2. Constriction Injuries
   3. Testicular Injuries
   4. Skin Injuries
   5. Female Genital Injuries

■ IMMEDIATE MANAGEMENT OF LIFE-THREATENING INJURIES

Genitourinary injuries occur in 10–20% of major trauma patients. Most of these injuries, with the exception of renal hilar disruption or shattered kidney, are not immediately life threatening. Because they are often accompanied by potentially life-threatening injuries to other organ systems, however, it is easy for the emergency physician to overlook and therefore miss signs or symptoms of urologic injury. Failure to diagnose and treat these injuries properly can result in significant long-term morbidity. Therefore, while evaluating the trauma patient, the physician needs to be aware of clues to genitourinary injury. These clues include (1) lumbar vertebral or lower rib fractures, (2) pelvic fractures, (3) flank pain or hematoma, (4) abnormal prostate on rectal exam, (5) blood at the urethral meatus, and (6) gross hematuria.

Immediate Treatment

For all patients with blunt or penetrating trauma, evaluate airway, breathing, circulation, and disability during the primary survey as per advanced trauma life support protocol (Chapter 10). During the secondary survey, evaluate for a boggy or high-riding prostate on rectal exam, perineal or scrotal hematoma, and any evidence of blood at the urethral meatus. If any of these

signs is present, perform a retrograde urethrogram before inserting a Foley catheter. If the signs are absent, insert a Foley catheter if indicated (ie, in unstable patients or those unable to urinate). Urethral studies should never delay diagnostic studies of, or treatment for, potentially life-threatening injuries. Figures 26–1, 26–2, and 26–3 provide algorithms for managing blunt, penetrating, and pediatric urologic injury.

Special Examinations & Procedures

Evaluation of the genitourinary system should be performed in a retrograde fashion: rule out urethral injury before bladder, then bladder before ureteral or renal injury.

A. CATHETERIZATION

A Foley catheter may be placed once physical examination supports the integrity of the urethra. If any signs of urethral injury are present, perform retrograde urethrogram first. If urethrogram is negative or not indicated, a 14–16F catheter should be placed using copious amounts of lubricating jelly and sterile technique. A folded 4- × 4-in gauze pad may be used to retract the foreskin in uncircumcised patients to prevent repeated unintended reduction of the foreskin over the glans with subsequent field and catheter contamination during placement. Any difficulty during placement warrants retrograde urethrography if urethral injury is a possibility. Gross or microscopic hematuria indicates possible urologic trauma, although the degree of micro-

477

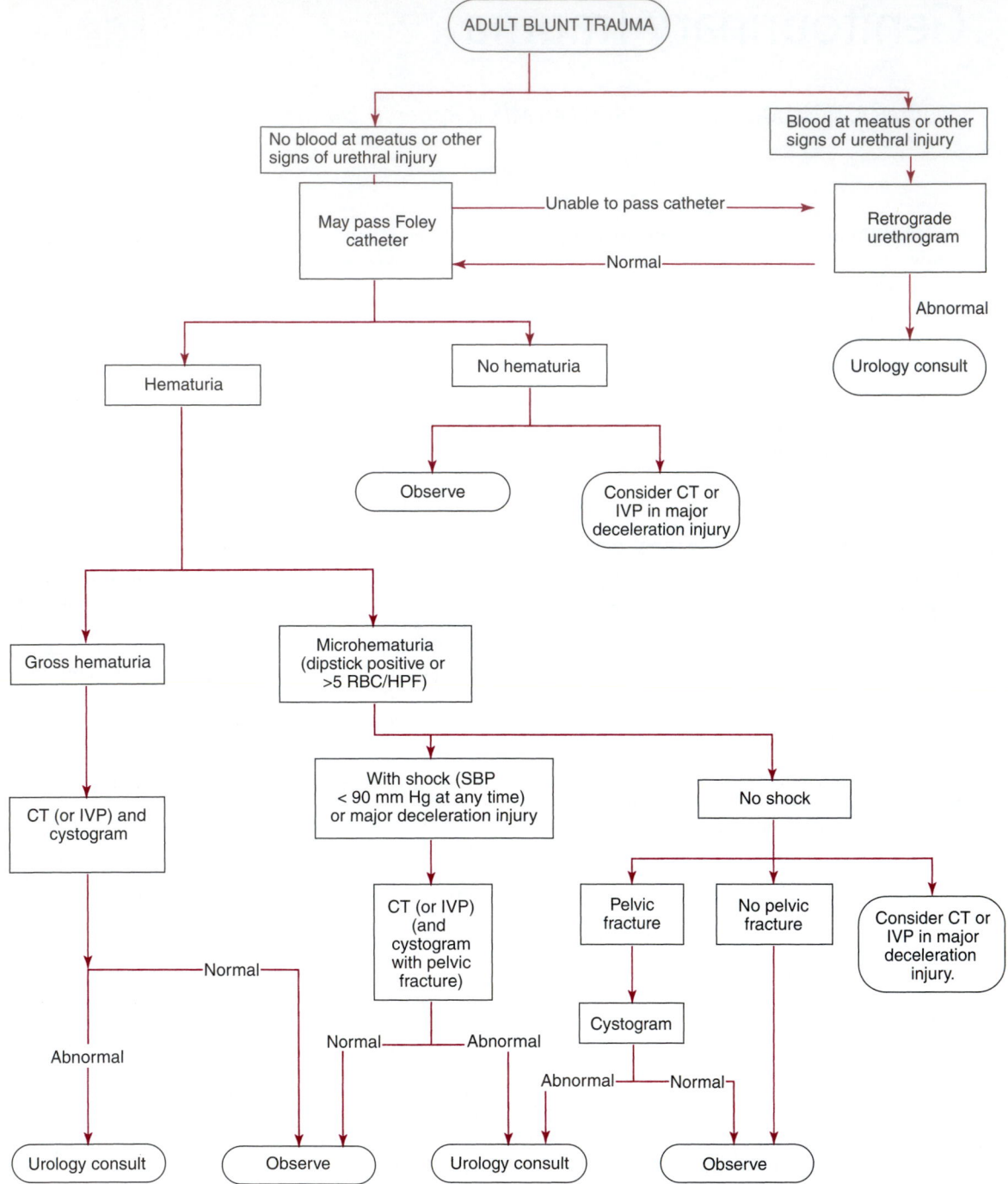

Figure 26–1. Algorithm for staging blunt trauma in the adult. IVP = intravenous pyelogram; RBC/HPF = red blood cells per high-power field; SBP = systolic blood pressure. (Modified and reproduced, with permission, from Tanagho EA, McAninch JW: *Smith's General Urology,* 13th ed. Appleton & Lange, 1992.)

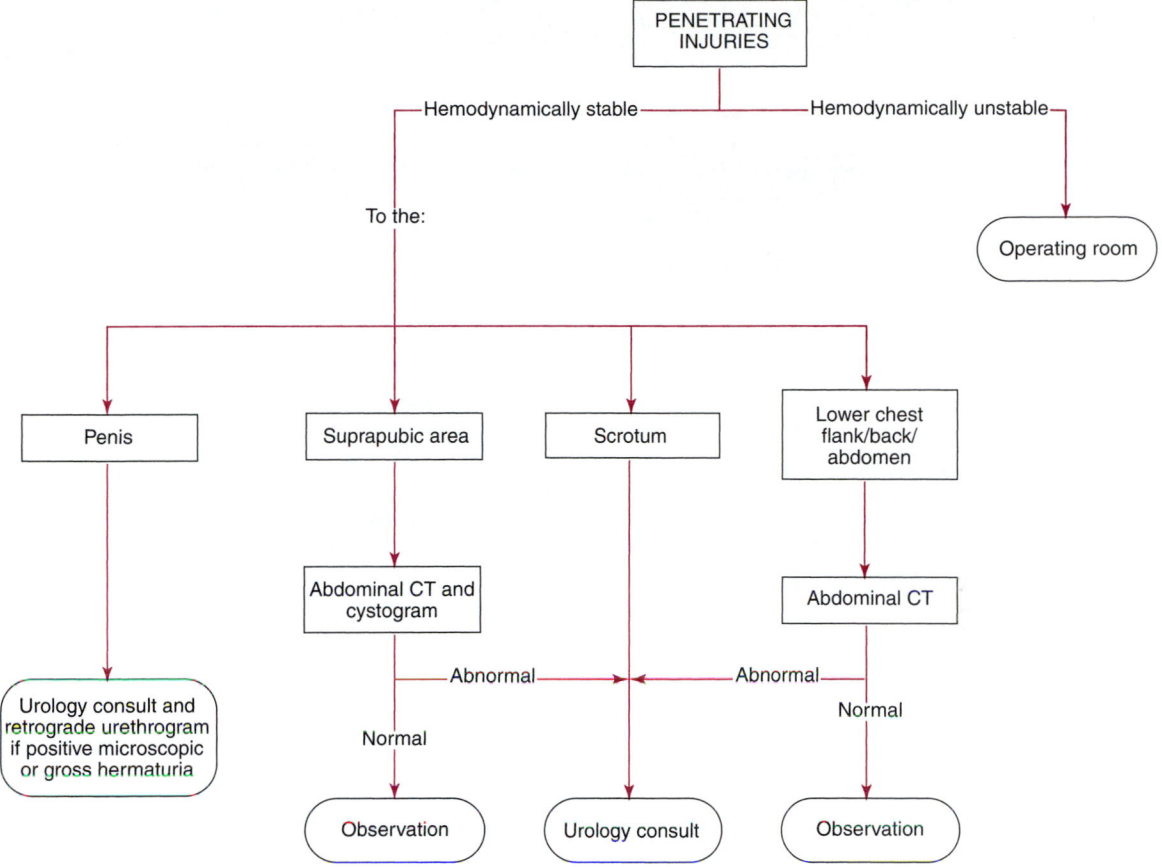

Figure 26–2. Algorithm for staging penetrating trauma in the adult. (Modified and reproduced, with permission, from Tanagho EA, McAninch JW: *Smith's General Urology,* 13th ed. Appleton & Lange, 1992.)

scopic hematuria does not correlate with the degree or location of injury.

In 1989, a 10-year prospective study established guidelines for evaluation and treatment of blunt renal trauma. Patients with gross hematuria require an imaging study. Patients with microscopic hematuria and a history of shock (systolic blood pressure < 90 mm Hg) or sudden deceleration injury should also have an imaging study performed. Those without shock or deceleration injury may be discharged home with outpatient urology follow-up to ensure that hematuria has cleared. Patients with penetrating injuries and more than 5 red blood cells per high-power field should undergo an imaging study, although the absence of hematuria does not eliminate the need for a study. With regard to penetrating trauma, the location of the wound is more important than the presence of hematuria for predicting injury, because significant injuries (9% of patients in

one study) can be present even in the absence of hematuria. In pediatric patients, the kidney is the most commonly injured intra-abdominal organ. As a result, even microscopic hematuria from trauma requires further workup (usually by computed tomography [CT] scan) in pediatric patients. Likewise, further evaluation is required for all patients with penetrating trauma and any degree of hematuria.

B. SUPRAPUBIC CATHETER PLACEMENT

Suprapubic catheter placement is indicated in trauma situations when Foley catheter placement is contraindicated, usually because urethral injury is suspected and cannot be confirmed with urethrogram or while awaiting surgical repair of a damaged urethra. Several commercial kits are available. Most of these kits utilize placement over a guidewire. If kits are unavailable, a single-lumen central venous catheter may be used.

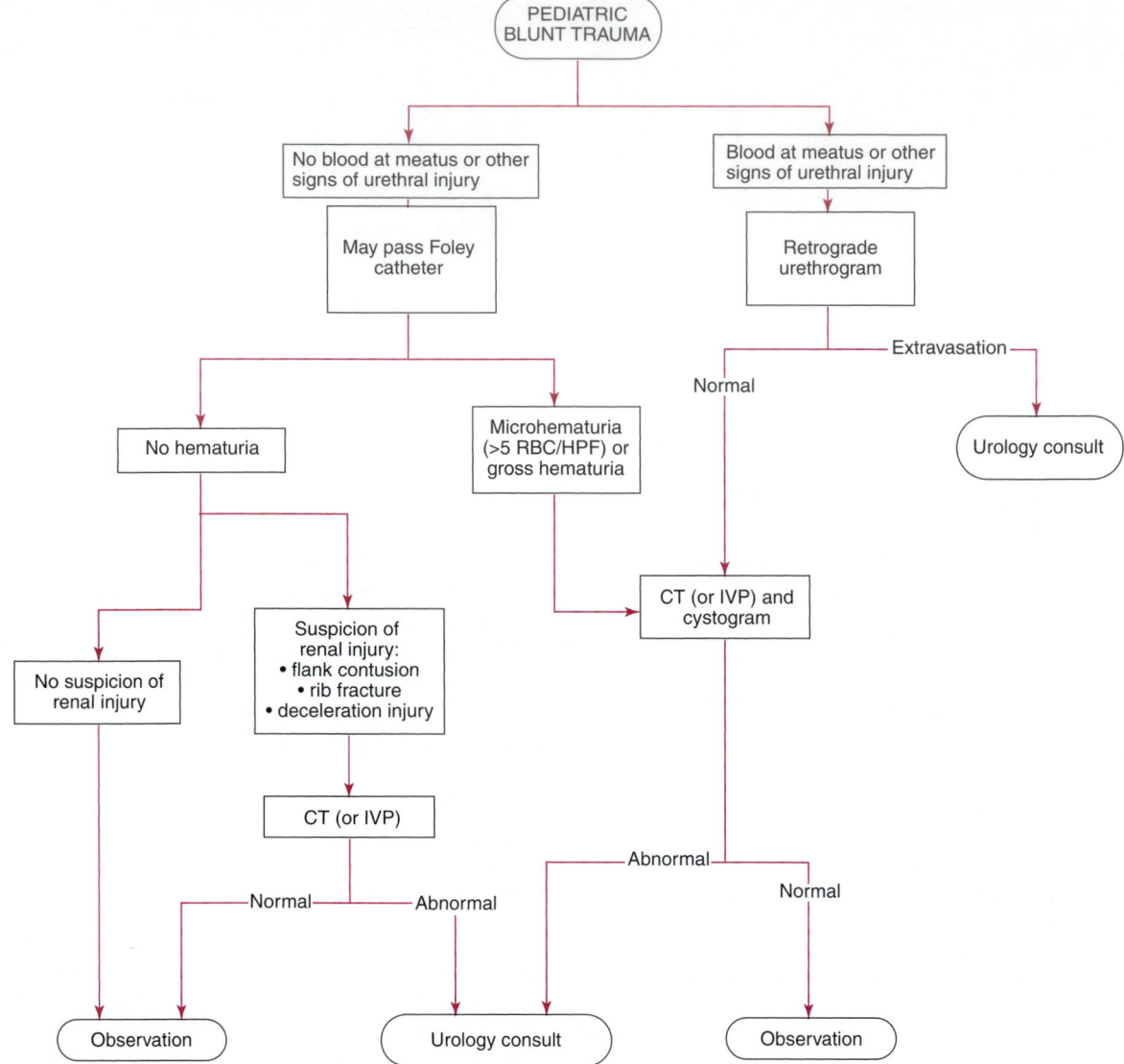

Figure 26–3. Algorithm for the evaluation of blunt trauma in children. IVP = intravenous pyelogram. (Modified and reproduced, with permission, from Tanagho EA, McAninch JW: *Smith's General Urology,* 13th ed. Appleton & Lange, 1992.)

C. Intravenous Pyelogram

No longer the study of choice, the intravenous pyelogram (IVP) has been replaced by the helical CT scan, although it is useful at institutions not equipped with CT scanners. These studies should be performed with an intravenous bolus of contrast followed by serial nephrotomograms. "One-shot" IVP studies in the trauma room are no longer recommended as a screening exam because of an unacceptably high level of false

positives and negatives. If verification of 2 functioning kidneys is needed prior to surgical repair of a kidney, a simple IVP may be performed in the operating room.

D. Retrograde Urethrography

If urethral injury is suspected (eg, blood at the meatus, boggy or high-riding prostate, scrotal or perineal hematoma), urethrography should be performed prior to Foley catheter placement. After a preinjection abdominal x-ray is obtained, a Cooke adapter on a 60-cc syringe is gently inserted into the urethra and 60 cc of full- or half-strength water-soluble contrast is injected over 60 seconds; the x-ray is taken during the last 10 seconds of injection. Extravasation with bladder filling denotes partial urethral tear, and extravasation with no bladder filling denotes complete urethral tear.

E. Retrograde Cystography

Bladder evaluation is required for gross hematuria or microscopic hematuria with pelvic fractures or penetrating injury. After a preliminary KUB, up to 400 cc of full-strength water-soluble contrast is instilled under gravity through a urethral catheter to the point of bladder contraction; x-rays are taken with the bladder full and after complete voiding. These x-rays may show either intra- or extraperitoneal extravasation. Because of the effective sealing capabilities of the 3-layered bladder wall, false negatives may be encountered if less than the recommended age-appropriate amount of contrast is instilled.

F. CT Scan

Helical CT scan with intravenous contrast is the study of choice for evaluating ureteral or renal trauma. CT scan may also be used for retrograde cystography, although the same procedure outlined above should be followed. Clamping the Foley catheter during an intravenous contrast pelvic CT scan is not adequate to eliminate bladder injury, because of inadequate bladder pressures and dilute dye.

G. Ultrasound

Although used frequently in trauma situations to detect peritoneal blood, ultrasound does not have the sensitivity to reliably detect specific renal injuries and, therefore, is not recommended in the workup of renal trauma.

Ahn JH, Morey AF, McAninch JW: Workup and management of traumatic hematuria. Emerg Med Clin North Am 1998; 16:145. [PMID: 9496319]

Carlin BI, Resnick MI: Indications and techniques for urologic evaluation of the trauma patient with suspected urologic injury. Semin Urol 1995;13:9. [PMID: 7597359]

Dreitlein DA, Suner S, Basler J: Genitourinary trauma. Emerg Med Clin North Am 2001;19:569. [PMID: 11554276]

Goff CD, Collin GR: Management of renal trauma at a rural, level I trauma center. Am Surg 1998;64:226. [PMID: 9520811]

McAleer IM, Kaplan GW: Pediatric genitourinary trauma. Urol Clin North Am 1995;22:177. [PMID: 7855953]

McGahan JP et al: Use of ultrasonography in the patient with acute abdominal trauma. J Ultrasound Med 1997;16:653. [PMID: 9323670]

Miller KS, McAninch JW: Radiographic assessment of renal trauma: our 15-year experience. J Urol 1995;154:352. [PMID: 7609096]

Nagy KK et al: Routine preoperative "one-shot" intravenous pyelography is not indicated in all patients with penetrating abdominal trauma. J Am Coll Surg 1997;185:530. [PMID: 9404875]

Rubin GD, Silverman SG: Helical (spiral) CT of the retroperitoneum. Radiol Clin North Am 1995;33:903. [PMID: 7676014]

■ EMERGENCY TREATMENT OF SPECIFIC INJURIES

RENAL INJURIES

 ESSENTIALS OF DIAGNOSIS

- *Often accompanied by other abdominal injuries in blunt trauma.*
- *Nausea, vomiting, flank ecchymosis, lower rib or lumbar fractures suggest injury.*
- *No reliable markers for diagnosis, including hematuria.*
- *CT scan is study of choice.*

General Considerations

Renal injuries are the most common urologic injuries. The kidneys are not fixed in place but hang from their vascular attachments and perirenal fat and move with the diaphragm. They are susceptible to deceleration injury, with blunt injury 5 times more common than penetrating injury. Kidneys with preexisting abnormalities such as tumors or hydronephrosis may be damaged by seemingly inconsequential mechanisms.

The diagnosis of renal trauma is complicated by the frequent presence of other peritoneal injuries, as well as the absence of any accurate markers for renal injury. Hematuria may be absent with significant renal injury, and the degree of hematuria does not correlate with the degree of injury when present. Renal injuries are graded on a scale of 1 to 5 (Figure 26–4). Following a general trend for the nonoperative management of many solid organ intra-abdominal injuries, many renal injuries are increasingly being managed without routine surgical exploration. However, only a special subset of patients with high-grade renal injuries are candidates for observation without surgical repair or nephrectomy.

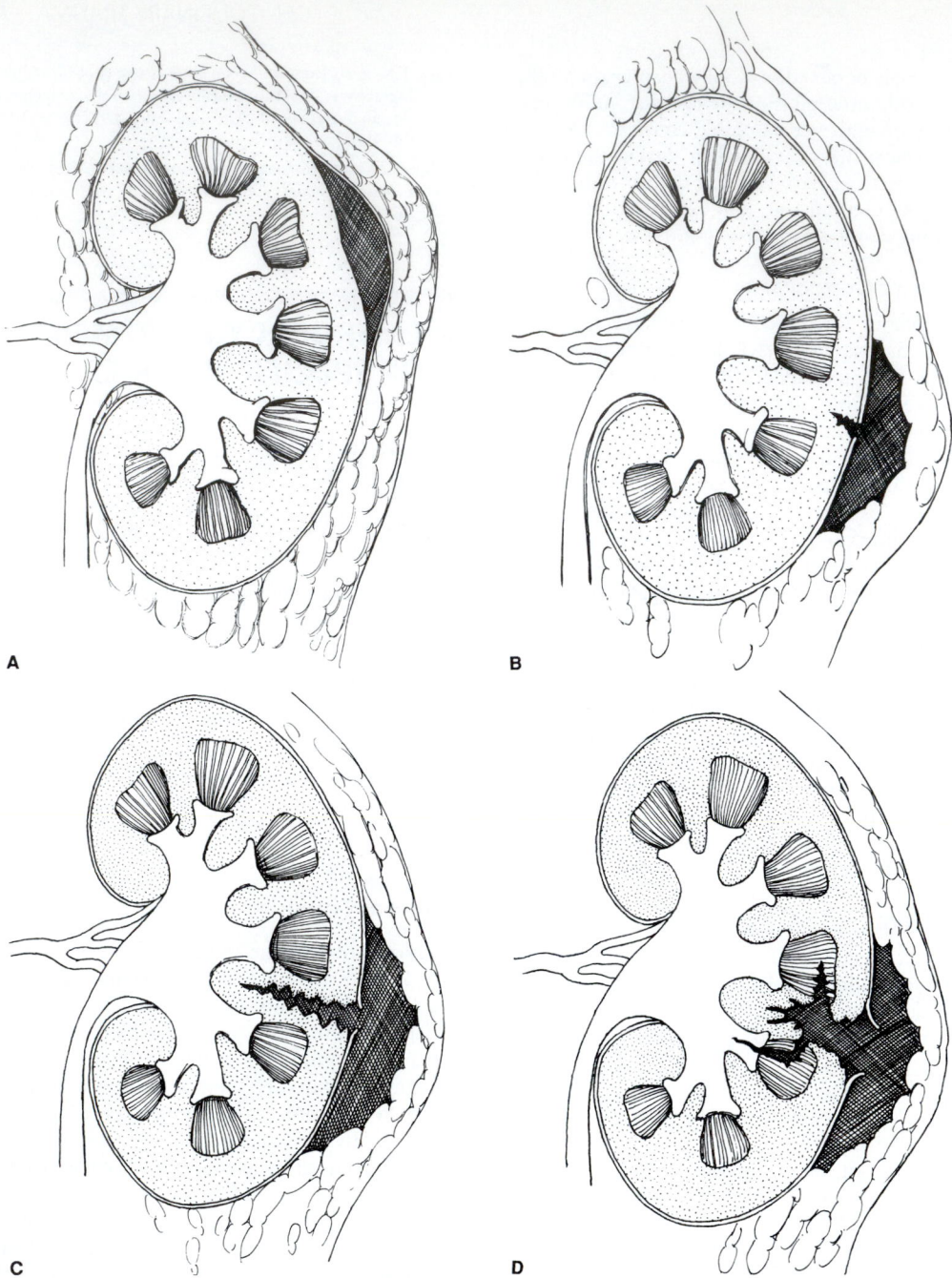

Figure 26–4. Classification of renal injuries. Grades I and II are minor. Grades III, IV, and V are major. **A:** Grade I—microscopic or gross hematuria; normal findings on radiographic studies; contusion or contained subcapsular hematoma without parenchymal laceration. **B:** Grade II—nonexpanding, confined perirenal hematoma or cortical laceration less than 1 cm deep without urinary extravasation. **C:** Grade III—parenchymal laceration extending more than 1 cm into the cortex without urinary extravasation. **D:** Grade IV—parenchymal laceration extending through the corticomedullary junction and into the collecting system. A laceration at a segmental vessel may also be present.

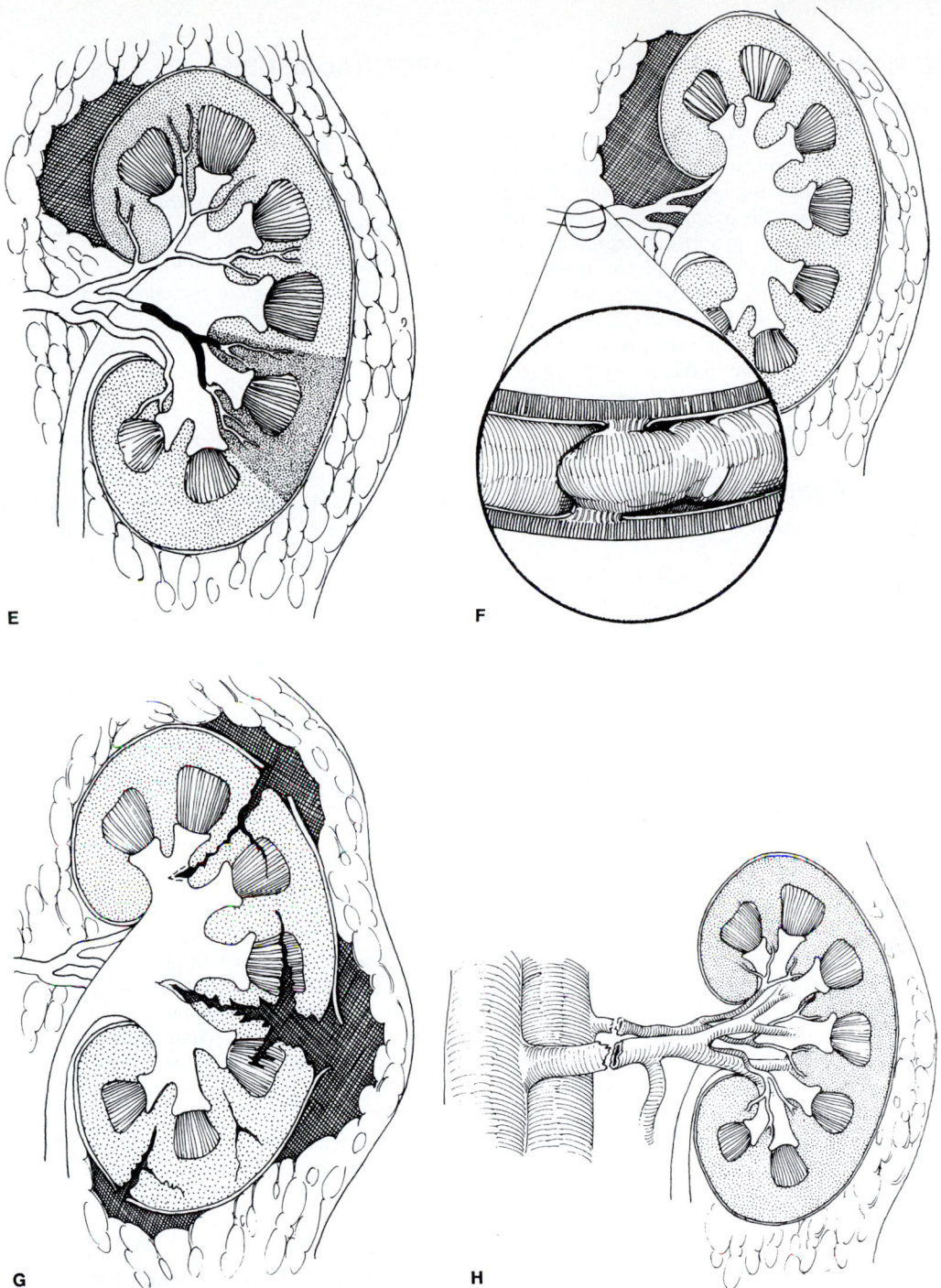

Figure 26–4, (continued). **E:** Grade IV—thrombosis of a segmental renal artery without a parenchymal laceration. Note the corresponding parenchymal ischemia. **F:** Grade V—thrombosis of the main renal artery. The inset shows the intimal tear and distal thrombosis. **G:** Grade V—multiple major lacerations, resulting in a "shattered" kidney. **H:** Grade V—avulsion of the main renal artery and/or vein. (Reproduced, with permission, from Tanagho EA, McAninch JW: *Smith's General Urology,* 16th ed. McGraw-Hill, 2004.)

Clinical Findings

A. Symptoms and Signs

Pain may be localized to one flank or over the abdomen, but visceral injury or pelvic fracture may obscure symptoms of renal injury. Nausea and vomiting, flank ecchymosis, lower rib fractures, or lumbar vertebral (especially transverse process) fractures may be noted. Urologic injury should be suspected in any penetrating wound to the flank or whose trajectory potentially crosses the paravertebral gutter. Extensive blood loss and shock may result from retroperitoneal bleeding. A palpable mass may indicate retroperitoneal hematoma or urinoma. If the retroperitoneum has been torn, hemoperitoneum will cause diffuse abdominal tenderness and ileus.

B. Laboratory Findings

Hematuria may or may not be present.

C. Imaging

The study of choice is helical CT scan of the abdomen and pelvis with intravenous contrast and immediate as well as delayed images (Figure 26–5). Under no circumstances should imaging delay necessary operative intervention. Surgical exploration should replace radiographic imaging in unstable patients who require immediate surgery. IVP is useful for diagnosing major renal injuries, although it will miss some smaller contusions and renal lacerations.

Treatment

Renal contusions (85% of blunt trauma renal injuries) and minor renal lacerations (12% of such injuries) can be managed expectantly and rarely require operative intervention. Outpatient urology follow-up is necessary to ensure that hematuria has cleared. Major lacerations (3% of blunt trauma renal injuries) may require operative intervention, although the trend is to manage these injuries conservatively when possible. Renal pedicle injuries, representing 1–2% of blunt injuries, often result in nephrectomy. Penetrating renal trauma usually requires surgical intervention. Absolute indications for surgical exploration include uncontrollable renal hemorrhage and shattered kidney or avulsion of the main renal vessels.

Goldman SM, Sandler CM: Upper urinary tract trauma—current concepts. World J Urol 1998;16:62. [PMID: 9542017]

Matthew LA, Smith EM, Spirnak JP: Nonoperative treatment of major blunt renal lacerations with urinary extravasation. J Urol 1997;157:2056. [PMID: 9146579]

Mee SL et al: Radiographic assessment of renal trauma: 10-year prospective study of patient selection. J Urol 1989;141:1095. [PMID: 2709493]

URETERAL INJURIES

 ESSENTIALS OF DIAGNOSIS

- *Usually from penetrating trauma.*
- *Patients with missed injuries may present with fever, abdominal pain, and mass.*
- *CT scan or retrograde pyelography are studies of choice.*

General Considerations

The least frequently injured portion of the genitourinary system is the ureter. The majority of these injuries (80–90%) result from penetrating trauma, although blunt trauma may cause injuries often accompanied by injuries to nonurologic systems. In children, ureteral injuries occur more commonly at the ureteropelvic junction, because of the increased mobility of the spine as well as the intra-abdominal rather than intrapelvic location of the bladder. Ureteral injuries are often diagnosed either intraoperatively or when complications arise later, because such injuries are infrequent, are difficult to diagnose, and frequently occur in the presence of other injuries.

Clinical Findings

A. Symptoms and Signs

Physical examination findings are nonspecific and usually related to associated intra-abdominal injuries, although pain similar to renal colic and a flank mass may be seen. Hematuria may be present but is often absent if complete ureteral transection has occurred. Use of intravenous indigo carmine dye during surgical exploration may help in the diagnosis of ureteral injury. Patients with a delay in diagnosis may present with abdominal pain, urinary urgency and frequency, fever, pyuria, and a palpable mass containing urine (urinoma) or blood.

B. Imaging

Both IVP and CT scan may miss ureteral injuries. If performed soon after injury and associated administration of resuscitative fluids, the extravasation of contrast from the ureter may show up only as a hazy, ground-glass appearance. If injuries are near the ureteropelvic junction, extension of fluid around the kidney may incorrectly lead to diagnosis of renal rather than ureteral injury. Because retrograde pyelography uses a more

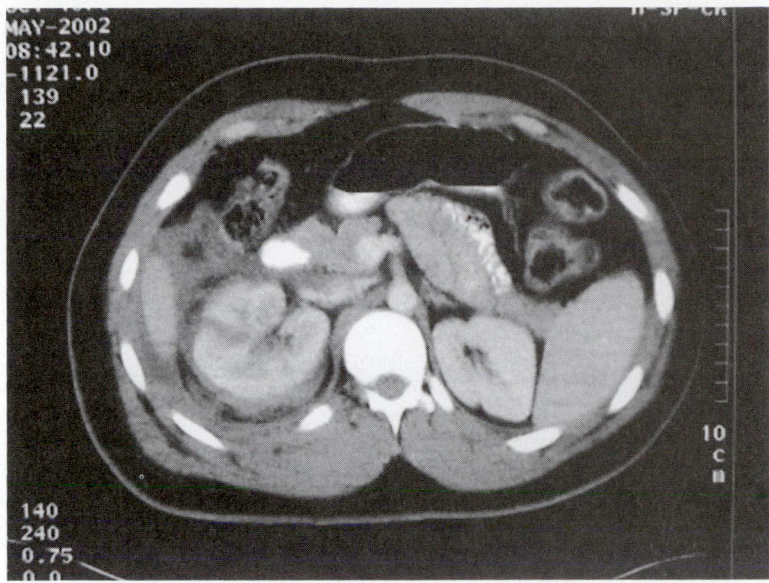

(1)

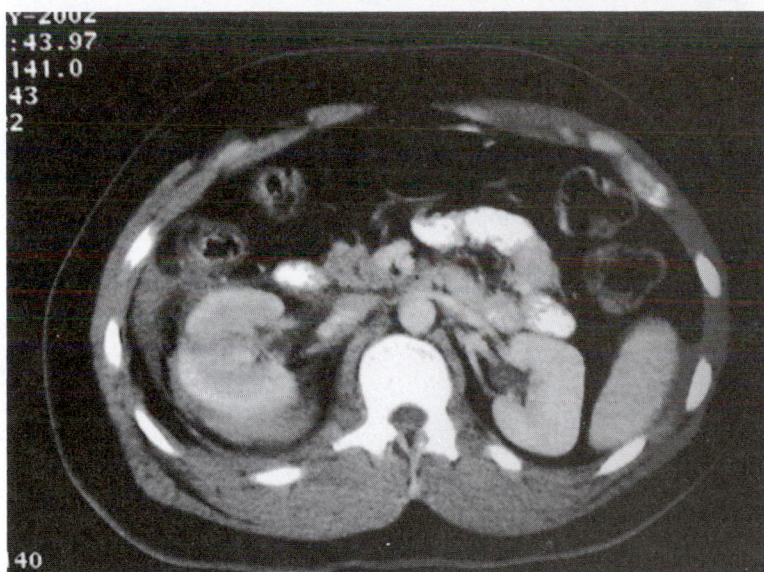

Figure 26–5. Adult blunt trauma patient with high-grade right renal laceration and perinephric hematoma. (Note the normal appearing left kidney.)

(2)

concentrated dye and fluoroscopy, this modality may pick up injuries missed by other methods.

Treatment

All ureteral injuries require operative repair. Delayed repair, although associated with increased incidence of infections, does not lead to increased rate of renal function loss.

Azimuddin K et al: Penetrating ureteric injuries. Injury 1998; 29:363. [PMID: 9813680]

Kotkin L, Brock JW: Isolated ureteral injury caused by blunt trauma. Urology 1996;47:111. [PMID: 8560642]

Medina D et al: Ureteral trauma: preoperative studies neither predict injury nor prevent missed injuries. J Am Coll Surg 1998;186:641. [PMID: 9632150]

BLADDER INJURIES

ESSENTIALS OF DIAGNOSIS

- *Usually due to blunt trauma or pelvic fractures.*
- *Gross hematuria and abdominal pain often present.*
- *Extraperitoneal rupture treated conservatively with Foley catheter.*
- *Intraperitoneal rupture requires surgical intervention.*
- *Retrograde cystogram is diagnostic study of choice.*

General Considerations

Bladder rupture most commonly occurs in association with blunt trauma and pelvic fractures, especially when the bladder is full. The rupture may occur into the intraperitoneal (Figure 26–6) or extraperitoneal space (Figure 26–7). The majority of ruptures (85%) occur into the extraperitoneal space and are often associated with pelvic fractures. Intraperitoneal ruptures are often caused by motor vehicle collisions during which a patient has a full bladder and are more likely to occur in patients with recent alcohol intake (predisposes to full bladders), women (thinner bladder musculature), and children (bladder not as protected by pelvis). Intraperitoneal bladder rupture generally occurs at the dome, the weakest area of the bladder.

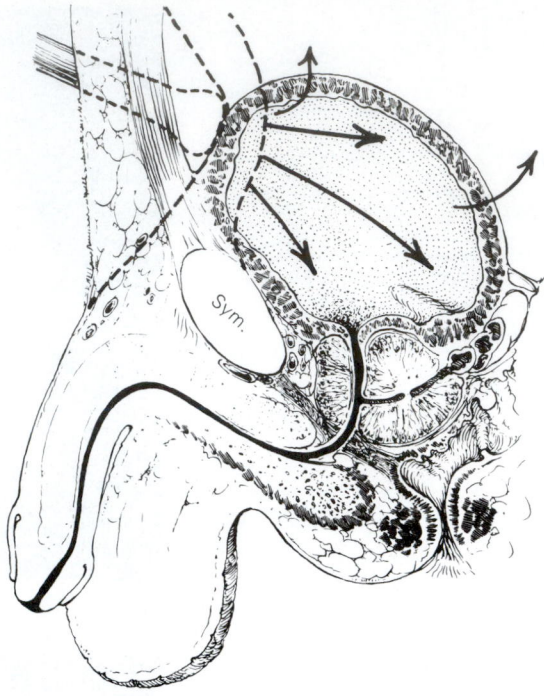

Figure 26–6. Mechanism of vesical injury. A direct blow over the full bladder causes increased intravesical pressure and intraperitoneal rupture. (Reproduced, with permission, from Tanagho EA, McAninch JW: *Smith's General Urology,* 16th ed. McGraw-Hill, 2004.)

Clinical Findings

A. SYMPTOMS AND SIGNS

Gross hematuria is the most frequent finding (98%), along with lower abdominal pain and inability to void.

B. IMAGING

Diagnosis of bladder injury is made by retrograde cystogram after urethral injury is ruled out by retrograde urethrogram. The bladder should be completely distended with 300–400 cc of water-soluble contrast material instilled through a Foley catheter. Radiographs are taken after complete distention is obtained and then repeated after the bladder has been drained completely. Intraperitoneal rupture will show contrast material extending into the abdomen, outlining loops of bowel wall with extension into the paracolic gutters. Extraperitoneal rupture will show a coarse, streaked pattern of extravasation adjacent to the bladder. A postvoid view should always be obtained and is helpful

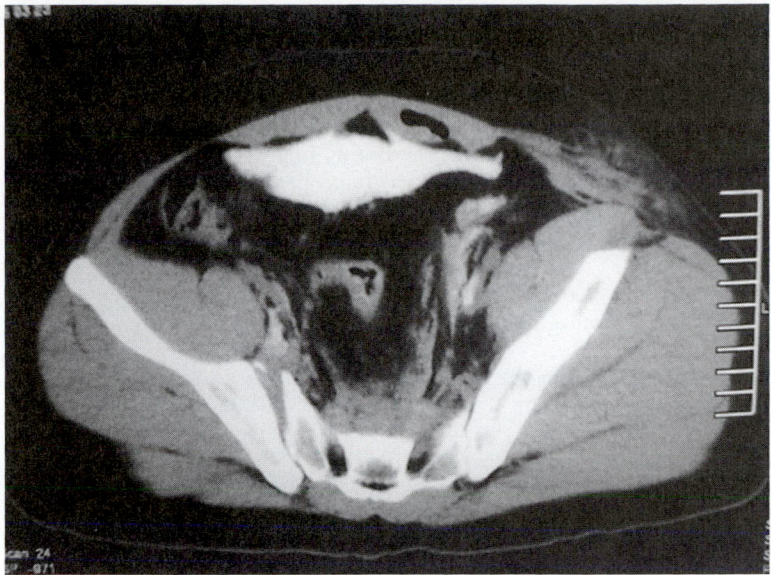

A

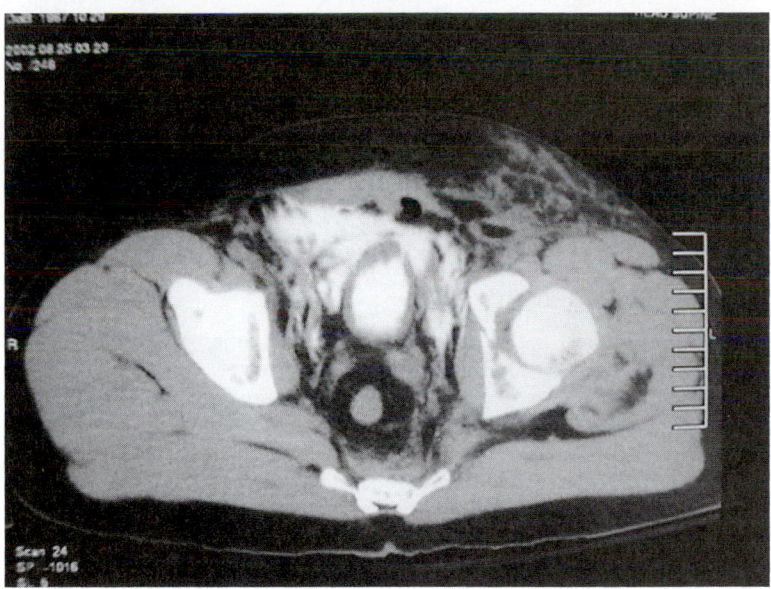

Figure 26–7. Adult blunt trauma patient with extraperitoneal bladder rupture. Note the contrast extravasation in the pelvis and along the left anterior abdominal wall. As evidence of significant pelvic trauma, note the right sacroiliac joint disruption (**A**) and the left acetabular fracture (**B**).

B

in diagnosing subtle injuries that may have been obscured on initial films.

Treatment

Intraperitoneal ruptures and all penetrating injuries to the bladder require surgical intervention. Extraperitoneal injuries can usually be managed nonsurgically with Foley catheter drainage, followed by repeat cystogram in 10–14 days. Simple contusions or incomplete lacerations can also be managed conservatively, with Foley catheter drainage and early urologic follow-up.

Ahn JH, Morey AF, McAninch: Workup and management of traumatic hematuria. Emerg Med Clin North Am 1998;16:145. [PMID: 9496319]

URETHRAL INJURIES

ESSENTIALS OF DIAGNOSIS

- *Significant injury because of frequent complications.*
- *Blood at urethral meatus and inability to void often seen.*
- *High-riding prostate on digital rectal exam.*
- *Retrograde urethrogram is best study.*

General Considerations

Urethral injuries are uncommon but are potentially the most debilitating because of the high rate of complications, such as incontinence, stricture formation, impotence, and chronic urinary tract infections. They occur most often in men secondary to blunt trauma. Urethral injuries in women are extremely rare and are usually associated with pelvic fractures.

If urethral injury is suspected, placement of a Foley catheter before a retrograde urethrogram is obtained is contraindicated, because it may cause further injury and worsen a partial tear. If a catheter has already been placed, it should not be removed, and a urethrogram should be performed around the catheter using a pediatric feeding tube and occluding the distal urethral meatus with gentle pressure on the glans.

A special injury of note is the traumatic removal of a Foley catheter, either while moving the patient or occasionally by the patient stepping on the catheter while ambulating. Significant injury can occur by this mechanism, and a urethrogram should be performed prior to reinsertion of any catheters.

1. Posterior Urethra

General Considerations

The posterior urethra, consisting of the prostatic and membranous portions, is injured most commonly during blunt trauma associated with bony pelvic injuries. The urethra is usually sheared off proximal to the urogenital diaphragm. The prostate then becomes displaced superiorly by the developing hematoma (Figure 26–8). Concomitant bladder injuries are associated with 35% of posterior urethral injuries.

Clinical Findings

A. SYMPTOMS AND SIGNS

Patients will complain of abdominal or perineal pain and an inability to void. Blood at the meatus is the most frequent sign of urethral injury. The prostate will be high-riding or boggy on rectal examination.

B. IMAGING

Retrograde urethrogram will show extravasation of contrast material superior to the urogenital diaphragm (Figure 26–9).

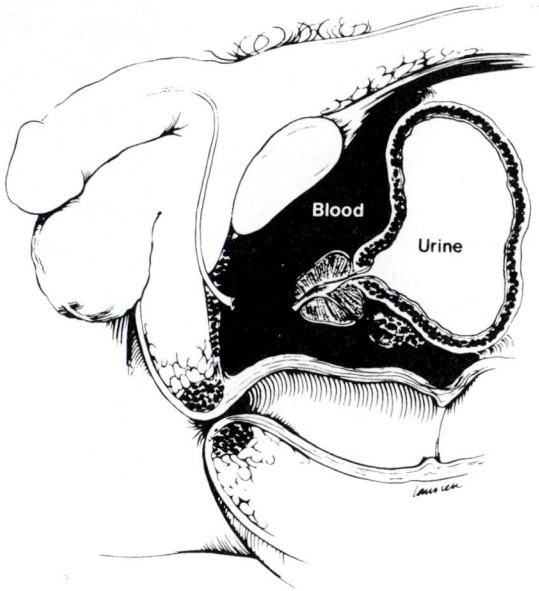

Figure 26–8. Injury to the posterior (membranous) urethra. The prostate has been avulsed from the membranous urethra secondary to fracture of the pelvis. Extravasation occurs above the triangular ligament and is periprostatic and perivesical. (Reproduced, with permission, from Tanagho EA, McAninch JW: *Smith's General Urology,* 16th ed. McGraw-Hill, 2004.)

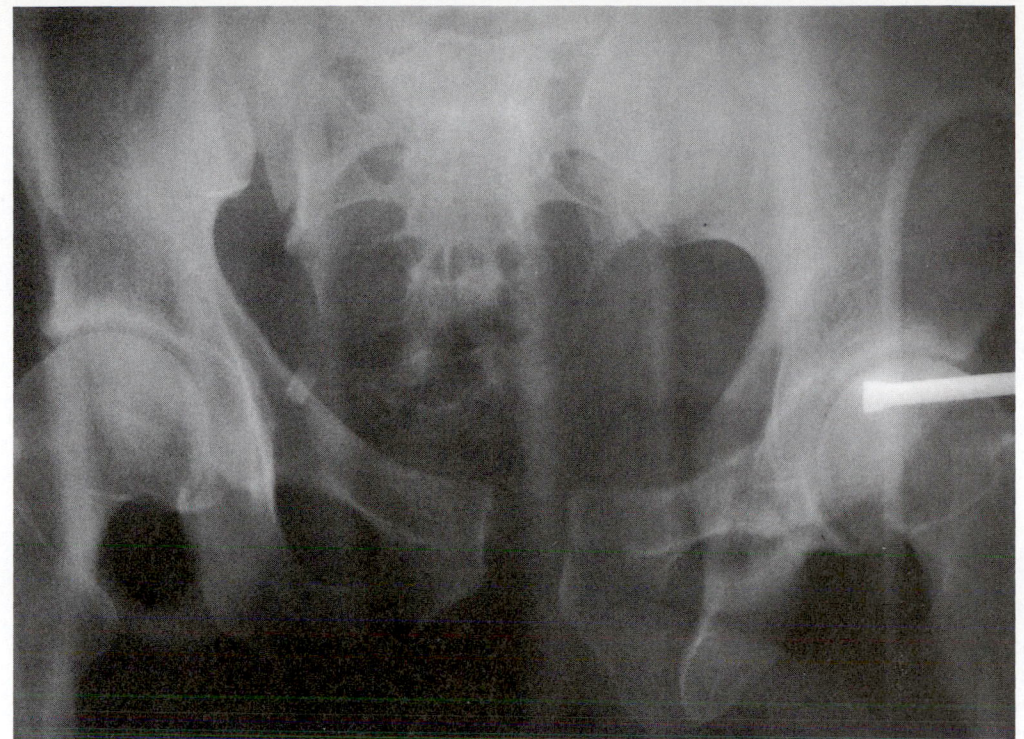

A

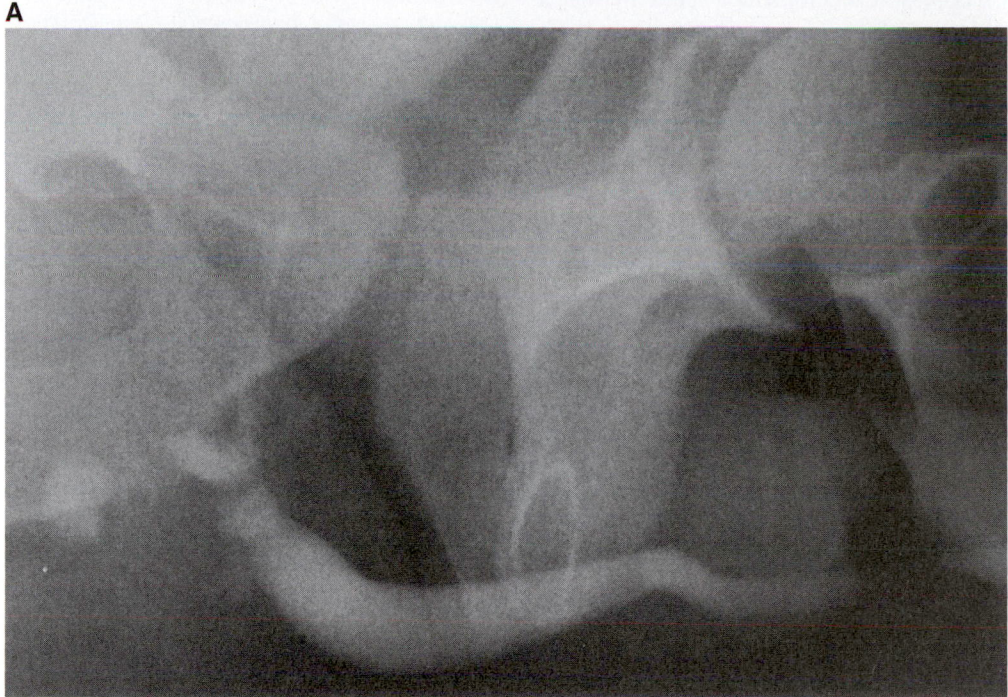

B

Figure 26–9. Adult male blunt trauma patient with prostatomembranous urethral injury. Pubic symphysis diastasis is noted (**A**). Free extravasation and failure of contrast to fill the bladder indicate a posterior urethral disruption (**B**).

Treatment

Initial management includes suprapubic cystostomy to provide urinary drainage. Definitive treatment options vary, and urologic consultation is essential.

2. Anterior Urethra

General Considerations

The anterior urethra, consisting of the bulbous and penile portions, is located below the urogenital diaphragm. Trauma to the anterior urethra is typically due to straddle injuries or a direct blow to the perineum, as well as from instrumentation or improper Foley catheter placement (Figure 26–10).

Clinical Findings

A. SYMPTOMS AND SIGNS

If Buck's fascia remains intact, extravasation of blood and urine will be confined to the penile shaft and perineum. With rupture of the Buck fascia, extravasation will extend along the abdominal wall, confined only by Colles' fascia, with resultant perineal "butterfly" hematoma.

B. IMAGING

Contrast extravasation will be seen on urethrogram (Figure 26–11).

Treatment

Long-term catheter drainage or direct reanastomosis are the most common treatment options.

Ahmed S, Neel KF: Urethral injury in girls with fractured pelvis following blunt abdominal trauma. Br J Urol 1996;78:450. [PMID: 8881960]

Boon TA, Van der Werken C: Urethral injuries revisited. Injury 1996;27:533. [PMID: 8994555]

Goldman SM et al: Blunt urethral trauma: a unified, anatomical mechanical classification. J Urol 1997;157:85. [PMID: 8976222]

Koraitim MM: Pelvic fracture urethral injuries: evaluation of various methods of management. J Urol 1996;156:1288. [PMID: 8808856]

EXTERNAL GENITAL INJURIES

ESSENTIALS OF DIAGNOSIS

- *Blunt trauma to erect penis may cause rupture with pain and deforming hematoma; evaluate for surgical repair.*
- *Blunt scrotal injuries require Doppler ultrasound studies.*
- *Genital burn injures require early Foley catheter placement to prevent edematous urethral obstruction.*

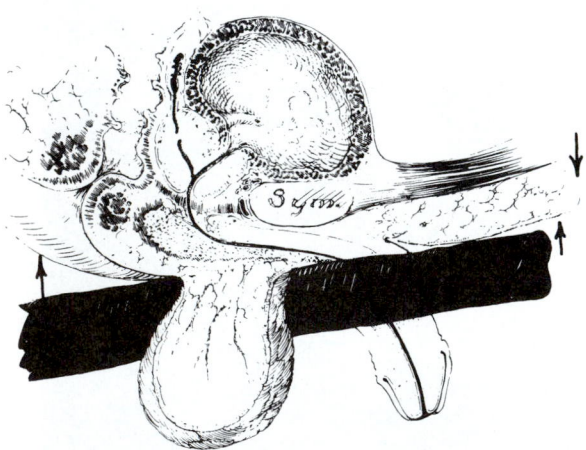
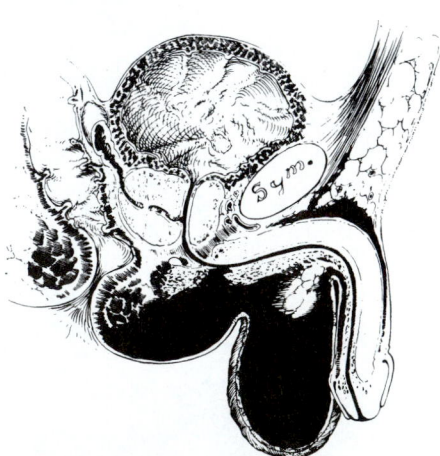

Figure 26–10. Injury to the bulbous urethra. *Left:* Mechanism: usually a perineal blow or fall astride an object; crushing of the urethra against inferior edge of pubic symphysis. *Right:* Extravasation of blood and urine enclosed within Colles' fascia. (Reproduced, with permission, from Tanagho EA, McAninch JW: *Smith's General Urology,* 13th ed. Appleton & Lange, 1992.)

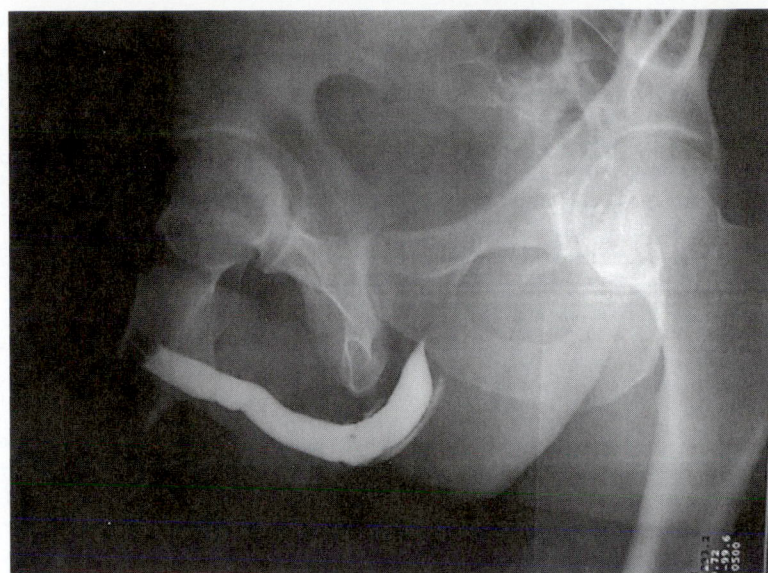

Figure 26–11. Adult male patient with straddle injury to perineum and blood at the urethral meatus. This positive retrograde urethrogram reveals extravasation in the bulbous portion of the urethra indicative of urethral injury.

• *Consider pelvic floor penetration and sexual assault with all vaginal lacerations.*

1. Penile Rupture

Penile fractures occur from blunt trauma to the erect penis causing rupture of the corpus cavernosum. The patient typically reports a loud "cracking" sound, immediate pain, and loss of erection.

Clinical Findings

A. SYMPTOMS AND SIGNS

A large hematoma will be visible on the shaft of the penis, and the axis of the shaft may be deviated.

B. IMAGING

Retrograde urethrogram may show extravasation if urethral injury is present.

Treatment

Immediate urologic consultation is indicated for surgical repair.

2. Constriction Injuries

Constriction injuries can occur from objects placed circumferentially around the penile shaft. Occasionally these injuries are from obstructive rings placed during sexual play in adults. They require immediate removal to prevent urethral injury or neurovascular compromise. In circumcised male infants, hair is a common culprit.

3. Testicular Injuries

Blunt trauma to the scrotum may result in testicular rupture by forcefully compressing the testis against the symphysis pubis or medial thigh.

Clinical Findings

A. SYMPTOMS AND SIGNS

Patients present with severe pain, nausea, vomiting, and extensive swelling due to hematoma formation, all of which make testicular examination difficult.

B. IMAGING

The diagnostic study of choice is ultrasound examination with Doppler flow studies.

Treatment

Simple hematomas can be managed conservatively with scrotal elevation and sitz baths. Larger hematomas may require surgical drainage. Testicular rupture and penetrating injuries should be explored and repaired surgically.

4. Skin Injuries

A degloving injury usually requires extensive surgical debridement and repair, and may require skin grafting. With zipper injuries, the trapped skin can be released by cutting the sliding portion of the zipper. Scrotal lacerations can be repaired in a layered fashion once testicular injury has been ruled out. Burn injuries deserve special consideration because of the massive edema that may develop, resulting in urethral obstruction. A urethral or suprapubic catheter should be placed early during the initial resuscitative phase.

5. Female Genital Injuries

If vaginal bleeding is present, perform a speculum examination to evaluate for vaginal lacerations in addition to any injuries noted to the external genitalia. Simple lacerations can be repaired using absorbable sutures. If unable to obtain hemostasis, operative repair is indicated. In all vaginal lacerations, it is important to rule out penetration of the pelvic floor, which may indicate significant organ and vascular damage. The possibility of sexual assault must always be considered, and follow-up with a gynecologist is recommended.

Goldman HB, Dmochowski RR, Cox CE: Penetrating trauma to the penis: functional results. J Urol 1996;155:551. [PMID: 8558658]

Goldman HB, Idom CB Jr, Dmochowski RR: Traumatic injuries of the female external genitalia and their association with urological injuries. J Urol 1998;159:956. [PMID: 9474191]

Kadish HA, Schunk JE, Britton H: Pediatric male rectal and genital trauma: accidental and nonaccidental injuries. Pediatr Emerg Care 1998;14:95. [PMID: 9583387]

Pantuck AJ, Kraus SL, Barone JG: Hair strangulation injury of the penis. Pediatr Emerg Care 1997;13:423. [PMID: 9435009]

Vertebral Column & Spinal Cord Trauma

27

Robert Casey Wilson, MD, & Louis J. Kroot, MD[1]

Immediate Management of the Patient with Suspected Spinal Injury

Further Evaluation of the Patient with Spinal Injury

Emergency Treatment of Specific Spinal Injuries

Vertebral Fractures without Spinal Cord Injury

Spinal Cord Injury with or without Vertebral Fractures

Whiplash (Hyperextension) Injuries (Cervical Spine Sprain)

■ IMMEDIATE MANAGEMENT OF THE PATIENT WITH SUSPECTED SPINAL INJURY

Suspect Spinal Cord Injury

Patients with blunt head injury or multiple injuries from blunt or penetrating trauma should be assumed to have cervical or thoracolumbar spine injuries until proved otherwise, unless they are fully alert and have no evidence of midline tenderness, focal neurologic defect, intoxication, or painful, distracting injury.

Immobilize Vertebral Spine

Immobilization of the vertebral spine is essential to prevent further injury to the spinal cord.

A. SUPINE POSITION

Optimal immobilization is obtained by placing the patient supine (face up) on a firm, flat surface (eg, rigid, long spine board) without a pillow and with lateral motion of the neck restricted by a rigid cervical collar (Philadelphia) and lateral neck rolls connected with tape across the forehead.

B. LATERAL POSITION

If the patient cannot lie supine for any reason (eg, vomiting), the lateral position with careful in-line cervical stabilization is acceptable. This immobilization should be maintained throughout resuscitation procedures, physical examination, and x-ray evaluation.

C. TECHNIQUE FOR MOVING THE PATIENT

If the patient must be moved, in-line spinal stabilization should be maintained and the head and trunk lifted or rolled as one unit (logroll).

Establish Airway & Maintain Ventilation

(See also Chapter 8.) Airway obstruction may be manifested by gurgling or sonorous respirations, ineffective respiration (chest movement without movement of air), apnea, or cyanosis. High cervical cord transection (above C2 or C3) results in apnea due to intercostal muscle and diaphragmatic paralysis; cervical cord transection (above C6) or injury at a lower level may still result in respiratory failure because of intercostal muscle weakness or paralysis.

Note: Neck alignment and immobility must be maintained during attempts to establish adequate ventilation.

A. GENERAL MEASURES

Using a tonsil tip sucker, clear mouth and upper airway of obvious foreign material. Position the head in neutral position, avoiding motion of the cervical spine. Insert nasal or oropharyngeal airway.

Provide supplemental oxygen by nasal cannula or mask if the patient is breathing, or support respiration with bag-mask combination (with supplemental oxygen) if hypoventilation is suspected.

Measure arterial blood gases as soon as possible to assess adequacy of ventilation, and monitor oxygen saturation using pulse oximetry, if available. Both the in-

---

[1]This chapter is a revision of the chapter by Henry M. Bartkowski, MD, PhD, from the 4th edition.

tercostal muscles and the diaphragm contribute to normal ventilation. In patients with cervical spinal cord injuries, loss of the intercostal muscle innervation may cause patients to tire easily, causing ineffective ventilation and progressively worsening hypoxemia and hypercapnia. Repeated arterial blood gas measurements are therefore essential to monitor any changes in ventilatory status.

B. ENDOTRACHEAL INTUBATION

If the measures described above fail to provide adequate ventilation or if hypoventilation or apnea is present, perform endotracheal intubation (Chapter 6). Endotracheal intubation should also be considered for airway control in the unconscious or obtunded patient with depressed gag and cough reflexes even if ventilation is adequate. If severe neck injury is accompanied by tracheal laceration, the trachea may be intubated directly through the wound.

When patients with suspected cervical spinal injuries require an emergent definitive airway, perform oral endotracheal intubation with in-line cervical immobilization. Designate an assistant to maintain this immobilization from the time the cervical collar is removed until it is replaced after the endotracheal tube has been taped in place. In general, rapid sequence intubation (unless contraindicated [Chapter 8]) is preferred as the least traumatic and most efficient method of achieving intubation. Cadaver studies have shown no significant movement of the cervical spine during orotracheal intubation using in-line cervical stabilization in contrast to simple cervical collar immobilization, in which significant movement occurs.

Nasotracheal intubation is an option only in the spontaneously ventilating patient. Because it is a blind technique, it occurs under less controlled intubating conditions that may predispose to emesis in patients with high likelihood of ileus or gastric atony. If time allows, fiberoptic intubation is a good alternative nontraumatic method in experienced hands.

C. CRICOTHYROTOMY

Rarely, in a patient with severe craniofacial trauma resulting in distorted normal anatomic relationships, it may be impossible to establish an orotracheal or nasotracheal airway. Also, conventional means of intubation are sometimes unsuccessful in the otherwise normal patient. In such cases, direct intubation of the trachea through cricothyrotomy or tracheostomy is indicated (Chapter 6).

D. SUCTIONING OF SECRETIONS

Patients with weak intercostal or diaphragmatic muscles cannot produce a strong cough and are therefore predisposed to progressive airway obstruction without any change in neurologic deficit. Frequent suctioning should be performed. An endotracheal airway may be required for patients with voluminous secretions.

Treat Pneumothorax & Tension Pneumothorax

See Chapter 24.

Establish Satisfactory Circulation

A. CARDIAC ARREST

If no pulse is detected, begin cardiopulmonary resuscitation (Chapter 7).

B. SHOCK OR HYPOTENSION

(See Chapter 9.) Shock (cool, pale skin; hypotension; abnormal mentation) or hypotension (systolic blood pressure < 90 mm Hg in an adult) may be due either to poor sympathetic tone below the level of the spinal cord lesion or to hypovolemia from other injuries. In most instances, hypovolemia is the cause. Sources of hypovolemia include hemorrhage into several compartments, such as the chest and the pelvis (evaluated by portable chest x-ray and anteroposterior view of the pelvis), the abdomen (evaluated by a focused assessment with sonography for trauma [FAST] exam [Chapters 6, 9, and 25], diagnostic peritoneal lavage [DPL], or computed tomography [CT] scan of the abdomen), or the femur (hemorrhage is usually obvious clinically). If open wounds are present, significant external hemorrhage may have occurred at the scene of the injury.

1. Hypovolemia—(See Chapter 9.) Insert 2 or more large-bore (≥ 16-gauge) intravenous catheters in an upper extremity; obtain blood for hematocrit, typing and cross-matching, electrolyte determinations, and renal function tests; and begin intravenous infusion of crystalloid solution to support blood pressure. Up to 3 L of crystalloid solution may be given before blood is required. *Caution:* Exercise care in fluid replacement, because patients with spinal cord injuries are at greater risk of heart failure than normal individuals.

If hypotension or shock is not quickly corrected by these methods, search for bleeding from other injuries (Chapter 10).

2. Poor sympathetic tone—Keep the patient supine and horizontal. Blood pressure in the normovolemic patient with spinal injury is usually normal as long as the patient is supine, because minimal sympathetic tone is required in this position. The use of low-dose dopamine, 5–10 µg/kg/min, may be necessary if no other source of hypotension has been identified and poor sympathetic tone is responsible for persistent hypotension despite supine patient positioning and crystalloid infusion.

C. Normal Blood Pressure

Avoid excess fluid administration, which may increase spinal cord swelling or precipitate heart failure.

D. Hypertension

Although hypertension is rarely caused by spinal cord injury itself, the resulting bladder or bowel distention and subsequent autonomic discharge of the mass reflex may cause hypertension. Rule out more likely causes, such as severe head injury or drug ingestion, before attributing hypertension to an injured spinal cord.

E. Head Injuries

Patients with altered mental status, seizures, or cranial nerve or other focal neurologic deficits require emergent imaging of the brain after the initial assessment and stabilization of the ABCs. A noncontrast CT scan of the head is the study of choice to identify intracranial injuries. If the patient has only a history of loss of consciousness and is alert and oriented in the emergency department, head CT scan can be delayed and accomplished in conjunction with other CT scans that may be required to evaluate the patient with possible spinal injury.

Minimize Neurologic Injury

A. Reduce Spinal Cord Swelling

Corticosteroids are useful in early treatment of spinal cord injury from blunt trauma, but only if begun within the first 8 hours after injury. Give methylprednisolone, 30 mg/kg as an intravenous bolus over 15 minutes; after a 45-minute delay, begin a maintenance infusion of 5.4 mg/kg/h for 24 hours in patients receiving treatment within the first 3 hours after injury. Patients receiving treatment 3–8 hours after injury should be maintained on steroid therapy for 48 hours. Initiation of steroid treatment greater than 8 hours after injury is probably of limited value and may increase morbidity and mortality secondary to nosocomial infections. Because of the often-limited information regarding time of injury in the initial emergency department evaluation, therapy should be instituted until injury time has been confirmed. Obtain neurosurgical consultation as soon as possible. Steroids play no role in the treatment of penetrating spinal cord injuries.

B. Give Antibiotics for Penetrating Injuries

Patients with penetrating spinal cord injury (eg, gunshot wound) should receive prophylactic antimicrobials. Nafcillin, 200 mg/kg/d intravenously in 4–6 divided doses, is widely recommended.

Treat Complications

A. Urinary Incontinence or Retention

Patients may not note bladder dysfunction after spinal trauma because of loss of sensation below the lesion. Insert an indwelling catheter whenever spinal trauma is verified, to prevent urinary retention and to aid in monitoring urine output.

B. Ileus

Paralytic ileus and gastric atony are common after spinal trauma. Give the patient nothing by mouth, and insert a nasogastric tube connected to intermittent low-pressure suction.

Take Additional Measures as Needed

A patient with spinal cord injury requires the same resuscitative measures customarily employed in major trauma. Insert an intravenous catheter and administer fluids and blood as required. Patients with spinal cord injury are particularly susceptible to exposure and should be covered with warm blankets in the emergency department to prevent hypothermia.

Perform a baseline laboratory evaluation, including complete blood count (CBC) with platelet estimate, coagulation panel, serum electrolyte concentrations, renal function tests, blood glucose concentration, blood typing and cross-matching, and urinalysis.

Treat other injuries. Evaluate and treat head injury and life-threatening conditions (eg, tension pneumothorax, cardiac tamponade, hemorrhagic shock) that take precedence over definitive treatment of vertebral and spinal cord trauma (Chapter 10). Maintain in-line spinal immobilization during resuscitation and treatment. If feasible, obtain cervical spine x-rays (anteroposterior and lateral) when the patient's condition permits. Even if no fractures are apparent, the spine may be unstable due to severe ligamentous injury. Maintain in-line immobilization until the patient can be reexamined free of distracting injury, intoxicants, or altered mental status.

Bracken MB et al: Administration of methylprednisolone for 24 or 48 hours or tirilazad mesylate for 48 hours in the treatment of acute spinal cord injury. JAMA 1997;277:1597. [PMID: 9168289]

Frohna WJ: Emergency department evaluation and treatment of the neck and cervical spine injuries. Emerg Med Clin North Am 1999;17:739. [PMID: 10584102]

Gerling MC et al: Effects of cervical spine immobilization technique and laryngoscope blade selection on an unstable cervical spine in a cadaver model for intubation. Ann Emerg Med 2000;36:293. [PMID: 11020675]

Goldberg W et al: Distribution and patterns of blunt traumatic cervical spine injury. Ann Emerg Med 2001;38:17. [PMID: 11423806]

■ FURTHER EVALUATION OF THE PATIENT WITH SPINAL INJURY

History

Patients with spinal cord injuries can usually provide an accurate history of the injury. For example, auto collisions often result in cervical spine injuries that are frequently associated with head injuries; people who fall from heights often land on their feet and sustain fractures of the feet, hips, thoracolumbar spine; and so on.

Complaints of back or neck pain should arouse a suspicion of spine injury. Stretching of the neck muscles, larynx, or esophagus in a hyperextension injury similar to whiplash may cause neck muscle pain and tenderness, hoarseness, or dysphagia. However, the absence of spinal pain does not eliminate the possibility of spinal injury, especially if the patient is under the influence of alcohol or other mind-altering drugs. Consider spinal injury in any patient with blunt head injury; a neurologic deficit anatomically consistent with injury at a particular spinal level; or a penetrating injury to the neck, chest, or abdomen.

General Physical Examination

A brief general physical examination should precede specific assessment of neurologic function. Obtain complete vital signs, including core temperature.

Carefully examine the head, chest, heart, abdomen, and extremities for other abnormalities. Remember that patients with spinal cord injuries may show few if any signs or symptoms of coexisting major injury because of anesthesia below the level of the lesion. Pain, guarding, rebound tenderness, and other signs may be absent despite the presence of fractured ribs, hemothorax, hemoperitoneum, peritonitis, and other major injuries. Examination of the genitals, rectum, and perineum may reveal priapism, decreased or absent rectal sphincter tone, or perineal sensation suggestive of spinal cord injury. Diligent, repeated examinations and laboratory tests (eg, CBC with differential, FAST exam, abdominal CT scan, DPL) are necessary to detect unsuspected injury.

Gently but thoroughly examine the neck and spine for deformity, edema, ecchymosis, muscle spasm, or tenderness indicating possible vertebral fracture; a palpable defect in the posterior neck ligaments may be the only clue to major spinal injury.

Neurologic Examination

The emergency department neurologic examination for spinal trauma must be more thorough than that for head injury, although the complete trauma evaluation and initial assessment of the Glasgow Coma Scale score remain mainstays of the evaluation (Chapter 10). Neurologic examination assesses the following functions: mentation, motor function, sensation, and brain-stem and spinal reflexes.

A. MENTATION

The spectrum of mentation includes all levels of consciousness ranging from alert to comatose:

1. An alert patient demonstrates an immediate and appropriate response to all external stimuli.
2. A patient in coma fails to respond normally to any external stimuli, including deep pain.
3. Gradation between these extremes is best described by specific responses to specific questions or sensory stimuli, for example, "Patient is sleepy but arouses to loud voice. Knows name and location, but not time or reason for being in the hospital." Avoid vague terms to describe states of consciousness (eg, obtunded, semicoma, semistupor, lethargy) in individual patients, because these terms may be subjective and less reliable, particularly when repeated examinations are performed by different people.

B. MOTOR FUNCTION

(See Tables 27–1 to 27–3.) Movement of extremities should be carefully assessed and graded as follows:

1. Normal movement means that the patient moves all extremities spontaneously, purposefully (ie, in response to specific commands), and with full strength and range of motion.
2. Paralysis denotes no movement of the extremity or muscle group, either spontaneously or in response to painful stimuli. (Stimuli should be applied both directly to the extremity and to the trunk, because failure to move may be secondary to hypesthesia of the extremity.) Failure to move at all, either spontaneously or in response to an unpleasant stimulus, may indicate paralysis due to a structural lesion (eg, fracture) or metabolic causes (eg, drug overdose). Often, failure to respond is simply due to an inadequately painful stimulus.
3. Gradation between these extremes should be described precisely, for example, "Patient extends right arm and leg, flexes left arm, and extends left leg in response to supraorbital pressure." Avoid broad descriptive terms such as "paraparesis" or "decerebrate posturing." Grade muscle strength from 0 (no movement) to 5 (full strength).

Table 27–1. Segmental motor innervation: upper extremity.[1]

Region	Muscle	C4	C5	C6	C7	C8	T1
Shoulder	Supraspinatus	----	----	----			
	Teres minor	----	----				
	Deltoid		----	----	----		
	Infraspinatus		----	----			
	Subscapularis		----	----	----		
	Teres major		----	----	----		
Arm	Biceps		----	----			
	Brachialis		----	----			
	Coracobrachialis		----	----	----		
	Triceps brachialis			----	----	----	
	Anconeus				----	----	
Forearm	Supinator longus		----	----			
	Supinator brevis		----	----	----		
	Extensor carpi radialis			----	----	----	
	Pronator teres			----	----		
	Flexor carpi radialis			----	----		
	Flexor pollicis longus				----	----	----
	Abductor pollicis longus				----	----	
	Extensor pollicis brevis			----	----	----	
	Extensor digitorum longus			----	----	----	
	Extensor indicis proprius			----	----	----	
	Extensor carpi ulnaris			----	----	----	
	Extensor digiti quinti			----	----	----	
Hand	Flexor digitorum sublimis				----	----	----
	Flexor digitorum profundus				----	----	----
	Pronator quadratus				----	----	----
	Flexor carpi ulnaris				----	----	----
	Palmaris longus				----	----	
	Abductor pollicis brevis			----	----	----	----
	Flexor pollicis brevis			----	----	----	
	Opponens pollicis				----	----	----
	Flexor digiti quinti			----	----	----	
	Opponens digiti quiniti			----	----	----	----
	Adductor pollicis					----	----
	Palmaris brevis					----	----
	Adductor digiti quinti				----	----	----
	Lumbricales					----	----
	Interossei					----	----

[1]Reproduced, with permission, from Chusid JG: *Correlative Neuroanatomy & Functional Neurology,* 19th ed. Lange, 1985.

4. Psychogenic paralysis rarely enters into the differential diagnosis of paralysis associated with trauma. See Chapter 16 for distinguishing features.

C. SENSATION

(See Figures 27–1 and 27–2 and Table 27–4.) Test as many sensory functions as possible in a patient with suspected spinal cord injury (in contrast to the more simple examination required for head trauma). Loss of some or all sensory functions below the lesion permits its precise anatomic localization. Perianal sensation should be tested; its presence eliminates the possibility of complete spinal cord transection and implies an improved prognosis.

1. Position, vibration, and light touch—The dorsal columns can be tested by determining response to vibration, light touch, and changes in position.

2. Pain and temperature—The ventral columns are tested by evaluating sensitivity to pain (pinprick) and temperature.

Table 27–2. Segmental motor innervation: lower extremity.[1]

	Muscle	L1	L2	L3	L4	L5	S1	S2
Hip	Iliopsoas	—	—	—				
	Tensor fasciae latae				—	—		
	Gluteus medius				—	—	—	
	Gluteus minimus				—	—	—	
	Quadratus femoris				—	—	—	
	Gemellus inferior				—	—	—	
	Gemellus superior					—	—	
	Gluteus maximus					—	—	—
	Obturator internus					—	—	
	Piriformis					—	—	
Thigh	Sartorius		—	—				
	Pectineus		—	—				
	Adductor longus		—	—				
	Quadriceps femoris		—	—	—			
	Gracilis		—	—	—			
	Adductor brevis		—	—	—			
	Obturator extemus			—	—			
	Adductor magnus			—	—			
	Adductor minimus			—	—			
	Semitendinosus				—	—	—	
	Semimembranosus				—	—	—	
	Biceps femoris				—	—	—	—
Leg	Tibialis anticus				—	—		
	Extensor hallucis longus				—	—		
	Popliteus				—	—	—	
	Plantaris				—	—	—	
	Extensor digitorum longus				—	—	—	
	Soleus					—	—	—
	Gastrocnemius					—	—	—
	Peroneus longus				—	—	—	
	Peroneus brevis				—	—	—	
	Tibialis posterior				—	—		
	Flexor digitorum longus					—	—	
	Flexor hallucis longus					—	—	
Foot	Extensor hallucis brevis				—	—	—	
	Extensor digitorum brevis				—	—	—	
	Flexor digitorum brevis					—	—	
	Abductor hallucis					—	—	
	Flexor hallucis brevis					—	—	—
	Lumbricales					—	—	—
	Adductor hallucis						—	—
	Adductor digiti quinti						—	—
	Flexor digiti quinti						—	—
	Opponens digiti quinti						—	—
	Quadratus plantaris						—	—
	Interossei						—	—

[1]Reproduced, with permission, from Chusid JG: *Correlative Neuroanatomy & Functional Neurology,* 19th ed. Lange, 1985.

Table 27–3. Motor function chart.[1]

Action to Be Tested	Muscle	Cord Segment	Nerves	Plexus
Shoulder Girdle and Upper Extremity				
Flexion of neck	Deep neck muscles (sternocleidomastoid and trapezius also participate)	C1–4	Cervical	Cervical
Extension of neck				
Rotation of neck				
Lateral bending of neck				
Elevation of upper thorax	Scaleni	C3–5	Phrenic	
Inspiration	Diaphragm			
Adduction of arm from behind to front	Pectoralis major and minor	C5–8, T1	Pectoral (thoracic; from medial and lateral cords of plexus)	Brachial
Forward thrust of shoulder	Seratus anterios	C5–7	Long thoracic	
Elevation of scapula	Levator scapulae	C3–5	Dorsal scapular	
Medial adduction and elevation of scapula	Rhomboids	C4, 5		
Abduction of arm	Supraspinatus	C4–6	Suprascapular	
Lateral rotation of arm	Infraspinatus	C4–6		
Medial rotation of arm	Latissimus dorsi, teres major, and subscapularis	C5–8	Subscapular (from posterior cord of plexus)	
Adduction of arm from front to back				
Abduction of arm	Deltoid	C5, 6	Axillary (from posterior cord of plexus)	
Lateral rotation of arm	Teres minor	C4, 5		
Flexion of forearm	Biceps brachii	C5, 6	Musculocutaneous (from lateral cord of plexus)	
Supination of forearm				
Adduction of arm	Coracobrachialis	C5–7		
Flexion of forearm				
Flexion of forearm	Brachialis	C5, 6		
Ulnar flexion of hand	Flexor carpi ulnaris	C7, 8; T1	Ulnar (from medial cord of plexus)	
Flexion of all fingers but thumb	Flexor digitorum profundus (ulnar portion)	C7, 8; T1		
Adduction of metacarpal of thumb	Adductor pollicis	C8, T1		
Abduction of little finger	Abductor digiti quinti	C8, T1		
Opposition of little finger	Opponens digiti quinti	C7, 8; T1		
Flexion of little finger	Flexor digiti quinti	C7, 8; T1		
Flexion of proximal phalanx, extension of 2 distal phalanges, adduction and abduction of fingers	Interossei	C8, T1		

(continued)

Table 27–3. Motor function chart.[1] (Continued)

Action to Be Tested	Muscle	Cord Segment	Nerves	Plexus
Shoulder Girdle and Upper Extremity (cont.)				
Pronation of forearm	Pronator teres	C6, 7	Median (C6, 7 from lateral cord of plexus; C8, T1 from medial cord of plexus)	
Radial flexion of hand	Flexor carpi radialis	C6, 7		
Flexion of hand	Palmaris longus	C7, 8; T1		
Flexion of middle phalanx of index, middle, ring, or little finger	Flexor digitorum superficialis	C7, 8; T1		
Flexion of hand				
Flexion of terminal phalanx of thumb	Flexor pollicis longus	C7, 8; T1		
Flexion of terminal phalanx of index or middle finger	Flexor digitorum profundus (radial portion)	C7, 8; T1		
Flexion of hand				
Abduction of metacarpal of thumb	Abductor pollicis brevis	C7, 8; T1	Median (C7, 8 from lateral cord of plexus; C8, T1 from medial cord of plexus)	Brachial
Flexion of proximal phalanx of thumb	Flexor pollicis brevis	C7, 8; T1		
Opposition of matacarpal of thumb	Opponens pollicis	C8, T1		
Flexion of proximal phalanx and extension of the 2 distal phalanges of index, middle, ring, or little finger	Lumbricales (the 2 lateral)	C8, T1	Ulnar	
	Lumbricales (the 2nd medial)	C8, T1		
Extension of forearm	Triceps brachii and anconeus	C6–8	Radial (from posterior cord of plexus)	
Flexion of forearm	Brachioradialis	C5, 6		
Radial extension of hand	Extensor carpi radialis	C6–8		
Extension of phalanges of index, middle, ring, or little finger	Extensor digitorum	C7–8		
Extension of hand				
Extension of phalanges of little finger	Extensor digiti quinti proprius	C6–8		
Extension of hand				
Ulnar extension of hand	Extensor carpi ulnaris	C6–8		
Supination of forearm	Supinator	C5–7	Radial (from posterior cord of plexus)	
Abduction of metacarpal of thumb	Abductor pollicis longus	C7, 8; T1		
Radial extension of hand				
Extension of thumb	Extensor pollicis brevis	C7, 8		
Radial extension of hand	Extensor pollicis longus	C6–8		
Extension of index finger	Extensor indicis proprius	C6–8		
Extension of hand				

(continued)

Table 27–3. Motor function chart.[1] (Continued)

Action to Be Tested	Muscle	Cord Segment	Nerves	Plexus
Trunk and Thorax				
Elevation of ribs	Thoracic, abdominal, and back	T1–L3	Thoracic and posterior lumbosacral branches	Brachial
Depression of ribs				
Contraction of abdomen				
Anteroflexion of trunk				
Lateral flexion of trunk				
Hip Girdle and Lower Extremity				
Flexion of hip	Iliopsoas	L1–3	Femoral	Lumbar
Flexion of hip (and eversion of thigh)	Sartorius	L2, 3		
Extension of leg	Quadriceps femoris	L2–4		
Adduction of thigh	Pectineus	L2, 3	Obturator	
	Adductor longus	L2, 3		
	Adductor brevis	L2–4		
	Adductor magnus	L3, 4		
	Gracilis	L2–4		
Adductor of thigh	Obturator externus	L3, 4		
Lateral rotation of thigh				
Abduction of thigh	Gluteus medius and mininus	L4, 5; S1	Superior gluteal	Sacral
Medial rotation of thigh				
Flexion of thigh	Tensor fasciae latae	L4, 5		
Lateral rotation of thigh	Piriformis	S1, 2	. . .	
Abduction of thigh	Gluteus maximus	L4, 5: S1, 2	Inferior gluteal	
Lateral rotation of thigh	Obturator intemus	L5, S1	Muscular branches form sacral plexus	
	Gemeli	L4, 5; S1		
	Quadratus femoris	L4, 5; S1		
Flexion of leg (assist in extension of thigh)	Biceps femoris	L4, 5; S1, 2	Sciatic (trunk)	Sacral
	Semitendinosus	L4, 5; S1		
	Semimembranosus	L4, 5; S1		
Dorsal flexion of foot	Tibialis anterior	L4, 5	Deep peroneal	
Supination of foot				
Extension of toes 2–5	Extensor digitorum lingus	L4, 5; S1		
Dorsal flexion of foot				
Extension of great toe	Extensor hallucis longus	L4, 5; S1		
Dorsal flexion of foot				

(continued)

Table 27–3. Motor function chart.[1] (Continued)

Action to Be Tested	Muscle	Cord Segment	Nerves	Plexus
Hip Girdle and Lower Extremity (cont.)				
Extension of great toe and the 3 medial toes	Extensor digitorum brevis	L4, 5; S1		
Plantar flexion of foot in pronation	Peroneus longus and brevis	L5, S1	Superficial peroneal	
	Gastrocnemius	L5, S1, 2	Tibial	
Plantar flexion of foot in supination	Tibialis posterior and triceps surae	L5, S1		
Plantar flexion of foot in supination	Flexor digitorum longus	S1, 2		
Flexion of terminal phalanx of toes II-V				
Plantar flexion of foot in supination	Flexor hallucis longus	L5, S1, 2		
Flexion of terminal phalanx of great toe				
Flexion of middle phalanx of toes II-V	Flexor digitorum brevis	L5, S1		
Flexion of proximal phalanx of great toe	Flexor hallucis brevis	L5, S1, 2		
Spreading and closing of toes	Small muscles of foot	S1, 2		
Flexion of proximal phalanx of toes				
Voluntary control of pelvic floor	Perineal and sphincters	S2–4	Pudendal	

[1]Modified from JC McKinley. Reproduced, with permission, from de Groot J: *Correlative Neuroanatomy*, 21st ed. Appleton & Lange, 1991.

3. Impaired mentation—When mentation is impaired, a pinprick or deep painful stimulation may be the only reliable sensory test.

D. Brain-Stem Reflexes

Brain-stem reflexes are usually intact except in the case of high cervical spinal cord injury, when nystagmus (midbrain, pons), facial hypalgesia (spinal nucleus of the trigeminal nerve), and hypoventilation (phrenic nerve, intercostals) may be present. ***Note:*** The presence of brain-stem signs should not be attributed to spinal cord injury until an intracranial lesion has been excluded.

E. Spinal Reflexes

Tendon jerks and plantar responses are usually absent below the level of an acute complete spinal cord transection (Table 27–5); asymmetry is also common. Spasticity or increased tone in muscle groups may occur with partial spinal cord injuries. Anal sphincter tone (reflex and voluntary) becomes flaccid following complete spinal cord transection. Priapism occurring soon after injury suggests immediate complete spinal cord lesion. Onset at a later time may indicate that the lesion has progressed from an incomplete to a complete stage. Sweating and skin vasomotor tone are absent below the level of a spinal cord lesion.

The bulbocavernosus reflex is dependent on an intact S1 and S2 spinal reflex. If the bulbocavernosus reflex is preserved in the presence of complete perineal sensory loss and flaccid paralysis of the lower extremities, it indicates that the period of spinal shock has passed and that the neurologic deficit is due to a lesion above the S1 segment. Absence of the bulbocavernosus reflex may indicate either the presence of spinal shock or a spinal cord lesion including the S1 and S2 segments. Spinal shock usually resolves within 24 hours and is accompanied by return of the bulbocavernosus reflex if the S1 and S2 segments are not directly involved in the spinal cord lesion.

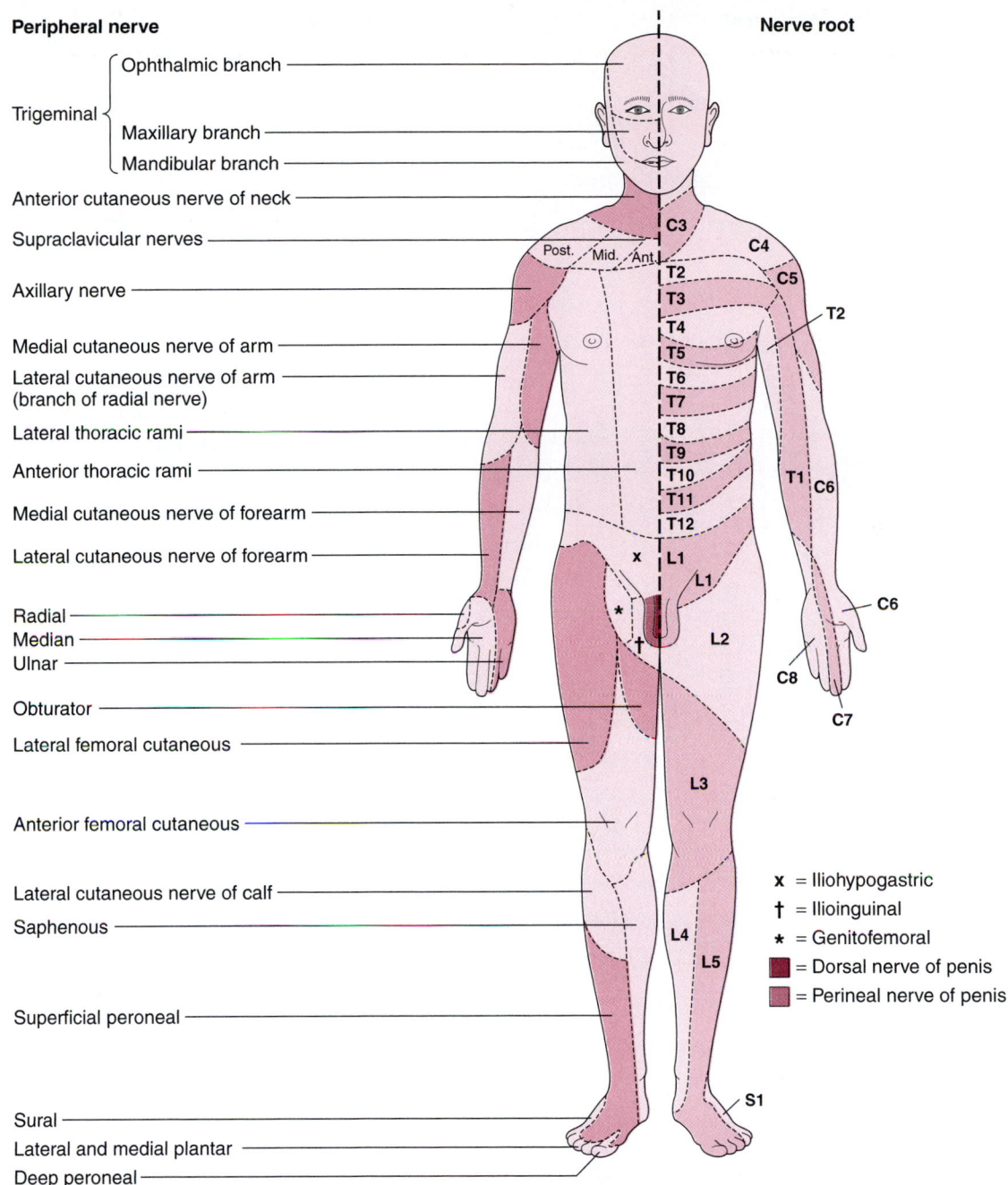

Peripheral nerve

Trigeminal
- Ophthalmic branch
- Maxillary branch
- Mandibular branch

Anterior cutaneous nerve of neck

Supraclavicular nerves

Axillary nerve

Medial cutaneous nerve of arm

Lateral cutaneous nerve of arm (branch of radial nerve)

Lateral thoracic rami

Anterior thoracic rami

Medial cutaneous nerve of forearm

Lateral cutaneous nerve of forearm

Radial
Median
Ulnar

Obturator

Lateral femoral cutaneous

Anterior femoral cutaneous

Lateral cutaneous nerve of calf

Saphenous

Superficial peroneal

Sural
Lateral and medial plantar
Deep peroneal

Nerve root

C3
Post. Mid. Ant.
C4
T2
C5
T3
T2
T4
T5
T6
T7
T8
T9
T10
T1 C6
T11
T12
L1
L1
C6
L2
C8
C7
L3

x = Iliohypogastric
† = Ilioinguinal
★ = Genitofemoral
■ = Dorsal nerve of penis
■ = Perineal nerve of penis

L4
L5

S1

Figure 27–1. **Cutaneous innervation.** (Reproduced, with permission, from Greenberg DA, Aminoff MJ, Simon RP: *Clinical Neurology*, 5th ed. McGraw-Hill, 2002.)

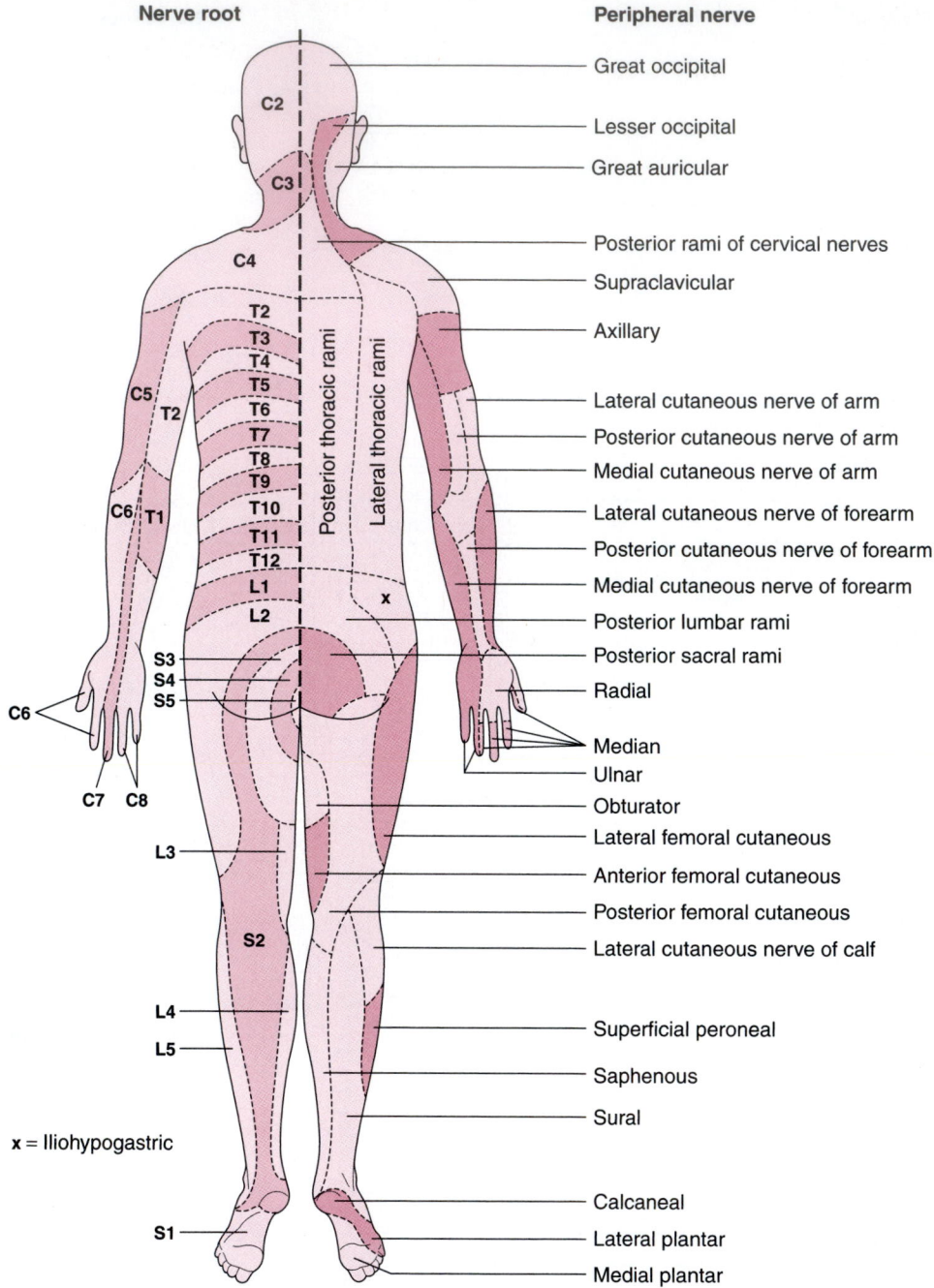

Figure 27–2. Cutaneous innervation. (Reproduced, with permission, from Greenberg DA, Aminoff MJ, Simon RP: *Clinical Neurology,* 5th ed. McGraw-Hill, 2002.)

Table 27–4. Commonly used landmarks for testing dermatomal sensation.

Location	Dermatome
Second rib	C4–T2
Nipple	T4
Lower rib border	T7–8
Umbilicus	T10
Inguinal ligament	T12–L1

Spinal Cord Syndromes

A. COMPLETE SPINAL CORD LESION

The absence of sacral sparing (perianal sensation, rectal sphincter tone) indicates a complete spinal cord lesion, with recovery unlikely if the condition persists longer than 24 hours. Sacral sparing suggests an improved prognosis.

Table 27–5. Summary of reflexes.[1]

Reflexes	Afferent Nerve	Center	Efferent Nerve
Superficial Reflexes			
Corneal	Cranial V	Pons	Cranial VII
Nasal (sneeze)	Cranial V	Brain stem and upper cord	Cranials, V, VII, IX, X, and spinal nerves of expiration
Pharyngeal and uvular	Cranial IX	Medulla	Cranial X
Upper abdominal	T7, 8, 9, 10	T7, 8, 9, 10	T7, 8, 9, 10
Lower abdominal	T10, 11, 12	T10, 11, 12	T10, 11, 12
Cremasteric	Femoral	L1	Genitofemoral
Plantar	Tibial	S1, 2	Tibial
Anal	Pudendal	S4, 5	Pudendal
Deep Reflexes			
Jaw	Cranial V	Pons	Cranial V
Biceps	Musculocutaneous	C5, 6	Musculocutaneous
Triceps	Radial	C6, 7	Radial
Periosteoradial	Radial	C6, 7, 8	Radial
Wrist (flexion)	Median	C6, 7, 8	Median
Wrist (extension)	Radial	C7, 8	Radial
Patellar	Femoral	L2, 3, 4	Femoral
Achilles	Tibial	S1, 2	Tibial
Visceral Reflexes			
Light	Cranial II	Midbrain	Cranial III
Accomodation	Cranial II	Occipital cortex	Cranial III
Ciliospinal	A sensory nerve	T1, 2	Cervical sympathetics
Oculocardiac	Cranial V	Medulla	Cranial X
Carotid sinus	Cranial IX	Medulla	Cranial X
Bulbocavernosus	Pudendal	S2, 3, 4	Pelvic autonomic
Bladder and rectal	Pudendal	S2, 3, 4	Pudendal and autonomics

[1]Reproduced, with permission, from deGroot J: *Correlative Neuroanatomy*, 21st ed. Appleton & Lange, 1991.

B. Partial Spinal Cord Lesions

1. Brown-Séquard syndrome—This syndrome is usually caused by penetrating injuries resulting in hemisection of the spinal cord. The findings include loss of distal ipsilateral position and vibration sense, distal ipsilateral motor loss and vasomotor paralysis, distal loss of pain and temperature sense below T12 on the contralateral side (including the genitals and perineum).

2. Central cord syndrome—This syndrome is usually due to cervical hyperextension, involving the central gray matter and the central parts of the lateral spinothalamic tracts. Quadriplegia may result, with minimal sacral sparing. The upper extremities are more involved than the lower extremities.

3. Anterior cord syndrome—This syndrome results from cervical hyperflexion injuries. Position and vibration (posterior column functions) are preserved, but motor function, temperature, and pain sensation are lost bilaterally below the lesion.

Reexamination

Neurologic examination is helpful only if it is repeated often enough to establish a diagnosis, suggest further diagnostic steps, or clearly establish a trend in neurologic function. The results of each examination may be seen as a point in a curve showing neurologic function with time. If successive examinations indicate improvement, further specialized testing may not be necessary. Failure to improve—verified by repeated examinations—indicates that additional studies are necessary, as does progressive deterioration from a baseline established by examination done on arrival in the emergency department. It is particularly important to note progressive neurologic dysfunction if injury involves the cervical spinal cord, because respiratory failure may result.

Laboratory Examination

Baseline studies required for all patients with suspected spinal cord injury include the following: CBC, urinalysis (specimen obtained by bladder catheterization), blood glucose concentration, serum electrolyte determinations, and renal function tests. Arterial blood gas measurements are necessary if ventilation is impaired or potentially threatened.

Imaging

Careful and correct interpretation of x-ray films is critically important in the treatment of spinal cord injury. Most spine abnormalities (eg, minor facet fractures and nondisplaced fractures) are more easily recognized by a radiologist, whose help should be sought in all cases. In a large study of blunt trauma patients, cervical spine injuries were identified in 2.4% of patients. Three-view cervical spine radiographs identified a cervical spine injury in 1.5% of the patients. Approximately 65% of all cervical spinal fractures and subluxations involve the lower vertebra (C5, C6, and C7). Radiographs were interpreted as normal in 0.9% of patients later found to have a cervical spine injury. *Note:* Normal spine x-rays do not exclude the presence of spinal cord injury. Spinal cord injury without radiographic abnormality is an uncommon but well-described condition, especially in children with flexible spinal columns and relatively larger head–to–body size ratios. In the NEXUS study, a large, observational, multicenter study, these injuries occurred in 0.07% of all blunt trauma patients and in 6% of all the patients with spinal injuries. Central cord syndrome (central hemorrhage) and spontaneously reduced dislocations can be associated with normal x-rays, as can ligamentous tears resulting from flexion-extension injuries (whiplash). A thorough physical examination and a careful repeated neurologic evaluation are therefore essential in all cases.

A. Chest, Skull, and Pelvis

Portable chest and pelvis radiographs are standard in the initial evaluation of the patient with blunt spinal injury. Associated head injuries are common, and spinal injury patients often require CT scan of the head to evaluate intracranial injuries.

B. Cervical Spine

Anteroposterior and lateral views of the cervical spine extending from C1 to T1 and an odontoid (open mouth) view are required if cervical cord injury is suspected. The lateral cervical spine view alone is only 79% sensitive in detecting cervical spine injuries. If the segments from C6 to T1 are not visible, a "swimmer's" view should be obtained by having the patient supine, with one upper extremity abducted and extended (arm raised above head) and the opposite upper extremity adducted and extended (arm kept at side of body). The shoulder of the adducted and extended extremity is then depressed by having a person stand at the foot of the bed and pull on the patient's hand. The x-ray is shot upward through the axilla of the abducted, extended extremity. Oblique views increase the sensitivity of the cervical spine series and are recommended by some in the evaluation of suspected cervical spinal injury. Standard oblique views require neck rotation; this can be avoided by performing a trauma oblique view, which is a modification of the oblique view. The trauma oblique view is obtained by aiming the x-ray beam at a 60-degree angle to the plane of the table with the patient supine (and immobilized).

Other diagnostic modalities must be used if all of the cervical vertebrae cannot be seen adequately with these techniques.

Flexion-extension views of the cervical spine have been recommended to evaluate ligamentous injuries in obtunded patients or in patients with persistent neck pain despite normal cervical spine radiographs. Recent studies have suggested little utility for flexion-extension views in children with normal initial cervical spine radiographs. In addition, flexion-extension views are discouraged for the acute evaluation of cervical instability because cervical spasm may temporarily stabilize the cervical spine despite significant ligamentous injuries.

Magnetic resonance imaging (MRI), with superior ability to visualize soft tissues, may begin to play a significant role in the evaluation of cervical spine ligamentous injuries. If a patient is suspected of having a ligamentous cervical spine injury, continuous immobilization with a well-padded, rigid cervical collar is recommended for 14–28 days until follow-up studies such as flexion-extension radiographs or MRI can be performed.

C. THORACIC AND LUMBOSACRAL SPINE

Indications for x-rays of the thoracic and lumbar spine follow the same criteria as those for the cervical spine. These criteria mandate that full radiographic evaluation be performed unless the patient is fully alert and has no evidence of midline bony tenderness; focal neurologic defect; intoxication; or painful, distracting injury. In addition, if a patient has a fracture in one portion of the spinal column, the entire spinal column must be imaged because the occurrence of an associated fracture at another level is relatively common.

D. SPECIAL STUDIES

1. CT scan—If a body scanner is available, the CT scan is the easiest and perhaps the best method of looking for vertebral column and spinal cord injury. MRI may be required for better visualization of the relationships between the spinal cord and the vertebral canal.

2. Tomography—Tomograms provide excellent detail of the spine, but they are more difficult to interpret (and no easier to perform) than CT scans.

3. MRI—MRI is indicated in patients with suspected spinal cord injuries and in patients with documented cord injuries. MRI provides a detailed view of the spinal cord, associated edema or hemorrhage, and surrounding soft tissues. With information obtained from MRI scans, injuries can be followed or operative interventions for cord decompression and spinal stabilization can be planned.

Hospitalization

Hospitalization is required for patients with neurologic deficit, an unstable or potentially unstable vertebral column (with or without fracture), fractures or subluxation of vertebral bodies, or severe pain requiring parenteral analgesics for relief.

Patients with uncomplicated fractures (ie, linear and undisplaced) of the transverse processes, sacrum, or coccyx and with normal results on neurologic evaluation and otherwise normal imaging studies do not require hospitalization. Provide symptomatic therapy as needed.

■ EMERGENCY TREATMENT OF SPECIFIC SPINAL INJURIES

Table 27–6 summarizes the mechanisms and common findings in many of the radiographically identifiable cervical spine injury patterns.

VERTEBRAL FRACTURES WITHOUT SPINAL CORD INJURY

Clinical Findings

In vertebral fractures without spinal cord injury, there is focal pain and tenderness over the vertebral column. Coughing or axial percussion of the head or feet may also cause pain that is referred to the fractured vertebral body. X-rays show fractures that may be in the vertebral body, the transverse processes, or the spinous processes. Coexisting dislocation or instability may be present. The neurologic examination is normal.

Treatment

Immobilize the patient on a firm surface (eg, rigid spine board), and use tape and lateral restraints (sandbags) or traction. Administer analgesia as needed.

Disposition

The only patients who do not require hospitalization are those with mildly symptomatic or asymptomatic, linear, nondisplaced, stable fractures of the spinous or transverse processes, or similar fractures of the sacrum or coccyx. Such patients may be given analgesics and a cervical collar for immobilization (if fractures are in the cervical vertebrae). A return visit should be scheduled within 1 week with an orthopedist or neurosurgeon.

All other patients should be hospitalized—specifically, those with displaced or unstable fractures; frac-

Table 27–6. Cervical spine injuries.[1]

Type of Injury	Injury Characteristics
Flexion-type injuries	
Simple wedge compression fracture	Anterior loss of height; intact posterior column; stable fracture.
Flexion teardrop fracture	Fracture of the anteroinferior aspect of the vertebral body; disruption of anterior, middle, and posterior columns; highly unstable injury.
Anterior subluxation	Disruption of posterior ligamentous complexes; potentially unstable.
Bilateral facet dislocation	Anterior displacement of more than half of the anteroposterior diameter of the vertebral body; highly unstable injury.
Clay shoveler's fracture	Fracture or avulsion of the spinous process; commonly seen in lower cervical vertebrae; stable injury.
Flexion-rotation injuries	
Unilateral facet dislocation	Anterior displacement of less than half of the anteroposterior diameter of the vertebral body; neurologic deficits can occur; rotation may be noted by malaligned spinous processes on anteroposterior film or off-set overlap of facets ("bow-tie sign") on lateral view; usually stable.
Rotary atlantoaxial dislocation	Type of unilateral facet dislocation; odontoid shows asymmetry of the lateral masses; unstable injury.
Extension-type injuries	
Hangman fracture	Fracture through pedicles of C2 secondary to hyperextension; spinolaminar disruption; unstable fracture.
Extension teardrop fracture	Displaced anteroinferior bony fragment; avulsion secondary to traction on anterior longitudinal ligament; highly unstable fracture.
Fracture of the posterior arch of C1	Odontoid view demonstrates no displacement of the lateral masses; stable injury.
Axial compression injuries	
Jefferson fracture	Lateral mass displacement of C1; significant prevertebral soft tissue edema; possibly unstable injury.
Burst fracture of the vertebral body	Disruption of the anterior and middle columns; mandates CT scan or MRI to evaluate retropulsion; if loss of height > 25%, neurologic deficit, or retropulsion occurs, then consider it to be an unstable fracture.
Complex mechanism injuries	
Atlantoaxial subluxation	Transverse ligament disruption; injury suspected if the predental space is > 3.5 mm (5 mm in children); unstable injury.
Atlanto-occipital dislocation	Complete disruption of all ligamentous relationships between atlas and occiput; death often occurs immediately; highly unstable.
Odontoid process fractures	Type I: Avulsion of tip of dens; stable fracture.
	Type II: Fracture at base of dens; unstable fracture.
	Type III: Fracture extends into body of C2; unstable fracture.

[1]Modified, with permission, from Hockberger RS, Kirshenbaum KJ: Spine. Page 332 in: Rosen P et al: *Emergency Medicine Concepts and Clinical Practice,* 5th ed., Vol. 3. 2002. Modified and reprinted with permission from Elsevier Science.

tures of cervical, thoracic, or lumbar vertebral bodies; open fractures; or multiple fractures.

SPINAL CORD INJURY WITH OR WITHOUT VERTEBRAL FRACTURES

Clinical Findings

Spinal cord injury with or without vertebral fractures is associated with neurologic symptoms and neurologic deficit. Findings are consistent with injury to the spinal cord (eg, sensory deficit ending circumferentially at T8). Bony injury to the vertebrae demonstrable on x-ray may or may not be apparent, because severe flexion-extension injuries and bony instability from ligamentous tears may cause serious or even fatal spinal cord injury without radiologically demonstrable abnormalities.

Treatment

A. ABCs

Check the airway, gag reflex, and adequacy of ventilation, because high cervical cord lesions may cause death from respiratory insufficiency. Provide ventilatory support with a bag-mask combination or endotracheal intubation, if necessary.

B. VERTEBRAL COLUMN STABILIZATION

Stabilize the vertebral column using a rigid cervical collar and lateral restraints (sandbags or head blocks) to minimize further injury to the spinal cord.

C. HYPOTENSION AND BLOOD LOSS

Correct hypotension and evaluate sources of blood loss such as hemorrhage into the chest, abdomen, pelvis, or femur. If no sources of hemorrhage are identified, judicious administration of intravenous crystalloid solutions (2–3 L) is indicated. If hypotension persists, low-dose dopamine, 5–10 μg/kg/min, is warranted to restore vasomotor tone.

D. OTHER MEASURES

Insert an indwelling urinary catheter and a nasogastric tube. Give nothing by mouth.

E. DRUG THERAPY

Spinal cord swelling from blunt trauma may be reduced by administering corticosteroids; however, the success of this treatment has not been proved. Give methylprednisolone in the dosing regimen previously discussed in this chapter.

F. CONSULTATION

Obtain emergency neurosurgical consultation.

Evaluation

Obtain standard radiograph of the entire spine and CT scans of the vertebrae likely to be injured based on the sensory level in a patient with a probable spinal cord injury. To further evaluate the specific spinal cord injury and to make decisions regarding operative treatment, MRI of the spine is indicated.

Disposition

Hospitalize all patients with neurologic deficit caused by spinal cord injury.

WHIPLASH (HYPEREXTENSION) INJURIES (Cervical Spine Sprain)

Clinical Findings

Patients with whiplash have a history of abrupt hyperextension of the neck (usually from a motor vehicle accident), usually without loss of consciousness. Injury from hyperflexion often occurs as well. Symptoms such as neck pain or muscle spasm, headache, hoarseness, and dysphagia often do not appear until 12–24 hours after injury. Neck pain may be referred to the arms or chest. Physical examination may show tenderness of anterior neck muscles and limited range of motion. Specifically, there is no evidence of neurologic deficit. By definition, whiplash does not cause fractures that are evident on cervical x-rays, although severe injuries may rupture the anterior disk fibers and result in widened disk spaces. X-rays are usually normal but may show reversal of the normal cervical lordosis. As previously mentioned, patients may have ligamentous instability despite normal cervical spine radiographs. For this reason, patients with persistent midline cervical spine tenderness should be immobilized in a well-padded, rigid collar 24 hours per day for 7–14 days until reexamined by a primary care physician or spine surgeon.

Treatment

Treatment consists of a rigid cervical collar, heat, and analgesics (narcotics are often required). Muscle relaxants may be indicated. At the time of reexamination, if a ligamentous injury is present, flexion-extension views will detect subluxation. MRI can be useful to identify ligamentous injuries in patients with possible cervical spine instability. If flexion-extension radiographs or MRI are abnormal, the patient should remain in the cervical collar and be referred to a spine surgeon to determine the significance of any subluxation.

Disposition

Hospitalization is rarely required. Refer the patient to a primary care physician or neurosurgeon for further evaluation.

Frohna WJ: Emergency department evaluation and treatment of the neck and cervical spine injuries. Emerg Med Clin North Am 1999;17:739. [PMID: 10584102]

Hoffman JR et al: Validity of a set of clinical criteria to rule out injury to the cervical spine in patients with blunt trauma. N Engl J Med 2000;343:94. [PMID: 10891516]

Mahadevan S et al: Interrater reliability of cervical spine injury criteria in patients with blunt trauma. Ann Emerg Med 1998; 31:197. [PMID: 9472180]

Mower WR et al: Use of plain radiography to screen for cervical spine injuries. Ann Emerg Med 2001;38:1. [PMID: 11423803]

Panacek EA et al: Test performance of the individual NEXUS low-risk clinical screening criteria for cervical spine injury. Ann Emerg Med 2001;38:22. [PMID: 11423807]

Pollack CV et al: Use of flexion-extension radiographs of the cervical spine in blunt trauma. Ann Emerg Med 2001;38:8. [PMID: 11423804]

Ralston ME et al: Role of flexion-extension radiographs in blunt pediatric cervical spine injury. Acad Emerg Med 2001;8:237. [PMID: 11229945]

Orthopedic Emergencies

28

Luis E. Rodriguez, MD, & John E. Gough, MD, FACEP

I. Immediate Management of Life-Threatening Injuries

II. Immediate Management of Limb-Threatening Injuries

Traumatic Amputations

Compartment Syndrome

III. General Orthopedic Principles

Fractures & Dislocations

Strains & Sprains

Splinting

Procedural Sedation

Child Abuse

IV. Management of Specific Orthopedic Injuries

Shoulder Girdle Injuries

Sternoclavicular Joint Dislocations

Clavicle Fractures

Acromioclavicular Joint Injuries

Scapula Fractures

Rotator Cuff Injuries

Shoulder Dislocations

Upper Extremity Injuries

Humerus Fractures

Supracondylar Fractures

Elbow Injuries

1. Olecranon Fractures
2. Radial Head Fractures
3. Elbow Dislocations
4. Subluxation of the Radial Head

Forearm Fractures

Wrist & Hand Injuries

1. Lunate or Perilunate Dislocations
2. Scapholunate Dislocations
3. Carpal Bone Fractures
4. Metacarpal Fractures
5. Phalanx Fractures & Dislocations
6. Subungual Hematoma
7. Boutonnière Deformity
8. Mallet Finger
9. Ulnar Collateral Ligament Rupture

Pelvic Girdle Injuries

Pelvic Fractures

Hip Injuries

1. Hip Fractures
2. Hip Dislocations

Lower Extremity Injuries

Femoral Shaft Fractures

Knee Joint Injuries

1. Patella Fractures
2. Patella Dislocations
3. Distal Femur Fractures
4. Tibial Plateau Fractures
5. Tibial Tuberosity Fractures & Osgood Schlatter Disease
6. Tibial Spine Fractures
7. Knee Dislocations
8. Knee Ligament Injuries: General Considerations
9. Knee Ligament Injuries: Collateral Ligaments
10. Knee Ligament Injuries: Cruciate Ligaments
11. Meniscal Tears
12. Tendon Ruptures

Tibial Shaft Fractures

Fibula Fractures

Ankle Joint Injuries

1. Lateral Malleolar Fractures
2. Medial Malleolar Fractures
3. Posterior Malleolar Fractures
4. Achilles Tendon Injuries
5. Peroneal Tendon Injuries
6. Ankle Dislocations
7. Ankle Sprains

Calcaneal Fractures

Talar Fractures

Subtalar Dislocations

Tarsal Injuries

Tarsometatarsal Injuries

Metatarsal Fractures

Phalangeal Injuries

Sesamoid Fractures

V. Common Pitfalls

■ I. IMMEDIATE MANAGEMENT OF LIFE-THREATENING INJURIES

All trauma patients presenting to the emergency department should be managed initially in the same manner, regardless of their underlying injuries. Orthopedic injuries may at times be grotesque in nature and can draw attention away from more critical elements of initial patient assessment and treatment. The emergency physician must remain objective and proceed with the primary survey, which consists of evaluating the airway, breathing, circulation, disability, and exposure (ABCDEs). Even some closed fractures can be associated with significant blood loss (Table 28–1).

Once the primary survey has been addressed (eg, intubation, tube thoracostomy), proceed to the secondary survey, which should be a thorough physical examination from head to toe with no system left unexamined. With cervical spine precautions in place, logroll the patient, assess the posterior scalp, and examine the entire spine for tenderness or step-off deformities. Perform a digital rectal examination to evaluate for sphincter tone, gross blood, or abnormal prostate position. When evaluating the pelvis for stability, apply gentle anteroposterior and lateral compression. Visualize and go through range of motion of all joints and document all lacerations, abrasions, and contusions. At this time, consider reduction of certain orthopedic emergencies such as a dislocated hip, knee, or any fracture or dislocation in which vascular compromise is present (Figure 28–1). Reduction should be done early, because complications such as avascular necrosis increase as time elapses. If possible, reduce fractures and dislocations with neurovascular compromise before transferring the patient to a trauma center for multisystem or severe injuries. If no immediate vascular compromise exists, the orthopedist may arrange to go to the operating room and reduce fractures or dislocations under general anesthesia.

■ II. IMMEDIATE MANAGEMENT OF LIMB-THREATENING INJURIES

TRAUMATIC AMPUTATIONS

 ESSENTIALS OF DIAGNOSIS

- *Sharp, guillotine injuries are best candidates for reimplantation.*
- *Keep amputated part clean, moisten with saline, and put on ice.*
- *Do not allow part to freeze.*
- *Cooling will help increase viability of amputated part up to 12–24 hours.*

General Considerations

Patients incurring traumatic amputations should be considered for reimplantation surgery. Young healthy patients with sharp, guillotine injuries without crushing or avulsion damage are the best candidates for successful reimplantation. However, it is best to consider all patients as potential candidates, care for the amputated part, and make appropriate consultations or arrange for transfer.

Clinical Findings

A. SYMPTOMS AND SIGNS

The patient presents with an amputated digit or limb.

B. X-RAY FINDINGS

Although this diagnosis is made clinically, x-rays often help delineate exactly where the injury occurred, or if underlying fractures or dislocations exist.

Treatment

The amputated part should be kept clean, wrapped in a sterile dressing, moistened with sterile saline, placed in a plastic bag, and put on ice. Do not use dry ice or allow the amputated part to freeze. Cooling the amputated part will increase the viability from 6–8 hours to approximately 12–24 hours. The injury should be treated as an open fracture, with appropriate use of antibiotics and tetanus prophylaxis.

Table 28–1. Potential blood loss from closed fractures.

Site	Amount (in L)
Pelvis	1–5+
Femur	1–4
Spine	1–2
Leg	0.5–1
Arm	0.5–0.75

Disposition

Patients with limb amputations usually require consultation with an orthopedic, plastic, or trauma surgeon. These patients should be admitted for further surgical management, neurologic and vascular evaluation, and monitoring of blood loss. Patients with small digit amputations may be managed in the emergency department and discharged with appropriate close follow-up.

COMPARTMENT SYNDROME

General Considerations

A potentially harmful complication of orthopedic injuries is the development of a compartment syndrome. Although predominantly occurring in the lower extremities, a compartment syndrome can potentially occur anywhere in the body including the abdomen and the orbits. The lower leg has four compartments: anterior, lateral, posterior, and deep posterior. Trauma below the knee can lead to progressive swelling with eventual decreased blood flow from vascular compression as well as neurologic compromise.

Clinical Findings

Classically the findings associated with compartment syndrome are pallor, pulselessness, pain, paresthesias, and poikilothermia. Decreased or absent pulses are a late finding, and the presence of a pulse does not exclude compartment syndrome. Due to alteration of normal mental status, delays in recognition of compartment syndrome are more likely to occur in sedated patients or in those with head injuries than in other patients. The diagnosis can be confirmed by measuring intracompartmental pressures with a Stryker needle or with a needle connected to an arterial line pressure monitor. Levels above 30 mm Hg are abnormal.

Treatment

Initially immobilization, elevation, cooling, and removal of any constricting bandages or splints are indicated. Intracompartmental pressures greater than 30 mm Hg generally require immediate intervention with fasciotomy. It is preferable to have a surgeon perform this procedure, if possible.

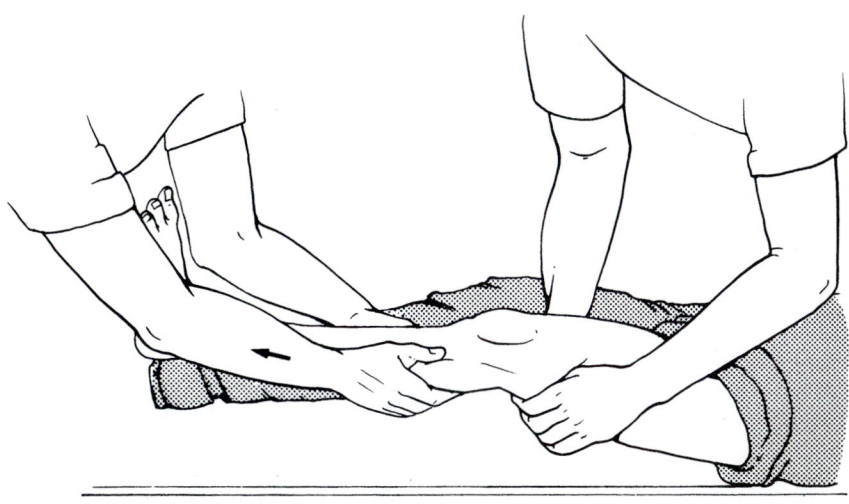

Figure 28–1. Technique of manual traction to align an angulated fracture and correct deformity.

Disposition

Patients with compartment syndrome require hospitalization for definitive surgical management.

■ III. GENERAL ORTHOPEDIC PRINCIPLES

FRACTURES & DISLOCATIONS

Fractures are disruptions in the continuity of bone and should be described with appropriate terminology. The terms *closed* or *open* designate important differences in the degree of skin breakdown at the fracture site. Degrees of displacement and angulation should be described in terms of the distal structure's relationship to the more proximal part of the body. For example, a posterior elbow dislocation describes the ulna in a posterior position relative to the distal humerus. Other descriptive terminology should be used, such as *comminuted* (fracture in more than two pieces), *impacted* (collapse of one fragment of bone onto another), *transverse* (fracture line at right angle to long axis of the bone), *oblique* (fracture line with angle other than right angle), and *spiral* (fracture line encircles bone secondary to rotational forces, often associated with child abuse). An *avulsion fracture* occurs when a ligament pulls a fragment of bone away. *Pathologic fractures* occur in weakened areas of bone as seen with osteomalacia, cysts, carcinomas, and Paget disease. When fractures occur with minimal trauma, consider the possibility of a pathologic fracture. *Stress fractures* occur most commonly in the lower extremity and are seen with repetitive trauma (eg, from prolonged marching or running). Stress fractures may be subtle and missed on initial radiographs. A bone scan may be necessary to make the diagnosis.

Dislocations are disruptions in the normal relationship of the articular surfaces of the bones making up a joint. They may be associated with fractures. Dislocations should be described by the relationship of the distal bone to the more proximal bone (ie, anterior-posterior, medial-lateral). A *subluxation* is an incomplete dislocation.

When pediatric fractures are evaluated, specific descriptions such as *greenstick, torus* or *buckle,* and *plastic deformity* may need to be used. Growth plate injuries in children are described by the Salter-Harris classification (Figure 28–2).

Type I Injuries

The epiphysis is separated from the metaphysis without radiographic evidence of metaphyseal or epiphyseal fracture. Type I injuries are more common in younger children and may be seen with birth trauma. Historically these lesions were associated with scurvy and rickets. If significant displacement is not present, Type I injuries may be difficult to diagnose on initial radiographs. Thickening of the growth plate and soft tissue swelling may be the only signs evident on x-rays. If an injury is suspected but cannot be identified on the initial films, immobilization and orthopedic follow-up are recommended.

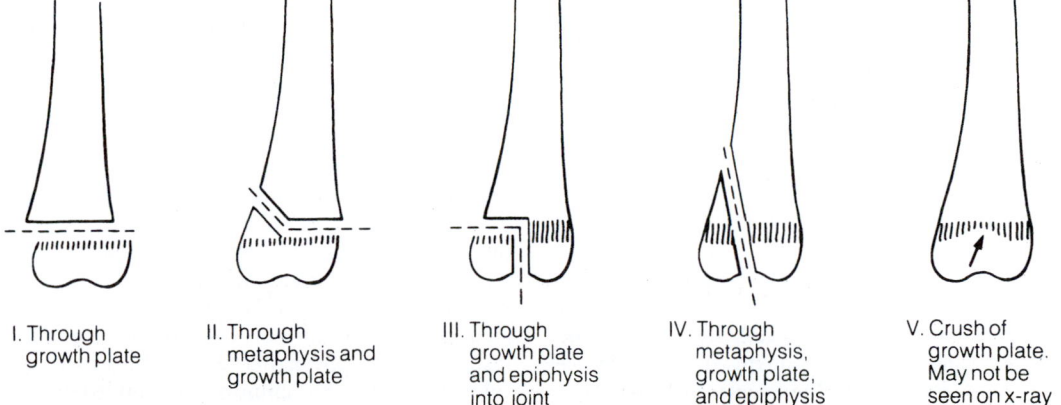

I. Through growth plate

II. Through metaphysis and growth plate

III. Through growth plate and epiphysis into joint

IV. Through metaphysis, growth plate, and epiphysis into joint

V. Crush of growth plate. May not be seen on x-ray

Figure 28–2. Salter-Harris classification of growth plate injuries.

Type II Injuries

Type II injuries are the most common physeal injuries and are most often seen in older children (> age 10 years). The fracture line travels through the physis and is associated with an oblique fracture of the metaphysis on the opposite side from where the force was applied. The metaphyseal fragment is referred to as the Thurston-Holland sign.

Type III Injuries

Type III injuries comprise a vertical fracture of the epiphysis perpendicular to the physis, extending into the growth plate. This type of injury is uncommon and most frequently occurs at the distal tibial epiphysis. To avoid the potential of growth plate arrest, the fracture must be appropriately reduced to maintain proper blood supply. Reduction is accomplished most commonly with operative fixation. If surgery is not performed, frequent rechecks and follow-up radiographs are recommended to ensure that the fracture does not become displaced after immobilization.

Type IV Injuries

Unlike Types I–III, Type IV injuries are the result of compressive rather than rotational or shearing forces. Vertical splitting of the epiphysis occurs, extending through the physis and metaphysis. Type IV injuries require surgical repair, and growth plate arrest may occur even with operative fixation.

Type V Injuries

Type V injuries, which are rare, are the result of severe crushing forces applied to the epiphysis at the area of the physis. When seen, they occur most often at the distal tibia and the knee. Because no fracture is visible, these injuries are frequently missed on initial radiographs. Often they are diagnosed on follow-up visits after the shortening and angular deformity secondary to growth plate arrest is evident. Nontraumatic causes include osteomyelitis and epiphyseal aseptic necrosis.

Eponyms

Even though emergency physicians are likely to be comfortable using the many eponyms that exist to describe fractures (eg, Colles, Monteggia, Galeazzi), it is probably more efficient to provide orthopedic consultants with an anatomic description using the above terminology. For example, merely stating that the patient has a Colles' fracture does not convey whether the injury requires simple splinting and follow-up versus acute open or closed reduction.

SPRAINS & STRAINS

Sprains are injuries to ligaments and may be associated with a fracture. The following grading system is used to describe the severity of the injury:

- Grade I: incomplete tear. Swelling and ecchymosis may be present. Immobilization and conservative care are indicated.
- Grade II: significant incomplete tear. Swelling and ecchymosis are usually present as is some laxity in the joint. Immobilization and orthopedic follow-up are indicated.
- Grade III: complete disruption. The joint is unstable. Orthopedic consultation is indicated for possible surgical repair.

When assessing joint instability, remember that joint effusions, guarding, and muscle contractions may complicate the initial clinical exam. If there is any question, a period of immobilization and follow-up examination are indicated. A strain is an injury to the muscle-musculotendinous unit. Strains are also graded according to severity. Most require immobilization and conservative management; however, surgical repair may be necessary, and orthopedic consultation or referral should be obtained if indicated.

SPLINTING

Splints are a basic part of orthopedic care. They are used to stabilize the injury, provide some amount of pain relief, and help prevent further injury. Some splints are designed to be temporary, such as those applied in the field by emergency medical services personnel. These splints should ideally stabilize the joint above and below the suspected injury. Emergency medical services personnel are generally taught to "splint it as it lies," and this concept also should apply initially in the emergency department. Attempting to correct deformities before obtaining radiographs is not recommended, unless vascular compromise is suspected.

Splints are often applied in the emergency department before the patient is discharged or admitted and are left in place until more definitive orthopedic care is instituted. All physicians should be experienced in splinting. Even if the splint is to be applied by a technician, the physician should ensure that the splint is adequately padded and the limb is stabilized in an appropriate position before the patient is discharged. In addition, the physician should reevaluate and document the limb's neurovascular status after any reduction or splinting procedure. Use of circumferential plaster (ie, casts) is greatly discouraged in the emergency department. In almost all orthopedic injuries, soft tissue swelling worsens after discharge, potentially leading to significant neurovascular compromise if a cast has been applied in the emergency department. Specific splinting instructions are provided below for each injury.

PROCEDURAL SEDATION

Before a fracture or dislocation is reduced, adequate analgesia and muscle relaxation must be provided. The best way to accomplish fracture or dislocation reduction is with sedation using either intravenous or intramuscular agents. Emergency departments should have specific policies in place for the administration and monitoring of patients undergoing sedation. The goal is to provide sufficient sedation for the procedure without having to administer general anesthesia.

Before sedating a patient, ensure that the patient has fasted for 4–6 hours prior to the procedure. Necessary equipment includes at least one functioning venous catheter, continuous pulse oximetry, a suction catheter, airway intubation equipment, and a bag-valve-mask. Mallampati oropharynx assessment and consideration of the patient's American Society of Anesthesiologists (ASA) categorization should be determined before beginning the procedure to ensure that the emergency physician can manage any potential airway complications resulting from sedation. In general, only ASA Class I or II patients (those without serious systemic comorbid diseases) should undergo procedural sedation in the emergency department. ASA Class III or IV patients should optimally receive treatment in the operating room.

Patients being sedated in the emergency department should receive supplemental oxygen regardless of initial oxygen saturation, and saturations should be maintained above 90% at all times. Medications should be short acting. Numerous medication combinations are available. We prefer using etomidate, 0.15 mg/kg intravenously. Etomidate has a profound and short-lived action, which should be sufficient for most procedures. Etomidate is currently not approved for use in children. It has been reported to cause adrenal suppression, the clinical significance of which is unknown. As with any sedative, airway support through airway maneuvers or assisted ventilation may be needed. An alternative is the combination of agents such as midazolam and fentanyl. Be aware that a potential side effect of fentanyl is chest wall rigidity (at higher doses or with rapid boluses), which may prohibit bag-mask ventilation and may necessitate paralyzation and intubation. Adequate documentation by trained nursing staff is a must, and sedated patients should be monitored until they can ambulate and tolerate fluids by mouth.

CHILD ABUSE

Unfortunately, child abuse remains a major problem in our society, with physical abuse affecting 2–5% of children in the United States. Skeletal injuries sometimes occur with abuse and may represent significant morbidity to the patient. Abuse should remain high on the list of differential diagnoses whenever injured children receive treatment, particularly if fractures are found in very young patients (ie, younger than age 3 years).

Clinical Findings

The approach to diagnosis should be the same as for all trauma patients. Keys to potential abuse may be evident in the history, such as history inconsistent with the injuries seen or delays in seeking care (may be evidenced by callus formation at a fracture site seen on x-rays). Physical findings may include pattern injuries, old bruises, and multiple fractures in various stages of healing.

Remember that significant force is required to produce fractures in the spine, scapula, and sternum. Rib fractures are uncommon in children except in the setting of abuse, and chest radiographs should be examined carefully to identify these injuries. Spiral fractures have long been identified as red flags to alert the emergency physician of possible abuse. This is particularly true of humeral and femoral fractures (particularly in patients less than age 3 years); however, spiral fractures of the tibia may be seen with accidental injuries. Pulling and twisting forces may also result in a tearing of the periosteum and cartilage at the growth plate of long bones, scapulae, and clavicles. These corner fractures may also have a "bucket-handle" loop associated with them, which may be seen on plain x-rays.

Treatment

Treatment of specific injuries is described below. Careful documentation is encouraged.

Disposition

Obtain appropriate pediatric, orthopedic, and social services consultations while the patient is still in the emergency department. All physicians are required to report suspected child abuse.

■ IV. MANAGEMENT OF SPECIFIC ORTHOPEDIC INJURIES

SHOULDER GIRDLE INJURIES

STERNOCLAVICULAR JOINT DISLOCATIONS

ESSENTIALS OF DIAGNOSIS

- Chest wall deformity.
- Sternoclavicular tenderness.
- Sternal x-rays or computed tomography aids in diagnosis.
- May be associated with mediastinal injuries.

General Considerations

Dislocations of the sternoclavicular joint (SCJ) are the least common dislocations of a major joint. SCJ dislocations are frequently associated with motor vehicle collisions but also occur from sports injuries (eg, football, rugby). Anterior dislocations are most common and occur secondary to anterolateral force applied to the shoulder. Posterior dislocations are associated with crushing forces applied to the chest, and 25% of posterior dislocations are associated with injuries to the superior mediastinal structures. The severity of the injury may be graded as follows:

- Grade I: mild sprain of the sternoclavicular and costoclavicular ligaments. May be treated with analgesia and sling and swathe.
- Grade II: subluxation of the SCJ, may be anterior or posterior. Associated with rupture of the sternoclavicular ligament. Treatment is the same as with Grade I injury; however, the joint must be immobilized for a longer period of time.
- Grade III: complete dislocation.

Clinical Findings

A. SYMPTOMS AND SIGNS

The diagnosis can often be made clinically. Tenderness, swelling, and deformity to the SCJ will be present. Patients typically use the unaffected arm to support the affected arm across the chest.

B. X-RAY FINDINGS

Plain radiographs, including anteroposterior, oblique, and 40-degree cephalic tilt views aid in the diagnosis. A computed tomography (CT) scan may be necessary and is indicated in all cases of posterior dislocations to evaluate for mediastinal injuries.

Treatment

Obtain orthopedic consultation for both anterior and posterior dislocations. Anterior dislocations may be reduced in the emergency department using procedural sedation by placing a rolled towel or sheet between the scapulae and applying traction to the affected arm. A posterior dislocation may need operative repair, and early orthopedic or trauma surgery consultation is appropriate because compression of critical upper mediastinal structures such as the great vessels and trachea may occur.

Disposition

Patients with anterior dislocations may be discharged in a sling and swathe. Even if the reduction is successful, the joint is often unstable and the clavicular head may dislocate again. However, because the purpose of the reduction is often more cosmetic than functional, even if reduction is unsuccessful the patient may be discharged with immobilization in a sling and orthopedic follow-up. Posterior dislocations may be reduced with traction and adduction; however, patients with posterior dislocations should be managed in consultation with a specialist and most likely will require admission.

CLAVICLE FRACTURES

ESSENTIALS OF DIAGNOSIS

- Clavicle deformity.
- X-rays confirm diagnosis.
- Most heal with conservative management.

Clinical Findings

A. SYMPTOMS AND SIGNS

Often the clavicle is deformed, and some swelling, tenderness, and occasionally crepitus are present.

X-RAY FINDINGS

Most clavicle fractures are easily seen with a clavicle series.

Treatment

Treat open fractures with antibiotics and orthopedic consultation. For closed clavicle fractures, treatment typically involves a sling, or sling and swathe.

Disposition

Patients with closed fractures may be discharged with orthopedic follow-up. Patients with open fractures require hospitalization for further management.

ACROMIOCLAVICULAR JOINT INJURIES

 **ESSENTIALS OF DIAGNOSIS**

- *Deformed and tender acromioclavicular joint.*
- *May be confused with clavicle injury.*
- *X-ray confirms diagnosis.*

General Considerations

Acromioclavicular joint (ACJ) injuries most commonly result from a direct fall onto the shoulder. ACJ injuries account for 25% of all dislocations within the shoulder girdle. These injuries are graded according to severity:

- Grade I: sprain, minimal tear of the acromioclavicular (AC) ligament
- Grade II: small tear of AC ligament, no change with weight bearing
- Grade III: complete disruption of AC ligament, coracoclavicular ligament, and muscle attachments

Clinical Findings

A. Symptoms and Signs

Patients should be examined in the sitting position. Often a deformity at the AC joint will be present, with swelling, tenderness, and occasionally crepitus.

B. X-ray Findings

X-rays should include anteroposterior, axillary, and 15-degree cephalic tilt views. Stress views are no longer recommended. Classically, separation between the acromion and the clavicle is seen.

Treatment

Type I and II injuries are treated conservatively with a sling. Type III injuries have traditionally been treated with surgical repair; however, conservative management has been used more recently with good results.

Disposition

Most patients may be discharged home. All patients should receive orthopedic referral for follow-up examination.

SCAPULA FRACTURES

 ESSENTIALS OF DIAGNOSIS

- *Pain and tenderness over scapula.*
- *May be associated with more severe intrathoracic injuries.*
- *X-ray (with axillary views) confirms diagnosis.*

General Considerations

Fractures of the scapula are uncommon, accounting for approximately 1% of all fractures. Fractures usually are secondary to direct blows (eg, falls, motor vehicle collisions) or to crush injuries. Because the scapula is well protected by muscle, the presence of a fracture indicates a significant mechanism of injury and warrants evaluation for other potential injuries. Associated injuries to the lung, chest wall, humerus, and clavicle often are present. Scapula fractures can be classified as follows:

- Type I: fracture of coracoid process, acromion process, or scapular spine
- Type II: fracture of the scapular neck
- Type III: intra-articular fracture involving the glenoid fossa
- Type IV: fracture of the body of the scapula (most common)

Clinical Findings

A. Symptoms and Signs

The patient will present with pain and tenderness over the scapula. A hematoma and crepitus may also be appreciated. The patient will usually hold the affected arm close to the body.

B. X-ray Findings

Fractures may be subtle on plain radiographs. Always obtain an axillary view to help identify fractures involving the glenoid, acromion, and coracoid processes. In some instances CT scanning may be necessary to identify subtle or intra-articular fractures. In children, the physis of the acromion may be seen on x-rays. In approximately 3% of individuals this structure remains unfused (os acromiale) and can be mistaken for a fracture.

Treatment

The majority of isolated scapula fractures are managed conservatively with a sling and swathe and pain management.

Disposition

Significantly displaced fractures rarely may require surgical repair; patients with such fractures should be admitted. Patients with isolated scapular fractures may be discharged with close follow-up.

ROTATOR CUFF INJURIES

ESSENTIALS OF DIAGNOSIS

- Pain and decreased motion of shoulder.
- Positive drop-arm test.
- Plain X-ray of little value.
- Arthrogram or magnetic resonance imaging will confirm diagnosis.

General Considerations

The rotator cuff comprises four muscles: the subscapularis (internal rotation), the infraspinatus and teres minor (external rotation), and the supraspinatus (adduction). Acute tears are commonly seen with falls, either directly onto the shoulder or on an outstretched hand, but may also occur in the setting of lifting heavy objects. Tears occur more commonly in middle-aged to elderly males and usually involve the dominant arm.

Clinical Findings

A. SYMPTOMS AND SIGNS

The patient complains of pain and decreased motion. Point tenderness over the greater tuberosity or a palpable defect may be seen. Tears may be evaluated by passively abducting the arm to 90 degrees and then applying pressure to the distal forearm. With significant acute tears, this will cause the patient to drop his or her arm (drop-arm test).

B. X-RAY FINDINGS

Plain radiographs are usually of little use but should be obtained to rule out occult fractures. Superior displacement of the humeral head may be seen but is not diagnostic.

Treatment

Provide adequate analgesia and a sling for comfort.

Disposition

Outpatient follow-up with scheduling of an arthrogram or magnetic resonance imaging (MRI) scan may be necessary to confirm the diagnosis. Patients may be discharged with orthopedic follow-up.

SHOULDER DISLOCATIONS

ESSENTIALS OF DIAGNOSIS

- Shoulder deformity, pain, and decreased movement.
- Majority are anterior dislocations.
- Anteroposterior, Y and axillary view X-rays confirm diagnosis.
- Perform thorough nerve exam.

General Considerations

The shoulder is the most commonly dislocated major joint in the body. Most (~95%) of these injuries are anterior dislocations and are often easily diagnosed clinically; however, in muscular individuals the clinical presentation may be less obvious. Posterior dislocations are much less common and are usually associated with violent muscle contractions as seen with seizures and electrocutions but may also occur with falls on a flexed, internally rotated arm. Posterior dislocations are often missed clinically and may also be difficult to identify on standard anteroposterior x-rays.

Clinical Findings

A. SYMPTOMS AND SIGNS

The patient usually holds the arm in adduction and the elbow flexed close to the body. Pain occurs with the least amount of movement. The glenoid fossa may be palpable. A complete neurologic and vascular exam of the extremity is of paramount importance. Assess the lateral aspect of the shoulder for sensation in the distribution of the axillary nerve. Examine radial, ulnar, and median nerve distributions thoroughly prior to sedation and reduction. Document brachial and radial pulses. Luxatio erecta is an uncommon form of anterior dislocation in which the humeral head is forced out of the glenoid fossa secondary to a hyperadduction injury and comes to rest against the coracoid or subglenoid fossa. Clinically, the arm will be adjacent to the head with the forearm flexed over the head. Luxatio erecta may also be associated with injury to the axillary artery.

With posterior dislocations the affected arm is usually held against the chest in adduction and is internally rotated. Abduction and external rotation are severely limited. The posterior shoulder may be prominent when viewed from above; however, this finding may be difficult to recognize, particularly in muscular individuals.

B. X-RAY FINDINGS

Obtain a shoulder series, including a Y-view (Figure 28–3), which can help diagnose the direction of dislocation. Axillary views are often the most helpful if any doubt exists about the diagnosis. X-rays will also help identify associated fractures. A Hill-Sachs deformity (impaction of the posterolateral humeral head) may occur with dislocation. A fracture of the anteroinferior glenoid rim (Bankart fracture) may be seen with anterior dislocations. Bankart fractures may be subtle and identified only on CT scans.

Treatment

Some controversy exists over the need to obtain x-rays prior to reduction of shoulder dislocations. We do not generally recommend bypassing x-rays at this time unless vascular compromise is present. In patients with chronic recurrent dislocations, the dislocations may occur without significant trauma (eg, reaching backward, rolling over in bed); in this setting, consider reducing the shoulder before obtaining radiographs.

Emergency physicians should be comfortable with numerous reduction methods. The patient will often require sedation prior to the procedure. We prefer the external rotation–adduction technique for reduction. With the patient in an upright position, the extremity is externally rotated while gentle traction and adduction are applied at the elbow. This technique is associated with a low risk of injury and does not require a great deal of force, as do the other methods. The traction-countertraction method—in which an assistant applies countertraction with a sheet and inline traction of the upper extremity—requires some physical strength (Figure 28–4). Do not try to pull the humerus into place. Instead place traction on the arm until the muscles fatigue and the humeral head slides in. After reduction, reevaluate neurovascular status and immobilize the shoulder with a sling and swathe. Obtain postreduction x-rays.

Disposition

Discharge patients with adequate analgesia such as nonsteroidal anti-inflammatory drugs or opiates and orthopedic follow-up in 2–3 days. If any neurologic findings are present, such as a wrist drop, obtain orthopedic consultation while the patient is still in the emergency department. Most of these neurologic findings are caused by a neuropraxia and usually improve over time.

Kocher MS, Waters PM, Micheli LJ: Upper extremity injuries in the pediatric athlete. Sports Med 2000;30(2):117. [PMID: 10966151]

Owens S, Itamura JM: Differential diagnosis of shoulder injuries in sports. Orthop Clin North Am 2001;32(3):393. [PMID: 11888134]

Ruotolo C, Nottage WM: Surgical and nonsurgical management of rotator cuff tears. Arthroscopy 2002;18(5):527. [PMID: 11987065]

UPPER EXTREMITY INJURIES

HUMERUS FRACTURES

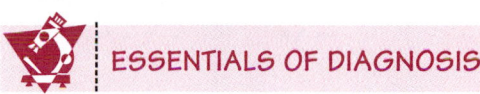

ESSENTIALS OF DIAGNOSIS

- *Frequent in elderly patients.*
- *Pain, deformity, and decreased mobility at shoulder.*
- *X-ray confirms diagnosis.*
- *Conservative management.*

General Considerations

Humerus fractures frequently occur in elderly women with a history of osteoporosis who fall on an outstretched hand (FOOSH). Consider pathologic fractures in younger patients without significant mechanisms, such as a 20-year-old baseball player who develops shoulder pain after pitching.

Clinical Findings

A. SYMPTOMS AND SIGNS

The patient usually presents with deformity at the shoulder and ecchymosis. It is important to assess vascular status because the brachial artery lies in proximity to the distal humeral shaft and associated arterial injury may be present. Assess for radial nerve injury and wrist drop, particularly with humeral shaft fractures. Children who FOOSH usually sustain supracondylar humeral fractures, which are described below.

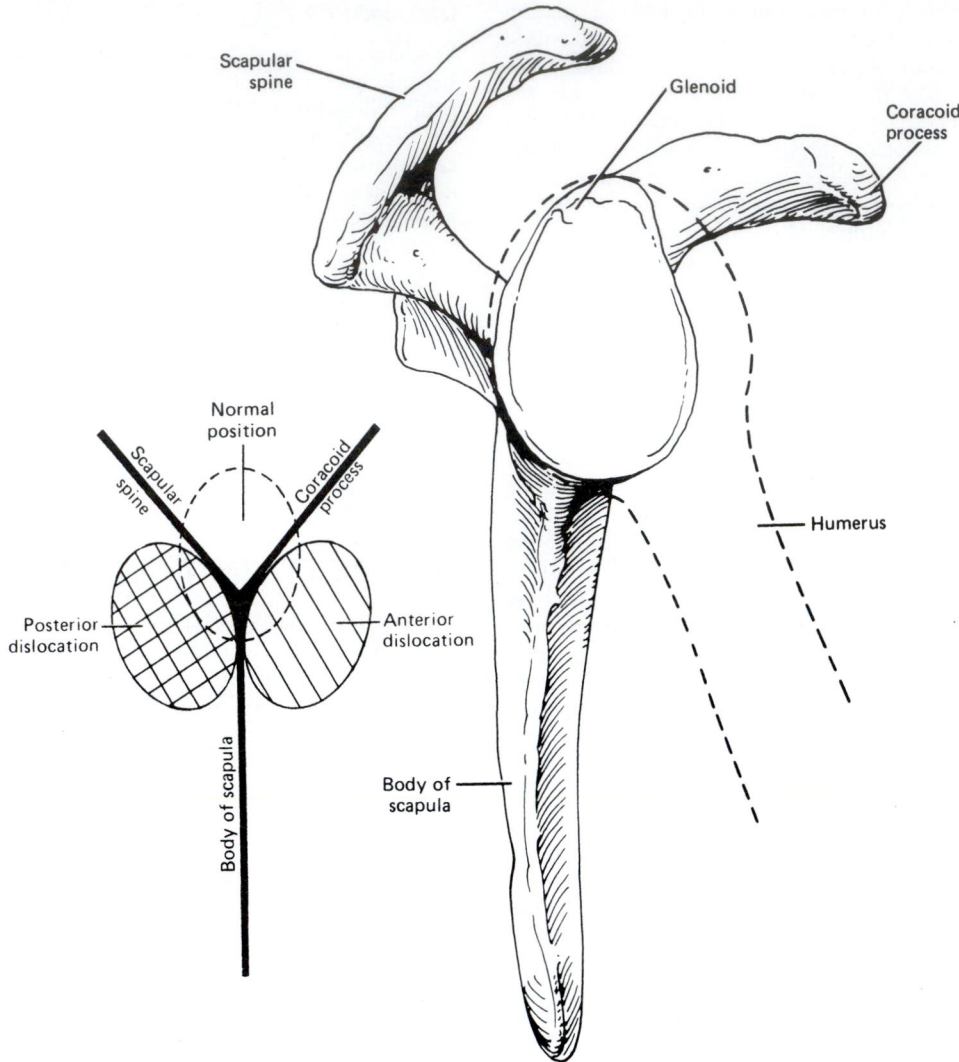

Figure 28–3. Sketch of view on tangential lateral x-ray shows the body of the scapula in its narrowest aspect. If the patient is poorly positioned, the medial and lateral borders are not superimposed. Normally the humeral head shadow lies directly over that of the glenoid, which may be hard to see. The position of the glenoid is indicated by the confluence of the scapular spine, the body of the scapula, and the coracoid process. A dislocated humeral head lies anterior or posterior to this point.

B. X-RAY FINDINGS

X-rays show these injuries clearly. Proximal humerus fractures with some impaction are the most common type. In younger patients, look for signs of a unicameral cyst or other pathologic causes of fracture.

Treatment

Conservative management is generally the rule, especially in the elderly. These patients do well with a splint, sling, and swathe (Figure 28–5), or sling and swathe alone, and adequate analgesia.

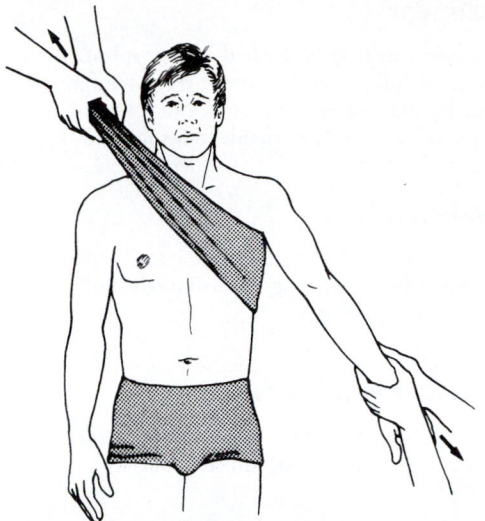

Figure 28–4. Method of producing traction on dislocated humerus and countertraction on thorax for reduction of shoulder dislocation.

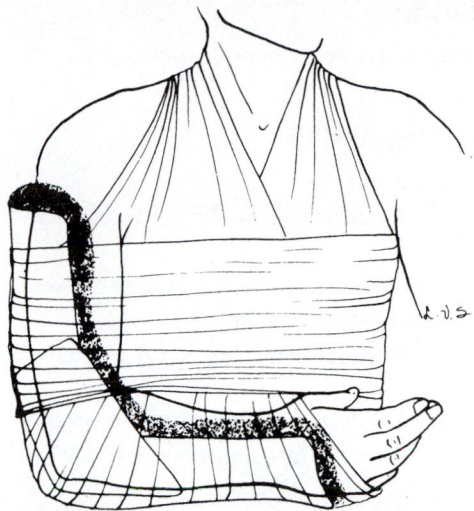

Figure 28–5. Posterior plaster splint with sling and swathe for immobilization of elbow or forearm injuries. Abundant cast padding is first wrapped around the arm. The posterior plaster must be reinforced medially and laterally to the elbow, but neither padding nor plaster should constrict the antecubital fossa.

Disposition

Patients should have orthopedic follow-up in 3–4 days. We recommend obtaining orthopedic consultation for any young person with humeral or humeral shaft fractures while the patient is still in the emergency department. If there is displacement of a humeral shaft fracture, a hanging or gravity splint may be applied. Occasionally these patients may undergo open reduction and internal fixation (ORIF).

SUPRACONDYLAR FRACTURES

ESSENTIALS OF DIAGNOSIS

- *Occurs after FOOSH.*
- *Elbow deformity, pain, and decreased mobility.*
- *Posterior fat pad on lateral x-ray is highly suggestive.*
- *May have high morbidity.*
- *Mandatory orthopedic consultation.*

General Considerations

Supracondylar fractures are of the distal humerus and classically occur in children. They are usually the result of a FOOSH. If not managed properly, supracondylar fractures may predispose to serious morbidity, including complications such as Volkmann ischemic contracture.

Clinical Findings

A. Symptoms and Signs

Patients usually present complaining of elbow pain and arm swelling. A neurologic and vascular exam is important and must include notation of the anterior interosseous nerve sensory distribution.

B. X-ray Findings

Supracondylar fractures may be subtle and at times may be suspected only by the presence of a posterior fat pad sign on a lateral elbow x-ray. Comparison views of the uninjured elbow may be of benefit if a fracture is suspected but not immediately apparent.

Treatment

All supracondylar fractures require orthopedic consultation. We recommend that these fractures not be reduced by emergency physicians.

Disposition

Disposition is as per orthopedic consultation.

ELBOW INJURIES

 ESSENTIALS OF DIAGNOSIS

- *Deformity, pain, and decreased range of motion.*
- *Assess for ulnar nerve injury.*
- *Anteroposterior and lateral x-rays are confirmatory.*
- *Consider fracture if posterior fat pad is present.*
- *No x-ray needed for a simple nursemaid's elbow.*

General Considerations

Elbow injuries usually occur from a direct blow to the elbow, causing immobility at the elbow joint. The patient generally holds the arm in flexion, and a moderate amount of swelling is present. Both fractures and dislocations may occur. It is important to assess neurologic function of the hand (especially in the ulnar nerve distribution because of its proximity to the elbow).

X-rays should include anteroposterior and lateral views. Always look for the presence of fat pads. A small anterior fat pad can sometimes be normal; however, the presence of a posterior fat pad is abnormal and should alert the clinician to a fracture, such as a radial head fracture in adults or a supracondylar fracture in children. *Even if a fracture is not visualized, treat the injury as though an occult fracture is present.*

1. Olecranon Fractures

Olecranon fractures may occur by direct trauma or less commonly by contraction of the triceps while the elbow is flexed.

Clinical Findings

A. SYMPTOMS AND SIGNS

Pain, limited range of motion, and a palpable defect or crepitus may be present.

B. X-RAY FINDINGS

Plain x-rays should be sufficient to confirm the diagnosis.

Treatment

Most fractures may be treated with a splint, sling, and orthopedic follow-up. Displaced fractures (greater than 2 mm separation) or the presence of an ulnar nerve injury mandates acute orthopedic consultation.

Disposition

Patients who do not meet criteria for surgery may be discharged home as long as orthopedic follow-up can be obtained in 1–2 days.

2. Radial Head Fractures

Radial head fractures may occur by either direct trauma or more commonly by an indirect mechanism such as a FOOSH.

Clinical Findings

A. SYMPTOMS AND SIGNS

The patient presents with pain, particularly on supination or pronation, and with limited range of motion. Elbow extension may be limited by joint effusion.

B. X-RAY FINDINGS

It is often difficult to see a definitive fracture on plain x-rays. As mentioned previously, the presence of a fat pad (especially posterior) should raise suspicion for an occult fracture.

Treatment

Simple radial head fractures are treated conservatively with analgesics and a simple sling. We recommend contacting an orthopedist for comminuted radial head fractures.

Disposition

Patients may be discharged with orthopedic follow-up in 3–5 days.

3. Elbow Dislocations

The elbow is second only to the shoulder as the most commonly dislocated major joint. Generally the radius and ulna are displaced together and the dislocation is described as the relationship of the ulna to the humerus (ie, posterior [most common], anterior, medial, or lateral). The most common mechanism is a fall, and associated fractures occur frequently.

Clinical Findings

A. SYMPTOMS AND SIGNS

The patient often holds the elbow in 45 degrees of flexion, and a deformity at the olecranon is usually visible. Because of the location of the brachial artery and median nerve, the patient's neurovascular status should be assessed and documented initially and reassessed frequently.

B. X-RAY FINDINGS

Examine plain radiographs for the presence of associated fractures.

Treatment

If neurovascular compromise is present, perform reduction as soon as possible. Dislocations may be reduced by applying traction to the wrist while the humerus is stabilized (Figure 28–6). Another technique involves applying traction at the wrist while the patient lies on his or her abdomen with the affected limb hanging off the bed. After appropriate analgesia and sedation, most dislocations can be reduced in a few minutes. These injuries should be reassessed for neurovascular injury and then placed in a long arm splint and sling (see Figure 28–5).

Disposition

Most patients may be discharged with adequate analgesia and orthopedic follow-up within 48 hours.

4. Subluxation of the Radial Head

Radial head subluxation (nursemaid's elbow) is a common injury, accounting for as many as 25% of elbow injuries in children. This injury usually occurs in the 1- to 3-year-old age group but may be seen up to school age and rarely in early teenagers. Subluxation occurs secondary to longitudinal traction on the arm while the elbow is extended and the arm pronated. This allows fibers of the annular ligament to slip between the radial head and the capitellum.

Clinical Findings

A. SYMPTOMS AND SIGNS

Generally no deformity is seen. Some tenderness is present over the radial head, and the child characteristically refuses to use the arm. Although subluxation of the radial head is a common injury, obtain a thorough history to allay concerns about potential child abuse.

B. X-RAY FINDINGS

Some authors suggest that if the clinician is confident with the mechanism of injury and the physical exam, radiographs need not be obtained prior to reduction. However, others assert that x-rays should always be obtained to rule out other potential injuries.

Treatment

Once the diagnosis is made, reduction is usually easily performed by stabilizing the elbow with one hand and, while applying gentle pressure on the radial head, supinating the forearm and flexing the elbow. Often a click or snap will be heard. The majority of patients regain normal use of the arm within minutes. Immobilization with a sling has been suggested; however, most patients will not comply, and if the reduction is successful, the sling likely will not make much difference.

Disposition

Unsuccessful or recurrent subluxations require outpatient orthopedic consultation.

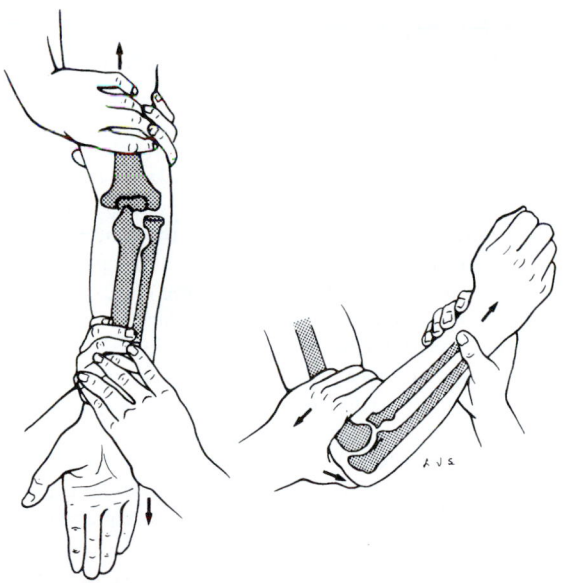

Figure 28–6. Reduction of posterior elbow dislocation by applying manual traction on the forearm while an assistant stabilizes the humerus. If radial or lateral displacement is present, it must be corrected before reduction is completed by flexion of the elbow.

FOREARM FRACTURES

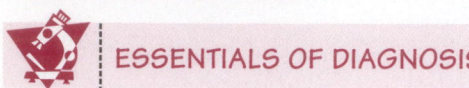

ESSENTIALS OF DIAGNOSIS

- *Pain and deformity present.*
- *X-rays are confirmatory.*
- *Assess for concomitant dislocations.*

General Considerations

Forearm fractures may occur secondary to varied mechanisms but are commonly seen with direct blows or a FOOSH. The site of injury determines the physical findings. Carefully examine the patient for function of the radial, median, and ulnar nerves. Assess, document, and later reassess distal pulses and tendon function. Development of a compartment syndrome should always be suspected and appropriate assessment performed. As noted earlier in this chapter, it is probably more useful to describe the injury anatomically; however, the forearm is an area where many common eponyms for fractures exist, for example,

- Colles' fracture: transverse fracture of distal radius with dorsal angulation
- Smith fracture: transverse fracture of distal radius with volar displacement
- Barton fracture: oblique, intra-articular fracture of the distal radius, with dorsal displacement of the distal fragment along with dorsal carpus subluxation
- Hutchinson (chauffeur's) fracture: intra-articular fracture of the radial styloid
- Monteggia fracture: ulna fracture with radial head dislocation
- Galeazzi fracture: fracture of distal third of radius associated with dislocation of the distal radioulnar joint

Treatment

Nondisplaced fractures are generally treated conservatively with a sugar-tong (U-shaped) splint (volar and dorsal splint from distal metacarpals going around the elbow) and orthopedic follow-up.

Disposition

Displaced fractures warrant orthopedic consultation to determine the appropriate method (open versus closed) and timetable for reduction. Displaced forearm fractures in children should be seen by the orthopedist in the emergency department.

Ring D, Jupiter JB, Zilberfarb J: Posterior dislocation of the elbow with fractures of the radial head and coronoid. J Bone Joint Surg Am 2002;84-A(4):547. [PMID: 11940613]

WRIST & HAND INJURIES

1. Lunate or Perilunate Dislocations

ESSENTIALS OF DIAGNOSIS

- *Occurs after FOOSH.*
- *Wrist swelling, pain, and tenderness.*
- *Anteroposterior and lateral x-rays of wrist are confirmatory.*
- *Look for "piece-of-pie" and "spilled teacup" signs.*

General Considerations

Lunate or perilunate dislocations usually occur from a fall on an outstretched upper extremity. It is believed to be part of a spectrum of injury associated with perilunate dislocation and occasionally a fracture.

Clinical Findings

A. SYMPTOMS AND SIGNS

Usually the patient presents with a swollen wrist, decreased mobility, and severe pain. Median nerve injuries may be seen on exam.

B. X-RAY FINDINGS

The lateral wrist view is the most important x-ray with these injuries. A line drawn through the center shaft of the radius normally bisects the lunate and capitate (Figure 28–7A). In a lunate dislocation the radius and capitate are bisected and the lunate is displaced either dorsal or volar, giving what is sometimes referred to as a spilled teacup appearance (Figure 28–7B and C). The anteroposterior view shows a triangular-shaped lunate bone with the apex pointing toward the fingers, which is commonly referred to as the piece-of-pie sign. A perilunate dislocation occurs when the line drawn through the radius bisects the lunate only and the capitate is displaced.

Treatment

This injury should be managed by providing analgesia and splinting temporarily for comfort in the emergency department. Consult with an orthopedic surgeon for anatomic realignment.

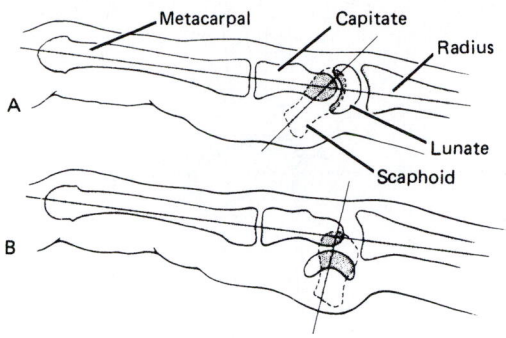
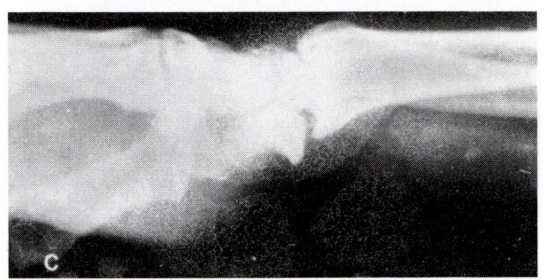

Figure 28–7. **A:** Normal anatomy of the wrist. Note that the proximal end of the capitate rests in the lunate concavity. A straight line drawn through the metacarpal and capitate into the radius should bisect the lunate. The scaphoid makes an angle of 45 degrees with the long axis of the radius. **B:** Lunate dislocation. Lunate dislocates volarly. The angle between the scaphoid and the long axis of the radius is 90 degrees instead of the normal angle of 45 degrees. **C:** X-ray of volar dislocation of lunate. (Reproduced, with permission, from Way LW [editor]:*Current Surgical Diagnosis & Treatment,* 9th ed. Appleton & Lange, 1991.)

Disposition

Patients undergoing ORIF should be admitted until the surgeon addresses the injury. Patients with reducible injuries may be given a long arm splint and sent home after arranging a treatment plan in conjunction with a surgeon.

2. Scapholunate Dislocations

 ESSENTIALS OF DIAGNOSIS

- *Frequently missed injury.*
- *Anteroposterior hand x-ray confirms diagnosis.*
- *"Terry Thomas" sign (greater than 3-mm scapholunate joint space).*

General Considerations

Usually occurring from a FOOSH, a scapholunate dislocation is a commonly missed hand injury.

Clinical Findings

A. Symptoms and Signs

The patient may present with wrist swelling and decreased mobility. Tenderness over the wrist may be present.

B. X-ray Findings

An anteroposterior view of the hand normally reveals a space between the scaphoid and lunate bone of less than 3 mm. If the distance is greater than 3 mm, then a dislocation injury is present.

Treatment

A scapholunate dislocation may temporarily be treated with analgesics and a radial gutter splint.

Disposition

Refer the patient to an orthopedic surgeon for definitive repair.

3. Carpal Bone Fractures

 ESSENTIALS OF DIAGNOSIS

- *Maintain high index of suspicion.*
- *Consider scaphoid view x-rays.*
- *Treat as fracture based on clinical findings even if x-ray findings are negative.*

General Considerations

Carpal bone fractures are often missed in the emergency department and require a high index of suspicion. Usually they occur after a fall on an outstretched upper extremity. Often, even if a fracture is not seen, the injury should be treated as a fracture in order to prevent long-term sequelae such as avascular necrosis seen with scaphoid or lunate (Kienböck disease) fractures due to the tenuous blood supply of these bones.

Clinical Findings

A. SYMPTOMS AND SIGNS

Carpal bone fractures usually lead to wrist and hand swelling with decreased mobility and pain. Tenderness is often seen over the injured area. If tenderness is present in the anatomic snuffbox, consider a scaphoid fracture, regardless of x-ray findings, and treat the injury appropriately.

B. X-RAY FINDINGS

Scaphoid and other carpal fractures may be seen on anteroposterior or dedicated scaphoid views. A triquetral fracture can often be seen on a lateral hand view as a small dorsal avulsion. Repeat x-rays in 1–2 weeks may often reveal a fracture that was not initially seen.

Treatment

Scaphoid fractures may be treated with a thumb spica splint (Figure 28–8); other fractures may be treated with a volar wrist splint (Figure 28–9).

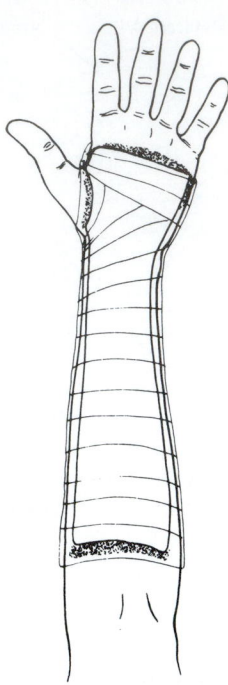

Figure 28–9. Volar splint for immobilization of wrist injuries.

Disposition

Patients may be discharged with analgesics and follow-up with an orthopedist in 2–3 days.

4. Metacarpal Fractures

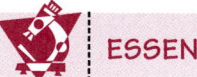 **ESSENTIALS OF DIAGNOSIS**

- Hand swelling and pain.
- Anteroposterior and lateral hand x-rays confirm diagnosis.
- Assess for angulation and rotation.

General Considerations

The most common metacarpal fracture, known as a boxer's fracture, is through the neck of the 5th metacarpal and occurs from punching an object or person. A Bennet fracture refers to an intra-articular fracture at the base of the first metacarpal. If the fracture is

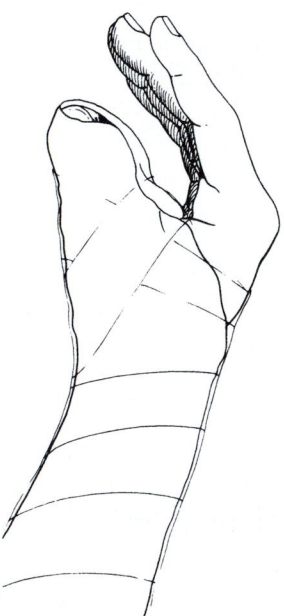

Figure 28–8. Thumb spica splint: A slab of plaster is applied over adequate padding and secured with a loose elastic bandage.

comminuted, then it is usually called a Rolando fracture.

Clinical Findings

A. SYMPTOMS AND SIGNS

The patient presents with hand swelling, particularly over the dorsal surface, and tenderness over the affected bone. Assess for rotational injury by having the patient attempt to close his or her fist. The presence of open wounds should raise the suspicion that the injury resulted from hitting teeth. These wounds should be treated as human bites, with copious irrigation and antibiotics.

B. X-RAY FINDINGS

Most metacarpal fractures should be visible on an anteroposterior or lateral view of the hand. Angulation of the fracture must be assessed in order to determine management.

Treatment

If any manipulation is needed, give the patient appropriate analgesics; local lidocaine infiltration may suffice. Correct any rotational deformity by gentle traction. If angulation of the metacarpal neck requires correction, it may be accomplished with gentle traction. The easiest way to remember angulation is the 10-20-30-40 rule. These are the maximum permissible degrees that may be tolerated in the 2nd, 3rd, 4th, and 5th metacarpals, respectively. Fractures involving the 2nd, 3rd, and 4th metacarpals may be treated with a volar wrist splint (Figure 28–10). After reduction, boxer's fractures may be placed in an ulnar gutter splint (Figure 28–11) and Bennet fractures in a thumb spica splint (see Figure 28–8).

Disposition

After the injury is splinted, the patient may be sent home with adequate analgesia. We recommend arranging follow-up specifically for 1st metacarpal base fractures because they require operative repair.

5. Phalanx Fractures & Dislocations

ESSENTIALS OF DIAGNOSIS

- Finger pain, deformity, and limited mobility.
- Finger x-rays are confirmatory.

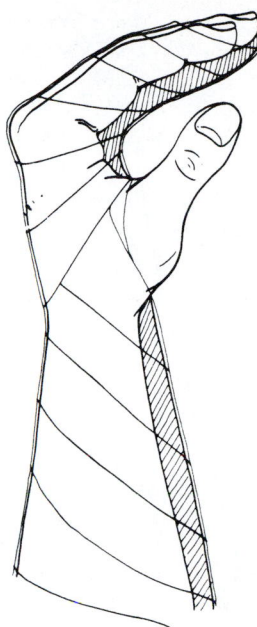

Figure 28–10. Volar wrist and hand splint for immobilization of metacarpal shaft fractures and wrist injuries. A plaster slab is applied over adequate padding and secured with a loose elastic bandage.

General Considerations

Phalanx fractures and dislocations often result from a direct blow to the affected digit. They may have rotational deformities as well as angulation.

Clinical Findings

A. SYMPTOMS AND SIGNS

With dislocations, an obvious deformity usually is seen. Patients with fractures may present with swelling, pain, decreased mobility, ecchymosis, and tenderness. Assess for capillary refill and sensation with 2-point discrimination as well as for rotational injury.

B. X-RAY FINDINGS

Plain x-rays of the hand, including anteroposterior and lateral views, often suffice. Occasionally a specific finger x-ray may be performed.

Treatment

Local anesthesia or digital blocks may be administered before manipulation. Reduction of dislocations and fractures can be managed with simple gentle traction. Splint these injuries with aluminum finger splints.

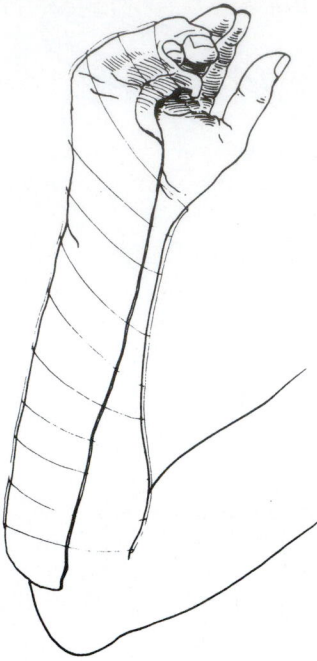

Figure 28–11. Ulnar gutter splint for immobilization of injuries to the metacarpals of the 4th and 5th fingers. A plaster slab is applied to the ulnar border of the forearm and hand over adequate padding and is then secured with a loose elastic bandage.

Disposition

The patient may be discharged with analgesics and hand surgeon follow-up in 3–4 days.

6. Subungual Hematoma
(See also Chapter 29.)

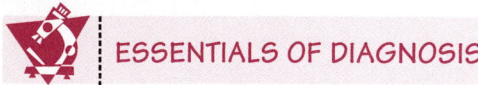

ESSENTIALS OF DIAGNOSIS

- *Painful fingernail and hematoma under nail.*
- *May be associated with tuft fracture.*

General Considerations

Subungual hematomas usually occur from a direct blow to the nail, such as from a hammer.

Clinical Findings

A. SYMPTOMS AND SIGNS

The patient presents with a painful digit. A hematoma is easily seen under the nail.

B. X-RAY FINDINGS

Anterioposterior and lateral views of the affected digit often show a distal tuft fracture.

Treatment

If the hematoma is in excess of 25% of the nail surface, consider removing the nail for inspection of the nail bed. If less than 25% is present, then simple nail trephination may be performed for immediate relief of pain. Trephination is performed by using an electric cautery device or a heated paper clip perpendicular to the nail.

Disposition

Antibiotics are needed if a nailbed injury is present with an open fracture; orthopedic follow-up should occur in 2–3 days. Simple hematomas may be followed up by a primary care provider in 1 week.

7. Boutonniere Deformity
(See also Chapter 29.)

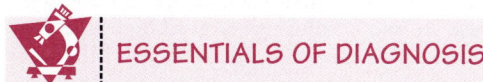

ESSENTIALS OF DIAGNOSIS

- *Swan neck deformity of finger.*
- *May have avulsion fracture on x-ray.*

General Considerations

A boutonniere deformity often occurs from forced flexion at the proximal interphalangeal joint with rupture of the central slip of the extensor tendon, causing the classic deformity.

Clinical Findings

A. SYMPTOMS AND SIGNS

The patient presents with obvious swan neck deformity. Decreased mobility and pain may also be present.

B. X-RAY FINDINGS

Occasionally an avulsion fracture of the middle phalanx may be seen on a lateral finger view.

Treatment

Splint the proximal interphalangeal joint in full extension for 4 weeks. Do not immobilize the distal joint.

Disposition

Discharge the patient with follow-up with a hand surgeon in 1 week. Give analgesics as needed.

8. Mallet Finger
(See also Chapter 29.)

 ESSENTIALS OF DIAGNOSIS

- *Flexion of distal phalanx.*
- *May have small avulsion fracture.*

General Considerations

Mallet finger often occurs as a sports-related injury when the distal phalanx receives a direct blow. The injury is a disruption of the extensor tendon at the site of insertion on the distal phalanx, with subsequently unopposed flexion of the distal phalanx.

Clinical Findings

A. Symptoms and Signs

Pain is present at the distal interphalangeal joint, and the classic mallet deformity occurs, in which the distal phalanx is flexed.

B. X-ray Findings

Occasionally a small avulsion fracture of the dorsal surface of the distal phalanx may be seen.

Treatment

Finger splint the distal interphalangeal joint in slight hyperextension. Commercially available splints can be used to reproduce this alignment. Splinting is required for at least 4–8 weeks.

Disposition

Discharge the patient with orthopedic follow-up within 3–4 days.

9. Ulnar Collateral Ligament Rupture

 ESSENTIALS OF DIAGNOSIS

- *Consider in a fall while holding a ski pole.*
- *Pain and swelling at 1st metacarpophalangeal joint.*
- *X-ray may show small avulsion fracture of proximal phalanx.*

General Considerations

Also known as gamekeeper's or skier's thumb, ulnar collateral ligament rupture occurs after a forceful dislocation radially of the proximal phalanx of the thumb with spontaneous relocation that results in rupture of the ulnar collateral ligament. This injury most commonly results from falling with a ski pole in hand.

Clinical Findings

A. Symptoms and Signs

Pain and swelling are present over the ulnar aspect of the proximal phalanx and metacarpal of the thumb. Weak pinching ability may be present. On exam there is tenderness with no end point on stress testing of the metacarpophalangeal joint (Figure 28–12). Stress testing in the emergency department is usually not possible in an acute injury.

B. X-ray Findings

Occasionally an avulsion fracture of the proximal phalanx may be seen.

Treatment

Apply a thumb spica splint and provide analgesics. Complete tears ultimately require surgical repair.

Disposition

Discharge the patient after immobilization; orthopedic follow-up is needed in 3–4 days for further repair.

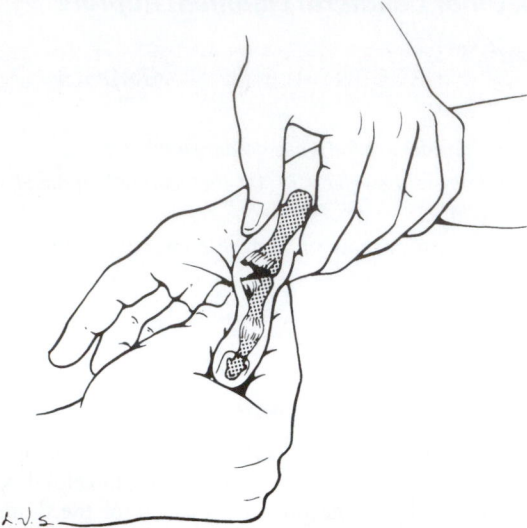

Figure 28–12. Stress examination of the thumb metacarpophalangeal collateral ligament. The ulnar side is injured more frequently. Test both sides in extension and 30 degrees of flexion. Compare the injured digit with the uninjured thumb. Feel for a firm end point and absence of excessive laxity.

PELVIC GIRDLE INJURIES

PELVIC FRACTURES

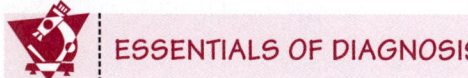

ESSENTIALS OF DIAGNOSIS

- *High degree of mortality.*
- *May have large amount of bleeding.*
- *Consider if scrotal hematoma, urethra blood, or abnormal prostate are present.*
- *Anteroposterior films are usually confirmatory.*

General Considerations

Pelvic fractures can be devastating injuries associated with significant mortality. The mechanism of injury in the majority of fractures is a high-velocity trauma as seen in motor vehicle collisions or when pedestrians are struck by cars. Fractures may also occur with low-velocity trauma such as crush injuries and simple falls, often seen in elderly individuals with osteoporosis. Much of

the high degree of mortality may be related to the incidence of significant associated injuries (eg, head, thoracic, abdominal trauma). High-energy injuries that significantly disrupt the pelvic ring commonly tear pelvic veins and arteries. Bleeding associated with these injuries is frequently massive with the potential for exsanguination (see Table 28–1). The mortality rate for patients presenting with hypotension associated with pelvic fractures is approximately 50%. The mechanism and associated injuries determine the patient's presentation.

Clinical Findings

A. SYMPTOMS AND SIGNS

All patients should receive a digital rectal examination to look for the presence of blood, to determine the position of the prostate, and for palpation of obvious fractures. Examination of the penis and testes or the vagina is necessary to evaluate for associated urologic and gynecologic injuries. If a urethral injury is suspected, do not place a urinary catheter; obtain a retrograde cystogram. If a urethral injury is present, consult with a urologist to place a suprapubic or Foley catheter (see Chapter 26). Compression to determine pelvic stability should be accomplished with gentle anteroposterior and lateral pressure (Figure 28–13).

B. X-RAY FINDINGS

X-rays should initially include an anteroposterior view. Inlet and outlet views may be helpful; however, CT scanning should be obtained to classify the extent of injury and to plan for treatment.

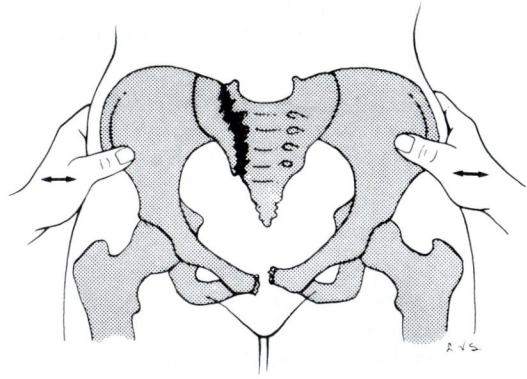

Figure 28–13. Compression-distraction test for stability of the pelvic ring. If the iliac crests can be pressed together or pulled apart, the pelvis is unstable. With more severe instability, one hemipelvis may be displaced proximally.

Treatment

Fractures associated with disruption of the symphysis pubis (open book fractures) are frequently associated with massive bleeding into the pelvis. The patient should be monitored continuously with attention to the circulatory status and adequate volume replacement. Application of military antishock trousers may be initiated in the prehospital setting and needs to be continued in the emergency department. A sheet wrapped around the pelvis may also be used in an attempt to stabilize the fracture, decrease the volume of the pelvis, and help tamponade bleeding. In some cases the orthopedist may opt to place an external fixator device in the emergency department. Some patients may need emergent ORIF or need to be transferred to radiology for arteriography and embolization.

Disposition

Obtain orthopedic consultation in all cases. Most patients will require hospitalization. Simple nondisplaced fractures of the pubic rami may be managed conservatively on an outpatient basis. Consultation with trauma surgery, urology, and gynecology may also be necessary.

HIP INJURIES

General Considerations

Hip injuries include various fractures and dislocations. As with pelvic fractures, hip injuries in young individuals are associated with high-energy trauma (eg, motor vehicle collisions, falls from height) and may be seen with direct (falls) or indirect (knee-to-dashboard) forces. Elderly patients frequently sustain hip injuries with lower forces such as a fall from standing.

1. Hip Fractures

ESSENTIALS OF DIAGNOSIS

- *Frequent in elderly patients.*
- *Hip pain and tenderness.*
- *Frequently limb is shortened and externally rotated.*
- *Anteroposterior and lateral films are usually confirmatory.*
- *Consider CT scan or MRI if x-rays are negative and diagnosis is still suspected.*

General Considerations

Hip fractures are described anatomically as they may occur through the femoral neck, intertrochanteric, or subtrochanteric.

Clinical Findings

A. SYMPTOMS AND SIGNS

The patient usually complains of groin pain. Shortening of the affected leg, with abduction and external rotation, is common but may not be obvious in cases of nondisplaced fractures.

B. X-RAY FINDINGS

Radiographs should include anteroposterior (with the legs in internal rotation) and lateral views. CT scanning may be necessary, particularly if acetabular involvement is suspected.

Treatment

Immobilize the affected leg. If the fracture is closed and no neurologic deficits are present, inline traction may be applied. This immobilization is often initiated in the prehospital setting.

Disposition

Monitor the patient for potential ongoing blood loss. Because of the risk of avascular necrosis of the femoral head, which occurs in 20% of these injuries, early orthopedic consultation is needed. Orthopedic consultation and admission for ORIF is warranted in the evaluation of all hip fractures.

2. Hip Dislocations

ESSENTIALS OF DIAGNOSIS

- *Pain and deformity at hip.*
- *Posterior dislocation is most common.*
- *Hip or pelvic x-rays are confirmatory.*
- *Patient's lower extremity is usually internally rotated and shortened.*

General Considerations

Hip dislocations are described by the relationship of the femoral head to the acetabulum. Dislocations may be accompanied by fractures of the acetabulum or femoral head. The vast majority (80–90%) of dislocations are posterior and are typically seen by indirect forces such as knee-to-dashboard injuries in motor vehicle collisions. Anterior dislocations are less common (10–15%) and may be seen slightly more frequently in patients with hip prostheses. Central dislocation refers to the femoral head being forced through a comminuted fracture of the acetabulum. Inferior dislocations are rare and occur almost exclusively in young children. Dislocations of the hip are generally the result of significant force, and potential associated injuries should be sought.

Clinical Findings

A. Symptoms and Signs

Clinical examination in posterior dislocations generally reveals a slightly shortened extremity, adduction, and internal rotation, with the hip and knee in flexion. With anterior dislocations, findings include abduction, external rotation, and flexion of the hip.

B. X-ray Findings

Obtain anteroposterior and lateral views to confirm the diagnosis and rule out associated fractures.

Treatment

Hip dislocations require urgent reduction to decrease the risk of avascular necrosis and neurologic sequelae. Posterior hip dislocations are commonly reduced by the Allis technique (Figure 28–14). After adequate sedation, the patient is placed supine and an assistant stabilizes the pelvis. The hip and knee are flexed to 90 degrees while upward traction and slight rotation are applied. Once the dislocation is reduced, the leg is extended.

An alternative method is the Stimson technique. The patient is placed prone with the leg extended over the edge of the bed. With an assistant stabilizing the pelvis, downward traction is applied with gentle rotation. The assistant then applies pressure over the greater trochanter toward the acetabulum.

Disposition

Once the dislocation is reduced by either method, the leg should be extended and placed in traction until postreduction x-rays can be obtained. Obtain orthopedic consultation for all hip dislocations.

Brooks RA, Ribbans WJ: Diagnosis and imaging studies of traumatic hip dislocations in the adult. Clin Orthop 2000; 377:15. [PMID: 10943181]

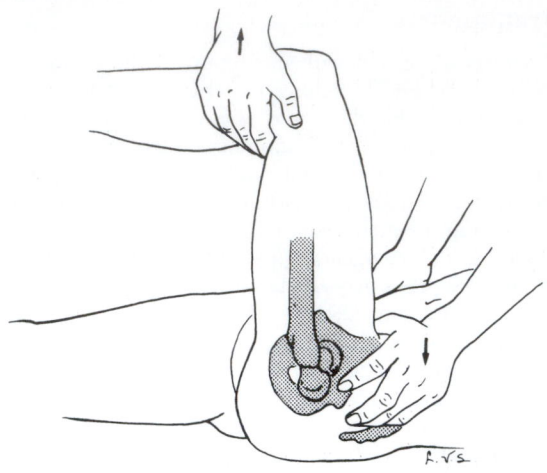

Figure 28–14. The Allis technique for reduction of posterior hip dislocation. Both hip and knee are flexed 90 degrees. An assistant stabilizes the pelvis while the operator pulls the femur anteriorly, rotating it slightly internally and externally to aid reduction, which is achieved mainly by deliberate, steady traction.

Yang EC, Cornwall R: Initial treatment of traumatic hip dislocations in the adult. Clin Orthop 2000;377:24. [PMID: 10943182]

LOWER EXTREMITY INJURIES

FEMORAL SHAFT FRACTURES

 ESSENTIALS OF DIAGNOSIS

- *Pain and deformity of femur.*
- *May lose large amount of blood in thigh.*
- *Anteroposterior and lateral x-rays of femur are confirmatory.*

Clinical Findings

Fractures of the femoral shaft occur most commonly with high-energy trauma. Fractures occurring with minimal trauma should alert the emergency physician to the possibility of a pathologic fracture.

A. Symptoms and Signs

As noted earlier, significant bleeding may occur secondary to femoral shaft fractures (see Table 28–1). The patient typically presents with tenderness and deformity of the thigh. Evaluate and document the neurovascular status. Although not as common as with lower leg fractures, significant soft tissue swelling can occur; therefore, frequent reexaminations should be performed to assess for the development of compartment syndrome.

B. X-RAY FINDINGS

Anteroposterior and lateral views should confirm the diagnosis. Adequate visualization of the knee and hip on these films is important because associated fractures are common.

Treatment

Adequate pain control and fluid resuscitation is indicated. Inline traction, either skeletal traction or an external traction device, should be applied to the leg.

Disposition

Obtain orthopedic consultation for admission and ORIF (usually with an intramedullary rod).

KNEE JOINT INJURIES

The knee is a large synovial hinge joint and is the most commonly involved joint in orthopedic injuries seen in the emergency department. The knee has a complex architecture of bone, muscle, ligament, and cartilage. The bones of the knee joint include the distal femur, proximal tibia, and patella. The fibula is not a part of the knee joint but serves as the attachment point for the lateral collateral ligament. The bones offer little stability to the joint, and the knee relies on the soft tissue components for proper function.

The medial collateral ligament originates from the medial femoral epicondyle and inserts on the medial aspect of the tibia just distal to the tibiofemoral joint. The medial collateral ligament provides stability to valgus stresses (Figure 28–15A) and helps stabilize the medial meniscus. The lateral collateral ligament originates from the lateral femoral epicondyle and inserts onto the proximal fibula, providing resistance to varus forces (Figure 28–15B). The cruciate ligaments are located within the intercondylar notch and are named anterior and posterior by their attachment to the tibia at the tibial spines. The cruciate ligaments protect against anterior and posterior displacement of the knee.

The menisci are cartilages positioned on the tibia. The menisci help dissipate forces within the knee joint and help prevent abnormal movement of the tibia and femur. The hamstring muscles (semitendinous, semimembranous, and the two heads of the biceps femoris)

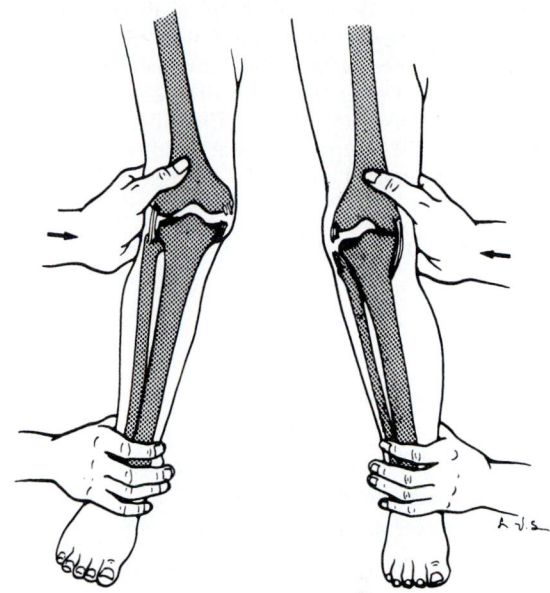

Figure 28–15. Valgus (**A**) and varus (**B**) stress tests for rupture of the medial and lateral collateral ligaments of the knee. More laxity than in the uninjured knee or lack of a firm end point constitutes a positive test. Pain and muscle guarding may make interpretation difficult.

are the main flexors of the knee. The quadriceps muscles (vastus medialis, vastus lateralis, vastus intermedius, rectus femoris) combine to form the quadriceps tendon, which inserts onto the superior patella and the retinaculum of the joint capsule and functions in extension of the knee joint.

The vasculature around the knee joint merits special attention. The collateral circulation is tenuous, and the popliteal artery is responsible for the blood supply to the lower leg. The popliteal artery is tethered above at the hiatus of the adductor magnus and below at the soleus muscle. This tethering makes the popliteal artery susceptible to injury from traction forces as seen with dislocations as well as disruption from fractures or penetrating wounds.

The emergency department evaluation of an acute knee injury frequently involves obtaining plain x-rays, with anteroposterior, lateral, and sunrise view. Several clinical decision rules exist to aid the emergency physician in determining which patients need x-rays acutely. The Pittsburgh rules note that mechanism of injury (such as blunt trauma and falls), patient age (greater than 55 years or less than 12 years), and inability to walk at least 4 weight-bearing steps are predictors of fractures that require radiographic evaluation. The Ottawa rules identify 5 indications for radiographs of the knee: age greater than 55 years, isolated tenderness of the patella, tenderness of the head of the fibula, inability to flex the knee to 90 degrees, and inability to transfer weight for 4 steps. Both sets of rules have demonstrated high sensitivity in predicting injuries and may be helpful to the emergency physician in the evaluation of the acutely injured knee.

1. Patella Fractures

ESSENTIALS OF DIAGNOSIS

- *May be secondary to direct blow or traction injury.*
- *Pain and tenderness are commonly seen.*
- *May disrupt extensor mechanism.*
- *Plain x-rays are usually sufficient.*
- *Bipartite patella may be misinterpreted as fracture.*

General Considerations

The patella is the largest sesamoid bone in the body and may be fractured by direct forces such as falls and by indirect forces. Forceful contraction of the quadriceps muscles may result in a transverse fracture of the patella. Significant fractures of the patella may disrupt the extensor mechanism of the knee.

Clinical Findings

A. Symptoms and Signs

Examination of the patient reveals pain and tenderness over the patella. A joint effusion may be present. If the patella is displaced significantly, a patellar defect may be palpable.

B. X-ray Findings

Plain radiographs including anteroposterior, lateral, and sunrise views are usually sufficient to identify the fracture; however, CT scanning or MRI may be necessary to identify occult injuries. Bipartite or multipartite patellae are congenital findings that may be confused with acute fracture.

Treatment

Obtain orthopedic consultation. Simple fractures may be treated with immobilization of the knee in extension.

Disposition

Patients with simple fractures may be discharged with outpatient follow-up. Open and displaced fractures require surgical repair.

2. Patella Dislocations

ESSENTIALS OF DIAGNOSIS

- *Common in adolescents.*
- *Almost always displaces laterally.*
- *Obvious deformity, restriction of motion.*
- *Plain x-rays are usually sufficient for diagnosis.*

General Considerations

The patella may be dislocated or subluxed by direct forces or a hyperflexion injury. The patella almost always displaces laterally. This injury occurs most commonly in adolescents. Often the patient gives a history of prior subluxations that resolved spontaneously.

Clinical Findings

A. Symptoms and Signs

Tenderness is present on physical examination, and a deformity is usually easily seen. A joint effusion may be present.

B. X-ray Findings

Plain radiographs are usually sufficient to confirm the injury.

Treatment

Management consists of closed reduction with appropriate sedation. This is accomplished by applying medial force to the patella while the knee is being extended.

Disposition

Immobilize the knee, give the patient crutches, and provide orthopedic referral for follow-up. Recurrent subluxations or dislocations may require surgical repair.

3. Distal Femur Fractures

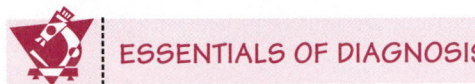

ESSENTIALS OF DIAGNOSIS

- *Generally represent high-energy injuries.*
- *Associated hip and patella injuries are common.*
- *Plain x-rays are usually sufficient.*
- *Obtain arteriogram if vascular injury is suspected.*

General Considerations

Fractures in the distal one third of the femur are typically described by the relationship of the fracture line to the femoral condyles. Distal femur fractures generally represent high-energy injuries.

Clinical Findings

A. SYMPTOMS AND SIGNS

Pain and deformity are usually present. Associated patella and hip injuries sometimes occur.

B. X-RAY FINDINGS

Diagnosis can usually be made with standard anteroposterior and lateral views. Oblique views and CT scanning may also be needed. If vascular compromise is suspected, obtain an arteriogram.

Disposition

Distal femur fractures are significant injuries that require orthopedic consultation in the emergency department. Skeletal traction and surgical repair are frequently required.

4. Tibial Plateau Fractures

ESSENTIALS OF DIAGNOSIS

- *Usually occur to lateral aspect.*
- *May be associated with peroneal nerve and popliteal artery injuries.*
- *CT scan is helpful in planning treatment.*
- *High suspicion for compartment syndrome.*

General Considerations

Tibial plateau fractures may result from axial loading and varus or valgus forces. The lateral portion of the tibia is most commonly involved. The fracture significantly impairs the function of the knee joint. Popliteal artery and peroneal nerve injuries may be seen, and the neurovascular status should be monitored continuously and documented.

Clinical Findings

A. SYMPTOMS AND SIGNS

Pain and tenderness are usually easily elicited. A hemarthrosis may be present, and the incidence of associated ligamentous injuries is significant.

B. X-RAY FINDINGS

Diagnosis is usually made on anteroposterior and lateral x-rays. CT scanning is often used to delineate the extent of the injury. Tomograms and MRI may also be used. If vascular injury is suspected, obtain an arteriogram.

Treatment & Disposition

Obtain orthopedic consultation to determine appropriate management. A compartment syndrome may accompany tibial plateau fractures, and compartment pressures should be measured if indicated.

5. Tibial Tuberosity Fractures & Osgood Schlatter Disease

ESSENTIALS OF DIAGNOSIS

- *Usually avulsion fracture of patella tendon.*
- *Obtain orthopedic consultation to determine treatment.*

General Considerations

These fractures generally occur secondary to strong flexion or extension of the knee against resistance. Fractures usually occur prior to closure of the epiphysis and represent an avulsion fracture caused by the patella tendon.

Clinical Findings

Tenderness is present and, based on the mechanism of injury, an effusion may be seen. Diagnosis is confirmed with plain radiographs. In adolescents, Osgood-Schlatter disease must be in the differential diagnosis. Osgood-Schlatter disease is most commonly seen in males aged 10–13 years. It represents a chronic traction injury to the tibial tuberosity and commonly occurs in adolescents engaging in sporting activities. Radiographic findings may be difficult to differentiate from an acute fracture. A careful history and exam will help delineate an acute injury. A hemarthrosis is not associated with Osgood-Schlatter.

Treatment & Disposition

Orthopedic consultation is necessary because tibial tuberosity fractures may require open reduction. Osgood-Schlatter disease is treated with immobilization and, in rare cases, surgery.

6. Tibial Spine Fractures

ESSENTIALS OF DIAGNOSIS

- *Not common; usually seen in children.*
- *Usually avulsion injury from cruciate ligament.*
- *Suspect associate ligament injury.*

General Considerations

Fractures of the tibial spines are not commonly seen. These fractures usually represent an avulsion injury by one of the cruciate ligaments. They are more commonly seen in children and most often involve the anterior tibial spine.

Clinical Findings

A. SYMPTOMS AND SIGNS

Localized pain and a hemarthrosis may be present. If a significant ligamentous injury has occurred, instability of the knee may be seen.

B. X-RAY FINDINGS

The presentation may be subtle and may be noted only as an incidental finding on the x-ray. Plain films will usually identify the injury. CT scanning, MRI, or arthroscopy may be needed to identify associated injuries such as cruciate ligament ruptures.

Treatment

Simple fractures are usually treated with immobilization.

Disposition

If significant ligamentous injury is present, surgery may be necessary.

7. Knee Dislocations

ESSENTIALS OF DIAGNOSIS

- *May be seen with high- or low-velocity injuries.*
- *Tenderness and joint effusion are usually present.*
- *Assess for associated popliteal artery injury.*

General Considerations

Dislocations involving the tibiofemoral joint (as opposed to patellar dislocations) are an orthopedic emergency and may represent a limb-threatening injury. They are commonly seen in high-energy trauma but may also be seen with low-velocity injuries such as from falls or jumping on a trampoline. The presence of a dislocation represents significant trauma to the soft tissues (ie, ligaments, menisci, and joint capsule). As noted above, the location and anatomy of the popliteal artery places it at significant risk of injury, particularly with posterior dislocations. Tenderness and joint effusion are generally present.

Clinical Findings

A. SYMPTOMS AND SIGNS

Visual deformity may be obvious, but some dislocations may reduce prior to evaluation. Careful attention to the neurovascular status is indicated, and the presence of a pulse does not rule out an arterial injury.

B. X-RAY FINDINGS

Plain radiographs help confirm the diagnosis. Traditionally, arteriography was recommended in all cases to identify arterial injuries such as intimal tears, which may be clinically subtle but progress to occlusion and ischemia. Some authors recommend that serial exams may be sufficient in low-velocity trauma. However, if arterial trauma is a possibility, arteriography or Doppler studies should be obtained.

Treatment

Management includes emergent reduction by inline longitudinal traction. The neurovascular status should be monitored continuously and reassessed frequently.

Disposition

Orthopedic consultation is necessary, and vascular surgical consultation may be needed. Patients for whom arteriography has not been obtained should be admitted for observation.

8. Knee Ligament Injuries: General Considerations

 ESSENTIALS OF DIAGNOSIS

- *Guarding and joint effusions may make diagnosis difficult in acute setting.*
- *Patient may need immobilization and follow-up examination.*

Knee ligament injuries may range from minor sprains to complete disruptions. The more subtle injuries may be difficult to assess acutely because guarding and joint effusions may make determination of joint instability problematic. If possible, the unaffected knee should be examined before the injured knee in order to determine the patient's baseline, because some degree of laxity may be normal for an individual. After initial clinical and radiographic assessment, it is often prudent to treat the injury with a period of immobilization and crutches and to arrange for a follow-up examination. Depending on the patient's clinical situation and associated injuries, it is sometimes helpful to have the orthopedic consultant examine the patient under general anesthesia.

9. Knee Ligament Injuries: Collateral Ligaments

The medial collateral ligament is the most commonly injured ligament in the knee. The mechanism of injury often involves sporting events. The lateral collateral ligament is less commonly involved and occurs more often in high-energy trauma such as motor vehicle collisions.

Clinical Findings

A. Symptoms and Signs

The patient usually presents with tenderness along the distribution of the ligament. Evaluate the ligament's stability by placing varus and valgus stresses (see Figure 28–15) with the knee in extension and with 30 degrees flexion.

B. X-ray Findings

Plain radiography is of limited use but should be obtained initially to rule out associated fractures. MRI has emerged as a useful modality to evaluate these injuries. Orthopedic follow-up should be arranged.

Treatment

Simple strains may be treated conservatively with immobilization and follow-up examination.

Disposition

Unstable joints will need further evaluation (eg, MRI, arthroscopy) and eventual surgical repair.

10. Knee Ligament Injuries: Cruciate Ligaments

Injuries to the cruciate ligaments usually result from direct anterior or posterior forces to the knee. Rotational forces may also injure the cruciate ligaments and are usually associated with other injuries (ie, menisci, collateral ligaments). Injuries may be associated with high- or low-energy trauma. The anterior cruciate ligament is the one most commonly injured.

Clinical Findings

A. Symptoms and Signs

Joint effusions are common, and hemarthrosis may be seen particularly with anterior cruciate ligament injuries. Stability of the anterior cruciate ligament is assessed clinically by the Lachman (Figure 28–16), pivot shift, or anterior drawer tests. Stability of the posterior cruciate ligament is evaluated by Sag sign (Figure 28–17).

B. X-ray Findings

Plain radiography may be unrevealing. Avulsion fractures of the tibial spines suggest a cruciate ligament tear. If the clinical examination does not reveal significant instability, outpatient follow-up examination may include MRI.

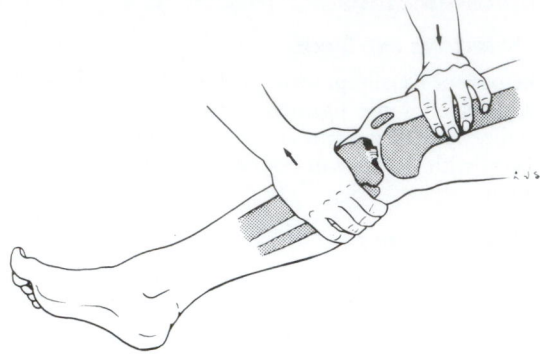

Figure 28–16. The Lachman test for rupture of the anterior cruciate ligament. Attempt to pull the tibia forward relative to the femur while the knee is slightly flexed. Any increase in laxity compared with the uninjured knee signifies injury.

Treatment

Immobilize the knee and give the patient crutches and non-weight-bearing status instructions.

Disposition

Orthopedic follow-up is indicated for all significant injuries, and arthroscopy may be performed for both diagnosis and treatment.

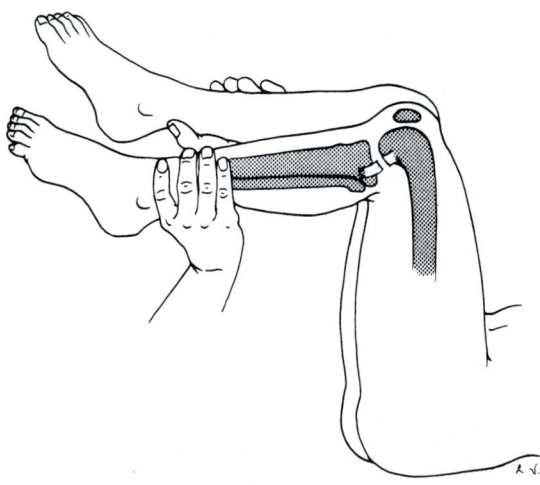

Figure 28–17. Rupture of the posterior cruciate ligament is a likely diagnosis when the tibia of the injured knee sags posteriorly below the distal femur when the legs are held flexed 90 degrees at the hip and knee.

11. Meniscal Tears

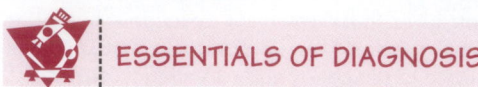 ESSENTIALS OF DIAGNOSIS

- *Medial meniscus most commonly affected.*
- *Patient may complain of knee locking.*
- *MRI or arthroscopy may be necessary for diagnosis.*

General Considerations

Meniscal tears usually occur when a rotational force is applied to the knee while the foot is planted. Because of degenerative process, the injury producing the acute tear may not be significant. The medial meniscus is most commonly affected.

Clinical Findings

A. SYMPTOMS AND SIGNS

The patient may complain of hearing a pop, but this finding is not specific. Joint line tenderness is usually present, and the patient may complain that the knee "locks." This locking is usually seen with a "bucket-handle" tear of the meniscus when the free central portion becomes lodged in the intercondylar notch. Clinical diagnosis is evaluated by use of the McMurray and Apley tests.

B. X-RAY FINDINGS

Plain films will not identify the tear but may be useful if associated bony injuries are suspected.

Treatment

Treatment involves knee immobilization, crutches, and pain control.

Disposition

Patients may be discharged from the emergency department with immobilization and orthopedic follow-up. Outpatient MRI is commonly used to make the diagnosis. Arthroscopy may be diagnostic and used to perform meniscectomy.

Roberts DM, Stallard TC: Emergency department evaluation and treatment of knee and leg injuries. Emerg Med Clin North Am 2000;18(1):67. [PMID: 10678160]

Seaburg DC et al: Multicenter comparison of two clinical decision rules for the use of radiography in acute, high-risk knee injuries. Ann Emerg Med 1998;32(1):8. [PMID: 9656942]

Swenson TM: Physical diagnosis of the multiple-ligament-injured knee. Clin Sports Med 2000;19(3):415. [PMID: 10918957]

12. Tendon Ruptures

- *May disrupt extensor mechanism.*
- *Quadriceps tendon is more commonly affected.*
- *CT scan or MRI may be needed to confirm diagnosis.*

General Considerations

Complete rupture of the quadriceps or patella tendon will disrupt the extensor mechanism of the knee. Injuries can occur with high-energy injuries or may be seen with low-energy trauma, particularly in the elderly. The quadriceps tendon is more commonly ruptured compared to the patella tendon.

Clinical Findings

A. SYMPTOMS AND SIGNS

The patient presents with a swollen and tender knee and is unable to extend the knee against resistance. A palpable defect may be appreciated.

B. X-RAY FINDINGS

Plain films may demonstrate an abnormal position of the patella. CT scanning and MRI confirm the diagnosis.

Treatment

Place the patient in a knee immobilizer until consultation is obtained.

Disposition

Management depends on the extent of the injury. Complete ruptures require surgical repair.

TIBIAL SHAFT FRACTURES

- *Most common long bone fracture.*
- *Open fractures sometimes occur.*
- *Plain x-rays are usually sufficient for diagnosis.*
- *Assess for compartment syndrome.*

General Considerations

The tibia is the most common site of long bone fractures. The majority of these fractures will occur with associated fracture of the fibula. The tibia can be injured by a variety of forces.

Clinical Findings

A. SYMPTOMS AND SIGNS

Because little soft tissue is found around the tibia anteriorly, open fractures are common. Pain, swelling, and deformity are usually present. Compartment syndrome sometimes occurs with tibial injuries, and frequent reassessments should be performed.

B. X-RAY FINDINGS

Plain films are usually adequate to identify the fracture. As with all suspected long bone injuries, the joints above and below should be adequately visualized on the radiographs.

Treatment

Measure compartment pressure if a compartment syndrome is suspected clinically. Simple nondisplaced fractures may be treated with a long leg posterior splint and crutches with orthopedic follow-up.

Disposition

Open, displaced, and comminuted fractures require orthopedic consultation because they require operative management.

FIBULA FRACTURES

- *Isolated fibula fractures are uncommon.*
- *Patient may be able to bear weight.*
- *Assess for Maisonneuve fracture.*

General Considerations

Isolated fibular fractures are uncommon because they are usually seen with an associated tibia fracture. They may occur by direct blow or with rotational forces. Of particular importance is a Maisonneuve fracture, which is a fracture of the proximal fibula with an associated medial malleolus ankle fracture or ligamentous disruption of the ankle without a fracture.

Clinical Findings

A. SYMPTOMS AND SIGNS

The patient usually complains of pain and tenderness, and a deformity can usually be palpated. If the fracture is an isolated fibular shaft fracture, the patient may be able to walk.

B. X-RAY FINDINGS

Plain x-rays should be sufficient for the diagnosis.

Treatment

Splints or compressive dressing may be applied for comfort. A Maisonneuve fracture represents an unstable ankle injury, and orthopedic consultation is needed to determine definitive management.

Disposition

With isolated, uncomplicated fibula fractures, the patient may be discharged with instructions to advance from non-weight-bearing status to weight-bearing status as tolerated.

ANKLE JOINT INJURIES

The bones of the ankle include the distal tibia, distal fibula, and the talus. The ankle mortise is formed by the medial and lateral malleoli and the plafond (the articular surface of the distal tibia). As with the knee, the ankle relies on articular cartilage, joint capsule, and ligaments to provide joint stability. Management of ankle injuries is based largely on the joint's stability.

The ligaments are divided into three sets: the syndesmotic (anterior and posterior tibiofibular ligaments); the lateral collateral (calcaneofibular, anterior talofibular, and lateral tibiocalcaneal ligaments); and the medial collateral or deltoid ligaments, which are further divided into four parts (posterior tibiotalar, tibiocalcaneal, anterior tibiotalar, and tibionavicular). Ankle injuries are common and often involve a combination of bony and ligamentous injuries.

As with knee injuries, clinical decision rules aid the emergency physician in determining whether plain radiography is needed in the evaluation of ankle or foot injuries. The Ottawa ankle rules state that ankle x-rays should be obtained if there is pain at the malleoli, inability to bear weight for 4 steps, and tenderness posteriorly or inferiorly at the malleoli. Ottawa foot rules recommend that x-rays be obtained if there is inability to bear weight for 4 steps and tenderness at the base of the fifth metatarsal or over the navicular bone. The sensitivity of the Ottawa ankle rules is 98–100%.

Pijnenburg AC et al: Radiography in acute ankle injuries: The Ottawa ankle rules versus local diagnostic decision rules. Ann Emerg Med 2002;39:599. [PMID: 12023701]

1. Lateral Malleolar Fractures

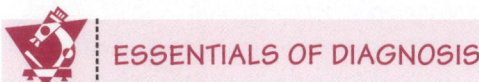 ESSENTIALS OF DIAGNOSIS

- *Inversion injury.*
- *May include minor avulsion fractures to complete joint disruption.*
- *Plain x-rays are usually sufficient for diagnosis.*

General Considerations

Lateral malleolar fractures may range from simple avulsion fractures seen with inversion to displaced fractures with mortise disruption.

Clinical Findings

A. SYMPTOMS AND SIGNS

The patient usually presents with point tenderness, swelling, and difficulty ambulating.

B. X-RAY FINDINGS

Plain radiographs are usually sufficient to make the diagnosis.

Treatment

Simple fractures may be treated with a posterior short leg splint with stirrups (Figure 28–18), crutches with no weight bearing, and orthopedic follow-up.

Disposition

Open or displaced fractures require orthopedic consultation for operative management.

2. Medial Malleolar Fractures

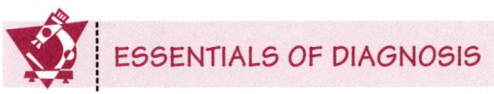 ESSENTIALS OF DIAGNOSIS

- *Eversion injury.*
- *Often associated with deltoid ligament injury.*
- *Plain x-rays are usually sufficient for diagnosis.*

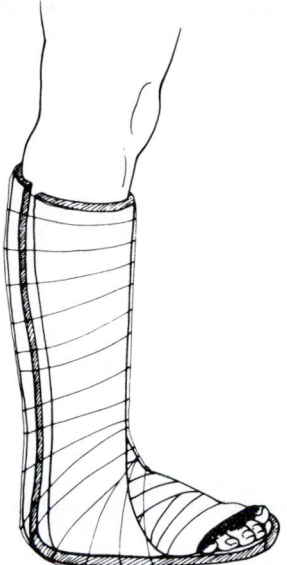

Figure 28–18. Combined sugar-tong splint and posterior-plantar plaster slab with padding for ambulatory (non-weight-bearing) patient with foot injuries.

General Considerations

Medial malleolar fractures result from eversion injuries or external rotation. These fractures are frequently associated with injuries to the deltoid ligament.

Clinical Findings

A. SYMPTOMS AND SIGNS

Pain, swelling, and difficulty in ambulating are usually present. Palpate the proximal fibula to determine whether a Maisonneuve fracture is present.

B. X-RAY FINDINGS

Plain films will usually suffice for the diagnosis.

Treatment

Management is similar to that for lateral malleolar fractures; however, if significant injury to the deltoid ligament has occurred, the rehabilitation period will be longer.

Disposition

Patients with closed injuries may be discharged with a posterior short leg splint with stirrups (Fig 28–18), crutches with no weight bearing, and orthopedic follow up in 2–3 days.

3. Posterior Malleolar Fractures

 ESSENTIALS OF DIAGNOSIS

- *Rare injury.*
- *Usually avulsion from posterior talofibular ligament.*
- *May represent significant joint instability.*

General Considerations

Fractures involving only the posterior malleoli are rare. They usually result from an avulsion injury involving the posterior tibiofibular ligament. If isolated they may be managed conservatively as above. If these fractures are associated with other injuries or joint instability, orthopedic consultation is indicated. Bimalleolar and trimalleolar fractures should be considered unstable and mandate orthopedic consultation for surgical management.

4. Achilles Tendon Injuries

 ESSENTIALS OF DIAGNOSIS

- *May occur from direct or indirect forces.*
- *Use Thompson test.*
- *Orthopedic consultation is necessary.*

General Considerations

Rupture of the Achilles tendon is often seen in middle-aged individuals participating in sporting activities. It may be secondary to a direct blow or can occur with indirect forces as with forced dorsiflexion. The patient frequently reports hearing a pop.

Clinical Findings

A. SYMPTOMS AND SIGNS

Localized pain and weakness in plantarflexion are present, and a deformity may be appreciated. The clinical diagnosis is based on history and clinical examination. To determine if the tendon has been ruptured, the emergency physician can squeeze the calf muscles with the patient prone and the knee flexed to 90 degrees (Thompson test) or alternatively squeeze the calf muscles with the patient kneeling on a chair with both

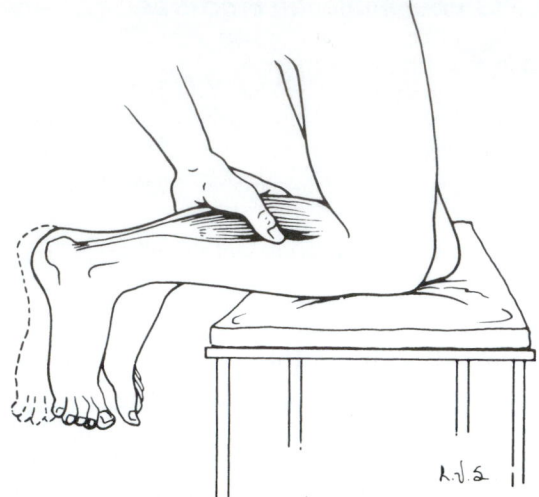

Figure 28–19. Test for Achilles tendon continuity. Squeeze the relaxed calf while observing the amount of ankle plantarflexion thus produced. If the tendon is ruptured, less motion occurs compared with that on the uninjured side.

knees flexed (Figure 28–19). Absence of plantarflexion or decreased plantarflexion compared to the unaffected side suggests rupture.

B. X-ray Findings

X-rays may show thickening of the tendon. MRI will confirm the diagnosis.

Treatment

A temporary long leg or stirrup splint may be placed until consultation with orthopedics.

Disposition

Orthopedic consultation should be obtained because Achilles tendon injuries may be managed surgically or nonoperatively.

5. Peroneal Tendon Injuries

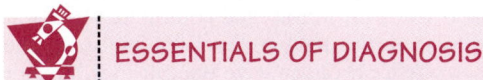
ESSENTIALS OF DIAGNOSIS

- *Usually results from forced dorsiflexion.*
- *Tenderness posterior to lateral malleolus.*

• *CT scan or MRI may be needed to confirm diagnosis.*

General Considerations

The peroneal tendons function in eversion, pronation, and plantarflexion. These tendons can become subluxed or dislocated by tearing of the superior retinaculum attachment on the fibula. The injury usually results from forced dorsiflexion.

Clinical Findings

A. Symptoms and Signs

The patient presents with pain, swelling, and weakness on eversion. Tenderness posterior to the lateral malleolus is present.

B. X-ray Findings

A small avulsion fracture of the lateral malleolus is pathognomonic of this injury. A CT or MRI scan may be needed to confirm the diagnosis.

Treatment

Treatment involves use of a posterior mold, crutches with no weight bearing, and analgesics.

Disposition

Orthopedic consultation is necessary to determine appropriate management. Patients with these injuries may be discharged with appropriate follow-up, but peroneal tendon injuries often need surgical repair.

Kibler WB: Diagnosis, treatment and rehabilitation principles in complete tendon ruptures in sports. Scand J Med Sci Sports 1997;7:119. [PMID: 9211613]

6. Ankle Dislocations

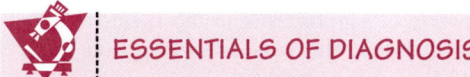
ESSENTIALS OF DIAGNOSIS

- *Associated fracture often present.*
- *Assess neurovascular status.*
- *Dislocation may require reduction before x-rays are obtained.*

General Considerations

An ankle dislocation represents displacement of the talus and foot from the tibia. Dislocations are described by the relationship of the talus to the tibia. They may be open or closed, and an associated fracture frequently occurs. Dislocations occur from axial loading to the foot in plantarflexion and are seen in sporting injuries and in high-energy trauma such as motor vehicle collisions.

Clinical Findings

A. SYMPTOMS AND SIGNS

The neurovascular status should be determined quickly. The patient will have gross deformity of the ankle joint.

B. X-RAY FINDINGS

Reduction is often performed prior to obtaining radiographs.

Treatment

Once the dislocation has been reduced, reassess the neurovascular status, splint the ankle, and obtain radiographs and orthopedic consultation.

Disposition

These patients will frequently be admitted and should not be discharged without consultation from an orthopedist.

7. Ankle Sprains

ESSENTIALS OF DIAGNOSIS

- Anterior talofibular ligament is affected most commonly.
- Swelling, ecchymosis, point tenderness.
- Assess for instability of ligaments.
- Ankle rules may help in determining need for x-rays.
- Most are managed conservatively.

General Considerations

Ankle sprains most often occur secondary to significant force applied as inversion and plantarflexion. The ligament most commonly affected is the anterior talofibular ligament, accounting for approximately two thirds of ankle sprains. The next most commonly affected ligament is the calcaneofibular ligament, and in 20% of cases the calcaneofibular and anterior talofibular are involved. The deltoid ligament located medially is injured less often (~5% of sprains). Eversion forces may initiate this injury, and sprains of the deltoid ligament typically require extended rehabilitation periods compared to the more common anterior talofibular or calcaneofibular ligament sprains. Deltoid ligament ruptures may be seen with medial malleolar fractures.

Clinical Findings

A. SYMPTOMS AND SIGNS

The patient typically presents with a history of a fall or twisting injury. Often swelling, ecchymosis, and point tenderness are present. Grading of sprains is described earlier in this chapter. Always assess for associated injuries such as a Maisonneuve fracture or Achilles tendon rupture.

Physical examination may include the anterior drawer test. With the patient seated, the knee flexed to 90 degrees, and the ankle in neutral position or 10 degrees of plantarflexion, gently pull forward on the heel while pushing the lower leg posteriorly. Visualize for any deformity or feel for a clunk. This test examines the integrity of the anterior talofibular ligament. The talar tilt-test assesses the anterior talofibular and calcaneofibular ligaments. With the knee flexed to 90 degrees and the ankle in a neutral position, invert the heel and assess for displacement of the talar head or laxity. The external rotation test is used to evaluate the distal talar syndesmotic ligaments. With the foot in neutral position and the knee flexed to 90 degrees, rotate the foot and assess for laxity and pain laterally.

B. X-RAY FINDINGS

Use history, physical findings, and Ottawa ankle rules to determine whether radiographs are necessary. X-rays will be negative for fracture but may demonstrate soft tissue swelling. In significant ligament sprains and ruptures, the mortise may be affected.

Treatment

Most ankle sprains may be treated conservatively on an outpatient basis. The RICE (**r**est, **i**ce, **c**rutches, and **i**mmobilization) treatment is usually indicated. For minor injuries, immobilization with an elastic bandage and crutches may be all that is necessary. For more significant injuries, a sugar-tong or posterior plaster splint may be applied. A plaster cast should never be applied acutely because of the risk of further swelling leading to increased pain and vascular compromise. Aircasts and other commercial devices may be useful. Crutches should be used (with no weight bearing initially and progressing to weight-bearing status as tolerated). Prescribe appropriate analgesics. Depending on the severity of injury, the patient may return to normal function in as little as a few days; however, it may be several weeks until proper function is restored.

Disposition

For minor injuries, treatment should be initiated as above. Follow-up may not be necessary. Patients may consider follow-up with a primary care provider for further evaluation in minor cases. Patients with significant sprains should receive treatment with immobilization and crutches as above and should be referred to an orthopedist within 1 week.

CALCANEAL FRACTURES

ESSENTIALS OF DIAGNOSIS

- *Most common tarsal bone fractures.*
- *Axial loading, often associated with vertebral fractures.*
- *The Boehler angle may detect subtle fractures.*
- *Orthopedic consultation is necessary.*

General Considerations

The calcaneus is the largest of the tarsal bones and the one most commonly fractured. The most common mechanism is axial loading from a fall. A high association exists between calcaneal fractures and other lower extremity and vertebral fractures.

Clinical Findings

A. SYMPTOMS AND SIGNS

The patient complains of severe pain in the heel and inability to bear weight. Ecchymosis and deformity may be present.

B. X-RAY FINDINGS

Obtain plain radiographs including anteroposterior, lateral, and axial views. Measurement of the Boehler angle on the lateral view may help to identify subtle fractures. The Boehler angle is formed by the intersection of lines drawn from the anterior and posterior elements of the superior portion of the calcaneus. The normal angle is 20–40 degrees; an angle of less than 20 degrees suggests a calcaneal fracture.

Treatment

A posterior leg splint or Jones wrap may be applied and the patient given crutches and non-weight-bearing status instructions.

Disposition

Orthopedic consultation is necessary to determine operative versus nonoperative management.

TALAR FRACTURES

ESSENTIALS OF DIAGNOSIS

- *No muscle attachment on talus.*
- *Tenuous blood supply.*
- *CT scan or MRI may be necessary to detect subtle fractures.*

General Considerations

The talus is the second largest tarsal bone and is the second most commonly injured bone after the calcaneus. The talus is the only bone in the foot with no muscle attachment; it is held in place by the malleoli and ligaments. The talus has a somewhat tenuous blood supply, and avascular necrosis is a potential with significant fractures. Fractures may result from plantarflexion, dorsiflexion, or inversion forces. Talus fractures usually result from high-energy trauma, and associated injuries are common.

Clinical Findings

A. SYMPTOMS AND SIGNS

Pain and swelling are common. Inversion and eversion are usually quite painful.

B. X-RAY FINDINGS

Plain radiographs may miss subtle fractures, and CT scanning or MRI may be necessary.

Treatment

Simple fractures are treated conservatively. Major fractures often require open reduction or prolonged non-weight-bearing immobilization.

Disposition

Patients should be admitted for further operative management.

SUBTALAR DISLOCATIONS

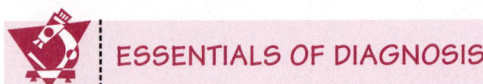

ESSENTIALS OF DIAGNOSIS

- *Uncommon injury.*
- *Associated with talocalcaneal and talonavicular ligament ruptures.*
- *Plain x-rays should be sufficient for diagnosis.*
- *Rapid reduction is indicated.*

General Considerations

Subtalar dislocations are rare injuries and occur secondary to severe rotational forces that rupture the talocalcaneal and talonavicular ligaments. The dislocation is usually lateral or medial, although anterior and posterior dislocations may occur.

Clinical Findings

A. SYMPTOMS AND SIGNS

A deformity is usually visible.

B. X-RAY FINDINGS

Plain radiographs including an anteroposterior view of the foot should determine the diagnosis.

Treatment

The dislocation should be reduced quickly, usually via closed reduction under adequate sedation. Inline longitudinal traction should be applied to the foot and then appropriate directional force applied to correct the deformity.

Disposition

After reduction, immobilization in a splint and orthopedic referral are indicated.

TARSAL INJURIES

ESSENTIALS OF DIAGNOSIS

- *Isolated dislocations are rare.*
- *Navicular fractures are most common, after calcaneal and talar fractures.*
- *Local tenderness and swelling are common.*
- *Plain x-rays are usually sufficient for diagnosis.*

General Considerations

Fractures and dislocations can occur in the other tarsal bones (ie, navicular, cuboid, and the cuneiforms). Isolated dislocations are rare injuries. Fractures of the navicular are the most common in this portion of the foot. Avulsion fractures of the navicular occur when eversion stresses are exerted on the deltoid and talonavicular ligaments.

Clinical Findings

Local pain and swelling are common. Plain radiographs may identify the injury; bone scans and tomography may be used to identify subtle injuries.

Treatment

Immobilization with a posterior short leg splint and orthopedic referral are indicated.

TARSOMETATARSAL INJURIES
(Lisfranc Injuries)

ESSENTIALS OF DIAGNOSIS

- *Uncommon injury; large amount of force is required.*
- *Lisfranc joint.*
- *Plain x-rays are usually sufficient for diagnosis.*

General Considerations

The tarsometatarsal joint comprises the articulation of the first 3 metatarsals with the medial, middle, and lateral cuneiform bones, as well as the articulation of the 4th and 5th metatarsals with the cuboid. The tarsometatarsal joint separates the forefoot from the midfoot and is commonly referred to as the Lisfranc joint. It functions in supination and pronation of the foot. Injuries to this joint are uncommon and generally are the result of a large force applied to the foot. Dislocations can occur in part or all of this joint and are frequently associated with metatarsal and tarsal fractures.

Clinical Findings

A. SYMPTOMS AND SIGNS

Pain and obvious deformity over the joint are generally present.

B. X-RAY FINDINGS

Plain films usually suffice; a lateral weight-bearing view may detect subtle injuries but is not indicated in the emergency department.

Treatment

These injuries are often managed with closed reduction and percutaneous wires.

Disposition

Orthopedic consultation is necessary.

Perron AD, Brady WJ, Keats TE: Orthopedic pitfalls in the ED: Lisfranc fracture-dislocation. Am J Emerg Med 2001;19:71. [PMID: 11146025]

METATARSAL FRACTURES

 ESSENTIALS OF DIAGNOSIS

- *Common; result from crush or twisting injuries.*
- *Most common at base of 5th metatarsal (Jones fracture).*
- *Treat with posterior splint.*

General Considerations

Metatarsal fractures are common, accounting for approximately one third of foot fractures. They may occur as a result of crush injuries or twisting forces.

Clinical Findings

A. SYMPTOMS AND SIGNS

A visible deformity may be present, along with tenderness and swelling.

B. X-RAY FINDINGS

A fracture involving the base of the 5th metatarsal is the most common fracture. Plain radiographs should be sufficient to make the diagnosis. Care should be taken to examine the x-rays for subtle abnormalities in the Lisfranc joint.

Treatment

Avulsion fractures involving the tuberosity of the proximal 5th metatarsal can be splinted for comfort, or the patient may be allowed to bear weight in a hard-soled shoe. Fractures involving the metaphysis of the proximal 5th metatarsal are more prone to complication (ie,

nonunion) and should be immobilized in a posterior splint (see Figure 28–18).

Disposition

Discharge the patient with orthopedic follow-up within a few days.

PHALANGEAL INJURIES

 ESSENTIALS OF DIAGNOSIS

- *Fractures and dislocations are common.*
- *Pain, obvious deformity.*
- *X-rays may be bypassed in minor injuries.*
- *Treatment involves buddy taping.*

General Considerations

Injuries to the toes are common and include both fractures and dislocations. Fractures of the phalanges are the most common fractures in the foot and frequently involve the 5th phalanx. Dislocations are rare; when seen, they most commonly occur in the metatarsophalangeal joint of the great toe.

Clinical Findings

A. SYMPTOMS AND SIGNS

Pain, swelling, and deformity are usually seen.

B. X-RAY FINDINGS

X-rays usually reveal the injury. Radiographs may not be obtained for minor injuries.

Treatment

Conservative management and immobilization by taping to the adjacent toe (buddy taping) are instituted. Dislocations are usually easily reduced with adequate sedation or a digital nerve block.

Disposition

Patients with simple fractures do not require orthopedic follow-up. Complicated fractures and dislocations should be immobilized with buddy taping; patients with complicated fractures and dislocations should be referred for outpatient orthopedic follow-up.

SESAMOID FRACTURES

 ESSENTIALS OF DIAGNOSIS

- *Seen most commonly in flexor hallucis brevis tendon.*
- *May be difficult to see on plain x-rays.*

General Considerations

Sesamoid bones commonly occur in the tendon of the flexor hallucis brevis. Fractures are not common and are usually the result of direct forces or hyperextension of the great toe.

Clinical Findings

A. SYMPTOMS AND SIGNS

Local pain is present.

B. X-RAY FINDINGS

Sesamoid bones are frequently unexpected findings on radiographs obtained to rule out other injuries. Sesamoid bones are not of uniform appearance, and sometimes fractures are difficult to recognize.

Treatment

Treatment is with immobilization, analgesia, and weight bearing as tolerated.

Disposition

These fractures generally do not require orthopedic evaluation; patients may be discharged to home.

■ V. COMMON PITFALLS

Missed orthopedic injuries are among the common malpractice claims in emergency medicine. Commonly missed injuries are carpal bone fractures, especially of the scaphoid. Other frequently missed injuries are posterior shoulder dislocations, hip and pelvic fractures in elderly patients, tarsometatarsal fracture dislocations, patellar tendon injuries, and compartment syndromes. Children may sustain injuries to growth plates with no radiographic evidence of injury on initial presentation. For this reason, emergency physicians should have a low threshold for immobilizing children with pain or tenderness near joints despite initially negative radiographs. Follow-up in 7–10 days should be arranged for reexamination out of the splint and possibly repeat x-rays. Patients should be advised that some nondisplaced fractures are not evident on initial radiographs and that outpatient follow-up and repeat radiographs may be indicated if pain or tenderness persists.

Hand Trauma

Adam Saperston, MD, MS[1]

29

Emergency Evaluation & Treatment
Examination of the Hand & Assessment of Function
Equipment & Materials for Treatment
Management of Specific Types of Hand Injuries
  Lacerations
  Fingertip Injuries
    1. Fingertip Amputations
    2. Subungual Hematoma
    3. Avulsion of Nail
  Distal Extensor Tendon Injuries
    1. Laceration of Extensor Tendons
    2. Mallet Finger
    3. Boutonniere Deformity
  Bone & Joint Injuries
  Infections
    1. Paronychia & Eponychia
    2. Herpetic Whitlow
    3. Felon
    4. Deep Fascial Space Infections
    5. Cellulitis (Including Human & Animal Bites)

    6. Suppurative Tenosynovitis
    7. Disseminated (Hematogenous) Gonococcal Infection
Minor Constrictive Problems
Thermal Injuries
    1. First-Degree Burns
    2. Second-Degree Burns
    3. Third-Degree Burns
    4. Electrical Burns
    5. Frostbite
Foreign Bodies
Complex Hand Injuries
    1. Amputations
    2. Flexor & Extensor Tendon Injuries
    3. Nerve Injuries
    4. High-Pressure Injection Injuries
    5. Closed Compartment Syndromes
    6. Mangling Injuries
Special Emergency Department Problems
    1. Removal of Rings
    2. Snakebite

ABBREVIATIONS USED IN THIS CHAPTER

CM	Carpometacarpal
DIP	Distal interphalangeal
IP	Interphalangeal
LET	Lateral extensor tendon
MET	Middle extensor tendon
MP	Metacarpophalangeal
PIP	Proximal interphalangeal
TET	Terminal extensor tendon

[1]This chapter is a revision of the chapter by Eugene S. Kilgore, Jr, MD, FACS, & William L. Newmeyer, MD, from the 4th edition.

■ EMERGENCY EVALUATION & TREATMENT

Hand injuries are one of the more common reasons for emergency department visits. Hand injuries may be isolated or part of multiple trauma. These injuries are seldom life threatening but can result in significant disability, threatening a patient's livelihood and lifestyle. These injuries can have significant economic impact with possible loss of occupation and lost time from work. Systematic examination and initial care has a direct effect on the ultimate consequence of any hand injury. Overall it is far better to undertreat and refer than to overtreat and cause avoidable iatrogenic injury or disability. The course of recovery depends on initial management.

Position the Patient

Ideally the patient can be seated facing directly opposite the examiner, or the patient may be placed supine. The hand should be placed on a firm support that can be positioned against or attached to the table. Clothing around the arm should be removed to the shoulder. Lighting should be good, preferably wall or ceiling mounted.

Control Bleeding

Bleeding is controlled by direct pressure with sterile gauze packs, elevation, and, if necessary, an arterial tourniquet (eg, blood pressure cuff inflated above systolic blood pressure). *Do not use clamps unless all other measures fail.* Blind clamping of vessels can lead to further injury.

Obtain History

A. Current Injuries

Ascertain the mechanism of injury by questioning the patient or others. An exact description of how the injury occurred will help determine the need for x-ray, antibiotics, urgent consultation, or no consultation. It is important to document the mechanism of injury, the time at which it occurred, and the environment in which it occurred. Ask about the following details associated with the mechanism of injury:

- Type of injury: crush, exploding, or simple amputation
- Lacerations: exactly what device was involved and how the lacerations were caused
- Position of the hand at the time of the injury (ie, fingers extended or flexed)
- Presence of pain, numbness, paresthesias, weakness, discoloration, coldness, clumsiness or poor coordination, or crepitus
- Circumstances surrounding open wounds: environment, whether inflicted in a dirty environment (ie, sewer or barnyard) or in a specific situation (ie, fight-clenched fist)

B. Relevant History

- History of prior or existing hand or upper extremity injuries or disorders. Dupuytren fasciitis, arthritis, and benign tumors are the most common nontraumatic problems noted.

- Bleeding disorders likely to influence hemostasis (eg, hemophilia).
- Factors that might impair wound healing (eg, use of corticosteroids).
- Tetanus immunization status (Chapter 30).
- Any allergies.
- General state of health, medications, and ongoing treatments.

Examine the Hand

Examination of the hand is started while the history is being taken. In the event of an open wound, proper instruments and sutures must be made ready. Sterile technique is essential at all stages of the examination and early treatment of hand injuries. A sensory examination should be done with a fine needle before anesthesia is used. Before beginning active examination, anesthetize the injured area of the hand, and apply and inflate a tourniquet.

A. Anesthesia

Anesthesia must be used if a wound is to be explored or sutured. The preferred anesthetic is 1% lidocaine *without* epinephrine. Never use epinephrine with local anesthetics in hand injury, because it may constrict the vessels and interfere with blood flow.

1. Digital block or wrist block—(See Figures 29–1 and 29–2.) Digital blocks are preferred for procedures done distal to the PIP joint. Half-inch (1.5-cm) needles of 25, 27, or 30 gauge should be used with small volumes of 1% lidocaine. In a digital block, use about 0.5–1.0 mL around the digital nerve. The injection should never render the tissues tense nor be circumferential.

In blocking peripheral nerves, the surgeon must be familiar with the anatomy of nerve distribution and the surrounding tissues. To avoid intravascular injection, always aspirate before injecting the anesthetic agent.

2. Local infiltration—(See Chapter 30; Figure 30–1.) Wounds can be infiltrated locally as long as the amount of anesthetic injected does not make the tissues tense.

3. Amount of solution—Systemic toxicity from overdosage may occur when large areas are anesthetized. This can be avoided by calculating the number of milligrams of drug in the volume of solution that may be required and then limiting the volume of injection so as to avoid giving a toxic dose (see Table 30–1).

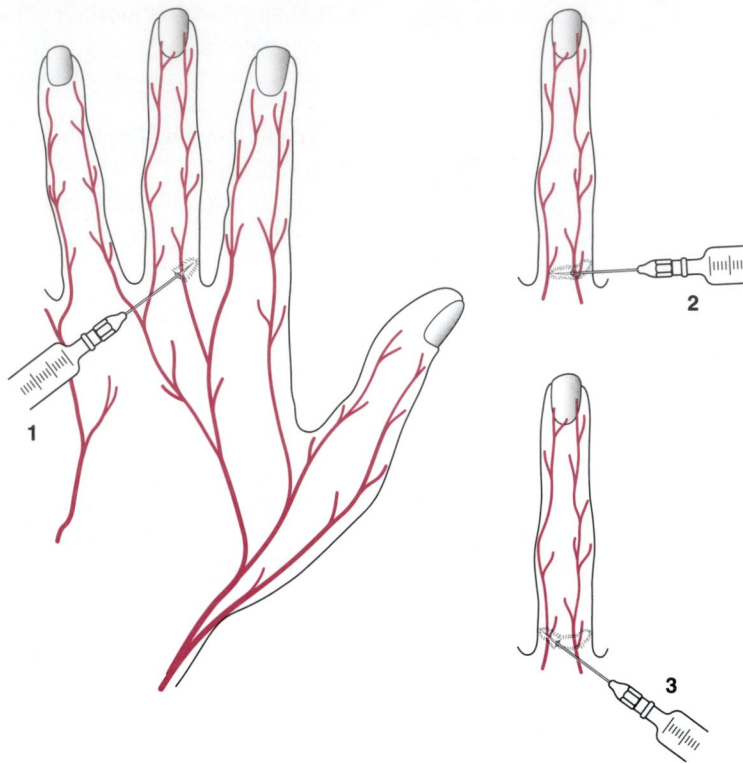

Figure 29–1. Digital block. (**1**) Use ½-inch (1.5-cm) needles of 25, 27, or 30 gauge with small volume of 1% lidocaine. (**2**) Use about 0.5–1.0 mL around the digital nerve. (**3**) The injection should never render the tissues tense nor be circumferential.

4. Inflamed areas—Anesthetic solutions should not be injected into inflamed areas unless these directly overlie an abscess that is to be drained. Such injections impair local tissue resistance to infection, may result in rapid systemic absorption because of the increased vascularity of inflamed tissues, and may be ineffective if the local tissue pH is low enough to reduce the anesthetic agent's ionic dissociation, which is essential for anesthetic activity.

B. APPLICATION OF TOURNIQUET

An arm tourniquet should always be in place on the arm when hand wounds are examined or treated. A blood pressure cuff can be used but should be inverted so that the tubes extend cephalad and out of the way. When the cuff is in place, it should be wrapped with cast padding to keep it from unwrapping when inflated.

When the anesthetic has taken effect and examination of the wound is about to start, the arm is elevated for 30 seconds and held there while the cuff is inflated to 275–300 mm Hg and the tubes clamped with Kelly clamps to prevent deflation. This procedure is well tolerated by most patients for at least 15–20 minutes.

C. EXAMINATION SEQUENCE

By dividing the examination into 4 distinct steps, much useful information can be gained rapidly.

1. Observe the posture of the hand lying supine and at rest upon the examining table. Any marked variation from the normal stance should alert the examiner to the possibility of deforming injury.

2. Observe active function of the various musculotendinous units and skeletal structures within the areas of injury.

3. Assess loss of sensibility by testing for sweat and for awareness of pain by using a fine needle in areas of suspected nerve injury. Two-point dis-

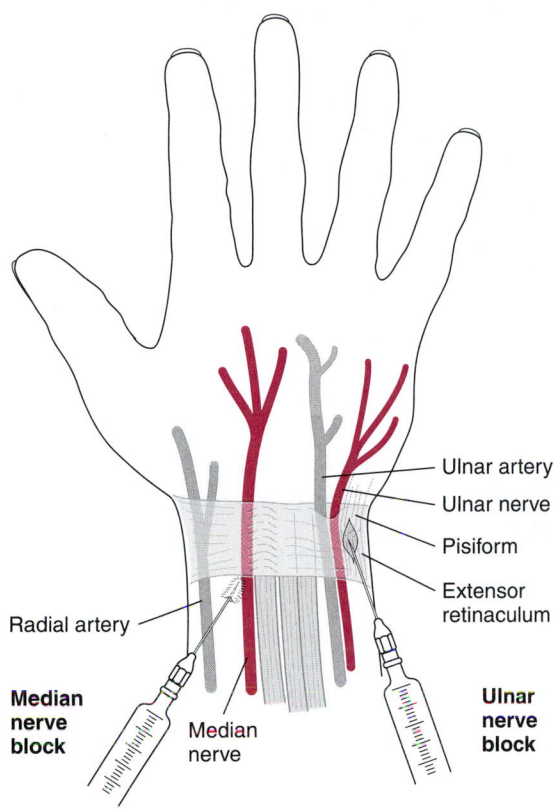

| Ulnar artery
| Ulnar nerve
| Pisiform
| Extensor retinaculum

Radial artery

Median nerve block

Median nerve

Ulnar nerve block

Figure 29–2. **A:** Median and ulnar nerve block.

crimination is a sensitive, objective measure of sensory deficit. This may be difficult to do accurately, and the character and location of a wound may be more helpful than sensory nerve testing in determining nerve injury. Sensory testing must be performed before application of a tourniquet and administration of anesthetics.

4. Inspect the wound, in a sterile, bloodless field with a simple 2-power magnifying loupe, if available. A tourniquet should be in place but should *not* be inflated until the anesthetic has become effective unless there is uncontrollable hemorrhage (see above). The examination must proceed concurrently with early treatment such as cleansing and debridement (Chapter 30) before definitive emergency treatment and suturing are done. ***Note:*** In handling and examining tissue, remember that removal of blood clots and careful manipulation of tissues to preserve the microcirculation are far more important in avoiding infection than the type of antiseptic wound preparation used.

■ EXAMINATION OF THE HAND & ASSESSMENT OF FUNCTION (See Figures 29–3 & 29–4.)

The hand is a highly mobile organ of extraordinary sensibility and remarkable adaptability, but it can be rendered useless or worse than useless by injury causing permanent stiffness, pain, or loss of sensibility. Prevention of permanent damage requires a sound knowledge of functional hand anatomy.

Terminology

(See Figure 29–5.) The hand and each finger have ulnar and radial sides and palmar and dorsal surfaces. There are 5 digits numbered and named as follows: I (thumb), II (index), III (long or middle), IV (ring), and V (small [little]). Commonly used abbreviations for the joints of the hand are shown in the box at the beginning of the chapter. Always specify which hand is injured, and note whether it is the dominant or nondominant hand.

Skin & Circulation

The skin of the palm sweats freely and is thick, tough, tethered by fascia, highly innervated, and well cushioned by fat. The dorsal skin, by contrast, is thin, very mobile, and less well supplied with sensory nerves. The arterial supply is mainly palmar. Venous and lymphatic drainage is mainly dorsal and can be impeded by dorsal injury, constriction, or taut skin.

Twelve Extrinsic Flexors

See Figure 29–3.

A. ANATOMY

1. Wrist flexors—There are 3 wrist flexors: the flexor carpi ulnaris (innervated by the ulnar nerve), the palmaris longus (median nerve), and the flexor carpi radialis (median nerve).

2. Digital flexors—There are 9 digital flexors (one for each IP joint). The flexor pollicis longus (innervated by the median nerve) flexes the thumb IP joint. Flexor digitorum superficialis (sublimis) moves each PIP joint (all median nerve). Each superficialis is generally able to contract independently, because the muscles are independent for each digit.

A flexor digitorum profundus moves each DIP joint (median nerve to index and long fingers; ulnar nerve to ring and small fingers). The 3 ulnar profundi have a

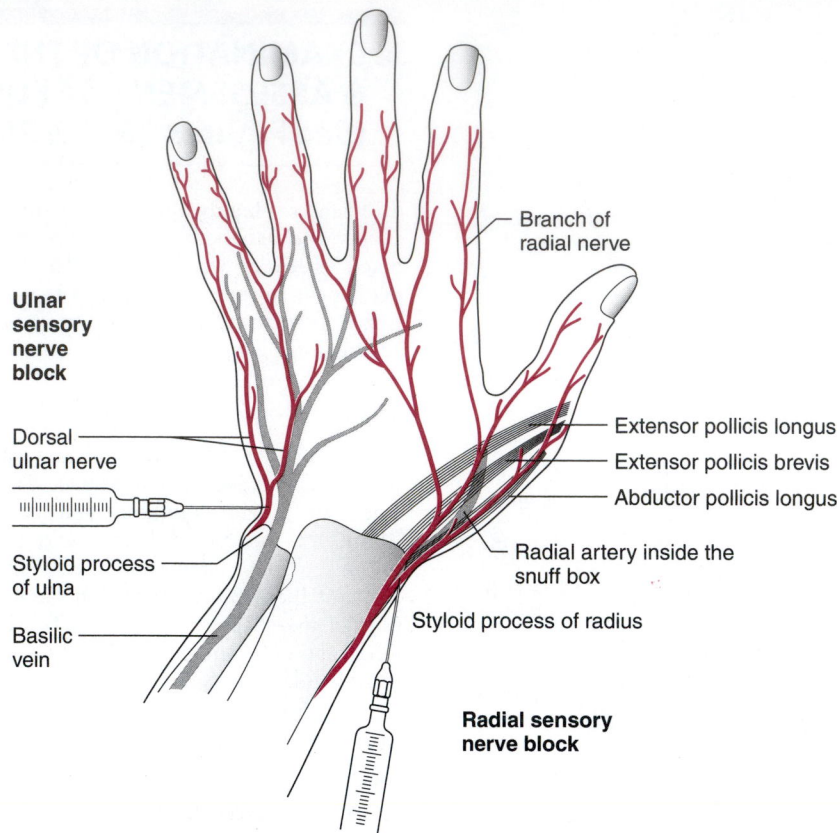

Figure 29–2. **B:** Radial and ulnar sensory nerve block.

common muscle mass, and therefore one cannot contract and move one of these digit tips independently.

B. Testing of Flexors

1. Flexor carpi radialis—The flexor carpi radialis is tested by having the patient flex the wrist; the flexor carpi ulnaris is tested by spreading the fingers. The palmaris longus is tested by having the patient spread the fingers while flexing the wrist.

2. Superficialis flexors—The superficialis flexors are tested by holding 3 digits not being tested in full extension and directing the patient to flex the fourth one. PIP flexion indicates an intact superficialis to that finger.

3. Profundus flexors—The profundus flexors are tested by asking the patient to actively flex all of the fingers so that the distal pads of the fingers meet the distal palm.

4. Flexor pollicis longus—The flexor pollicis longus is tested by having the patient actively flex the terminal phalanx of the thumb.

Twelve Extrinsic Extensors

(See Figure 29–4.) All extensors are innervated by the radial nerve.

A. Anatomy

1. Central wrist extensors—The extensor carpi radialis longus and extensor carpi radialis brevis insert into the bases of the second and third metacarpals, respectively.

2. Extensor and ulnar deviator—The extensor carpi ulnaris inserts into the base of the fifth metacarpal.

3. Abductor pollicis longus—The abductor pollicis longus deviates the wrist radially and stabilizes the base of the thumb (first metacarpal). It is tested by abducting the thumb radially.

4. Two thumb extensors—The extensor pollicis brevis acts mainly at the MP joint; the extensor pollicis longus acts at the IP joint in concert with the intrinsics

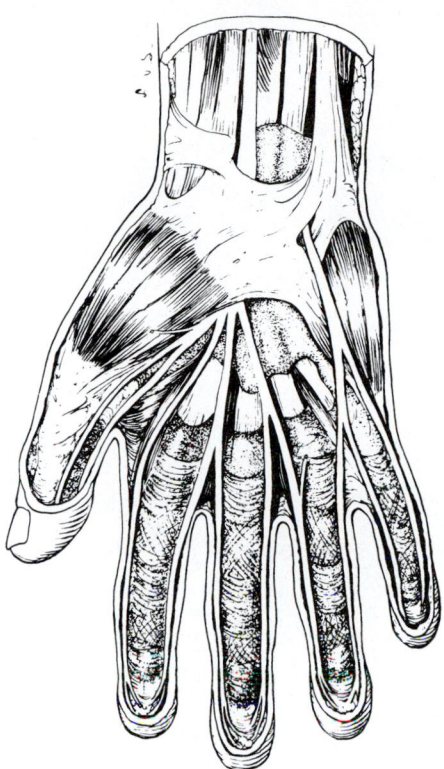

Figure 29–3. Palmar hand with skin removed reveals flexor tendons with their sheaths and the median and ulnar nerves with their terminal sensory branches. (Modified and reproduced, with permission, from Way LW [editor]: *Current Surgical Diagnosis & Treatment,* 9th ed. Appleton & Lange, 1991.)

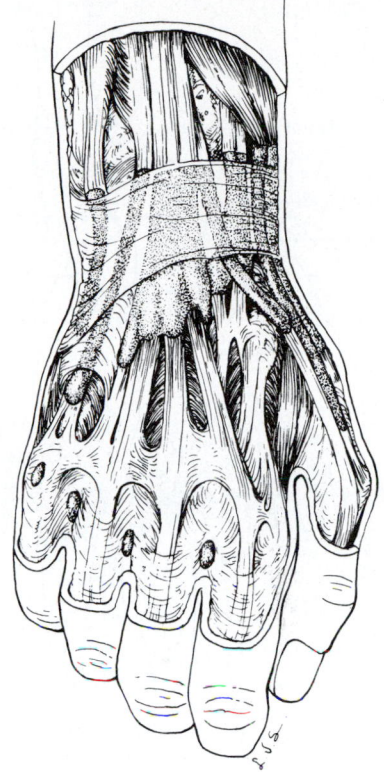

Figure 29–4. Cutaway view of the dorsal hand demonstrates that the extensor tendons are ensheathed only at wrist level. (Modified and reproduced, with permission, from Way LW [editor]: *Current Surgical Diagnosis & Treatment,* 9th ed. Appleton & Lange, 1991.)

but, unlike the intrinsics, can extend the joint with much force and can even hyperextend it.

5. Four finger extensors—An extensor digitorum communis to each finger forms the central slip (middle extensor tendon) of the extensor hood.

6. Index and small fingers—The index and small fingers have independent (proprius) extensor tendons as well. These extend these fingers when the long and ring fingers are flexed.

B. TESTING OF EXTENSORS

Test the extensors by asking the patient to extend the fingers at the MP joint and to extend the IP joints. The latter is achieved by action of the extensor in conjunction with the intrinsic tendons in the extensor hood. The proprius tendons of the index and small fingers al-

ways lie ulnar to the extensor digitorum communis of each.

Twenty Intrinsic Muscles

A. ANATOMY

Of 20 intrinsics, 15 are innervated by the ulnar nerve and 5 by the median nerve. In conjunction with the extensor tendon, they form the extensor hood mechanism, which is a proximally based triangular sheet of 3 interconnected tendons. The lateral margins ("lateral bands") are the small lateral extensor tendons (LETs) from the intrinsic muscles. The central large tendon ("central slip") from the extrinsic extensors is called the middle extensor tendon (MET), which inserts on the middle phalanx of each finger. The terminal extensor tendon (TET) is made up of a coalescence of METs

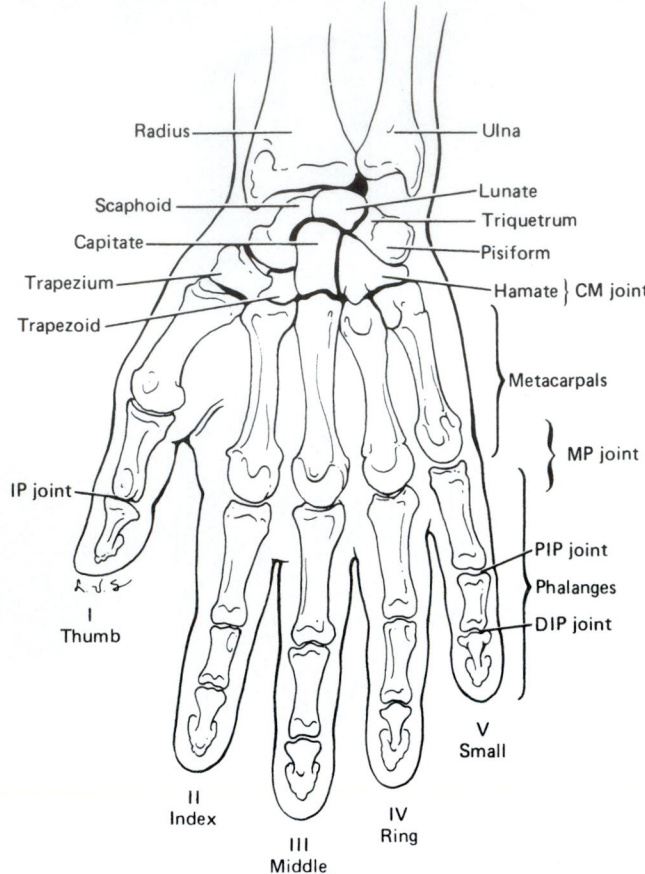

Figure 29–5. Terminology of bones and joints of the hand.

and LETs into a very thin tendon that inserts on the distal phalanx. In the case of the thumb, which has only 2 phalanges, the equivalent of the MET is the extensor pollicis brevis; the equivalent of the TET is the extensor pollicis longus. The intrinsics flex the MP and extend the IP joints and abduct and adduct the digits. Working all together, they cup the palm.

B. Testing of Intrinsics

1. Thenar and hypothenar intrinsics—The thenar and hypothenar intrinsics act to pronate the thumb and little finger and thereby cup the palm. Have the patient make the distal fat pads of the thumb and small finger meet.

2. Other intrinsics—Have the patient abduct the extended second through fifth digits; then flex these digits at the MP joints while extending the PIP and DIP joints.

Examination of Nerve Injuries

The 3 major nerves to the hand are the radial, median, and ulnar nerves.

A. Radial Nerve

The radial nerve innervates all extensors.

1. Motor testing—Muscle testing is done by having the patient extend the wrist and digits (Figure 29–6C).

2. Sensory examination—The radial nerve gives off a sensory branch that provides sensibility for the dorsal-radial aspect of the hand (Figure 29–6A and B).

B. Median Nerve

The median nerve innervates 9 of 12 extrinsic flexors, the lumbricals to the index and long fingers, and the 3 muscles of the thenar eminence, which are mainly concerned with opposition.

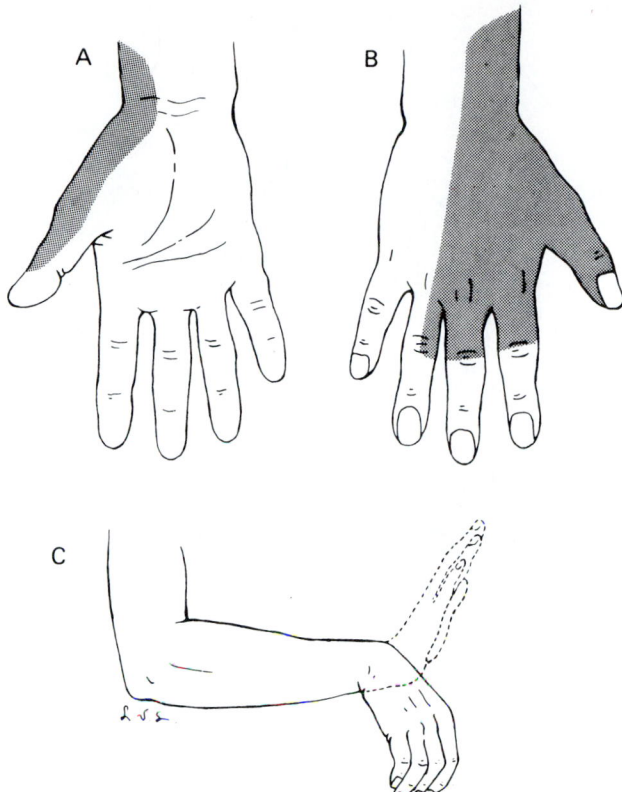

Figure 29–6. Palmar (**A**) and dorsal (**B**) areas of autogenous radial nerve sensibility. Loss of radial sensibility is not critical. A simple test for main trunk radial paresis is shown in **C**.

1. Motor testing—

a. High median nerve—Testing for high median nerve injuries is done by flexing the DIP joint of the index finger and the IP joint of the thumb (Figure 29–7).

Have the patient passively hold the fourth and fifth fingers fully flexed into the palm and follow this by full active flexion of the second and third fingers (Figure 29–7C).

Have the patient flex the thumb to touch the distal palm at the base of the fifth finger (Figure 29–7D).

b. Low median nerve—To test for low median nerve loss (eg, at the wrist), have the patient pronate the thumb, pressing the distal fat pad of the thumb against that of the ring finger. Then feel for a firm, contracted adductor pollicis brevis alongside the thumb metacarpal.

2. Sensory examination—The median nerve provides sensibility to the radial two-thirds of the palm and the palmar surfaces of the thumb, the index and long fingers, the radial side of the ring finger, and the dorsal surface of the middle and distal phalanges of these fingers (Figure 29–7A and B). Because of the importance of this zone of sensibility, the median nerve is called the "eye of the hand."

C. ULNAR NERVE

The ulnar nerve innervates 15 of the 20 intrinsic muscles and only 3 extrinsic muscles.

1. Motor testing—The intrinsics are tested by any of the following maneuvers: With the palm flat on the table, have the patient abduct and adduct the fingers, cross the fingers, or forcefully move the pointed index finger in a radial direction.

The extrinsics are tested as follows: Forcefully flex the tips of the ring and small fingers to meet the distal palm to evaluate their profundi (Figure 29–8C); then forcefully spread the fingers apart and palpate for a tensed flexor carpi ulnaris tendon at the wrist.

2. Sensory examination—The ulnar innervates the radial and ulnar halves of the pads of the small finger, the ulnar half of the pads of the ring finger, and the ulnar side of the hand (Figure 29–8A and B). The additional loss of sensibility on the dorsoulnar aspect of the body of the hand signifies a high lesion well proximal to the wrist.

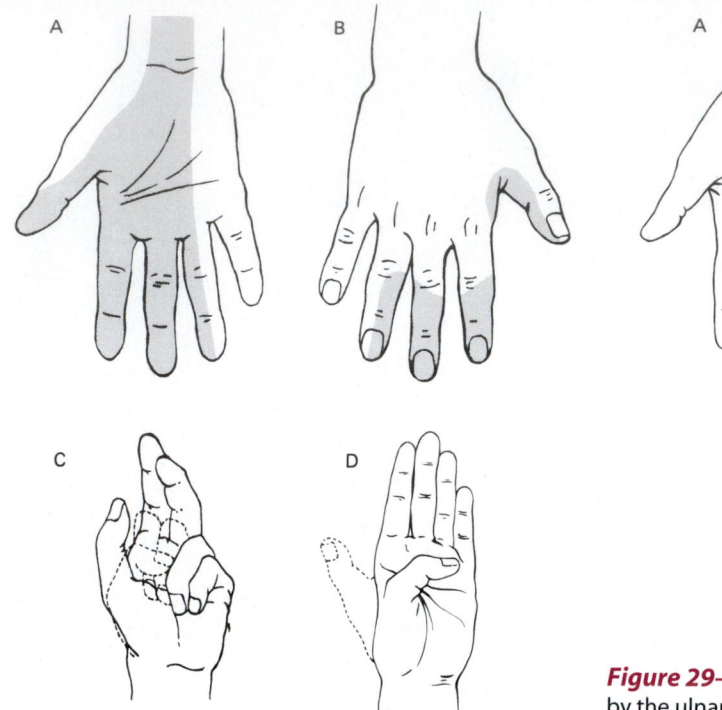

Figure 29–7. **A** and **B:** Autogenous median nerve sensibility is indicated by the shaded areas. The profundi of the index and long fingers (**C**) are innervated by the median nerve, as is the flexor pollicis longus (**D**).

X-ray Examination

Any severe injury to the hand requires x-rays to detect fractures, dislocation, and opaque foreign material or gas. Special positions should be requested, depending on the site and direction of trauma. If there is any doubt about the normalcy of the skeleton, comparable views of the opposite side should be taken for comparison.

■ EQUIPMENT & MATERIALS FOR TREATMENT

Instruments, Antiseptic Solutions, & Sutures

A. NEEDLES

Suturing should be carefully done with fine-pointed and very sharp cutting needles (eg, Ethicon P-1, P-3).

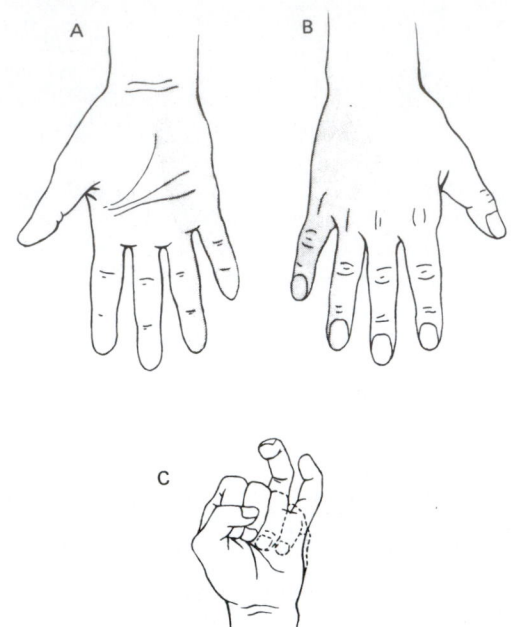

Figure 29–8. **A** and **B:** The shaded area is innervated by the ulnar nerve. **C:** Terminal phalangeal flexion of ring and small fingers is by profundi innervated by the ulnar nerve.

B. SUTURING MATERIAL

Fine (4-0, 5-0, or 6-0) monofilament polypropylene suture material is preferred for skin closure. Only in infants and children should an absorbable suture such as 5-0 or 6-0 chromic or plain catgut be used.

C. INSTRUMENTS

Fine plastic surgery forceps, retractors, clamps, and needle holders are required.

D. SKIN AND WOUND PREPARATION

The skin around the wound may be sterilized as described in Chapter 30. Take care not to splash disinfectants in the wound itself. The hand and wound may be irrigated with normal saline or even tap water (hydrogen peroxide can be toxic and is less preferable). Avoid prolonged soaking.

Dressings, Splints, & Antibiotics

A. INNER DRESSINGS

Petrolatum-impregnated gauze followed by a surgical gauze sponge saturated with water (tap water or sterile saline solution) is applied over the wound as the "core" dressing. The wetness draws blood from the wound and prevents dead space. None of this goes circumferentially around the digit, hand, or forearm.

A foam pad such as a Reston pad with an adherent surface on one side (or comparable substitute) is then applied over the core dressing.

Soft elastic gauze (Kerlix, Kling) or cast padding to form a soft, well-padded dressing is applied over the foam pad and may go circumferentially around the part.

B. SPLINT

The wrist is the most important joint to splint for all major hand injuries, even if only one digit is injured. Well-padded plaster as a splint protects the hand.

For isolated pain-free dorsal injuries at the DIP or PIP joint, a tongue blade cut to the length of 2 phalanges and padded with gauze or foam rubber makes an excellent splint. If there is a wound over the joint, such a splint should be placed on the palmar side; if not, it is placed on the dorsum.

The most useful palmar splint consists of 10–12 layers of plaster cut to fit the involved digit or digits and extending halfway up the volar surface of the forearm. It is padded with a thin foam pad (eg, Reston) and held in place with a loosely wrapped roll of plaster of paris, bias-cut stockinet, or elastic bandage. The hand generally should be in the "position of function," that is, slight wrist extension and MP flexion, with the PIP and DIP joints in partial extension and the thumb web open (Figure 29–9). Modification must be applied to take tension off a specific wound.

C. SLING

No patient should leave the emergency department without a sling to hold the hand at the level of the heart or higher to promote venous and lymphatic drainage. Slings that hold the hand lower than the heart encourage the development of tissue edema. To avoid a tourniquet effect, the extremity should usually be outside of a sleeve.

■ MANAGEMENT OF SPECIFIC TYPES OF HAND INJURIES

LACERATIONS

Small Lacerations

Simple lacerations (superficial lacerations not extending into subcutaneous fat and not perpendicular to skin tension lines) can be closed by sterile surgical tapes (ie, Steri-Strips) or tissue adhesives. Wounds that require

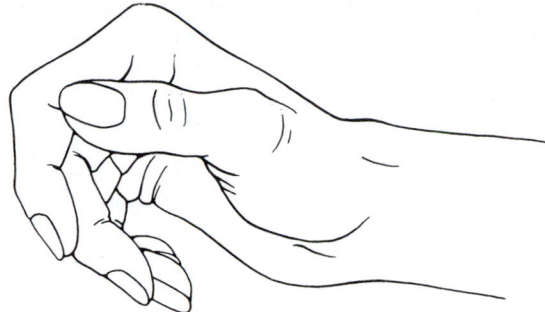

Figure 29–9. Position of function of the hand. Note graded flexion of fingers and slight dorsiflexion of wrist.

sutures (lacerations that are parallel to skin tension lines or into subcutaneous fat) should be evaluated in a sterile, bloodless field. Splinting and elevation of the limb can help healing and reduce pain. Splinting is also important for wounds that cross joints to prevent joint stiffness or contracture from wound scarring. Follow-up with a primary care physician in 7–10 days for suture removal is appropriate.

Extensive Lacerations

Wounds should be carefully evaluated in a sterile, bloodless field. Irrigation and cleaning with tap water or sterile saline is the next step. Careful handling of tissues is essential. Approximate the wound margins with sutures. If the wound is dirty, do not close under tension. If the edges cannot be easily approximated, the wound may be left open and the patient referred to a hand surgeon for primary or delayed split-thickness grafting. Consider the need for local and systemic antibiotics and tetanus prophylaxis.

FINGERTIP INJURIES

1. Fingertip Amputations

Clinical Findings

Fingertip amputations are the most common type of amputation of the upper extremity. The location and size of the defect have to be considered. Depending on the location of the amputation, fingertip injuries can be classified into 4 zones. The zones have been designed to define the type of pulp damage and the existence of associated lesions of the nail bed and bone. The Zone 1 lesion is a distal amputation located far from the distal phalanx tubercle. Usually the lesion is less than 1 cm in area and does not affect the nail bed or bone. Zone 2 lesions involve the nail bed and usually partial phalangeal bone disruption and exposure. In Zone 3 the nail matrix is involved so that the nail growth will be followed by curved deformation. Zone 4 defines an amputation at the level of the distal phalanx, near the distal interphalangeal joint. Despite the intact distal attachment of the extensor and flexor tendons at the distal phalanx, the active motion of the distal remnant is limited.

Important information to be obtained from the patient includes age, the digit injured, mechanism and time of injury, occupation, location of the wound, and hand dominance. The digit injured influences management. Most hand surgeons want to maintain length of the thumb. The index finger is considered the next priority before other fingers. An intact pulp-to-pulp pinch mechanism is the goal.

Treatment & Disposition

For Zone 1 injuries with pad loss of less than 1 cm, healing by secondary intention is the simplest and often best approach. Large dorsal wounds also heal well with this technique. It is the treatment of choice for pediatric fingertip amputations, especially when there is no bone exposure. Initial treatment includes wound cleansing, a nonadherent sterile dressing, appropriate tetanus prophylaxis, splinting, and a bulky dressing to protect the tip. Amputations that expose the distal phalanx are usually treated as contaminated open fractures with an initial intravenous dose of a cephalosporin followed by an oral course. Patients should have appropriate follow-up care in 1–3 days for wound care check.

Fingertip amputations that have significant pad loss or bone loss (Zones 2–4) usually require the expertise of a hand surgeon. Surgical options include primary closure, full- or partial-thickness skin grafts, composite grafts, flaps, and replantation. If the amputated fingertip pad has been retained, is clean, and is in good condition, it may be reattached as a full-thickness skin graft.

2. Subungual Hematoma

Clinical Findings

Hematoma from blunt trauma (ie, a hammer blow) or crush injury that ruptures subungual blood vessels causes pain and dark red to black discoloration of the nail bed. An x-ray will rule out a fractured phalanx.

Treatment

Large subungual hematomas cause significant pain and should be evacuated via nail trephination (making a hole in the nail) with a high-temperature microcautery device or an 18-gauge needle or via complete removal of the nail. Use of heated paper clips may introduce

carbon particles known as "lampblack" into the nail bed. Anesthesia is not usually required for trephination, and pain relief is immediate following decompression. Large subungual hematomas are often associated with significant nailbed lacerations. Many authors recommend removal of the nail and repair of nail bed lacerations for large subungual hematomas to promote optimal healing and normal nail growth. When the nail is removed, it should be cleaned and placed back into position, secured with sutures to function as a splint for the nail bed and to keep the proximal nail fold open.

A fracture of the distal phalanx on radiographs may technically be called an open fracture, although these injuries usually heal without complication. Osteomyelitis is not often associated with ungual tuft fractures. The risk of infection with an open fracture of the phalanx proper should be considered, and a broad-spectrum antibiotic and close follow-up are recommended.

Disposition

Patients with a subungual hematoma may be discharged from the emergency department after treatment (trephination, nail removal with or without nail bed repair). All patients with subungual hematoma should be informed about the possibility of nail loss or deformity. Antibiotics are recommended for hematomas associated with tuft fractures.

3. Avulsion of Nail

Clinical Findings

Avulsion of the nail results from a force elevating the tip of the nail and ripping it off its bed, or from a downward crushing force sufficient to tear the base of the nail out of the eponychial sulcus, ripping open the nail bed, and carrying the nail plate on a palmar-based pedicle flap.

Treatment

Nails avulsed at the base should be completely removed. If such a nail is left in place, a badly lacerated nail bed that requires repair may inadvertently be overlooked. The nail also creates a dead space that promotes scarring and infection.

A. REMOVAL OF NAIL

Anesthetize by digital block. Remove the avulsed nail by inserting a clamp under the distal attached portion of the nail and advancing it proximally, removing the nail by spreading the clamp. The exposed nail bed should be covered with either the original nail (as described above) or with sterile petrolatum gauze and a portion of the gauze tucked into the nail sulcus. A lacerated nail bed should be meticulously closed with 5-0 or 6-0 absorbable suture.

B. REATTACHMENT OF DISTAL TORN FINGER FLAP

If the distal portion of the finger has been torn off with the nail and has been left attached to the finger by a volar pedicle, the flap should be anatomically reduced and held with strips of paper tape (eg, Steri-Strips), or it should be sutured back in position with 6-0 absorbable suture. Antibiotics should be administered.

C. MANAGEMENT OF FRACTURES

Open fractures of the distal phalanx are reduced and held by soft tissue suturing. If the fracture is displaced, internal fixation with a Kirschner wire may be necessary.

Disposition

The patient should follow up in 2–3 days for wound check and dressing change. Complicated problems should be referred to a hand surgeon and an immediate appointment made.

DISTAL EXTENSOR TENDON INJURIES[2]

1. Laceration of Extensor Tendons

Clinical Findings

Dorsal finger and hand wounds frequently result in a partially or completely lacerated extensor tendon or extensor tendon hood mechanism. The extent of injury can be determined only by adequate exposure and direct examination. Accurate assessment of a tendon can be difficult because a 90%-lacerated tendon can still retain function. A partial tendon laceration can often be discovered by testing the tendon against resistance. Strength against resistance is diminished if a partial tendon laceration exists. Description using the 8 zones of extensor tendon injuries will help assess and guide treatment (Figure 29–10).

Treatment

Treatment of a partial tendon laceration that is less than 50% requires no repair and is treated with a protective splint. Extensor tendon repair can be performed in the emergency department after careful irrigation, inspection, and debridement or later by the consultant.

---

[2]Flexor and proximal extensor tendon injuries are discussed with flexor tendon injuries later in this chapter.

If the tendon ends can be retrieved easily with minimal extension of the wound or by slight stretching of the skin, the tendon should be repaired in the emergency department by a simple figure-of-eight suture or a crisscross suture technique with 4-0 or 5-0 suture (in infants, 6-0 nylon) (Figure 29–11). A padded plaster forearm splint is then applied with the digit and hand positioned so that the repair is relaxed as much as possible. No individual joint should be hyperextended, nor should all joints be simultaneously extended. The MP joint should not be immobilized in full extension, because contraction of collateral ligaments may result in fixation of the joint in extension. One or more neighboring fingers should always be immobilized with the injured digit.

Disposition

If the tendon ends are not easily retrieved, notify a hand surgeon immediately and make arrangements for repair as soon as possible.

In the interim, administer antibiotics for 2–3 days (see discussion of cellulitis, below).

2. Mallet Finger

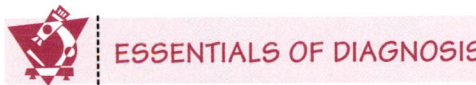

ESSENTIALS OF DIAGNOSIS

- *Suspect if bruising is present at DIP joint.*
- *X-ray may be normal or show an avulsed chip at DIP joint.*
- *Carefully test extension of DIP joint.*
- *If left untreated, swan neck deformity will occur.*

Clinical Findings

Mallet finger is caused by laceration or avulsion of the extensor tendon at its insertion at the dorsum of the distal phalanx. A mallet finger commonly occurs after the distal finger is forcibly flexed such as from a sudden blow to the tip of the extended finger. Clinically, there may be ecchymosis at the DIP joint, but tenderness and swelling may be absent. An x-ray may be normal or demonstrate an avulsed chip fragment at the dorsum of the DIP joint. If the articular fracture involves more than 40% of the joint surface, referral to a hand specialist for open reduction is required. The extensor lag may not be present on the initial emergency department evaluation. Careful testing of extension at the DIP is important in identifying this problem. If left untreated,

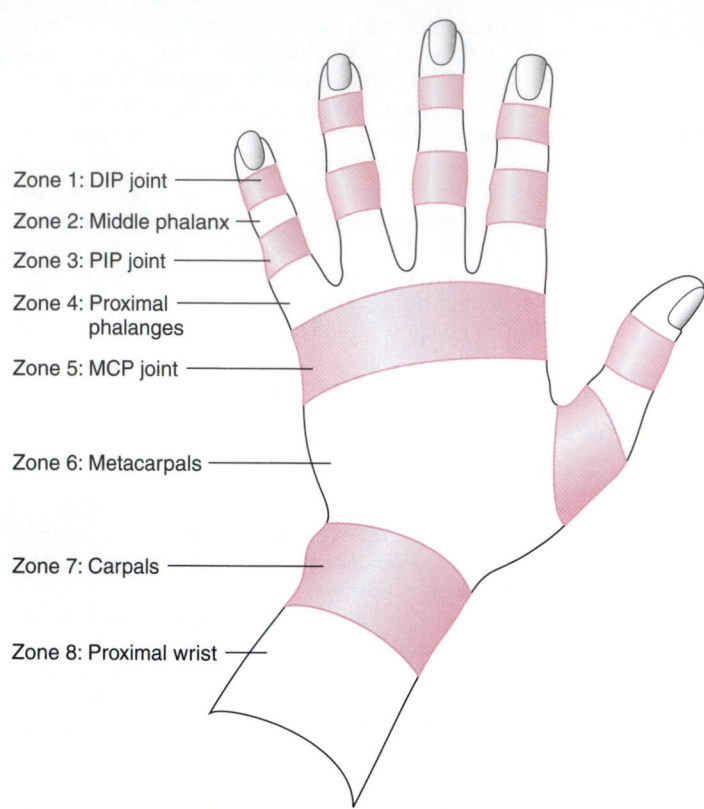

Zone 1: DIP joint
Zone 2: Middle phalanx
Zone 3: PIP joint
Zone 4: Proximal phalanges
Zone 5: MCP joint
Zone 6: Metacarpals
Zone 7: Carpals
Zone 8: Proximal wrist

Figure 29–10. Zones of extensor tendon injury.

a flexion deformity at the DIP joint will develop followed by hyperextension at the PIP joint (swan neck deformity) (Figure 29–12).

Treatment

A. OPEN MALLET INJURIES

Open injures are treated by tenorrhaphy and intramedullary fixation of the DIP joint by a hand surgeon. Give prophylactic antibiotics (see discussion of cellulitis, below).

B. CLOSED MALLET INJURIES

Closed injuries may be treated by continuous dorsal external padded splint fixation of the DIP joint in full extension for 6–8 weeks. During splint changes the joint should be held up in extension. The digit should be kept dry to prevent maceration of the skin.

Disposition

The patient should follow up with a hand surgeon.

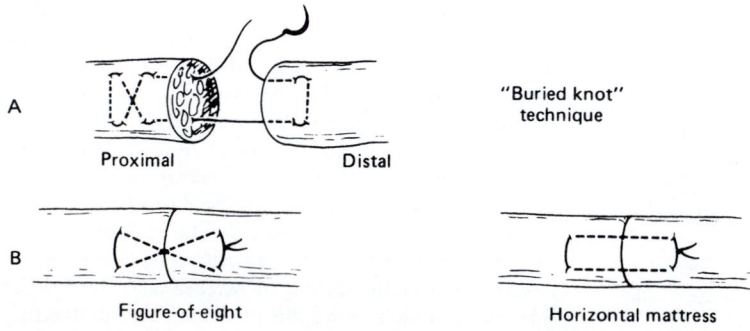

A

Proximal   Distal

B

Figure-of-eight

"Buried knot" technique

Horizontal mattress

Figure 29–11. Methods of tenorrhaphy. **A:** For large-caliber tendons. **B:** These suture techniques are best for thin tendons with limited separation of stumps (eg, digital extensors). (Reproduced, with permission, from Schrok TR [editor]: *Handbook of Surgery,* 7th ed. Jones Medical Publications, 1982.)

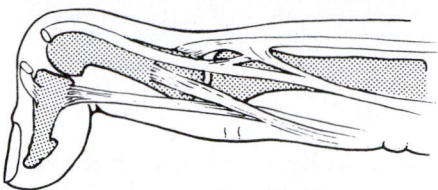

Figure 29–12. Mallet finger with swan-neck deformity. Rupture, laceration, or avulsion of the insertion of the extensor mechanism results in mallet finger. (Modified and reproduced, with permission, from Way LW [editor]: *Current Surgical Diagnosis & Treatment,* 9th ed. Appleton & Lange, 1991.)

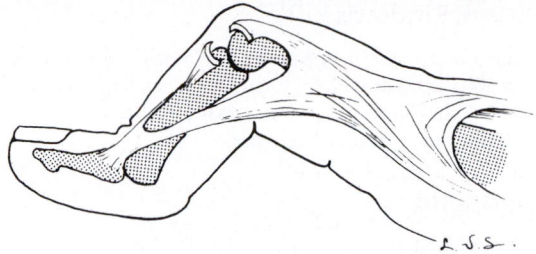

Figure 29–13. Boutonniere deformity. Avulsion or laceration of the central extensor mechanism results in a flexion deformity at the PIP joint and hyperextension of the DIP joint—the boutonniere, or buttonhole, deformity. (Modified and reproduced, with permission, from Way LW [editor]: *Current Surgical Diagnosis & Treatment,* 9th ed. Appleton & Lange, 1991.)

3. Boutonniere Deformity

ESSENTIALS OF DIAGNOSIS

- *Suspect when trauma causes a painful, swollen PIP joint.*
- *X-rays are usually normal.*
- *Deformity is rarely clinically identifiable immediately after the event.*

Clinical Findings

Early diagnosis of a closed middle extensor tendon rupture or avulsion is difficult before the boutonniere (buttonhole) deformity has occurred. High suspicion is needed when the patient presents with trauma and a painful, swollen PIP joint. Although uncommon, volar dislocations of the PIP joint can cause MET rupture. Unless a dislocation is present, radiographs are usually normal.

In boutonniere deformity, the distal joint is hyperextended and the PIP joint of the finger (the MP joint of the thumb) is flexed (Figure 29–13). Extensor hood integrity is lost at the apex of the PIP joint of the finger (MP joint of the thumb) as a result of laceration or blunt trauma to the dorsum of the joint. The deformity is rarely manifest immediately after trauma and comes on insidiously as a result of gradual stretching of the injured hood. The underlying head of the bone protrudes through the hood, pushing aside the MET (extensor pollicis brevis of the thumb), which recedes, and the LETs, which slip volarly to become flexors of the joint and hyperextensors of the distal joint.

Treatment

A. OPEN INJURIES

Open injuries should be repaired (by a hand surgeon) as soon as possible with figure-of-eight nylon sutures and the joint splinted in full extension for 4 weeks with a palmar digital splint.

B. CLOSED INJURIES

Closed injuries must be suspected if there is a history of a direct blow to the dorsum of the joint followed by swelling. Treatment consists of 4 weeks of PIP (thumb MP) splinting in extension to avoid boutonniere deformity, which rarely occurs if prompt treatment is provided.

Secondary reconstruction of this deformity is very difficult and may never restore full motion of the IP joints.

Disposition

Open injuries should be irrigated and covered and the patient sent to a hand surgeon at once. Patients with suspected closed middle extensor tendon injuries should get early referral to a hand surgeon. The hand should be splinted with the PIP joint in extension, leaving the MP and DIP joints mobile.

BONE & JOINT INJURIES

Bone and joint injuries are discussed in more detail in Chapter 28, but a few general principles are emphasized here.

Clinical Findings

If there is any question of bone or joint injury on x-ray, obtaining added views in other planes and identical views of the opposite extremity or a follow-up view in 7–10 days may resolve the issue.

Treatment

A. SPLINTING

The wrist joint is the principal joint governing movement and comfort of an immobilized fracture. Therefore, it should be splinted initially. In addition, to splint one finger well, an adjacent finger should be splinted with it. The thumb may be immobilized alone. The preferred position should be that of wrist extension, functional finger flexion, and opposition of the thumb. If there is throbbing pain at any time, it must be relieved promptly by loosening the bandages that secure the splint.

B. STABLE INJURIES

Stable dislocations or fractures can usually be treated in the emergency department by reduction and splinting, with appropriate anesthesia. Force should never be used. In lieu of force, open reduction is preferred.

C. OPEN OR UNSTABLE INJURIES

Open or unstable injuries require a specialist's skill. The patient should be given a temporary splint and dressing and referred to a hand surgeon immediately. Give prophylactic antibiotics (see discussion of cellulitis, below).

Disposition

Patients with closed, stable injuries should follow up with an orthopedic surgeon or hand specialist in 7–10 days for assessment of comfort and integrity of the splint. Patients with open joint injuries, unstable injuries, or injuries that cannot be reduced easily must be referred early to a specialist experienced in hand surgery.

Aronowitz E, Leddy J: Closed tendon injuries of the hand and wrist in athletes. Clin Sports Med 1998;17(3):449. [PMID: 9700414]

Harrison BJ, Hilliard MW: Emergency department evaluation and treatment of hand injuries. Emerg Med Clin North Am 1999;17(4):793. [PMID: 10584103]

Patel J et al: Hand lacerations—an audit of clinical examination. J Hand Surg [Br] 1998;23(4):482. [PMID: 9726549]

Perron AD et al: Orthopedic pitfalls in the emergency department: Closed tendon injuries of the hand. Am J Emerg Med 2001;19:76. [PMID: 11146026]

Roser S, Gellman H: Comparison of nail bed repair versus nail trephination for subungual hematomas in children. J Hand Surg [Am] 1999;24(6):1166. [PMID: 10584937]

Wilhelmi B et al: Epinephrine in digital blocks: revisited. Ann Plast Surg 1999;43(5):572. [PMID: 10560879]

INFECTIONS

Infections of the hand are frequently encountered in emergency departments. Nearly all infections result from neglect following trauma and are fostered by venous congestion and tissue edema.

Careful handling of tissue, elimination of dead space, immobilization and elevation of the arm immediately after injury, and avoidance of constriction by snug clothing or jewelry are far more important in preventing infection than any type of wound preparation or antibiotic prophylaxis. The objective of treatment of all infections is to reverse congestion and restore normal circulation. If there is a possibility of serious infection, immobilize the hand in a splint. Applying zinc oxide ointment next to the skin in the inner (core) dressing promotes drainage by preventing drying, caking, and sealing off of the wound.

All existing or potential infections should be monitored closely, for example, hourly or daily depending on the severity. Infections that may be treated in the emergency department include those of the nail folds, felons, simple abscesses, and cellulitis. Patients with other infections should be immediately referred.

1. Paronychia & Eponychia

 ESSENTIALS OF DIAGNOSIS

- Swelling and collection of pus inside or around nail fold.
- Consider X-ray to rule out foreign body or osteomyelitis.
- Consider antibiotics if extensive cellulitis or lymphangitis is present.

Clinical Findings

Inflammation leading to a collection of pus inside the nail fold is seen after trauma and often as a consequence of stress (Figure 29–14A). If neglected, it may extend around the entire nail margin and cause a floating nail. The usual cause is *Staphylococcus aureus*. Cultures are rarely necessary. Chronic paronychia is found in patients with occupational exposure to moisture or cleaning solutions (ie, housekeepers or dishwashers) and is most often caused by *Candida albicans*.

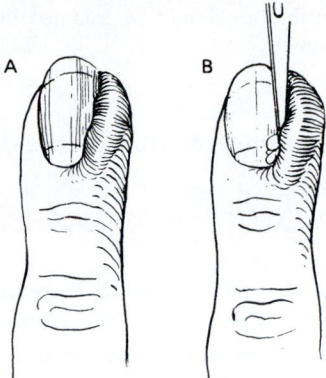

Figure 29–14. Incision and drainage of paronychia. (Modified and reproduced, with permission, from Way LW [editor]: *Current Surgical Diagnosis & Treatment,* 9th ed. Appleton & Lange, 1991.)

An x-ray should be considered to rule out the presence of a foreign body or distal phalangeal osteomyelitis.

Treatment

Treatment consists of simple elevation of the nail fold with a No. 11 scalpel at the site of maximum tenderness or pus (Figure 29–14B). Generally, there is no pain if an abscess is already pointing and no blood is drawn with the scalpel. If the scalpel causes any pain, administer a digital block anesthetic.

Antimicrobial agents are not indicated unless extensive cellulitis or lymphangitis is present. Chronic paronychia treatment may require nail removal, marsupialization of the eponychial fold, oral antibiotic, and topical antifungal ointment.

Disposition

As with any hand infection, the patient should keep the hand elevated and follow up in 24–48 hours. A common complication is osteomyelitis of the distal phalanx. Chronic paronychia requires referral to a hand surgeon for possible marsupialization.

2. Herpetic Whitlow

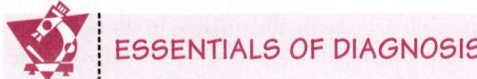 **ESSENTIALS OF DIAGNOSIS**

- *Collection of grouped vesicles with erythematous base on the fingertip.*

- *Use oral acyclovir in immunocompromised individuals.*

Herpetic whitlow is the most common viral infection of the hand, a self-limited herpes simplex viral infection of the distal finger. It classically presents as grouped vesicles with an erythematous base on the fingertip. Treatment is supportive; oral acyclovir is used in immunocompromised patients.

3. Felon

 ESSENTIALS OF DIAGNOSIS

- *Patient has a painful and swollen distal phalanx fat pad.*
- *Staphylococcus aureus is the most common cause.*
- *Most felons can be drained where the abscess points—usually mid pad with a central longitudinal incision.*

Clinical Findings

A felon is an abscess of the distal phalanx fat pad. *S aureus* is the most common pathogen. The patient usually presents with a painful and swollen distal pulp space.

Treatment & Disposition

Classic treatment of felons emphasized the need for early and complete incision through the septa via fish-mouth incisions to provide adequate drainage and to relieve pressure (Figure 29–15). But complications include damage to nerves and blood vessels as well as unstable finger pads, and painful neuromas or anesthetic fingertips may result. Most felons can be drained where they point—usually in the mid pad—by a central longitudinal incision that does not cross the distal flexion crease. Felons can also be drained by a single lateral incision. The incision should be made along the ulnar aspect of digits II–IV and the radial aspects of digits I and V, avoiding pincher surfaces. The incision is started 0.5 cm distal to the DIP joint crease and dorsal to the neurovascular bundle of the fingertip. Irrigate and loosely pack the wound, and then immobilize the finger. Treat empirically with antistaphylococcal oral antibiotics for

A

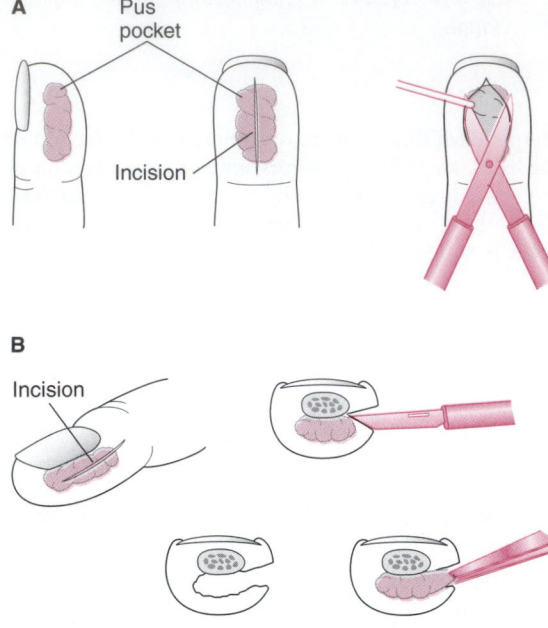

B

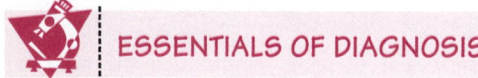

Figure 29–15. Incision and drainage of felon. **A:** Central longitudinal incision—the recommended approach. **B:** Classic lateral or fishmouth incision, which has greater risk of complication.

5 days and arrange follow-up in 1–3 days for wound care check.

4. Deep Fascial Space Infections

ESSENTIALS OF DIAGNOSIS

- All deep space abscesses require referral to a hand surgeon.
- Antibiotics should be started in the emergency department.

The 4 potential deep fascial space infections of the hand are the subfascial web space, the dorsal subaponeurotic space (collar button abscess), a midpalmar space abscess, and the thenar space. Deep space abscesses are frequently seeded with *S aureus,* streptococci, and coliforms. All deep space infections require referral to a hand surgeon for operative exploration and

drainage. Antibiotics should be initiated in the emergency department.

5. Cellulitis (Including Human & Animal Bites)

ESSENTIALS OF DIAGNOSIS

- A progressive cellulitis caused by Pasteurella multocida *is easily seen in the first 24 hours.*
- Cellulitis due to other pathogens usually takes 2–3 days to become clinically evident.
- Another pathogen, Capnocytophaga canimorsus, *associated with animal bites, can cause overwhelming sepsis in immunocompromised individuals.*
- Have a high suspicion for closed-fist bite wound when caring for patient with open wound over the MP joint following an altercation. Patients with these seemingly small wounds often present later with significant infections.

Treatment

A. UNCOMPLICATED CELLULITIS AND ANTIBIOTIC PROPHYLAXIS

Wounds with an increased risk of infection (ie, human or animal bites, crush wounds, or contaminated wounds) should have antibiotic coverage for *S aureus* or *Streptococcus pyogenes.* Treatment recommendations include a first-generation cephalosporin such as cephalexin for oral use or cefazolin for intravenous use, or a penicillinase-resistant penicillin such as dicloxacillin for oral use or nafcillin or oxacillin for intravenous use. Trimethoprim-sulfamethoxazole (TMP-SMZ) or erythromycin may be effective in penicillin-allergic patients. Special consideration for polymicrobial coverage and possible admission are needed for diabetic patients and drug abusers.

B. ANIMAL BITES

Infections caused by animal bites (ie, dog or cat) are often caused by *P multocida,* which causes a rapidly progressive cellulitis, easily identifiable in 24 hours. Infections from other pathogens are not usually evident for 2–3 days. Another common pathogen, *C canimorsus* (formerly known as DF-2), is a fastidious gram-negative rod that can cause overwhelming sepsis in immunocompromised individuals. Treatment for animal bites includes amoxicillin-clavulanate, clindamycin plus a fluoroquinolone in penicillin-allergic adults, or clindamycin plus TMP-SMZ in children. Do not close these wounds.

C. HUMAN BITES

A wound over the MCP joint (especially of the dominant hand) is likely to represent a closed-fist bite wound sustained during an altercation. These wounds have a high likelihood for infection. Patients often present with infected "fight-bite" wounds several days after suffering a seemingly minor injury during a fight. Perform a thorough examination of these wounds, looking for injuries to the extensor tendon or joint capsule. Any violation of these structures mandates orthopedic consultation. Wounds that do not involve the joint capsule or the extensor tendon should be thoroughly irrigated and any devitalized tissue debrided.

Some authors have recommended mandatory admission at the time of initial evaluation even without any signs of infection or tendon or joint involvement, whereas others advocate outpatient therapy with oral antibiotics and close follow-up. Infections from human bites involve mixed anaerobes, streptococci, *S aureus*, and *Eikenella corrodens* and should be treated in the hospital. Antibiotic treatment options include amoxicillin-sulbactam, cefoxitin, and ticarcillin-clavulanate. Penicillin-allergic patients may receive clindamycin plus TMP-SMZ, or clindamycin plus fluoroquinolone. Prophylactic antibiotics for human bite wounds include amoxicillin-clavulanate or a second-generation cephalosporin. Given the propensity of these wounds to become infected, fight bites should never be sutured.

Disposition

Hospitalization under the care of a hand specialist is required for severe cases (extensive cellulitis, involvement of tendons or joints, infections of the palmar space, systemic symptoms, or unusual pathogens) or if the patient is unreliable or unable to take oral antibiotics. Patients with cellulitis managed as outpatients should be seen every day and hospitalized if the process continues.

6. Suppurative Tenosynovitis

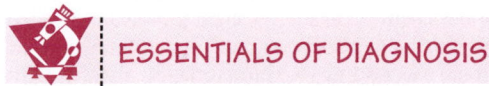

ESSENTIALS OF DIAGNOSIS

- Swelling, erythema, and tenderness along the tendon sheath.
- Exquisite pain on passive movement of tendon.

- Consider gonococcal infection in young adults without an open wound.

Clinical Findings

Suppurative tenosynovitis (nongonococcal) is characterized by swelling, erythema, and tenderness along the tendon sheath and, most important, exquisite pain on passive movement of the flexor tendon in the digit or the extensor tendon crossing the wrist. In flexor tenosynovitis, passive movement is definitely achieved by holding the fingernail alone and prying it dorsally to extend the distal joint. The infection may have occurred because of an open wound contiguous to the involved tendon.

Treatment & Disposition

In selected reliable patients with a confirmed diagnosis, outpatient therapy with close follow-up may be possible. Whenever there is inflammation with significant swelling, immediate hospitalization under the care of a hand specialist is required for open surgical drainage and parenteral antibiotic therapy. After obtaining appropriate specimens for culture, begin a cephalosporin (eg, cefazolin, 100 mg/kg/d in 3 divided doses) intravenously without waiting for the results of cultures. Immobilize the wrist and hand in a splint, and support the arm in a sling until operation can be performed.

7. Disseminated (Hematogenous) Gonococcal Infection

The diagnosis and treatment of gonococcal infection are discussed in Chapter 40. In young adults, tenosynovitis is often caused by gonococcal infection. The tenosynovitis is not associated with an open wound near the involved tendon sheath but is frequently associated with pustular skin lesions typical of gonococcal infection. Hospitalization for intravenous antibiotic therapy is usually indicated. In selected reliable patients whose diagnosis is confirmed, outpatient therapy with close follow-up may be possible. See Chapter 40 for recommended treatment.

Perron AD, Miller MD, Brady WJ: Orthopedic pitfalls in the ED: fight bite. Am J Emerg Med 2002;20(2):114. [PMID: 11880877]

Talan DA et al: Bacteriologic analysis of infected dog and cat bites. New Engl J Med 1999;340(2):85. [PMID: 9887159]

MINOR CONSTRICTIVE PROBLEMS

Clinical Findings

The 3 common constrictive problems described here are often seen in the emergency department. Only the first is usually a true emergency.

A. Carpal Tunnel Syndrome (Compression of the Median Nerve)

Carpal tunnel syndrome is characterized by aching and numbness over the distribution of the median nerve (see Figure 29–7), with sparing of the small finger. These symptoms often awaken the patient from sleep and may be elicited by full flexion of the wrist for 30 seconds (Phalen maneuver). Tapping over the median nerve at the wrist crease may feel like an electric shock (Tinel sign). Patients with this nerve compression may present with rapid onset of acute edema and progressive loss of feeling after trauma, inflammation, or allergy, and it requires urgent consultation with a hand specialist.

B. Stenosing Flexor Tenosynovitis (Trigger Thumb or Trigger Finger)

Stenosing flexor tenosynovitis is characterized by local tenderness over the proximal tendon pulley at the MP joint, with pain referred to the PIP joint and a snapping when the finger or thumb goes through an active range of motion. Usually a history of repetitive strain is involved.

C. De Quervain Tenosynovitis

De Quervain tenosynovitis is characterized by pain and tenderness when tendons in the first dorsal compartment on the radial side of the wrist are actively or passively stretched; specifically, when the fist is clenched over the thumb while the wrist is put into marked ulnar deviation (Finkelstein test).

Treatment

A. Carpal Tunnel Syndrome

Initial treatment involves wrist splinting and the use of nonsteroidal anti-inflammatory drugs. Activity modification and therapeutic exercises may also improve symptoms. The next step in treatment is injection of the carpal canal using 1 mL of steroid and 2–3 mL of lidocaine. Never inject into the substance of median or ulnar nerves.

B. Flexor Tenosynovitis

Administration of nonsteroidal anti-inflammatory agents may be started in lieu of injection therapy. Steroids should not be injected if an infectious process is suspected. About 0.5 mL each of steroid and lidocaine should be injected into the synovial bursa through the tendon flexor pulley at the base of the digit. The finger should be splinted in extension.

C. De Quervain Tenosynovitis

Nonsurgical treatment involves rest, splinting with a thumb spica splint, anti-inflammatory medications, stretching exercises, and corticosteroid injections. If injecting, use about 0.5 mL each of steroid and lidocaine at the radial styloid process but avoid the radial nerve.

Disposition

Referral to a hand surgeon is advised because multiple injections or surgical release of the tight ligament or sheath may be required.

THERMAL INJURIES
(See also Chapter 43.)

1. First-Degree Burns

Clinical Findings & Treatment

Simple burns (redness without blistering) are treated with cold tap water rinse and analgesia. Comfort may be augmented by a soft nonirritative wrap to protect and immobilize the hand. Elevation and avoidance of constriction by snug garments are also advised.

Disposition

The patient should return or telephone for follow-up after 1–2 days.

2. Second-Degree Burns

Clinical Findings & Treatment

Blisters signify partial-thickness (second-degree) burns, which always retain cutaneous sensation even though they are variable in depth. Although this treatment is controversial, large blisters should be aspirated or unroofed and debrided. Small blisters may be left intact. Silver sulfadiazine (Silvadene) cream may be applied topically. For sulfa-allergic patients, bacitracin may be used instead. Second-degree burns may be dressed with a bulky dressing and the hand splinted in the position of function. Tetanus prophylaxis must be current (Chapter 30). In the case of burns caused by hot tar, the tar may be removed as described in Chapter 43.

Disposition

Patients with extensive burns or marked edema should be immediately referred to a hand specialist for evaluation and possible hospitalization. Patients with lesser involvement should be seen every 1–3 days for a dressing change, especially once blister debridement is started.

3. Third-Degree Burns

Clinical Findings & Treatment

Full-thickness (third-degree) burns require bulky, loose sterile dressings with an anti-infective agent such as silver sulfadiazine. Appropriate elevation and splinting are also advised. Tetanus prophylaxis must be current (Chapter 30).

Disposition

If the burn is extensive (eg, > 1–2 cm^2 [⅜–¾ in^2]) or is over the dorsum of a joint, refer the patient immediately to a hand specialist for decisions about the need for debridement and grafting.

4. Electrical Burns
(See also Chapter 44.)

Burns from electricity are of 2 kinds: crossed circuit, producing arc heat; and conduction of high-voltage current within the tissues. Arc heat is often more frightening than extensively injurious to tissues. There is generally blackening of the skin owing to deposit of carbon. The burn may be anywhere from first-degree to third-degree in severity but is usually localized. The treatment of arc heat burns is the same as that of other thermal burns.

High-voltage conduction burns involve a point of entry and another point of exit. The deep tissues are often coagulated out of proportion to surface skin changes. Blood vessels and nerves are the pathways of conduction and therefore most vulnerable. Immediate irreversible ischemia and paralysis are common. Such cases require hospitalization under the care of a hand specialist for urgent fasciotomy where prophylactically indicated and for observation for systemic effects of the electrical shock. Appropriate debridement (even amputation), grafting, and reconstruction will follow. Extremity destruction is sometimes overwhelming.

If the electrical conduction pathway within the body is not limited to the hand but also involves other areas, consideration should be given to possible myocardial injury. An electrocardiogram and cardiac isoenzymes (CK-MB and troponin) measurement should be obtained. Cardiac monitoring is necessary if myocardial injury is suspected.

5. Frostbite
(See also Chapter 44.)

Exposure to cold may result in superficial or deep frostbite depending on the windchill factor and duration of exposure. Measures to prevent this vasoconstrictive disorder and the irreversible microvascular thrombotic events that lead to gangrene include the following: (1) avoiding exposure to wind, cold metal, snow, and ice by wearing protective gloves; (2) preserving the total body heat by wearing suitable clothing and head gear and avoiding sweat-producing physical effort or alcohol consumption; (3) ensuring adequate caloric intake, high in fat and carbohydrate; and (4) refraining from smoking.

Superficial frostbite is limited to the skin. It exists when the discomfort of fingers exposed to cold is replaced by numbness. Reversal by warming is urgently required and is usually heralded by a warm tingling sensation.

Deep frostbite is signaled by pain and swelling of the entire hand, followed by extensive blister formation and dysesthesia. Deep frostbite requires hospitalization under the care of a hand specialist. Cryofibrinogenemia aggravates the problem and is worsened by the use of heparin, which facilitates precipitation of cryofibrinogen. Treatment consists of rest and warming the patient and the hands. Immersion in water at 37–40 °C (98.6–104 °F) for a short time (eg, 20 minutes) may be beneficial. Blisters must be debrided and dressed with sterile dressings. Sympathetic blockade should be considered.

Luce E: The acute and subacute management of the burned hand. Clin Plast Surg 2000;27(1):49. [PMID: 10665355]

Smith MA, Munster AM, Spence RJ: Burns of the hand and upper limb—a review. Burns 1998;24(6):493. [PMID: 9776087]

FOREIGN BODIES

Fishhooks, splinters, and other objects may have barbs or barblike projections that prevent withdrawal from the wound in the normal retrograde way. Removal is possible by pushing the foreign body along the direction of entry and removing it via a counterincision where it presents under the tented skin. Nerve block or other anesthesia and tourniquet ischemia are necessary before extraction is attempted. Prophylactic antibiotics and tetanus immunization are often necessary.

Foreign bodies embedded in the hand may be difficult to locate and remove. The diagnosis is based on the history and examination, and x-rays are almost always useful in the case of glass or metal. Modalities such as computed tomography, magnetic resonance imaging, and ultrasound can be helpful in finding nonradiopaque foreign bodies. If immediate accessibility and easy removal seem possible, an attempt can be made to remove the foreign body using regional anesthesia, a tourniquet, and sterile technique with loupe magnification. Typically, however, the discoloration of tissues by blood precludes the immediate search for a foreign body, which will be found much more easily after 3–4 weeks when phagocytosis has cleared the blood. Before starting the procedure, tell the patient that if search and removal prove at all difficult (eg, longer than 10–15 minutes), the procedure will be abandoned and referral made to a hand specialist.

Consider leaving an entry wound open by inserting a loose drain, applying an appropriate dressing, and elevating and immobilizing the part. Give prophylactic local or systemic antibiotics and tetanus prophylaxis (Chapter 30). The patient can usually be assured that retrieval of small deep foreign bodies is not urgent, because they do not travel in the body, and that it is often contraindicated by the difficulty and risk of removal.

Blankstein A et al: Localization, detection and guided removal of soft tissue foreign bodies in the hands using sonography. Arch Orthop Trauma Surg 2000;120(9):514. [PMID: 11011671]

COMPLEX HAND INJURIES

Classification

Complex injuries include the following: amputations, serious tendon injuries, nerve injuries, high-pressure injection injuries, closed compartment syndromes, mangling injuries, and gunshot wounds.

Evaluation & Initial Management

In complex injuries, emphasis should be placed on early, rapid diagnosis and institution of supportive therapy. Many complex injuries require referral to a hand specialist immediately or early. In all cases, use conservative measures as outlined below.

A. Avoid Manipulation

Once the decision has been made to transfer or hospitalize the patient, the extremity should not be handled, probed, manipulated, or otherwise disturbed unless absolutely necessary. Foreign material that can be easily lifted out should be removed. Protect with a sterile dressing and, if necessary, a loosely applied splint pending definitive management.

B. Prepare for Possible Urgent Surgery

If there is a reasonable likelihood of surgery within 8–10 hours, give nothing by mouth. An intravenous infusion should be started in the uninjured limb and laboratory work ordered.

C. Give Antibiotics

In the case of open or penetrating wounds, antibiotics should be given parenterally (preferably intravenously in the uninjured extremity) as soon as possible; the earlier they are started, the more effective they are. Give cefazolin, 1–2 g intramuscularly or intravenously every 6–8 hours (adult dose) or 25–100 mg/kg/d intramuscularly or intravenously, divided every 4–8 hours (for children aged > 1 month).

1. Amputations

Clinical Findings

Amputations account for about 1% of hand injuries. The diagnosis of amputation is obvious on inspection of the part. Amputations are generally classified as partial (incompletely severed part) or complete.

Generally, tidy amputations at the level of the middle phalanx or the wrist or distal forearm have the best chance of functionally successful replantation. In the case of single-digit amputation, surgeons are much more inclined to favor replantation of a thumb than of a single finger. Discussions with the patient or relatives regarding the feasibility of replantation should be left to the hand surgeon.

Treatment & Disposition

A. Replantation Possible

Place the amputated member in gauze moistened with saline and then place it in a sealed plastic bag or container that is maintained at 4 °C (39.2 °F) (eg, on wet ice). *Do not freeze the amputated part*, because this destroys its viability.

After starting appropriate supportive measures, if the treating facility is not capable of providing the microsurgical specialized care required for replantation, arrange promptly for referral to a capable facility. The treating physician must contact a microsurgical specialist at the hospital to which he or she would like to refer the patient in order to obtain the specialist's permission for transfer. Failure to do so could be considered a violation of the law (COBRA-EMTLA; see Chapter 5) and might subject the referring physician and hospital to significant financial penalties.

B. Replantation Impossible

If the amputated member either is not recovered or is clearly not salvageable, appropriate in-house or emergency department surgery should be undertaken to close the stump. Except for the simple fingertip pad amputation (discussed above), these injuries should almost always be referred to a hand specialist.

2. Flexor & Proximal Extensor Tendon Injuries

 ESSENTIALS OF DIAGNOSIS

- First suspect that tendon injury may exist; impairment may not become evident until hours, days, or weeks later.
- Check strength of digit against resistance.
- Direct visualization and examination of open wound in sterile, bloodless field is indicated.

General Considerations

Almost all flexor tendon injuries, and those extensor injuries in which the proximal tendon has retracted out of reach, are considered complex injuries. Management of easily accessible extensor tendon injuries is discussed earlier in this chapter.

Clinical Findings

A crucial step in the emergency management of any flexor or proximal extensor tendon injury is to suspect that it may exist and make the proper diagnosis. Impairment of a partially divided tendon (sometimes subtotally or even totally divided) may be functionally masked at the outset, only to become evident hours, days, or weeks later.

In open injuries, tendon lacerations can often be diagnosed by the abnormal stance of the involved part of the hand and almost always by careful functional examination. If the diagnosis is not obvious, but the location of the wound raises the possibility of tendon injury, direct examination of the wound is indicated. Visualization of flexors can be difficult anywhere, whereas visualization of extensors is difficult mainly when they lie proximal to the metacarpal necks.

Occasionally the emergency physician will see a closed profundus tendon rupture. Such an injury almost always follows sudden violent stretch of the flexor, after which the patient is unable to flex the distal phalanx.

Treatment

Obtain immediate consultation with a hand specialist. Dress the wound after irrigation, and splint the wrist

and hand. Remove jewelry and snug garments, and elevate the extremity until definitive treatment can be given. Flexor tendon repair may be delayed as long as 10 days without compromising the eventual outcome. If tendon repair is to be delayed, the wound should be sutured and appropriate antibiotics administered (eg, cefazolin, 1–2 g intravenously, followed by cephalexin, 500 mg orally 4 times daily for 3–5 days).

Disposition

Visualization of a lacerated tendon sheath is reason for referral unless the entire course of the tendon gliding beneath the laceration is observed to be intact. If in doubt, refer immediately, because neglected partial tendon lacerations can go on to rupture.

3. Nerve Injuries

Clinical Findings

Early diagnosis is crucial. The cause and nature of injury, the symptoms, or the location and depth of a laceration may suggest possible nerve injury. If careful motor, sweat, and sensory examination is performed and sometimes repeated more than once for the sake of consistency in appropriate cases (Figures 29–16 and 29–17), few significant nerve injuries will be missed.

Treatment

Appropriate dressing and splinting should be applied when indicated and the patient warned about injury to anesthetized skin until definitive treatment can be given.

Disposition

Refer the patient to a hand surgeon, and determine when the patient is to be transferred for definitive care.

4. High-Pressure Injection Injuries

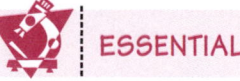 **ESSENTIALS OF DIAGNOSIS**

- Initial appearance of hand may show only pinpoint portal of entry and look deceptively normal.
- Obtain an X-ray.
- Ask about the type, amount, and velocity of the injected material.

Clinical Findings

High-pressure jets of a variety of hot and cold fluids (eg, grease, water, plastics, organic solvents) and gases

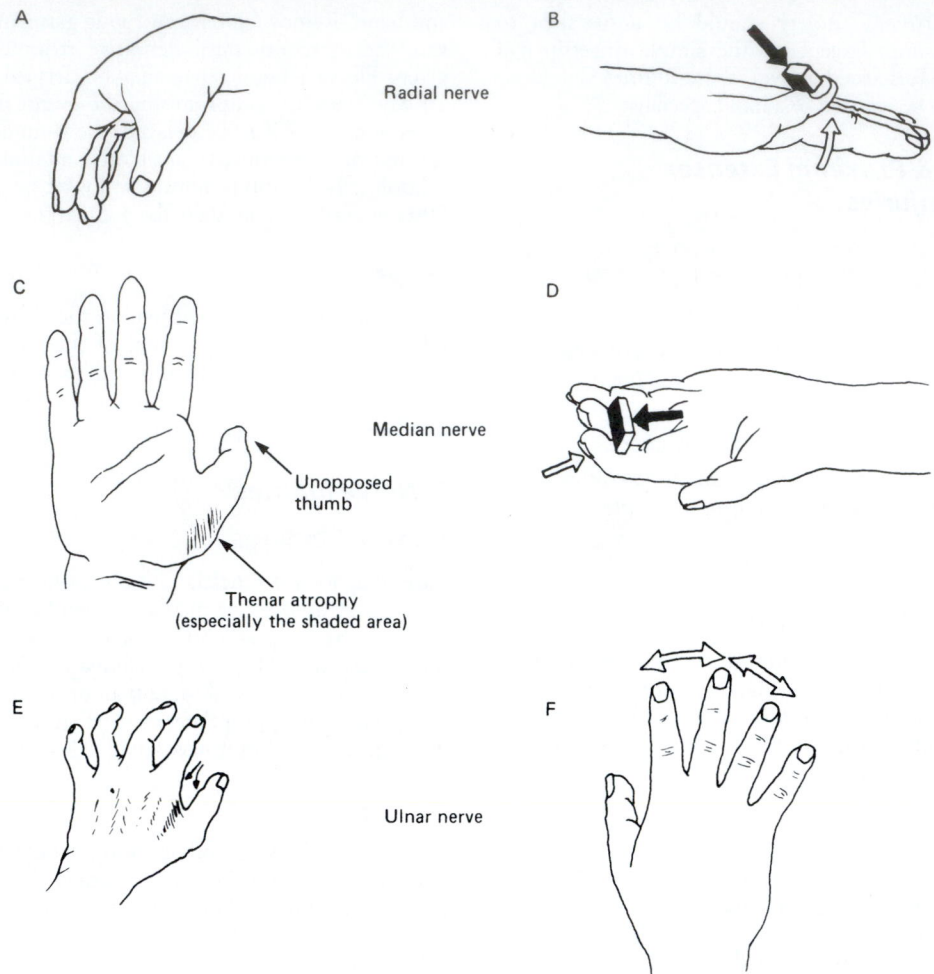

Figure 29–16. Assessing nerve injury. **A:** Wrist drop in radial injury. **B:** Forceful extension of thumb tip is lost in radial nerve injury. **C:** "Ape hand" deformity in median nerve injury. **D:** Forceful flexion of tip of index finger is lost in high median nerve injury. **E** and **F:** Thumb web atrophy and clawing of ring and small fingers, and loss of abduction and adduction in ulnar nerve injury. (Reproduced, with permission, from Schrok TR [editor]: *Handbook of Surgery,* 7th ed. Jones Medical Publications, 1982.)

are widely used in industry. Accidental penetration of the skin through a pinpoint portal of entry may result in devastating damage, even though the initial (postinjection) appearance of the hand or other body part is usually deceptively normal. This is because the foreign material spreads instantly along tissue planes and is widely distributed in the hand or other part. Spread of material up a flexor tendon sheath after penetration of a digital pad is quite common. An x-ray should be obtained, because some injected materials are radiopaque (eg, lead-based paint). When a chemical, inflammatory,

or thermal response becomes manifest 4–12 hours after injury, extensive ischemia and tissue necrosis may be seen. Important historical factors are the type, amount, and velocity of the injected material and the anatomic location. The type of material injected is the most important clue to the severity of the injury.

Treatment & Disposition

Give analgesics for pain if necessary, and splint the extremity in a sling for comfort. Digital blocks are con-

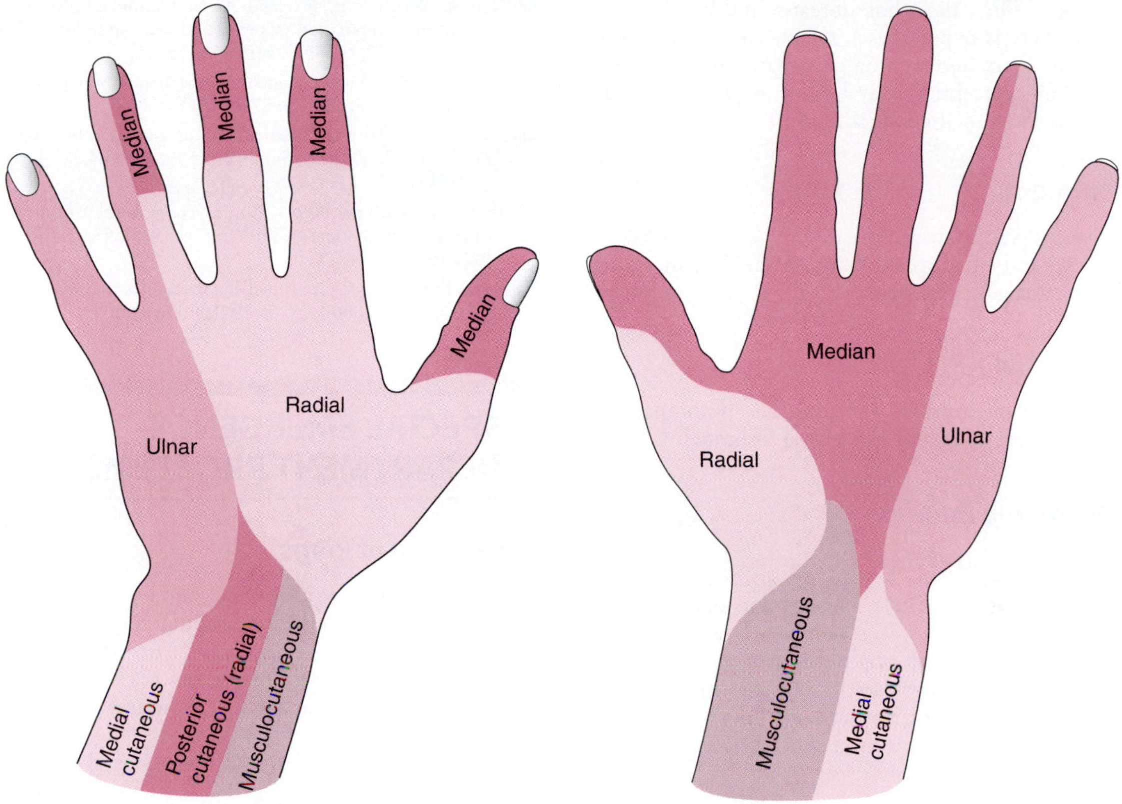

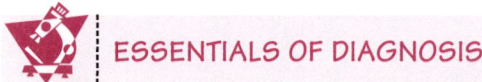

Figure 29–17. Sensory distribution of the hand.

traindicated due to the possibility of increased tissue pressure and vascular compromise. Obtain x-rays.

Give nothing by mouth, and consult a hand surgeon immediately regarding referral. Prompt tetanus prophylaxis, systemic antibiotics, and decompressive surgery (eg, fasciotomy) must be arranged in most cases. Even so, the prognosis for maintaining circulation and salvaging function is often dismal.

5. Closed Compartment Syndromes

ESSENTIALS OF DIAGNOSIS

- History of progressive pain and rock-hard compartment.
- Pain on passive movement.
- Hypoesthesia or paralysis of the digits.

General Considerations

A compartment syndrome (eg, congestion progressing to various degrees of ischemia) can occur in any space of the digit, hand, forearm, or arm. It may involve a single space (eg, extensor and flexor compartments of the forearm and intrinsic muscle compartments of the hand). Obstructed venous flow leads to microvascular stagnation and death of muscle, fat, and nerves. Compartment syndrome may result from external compression (eg, a tight cast, prolonged pressure against an extremity of a comatose patient) or from internal swelling (eg, from severe bleeding, crush injury, burn, fracture, allergy, or infectious inflammatory reaction). The fate of a neglected case in which surgical decompression has not been performed is late fibrosis and severe functional impairment.

Clinical Findings

The typical patient presents with a history of progressive severe pain (eg, throbbing) and a rock-hard compartment. When the whole forearm and hand are involved, there is hypoesthesia, reluctance or inability to move the digits, and pain on passive extension of flexed digits. Pain perception may be lost as pressure on the nerves destroys their conducting ability.

Treatment

Treatment is supportive until definitive surgical decompression can be performed. Support the limb in a sling, and give analgesics for pain.

Disposition

Urgent hospitalization for surgical decompression under the care of a hand specialist is indicated.

6. Mangling Injuries

Clinical Findings

Mangling injuries include gunshot and blast wounds, severe open crush wounds, severe bites by large animals, and a large variety of ripping or tearing injuries (ie, lawnmower- or snowblower-associated injuries). The common denominator is multitissue involvement, distortion, and significant wound contamination.

Treatment

Rapid initiation of supportive measures; loose, bulky, sterile dressing and splinting; immediate administration of antibiotics (eg, cefazolin, 50–100 mg/kg/d intravenously or intramuscularly in 2–3 divided doses); and definitive surgical treatment are important to a successful outcome.

Disposition

All such injuries require immediate hospitalization and referral to a hand specialist for operative debridement and repair.

Arellano A, Wegener E, Freeland A: Mutilating injuries to the hand: early amputation or repair and reconstruction. Orthopedics 1999;22(7):683. [PMID: 10418865]

Chin G et al: Snowblower injuries to the hand. Ann Plast Surg 41(4):390, 1998. [PMID: 9788219]

Lewis HG et al: A 10-year review of high-pressure injection injuries to the hand. J Hand Surg [Br] 1998;23(4):479. [PMID: 9726548]

Martin C, Gonzalez del Pino J: Controversies in the treatment of fingertip amputations. Clin Orthop 1998;353:63. [PMID: 9728160]

Vasilevski D et al: High-pressure injection injuries to the hand. Am J Emerg Med 2000;18:820. [PMID: 11103737]

■ SPECIAL EMERGENCY DEPARTMENT PROBLEMS

1. Removal of Rings

All rings, bracelets, wristwatches, and snug shirt sleeves and coat sleeves should be prophylactically removed whenever injury, surgery, infection, or other cause of acute swelling of any part of the hand exists. Failure to do so may lead to serious congestion and unnecessary complications.

A ring on a swollen finger can be removed in 3 ways:

1. Lubricate the skin with soap, and carefully slip off the ring.

2. Wrap the digit snugly with a string from the distal tip to just below the ring, and in that way "milk" edema out of the digit so that the ring can be removed over the string.

3. Cut the ring with a commercial ring cutter, spread it with 2 pairs of pliers, and remove it. This is the preferred method when there is significant digital injury or swelling distal to the ring.

2. Snakebite

See Chapter 44 for treatment.

Wound Care

Louis J. Kroot, MD, & David Hurst, MD[1]

Emergency Management of Life-Threatening Problems
Hemostasis
Wound Assessment
History
Examination
Anesthesia
Cleaning & Debridement
Wound Closure
1. Suture Selection
2. Wound Tapes
3. Wound Staples
4. Tissue Adhesives
5. Choice of Closure Technique
6. Drainage of the Wound
Postoperative Wound Care & Dressings
1. Potential Infections & Antimicrobials

2. Tetanus Prophylaxis
3. Rabies Prophylaxis
4. Follow-up Care of the Wound
5. Suture Removal
Emergency Treatment of Specific Types of Wounds
Facial Lacerations
Intraoral Lesions
Blast Injuries
High-Pressure Injection Injuries
Degloving Injuries
Amputations
Bites
1. Dog Bites
2. Cat Bites
3. Human Bites
Puncture Wounds

■ EMERGENCY MANAGEMENT OF LIFE-THREATENING PROBLEMS

All patients with open wounds should be examined thoroughly for evidence of serious or life-threatening injuries that may not be obvious on initial presentation. Treat life-threatening conditions immediately. If necessary, institute cardiopulmonary resuscitation (CPR) at once (Chapter 7). Ensure adequate ventilatory status, and treat shock (Chapter 9) and hemorrhage prior to wound assessment. Consider the possibility of internal bleeding.

When facial and scalp injuries are present, look closely for evidence of intracranial or cervical spine injury. If cervical spine injury is suspected, immobilize the neck before performing radiologic evaluation. Serial neurologic examinations are crucial to the evaluation of any head injury.

HEMOSTASIS

Prior to wound closure, establish absolute hemostasis to prevent hematoma formation and further blood volume depletion. Hemostasis is accomplished by direct and indirect methods. The use of indirect methods first is preferred in order to carefully assess the wound, avoid possible injury to important structures, and allow time for replacement of significant blood loss.

Indirect Hemostasis

Indirect methods of achieving hemostasis in the acute wound include elevation, pressure, application of vasoconstrictive agents, and chemical promoters of clotting. These methods are usually effective in the control of diffuse vascular oozing and lymph extravasation.

A. ELEVATION

Elevation of the injured part above the level of the heart is least damaging to the tissues and markedly diminishes capillary oozing. Caution is required in elderly patients with arteriosclerotic vascular disease, because elevation of the lower extremity may induce tissue hypoxia.

---

[1]This chapter is a revision of the chapter by Robert L. Walton, MD, W. Earle Matory, Jr., MD, FACS, & Steven H. Turkeltaub, MD.

B. PRESSURE

Pressure can be used in various ways to effect hemostasis. Direct pressure over a vigorously bleeding wound is perhaps the most common method for rapid control of blood loss. In extremity wounds, a proximally placed blood pressure cuff is frequently used to control bleeding of distal wounds. In either case, take care to avoid the potential sequelae arising from excessive pressure.

Simple cutaneous lacerations are usually manifested by a diffuse capillary ooze that can be an annoying interference with inspection and repair. A simple pressure dressing applied to the wound for 20 minutes will usually control oozing. Ideally, pressure should not exceed capillary pressure (30 mm Hg) and should not impede vascular flow to distal parts. For proximal extremity wounds, apply pressure in graded fashion from the distal aspect of the extremity to the wound to avoid the tourniquet effect of the dressing. The graded pressure is accomplished with bulky dressings and elastic bandages. Assess capillary flow and sensibility of distal parts frequently to avoid ischemic injury.

Reserve the use of tourniquets for isolated digital injuries or for complex injuries associated with excessive blood loss or requiring specialized examination. The tourniquet is placed proximal to the wound (usually the upper arm) and is inflated to 20–30 mm Hg above systolic pressure. Most patients can tolerate the ischemia resulting from this maneuver for 15–20 minutes. However, the ischemia produces a reactive vasodilatation upon release of the tourniquet and may result in resumption of bloody oozing or hematoma formation.

C. VASOCONSTRICTION

Epinephrine-containing solutions are frequently used in acute wounds to control capillary oozing. Concentrations of 1:400,000–1:100,000 units are used for these purposes. After infiltration, a full 7 minutes is required for maximal vasoconstrictive effect. *Caution:* Epinephrine decreases local wound defense mechanisms and should not be used in contaminated wounds because of the increased risk of infection. Although it will not affect the viability of acute random cutaneous flaps, epinephrine can induce vasospasm that may lead to necrosis of tissues supplied by an end-arterial circulation. For this reason, epinephrine is contraindicated in the management of wounds of the penis, of any digit, of the tip of the nose, or in any tissue with circulation compromised by the trauma.

D. CHEMICAL HEMOSTATIC AGENTS

Avoid using hemostatic agents, such as Avitene, Gelfoam, or Surgicel, in the emergency department setting; these agents have been shown to potentiate infections in contaminated wounds.

Topical bovine thrombin can cause an allergic or anaphylactic reaction, intravascular coagulation, or death.

Direct Hemostasis

Direct methods of hemostasis include ligation and electrocauterization of the cut vessel ends. Use direct hemostasis for bleeding that cannot be controlled by indirect methods. An exception to this rule is injury to major vascular tributaries (eg, ulnar, femoral, brachial artery). Further injury to the cut vessel end resulting from attempts at direct hemostasis may preclude successful repair. In these situations, it is wise to apply firm pressure to the wound and consult a vascular surgeon.

A. LIGATION

Simple tying or suture ligation is indicated for most vessels more than 2 mm (1/16 in) in external diameter. To avoid excessive tissue trauma, one must precisely identify and clamp the vessel end prior to ligation. Cut arteries usually require only simple tying. Veins, however, do not hold ligatures well, and suture ligation is preferable. Suture ligation may be performed by passing the suture needle through a portion of the vessel wall and then circumferentially tying the vessel. This method prevents slippage of the ligature. *Caution:* Do not ligate arteries and veins en masse, because this may predispose to arteriovenous fistula formation. Absorbable sutures are preferred for tying and suture ligation in the acute wound. Synthetic absorbable sutures (polyglycolic acid [Dexon] and polyglactin [Vicryl]) are advantageous because of their low reactivity and high friction coefficients. Chromic catgut is also satisfactory.

B. ELECTROCAUTERY

Damped electric current is effective in coagulating small vessel ends. Monopolar cautery causes approximately 3 times as much tissue necrosis as bipolar coagulation. Pinpoint coagulation is preferred, with delivery of the least amount of current needed for vessel thrombosis. *Caution:* Some surgeons use undamped electric current for cutting tissues during debridement of the acute wound. Although quite effective in diminishing blood loss, cutting current inflicts significant thermal injury to the surrounding tissues and increases their susceptibility to infection. This technique is not recommended for wound debridement or hemostasis.

C. CHEMICAL CAUTERY

Caution: Silver nitrate and other caustics achieve hemostasis through tissue coagulation but are not recommended for wound hemostasis because of the amount of tissue necrosis they produce.

■ WOUND ASSESSMENT

HISTORY

A detailed, thorough history is essential for assessing the extent of injury and for organizing appropriate wound management. Three basic questions are used to reconstruct the history of the injury.

A. WHEN DID THE INJURY OCCUR?

The time of injury is important for determining the interval between injury and treatment. Most civilian injuries contain fewer than 10^5 bacteria per gram of tissue in the first 6 hours and are therefore relatively safe to close. After the first 6 hours, bacteria may proliferate and increase the risk of infection if the wound is surgically closed. Exceptions to the 6-hour limit vary depending on the degree of wound contamination, the mechanism of injury, and the location of the wound. As a rule, local tissue resistance is directly proportionate to blood supply. Facial lacerations may often be closed safely within 24 hours of injury, owing to the abundant blood supply in that area.

B. WHERE DID THE INJURY OCCUR?

What were the possible contaminants associated with the injury? Contact with feces, pus, saliva, or soil greatly increases the risk of infection and precludes primary closure.

C. HOW DID THE INJURY OCCUR?

The mechanism of injury and the type of instrument inflicting the wound influence subsequent management. Knowing the type of instrument that inflicted the wound will aid in assessing the extent of injury as well as the need for further diagnostic studies. The degree of wound contamination depends in part of the state of cleanliness of the instrument inflicting the injury.

Types of Injuries

A. LACERATIONS

Lacerations cause minimal tissue injury and are relatively resistant to infection.

B. PUNCTURE WOUNDS

Puncture wounds may become infected, especially if they are contaminated or if a foreign body is present.

C. STRETCH INJURIES

Stretch injuries can produce damage to blood vessels, nerves, ligaments, or tendons that is not visible superficially.

D. COMPRESSION OR CRUSH INJURIES

Compression or crush injuries result in the greatest amount of tissue necrosis. Hemorrhage into the soft tissues is common, resulting in ecchymosis and hematoma formation. The crushed tissue has a markedly impaired ability to heal and resist infection.

E. BITES

Bites are heavily contaminated and may require delayed closure.

Tetanus Immunization Status

It is important to ascertain the tetanus immunization status of patients who have sustained open wounds. Determine the date of the patient's most recent booster shot.

Allergies

The existence of any allergies or adverse reactions should always be elicited before treatment is started. Ask the patient specifically about past problems with anesthetics, antibiotics, or analgesics. Such questioning may remind the patient of a forgotten allergic or adverse reaction.

EXAMINATION

Careful inspection of the wound is imperative for proper management. Inspection should be conducted in an emergency care or surgical facility where adequate lighting and equipment are available. Sterile technique and gentle handling of tissues are mandatory to avoid additional tissue injury or contamination.

Definitive wound evaluation requires a cooperative patient. If the patient is uncooperative, it is perhaps wise to consider restraints, sedation, or local (see below) or general anesthesia—or even to postpone the examination, if possible, until more favorable conditions exist.

Assess Type & Extent of Injury

In assessing the type and extent of injury, consider the following questions:

- Is there loss of function in the injured part?
- Are important underlying structures involved, such as nerves, major blood vessels, ducts, ligaments, bones, or joints?
- What is the level of contamination in the wound?
- Are any foreign bodies present?
- What is the viability of the injured parts? Are any parts missing?

Examine for Avulsion Flaps

Avulsion flaps may result in a sizable amount of nonviable tissue that may not be apparent initially. Distally located flaps result in greater tissue destruction than do proximally located flaps. Venous congestion is a sure sign of ultimate tissue death.

Amputated tissue may be reattached in some cases. Seal the parts in a dry, sterile container and cool them on ice. If replantation is considered a possibility, consult a microsurgeon or appropriate specialist immediately.

Consider Location of Wound

A. HEAD AND NECK

Deep injuries to the head and neck frequently involve important underlying structures (Chapter 23). These complex anatomic areas cannot be extensively debrided without major functional or cosmetic loss. Wound evaluation and repair are often best done in the operating room by a maxillofacial or general surgeon. The importance of serial evaluations of the central nervous system and cervical spine in the presence of major head and neck trauma cannot be overemphasized.

B. CHEST AND ABDOMEN

Wounds of the chest and abdomen must be evaluated for possible communication with a body cavity as well as internal organ injury (Chapters 24 and 25).

C. EXTREMITIES

Deep wounds in the extremities must be carefully examined and anatomic landmarks visualized. Pulse deficits or bruits may be present, and an arteriogram may be indicated if the path of injury passes close to a major blood vessel (Chapter 38). Injuries to the extremities require detailed examination of nerve, tendon, and circulatory function (Chapter 29). Avoid extending the injury by inadvertent manipulation or haphazard probing. Make sure that no tourniquet is inadvertently left in place where a dressing is applied. Adequate lighting, exposure, and selection of instruments are mandatory. Most tendon and nerve repairs and all vascular repairs should be performed in an operating room.

Prepare for Definitive Care

After initial assessment, cover the wound with a sterile dressing until definitive management or further evaluation can be performed. Obtain any necessary x-rays only after the wound has been protected from the possibility of additional contamination. If considerable delay in definitive evaluation and management is anticipated, the wound should be cleaned, conservatively debrided, and temporarily closed or covered. Extensive wounds—or minor ones involving major structures—are best evaluated and managed in the operating room.

ANESTHESIA

Preliminary Examination

Perform a careful sensory and motor neurologic examination before administering anesthetic.

Choice of Agent

Local and infiltrative anesthetics have varying attributes with regard to safety, potency, duration of action, and effects on the local wound milieu (Table 30–1). Lidocaine is perhaps the safest local anesthetic, because allergic reactions are rare. The major problem with all local anesthetics is systemic absorption resulting in cardiovascular and central nervous system toxicity. For an adult, the maximum safe dose of 1% lidocaine without epinephrine is 5 mg/kg (do not exceed 300 mg); for 1% lidocaine with epinephrine, 7 mg/kg (do not exceed 500 mg). For children, the safety and efficacy of lidocaine and mepivacaine are known; child safety and efficacy of the other drugs in Table 30–1 are not known.

Topical Anesthesia

Topical anesthesia is especially useful in the management of small wounds in children who do not tolerate local infiltration. A commonly used combination solution is LET (lidocaine, epinephrine, and tetracaine). To apply the solution, soak a gauze pad in it and place the pad directly over the wound for 20 minutes. Do not use over mucous membranes or areas with end-arterial circulation (fingers, toes, nose, penis). Anesthesia can often be judged by the appearance of blanching at the wound site. Use the minimal amount of anesthetic necessary.

Inhalation Anesthesia

Inhalation anesthesia with nitrous oxide administered by experienced personnel can be a useful adjunct, especially for children.

Local Infiltration

A. METHOD OF INJECTION

Infiltration of a local anesthetic agent is performed gently near the edge of the wound or directly into the wound with a small (No. 25–30) needle (Figure 30–1). Pain associated with local infiltration is partly due to the stretching of sensitive nerve endings in the dermis and may also be due in part to the difference in acidity

Table 30–1. Drugs used for local anesthesia.[1]

	Cocaine	Procaine (Novocain)	Tetracaine[2] (Pontocaine)	Lidocaine (Xylocaine, Many Others)	Bupivacaine[2] (Marcaine, Sensoricaine)	Mepivacaine (Carbocaine)
Potency (compared to procaine)	3	1	10	2–3	9–12	1.5–2
Toxicity (compared to procaine)	4	1	10	1–1.5	4–6	1–1.5
Stability at sterilizing temperature	Unstable	Stable	Stable	Stable	Stable	Stable
Total maximum adult dose	100–200 mg	500 mg	50–100 mg	300 mg	175 mg	400 mg
Total maximum pediatric dose	. . .	. . .	. . .	4 mg/kg	. . .	5 mg/kg
Infiltration Concentration[3] Onset of action Duration	. . . .	0.25–1% 5–15 min 45–60 min	0.05–0.1% 10–20 min 1½–3 h	0.5–1% 3–5 min 30–60 min	0.25% 5–10 min 1½–2 h	0.5% 5–10 min 1¼–2½ h
Nerve block Concentration[3] Onset of action Duration	. . . .	1–2% 5–15 min 45–60 min	0.1–0.2% 10–20 min 1½–3 h	1–2% 5–10 min 1–1½ h	0.25–0.5% 7–21 min 2–6 h	1–2% 5–10 min 1¼–2½ h

[1]Addition of vasopressor prolongs duration by 25–50%; exercise care when used topically, to avoid excessive systemic absorption.
[2]Not recommended for children.
[3]0.5% solution = 5 mg/mL; 1% solution = 10 mg/mL; 2% solution = 20 mg/mL.

of some anesthetics (the pH of commercial preparations of lidocaine is 5.0–7.0). Associated pain can be reduced by using smaller amounts of more concentrated anesthetic solutions and slower infiltration rates or, in the case of lidocaine, by preparing it as a buffered solution (9 mL of 1% lidocaine, to which 1 mL of sodium bicarbonate solution, 44 mEq/50 mL, is added). Restrict the dose of anesthetic to the least amount that will provide

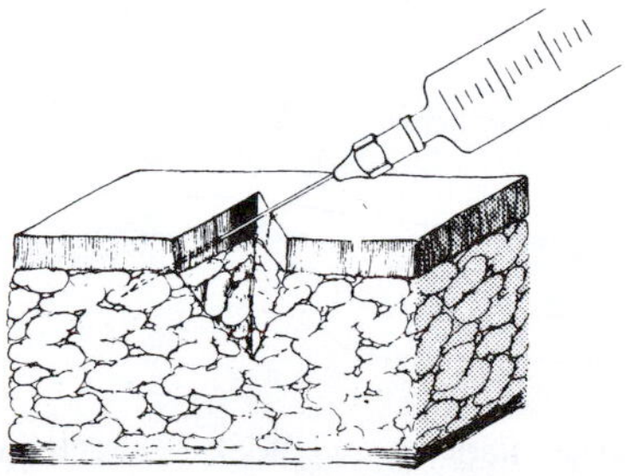

Figure 30–1. Injection of local anesthetic for wound closure. (Reproduced, with permission, from Dunphy JE, Way LE [editors]: *Current Surgical Diagnosis & Treatment*, 5th ed. Lange, 1981.)

adequate anesthesia. This is particularly true for facial lacerations, where infiltration distorts important landmarks and makes precise matching of wound edges difficult. Infiltration of anesthetic directly into the wound is less painful but may spread infection in heavily contaminated wounds.

B. Epinephrine Hemostasis

Lidocaine and similar agents cause relaxation of spastic vessels, and bleeding may start again following local anesthesia. Addition of epinephrine overcomes this tendency and also prolongs the anesthetic effect. The concentration of epinephrine does not need to be higher than 1:400,000, and at least 7 minutes should be allowed for the full vasoconstrictive effect. Use a fresh vial of 1:1000 epinephrine, and dilute it with plain 1% or 2% lidocaine. Premixed solutions of epinephrine-containing local anesthetics may lose their potency during prolonged storage.

Although epinephrine has been shown to have little adverse effect on survival of experimental cutaneous flaps, its use in patients with traumatically elevated skin flaps or in tissues with questionable viability is not recommended. Never administer epinephrine in areas where segmental blood supply is critical (eg, fingers and toes). Epinephrine is contraindicated in heavily contaminated wounds, because it severely compromises local wound defense mechanisms. Consider the systemic side effects of epinephrine in patients with cardiovascular and peripheral vascular disease.

Regional Anesthesia

Regional anesthesia (sensory nerve blockage at a site proximal to the wound) is more difficult to achieve than local anesthesia, but it provides a larger anesthetic area and allows more extensive exploration and manipulation of the tissues. Because local wound anatomy is not distorted by regional block, more precise alignment of wound edges is possible. Onset of anesthesia is a function of the type of agent used and how close to the nerves the agent is injected. The duration of anesthesia can be prolonged with epinephrine; however, epinephrine should not be used for digital nerve blocks. Regional anesthesia is particularly applicable in extremity injuries complicated by heavy contamination or in extensive injury requiring long operating times for repair. It is also used in patients who are not good candidates for general anesthesia.

A. EXAMPLES

Examples of regional nerve blocks include axillary block; isolated ulnar, median, and radial nerve blocks; digital nerve blocks; trigeminal nerve blocks; sciatic and femoral nerve blocks; and spinal anesthesia. Digital, infraorbital, and submental blocks are commonly performed in the emergency department. Isolated ulnar, median, and radial nerve blocks should be performed only by an experienced physician.

B. PITFALLS

Pitfalls of regional anesthesia include difficulty in placing the anesthetic close to the supplying sensory nerve; loss of valuable time in waiting for it to take effect; and risk of permanent injury to the nerve from direct infiltration of anesthetic into the nerve.

Common Regional Blocks for Hand Surgery

Several techniques for regional blocks in hand surgery are described below. Whatever the method used, a thorough understanding of anatomy is crucial. Avoid probing for paresthesias. Attempt to infiltrate the anesthetic without penetrating the nerve sheath, because this may injure the nerve.

Use a 25- or 27-gauge needle; larger needles may cause significant nerve injury. Wait about 10 minutes for the full anesthetic effect in digital blocks and 20 minutes for wrist blocks.

A. DIGITAL BLOCK

The technique requires 2 separate needle sticks with 4 injections of 1 mL of 1% lidocaine next to the nerve bundle of all 4 digital nerves. The needle is first inserted dorsally to block the dorsal digital nerve and is then redirected without removal toward the volar nerve and the anesthetic is injected. The procedure is repeated on the opposite side of the digit.

B. RADIAL NERVE BLOCK

The radial sensory nerve emerges beneath the brachioradialis tendon (Figure 30–2) about 6 cm (2⅜ in) above the Lister tubercle. Inject about 4 mL of lidocaine in a 2-cm (¾-in) wide band 4 cm (1⁹⁄₁₆ in) above the Lister tubercle.

C. MEDIAN NERVE BLOCK

The median nerve at the wrist lies just radial and deep to the palmaris longus tendon and the transverse carpal ligament (Figure 30–3). The palmaris longus, when present, is easily identified by having the patient make a fist and flex the wrist. Insert the needle dorsally and distally between the palmaris longus and flexor carpi radialis, and inject 4 mL. The lidocaine can be milked into the carpal tunnel to achieve the maximum blocking effect.

D. ULNAR NERVE BLOCK

The ulnar nerve and artery course just dorsal to the flexor carpi ulnaris at the wrist (Figure 30–4). Avoid inadvertent injection of anesthetic into the artery by aspirating as the needle is advanced. Inject 2 mL on the ulnar side of the flexor carpi ulnaris. An additional 2 mL should be injected on the radial side to achieve a total block.

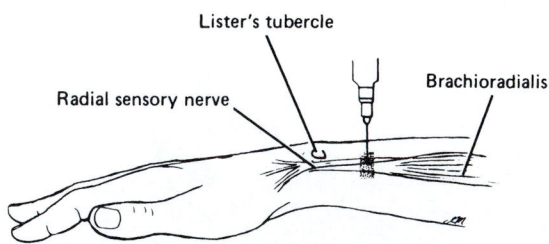

Figure 30–2. Radial nerve block, in which anesthetic is injected in a 2-cm (¾-in) wide band 4 cm (1⁹⁄₁₆ in) proximal to the Lister tubercle on the radial aspect of the forearm. (Modified and reproduced, with permission, from Newmeyer WL: *Care of Hand Injuries.* Lea & Febiger, 1979.)

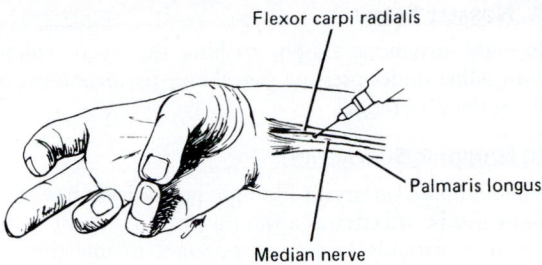

Figure 30–3. Median nerve block. Inject anesthetic around the median nerve just proximal to the wrist. The nerve is located between the tendons and the palmaris longus and flexor carpi radialis. (Modified and reproduced, with permission, from Newmeyer WL: *Care of Hand Injuries.* Lea & Febiger, 1979.)

Common Regional Blocks for Facial Surgery

A. INFRAORBITAL NERVE BLOCK

The infraorbital foramen can be easily palpated along the anterior maxilla and lies along a line drawn between the pupil and the maxillary canine. Inject about 1–2 mL as the needle is advanced from a lateral to a medial direction (Figure 30–5). Avoid penetrating the nerve by being careful not to enter the foramen. An intraoral approach may also be used. Wait for symptoms of numbness of the upper lip. Infraorbital nerve block provides anesthesia of the cheek, upper lip, and parts of the nose.

B. SUPRAORBITAL NERVE BLOCK

The exit of the supraorbital nerve from the orbit is readily identified by palpating the supraorbital notch. Inject a total of 1–2 mL of anesthetic about 0.5 cm (³⁄₁₆ in) above the orbital rim (Figure 30–6). Advance

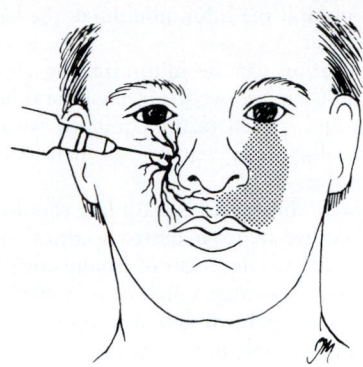

Figure 30–5. Infraorbital nerve block. Intraoral or percutaneous injection around the palpable infraorbital foramina will result in anesthesia within the stippled area.

the needle from a lateral to a medial direction, and avoid penetrating the nerve. If both supraorbital and infratrochlear blocks are needed, the wheal should be extended medially toward the midline. Supraorbital block is helpful in anesthetizing the forehead.

CLEANING & DEBRIDEMENT

Hair Removal

Wounds in hairy areas are difficult to debride and suture, and hair in a wound acts as a foreign body, delaying healing and promoting infection. Shaving hair around wound edges facilitates management but invites

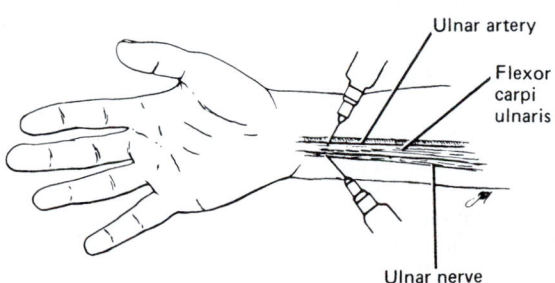

Figure 30–4. Ulnar nerve block. Inject anesthetic around the ulnar nerve just proximal to the wrist on either side of the flexor carpi ulnaris. (Modified and reproduced, with permission, from Newmeyer WL: *Care of Hand Injuries.* Lea & Febiger, 1979.)

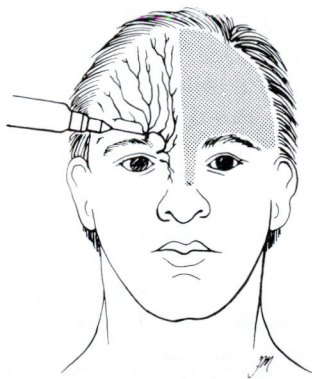

Figure 30–6. Supraorbital nerve block. Inject anesthetic slightly superior to the orbital ridge at the supraorbital notch. Stippling shows area of anesthesia from ipsilateral injection.

wound infection if the infundibulum of the hair follicle is injured.

Contamination can be minimized by clipping the hair 1–2 mm (⅟₁₆ in) above the level of the skin. Depilatory agents and special razors equipped with recessed blades also allow safe removal of hair without infundibular injury.

Caution: Eyebrow and eyelash hair should never be removed, because removal destroys critical landmarks and makes accurate alignment of wound edges difficult. Misalignments may cause notch or step-off deformities in the brow line. Eyebrow hair also regrows slowly, creating a cosmetic problem.

Mechanical Cleansing

As an adjunct to surgical debridement, mechanical cleansing of the wound by irrigation or scrubbing is quite effective. Soaps and detergents should not be used in the open wound in conjunction with mechanical cleaning.

A. Irrigation

To be effective, irrigating solutions must be delivered under pressure. The danger of tissue injury with high-pressure irrigation must be weighed against the benefits of decontamination.

Numerous devices are available for high-pressure irrigation, but the simplest and least expensive is syringe irrigation. A 35- or 50-mL syringe and a 19-gauge or blunt needle connected to a reservoir of irrigating fluid by a 3-way stopcock are most suitable. Bulb syringe irrigation has been shown to be no more effective in preventing wound infection than no irrigation at all.

Normal saline (or similar balanced crystalloid solution) is forcefully injected close to the wound surface and perpendicular to the surface of the skin. The amount of irrigant used depends on the size of the wound and the suspected extent of contamination.

B. Mechanical Scrubbing

1. Sponge—Mechanical scrubbing of the wound surface is usually best performed with a highly porous sponge. Sponges routinely used for hand washing work well. Brushes and low-porosity sponges decrease the wound's resistance to infection.

2. Brush—"Abrasion tattooing," in which debris is embedded in the skin, requires vigorous scrubbing or dermabrasion to remove embedded debris. Soaps and detergents should not be used.

Skin & Wound Cleansers

Cleanse the wound and surrounding skin to remove transient microflora, gross debris, coagulated blood, and the like.

A. Normal Saline

In most instances, simply washing the open wound with saline under pressure (see above) removes most of the surface bacteria.

B. Nonionic Surfactant

The nonionic surfactant Pluronic polyol F-68 has been shown to be effective as a wound cleansing agent without demonstrably impairing resistance to infection or wound healing.

C. Hydrogen Peroxide

The foaming action of hydrogen peroxide is frequently used to remove particulate debris and recently clotted blood from wounds. *Caution:* For these purposes, dilute solutions of hydrogen peroxide (1% or less) must be used to reduce the potential for tissue injury associated with oxidation. In most cases, a less toxic means of wound cleansing may be preferred.

D. Ionic Soaps and Detergents

Ionic soaps and detergents (eg, pHisoHex) should *not* be used for wound cleansing, because they are extremely irritating to tissues and increase the potential for infection if used directly on the wound. They may be used for cleansing of intact skin surrounding the wound, although they have not been shown to be superior to ordinary soap or other agents for this purpose. After application, they should be removed by thorough rinsing with water. Prolonged use of agents containing hexachlorophene (particularly in children) is associated with severe toxicity, including neurologic damage and even death.

E. Skin Disinfectants and Antimicrobials

Skin disinfectants and antimicrobials vary in their microbicidal effects in wounds. Most are irritating to normal tissues, and some may cause severe toxicity by their systemic absorption (eg, chlorhexidine, antimicrobial powders). Although a 1% solution of povidone-iodide is considered nontoxic, there is conflicting evidence regarding its efficacy in preventing wound infection. Tincture of iodine has been shown to potentiate wound infection, and its use can also result in elevation of blood iodine levels. Irrigation of wounds with antibiotic solutions is associated with a decreased rate of wound infection.

Debridement

Remove retained debris and devitalized tissue by surgical excision and mechanical cleansing.

Surgical debridement consists of excising devitalized or severely contaminated tissues and irregular areas that interfere with wound closure. Use a stainless steel scalpel blade for debridement.

A. Total Excision of the Wound

The simplest method of debridement is total excision of the wound, creating a surgically clean area. ***Caution:*** Total excision is appropriate only for wounds that do not involve specialized structures (eg, injuries of the abdominal wall and thighs). More selective debridement is indicated for wounds on the hand or face.

1. Special gauze pack and closure—It is often helpful to pack the wound with gauze, close with sutures, and excise the entire mass as a tumor, leaving a cuff of normal tissue attached. Take care to avoid exposure of the gauze during dissection.

2. Vital staining—An alternative method of debridement is to stain the wound with a vital dye such as methylene blue, close, and excise the entire stained area.

B. Selective Debridement

In most situations, it is best to mechanically cleanse the wound (see above) and then perform selective debridement of all grossly nonviable tissue. Because a reliable laboratory test for tissue viability is not available, tissue viability must be assessed by careful inspection. Signs of tissue necrosis include gray or black color and lack of bleeding when the tissue is incised. Remove all nonviable portions except certain fibrous tissue remnants. Mangled, irregular wound edges imply severe local tissue injury and should be sharply debrided. If, on initial or subsequent evaluation, it appears that adequate debridement would prevent tension-free simple closure, consult an experienced surgeon for wound management.

The potential viability of attached soft tissue parts depends on vascular supply and on the extent of injury. Venous effluent is the most critical component of vascularization. Assess traumatically elevated skin flaps for capillary refill and the presence of venous congestion. Rapid capillary refill or cyanosis in the flap indicates venous obstruction. If a sharp demarcation is seen between normal and abnormal perfusion of the flap, excision of the abnormal portion is indicated. If the area of perfusion is not well demarcated, clean and closely observe the wound. Consultation with a surgeon may be warranted.

Excision procedures on the face, particularly of specialized structures such as the ear or nose, require a conservative approach. The facial area has an abundant blood supply that enables tissues to survive on surprisingly small pedicles. In these cases, observation and expectant treatment are warranted. Obtain surgical consultation before performing any major debridement or debridement of a specialized part.

WOUND CLOSURE

After the wound has been examined, anesthetized, cleaned and debrided, and reexamined, the physician must decide whether to close it. Primary wound closure is preferable because of faster healing, less scarring, improved hemostasis, and better aesthetic and functional results. All foreign bodies should be removed to minimize the chance of infection.

Contraindications to Wound Closure

Several factors affect the risk of infection with wound closure and determine whether closure is justified.

A. Heavy Bacterial Colonization

A prolonged interval (more than 6 hours) between injury and attempted closure is usually a contraindication to wound closure. In a generously vascularized area such as the face, wound closure may be attempted up to 24 hours after injury.

Heavily contaminated wounds (eg, bites) should be left open. Active wound infection at the time of the emergency department visit contraindicates closure of the wound.

B. Major Tissue Defects

Closure is contraindicated if the wound cannot be closed without excessive tension.

C. Other Factors

Closure is contraindicated if there are retained foreign bodies, devitalized tissue, or tissue with borderline adequate perfusion (high likelihood of infection).

Primary Closure

A. Objectives

The objectives of primary wound closure are (1) precise alignment of injured parts to facilitate rapid healing, return of function, and a good cosmetic result; and (2) avoidance of tissue injury (eg, excessive electrocautery, strangulating sutures), hematoma formation, and wound tension.

B. Delayed Primary Closure

Contaminated wounds, if properly debrided, will gain resistance to infection if left open. After 48–96 hours, these wounds can then be closed with essentially no loss in wound healing time. Consider delayed primary closure in the case of wounds contaminated by feces, pus, a foreign body, or saliva in the case of bite wounds. Crush and blast injuries and avulsion injuries are markedly susceptible to infection and necrosis and should also be considered for delayed closure.

After initial debridement, dress the open wound with fine-mesh gauze and a sterile dressing. It should be left undisturbed for the next 4 days unless unexplained fever develops. After this time, the wound is closed using sterile technique.

If delayed closure is elected, the patient should be hospitalized (for large or serious wounds) or seen daily on an outpatient basis.

1. Suture Selection

All sutures represent foreign bodies in the wound. For this reason, use the smallest size and the least amount of suture that will achieve adequate tissue apposition. Do not use sutures in contaminated wounds unless they are absolutely necessary to maintain alignment of tissue parts.

The choice of needle and suture size is generally dictated by the size and location of the wound and the desired precision of closure.

Atraumatic needles (round, tapered) are used for closing fascia, muscle, and subcutaneous tissues as well as for repairing lacerated vessels and nerves. Cutting needles are used primarily for dermal and epidermal closure, where the tough collagen fibers must be "cut" by the needle to allow easy passage of the suture.

Large-diameter suture materials (2-0, 3-0) are best for closing major fascial layers and tissues subjected to strong tensile forces (eg, knee and elbow wounds). The effective strength of a suture material is only as great as the strength of the tissue being sutured: fine sutures placed in wounds subject to mechanical stresses may result in disruption of the wound if the fine suture material pulls through the wound.

Generally, fine sutures are used in wounds (or their parts) requiring precise alignment; 5-0 and 6-0 sutures are preferred for closure of facial lacerations. Layered closure (fascia, dermis) of any wound allows placement of fine epidermal sutures anywhere on the body. The epidermis itself has little tensile strength, and sutures are placed in this layer only to achieve accurate alignment of wound edges.

Percutaneous closure of the epidermis and dermis in regions other than the face is best managed by the use of 3-0 or 4-0 suture material. Suture marks are the result of tension in the tied suture and the length of time the suture is left in place.

Absorbable Sutures

Absorbable sutures are biodegraded and lose their tensile strength in 2–6 weeks.

A. Gut Sutures

Sutures derived from sheep submucosa or beef serosa are digested by proteolytic enzymes in the wound. They are more rapidly degraded in the presence of infection.

The knot-holding ability of plain gut is rather inconsistent; chromic gut seems to be better in this regard.

1. Plain gut—Plain gut incites an intense inflammatory reaction in the wound and loses its tensile strength within 2 weeks.

2. Chromic gut—Treatment of gut with chromium salts decreases its tissue reactivity and prolongs its survival to about double that of plain gut. In some studies, however, it has been shown to potentiate infection more than plain gut.

B. Synthetic Sutures

Polyglycolic acid (Dexon), polyglactin (Vicryl), and polydioxanone (PDS) produce minimal tissue reaction in the wound and are most commonly used for dermal and subcutaneous closures and vascular ligation.

1. Degradation—Polyglycolic acid and polyglactin are degraded by hydrolysis and lose 50% of their tensile strength in 14–20 days and about 90% by the fourth week (comparable to chromic catgut). Polydioxanone, a third-generation synthetic absorbable suture, loses 50% of its tensile strength in 5 weeks and 90% at 2 months.

2. Tying qualities—Although similar to silk in their handling characteristics, polyglycolic acid and polyglactin sutures do not hold knots quite as well. Polydioxanone looks, feels, and handles like monofilament nylon or polypropylene.

3. Use in acute wounds—Absorbable synthetic sutures are probably superior to gut sutures in acute wounds because of their low tissue reactivity and resistance to degradation in the presence of infection. The monofilament characteristics of polydioxanone make it almost the ideal synthetic absorbable suture.

Nonabsorbable Sutures

Nonabsorbable sutures are degraded very slowly or not at all in the tissues.

A. Silk

Silk sutures represent the most common type of natural fiber suture. Silk gradually loses its tensile strength and is classified as a slowly absorbable suture material. The tissue reactivity of silk is the greatest of all nonabsorbable sutures, and its use in acute wounds has generally been abandoned.

B. Stainless Steel and Metallic Clips or Staples

Stainless steel sutures and metallic clips have been used for years because of their presumed inertness. These materials have been shown to increase infection rates significantly in contaminated wounds. The increase is probably the result of mechanical irritation resulting from their rigidity and not to corrosion. The stiffness of metallic sutures makes tying quite cumbersome.

Many types of disposable skin staple devices are available. The staple configurations vary but are primarily designed to approximate wound edges with minimal tissue trauma. Some staples project above the skin surface to avoid staple marks. As with wound tapes, precise epidermal alignment is difficult to achieve with a skin staple, and these devices should not be used for cosmetic skin closures. Because a stapled wound usually does not contain dermal sutures, its tensile strength depends on the presence of the staple, and this must be kept in mind when considering staple closure of wounds subjected to increased tension (eg, joint surfaces, mobile parts). If early removal of the staple is contemplated, the wound should be supported by skin tapes until the wound gains sufficient tensile strength to withstand local biomechanical forces. The time required varies from 1 to 2 weeks depending on the wound's location.

C. Synthetic Sutures

1. Dacron—Dacron is a polyester that elicits less tissue reaction than silk. Because of its high friction coefficient, it is as difficult to handle as a suture. The friction injury imposed on the tissues by Dacron can be overcome by coating it with Teflon.

2. Nylon—Nylon causes less tissue reactivity than Dacron, and its use in contaminated wounds results in lower wound infection rates. Monofilament nylon sutures lose approximately 20% of their tensile strength within a year after placement in a wound. The monofilament form of nylon is quite stiff and does not hold knots well. Multifilament nylon sutures completely lose their tensile strength in the wound after 6 months, but they are easier to tie than monofilament sutures.

3. Polypropylene and polyester—Polypropylene and polyester materials cause the least reactivity of all suture materials. They maintain their tensile strength indefinitely and are the suture material of choice for closure of contaminated wounds. These materials are used most commonly for fascia and skin closure. They are also advantageous in the repair of vascular, nerve, and tendon injuries. Because of their softer consistency, these materials generally hold knots better than does nylon.

2. Wound Tapes

Sutureless closure of the acute wound provides maximum resistance to infection. Various tape materials have been used and have resulted in significantly diminished wound infection rates compared to those in suture closure. Tape closure is most advantageous in the contaminated wound but is also useful in superficial clean and tidy wounds, wounds in children, and wounds in obese patients.

Tape closure is inferior to suture closure in maintaining precise wound edge alignment and eversion, requisites for cosmetically acceptable closure. However, tape closure is often used after early removal of sutures in order to minimize suture marks and to provide additional splinting of the wound until tensile strength is sufficient to resist local forces tending to pull the edges of the wound apart.

Attributes of Wound Tapes

A. Strength

To be effective, skin tapes must be strong enough to support the wound edges in close apposition until sufficient healing has occurred.

B. Adherence

The tapes must have excellent skin adherence and should not macerate the underlying skin surface. Removing all moisture and using a defatting agent (eg, acetone) enhances adhesiveness to the skin, and tapes so applied will adhere for up to 2 weeks. Although tincture of benzoin is occasionally used to increase adhesiveness and may initially enhance tape adhesion, it is solubilized by skin oils and rapidly loses its effectiveness.

C. Types

Microporous, rayon-reinforced wound tapes satisfy the requirements for wound tapes quite well and are used most often (eg, Steri-Strips; Figure 30–7). Simple wound tapes can be fashioned from plain microporous 1.25-cm (½-in) paper tape and should be sterilized by applying iodine to the central area of the tape touching the wound.

Wound Tapes over Deep Sutures

Suture closure in irregular lacerations and crush injuries allows for better approximation of skin edges than does tape closure. Moreover, tape only approximates the superficial portion of the wound, leaving the deeper wound layers more vulnerable to local biomechanical stresses and resulting in a weak, unsightly scar. In clean wounds, it is sometimes preferable to close the deeper layers with sutures and then approximate the superficial layers with tape.

3. Wound Staples

Stainless steel wound staples (Ethicon, 3M, Deknatel, others) are occasionally used in the emergency department. Wounds—especially long, linear lacerations—can be closed more quickly with staples than with sutures. In some cases, when the costs of suture instrument sets,

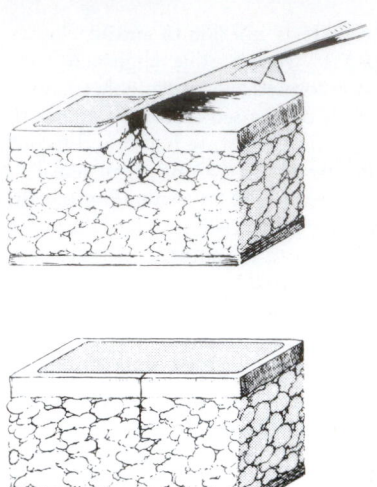

Figure 30–7. Epidermal closure with tape. **Top:** Gentle traction is applied on the Steri-Strip to approximate the edges. **Bottom:** Closure of the wound. (Reproduced, with permission, from Dunphy JE, Way LE [editors]: *Current Surgical Diagnosis & Treatment,* 5th ed. Lange, 1981.)

suture material, and labor are considered, stapling a wound may be considerably less costly. However, crushed or ischemic tissue may cause point necrosis and infection at the staple tip and produce a less cosmetically satisfactory result. Thus, staples should probably be limited to areas of less cosmetic importance, such as on the scalp or trunk.

4. Tissue Adhesives

Cyanoacrylate tissue adhesives (Dermabond) are now available for use in the United States. Cyanoacrylate adhesives polymerize rapidly when applied to tissues and form an adhesive layer on top of intact epithelium to hold the wound edges together. These adhesives cause an intense inflammatory reaction and should be used only on minor superficial lacerations. They should not be used near the eye, on mucous membranes or mucosal surfaces, on moist areas, or on areas with dense hair. Tissue adhesives should not be used for infected wounds.

Tissue adhesives are useful for minor wounds, those less than 5 cm in length and with separated wound edges less than 0.5 cm; they are most beneficial for wounds that would close spontaneously. Wounds greater than 5 cm in length and 0.5 cm in separation have increased tensile forces that may lead to poor wound edge approximation and a poor cosmetic outcome. Subcutaneous sutures may be useful in decreasing wound edge tension and may lead to a far better cosmetic result.

Preparation of wounds for closure with tissue adhesives is the same as for sutures. Thoroughly cleanse the wound and control bleeding before applying tissue adhesive. Hold the wound edges together and slightly everted with tissue forceps. Apply the adhesive by lightly wiping the applicator tip in the direction of the long axis. Apply a few layers quickly and then hold the wound edges together for about 60 seconds to ensure adequate bonding. Once applied, tissue adhesives should not be covered with ointment or dressing. If any adhesive is applied to unwanted areas, it can be removed with petroleum jelly or acetone (nail polish remover). Many tissue adhesives are commercially available, with many different applicator sizes and applicator tips. Also available are accessories to assist with the entire procedure, from wound cleansing devices to tissue forceps of various sizes and shapes for any size or shape wound.

Among the benefits of tissue adhesives is better cosmetic appearance, if used appropriately. Even more beneficial is the decreased risk of wound infection. The manufacturer of Dermabond states that the incidence of wound infection with this product is 3.6% and the incidence of dehiscence requiring retreatment is 2.2%; neither finding was statistically different by comparison with wounds closed with sutures.

5. Choice of Closure Technique

The choice of an appropriate material for wound closure is based on biologic and mechanical properties of the material and the characteristics of the wound. Decisions about layers to be closed are based on several factors, the most important of which are stress, dead space, and skin approximation.

Fascia

In soft tissue wounds that do not involve the face, the strength of closure depends on the fascia. Because fascia heals slowly, the suture material should be capable of maintaining its strength for a long time. Synthetic nonabsorbable sutures are best for this purpose.

Muscle & Fat

Muscle and fat do not hold sutures well, and closure is performed primarily to obliterate dead space. Dead space results from traumatic tissue loss, debridement, or gaping of subcutaneous layers. Suturing of dead space invariably produces additional tissue trauma and necrosis and is contraindicated in the closure of contaminated wounds. When such suturing is performed, it should be accomplished with the fewest possible loosely placed sutures. Chromic gut or one of the synthetic absorbable sutures should be used for this purpose.

Skin

Skin closure may be accomplished by layers, full-thickness percutaneous sutures, skin tapes, or a combination of these methods. The type of skin closure method chosen depends on the forces tending to open the wound and how good a cosmetic result is desired. The width of the scar that will result from healing will be influenced by the local stresses of the surrounding tissues. The direction of maximum force of skin tension is usually parallel to the skin wrinkles. Wounds oriented in the same direction as local stresses are subjected to less tension during healing and consequently produce a less visible scar. Examples include transverse lacerations of the forehead and vertical lacerations of the upper lip. Wounds that cross lines of maximal skin stress will be subjected to increased tension during healing. These wounds frequently widen with time and have a tendency to form hypertrophic scars. Examples are transverse lacerations of the cheek and axial lacerations over the elbows.

The propensity of a scar to hypertrophy is also influenced by factors unrelated to its location or technique of closure. The tendency of children and adolescents to form hypertrophic scars is notorious and is probably influenced by elevated levels of growth hormone or other growth factors. Pregnant women have an increased incidence of hypertrophic scar formation that decreases with the resumption of normal menses after delivery; this tendency is often associated with a parallel increase in pigmentation coinciding with pregnancy. Some investigators have postulated that hypertrophic scars and pigmentation are under similar hormonal influences. An increased incidence of hypertrophic scar and keloid formation is also found in blacks and other dark-skinned races. These specific groups of patients will demonstrate an exaggerated scar formation response that can be controlled only by manipulation of the wound in ways beyond the technical aspects of closure. Not all patients in these groups will form hypertrophic scars, however, and it is impossible to predict which patients might, except perhaps in the case of patients who have a history of hypertrophic scar formation. In these patients, precise wound closure using fine suture materials and atraumatic technique may lessen the degree of hypertrophic scarring that might otherwise result. Other methods of wound control include prolonged splinting, pressure bandages, corticosteroid therapy, and radiation therapy. In the acute wound, however, primary consideration is given to the location and orientation of the wound and its method of closure.

A. HIGH-STRESS WOUNDS

Layered wound closure is used to support wounds subjected to high skin tensions. The dermis is approximated with interrupted sutures, usually absorbable synthetics (Figure 30–8A–C). These sutures should not involve the epidermis, because of the risk of epithelial cyst formation. The epidermal layers are then adjusted with fine nonabsorbable sutures or tapes (Figure 30–8D and E). This method of skin closure is commonly used for facial lacerations.

B. LOW-STRESS WOUNDS

Percutaneous sutures are used for most other sites. It is important to evert the wound edges and to effect precise epidermal approximation to achieve the best results (Figure 30–9). Monofilament synthetic nonabsorbable sutures are the materials of choice for this type of closure. The size of suture material is not as important as the tightness of closure and the length of time the suture is left in place. These sutures should be removed by the seventh day to avoid epithelialization of the suture tracts. If additional support of the closure is required, as in wounds subjected to increased tension, skin tapes can be applied.

6. Drainage of the Wound

Drains constitute foreign bodies, produce tissue necrosis, serve as conduits for bacterial contamination of the wound, and are not very effective in preventing hematoma formation. If sound principles of management have been carefully followed, drains are usually unnecessary in the acute wound. If oozing cannot be controlled, it is preferable to delay wound closure. Drains, however, may be effective in evacuating pus and necrotic exudates that might be found in heavily contaminated or already infected wounds.

POSTOPERATIVE WOUND CARE & DRESSINGS

Postoperative wound care should provide an ideal environment for wound healing. This is accomplished primarily through the use of dressings. A dressing serves one or more of 7 different functions: protection, immobilization, control of edema (compression), absorption, debridement, delivery of topical medications (antibiotics), and cosmetic appearance.

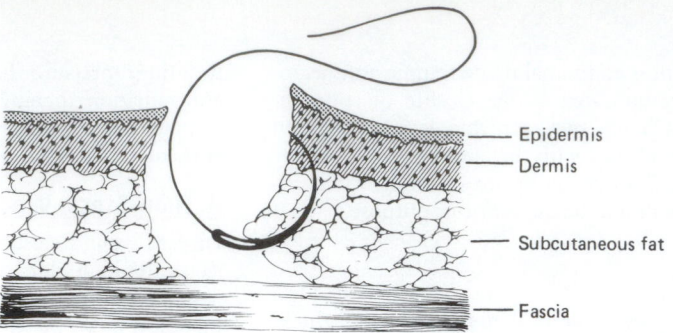

Epidermis

Dermis

Subcutaneous fat

Fascia

A. The strength of the closure lies in the dermis. Occasionally the subcutaneous fat is incorporated to obliterate dead space.

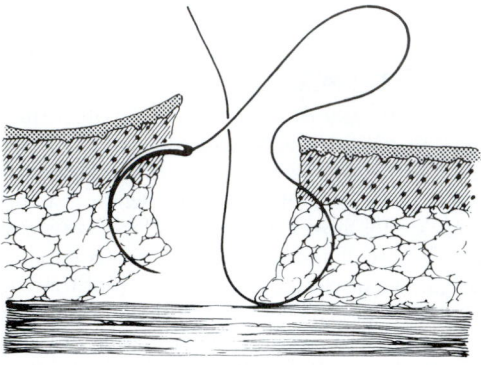

B. The suture is placed so that the knot will lie in the deepest part of the wound. Take care to avoid incorporating the epidermis with this suture, since epithelial cysts will form and result in suture extrusion.

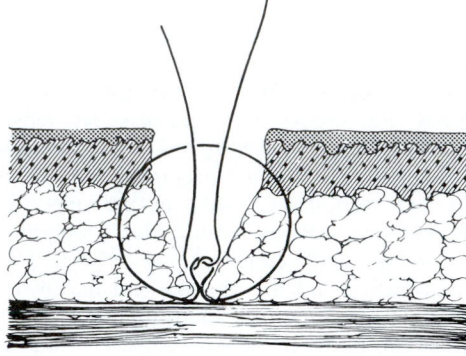

C. The dermal suture is tied just tightly enough to approximate the wound margins. Synthetic absorbable sutures are most commonly used for closure of the dermis.

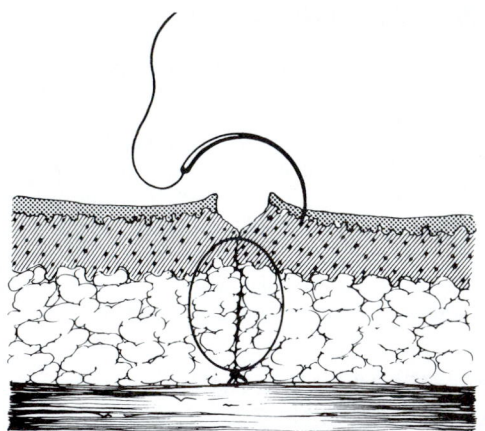

D. After the dermis is approximated, a fine "epidermal" suture is placed to align the wound edges. This suture adds little to the tensile strength of the wound closure.

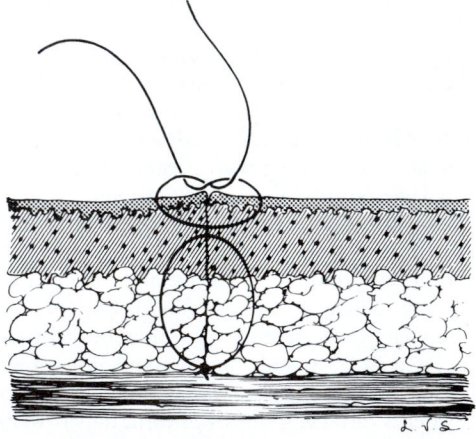

E. The epidermal suture is tied just tightly enough to approximate the epidermal edges of the wound. Since the strength of this closure lies in the dermis, the epidermal suture can be removed after 2–3 days. Skin tapes are often used to support the wound for an additional 7–10 days.

Figure 30–8. Layered cutaneous closure.

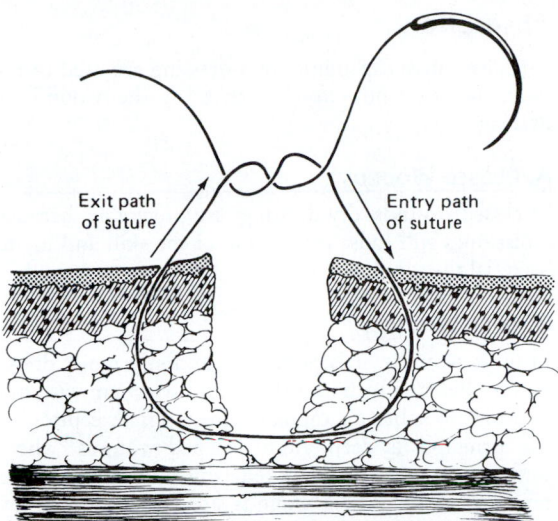

Exit path
of suture

Entry path
of suture

Figure 30–9. Percutaneous suture. Ideal placement of the suture everts the wound margins. This is accomplished by directing the needle away from the wound margin at the entrance point and toward the wound margin at the exit point. The path of a properly placed percutaneous suture will be wider at its base than at the skin entry and exit points.

Protection

Wounds closed by percutaneous sutures are susceptible to surface bacterial invasion for the first 48 hours after closure. During this time, the wound should be protected with sterile dressings or frequent suture line care.

A. DRESSINGS

If dressings are used, nonadherent materials (eg, Telfa, petrolatum-impregnated gauze) are favored because removal is easy and does not disturb sutures or coated wound edges.

Petrolatum-impregnated dressings have been shown to decrease the rate of epithelialization in partial-thickness wounds. For this reason, ointment-impregnated dressings (eg, bacitracin, combined neomycin sulfate and polymyxin B sulfate [Neosporin]) or nonadherent occlusive dressings (Op-Site) are preferred for this particular type of wound.

Occlusive or semiocclusive polyurethane, methacrylate, silicone polymer, or gel dressings provide excellent protection, and most do not alter the rate of normal epithelialization. If the wound contains residual necrotic debris or significant levels of bacterial contamination, however, the risk of wound infection is increased with these dressings.

B. UNDRESSED WOUNDS

Suture line care without a dressing is commonly used for facial wounds and involves frequent meticulous cleansing with saline or dilute hydrogen peroxide solution. Cleansing removes the adherent coagulum from the suture-skin juncture, decreasing the likelihood of stitch abscess formation. After cleansing, the wound is dressed with an antibiotic cream or ointment (eg, bacitracin-neomycin).

C. TAPE DRESSINGS

Taped wounds are quite resistant to surface bacterial contamination. They usually require no protection other than that provided by the tape itself. These wounds should be checked frequently for wound drainage beneath the tape. Excessive drainage can cause maceration of the wound edge and thereby provide an excellent medium for bacterial proliferation.

Immobilization

Immobilization of the wound enhances resistance to infection and may accelerate healing.

A. MATERIALS

Immobilization is accomplished with splints, bulky dressings, skin tapes, or combinations of these methods.

B. DURATION OF IMMOBILIZATION

Ideally, immobilization of the wound should be continued until it is no longer vulnerable to infection and has gained sufficient strength to withstand the stresses of motion and skin tension. Wounds become resistant to infection within a week, but development of maximal strength requires about 6 weeks. Protracted immobilization will defeat its possible advantages, for example, possibly producing permanent joint contractures in elderly persons. The advantages of wound immobilization must be weighed against the undesirable consequences. Extended immobilization is advisable for wounds of the face or whenever a good cosmetic result is desired. Areas such as the jaw line, chin, shoulder, and knee are subjected to more severe tissue stresses than are other areas and frequently require support for up to 3 months to achieve the best result. Extended wound support is also necessary in patients with neoplasms or immunodeficiency.

Control of Edema

Edema slows down the repair mechanisms and increases fibrous tissue proliferation. The wound with minimal edema will proceed to earlier complete healing and return of function. Peak wound edema occurs by 48 hours and gradually resolves over the next 4–6 days.

Persistent tissue edema after 7 days suggests inflammation or infection. In most cases, a compression dressing is beneficial during the first week of wound healing. In wounds that are prone to hypertrophic scarring, edema persists locally for up to 2 years. In these wounds, continued pressure may be beneficial in controlling the extent of hypertrophic scarring. Custom-made elastic pressure garments are excellent adjuncts in this regard; otherwise, simple elastic bandages are equally effective.

A. Elevation

Elevation of the wound above the level of the heart is the simplest way to limit the amount of excess tissue fluid in the wound. In the ambulatory patient, the common triangular bandage sling or "yoke" sling serves these purposes well. Slings, like any other dressing, are only as good as patient compliance; instruction in their use is important if the goal is to be achieved.

B. Pressure Dressing

In certain situations, it is advantageous to apply pressure over the wound along with elevation by using bulky pressure dressings.

Caution: Compression dressings should not be used in crush injuries or in injuries that tend to develop into compartment syndromes (eg, severe injuries of the forearm or leg). Continued pain or diminished sensitivity necessitates removal of the dressing and careful examination of the wound. Although these dressings are often used to absorb bloody oozing at the operative site, they should not be used as a substitute for diligent hemostasis.

Avoid constriction of proximal parts with these dressings, because venous and lymphatic congestion will occur as result of the tourniquet effect.

Bony prominences must be carefully padded, with generous use of bulk. To ensure uniform compression throughout and to avoid constriction and pressure-point injury, smooth, even wrapping that avoids lumps is necessary when compression dressing is applied.

In managing hand wounds, it is important to place 1 or 2 layers of gauze between the fingers to prevent maceration by sweat. The toes and fingertips should be exposed so that the physician can assess sensibility and capillary refill.

Rolled gauze or bias-cut stockinet is preferred over elastic bandages, which are often too constricting. The finished dressing should be firm but not strangulating.

In extremity injuries, compression dressing should extend proximally from the most distal point. For example, a wound of the forearm requiring a compression dressing is managed by applying the dressing starting from the fingers to above the wound.

Absorption

The absorptive capabilities of a dressing are used to remove bloody and serous ooze from the wound or drainage site.

A. Closed Wounds

In closed wounds, dry dressings are preferable, because moist ones will cause maceration of the skin and invite bacterial invasion.

B. Open Wounds

In open wounds, it is preferable to apply moist dressings to the open wound surface and back them with dry dressings to achieve a capillary effect. The exception to this principle is deep, tunnel-shaped wounds, where surface evaporation is limited, thus diminishing the capillary effect. These wounds are best managed by packing with dry gauze to achieve maximum absorption.

C. Materials

In all instances, absorptive dressings should be composed of fine-mesh gauze or spun fabric.

Caution: Cotton meshes and synthetic equivalents become incorporated into the wound as foreign bodies that incite tissue inflammation and cause subsequent bacterial proliferation.

Dextran polymers (eg, Debrisan wound-cleaning beads) have remarkable hygroscopic properties and serve well as absorbent dressings. They are quite effective in removing bacterial toxins and serous effluents from the wound surface. Wound healing is not significantly altered by their use.

Debridement

Dressings are frequently used for mechanical debridement of the open wound. The traditional wet-to-dry method utilizes avulsion of adherent tissues to remove devitalized remnants from the wound surface. Unfortunately, this method does not discriminate between viable and nonviable elements and reinjures the wound with each dressing change. Although painful and detrimental to wound healing, this method is effective in removing fine tenacious material from the wound surface. It should be discontinued as soon as the desired effect has been achieved.

The technique is as follows: Several layers of moist gauze are applied to the wound surface and allowed to dry. After about 4 hours, the adherent dressing is removed. Moistening the dry dressing before removal to loosen the dressing and lessen the pain of removal (as may be done by a sympathetic hospital attendant) defeats the purpose.

Delivery of Topical Antibiotics

The most common medicaments used in a dressing are antibacterials. Topical antibacterials are used to control bacteria that cannot be reached by systemic agents. They are *not* a substitute for adequate debridement.

A. AGENTS

Mafenide (Sulfamylon) and silver sulfadiazine (Silvadene) are most effective in this regard. These agents are also useful in partial-thickness injuries or marginally viable tissues (eg, abrasions, burns, crush injuries). By decreasing the potential for bacterial invasion, they diminish the likelihood of infection and the resulting tissue necrosis.

B. ADVERSE REACTIONS

Use of these agents must be monitored closely, because excessive amounts may cause acid-base imbalances (mafenide) or leukopenia (silver sulfadiazine). Both agents retard wound epithelialization and should be discontinued when the necrotic debris has been removed and wound bacterial counts are fewer than 10^5 organisms per gram of tissue.

Cosmetic Appearance

To the patient or casual observer, the sight of a wound is abhorrent and may be an occasion for adverse response. A dressing hides the wound and allows the patient to proceed with the process of rehabilitation without that distraction. In addition, a carefully applied, neat-appearing dressing reassures the patient that good wound care has been provided.

1. Potential Infections & Antimicrobials

Antimicrobials may be effective in preventing wound infection, particularly when the wound has fewer than 10^6 organisms per gram of tissue before treatment is started. Wounds with more than 10^6 organisms per gram of tissue often become infected despite antibiotic prophylaxis and should be left open. Systemic antibiotics, to be effective, must be started as soon as possible following injury, preferably within 4 hours. Topical antibiotics are commonly used to suppress bacterial growth, although their efficacy at preventing subsequent infection is probably low.

The likelihood of wound infection must be judged by the mechanism of injury, the level of contamination, the adequacy of debridement, and the patient's general status.

Small inocula will result in infection if necrotic debris, foreign bodies, or altered tissue defense mechanisms (as occur in crush or contused wounds) are present. If adequate wound management must be delayed for any reason, then consider systemic antimicrobial prophylaxis.

Sharp lacerations are markedly resistant to infection and in most instances will not require chemoprophylaxis. Open wounds, by virtue of their inflammatory response and resistance to bacterial dissemination, rarely become infected unless the initial level of contamination is great and cannot be reduced by cleansing and debridement. Furthermore, the fibrinous coagulum in these wounds limits the possible effectiveness of systemic antimicrobials on bacterial contaminants, thus making their use impractical.

Deep wounds or those that involve poorly vascularized structures such as bone, tendon, ligament, or fascia should be treated with systemic antibiotics prophylactically.

Oral mucosal lacerations rarely require systemic antibiotic prophylaxis, because the infection rate is low and randomized trials have not demonstrated a benefit from such treatment.

Grossly contaminated wounds such as those that come in contact with feces, pus, or saliva should not be closed. Systemic antimicrobial therapy is mandatory. The choice of drug is based on the suspected predominant pathogen (Table 30–2).

2. Tetanus Prophylaxis

Tetanus prophylaxis is virtually 100% effective if used properly. Overuse of tetanus toxoid may induce serious allergic reactions.

Investigate Previous Active Immunization

A history of standard primary immunization with tetanus toxoid (or diphtheria-tetanus-pertussis vaccination) followed by boosters every 10 years virtually guarantees immunity from tetanus. In the United States, nearly all individuals over age 2 years have had primary immunization (3 doses at 4–week intervals followed by one booster), and this too nearly guarantees immunity. Even individuals with only 2 previous tetanus toxoid immunizations will develop antibody rapidly enough following a tetanus toxoid booster so that passive immunization will be unnecessary in most cases. Patients

Table 30–2. Choice of antimicrobials for prevention of infection in specific types of wounds.[1]

Type of Wound	Antimicrobial of Choice	Alternative
Human bite	Amoxicillin/Clavulanate 875/125 mg BID	Cefuroxime 250–500 mg BID
Animal bites	Amoxicillin/Clavulanate 875/125 mg BID	Clindamycin 150–450 mg QID plus Ciprofloxacin 500 mg BID
Other wounds	Amoxicillin/Clavulanate 875/125 mg BID	Clindamycin 150–450 mg QID or Cephalexin 500 mg QID

[1]These recommendations apply only to wounds *without* evidence of infection at the time of examination and should be given for 3–5 days.

over age 50 years, foreign-born patients, or patients unable to provide a history of tetanus immunization must be assumed to have incomplete immunization and should be given tetanus prophylaxis (Table 30–3).

Determine Risk of Tetanus

The risk of tetanus is greater with wounds that are heavily contaminated by soil or feces, those involving crush injury of surrounding tissue, and those coming to medical attention after a delay of more than 24 hours.

Table 30–3. Guide to tetanus prophylaxis in wound management.[1]

History of Tetanus Immunization (Doses)	Clean Minor Wounds		All Other Wounds	
	Td[2]	TIG[2]	Td[2]	TIG[2]
Uncertain	Yes	No	Yes	Yes
0–1	Yes	No	Yes	Yes
2	Yes	No	Yes	No[3]
3 or more	No[4]	No	No[4]	No

[1]Adapted from *MMWR* 1991;40:1.
[2]Td = tetanus and diphtheria toxoids, adult type, for persons over 7 years of age. DTP for children under 7 years of age. TIG = tetanus immune globulin.
[3]Unless wound is more than 24 hours old.
[4]Unless it has been more than 10 years since last dose.

Select Active or Passive Immunizations

Table 30–3 shows the U.S. Public Health Service recommended tetanus immunization schedules. Td (tetanus toxoid combined with adult-dose diphtheria toxoid) is preferable to tetanus toxoid alone. If passive immunization is required, human tetanus immune globulin is preferred over horse serum. The recommended dose is 250 units intramuscularly. If equine tetanus antitoxin must be used, inquire about and test for horse serum allergy before administering. The usual dose is 3000–5000 units. If both Td and tetanus immune globulin or antitoxin are given, they should be administered in separate sites using separate syringes.

3. Rabies Prophylaxis

Assess Risk of Rabies Exposure

See Figure 30–10.

A. Species of Biting Animal

Carnivorous animals (especially skunks, foxes, badgers, bobcats, coyotes, raccoons, dogs, and cats) and bats are more likely to be infected. Rabbits, squirrels, hamsters, guinea pigs, gerbils, chipmunks, rats, mice, and other rodents rarely transmit rabies in the United States.

B. Determine if Animal Is Rabid (if Possible)

(*Note:* Behavior is *not* a reliable sign of the rabid state.) If examination of the animal's brain for rabies is negative, it can be assumed that the animal's saliva did not contain rabies virus.

Healthy domestic dogs and cats should be observed for 10 days by a veterinarian. If signs of rabies develop, the animal should be killed and its brain examined for rabies virus at the local public health laboratory.

Stray or unwanted dogs and cats that cause bites should be killed immediately and examined for rabies. Wild animals that cause bites should be killed immediately and the brain examined for rabies.

C. Circumstances of Biting Incident

Unprovoked attacks are more likely to mean that the animal is rabid. Bites from apparently healthy animals that are fighting or feeding or that have been picked up or petted should be considered *provoked* and so have a low likelihood of causing rabies.

D. Types of Exposure

Any penetration of skin by teeth is regarded as a bite. Nonbite exposure consists of contamination of scratches, abrasions, mucous membranes, or previous wounds with infected animal saliva.

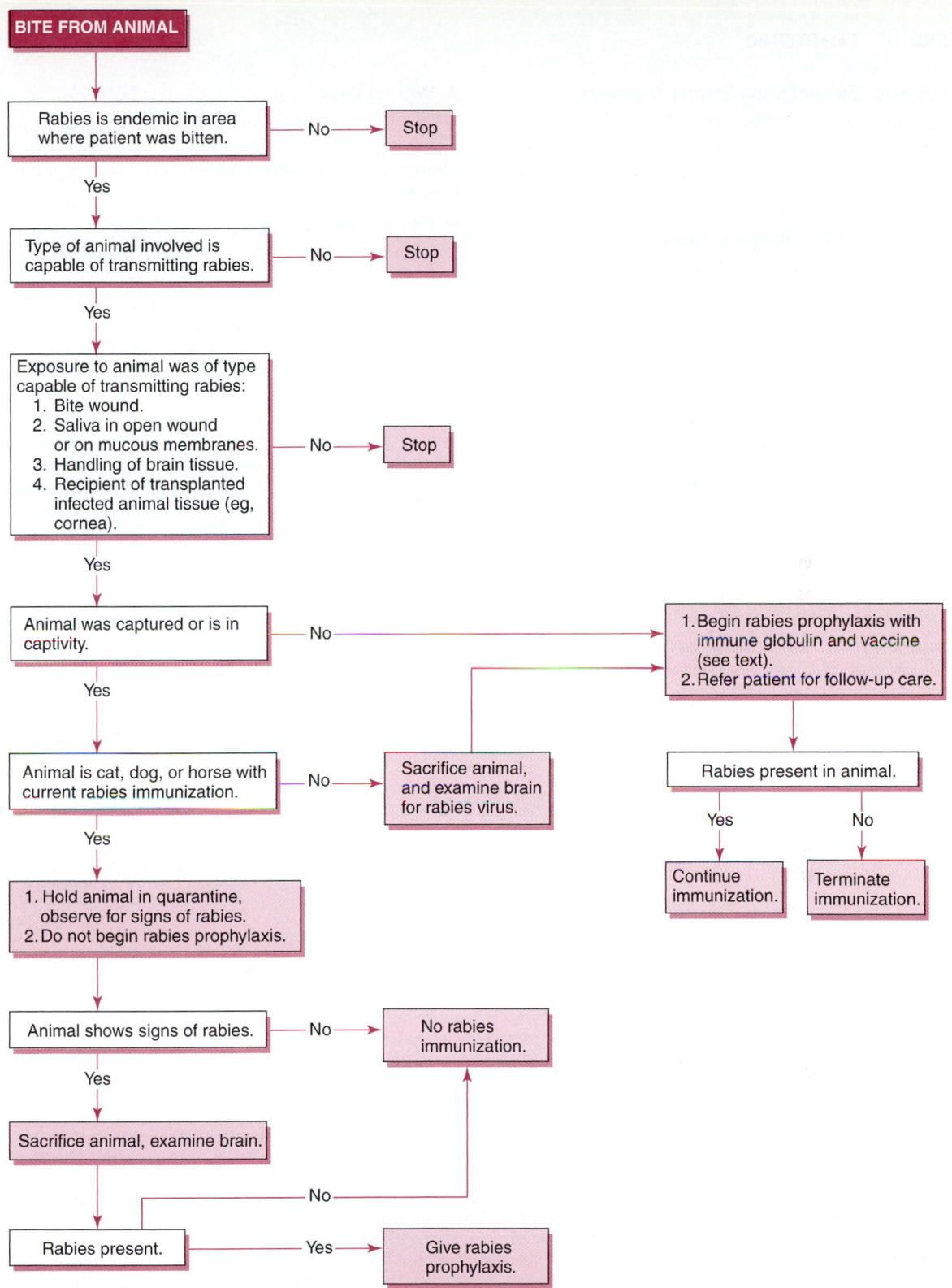

Figure 30–10. Algorithm for management of possible rabies exposure.

E. RABIES IMMUNIZATION STATUS OF ANIMAL

Vaccines are effective for cats and dogs but are *not* effective in preventing rabies in other animals, especially wild animals that have been domesticated (eg, pet skunks, foxes).

F. PREVALENCE OF RABIES IN REGION

Certain areas are devoid of rabies (eg, San Francisco, Great Britain). Some rural areas are considered at high risk for rabies (eg, Texas-Mexico border).

Management of Patients at High Risk

Provide tetanus prophylaxis (see above), and give antibiotics if indicated (see above). *Quickly* administer appropriate postexposure rabies prophylaxis (see Figure 30–10 and Tables 30–4 and 30–5).

Act quickly! The sooner antirabies measures are instituted, the more effective they are.

A. WOUND CARE

(This is the most important step.) Wash the wound copiously with 20% green soap tincture and water. *Note:* Quaternary ammonium compounds and alcohol are no longer recommended.

B. PASSIVE IMMUNIZATION

1. Rabies immune globulin USP—This neutralizing antibody should be given to all patients except those previously immunized who have documented antibody titers or those who have received preexposure human diploid cell rabies vaccine prophylaxis or a full course of human diploid cell rabies vaccine. Give 20 IU/kg at the onset of rabies therapy; rabies immune globulin can be given as late as the eighth day if necessary. Recommendations from the CDC in 1999 indicate that, if anatomically feasible, the full dose of rabies immune globulin should be thoroughly infiltrated in and around the wound; any remaining rabies immune globulin should be injected intramuscularly at a site distant from

Table 30–4. Rabies postexposure prophylaxis guide.[1]

The following recommendations are only a guide. In applying them, take into account the species involved, the circumstances of the bite or other exposure, the vaccination status of the animal, and the presence of rabies in the region. Local or state public health officials should be consulted if questions arise about the need for rabies prophylaxis.

Animal Species	Condition of Animal at Time of Attack	Treatment of Exposed Person[2]
Domestic Dog and cat	Healthy and available for 10 days of observation.	None, unless animal develops rabies.[3]
	Rabid or suspected rabid.	RIG[4] and HDCV.[5]
	Unknown (escaped).	Consult public health officials. If treatment is indicated, give RIG[4] and HDCV.[5]
Wild Skunk, bat, fox, coyote, raccoon, bobcat, and other carnivores	Regard as rabid unless proved negative by laboratory tests.[6]	RIG[4] and HDCV.[5]
Other Livestock, rodents, and lagomorphs (rabbits and hares)	Consider individually. Local and state public health officials should be consulted on questions about the need for rabies prophylaxis. Bites of squirrels, hamsters, guinea pigs, gerbils, chipmunks, rats, mice, other rodents, rabbits, and hares almost never call for antirabies prophylaxis.	

[1]Adapted from *MMWR* 1999;48:1.

[2]All bites and wounds should immediately be thoroughly cleansed with soap and water. If antirabies treatment is indicated, both rabies immune globulin (RIG) and human diploid cell rabies vaccine (HDCV) should be given as soon as possible, regardless of the interval from exposure.

[3]During the usual holding period of 10 days, begin treatment with RIG and vaccine (preferably with HDCV) at first sign of rabies in a dog or cat that has bitten someone. The symptomatic animal should be killed immediately and tested.

[4]If RIG is not available, use antirabies serum, equine (ARS). Do not use more than the recommended dosage.

[5]If HDCV is not available, use duck embryo vaccine (DEV) or other rabies vaccine. Local reactions to vaccines are common and do not contraindicate continuing treatment. Discontinue vaccine if fluorescent antibody tests of the animal are negative.

[6]The animal should be killed and tested as soon as possible. Holding for observation is not recommended.

Table 30–5. Rabies immunization regimens.[1]

Preexposure				
Preexposure rabies prophylaxis for persons with special risks of exposure to rabies, such as animal care and control personnel and selected laboratory workers, consists of immunization with either human diploid cell rabies vaccine (HDCV) or duck embryo vaccine (DEV), according to the following schedule, followed by a booster dose every 2 years.				
Rabies Vaccine	**Number of 1-mL Doses**	**Route of Administration**	**Intervals Between Doses**	**If No Antibody Response to Primary Series, Give:[2]**
HDCV	3	Intramuscular	1 week between first and second: 2–3 weeks between second and third.[3]	1 booster dose.[3]
Postexposure				
Postexposure rabies prophylaxis for persons exposed to rabies consists of the immediate, thorough cleansing of all wounds with soap and water, administration of rabies immune globulin (RIG) or, if RIG is not available, antirabies serum, equine (ARS), and the initiation of either HDCV or DEV, according to the following schedule.				
Rabies Vaccine	**Number of 1-mL Doses**	**Route of Administration**	**Intervals Between Doses**	**If No Antibody Response to Primary Series, Give:[2]**
HDCV	5[4]	Intramuscular	Doses to be given on days 0, 3, 7, 14, and 28.	An additional booster dose.[5]

[1]Adapted from *MMWR* 1999;48:1.
[2]If no antibody response is documented after the recommended additional booster dose(s), consult the state health department or CDC.
[3]Serum for rabies antibody testing should be collected 2–3 weeks after the last dose only in immunocompromised patients.
[4]The World Health Organization recommends a sixth dose 90 days after the first dose.
[5]An additional booster dose should be given only to immunocompromised patients.

vaccine administration. Because rabies immune globulin may partially suppress the antibody response to vaccine, no more than the recommended dose should be given.

2. Equine rabies immune globulin—This preparation should be used only when the human (USP) product is not available. Check for allergy to horse serum. The product contains 1000 IU/vial (about 5 mL). The dose is 40 IU/kg.

C. ACTIVE IMMUNIZATION

Human diploid cell rabies vaccine is an inactivated virus vaccine prepared from rabies virus grown on human diploid fibroblasts. Give five 1-mL doses intramuscularly on specified days. The first dose is given as soon as possible after the bite; subsequent doses are given on days 3, 7, 14, and 28. No booster dose is needed.

If preexposure human diploid cell rabies vaccine prophylaxis and adequate booster doses have been given (because of occupation as a veterinarian, for example), only two 1-mL intramuscular doses of human diploid cell rabies vaccine are needed, one as soon as possible after the bite and the other 3 days later.

Routine serologic testing after treatment with human diploid cell rabies vaccine is not necessary unless the patient is immunocompromised or is taking corticosteroids. Individuals taking steroids should discontinue the medication while receiving antirabies treatment.

4. Follow-up Care of the Wound

After initial wound management, provisions must be made for follow-up and local wound care. Instruct the patient in how to recognize signs and symptoms of wound complications. A specific appointment for return should be made before discharge from the emergency department. It is helpful to supply patients with a printed list of danger signals and directions on wound care.

Simple instructions giving specific details about wound care are useful in these situations. Patients want to know about limitations on activity, when they can bathe or shower, the type and frequency of dressing changes, when sutures will be removed, and precautions after suture removal.

The changes that occur in a wound during the course of normal wound healing may cause anxiety, particularly if the wound is on the face and other exposed areas. The patient should be told that thickening of the area surrounding a scar usually abates by 3 months. Redness of the scar usually persists for 3–6 months. The scar may assume various shades of blue depending on the environmental conditions. If the patient is prone to develop hypertrophic scars or keloids, it is wise to mention this possibility (particularly in children, adolescents, individuals of more heavily pigmented races, and pregnant women and in wounds of the shoulders, anterior chest, elbows, and knees).

The fate of any wound as forming a "good" or "bad" scar is unpredictable. It is best to advise the patient that the ultimate appearance of the scar will not be known for at least 9 months. Evaluation for possible scar revision should be delayed until after that time.

5. Suture Removal

The timing of suture removal depends on many factors such as location; type of wound closure; presence of infection; and the patient's age, health, and compliance. Table 30–6 is a general guideline for suture removal in healthy adults with uncomplicated wounds. Modifications of these recommendations should be tailored to individual patterns.

Abenavoli FM: Using Dermabond. Plast Reconstr Surg 2001; 108:269. [PMID: 11420548]

Bruns TB et al: Using tissue adhesive for wound repair: a practical guide to Dermabond. Am Fam Physician 2000;61:1383. [PMID: 10735344]

Diphtheria, tetanus, and pertussis: recommendations for vaccine use and other preventive measures. Recommendations of the Immunization Practices Advisory Committee (ACIP). MMWR Recomm Rep 1991;40(RR-10):1. [PMID: 1865873]

Hollander JE: Laceration management. Ann Emerg Med 1999; 34:356. [PMID: 10459093]

Hsu SS et al. Tetanus in the emergency department: a current review. J Emerg Med 2001;20:357. [PMID: 113488]

Human rabies prevention—United States, 1999. Recommendations of the Advisory Committee on Immunization Practices (ACIP). MMWR Recomm Rep 1999;48(RR-1):1. [PMID: 10077411]

Table 30–6. Timing of suture removal.

Location	Time (Days)
Eyelid	3
Cheek	3–5
Nose, forehead, neck	5
Ear, scalp	5–7
Arm, leg, hand, foot	7–10+
Chest, back, abdomen	7–10+

Leach J: Proper handling of soft tissue in the acute phase. Facial Plast Surg 2001;17:227. [PMID: 11735055]

Thompson WL et al: Peripheral nerve blocks and anesthesia of the hand. Mil Med 2002;167:478. [PMID: 12099083]

Singer AJ et al: Closure of lacerations and incisions with octylcyanoacrylate: a multicenter randomized controlled trial. Surgery 2002;131:270. [PMID:1189403]

■ EMERGENCY TREATMENT OF SPECIFIC TYPES OF WOUNDS

FACIAL LACERATIONS (See Chapter 23.)

INTRAORAL LACERATIONS

Lacerations of the oral mucosa and tongue may not require closure if they are small. The rich blood supply promotes rapid healing, and cosmetic considerations are minimal. However, large or gaping wounds, through-and-through lacerations, and lacerations involving important deep structures, such as muscle or bone, require repair. In such wounds, after irrigation with saline, disrupted muscle should first be approximated with absorbable suture (eg, 5-0 Vicryl) and the mucosa closed with absorbable suture (eg, 5-0 chromic gut or Vicryl). It is best to use the minimum number of sutures that will allow approximation of the wound edges.

Through-and-through lacerations of the lip merit special attention:

1. Irrigate the wound thoroughly, inside and out. A dry gauze roll between the lip and teeth will help prevent recontamination of the irrigated wound.
2. Close the mucosal laceration with absorbable suture (eg, 5-0 chromic gut or Vicryl).
3. Irrigate the wound again from the outside. The sutured mucosa will prevent reentry of saliva.
4. If the orbicularis oris muscle is disrupted, approximate it with absorbable suture (eg, 5-0 Vicryl).
5. Close the external skin with interrupted sutures of 6-0 monofilament nylon. Take extreme care to line up the opposing vermilion borders of the lip.
6. Examine the adjacent teeth that produced the wound; they may be fractured or avulsed.

BLAST INJURIES

Clinical Findings

Wounds resulting from high-velocity missiles and shotgun blasts are among the most severe wounds encountered in civilian practice. Extensive tissue destruction is incurred locally, with loss or disruption of the wound parts to form a cavity. Sites distant from the point of impact may be injured as a result of shock waves transmitted through tissues. The extent of injury of these complex wounds is difficult to assess.

Treatment

Initial care is directed at hemostasis, cleansing, and minimal debridement. It is wise not to close the wound primarily.

Repeated staged exploration at first presentation and then again 24 hours and 48 hours apart is used to remove necrotic or devitalized tissues.

Antibiotic prophylaxis is recommended. Cefazolin, 1 g intravenously every 8 hours, is satisfactory.

The wound is then closed secondarily, with priority given to reestablishment of bony relationships, followed by soft tissue coverage.

Disposition

Hospitalize all patients for management.

HIGH-PRESSURE INJECTION INJURIES

General Considerations

High-pressure injection equipment is used in industry to force liquids such as paint, paint thinner, oil, or grease through a small nozzle under high pressure, sometimes at pressure exceeding several thousand psi. If the nozzle is held against or close to the skin, it is possible for the liquid stream to be injected through the skin and into the subcutaneous tissues.

Clinical Findings

These injuries have the potential for severe sequelae usually resulting from direct trauma and intense inflammation incited by the injected liquid. The edema that develops from the resulting inflammation can lead to increased tissue compartment pressures and may lead to compartment syndrome. The type of injected material and amount and pressure velocity will determine the degree of inflammation and severity of injury.

Patients with these types of injuries usually have small puncture wounds that are usually isolated to the extremities. Patients often present with pain out of proportion to the appearance of the wound and, if early, often with only minimal swelling. Because the material is injected at great force, the distance it can be injected into the tissues from injection site can be significant.

Treatment & Disposition

Carefully assess neurovascular function at the time of presentation and attempt appropriate pain control via parenteral analgesics. Avoid digital blocks because of the resulting increase in pressure. Parenteral antibiotics should also be initiated at first presentation, directed at normal skin flora (*Staphylococcus* and *Streptococcus*). Appropriate radiographs should be obtained because some materials are radiopaque and may demonstrate the extent of subcutaneous spread and may also show the presence of subcutaneous emphysema. Early consultation with a hand specialist or other surgical specialist for early surgical debridement and follow-up is recommended.

DEGLOVING INJURIES

Clinical Findings

Separation of the skin and subcutaneous tissues from the underlying musculofascial planes constitutes a degloving injury. For flaps attached by a pedicle, the determinant of survival is their circulation.

Treatment & Disposition

All but trivial degloving injuries require hospitalization. Plastic surgical consultation is advisable.

AMPUTATIONS

Clinical Findings

The greater the degree of ischemic injury resulting from interruption of blood flow, the less the chances for survival of the amputated part. Six hours is probably the longest time an amputated part can be deprived of its blood supply without cooling and still survive. Immediate cooling increases the tolerable ischemic time of the amputated part to 12–24 hours. This is particularly important when replantation must be delayed while the patient is transferred to a hospital where a surgical team skilled in replantation is available.

Contraindications to replantation are the presence of significant associated injuries that may be life threatening, severe degloving or crush injuries of the amputated part, and major systemic disease.

Treatment

To ensure the most expeditious management, every emergency department should know the location of the nearest microvascular replantation center before arranging for patient transfer. Initial treatment is outlined here:

1. Gently cleanse the amputated part of gross contaminants; dry it; and place it in a clean, dry poly-

ethylene bag. Place the bag in regular (wet) ice or in a refrigerator at 4 °C (about 40 °F).

2. Control hemorrhage by pressure or elevation, or by tourniquet if the other methods are not successful. Gently cleanse the wound and cover it with a sterile dressing.

3. Consider antimicrobial and tetanus prophylaxis in most instances. A parenteral cephalosporin is commonly used for these purposes (eg, cefazolin, 1 g intravenously).

4. Reestablish normal blood volume. Blood transfusion may be necessary, because these injuries are occasionally associated with major blood loss.

Disposition

Immediately refer the patient to a facility where limb replantation can be done by experts in that procedure.

BITES

Most nonprimate mammalian bite wounds are minor, and only about 10% require suturing. The rare patient with major injuries sustained in an animal attack should be evaluated and receive treatment as any other patient with severe trauma.

Meticulous wound care is the cornerstone of therapy for bite wounds and is the most important factor in preventing infection. The wound should be cleansed, debrided, and copiously irrigated. Treat all bite wounds on the extremities aggressively, with antibiotics and elevation and immobilization of the affected part.

Routine cultures in the absence of infection need not be obtained, because there is no useful correlation between positive cultures and wounds that later develop clinical signs of infection.

Antimicrobial prophylaxis (see Table 30–2) is recommended for all human and most cat bites but only for high-risk dog bites (below). The need for tetanus and rabies prophylaxis (Tables 30–3 and 30–4) should also be evaluated.

1. Dog Bites

Dog bites cause open wounds, often with tissue necrosis secondary to crush injury. Treat by prompt excisional debridement within 6 hours. If the extent of the wound or the length of time since injury precludes primary closure, the wounds should be irrigated, debrided, and left open or loosely sutured. Infection is unusual, and antimicrobial prophylaxis is not indicated in routine cases.

Dog bites associated with a high risk of infection are those of the hand, puncture wounds, and injuries more than 6–12 hours old. These wounds should be treated with vigorous local care and left unsutured. Antibiotic prophylaxis is recommended; amoxicillin/clavulante 875/125 mg BID is the treatment of choice. An alternative is clindamycin 150–450 mg QID plus ciprofloxacin 500 mg BID. A three to five-day course is recommended. Low-risk bites do not require prophylactic antibiotics and may be sutured after appropriate wound care. Hospitalization is rarely indicated unless injuries are multiple or extensive or infection is present.

Infected bites should be cleansed and debrided and the affected limb immobilized and elevated. A parenteral dose of a first-generation cephalosporin (eg, cefazolin, 1 g for adults, 8–17 mg/kg for children, intravenously) should be administered in the emergency department and the patient discharged with oral antibiotics (same as those for prophylaxis, above) for 7–10 days. Patients should receive follow-up care within 1–2 days and be instructed to return earlier if their condition worsens. Hospitalize patients who have symptoms of sepsis.

2. Cat Bites

Cat bites cause deep puncture wounds with little crush injury and are associated with a high risk of infection, mainly with *Pasteurella multocida*. Wounds caused by cat claws are considered equivalent to bites. Treatment includes local cleansing, debridement, and prophylactic antibiotics for all significant bites. Amoxicillin-clavulanate is the treatment of choice (Table 30–2).

Cat bite infections occurring within 24 hours are due to *P multocida* and should be treated as above. Wounds becoming infected after 24 hours should be treated with a first-generation cephalosporin or amoxicillin/clavulante (see Dog Bites, above) for 7–10 days.

Hospitalization is rarely indicated unless infection is severe or involves the hand. Primary closure should not be performed except in low-risk, cosmetically disfiguring facial bites.

3. Human Bites

General Considerations

Adult human bites are more serious than dog or cat bites. They are characterized by crush and tear injuries and are commonly located over the knuckles or the dorsum of the hand, frequently involving the tendons or joints. Inoculation of large numbers of bacteria from dental plaque also occurs. (Bites by children appear to carry a low risk of infection because of fewer mouth bacteria and less biting force.) Despite their rather innocuous initial appearance, these wounds are extremely dangerous, because they are prone to severe necrotizing infection.

Treatment & Disposition

Hospitalize patients with suspected tendon, joint, or cartilage involvement (eg, bites of the hand or ear) for vigorous irrigation, debridement, and parenteral antimicrobials (high-dose penicillin or clindamycin). Wounds of this type are never closed. Bites of other structures may be treated with vigorous irrigation and debridement in the emergency department, followed by antimicrobial prophylaxis (see Table 30–2). The injured part should be elevated, immobilized, and checked frequently to assess the possible spread of infection. The patient should be reexamined within 6–18 hours and subsequently at 1- to 2-day intervals for a week.

Signs of necrotizing infection are progressive erythema, blistering, and frank necrosis. If these signs are already present at the time of initial evaluation, hospitalization is indicated for wide debridement of the involved parts and parenteral antimicrobial therapy.

PUNCTURE WOUNDS

General Considerations

Puncture wounds are at risk of becoming infected, especially if dirty, contaminated, or containing foreign materials. Wounds associated with penetration through the soles of shoes (especially sneakers) often contain particles of debris and are particularly susceptible to infection. If joint capsule or bone is penetrated, septic arthritis and osteomyelitis can occur. *Pseudomonas* species are common pathogens.

All puncture wounds should be probed gently with forceps or a long (6.5-cm or 2.5-in), 22-gauge needle for the presence of foreign bodies; control pain as needed with 1% lidocaine anesthetic. Obtain soft-tissue x-rays of all wounds for which the history or mechanism of injury suggests retention of a foreign body (eg, broken glass, flying piece of metal), even if results of the wound probe are negative.

Treatment & Disposition

A. WOUND CLEANSING AND EXPLORATION

Irrigate the wound with normal saline under pressure and cleanse it with 1% povidone-iodine solution. Probe gently and remove foreign materials. Local infiltration with 1% lidocaine and slight enlargement of the wound may be necessary for adequate exploration. Extensive dissection in the emergency department to search for small or deeply embedded objects is not recommended.

B. TETANUS AND ANTIBIOTICS PROPHYLAXIS

Ensure that tetanus prophylaxis is up to date (see Table 30–3). Treat dirty or deep wounds (especially those with possible joint or bone involvement) with prophylactic antibiotics (Table 30–2). If penetration occurred through the sole of a sneaker (unless very superficial), consider prophylaxis against the high risk of *Pseudomonas* infection with antipseudomonal cephalosporin as a single parenteral dose (eg, ceftazidime, 1 g intramuscularly) or ciprofloxacin 500 mg BID for 3–5 days.

C. ELEVATION AND FOLLOW-UP

Instruct patients to elevate any involved extremity and, in foot injuries, to bear no weight for 3–5 days. Except in the case of superficial punctures, patients should be reexamined in 5–7 days or earlier if increased pain, redness, red streaking, or pus is noted.

D. OSTEOMYELITIS

Patients with pain persisting longer than 5–7 days or with an abnormal erythrocyte sedimentation rate may have osteomyelitis. In either case, obtain x-rays of the affected area and, if normal, consider limited bone scan of the area. Refer patients with osteomyelitis to the specialist appropriate to the area of involvement.

E. RETAINED FOREIGN BODIES

Retained foreign bodies in critical areas (eg, eye) require urgent specialty consultation. Refer patients with possible retained foreign bodies in noncritical areas for outpatient surgical removal in 2–3 weeks.

Armstrong BD: Lacerations of the mouth. Emerg Med Clin North Am 2000;18:471. [PMID: 10967735]

Baldwin G et al: Puncture wounds. Pediatr Rev 1999;20:21. [PMID: 9919048]

Bower MG: Evaluating and managing bite wounds. Adv Skin Wound Care 2002;15:88. [PMID: 11984053]

Chrisodoulou L et al: Functional outcome of high-pressure injection injuries of the hand. J Trauma 2001;50:717. [PMID: 1303170]

Goldstein EJ: Current concepts on animal bites: bacteriology and therapy. Curr Clin Top Infect Dis 1999;19:99. [PMID: 10472482]

Howes DS et al: Triage and initial evaluation of the oral facial emergency. Emerg Med Clin North Am 2000;18:371. [PMID: 10967730]

Lewis HG et al: A 10-year review of high-pressure injection injuries to the hand. J Hand Surg [Br] 1998;23:479. [PMID: 9726548]

Markal N et al: Compression neuropathy of the hand after high-pressure air injection. Ann Plast Surg 2000;44:680. [PMID: 10884095]

Mizani MR et al: High-pressure injection injury of the hand. The potential for disastrous results. Postgrad Med 2000;108:183. [PMID: 0914127]

Presutti RJ: Prevention and treatment of dog bites. Am Fam Physician 2001;63:1567. [PMID: 11327433]

Schnall SB et al: High-pressure injection injuries to the hand. Hand Clin 1999;15:245. [PMID: 10361635]

Soucacos PN: Indications and selection for digital amputation and replantation. J Hand Surg [Br] 2001;26:572. [PMID: 11884116]

Vasilevski D et al: High-pressure injection injuries to the hand. Am J Emerg Med 2000;18(7):820. [PMID: 11103737]

Wrightman JM et al: Explosions and blast injuries. Ann Emerg Med 2001;37:664. [PMID: 11385339]

SECTION IV
Nontrauma Emergencies

Eye Emergencies

31

William R. Dennis, Jr, MD, & Alia M. Dennis, MD[1]

I. Emergency Evaluation of Important Ocular Symptoms
Evaluation of the Red or Painful Eye
Evaluation of Acute Unilateral Visual Loss
II. Ocular Conditions Requiring Immediate Treatment
Acute Angle-Closure Glaucoma
Central Retinal Artery Occlusion
Orbital Cellulitis
Cavernous Sinus Thrombosis
Endophthalmitis
Retinal Detachment
Toxic Causes of Blindness
III. Nontraumatic Ocular Emergencies
Acute Dacryocystitis
Acute Dacryoadenitis
Acute Hordeolum (Sty)
Eyelid Infections (Preseptal Cellulitis)
Spontaneous Subconjunctival Hemorrhage
Conjunctivitis
Bacterial Corneal Ulcer
Viral Keratoconjunctivitis
Acute Hydrops of the Cornea
Hyphema
Uveitis (Iritis & Iridocyclitis)

Vitreous Hemorrhage
Retinal Hemorrhage
Central Retinal Vein Occlusion
Optic Neuritis
IV. Ocular Burns & Trauma
Ocular Burns
 Alkali Burns
 Acid Burns
 Thermal Burns
 Burns Due to Ultraviolet Radiation
Mechanical Trauma to the Eye
 Penetrating or Perforating Injuries
 Blunt Trauma to the Eye, Adnexa, & Orbit
  1. Ecchymosis of the Eyelids (Black Eye)
  2. Lacerations of the Eyelids
  3. Orbital Hemorrhage
  4. Fracture of the Ethmoid Bone
  5. Blowout Fractures of the Floor of the Orbit
  6. Corneal Abrasions
  7. Corneal & Conjunctival Foreign Bodies
V. Equipment & Supplies
VI. Common Techniques for Treatment of Ocular Disorders
VII. Common Pitfalls to Be Avoided in the Management of Ocular Disorders

---

[1]This chapter is a revision of the chapter by Kalid F. Tabbara, MD, from the 4th edition.

■ I. EMERGENCY EVALUATION OF IMPORTANT OCULAR SYMPTOMS

EVALUATION OF THE RED OR PAINFUL EYE
(See Figure 31–1 and Table 31–1.)
History & Examination

Historical factors are important in determining the cause of ocular complaints. History, when correlated with characteristic ocular findings, usually makes the diagnosis. A complete eye examination includes the following:

A. VISUAL ACUITY

Test corrected visual acuity using a standard acuity chart (Snellen). Abnormal acuity in a patient who normally has 20/20 vision usually indicates disease of the eyeball or visual pathway. Pain and decreased acuity indicate corneal disease, acute angle-closure glaucoma, or iritis.

B. INSPECTION

Inspect external lids, lashes, lacrimal ducts, orbit, and periorbital area for any signs of trauma, infection, exudate, and the like.

C. PUPILLARY FUNCTION

Check for symmetrical pupils and reactivity to light and accommodation.

D. EXTRAOCULAR MOTILITY

Check for integrity of extraocular muscles and note any abnormalities.

E. VISUAL FIELDS

Check for abnormalities in the visual fields.

F. SLIT LAMP EXAMINATION

Slit lamp examination should be done before and after fluorescein staining.

G. INTRAOCULAR PRESSURE

Intraocular pressure can be tested with a Tono-Pen or Schiotz tonometer (described later in this chapter).

H. FUNDUSCOPY

Funduscopy is used to check the retinal field.

I. OTHER STUDIES

Further diagnostic studies including laboratory specimens, plain x-rays, computed tomography (CT) scan, or magnetic resonance imaging of the orbits may be needed to establish the diagnosis.

Disposition

Patients thought to have ocular conditions that may permanently decrease visual acuity (eg, acute angle-closure glaucoma) should be hospitalized. Patients with other conditions may receive treatment and be discharged if close follow-up evaluation is ensured.

EVALUATION OF ACUTE UNILATERAL VISUAL LOSS
(See Figure 31–2.)
Look for Trauma

Exclude trauma as a cause of visual loss. Both blunt and penetrating ocular injuries may result in blindness.

History & Examination

Obtain a history from the patient (rate of onset of visual loss; whether it is unilateral or bilateral, painful or painless, with or without redness). Ophthalmologic examination should emphasize visual acuity and visual field testing.

A. INABILITY TO VISUALIZE RETINA

Cloudy media will completely obscure the retina (red reflex absent) or will make it impossible to visualize retinal landmarks such as the optic disk. Chronic causes of hazy media are common (eg, cataracts) and should not be confused with whatever is causing acute visual loss.

B. ABNORMAL VISUAL FIELDS

Grossly abnormal visual fields are usually caused by central nervous system disease and thus generally affect both eyes (not always to the same degree). The retinas are usually normal on ophthalmoscopic examination.

1. Hemianopia—Hemianopia is usually due to postchiasmal neurologic disorders (eg, tumor, aneurysm, migraine, stroke), in which case other acute neurologic lesions are present as well. Rarely, it is psychogenic in origin.

2. Central scotoma—A central scotoma indicates isolate macular involvement typical of retrobulbar neuritis and may or may not be associated with pain.

3. Tubular vision—Tubular vision not in conformity with the laws of optics is characteristic of psychogenic visual loss.

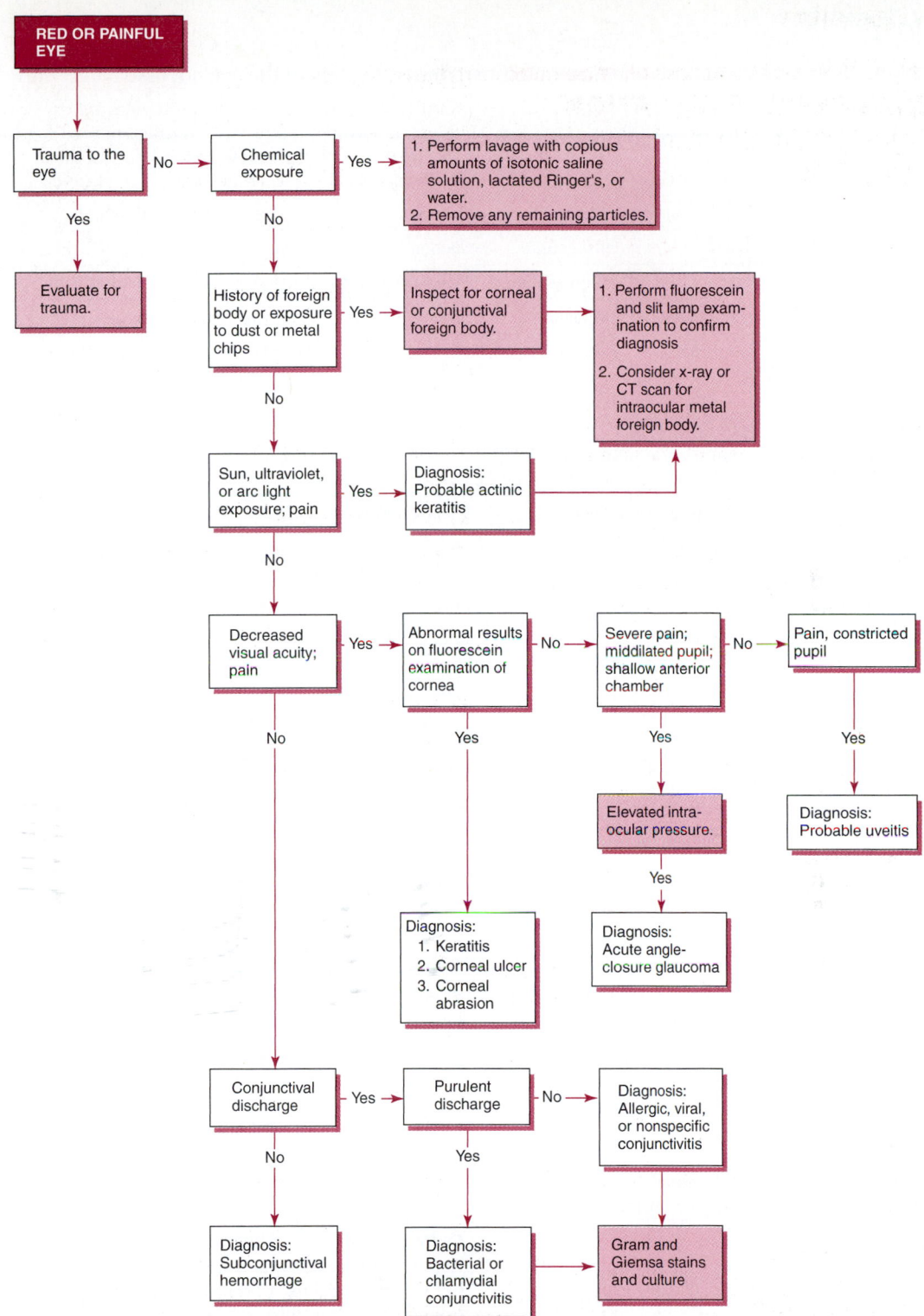

Figure 31–1. Assessment of the red or painful eye.

Table 31–1. Differential diagnosis of unilateral acute redness and pain of the eye not associated with trauma.[1]

History and Clinical Findings	Conjunctivitis	Iritis[2]	Acute Glaucoma	Corneal Infection (Bacterial Ulcer)	Corneal Erosion
Incidence	Extremely common.	Common.	Common.	Common.	Common.
Onset	Insidious.	Insidious.	Sudden.	Slow.	Sudden.
Vision	Normal.	Slightly blurred.	Markedly blurred.	Usually blurred.	Blurred.
Pain	None to moderate.	Moderate.	Severe.	Moderate to severe.	Severe.
Photophobia	None to mild.	Severe.	Minimal.	Variable.	Moderate.
Nausea and vomiting	None.	None.	Occasional.	None.	None.
Discharge	Moderate to copious.	None.	None.	Watery.	Watery.
Ciliary injection	Absent.	Present; circumcorneal.	Present.	Present.	Present.
Conjunctival injection	Severe; diffuse in fornices.	Minimal.	Minimal, diffuse.	Moderate, diffuse.	Mild to moderate.
Cornea	Clear.	Usually clear.	Steamy.	Locally hazy.	Hazy.
Stain with fluorescein	Absent.	Absent.	Absent.	Present.	Present.
Hypopyon	Absent.	Occasional.	Absent.	Occasional.	Absent.
Pupil size	Normal.	Constricted.	Middilated, fixed, and irregular.	Normal.	Normal or constricted.
Intraocular pressure	Normal.	Normal.	Elevated.	Normal.	Normal.
Gram-stained smear	Variable; depending on cause.	No organisms.	No organisms.	Organisms in scrapings from ulcers.	No organisms.
Pupillary light response	Normal.	Poor.	None.	Normal.	Poor to normal.

[1]The most helpful findings are shaded.
[2]Acute anterior uveitis.

C. ABNORMAL RETINA

An abnormal retina, usually in the eye with visual loss, is characteristic of several rare but serious conditions.

1. Central retinal artery occlusion—In central retinal artery occlusion, the fundus is usually pale with a cherry-red fovea. *This is a medical emergency.* (See below.)

2. Central retinal vein occlusion—Central retinal vein occlusion is associated with multiple widespread retinal hemorrhages.

3. Retinal hemorrhage—Retinal hemorrhage from other causes (eg, anticoagulation) may produce visual loss.

4. Retinal detachment—Retinal detachment produces visual loss preceded by visual flashes. If visual acuity is affected, detachment is large and easily visible on direct ophthalmoscopy; however, small detachments may require indirect ophthalmoscopy for visualization. Flashes of light may also occur in patients with migraine or as a result of posterior vitreous detachment.

Differential Diagnosis

Causes of acute visual loss are listed below and discussed on subsequent pages.

A. ACUTE ANGLE-CLOSURE GLAUCOMA

Acute angle-closure glaucoma causes corneal edema, but the more striking findings are eye pain; pupils fixed in mid position or dilated, often with irregular margins; a shallow anterior chamber angle (Figure 31–3); and greatly increased intraocular pressure. *Acute angle-closure glaucoma is a medical emergency.* (See below.)

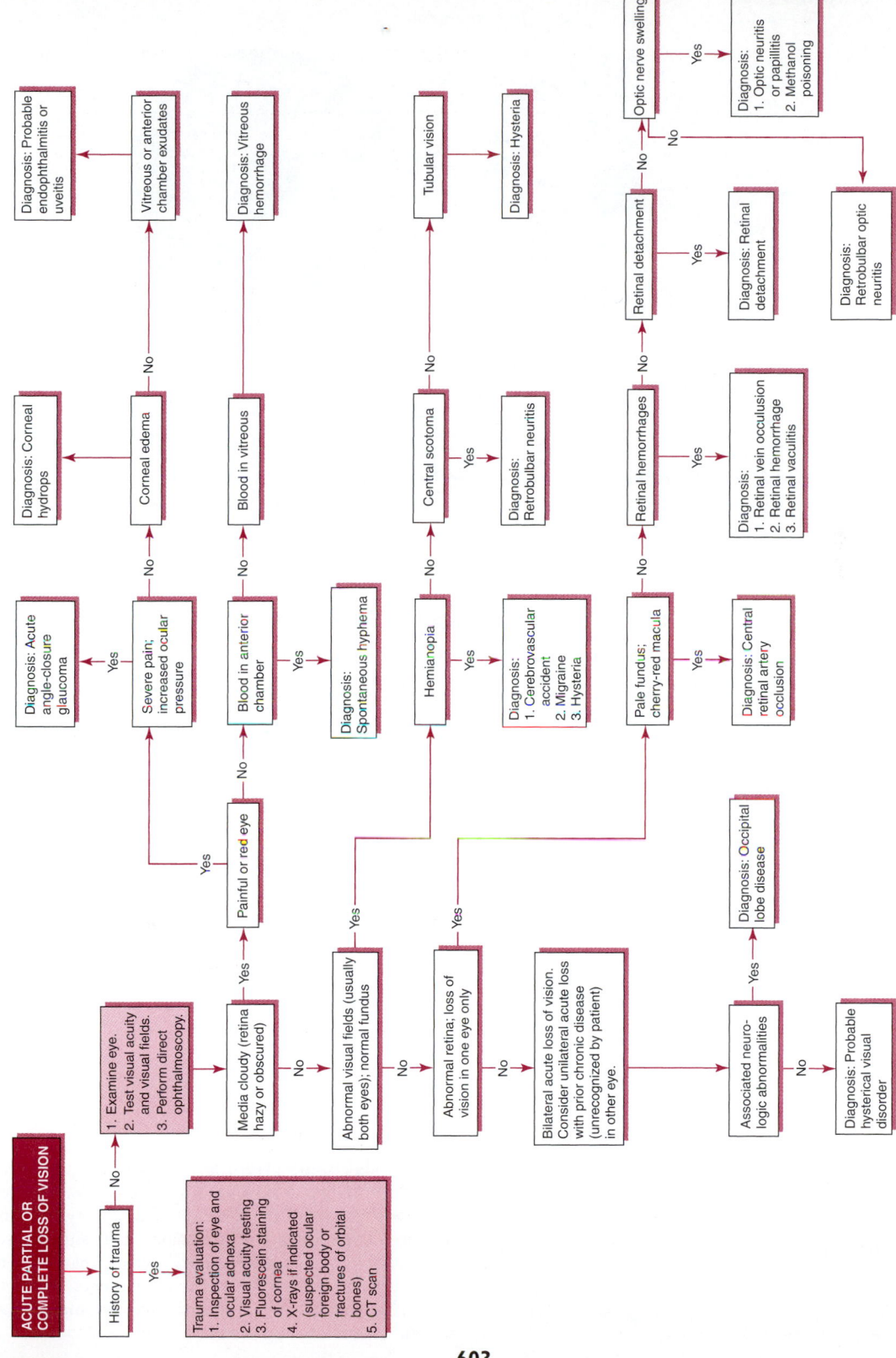

Figure 31–2. Assessment of acute partial or complete loss of vision.

603

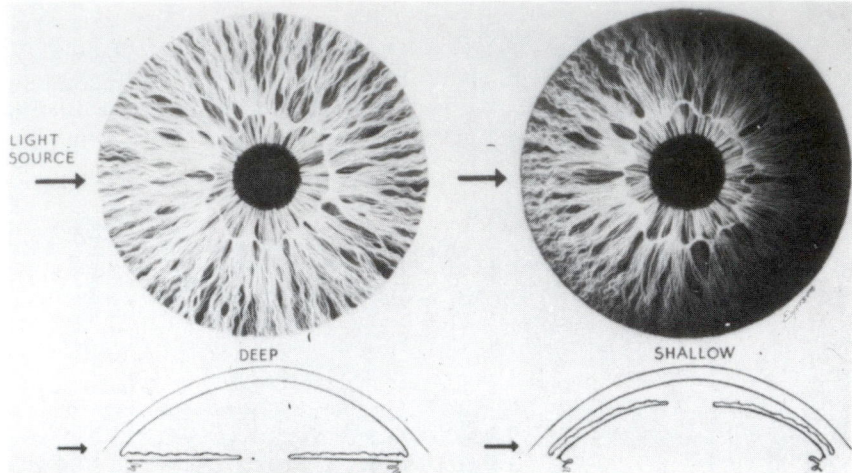

Figure 31–3. Estimation of depth of anterior chamber by oblique illumination. (Courtesy of R Shaffer.) (Reproduced, with permission, from Riordan-Eva P, Whitcher JP: *Vaughan & Asbury's General Ophthalmology,* 16th ed. McGraw-Hill, 2004.)

B. CORNEAL EDEMA

Severe corneal edema of diverse causes (eg, abrasion, keratitis) may cause visual loss with eye pain.

C. HYPHEMA

Hyphema is associated with blood in the anterior chamber on inspection.

D. VITREOUS HEMORRHAGE

Vitreous hemorrhage causes painless visual loss, which is often total. The anterior chamber is clear. The red reflex is often absent.

E. ENDOPHTHALMITIS

Endophthalmitis (intraocular infection) is a rare condition usually associated with eye pain and decreased visual acuity. Eye examination will disclose pus in the anterior chamber or vitreous.

Disposition

All patients with sudden visual loss due to ocular disease should be seen by an ophthalmologist before being discharged from the emergency department.

Leibowitz HM: The red eye. N Engl J Med 2000;343:345. [PMID: 10922425]

Markoff DD et al: Common ophthalmologic emergencies: examination, differential diagnosis, and therapeutic management. Emerg Med Rep 1999;20:1.

■ II. OCULAR CONDITIONS REQUIRING IMMEDIATE TREATMENT

ACUTE ANGLE-CLOSURE GLAUCOMA

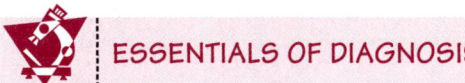 ESSENTIALS OF DIAGNOSIS

- *Severe pain, blurred vision, nausea and vomiting.*
- *Red, nonreactive mid-dilated pupil.*
- *Increased intraocular pressure confirms diagnosis.*

General Considerations

Acute angle-closure glaucoma results from sudden increase in intraocular pressure owing to blockage of the outflow channels in the anterior chamber angle by the iris root. The sudden rise in intraocular pressure causes intraocular vascular insufficiency, which may lead to optic nerve or retinal ischemia. If the acute attack of angle-closure glaucoma is not managed promptly, permanent vision loss may result.

Clinical Findings

Acute angle-closure glaucoma is characterized by severe pain, halos around lights, blurred vision, photophobia, and nausea and vomiting. The affected eye is red, with a nonreactive middilated pupil (often with irregular margins), a hazy cornea, and a shallow anterior chamber angle. Intraocular pressure is usually markedly increased (see below for the technique of tonometry). The patient may have hyperopia (farsightedness).

Differential Diagnosis

See Figure 31–2 and Table 31–1. In iridocyclitis (iritis), intraocular pressure is normal and the pupil is small and constricted. In conjunctivitis, intraocular pressure is normal and the pupil is not affected. Corneal ulcer is diagnosed by fluorescein staining of the cornea.

Treatment

Acute angle-closure glaucoma is an emergency. Failure to provide prompt treatment may result in permanent blindness. Hospitalize the patient, and obtain immediate ophthalmologic consultation for management.

Reduce the intraocular pressure by one or more of the following means:

- Timolol, 0.5%, 1 drop in the affected eye
- Pilocarpine, 2% eye drops, 2 drops every 15 minutes for 2–3 hours
- Mannitol, 20%, 250–500 mL intravenously over 2–3 hours
- Acetazolamide, 500 mg orally or 250 mg intravenously
- Glycerin, 1g/kg orally in cold 50% solution mixed with chilled lemon juice

Give sedation and analgesics as necessary to control pain and agitation.

Disposition

Acute angle-closure glaucoma calls for urgent referral to an ophthalmologist and hospitalization for initial medical treatment, followed by definitive surgical therapy.

CENTRAL RETINAL ARTERY OCCLUSION

ESSENTIALS OF DIAGNOSIS

- *Sudden, painless complete loss of vision.*
- *Exam shows pallor of disk, retinal edema, and "boxcar" appearance of retinal veins.*
- *Treatment must be initiated immediately.*

General Considerations

Central retinal artery occlusion is most commonly embolic in origin. The retina is completely without blood as long as the artery is occluded, and visual receptors in the retina will degenerate within 30–60 minutes if blood flow is not restored.

Clinical Findings

There is a typical history of sudden, complete, painless loss of vision in one eye, usually in an older person. Ophthalmoscopic examination discloses pallor of the optic disk, edema of the retina, cherry-red fovea, bloodless constricted arterioles that may be difficult to detect, and "boxcar" segmentation of blood in the retinal veins.

Treatment

Central retinal artery occlusion is an emergency. If occlusion has persisted for over 1 hour without treatment, vision has most likely been lost permanently; however, aggressive treatment should still be started. Visual recovery has occurred up to 3 days after central retinal artery occlusion. It is recommended that treatment be started if the patient is seen within 24 hours after onset of symptoms.

Treatment measures consist of ocular massage (moderate pressure for 10 seconds and release for 5 seconds), anterior chamber paracentesis, intravenous acetazolamide, or inhaled carbogen (oxygen–carbon dioxide mixture of 95% oxygen and 5% carbon dioxide). Other modalities to be considered by ophthalmology are direct infusion of tissue plasminogen activator (t-PA) or urokinase in the ophthalmic artery.

Disposition

All patients should be hospitalized on an emergent basis for treatment by an ophthalmologist.

ORBITAL CELLULITIS

ESSENTIALS OF DIAGNOSIS

- *Redness around the orbit.*
- *Pain with extraocular movement.*
- *Intravenous antibiotics and emergent consultation for admission.*

General Considerations

Acute infection of the orbital tissues is commonly caused by *Streptococcus pneumoniae,* other streptococci,

Staphylococcus aureus, and (chiefly in children) *Haemophilus influenzae.* Less frequently, certain fungi of the Phycomycetes group may cause orbital infections in diabetic patients (rhinoorbitocerebral mucormycosis). Most causative organisms enter the orbit by direct extension from the paranasal sinuses (especially through the ethmoid sinus) or through the vascular channels draining the periorbital tissues. Rarely, infection may spread to the cavernous sinus or meninges.

Clinical Findings

There is a history of sinusitis or periorbital injury, pain in and around the eye, and sometimes reduced visual acuity. Examination discloses swelling and redness of the eyelids and periorbital tissues, chemosis of the conjunctiva, exophthalmos, and limitation of movement of the eye in all fields of gaze. Disk margins may be blurred, and fever is commonly present. There may be x-ray evidence of sinusitis. CT scan shows soft tissue orbital infiltration.

Patients with invasive infection due to fungi of the Phycomycetes group (*Mucor, Rhizopus,* and other genera) may present with rapidly progressive orbital cellulitis, often with cavernous sinus thrombosis. Diabetic and immunocompromised patients are at increased risk. Examination often reveals coexisting maxillary and/or ethmoid sinusitis and palatal or nasal mucosal ulceration.

Treatment & Disposition

Obtain cultures of blood and periorbital tissue fluid. Patients should be admitted and appropriate broad-spectrum intravenous antibiotics started (clindamycin and ceftazidime). Obtain immediate otolaryngologic (ENT) or ophthalmologic consultation. Obtain CT scan of the orbit to rule out orbital abscess and intracranial involvement. Patients with orbital phycomycosis are given intravenous amphotericin B and require surgical intervention for debridement of infected tissue. Neurosurgical consultation is required to rule out intracranial involvement.

CAVERNOUS SINUS THROMBOSIS

 **ESSENTIALS OF DIAGNOSIS**

- *Complication from facial or sinus infections.*
- *Headache, nausea, pain, and decreased vision are nonspecific symptoms.*

- *Intravenous antibiotics early.*

General Considerations

Cavernous sinus thrombosis is usually associated with orbital and ocular signs and symptoms. The disease results from hematogenous spread of infection from a distant focus or from extension from a throat, facial, paranasal sinus, or orbital infection. Cavernous sinus thrombosis starts as a unilateral infection and commonly spreads to involve the other cavernous sinus.

Clinical Findings

The patient complains of chills, headache, lethargy, nausea, pain, and decreased vision. Fever, vomiting, and other systemic signs of infection are present. Ophthalmologic examination discloses unilateral or bilateral exophthalmos, absent pupillary reflexes, and papilledema. Involvement of the third, fourth, and sixth cranial nerves or of the ophthalmic branch of the fifth nerve leads to limitation of ocular movement and decrease in the corneal sensation.

Treatment & Disposition

Hospitalize the patient immediately, and send blood to the laboratory for culture and sensitivity studies and start appropriate antibiotics. Seek ophthalmologic, neurologic, and medical consultation early. Obtain CT scan of the head and orbit.

ENDOPHTHALMITIS

 ESSENTIALS OF DIAGNOSIS

- *Pus in anterior chamber is diagnostic.*
- *Obtain emergent ophthalmology consultation for drainage and antibiotic treatment.*

General Considerations

Endophthalmitis is an acute microbial infection confined within the globe. Infection involving the sclera as well as other intraocular structures is called panophthalmitis. Infections of the globe can be exogenous or endogenous. Exogenous infection results from penetrating injury or may follow intraocular surgery or a ruptured corneal ulcer. Endogenous infection by the hematogenous route is less common and may be accompanied by fever and chills.

Clinical Findings

The patient complains of pain, blurred vision, and photophobia. Examination discloses redness of the eye, chemosis of the conjunctiva, swelling of the eyelid, hypopyon (pus in the anterior chamber), and cloudy media (fundus hazily seen, or absent red reflex).

Treatment & Disposition

Send blood (2 specimens) for culture and sensitivity studies. Obtain emergent ophthalmologic consultation. Give sedation and analgesics.

The patient may have to undergo anterior chamber tap and vitreous aspiration (by an ophthalmologist). Send specimens thus obtained for staining with Giemsa and Gram stains and for cultures on appropriate media.

Check stained smears of ocular fluid, and if no organisms are seen, give empiric subconjunctival and systemic antibiotics while results of culture are pending.

RETINAL DETACHMENT

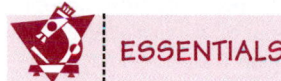

ESSENTIALS OF DIAGNOSIS

- *Painless decrease in vision.*
- *History of flashes of light, then "curtain" in front of eye.*
- *Urgent consultation for surgical repair.*

General Considerations

Detachment of the retina is actually separation of the neurosensory layer from the retinal pigment epithelium. Subretinal fluid accumulates under the neurosensory layer. Detachment may become bilateral in one fourth of cases. Retinal detachment is more common in older people and in those who are highly myopic. Hereditary factors may also play a role. Three types of primary retinal detachment are recognized: (1) rhegmatogenous detachment, from retinal holes or breaks, (2) exudative detachment, usually from inflammation, and (3) traction detachment, which occurs when vitreous bands pull on the retina. Minimal to moderate trauma to the eye may cause retinal detachment, but in such cases predisposing factors such as changes in the vitreous, retina, and choroid play an important role in pathogenesis. Severe trauma may cause retinal tears and detachment even if there are no predisposing factors.

Clinical Findings

The patient complains of painless decrease in vision and may give a history of flashes of lights or sparks. Loss of vision may be described as a curtain in front of the eye or as cloudy or smoky. Central vision may not be affected if the macular area is not involved; this frequently causes a delay in seeking treatment. Patients in whom the macula is detached present to the emergency department with sudden deterioration of vision.

Intraocular pressure is normal or low. The detached retina appears gray, with white folds and globular bullae. Round holes or horseshoe-shaped tears may be seen by indirect ophthalmoscopy in the rhegmatogenous detachment. Vitreous bands or other changes may be seen in the traction type of detachment.

Differential Diagnosis

Primary retinal detachment should be differentiated from detachment secondary to other causes, for example, from preeclampsia-eclampsia or tumors of the choroid.

Treatment & Disposition

Arrange for immediate referral to an ophthalmologist. If the macula is attached and central visual acuity is normal, the condition should be urgently treated by an ophthalmologist.

Retinal reattachment can be accomplished only by surgery, which is successful in about 80% of cases. If the macula is detached or threatened, operation should be scheduled on an urgent basis, because prolonged detachment of the macula results in permanent loss of central vision.

TOXIC CAUSES OF BLINDNESS

A wide variety of organic chemicals may lead to visual deterioration. Ingestion of chemicals that cause corneal or lenticular opacities usually leads to insidious onset of visual loss. Ingestion of compounds that cause damage to nervous tissue may lead to slow or rapid deterioration of vision. Exposure to toxic doses of methanol, halogenated hydrocarbons (eg, methyl chloride), arsenic, and lead may cause permanent visual damage. Acute or chronic administration of drugs such as ethambutol, chloramphenicol, quinine, and salicylates may also cause optic neuritis and loss of vision.

By far the most common toxic cause of blindness is methanol (methyl alcohol). Ingestion of only a few milliliters may cause permanent blindness. Acute methanol poisoning causes nausea and vomiting and abdominal pain. Headache, dizziness, and delirium may occur. Loss of vision may be complete and sudden a few hours after drinking methanol or may occasionally be noted about 3 days after exposure. Pupillary reflexes are sluggish. Ophthalmoscopic examination shows swelling and hyperemia of the optic nerve head, distention of the veins, and peripapillary edema of the retina.

Hospitalize the patient immediately. See Chapter 45 for details of evaluation and treatment.

Banker AS et al: Retinal detachment. Ophthalmol Clin North Am 2001;14:695. [PMID: 11787748]

Beatty S et al: Acute occlusion of the retinal arteries: current concepts and recent advances in diagnosis and management. J Accid Emerg Med 2000;17:324. [PMID: 11005400]

Danis RP: Endophthalmitis. Ophthalmol Clin North Am 2002;15:243. [PMID: 12229241]

Hitchings RA: Glaucoma in the new millennium. Ophthalmol Clin North Am 1999;12:519.

Jain A et al: Orbital cellulitis in children. Int Ophthalmol Clin 2001;41:71. [PMID: 11698739]

McGuigan ME: Poisoning potpourri. Pediatr Rev 2001;22:295. [PMID: 11533378]

Migirov L, Eyal A, Kronenberg J: Treatment of cavernous sinus thrombosis. Isr Med Assoc J 2002;4:468. [PMID: 12073429]

Sharma S et al: Retinal artery occlusions. Ophthalmol Clin North Am 1998;11:591.

■ III. NONTRAUMATIC OCULAR EMERGENCIES

ACUTE DACRYOCYSTITIS

ESSENTIALS OF DIAGNOSIS

- *Swelling, redness, and tenderness over the lacrimal sac.*
- *Warm compresses and systemic antibiotics for treatment.*

General Considerations

Acute infection of the lacrimal sac occurs in children and adults as a complication of nasolacrimal duct obstruction. The most frequently encountered causative organism is *S pneumoniae*.

Clinical Findings

The patient complains of pain. There may be a history of tearing and discharge. Examination discloses swelling, redness, and tenderness over the lacrimal sac (Figure 31–4).

Pus should be collected, for Gram-stained smear and culture, by applying pressure over the lacrimal sac.

Treatment

Prescribe warm compresses 3–4 times daily. Begin appropriate systemic antibiotic therapy with first-generation cephalosporin or amoxicillin-clavulanate, until culture results are reported. Results of Gram-stained smears of purulent exudate may be helpful in guiding empiric therapy. Topical sulfacetamide, 10% eye drops, may be given every 2 hours, and erythromycin ophthalmic ointment, 0.5% (5 mg/g), may be used at bedtime.

Massage of the nasolacrimal sac to express purulent discharge through the punctum is helpful in infants. The technique is to apply pressure over the lacrimal sac with a cotton swab (Q-tip). Irrigation of the lacrimal sac with diluted antibiotics should be done by an ophthalmologist.

Disposition

The patient can be discharged to home care with a prescription for systemic antibiotics and instruction in how to apply warm local compresses. Consult an ophthalmologist for consideration of surgical correction. The patient should be seen again within 3–4 days.

ACUTE DACRYOADENITIS

ESSENTIALS OF DIAGNOSIS

- *Swelling and pain over temporal aspect of upper eyelid.*

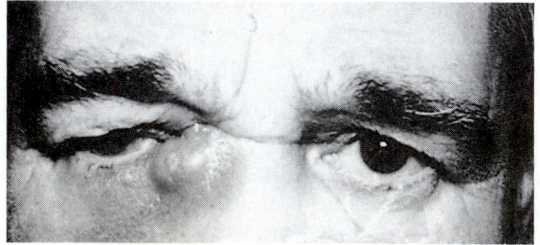

Figure 31–4. Acute dacryocystitis. (Reproduced, with permission, from Vaughan D, Asbury T, Tabbara KF: *General Ophthalmology*, 12th ed. Appleton & Lange, 1989.)

Clinical Findings

Infection and inflammation of the lacrimal gland is characterized by swelling, pain and tenderness, and redness over the upper temporal aspect of the upper eyelid.

Differential Diagnosis

Acute dacryoadenitis must be differentiated from viral infection (mumps), sarcoidosis, Sjögren syndrome, tumors, leukemia, and lymphoma.

Treatment

Purulent bacterial infections should be treated by incision and drainage of localized pus collections, antibiotics, warm compresses, and systemic analgesics. Viral dacryoadenitis (mumps) is treated conservatively.

Disposition

The patient should be referred to an ophthalmologist for follow-up care in 2–3 days.

ACUTE HORDEOLUM (Stye)

 ESSENTIALS OF DIAGNOSIS

- *Pain and redness with swelling over the eyelid.*
- *Warm compresses and topical antibiotic 3 times daily are key to treatment.*

General Considerations

Acute hordeolum is a common infection of the lid glands: the meibomian glands (internal hordeolum) and the glands of Zeis or Moll (external hordeolum). The most frequent causative organism is *S aureus.*

Clinical Findings

A stye is characterized by pain and redness with variable swelling over the eyelid. A large hordeolum may rarely be associated with swelling of the preauricular lymph node on the affected side, fever, and leukocytosis.

Treatment

If pus is localized and pointing out to the skin or conjunctiva, a horizontal incision is made through the skin or a vertical incision through the conjunctiva. (This procedure should be performed by an ophthalmologist.)

Disposition

The patient can be discharged to continue treatment with warm compresses 3 times daily and topical antibiotic ointment (erythromycin or tetracycline) twice daily at home.

EYELID INFECTIONS (Preseptal Cellulitis)

 ESSENTIALS OF DIAGNOSIS

- *Tenderness and pain with erythema surrounding the eye.*
- *Key to diagnosis is no pain with ocular movement.*
- *Antibiotic treatment and daily follow-up to ensure the infection doesn't progress to orbital cellulitis.*

General Considerations

Preseptal cellulitis is an infectious or inflammatory process of the eyelid. Common causative organisms are S aureus, streptococci, and *H influenzae.* Viral causes should be considered if associated with a skin rash (eg, herpes zoster).

Clinical Findings

There is tenderness, erythema, and edema of the eyelid. No proptosis, no pain with ocular movement, and no restriction of extraocular motility is present. If any of these are present, consider orbital cellulitis.

Treatment

Give amoxicillin-clavulanate for 10 days. Antivirals may be considered if herpes zoster is suspected. Incision and drainage may be needed in more severe cases.

Disposition

The patient can be discharged with daily follow-up with ophthalmology or otolaryngology. If the patient returns with failure of antibiotics or worsening symptoms, start intravenous antibiotics and obtain emergent ophthalmology or ENT consult.

SPONTANEOUS SUBCONJUNCTIVAL HEMORRHAGE

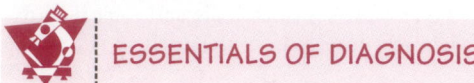

ESSENTIALS OF DIAGNOSIS

- *Painless.*
- *Vision is not affected.*

General Considerations

Rupture of conjunctival or episcleral blood vessels may occur spontaneously or in association with minimal trauma, violent coughing, or retching. The possibility of coagulopathies and systemic hypertension must be investigated in recurrent subconjunctival hemorrhage.

Clinical Findings

The conjunctiva suddenly becomes bright red in blotchy distribution. There is no pain, and vision is not affected. Severe cases may be characterized by chemosis and subconjunctival accumulation of blood clots. Check for hypertension, and obtain a complete blood count with differential and coagulation panel (prothrombin time, partial thromboplastin time, and platelet count) if hemorrhage recurs or if there is any other evidence of bleeding diathesis.

Treatment & Disposition

Treat with cold compresses within the first 12 hours after onset; later, use warm compresses for 10–15 minutes 3 times daily. The patient can be discharged to private care or a clinic and should be seen within 2–3 days for follow-up examination and care if needed.

CONJUNCTIVITIS

ESSENTIALS OF DIAGNOSIS

- *Most frequent cause of red eye.*
- *Purulent drainage and conjunctival hyperemia help with diagnosis.*

General Considerations

Conjunctivitis is a frequent cause of red eye. It should be dealt with as an urgent medical problem until it is certain that the process is under control.

Causes of Acute Conjunctivitis

A. INFECTION

Acute conjunctivitis may be caused by bacterial, viral, parasitic, fungal, or chlamydial infection.

B. CHEMICAL IRRITATION

Chemical irritations causing acute conjunctivitis include chlorine gas and tear gas.

C. ALLERGY

Allergic causes of acute conjunctivitis include vernal keratoconjunctivitis and hay fever.

D. SKIN DISORDERS

Skin disorders such as Stevens-Johnson syndrome, acne rosacea, Lyell disease, Kawasaki disease, and psoriasis may cause acute conjunctivitis.

E. SYSTEMIC DISORDERS

Sjögren syndrome and vitamin A deficiency may cause acute conjunctivitis.

Clinical Findings

See Table 31–2. The patient complains of a "scratchy" sensation or pain, with conjunctival discharge. One or both eyes may be affected. Adherence of the eyelids upon awakening is common in bacterial conjunctivitis.

Examination discloses conjunctival hyperemia, purulent or mucopurulent discharge, and variable degrees of lid swelling. Material should be taken from the conjunctival sac for smear (Gram and Giemsa stains) and for culture on blood and chocolate agar. Viral cultures may also be indicated.

Treatment

Until laboratory reports are received, prescribe topical sulfacetamide, 10% eye drops, or ciprofloxacin, 0.3% eyedrops (an alternative to ciprofloxacin is ofloxacin), 4 times daily; and erythromycin or tetracycline ophthalmic ointment at bedtime for suspected bacterial conjunctivitis.

For suspected chlamydial infection (eg, history of urethritis), prescribe topical and systemic tetracycline or erythromycin. Give 0.5 g 4 times daily for 21 days (adult dose). Doxycycline, 100 mg twice daily, may be substituted for tetracycline. Consider treatment for gonorrhea.

Disposition

Discharge patients to home care with instructions to return for follow-up in 48–72 hours. Patients who do not respond to treatment should be referred to an ophthalmologist.

Table 31–2. Differential diagnosis of conjunctivitis.

Clinical Features	Bacterial	Chlamydial	Viral	Allergic	Irritant
Onset	Acute.	Acute or subacute.	Acute or subacute.	Recurrent	Acute.
Pain	Moderate.	Mild to moderate.	Mild to moderate.	None.	None to mild.
Discharge	Copious, purulent.	Moderate, purulent.	Moderate, seropurulent.	Moderate, clear.	Minimal, clear.
Gram-stained smear	PMNs, bacteria.	PMNs, monocytes, no bacteria.	PMNs, monocytes, no bacteria.	Eosinophils present.	Negative.
Routine culture	Usually *Staphylococcus aureus*, pneumococci.	Negative.	Negative.	Negative.	Negative.
Special culture	. . .	*Chlamydia.*	Adenoviruses; occasionally enteroviruses; rarely others.	Negative.	Negative.
Preauricular adenopathy	Common.	Common.	Common.	No.	Rare.

PMNs = polymorphonuclear neutrophils.

BACTERIAL CORNEAL ULCER

 ESSENTIALS OF DIAGNOSIS

- *Exam with fluorescein aids in diagnosis.*
- *Antibiotic treatment and close follow-up are mandatory.*
- *Common in contact lens wearers.*

General Considerations

Corneal infections may be due to bacteria, viruses, chlamydiae, or fungi. The conjunctiva may or may not be involved. Bacterial corneal ulcers are serious, because rapid perforation of the cornea and loss of aqueous humor may occur; bacterial endophthalmitis may occur if bacterial ulcers are not properly treated.

Clinical Findings

The patient complains of pain and photophobia, blurring of vision, and eye irritation. Examination discloses conjunctival hyperemia and chemosis, corneal ulceration, or whitish-yellowish infiltration. The examination is facilitated by fluorescein staining and inspection with ultraviolet light. Hypopyon may be present. Scrapings from the cornea should be taken for culture and staining with Gram and Giemsa stains.

Differential Diagnosis

See Table 31–1.

Treatment & Disposition

Management of bacterial corneal infections causing corneal ulcers must be instituted as early as possible. The patient should be seen by an ophthalmologist before discharge from the emergency department. Hospitalization may be necessary, especially if hypopyon is present.

VIRAL KERATOCONJUNCTIVITIS

 ESSENTIALS OF DIAGNOSIS

- *Redness and pain with palpebral conjunctival follicles in one eye.*
- *Adenovirus is most common; however, sulfacetamide is used.*

Clinical Findings

Viral keratoconjunctivitis is an acute conjunctivitis and keratitis caused most frequently by adenovirus (types 8 and 19). The patient complains of redness of the eye associated with tearing and moderate pain. The onset is often in one eye only, and this eye is more severely affected. Sensitivity to light (photophobia) may be noted

5–14 days after onset. Examination discloses swelling of the eyelids and bulbar conjunctival hyperemia, with follicles noted over the palpebral conjunctiva. A pseudomembrane may be noted over the palpebral conjunctiva. A tender preauricular lymph node can be palpated. Subconjunctival hemorrhage may occur within 48 hours. Corneal epithelial keratitis accompanies the conjunctivitis, but subepithelial opacities are not seen until 5–14 days after onset of symptoms.

In adults, the disease is confined to the external eye. Children may have fever, pharyngitis, and diarrhea (pharyngoconjunctival fever). Staining of conjunctival scrapings with Giemsa stain demonstrates a predominantly mononuclear inflammatory reaction. When pseudomembranes occur, polymorphonuclear neutrophils may be seen. Culture for adenovirus is usually positive in the first 2 weeks after onset. Chlamydial conjunctivitis should always be considered in the differential diagnosis.

Treatment

Treatment is symptomatic. Topical decongestants may be helpful. Dark glasses may relieve photophobia. If the diagnosis is uncertain, send material for culture for bacteria, and start sulfacetamide, 10% eye drops, 4 times daily; and tetracycline, 1% (10 mg/g) ointment twice daily, while awaiting laboratory results.

Because epidemics have been caused by spread of the viral agent by physicians and nurses, handwashing between examinations and complete sterilization of tonometer footplates are mandatory preventive measures.

Disposition

The patient should be discharged with instructions to seek a medical appointment in 2–3 days. Patients should take care to avoid spread of virus from ocular secretions to other family members, and they should preferably stay home from work for a few days to avoid spread of the infection.

ACUTE HYDROPS OF THE CORNEA

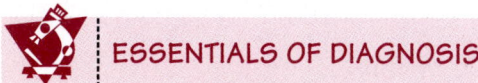

ESSENTIALS OF DIAGNOSIS

- Sudden, painless decrease in vision.
- Unaffected eye shows keratoconus.
- Follow-up with ophthalmologist in 24–72 hours.

General Considerations

Acute hydrops of the cornea may occur in patients with keratoconus who develop rupture of Descemet's membrane, with resulting infiltration of the corneal stroma by aqueous humor. This may occur suddenly, resulting in corneal clouding.

Clinical Findings

The typical presentation is of sudden, painless, marked decrease in visual acuity in a patient with keratoconus. There may be mild eye irritation, and the cornea is cloudy as a result of corneal edema. The patient usually has keratoconus in the other eye. Bacterial or viral keratitis must be ruled out.

Treatment

Hypertonic eye drops, for example, sodium chloride, 2% or 5% solution, should be instilled 4 times daily for 1 week. Apply a stream of hot air twice daily by hair dryer to speed dehydration of the cornea. Avoid rubbing the eye.

Disposition

Refer the patient to an ophthalmologist within 24–72 hours.

HYPHEMA

ESSENTIALS OF DIAGNOSIS

- Sudden decrease in visual acuity.
- Sitting the patient up can aid in the diagnosis, because blood will accumulate inferiorly.
- Must check intraocular pressure.

General Considerations

Hyphema (blood in the anterior chamber) is usually caused by nonperforating trauma to the eye. In rare instances, hyphema may occur spontaneously as a complication of an ocular or systemic disorder.

Clinical Findings

Hyphema is characterized by sudden decrease in visual acuity. If the intraocular pressure is elevated, there may be pain in the eye with or without headache.

The whole anterior chamber may be filled with blood, or a blood level may be seen. The conjunctiva is hyperemic with perilimbal injection.

Treatment

Elevate the patient's head 30 degrees. Cover the affected eye with a shield. If intraocular pressure is elevated, immediate ophthalmologic consultation is needed for surgical evacuation of blood.

Recently, intracameral injection (performed by an ophthalmologist) of 25 μg of t-PA has been shown to expedite the resorption of blood clots in the anterior chamber. Aminocaproic acid can be used topically to stabilize the clot and decrease the rate of rebleeding.

Disposition

Acute care and evaluation by an ophthalmologist is essential. Operative evacuation of nonabsorbed blood clots may be required. Recurrence of bleeding on the third to fifth days following injury is not uncommon. Disposition should be determined by the ophthalmologist. All patients with hyphema should be examined every day for 5 days and then as directed by the ophthalmologist.

UVEITIS
(Iritis & Iridocyclitis)

 ESSENTIALS OF DIAGNOSIS

- *Photophobia, pain, and constricted pupil secondary to ciliary spasm.*
- *Mydriatics are key to treatment.*

General Considerations

The uvea consists of the iris, ciliary body, and choroid. Anterior uveitis is inflammation of the iris and ciliary body, or iridocyclitis. Inflammation of all 3 structures is called panuveitis.

Clinical Findings

See Table 31–1. The patient complains of blurred vision, photophobia, and headache or ocular pain. Ciliary injection may be present around the limbus, and conjunctival injection may be minimal. Intraocular pressure may be elevated. There is no conjunctival discharge.

Treatment

Instill prednisolone acetate, 1% eye drops, 5 times daily. More frequent applications may be required in certain severe cases of anterior uveitis. Instill a cycloplegic mydriatic agent, such as tropicamide or cyclopentolate, 1% eye drops, 1 drop every 8 hours. If intraocular pressure is elevated, give acetazolamide, 250 mg orally every 6 hours.

Disposition

Patients with uveitis should be seen the next day for follow-up care. Continuing care should be by an ophthalmologist. The cause of uveitis should be investigated.

VITREOUS HEMORRHAGE

 ESSENTIALS OF DIAGNOSIS

- *Sudden, painless loss of vision.*
- *Patient complains of seeing "floaters."*
- *Secondary to trauma, retinal detachment, or diabetic retinopathy.*
- *Urgent ophthalmology consultation is needed.*

General Considerations

Spontaneous hemorrhage into the vitreous body may result from local factors in the eye (eg, retinal tears, tumors, inflammation, venous occlusion, retinal detachment) or from associated systemic disorders (eg, hematopoietic diseases, diabetes mellitus, hypertension) (Table 31–3). Blood in the vitreous body clots rapidly, and removal of red blood cells is retarded because of the network of collagen fibers and hyaluronic acid.

Table 31–3. Some known causes of spontaneous vitreous hemorrhage not associated with trauma.

Diabetic retinopathy
Retinal tear
Posterior vitreous detachment
Retinal vein occlusion
Retinal detachment
Sickle cell disease
Ocular toxocariasis
Hypertension

Clinical Findings

Vitreous hemorrhage is characterized by sudden, painless loss or deterioration of vision in the affected eye. The eye is not red. The red reflex of the fundus is hazy or faint or becomes black. Details of the retina and optic nerve are obscured by the cloudy vitreous.

Treatment & Disposition

The patient should be evaluated immediately by an ophthalmologist. Partial or total vitrectomy may have to be considered later if absorption of blood does not occur or if vitreous clouding occurs secondary to organization of the blood clot. Photocoagulation of the neovascular network (ie, new blood vessel formation, as occurs in diabetic or sickle cell retinopathy), when present, may be considered in some cases as a prophylactic measure.

Recent studies have shown that intravitreal injection of 25 μg of t-PA may be considered in selected patients with traumatic vitreous hemorrhage.

RETINAL HEMORRHAGE

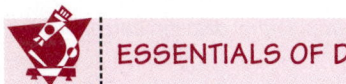 **ESSENTIALS OF DIAGNOSIS**

- *Painless loss of vision occurs if the hemorrhage is in the macular area.*
- *May have no symptoms.*

General Considerations

Retinal hemorrhage may be due to trauma, local ocular disease, or systemic disorders (Table 31–4). Hemorrhages may occur in superficial or deep layers of the retina or in the preretinal or subhyaloid space.

Clinical Findings

The patient may complain of sudden decrease in vision when hemorrhage occurs in the macular or perimacular area. Small peripheral retinal hemorrhages cause no symptoms. Superficial retinal hemorrhages occurring in the nerve fiber layer are bright red and flame-shaped on ophthalmoscopic examination. Deep retinal hemorrhages are round and have a dark red color. Subhyaloid hemorrhage occurs in the space between the vitreous body and the internal limiting membrane and may have a boat-shaped appearance. A neovascular network may rupture and cause retinal or vitreous hemorrhage.

Table 31–4. Systemic conditions associated with retinal hemorrhage.

Hypertension
Atherosclerosis
Diabetes mellitus
Hemoglobinopathies (eg, sickle cell disease)
Anemia
Subacute infective endocarditis
Leukemia, lymphoma
Hyperviscosity syndromes
Cancer (rarely) (eg, breast, eye)
Giant cell arteritis, Takayasu arteritis
Infections (eg, cytomegalovirus)
Autoimmune disease (eg, lupus erythematosus, polyarteritis nodosa)
Intracranial tumor
Anticoagulation

Treatment & Disposition

Treatment depends on the cause; there is no specific treatment. The patient should be referred to an ophthalmologist for further care, for example, photocoagulation of new vessels associated with local or systemic conditions (eg, diabetes) to prevent recurrences.

CENTRAL RETINAL VEIN OCCLUSION

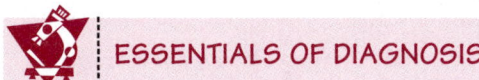 **ESSENTIALS OF DIAGNOSIS**

- *Unilateral, painless loss of vision.*
- *Often in elderly with glaucoma or hypertension.*

General Considerations

Central retinal vein occlusion occurs most frequently in elderly patients with glaucoma or hypertension. The incidence is increased also in diabetes mellitus, autoimmune diseases, Waldenström macroglobulinemia, cryoglobulinemia, sickle cell disease, polycythemia vera, and leukemia.

Clinical Findings

The patient complains of sudden painless loss of vision in one eye. Ophthalmoscopy reveals dilated and tortuous veins, retinal and macular edema, multiple or diffuse retinal hemorrhages, and attenuated arterioles.

Treatment & Disposition

There is no specific therapy. Refer the patient to an ophthalmologist within 24 hours for assessment of possible glaucoma or associated systemic disease. If local predisposing factors such as glaucoma are ruled out, patients with occlusion should have a complete medical evaluation.

OPTIC NEURITIS

ESSENTIALS OF DIAGNOSIS

- *Painful unilaterally, especially with movement.*
- *Afferent pupillary defect.*
- *Many causes: case should be discussed with ophthalmology or neurology consult.*

General Considerations

Optic neuritis may be due to a variety of causes, including demyelinating diseases; systemic infections; nutritional and metabolic disorders; exposure to toxic substances (eg, arsenic, methanol, lead, tobacco); vascular insufficiency; and local extension of infection from intraocular structures, sinuses, or meninges. Optic neuritis includes retrobulbar neuritis (inflammation of the optic nerve posterior to the globe), in which there are by definition no ophthalmoscopic findings.

Clinical Findings

The patient complains of decreased vision in one eye and sometimes pain on moving the eye. The pupillary reflex is sluggish. Ophthalmoscopic examination in optic neuritis shows hyperemia of the optic nerve head (may not be present in retrobulbar neuritis), congestion of the large veins, blurring of the disk margin, peripapillary retinal edema, and flame-shaped hemorrhages near the optic nerve head. Visual field testing discloses a central scotoma.

Treatment & Disposition

Treatment depends on the cause. Systemic corticosteroids may be helpful in cases associated with demyelinating disease. The patient should be referred to an ophthalmologist or neurologist for further care within 1–2 days.

Benson WH, Lanier JD: Current diagnosis and treatment of corneal ulcers. Curr Opin Ophthalmol 1998;9:45. [PMID: 10387468]

Bhagat N: Central retinal vein occlusion: review of management. Eur J Ophthalmol 1999;9:165. [PMID: 10544972]

Crouch ER: Topical aminocaproic acid in the treatment of traumatic hyphema. Arch Opthalmol 1997;115:1106. [PMID: 9298049]

Curl A: Seeing red. A review of subconjunctival hemorrhage. Adv Nurse Pract 1999;7:77. [PMID: 10373806]

Grewal S et al: Acute hydrops in the corneal ectasias: associated factors and outcomes. Trans Am Ophthalmol Soc 1999;97:187. [PMID: 10703124]

Hamill MB: Current concepts in the treatment of traumatic injury to the anterior segment. Ophthalmol Clin North Am 1999; 12:457.

Hochman MA et al: Pathophysiology and management of subretinal hemorrhage. Surv Ophthalmol 1997;42:195. [PMID: 9406367]

Kaufman HE: Treatment of viral diseases of the cornea and external eye. Prog Retin Eye Res 2000;19:69. [PMID: 10614681]

Lederman C et al: Hordeola and chalazia. Pediatr Rev 1999;20: 283. [PMID: 10429150]

Mawn LA et al: Preseptal and orbital cellulitis. Opthalmol Clin North Am 2000;13:633.

Shields SR: Managing eye disease in primary care. Part 2. How to recognize and treat common eye problems. Postgrad Med 2000;108:83. [PMID: 11043082]

Spraul CW et al: Vitreous hemorrhage. Surv Ophthalmol 1997; 42:3. [PMID: 9265701]

Tolls DB: Peripheral retinal hemorrhages: a literature review and report on thirty-three patients. J Am Optom Assoc 1998;69: 563. [PMID: 9785731]

Van Stavern GP: Management of optic neuritis and multiple sclerosis. Curr Opin Ophthalmol 2001;12:400. [PMID: 11734679]

Weinberg RS: Uveitis. Update on therapy. Ophthalmol Clin North Am 1999;12:71.

Yeatts RP: Acquired nasolacrimal duct obstruction. Ophthalmol Clin North Am 2000;13:719.

■ IV. OCULAR BURNS & TRAUMA

OCULAR BURNS

ESSENTIALS OF DIAGNOSIS

- *History and physical examination.*
- *Copious irrigation with normal saline, lactated Ringer's, or water after topical anesthetic is placed.*
- *Check pH after irrigation; should be 6.8–7.4.*

- *Immediate ophthalmology consultation is needed.*

General Considerations

Apart from the history, the diagnosis of chemical burns is usually based on the presence of swollen eyelids with marked conjunctival hyperemia and chemosis. The limbus may show patchy balanced areas with conjunctival sloughing, especially in the interpalpebral area. There is usually corneal haze and diffuse edema, with wide areas of epithelial cell loss and corneal ulcerations. Corneal ulcerations can be better visualized with blue light following instillation of fluorescein.

ALKALI BURNS

Clinical Findings

Alkali burns (especially particulate alkali such as lime) are very serious, because even after apparent removal of the offending agent, tiny particles may remain lodged within the cul-de-sac and cause progressive damage to the eye.

Treatment

Instill a topical anesthetic *immediately* (proparacaine, 0.5%; or tetracaine, 0.5%), and then copiously irrigate the eye with 2–3 L isotonic saline solution, water, or lactated Ringer's solution. A lid retractor may be useful.

Double eversion of the eyelids (Figure 31–5) should be performed to look for and remove material lodged in

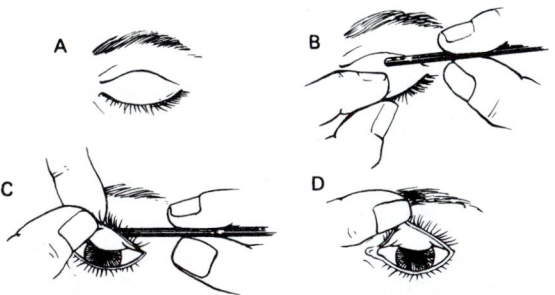

Figure 31–5. Eversion of the upper lid. **A:** The patient looks downward. **B:** The fingers pull the lid down, and a rod is placed on the upper tarsal border. **C:** The lid is pulled up over the rod. **D:** The lid is everted. (Redrawn and reproduced, with permission, from Liebman SD, Gellis SS [editors]: *The Pediatrician's Ophthalmology.* Mosby, 1966.)

the cul-de-sac. Solid particles of alkali should be removed with forceps or a moist cotton swab. After particles have been removed, irrigate again.

Do not attempt to neutralize the alkali with acid, because the heat generated by the chemical reaction may cause further injury.

Instill topical mydriatic eye drops and antibiotic ointment. After irrigation, the pH of the eye should be checked and the range should be 6.8–7.4. If the pH is still high, continue with irrigation. Parenteral narcotic analgesia is often required for pain relief (eg, morphine, 10 mg subcutaneously).

Disposition

Obtain immediate ophthalmologic consultation.

ACID BURNS

Clinical Findings

Acid burns as a rule cause damage more rapidly but are generally less serious than alkali burns, because they do not cause progressive destruction of ocular tissues (as do alkali burns).

Treatment

Immediately after exposure, irrigate the eyes copiously with sterile isotonic saline solution, lactated Ringer's, or tap water. Topical anesthetic (proparacaine, 0.5%) may be instilled to minimize pain during irrigation. Do not attempt to neutralize the acid with alkali.

Parenteral or oral narcotic analgesics may be necessary. Patch the eye if corneal defects are present.

Disposition

Obtain immediate ophthalmologic consultation.

THERMAL BURNS

Clinical Findings

Injury due to thermal burns of the eyelids, cornea, and conjunctiva may range from minimal to extensive. Superficial corneal burns have a good prognosis, though corneal ulcers may occur as a result of loss of corneal epithelium.

Thermal burns of the skin of the eyelids may be first, second, or third degree. Conjunctival hyperemia is noted. The cornea may show diffuse necrosis of the exposed corneal epithelium in the interpalpebral area.

Corneal haze due to corneal edema is frequently seen in thermal burns of the cornea and may lead to decrease in vision.

Treatment

The treatment of ocular burns is similar to the treatment of burns occurring elsewhere on the body (Chapter 43). Provide systemic analgesia. Instill proparacaine, 0.5%, or tetracaine, 0.5%, to minimize pain during manipulation. In cases of corneal burns, instill a mydriatic agent.

Disposition

Hospitalize patients with severe burns for local care and administration of systemic analgesia. Obtain ophthalmologic consultation.

BURNS DUE TO ULTRAVIOLET RADIATION

Destruction of the corneal epithelium by ultraviolet light is know as actinic keratitis, snow blindness, and welder's arc burn (flash burn), depending on the source of ultraviolet radiation.

Clinical Findings

The patient complains of pain and gives a history of exposure to ultraviolet light 6–12 hours earlier (eg, skiing, sunlamp). Examination discloses tearing, conjunctival hyperemia, and corneal haziness. There may be a superficial punctate staining of the cornea seen with fluorescein and with magnification (eg, slit lamp). Exposure to a welder's arc without protective filters produces keratitis similar to that resulting from ultraviolet radiation.

Treatment

Topical anesthetic should be instilled during the eye examination only. Do not give the patient a topical anesthetic to use at home. Instill a mydriatic agent and an antibiotic ointment. Recovery occurs within 12–36 hours. Provide systemic analgesics for pain (aspirin and codeine or equivalent).

Disposition

Patients with severe burns should be hospitalized. All other patients should be seen for follow-up the next day (by an ophthalmologist, if possible).

MECHANICAL TRAUMA TO THE EYE

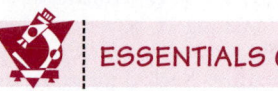 **ESSENTIALS OF DIAGNOSIS**

- *History is key to diagnosis.*
- *Full exam is paramount to treatment and diagnosis.*

General Considerations

Ocular trauma may be classified as penetrating or nonpenetrating. Trauma can lead to serious damage and loss of vision. Eye injuries are common in spite of the protection afforded by the bony orbit and the cushioning effect of orbital fat. More widespread use of safety goggles would prevent most serious injuries to the eye.

Evaluation

Obtain a history of the injury from the patient or someone who knows what happened. Measure and record visual acuity with and without eyeglasses and through a pinhole aperture. Inspect the eyelids, conjunctiva, cornea, anterior chamber, pupils, lens, vitreous, and fundus for breaks in tissue and hemorrhage. Search for corneal lesions (eg, abrasion) by instilling fluorescein dye and examining the eye using a light with a light-blue filter.

X-ray examination (orbital soft tissue film with contact lens localizer) or CT scan may be indicated to rule out radiopaque foreign bodies and to look for fractures of orbital bones.

Treatment & Disposition

Hospitalize patients with severe injuries, and consult an ophthalmologist immediately. Avoid causing further damage by manipulation. For more detailed discussion of treatment and disposition, see below under the specific type of injury.

For severe pain, photophobia, or foreign body sensation, instill a topical anesthetic (eg, proparacaine, 0.5%, 1–2 drops once or twice). Systemic analgesics may be required. Cover the eye with an eye shield.

PENETRATING OR PERFORATING INJURIES

General Considerations

Penetrating or perforating ocular injuries require immediate careful attention and prompt surgical repair to prevent possible loss of the eye.

Many facial injuries, especially those occurring in automobile accidents, are associated with penetrating ocular trauma. Some injuries may be concealed and inapparent because of eyelid swelling or because the patient's other injuries have dominated the attentions of the emergency department team. Such injuries, if not promptly attended to and adequately managed by an ophthalmologist, may lead to loss of vision.

Evaluation

Obtain and record a description of how the injury occurred. Examine the eye and ocular adnexa, including vision testing if the patient's condition permits. Do not apply pressure on the globe. CT scan is indicated to rule out intraocular radiopaque foreign body and to look for fractures of orbital bones.

Clinical Findings

Penetrating injuries are those that cause disruption of the outer coats of the eye (sclera, cornea) without interrupting the anatomic continuity of that layer, thus preventing prolapse or loss of ocular contents. Perforating injuries are those resulting in complete anatomic disruption (laceration) of the sclera or cornea. Such wounds may or may not be associated with prolapse of uveal structures. Wounds of the sclera or cornea are often associated with intraocular or intraorbital foreign bodies.

Treatment

The objectives of emergency management of ocular penetrating or perforating injuries are to relieve pain, preserve or restore vision, and achieve a good cosmetic result. *Avoid needless examination.*

Relieve pain with systemic analgesia, as needed. A sedative may be required. Cover the eye with an eye shield. Patch the uninjured eye also to minimize ocular movements. Do not manipulate the eye, instill eye drops, or apply antibiotic treatment.

Give tetanus prophylaxis if needed (Chapter 30.) Prohibit oral intake until the patient is examined by an ophthalmologist, because urgent surgery may be required. Provide hydration with intravenous fluids (eg, 5% dextrose in half-normal saline given at a rate of 125 mL/h for an adult).

Give parenteral antibiotics directed against gram-negative and gram-positive organisms. Give antiemetic agents to prevent further injury from intraocular pressure increase.

Disposition

The patient should be seen by an ophthalmologist for management of severe injuries, investigation of intraocular foreign bodies, and immediate surgical repair as required. Prompt repair of uveal prolapse decreases the risk of sympathetic ophthalmia in the uninjured eye. Delay in management of corneal lacerations may increase the risk of surgical and postoperative complications.

BLUNT TRAUMA TO THE EYE, ADNEXA, & ORBIT

Contusions of the eyeball and ocular adnexa result from blunt trauma. The outcome of such an injury cannot always be determined, and the extent of damage may not be obvious upon superficial examination. Careful eye examination is needed, along with x-ray examination or CT scan when indicated.

Types of Injury

A. EYELIDS

Check the eyelids for ecchymosis (see below), swelling, laceration, and abrasions.

B. CONJUNCTIVA

Check the conjunctiva for subconjunctival hemorrhages or laceration of the conjunctiva.

C. CORNEA

Check the cornea for edema, laceration, or rupture.

D. ANTERIOR CHAMBER

Check the anterior chamber for hyphema, recession of angle, or secondary glaucoma.

E. IRIS

Check the iris for iridodialysis, iridoplegia, rupture of iris sphincter, iris prolapse through corneal or scleral lacerations, or iris atrophy (later).

F. CILIARY BODY

Check the ciliary body for hyposecretion of aqueous humor or for ciliary body prolapse through scleral lacerations.

G. LENS

Check the lens for dislocation or cataract (later).

H. VITREOUS

Check the vitreous for hemorrhage or prolapse.

I. CILIARY MUSCLE

Check the ciliary muscle for paralysis or spasm.

Treatment & Disposition

Injury severe enough to cause intraocular hemorrhage (eg, vitreous hemorrhage or hyphema) involves the danger of delayed secondary hemorrhage from a damaged uveal vessel, which may cause intractable glaucoma and permanent damage to the eyeball. In such cases, immediate ophthalmologic consultation is necessary to rule out other eye injuries.

Except for rupture of the eyeball itself, contusions do not usually require immediate definitive treatment. Apply an eye shield if the globe has been perforated and consult ophthalmology immediately.

Use atropine, 1% eye drops, twice daily. Acetazolamide, mannitol, or other systemic agents may be necessary to lower intraocular pressure. Give systemic analgesia.

Refer all patients to an ophthalmologist.

1. Ecchymosis of the Eyelids (Black Eye)

Clinical Findings

Blood in the periorbital tissues may occur from direct trauma or a blow to adjacent areas (eg, nose). The loose subcutaneous tissue around the eye permits blood to spread extensively. The diagnosis is usually obvious. Always rule out trauma to the eye itself (hyphema, blowout fracture, or retinal detachment).

Treatment

Apply cold compresses to decrease swelling and help stop bleeding. Twenty-four hours later, apply warm compresses to accelerate absorption of the hematoma. Exclude more serious ocular injury by careful examination.

Disposition

If the eye itself is uninjured, no follow-up contact is necessary.

2. Lacerations of the Eyelids

Clinical Findings

Lacerations or other wounds of the eyelids may be associated with serious ocular injuries not apparent at first examination, for example, injury to the lacrimal system, levator muscle, or optic nerve. A meticulous search for such injuries is mandatory in every patient with eyelid lacerations.

Treatment & Disposition

Patients with lacerations of the eyelids require suturing and then complete ophthalmologic evaluation. Lacerations involving the tarsal plate, the upper eyelids, or medial canthal area should be repaired by an ophthalmologist.

3. Orbital Hemorrhage

Clinical Findings

Exophthalmos and subconjunctival hemorrhage in a patient with a history of blunt trauma to the face suggest rupture of orbital blood vessels. There may be conjunctival chemosis or ecchymosis of the eyelids.

Treatment & Disposition

Apply cold compresses, and obtain urgent ophthalmologic consultation. Hospitalize the patient for observation if severe injury has occurred.

4. Fracture of the Ethmoid Bone

The ethmoid bone is part of the medial wall of the orbit. Fracture of the ethmoid bone most frequently occurs with blunt trauma to the orbit.

Clinical Findings

Fracture of the ethmoid bone is manifested by subcutaneous emphysema of the eyelids. There may or may not be ecchymosis of the eyelids. X-ray reveals air in the orbit. Fractures of other orbital bones should be ruled out by radiography.

Treatment

Fractures of the ethmoid bone usually do not require operative reduction. Provide analgesia as needed. Apply cold compresses. Give systemic antibiotic. Instruct the patient to avoid sneezing or blowing the nose.

Disposition

Refer the patient to an ophthalmologist within 1–2 days.

5. Blowout Fractures of the Floor of the Orbit

Clinical Findings

Blowout fracture may be associated with enophthalmos and hypotropia (visual axis of the injured eye is displaced downward in comparison to that of the sound eye), diplopia in the primary position or in upward gaze, limitation of ocular movement in upward gaze, and decreased or absent sensation over the maxilla. CT scan of the orbit shows orbital floor displacement.

Treatment

Provide analgesia as needed. Apply a topical antibiotic ointment such as gentamicin, 0.3%. Apply cold compresses and a sterile eye patch.

Disposition

Hospitalize the patient, and seek early consultation with an ophthalmologist and otolaryngologist because of possible fractures of the maxilla or zygoma. Obtain CT scan of the orbit.

6. Corneal Abrasions

 ESSENTIALS OF DIAGNOSIS

- *Pain, photophobia, blurring vision.*
- *Fluorescein stain is key to diagnosis.*
- *Always rule out globe perforation.*

Clinical Findings

The patient complains of pain, photophobia, and blurring of vision. There is usually a history of trivial trauma. Patients with severe pain and blepharospasm may require proparacaine, 0.5%, instilled in the eye to facilitate eye examination. In severe cases, the eye is red and the corneal surface is irregular and loses its normal luster. Staining with fluorescein reveals a defect in the corneal epithelium. Always rule out infection or perforation of the globe.

Treatment

Irrigate the eye gently with sterile saline solution to remove the debris and loose foreign bodies. In severe cases, instill 2 drops of either atropine, 1%, or homatropine, 5%, to relax the ciliary muscle and relieve pain. Instill ophthalmic antibiotic ointment. ***Caution:*** Do not use ointment containing corticosteroids.

Provide analgesia as needed, for example, acetaminophen with codeine, 30 mg, orally. Avoid giving the patient topical anesthetics, which may lead to irreversible corneal damage.

Disposition

Refer patients for daily outpatient follow-up care. Ophthalmologic consultation should be obtained for corneal abrasions that fail to resolve in 48–72 hours.

7. Corneal & Conjunctival Foreign Bodies

 ESSENTIALS OF DIAGNOSIS

- *Pain, foreign body sensation.*
- *Use fluorescein; make sure to look under lids.*
- *May need to rule out intraocular foreign body.*

Clinical Findings

There may be a history of working with high-speed tempered steel tools (eg, drilling), or there may be no history of trauma to the eye and the patient may even be unaware of a foreign body in the eye. In most cases, however, the patient complains of a foreign body sensation in the eye or under the eyelid, or just irritation in the eye. A corneal foreign body can be seen with the aid of a loupe and well-focused diffuse light. Conjunctival foreign bodies often become embedded in the conjunctiva under the upper eyelid. The lid must be everted (see Figure 31–5) to facilitate inspection and removal.

Sterile fluorescein should be instilled to visualize minute foreign bodies not readily visible with the naked eye or loupe. Rule out intraocular foreign body (in certain cases, soft tissue x-ray or CT scan may be required for this purpose).

Treatment

Some loose foreign bodies can be removed with a moist cotton swab. Foreign bodies superficially embedded can be removed with the tip of a hypodermic needle or blunt spud. Anesthetize the cornea first with proparacaine or tetracaine solution, 0.5%. Instill ophthalmic antibiotic ointment (gentamicin, 0.3%; or sulfacetamide, 10%).

Disposition

After the foreign body has been removed, the patient should be seen again in 24 hours to make certain that infection has not occurred. Refer the patient to an ophthalmologist if foreign bodies are deeply embedded in the cornea, because they may have to be removed in the operating room under magnification.

Brady SM et al: The diagnosis and management of orbital blowout fractures: Update 2001. Am J Emerg Med 2001;19:147. [PMID: 11239261]

Hamill MB: Current concepts in the treatment of traumatic injury to the anterior segment. Ophthalmol Clin North Am 1999; 12:457.

Harlan JB Jr et al: Evaluation of patients with ocular trauma. Ophthalmol Clin North Am 2002;15:153. [PMID: 12229230]

Kuckelkorn R: Emergency treatment of chemical and thermal eye burns. Acta Ophthalmol Scand 2002;80:4. [PMID: 11906296]

Mester V et al: Intraocular foreign bodies. Ophthalmol Clin North Am 2002;15:235. [PMID: 12229240]

Reich J: Investigating a foreign body. Part 1—Where and how to look. Aust Fam Physician 2000;29:974. [PMID: 11059088]

Reich J: Investigating a foreign body. Part 2—Removal. Aust Fam Physician 2000;29:1086. [PMID: 11127070]

Reppucci VS et al: Current concepts in the treatment of traumatic injury to the posterior segment. Ophthalmol Clin North Am 1999;12:465.

Schrage RF: Eye burns: an emergency and continuing problem. Burns 2000;26:689. [PMID: 11024601]

V. EQUIPMENT & SUPPLIES

Basic Equipment

A great many specialized instruments have been devised for the investigation of eye disorders. Most emergency conditions can be diagnosed with the aid of a few relatively simple instruments. The following should be available in the emergency department:

- Hand flashlight with fresh batteries
- Slit lamp
- Ophthalmoscope (preferably with lens that has a blue filter)
- Visual acuity chart (Snellen)
- Tonometer
- Pinhole and occluder
- Eye shield (plastic or metal) and tape

Basic Medications

See Table 31–5.

A. LOCAL ANESTHETICS

Proparacaine, 0.5%, or tetracaine, 0.5%, may be used.

B. DYES

Sterile fluorescein papers should be on hand.

C. MYDRIATICS

Tropicamide ophthalmic solution, 0.5% or 1%, is a satisfactory mydriatic when the examiner wishes to obtain a clear view of the lens, vitreous, or ocular fundus. Eye drops (atropine, 1%; or homatropine, 5%) may be used in patients with iritis.

D. MIOTICS

The miotic agent pilocarpine, 1% or 2%, should be on hand.

E. ANTIBACTERIAL AGENTS

Antibacterial agents include tetracycline, 1% ophthalmic ointment; polymyxin B-bacitracin ophthalmic ointment; sulfacetamide, 10% ophthalmic solution or ointment; or gentamicin, 0.3% ointment.

VI. COMMON TECHNIQUES FOR TREATMENT OF OCULAR DISORDERS

Eversion of the Upper Eyelid

See Figure 31–5. The patient is instructed to look down. Grasp the eyelashes at the outer margin of the lid with the thumb and forefinger of one hand, and gently and slowly draw the lid downward and outward. Using a cotton swab, press against the upper edge of the tarsus over the center of the lid while turning the lid margin rapidly outward and upward over the applicator. With the lashes thus held against the upper orbital rim, the exposed palpebral conjunctiva can be inspected closely. After the examination is completed and the foreign body removed (if possible), when the patient looks up, the lid returns to its normal position.

Eye Drops

The patient should sit with both eyes open and looking up. Pull down slightly on the lower lid, and place 2 drops in the lower cul-de-sac. The patient is then asked to look down while finger contact on the lower lid is maintained. Do not let the patient squeeze the eye shut. Do not touch the eye or the eyelid with the applicator; likewise, do not instill eye drops with the dropper held far away from the eye.

Ointments

Ointments are instilled in the same way as liquids. While the patient is looking up, lift out the lower lid to trap the medication in the conjunctival sac. The lids

Table 31–5. Commonly used ophthalmic medications.

Antimicrobials	Uses	Dosage & Dosage Forms
Bacitracin Polysporin (bacitracin and polymyxin B)	Gram-positive and gram-negative organisms	Ophthalmic ointment: place ointment 4 times daily for 7–10 days.
Chloramphenicol (Chloroptic)	Gram-positive and gram-negative organisms	0.5% solution, 1% ointment: 1–2 drops or place ointment 3–6 times daily for 7–10 days.
Ciprofloxacin (Ciloxan) Norfloxacin (Chibroxin) Ofloxacin (Ocuflox)	Gram-positive and gram-negative organisms; covers *Pseudomonas*	0.3% solutions for conjunctivitis: 1–2 drops every 2 hours for 2 days, then every 4 hours for 5 days. For ulcer, 2 drops every 15 minutes for 6 hours, then 2 drops every 30 minutes for the next 18 hours; day 2, use 2 drops every hour; days 3–14, use 2 drops every 4 hours.
Erythromycin (Ilotycin)	Gram-positive organisms, *Chlamydia*	0.5 mg 4 times a day for 5–7 days.
Gentamicin (Genoptic, Garamycin) Tobramycin (Tobrex) Neomycin (Neosporin with bacitracin and polymyxin B)	Gram-positive and gram-negative organisms; covers *Pseudomonas*	Gentamicin and tobramycin as 0.3% solution and 0.3% ointment. Neomycin, 1–2 drops every 2–4 hours 10 days; for ointment, use 2–4 hours for 7–10 days.
Polymyxin B & trimethoprim (Polytrim)	Gram-positive organisms	Ophthalmic solution: 1 drop every 3 hours for 7–10 days.
Sulfacetamide sodium (Bleph-10, Sulamyd)	Gram-positive and gram-negative organisms; does not cover *Pseudomonas*	10%, 15%, 30% solutions: 2 drops every 2–3 hours for 7–10 days. 10% ointment: place ointment every 3–4 hours for 7–10 days.
Trifluridine (Viroptic)	Herpes	1% solution: 1 drop every 2 hours while awake with maximum 9 drops per day. After reepithelialization, decrease to 1 drop every 4 hours for 7 days.
Mydriatics		
Atropine sulfate	Dilation, uveitis, cycloplegia	0.25–2% solution; lasts 2 weeks.
Cyclopentolate (Cyclogyl)	Dilation, cycloplegia	2–5% solution; lasts 48 hours.
Phenylephrine (Neo-Synephrine)[1]	Dilation, no cycloplegia	2.5–10% solution; lasts 2–3 hours.
Scopolamine (Hyoscine)	Dilation, cycloplegia	0.25% solution; lasts 7 days.
Anesthetics[2]		
Proparacaine (Ophthetic Ophthaine)	Local anesthesia	0.5% solution
Tetracaine (Pontocaine)	Local anesthesia	0.5% solution

[1]Cardiac patients should not use phenylephrine.
[2]Anesthetics should not be prescribed for unsupervised use.

should be kept closed for at least 1 minute to allow the ointment to melt. Tubes of ointment may be warmed with warm water before the ointment is instilled in the lower fornix.

Warm Compresses

Use a clean towel or washcloth soaked in warm tap water well below the temperature that will burn the thin skin covering the eyelids. Warm compresses are usually applied to the area for 15 minutes 4 times daily. The therapeutic rational is to increase blood flow to the affected area and decrease pain and inflammation.

Removal of Superficial Corneal Foreign Body

The main considerations are good illumination, magnification, anesthesia, proper positioning of the patient, and sterile technique. If possible, the patient's visual acuity should be recorded first.

The patient may be sitting or supine. A loupe should be used unless a slit lamp is available. (A loupe must be used if the patient is supine.) An assistant should direct a strong flashlight into the eye at an oblique angle. The examiner may then see the corneal foreign body and remove it with a moist cotton swab. If this is not successful, the foreign body may be removed with a metal spud while the lids are held apart with the other hand to prevent blinking. An antibacterial ointment is instilled after the foreign body has been removed.

Note: It is essential to see the patient the next day to be certain infection has not occurred and healing is under way.

Home Medication

At home, the same techniques should be used as described above except that drops should be instilled with the patient lying supine. Experienced patients (eg, those with glaucoma) are usually quite skillful in self-administration of eye drops.

Tonometry

Tonometry is the determination of intraocular pressure using a special instrument that measures the amount of corneal indentation produced by a given weight. Tonometry readings should be taken on any patient suspected of having increased intraocular pressure.

A. PRECAUTIONS

Tonometry should be done with great caution on patients with corneal ulcers. It is extremely important to clean the tonometer before each use by carefully wiping the footplate with a cotton swab moistened with sterile solution (be sure it is dry before using) and to sterilize the instrument once a day (dry heat). The tonometer should be sterilized by flame or in a hot-air tonometer sterilizer after use on an inflamed eye.

Corneal abrasions are rarely caused by tonometry. Epidemic keratoconjunctivitis can be spread by tonometry, and this can be prevented if the tonometer is cleaned before each use and the principle of handwashing between patients is meticulously observed.

B. TECHNIQUE

Anesthetic solution (tetracaine, 0.5%; or proparacaine, 0.5%) is instilled into each eye. The patient lies supine and is asked to stare at a spot on the ceiling with both eyes or at a finger held directly in the line of gaze overhead. The lids are held open without applying pressure on the globe. The tonometer is then placed on the corneal surface of each eye and the scale reading taken from the tonometer. The intraocular pressure is determined by referring to a chart that converts the scale reading to millimeters of mercury for a Schiotz tonometer. If the scale reading is 4 or less, the 7.5-g and 10-g weights are added separately to gain further information concerning the intraocular pressure. Normal intraocular pressure is 12–20 mm Hg.

C. INTERPRETATION OF ABNORMALITIES

If the intraocular pressure is 20 mm Hg or more, further investigation is indicated to determine whether glaucoma is present. Tonometry is an effective screening device to select patients for glaucoma testing. Visual field testing and ophthalmoscopic examination should be done and tonometry repeated several times at different hours of the day or on different days before a diagnosis of glaucoma is warranted. If the pressure remains high on successive readings and there is a visual field defect or cupping of the optic disks, the diagnosis of glaucoma is established. In borderline cases, tonography may be helpful in establishing the presence or absence of glaucoma.

Corneal Staining

Corneal staining consists of instillation of fluorescein into the conjunctival sac to outline irregularities of the corneal surface. Staining is indicated in corneal trauma or other corneal disorders (eg, herpes simplex keratitis) when examination with a loupe or slit lamp in the absence of a stain has not been satisfactory.

A. PRECAUTIONS

Because the corneal epithelium—the chief barrier to corneal infection—is usually interrupted when corneal staining is indicated, be certain that whatever dye is used (particularly fluorescein) is sterile.

B. EQUIPMENT AND MATERIALS

Note: Fluorescein must be sterile. Fluorescein papers or sterile individual dropper units are safest. Fluorescein solution from a dropper bottle may be used, but there is a substantial risk of contamination.

C. TECHNIQUE

The individually wrapped fluorescein paper is wetted with sterile saline or touched to the wet conjunctiva so that a thin film of fluorescein spreads over the corneal surface. Any irregularity in the cornea is stained by the fluorescein and is thus more easily visualized using a light with a blue filter.

D. NORMAL AND ABNORMAL FINDINGS

If there is no superficial corneal irregularity, a uniform film of dye covers the cornea. If the corneal surface has been altered, the affected area absorbs more of the dye and will stain a deeper green. It is customary to sketch the staining area on the patient's record for later comparison to show the progress of healing.

Estimation of Anterior Chamber Depth

See Figure 31–3. Using a hand flashlight, shine the light obliquely and parallel to the plane of the iris across the cornea and anterior chamber. A normal anterior chamber will be fully illuminated. With a shallow anterior chamber (as in angle-closure glaucoma), the anteriorly displaced iris will cast a shadow.

■ VII. COMMON PITFALLS TO BE AVOIDED IN THE MANAGEMENT OF OCULAR DISORDERS

Dangers in the Use of Local Anesthetics

Unsupervised self-administration of local anesthetics is dangerous, because the patient may further injure an anesthetized eye without knowing it. Furthermore, most anesthetics delay healing. This is particularly true

of butacaine, which also elicits a high incidence of allergic responses. Therefore, patients should not be given local anesthetics to take home. Eye pain should be controlled by systemic analgesics.

Errors in Diagnosis

The most common mistaken ophthalmologic diagnosis is conjunctivitis when the correct diagnosis should be iritis (anterior uveitis), glaucoma, or corneal ulcer (especially herpes simplex ulcer). The differentiation between iritis and acute glaucoma may be difficult also.

Misuse of Atropine

Atropine must never be used in routine diagnosis. It causes cycloplegia (paralysis of the ciliary muscle) of about 14 days' duration and can precipitate an attack of glaucoma if the patient has a narrow anterior chamber angle.

Dangers of Local Corticosteroid Therapy

Local ophthalmologic corticosteroid preparations (eg, prednisolone) are often used for their anti-inflammatory effect on the conjunctiva, cornea, and iris. Although a patient with conjunctivitis, corneal inflammation, or iritis can be made more comfortable with topical corticosteroids, it must be stressed that the corticosteroids are associated with 4 very serious complications when used in the eye: herpes simplex keratitis, open-angle glaucoma, cataract formation, and fungal infection.

The most common complications are herpes simplex keratitis and glaucoma. Corticosteroids enhance the pathogenicity of herpes simplex virus, apparently by increasing the destructive effect of collagenase on the collagen of the cornea. This is evidenced by the fact that perforation of the cornea occasionally occurs when corticosteroids are used during the more active stage of herpes simplex cornea infection. Corneal perforation was a rare complication of dendritic keratitis before corticosteroids came into general use. In the treatment of any corneal inflammation, particularly if the corneal epithelium is not intact, the prolonged use of corticosteroids is sometimes complicated by fungal infection, and this may lead to loss of the eye. Topical corticosteroids can cause or aggravate open-angle glaucoma and, less commonly, can produce cataracts.

For these reasons, although corticosteroids are valuable in the treatment of ocular disease, any patient on whom they are being used should be watched carefully for the development of complications. Corticosteroids should not be used unless specifically indicated (eg, in iritis, certain types of keratitis, and acute allergic disorders), and patients using prescribed topical corticosteroids should always see an ophthalmologist for follow-up examination.

Use of Contaminated Eye Medications

The external coats of the eye, including the sclera and the corneal epithelium, are resistant to infection. However, once the corneal epithelium or sclera is broken by trauma, the tissues become markedly susceptible to bacterial infection. For this reason, ophthalmic solutions that may be used in injured eyes must be prepared with the same degree of caution as fluids intended for intravenous administration.

Sterile, single-use disposable units of the common ophthalmic solutions should be used whenever liquid medication is instilled into an injured eye. For routine use in intact eyes, nearly all eye medications are now available in small plastic containers. It is safe to use these medications provided they are not kept a long time after opening (eg, > 1 month) and are not contaminated accidentally.

Overtreatment

Some patients with chronic conjunctivitis or keratitis may be made worse by overtreatment with topical medications. These patients should be evaluated by an ophthalmologist.

Liu GT et al: The neuro-ophthalmologic examination (including coma). Ophthalmol Clin North Am 2001;14:23. [PMID: 11370569]

ENT Emergencies: Disorders of the Ear, Nose, Sinuses, Oropharynx, & Mouth

32

David C. Van, MD, MS

I. Immediate Management of Potentially Harmful Problems

    Ear Pain
    Hearing Loss
    Vertigo
    Epistaxis
    Nasal Obstruction
    Sore Throat
    Tooth Fracture
    Tooth Subluxation or Avulsion
    Postextraction Tooth Hemorrhage

II. Management of Specific Disorders

  Disorders of the Ear
    Cerumen Impaction

    Frostbite
    Chronic (Suppurative) Otitis Media
  Disorders of the Sinuses (Sinusitis)
  Disorders of the Oropharynx
    Peritonsillitis (Peritonsillar Cellulitis & Abscess)
    Epiglottitis
    Croup
  Disorders of the Mouth
    Tooth Anatomy
    Tooth Pain
    TMJ Pain
    TMJ Dislocation

■ I. IMMEDIATE MANAGEMENT OF POTENTIALLY HARMFUL DISORDERS

EAR PAIN

The complaint of ear pain is more common among children than adults and usually relates to an infectious process. Though some conditions are serious, patients with most ear pain conditions can receive treatment and be discharged by the emergency physician without consultation (Table 32–1).

Clinical Findings

A. HISTORY

Ask patients about history of trauma, surgery, or recurrent infections involving the ear. Also ask about specific symptoms (eg, recent fever, upper respiratory infection, or canal discharge) and pain quality (eg, pain, pressure, itching, or "buzzing" sounds). Have the patient identify the exact location of the pain. A narrow differential diagnosis can be explored based on these historical characteristics.

B. PHYSICAL EXAMINATION

Palpate the area surrounding the ear to identify lymph nodes or a bony prominence. Tender nodes are common in infections of the middle and external ear. Pain, swelling, and erythema at the mastoid process should prompt the clinician to consider mastoiditis. If the pain relates to the canal, examine its external orifice for evidence of discharge. Next, view the canal and tympanic membrane. Make careful note of the appearance of the tympanic membrane regarding color; reflectivity; visibility of landmarks; and presence of fluid, air bubbles behind the membrane, or perforations. Check tympanic membrane motility by insufflation. Compare to the normal ear. If the ear exam is normal, look to the upper teeth and temporomandibular joint as possible causes.

Table 32–1. Diagnosis and treatment of ear pain.

Diagnosis	Diagnostic Clues	Treatment	Comments
Acute mastoiditis	Fever or chills; pain, swelling, and erythema at mastoid process. Typically an extension of acute otitis media. Normal canal and findings of concurrent otitis media.	ENT consultation, admission, IV antibiotics, possible necessity for surgical intervention. Cefotaxime, 1 g IV q 24 h, or ceftriaxone, 1–2 g IV q 24 h.	Relatively rare. Usually *S pneumoniae, S pyogenes, S. aureus*. If it develops after resolved otitis media: acute coalescent mastoiditis.
Bullous myringitis	Severe ear pain. TM: bullae on TM surface, with surrounding erythema. Middle ear space not affected.	Erythromycin (EES, adult: 400 mg qid; child: 10 mg/kg qid), doxycycline, azithromycin.	*Mycoplasma* (or viral).
Chrondritis, perichondritis	Pain or swelling to the external (cartilaginous) ear. Recent ear trauma. Warm, erythematous, tender auricle, pinna skin. Evidence of recent trauma or piercing. If ear is deformed, suspect chondritis (cartilage infection).	Remove foreign bodies, irrigate wounds. Warm soaks and oral cephalexin. Outpatient ENT follow-up. If evidence of cartilage involvement, ENT consultation, admission, IV antibiotics.	
Foreign body	Usually young child, witnessed insertion. Foreign body in canal.	Removal is typically uncomfortable. Tailor method to the characteristics of the foreign body (Frazier suction, alligator forceps, curette). Prep with topical anesthetic. Children may require restraint or sedation.	If canal trauma is present, treat as for otitis externa, outpatient follow-up.
Infected sebaceous cyst	Pain in canal. No discharge. Erythematous, cystic canal surface. Pain with pinna traction.	Incise and drain cysts. Cephalexin or dicloxacillin. Outpatient ENT follow-up.	May prevent recurrence with selenium sulfide (Selsun) or ketoconazole/steroid shampoo.
Insect in canal	Buzzing or movement sensation. Insect in canal or on TM.	Immobilization will relieve the discomfort. Instill lidocaine in the canal with a syringe and flexible catheter. Flush out when patient is calm.	Alternatively, may remove a large insect with narrow alligator forceps through the otoscope.
Otitis externa (swimmer's ear)	Common in regular swimmers. Ear pain, itching. Purulent discharge, erythematous canal, pain with pinna traction. Canal may be occluded by wall edema. Normal hearing unless canal is occluded.	Place a cotton wick through an obstructed or near-obstructed canal. Treat with topical steroid and antibiotic preparations: hydrocortisone-polymyxinneomycin (Cortisporin Otic), 4 drops qid, or hydrocortisone-ciprofloxacin (Cipro HC Otic), 3 drops bid.	Typically *Pseudomonas*. Outpatient follow-up within 3 days. Reduce recurrence risk with drying rubbing alcohol drops following water exposure. Consider malignant variant in diabetic, immunocompromised, or elderly patients.
Otitis externa (malignant)	Elderly, immunocompromised, or diabetic patient with findings of otitis externa. Physical findings as above.	ENT consultation, admission, IV antibiotics (imipenem-cilastatin, 500 mg IV q 6 h; ciprofloxacin, 400 mg IV q 12 h or 750 mg PO q 12 h).	*Pseudomonas* can cause rapidly progressing, necrotizing disease among vulnerable patients. Outpatient treatment may be acceptable in early disease. CT scan if mastoid osteomyelitis is suspected.

(continued)

Table 32–1. Diagnosis and treatment of ear pain. (Continued)

Diagnosis	Diagnostic Clues	Treatment	Comments
Serous/secretory otitis media	Preceding upper respiratory infection or otitis media. Unilateral hearing loss, pain, pressure, or bubbling sound (all of variable severity). Normal canal. TM not erythematous, but decreased motility and light reflex. Landmarks visible. Air-fluid levels behind TM.	Decongestant for 14 days.	Not infectious. Relates to eustachian canal obstruction. Obtain ENT evaluation if it doesn't resolve in 2 weeks. Some clinicians differentiate serous (mobile fluid) from secretory (thick, nonmotile fluid) otitis, but treatment is the same.
Suppurative otitis media	Common in children. Preceding upper respiratory infection. May lead to TM rupture (severe pain followed by rapid, spontaneous relief). Normal canal. TM is erythematous, dull light reflex, limited motility (most specific), landmarks not visible. Compare to other side. Make note of TM rupture, if present. Decreased hearing on affected side.	Amoxicillin (adults: 500 mg tid × 10 d; children: 15 mg/kg tid × 10 d). If child has had abscess in past month: high-dose amoxicillin (30 mg/kg tid × 10 d). If recent treatment failure: amoxicillin-clavulanate (Augmentin, 25–30 mg/kg tid × 10 d). Other options: trimethoprim/sulfamethoxazole, cefuroxime, ceftriaxone IM.	Typical organisms: *S pneumonia, H influenzae* (children). Ruptured TM will require follow-up every 2–4 weeks to ensure healing.

TM = tympanic membrane.

C. Other Studies

If history and physical examination suggest mastoiditis, computed tomography (CT) scan should be obtained.

Treatment

Each condition requires a specific treatment (see Table 32–1).

HEARING LOSS

Sudden hearing loss is a deficit of less than 3 days duration and may be partial or complete. Diagnoses can be categorized as conductive (external or middle ear cause) or sensorineuronal (inner ear or cochlear nerve–central nervous system cause). Medication-related injuries are usually dose and duration related, which should be considered when determining which patients are at risk for this complication. Many potential causes must be considered (Table 32–2).

Table 32–2. Causes of sudden hearing loss.

Conductive
Foreign body or mass (U)
Otitis externa with obstruction (U)
Otitis media (U)
Otosclerosis (U)
Tympanic membrane rupture (U)
Infectious
Herpes (simplex, zoster) (B)
Mononucleosis (Epstein-Barr virus, cytomegalovirus) (B)
Mumps (B)
Syphilis (B)
Hematologic
Berger disease (B)
Leukemia (B)
Polycythemia (B)
Sickle cell anemia (B)
Metabolic
Diabetes mellitus (B)
Hyperlipidemia (B)
Medication
Aminoglycosides (B)
Loop diuretics (B)
Salicylates (B)
Other
Acoustic neuroma (U)
Acoustic trauma (loud noise) (U or B)
Meniere disease (U or B)

Note: All are sensorineuronal except in the conductive category. U = unilateral; B = bilateral (typically).

SENSINEURONAL

Clinical Findings

A. History

The patient's account of precipitating events (trauma or recent activities) and the duration of symptom onset (seconds, hours, days) should help narrow the focus on possible causes. Unilateral deafness should increase the suspicion for a conductive process (or acoustic neuroma), whereas bilateral symptoms would suggest a systemic (metabolic or drug-related) problem. Take a careful medication history. Severity (partial versus complete loss of hearing) also should be assessed. Finally, the presence of tinnitus, vertigo, or neurologic symptoms should alert the clinician to the likelihood of a sensorineuronal cause.

B. Physical Examination

Look at the canals and tympanic membranes to rule out foreign body obstruction, infection, or injury. The cranial nerves should be examined. Weber and Rinne tests are useful for differentiating between conductive and sensorineuronal causes. The Webber test is performed by placing a vibrating 512-Hz tuning fork on the midparietal head (Figure 32–1). In unilateral conductive hearing loss, sound is heard more loudly in the impaired ear (it is more sensitized from previous decreased stimulus from the air). The Rinne test requires the base of a vibrating fork to be placed on the mastoid process. At the point when the patient cannot hear the sound, it is quickly moved off the bone and the tines placed at

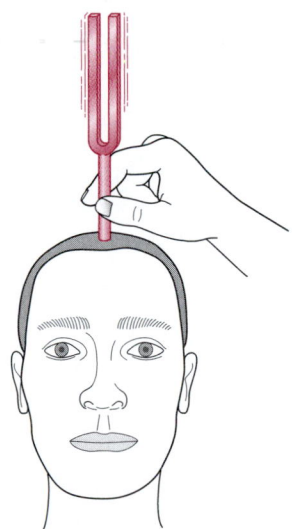

Figure 32–1. In the Webber test, vibrations are louder on the side with a conductive deficit.

the ear canal (Figure 32–2). Repeat on each side. Normally, the patient can hear through the air longer than with bone conduction, but a pronounced difference indicates sensorineural loss. A conductive deficit in either ear will make bone conduction louder than air on the affected side.

C. OTHER STUDIES

Bloodwork is helpful if infectious or metabolic causes are being considered. CT scan is appropriate for a suspected acoustic neuroma.

Treatment

Treatment should be directed toward the underlying disorder. Rapid follow-up by the appropriate provider (ie, otolaryngologist, neurologist) is recommended.

VERTIGO
— Ear canal — nystagmus
— TM
— CN
— CNS

True vertigo (room spinning, exaggerated or fictitious sensation of motion) can be quite disconcerting to patients, some of whom present in dramatic discomfort.

Clinical Findings

A. HISTORY

The most important determination is between central (central nervous system) and peripheral (relating to the 8th cranial nerve or the inner ear apparatus) causes. This classification usually can be resolved on the basis of history alone (Table 32–3). Symptoms that are severe, of recent or sudden onset, and related to head movement typically relate to a peripheral disorder. Ask about recent use of potentially vestibulotoxic drugs:

aminoglycosides, vancomycin, phenytoin, quinidine, and minocycline have been implicated. Caffeine, nicotine, and alcohol are known to exacerbate symptoms. Head trauma can occasionally lead to semichronic symptoms (lasting months to years). Specific causes of peripheral vertigo are described in Table 32–4.

B. PHYSICAL EXAMINATION *CN-8 — AUDITORY*

Examine the ear canal, tympanic membrane, cranial nerves, and cerebellar function. All patients with vertigo may have difficulty with the tandem walk exercise, but the presence of focal cerebellar exam findings (rapid alternating movements, heel-shin slide, or finger-to-nose pointing tests) should raise suspicion for a central cause. Indentifying nystagmus, especially with head movement and extreme left and right lateral gaze, is a crucial part of narrowing the differential diagnosis. The Dix-Hallpike test can help elicit the vertigo symptoms and nystagmus if they are not present at rest. In this test, the examiner places a hand on the patient's occiput, and the patient is rapidly reclined from an upright position onto a flat surface. The head should extend off the back edge so that the neck can be somewhat hyperextended. The test can be repeated with the head rotated to each side. A positive result occurs when nystagmus is observed after the movement, or if the patient reports an acute worsening of the vertigo. Nystagmus relating to a peripheral cause typically starts 1–3 seconds and diminishes over 5–30 seconds after head movement. The examiner must quickly observe the eyes after moving the patient. On occasion the symptoms improve by the time of evaluation, and these characteristic signs may be difficult to elicit. Ask family members if they observed unusual eye movements during earlier attacks.

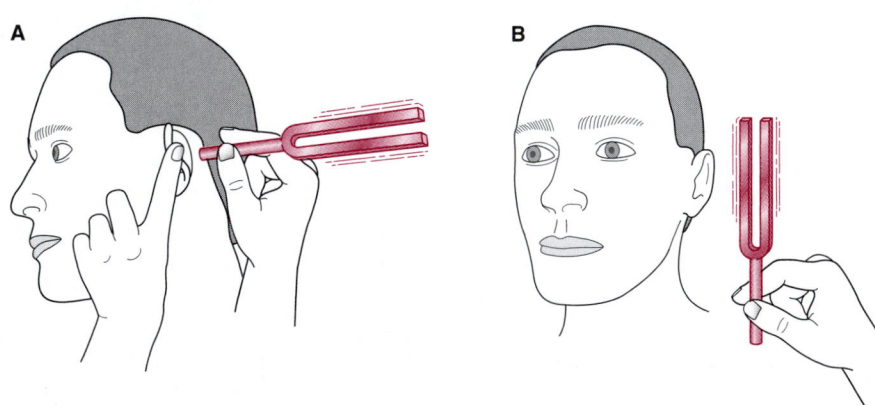

Figure 32–2. Bone vibration that is longer than air vibration indicates a conductive problem. In a sensorineural deficit, air conduction is significantly longer than bone conduction.

Table 32–3. Central versus peripheral vertigo.

Symptom or Examination Finding	Peripheral Causes	Central Causes
Duration of onset	Minutes to hours.	Weeks to months.
Intensity	Severe.	Moderate.
Nausea, vomiting	Typical.	Often absent.
Relation to head movement	Movement exacerbates symptoms.	Often symptoms unrelated to movement.
Patient age	Any; often young.	Usually elderly.
Nystagmus	Always horizontal or rotatory. Worse with head movements and fatigues over 5–30 seconds.	Presence is variable. May be vertical or horizontal with no fatigue.
Cranial nerve or cerebellar deficits	Absent.	Often present (especially ataxia—usually with slow onset; sudden onset suggests cerebellar hemorrhage).
Hearing	Often decreased (unilateral) or with tinnitus.	Usually normal.
Causes	Ménière disease. Labyrinthitis (viral or bacterial). (Benign) positional vertigo. Canal foreign body or otitis media. Acoustic neuroma.	Drugs. Cerebellar mass or stroke. Encephalitis or brain abscess. Vertebral basilar artery insufficiency. Temporal lobe epilepsy. Multiple sclerosis.

Table 32–4. Causes of peripheral vertigo.

Condition	Diagnosis	Comments
Acoustic neuroma	Gradual (days to weeks) onset; unilateral hearing loss and tinnitus. Initially mimics vestibular neuronitis, but symptoms worsen over weeks as tumor progresses centrally. Central signs and symptoms (decreased corneal reflex, ataxia) later in course. Diagnosis by CT scan.	Schwann cell tumor. Recovery correlated with early surgery.
Benign paroxysmal (positional) vertigo	Symptoms and nystagmus associated with head movement—often subsiding gradually several minutes after movement.	Most common cause of peripheal vertigo. Typically no specific cause.
Ménière disease (paroxysmal labyrinthine vertigo)	Associated with unilateral hearing loss and tinnitus. Vertigo with sudden onset and short (1–24 hours) duration. Intense, recurrent, associated with vomiting and distress. Ear pressure. Nystagmus during the attacks, not between or positional.	Sometimes associated with high salt intake; may improve with low-sodium diet.
Suppurative labyrinthitis	Prominent hearing loss and vertigo. Temporally related to recent bacterial infection of middle or inner ear. Diagnosis by CT scan.	CT scan to evaluate for mastoiditis. Requires inpatient treatment with intravenous antibiotics or surgery.
Vestibular neuronitis	Symptom onset over 1–2 hours. Nystagmus and discomfort associated with head movement. No hearing loss.	Lasts 3–7 days, but mild symptoms may persist for weeks. Thought to be related to viral labyrinthitis.

C. OTHER STUDIES

Imaging (by CT scan or magnetic resonance imaging [MRI]) is warranted for patients with a suspected central cause or elderly patients with equivocal findings. MRI provides superior resolution of the cerebellum, though CT scan will typically rule out large lesions.

Treatment

Patients with prolonged nausea and poor fluid intake will often require intravenous hydration. Pharmacotherapy is more successful in peripheral-type vertigo. It is directed at relief of symptoms and does not affect the duration of the illness. The first-line agent is oral meclizine, 25–50 mg every 8–12 hours, but patients unable to manage oral fluids are better off with intravenous normal saline and diazepam, 5–10 mg intravenously (2–4 mg intravenously for the elderly), or transdermal scopolamine (0.5-mg patch). In general, drugs with anticholinergic effects are useful. These include diphenhydramine, 50 mg intramuscularly or orally every 6–8 hours; dimenhydrinate, 50–100 mg intramuscularly or orally every 4 hours; cyclizine, 50 mg orally every 6 hours; promethazine, 25 mg orally, rectally, or intravenously every 6–8 hours; or droperidol, 2.5–5 mg intravenously. Patients with peripheral vertigo can be discharged after moderate improvement of symptoms and ability to take oral liquids. Depending on the cause, symptoms are likely to last several hours to 1 week but may persist for 4–5 weeks. Many patients with central vertigo will require inpatient management targeted at the underlying cause, though those who are comfortable after treatment and have firm follow-up can be discharged.

Alternatively, the particle repositioning (Epley) maneuver can be tried if positional vertigo is suspected. It is based on the belief that moving the canalith to the utricle area of the inner ear will prevent it from stimulating the sensory mechanism. After determining the affected side (this is the nystagmus fast-component direction), perform the Dix-Hallpike test if necessary. It involves rather extreme extension and rotational movements of the neck, and its success depends partly on the patient's ability to tolerate these positions. All motions should be done slowly, such that each full cycle of the maneuver takes 2 minutes. Place the patient in a sitting position, turn the head 45 degrees toward the affected side, lay the patient down and allow the head to extend 45 degrees beyond neutral while hanging off the top edge of the bed. Rotate the extended head to the midline and then 90 degrees away from the affected side (total rotation: 135 degrees). Then flex the neck to neutral, sit the patient up and rotate the head back to midline. The maneuver often must be repeated several times to be successful.

EPISTAXIS

Most episodes of epistaxis do not result in significant blood loss, are not life threatening, and can be managed with minimally invasive measures. However, the clinician will generally be well advised to start with an assessment of hemodynamic stability and provide support (intravenous fluids or blood products) when appropriate. The typical bleeding site is the Kiesselbach area of the anteromedial nostril, an area at risk due to the anastomoses of three separate arteries (Figure 32–3). Though predominantly due to trauma or environmental exposure, epistaxis can rarely be the first symptom of a growing nasal or sinus malignancy.

Clinical Findings

A. HISTORY

Many patients will be predisposed to bleeding, due to warfarin, platelet-inhibiting medications, renal failure, or hemophilia. These conditions require early identification so that a workup can be initiated. Blunt nose trauma or nose picking are common causes of bleeding. In cold seasons, the dry conditions created by noncirculated, heated indoor air can dehydrate the airways, predisposing the nasal mucosa to cracking. The repeated blowing and wiping of a nose in the setting of upper respiratory infection or allergic rhinitis can abrade and injure the mucosal surface. The absence of a sensation of blood in the oropharynx suggests anterior bleeding. Finally, epistaxis risk is increased in pregnancy, and identification of possible pregnancy is relevant for selection of pharmacologic adjuncts to treat the epistaxis.

B. PHYSICAL EXAMINATION

Hemodynamically stable patients are best examined sitting upright. In this position, most blood will exit the anterior nose and ingestion or aspiration will be mini-

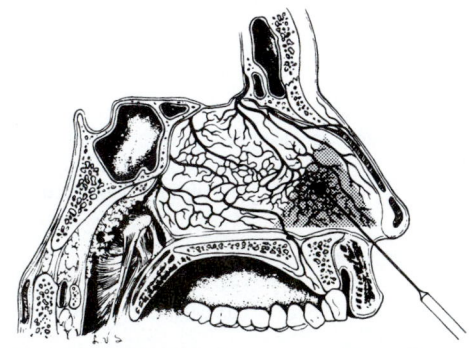

Figure 32–3. Cauterization of bleeding at the Kiesselbach plexus.

mized. If the bleeding is active, the patient should be told to clear each nostril of clots and then be shown how to pinch the entire cartilaginous portion of the nose for 15 minutes. This is sometimes all that is required to stop the bleeding (however, the nose should always be reexamined to confirm hemostasis). During this time, the clinician should don protective clothing and eyewear and set up a headlamp illuminator, a nasal speculum, and a Frazier suction device. The nasal speculum is inserted such that squeezing the handle pushes on the upper and lower margins of the nostril. Both sides of the nose should be examined for bleeding and the integrity of the septum confirmed. Observe the posterior oropharynx for 10–15 seconds to confirm whether fresh blood is flowing down the back wall. A predominance of fresh blood in the oropharynx compared to the anterior nose suggests a posterior source.

Treatment

A. ANTERIOR EPISTAXIS

Epistaxis from an anterior source can usually be controlled without otolaryngologic (ENT) consultation. In general, minimally invasive and technically simple methods are preferred, but refractory bleeding requires escalation to more invasive procedures. Some patients may benefit from gentle opiate or benzodiazepine sedation. While using the Frazier suction device to keep the field clear of blood, apply 1% phenylephrine, 4% cocaine, or 2% lidocaine-epinephrine solution with a cotton swab or pledget for vasoconstriction and local anesthesia. Alternatively these solutions may be sprayed onto the mucosal surface. When the bleeding site can be seen, simple cautery with silver nitrate is often all that is required (see Figure 32–3). Exercise care to use only unilateral, brief applications only to the bleeding site. Rolling the material a short distance from above and over the bleeding site will prevent too much interference from blood flowing downward.

Bleeding that persists should be treated with packing. Several options are available. Lidocaine-epinephrine-, phenylephrine-, or cocaine-soaked pledgets (dilute the latter 2 agents 1:1 with normal saline to minimize systemic effects) can be placed in the inferior nostril via narrow forceps, then successively pushed superiorly until the nostril is packed. Commercial nasal tampons (Merocel) are simple to place after lubrication with a petrolatum-based ointment (Figure 32–4A). They are inserted blindly along the inferior (floor) surface of the nostril to a depth of 8 cm and then expanded with the application of saline or 1:1 dilutions of the vasoconstricting agent. Take care not to injure the lateral turbinates. As the material expands, pressure is uniformly applied to the inner walls, tamponading bleeding. Pro-coagulant products (Surgicel, Gelfoam)

may be used alone or in conjunction with other materials to augment the hemostatic effect.

If none of these methods is successful, a formal anterior pack with petroleum jelly gauze strip material may be necessary. It is placed in a similar fashion to the pledgets: the end of a continuous strip is placed inferiorly and far back in the nose, then pushed up to tamponade the upper surfaces and make room for successive strips. The nostril must be fairly tightly packed, and most clinicians repeat the procedure on the other side if bleeding persists. All patients with nasal packs should receive prophylaxis against bacterial sinusitis: amoxicillin-clavulanate, 875 mg twice daily for adults, 40 mg/kg/d divided 2–3 times daily for children. Packing material should be removed by an otolaryngologist in 3–5 days. Patients with anterior packs can be discharged to home.

B. POSTERIOR EPISTAXIS

Posterior bleeding more typically arises from an arterial source and will not respond to the methods described above. Treatment of this entity requires the use of a Foley catheter or nasal balloon device (Epistat, Nasostat) (Figure 32–4B). In addition to a posterior balloon, the specialized devices have an anterior tamponade apparatus (balloon or expanding tampon) that can be inflated or expanded independently. To prevent ischemia of the anterior nasal mucosa, the anterior portion is intended to exert less pressure than the posterior balloon. Insert it into the nostril such that the balloon is in the posterior portion of the nose. Then inflate the posterior balloon with saline until the point of discomfort. Properly placed, the posterior balloon may be all that is required to stop the bleeding. Usually, though, the anterior nose should be packed with petrolatum gauze (or the anterior balloon or tampon inflated to low pressure with the commercial devices) for tamponade. Patients with posterior packs should be admitted for airway observation, prophylactic antibiotics, and ENT consultation.

NASAL OBSTRUCTION

Most patients who present to the emergency department will have an acute obstruction (foreign body, trauma). Rarely, the problem is a complication of a chronic obstructive condition, such as an infection relating to a tumor or deviated septum.

Clinical Findings

A. HISTORY

Ask the patient how long the symptoms have been present and whether there were any precipitating events. In children, the most common cause of obstruction is a foreign body, often a colorful bead or a piece of food,

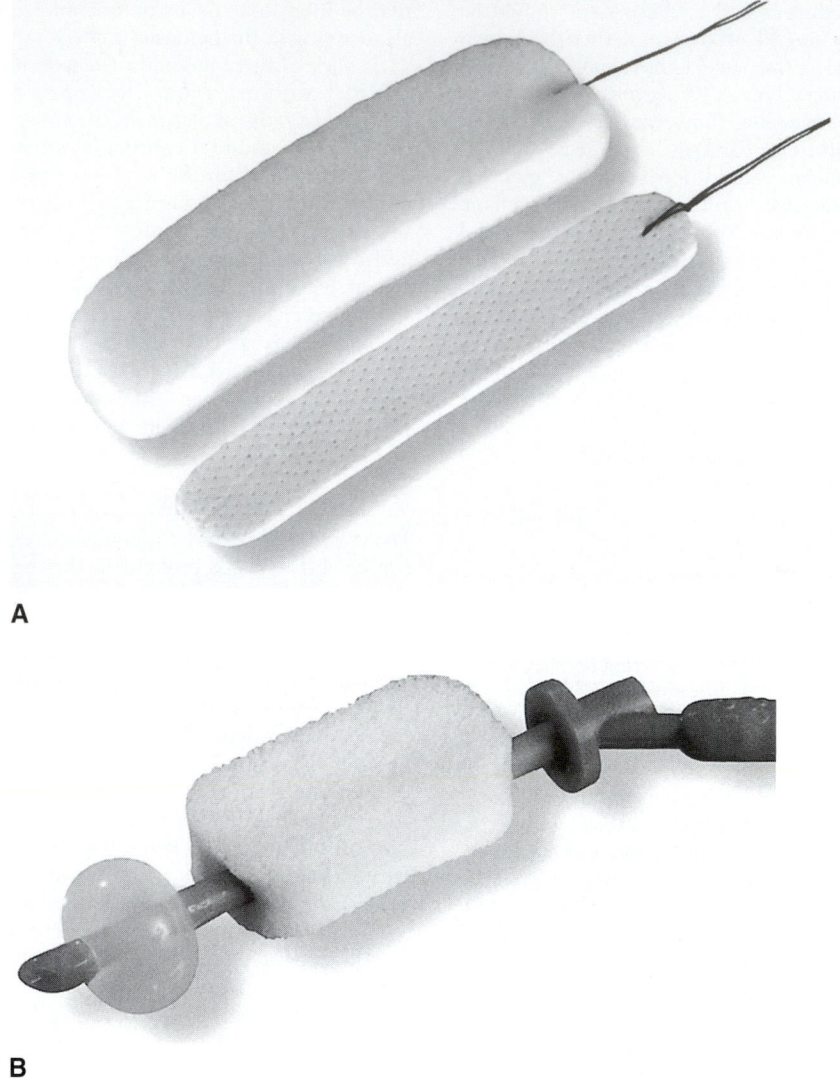

A

B

Figure 32–4. The Xomed Merocel Pope (**A**) and Epistat II (**B**) products.

and the history and diagnosis will be straightforward. Patients should also be queried regarding presence of a discharge. Purulent or foul-smelling liquids suggest an infection component—possible accompanying an established foreign body. Nearly all cases of nasal obstruction will involve one side, negating the risk of airway compromise and allowing for outpatient workup of cases that defy emergency department management.

B. PHYSICAL EXAMINATION

Look into each nostril with the otoscope or a nasal speculum. Most conditions can be characterized and treatment initiated based on direct inspection (Table 32–5).

SORE THROAT

Many conditions lead to the common symptom of throat pain, and although most are relatively benign, several can result in airway compromise and require heroic interventions. The patient who presents with drooling, severe difficulty swallowing, stridor, or difficulty moving air should be examined in a setting where airway equipment is close by. The evaluation of persons

Table 32–5. Diagnosis and treatment of nasal obstruction.

Diagnosis	Diagnostic Clues	Treatment
Abscess	Red, tender, fluctuant mass.	Incise, drain, place temporary wick, or pack inside to prevent recurrence.
Choanal atresia	Neonates only. Nasal tube will be difficult to pass on affected side.	ENT consultation in emergency department.
Deviated septum	Chronic symptoms, though may be acutely worsened by local or sinus infection. Outpatient CT scan will demonstrate extent.	Treat sinusitis, if present. ENT referral.
Foreign body	Typically infants, small children. Objects evident by inspection of the nostril. Purulent discharge may indicate concurrent sinusitis.	Remove with forceps. Alternatively, insert small Foley catheter past the object, inflate balloon, and pull out.
Hematoma	Usually recent history of trauma. Mass is anterior, usually on septum. Examine by transilluminating the septum with bright light.	Incise, drain completely, pack loosely to ensure that mucosal layer is in contact with underlying cartilage.
Polyps	Usually painless, small. Cause minimal obstruction. May be directly visible through nostrils.	ENT referral.
Rhinitis (allergic, viral)	Clear discharge, bilateral symptoms. Allergic rhinitis is usually seasonal or related to environment change or pet exposure. Often with eye involvement. Viral rhinitis has concurrent upper respiratory symptoms.	Symptomatic: decongestants, antihistamines.
Tumor	Gradually progressive symptoms to critical point of emergency department presentation. Discharge may be blood streaked. Mass is nonfluctuant.	ENT referral. Emergency department ENT consultation if bilateral.

with obstructive airway symptoms requires balancing the need for examination and imaging studies with their safety, because certain conditions may worsen with time. If a lateral soft tissue neck x-ray can be safely obtained, it should precede the examination of pediatric patients. It will help rule out epiglottitis and pharyngeal abscess. In some cases, it may be prudent for a person skilled in airway management to observe the patient while x-rays are obtained. In general, children with these symptoms should remain with a parent throughout the preliminary workup, because any distress from parental separation may worsen the condition.

Clinical Findings

A. History

In children, a careful immunization history may help identify those at risk for *Haemophilus influenzae* type B (Hib) infections. Although the incidence of pediatric epiglottitis has fallen dramatically as a result of the Hib vaccine, it is not zero. Over what time course did the problem develop? The rapid development of severe symptoms requires a prompt workup and treatment. Is there associated odynophagia (pain with swallowing) or dysphagia (difficulty swallowing)? These symptoms should prompt the examiner to consider imaging the neck. Fever, cough, or sputum should prompt consideration of infectious causes, and widespread symptoms (eg, headache, body aches, chest and joint pains, diarrhea) suggest a viral source. Sore throat without a cough is more likely to be from a bacterial infection.

B. Physical Examination

Patients with significant airway swelling and compromise (epiglottitis, abscesses) voluntarily sit straight up with the neck slightly extended. Such a general appearance is ominous. Examine the floor of the mouth, looking for focal elevations and tongue displacement. Look at the gingiva for evidence of abscess. Examine the uvula, tonsillar pillars, and entrance of the oropharynx for swelling, exudate, or erythema. Asymmetry should increase the suspicion for an abscess (Figure 32–5). Examine the anterior neck for evidence of lymph node enlargement, other masses, or asymmetry.

C. Other Studies

Lateral and anteroposterior soft tissue neck x-rays can be useful for identifying epiglottis or retropharyngeal abscesses (Figure 32–6). Stable patients will benefit

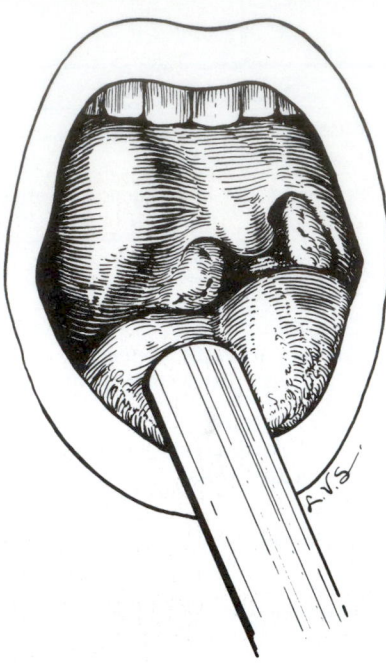

Figure 32–5. Asymmetric tonsillar pillar swelling and uvular displacement are typical of peritonsillitis.

from intravenous contrast CT scan to delineate the exact location and extent of any mass or abscess.

Treatment

Each condition requires specific treatment (Table 32–6). Simple pharyngitis is by far the most common cause of sore throat among children and adults, and viral infections predominate (90%). Recent investigations suggest that differentiating bacterial from viral causes is difficult to accomplish by appearance alone. Yet untreated pediatric group A streptococcal infections are associated with acute rheumatic fever and valvular heart disease. The broad application of antibiotics will inevitably lead to emergence of resistant strains. The combination of throat pain, fever, and tender anterior cervical lymph nodes and the absence of a cough suggest strep and might reasonably be treated immediately. Otherwise, astute clinicians often rely on rapid strep tests or culture to determine which patients need antibiotics. This approach requires a reliable follow-up mechanism to be successful. Anxious parents can usually be convinced of the wisdom of this strategy because it avoids unnecessary antibiotics and their occasional concomitant allergic reaction and other side effects. Among sicker children and adults, the need for admis-

sion will in many cases depend on serial assessment of breathing comfort and ability to take oral liquids.

Refer to the "Oropharynx" section, below, for specific details related to peritonsillitis (peritonsillar cellulitis and abscess) and epiglottitis.

TOOTH FRACTURE

Tooth fractures are graded by the Ellis classification system (Figure 32–7). Fractures of the enamel alone (Ellis class I) require no urgent treatment (save gentle smoothing of any rough edges with sandpaper). An office dentist can fill in the defect later to satisfy cosmetic needs, but there is no risk of long-term damage to the tooth. Class II fractures are deeper and expose the dentin. Such injuries are characterized by a patch of yellow in the middle of the tooth defect. The dentin is vulnerable to bacteria, and prompt covering is essential for long-term preservation of the tooth. The wound should be irrigated with sterile saline, dried, and covered with calcium hydroxide paste or a foil or equivalent dressing. Because the permanent teeth in children have relatively thin dentin layers, bacterial penetration to the pulp is a greater risk in Ellis II fractures and dental consultation is appropriate. If unavailable, apply a dressing and refer the patient for prompt follow-up. Identification of blood or a pink spot in the defect indicates exposure of the pulp and an Ellis class III injury. Typically, this portion of the tooth is quite sensitive, making most class III fractures quite painful. Sterile saline irrigation and emergency department dental consultation are standard. Consider applying a local anesthetic block for management of pain.

TOOTH SUBLUXATION OR AVULSION

Subluxation is a traumatic injury, and results in a tooth that is, to varying degrees, loose in the socket. Gentle pressure alternating from the lingual and buccal aspects of the tooth with a cotton swab will demonstrate the extent of movement and is a necessary part of the evaluation. Primary teeth require no treatment. Patients with minimal laxity (up to 2 mm at tip) can be discharged with advice to eat only liquid or soft foods and follow-up with a dentist. Moderate mobility (more than 2 mm) or teeth that appear partly extruded from the socket depth will require socket reseating and a splint to prevent further injury to the vascular supply and fibrous cementum connections with the underlying alveolar bone. Immobilizing the tooth will maximize its long-term viability. Various materials are available for this purpose, and are generally placed by the dentist in the emergency department. If the emergency physician has access to these materials, he or she may apply the splint

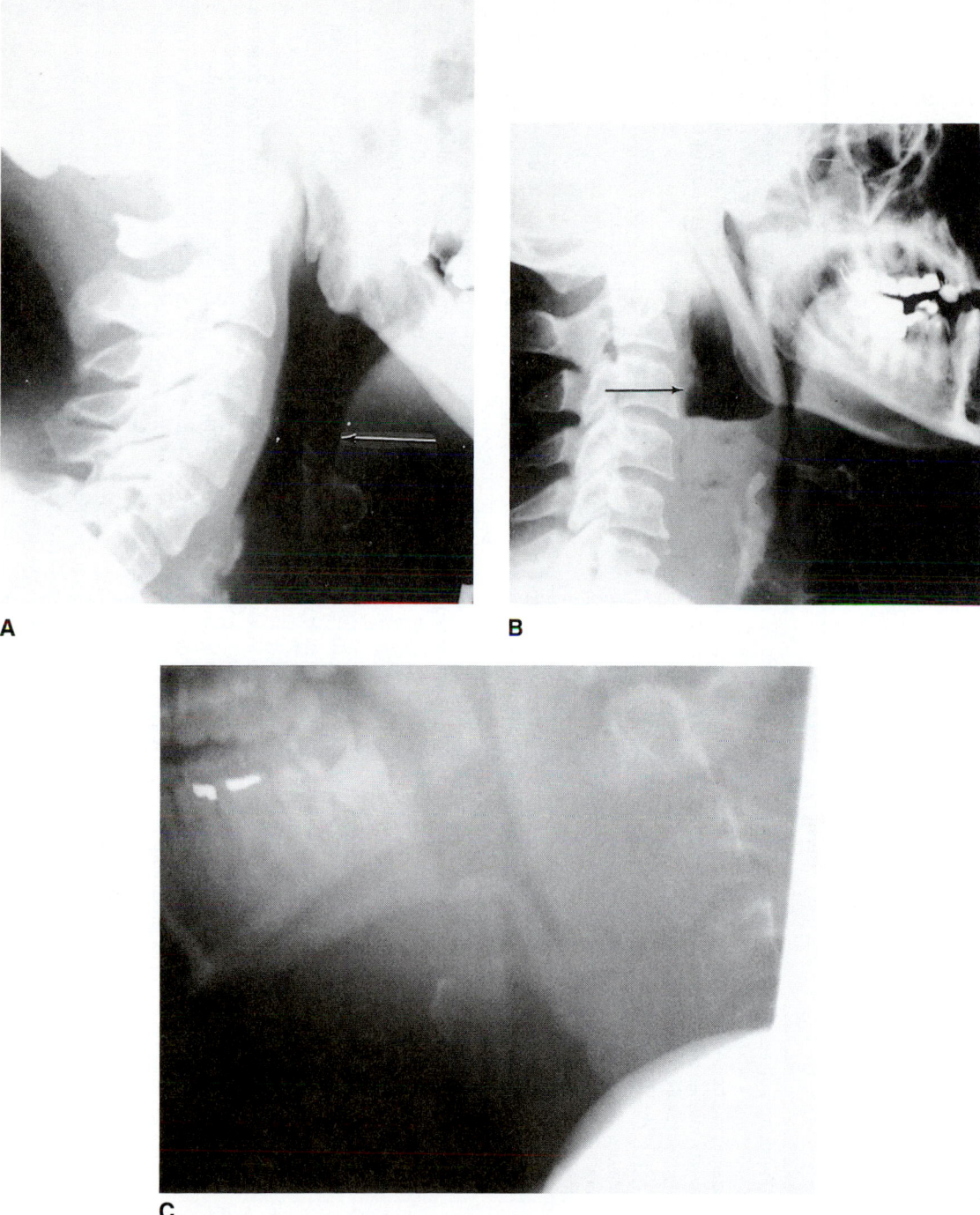

A

B

C

Figure 32–6. Soft-tissue lateral x-rays. **A:** A normal soft tissue lateral x-ray demonstrating no enlargement of the epiglottis or tissues between the airway and cervical vertebrae. **B:** Retropharyngeal abscess in an adult. The airway is displaced anteriorly by a mass that contains an air-fluid level. **C:** Epiglottitis in a child. The epiglottis is enlarged and has a "thumbprint" shape.

Table 32–6. Diagnosis and treatment of sore throat.

Diagnosis	Diagnostic Clues	Treatment	Comments
Allergic reaction	Often history of recent food intake. May progress over 5–30 minutes, when severe. Quality of voice may help identify location of the swelling (hoarse: supraglottic airway; muffled or nasal: oropharynx). Edematous mucosa (uvula, soft palate) may be visible by direct oropharynx inspection.	Epinephrine, 0.3 mg SQ; diphenhydramine, 50 mg IM; methylprednisolone, 125 mg IV/IM. Histamine blockers (famotidine, ranitidine) are controversial. Intubate if severe obstruction is present.	Multiple possible routes of antigen entry, though most are ingestion or inhalation. May be accompanied by hives or ana-phylaxis. Throat pain may be the minor complaint.
Anaerobic phar-yngitis (Vin-cent angina)	May involve mouth and pharynx, associated with poor oral hygiene. Mucosal ulceration, pseudomembranes, foul breath.	Hydrogen peroxide rinses and oral penicillin or doxycycline.	Clinical diagnosis.
Bacterial pharyngitis	Common. Fever; sore throat without cough; bilateral tonsillar swelling; and white, tender cervical lympha-denopathy. Often difficult to differentiate from viral pharyngitis on clinical grounds. Culture.	Although streptococci predominate in children, other organisms (*Mycoplasma, Chlamydia*) may cause some adult illness. Benzathine penicillin, 1.2 million units IM (300,000–600,000 units if <27 kg) affords good compliance.	Consider epiglottitis. Uncommonly causes airway obstruction, but admit patient if oral secretions are difficult to control. Penicillin has a 10–20% failure rate. Use erythromycin or equivalent if treatment failure. Untreated group A streptococcal infection is associated with acute rheumatic fever.
Diphtheria	Ill appearing. Fever, dysphagia common. Prominent gray pseudomembrane over tonsillar pillars. Diphtheria culture of throat swabs.	Give antitoxin, observe for allergic reaction. Erythromycin or penicillin. Admit with respiratory isolation.	Uncommon in United States. Occasional toxic systemic sequelae.
Epiglottitis	Fever, voice hoarseness, severe pain, worse with swal-lowing. Drooling and sniffing position when swelling is severe. Condition is now as or more prevalent in adults, who may have lss acute presentations. Useful studies: soft tissue neck x-ray (enlarged epiglottis—"thumbprint" sign), fiberoptic laryngoscopy (red, swollen only at bedside in stable adults).	Immediate airway intervention in unstable pa-tients or ENT consultation and operating room intubation in less acute children. Consider blood cultures and early IV antibiotics (ceftriaxone, 50 mg/kg IV q 12 h). All patients need admission.	Routine use of the *H influenzae* vaccine has sharply decreased the incidence among children. Epiglottitis in a vaccinated indi-vidual should prompt consideration of an antibiotic with *S aureus* and streptococci coverage.
Gonococcal, chlamydial pharyngitis	Variable exudate, symptoms sometimes mild. Culture of DNA testing of oropharyngeal swabs. Requires genital exam and testing.	Similar to genital infections, though more failures occur with oral form. Ceftriaxone, 125 mg IM × 1 dose, and doxycycline, 100 mg q 12 h × 10 d. Test sex contacts.	Results from orogenital contact. Symptoms may be mild and chronic.

Condition	Clinical features	Management	Comments
Herpes pharyngitis	Vessicles in oropharynx and mouth, exudate, fever. Laboratory examination of lesion scrapings permits confirmation.	Acyclovir, famciclovir, or valacyclovir are indicated in immunocompromised patients and may shorten the course for others.	Typically history of orogenital contact.
Infectious mononucleosis	Fever, pale exudates on tonsillar pillars. Generalized lymphadenopathy, splenomegaly. Monospot and liver function tests. Blood count differential: atypical mononuclear cells.	Supportive care. Consider steroids, IV fluids, and admission for patients with severe swelling and dehydration.	Typically ages 15–30 years.
Ludwig angina	Fever, dysphagia, mouth floor and neck swelling, pain. Often associated with voice change. Typically follows poor dental care or recent lower molar extraction. Elevation and firm, tender floor of mouth—often unilateral. Trismus and firm, tender upper neck often present. CT scan most useful to confirm diagnosis in stable patients.	Position patient upright and protect airway as dictated by clinical appearance. When indicated, fiberoptic intubation is preferred. IV antibiotics for polymicrobial and anaerobic flora: ticarcillin-clavulanate or piperacillin-tazobactam with clindamycin or metronidazole. All patients need admission.	Surgery is required for patients who do not respond to antibiotics. Dental examination and removal of affected teeth. High aspiration complication rate.
Peritonsillar cellulitis and abscess	Most common deep-space infection in throat. A progression of bacterial tonsillitis. Most common in young adults. Fever, difficulty and pain with swallowing, "hot potato" voice, and foul-smelling breath. Trismus is typical, and the exam reveals unilateral soft palate swelling and uvular deviation. Consider CT scan.	Typically responds to incision and drainage, though multiple (3–4) punctures with an 18-gauge needle and aspiration have been advocated. Penicillin and clindamycin. Patients with mild cases and no airway compromise can be discharged with ENT follow-up.	To prevent uncontrolled rupture, use only gentle intraoral pressure on the peritonsillar mass. The carotid artery is 2.5 cm posterior and lateral to the peritonsillar tissue. Avoid deep penetration of the abscess with sharp instruments.
Retropharyngeal, prevertebral abscess	Mainly affects children aged < 6 years. Fever, pain, and difficult swallowing; voice change (described as a "duck quack" sound). Stridor if severe. Pain with forced side-to-side movement of the thyroid cartilage. Lateral neck x-rays demonstrate anterior displacement of trachea by diffuse soft tissue mass. CT scan with IV contrast if plain x-rays not definitive.	Stabilize airway, ENT consultation, IV antibiotics to cover mixed oral and anaerobic infection (see Ludwig angina), admission. Large abscesses will require incision and drainage.	Abscess may rupture into mediastinal or pleural spaces. Presence of trismus and a tender, firm swelling in the anterior neck triangle should increase suspicion for parapharyngeal abscess.

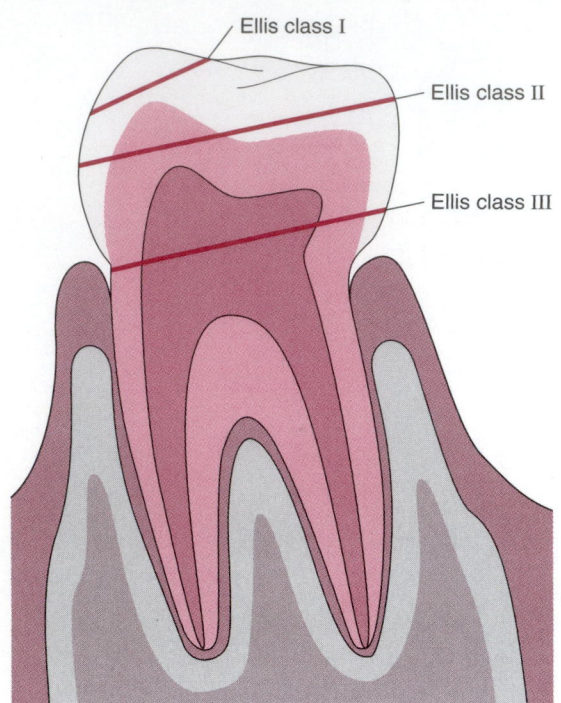

Ellis class I

Ellis class II

Ellis class III

Figure 32–7. The Ellis tooth fracture classification system.

and discharge the patient with dental follow-up. At the very least, a foil-like material can be pressed over the loose tooth and its neighbors to anchor it.

Total avulsion is a somewhat more urgent matter, because the chance for tooth survival falls with every minute it is out of the socket. If the tooth cannot be found, the possibility of tracheal aspiration should be investigated. Hanks' solution is the ideal storage and transportation medium for avulsed teeth, but because it is rarely available outside the hospital, patients who call ahead should be told to put the teeth in milk. Saliva and normal saline are less ideal options, and plain water or a dry surface are to be avoided for reasons of osmolality and cellular desiccation. Dry teeth will benefit from a brief soak in Hanks' Balanced Salt Solution (HBSS) or normal saline, but there should be little delay before replanting them directly into the socket. This procedure cannot wait for the dental consultant and can be done by the first clinician to make contact with the patient. When handling the tooth, touch only the crown (enamel) surface, because the cementum is fragile. After irrigation with HBSS or saline, place the tooth firmly into the socket. Compare to the shape of mirror-image teeth on the other side of the mouth to

clarify proper orientation if multiple teeth are out. Splinting (see above) will ensure that the tooth remains securely in place. This may require consulting the dentist. A short course (5 days) of prophylactic antibiotics should be given and dental follow-up arranged.

POSTEXTRACTION TOOTH HEMORRHAGE

Bleeding from the site of a recently extracted tooth may result from the simple dislodgment of clot from the base of the socket or may be a sign of an underlying blood dyscrasia. Patients should be asked about a history of hemophilia or use of antiplatelet or anticoagulant drugs. Laboratory testing may be necessary to evaluate the coagulation status. Initial management should entail placing rolled cotton gauze in the socket and asking the patient to bite down for 20 minutes. As an adjunct, lidocaine-epinephrine can be injected into the gingiva at the bleeding site prior to gauze pressure. Bleeding that does not respond to these measures will require dental consultation for revision of the socket.

Barrett EJ et al: Avulsed permanent teeth: a review of the literature and treatment guidelines. Endod Dent Traumatol 1997; 13:153. [PMID: 9550040] (A primer aimed at primary care dentists for optimal care of tooth avulsion.)

Bisno AL: Acute pharyngitis. N Engl J Med 2001;18:205. [PMID: 11172144] (Review of current recommendations of expert advisory committees.)

Bluestone CD: Clinical course, complications and sequelae of acute otitis media. Pediatr Infect Dis J 2000;19(5 Suppl):S37. [PMID: 10821471] (Description of the uncommon but malignant bony and intracranial extensions of suppurative middle ear infections.)

Chopra R: Epistaxis: A review. J R Soc Health 2000;120:31. [PMID: 10918781] (Review of epistaxis and its management.)

Corneli HM: Rapid strep tests in the emergency department: an evidence-based approach. Pediatr Emerg Care 2001;17:272. [PMID: 11493831] (Discussion of integration of various forms of the rapid strep test commonly used in emergency and primary care settings into a logical diagnostic strategy.)

Dewhurst SN et al: Emergency treatment of orodental injuries: a review. Br J Oral Maxillofac Surg 1998;36:165. [PMID: 9678879] (Review of treatment strategies for a variety of traumatic situations, with an emphasis on management in children.)

Donly KJ: Management of sports-related crown fractures. Dent Clin North Am 2000;44:85. [PMID: 10635470] (Discussion specific to the problem of tooth fracture.)

Hilton M et al: The Epley (canalith repositioning) manoeuvre for benign paroxysmal positional vertigo. Cochrane Database Syst Rev 2002;CD003162. [PMID: 11869655] (Review of randomized trials evaluating the efficacy of the canalith repositioning [Epley] maneuver.)

Jacobs RF: Judicious use of antibiotics for common pediatric respiratory infections. Pediatr Infect Dis J 2000;19:938. [PMID: 11001130] (Outlines recommendations of a CDC/American

Academy of Pediatrics panel on treatment of common pediatric respiratory infections including the common cold, otitis media, sinusitis, and tonsillopharyngitis. Addresses principles for containment of antimicrobial resistance.)

Kalan A et al: Foreign bodies in the nasal cavities: a comprehensive review of the aetiology, diagnostic pointers, and therapeutic measures. Postgrad Med J 2000;76:484. [PMID: 10908376]

Klein JO: Review of consensus reports on management of acute otitis media. Pediatr Infect Dis J 1999;18:1152. [PMID: 10608648] (Two comprehensive summaries of practice guidelines for this commonly overtreated condition.)

Layug ML et al: Interim storage of avulsed permanent teeth. J Can Dent Assoc 1998;64:357. [PMID: 9648418] (Review of the evidence for various preservation techniques. A literature review leads to debunking of various myths regarding treatment of the avulsed tooth.)

Lippincott LH et al: ENT issues in pregnancy. J La State Med Soc 1999;151:350. [PMID: 10474980] (Addresses common ENT disorders and the physiologic changes in pregnancy that may predispose patients to develop them. Outlines safe treatments for epistaxis and other common ENT conditions.)

Marais J et al: Bullous myringitis: a review. Clin Otolaryngol 1997;22:497. [PMID: 9466056] (Review of the treatment of bullous myringitis.)

McCracken GH Jr: Diagnosis and management of acute otitis media in the urgent care setting. Ann Emerg Med 2002; 39:413. [PMID: 11919528]

Osguthorpe JD et al: Frontal sinus malignancies. Otolaryngol Clin North Am 2001;34:269. [PMID: 11344078] (Review of paranasal tumors and their management.)

Peyvandi F et al: Rare coagulation disorders. Thromb Haemost 1999;82:1207. [PMID: 10544899] (Review of the presentation and management of various factor-deficiency conditions that may complicate epistaxis.)

Pichichero ME et al: Controversies in the medical management of persistent and recurrent acute otitis media. Recommendations of a clinical advisory committee. Ann Otol Rhinol Laryngol (Suppl) 2000;183:1. [PMID: 10963616] (Review of recommendations for management of chronic otitis media.)

Pond F et al: Epistaxis: strategies for management. Aust Fam Physician 2000;29:933. [PMID: 11059081] (Review of epistaxis and its management.)

Schapowal A: Otitis externa: a clinical overview. Ear Nose Throat J 2002;81:21. [PMID: 12199185]

Schulze SL et al: Pediatric external auditory canal foreign bodies: a review of 698 cases. Otolaryngol Head Neck Surg 2002; 127:73. [PMID: 12161734]

Stollerman GH: Rheumatic fever in the 21st century. Clin Infect Dis 2001;33:806. [PMID: 11512086] (Review of the pathogenesis of acute rheumatic fever and acute glomerulonephritis, with diagnosis and treatment recommendations.)

Thompson LD et al: Extracranial sinonasal tract meningiomas: a clinicopathologic study of 30 cases with a review of the literature. Am J Surg Pathol 2000;24:640. [PMID: 10800982] (Review of paranasal tumors and their management.)

Tusa RJ: Vertigo. Neurol Clin 2001;19:23. [PMID: 11471767] (Thorough review of diagnostic and management strategies for vertigo. Includes discussion of nonpharmacologic modalities.)

Wang NE et al: Mastoiditis: a case-based review. Pediatr Emerg Care 1998;14:290. [PMID: 9733257] (Review.)

Zadeh MH et al: Evaluation of hearing impairment. Compr Ther 2001;27:302. [PMID: 11765688] (Review of the approach to identifying and treating causes of sudden and semiacute hearing loss.)

■ II. MANAGEMENT OF SPECIFIC DISORDERS

DISORDERS OF THE EAR

Please refer to the "Immediate Management" section and Table 32–1 for discussion of the following conditions: otitis externa, malignant otitis externa, foreign body or insect in canal, infected sebaceous cyst, chondritis, perichondritis, suppurative and serous otitis media, bullous myringitis, and acute mastoiditis.

CERUMEN IMPACTION

 ESSENTIALS OF DIAGNOSIS

- *Readily apparent by direct otoscope inspection.*

Clinical Findings

The walls of the ear canal possess a secretory mechanism that results in a coating of the familiar waxy substance, cerumen. Over months, this material can collect and result in canal obstruction. Rarely does the material need to be emergently removed, but its presence can lead to mild pressure, vertigo, or hearing loss symptoms, and it may obscure inspection of the tympanic membrane.

Treatment

Two methods are available for evacuation: blunt removal and irrigation. Blunt removal entails use of a plastic curette, and care must be taken not to puncture the drum or injure the walls of the canal. Large, hard impactions may defy easy removal by this method and are better suited to removal by irrigation. Blunt removal should be discontinued if it becomes clear that the drum is perforated. For irrigation, a warm solution of equal parts 3% hydrogen peroxide and water is directed at the mass with a flexible catheter. Cut the catheter of a butterfly needle and attach the remaining tubing to a 30 cc syringe. The flexible tubing can be inserted directly into the canal by the patient or clinician with little risk of injuring the walls or tympanic membrane. Repeated emergency department irrigation at 15-minute intervals will remove all but the hardest masses. If this method does not work, continued home treatments (5–10 per day) will soften and clear the remaining obstruction within a few days. Care should be taken with either method in elderly or diabetic patients because canal trauma may predispose the patient to malignant otitis externa.

FROSTBITE

 ESSENTIALS OF DIAGNOSIS

- *Protruding appendages (ie, nose, ears, fingers, toes) are affected most often.*
- *Pale color, insensate.*
- *Injury borders may not be apparent for several hours.*

Clinical Findings

The nose and auricle are particularly vulnerable to injury from cold exposure. Superficial skin injuries are red and tender in the emergency department, but moderate and severe cases will appear pale and lack sensation prior to warming. Pain may not develop until later. After warming, the skin appearance will provide clues to the severity and extent of the damage. In the emergency department, the affected areas should be warmed with saline of slightly more than body temperature (100–105 °F). Inspect the lips, nose, and auricle regarding shape and contours, sensation, edema, skin color, and lesions. It may be helpful to draw a diagram showing the borders of injury. The distal edges of the auricle and tip of the nose are typically the first to be affected by cold exposure, with injury progressing proximally after prolonged exposure.

Grading the Injury

Accurate grading of cold exposure injuries can be attempted 1–2 hours after rewarming, but serious cases may require 1–2 days of observation for full assessment. Frostnip is a mild form of injury, characterized by pain,

pallor, and numbness and resolves with no permanent injury after rewarming. Frostbite is graded in 4 levels of severity:

1. First-degree injuries demonstrate hyperemia and edema, with eventual return of most sensation.
2. Second-degree injuries are similar to first-degree injuries but involve blisters. Recovery of sensation is variable.
3. Third-degree injuries exhibit deeper skin and cartilaginous tissue damage, with smaller, hemorrhagic, blisters. There is significant permanent sensory deficit.
4. Fourth-degree injuries remain pale, insensate, develop no blisters, and have permanent skin and cartilage breakdown. There is eventual full-thickness necrosis and deformity.

Patients should be assessed for systemic cold injury and receive treatment for core hypothermia if necessary. Significant cold exposure causes a physiologic diuresis, and persons with prolonged exposure should receive warmed intravenous fluids. The ear should be covered (usually with a head wrap) with care taken to preserve the inherent shape and projection of the pinna. Gauze padding may be loosely placed in and behind the ear to preserve its shape until it has healed. The full extent of injury may take days to become apparent, and hospitalization for wound care is appropriate for severe (third- or fourth-degree) injuries. Update the tetanus toxoid. Recovered areas will remain abnormally cold-sensitive and prone to injury, because the tissues rarely heal completely. Encourage patients to avoid future cold exposure.

CHRONIC (SUPPURATIVE) OTITIS MEDIA

 ESSENTIALS OF DIAGNOSIS

- *Persistent ear pain and discharge despite antibiotics.*

Chronic otitis media refers to persistent discharge of purulent fluid through a tympanic membrane perforation. Ordinary ruptures of the tympanic membrane heal in 1–2 weeks, and persistent defects should prompt close scrutiny. Accumulations of keratin result in formation of a cholesteatoma, which can contribute to injury to the bony structures of the middle ear. Persistent infections of the middle ear have a low incidence association with meningitis (from hematogenous spread) as well as mastoiditis. CT scan will reveal the latter condition, and clinical judgment should be used to determine which patients need a lumbar puncture. Management of mastoiditis is usually surgical. Infections limited to the middle ear should be treated with antibiotics (see Table 32–1) and prompt outpatient ENT evaluation.

DISORDERS OF THE SINUSES (SINUSITIS)

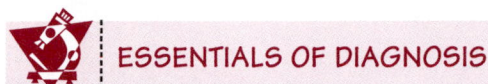 **ESSENTIALS OF DIAGNOSIS**

- Midface pain associated with fever and purulent nasal discharge.
- Often recurrent.

General Considerations

The paranasal sinuses (maxillary, frontal, ethmoid, and sphenoid) are ordinarily air filled and communicate with the nasal passages through small ostia. Most bacterial infections occur in the setting of functional or anatomic obstruction, inflammation, impaired drainage, and bacterial overgrowth. The sinus fills with purulent fluid. Chronic sinusitis occurs with infections that persist for more than 3 months—often in a setting of irreversible obstruction or resistant bacteria and sometimes requires surgical drainage.

Clinical Findings

A. HISTORY

Sinusitis universally causes pain and pressure to the upper face, which may be perceived as a frontal headache. Fever, chills, and nasal discharge are common. When nasal discharge is present, determine the side of the discharge. Maxillary sinusitis commonly causes pain in the upper teeth. Symptoms typically worsen over 1–3 days and may follow an upper respiratory infection. Some patients with structural anomalies are predisposed to these infections and may give a history of similar previous episodes.

B. PHYSICAL EXAMINATION

Fever may be present. Classically, pressure or gentle tapping over the affected sinus will reveal tenderness on one side. The maxillary sinus is most often affected and

can be examined by applying bilateral thumb pressure to the inferior aspect of the zygotic prominence above the corners of the mouth. Transillumination of the maxillary sinus can be accomplished in a darkened room by placing the otoscope light source directly against the zygoma and observing transmission of light through the anterior hard palate (behind the upper incisors). Though this test is less sensitive than x-ray, the presence of purulent fluid in the maxillary sinus will often obscure the light on one side. Plain sinus x-rays will reveal the presence of large sinus fluid collections (Figure 32–8A and B), but CT scan is the most sensitive test and will reveal anatomic anomalies such as small tumors or a deviated septum (Figure 32–8C). Typically this study can be done on an outpatient basis if the diagnosis remains in question or if the infection has failed to improve with a course of antibiotics.

Treatment

Culturing the sinus fluid directly is not practical in the emergency department. Empiric antimicrobial therapy should cover *H influenzae, Moraxella catarrhalis,* and gram-positive bacteria. Therapy should be continued for 12 days. Amoxicillin-clavulanate, 875 mg twice daily, covers β-lactamase-resistant strains and the mixed flora typical of these infections. Trimethoprim-sulfamethoxazole and cefuroxime are alternatives for penicillin-allergic patients. Nasal decongestant pills and sprays can sometimes reduce swelling around the sinus ostia and promote drainage. Often the infection in the sinus is related to a mass (tumor, polyp, deviated septum, turbinate anomaly) or inadequate drainage (middle meatus obstruction), and patients should be referred to a primary care clinician or otolaryngologist for an evaluation after resolution of the acute episode. Occasionally surgical correction may be necessary.

Chronic sinusitis has been associated with *Staphylococcus aureus* infections, but lasting resolution will often follow only surgical drainage and correction of the anatomic obstruction. Immunocompromised persons are at risk for *Pseudomonas aeruginosa* and fungal infections. Treatment recommendations continue to evolve for chronic, recurrent sinusitis, largely in response to poor long-term success rates among some patient groups.

Complications

Several conditions related to sinus infection have been described. Direct extension of the infection to surrounding tissues can lead to frontal osteomyelitis, facial cellulitis, periorbital cellulitis, or periorbital abscess. For this reason, high fever, ocular movement problems,

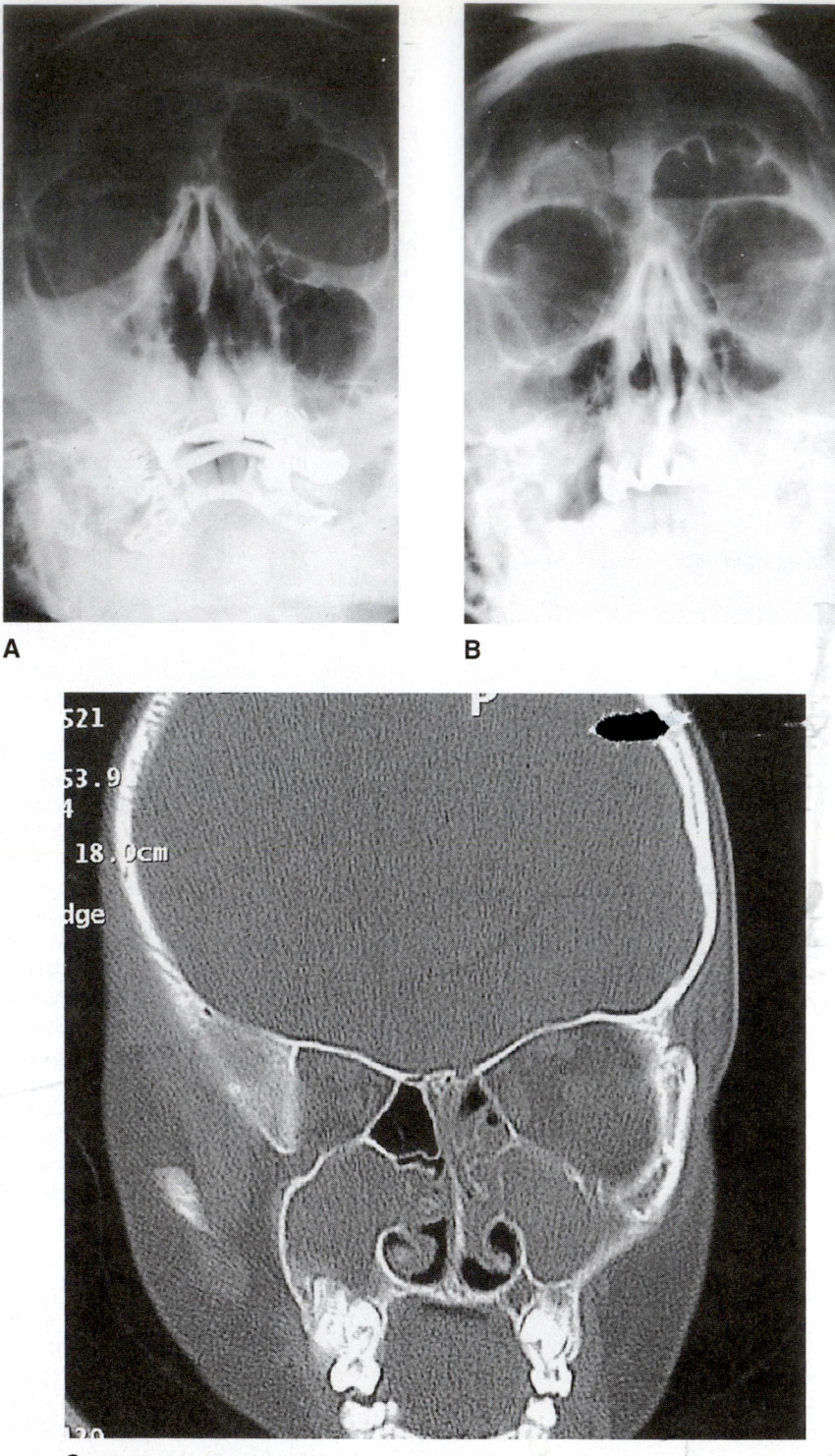

Figure 32–8. Sinus imaging. **A:** Frontal sinusitis. **B:** Maxillary sinusitis. The affected air spaces are opacified due to being filled with fluid. **C:** CT scan demonstrating bilateral maxillary sinus and one ethmoid sinus opacification consistent with sinusitis.

enophthalmos, diplopia, facial skin swelling, erythema, or extreme tenderness should be studied by CT scan. Intracranial extension can lead to meningitis, cavernous sinus thrombosis, brain abscess, or subdural empyema. Therefore, prominence of a headache or neurologic findings should prompt examination with CT scan or lumbar puncture.

DISORDERS OF THE OROPHARYNX

Please refer to the "Immediate Management" section and Table 32–6 for discussion of epiglottitis, Ludwig angina, and other causes of throat pain. What follows is a more detailed discussion regarding the pathophysiology and treatment of airway deep space infections.

PERITONSILLITIS (PERITONSILLAR CELLULITIS & ABSCESS)

 ESSENTIALS OF DIAGNOSIS

- Extensive swelling does not typically obstruct the airway.
- "Hot potato" voice.
- Fever, severe pain.
- Systemic dehydration typical.

General Considerations

Peritonsillitis, peritonsillar cellulitis, and abscess (also known collectively as *quinsy*) are extensions of mixed-flora bacterial infections of the tonsils. The differentiation between cellulitis and abscess is difficult to make on clinical grounds and is determined by identification of an abscess by intravenous contrast CT scan or more commonly by drainage of pus after aspirating or incising the mass. Therefore, the initial treatment of each is the same. See Table 32–6 for a review of typical symptoms and a differential diagnosis. Once the diagnosis is made, most peritonsillar masses should be treated with intravenous antibiotics and a drainage procedure in the emergency department.

Drainage Procedure

A. PREPARATION

First, make certain that the patient does not have obstructive airway issues. Patients with impending airway collapse should receive an emergency artificial airway prior to decompression of the mass. The patient should be placed sitting upright in a dental chair with a headrest supporting the occiput. The upright position makes handling of oral secretions easier, and the headrest helps the patient relax and restricts movement during the procedure. The tonsillar mass should be palpated gently with a cotton swab to confirm fluctuance. A pulsatile mass should prompt the clinician to order an intravenous contrast enhanced CT scan to confirm the diagnosis and rule out the possibility of carotid artery aneurysm. For the drainage procedure to be successful, patients must not have extreme trismus and they should be cooperative and well anesthetized. Patients will generally be more cooperative when premedicated with a moderate dose of intravenous or oral opiate analgesic. Next, use a topical anesthetic spray such as Benzocaine-tetracaine, followed by an injection of 1–2 ml of 2% lidocaine-epinephrine into the mucosal layer of the abscess. Frazier suction should be made ready for control of secretions and any pus or blood that result from the procedure.

B. NEEDLE DRAINAGE

Place an 18-gauge needle on a 10-mL syringe. The tip of the plastic needle cap should be cut off such that when placed back on the needle, 0.5 cm of the needle protrudes beyond the end. This will prevent accidental deep penetration of the mass. Insert the needle on an axis level with the tongue into the superior pole of the peritonsillar mass (the most common site for fluid) and aspirate (Figure 32–9). Remove and culture as much fluid as possible. Next, aspirate from the middle pole, then the inferior pole. Take care to avoid directing the needle in a lateral direction, so as to avoid puncturing the carotid artery. Because the needle may have missed the pocket of fluid, or the fluid may have been too thick to flow through the needle, a negative aspirate procedure does not rule out an abscess. Opening the pocket with a scalpel blade (see below) at the location where pus was aspirated is optional but will minimize the risk of recurrence.

C. OPEN DRAINAGE

Though many clinicians advocate needle aspiration (with antibiotics) as a safer and more comfortable method, incision and drainage with a scalpel blade appears to minimize recurrence risk. Some authors have suggested incising the mass at the location where pus has been aspirated by needle to minimize risk of both injury and infection recurrence. After anesthetizing the upper pole of the mass (see above), tape should be wrapped around the proximal aspect of the blade to

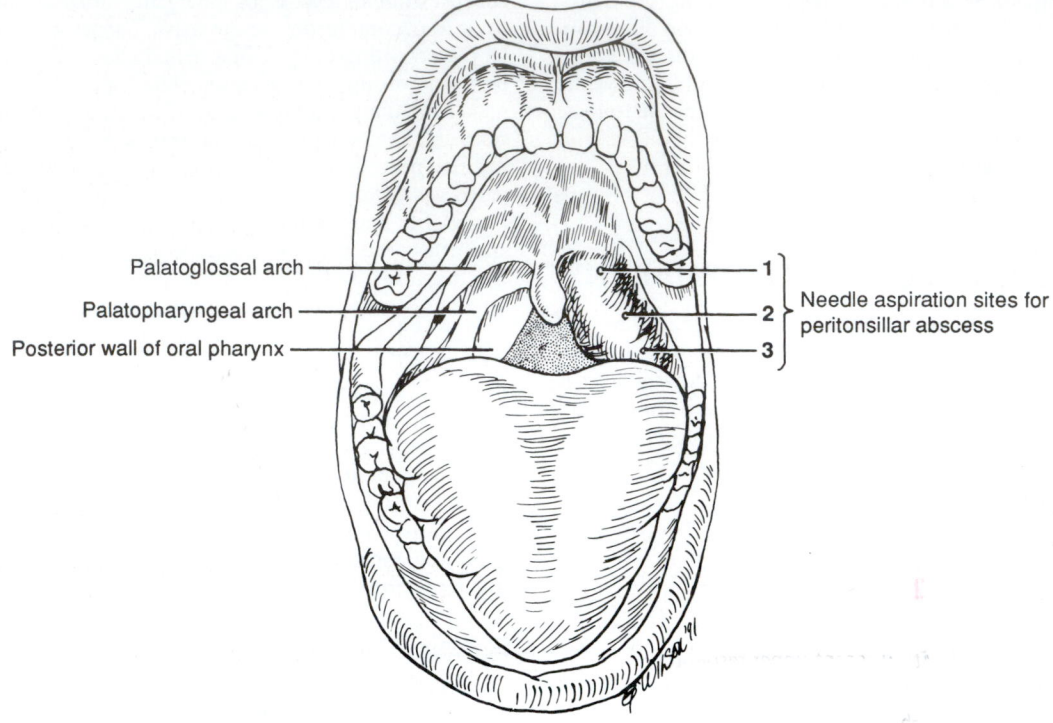

Palatoglossal arch

Palatopharyngeal arch

Posterior wall of oral pharynx

1
2
3

} Needle aspiration sites for peritonsillar abscess

Figure 32–9. Needle drainage sites for peritonsillar abscess.

prevent it from being inserted deeper than 0.5 cm. A single stab of depth 0.5 cm is made into the superior pole and extended no more than 0.5 cm in an inferolateral direction. Place the suction device tip into the incised area to remove any pus. Any bleeding that develops will usually resolve after the patient gargles with diluted hydrogen peroxide or salt water.

Patients should be observed for at least 1 hour following the procedure. Most are dehydrated and will benefit from intravenous fluids. Those able to take oral fluids and pills can be discharged with oral antibiotics. The preferred regimen is penicillin, 2–4 million units intravenously followed by 500 mg orally 4 times daily, or cephalosporins (eg, cefazolin, 1 g intravenously, followed by cephalexin, 500 mg 4 times daily for 10 days). Most patients will need oral nonsteroidal anti-inflammatory agents and opiate analgesics for pain control. ENT follow-up in 2–3 days should be arranged. Patients with high fever, those unable to take oral fluids, and immunocompromised patients should be admitted for intravenous fluids and antibiotics. Some authors have advocated admitting patients with negative aspirates as well, for intravenous antibiotics and close observation.

EPIGLOTTITIS

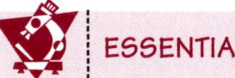

ESSENTIALS OF DIAGNOSIS

- *Fever, throat pain, swallowing pain.*
- *Decreased prevalence in children.*
- *Adults appear nontoxic.*
- *Definitive diagnosis by endoscopy.*

Due to widespread use of the Hib vaccine, epiglottitis is now more common among adults than children. Children with epiglottitis have high fever and varying levels of toxicity by appearance (see Table 32–6). In children suspected of having epiglottitis, flexible fiberoptic or direct laryngoscopy must be done to make or rule out the diagnosis. First, a skilled pediatric airway specialist must be called (this may be the emergency physician, otolaryngologist, or anesthesiologist). If patient stability permits, this clinician can accompany the child and parent while a lateral soft tissue neck x-ray is obtained. This, alone, may demonstrate the enlarged epiglottis (see Figure 32–6C). If the diagnosis remains uncertain, or the child is too unstable to have an x-ray, the patient should be accompanied to the operating room, where laryngoscopy or endotracheal intubation can be accomplished in a setting where a surgical airway can be easily done if the orotracheal method fails. All pediatric patients found to have epiglottitis should ultimately be intubated for airway protection and admitted.

Adults with epiglottitis usually present with 2–3 days of steadily worsening throat pain, difficulty swallowing, and fever. The potential for rapid loss of airway patency is lower among adults, and most patients can have x-ray and emergency department flexible fiberoptic laryngoscopy without concern for rapid airway collapse. Those with epiglottitis should be admitted and receive intravenous antibiotics such as ceftriaxone, 1 g intravenously or intramuscularly every 24 hours.

CROUP

 ESSENTIALS OF DIAGNOSIS

- *Associated with a recent upper respiratory infection.*
- *"Barking" cough.*
- *Often quick resolution.*

General Considerations

Croup (laryngotracheobronchitis) is exclusively a disease of children, affecting mainly those aged 6 months to 3 years. It is the most common cause of stridor among young children presenting to the emergency department. Unlike the supraglottic swelling of epiglottitis, croup leads to obstruction of the subglottic trachea (below the cords, mainly at the level of the cricoid cartilage).

Clinical Findings

A. HISTORY

The predominant cause is parainfluenza virus, and its peak incidence is fall and winter. The children are typically brought in at night, having recently developed a barking cough preceded by 2–3 days of a viral-type respiratory infection. The stridulous breathing is noisy and high-pitched, a result of air traveling through a severely narrowed airway. On occasion the symptoms will have improved by the time of arrival at the emergency department—possibly related to cold or moist night air. Because an aspirated airway foreign body could mimic the symptoms of croup, parents should be questioned regarding this possibility.

B. PHYSICAL EXAMINATION

Children with croup usually appear nontoxic. When present, fever is usually low grade, reflecting an underlying viral infection. With exertion or crying, rapid air movement through the small subglottic aperture becomes difficult and respiratory distress worsens. In extreme cases, cyanosis may occur. Because the lungs are not affected, the oxygen saturation is typically normal. Oropharyngeal exam is normal or may reveal the bilateral nonspecific erythema and swelling associated with a viral upper respiratory infection. Any unilateral swelling or tonsillar exudates should prompt consideration of bacterial surface or closed-space infections. Transmitted airway noise may obscure auscultation of lung sounds, which are normal in croup. An anteroposterior soft tissue neck x-ray will demonstrate the steeple sign of upper tracheal narrowing (Figure 32–10A). The serum white blood count may be elevated, but this is not specific for croup and has little value for differentiating croup from other processes. Occasionally, older children will present with a barking cough and the appearance of croup. An anteroposterior soft tissue neck x-ray will confirm the diagnosis (Figure 32–10B). The underlying cause is more likely to be bacterial among children older than 6 years.

Treatment

Consideration should be given to the stability of the patient's airway. Croup rarely leads to complete airway obstruction, and mild epiglottitis can present with symptoms similar to croup (see "Epiglottitis" section, above). The initial therapy is nebulized saline, which can be delivered by face mask or by having the parent direct the mist at the child's mouth ("blow-by"). Nebulized racemic epinephrine should be used for patients who do not improve promptly: place 10 drops of 2.25% solution and 2–3 mL of saline in a nebulizer. The treatment may be repeated every 20–30 minutes. Dexamethasone, 0.6 mg/kg intramuscularly, is a useful adjunct for refractory croup. Serial clinical evaluations of patient comfort will help identify the small percentage of children who will require admission for observation and further therapy. Typically the symptoms improve within 1–2 hours in the emergency department, and the children can be discharged.

DISORDERS OF THE MOUTH

Though myriad disorders involve the teeth and periodontal tissues, patients typically present to the emergency department with acute processes in the mouth such as pain. Careful examination of the mouth is the key to correct diagnosis.

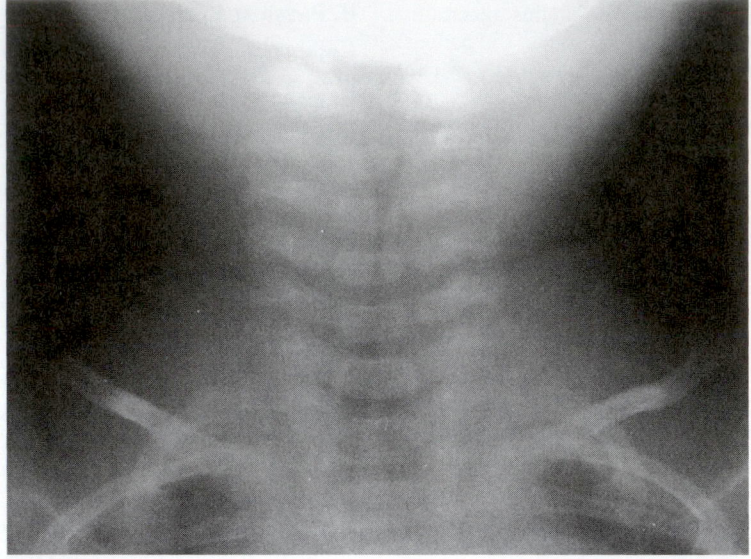

A

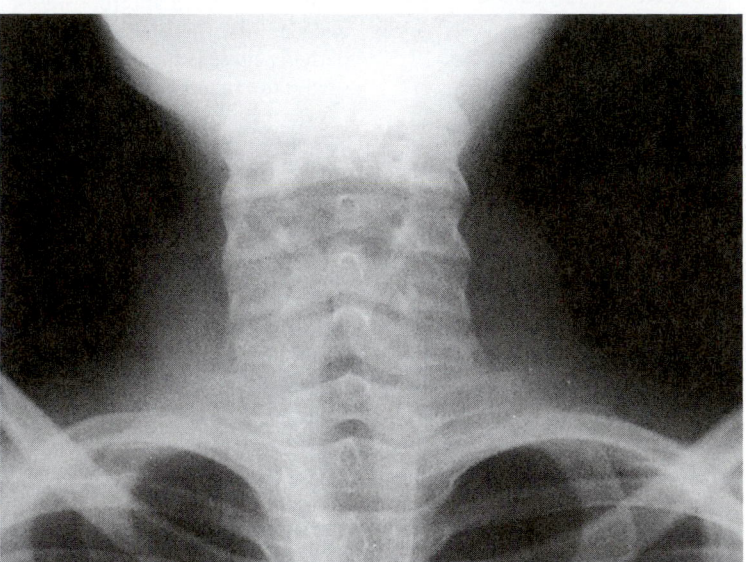

B

Figure 32–10. The "steeple" sign of croup in a 1-year-old (**A**) and a 12-year-old (**B**).

TOOTH ANATOMY

Teeth consist of a central pulp tissue, which is innervated by pain fibers and produces dentin (Figure 32–11). The dentin surrounds the pulp; makes up the bulk of the tooth mass; and is coated with enamel, a hard material that forms the outer surface of the tooth. The tooth surface of the root portion comprises cementum, which is less dense than enamel and not designed to withstand exposure to mouth flora and acids. Each tooth is embedded in periodontium, which consists of a bony support (alveolar bone) that is contiguous with

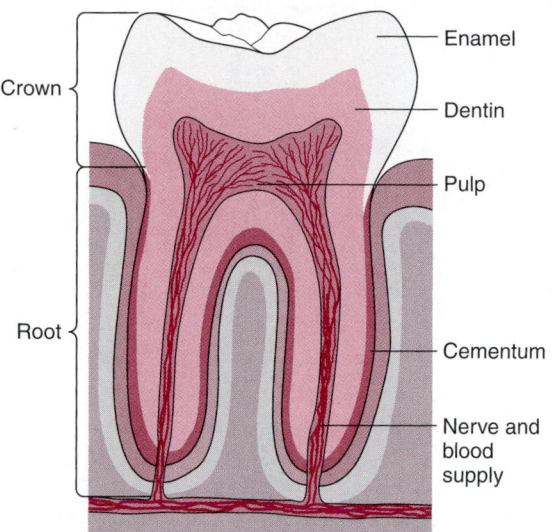

Figure 32–11. Tooth anatomy.

underlying mandible and maxilla. The gingiva is the highly vascular mucosal tissue (gums) that covers the alveolar bone.

TOOTH PAIN
(See Table 32–7.)

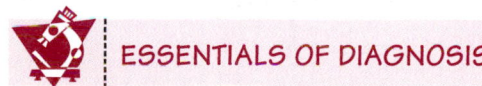 ESSENTIALS OF DIAGNOSIS

- *Commonly associated with prior tooth injury or cavity.*
- *Differentiate simple infection from abscess.*

Clinical Findings

A. HISTORY

Because dental caries are the most common source of tooth pain, ask patients about their cleaning habits and frequency of dentist visits. Duration and rate of pain onset may be useful clues to a subacute process, whereas recent trauma or dental instrumentation would suggest a noninfectious problem. Is the pain limited to one tooth or a particular area of the mouth? Pain that worsens with chewing implicates a local tooth problem.

B. PHYSICAL EXAMINATION

The focus of the examination should be the area said to be painful. Tap on suspect teeth with a tongue blade:

This will elicit tenderness from infections inside the tooth (pulpitis) and at the tooth root (periapical abscesses). A high degree of tenderness suggests the latter, and a Panorex film is useful for confirming the diagnosis. A thorough viewing of the tooth and surrounding periodontium from all sides (use a warmed mirror to look at the lingual aspect) may demonstrate the cavity or any swelling. Focal erythema, swelling, and fluctuance would suggest a periodontal abscess. Examine the gingiva for ulcerations and pseudomembranes (acute necrotizing ulcerative gingivitis). The presence of blood can indicate poor periodontal health or may have resulted from recent trauma or instrumentation. Examine the tongue and floor of the mouth. Extension of dental infections into the soft tissues of the mandible can lead to Ludwig angina, characterized by a firm, boardlike mouth floor and tongue elevation (see Table 32–6).

Treatment

Because most conditions are best treated definitively in a fully equipped dental office, oral analgesics and discharge with dental follow-up are usually indicated. Most patients benefit from anti-inflammatory agents such as ibuprofen or naproxen, or oral opiate analgesics such as codeine or hydrocodone as an adjunct. Application of a tooth block with a long-acting local anesthetic can provide hours of relief for those with severe pain and can reduce the reliance on oral analgesics. The anesthetic must be injected to the depth of the root tip to be effective. Place a block by injecting a 25-gauge needle parallel to the tooth to a depth of 0.5–0.8 cm (from the tooth-gingival interface) and infiltrate with 0.75% bupivacaine.

Because dental pain is a favored complaint of drug seekers, a small portion of those presenting with toothache will have fictitious pain. Short courses (2–3 days) of opiates are advisable when the presentation seems implausible. Some authors have suggested that the absence of relief from a well-placed block suggests an ulterior motive.

Most painful tooth conditions also require therapy with an antibiotic. Oral penicillin, 500 mg 4 times daily, is the treatment of choice for typical tooth and periodontal infections, but immunocompromised patients and those with high fever or severe illness should have parenteral penicillin, 15–20 million units/d, or a cephalosporin as well as clindamycin for anaerobic (mainly *Bacteroides fragilis*) coverage. Amoxicillin-clavulanate is a single oral agent that covers these organisms.

TMJ PAIN

TMJ pain (also broadly labeled temporomandibular disorder) is an inflammatory process of the temporo-

Table 32–7. Diagnosis and treatment of tooth pain.

Diagnosis	Diagnostic Clues	Treatment	Comments
Acute necrotizing ulcerative gingivitis (trench mouth)	Diffuse gingival pain, tenderness. May be accompanied by fever. Gingival tissues are ulcerated and may be covered with a gray pseudomembrane. Mouth has a foul odor.	Requires meticulous oral hygiene: saltwater or hydrogen peroxide rinses, frequent brushing. Topical and systemic oral analgesics. Oral antibiotics. Dental follow-up.	Represents an infection of the gingiva by native mouth flora. More common in immunocompromised persons but mostly associated with poor oral hygiene.
Aphthous stomatitis	Formation of small (2–3 mm) white plaques on mucosal surfaces of the mouth. Tender to touch, may bleed if scraped. Surrounding erythema suggests secondary infection.	Topical analgesics and oral rinses (hydrogen peroxide). Oral antibiotics for superinfected lesions.	Onset often relates to stress or poor nutrition.
Periapical abscess	Signs and symptoms of simple caries but with fever and extreme sensitivity to tooth percussion. Panorex film to demonstrate abscesses.	Incision and drainage, usually by a dental consultant. Intravenous antibiotics in the emergency department, followed by oral antibiotics at home.	Extension of the pulp infection into the root and periodontium, with resultant formation of an abscess.
Periodontal abscess	Focal gingival swelling, erythema, fluctuance. Tender to pressure.	Incision and drainage. Procedure is simpler than for a periapical abscess, because pocket is superficial. Anesthetize with lidocaine-epinephrine prior to stab incision.	Advisable to suture a small piece of Penrose drain or iodoform tape into the cavity to keep open for 2–3 days (until follow-up). Frequent saltwater rinses.
Postextraction pain	Pain immediately following removal of a tooth. Rarely, pain will develop 3 days following the procedure, and examination of the socket reveals the foul odor and localized erythema consistent with a periodontal socket infection.	For immediate pain: oral analgesics. Socket infections require opiate analgesics or tooth block. The socket should be irrigated and oral antibiotics given. Dental consultation is preferable, as the socket can be packed with dental paste for prompt pain relief.	If dental consultation is not available in the emergency department, patients with socket infection should be referred to the dentist for prompt follow-up.

Condition	Signs and symptoms	Treatment	Comments
Pulpitis	Poor dental care (by patient history or examination of mouth). Defect in tooth enamel may be visible. No fever. Pain localized to 1–2 teeth, which are tender to tapping.	Oral analgesics, antibiotics. Consider tooth block (see text).	Prompt (1–2 d) dental follow-up: tooth may need removal. Simple caries are painless. Presence of pain implies extension of the defect into pulp, with resultant inflammation.
Root canal pain	Pain in a tooth following a root canal procedure. Tender with pressure and chewing. Tooth may appear to sit higher above the gingival ridge than appropriate.	Dental consultation. Build-up of gas or fluid at the tooth apex may require release.	Pain may respond poorly to systemic or tooth block analgesia.
Subluxation or avulsion	Loose (subluxation) or absent (avulsion) tooth.	Replace, splint (see text).	Tooth survival correlates with subluxation severity and time the tooth is out of the socket.
Tooth eruption	Infants aged 6 months to 3 years: primary teeth. Associated with low-grade fever and (infrequently) diarrhea. Secondary teeth begin to appear at age 5 years. Third (wisdom) molars can become impacted, causing inflammation and pain with chewing. Occasional periodontal abscess.	Treat dehydration, if present. In infants and children: topical anesthetics, oral ibuprofen. For third molar impaction, drain abscess (if present), oral analgesics, antibiotics.	Third molars may require removal, and these patients should be referred for prompt dental follow-up.
Tooth fracture	History of a blow to the mandible or recent dental procedure or hardware. Pain with chewing. Fissure in tooth may be visible.	Oral analgesics.	Need prompt dental follow-up.

mandibular joint, which often relates to overuse, trauma, or various arthritides.

Clinical Findings

The joint area is tender to pressure on one or both sides, and pain is elicited with biting down on a tongue blade and mandible manipulation. The examiner can grip the chin and lower incisors and gently rock the mandible from side to side to elicit TMJ tenderness. Except in cases of recent trauma, x-ray images are rarely indicated in the acute setting.

Treatment & Disposition

The usual therapy is for the patient to reduce the forceful use of the joint by avoiding hard foods and to use anti-inflammatory medications for 1–2 weeks. Follow-up with a dental professional for persistent pain is recommended, at which point chewing and biting habits can be explored. Occasionally, corrective appliances are used to promote correct positioning and use of the jaw.

TMJ DISLOCATION

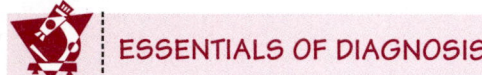

ESSENTIALS OF DIAGNOSIS

- *Inability to close mouth.*
- *Onset sudden, associated with a "click."*

One of the most satisfying procedures encountered in the emergency department is reduction of a TMJ dislocation. Typically the patient gives a history of wide mouth opening (typically a yawn or laughter) followed by an inability to close the mouth after feeling a click. Often, these patients are intoxicated. They present with mouth open, are unable to speak clearly, and are sometimes distressed due to masseter spasm and pain. If the examination reveals deviation of the mandible to one side, the dislocation may be unilateral.

The solution is easy and elegant. The clinician sits the patient on a stretcher with the back up to support the head (alternatively, the patient can be placed sitting on the floor with his or her back against the wall). The clinician faces the patient, and after padding the thumbs with layers of gauze, places them on the posterior lower molars and grips the underside of the mandible angle with the fingers. Steady, forceful downward pressure is applied onto the rear molars. Successful reduction is characterized by a sudden snapping of the mandible back into place, which can put the examiner's digits at risk of a bite injury if he or she is not

prepared. The patient will have immediate relief. If severe masseter spasm is present, a muscle relaxant (eg, diazepam or midazolam intravenously) will make for an easier reduction. Patients who sustain this injury are at increased risk for developing it again and should be warned to avoid wide mouth openings in the future.

American Academy of Pediatrics Subcommittee on Management of Sinusitis and Committee on Quality Improvement: Clinical practice guideline: Management of sinusitis. Pediatrics 2001; 108:798. [PMID: 11533355] (Practice guidelines addressing the choice of optimal antibiotics and the identification of patients who will require them.)

Blotter JW et al: Otolaryngology consultation for peritonsillar abscess in the pediatric population. Laryngoscope 2000;110: 1698. [PMID: 11037828] (Review of 102 pediatric peritonsillitis cases treated with admission, intravenous antibiotics, and either discharge or tonsillectomy in the operating room, depending on response to 24 hours of therapy.)

Hartmann RW Jr: Ludwig's angina in children. Am Fam Physician 1999;60:109. [PMID: 10414632] (Review.)

Hebert PC et al: Adult epiglottitis in a Canadian setting. Laryngoscope 1998;108:64. [PMID: 9432069] (Retrospective review of 813 cases in 2 centers reveals a case fatality rate of 1.2%.)

Luhmann JD et al: Sedation for peritonsillar abscess drainage in the pediatric emergency department. Pediatr Emerg Care 2002; 18:1. [PMID: 11862127] (Review of an institutional experience with conscious sedation for incision and drainage treatment in 42 children over a 3.5-year time period.)

Murphy JV et al: Frostbite: pathogenesis and treatment. J Trauma 2000;48:171. [PMID: 10647591] (Review of recent developments in the understanding of pathophysiology and treatment of cold-induced injury.)

Newton-John T et al: Chronic idiopathic orofacial pain: II. What can the general dental practitioner do? Br Dent J 2001;191: 72. [PMID: 11508414] (Review of the scope of treatment options for new and chronic temporomandibular disorder pain.)

Reamy BV: Frostbite: review and current concepts. J Am Board Fam Pract 1998;11:34. [PMID: 9456445] (Review of recent developments in the understanding of pathophysiology and treatment of cold-induced injury.)

Rosekrans JA: Viral croup: current diagnosis and treatment. Mayo Clin Proc 1998;73:1102. [PMID: 9818047] (Review.)

Snow V et al: Principles of appropriate antibiotic use for acute sinusitis in adults. Ann Intern Med 2001;134:495. [PMID: 11255527] (Review of appropriate antibiotic use in sinusitis.)

Steed PA et al: Temporomandibular disorders—traumatic etiology vs. nontraumatic etiology: a clinical and methodological inquiry into symptomatology and treatment outcomes. Cranio 2001;19:188. [PMID: 11482831] (Multicenter observational study evaluating the demographic distribution, symptom characteristics, and outcomes of 1842 patients with temporomandibular disorders.)

Stroud RH et al: An update on inflammatory disorders of the pediatric airway: epiglottitis, croup, and tracheitis. Am J Otolaryngol 2001;22:268. [PMID: 11464324] (Review of pediatric airway conditions requiring management in the emergency department.)

Pulmonary Emergencies

33

Christopher R. Pund, MD, & C. Keith Stone, MD[1]

Immediate Management of Life-Threatening Problems
   Hemoptysis
   Pneumothorax
   Asthma & Chronic Obstructive Pulmonary Disease
   Acute Pulmonary Embolism
Emergency Management of Specific Conditions
   Pneumomediastinum & Subcutaneous
      Emphysema
   Pleurodynia

Pleural Effusion
Atelectasis
Pneumonia & Bronchitis
Pulmonary Tuberculosis
Pulmonary Aspiration Syndrome
Acute Lung Injury & Acute Respiratory Distress
   Syndrome
Cystic Fibrosis
Interstitial Pulmonary Disease

■ IMMEDIATE MANAGEMENT OF LIFE-THREATENING PROBLEMS (See also Chapter 11.)

HEMOPTYSIS

General Considerations

Hemoptysis is the expectoration of blood originating from the bronchopulmonary tree. It is a common condition with diverse causes ranging from benign to life-threatening disorders (Table 33–1). Morbidity and mortality depend primarily on the cause and severity of the bleeding. Massive hemoptysis is defined as coughing up of more than 200 mL of blood in a 24-hour period or, more practically, as any amount that becomes hemodynamically significant or threatens ventilation. Massive hemoptysis requires prompt evaluation and treatment in order to prevent death from asphyxiation or hypovolemic shock. If a patient has active moderate hemoptysis, consisting of small volumes (less than 20 mL) of gross blood, or hemoptysis by history alone, management can proceed in a similar but more leisurely manner.

Clinical Findings

History and physical examination are vitally important in identifying patients at high risk for pulmonary hemoptysis and to rule out nonpulmonary sources of hemorrhage (see Table 33–1).

A. HISTORY

Inquire about associated signs and symptoms. Hemoptysis can occur with an acute onset of fever, productive cough (pneumonia or bronchitis), a chronic productive cough (bronchiectasis or chronic bronchitis), or an acute onset of dyspnea and pleuritic chest pain (pulmonary embolism). Ask about weight loss, fevers, and night sweats (tuberculosis); underlying chronic lung disease (Goodpasture syndrome or vasculitis); and especially a history of tobacco use (cancer).

B. PHYSICAL EXAMINATION

Evaluate vital signs and assess patient for possible hemodynamic instability. Any significant hypoxia, tachypnea, tachycardia, or hypotension should be considered crucial in these patients. Do not continue the physical examination until the airway, breathing, and circulation (ABCs) have been stabilized. The examination should be aimed at grossly localizing the hemoptysis to a cardiac, pulmonary, or otolaryngologic source. Evaluate the lungs for evidence of disease, such as wheezing, rales, rhonchi, egophony, or hyperresonance of the chest wall. Also, assess the nose and mouth for possible nonpulmonary sources of bleeding and perform careful cardiac auscultation for the opening snap or diastolic rumble associated with mitral stenosis.

---

[1]Portions of this chapter were revised from the chapter by John Mills, MD, & John M. Luce, MD, from the 4th edition.

Table 33–1. Conditions causing hemoptysis.

Pulmonary hemoptysis
  Pulmonary parenchymal disease
    Bronchitis
    Bronchiectasis
    Tuberculosis
    Lung abscess
    Pneumonia
    Fungal infection of old cavities (eg, aspergilloma)
    Lung parasites (ascariasis, schistosomiasis, etc)
    Pulmonary neoplasms
    Pulmonary infarction
    Trauma (Chapter 18)
    Arteriovenous malformations
    Pulmonary vasculitis
    Goodpasture's syndrome
  Extrapulmonary disease
    Thrombocytopenia
    Other coagulopathies
    Heart failure
    Mitral stenosis
Nonpulmonary hemoptysis
  Aspiration of blood from nasal, oropharyngeal, gastrointestinal, or other bleeding site
Pseudohemoptysis
  Production of red-tinged sputum not due to blood

C. Laboratory Evaluation

The laboratory evaluation should include complete blood count with differential, prothrombin and partial thromboplastin times, chest x-ray, electrocardiogram, and arterial blood gases (if severe bleeding or respiratory difficulties are present). Type and cross-match blood if anemia or hypotension is present. Occasionally renal function studies and urinalysis may be appropriate. As time permits, it may be reasonable to send sputum for bacterial and fungal cultures and for an acid fast bacillus stain for tuberculosis if suspected.

Treatment

Treatment depends primarily on severity and duration of hemoptysis. Immediate attention must be given to the ABCs.

A. Maintain Airway, Oxygenation, and Ventilation

Emergently protect the airway with vigorous suctioning, postural drainage, and endotracheal intubation as necessary to prevent asphyxiation. A large, 8.0-mm endotracheal tube should be used to facilitate suctioning and allow bronchoscopy as needed. Supplemental oxygen should be given to maintain oxygen saturation at greater than 95% by applied pulse oximetry. The hemithorax suspected as the source of bleeding should be kept in a decubitus and dependent position. In this position, the contralateral, well-ventilated lung field is kept free from any obstruction by blood. Monitor ventilation periodically with repeat arterial blood gases.

B. Maintain Circulation

After airway and breathing are secured, 2 large-bore (≥ 16-gauge) intravenous catheters should be placed along with cardiac monitoring and a noninvasive blood pressure cuff. Initiate infusion of crystalloid solution (normal saline or lactated Ringer's). Assess the patient for signs and symptoms of hypovolemic shock (ie, pale, cool skin; altered mental status; hypotension; tachycardia). Treat shock with rapid intravenous crystalloid infusion (up to 2 L) followed by packed red blood cells as needed. Patients who have thrombocytopenia should receive platelets. Patients with coagulopathy or who are taking Coumadin should receive fresh frozen plasma. Place a Foley catheter to monitor urine output if the patient is showing signs of hypovolemic shock.

C. Provide Other Treatments

If the bleeding continues and the patient remains unstable, urgent bronchoscopy should be performed. This allows suctioning of the airway, visualization of the bleeding, and temporary endobronchial tamponade through a balloon-tip catheter. If the bleeding source is clearly identified and the patient appears to be an acceptable surgical candidate, surgical resection can be considered by the cardiothoracic surgeon. However, if the patient is a poor surgical candidate, selective arteriography followed by bronchial artery embolization can be used. This procedure can be performed with or without bronchoscopy and is considered significantly safer than surgical resection, with much lower morbidity and mortality rates.

Disposition

Admit all patients with massive, moderate, or ongoing hemoptysis, and seek immediate consultation with either a pulmonologist or a thoracic surgeon to discuss immediate diagnostic and therapeutic options. These patients are most often admitted to the intensive care unit for close observation until bleeding resolves and hemodynamic status is stabilized. Hospitalize other patients if initial evaluation discloses severe disorders requiring prompt treatment and evaluation (eg, heart failure, tuberculosis). Most patients with minimal hemoptysis can be discharged to home with internist or specialist follow-up in 3–7 days. Treat any underlying conditions (eg, pneumonia, bronchitis) as deemed necessary.

Haponik EF, Fein A, Chin R: Managing life-threatening hemoptysis: has anything really changed? Chest 2000;118:1431.

[PMID: 11083697] (Results of a survey on clinicians' approaches to management of life-threatening hemoptysis. Respondents were physicians attending the 1998 American College of Chest Physicians Annual Scientific Assembly.)

Jean-Baptiste E: Clinical assessment and management of massive hemoptysis. Crit Care Med 2000;28(5):1642. [PMID: 10834728] (Overview of current evaluation and treatment of massive hemoptysis.)

Lee TW et al: Management of massive hemoptysis: a single institution experience. Ann Thorac Cardiovasc Surg 2000;6:232. [PMID: 11042478] (Retrospective study evaluating the outcome of conservative and surgical treatment for patients presenting with massive hemoptysis.)

PNEUMOTHORAX
(See also Chapters 11 and 24.)

 ESSENTIALS OF DIAGNOSIS

- *Acute-onset dyspnea, pleuritic chest pain.*
- *Hyperresonance on percussion, decreased breath sounds on affected side.*
- *Triad of tension pneumothorax: decreased breath sounds, hypotension, jugular venous distension.*

General Considerations

Pneumothorax is the abnormal collection of air within the pleural space. This condition may be classified as either spontaneous (primary or secondary) or traumatic (penetrating or blunt chest trauma, iatrogenic).

Primary spontaneous pneumothoraces occur in patients without clinically apparent lung disease (often young, tall men, aged 20–40 years, who usually smoke). Secondary pneumothoraces are a complication of preexisting underlying pulmonary disease (usually chronic obstructive pulmonary disease [COPD], pneumonia, cystic fibrosis, asthma, tuberculosis, or *Pneumocystis carinii* pneumonia infection).

Traumatic pneumothoraces are common and must always be considered in trauma patients or in patients following any invasive procedure such as subclavian line placement, thoracocentesis, lung or pleural biopsies, or even barotrauma from positive-pressure ventilation. Tension pneumothorax is produced if air continues to enter the pleural space through a defect acting as a one-way valve. As this pressure within the pleural space becomes greater than atmospheric pressure, it can cause a shift of the mediastinum toward the contralateral side. This shift leads to compression on the vena cava with resultant decreased venous return to the heart, hypoxia, decreased cardiac output, and ultimately death if not treated quickly.

Clinical Findings

A. Symptoms and Signs

Patients may be asymptomatic but usually present with any combination of pleuritic chest pain, tachypnea, and tachycardia. Percussion and auscultation will reveal hyperresonance and decreased breath sounds, respectively, on the affected side of the chest. In a tension pneumothorax with a significant amount of accumulated air, the trachea may be shifted away from the collapsed side with severe tachycardia, hypotension, cyanosis, and distended neck veins.

B. Imaging and Laboratory Findings

Chest x-ray will reveal most significant pneumothoraces except those localized to the anterior pleural space in supine patients. An upright chest x-ray or expiratory film may help with the diagnosis in these cases. Chest computed tomography (CT) scan is not routinely recommended for patients with first-time pneumothorax but may be indicated to evaluate suspected pulmonary disorders, trauma, and recurrent pneumothorax or while managing persistent air leaks. Assess the degree of respiratory insufficiency with arterial blood gases (PCO_2, PO_2).

Treatment & Disposition

Immediately ensure that the patient has an intact airway. If the airway is not intact, perform suctioning and endotracheal intubation as necessary. Provide supplemental oxygen if intubation is not needed. Treatment and management options depend primarily on the cause and size of the pneumothorax and on the patient's stability. Patients are generally considered stable if their respiratory rate is less than 24 breaths/min, heart rate is between 60 and 120 beats/min with normal blood pressure, and oxygen saturation is greater than 90% and if the patient can speak in whole sentences between breaths. Otherwise, patients may be deemed unstable.

A. Primary Spontaneous Pneumothorax

Clinically stable patients with small pneumothoraces may be observed in the emergency department for 3–6 hours and discharged to home if repeat chest x-ray excludes progression of the pneumothorax. Aspiration is appropriate only if the pneumothorax enlarges. Admission is indicated for patients who cannot reliably have follow-up within 12–48 hours with repeat chest x-ray. Patients who are unstable or stable with a large pneumothorax should undergo reexpansion of the lung with a 16–22F catheter (pigtail) attached to a Heimlich valve–water seal device or undergo tube thoracostomy and be hospitalized. If a bronchopleural fistula is suspected or the patient may require positive-pressure ventilation, a 24–28F standard chest tube may be used.

B. SECONDARY SPONTANEOUS PNEUMOTHORAX

Although somewhat controversial, it is now recommended that even clinically stable patients with small secondary pneumothoraces should be admitted rather than managed in the emergency department and discharged to home. Patients should be stabilized with simple aspiration or tube thoracostomy and hospitalized. Clinically stable patients with large pneumothoraces or unstable patients should undergo chest tube placement and be hospitalized. Refer these patients for medical or surgical intervention to prevent recurrence.

C. TENSION PNEUMOTHORAX

Immediate needle thoracostomy (with a 14- to 16-gauge needle in the second intercostal space at the midclavicular line) should be performed if tension pneumothorax is suspected clinically. Do not wait for x-ray confirmation if the patient is unstable. Definitive tube thoracostomy should then be performed as soon as possible. The patient should be admitted for symptomatic treatment of chest pain and cough with serial chest x-rays until the pneumothorax resolves.

D. TRAUMATIC PNEUMOTHORAX

Immediately assess for and treat tension pneumothorax if suspected as noted above. If the pneumothorax is secondary to blunt or penetrating injury with a high suspicion of hemothorax, a large-bore (32–36F) chest tube should be used to allow drainage of air and blood. If the pneumothorax is not highly suspect for hemothorax, a tube sized 28F or greater is appropriate.

Baumann MH et al: Management of spontaneous pneumothorax. An American College of Chest Physicians Delphi consensus statement. Chest 2001;119(2):590. [PMID: 11555554] (Evidence-based multidisciplinary expert panel consensus recommendations for management of adults with primary and secondary pneumothoraces.)

ASTHMA & CHRONIC OBSTRUCTIVE PULMONARY DISEASE

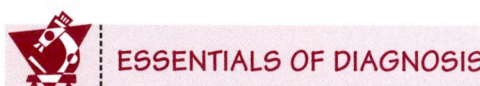 ESSENTIALS OF DIAGNOSIS

Asthma

- *Cough, wheezing, chest tightness, often worse at night.*
- *Physical exam: prolonged expiratory phase or bilateral wheezing, tachypnea, tachycardia, hypoxia.*
- *Reversible with bronchodilators.*

Chronic Obstructive Pulmonary Disease

- *Smoker with chronic productive cough complains of dyspnea.*
- *Increased sputum production, bilateral wheezing, rales, rhonchi.*

General Considerations

COPD is an umbrella term used to describe a group of lung conditions characterized primarily by chronic or recurrent airflow obstruction. The individual conditions are chronic bronchitis, emphysema, and asthma. Although each entity varies in its distinct anatomic and clinical features, patients share a common major complaint of dyspnea. Patients with these disorders present to the emergency department with severe respiratory distress, life-threatening hypoxia, and a need for emergent management. Because of the underlying airflow obstruction, these entities are evaluated in a similar manner to one another and share some basic treatment strategies.

Asthma is a chronic but reversible inflammatory disorder of both the large and small airways. It is characterized by airway obstruction caused by periodic bronchospasm and hypersecretion of mucus. With chronic disease and prolonged attacks, smaller airways can become blocked secondary to increased hypertrophy of bronchial smooth muscle or mucus glands, progressive mast cell activation, and inflammatory cell infiltration. This clinical picture leads to air trapping, ventilation-perfusion mismatches, and resultant hypoxemia and respiratory failure.

Chronic bronchitis and emphysema are both partially reversible but generally progressive diseases of airway obstruction. Both entities are highly correlated with tobacco smoking and are often associated with bronchospastic coughing, wheezing, and severe airway hyperreactivity. Chronic bronchitis is a clinical diagnosis and is present in any patient with a daily productive cough for at least 3 months in at least 2 consecutive years. Its hallmark is hypersecretion of mucus in the large airways resulting from chronic irritation of inhaled substances and chronic infections. Emphysema is defined as destruction of lung parenchyma with abnormal coalescence of the airways distal to the terminal bronchioles.

Many conditions are commonly associated with asthma and COPD exacerbations and are listed in Table 33–2. Some of these conditions are treatable, and the clinician should ask about them specifically while taking the patient's history.

Table 33–2. Common precipitating factors in acute asthma and exacerbations of chronic obstructive pulmonary disease.

Infection (especially upper respiratory tract viral infections)
Drugs (aspirin, nonsteroidal anti-inflammatory agents, food coloring, β-blockers)
Exercise
Emotional stress
Inhaled irritants (eg, air pollution, cigarette smoke)
Occupational exposure to dusts, gases, etc
Aeroallergens (pollens, grasses, molds, animal dander)
Gastroesophageal reflux disease
Weather changes (especially cold)
Menses (catamenial asthma)
Uncompensated congestive heart failure (cardiac asthma)
Noncompliance

Clinical Findings

A. ASTHMA

1. History—The most common clinical characteristics include chronic or episodic wheezing, cough, and dyspnea. Diagnosis depends on a prolonged history of asthmatic symptoms (as described above) associated with known precipitating factors (see Table 33–2) and a sufficient, often immediate, response to bronchodilators. There may be associated chest tightness or pain, allergic symptoms (such as rhinitis, sneezing, nasal obstruction, conjunctivitis) or symptoms of purulent bronchitis or sinusitis. Presentations, signs, and symptoms vary widely and can change over time. Although diffuse wheezing is the hallmark of asthma, nonproductive cough may occur without wheezing. Asthma attacks can occur spontaneously without known precipitating factors.

2. Physical examination—Patients will show some degree of respiratory distress and usually demonstrate periodic symptoms of coughing.

a. Mild exacerbations—Patients with mild exacerbations typically present with tachypnea, normal mental status, oxygen saturation greater than 95%, the ability to speak in full sentences, and only expiratory wheezing with prolonged expiratory phase on auscultation.

b. Moderate exacerbations—Patients with moderate exacerbations get breathless while talking in short phrases, prefer sitting up, may appear somewhat agitated, commonly have increased respiratory rate with moderate use of accessory respiratory muscles, are tachycardic with oxygen saturation of 91–95% and a near normal PCO_2, and have both inspiratory and expiratory wheezing.

c. Severe exacerbations—Patients with severe exacerbations present with breathlessness at rest, ability to say only occasional words, inability to recline, respiratory rate greater than 30 breaths/min, oxygen saturation less than 91%, PaO_2 less than 60 mm Hg, $PaCO_2$ greater than 40, significant use of accessory muscles with nasal flaring, heart rate greater than 120 beats/min, pulsus paradoxus often greater than 10–20 mm Hg, agitation, and poor air movement with nearly inaudible breath sounds.

d. Impending respiratory failure—Patients with impending respiratory failure are unable to speak, have paradoxical thoracoabdominal movements, relative bradycardia, little air movement, and are confused or drowsy secondary to increasing levels of carbon dioxide.

Although an obvious relationship exists between symptoms and airflow obstruction, clinical findings alone are not reliable indicators of severity. Because many patients and physicians will underestimate the severity of airflow limitations, objective measurements such as peak expiratory flow (PEF) measurements should be obtained when feasible.

B. CHRONIC BRONCHITIS

1. History—Patients with acute exacerbations of chronic bronchitis are smokers who complain of increased sputum production in addition to worsening dyspnea on exertion. They come to the emergency department for treatment of worsening symptoms and any underlying complications (eg, pneumonia, congestive heart failure, pneumothorax).

2. Physical examination—These patients were labeled in the past as "blue bloaters," meaning they are frequently cyanotic and overweight, with peripheral edema, but often appear comfortable at rest. These patients begin to present in their late 30s or early 40s with a history of multiple past lung infections. The dyspnea is usually mild, whereas peripheral edema may be marked, and the patient quickly notes limitations with exercising. Examination of the chest reveals bilateral wheezing, rales, and rhonchi.

C. EMPHYSEMA

1. History—These patients always have an extensive smoking history and complaints of worsening dyspnea on exertion, often with more severe coughing. As the severity and duration of disease progress, dyspnea may also occur at rest.

2. Physical examination—These patients have been called "pink puffers." They are typically thin smokers who are not cyanotic but appear quite uncomfortable and have significant complaints of dyspnea. They are usually over age 50 and have a chronic hacking cough (usually productive of scant, clear sputum). Dyspnea is often severe with obvious use of accessory muscles of respiration. The chest walls are barrel shaped and very quiet on examination, without adventitious sounds noted.

Evaluation

A. MEDICAL HISTORY

Duration, severity, and comparison with previous attacks (ie, more or less severe than usual) should be sought, along with recent exposure to common precipitating factors of disease. Identify precisely all medications being taken, with dosages and times of administration. Document any past or current home oxygen use; any recent completion of corticosteroids; and any previous hospitalizations including intensive care unit stays and especially intubations.

B. LABORATORY AND OTHER FINDINGS

1. Arterial blood gases—An arterial blood gas is a direct measure of cardiopulmonary function. Although not routinely necessary for asthma patients, arterial blood gases should be part of the evaluation of every severe asthma attack and are virtually mandatory for patients with exacerbations of COPD. Symptoms and physical findings cannot be used to predict blood gas values accurately. All patients with acute exacerbations of asthma and COPD will have some degree of hypoxemia, even those with minimal bronchospasm undetectable by auscultation. Most asthma patients are hypocapnic as a result of reflex hyperventilation, whereas COPD patients may have low, normal, or even elevated arterial PCO_2.

During a severe asthma attack, as airway resistance increases significantly, poor gas exchange develops with worsening hypoxemia and rising PCO_2 levels. Thus, a normal or elevated PCO_2 with concomitant respiratory acidosis indicates a very sick patient with impending respiratory failure.

Patients with chronic bronchitis and emphysema compensate for the acid load of chronic hypercapnia by bicarbonate retention (chronic respiratory acidosis with metabolic compensation), producing a relatively normal arterial blood pH. Therefore, a markedly lowered arterial blood pH in conjunction with hypercapnia indicates that the carbon dioxide retention is probably of recent onset (within 1–2 days) or that acidosis has a metabolic component. The new arterial blood gas must be compared with prior blood gas values and the current clinical condition to accurately evaluate the significance of the test.

2. Chest x-ray—The chest x-ray in routine cases of asthma will be normal or demonstrate mild thoracic hyperinflation. However, it may be beneficial in revealing complications such as pneumonia, pneumothorax, or foreign body in young children (unilateral hyperinflation). In general, unless there is a reason to suspect another diagnosis or complications of asthma, a chest x-ray is not necessary for mild to moderate asthma.

By contrast, patients with COPD will often have chest x-ray findings, which may lead to changes in patient management. These findings include complications of COPD and findings consistent with congestive heart failure, lung cancer, tuberculosis, and pleural effusions. Therefore, it is recommended that a chest x-ray be ordered for all patients evaluated in the emergency department for an acute exacerbation of COPD.

3. Peak expiratory flow measurement—Physicians and patients often underestimate the severity of asthmatic disease. PEF is a useful measurement for judging severity and monitoring the response to therapy in cases of mild to moderate asthma exacerbations. However, it is not helpful in severe asthma attacks, young children, or other difficult patients who are often unable or unwilling to cooperate. PEF should be compared with the patient's personal best or predicted peak flow values, which are based on age, sex, and height. PEF less than 50% of predicted indicates a severe exacerbation.

Initially considered extremely helpful for COPD exacerbations, it is now recommended that PEF should not be used to diagnosis exacerbations nor determine their severity.

4. Pulse oximetry—Pulse oximetry is used primarily to evaluate for hypoxemia. It is useful for monitoring oxygenation but provides no information on ventilation, hence, arterial blood gases are needed.

5. Electrocardiogram—Look for evidence of supraventricular and ventricular arrhythmias, myocardial ischemia or infarct, and cor pulmonale (right ventricular hypertrophy, right atrial hypertrophy).

6. Complete blood count and differential—Leukocytosis is common (especially in children) as a result of demargination induced by endogenous and exogenous epinephrine and corticosteroid use. Therefore, the white blood cell count is not a reliable indicator of infection; however, a shift to the left (to more immature leukocytes) may suggest infection. Marked eosinophilia occurs in some patients and does not indicate that asthma is due to allergy.

7. Electrolytes—Serum electrolytes are of little benefit but may demonstrate hypokalemia (especially if the patient is taking diuretics) or dehydration.

8. Microscopic examination of sputum—Sputum examination is usually not helpful in asthma patients unless an associated pneumonia triggered the exacerbation.

Patients with COPD have chronically infected airways, but the amount of sputum and degree of purulence often increase during these exacerbations. Gram-stain samples may confirm the presence of significant infection (abundant polymorphonuclear neutrophils) and may help guide antimicrobial therapy, if needed.

9. Theophylline levels—Serum concentrations should be obtained if the patient is currently taking theophylline. Theophylline has a narrow therapeutic index, and even when levels are toxic, the clinical examination cannot predict the level.

Differential Diagnosis

Patients with many other conditions can present with wheezing, cough, shortness of breath, or any combination of the 3.

A. ADULTS

Adults can present with wheezing with many other conditions besides asthma and COPD. Some of these conditions include pulmonary embolus (tachycardia, tachypnea, hypoxia, chest pain), anaphylaxis (new medications, fish, allergens, angioedema), inhalation injury (history of exposure), uncompensated congestive heart failure (rales, distended neck veins, dependent edema, dyspnea), pneumonia (fever, cough, chills, infiltrate on x-ray), foreign body (elderly patients, oropharyngeal cancer, stroke), bronchiolitis obliterans, laryngotracheal masses, or vocal cord paralysis and dysfunction.

B. CHILDREN

In young patients with a long history of recurrent wheezing, there is little doubt about the diagnosis. In patients with their first attack of wheezing, look closely for other causes such as epiglottitis (any age, abrupt onset of fever, sore throat, inspiratory stridor, dysphagia, drooling, toxic appearance), croup (usually aged 6 months to 3 years, 2–3 days of upper respiratory symptoms, "barking" cough worse at night, fever), bronchiolitis (usually respiratory syncytial virus, younger than age 2 years), foreign body aspiration (no previous history of wheezing, unilateral wheezing, unilateral atelectasis on chest x-ray, no response to bronchodilators). Other possibilities include cystic fibrosis, bronchopulmonary dysplasia, immunodeficiency syndromes, or congenital cardiovascular anomalies.

Treatment

The initial approach to treatment of asthma and COPD exacerbations revolves around 3 goals: (1) correcting hypoxemia rapidly, (2) reversing airway obstruction, and (3) taking steps to reduce recurrence of airflow obstruction. These goals can be accomplished by providing supplemental oxygen, bronchodilators, and systemic corticosteroids as needed. The level of care is determined by the severity of disease. All patients should be placed on noninvasive blood pressure monitoring and pulse oximetry. Any patient having a moderate to severe attack also must be placed on a cardiac monitor, and peripheral venous access should be established as soon as possible.

A. MILD EXACERBATIONS

1. Respiratory support—Correct hypoxemia with supplemental oxygen by nasal cannula. Maintain oxygen saturations greater than 90%. In asthma patients, obtain PEF (usually greater than 50% predicted).

2. β-Adrenergic agonists—These medications are the mainstay of treatment for asthma and COPD. The ones most commonly used are the short-acting β_2-selective agents. These agents cause rapid relaxation of bronchial smooth muscles, resulting in bronchodilation and reducing airflow obstruction. Albuterol, levalbuterol (the R-isomer of albuterol), and metaproterenol are used most often. Inhalation, through metered-dose inhalers (MDIs) or nebulizers, has been shown to be faster and to deliver higher concentrations of medication to the lungs with fewer systemic side effects than oral preparations. However, MDIs require coordination and a cooperative, alert patient who can hold his or her breath for 5–10 seconds. Therefore, passive nebulized β_2-agonists are more often used in moderate and severe exacerbations. For mild disease, albuterol MDI dosing is 4–6 puffs every 20 minutes (up to 4 hours), and nebulized solutions should be given at 2.5 mg every 20–30 minutes for 3 doses as needed for dyspnea. Monitor patients for side effects such as tachycardia, especially if a history of underlying cardiovascular disease is present. An inhaled β_2-adrenergic agonists may need to be continued every 4 hours for 24–48 hours.

3. Systemic corticosteroids—Steroids are well known to inhibit both inflammatory cell recruitment and the release of inflammatory mediators into the airways. Many patients with moderate to severe obstructive airway disease take chronic steroids. Although steroids do not initially change emergency department management, these medications are crucial to reduce the rate of relapse in moderate to severe exacerbations. They can also be helpful in mild attacks if the patient is not responding well to initial bronchodilator treatments. Consider steroids if the patient is taking oral or inhaled steroids, has had prolonged symptoms, or recently completed a steroid taper. The patient should continue steroids for 3–10 days after discharge to prevent a recurrence (adults: prednisone, 60 mg first day, then

40 mg/d after discharge; children: prednisone, 2 mg/kg first day, then 1 mg/kg/d after discharge).

4. Anticholinergics—Ipratropium bromide, an atropine-like compound, is available as a MDI (Atrovent) and can be used to reverse vagally mediated bronchospasm without the unwanted anticholinergic side effects. If the asthma patient has known previous improvement with Atrovent, it should be added to initial therapy. Otherwise, it should be reserved for more severe disease. COPD patients, by contrast, should be started on anticholinergic nebulized or MDI treatment. Anticholinergics have proven additive bronchodilatory effects when used with β_2-adrenergic medications in this population.

5. Antibiotics—Antibiotics are typically not indicated for mild asthma or COPD exacerbations unless evidence of infection is present on physical examination or chest x-ray. Patients with an acute exacerbation of COPD, presenting with worsening dyspnea and increased cough and sputum production, may have underlying pneumonia and should receive antibiotics.

B. MODERATE EXACERBATIONS

1. Respiratory support—Give supplemental oxygen by nasal cannula. Titrate to keep oxygen saturation greater than 90%. Higher levels of functional inspired oxygen concentration (FIO_2) in patients with COPD may be associated with worsening hypercapnia or apnea. This occurs because they tend to have baseline carbon dioxide elevations with a hypoxic ventilatory drive, and as they lose this hypoxic drive, apnea can occur. If the patient appears to be deteriorating, repeat arterial blood gases should be obtained after 30 minutes to reassess ventilation. However, clinical examination of the patient, not the arterial blood gas level, should direct the need for intubation.

2. β-Adrenergic agonists—Give albuterol, nebulized solution 2.5 mg every 20–30 minutes for 3 doses, or MDI with spacer 6–12 puffs every 20 minutes (up to 4 hours as needed).

3. Systemic corticosteroids—Adults: prednisone, 60 mg orally, or methylprednisolone, 60–125 mg intramuscularly or intravenously (if patient is unable to tolerate oral form); children: prednisone, 2 mg/kg first dose should be administered immediately. Discharge the patient to home with a steroid burst (adults: prednisone, 40 mg/d; children: 1 mg/kg, for 3–5 days) or taper (10–14 days) depending on severity.

4. Anticholinergics—Ipratropium MDI or nebulized treatment should be given to asthma patients with known response to this medication. All COPD patients should receive ipratropium MDI (2–6 puffs every 4–6 hours) with albuterol or via nebulized treatment if unable to cooperate with inhalers.

5. Antibiotics—Antibiotics are not indicated for patients with moderately severe asthma exacerbations unless evidence of infection is present on physical examination or chest x-ray. However, antibiotics are recommended for patients with an acute exacerbation of COPD. The macrolides and newer fluoroquinolones provide excellent monodrug therapy.

6. Positive airway pressure—If the patient continues to deteriorate without significant improvement from the above measures, bilevel positive airway pressure (BiPAP) or continuous positive airway pressure (CPAP) can be administered in an attempt to avoid intubation.

C. SEVERE OR LIFE-THREATENING EXACERBATIONS

1. Respiratory support—These patients can decompensate quickly; therefore, treatment should precede history taking. These patients often present with near-fatal asthma or COPD (evidence of respiratory failure or respiratory arrest), status asthmaticus (severe bronchospasm that does not respond to aggressive therapies within 30–60 minutes), or lethargy and disorientation. Immediate attention should be given to rapid correction of hypoxemia with 100% supplemental oxygen by face mask to keep saturations greater than 90%.

2. Intubation and mechanical ventilation—Because patients may die without assisted ventilation, consider intubation if the patient appears exhausted, confused, or cyanotic. The clinical evaluation over time will dictate the need for intubation. Rapid-sequence intubation may need to be performed, but overwhelming exhaustion often makes this step unnecessary. Large endotracheal tubes should be used that facilitate suctioning and bronchoscopy, if needed. Ventilatory settings should allow an FIO_2 of 100% with hypoventilation (respiratory rate = 8–10 breaths/min), known as permissive hypercapnia. This hypercapnia, along with lower tidal volumes (6–8 mL/kg), helps to decrease overdistention, air trapping, and resultant barotrauma.

3. β-Adrenergic agonists—Give continuous albuterol nebulized treatment for 1 hour at high doses (5 mg every 20–30 minutes for 3 doses) to maximize results.

4. Systemic corticosteroids—Methylprednisolone, 60–125 mg intravenously for adults, or 2 mg/kg for first pediatric dose, should be administered immediately. Lower doses (0.5 mg/kg–1.0 mg/kg) can continue, scheduled every 6–8 hours during hospitalization, with a 10- to 14-day oral taper on discharge.

5. Anticholinergics—Ipratropium nebulized solution, 0.5 mg every 20–30 minutes for 3 doses, mixed with albuterol nebulized treatment should be given and then scheduled every 4–6 hours during hospitalization.

6. Antibiotics—For patients with COPD, start intravenous antibiotics in the emergency department if they cannot tolerate oral antibiotics. Inpatient antibiotic coverage for pneumonia will include a combination of a fluoroquinolone, a β-lactam/β-lactamase inhibitor, a macrolide, or a third-generation cephalosporin. If the exacerbation is due primarily to asthma, antibiotics may be withheld.

D. Other Known Treatment Modalities

1. Magnesium sulfate—Magnesium has a direct relaxing effect on bronchial smooth muscle and also helps to stabilize many inflammatory mediators. For patients with severe asthma, magnesium (in conjunction with ongoing treatment) may help improve airway obstruction and avoid intubation. The dosing is 2–3 g intravenously, infused at 1 g/min, with close monitoring of blood pressure. The infusion should stop if hypotension, respiratory depression, or decreased deep tendon reflexes occurs.

2. Methylxanthines—Theophylline (oral) or aminophylline (intravenous) are moderately effective bronchodilators that may be considered in severe asthma in conjunction with other treatments if the disease is refractory. However, they have a very narrow therapeutic margin. Toxicity may be manifested by tachydysrhythmias, gastrointestinal upset, and central nervous system irritability. These medications are no longer recommended for the treatment of acute exacerbations of COPD.

3. Ketamine—Ketamine has been shown to be a significant bronchodilator and should be the agent of choice during sedation for intubation of severely agitated patients with refractory disease (status asthmaticus). Usual anesthetic induction dose is 1–2 mg/kg intravenously or 4 mg/kg intramuscularly.

Disposition

A. Asthma

Asthma patients who demonstrate a good response (PEF > 70% of predicted) and whose symptoms resolve can be discharged home. Those with an incomplete response to treatment (PEF 50–70% of predicted) with improved symptoms and no hypoxia can be discharged if close follow-up and correct use of inhalers can be demonstrated. All others, including patients seen in an emergency department within the past 3 days, those with a change in mental status, or those having a significant complication should be hospitalized for further treatment and observation for deterioration. Severe attacks should be treated in the intensive care unit.

B. Acute Exacerbations of COPD

Acute exacerbations of COPD should be treated with admission in patients who remain symptomatic, have significant comorbidities, develop mental status changes, are unable to perform activities of daily living without assistance, are unresponsive to treatment, or have a treatable complication such as congestive heart failure or pneumothorax. Patients with impending respiratory failure should receive treatment in the intensive care unit. If these patients have responded to emergency department treatment, are reliable with good follow-up, and feel they are back to their baselines, they can be discharged to home.

Li JT et al: Algorithm for the diagnosis and management of asthma: a practice parameter update: Joint Task Force on Practice Parameters, representing the American Academy of Allergy, Asthma, and Immunology, the American College of Allergy, Asthma, and Immunology, and the Joint Council of Allergy, Asthma, and Immunology. Ann Allergy Asthma Immunol 1998;81:415. [PMID: 9860033] (A thorough and complete update of the previously published practice parameters for the diagnosis and treatment of asthma.)

National Asthma Education and Prevention Program: Practical Guide for the Diagnosis and Management of Asthma Based on the *Expert Panel Report 2: Guidelines for the Diagnosis and Management of Asthma.* National Institutes of Health Consensus Development Conference Consensus Statement. 1997;(Suppl. 4). [PMID: 974051] (Evidence-based, expert panel consensus recommendations for the diagnosis and management of asthma.)

Snow V et al: The evidence base for management of acute exacerbations of COPD: clinical practice guidelines, part 1. Chest 2001;119(4):1185. [PMID: 11296188] (A joint expert panel formed by the American College of Physicians, American Society of Internal Medicine, and American College of Chest Physicians has developed evidence-based management recommendations for acute exacerbations of COPD from research centered primarily on emergency department and inpatient treatment settings.)

ACUTE PULMONARY EMBOLISM

 ESSENTIALS OF DIAGNOSIS

- *Acute onset of dyspnea, pleuritic chest pain, tachypnea, tachycardia.*
- *Hypoxemia with widened A-a gradient.*
- *Pulmonary angiogram is gold standard.*

General Considerations

A variety of clinical conditions may cause clots to form in the venous system that when dislodged will cause pulmonary emboli (Table 33–3). Venous thrombosis may result from a generalized hypercoagulable state, venous endothelial injury, or local stasis (Virchow triad). Clots that cause clinically significant pulmonary emboli form most commonly in the iliofemoral and pelvic venous beds. Pulmonary embolization, from veins of the upper extremities or distal lower extremities, is rare.

When embolization occurs, the consequences and manifestations depend on the size of the embolism, the patient's underlying cardiorespiratory status, and whether subsequent infarction of pulmonary tissue occurs. With small- to medium-sized emboli, obstruction of a localized portion of the pulmonary vascular tree causes local atelectasis with resulting ventilation-perfusion (V/Q) abnormalities and hypoxemia. Reflex hyperventilation with resultant hypocapnia and tachycardia also occurs. With massive embolization (obstructing over 60% of the vascular bed), acute pulmonary hypertension, right heart strain, systemic hypotension, and shock may also occur. Fragmentation of large emboli with distal migration of clot or further embolization may result in stepwise changes in clinical status. Death may occur suddenly.

Clinical Findings

Patients should initially be categorized into pretest clinical categories (low, moderate, or high risk) following the history, physical examination, and clinical findings.

Table 33–3. Conditions that predispose to pulmonary embolization.

Venous stasis
  Prolonged immobility (eg, bed rest, stroke)
  Chronic obstructive pulmonary disease
  Congestive heart failure
Venous endothelial damage
  Surgery within past 3 months
  Fractures of long bones or hip
  Burns
  Lower extremity trauma
Hypercoagulability
  Malignant neoplastic disease
  Use of oral contraceptives
  Marked obesity
  Protein C or S deficiency
Antithrombin III deficiency
Presence of factor V Leiden
Previous history of deep venous thrombosis or pulmonary
  embolism

This pretest probability will aid in directing further evaluation.

A. Symptoms and Signs

The illness often begins abruptly, and a predisposing underlying condition is almost always present (see Table 33–3). Dyspnea, cough, anxiety, and chest pain occur in varying combinations. Hemoptysis may occur, and syncope is rare. Tachycardia and tachypnea are commonly noted on examination. Low-grade fever, hypotension, cyanosis, signs of deep venous thrombosis, pleural friction rub, and signs of pulmonary consolidation may be present.

B. Laboratory and Other Findings

1. Chest x-ray—Although the chest x-ray is abnormal in most patients with pulmonary embolization with infarction, the abnormalities are often nonspecific (eg, atelectasis, pleural effusions, small infiltrates). The Westermark sign (dilated pulmonary vasculature proximal to embolus with oligemia distal) and Hampton's Hump (a pleural-based density with a rounded border facing the hilum) are specific though uncommon findings in pulmonary emboli.

2. Electrocardiogram—The electrocardiogram is often abnormal, usually demonstrating tachycardia or diffuse nonspecific ST-T abnormalities. The classic finding of acute right heart strain (S1/Q3/T3; T-wave inversion in leads V1–V3) is more specific but somewhat uncommon. In massive pulmonary emboli, there may be findings of myocardial ischemia (leading to mistaken diagnosis of myocardial infarction without realization of the underlying cause).

3. Arterial blood gases—A clinically significant pulmonary embolism is almost always associated with hypoxemia (oxygen saturation < 90%; PO_2 < 80 mm Hg); however, this finding may be partially obscured by the reflex hyperventilation and hypocapnia that occur in most patients.

4. D-Dimer—The serum levels of D-Dimer (a degradation product of cross-linked fibrin) measured via an enzyme-linked immunoassay (ELISA) technique have been shown to be a highly sensitive (95%) screening examination in the assessment for acute thrombus formation. Therefore, if ELISA D-Dimer is negative, it can be helpful to avoid invasive procedures such as pulmonary angiogram or CT angiography in low-risk patients. However, be cautious with this test. If the patient has been given a moderate to high pretest probability for pulmonary embolus, then a definitive test (CT scan or angiogram) must be performed. Also, many hospitals have only the latex agglutination D-Dimer assay, which has not been shown to have the same sensitivity and should not be used alone (or with indeterminate V/Q scans) to rule out acute thrombus. For this reason, the test remains controversial, and many institutions do not incorporate D-Dimer testing into their management strategies.

C. Diagnostic Imaging

1. Ventilation-perfusion radionuclide lung scans—

a. Normal V/Q scan—A normal scan excludes significant embolization and the need for further testing because it is a highly sensitive screening examination in patients without known cardiopulmonary disease. However, a variety of other conditions (most commonly COPD) can result in an abnormal V/Q scan, making many results nonspecific (indeterminate). Therefore, in patients with known cardiopulmonary disease, a spiral CT angiogram may be a wiser first step in the evaluation of pulmonary emboli.

b. High probability V/Q scan—A high probability V/Q scan is defined as a large perfusion defect in areas of normal ventilation and is highly specific (but insensitive) for acute pulmonary emboli. As a result, a high probability scan is sufficient to confirm diagnosis of pulmonary emboli.

c. Indeterminate V/Q scan—An indeterminate V/Q scan (also reported as nondiagnostic, low probability, or intermediate probability) is more difficult to use clinically (and more confusing) and requires previously assessed pretest clinical suspicion.

If the V/Q scan was indeterminate with a low to moderate clinical suspicion of pulmonary embolism, then perform ELISA D-Dimer (if negative: seek alternative cause; if positive: perform spiral CT angiography or duplex Doppler ultrasound—some hospitals go directly to spiral CT or Doppler without D-Dimer).

Alternatively, if the V/Q scan was indeterminate with a high clinical suspicion of pulmonary embolism, perform a lower extremity venous Doppler ultrasound (if positive: treat pulmonary embolism or deep venous thrombosis, if negative: perform spiral CT angiography; if CT is positive: treat pulmonary embolism or deep venous thrombosis, if CT is negative: obtain pulmonary angiogram).

2. Helicospiral CT angiography—

Contrast-enhanced spiral CT scan allows for rapid evaluation but requires proper technique and expert radiographic interpretation. Although it is a very sensitive test for central pulmonary emboli, it may miss isolated subsegmental emboli. A spiral CT can also offer clues to alternative diagnoses if there is no evidence of pulmonary emboli. Most protocols for pulmonary emboli evaluation will also scan the pelvis and lower extremities as well as the chest in order to simultaneously evaluate for deep venous thrombosis (therefore, duplex Doppler may be unnecessary). Spiral CT scan is the initial study of choice to evaluate for pulmonary emboli in patients with underlying cardiopulmonary disease or an abnormal chest x-ray.

If the spiral CT scan is positive for pulmonary emboli or demonstrates an alternative diagnosis, then provide treatment as indicated. If the CT scan is negative or indeterminate with symptoms of deep venous thrombosis or moderate to high pretest clinical suspicion, then a Doppler ultrasound of the lower extremities is indicated (if positive: treat deep venous thrombosis or pulmonary emboli; if negative: obtain pulmonary angiogram for definitive diagnosis). If the CT scan is negative with low pretest clinical suspicion, then seek an alternative cause for the symptoms.

3. Venous Doppler ultrasound—

Doppler ultrasound is a noninvasive test used to evaluate for deep venous thrombosis. It is an operator-dependent procedure, and the results are often difficult to assess in patients with previous deep venous thrombosis. It is otherwise highly sensitive and specific for the diagnosis of deep venous thrombosis. This test is most useful in patients without evidence of deep venous thrombosis but with high clinical suspicion for acute pulmonary emboli or indeterminate V/Q or spiral CT scans.

If the duplex Doppler is positive, use anticoagulation to treat for acute deep venous thrombosis or pulmonary emboli. If the test is negative in low-risk patients, then repeat it in 5–7 days. If the test is negative in moderate- to high-risk patients, then perform spiral CT angiography or pulmonary angiogram for a definitive diagnosis.

4. Pulmonary angiogram—

Pulmonary angiogram is the gold standard because of its high sensitivity and specificity. It is expensive and invasive, difficult to obtain, requires radiographic expertise, and can be associated with severe complications. Angiogram is most effective when diagnosis of pulmonary emboli must be established with certainty (eg, in patients in whom anticoagulation carries a high risk of adverse effects, in patients who will receive long-term anticoagulation, and in patients who will receive thrombolytic therapy).

Treatment

A. Respiratory Support

Correct hypoxemia with oxygen, 5–10 L/min, by nasal cannula or mask. If hypercapnia is present on admission, arterial blood gas measurements should be repeated within 15–20 minutes. Continuously monitor oxygen saturation by pulse oximetry. Worsening hypercapnia with progressive obtundation is an indication for emergent intubation.

B. Anticoagulation Therapy

Use unfractionated heparin (UFH) or low-molecular-weight heparin (LMWH) as soon as possible to prevent further clot formation in patients with high clinical likelihood for pulmonary emboli or with diagnosed pulmonary emboli. Use UFH with an initial 80 IU/kg bolus followed by 18 IU/kg/h infusion or LMWH (enoxaparin or dalteparin) to initiate anticoagulation. LMWH is at least as effective and safe as UFH and is more convenient. Compared with UFH, LMWH is more expensive but may reduce the total hospital cost and length of stay because activated partial thromboplastin time levels need not be followed in these patients. Evaluate patients for contraindications to anticoagulation prior to administration.

C. Thrombolytic Therapy

Although anticoagulation is sufficient treatment for most patients with pulmonary emboli, a few patients present with right heart dysfunction, hemodynamic compromise, or cardiogenic shock and may benefit from clot removal from the pulmonary artery. Thrombolytic agents such as streptokinase, urokinase, and tissue plasminogen activator achieve such lysis and may also may prevent damage to the pulmonary vascular bed and decrease the morbidity and mortality associated with pulmonary emboli. Thrombolytic therapy may be associated with severe bleeding and cannot be used in patients with recent trauma, cerebral vascular accident, or gastrointestinal tract hemorrhage (see contraindications to thrombolytic therapy in Chapter 34). Before thrombolytic therapy is started, standard protocol must be followed: discontinue heparin and ensure that the thrombin time, prothrombin time, or activated partial thromboplastin time is less than twice the normal value. For the strict dosing and administration criteria of these thrombolytic agents, consult the package inserts. Thrombolytic agents should be discontinued if significant bleeding occurs; the actions of these drugs can be reversed with fresh frozen plasma. Reinstate heparin treatment after thrombolytic therapy has been completed.

D. Surgical Treatment

A transvenous catheter embolectomy or open surgical embolectomy may be a life-saving maneuver in a patient with massive emboli and refractory hypotension or in patients with contraindications to or failure of thrombolytics. A Greenfield filter may also be introduced to capture further emboli.

Disposition

Hospitalize all patients for continued anticoagulation and supportive care. Patients with large emboli or hemodynamic impairment, or those receiving thrombolytics, should be monitored in the intensive care unit.

Patients in whom pulmonary embolism is strongly suspected should be hospitalized for anticoagulation (if no contraindications are present) until a definitive diagnosis can be made.

Arcasoy SM: Thrombolytic therapy of pulmonary embolism: a comprehensive review of current evidence. Chest 1999;115 (6):1695. [PMID: 10378570] (Extensive review of medical research from 1966 to 1998 with the development of evidence-based guidelines for the use of thrombolytics in the treatment of acute pulmonary emboli.)

Bloomgarden DC: Newer diagnostic modalities for pulmonary embolism. Pulmonary angiography using CT and MR imaging compared with conventional angiography. Emerg Med Clin North Am 2001;19(4)975. [PMID: 11762283] (Provides an in-depth, evidence-based review of the benefits of CT pulmonary angiography as a first-line diagnostic modality in evaluation for pulmonary emboli and a brief overview of the future use of magnetic resonance angiography.)

Edlow JA: Emergency department management of pulmonary embolism. Emerg Med Clin North Am 2001;19(4):995. [PMID: 11762284] (Thorough evidence-based review of current evaluation, diagnosis, and treatment of acute pulmonary embolism in the emergency department.)

Holbert JM: Role of spiral computed tomography in the diagnosis of pulmonary embolism in the emergency department. Ann Emerg Med 1999;33(5):520. [PMID: 10216328] (Reviews advantages and disadvantages of all current diagnostic modalities for acute pulmonary emboli with a suggested algorithm for emergency department evaluation.)

Wolfe TR, Hartsell SC: Pulmonary embolism: making sense of the diagnostic evaluation. Ann Emerg Med 2001;37(5):504. [PMID: 11326187] (Review of large prospective studies with a proposed evidence-based diagnostic algorithm for the evaluation of suspected pulmonary embolism.)

■ EMERGENCY MANAGEMENT OF SPECIFIC CONDITIONS

PNEUMOMEDIASTINUM & SUBCUTANEOUS EMPHYSEMA

 ESSENTIALS OF DIAGNOSIS

- Soft tissue swelling, subcutaneous emphysema.
- Hamman's crunch, air in the mediastinum on chest x-ray.

General Considerations

Pneumomediastinum is commonly associated with pneumothorax (air in the mediastinum). It most commonly occurs from rupture of an overdistended alveolus or a collection of such alveoli ("bleb") into the peri-bronchovascular interstitial space with dissection backward along the bronchi to the mediastinum (Macklin effect). Because the mediastinal pleura is weaker than the pleura surrounding the lung, air may dissect into the mediastinum before entering the pleural space.

Pneumomediastinum may occur without pneumothorax; air also may dissect through contiguous fascial planes into the neck and other soft tissues, causing subcutaneous emphysema. Occasionally pneumomediastinum is due to rupture of the esophagus (Boerhaave syndrome), and this diagnosis should be considered if the patient is acutely ill and has a history of vomiting. Pneumomediastinum also may have iatrogenic (mechanical ventilation, laparoscopy, biopsy) or posttraumatic causes or may result from asthma, Valsalva maneuver (smoking crack cocaine or marijuana, active labor, coughing), gas-producing bacterial mediastinitis, oral trauma (hypopharynx), or acute decompression injury (diving).

Clinical Findings

Chest pain, aggravated by respiration, moving, and position changes, is a common symptom of pneumomediastinum. Diagnosis is made by hearing a mediastinal "crunch" (Hamman's crunch, a crunching sound heard over the heart during systole) on auscultation and seeing air in the mediastinum on chest x-ray. Subcutaneous emphysema presents as soft tissue swelling, especially in the neck. A crackling sound is heard when the tissues are compressed.

Treatment & Disposition

No specific treatment is indicated unless esophageal rupture is present (Chapter 24). Associated conditions such as pneumothorax should be corrected. Analgesics may be required.

Hospitalize patients with severe pneumomediastinum with cardiovascular compromise (extensive spread of mediastinal air), for patients with pneumomediastinum complicated by other disorders (eg, mediastinitis, systemic air embolus, or pneumopericardium), or for patients who require narcotics for pain relief.

McHugh TP: Pneumomediastinum following penetrating oral trauma. Pediatr Emerg Care 1997;13(3):211. [PMID: 9220508] (A review of the pathophysiology and treatment of pneumomediastinum with a case report of a toddler developing pneumomediastinum after falling with a spoon in his mouth.)

Richard HM III et al: Pneumothorax and pneumomediastinum after laparoscopic surgery. Clin Imaging 1997;21(5):337. [PMID: 9316753] (Study evaluating the incidence and significance of pneumomediastinum after laparoscopic surgeries, noting this finding was not associated with significant morbidity and mortality.)

Wintermark M, Schnyder P: The Macklin effect: a frequent etiology for pneumomediastinum in severe blunt chest trauma. Chest 2001;120(2):543. [PMID: 11502656] (A review of the pathophysiology of pneumomediastinum with a retrospective analysis of patients with this diagnosis in one hospital, directly relating the presence of the Macklin effect to the length of intensive care unit stay.)

PLEURODYNIA

 ESSENTIALS OF DIAGNOSIS

- *Self-limited viral illness of skeletal muscle.*
- *Severe pleuritic pain in ribs.*
- *Low-grade fever, malaise.*

General Considerations

Pleurodynia (*pleura,* side; *odyne,* pain) is an acute, self-limited, and benign (though uncomfortable) viral illness of the skeletal muscle, not of the pleura or peritoneum. Most cases occur in epidemics during summer or early fall in young adults and children. It is caused primarily by group B coxsackieviruses and echoviruses.

Clinical Findings

Systemic symptoms are mild (low-grade fever, malaise), but pleuritic pain in the lower ribs is severe (hence the name "devil's grip"). Examination may disclose low-grade fever and a pleural rub in some cases, although the physical examination is normal in many patients. Chest x-ray usually shows no abnormalities, but there may be a small amount of pleural friction fluid, a small pulmonary infiltrate, or both. The leukocyte count and the erythrocyte sedimentation rate are usually normal or only minimally elevated. Pleurodynia may sometimes be accompanied by pericarditis, which may be diagnosed by a friction rub on auscultation or an enlarged cardiac silhouette on chest x-ray. Serious thoracic and abdominal pathology must also be ruled out.

Treatment

No specific therapy is available. For symptomatic relief, nonsteroidal anti-inflammatory agents may be effective. Aspirin is said to be less effective. Narcotic analgesics may be needed.

Disposition

Hospitalization is necessary only for patients who require parenteral analgesics or who also have pericarditis.

Pichichero ME et al: Clinical and economic impact of enterovirus illness in private pediatric practice. Pediatrics 1998;102(5): 1126. [PMID: 9794944] (Prospective multicenter study from pediatric practices in New York, Arizona, and California evaluating the diagnosis and morbidity of enterovirus infections [including pleurodynia] for patients and its direct economic impact on the medical community, including the emergency department.)

PLEURAL EFFUSION

 ESSENTIALS OF DIAGNOSIS

- *Pleuritic chest pain, dyspnea with or without fever, cough.*
- *Decreased breath sounds, decreased tactile fremitus on affected side.*
- *Thoracentesis is definitive diagnostic and often therapeutic procedure.*

General Considerations

Pleural effusions are an abnormal collection of fluid between the parietal and visceral pleura as a result of a local disease process or inflammation. Normally 5–15 mL of serous fluid is present in the pleural space. An effusion can be classified as either an exudate or transudate to help in differential diagnosis. Exudative fluid analysis reveals (1) pleural fluid protein–to–serum protein ratio greater than 0.5, (2) pleural fluid lactate dehydrogenase (LDH)–to–serum LDH ratio greater than 0.6, and (3) pleural fluid LDH greater than two thirds of the upper limit of normal serum LDH. Exudates are associated with direct disease of the pleura itself usually from infection, inflammation, or malignancy. Transudates do not have the above characteristics and are most commonly caused by congestive heart failure, cirrhosis with ascites, or nephrotic syndrome. Every patient with a newly diagnosed pleural effusion requires prompt evaluation to determine the cause so that early and appropriate therapy can be given.

Clinical Findings

A. SYMPTOMS AND SIGNS

The patient may complain of pleuritic or nonpleuritic chest pain or dyspnea. Chest examination discloses dullness, decreased breath sounds, and decreased tactile fremitus on the involved side.

B. IMAGING

Upright posteroanterior and lateral chest x-rays can demonstrate pleural fluid in most cases if more than

250 mL of fluid is present (eg, blunting of costophrenic angles). Decubitus films are useful to differentiate pleural fluid from pleural scarring and to determine whether the fluid is loculated. Bilateral decubitus films may be necessary to demonstrate fluid in the case of very small effusions. X-rays or CT scans may be helpful in differentiating effusions from lung abscess adjacent to the pleura.

Treatment

A. OXYGEN

If dyspnea is present, obtain pulse oximetry or arterial blood gas measurements, and begin supplemental oxygen by mask or nasal cannula.

B. THORACENTESIS

If chest examination or chest x-ray shows a massive fluid accumulation (ie, most of one hemithorax), or the patient is in respiratory distress, prompt thoracentesis with removal of 500–1000 mL of fluid should be considered for relief of symptoms. Remove the fluid over 30–90 minutes to prevent pulmonary edema in the reinflated lung. Recovered fluid should be sent for differential white blood cell count; determination of protein, LDH, and glucose content; cytologic study; cultures; and pleural fluid pH. If the patient is not in distress, thoracentesis should be deferred until after hospital admission.

Disposition

All patients with unexplained pleural fluid accumulations should be hospitalized for diagnosis and treatment. Stable patients with recurrent fluid of known cause (eg, metastatic cancer or heart failure) should be referred to their regular source of medical care or given treatment in the emergency department (eg, by thoracentesis) and discharged unless the underlying illness requires hospitalization.

Light RW: Management of pleural effusions. J Formos Med Assoc 2000;99(7):523. [PMID: 10925561] (Review of current diagnostic, therapeutic, and prognostic strategies for pleural effusions.)

ATELECTASIS

 ESSENTIALS OF DIAGNOSIS

- *Decreased breath sounds or dullness to percussion over affected lung fields.*
- *Evidence of lung collapse on chest x-ray.*

General Considerations

Collapse of alveoli and small airways in a portion of the lung may result from extrinsic compression (pneumothorax, hydrothorax) or intrinsic abnormalities (hypoventilation, bronchial obstruction). Only intrinsic (resorption) atelectasis is discussed here. In the emergency department, intrinsic atelectasis may be seen in conditions causing hypoventilation (secondary to drug overdose or severe pleuritic pain from blunt chest trauma, tracheal trauma, or pulmonary embolism) or bronchial obstruction (asthma, foreign body, bronchial tumor, or aspiration).

Clinical Findings

A. Symptoms and Signs

There are usually no findings other than those of the underlying disease, although patients with extensive atelectasis may experience chest pain, cough, or dyspnea. Physical findings may be absent but when present are nonspecific dry crackles, decreased breath sounds, or dullness to percussion over the affected lung. History of recurrent pneumonia in the same lobe may suggest airway obstruction.

B. Imaging and Laboratory Findings

Chest x-ray shows areas of lung collapse. Coexisting signs may include depression or elevation of the hilum, elevation of a hemidiaphragm, or compensatory hyperinflation of other parts of the involved lung (often seen only on forced expiratory chest x-rays). CT scan may demonstrate location of an obstruction. Bronchoscopy is the definitive study, especially if tumor or foreign body is suspected.

Arterial blood gases should be measured to assess respiratory function; hypoxemia and hypocapnia may be present.

Treatment

Emergency treatment should include hemodynamic monitoring with supplemental oxygen, chest physical therapy, meticulous pulmonary toilet, and treatment of underlying conditions (eg, aspiration of gastric contents, drug overdose, pain).

Disposition

Almost all patients with atelectasis must be hospitalized for evaluation and treatment of the underlying cause. The only exceptions are patients with chronic atelectasis of known cause who have not responded to vigorous therapy in the past (eg, carcinomatous bronchial obstruction) and those with very mild degrees of atelecta-sis (subsegmental) clearly due to self-limited disease (drug overdose, pleurisy).

Rabinowitz RP: Management of infections in the trauma patient. Surg Clin North Am 1999;79(6):1373. [PMID: 10625984] (Thorough discussion of the common types of infection in the trauma patient and the initial approach to the febrile trauma patient.)

van der Jagt EW: Contemporary issues in the emergency care of children with asthma. Immunology and Allergy Clinics of North America 1998;18(1). (Extensive literature review including pathophysiology and treatment of asthma and its complications.)

PNEUMONIA & BRONCHITIS

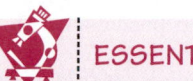 ESSENTIALS OF DIAGNOSIS

Pneumonia

- *Fever, productive cough, dyspnea, pleuritic chest pain.*
- *Rales, rhonchi, wheezing, or hemoptysis.*
- *Decreased breath sounds or dullness to percussion over affected lobe.*
- *Infiltrate on chest radiograph.*

Bronchitis

- *Cough associated with midline chest pain or burning.*
- *Fever, dyspnea.*

General Considerations

Pneumonia and acute bronchitis are common emergency department entities, and they can be difficult to differentiate from one another. Suspect pneumonia or bronchitis in any patient presenting with fever, cough (with or without productive sputum), or dyspnea. Differentiation is important because treatment, disposition, and prognosis can differ significantly.

Clinical Findings

A. Acute Bronchitis

Diagnosis is based primarily on history and physical examination. Patients complain of cough, fever, and constitutional symptoms. The cough is initially dry (due to bronchospasms) but can become productive and is often associated with a midline chest pain or burning. Hemoptysis, wheezing, rhonchi, and rales may also be present. Laboratory tests are typically not helpful in making the diagnosis. Chest x-ray will show no evidence of infiltrate and is not indicated unless patients are dyspneic, hypoxic, or have significant comorbidities (eg, COPD, dementia). The cause is primarily viral (90%).

B. PNEUMONIA

Patients present with fever, dyspnea, cough, pleuritic chest pain, and increased sputum production. Evidence of an infiltrate will appear on the chest x-ray. Other signs noted on physical examination include rales or rhonchi on chest auscultation, often with locally decreased breath sounds and dullness to percussion.

The primary goal of the history and physical examination should be to identify patients at high risk for significant morbidity and mortality. If pneumonia is suspected, check pulse oximetry and obtain a chest x-ray to aid in diagnosis and help rule out other conditions. Use clinical judgment to determine the need for further testing. The necessity of blood and sputum cultures and Gram stains in patients well enough to be discharged has been debated, but these tests should always be obtained in patients who will be admitted. Microbiologic testing will not change the initial emergency department treatment of community-acquired pneumonia but in a small number of cases may alter the choice of antimicrobials after admission. The leukocyte count is not associated with increased morbidity and mortality and therefore should not be used in guiding patient management.

Some helpful tests may include arterial blood gas measurements (hypoxia), hemoglobin and hematocrit (anemia), and a basic metabolic panel (dehydration, renal insufficiency) and may also include HIV screening, tuberculosis screening, and screening for *Legionella* and *Mycoplasma* pneumonia for hospitalized patients at high risk for these diseases.

Treatment

A. ACUTE BRONCHITIS

This condition rarely needs aggressive management in the emergency department. Administer supplemental oxygen to hypoxic patients or intravenous fluids to patients who appear to be dehydrated. Otherwise, use symptomatic treatment with antipyretics and cough suppressants as needed. β-Adrenergic MDIs (albuterol) are used to suppress cough secondary to bronchospasm. Antibiotics are not recommended because the primary cause is likely viral (unless the course is prolonged or the patient has significant underlying comorbidities).

B. PNEUMONIA

Patients well enough to be discharged home should be given instructions for antipyretic use and cough suppressants as needed, and they should be started on an-

tibiotics. Doxycycline, a newer-generation fluoroquinolone, or a macrolide are equally appropriate antimicrobial choices. Each should be given for 7–10 days (except azithromycin, which is used for only 5 days). Patients who will be admitted can be started on initial antibiotics, which include (1) a newer-generation fluoroquinolone or (2) a macrolide plus a β-lactam/β-lactamase inhibitor.

The initial antibiotic choices for patients admitted to the intensive care unit typically include either a newer-generation fluoroquinolone or macrolide plus either cefotaxime or a β-lactam/β-lactamase inhibitor. All patients should receive supplemental oxygen and intravenous fluids if dehydrated. See Chapter 40 for more specific pneumonia treatment recommendations.

Disposition

Patients with acute bronchitis can be discharged home with the above treatment if they are not hypoxic and do not have significant underlying cardiopulmonary disease. Pneumonia patients who are younger than age 50 years without comorbidities or altered physical examination findings can be safely discharged to home with antibiotics and follow-up in 72 hours unless they are immunocompromised, are unable to tolerate oral intake, have psychiatric illness, are alcohol or drug abusers, are homeless, or lack social support. Most patients who fall into one of these categories will be hospitalized. If the patient has significant comorbidities, has altered mental status, or is hemodynamically unstable, intensive care unit admission and possible intubation are appropriate. Although cultures should be drawn expeditiously, they should not delay administration of antibiotics.

Bartlett JG et al: Practice guidelines for the management of community-acquired pneumonia in adults. Infectious Diseases Society of America. Clin Infect Dis 2000;31(2):347. [PMID: 10987697] (Evidence-based practice guidelines for the diagnosis and treatment of community-acquired pneumonia in adults.)

DeBlieux PM, Slaven EM: Community-acquired pneumonia: deciding whom to admit and which antibiotics to use. Emergency Medicine Practice 1999;1(4):1. (Review of the most recent published guidelines for the management of community-acquired pneumonia with specific indications for admission and recommendations for antibiotic choice in the emergency department.)

Fine MJ et al: A prediction rule to identify low-risk patients with community-acquired pneumonia. N Engl J Med 1997;336 (4):243. [PMID: 8995086] (Based on an extensive analysis of nearly 15,000 inpatients and validated by the pneumonia PORT cohort study, the authors have developed a 2-step algorithm for risk stratification of patients with community-acquired pneumonia that is used to help physicians make evidence-based decisions regarding hospitalization.)

Gonzales R et al: Principles of appropriate antibiotic use for treatment of uncomplicated acute bronchitis: background. Ann Emerg Med 2001;37(6):720. [PMID: 11385346] (Multidisciplinary expert panel formed by the Centers for Disease Control and Prevention, which developed evidence-based recommendations on the management of patients with acute bronchitis.)

PULMONARY TUBERCULOSIS

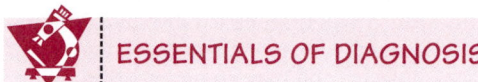 **ESSENTIALS OF DIAGNOSIS**

- *Fever, weight loss, hemoptysis, night sweats.*
- *Chest x-ray notes hilar adenopathy with parenchymal infiltrates, often upper lobes or apical.*
- *Positive purified protein derivative (PPD) skin test with positive acid fast bacilli on sputum smear.*
- *Sputum culture for M tuberculosis is definitive diagnosis.*

General Considerations

Tuberculosis remains the world's leading infectious cause of death and reestablished itself as a major concern in the mid 1980s as the incidence rose sharply in the United States. Since 1993, the incidence has once again declined after significant federal funding was released for statewide tuberculosis control programs. These programs are aimed at controlling the major causes for this initial resurgence, including the HIV epidemic, immigrants with undiagnosed tuberculosis from high-risk countries (ie, those with multidrug-resistant tuberculosis), previously established suboptimal antimicrobial regimens, and patient noncompliance. HIV is the most important risk factor for infection with tuberculosis.

Pulmonary infection is caused when susceptible individuals inhale aerosolized droplets infected with *Mycobacterium tuberculosis*. Susceptible populations include HIV-positive individuals; those with close exposure to known infected persons; immigrants from Asia, Africa, or Latin America; medically underserved urban populations; the elderly; residents of nursing homes or correctional facilities; homeless populations; and health care workers.

In immunocompetent hosts, primary tuberculosis is usually asymptomatic and is often identified only when a patient has a positive tuberculosis skin test. Initially the organisms either are killed by alveolar macrophages or persist and replicate within inactivated macrophages that can gain access to regional lymph nodes and disseminate into the bloodstream. Dissemination to the lungs (miliary tuberculosis) or to the kidneys, lymphatics, pleura, meninges, or bone (extrapulmonary tuberculosis) can also rarely occur. Eventually the organism lies dormant, walled off within granulomas, and may never again cause infection. However, depending on the host immune response, dormant organisms may become reactivated (reactivation tuberculosis). Risk factors for reactivation tuberculosis include HIV, recent tuberculosis infection (within 2 years), intravenous drug abuse, diabetes mellitus, prolonged steroid use, endstage renal disease, or chronic malabsorption syndromes. The goal in the emergency department is to recognize patients at high risk for disease; initiate early diagnosis, treatment, and referral for these patients; and protect hospital staff via early patient isolation.

Clinical Findings

Many patients will know if they have had or been exposed to tuberculosis in the past. All patients with pulmonary symptoms should be questioned about the above-stated known risk factors for tuberculosis.

A. SYMPTOMS AND SIGNS

The most common symptom of tuberculosis is cough, initially dry, often becoming purulent with or without hemoptysis. Fever is also very common, especially during the day with resolution at bedtime; night sweats are a major complaint. Fatigue, malaise, weight loss with anorexia, and occasionally pleuritic chest pain may be reported. Patients may appear chronically ill, with mental status changes (central nervous system disease), lymphadenopathy, rales on chest auscultation, and often a normal chest examination.

B. X-RAY FINDINGS

Primary tuberculosis may appear on chest x-ray as parenchymal consolidation, atelectasis, pleural effusion, or possible paratracheal lymphadenopathy. A calcified Ghon complex may be evidence of healed primary infection. Reactivation tuberculosis often has a predilection for the upper lobes. Immunocompromised patients, especially HIV patients, may present with myriad changes on the chest x-ray.

C. LABORATORY FINDINGS

1. Cultures and serologic testing—Many new methods (direct amplification tests, high-performance liquid chromatography, DNA fingerprinting with polymerase chain reaction technique, and serologic tests using ELISA) have been used to more rapidly identify *M. tuberculosis*. However, definitive diagnosis still depends on sputum cultures (which may take weeks). Now, with the emergence of multidrug-resistant tuberculosis, cultures are the standard of care because proper treatment depends on the susceptibility results. In the emergency department, acid fast staining of sputum can be performed and may be helpful in aiding diagnosis.

2. Tuberculosis skin testing—If a patient is suspected of having tuberculosis, an intradermal purified protein derivative (PPD) skin test should be administered. Because these tests are not completed and read until 48–72 hours after administration, they are not very useful in the emergency department. A positive test (varying diameters of circumferential skin induration depending on risk factors for the disease) indicates previous infection or active tuberculosis infection. Positive PPD tests should be followed with chest x-ray to evaluate for new or active disease. Severely immunocompromised patients or HIV patients may be anergic and require an anergy skin test panel.

Treatment

A. Confirmed or Suspected Tuberculosis

Because more than 4% of isolates are resistant to isoniazid in most of the United States, it is now recommended that all patients with confirmed or suspected tuberculosis be started on 4-drug therapy. The initial regimen consists of the following drugs: isoniazid, rifampin, pyrazinamide, and either ethambutol or streptomycin. All drugs should be continued until the susceptibility results from the sputum cultures are available. If the isolates are susceptible to isoniazid, rifampin, and pyrazinamide, then the fourth drug can be discontinued. A 6-month treatment course has been proven to be effective. Isoniazid and rifampin should be continued throughout this period, whereas pyrazinamide and ethambutol or streptomycin can usually be discontinued after 2 months, if there is no evidence of multidrug-resistant, miliary, or extrapulmonary tuberculosis. If any of these forms are present, a 12-month treatment course should continue.

B. Latent Tuberculosis

Patients who have had positive PPD tests but negative chest x-ray and sputum (latent tuberculosis) and are at risk of reactivation tuberculosis should be given 9 months of isoniazid or 2 months of rifampin plus pyrazinamide. In children, only 9 months of isoniazid is recommended. Isoniazid is not recommended for pregnant patients. Patients with latent tuberculosis do not need treatment if they can prove or are certain that they already received treatment.

C. Reporting Requirements

The local health department must be informed of all cases of tuberculosis to ensure adequate care, availability of treatment resources, and compliance with therapy.

D. Respiratory Isolation

Any patient suspected or known to have tuberculosis must be immediately placed in designated respiratory isolation rooms designed for the emergency department and hospital wards. Emergency department staff should quickly assess and triage these individuals and apply masks to patients and distribute respirators approved by the Occupational Safety and Health Administration to physicians and nursing teams. Patients should remain in isolation, either within the hospital setting, or in their own house, until proven to be noninfectious.

E. HIV Testing

All patients with newly diagnosed tuberculosis should be offered HIV testing because a significant number of patients are coinfected and have an increased risk of opportunistic infections and death.

F. Infants, Children, and Adolescents

This population of patients with active, culture-proven *M. tuberculosis* should receive essentially the same treatment as adults. Latent tuberculosis in children is treated with 9 months of isoniazid only. Diseases are more likely to disseminate in children younger age 4 years. Avoid ethambutol in children because of secondary ocular toxicity.

G. Pregnant Patients

Pregnant women with tuberculosis can still receive rifampin, isoniazid, and pyrazinamide. However, ethambutol and streptomycin should be avoided because of the risk of ocular toxicity and congenital deafness, respectively. Mothers can still breast feed if taking these medications.

Disposition

Most patients are usually admitted for full work-up and evaluation after the initial diagnosis is confirmed. However, many patients can safely receive treatment at home with specific home isolation precautions along with screening and prophylactic treatment for family members and household contacts. Patients must fully understand the importance of adherence to their therapeutic regimens. If adherence cannot be confirmed, directly observed therapy will be provided and enforced by a public health official. Report all new diagnoses to the health department and ensure immediate primary care or infectious disease follow-up.

All patients with multidrug-resistant tuberculosis, patients who are significantly ill or immunocompromised, those who are unable to care for themselves, homeless patients, those living in an institution (eg, nursing home, prison), the elderly, those with multiple comorbidities, and those coinfected with HIV should be hospitalized with respiratory droplet precautions. Hospitalization ensures that these patients remain in respiratory isolation, receive therapy daily, and are observed closely for adverse effects of antituberculosis medications.

Advisory Council for the Elimination of Tuberculosis (ACET). Tuberculosis elimination revisited: obstacles, opportunities, and a renewal commitment. MMWR 1999;48(RR-9):1. [PMID: 10485562] (The Centers for Disease Control and Prevention and ACET have reviewed their 1989 strategic plan to eradicate tuberculosis and have added new recommendations for diagnosis, treatment, and prevention based on the latest technology.)

PULMONARY ASPIRATION SYNDROME

 ESSENTIALS OF DIAGNOSIS

- *High-risk patients with drug or alcohol intoxication, seizures, or swallowing disorders; obtunded patients.*
- *Immediate respiratory difficulty due to chemical burn, hypoxemia, rales, wheezing (often unilateral).*
- *Chest x-ray can be negative initially.*

General Considerations

Acute aspiration of gastric contents (Mendelson syndrome) may produce significant lung injury by acid corrosion, bronchial obstruction with food particles, or induction of chemical pneumonitis that is later complicated by bacterial pneumonia. Aspiration of gastric acid (pH < 2) produces immediate pulmonary injury that pathophysiologically is a form of acute respiratory distress syndrome. Aspiration of neutral gastric secretions admixed with food produces a more delayed injury; retained food particles may cause bronchial obstruction with atelectasis. All of these conditions are included in the term *pulmonary aspiration syndrome.*

By contrast, aspiration of oropharyngeal secretions, especially in individuals with poor dental hygiene and large amounts of dental plaque, causes bacterial pneumonia (so-called aspiration pneumonia). This necrotizing process may be acute or subacute in onset and commonly results in lung abscess.

Clinical Findings

Pulmonary aspiration occurring in the hospital may occur during anesthesia, cardiopulmonary resuscitation, or other procedures. Community-acquired cases are usually associated with drug (including alcohol) intoxication, seizures, disorders of swallowing, or gastroesophageal sphincteric incompetence. Within minutes to hours after aspiration, the patient develops productive cough; dyspnea; fever; leukocytosis; and signs of consolidation, pulmonary rales, or dullness. Chest x-ray shows pulmonary infiltrate without a characteristic pattern, although dependent segments of the lung (especially the right lower lobe) are more commonly involved.

Sputum shows abundant leukocytes but no bacteria (or scant normal flora) on microscopic examination. Cultures are sterile or show scant normal flora. Food particles may be present on gross examination of sputum.

Arterial blood gas and pH measurements must be made to assess ventilatory status. Pulse oximetry may suffice as a guide to arterial oxygenation if the saturation is high (> 90%).

Treatment

Provide respiratory support (eg, supplemental oxygen) as necessary on the basis of arterial blood gas measurements (or pulse oximetry) and clinical findings (Chapter 11). If the patient has significant dyspnea or respiratory distress, immediately establish airway control with intubation and mechanical ventilation.

Witnessed aspirations should be treated by prompt oropharyngeal and tracheal suctioning. Acute obstruction of the upper airway should be treated immediately with the Heimlich maneuver. Retained, aspirated foreign bodies (greatest risk in children) often necessitate bronchoscopy for final diagnosis and removal.

Corticosteroids have not been demonstrated to be helpful and may increase susceptibility to infection. Antibiotics for aspiration pneumonia should be given only if infection occurs and not as prophylaxis following an episode of aspiration.

Disposition

All patients should be hospitalized for observation and treatment as necessary.

Young MA, Reynolds JC: Respiratory complications of gastrointestinal diseases. Gastroenterol Clin North Am 1998;27(4): 721. [PMID: 9890112] (Evidence-based review of gastroesophageal reflux disease and the management of the extraesophageal manifestations of the disease, including pulmonary aspiration.)

ACUTE LUNG INJURY & ACUTE RESPIRATORY DISTRESS SYNDROME (See Table 33–4.)

 ESSENTIALS OF DIAGNOSIS

- *Recent known exposure to high-risk systemic or pulmonary etiologic agent.*

Table 33–4. Selected clinical causes of acute lung injury and acute respiratory distress syndrome.

Pulmonary disorders
  Pneumonia (Chapter 33)
  Aspiration of gastric contents (Chapter 33)
  Near-drowning (Chapter 38)
  Toxic gas inhalation or smoke inhalation (Chapter 43)
  Pulmonary contusions (Chapters 10, 24)
  Embolic disease (thombus, Chapter 33; fat, Chapter 28; amniotic fluid, Chapter 36)
  High-altitude pulmonary edema (Chapter 44)
Extrapulmonary disorders
  Trauma (Chapter 24)
  Pancreatitis (Chapter 13)
  Drug overdose (eg, narcotics, salicylates, nitrofurantoin, hydrocarbons) (Chapter 45)
  Uremia (Chapter 37)
  Disseminated intravascular coagulation/thrombotic thrombocytopenic purpura (Chapter 39)
  Multiple transfusions (Chapter 39)
  Shock (septic shock most common cause) (Chapter 9)
  Cardiopulmonary bypass (Chapter 34)

- *Acute-onset respiratory failure ($Pao_2 < 60$ mm Hg with $FIO_2 > 50\%$).*
- *No chemical evidence of cardiogenic or volume overload pulmonary edema (pulmonary capillary wedge pressures < 18 mm Hg).*
- *Chest x-ray shows diffuse bilateral infiltrates with normal heart size.*

General Considerations

Acute lung injury is a clinical syndrome composed of acute respiratory failure with impaired oxygenation secondary to overwhelming noncardiogenic pulmonary edema (bilateral pulmonary infiltrates on chest x-ray without clinical evidence of cardiogenic or volume overload pulmonary edema). Acute respiratory distress syndrome (ARDS), formerly called adult respiratory distress syndrome, is the most severe form of acute lung injury. Both entities are associated with significant mortality (30–40% or much higher if associated with sepsis) and are characterized by diffuse pulmonary capillary endothelial cell and alveolar epithelial cell damage with resultant pulmonary edema. Diverse specific pulmonary and extrapulmonary insults have been associated with the development of acute lung injury and ARDS (see Table 33-4). Without early diagnosis, intervention, and treatment of the underlying cause, most patients will die of multiorgan system failure.

Clinical Findings

A. SYMPTOMS AND SIGNS

Patients will present with dyspnea (usually 12–48 hours after the inciting event), which can rapidly progress to respiratory failure requiring intubation and positive-pressure ventilation. Symptoms of the underlying disorder may also be present (fever, trauma, burns), and some patients may have wheezing or cough productive of frothy or blood-tinged nonpurulent sputum. Rales are almost always present.

B. IMAGING AND LABORATORY FINDINGS

Hypoxemia is universal and early arterial blood gases may demonstrate decreased Pco_2 secondary to hyperventilation. As impending respiratory failure and fatigue set in, resultant hypercapnia develops. Chest x-ray will demonstrate diffuse bilateral infiltrates but may be variable in patients with underlying pulmonary disease. Although not routinely recommended for diagnosis, a pulmonary artery catheter may be required to help differentiate noncardiac pulmonary edema from a cardiac cause. Pulmonary artery occlusion pressures (pulmonary capillary wedge pressures) less than or equal to 18 mm Hg are consistent with acute lung injury.

Treatment

A. PROVIDE RESPIRATORY SUPPORT

1. Supplemental oxygen—Provide high initial oxygen concentration ($FIO_2 = 50$–100%), continue to monitor oxygen saturation with pulse oximetry, and titrate to the lowest possible FIO_2 to keep oxygen saturation greater than 90%.

2. Intubation and mechanical ventilation—Mechanical ventilation is the central supportive intervention. Clinicians have implemented numerous ventilation strategies, but most support the use of high positive end-expiratory pressure (PEEP) with low tidal volumes to limit peak airway pressures and resultant barotraumas. Besides PEEP, other maneuvers are also used to help open collapsed alveoli. The most important of these maneuvers is prone positioning, which redistributes blood flow and ventilation, decreases atelectasis, and therefore improves oxygenation.

B. MAINTAIN CIRCULATION

Avoid both dehydration and vigorous hydration. Keep the pulmonary capillary wedge pressure as low as possible while maintaining an adequate cardiac index. This may be extremely difficult and may require internal monitoring via a Swan Ganz catheter.

C. TREAT UNDERLYING CLINICAL CAUSE

Prompt evaluation with rapid identification of the underlying cause is paramount for the survival of these patients. Specific treatment for the inciting disorder (most commonly sepsis) should begin as soon as possible in the emergency department. See Table 33–4 for causes, and refer to listed chapters for specific therapies of each cause.

Disposition

Hospitalize all patients for therapy in the intensive care unit. Very rarely noncardiac pulmonary edema due to a specifically treatable condition (eg, high altitude, narcotics) will resolve rapidly and completely in a few hours, allowing the patient to be discharged from the emergency department.

Brower RG: Treatment of ARDS. Chest 2001;120(4):1347. [PMID: 11591581] (An exhaustive review of the currently published literature and a summary of past, present, and future evidence-based management options for patients with acute lung injury or ARDS.)

Steinberg KP: Acute lung injury and acute respiratory distress syndrome. The clinical syndrome. Clin Chest Med 2000;21(3): 401. [PMID: 11019717] (A thorough review of definitions, pathophysiology, risk factors, clinical manifestations, and prognosis of acute lung injury or ARDS.)

Weinacker AB: Acute respiratory distress syndrome: physiology and new management strategies. Annu Rev Med 2001;52:221. [PMID: 21091756] (Review of the clinical and pathologic features of ARDS and current treatment strategies to prevent lung injury and improve survival.)

CYSTIC FIBROSIS

Clinical Findings

Cystic fibrosis is an autosomal recessive disease with an abnormal transmembrane protein, which causes thick and viscous mucus with subsequent obstruction and damage to organs with exocrine function. Patients will have a history of chronic lung disease (especially bronchiectasis), pancreatic insufficiency, and gastrointestinal complaints. Most symptoms of disease and many complications develop at an early age (2–20 years), often with a history of cystic fibrosis in relatives. Other common findings include increased sweat chloride tests, failure to thrive (infants), ileus, azoospermia (male infertility), gallstones, biliary cirrhosis, intussusception, steatorrhea, nasal polyps, sinusitis, recurrent pneumonia with digital clubbing, and eventually cor pulmonale.

Treatment

A. PULMONARY INFECTIONS

Cystic fibrosis patients are often hospitalized for acute pulmonary infections. They require supplemental oxygen, vigorous hydration (to mobilize mucus plugs), chest physiotherapy (percussion and postural drainage), and antimicrobial treatment. Antibiotics should be based on initial Gram stain of sputum and culture. Because *Staphylococcus aureus* (even multidrug-resistant *S. aureus*) and *Pseudomonas aeruginosa* are commonly present, combination therapy with an antipseudomonal penicillin (eg, ticarcillin) and an aminoglycoside (tobramycin) can be used.

B. COMPLICATIONS

All complications should also be treated, including pneumothorax (thoracostomy), intussusception (barium enema), right heart failure (diuretics), and hyperglycemia (insulin).

C. FUTURE TREATMENTS

The most promising future treatments for cystic fibrosis include multiple gene therapy vectors used to replace the patient's defective copy for the abnormal protein.

Disposition

Hospitalization is often required for evaluation and treatment of new respiratory symptoms or complications of disease. However, because nosocomial infections can be detrimental to these patients and many patients are already taking chronic maintenance antibiotics, consultation with the pulmonologist should be obtained to assist with the final treatment decision.

Koch C, Hoiby N: Diagnosis and treatment of cystic fibrosis. Respiration 2000;67(3):239. [PMID: 10867591] (Review of current diagnostic aspects of cystic fibrosis and treatment with both intensive antimicrobial regimens and anti-inflammatory medications.)

Lees CM, Smyth RL: The current management of cystic fibrosis. Int J Clin Pract 2000;54(3):171. [PMID: 10829360] (Evidence-based review of the most current treatment strategies for patients with cystic fibrosis.)

INTERSTITIAL PULMONARY DISEASE

General Considerations

A variety of conditions may produce diffuse progressive pulmonary interstitial inflammation and fibrosis, including drugs, pneumoconioses, collagen diseases, sarcoidosis, organic and inorganic dusts, and illnesses of unknown cause with pathologic features involving chiefly the lungs (eg, idiopathic interstitial fibrosis). Aside from the pneumoconioses and sarcoidosis, these illnesses are relatively uncommon. The principal feature of all of them is that dyspnea begins gradually and seldom occurs acutely without a background of increasing shortness of breath. When dyspnea of acute onset does occur, it is often due to intercurrent illness (eg, pulmonary infection). Patients also have pulmonary function tests that demonstrate restrictive lung dysfunction and impaired gas exchange.

Clinical Findings

Many patients with interstitial pulmonary disease will know their diagnosis; if not, it can seldom be made with certainty in the emergency department setting, because lung biopsy or bronchoalveolar lavage are often required.

A. Symptoms and Signs

Gradually increasing dyspnea, especially on exertion, is the only reliable symptom. Chest pain, cough, sputum production, and other symptoms may occur but are inconsistent. Physical findings are variable, but dry crackles (rales) at the bases of the lungs are common. Cyanosis and clubbing may be present as well.

B. Imaging

Chest x-ray usually shows interstitial infiltrates, although this may be a subtle finding. High-definition CT scans of the chest are also helpful in assessing these patients. Other changes may be present depending on the disease process (eg, hilar adenopathy in sarcoidosis, conglomerate fibrosis in silicosis).

Treatment & Disposition

Provide respiratory support as needed, and treat intercurrent disease (eg, infection). Hospitalize patients with respiratory failure or recent marked worsening of symptoms or those in whom acute infection is suspected. Refer all patients not already under care to a pulmonary disease specialist. Early lung transplantation offers a surgical therapeutic option for selected patients.

Gross TJ, Hunninghake GW: Idiopathic pulmonary fibrosis. N Engl J Med 2001;345(7):517. [PMID: 11519507] (Review of the pathophysiology, current symptomatic and investigational treatments, and need for early referral of patients with interstitial pulmonary fibrosis to specialists for enrollment in clinical trials or for lung transplantation.)

Cardiac Emergencies[1]

34

Roger L. Humphries, MD, & C. Keith Stone, MD[2]

<table>
<tr><td>

Acute Coronary Syndrome
  Acute Myocardial Infarction (Coronary Occlusion)
  Complications of Myocardial Infarction
  1. Shock (Cardiogenic Shock)
  2. Congestive Heart Failure
  3. Acute Mitral Regurgitation & Ventricular Septal Rupture
  4. Myocardial Rupture
  5. Systemic or Pulmonary Embolization
  6. Pericarditis
  Angina Pectoris
Heart Failure
  Severe Heart Failure, Including Pulmonary Edema
  Mild to Moderate Heart Failure

</td><td>

Hypertension & Hypertensive Crisis
Pericarditis, Pericardial Effusion, & Cardiac Tamponade
  Pericarditis & Pericardial Effusion
  Cardiac Tamponade
Myocarditis & Cardiomyopathy
Aortic Aneurysms & Dissections
Congenital Heart Disease
  Cyanosis
  Anoxic Spells
  Heart Failure
  Pulmonary Hypertension
  Coarctation of the Aorta

</td></tr>
</table>

Immediate Management

Cardiac disease is usually manifested by symptoms of chest pain, dyspnea or respiratory distress, cardiac arrest or syncope, or shock. Because these symptoms are so commonly encountered in the emergency department and because they may result from disease in many organs other than the heart, they are discussed separately (Chapters 7, 9, 11, 12, and 17). Because almost any cardiac disease is at least potentially life threatening, no attempt has been made in this chapter to categorize disorders on the basis of severity or to assign priorities in treatment.

■ ACUTE CORONARY SYNDROME

Acute coronary syndrome refers to a spectrum of conditions that develop from blood flow that is insufficient to meet the metabolic needs of the myocardium. Patients with an acute coronary syndrome exist on a clinical continuum from unstable angina to non-ST-segment-elevation myocardial infarction to ST-segment-elevation myocardial infarction.

ACUTE MYOCARDIAL INFARCTION (Coronary Occlusion)

Myocardial infarction results when arterial blood flow to the myocardium is suddenly decreased or interrupted. It is usually due to atherosclerotic coronary artery disease with plaque rupture and sudden occlusion by thrombus; vasculitis or emboli are less common causes. Complete occlusion, most often with thrombus, is found in 80–90% of patients with chest pain and ST segment elevation who are studied by coronary angioplasty within several hours of onset. Rarely, patients dying of myocardial infarction are found to have normal coronary arteries, and infarction in such cases is presumably due to spasm of a coronary artery or thrombosis with complete lysis. Cocaine use has been associated with acute myocardial infarction, probably as a result of coronary spasm with or without intravascular thrombus formation. In myocardial infarction, severely ischemic and infarcted muscle contracts and relaxes poorly or not at all; if infarction is extensive, decreased cardiac output with heart failure or shock may result. After myocardial in-

[1]See also Chapter 35 for emergencies due to cardiac arrhythmias.
[2]This chapter is a revision of the chapter by Melvin D. Cheitlin, MD, & Joseph A. Abbott, MD, from the 4th edition.

farction, the ventricle may become aneurysmal or may even rupture. If conducting tissue is ischemic or infarcted, conduction abnormalities may occur. The infarcted endocardium attracts platelets and fibrin that may form mural clots, which can subsequently embolize. During acute myocardial infarction, the myocardium is electrically unstable, resulting in ventricular arrhythmias that are frequently life threatening.

Upon occlusion of a coronary artery, necrosis occurs in a time-dependent course, proceeding from endocardium to epicardium, generally over 4–6 hours. When residual perfusion by collateral vessels is present or lysis or thrombus occurs—either spontaneously or as a result of therapy—there will be salvage of myocardium. The earlier the reperfusion, the more myocardium is salvaged.

Clinical Findings

A. Symptoms and Signs

Most patients with myocardial infarction have chest discomfort that is typically substernal and may radiate to the neck or left arm. Occasionally, pain occurs in atypical areas such as the right arm, shoulders, back, or epigastrium. The pain is usually oppressive or squeezing in character and may be associated with anxiety, restlessness, nausea and vomiting, abdominal bloating, dyspnea, and diaphoresis. It commonly begins at rest, worsens gradually, and frequently persists for hours. Occasionally, myocardial infarction is painless—especially in elderly or diabetic patients—and is manifested by the acute onset of left heart failure, hypotension, or cardiac arrhythmias. Up to 25% of patients with an acute myocardial infarction may not develop any significant symptoms that would prompt the patient to seek medical attention.

Physical findings vary, and none are specific or diagnostic of myocardial infarction. An S_4 gallop or at times an S_3 gallop may be present. Occasionally, an apical systolic murmur or mitral insufficiency due to papillary muscle and left ventricular dysfunction is present. In patients with uncomplicated myocardial infarction, there may be no abnormal findings on physical examination. When cardiopulmonary physical findings are present, they tend to reflect the presence of complications (see below).

B. Electrocardiographic Findings

The electrocardiogram (ECG) shows signs of infarction (eg, high-voltage T waves, elevated ST segments, ST-segment-elevation myocardial infarction, abnormal Q waves) in about half of patients. Other patients may have T wave inversions (non-ST-segment-elevation myocardial infarction). In the remainder, the initial ECG shows only nonspecific ST or T wave changes, or may be normal. **Note:** A normal ECG *does not* rule out the possibil-

ity of myocardial infarction. Continuous ST segment monitoring or serial ECGs provide additional information and may demonstrate an evolving acute coronary syndrome in patients with initially nondiagnostic ECGs.

C. Laboratory Findings

A detailed discussion of all markers of cardiac ischemia is beyond the scope of this chapter. Elevation of the CK-MB isoenzyme is still considered by the World Heath Organization as one of the criteria used to diagnosis acute myocardial infarction. Because CK-MB is found not only in the myocardium but also in brain and skeletal muscle, it is less specific for a myocardial ischemic event than are some other markers. The CK-MB serum level elevates usually within 4–6 hours after the onset of an acute myocardial infarction and peaks within 12–24 hours. Levels return to baseline generally within 2–3 days of an acute myocardial infarction. Within 6 hours of an acute myocardial infarction, the sensitivity and specificity of elevations in the serum CK-MB levels are 17–62% and 92–100%, respectively.

Troponin is a complex of three specific proteins found in striated muscle. Two of the subunits, cardiac troponin T (cTnt) and I (cTni), are useful as clinical markers of myocardial injury. Because these cardiac proteins are genetically unique, cTnt and cTni are the most cardiac-specific biochemical markers. With recent improvements in the assay, microinfarctions are diagnosed when elevations in cTnt or cTni occur without elevations in the CK-MB levels. After an acute myocardial infarction, cardiac troponin serum levels generally elevate within 2–6 hours, peak at 12–24 hours, and may stay elevated for 7–10 days. The sensitivities of elevations of cTnt and cTni within 6 hours of an acute myocardial infarction are 50–59% and 6–44%, respectively. The specificities of elevations of cTnt and cTni within 6 hours of an acute myocardial infarction are 74–96% and 93–99%, respectively.

One of the first cardiac markers used clinically, myoglobin, is still used by some today. Myoglobin is the most sensitive early marker of cardiac injury. After an acute myocardial infarction, elevations occurs within 1–3 hours, levels peak within 4–12 hours, and levels remain elevated for 12–36 hours. The sensitivity and specificity of myoglobin for detecting myocardial infarction within 6 hours of symptom onset are 55–100% and 76–98%, respectively.

Differential Diagnosis

For a complete differential diagnosis of chest pain, see Chapter 12. Aortic dissection, pericarditis, and gastrointestinal disorders (eg, peptic ulcer disease, pancreatitis) must be excluded in patients being considered for thrombolytic therapy.

Note: The diagnosis of myocardial infarction is suggested by the history, and a decision to admit the patient to the coronary care unit immediately should be based on this information alone. Because of the relatively benign course of patients admitted with a good history suggesting myocardial infarction and a normal initial ECG, in some institutions these patients are admitted to a monitored intermediate care unit rather than a coronary care unit. No amount of laboratory data obtained in the emergency department will definitely rule out myocardial infarction.

Treatment

Patients experiencing acute cardiac syndrome should receive aggressive treatment with the goal of rapidly reperfusing ischemic myocardium. The two methods currently available are pharmacologic thrombolysis via plasminogen activators and procedural coronary intervention. The effectiveness of either modality in reducing mortality and myocardial damage depends on how early it is given after the onset of symptoms.

A. IMMEDIATE MEASURES

Begin intravenous infusion of 0.9% normal saline through a secure intravenous catheter. Use microdrip infusion to minimize volume overload. Start 2–3 peripheral venous lines in patients receiving thrombolytic agents. Begin oxygen, 2–5 L/min, by nasal cannula or mask.

Start electrocardiographic monitoring, and obtain a 12-lead ECG. If chest pain is present, give nitroglycerin, 0.5 mg sublingually or one puff delivered to the oral mucosa. Repeat if no effect occurs in 5 minutes. If chest pain returns and systolic blood pressure is above 100 mm Hg, start intravenous nitroglycerin at 10 μg/min and increase by 5 μg/min every 3–5 minutes until systolic blood pressure falls by 10% or chest pain is relieved. The systolic blood pressure should not drop below 90 mm Hg.

Give a narcotic analgesic (eg, morphine, 2–8 mg intravenously) if chest pain persists. Give furosemide, 40 mg by intravenous bolus injections, if the patient has pulmonary edema. Give the patient a 160- to 325-mg non-enteric-coated aspirin tablet to chew.

In the absence of contraindications for β-blockers (heart rate < 55/min, systolic blood pressure < 90 mm Hg, moist rales above the lower third of the lung fields, advanced atrioventricular block, or history of asthma), give 15 mg of metoprolol in three 5-mg intravenous injections at 2-minute intervals.

B. ADDITIONAL MEASURES

Establish a laboratory test data base: complete blood count (CBC) with differential, serum creatinine and electrolyte measurements, blood urea nitrogen determinations, enzyme levels (preferably CK isoenzymes, cTni or cTnt, etc). Platelet count, prothrombin time, partial thromboplastin time, and blood for typing (and cross-matching if needed) should be obtained for patients to be given thrombolytic therapy. Monitor urine output.

C. OPTION 1: THROMBOLYTIC THERAPY

If the duration of chest discomfort is at least 30 minutes and less than 4–6 hours and no contraindications are present, pharmacologic revascularization is indicated. Many thrombolytic agents are available, including streptokinase, anistreplase (APSAC), alteplase (tissue plasminogen activator: t-PA), reteplase (r-PA), and tenecteplase (TNK). Thrombolytics should be initiated in the emergency department because the benefit of pharmacologic thrombolysis decreases with each passing hour after myocardial infarction. Some patients with myocardial infarction may benefit from thrombolytics up to 12 hours after the onset of chest pain, although 6 hours is generally considered the cutoff. Alteplase administration over 90 minutes improved survival when compared to streptokinase or 3-hour alteplase infusion. Even though intracranial bleeding events increased, alteplase demonstrated a long-term survival advantage presumably secondary to earlier thrombolysis and reperfusion of thrombosed coronary arteries. Compared to alteplase, TNK may offer advantages of a single bolus administration and fewer intracranial hemorrhage complications. Intracranial hemorrhage is the most devastating complication of thrombolytic therapy, occurring in 0.5–3.3% of patients.

1. **Indications**—The indications for pharmacologic revascularization are as follows:

- ST segment elevation of at least 0.1 mV in 2 or more leads (II, III, aVF or V1–V6, I, aVL) suggests acute injury in the absence of left bundle branch block. An acute true posterior myocardial infarction (with ST depression in leads V1–V4) is also an indication for thrombolysis. Patients with ongoing chest pain and a new (or not known to be old) left bundle branch block should also be considered for pharmacologic reperfusion.

- Both chest pain and ST elevation are not relieved by 2–3 sublingual nitroglycerin tablets.

- Patient is alert and oriented, or a family member or friend familiar with the patient's medical history is present.

- No contraindications to thrombolytic therapy or anticoagulation therapy are present (see below).

2. Contraindications—

a. Absolute contraindications—Absolute contraindications are as follows:

- History of any hemorrhagic cerebrovascular event (stroke, arteriovenous malformation, or aneurysm) or any nonhemorrhagic cerebrovascular event or transient ischemic attack (within the last year)
- Any intracranial neoplasm
- Active, internal bleeding (eg, serious gastrointestinal bleeding) excluding menses
- Suspected aortic dissection

b. Relative contraindications—In the following conditions, the risks associated with thrombolytic therapy may be increased, and clinical judgment should be used in evaluating expected benefits:

- Recent (within 10 days) puncture of a noncompressible blood vessel
- Poorly controlled hypertension of several years' duration or severe, uncontrolled arterial hypertension (diastolic blood pressure greater than 110 mm Hg or systolic blood pressure greater than 180 mm Hg)
- Diabetic hemorrhagic retinopathy or hemorrhagic ophthalmic condition
- Current treatment with an anticoagulant with international normalized ratio greater than 2–3 or other bleeding diathesis
- Pregnancy
- Any other condition associated with a predisposition to bleeding (eg, ulcerative colitis, active peptic ulcer disease, polycystic kidneys, gastrointestinal arteriovenous malformation, vascular tumors) or bleeding within 4 weeks
- Prolonged (> 5 minutes) or traumatic external cardiac compression or traumatic endotracheal intubation
- History of nonhemorrhagic cerebrovascular accident beyond 1 year
- Recent (within 4 weeks) trauma or major surgery at a noncompressible site (eg, coronary artery bypass surgery, organ biopsy, intra-abdominal surgery, or obstetric delivery)

3. Dosages—If indicated, the following dosage regimens are recommended:

a. Streptokinase—The recommended dosage is 1.5 million units in 250 mL of 5% dextrose in water, given intravenously over 1 hour. Because of the risk of serious allergic reactions, streptokinase is contraindicated in patients who have ever received streptokinase previously.

b. Alteplase—The recommended dosage is 15 mg intravenous bolus followed by 0.75 mg/kg (maximum 50 mg) intravenous infusion over 30 minutes and then 0.5 mg/kg (maximum 35 mg) over 60 minutes. Alteplase has a very short half-life (5 minutes); therefore, unfractionated heparin must be used to prevent reocclusion. Heparin should be started as a bolus of 60 units/kg at the start of the alteplase infusion followed by a maintenance dose of 12 units/kg. The reduction in mortality with alteplase thrombolysis (if used within 6 hours of symptom onset) is 23–30%.

c. APSAC—The recommended dosage is 30 mg intravenously infused slowly over 5 minutes. Because of the risk of serious allergic reaction, patients who have received streptokinase or APSAC previously cannot be given the drug again.

d. Urokinase—The recommended dosage is a loading dose of 0.5 million units over a 10-minute period. This is followed by infusion doses of 1.6–4.5 million units over 18–24 hours.

e. Reteplase—r-PA, a variation of t-PA, has a half-life of 13–16 minutes and is simpler to administer than t-PA. The dose is two 10-unit intravenous boluses over 2 minutes, with 30 minutes between each dose.

f. Tenecteplase—TNK is a third-generation variation of t-PA. It has improved fibrin specificity and a longer half-life, allowing single bolus administration. The dose is based on weight, ranging from 30 mg to 50 mg rapid bolus. Overall mortality compared to t-PA was equal; however, in patients presenting later in the course of an acute myocardial infarction, those given TNK had fewer episodes of nonintracranial bleeding.

Excellent evidence indicates that myocardial reperfusion salvages myocardium—resulting in better ventricular function than conventional management—and improves survival if reperfusion occurs within 6 hours after the onset of symptoms of myocardial infarction. Thrombolytic therapy may be beneficial in patients with persistent chest pain for up to 24 hours after onset of symptoms. t-PA results in a higher percentage of vessel patency (60–80%) than does streptokinase (30–60%) within the first hour with an associated improvement in survival.

4. Heparin—Heparin should be used in conjunction with any thrombin-specific thrombolytic agent such as alteplase. Because of the systemic fibrinolysis achieved by streptokinase or APSAC, anticoagulation with heparin is not indicated. Intravenous heparin, 60 units/kg bolus followed by 12 units/kg/h, should be given in a separate line while alteplase is infusing because of the short half-life of alteplase and because of the danger of recurring thrombosis. Heparin should be continued for 48 hours or longer, maintaining activated partial thromboplastin time at twice normal.

5. Monitoring—Transfer patients given thrombolytic therapy to an intensive care unit as soon as possible after initiation of treatment. Monitor the following:

- Blood pressure every 15 minutes during infusion and every 30–60 minutes thereafter.
- ECG rhythm strip for reperfusion arrhythmias and ST segment changes.
- Bleeding complications and changes in neurologic status. Avoid venous or arterial punctures and unnecessary trauma.
- Twelve-lead ECG 4 hours after the start of therapy and as needed (eg, for recurrence of chest pain).
- CK with isoenzymes and cTni or cTnt 4 hours after initiation of treatment and at 4-hour intervals for 24 hours.

D. OPTION 2: PERCUTANEOUS CORONARY INTERVENTION

Formerly termed angioplasty, percutaneous coronary intervention (PCI) involves cardiac catheterization and various techniques to assess and restore vessel patency emergently. Coronary artery stenting has become the procedure of choice. When performed early in the course of an acute myocardial infarction, PCI has demonstrated improved survival rates over pharmacologic thrombolysis. Increased rates of normal flow and decreased rates of reocclusion in the infarct-related artery are much more likely when PCI is chosen over pharmacologic thrombolysis. In addition, early definition of coronary anatomy can be used to tailor therapy and improve risk stratification. One study comparing PCI with t-PA found a reduction in mortality of 4% with PCI. Major complications associated with thrombolytics such as intracranial bleeding do not occur with PCI. In patients with contraindications to thrombolytics, PCI is the only option available to restore perfusion and salvage myocardium. Rescue PCI is useful for patients who have received thrombolytics but whose chest pain or ST segment elevation has failed to resolve. Unfortunately, PCI is not widely available; fewer than 18% of U.S. hospitals are equipped to perform the procedure.

Disposition

Hospitalize all patients with clinical histories suggesting myocardial infarction, and start electrocardiographic monitoring (in a coronary care unit, if possible). Patients with suspected myocardial infarction and normal initial ECGs and initial cardiac enzymes may be admitted to a monitored intermediate care unit.

COMPLICATIONS OF MYOCARDIAL INFARCTION

About 10–15% of patients reaching the hospital with myocardial infarction die during hospitalization. One or more complications occur in over half of all patients with myocardial infarction.

1. Shock (Cardiogenic Shock)

Shock complicating myocardial infarction occurs in 7–8% of patients and may be caused by extensive myocardial infarction with decreased cardiac output (most common), inappropriate reflex peripheral vasodilatation, arrhythmias, hypovolemia, right ventricular infarction, and mechanical complications such as ruptured ventricular septum and severe mitral regurgitation. Free-wall myocardial rupture results in tamponade and shock. The mortality rate is as high as 70–80% among patients with cardiogenic shock as a complication of acute myocardial infarction.

Clinical Findings

Hypotension accompanied by confusion, obtundation or restlessness, cool skin, oliguria, and metabolic acidosis suggests shock. Mild to moderate hypotension alone is common in myocardial infarction and does not itself indicate shock. Shock in myocardial infarction may be due to many causes (see Table 9–1), which may be difficult to differentiate noninvasively (Table 34–1).

Treatment

Use any or all of the measures discussed here as necessary. (See also Chapter 9.)

A. AIRWAY MANAGEMENT

Give oxygen, 5–10 L/min, by mask or nasal cannula. Patients in shock with respiratory failure require endotracheal intubation.

B. VENOUS PRESSURE MONITORING

Monitor central pressure with a Swan-Ganz pulmonary artery catheter (or, far less desirably, a central venous pressure catheter, since in acute myocardial infarction, left ventricular filling pressure can be markedly elevated with normal right ventricular filling pressure, and vice versa). Use an arterial line to measure blood pressure. If possible, defer insertion of these catheters until the patient has been hospitalized.

C. OTHER MEASURES

Give a fluid challenge (200 mL of saline intravenously over 20 minutes) if the patient is not in congestive heart failure (ie, no rales, no pulmonary edema on chest x-ray). Repeat as needed if congestive heart failure does not develop. Correct arrhythmias (see below). Insert a Foley catheter, and measure urine output hourly.

D. DRUG THERAPY

Give dopamine (or dobutamine), 2.5–20 µg/kg/min by continuous intravenous infusion. Use the smallest effec-

Table 34–1. Differential diagnosis by hemodynamics of heart failure and hypotension after myocardial infarction.

Arterial Pressure	Central Venous Pressure	Pulmonary Arterial Wedge Pressure	Stroke Volume Index	Diagnosis	Treatment
→	→ or ↑	↑	→ or ↓	Heart failure	Diuretics; preload and afterload reduction
→ or ↓	→ or ↓	↓	↓	Hypovolemia	Saline volume loading
→ or ↓	↑	→ or ↓	→ or ↓	Pulmonary embolism Right ventricular myocardial infarction	Ventilation/perfusion scan; saline or dextran; volume loading; *no* diuretics
↓	→ or ↑	↑	↓	Cardiogenic shock	Inotropic agents; diuretics; preload and afterload reduction if arterial pressure can be maintained; counterpulsation

→ = Normal; ↓ = Decreased or low; ↑ = Elevated or high.

tive dose, guided by hemodynamic response. When shock is caused by inappropriate vasodilatation (rare), α-adrenergic drugs such as norepinephrine are useful.

E. Percutaneous Coronary Intervention

Evidence indicates that acute revascularization by PCI might be particularly effective in patients who develop cardiogenic shock early (within 3–6 hours) after onset of myocardial infarction. PCI acutely should be seriously considered in such patients because thrombolytics are ineffective in cardiogenic shock associated with an acute myocardial infarction.

Disposition

All patients with cardiogenic shock must be hospitalized, preferably in an intensive care unit. Therapy is directed at the likely causes of shock (eg, fluid administration to patients with right ventricular infarction). Intra-aortic balloon pump (IABP) counterpulsation can increase cardiac output and improve both coronary and systemic perfusion. IABP counterpulsation is most commonly used to support the patient with cardiogenic shock during PCI.

2. Congestive Heart Failure

Congestive heart failure is caused by extensive myocardial infarction, volume overload, arrhythmias, acute mitral regurgitation, or ventricular septal rupture.

Clinical Findings

Symptoms and signs of congestive heart failure include dyspnea, anxiety, tachypnea, tachycardia, pulmonary rales or frank pulmonary edema, jugular venous distention, hypoxemia, and typical findings on chest x-ray (cardiomegaly, pulmonary vascular plethora, Kerley B lines, pleural effusion, or pulmonary infiltrates consistent with pulmonary edema). Wheezing may also be a sign of congestive heart failure (cardiac asthma). Suspect right ventricular infarction in inferior myocardial infarction if signs of right heart failure (right ventricular gallops, elevated central venous pressure, hepatomegaly, peripheral edema) are prominent in the absence of signs of left heart failure (dyspnea, rales, pulmonary congestion on chest x-ray).

Treatment

A. Airway Management

Give oxygen, 5–10 L/min, by mask or nasal cannula. Obtain arterial blood gas measurements. Treat respiratory failure if present.

B. Drug Therapy

1. Furosemide—Give furosemide, as an intravenous bolus of at least the patient's normal total daily dose. If the patient is not already taking furosemide, administer a 40-mg intravenous bolus initially, and observe the diuretic response by monitoring the patient's symptoms and urine output. Diuretics are contraindicated if right ventricular infarction is suspected.

2. Morphine—Give morphine, 2–8 mg intravenously.

3. Nitroglycerin—Apply nitroglycerin ointment, 1.25–2.5 cm (½–1 in), under an occlusive dressing if symptoms are mild. For severely symptomatic patients, a nitroglycerin infusion will benefit patients because both preload and afterload are reduced. In patients with inferior or right ventricular acute myocardial infarction, nitrates are relatively contraindicated because they may precipitate profound hypotension. Hypotension related to nitrates is treated with reduction or discontinuation of the infusion depending on the degree of symptomatic hypotension. Intravascular volume expansion with intravenous fluid infusions will often quickly correct hypotension.

Disposition

Treatment of congestive heart failure in the emergency department is directed at reducing the intravascular volume through diuretics or vasodilation. Patients with respiratory failure may require intubation in the emergency department. Hemodynamic monitoring with a pulmonary artery catheter may assist in assessing volume status. In the setting of an acute myocardial infarction, patients with congestive heart failure should be closely monitored in an intensive care unit.

3. Acute Mitral Regurgitation & Ventricular Septal Rupture

Mechanical failure of infarcted tissue (eg, rupture of the ventricular septum or of papillary muscle supporting the chordae tendineae) is a common cause of acute mitral regurgitation and ventricular septal rupture. Minimal-to-moderate mitral regurgitation is common after myocardial infarction as a result of papillary muscle and left ventricular wall dysfunction. Severe degrees of mitral regurgitation can result from marked ischemia with little or no infarction and can be completely reversed with revascularization.

Clinical Findings

Abrupt, severe congestive heart failure with pansystolic regurgitation murmur suggests acute mitral regurgitation or ventricular septal rupture. Echocardiography to detect mitral regurgitation or the abnormal velocity jet of a ventricular septal defect can establish the diagnosis.

Treatment

A. Immediate Measures

To be truly effective the following measures must be instituted in an intensive care unit:

- Treat heart failure with diuretics, morphine, and nitroglycerin ointment (usually of minimal effectiveness).
- Obtain urgent cardiologic and cardiac surgical consultation.
- IABP is a useful temporizing measure while the patient is being prepared for surgery.

B. Follow-Up Measures

The only life-saving treatment for most patients is emergency cardiac catheterization followed by surgery.

Disposition

Hospitalize all patients for treatment and surgery.

4. Myocardial Rupture

The chief cause of myocardial rupture is mechanical failure of an infarcted ventricular wall.

Clinical Findings

Myocardial rupture is an uncommon cause of sudden death during acute myocardial infarction; it is responsible for only about 5% of deaths. Myocardial rupture is suggested by abrupt onset of hypotension with increased venous pressure (ie, cardiac tamponade). Pulseless electrical activity often occurs.

Treatment & Disposition

If echocardiography or bedside emergency ultrasound demonstrates a pericardial effusion, pericardiocentesis is indicated and can be performed under ultrasound guidance (Chapter 6). When emergent ultrasound is not available to assess a patient for possible pericardial tamponade, blind pericardiocentesis may be life saving.

Obtain emergency cardiac surgical consultation for immediate cardiac surgery. This is successful in the few cases in which rupture has been minimal with slow intrapericardial hemorrhage.

5. Systemic or Pulmonary Embolization (See also Chapter 33.)

Systemic or pulmonary embolization is commonly caused by intracardiac mural thrombosis or phlebothrombosis.

Clinical Findings

The most common findings in pulmonary embolism are sudden unexplained dyspnea and tachycardia. Occasionally, pleuritic pain, signs of right heart strain, or abnormal chest x-ray may occur. Patients at greatest risk are those with thrombus visualized in the left or right ventricle by 2-dimensional echocardiography. The diagnosis may be confirmed by computed tomography (CT) scan of the chest, lung scan, or arteriography (Chapter 33). Systemic embolization is suspected when symptoms and signs of arterial occlusion occur. The clinical picture depends on the artery occluded, for example, flank pain and hematuria with renal artery embolism; pallor, pain, and loss of pulse with brachial or femoral artery embolism; stroke with cerebral artery embolism.

Treatment & Disposition

Give oxygen, draw blood for determination of prothrombin and partial thromboplastin times, and then begin systemic anticoagulation with heparin, 80 units/kg bolus followed by 18 units/kg/h infusion, or a low-molecular-weight heparin such as enoxaparin, 1 mg/kg subcutaneous administration every 12 hours. Pericarditis is a relative contraindication to anticoagulation because of the risk of bleeding into the pericardial sac, with resulting cardiac tamponade. Heparin is also contraindicated in patients with recent stroke, active duodenal ulcer, or active bleeding that cannot be controlled by direct pressure. Even though it does not cross the placenta, heparin must be used with caution in pregnant patients, especially during the third trimester. (Acute myocardial infarction during pregnancy is quite rare.)

With a massive pulmonary embolism with right heart failure or shock, intravenous fibrinolysis with streptokinase, urokinase, or t-PA has been recommended in doses similar to those given for acute myocardial infarction. Occasionally, mechanical disruption of the embolic thrombus by a catheter has been life saving.

Seek appropriate surgical consultation (with a thoracic, general, or vascular surgeon) for patients with persistent hypotension, contraindications to thrombolytic therapy, or systemic embolization who may benefit from surgical intervention (eg, angioplasty and embolectomy for a pulseless and ischemic extremity).

All patients should be hospitalized in the coronary care unit.

6. Pericarditis

When transmural myocardial infarction causes pericardial inflammation over the area of necrosis, pericarditis may occur within the first week. Pericarditis occurring more than 1 week after myocardial infarction may be the result of Dressler syndrome, an autoimmune reaction.

Clinical Findings

Pericarditis usually does not appear until 2–3 days after the onset of myocardial infarction. The appearance of a friction rub is often the only manifestation; pain and electrocardiographic changes are often absent. Frequently, a small pericardial effusion may be detected by echocardiography. If a pericardial friction rub is heard in the first 24 hours after onset, suspect pericarditis as a primary diagnosis rather than as being due to acute myocardial infarction. Early ECG signs of pericarditis include diffuse ST segment elevation (with a concave upslope and indistinct J point) and diffuse PR segment depression (except in AVR, where the PR segment is elevated).

Treatment

Treat pain with a nonsteroidal anti-inflammatory agent such as indomethacin, 25–50 mg orally 3 times a day. If pain is severe, give morphine, 2–4 mg intravenously every 5–10 minutes, and repeat as necessary.

Disposition

Hospitalize the patient in a coronary care unit for pain control and monitoring for possible cardiac tamponade (rare).

ANGINA PECTORIS

General Considerations

Myocardial ischemia (with attendant angina pectoris) results from an imbalance between myocardial oxygen supply and demand. Clinical findings vary depending on the severity of ischemia and on the frequency, duration, and rapidity of onset of ischemic episodes. If the demand for myocardial blood flow exceeds the capacity of the obstructed coronary arterial tree to supply it, the discomfort (angina pectoris) lasts until the excessive demand for coronary flow is reduced.

Discomfort is more intense and lasts longer when coronary blood flow decreases markedly, as occurs with sudden marked increase in coronary artery obstruction resulting from abrupt development of thrombus over an atherosclerotic plaque, embolization to a coronary artery, or sudden occlusion by coronary artery spasm. If myocardial necrosis then occurs, the condition is termed myocardial infarction; otherwise, the episode is one of acute coronary insufficiency, or preinfarction angina.

If obstruction is so severe that coronary blood flow is barely adequate to meet resting demands, even small increases in myocardial oxygen demand may cause angina. In addition, small aggregations of platelets on a ruptured plaque, spasm, or increased vasomotor tone can cause minor changes in the caliber of the severely obstructed coronary artery and precipitate angina.

Myocardial ischemia can exist in the absence of any chest discomfort. In patients with severe ischemia, 24-hour electrocardiographic monitoring shows that 80% of the episodes of ST segment depression lasting for a minute or more are present without angina (so-called silent ischemia). Painless myocardial infarction is not unusual in elderly or diabetic patients.

Clinical Findings

A. STABLE ANGINA (ANGINA OF EFFORT)

By definition, the pattern of discomfort, its frequency of occurrence, and precipitating factors have remained the same for 3 or more months.

Discomfort is usually substernal but may originate in other areas (eg, elbow, forearm, shoulder, neck interscapular region, or jaw), although substernal discomfort eventually occurs. It is usually precipitated by activities that increase myocardial oxygen consumption (eg, exercise, eating, or emotional upset), lasts longer than 1 minute and usually less than 15 minutes, and is usually relieved by rest or nitroglycerin. Pain that meets these criteria usually indicates the presence of fixed coronary obstruction. The most important feature suggesting the diagnosis of angina pectoris is discomfort precipitated by exercise or emotion.

B. UNSTABLE ANGINA

Anginal pain that begins in a patient previously free of pain (ie, pain of less than 1 month's duration) is called new-onset angina. Unstable angina is that which has changed in pattern, becoming more frequent (crescendo angina) and longer lasting. It is precipitated by a lesser degree of activity and may respond less to rest and nitroglycerin than does stable angina. Angina that occurs at rest without any obvious precipitating factor (rest angina) is the most serious form of unstable angina.

Sudden changes in angina not associated with increased myocardial oxygen demand (eg, increased blood pressure or heart rate) are presumed to be caused by a change in the anatomy of the coronary artery, for example, new vessel obstruction caused by progression of heart disease, development of thrombus, or other factors such as platelet aggregation or coronary spasm.

C. ATYPICAL ANGINA, OR PRINZMETAL (VARIANT) ANGINA

Prinzmetal angina occurs as a result of a sudden, reversible, severe coronary artery obstruction (coronary artery spasm). It may occur in patients with fixed atherosclerotic coronary lesions and less often in those with minimal or no fixed coronary obstruction. Chest discomfort usually occurs without a precipitating cause. It frequently occurs at rest or awakens the patient at night. The discomfort frequently lasts longer than the usual episode of angina and is often accompanied by ST segment elevation (current of injury) that is transient and reversed in minutes after administration of nitroglycerin. With lesser degrees of spasm, ST segment depression may occur. Ventricular ectopy and ventricular tachyarrhythmias may also occur.

Differential Diagnosis

See Chapter 12.

Treatment & Disposition

A. STABLE ANGINA

Nitroglycerin, 0.4 mg sublingually, is the drug of choice when pain starts. It may also be taken prophylactically several minutes before activities that regularly precipitate angina. Pain is usually relieved in 1–2 minutes. Nitroglycerin tablets deteriorate in about 6 months; headache and sublingual tingling are common side effects of active tablets.

Patients with stable angina that has exhibited a set pattern of frequency and precipitating factors over 3 or more months do not require hospitalization and should be referred for evaluation on an outpatient basis.

B. UNSTABLE ANGINA, REST ANGINA, AND PRINZMETAL ANGINA

1. Immediate measures—Give oxygen, 5-10 L/min, by mask or nasal cannula. Hospitalize the patient immediately in the coronary care unit, and obtain daily ECGs and myocardial enzyme determinations (CK isoenzymes and cTni or cTnt) to detect possible myocardial infarction.

2. Morphine—Give morphine, 2–3 mg intravenously every 5–10 minutes, to relieve prolonged pain. Monitor blood pressure.

3. Nitroglycerin—Apply nitroglycerin paste, 1.25 cm (½ in), to the skin under an occlusive dressing every 4 hours, or transdermal nitroglycerin patches may be substituted. Topical nitroglycerin can be used if the patient is pain free. If the pain persists, an intravenous infusion of nitroglycerin is indicated at an initial rate of 10 μg/min.

4. β-Blockers—Add a β-adrenergic blocking agent (eg, metoprolol, 5 mg intravenously over 2 minutes, every 5–10 minutes until a total dose of 15 mg has been administered) unless contraindicated (heart rate less than 60 beats/min, atrioventricular block, severe asthma, or chronic obstructive pulmonary disease).

5. Aspirin—Start non-enteric-coated aspirin, 160–325 mg orally. Aspirin has been shown to reduce the incidence of myocardial infarction and death by about 50%.

6. Anticoagulation—Antiocoagulation may also be helpful in these patients. Use unfractionated heparin at 80 units/kg intravenous bolus followed by 18 units/kg/h intravenous infusion or a low-molecular-weight heparin such as enoxaparin, 1 mg/kg administered subcutaneously every 12 hours. Compared to unfractionated heparin, enoxaparin was associated with decreased mortality in patients with acute myocardial infarction or recurrent angina.

7. Other drug therapies—Glycoprotein IIB/IIIA receptor antagonists such as tirofiban and eptifibatide are the newest agents to be approved for use in patients with unstable angina. These agents block platelet binding at the receptor site that cross links fibrinogen to the platelets. Although these agents have shown promise when used in conjunction with PCI, their role in unstable angina is still being defined.

8. Percutaneous coronary intervention—If pain continues despite treatment, consider PCI. If acute myocardial infarction has occurred and pain continues despite optimal medical management or thrombolytics, PCI must be considered. Percutaneous aortic balloon counterpulsation may also be useful in patients with cardiogenic shock.

American College of Cardiology: 1999 Update: ACC/AHA guidelines for the management of patients with acute myocardial injury. Accessed at http://www.acc.org/clinical/guidelines/nov96/1999/index.htm

Antman EM: Decision making with cardiac troponin tests. N Engl J Med 2002;346:2079. [PMID: 12087146]

Braunwald E et al: ACC/AHA 2002 guidelines update for the management of patients with unstable angina and non-ST-segment elevation myocardial infarction—summary article. J Am Coll Cardiol 2002;40:1366. [PMID: 12383588]

Brown M et al: Acute interventions for myocardial reperfusion. Emerg Med Clin North Am 1998;16:565. [PMID: 9739775]

Char DM, Israel E, Ladenson J: Early laboratory indicators of acute myocardial infarction. Emerg Med Clin North Am 1998;16:519. [PMID: 9739773]

Diop D, Aghababian RV: Definition, classification, and pathophysiology of acute coronary ischemic syndromes. Emerg Med Clin North Am 2001;19:259. [PMID: 11373977]

Hayes OW: Emergency management of acute myocardial infarction: focus on pharmacologic therapy. Emerg Med Clin North Am 1998;16:541. [PMID: 9739774]

Karras DJ, Kane DL: Serum markers in the emergency department diagnosis of acute myocardial infarction. Emerg Med Clin North Am 2001;19:321. [PMID: 11373981]

Lee TH, Goldman L: Evaluation of the patient with acute chest pain. N Engl J Med 2000;342:1187. [PMID: 10770985]

Llevadot J, Giugliano RP, Antman EM: Bolus fibrinolytic therapy in acute myocardial infarction. JAMA 2001;286:442. [PMID: 11466123]

McPherson JA, Gibson RS: Reperfusion therapy for acute myocardial infarction. Emerg Med Clin North Am 2001;19:433. [PMID: 11373988]

Shannon AW, Harrigan RA: General pharmacologic treatment of acute myocardial infarction. Emerg Med Clin North Am 2001;19:417. [PMID: 11373987]

■ HEART FAILURE

Heart failure is the expected outcome of many cardiac diseases. The basic abnormality is inability of the heart to maintain cardiac output sufficient to meet systemic demands. Compensatory mechanisms include (1) dilatation of the ventricle to maintain normal stroke volume (Frank-Starling mechanism); (2) retention of sodium and water by the kidneys to maintain intravascular volume; (3) increased activity of the sympathetic nervous system, leading to tachycardia and increased systemic vascular resistance; and (4) increased serum renin and angiotensin, which stimulate aldosterone output and cause retention of sodium and water as well as increased systemic vascular resistance. Cardiac output is usually maintained at normal levels or below, but at the expense of increased ventricular volume and filling pressure. The increased ventricular filling or diastolic pressures result in increased pulmonary or systemic venous pressures, with consequent pulmonary or peripheral edema. Tissue and organ dysfunction may result from increased venous pressure, decreased cardiac output, and edema.

Recently, it has been recognized that heart failure may occur primarily because of diastolic dysfunction where the ventricle appears to be noncompliant; therefore, even with normal diastolic volumes the high filling pressure results in pulmonary congestion. This type of heart failure is seen in hypertension, especially in elderly patients; in hypertrophic cardiomyopathy; and in myocardial ischemia. In many patients, both systolic and diastolic dysfunction are present. An echocardiographic-Doppler study should be performed in all patients with congestive heart failure to help determine the cause of the failure and the degree of systolic and diastolic dysfunction. The echocardiographic-Doppler study need not be done in the emergency department or at the first visit.

Although the distinction between mild to moderate heart failure and severe heart failure is not absolute, it has practical therapeutic implications.

SEVERE HEART FAILURE, INCLUDING PULMONARY EDEMA

Clinical Findings

A. SYMPTOMS AND SIGNS

Frank pulmonary edema may occur with severe left heart failure. Patients experience dyspnea at rest (Chapter 11) and in severe cases may be cyanotic and cough up frothy sputum. Peripheral edema may or may not be present; edema may be severe (anasarca) in severe right heart failure. Pulmonary edema may be accompanied by wheezing, and a loud S_3 sound is usually present. Loud rhonchi and rales may interfere with more detailed evaluation.

B. X-RAY FINDINGS

Chest x-ray may show pulmonary edema, pleural effusions, or cardiomegaly.

C. LABORATORY FINDINGS

Arterial blood gas measurements show hypoxemia; pH and PCO_2 vary, but hypocapnia and metabolic acidosis are common. With exhaustion, hypercapnia may occur, in which case intubation and mechanical ventilation are required. Recently the serum level of a neuropeptide, B-type natriuretic peptide (BNP), has been used clinically as a good marker for congestive heart failure. BNP is released from the ventricular myocardium in response to increases in ventricular wall tension. Above a BNP cutoff level of 100 pg/mL, the sensitivity and specificity are 90% and 76%, respectively, for differentiating congestive heart failure from other causes of dyspnea.

D. ELECTROCARDIOGRAPHIC FINDINGS

Sinus tachycardia is common in patients with severe heart failure. In patients with hypertensive heart disease, left ventricular hypertrophy may be evident. In addition, obtain an ECG to detect the presence of ischemia.

The differential diagnosis is discussed in Chapters 11 and 12.

Of paramount importance is the establishment of the cause of the heart failure. Specific causes have specific therapies, for example, valve replacement for pulmonary edema from severe aortic stenosis, or lowering of blood pressure for hypertension.

Note: Acute myocardial infarction or ischemia must be considered in all patients with sudden onset of congestive heart failure.

Treatment

A. OXYGENATION AND VENOUS ACCESS

Begin oxygen, 2–4 L/min, by mask or nasal cannula while awaiting the results of blood gas measurements. Insert a peripheral intravenous catheter, and give 0.9% normal saline by microdrip infusion to keep the catheter patent.

B. MORPHINE

Give morphine, 2–4 mg intravenously. Repeat every 20–30 minutes as needed for dyspnea, but stop if somnolence or hypercapnia supervenes.

C. FUROSEMIDE

Give furosemide, 40 mg as an intravenous bolus. If the patient is not already taking oral furosemide, 40 mg intravenously is a common initial dose. For patients already taking oral furosemide, administer at least the daily dose as an intravenous bolus. If the patient fails to respond in 10 minutes, repeat the dose once.

C. NITROGLYCERIN

Nitroglycerin, being a potent vasodilator, is useful in severe congestive heart failure because it reduces preload and afterload. The dose is 10 µg/min initially. Severe hypotension can develop, especially in the setting of an acute inferior or right ventricular infarction.

D. NITROPRUSSIDE

If the cause of severe congestive heart failure is directly related to hypertensive emergency, administer nitroprusside, 2–20 µg/kg/min as a continuous infusion. While the patient is monitored carefully (arterial pressure monitor is recommended), the dose can be titrated to achieve the desired blood pressure.

E. NESIRITIDE

Just as the measurement of BNP is useful for the diagnosis of congestive heart failure, the administration of BNP (nesiritide) improves hemodynamics and dyspnea in patients with severe decompensated congestive heart failure. Nesiritide is administered as a 2 µg/kg bolus over 1 minute, followed by a continuous infusion of 0.01 µg/kg/min generally for 12–24 hours. The major side effect of nesiritide is hypotension, which generally resolves quickly when the infusion is reduced or stopped.

Disposition

Hospitalize all patients with severe heart failure. Search for the reason behind the recurrent pulmonary edema, for example, noncompliance with regard to prescribed diet and medications, paroxysmal arrhythmias, institution of a medication with a negative inotropic effect, pulmonary emboli, or complicating disease.

MILD TO MODERATE HEART FAILURE

Clinical Findings

A. SYMPTOMS AND SIGNS

Nocturnal cough or dyspnea, orthopnea, dyspnea on exertion, and ankle swelling are common. The patient is not in distress at rest. Cardiomegaly is almost always found and is usually associated with some symptoms or sign of underlying cardiac disease (eg, angina or findings characteristic of aortic stenosis). Other important signs include increased venous pressure, hepatojugular reflux, pulmonary rales or pleural effusion, sacral or peripheral edema, and S_3 gallop.

Because hypertension is one of the most common causes of heart failure, record the blood pressure reading in both arms with the patient supine and sitting.

B. X-RAY FINDINGS

Chest x-ray may demonstrate cardiomegaly and pulmonary congestion.

C. ELECTROCARDIOGRAPHIC FINDINGS

Although there are no specific electrocardiographic manifestations of heart failure, it is nonetheless helpful to obtain an ECG.

D. LABORATORY FINDINGS

Obtain serum electrolyte determinations, renal function tests, and blood urea nitrogen and serum creatinine measurements. When renal blood flow is decreased, a rise in blood urea nitrogen out of proportion to the rise in serum creatinine is common (prerenal azotemia). Recently, measurement of serum BNP (as mentioned in the previous section) has been shown to improve accuracy in the diagnosis of congestive heart failure.

Treatment

Provide the patient with instructions for a low-sodium (1–2 g/d) diet. Prescribe a diuretic. A thiazide diuretic (eg, hydrochlorothiazide, 25 mg orally twice daily with potassium supplementation) should be sufficient initial therapy for most patients. Control hypertension if present (see below).

Disposition

By definition, hospitalization is not required for patients with mild heart failure per se, although it may be prudent to hospitalize some patients (eg, unreliable patients, those with other underlying illnesses or new-onset symptoms). All patients should be referred for long-term care and should be seen again within 1 week after their visit to the emergency department. Most of these patients will be candidates for medical therapy with angiotensin-converting enzyme inhibitors (eg, captopril or enalapril) or β-blockers. These agents have been shown to improve symptoms in patients with moderate congestive heart failure.

Colucci WS et al: Intravenous nesiritide in the treatment of decompensated congestive heart failure: Nesiritide Study Group. N Engl J Med 2000;343:246. [PMID: 10911006]

■ HYPERTENSION & HYPERTENSIVE CRISIS

Clinical Findings

The emergency physician evaluates patients with elevated blood pressures on a daily basis. The urge exists to treat all abnormal vital signs. Emergency physicians should avoid reflexly treating all elevated blood pressures without considering the patient in light of the clinical setting. For example, a patient experiencing pain or anxiety may be hypertensive in the emergency department simply as an adrenergic reflex. Aggressive treatment of asymptomatic hypertension in the emergency department may not be benign because it may lead to hypoperfusion and precipitate cerebrovascular ischemic events. When hypertension acutely causes symptoms, the organs most commonly affected include the brain, heart, and kidneys. Two categories of hypertension seen in emergency department patients merit further discussion: hypertensive urgency and hypertensive emergency.

A. HYPERTENSIVE URGENCY

Hypertensive urgency is classically defined as a severely elevated blood pressure in a patient with no symptoms, signs, or laboratory findings of end organ damage. Typical screening studies include serum creatinine (acute elevation), urinalysis (proteinuria, red blood cells, or red cell casts), chest x-ray (pulmonary edema or thoracic aortic dissection), and ECG (cardiac ischemia).

B. HYPERTENSIVE EMERGENCY

Hypertensive emergency occurs when elevated blood pressure is responsible for symptoms, signs, or laboratory evidence of end organ damage, such as mental status changes (hypertensive encephalopathy), cardiac ischemia or congestive heart failure, or acute renal failure.

Treatment

A. CATEGORIES OF MANAGEMENT

1. Hypertensive urgency—If history, physical exam, and screening tests do not reveal any end organ damage, blood pressure should be controlled within 24–48 hours. Reliable patients can be discharged home with rapid follow-up with a primary care physician for blood pressure recheck and initiation or adjustment of antihypertensive therapy if blood pressure remains elevated. If therapy is used, oral agents are appropriate. Clonidine, 0.2 mg by mouth followed by 0.1 mg every hour until the blood pressure is adequately controlled; captopril, 12.5–25 mg by mouth; or sublingual or oral labetalol, 200–400 mg, may be used.

2. Hypertensive emergency—Treatment involves rapid but controlled reduction in blood pressure using intravenous medications. The goal is to reduce the mean blood pressure by 25% within 1 hour of presentation. If the initial reduction is well tolerated by the patient, reduction to normal levels can be achieved over the ensuing 24 hours.

B. DRUGS USED TO TREAT HYPERTENSIVE EMERGENCIES

Caution: Avoid rapid, severe drops in blood pressure, because watershed cerebral infarction can occur. Blood pressure should be lowered gradually to the 160–180 mm Hg range acutely and then lowered further only gradually over a period of days with oral therapy.

1. Nitroprusside—Nitroprusside is a potent vasodilator. Give by continuous intravenous infusion at a rate of 2–20 μg/kg/min. This drug lowers blood pressure in seconds; stopping the infusion results in rapid return of blood pressure to the previous level. Hospitalization in an intensive care unit and intra-arterial pressure monitoring are usually required.

2. Labetalol—Labetalol is a combination α- and β-blocker useful in hypertensive emergency. The dose is 20 mg intravenously over 2 minutes. The dose can be doubled every 10 minutes until blood pressure reduction is achieved. The maximum total dose is 300 mg.

3. Hydralazine—Hydralazine is a vasodilator used mainly in pregnancy because it also increases uterine blood flow. The dose is 10–40 mg intravenously every 15–30 minutes. If a continuous infusion is required, the dose is 1.5–5.0 μg/kg/min.

4. Fenoldopam—Fenoldopam is particularly useful in patients with renal insufficiency or failure as an alternative to nitroprusside, which has been associated with cyanide toxicity. The initial dose is 0.1–1.6 μg/kg/min.

5. Enalaprilat—Enalaprilat is an intravenous angiotensin-converting enzyme inhibitor. It is useful in congestive heart failure or for stroke patients as an alternative to nitroprusside. The dose is 1.25–5.0 mg per dose over 5 minutes every 6 hours.

Disposition

Patients with hypertensive crisis require immediate hospitalization. Patients with hypertensive urgency should be referred to a primary care physician within 12–24 hours. Evidence-based recommendations do not exist for the optimal timing and degree of blood pressure control in hypertensive urgency patients.

Bisognomo JD: Malignant hypertension. Emedicine; www.emedicine.com/med/topic1107.html

Cherney D, Straus S: Management of patients with hypertensive urgencies and emergencies. J Gen Intern Med 2002;17:937. [PMID: 12472930]

Vidt DG: Emergency room management of hypertensive urgencies and emergencies. J Clin Hypertens 2001;17:158. [PMID: 11416701]

■ PERICARDITIS, PERICARDIAL EFFUSION, & CARDIAC TAMPONADE

PERICARDITIS & PERICARDIAL EFFUSION

General Considerations

Acute pericarditis may result from viral or bacterial infections (including tuberculosis), collage vascular diseases (especially rheumatic fever and disseminated lupus erythematosus), uremia, penetrating and nonpenetrating trauma, or myocardial infarction, and it may develop after pericardiotomy or irradiation of the mediastinum. It also may be associated with neoplasm (especially lymphomas such as Hodgkin disease). Pericarditis may also develop from annular or myocardial abscesses due to infective endocarditis. Pericardial effusion, and even cardiac tamponade, may develop in patients with acquired immunodeficiency syndrome (AIDS). Occasionally, drugs such as hydralazine or procainamide can cause an immune-response pericarditis. Varying degrees of myocarditis usually accompany pericarditis and account for the electrocardiographic changes. It is important to make an accurate etiologic diagnosis of pericarditis, if possible, because the specific cause may dictate the type of treatment required.

Clinical Findings

A. Symptoms and Signs

Fever and symptoms of the underlying disease may be present. Acute pericarditis usually causes persistent anterior chest pain that is frequently made worse by lying down and made better by sitting up and leaning forward. A pleuritic component is common. Radiation of pain to the neck, left shoulder, or arm occurs frequently.

1. Pericardial friction rub—The most common and most important diagnostic finding is pericardial friction rub with 2 or 3 components. The rub is frequently accentuated by having the patient breathe deeply or lean forward on hands and knees. A pericardial rub is absent in some cases, however.

2. Pleural friction rub—A pleural friction rub may be present as well.

3. Pericardial effusion—Pericardial effusion is rarely revealed on physical examination and is usually suspected on chest x-ray and confirmed by echocardiogram. With large effusions, heart sounds may be diminished, and pulmonary consolidation, rales at the base of the left lung, and dullness to percussion below the left scapula (Ewart's sign) may be present. Pericardial rub may lessen or disappear as pericardial effusion develops or may persist in the face of a large effusion. A rapidly accumulating effusion may cause cardiac tamponade (see below).

B. X-ray and Other Findings

1. Electrocardiogram—The ECG is usually abnormal in pericarditis, but the most common findings are nonspecific ST and T wave abnormalities. Initially, changes relatively specific for pericarditis are ST segment elevation in many leads (usually I, II, aVF, and V2–V6), with preservation of the normal concavity of the ST segment. Return of ST segments to the baseline on the ECG in a few days is followed by symmetric T wave inversion. Occasionally, the J junction elevation of ST segments seen as a normal variant may be confused with the electrocardiographic changes of pericarditis; however, in the normal variant, these changes do not evolve further. In pericarditis, moreover, the ST segment elevation is usually 25% or more of the T wave height in leads V5 or V6. Depression of the PR segment is highly indicative of pericarditis.

2. X-rays—No chest x-ray changes are specific for pericarditis. In some patients, hypoventilation resulting from pleuritic pain may be sufficiently severe to cause atelectasis. The chest x-ray is also an insensitive indicator of pericardial effusion, especially in the case of rapidly developing effusions that only minimally distend the pericardial sac. An enlarged cardiac silhouette with a "water-flask" contour may be seen in the case of large effusions that have developed gradually. At times, the presence of pericardial fluid may be suspected if a radiolucent line representing epicardial fat is seen on the lateral chest x-ray well inside the cardiac silhouette and separated from the sternum by pericardial fluid.

3. Echocardiography—Echocardiography is the most sensitive and specific noninvasive test for pericardial fluid and should be performed in all cases of suspected pericardial effusion or pericarditis.

Treatment

Begin electrocardiographic monitoring. Monitor blood pressure every 5–15 minutes. In patients with hemodynamic instability, insert a central venous pressure catheter (Chapter 6), and monitor central venous pressure to detect signs of possible cardiac tamponade (Table 34–2).

Draw blood for CBC, serum electrolyte measurements, and renal function tests. Relieve pain with morphine, 2–4 mg intravenously every 5–10 minutes, until pain is relieved; repeat as needed.

Obtain an echocardiogram as soon as possible to look for signs of pericardial effusion. Consider consultation with a cardiologist.

Table 34–2. Classification of cardiac tamponade.

	Blood Pressure	Heart Rate	Pulsus Paradoxus[1]	Central Venous Pressures
Normal hemodynamics (ie, pericardial effusion without cardiac tamponade)	Normal	Normal to increased	Not present (≤ 10 mm Hg)	Normal
Compensated cardiac tamponade	Normal	Normal to increased	Present (> 10 mm Hg)	Increased
Decompensated cardiac tamponade	Decreased; shock may be present	Increased	Present (> 10 mm Hg)	Increased

[1]Normal is defined as ≤ 10 mm Hg.

Consider pericardiocentesis (Chapter 6) to aid in etiologic diagnosis, especially if signs of infection (eg, fever) are present, suggesting pyogenic pericarditis or possible malignant pericarditis. If indicated, pericardiocentesis should be performed in an intensive care unit, cardiac catheterization lab with fluoroscopic guidance, or in the operating room. Pericardiocentesis in the emergency department should be done only to relieve decompensated cardiac tamponade and not to assist in etiologic diagnosis.

Disposition

Hospitalize most patients with acute pericarditis (with or without effusion), preferably in an intensive care or monitored intermediate care unit. Young patients with pericarditis who have had symptoms of several days' duration, who are hemodynamically stable with normal laboratory tests, and who are reliable often can be discharged with close follow-up in 1–3 days.

CARDIAC TAMPONADE

General Considerations

Accumulation of fluid in the pericardial space faster than the pericardium can accommodate it by distention results in compression of the heart, or cardiac tamponade. Pathophysiologic changes similar to tamponade may also result from constrictive pericarditis, although they are much more slowly progressive than tamponade resulting from rapidly accumulating pericardial fluid. The principal result of the cardiac tamponade is reduced diastolic filling of the ventricles, with resulting reduced cardiac output. Ultimately, shock and death supervene.

Clinical Findings

A. SYMPTOMS AND SIGNS

1. Coexisting or antecedent findings—There may be coexisting or antecedent signs or symptoms of pericarditis or pericardial effusion or of the disease process causing effusion. However, some patients develop cardiac tamponade without coexisting findings.

2. Tachycardia and hypotension—If cardiac tamponade progresses so that central venous pressure rises higher than 18 mm Hg, right ventricular filing decreases, causing subsequent decreases first in right ventricular and then in left ventricular stroke volume. Reflex tachycardia and increased systemic vascular resistance result to support systemic blood pressure. As cardiac tamponade worsens, these compensations fail, resulting in a sharp drop in cardiac output and blood pressure (decompensated cardiac tamponade). Because death follows rapidly if decompensated tamponade is not relieved, even slight hypotension or tachycardia occurring in patients with suspected pericardial effusion must be carefully monitored.

3. Pulsus paradoxus—In the normal healthy individual, systolic blood pressure drops no more than 8–10 mm Hg on normal inspiration. This change is exaggerated in cardiac tamponade, and palpable pulse volume may also decrease on inspiration. Pulsus paradoxus is common in cardiac tamponade resulting from pericardial effusion but is less common in tamponade associated with constrictive pericarditis.

4. Kussmaul's sign—During inspiration in cardiac tamponade there may be an increase in estimated central venous pressure (eg, by observation of jugular venous pulsation) rather than the normal decrease.

B. X-RAY AND OTHER FINDINGS

1. Echocardiography—Echocardiography is the most sensitive and specific noninvasive test for the presence of pericardial fluid and should be performed as soon as possible in all patients with suspected cardiac tamponade. With cardiac tamponade, there is marked swinging of the heart and collapse of the right atrial and ventricular chamber on expiration. In addition, diastolic collapse of the right ventricle is diagnostic of pericardial tamponade.

2. X-rays—Findings on chest x-ray usually are not helpful in the diagnosis of cardiac tamponade. A sudden marked increase in apparent heart size should suggest the possibility of pericardial effusion.

3. Electrocardiogram—In cardiac tamponade, the ECG may show electrical alternates either of the QRS complex alone or of the entire complex (P, QRS, and T waves). This finding is rare in pericardial effusion without tamponade.

C. CLASSIFICATION OF CARDIAC TAMPONADE

The severity of cardiac tamponade may be classified as set forth in Table 34–2.

Treatment

A. DECOMPENSATED CARDIAC TAMPONADE

Note: Decompensated cardiac tamponade is an immediate threat to life and requires emergent treatment.

1. Oxygenation and blood pressure support—Give oxygen, 5–10 L/min, by mask or nasal cannula. Insert a large-bore ($\geq$ 16-gauge) peripheral intravenous catheter, and infuse crystalloid solution to support blood pressure. In an adult, give 300–500 mL in 10–20 minutes, and then continue the infusion based on the blood pressure response.

2. Dopamine—Give dopamine, 2–20 μg/kg/min intravenously. Adjust dosage based on the blood pressure.

3. Pericardiocentesis—If available, emergent echocardiography or emergent bedside sonography in the emergency department can be diagnostic. In addition, pericardiocentesis can be performed under ultrasound guidance (Chapter 6). If ultrasound is not available and the patient is in extremis, blind pericardiocentesis can be life saving.

B. COMPENSATED CARDIAC TAMPONADE

Give oxygen, as described above. Monitor blood pressure every 5–15 minutes. Start continuous electrocardiographic monitoring. Insert a central venous pressure catheter, and monitor central venous pressure.

Insert a large-bore (≥ 16-gauge) peripheral intravenous catheter, and keep it patent with crystalloid solution. Confirm the presence of pericardial fluid or (rarely) pericardial thickening by bedside emergency ultrasound or echocardiography within 1 hour.

Caution: Do not administer diuretics or preload reduction (eg, nitrates) to control venous plethora (hypotension will result). Treatment of the pericardial tamponade is recommended before administering any general anesthetic. Anesthesia will cause withdrawal of sympathetic support to the heart and venous bed and will result in severe hypotension.

Disposition

Hospitalize all patients with suspected or documented cardiac tamponade, preferably in an intensive care unit, and obtain urgent cardiologic and cardiothoracic surgical consultation.

Bogolioubov A et al: Circulatory shock. Crit Care Clin 2001;17: 697. [PMID: 11525054]

Goyle KK, Walling AD: Diagnosing pericarditis. Am Fam Physician 2002;66:1695. [PMID: 12449268]

Soler-Soler J et al: Management of pericardial effusion. Heart 2001; 86(2):235. [PMID: 11454853]

■ MYOCARDITIS & CARDIOMYOPATHY

Many diseases affecting the myocardial muscle have heart failure as their ultimate outcome. Secondary cardiomyopathies may be classified as shown in Table 34–3.

In most patients, the cause is unknown. The most common cause of acute myocardial injury and heart failure is coronary artery disease with ischemia or infarction, and this diagnostic possibility must be considered in every patient who has sudden onset of congestive heart failure. Infectious causes of myocarditis include

Table 34–3. Classification of causes of secondary cardiomyopathy, with examples.

Infectious
  Viral disease (coxsackie B and arbovirus infections,
    poliomyelitis)
  Bacterial disease (diphtheria)
  Parasitic disease (Chagas disease)
  Rickettsial disease (scrub typhus)
Immunologic
  Rheumatic fever
  Systemic lupus erythematosus
Toxic
  Alcohol
  Emetine
  Doxorubicin
Muscular
  Pseudohypertrophic muscular dystrophy
Metabolic
  Hyperthyroidism
  Hypothyroidism
  Beriberi
  Glycogen storage disease
Infiltrative
  Amyloidosis
  Hemochromatosis
Neoplastic
  Lymphoma
Physical
  Hyperthermia
Peripartum

viruses (mainly enteroviruses, especially coxsackievirus B), bacteria, protozoa (*Trypanosoma cruzi* and *Borrelia burgdorferi*), and parasites (*Trichinella*).

Clinical Findings

Symptoms and signs may mimic those of almost any form of heart disease. Chest pain is common. Mild myocarditis or cardiomyopathy is frequently asymptomatic; severe cases are associated with heart failure, arrhythmias, and systemic embolization. Manifestations of the underlying disease (eg, Chagas disease) may be prominent. Most patients with biopsy-proven myocarditis report a recent viral prodrome preceding cardiovascular symptoms.

Electrocardiographic abnormalities are often present, although the changes are frequently nonspecific. A pattern characteristic of left ventricular hypertrophy may be present. Flat or inverted T waves are most common, often with low-voltage QRS complexes. Intraventricular conduction defects and bundle branch block, especially left bundle branch block, are also common.

An echocardiogram is useful to detect wall motion abnormalities or a pericardial effusion. Chest radiographs can be normal or show evidence of congestive heart failure with pulmonary edema or cardiomegaly.

In acute myocarditis, cardiac enzymes (CK-MB, cTni, or cTnt) may be elevated. Endomyocardial biopsy is diagnostic.

Treatment

Bed rest is widely recommended, and there is some evidence supporting its benefits. If the cause of the disease is known (eg, trichinosis, acute rheumatic fever), begin therapy recommended for the underlying disease. Complications of myocarditis include chest pain, arrhythmias, embolization, and heart failure; these should be treated appropriately.

Disposition

Hospitalization is indicated unless the condition is chronic and stable.

Pawsat DE, Lee JY: Inflammatory disorders of the heart: pericarditis, myocarditis and endocarditis. Emerg Med Clin North Am 1998;16:665. [PMID: 9739781]

■ AORTIC ANEURYSMS & DISSECTIONS

See Chapter 38.

■ CONGENITAL HEART DISEASE

The differential diagnosis of congenital heart disease is beyond the scope of this book. The general principles of management are outlined below as a guide for emergency physicians.

Classification

Classification of congenital heart disease is based on the hemodynamic effects produced or on specific anatomic abnormalities:

- Left-to-right shunts: interatrial septal defect, interventricular septal defect, patent ductus arteriosus
- Right-to-left shunts: cyanotic heart disease (eg, transposition of the great vessels, tetralogy of Fallot, pulmonary atresia, tricuspid atresia)

- Valvular stenosis, hypoplasia, and atresia: pulmonary valve and aortic valve stenosis, tricuspid atresia, pulmonary atresia, mitral and aortic atresia
- Abnormalities of position: dextrocardia, transposition of the great vessels, corrected transposition
- Abnormalities of great vessels: coarctation of the aorta, patent ductus arteriosus, arterial rings

Obviously, individual lesions may combine attributes from 2 or more categories. For example, tricuspid atresia is both a right-to-left shunt (owing to interatrial communication) and an atretic lesion.

Pathophysiology

Large left-to-right shunts cause increased blood flow through the lungs and volume overload of one or both ventricles. Right-to-left shunts cause systemic venous return to bypass the lungs and go directly into the arterial circulation. The resulting arterial desaturation (if severe) may cause cyanosis.

Valvular obstruction (aortic or pulmonary stenosis) and aortic obstruction (coarctation of the aorta) cause afterload abnormalities of the involved ventricles. Vascular rings around the trachea and esophagus cause symptoms resulting from obstruction (eg, dyspnea, cough, dysphagia).

CYANOSIS

All infants (under age 1 year) who have cyanotic heart disease are at risk for potential serious illness with sudden life-threatening complications. Lesions producing right-to-left shunts are frequently undetected until after the newborn period, because pulmonary blood flow is maintained by a patent ductus arteriosus. When the ductus arteriosus begins to close, cyanosis becomes manifest. If the ductus arteriosus is the major source of pulmonary blood flow—as may be the case in pulmonary atresia—the patient may become markedly cyanotic and die rapidly after the ductus arteriosus closes.

No matter how well these children do or how asymptomatic they appear, their entire ability to oxygenate blood may depend on the presence of a patent ductus arteriosus, which may close unpredictably at any time.

Clinical Findings

Cyanosis is most apparent in highly vascularized areas with superficial capillaries, for example, lips, oral and conjunctival mucosa, and nail beds. With more severe hypoxemia and desaturation, other areas of skin may appear cyanotic. The diagnosis may be confirmed by arterial blood P_{O_2} measurements.

Treatment & Disposition

All infants with cyanosis (intermittent or constant) should be hospitalized for immediate evaluation by a pediatric cardiologist, because emergency catheterization and angiocardiography may be necessary. Frequently, definitive diagnosis can be made by 2-dimensional echocardiography, with and without Doppler ultrasound.

Older children with stable cyanotic heart disease do not require emergency hospitalization but should be referred for evaluation. If other signs of cardiac disease are present (eg, heart failure, arrhythmias), hospitalization or treatment is indicated as appropriate.

ANOXIC SPELLS

Clinical Findings

Anoxic spells are common in patients with cyanotic heart disease and usually start after the infant is aged 3 months or older. They rarely occur after age 4–5 years. The spells frequently start with the infant becoming fussy and developing increasing cyanosis and tachypnea. The infant then suddenly goes limp. These spells often occur in the morning after a good night's rest or when the child becomes more active, usually during feeding or straining at stool, and they are associated with sudden marked increases in right-to-left shunting.

Treatment

Place the child in the knee-chest position, and quickly give morphine, 0.2 mg/kg intramuscularly or subcutaneously. Give 100% oxygen by face mask, and be prepared to perform immediate intubation. If pH is 7.1 or lower, give sodium bicarbonate, 1–2 mEq/kg, intravenously to correct acidosis. If hypoglycemia is present or suspected, give 10% glucose solution intravenously at a rate of 5–10 mL/kg/h, and monitor blood glucose concentration.

In children with anoxic spells and tetralogy of Fallot, propranolol, 0.01 mg/kg slowly intravenously, has been helpful. The dose may be repeated in 5 minutes.

Disposition

An unexplained episode of syncope, "lip spell," or convulsions in any child with known cyanotic heart disease should suggest anoxic spells. The child should be hospitalized immediately.

HEART FAILURE

Congestive heart failure in infancy is usually associated with large left-to-right shunts at the ventricular level (eg, ventricular septal defect) or arterial level (eg, patent ductus arteriosus). It may also be associated with obstructive lesions such as aortic stenosis, aortic or mitral atresia, and coarctation of the aorta. Rarely, the cause can be anomalous origin of the left coronary artery from the pulmonary artery. Congestive heart failure may occur in the infant with atrial tachycardia or atrial flutter with rapid ventricular response, with or without preexcitation syndromes. Underlying heart disease need not be present.

Clinical Findings

Congestive heart failure in infants is manifested by dyspnea on exertion just as it is in adults. Because the most common strenuous activity in which an infant engages is feeding, an infant with congestive heart failure will have to stop and breathe at the end of each swallow. Difficulty in taking the entire bottle in the usual 15–20 minutes may therefore be the principal manifestation of heart failure. In addition, the baby may be sluggish and fussy and have a weak cry.

Physical findings in these infants are those of the underlying lesion as well as those associated with congestive heart failure.

A. AORTIC MURMURS

In aortic murmurs (eg, pulmonary stenosis and coarctation of the aorta), systolic ejection murmurs are heard. They are frequently accompanied by ejection clicks. Patent ductus arteriosus or aortopulmonary windows are associated with continuous murmurs heard at the base of the heart. If stenosis is severe or if cardiac output is severely decreased, the murmur may not be loud.

B. TACHYPNEA AND TACHYCARDIA

Tachypnea and tachycardia are usually present.

C. SWEATING

Because of the increased activity of the sympathetic nervous system in children with congestive heart failure, profuse sweating is common.

D. BIVENTRICULAR FAILURE

Isolated left heart failure is unusual in infants. Biventricular failure with ventricular gallops, rales, hepatomegaly, and edema is more common.

E. VENOUS DISTENTION

Because of the short neck in infants, venous distention frequently cannot be detected.

F. HEPATOMEGALY

Hepatomegaly may develop within a few hours after the onset of congestive heart failure and may resolve just as quickly with therapy.

Disposition

A. IMMEDIATE HOSPITALIZATION

Any infant or child with newly diagnosed congestive heart failure—especially if it is associated with a systolic ejection murmur—must be hospitalized for immediate evaluation. The murmur may be due to aortic stenosis, pulmonary stenosis, or coarctation of the aorta, each of which requires prompt diagnosis and treatment.

B. OUTPATIENT CARE

Children with mild congestive heart failure due to stable, previously diagnosed congenital heart disease may be managed on an outpatient basis. Diuretics and digitalis (in older infants and children) are frequently effective.

PULMONARY HYPERTENSION

The child with a large ventricular septal defect or patent ductus arteriosus can develop significant irreversible changes in the pulmonary vascular bed within 2 years and must therefore be evaluated as soon as the problem is discovered.

Linear growth and weight gain may be slow. After age 2 years, compensatory mechanisms that decrease the size of the left-to-right shunt are frequent: for example, increased pulmonary vascular resistance, decreased pulmonary blood flow because of decreasing size of the ventricular septal defect, or development of infundibular pulmonary stenosis because of hypertrophy of the crista supraventricularis.

Prompt referral to a pediatric cardiologist is indicated if previously undiagnosed ventricular septal defect or patent ductus arteriosus is detected.

COARCTATION OF THE AORTA

The diagnosis of coarctation of the aorta is made by finding femoral pulses that are decreased or absent when compared to brachial pulses. If femoral pulses are present but faint, blood pressure taken with a cuff of the appropriate size in the upper and lower extremities should show lower blood pressure in the legs than in the arm if coarctation of the aorta exists. Prompt referral to a cardiologist is indicated.

Grifka RG: Cyanotic congenital heart disease with increased pulmonary blood flow. Pediatr Clin North Am 1999;46:405. [PMID: 10218083]

Nouri S: Congenital heart defects: cyanotic and acyanotic. Pediatr Ann 1997;26:92. [PMID: 9121846]

Waldman JD, Wernly JA: Cyanotic congenital heart disease with decreased pulmonary blood flow in children. Pediatr Clin North Am 1999;46:385. [PMID: 10218082]

Cardiac Arrhythmias

35

David A. Wald, DO

Tachyarrhythmias
Supraventricular Arrhythmias
1. Sinus Tachycardia
2. Paroxysmal Supraventricular Tachycardia
3. Atrial Fibrillation
4. Atrial Flutter
5. Multifocal Atrial Tachycardia
6. Preexcitation Arrhythmias
Ventricular Arrhythmias
1. Ventricular Tachycardia
2. Proarrhythmic Ventricular Arrhythmias
3. Polymorphic Ventricular Tachycardia (including Torsades de Pointes)
4. Ventricular Fibrillation
Bradyarrhythmias, Conduction Disturbances, & Escape Rhythms
Sinus Bradycardia
Sinus Arrest
Sinoatrial Block
1. First-Degree Sinoatrial Block
2. Second-Degree Sinoatrial Block (Mobitz Type I)

3. Second-Degree Sinoatrial Block (Mobitz Type II)
4. Third-Degree Sinoatrial Block
5. Sick Sinus Syndrome
Atrioventricular Block
1. First-Degree Atrioventricular Block
2. Second-Degree Atrioventricular Block (Mobitz Type I)
3. Second-Degree Atrioventricular Block (Mobitz Type II)
4. Third-Degree Atrioventricular Block (Complete Heart Block)
Idioventricular Rhythm
Atrioventricular Junctional Rhythm
Permanent Cardiac Pacemakers
Complications of Implantable Cardiac Pacemakers
Pacemaker Malfunction
Implantable Cardioverter Defibrillators
Complications of Implantable Cardioverter Defibrillators
Implantable Cardioverter Defibrillator Malfunction
Appendix: Commonly Encountered Cardiac Arrhythmias

Patients with cardiac arrhythmias often present to the emergency department. The patient's hemodynamic status determines the urgency with which the assessment and management should proceed. Patients with serious signs and symptoms (ie, shock, hypotension, congestive heart failure [CHF], severe shortness of breath, altered level of consciousness, ischemic chest pain, or acute myocardial infarction) require immediate treatment. With stable patients, more time is afforded for review of the 12-lead electrocardiogram (ECG) and rhythm strip to diagnose the cardiac arrhythmia. Review of available medical records, especially a prior ECG, may also assist in arrhythmia diagnosis. Examples of commonly encountered arrhythmias are presented in the appendix to this chapter.

■ TACHYARRHYTHMIAS

Immediate synchronized direct current (DC) cardioversion should be performed on all patients presenting with serious signs and symptoms. In the unstable patient, specific arrhythmia diagnosis (supraventricular or ventricular) does not need to be made immediately because the initial management is the same. Patients with polymorphic ventricular tachycardia (PMVT) of 30 seconds or more and all unstable patients should be treated with immediate asynchronous defibrillation.

In stable patients, the initial medical management will be guided by the underlying rhythm and findings of a detailed history and physical examination. In recent years, the more traditional approach to categorize patients as either stable or unstable has been modified. Hemodynamically stable patients can be further subdivided into those with preserved or impaired cardiac function. Findings of impaired cardiac function in a patient who is otherwise stable may alter the pharmacologic treatment.

SUPRAVENTRICULAR ARRHYTHMIAS

1. Sinus Tachycardia

Clinical Findings
(See Appendix, Figure 35–3.)

Sinus tachycardia occurs when the sinus rate is faster than 100 beats/min. Usually the rate is 101–160 beats/min. Young, healthy adults can accelerate their heart rate up to 180–200 beats/min, particularly during exercise. Young children have been noted to have sinus rates up to 220 beats/min. Sinus tachycardia should not be viewed as a primary arrhythmia but more as a response to an underlying illness or condition. It is often normal in infancy and early childhood but can occur as a result of a number of conditions including pain, fever, stress, other hyperadrenergic states, anemia, hypovolemia, hypoxia, myocardial ischemia, pulmonary edema, shock, and hyperthyroidism. Certain medications and illicit drugs can also cause tachycardia.

Treatment & Disposition

The treatment of sinus tachycardia is directed at the underlying cause. This may include correction of dehydration with intravenous fluids, analgesic or antipyretic administration, or supplemental oxygen to correct hypoxia. Treatment aimed at correcting the heart rate may be harmful if the tachycardia is compensatory and is supporting the cardiac output. Gradual slowing of the heart rate during carotid sinus massage may help to differentiate sinus tachycardia from other supraventricular arrhythmias. Further management, including the need for hospitalization, depends on the underlying condition.

2. Paroxysmal Supraventricular Tachycardia

Clinical Findings
(See Appendix, Figures 35–6 to 35–11.)

Paroxysmal supraventricular tachycardia (PSVT) is a general term that refers to a number of tachyarrhythmias that arise from above the bifurcation of the His bundle. Approximately 90% of these arrhythmias occur as a result of a reentrant mechanism; the remaining 10% occur as a result of increased automaticity.

Atrioventricular nodal reentrant tachycardia (AVNRT) is the most common form of PSVT, accounting for 50–60% of cases. The heart rate is usually 180–200 beats/min and is characterized by sudden onset and sudden termination. Because the reentrant mechanism occurs within the AV node itself, virtually simultaneous excitation of the atria and ventricles occurs. As a result, the P waves occur concurrent with the QRS complexes and are difficult to visualize on the ECG. Often, patients with AVNRT do not have underlying heart disease. Common precipitating factors include alcohol, caffeine, and sympathomimetic amines. Patients with AVNRT usually present in their third or fourth decade of life, and the majority (approximately 70%) are female.

Atrioventricular reciprocating tachycardia (AVRT) accounts for 30–40% of PSVT. In most cases, the impulse travels down the AV node and follows a retrograde path up the accessory bypass tract. Because activation of the ventricles occurs through normal conduction pathways, the accessory pathway is concealed, and the QRS morphology is normal. Consider AVRT if the heart rate is faster than 200 beats/min or if P waves are seen following the QRS complex.

Sinus node reentry and intra-atrial reentry are uncommon causes of PSVT, each accounting for approximately 5% of cases. In these arrhythmias, the heart rate is usually 130–140 beats/min. More often, patients with these arrhythmias have underlying heart disease.

Automatic atrial tachycardia is another uncommon arrhythmia, accounting for less than 5% of cases of PSVT. The heart rate is usually 160–250 beats/min but may be as slow as 140 beats/min. In this case, the underlying mechanism is increased automaticity rather than reentry. Automatic atrial tachycardia is commonly associated with underlying heart disease. This arrhythmia is difficult to treat and may be refractory to standard measures including cardioversion.

PSVT can be classified as AV nodal dependent or independent. This strategy may prove useful in formulating treatment options. AVNRT and AVRT are AV nodal dependent, meaning that the AV node is involved in the reentrant circuit. For these rhythms, pharmacologic management is designed to decrease conduction through the AV node.

Treatment

A. UNSTABLE PATIENTS

Patients with PSVT who are hemodynamically unstable require immediate synchronized DC cardioversion. Recommendations are to start with low energy levels (50 joules [J]) and then to increase the initial dose by

50 J as needed until sinus rhythm is restored. If clinical circumstances permit, administer intravenous sedatives. Avoid the common error of delaying emergent cardioversion to perform other patient care activities.

If immediate cardioversion is unavailable, physical maneuvers that cause vagal stimulation can be attempted. If unsuccessful, a trial dose of adenosine or a calcium-channel blocker may be administered. Note that calcium-channel blockers are contraindicated in patients with hypotension or severe CHF.

B. Stable Patients

Tachycardia associated with PSVT is usually well tolerated unless the patient has underlying heart disease or left ventricular dysfunction.

1. Physical maneuvers—In stable patients, physical maneuvers causing vagal stimulation can be attempted prior to medication administration. Maneuvers that stimulate the vagus nerve such as the Valsalva maneuver (expiration against a closed glottis), Mueller maneuver (deep inspiration against a closed glottis), cold water facial immersion, gagging, and carotid sinus massage are at times effective in terminating PSVT that results from AV nodal and sinoatrial (SA) nodal dependent mechanisms. Eyeball pressure may also cause vagal stimulation but is not recommended because of the possibility of ocular injury. Perform carotid sinus massage only after auscultation for carotid bruits.

2. Pharmacologic treatment—If vagal stimulation is ineffective, adenosine is considered first-line medical therapy for conversion of PSVT. In general, pharmacologic agents with AV nodal blocking properties such as adenosine, β-blockers, calcium-channel blockers, and digoxin are used for the acute management and prevention of AV nodal dependent PSVT. Other antiarrhythmic agents, such as procainamide and amiodarone, that exert effects at various levels of the cardiac conduction system are used for the management and prevention of AV nodal independent PSVT. Antiarrhythmic medications may be considered for conversion of PSVT when AV nodal blocking agents are unsuccessful.

a. Adenosine—Adenosine is an endogenous nucleoside that slows conduction through the AV node and is successful in terminating more than 90% of PSVTs resulting from AV nodal reentry mechanisms (AVNRT and AVRT). Adenosine may also be effective in terminating sinus node reentry tachycardia but is usually ineffective in terminating automatic atrial tachycardia. Often adenosine will cause a transient AV block, briefly exposing the underlying atrial activity. Administration of a medication with more prolonged effect on the AV node (β-blockers or calcium-channel blockers) may provide a more sustained reduction in ventricular rate.

Administer adenosine rapidly, and follow each dose immediately with a 20-cc saline flush. Administer an initial intravenous dose of 6 mg over 1–3 seconds. If this does not terminate the PSVT, a 12-mg dose can be administered in 2 minutes. The 12-mg dose can be repeated one additional time if necessary. Common side effects include facial flushing, hyperventilation, dyspnea, and chest pain. These side effects are often transient owing to the short half-life of adenosine (less than 5 seconds). The effects of adenosine are antagonized by caffeine and theophylline and potentiated by dipyridamole and carbamazepine. Heart transplant patients may be overly sensitive to the effects of adenosine; if necessary, use smaller doses. Because adenosine can provoke bronchospasm, use caution if it is being administered to patients with a history of reactive airway disease.

Adenosine can also be administered to a stable patient with a wide QRS complex tachycardia suspected to be supraventricular in origin. Adenosine is preferred over calcium-channel blockers in patients with hypotension or impaired cardiac function and in patients concomitantly receiving β-adrenergic blocking agents.

b. β-Adrenergic Blocking Agents—β-Blockers such as propanolol or esmolol slow SA node impulse formation and slow conduction through the AV node. These medications should be used with caution in patients with a history of reactive airway disease and CHF.

c. Propanolol—Propranolol is a nonselective β-adrenergic blocking agent. As an alternative to calcium-channel blockers, propranolol is administered intravenously at a dose of 1–3 mg over 1–3 minutes. If necessary, an additional dose can be administered in 2 minutes to a total dose of 0.1 mg/kg. Esmolol is an ultra-short-acting β_1-selective β-blocker that has the advantage of a brief half-life (~10 minutes) and a rapid onset of action. Administer a loading dose of 0.5 mg/kg over 1 minute. This is followed by a maintenance infusion of 50 µg/kg/min. If the response is inadequate, another dose of 0.5 mg/kg can be administered after 4 minutes and the maintenance infusion increased to 100 µg/kg/min. When heart rate control is achieved, reduce the maintenance infusion to 25 µg/kg/min.

d. Calcium-channel blockers—Calcium-channel blockers such as diltiazem or verapamil are effective in converting PSVT to sinus rhythm. The efficacy of diltiazem and verapamil in terms of conversion rates, rapidity of response, and safety profile appear similar. These medications decrease SA and AV node conduction and cause prolongation of the AV node refractory period. Calcium-channel blockers also decrease myocardial contractility and peripheral vascular resistance. Use calcium-channel blockers with caution in patients with left ventricular dysfunction or CHF. Avoid these medications in patients with wide complex tachycardia of unknown origin, ventricular tachycardia, or tachycardia with ventricular preexcitation. Hypotension is the most concerning side effect of intravenous administration and occurs in 10–15% of patients. Pretreatment with intravenous calcium has been recommended for patients with borderline hypotension as pretreatment to prevent further decline in the blood pressure after administration of intravenous calcium-channel blockers.

(1) Verapamil—The initial dose of verapamil is 5–10 mg administered intravenously over 1–2 minutes. Additional doses of 5–10 mg can be administered every 15 minutes as needed until the desired effect is achieved or a total of 30 mg has been administered.

(2) Diltiazem—The initial dose of diltiazem is 0.25 mg/kg administered intravenously over 2 minutes (20 mg for the average adult). If necessary, a dose of 0.35 mg/kg can be administered in 15 minutes. After conversion, a maintenance infusion can be started at 5–10 mg/h and can be increased to a maximum of 15 mg/h if needed. The hemodynamic effects of diltiazem are often less pronounced than those of verapamil.

e. Digoxin—Digoxin administration will increase vagal tone while reducing sympathetic activity. As a result, conduction through the AV node is slowed. Digoxin may be administered as an intravenous bolus dose of 0.5 mg. Additional doses of 0.25 mg may be given as needed every 2–4 hours, with a total dose not to exceed 1.25 mg in 24 hours. The immediate benefit of digoxin is lessened by its slow onset of action. When used in combination, digoxin may allow for lower doses of subsequently administered antiarrhythmic agents. Avoid digoxin in patients with atrial fibrillation with ventricular preexcitation.

f. Amiodarone—Amiodarone is a class III antiarrhythmic agent with sodium- and potassium-channel blocking properties and β-blocking and calcium-channel blocking properties. By virtue of its β-blocking and calcium-channel blocking properties, amiodarone slows conduction through the AV node. In patients with impaired cardiac function or CHF, treatment options narrow. Amiodarone has a solid safety profile and may be an effective alternative agent in this situation. Amiodarone can be administered as a slow intravenous infusion of 150 mg over 10 minutes. This is followed by a maintenance infusion of 1 mg/min for 6 hours and then 0.5 mg/min. Additional bolus doses of 150 mg can be repeated as needed for resistant or recurrent PSVT up to a total daily dose of 2 g.

g. Procainamide—Procainamide is a class IA antiarrhythmic agent with sodium-channel blocking properties. Procainamide will slow conduction through both the AV node and, if present, an accessory bypass tract. Procainamide can be considered for patients with PSVT refractory to AV nodal blocking agents. The recommended loading dose of procainamide is 17 mg/kg administered as a slow intravenous infusion at a rate of 20–30 mg/min (1 g for an average adult). Stop the initial infusion if the arrhythmia is suppressed, hypotension develops, or the QRS complex widens by more than 50% of its original duration. After arrhythmia suppression, start a maintenance infusion at 1–4 mg/min.

Disposition

Hospitalization is recommended for patients in PSVT with accompanying serious signs and symptoms, patients requiring emergent cardioversion, patients in PSVT with ventricular preexcitation, and patients with arrhythmias refractory to standard treatment. Outpatient follow-up care should be provided for the otherwise healthy patient with a transient episode of PSVT converted to sinus rhythm in the emergency department.

3. Atrial Fibrillation

Clinical Findings
(See Appendix, Figures 35–12 & 35–13.)

In atrial fibrillation (AF), the atrial rate is disorganized and is 400–650 beats/min. AF is characterized by an irregularly irregular ventricular rate with the absence of discernible P waves.

AF is the most common sustained cardiac arrhythmia in adults; the incidence is about 10–20 times that of atrial flutter. It is estimated that AF affects more than 2 million persons in the United States; its prevalence increases with age, approaching 10% in those over age 80 years. AF can occur in the absence of underlying heart disease or may be associated with a number of conditions, including chronic hypertension, valvular disease, cardiomyopathy, myocardial ischemia, myocarditis, pericarditis, or congenital heart disease. AF may also occur in the presence of other systemic disorders, including hyperthyroidism, pulmonary embolism, hypoxia, and excess consumption of alcohol or caffeine.

Patients with nonvalvular AF have approximately a 5% annual incidence of stroke as a result of a thromboembolic event. This risk increases 4-fold in patients with mitral stenosis and increases dramatically in older patients, approaching 30% in patients aged 80–89 years.

Treatment

Acute management of AF includes ventricular rate control and prevention of thromboembolic complications. Additional management considerations include restoration and maintenance of sinus rhythm.

A. Unstable Patients

Patients in AF with a rapid ventricular response who are hemodynamically unstable require immediate synchronized DC cardioversion. Recommendations are to start with 100 J and then to increase the dose by 50 J as needed until sinus rhythm is restored.

B. Stable Patients

In stable patients with a rapid ventricular response, the initial goal is rate control. This can usually be achieved with β-blockers, calcium-channel blockers, or digoxin. β-Blockers may prove most helpful in patients with hyperthyroidism but are relatively contraindicated in patients with CHF. Diltiazem and verapamil can often slow the ventricular rate and have the added benefit of antianginal effects and blood pressure control in hypertensive patients. In more than 90% of patients, a reduction in heart rate of at least 20% is noted. Diltiazem appears to be safe for use in patients with mild CHF. Digoxin can also help control the ventricular rate in patients with AF and may be useful in patients with left ventricular dysfunction. Its slower onset of action as compared to other agents makes it less useful for acute rate control. In patients with mild to moderate CHF, the administration of amiodarone may prove useful. Intravenous amiodarone can also be considered an alternative agent for rate control when the above agents fail. The specific medication choice will often be dictated by the urgency of the situation, the medication profile, physician preference, and the patient's underlying condition.

1. Anticoagulants—Prophylactic anticoagulation with warfarin has been shown to significantly reduce the incidence of stroke in patients with AF. If new-onset AF is of undetermined duration or greater than 48 hours' duration, initiation of anticoagulation is necessary. Current recommendations include anticoagulation for 3 weeks, followed by elective cardioversion and then continued outpatient anticoagulation for 4 more weeks. An alternative strategy is initial anticoagulation with unfractionated or low-molecular-weight heparin followed by transesophageal echocardiography to evaluate the left atrial appendage for the presence of clot. If no clot is identified, the patient may safely undergo cardioversion, followed by anticoagulation for 4 weeks. If a left atrial appendage clot is identified by transesophageal echocardiography, recommendations include anticoagulation for 3 weeks, followed by cardioversion and then continued anticoagulation for 4 additional weeks. In patients with AF of less than 48 hours' duration, anticoagulation is not recommended.

2. Antiarrhythmics—Various antiarrhythmic agents including amiodarone, procainamide, quinidine (class Ia), sotolol (class III), and ibutilide (class III) are used to chemically convert AF. Pharmacologic or electrical cardioversion may be considered in selected stable emergency department patients with AF of less than 48 hours' duration. Postponing cardioversion could lead to an increased resistance to attempts at conversion.

Disposition

Patients with chronic rate-controlled AF do not require hospital admission. In patients with new-onset AF, hospitalization is often required for ventricular rate control, initiation of anticoagulation, and sometimes for initiation of antiarrhythmic therapy. If a patient presents with thromboembolic complications, hospital admission will also be necessary.

4. Atrial Flutter

Clinical Findings
(See Appendix, Figure 35–14.)

In atrial flutter, the atrial rate is usually 250–350 beats/min. At times, the characteristic sawtooth flutter waves may be seen on ECG, particularly in lead II. Typically, atrial flutter will present with 2:1 atrioventricular (AV) conduction. For this reason, it is important to consider atrial flutter in the differential diagnosis of a regular tachycardia at approximately 150 beats/min even in the absence of flutter waves. Atrial flutter occurs less commonly than AF but is more often associated with underlying heart disease.

If atrial flutter is suspected in a patient with a nondiagnostic ECG, several options are available to better identify atrial activity. Vagal maneuvers or administration of an AV nodal blocking agent may briefly slow conduction through the AV node and unmask the flutter waves. At times, obtaining Lewis leads may also aid in uncovering P waves. To perform Lewis leads, the left and right arm electrodes are moved from the upper extremities to different positions on the anterior chest wall as lead I is monitored for evidence of P waves.

Treatment

Acute management of atrial flutter includes ventricular rate control and prevention of thromboembolic complications. Additional management considerations include restoration and maintenance of sinus rhythm.

A. Unstable Patients

Patients in atrial flutter with a rapid ventricular response who are hemodynamically unstable require immediate synchronized DC cardioversion. Recommendations are to start with 50 J and then increase the initial dose by 50 J as needed until sinus rhythm is restored.

B. Stable Patients

In stable patients with a rapid ventricular response, the initial goal is rate control. Adequate heart rate control can be achieved with the administration of either β-blockers or calcium-channel blockers. Digoxin is often less effective acutely because of its slow onset of action. Amiodarone or diltiazem are alternatives for rate control in the stable patient with impaired cardiac function or CHF.

The stroke risk for patients in atrial flutter appears to be similar to that of AF. Although controversial, some authors suggest using the same anticoagulation guidelines for atrial flutter as in AF.

Disposition

Patients with chronic rate-controlled atrial flutter do not require hospital admission. In patients with new-onset atrial flutter, hospitalization is often required for ventricular rate control, initiation of anticoagulation, and sometimes for initiation of antiarrhythmic therapy.

5. Multifocal Atrial Tachycardia

Clinical Findings
(See Appendix, Figure 35–15.)

In multifocal atrial tachycardia (MAT) the heart rate is typically 100–130 beats/min. The characteristic ECG finding is at least 3 different P wave morphologies. The rhythm often appears irregular and can at times be confused with AF. Varying PR intervals may also be noted. When the rate is slower than 100 beats/min, the term wandering atrial pacemaker is applied. Unless underlying aberrant conduction is present, the QRS complexes are narrow. Severe underlying chronic obstructive pulmonary disease accounts for approximately 60–85% of cases. Other causes include CHF, hypokalemia, hypomagnesemia, pulmonary hypertension, hypoxia, hypercapnia, and methylxanthine toxicity.

Treatment

The initial treatment of MAT is directed at correcting the underlying cause. As with AF, the initial goal of therapy is to achieve heart rate control. Because MAT does not respond to electrical cardioversion, pharmacologic intervention may be required.

Metoprolol can be a first-line agent for symptomatic patients who do not have contraindications to β-blockers. Metoprolol is a β$_1$-selective β-adrenergic blocking agent that slows conduction through the AV node. It is administered as a 5-to 10-mg intravenous bolus over 3 minutes. If necessary, the dose can be repeated in 10–15 minutes. Esmolol may be a reasonable alternative because of its short half-life.

Magnesium may be effective in converting MAT and can be administered as a 2-g intravenous bolus over 1 minute. This is followed by a 2 g/h infusion for 5 hours. Magnesium can still be effective if serum magnesium levels are in the normal range. Potassium repletion may be helpful in patients who are hypokalemic.

Amiodarone, digoxin, or diltiazem may be considered as alternative agents for rate control, especially when the patient exhibits findings of CHF.

Disposition

Patients with a new diagnosis of MAT do not necessarily require hospital admission. Patients may require hospitalization for MAT if the heart rate is difficult to control or for further management of the underlying condition.

6. Preexcitation Arrhythmias

Clinical Findings
(See Appendix, Figures 35–11 & 35–13.)

Preexcitation refers to ventricular preexcitation that occurs as a result of impulse conduction through an accessory AV pathway. The Wolf-Parkinson-White (WPW) syndrome is the most common form of ventricular preexcitation. On the ECG, a short PR interval (less than 120 ms) and the presence of a δ wave (initial upward slurring of the QRS complex) signify ventricular preexcitation. The Lown-Ganong-Levine syndrome is also considered in the class of preexcitation arrhythmias. This syndrome is characterized by a short PR interval, normal QRS morphology, and associated episodes of PSVT.

A variety of arrhythmias may occur in patients with WPW syndrome; the most common is orthodromic AVRT. In this case, the cardiac impulse travels down the AV node (antegrade conduction) and stimulates the ventricles through the normal conduction pathways. The accessory AV bypass tract serves as the retrograde limb of the circuit. In the absence of aberrant ventricular conduction or a fixed bundle branch block, the morphology of the QRS complex is narrow without evidence of ventricular preexcitation (absent δ wave).

Rarely, antidromic AVRT occurs whereby the accessory AV pathway acts as the antegrade limb of the circuit and the AV node as the retrograde limb. Antidromic AVRT will produce a wide QRS complex tachycardia and may masquerade as ventricular tachycardia (VT). The tachycardia may be extremely rapid, leading to ventricular fibrillation (VF) as a result of an R-on-T phenomenon.

AF is the second most common arrhythmia associated with WPW syndrome. AF with ventricular preexcitation has a high potential to precipitate hemodynamic compromise. AF with a rapid ventricular rate is characterized by an irregular tachycardia and a wide QRS complex resulting from ventricular preexcitation.

Treatment

Patients with orthodromic AVRT who are hemodynamically unstable require immediate synchronized DC cardioversion. Recommendations are to start with 50 J and then to increase the initial dose by 50 J as needed until sinus rhythm is restored. In patients with known WPW syndrome presenting with a narrow complex regular tachycardia, orthodromic AVRT can be assumed. In stable patients, the medical treatment will be the same as in AVNRT. Pharmacologic treatment with adenosine, β-adrenergic blocking agents, or calcium-channel blockers can be administered as deemed necessary and appropriate for the individual case. In general, the treatment of orthodromic AVRT with AV nodal blocking agents is safe. The risk of enhancing antegrade conduction down the bypass tract is very low.

Treatment of AF with ventricular preexcitation is different from that of orthodromic AVRT. If the patient is hemodynamically unstable, immediate synchronized DC cardioversion starting at 100 J is warranted. The use of AV nodal blocking agents, specifically β-blockers, calcium-channel blockers, and digoxin is contraindicated. If conduction through the AV node is slowed, conduction down the accessory pathway may be enhanced, possibly degenerating to VF. Because procainamide will slow conduction through both the AV node and the accessory pathway, it is the medication of choice when AF with a rapid ventricular response is associated with ventricular preexcitation. Procainamide is also the medication of choice in antidromic AVRT. Amiodarone can be used as an alternative agent in treating AF with ventricular preexcitation and findings of CHF.

Disposition

Hospitalization is not required for patients who are asymptomatic with evidence of ventricular preexcitation on the ECG (sinus rhythm, short PR, and a δ wave). Hospitalize all patients who have serious signs and symptoms or those requiring cardioversion. In addition, hospitalization is recommended for patients with AF and ventricular preexcitation or antidromic AVRT. Patients who present with stable orthodromic AVRT may be discharged with close outpatient follow-up after pharmacologic conversion in the emergency department.

Applegate TE: Atrial arrhythmias. Prim Care 2000;27:677. [PMID: 10918675] (Evaluation and management of atrial arrhythmias.)

Atkins DL et al: Treatment of tachyarrhythmias. Ann Emerg Med 2001;37:S91. [PMID: 11290974] (Overview and guidelines for the treatment of tachyarrhythmias.)

Chauhan VS et al: Supraventricular tachycardia. Med Clin North Am 2001;85:193. [PMID: 11233949] (Classification, mechanism, clinical presentation, and therapy of supraventricular tachycardia.)

Li H et al: Evaluation and management of atrial fibrillation in the emergency department. Emerg Med Clin North Am 1998;16:389. [PMID: 9621849]

Pelosi F et al: Evaluation and management of atrial fibrillation. Med Clin North Am 2001;85:225. [PMID: 11233947]

Trohman RG: Supraventricular tachycardia: implications for the intensivist. Crit Care Med 2000;28:129. [PMID: 11055681] (Diagnosis and management of supraventricular tachycardia.)

Xie B et al: Clinical difference of narrow complex QRS tachycardias. Emerg Med Clin North Am 1998;16:295. [PMID: 9621846] (Diagnostic approach to narrow complex QRS tachycardias.)

VENTRICULAR ARRHYTHMIAS

1. Ventricular Tachycardia

Clinical Findings
(See Appendix, Figures 35–16 & 35–17.)

VT is the most common cause of wide QRS complex tachycardia. The term VT is used when 6 or more consecutive ventricular beats occur. The ventricular rate is usually 180–250 beats/min, although rates slower than 160 beats/min may occur. Nonsustained VT is characterized by an episode lasting less than 30 seconds. Sustained VT is characterized by an episode lasting longer than 30 seconds, associated with hemodynamic compromise, or requiring therapeutic intervention for termination. Wide complex tachycardia (WCT) refers to a regular tachycardia with a QRS complex greater than 0.12 seconds (120 ms) in duration. WCT most often occurs as a result of either VT or SVT with aberrant conduction (underlying or rate-dependent bundle branch block). Very rarely, WCT will occur as a result of antidromic AVRT.

In approximately 85% of patients presenting in the emergency department with WCT, the underlying arrhythmia is VT. The presence of structural heart disease, coronary artery disease, prior myocardial infarction, or CHF strongly suggests VT. Certain ECG findings favor VT over SVT with aberrant conduction. These findings include a QRS complex wider than 160 ms, the presence of fusion beats, and evidence of AV dissociation. AV dissociation occurs in about 50% of patients with VT and confirms the diagnosis. An algorithm has been developed to assist clinicians in distinguishing VT from SVT with aberrant conduction (Figure 35–1). Proper application of this diagnostic tool may help decrease misclassification of WCT. A common clinical error that must be avoided is to assume that WCT is SVT with aberrant conduction. All cases of WCT of unknown origin should be managed as VT.

Treatment

A. UNSTABLE PATIENTS

Patients with VT or WCT of unknown origin who are hemodynamically unstable with serious signs and symptoms require immediate synchronized DC cardioversion. Recommendations are to start with 50–100 J and then increase the initial dose by 50 J as needed until sinus rhythm is restored. Some authors advocate

for cardioversion as an alternative to medical management in the patient with stable VT.

B. STABLE PATIENTS

Traditionally, patients with stable VT are administered an antiarrhythmic agent for chemical cardioversion. A number of medications are available. The choice for a particular patient is often based on physician preference and experience, findings of preserved or impaired cardiac function, and the underlying cause of the VT.

1. Lidocaine—Lidocaine is a class Ib antiarrhythmic with sodium-channel blocking properties. Because it can be administered rapidly with few side effects, some authors consider it the agent of choice for ventricular arrhythmias associated with acute myocardial ischemia or infarction. The recommended intravenous loading dose is 1.0–1.5 mg/kg. If required, a second bolus dose of 0.75–1.5 mg/kg can be administered in 5–10 minutes. If ventricular ectopy persists, an additional bolus dose of 0.5–0.75 mg/kg can be administered every 5–10 minutes to a maximum dose of 3 mg/kg. After rhythm suppression, start a maintenance infusion at

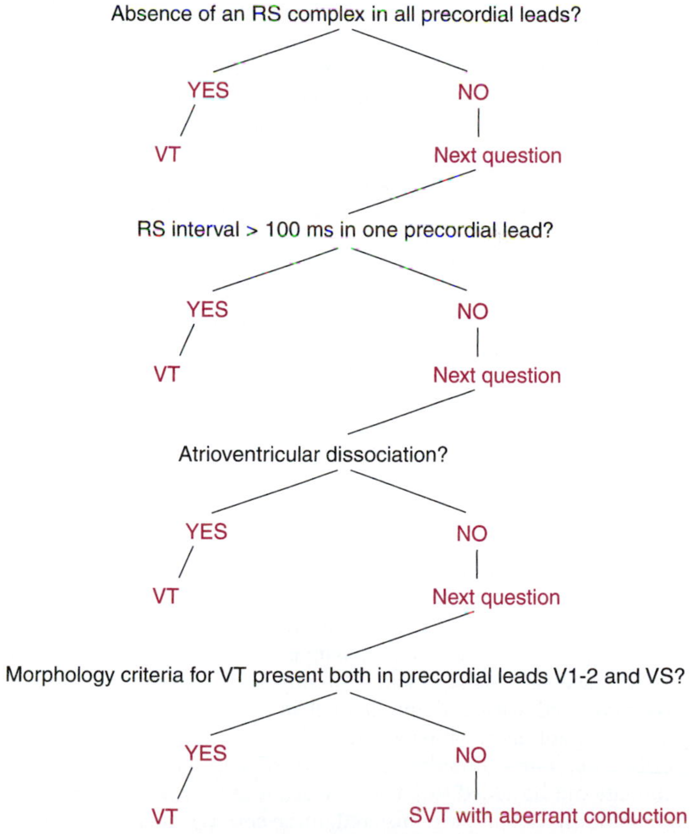

Figure 35–1. Algorithm for the diagnosis of tachycardia with a wide QRS complex. (Reproduced, with permission, from Brugada P et al: A new approach to the differential diagnosis of a regular tachycardia with a wide QRS complex. Circulation 1991;83:1649–1659. [PMID: 2022022])

2–4 mg/min. Lidocaine has the lowest incidence of toxicity of all currently used antiarrhythmic medications.

2. Other drugs—Procainamide is an alternative agent to lidocaine for the treatment of stable monomorphic VT. Bretylium is a class III antiarrhythmic that recently has become unavailable for use in the United States. Amiodarone may be preferable to other antiarrhythmic agents for ventricular tachycardia in patients with CHF. In comparison to other antiarrhythmic agents, amiodarone has greater efficacy and a lower incidence of proarrhythmic side effects. Dosing guidelines for amiodarone and procainamide are discussed in the section on PSVT.

Disposition

Hospitalization is recommended for all patients who present with VT.

2. Proarrhythmic Ventricular Arrhythmias

Clinical Findings

Proarrhythmia refers to the exacerbation of an existing arrhythmia or the development of a new arrhythmia during antiarrhythmic therapy. Most proarrhythmic episodes occur shortly after the initiation of antiarrhythmic therapy and can range from ventricular ectopy to intractable VT or VF.

Numerous medications have been implicated in causing ventricular arrhythmias. Digoxin toxicity has been associated with VT and carries a 60–65% mortality rate. Type I antiarrhythmic agents with sodium-channel blocking activity are associated with a 5–10% incidence of proarrhythmia. In addition, other medications that have sodium-channel blocking properties may be proarrhythmic in toxic doses. These medications include diphenhydramine, phenothiazines, propoxyphene, tricyclic antidepressants, and cocaine.

Treatment

Early recognition and discontinuation of the offending agent is an important aspect of care. As with other tachyarrhythmias, synchronized DC cardioversion is indicated for patients who are hemodynamically unstable.

Pharmacologic management of ventricular arrhythmias associated with sodium-channel blocking agents (ie, tricyclic antidepressants) is undertaken with sodium bicarbonate. Three ampules (150 mEq) of sodium bicarbonate can be added to 1 L of 5% dextrose in water. The solution can be administered intravenously at a rate of 2 mL/kg/h and titrated to a serum pH of 7.5–7.55. If VT occurs secondary to digoxin toxicity, the use of digoxin Fab fragments (Digibind) is indicated. Additional therapy may be warranted in specific clinical circumstances.

Disposition

Although uncommonly encountered in the emergency department, patients with proarrhythmic ventricular arrhythmias should be hospitalized for cardiac monitoring.

3. Polymorphic Ventricular Tachycardia (Including Torsades de Pointes)

Clinical Findings (See Appendix, Figure 35–18.)

Polymorphic ventricular tachycardia (PMVT) is a form of VT with varying QRS complex morphology. The rhythm is often irregular and hemodynamically unstable, and it can degenerate to VF.

Torsades de pointes is a form of PMVT associated with a prolonged QT interval on the baseline ECG. The rhythm is often described as having a twisting-on-point appearance and can be either paroxysmal or sustained. The heart rate is usually 200–250 beats/min. Long QT syndromes associated with torsades de pointes include Lange-Nielsen syndrome and Romano-Ward syndrome. Torsades de pointes may also occur as a result of numerous medication interactions. A complete list of medications that have been reported to prolong the QT interval is available at www.qtdrugs.org.

PMVT can also occur in the absence of a prolonged QT interval. In this case, cardiac ischemia or underlying structural heart disease is often the cause.

Treatment & Disposition

Patients with PMVT who are hemodynamically unstable with serious signs and symptoms require immediate defibrillation. Recommendations are to start with 200 J. To prevent recurrence, discontinue all agents that can prolong the QT interval.

Magnesium is the medication of choice for the management of torsades de pointes associated with congenital and acquired forms of long QT syndrome. It may be effective even when serum levels are normal. A 2-g intravenous dose can be administered as a slow push over 5 minutes. Follow the bolus dose by a maintenance infusion of 1–2 g/h. Consider supplemental potassium as an adjunctive therapy to maintain serum potassium levels in the high normal range. Temporary transvenous pacing at rates around 100 beats/min may be useful to prevent recurrences, especially in patients with bradycardia or pauses.

Hospitalization is recommended for all patients who present with PMVT.

4. Ventricular Fibrillation
Clinical Findings
(See Appendix, Figure 35–19.)

VF is characterized by an irregular ventricular rhythm with no discernible distinction between the QRS complex, ST segment, and T waves. VF is a common cause of sudden cardiac death and remains a significant contributor to mortality in the first 24 hours after an acute myocardial infarction. In the absence of early bystander cardiopulmonary resuscitation and initiation of advanced cardiac life support, including defibrillation, survival rates are poor.

Treatment & Disposition

Upon recognition of VF or pulseless VT, the immediate treatment is asynchronous defibrillation with 200 J. If required, administer a second shock with 200–300 J and a third at 360 J. Secure the patient's airway with endotracheal intubation. Pharmacologic therapy advocated in the 2000 American Heart Association guidelines includes vasopressin or epinephrine for persistent VF or pulseless VT after 3 stacked defibrillations. The antiarrhythmics, amiodarone or lidocaine, are used if the arrhythmia persists after 3 additional stacked defibrillations. All patients who have been successfully resuscitated from VF or pulseless VT should be started on a drip of the last antiarrhythmic administered and admitted to the intensive care unit for close observation. If an acute coronary syndrome is suspected as the cause of the arrest, the patient may require cardiac catheterization for evaluation and treatment. Chapter 7 offers a more in-depth discussion of the management of cardiac arrest.

Brady WJ et al: Wide QRS complex tachycardia: ECG differential diagnosis. Am J Emerg Med 1999;17:376. [PMID: 10452438] (Case presentations and discussion of wide QRS complex tachycardias.)

Brugada P et al: A new approach to the differential diagnosis of a regular tachycardia with a wide QRS complex. Circulation 1991;83:1649. [PMID: 2022022] (An algorithmic approach to the diagnosis of ventricular tachycardia.)

Chaudhry GM: Antiarrhythmic agents and proarrhythmia. Crit Care Med 2000;28:158. [PMID: 11055686] (Classes of antiarrhythmic agents and their proarrhythmic side effects.)

Flinders DC et al: Ventricular arrhythmias. Prim Care 2000;27:709. [PMID: 10918676] (Pathophysiology and clinical presentation of ventricular arrhythmias.)

Gupta AK et al: Wide complex tachycardias. Med Clin North Am 2001;85:245. [PMID: 11233948] (Differential diagnosis and management of WCTs.)

Miller MB: Arrhythmias associated with drug toxicity. Emerg Med Clin North Am 1998;16:405. [PMID: 9621850] (Complications and arrhythmias associated with medication toxicity.)

Passman R et al: Polymorphic ventricular tachycardia, long Q-T syndrome, and torsades de pointes. Med Clin North Am 2001;85:321. [PMID: 11233951] (Diagnosis and management of various forms of PMVT.)

Shah CP et al: Clinical approach to wide QRS complex tachycardias. Emerg Med Clin North Am 1998;16:331. [PMID: 9621847] (Diagnostic approach to wide QRS complex tachycardias.)

■ BRADYARRHYTHMIAS, CONDUCTION DISTURBANCES, & ESCAPE RHYTHMS

As in tachycardia management, if a bradycardic patient is hemodynamically unstable, immediate intervention is required regardless of the origin of the underlying arrhythmia (eg, SA block, AV block, ventricular escape rhythm). Transcutaneous cardiac pacing is the initial intervention of choice for patients with serious signs and symptoms that occur as a result of a bradyarrhythmia. In stable patients, or in patients with mild symptoms (eg, dizziness, lightheadedness), pharmacologic treatment is often initiated with or without standby pacing. Medical management can be initiated in patients with symptomatic bradycardia as a bridge to cardiac pacing, or may be initiated if emergency cardiac pacing is unavailable.

Primary conduction system disturbances account for 15% of bradyarrhythmias encountered in the emergency department setting. The remaining 85% occur as a result of various secondary causes such as acute coronary ischemia (40%), medications or toxicologic causes (20%), metabolic causes (5%), neurologic causes (5%), permanent pacemaker failure (2%), and other miscellaneous causes (13%). Symptomatic bradycardia resulting from AV conduction disturbances or sick sinus syndrome is more common in the elderly; the majority of patients present at age 65 years or older.

SINUS BRADYCARDIA
Clinical Findings
(See Appendix, Figure 35–4.)

Sinus bradycardia occurs when the sinus rate is slower than 60 beats/min. Usually the rate is 45–59 beats/min, but on rare occasion it may be as slow as 35 beats/min.

Sinus bradycardia is commonly associated with sinus arrhythmia and is often a normal finding in young, healthy, athletic individuals. Sinus bradycardia is often benign and does not necessarily indicate sinus node dysfunction. Although commonly physiologic, sinus bradycardia may be pathologic when patients experience symptoms of cerebral hypoperfusion or when the heart rate does not increase appropriately with activity or exercise. Certain underlying conditions have been associated with a slowing of the heart rate, including hypothermia, hypothyroidism, and increased intracranial pressure. In addition, a number of different medications, including β-blockers, calcium-channel blockers, clonidine, digoxin, and lithium, can cause bradycardia.

Treatment & Disposition

Usually no treatment is required for asymptomatic sinus bradycardia. When serious signs and symptoms are present, medical management, pacemaker placement, and hospital admission are indicated.

SINUS ARREST

Sinus arrest is defined as a failure of sinus node impulse formation. On the ECG, random periods of absent cardiac activity may be noted. Unless escape beats occur, lengthy pauses are noted. When pauses occur, patients may complain of dizziness or lightheadedness or may have syncope. If untreated, pauses longer than 2.5 seconds may progress to asystole.

SINOATRIAL BLOCK

SA block differs from sinus arrest in that SA block is a form of exit block rather than failure of impulse formation. Like sinus arrest, SA block may occur as a result of a number of conditions, including acute myocardial infarction, myocarditis, fibrosis of the SA node, excessive vagal tone, and digoxin toxicity. Analogous to AV block, SA block can be classified into first-, second-, and third-degree heart block.

1. First-Degree Sinoatrial Block

First-degree SA block does not produce any ECG changes. The diagnosis can be made only through electrophysiologic testing.

2. Second-Degree Sinoatrial Block (Mobitz Type I) (See Appendix, Figure 35–24.)

Second-degree Mobitz type I SA block, also known as SA Wenckebach, is characterized by PP intervals that gradually shorten while the PR interval remains constant. This cycle terminates with a blocked P wave. The length of the pause is shorter than twice the preceding PP cycle.

3. Second-Degree Sinoatrial Block (Mobitz Type II)

Second-degree Mobitz type II SA block is characterized by fixed pauses. On the ECG, the PP interval remains constant and is then followed by a blocked P wave. The PP interval, including the blocked P wave, will be twice the length of the normal PP interval.

4. Third-Degree Sinoatrial Block

Third-degree SA block may be difficult to distinguish from sinus arrest. Patients with either conduction disturbance present with variable pauses on the ECG until an escape rhythm occurs or sinus rhythm is restored.

5. Sick Sinus Syndrome

Clinical Findings

Sick sinus syndrome is a manifestation of sinus node dysfunction. Patients with the syndrome may present with a wide range of bradyarrhythmias. Numerous arrhythmias are associated with sick sinus syndrome, including marked sinus bradycardia, sinus pause, sinus arrest, and SA block. On occasion, patients may also present with ventricular or atrial tachyarrhythmias.

Treatment & Disposition

Treatment may be indicated when pauses of more than 2–3 seconds occur or if the patient is symptomatic. Administration of atropine or initiation of temporary cardiac pacing may be required. Symptomatic patients will require hospital admission, often for permanent pacemaker placement.

ATRIOVENTRICULAR BLOCK

AV block refers to a group of conduction disturbances within the AV junctional tissue. In general, AV block is characterized by prolonged conduction time or a failure to conduct impulses through the AV node. The conduction disturbance can be partial (first- or second-degree AV block) or complete (third-degree AV block). In general, the hemodynamic effects will depend on the ventricular rate and the presence of underlying heart disease. AV conduction blocks are traditionally classified as first-, second-, or third-degree heart block.

1. First-Degree Atrioventricular Block
(See Appendix, Figure 35–25.)

First-degree AV block is the most common conduction disturbance and is characterized by a PR interval that is prolonged greater than 0.2 seconds. In general, the PR interval is constant, and each atrial impulse is conducted to the ventricles. First-degree AV block can be a normal variant in young or athletic individuals due to excessive vagal tone. First-degree AV block is also common in elderly patients without underlying heart disease. It may occur in patients with myocarditis, mild digoxin toxicity, and inferior wall myocardial infarction secondary to AV nodal ischemia.

2. Second-Degree Atrioventricular Block
(Mobitz Type I)
(See Appendix, Figure 35–26.)

Second-degree Mobitz type I AV block is also known as Wenckebach AV block. This type of block is characterized by a progressive lengthening of the PR interval followed by a nonconducted P wave leading to a dropped QRS complex. Classically, the PP interval remains constant except when sinus arrhythmia is present. The RR interval will have a characteristic cycle throughout the conduction disturbance. The RR interval that includes the blocked P wave is the longest in duration. This is then followed by RR intervals that subsequently become shorter until the next P wave is blocked.

On a rhythm strip, grouped beating is often evident and can further help distinguish second-degree from third-degree AV block. The blocked P waves may occur frequently or periodically, and may or may not occur with regularity. Because Mobitz type I AV block is at the level of the AV node, the QRS complex is normal in configuration unless aberrant ventricular conduction or an underlying bundle branch block exists. In general, Mobitz type I AV block does not usually produce hemodynamically significant symptoms. It can be seen in patients with acute myocardial infarction (usually inferior wall) and does not commonly progress to complete heart block (CHB). If CHB does occur, the escape rhythm pacemaker is usually located in the AV junctional tissue and is often fast enough to maintain an adequate cardiac output.

3. Second-Degree Atrioventricular Block
(Mobitz Type II)
(See Appendix, Figure 35–28.)

Second-degree Mobitz type II AV block is characterized by a constant PR interval, either normal or prolonged, that is followed by a nonconducted P wave. In Mobitz type II AV block, the QRS complex is usually wide. This occurs because Mobitz type II AV block represents an infranodal block. At times, every other P wave is blocked. This is described as 2:1 AV conduction. When this occurs, one cannot distinguish between Mobitz type I or type II AV block (see Appendix, Figure 35–27). Mobitz type II AV block is common in patients with acute myocardial infarction (usually anterior wall) and can suddenly progress to CHB resulting in syncope.

4. Third-Degree Atrioventricular Block
(Complete Heart Block)

Clinical Findings
(See Appendix, Figures 35–29 to 35–31.)

Third-degree AV block, or CHB, is characterized by independent atrial and ventricular activity. As a result of complete AV block, no atrial impulses are conducted through the AV node. The ventricular rate is determined by the intrinsic escape rhythm, AV junctional escape (usually 45–60 beats/min), or an idioventricular escape rhythm (usually 30–40 beats/min). The atrial rate may be sinus in origin or may be from an ectopic atrial focus. In CHB the atrial rate is typically faster than the ventricular rate. As noted with second-degree AV block, the hemodynamic consequences depend on the ventricular rate and the presence of underlying heart disease. Syncope or CHF commonly accompany acute acquired CHB. Complete AV block is most commonly caused by coronary artery disease or by degeneration of the cardiac conduction system.

Treatment & Disposition

A. UNSTABLE PATIENTS

Emergency cardiac pacing is indicated for patients with hemodynamically unstable bradycardia, especially for patients who have failed medical therapy, patients with malignant escape rhythms, and patients in bradyasystolic arrest. Transcutaneous cardiac pacing is the initial intervention because of its ease of application, compared to temporary transvenous pacing. In unstable patients, medical management can be initiated, although at times its utility is only temporary.

B. STABLE PATIENTS

1. Atropine—Atropine is an anticholinergic medication with parasympatholytic properties leading to enhanced SA node automaticity and AV node conduction. The initial intravenous dose of atropine is 0.5–1.0 mg, which can be repeated every 5 minutes to a total dose of 0.04 mg/kg (3 mg for the average adult). The maximal dose produces complete vagal blockade. Atropine is recommended for, but not limited to, patients with symptomatic bradycardia or relative bradycardia, bradycardia with malignant escape rhythms, and asystole.

Rarely, a paradoxic reduction in heart rate has been observed in patients with advanced AV block after administration of atropine. Therefore, use atropine with caution in patients with infranodal AV block (Mobitz type II, and CHB with wide QRS complexes). Other rarely encountered side effects of atropine administration include worsening of cardiac ischemia in patients with an acute myocardial infarction, or the development of a ventricular tachyarrhythmia. These adverse effects are uncommon, but knowledge of such responses may assist with proper patient selection. Atropine is not effective in the management of the heart transplant patient with symptomatic bradycardia because of surgical denervation of the vagus nerve.

2. Isoproterenol—Isoproterenol is a nonspecific β-adrenergic agonist that causes an increase in heart rate and cardiac contractility. The combined effects lead to increases in cardiac output and systolic blood pressure and decreases in systemic and pulmonary vascular resistance and diastolic blood pressure. As a result, no significant change in mean arterial pressure occurs. Myocardial oxygen demand is increased as a result of the increased heart rate and contractility. In addition, isoproterenol causes smooth muscle relaxation and bronchodilation. Isoproterenol may be used to treat symptomatic bradycardia in heart transplant patients. The initial intravenous dose of isoproterenol is 1 μg/min, titrated slowly until the desired hemodynamic effects are achieved. The maximum infusion rate is 4 μg/min.

3. Dopamine—Dopamine is an endogenous catecholamine with dose-related effects. At doses of 3.0–7.5 μg/kg/min, it has β-agonist properties resulting in increased heart rate and cardiac output. The β-agonist effects are less pronounced than those of isoproterenol. Dopamine is the preferred catecholamine for symptomatic bradycardia refractory to atropine.

4. Aminophylline—Aminophylline, a methylxanthine derivative, is a competitive antagonist of adenosine. Conduction disturbances during an acute myocardial infarction may be partially mediated by the endogenous release of adenosine. Aminophylline can be administered intravenously at a dose of 5–6 mg/kg infused over 5 minutes. A maintenance infusion may be required and can be initiated at 0.5 mg/kg/h.

5. Glucagon—Glucagon stimulates cyclic adenosine monophosphate production. It may be beneficial in the treatment of bradycardia associated with β-blocker or calcium-channel blocker toxicity. An initial intravenous dose of 0.05–0.15 mg/kg is recommended, although optimal doses have not been determined.

Disposition

Hospitalize all patients who have symptomatic bradycardia. Discontinue medications with AV nodal blocking properties. Although some patients with advanced AV conduction blocks will be asymptomatic, it is recommended that all patients with newly diagnosed second-degree Mobitz type II AV block and CHB be hospitalized.

Often patients with Wenckebach AV block will be asymptomatic. Treatment is usually not necessary unless symptoms occur. In general, no treatment is necessary for patients with first-degree AV block. At times, hospitalization will be necessary to treat the underlying condition such as myocardial ischemia or digoxin toxicity.

■ IDIOVENTRICULAR RHYTHM

Clinical Findings
(See Appendix, Figure 35–22.)

Idioventricular rhythm refers to the occurrence of 6 or more consecutive ventricular escape beats. The rate of an idioventricular escape rhythm is usually 30–40 beats/min. The duration of the QRS complex often exceeds 0.16 seconds. The morphology of the QRS complex is similar to that in premature ventricular contractions (PVCs) but varies depending on the location of the ectopic ventricular focus. Escape rhythms often develop in response to severe bradycardia or an advanced AV block. If the rate is 50–100 beats/min, the rhythm is called accelerated idioventricular rhythm (AIVR). AIVR can also be seen after administration of thrombolytic therapy for acute myocardial infarction and may serve as a marker of reperfusion.

Treatment & Disposition

Treatment may be indicated if the ventricular escape rhythm is unable to maintain adequate cerebral perfusion or if the patient is unstable. If ventricular escape beats occur in response to advanced AV block, it could be dangerous to abolish the escape rhythm. In this case, the escape rhythm may be helping to maintain adequate perfusion. Management is directed at treating the underlying AV block. If AIVR occurs secondary to reperfusion, no treatment is generally needed. Because an idioventricular escape rhythm often occurs as a result of advanced AV block, the majority of patients will require hospitalization.

■ ATRIOVENTRICULAR JUNCTIONAL RHYTHM

Clinical Findings
(See Appendix, Figure 35–23.)

AV junctional escape rhythm refers to the occurrence of 6 or more consecutive junctional escape beats. The ventricular rate is usually 45–60 beats/min. AV junctional rhythm, like AV junctional premature beats, may originate from any location in the AV junctional tissue. Because the origin of the rhythm is the AV junctional tissue, the QRS complex is narrow unless the patient has a preexisting bundle branch block. If the junctional escape rhythm is faster than 60 beats/minute, the term AV junctional tachycardia is applied. If this rhythm is present, digoxin toxicity should be ruled out.

Treatment & Disposition

Patients with sinus bradycardia and occasional or intermittent AV junctional escape beats do not generally require intervention. Treatment including hospitalization will depend on the underlying cause of the cardiac arrhythmia.

Brady WJ: Diagnosis and management of bradycardia and atrioventricular block associated with acute cardiac ischemia. Emerg Med Clin North Am 2001;19:371. [PMID: 1137398] (Diagnosis and management of bradycardia and conduction disturbances.)

Brady WJ et al: Evaluation and management of bradyarrhythmias in the emergency department. Emerg Med Clin North Am 1998;16:361. [PMID: 9621848]

Kaushik V et al: Bradyarrhythmias, temporary and permanent pacing. Crit Care Med 2000;28:121. [PMID: 11055680] (Diagnosis of bradyarrhythmias and indications for cardiac pacing.)

■ PERMANENT CARDIAC PACEMAKERS
(See Appendix, Figures 35–32 to 35–37.)

It is estimated that more than 150,000 new patients have permanent cardiac pacemakers implanted in the United States annually. Emergency medicine physicians should be familiar with normal pacemaker function and be knowledgeable about common pacemaker malfunctions. It is estimated that permanent pacemakers have a 6% yearly incidence of malfunction. Although many of these malfunctions will be identified during routine evaluation, some malfunctions will occur unexpectedly, resulting in an emergency department visit.

Types of Pacemakers

Pacemakers are either single-chamber (atrium or ventricle) or dual-chamber (atrium and ventricle) devices. In single-chamber pacemakers, a single lead paces and senses in the same chamber, most often the right ventricle. In dual-chamber pacemakers, one pacing and sensing lead is in the right atrium, and the other is in the right ventricle. Some newer, more advanced devices have a third pacing lead placed in the coronary sinus enabling biventricular pacing.

Since 1990, almost all pacemaker leads are bipolar. Bipolar leads have 2 electrodes on the same pacing lead, a distal cathode, and a proximal anode located approximately 1 cm apart near the distal tip of the pacemaker lead. Bipolar leads produce a small electrical field between the 2 electrodes. This produces a small, sometimes barely noticeable pacing spike on the ECG. Older pacemaker leads were unipolar in design. The cathode was located at the distal end of the lead, and the pulse generator served as the anode. Unipolar leads produce a larger electrical field and give rise to larger pacemaker spikes on the ECG. Unipolar leads are more likely to sense noncardiac electrical events such as pectoralis muscle activity. This can result in inappropriate inhibition of pacemaker activity (myopotential inhibition). The introduction of bipolar leads has virtually eliminated this type of oversensing malfunction.

Pacemaker Codes & Settings

In April 2001, the North American Society of Pacing and Electrophysiology (NASPE) and the British Pacing and Electrophysiology Group (BPEG) revised and updated the generic pacemaker code (Table 35–1). The first position identifies which chambers are paced. The second position identifies the chambers in which the pacemaker senses cardiac depolarizations. The letter designation for the first and second positions is the same. The third position represents the pacemaker's response to a sensed cardiac event. In general, when a pacemaker senses spontaneous cardiac activity, it is either inhibited from firing or a pacemaker spike is triggered. The fourth position designates whether the pacemaker has the ability for rate-responsive (rate-modulation) functions. Pacemakers with this function can increase the pacemaker discharge rate during exercise or

Table 35–1. The 2001 revised NASPE/BPEG pacemaker code.[1]

Chamber(s) Paced	Chamber(s) Sensed	Response to Sensing	Rate Modulation	Multisite Pacing
O (None)	O	O	O	O
A (Atrium)	A	T (Triggered)	R (Rate modulation)	A
V (Ventricle)	V	I (Inhibited)		V
D (Dual A + V)	D	D (Dual T + I)		D

[1]Reproduced, with permission, from Bernstein AD et al: The revised NASPE/BPEG generic code for antibradycardia, adaptive-rate, and multisite pacing. Pacing Clin Electrophysiol 2002;25:260–264.

movement in an attempt to meet metabolic demands. The fifth position indicates the presence and location of multisite pacing (ie, biventricular pacing).

Although pacemakers may be programmed for many different modes, 4 common settings are likely to be encountered by the emergency physician: VVI, VVIR, DDD, and DDDR (Table 35–2). In patients with single-chamber pacemakers, VVI is the most commonly programmed pacing mode. In this mode, the pacemaker will pace and sense the right ventricle. If the pacemaker senses intrinsic ventricular activity, the pacemaker is inhibited from firing. If the intrinsic ventricular rate is slower than the programmed rate, ventricular pacing occurs at a fixed rate. A disadvantage of VVI pacing is its inability to increase the pacemaker rate when the patient is physically active. Patients with single-chamber ventricular pacemakers may develop pacemaker syndrome. This can occur as a result of the loss of AV synchrony, retrograde VA conduction, or an inability to increase the pacemaker rate with activity. Common symptoms include malaise, fatigue, shortness of breath, chest pain, dizziness, and near syncope. VVIR pacing provides for rate-responsive demand ventricular pacing.

Dual-chamber pacing can be used to counteract the effects of pacemaker syndrome by preventing the loss of AV synchrony. Dual-chamber pacemakers may function in a variety of modes depending on the underlying intrinsic rhythm. DDD pacing is the most common mode for dual-chamber pacemakers. This allows for dual-chamber pacing and sensing. The pacing stimulus can be inhibited or triggered depending on the intrinsic rhythm. Dual-chamber pacemakers will be programmed with both a lower rate limit and an upper rate limit. DDDR pacing provides for rate-responsive demand AV sequential pacing.

Table 35–2. Commonly used pacing codes.

Pacing Code	Chamber Paced	Chamber Sensed	Pacemaker Function
VVI	Ventricle	Ventricle	Demand ventricular pacing. If the intrinsic ventricular rate is faster than the programmed rate, the pacing stimuli is inhibited. If the intrinsic rate if slower than the programmed rate, asynchronous pacing occurs.
VVIR	Ventricle	Ventricle	Demand ventricular pacing with the added feature of rate responsiveness.
DDD	Atrium + ventricle	Atrium + ventricle	Dual-chamber atrioventricular pacing. Both atria and ventricle are paced and sensed.
DDDR	Atrium + ventricle	Atrium + ventricle	Dual-chamber atrioventricular pacing with the added feature of rate responsiveness.
VAT	Ventricle	Atrium	In this mode, the dual-chamber pacemaker senses the atrial activity, then proceeds to pace the ventricles at the same rate with an appropriate atrioventricular interval.
VOO	Ventricle	None	Asynchronous ventricular pacing. This is the mode that a single-chamber ventricular pacemaker reverts to when a magnet is applied.
DOO	Atrium + ventricle	None	Asynchronous atrioventricular pacing. This is the mode that a dual-chamber pacemaker reverts to when a magnet is applied.

COMPLICATIONS OF IMPLANTABLE CARDIAC PACEMAKERS

Venous Access

Although uncommon, the majority of venous access complications occur early after implantation. Venous access complications include bleeding, pneumothorax, hemothorax, and rarely air embolism. Venous thrombosis is another rare complication of pacemaker placement. Patients may present with unilateral upper extremity pain and swelling.

Pacemaker Pocket Site

Early pacemaker pocket site complications include bleeding with hematoma formation, wound dehiscence, or infection. Early pocket site infections are usually caused by *Staphylococcus aureus*. Late complications (greater than 30 days after implantation) can include pacemaker site erosion, keloid formation, pacemaker migration, and infection. Late infections are usually caused by *Staphylococcus epidermidis*. Approximately 6% of patients with permanent pacemakers develop pocket site infections.

Lead Complications

A number of complications can occur with endocardial pacemaker leads. Lead dislodgment is uncommon; rates are less than 2% for ventricular leads and less than 5% for atrial leads. If lead dislodgment is suspected, obtain posteroanterior and lateral chest radiographs and compare them with a prior chest x-ray. Lead fracture or insulation break may also occur. Lead fractures generally occur at three sites: (1) close to the pulse generator, (2) at the venous entry site, and (3) within the heart. Lead fractures may be diagnosed by chest x-ray or by pacemaker interrogation.

Cardiac perforation is another uncommon but potentially serious lead complication. Suspect perforation in the patient with a new paced right bundle branch block pattern on ECG, intercostal muscle or diaphragmatic contractions (hiccups), pericardial effusion, or tamponade. Cardiac perforation may also be identified by a plain chest radiograph demonstrating the tip of the pacemaker lead outside the cardiac silhouette. Echocardiography may be invaluable in diagnosing a pericardial effusion. Most cases (80%) of perforation occur within the first 4 days of pacemaker insertion. Another uncommon lead complication is Twiddler syndrome. This occurs when a patient wiggles or rotates the pacemaker generator, eventually dislodging the pacemaker leads.

PACEMAKER MALFUNCTION (See Appendix, Figure 35–37A and B)

General Considerations

The most common pacemaker malfunctions are sensing abnormalities. Sensing malfunctions are further subdivided into undersensing or oversensing. Undersensing occurs when the pacemaker fails to sense intrinsic electrical cardiac activity (P wave or QRS complex). On the ECG, a pacing spike is preceded by an intrinsic P wave or QRS complex. Oversensing is the inappropriate inhibition of a pacing stimulus. On the ECG, this is evident by a pause that is longer than the programmed pacemaker rate.

Other pacemaker malfunctions include failure to pace and failure to capture. Failure to pace is characterized by an absence of an appropriate pacing stimulus. Failure to capture occurs when a pacing stimulus fails to depolarize the myocardium. Physiologic failure to capture may occur if the pacing stimulus occurs during the ventricular refractory period (within 300 ms after a native depolarization). This is not a malfunction, but reprogramming may still be necessary.

Lead complications are common causes of pacemaker malfunction. An increase in the pacing threshold may also cause sensing malfunctions and failure to capture. This can occur as a result of fibrosis at the lead tip, hyperkalemia, hypoxemia, myocardial ischemia, and antiarrhythmic drug toxicity. Battery depletion or component failure may result in failure to pace or undersensing. Electromagnetic interference from electrocautery or magnetic resonance imaging (MRI) can lead to oversensing. Patients with implantable cardiac pacemakers should not undergo MRI. Variable effects have been documented, including pacemaker motion, function modification, heating of the pacemaker generator, and induction of voltage or current in the pacing leads.

Pacemaker mediated tachycardia (PMT) is an uncommon complication that can occur with dual-chamber pacemakers. PMT can be triggered by a PVC with ventricular-to-atrial (VA) conduction. Retrograde atrial activity triggers a ventricular paced beat. As the ventricular paced beat undergoes VA conduction, another ventricular paced beat is triggered and the cycle continues. PMT will be evident by sustained pacing at the upper limit of the programmed pacing rate (100–140 beats/min). The ECG will characteristically reveal a wide complex paced tachycardia. PMT is often not life threatening because the heart rate does not usually result in hemodynamic instability.

Runaway pacemaker is another rare cause of a wide QRS complex paced tachycardia. In this case, the malfunctioning pulse generator discharges at a rate above its preset upper limit.

Clinical Findings

Patients may present with a number of symptoms suggestive of pacemaker malfunction. These include dizziness, lightheadedness, near syncope, syncope, palpitations, shortness of breath, or chest pain. The symptoms most concerning are those associated with cerebral hypoperfusion. Patients may present after blunt chest trauma or external defibrillation leading to pacemaker malfunction. Bradycardia may be an indicator of malfunction because the lower limit of fixed rate pacing is typically 50–60 beats/min. This may occur as a result of oversensing or failure to pace. The upper limit of rate responsive pacemakers is generally 100–140 beats/min. A paced rhythm at this rate may or may not be pacemaker malfunction.

Evaluation of the patient suspected of having pacemaker malfunction includes a 12-lead ECG and rhythm strip. If available, a comparison ECG may be helpful. A chest radiograph should also be obtained. Serum electrolyte and antiarrhythmic levels may also be necessary.

A systematic approach to the evaluation of the 12-lead ECG and rhythm strip may help to identify pacemaker malfunction. The ECG should be evaluated to determine the presence or absence of appropriate pacing spikes. A normally functioning pacemaker should be inhibited from firing when the patient's intrinsic rate is faster than the programmed rate. Pacemaker function cannot be evaluated when the intrinsic rate is faster than the programmed rate. When properly inhibited, no pacing spikes are seen on the ECG.

Magnet application may provide information regarding battery depletion or malfunction. When applied correctly over the pacemaker generator, the magnet triggers a reed switch, which inactivates the sensing function. The pacemaker should revert to an asynchronous pacing mode at a rate (magnet rate) preset by the manufacturer (VOO or DOO mode). A magnet rate that is slower than the manufacturer's preset rate suggests battery depletion. If no pacemaker spikes occur after magnet application, lead fracture or another malfunction may be the cause. Because there is no industry standard, the response of a particular brand of pacemaker may be variable when a magnet is applied.

Treatment & Disposition

Treat venous access complications accordingly. Admit for parenteral antibiotics any patients suspected of having pocket site infections.

For patients presenting with pacemaker malfunction leading to symptomatic bradycardia, institute pharmacologic treatment or emergency pacing measures. If transcutaneous cardiac pacing is initiated, place the anterior pacing pad as far away from the pacemaker generator as possible. In the setting of symptomatic brady-cardia, a magnet can also be applied to revert to asynchronous pacing. If a patient requires synchronized DC cardioversion or defibrillation, place the paddles or pads as far from the pulse generator as possible.

In the emergency department, treatment of PMT may be undertaken by a number of different maneuvers. First, a magnet may be applied to terminate the tachycardia. If a magnet is unavailable or unsuccessful, chest wall stimulation using a transcutaneous pacemaker can be attempted. The required stimulus is usually 10–20 ma. This is less than the stimulus generally required for transcutaneous pacing. If unsuccessful, isometric exercises can be tried. Finally, chest thumps have had success in terminating PMT; no more than two are recommended. Each of the above techniques is designed to affect the sensing function of the pacemaker, inhibit ventricular pacing, and terminate PMT. If the above are unsuccessful, cardiology consultation for pacemaker interrogation and reprogramming will be necessary.

Runaway pacemaker is a rarely encountered problem. Pharmacologic intervention or magnet application can be attempted but will most likely be unsuccessful. Definitive treatment may require disconnecting the pacemaker leads or removal of the pulse generator.

Obtain cardiology consultation for patients suspected of having pacemaker malfunction. Unless the pacemaker can be interrogated in the emergency department, the majority of patients with suspected pacemaker malfunction will require hospitalization.

Bernstein AD et al: The revised NASPE/BPEG generic code for antibradycardia, adaptive-rate, and multisite pacing. Pacing Clin Electrophysiol 2002;25:260. [PMID: 11916002] (Position statement revising the pacemaker code.)

Cardiac pacemakers and EKG recordings. Online Journal of Cardiology; www.mmi.mcgill.ca/heart/ecgPindex.html

Glickson M et al: Cardiac pacing: a review. Med Clin North Am 2001;85:323. [PMID: 11233953]

Griffin J et al: Runaway pacemaker: a case report and review. J Emerg Med 2000;19:177. [PMID: 10903469]

Weinberger B et al: Pacemaker and automated internal cardiac defibrillator. eMedicine; http://www.emedicine.com/emerg/topic805.htm (Review of cardiac pacing and automated internal cardiac defibrillator.)

Xie B et al: Permanent cardiac pacing. Emerg Med Clin North Am 1998;16:419. [PMID: 96218551] (Review of cardiac pacing and its complications.)

■ IMPLANTABLE CARDIOVERTER DEFIBRILLATORS

Despite access to prehospital emergency care and early defibrillation, sudden cardiac death remains a significant health problem. It is estimated that more than

400,000 people have sudden cardiac death in the United States annually. Implantable cardioverter defibrillators (ICD) have dramatically reduced the incidence of sudden cardiac death resulting from life-threatening ventricular arrhythmias. Since becoming commercially available in the late 1980s, more than 250,000 ICDs have been implanted worldwide.

Since receiving U.S. Food and Drug Administration approval in 1985, ICDs have undergone significant technologic advances. Initially, devices were implanted in the abdominal wall and epicardial patches were sewn in place via a median sternotomy. Newer third-generation devices are smaller, and most are implanted in the subpectoral fascia using a transvenous lead system, similar to permanent pacemaker systems. As compared to earlier models, third-generation devices have more advanced tachycardia detection and termination features with longer battery life (7–8 years). The advanced tachycardia termination features include antitachycardia pacing, low-energy cardioversion, and high-energy defibrillation. Newer ICDs are also capable of rate-responsive dual-chamber back-up pacing.

COMPLICATIONS OF IMPLANTABLE CARDIOVERTER DEFIBRILLATORS

Venous access, ICD pocket site, and lead complications are all similar to the complications associated with permanent cardiac pacemaker systems. The most common lead complication is dislodgement, which is estimated to occur in up to 10% of cases.

IMPLANTABLE CARDIOVERTER DEFIBRILLATOR MALFUNCTION

Clinical Findings

Although uncommon, frequent or recurrent shocks may represent an ICD malfunction. An increased frequency of shocks may be caused by a number of conditions including an increased frequency of ventricular arrhythmias, device inefficacy, or an ICD sensing malfunction. The most common cause of an increased frequency of ICD shocks is an increased frequency of VT or VF. Ventricular arrhythmias can occur as a result of worsening left ventricular dysfunction, myocardial ischemia, or changes in antiarrhythmic therapy. An ICD sensing malfunction may lead to double counting of the T waves or inappropriate recognition of SVT as VT. Lead complications may also cause inappropriate ICD shocks.

Occasionally a patient may present with a sustained ventricular arrhythmia without ICD intervention. Although rare, this may occur as a result of a failure to detect the arrhythmia or exhaustion of therapies. In patients with ICDs, antibradycardia pacing malfunctions will be similar to those experienced by patients with implantable cardiac pacemakers.

MRI is contraindicated in patients with an ICD. The strong magnetic field may damage the ICD generator and interfere with antitachycardia therapy.

Treatment & Disposition

Temporary device deactivation may be necessary when frequent shocks occur. Similar to cardiac pacemakers, magnet application should trigger a magnetically activated reed switch. This disables all antitachycardia functions (antitachycardia pacing and shock therapies). Antibradycardia pacing functions are unaffected. Although most ICDs are immediately deactivated when a magnet is applied correctly, responses are somewhat manufacturer-dependent. Deactivation is not commonly performed, however, because the most common reason for frequent shocks is an increase in the frequency of VT or VF.

If recurrent ventricular arrhythmias result in frequent ICD shocks, antiarrhythmic administration and sedation may be necessary. If the ventricular arrhythmia is incessant, external cardioversion or defibrillation may be needed. Place the defibrillator pads or paddles as far from the ICD generator as possible. Older ICDs with epicardial electrodes have been reported to increase the defibrillation threshold by preventing externally applied current from passing into the myocardium. This may decrease the likelihood of successful defibrillation.

Pinski SL: Emergencies related to implantable cardioverter-defibrillators. Crit Care Med 2000;28:174. [PMID: 11055688] (Review of the complications of implantable cardioverter defibrillators.)

Shah CP et al: Implantable cardioverter defibrillators. Emerg Med Clin North Am 1998;16:463. [PMID: 9621852] (Review of implantable cardioverter defibrillators.)

GENERAL REFERENCES

Emergency cardiac care guidelines. Part 6: Advanced cardiac life support. Section 5: Pharmacology I: Agents for arrhythmias. Circulation 2000;102:112. [PMID: 10966669] (Pharmacology review of advanced cardiac life support medications.)

Emergency cardiac care guidelines. Part 6: Advanced cardiac life support. Section 7: Algorithm approach to ACLS emergencies. Circulation 2000;102:136. [PMID: 10966671] (Advanced cardiac life support guidelines.)

Wald DA: Therapeutic procedures in the emergency department patient with acute myocardial infarction. Emerg Med Clin North Am 2001;19:451. [PMID: 11373989] (Review of cardioversion, defibrillation, and temporary cardiac pacing.)

APPENDIX: COMMONLY ENCOUNTERED CARDIAC ARRHYTHMIAS

Normal Sinus Rhythm (Figure 35–2)

The heart rate is 60–100 beats/min. There is a constant and normal PR interval, and the P wave will be upright in lead II and inverted in lead aVR.

Sinus Tachycardia (Figure 35–3)

The heart rate is faster than 100 beats/min. Usually the rate is 101–160 beats/min. The P wave morphology is the same as in normal sinus rhythm.

Sinus Bradycardia (Figure 35–4)

The heart rate is slower than 60 beats/minute. Usually the rate is 45–59 beats/min. Sinus bradycardia is commonly associated with sinus arrhythmia. The P wave morphology is the same as in normal sinus rhythm.

Sinus Arrhythmia (Figure 35–5)

The heart rate is usually 45–100 beats/min. The P wave morphology is the same as in normal sinus rhythm. The PP or RR cycles vary by 0.16 s or more. Most commonly, sinus arrhythmia occurs in relation to the respiratory cycle. The sinus rate will gradually increase with inspiration and slow with expiration.

Automatic Atrial Tachycardia (Figure 35–6)

The heart rate is usually 160–250 beats/min but may be as slow as 140 beats/min. The P wave morphology is usually different from that of normal sinus rhythm.

The PP and RR cycles are regular in most cases. When the atrial rate is slower than 200 beats/min, 1:1 AV conduction is commonly noted. When the atrial rate is faster than 200 beats/min, the ventricular rate is often half the atrial rate because of the refractoriness of the AV node.

Atrioventricular Nodal Reentrant Tachycardia (Figures 35–7 to 35–10)

The heart rate is usually 180–200 beats/min. The P waves occur concurrent with the QRS complex and are often difficult to visualize on the ECG.

Atrioventricular Reciprocating Tachycardia (Figure 35–11)

The heart rate is usually faster than 200 beats/min. Because activation of the ventricle occurs through normal conduction pathways, the accessory pathway is concealed, and the QRS morphology is normal.

Atrial Fibrillation (Figures 35–12 & 35–13)

The atrial rate is disorganized and is 400–650 beats/min. The ventricular rate is irregularly irregular. No P waves are discernible on ECG.

Atrial Flutter (Figure 35–14)

The atrial rate is usually 250–350 beats/min. Characteristic sawtooth flutter waves may be seen on the ECG, particularly in lead II. Variable AV conduction may be noted. Typically, 2:1 AV conduction occurs, resulting in a ventricular rate of approximately 150 beats/min.

Multifocal Atrial Tachycardia (Figure 35–15)

The heart rate is typically 100–130 beats/min. The characteristic ECG finding is at least 3 different P wave morphologies. Varying PR intervals may also be noted.

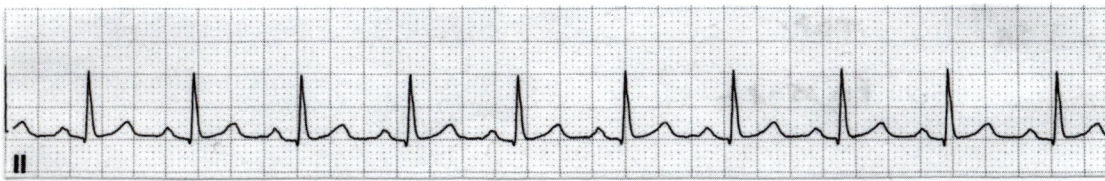

Figure 35–2. Normal sinus rhythm at a rate of 90 beats/min.

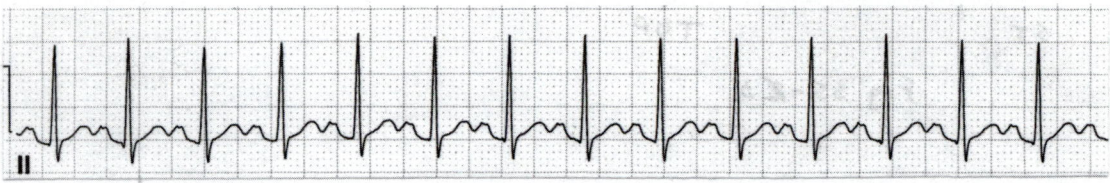

Figure 35–3. Sinus tachycardia at a rate of 130 beats/min.

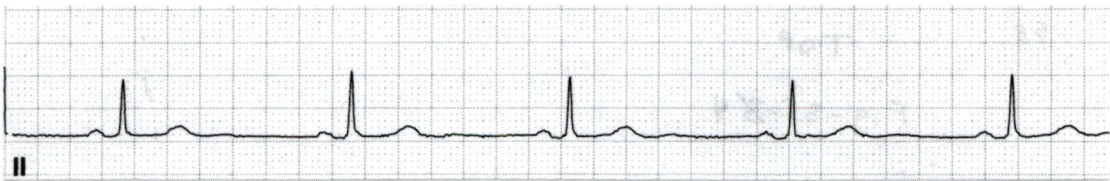

Figure 35–4. Sinus bradycardia at a rate of 45 beats/min.

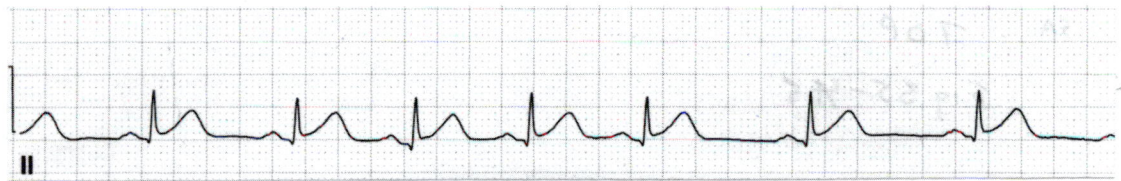

Figure 35–5. Sinus arrhythmia. The heart rate varies between 60 and 80 beats/min.

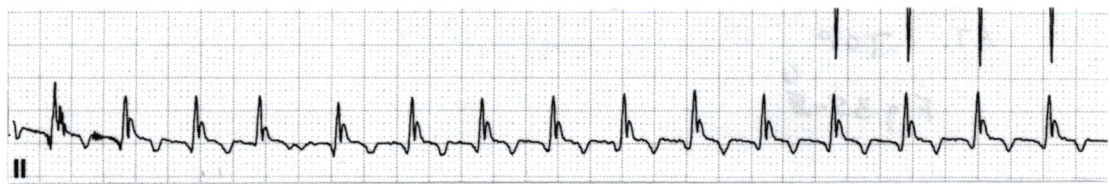

Figure 35–6. Automatic atrial tachycardia at a rate of 140 beats/min.

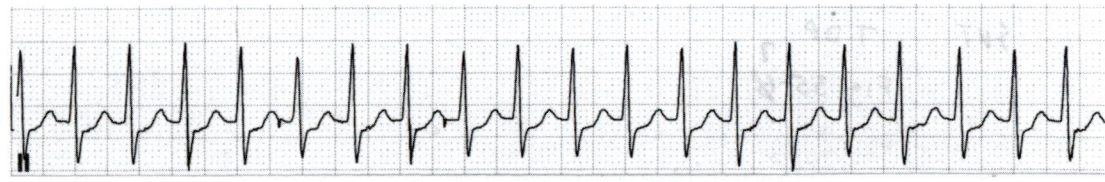

Figure 35–7. Atrioventricular nodal reentrant tachycardia at a rate of 175 beats/min. Note the absence of clearly discernible P waves.

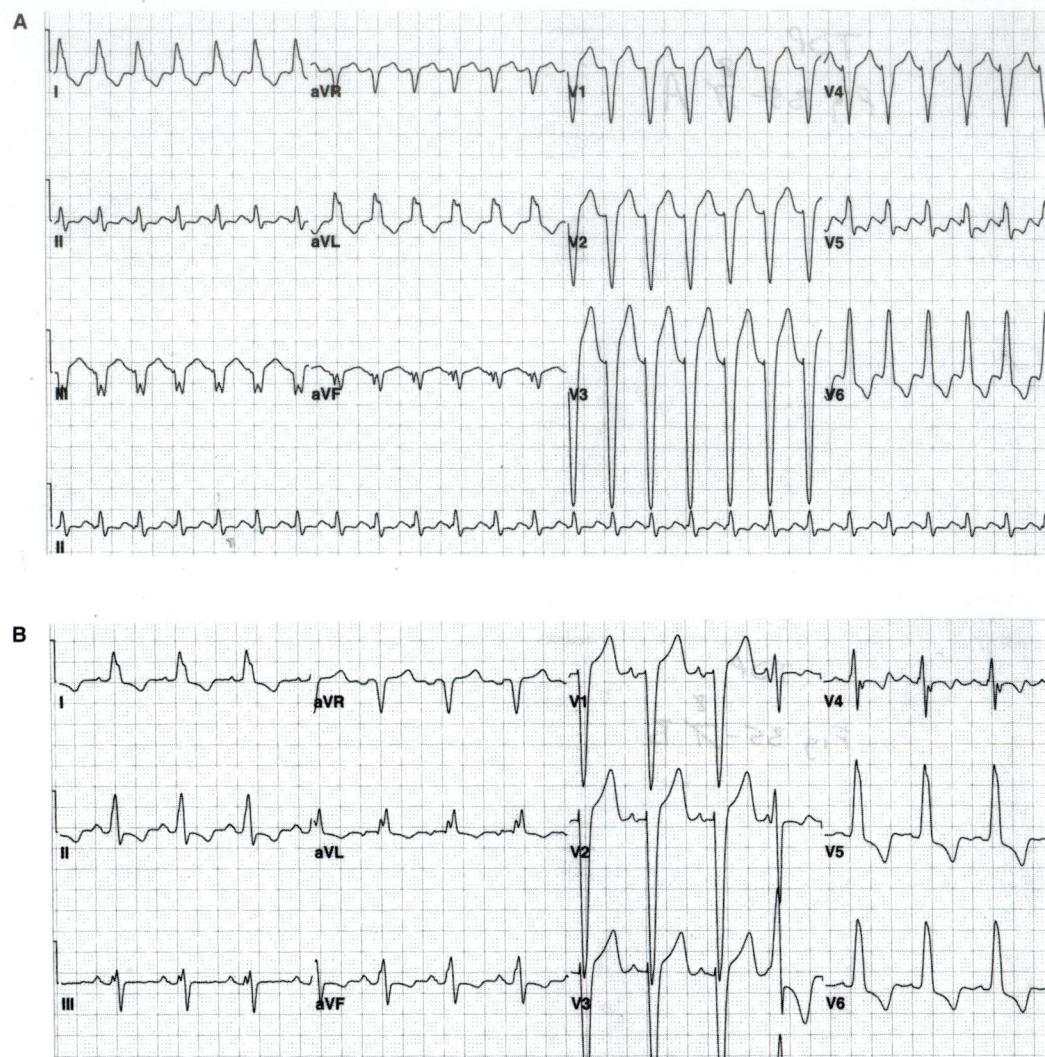

Figure 35–8. **A:** AV nodal reentrant tachycardia with a left bundle branch block (LBBB) at a rate of 155 beats/min. **B:** The baseline ECG in the same patient showing sinus rhythm with a LBBB at a rate of 95 beats/min. Note that the 11th beat is a premature ventricular contraction.

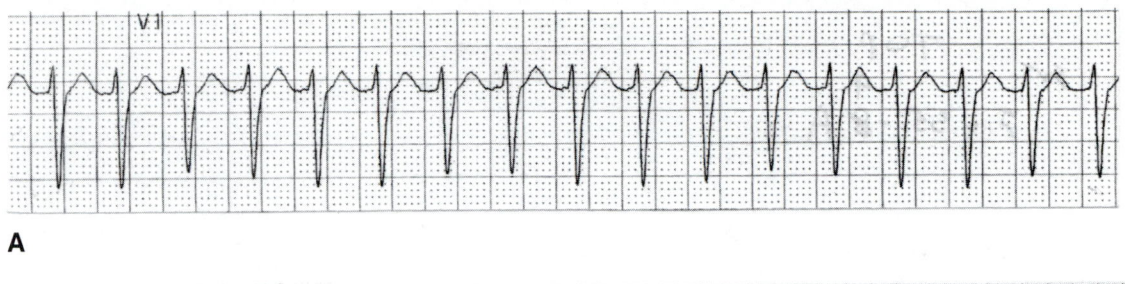

A

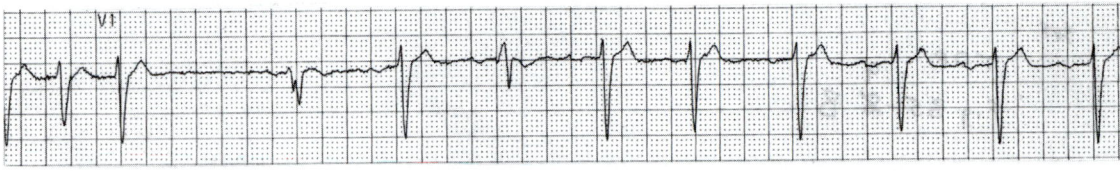

B

Figure 35–9. A: AV nodal reentrant tachycardia at a rate of 150 beats/min. **B:** Seconds later after the administration of adenosine, the same patient converts to sinus rhythm.

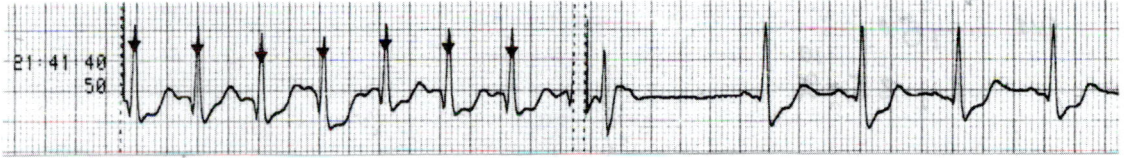

Figure 35–10. Paroxysmal supraventricular tachycardia at a rate of 150 beats/min in a patient who is hemodynamically unstable. After the 7th beat, the patient is cardioverted with 50 J to sinus rhythm.

A

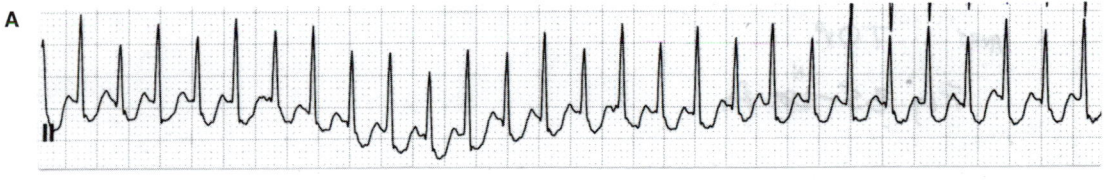

B

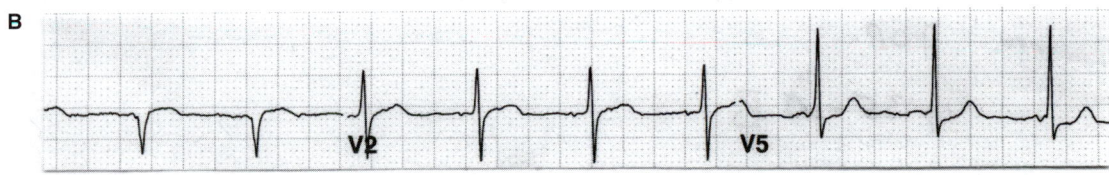

Figure 35-11. A: AV reciprocating tachycardia at a rate of 250 beats/min. **B:** The same patient after pharmacologic conversion showing sinus rhythm with ventricular preexcitation.

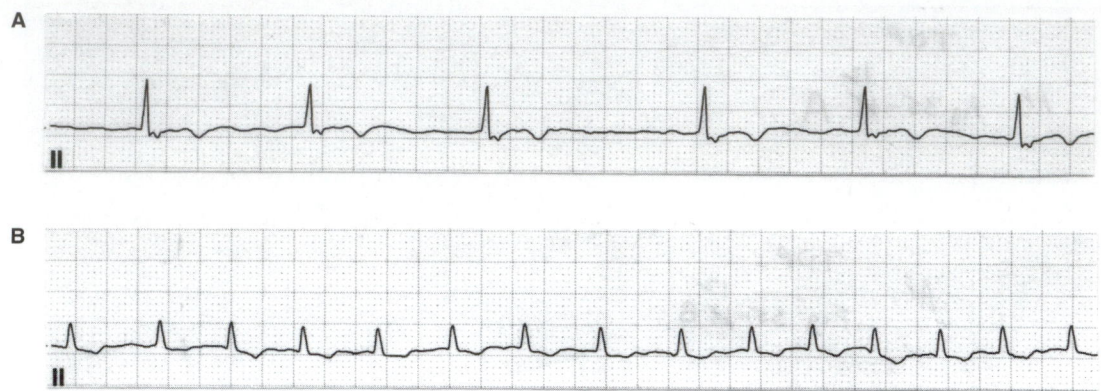

Figure 35–12. **A:** Atrial fibrillation with a controlled ventricular response. **B:** Atrial fibrillation at a ventricular rate of 130 beats/min.

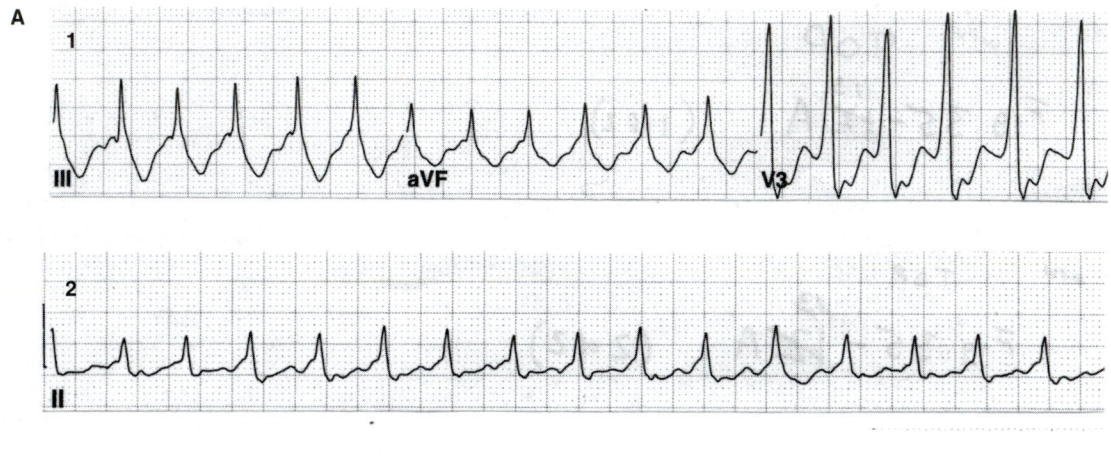

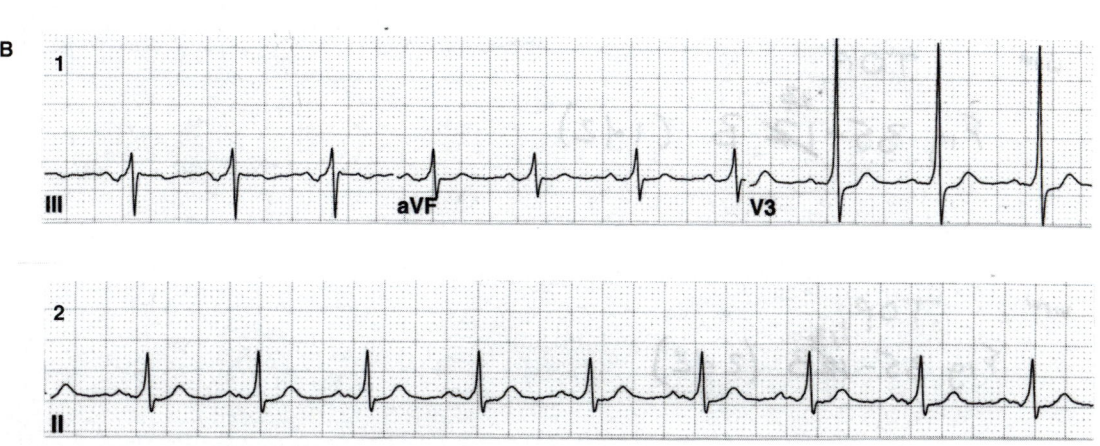

Figure 35–13. **A:** Atrial fibrillation with ventricular preexcitation. **B:** The same patient after pharmacologic conversion showing sinus rhythm with ventricular preexcitation.

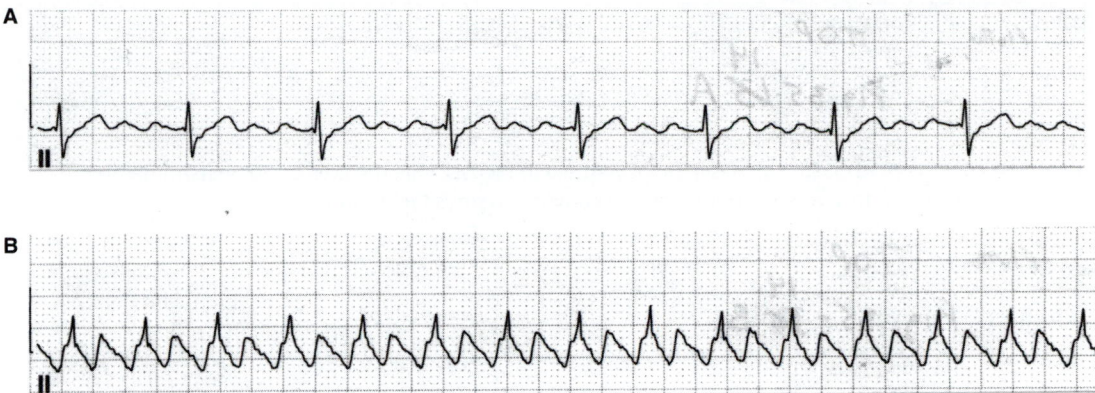

Figure 35–14. **A:** Atrial flutter with 4:1 AV conduction. **B:** Atrial flutter with 2:1 AV conduction. The ventricular rate is 145 beats/min.

Ventricular Tachycardia (Figures 35–16 & 35–17)

The ventricular rate is usually 180–250 beats/min, although rates slower than 160 beats/min may occur. The QRS complex is wide (greater than 0.12 s in duration) and often bizarre in appearance. Fusion beats or AV dissociation may be noted. If AV dissociation is present, the diagnosis of VT is confirmed.

Polymorphic Ventricular Tachycardia (Torsades de Pointes) (Figure 35–18)

The heart rate is usually 200–250 beats/min. Torsades de pointes is described as having a twisting-on-point appearance.

Ventricular Fibrillation (Figure 35–19)

VF is characterized by an irregularly irregular ventricular rhythm with no discernible distinction between the QRS complex, the ST segment, and T waves.

Premature Atrial Contractions (Figure 35–20)

A premature atrial contraction (PAC) may originate from anywhere in the atria except the sinus node. The P wave morphology is usually different from that of normal sinus rhythm. It is common to see a postectopic pause after a PAC. The QRS complex is narrow unless aberrantly conducted.

Premature Ventricular Contractions (Figure 35–21)

A PVC may originate from anywhere in the ventricles. The QRS complex is 0.12 s or longer in duration and resembles either a left or right bundle branch block. Uniform PVCs originate from the same foci and have the same appearance. Multiform PVCs have different morphology because they originate from different ventricular foci.

Idioventricular Rhythm (Figure 35–22)

The ventricular rate is usually 30–40 beats/min. The morphology of the QRS complexes will be similar to

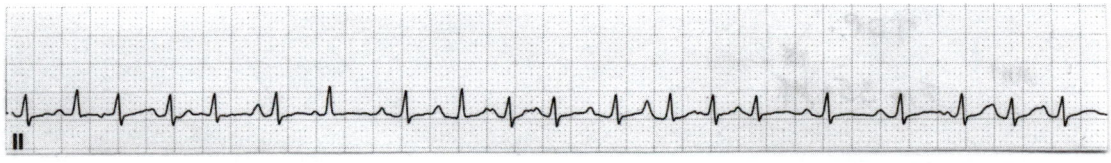

Figure 35–15. Multifocal atrial tachycardia at a rate of 145 beats/min. Note the different P wave morphologies.

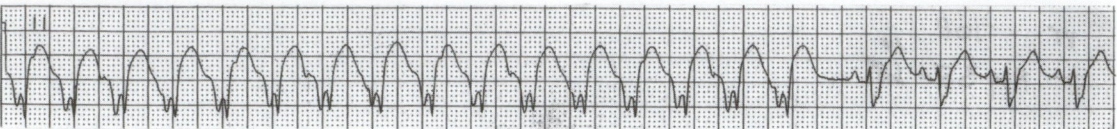

Figure 35–16. The rhythm strip shows a run of ventricular tachycardia; the rate is 150 beats/min. After 16 beats the ventricular tachycardia spontaneously converts to sinus tachycardia.

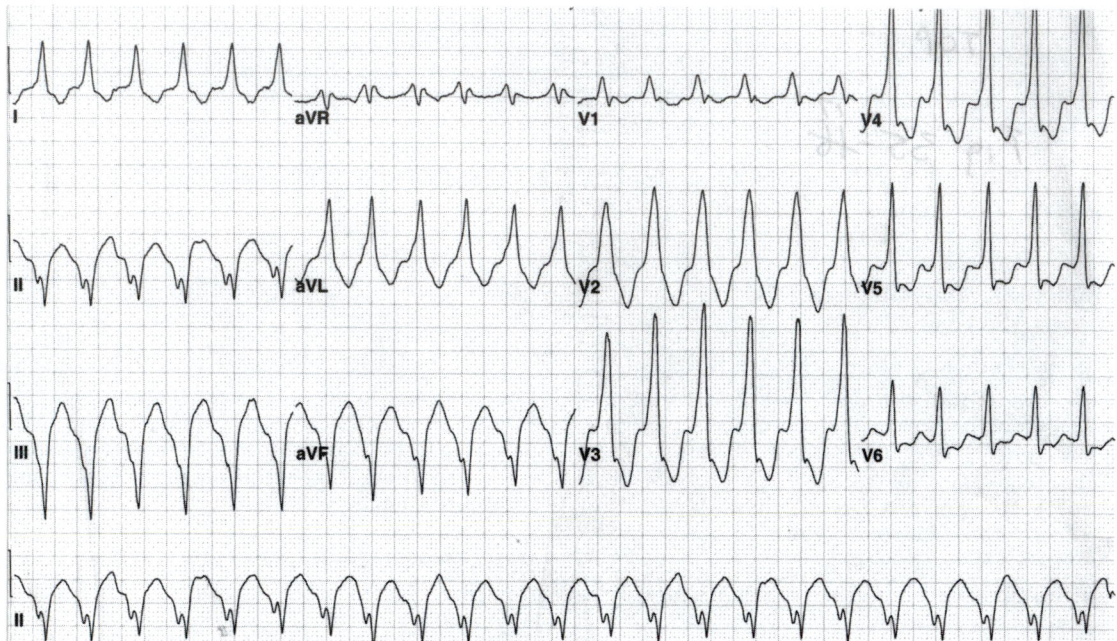

Figure 35–17. Ventricular tachycardia at a rate of 145 beats/min.

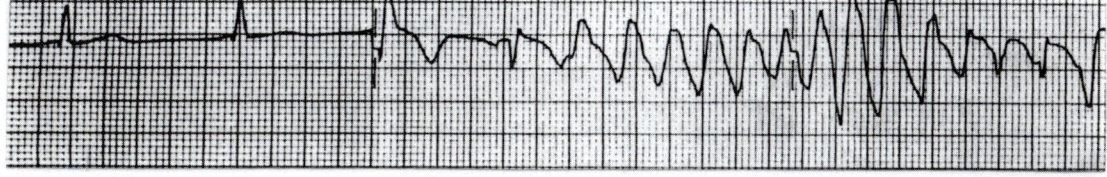

Figure 35–18. Polymorphic ventricular tachycardia.

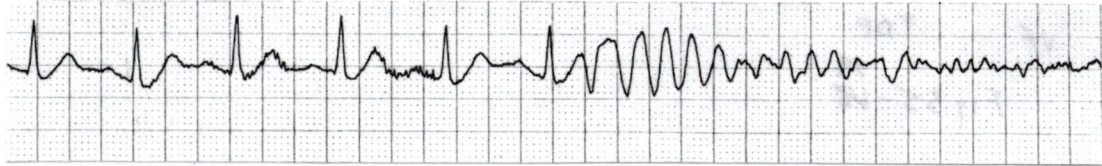

Figure 35–19. Ventricular fibrillation. After 6 beats, sinus rhythm degenerates into ventricular fibrillation.

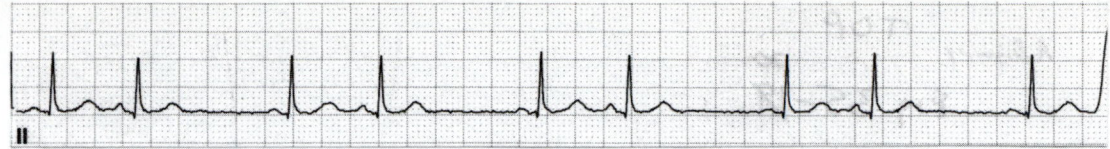

Figure 35–20. Sinus rhythm with premature atrial contractions in a bigeminal pattern. The configuration of the P waves of the premature atrial contractions are different from that of normal sinus rhythm.

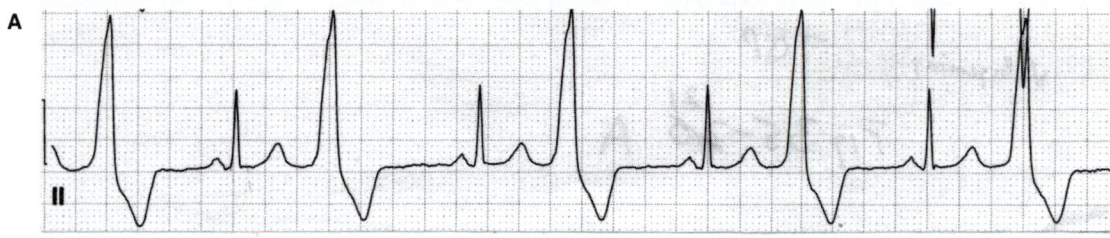

Figure 35–21. **A:** Sinus rhythm with frequent premature ventricular complexes in a pattern of bigeminy. **B:** Sinus rhythm with frequent premature ventricular complexes in a pattern of trigeminy.

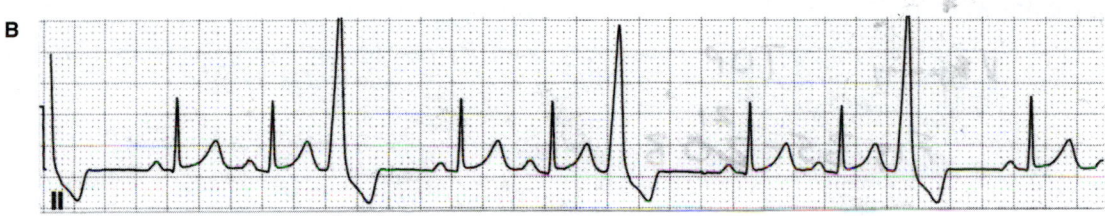

Figure 35–22. **A:** Atrial fibrillation with an idioventricular escape rhythm. **B:** Accelerated idioventricular rhythm at a rate of 50 beats/min.

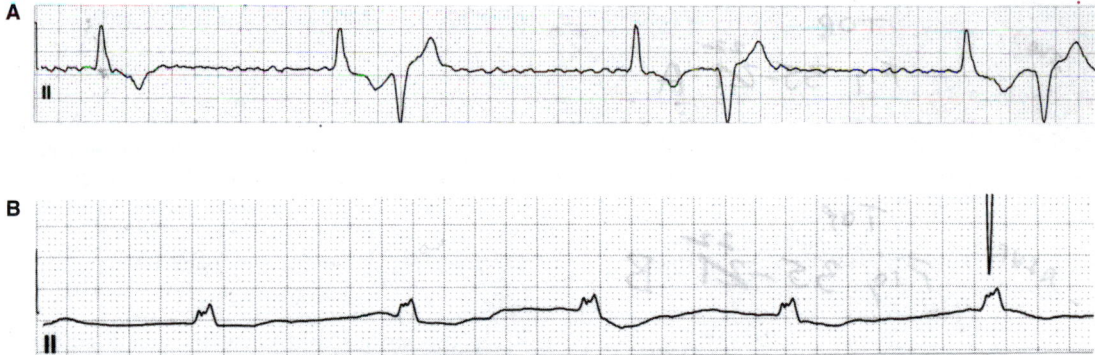

Figure 35–23. AV junctional rhythm at a rate of 40 beats/min.

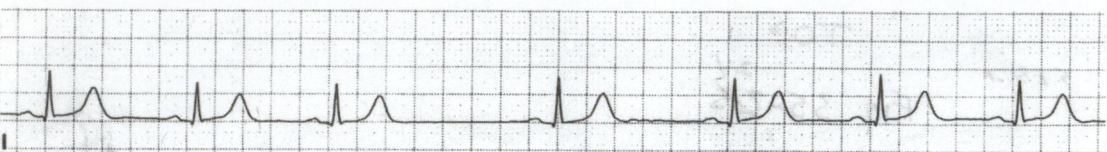

Figure 35–24. Sinus rhythm with second-degree Mobitz type I SA block. Note that the PP intervals gradually shorten, whereas the PR intervals remains constant. The cycle terminates with a blocked P wave. The length of the pause is shorter than twice the preceding PP cycle.

premature ventricular contractions but will vary depending on the location of the ventricular foci. If the ventricular rate is 50–100 beats/min, the rhythm is called accelerated idioventricular rhythm.

Atrioventricular Junctional Rhythm (Figure 35–23)

The ventricular rate is usually 45–60 beats/min. The QRS complex is narrow unless aberrantly conducted. If the junctional rhythm is faster than 60 beats/min, the term AV junctional tachycardia is applied.

Sinoatrial Block (Figure 35–24)

SA block is characterized by blocked P waves, evident by a long PP interval. The PP intervals before the blocked P wave may gradually shorten (SA Wenckebach), or the PP intervals may be constant (second-degree Mobitz type II SA block).

First-Degree Atrioventricular Block (Figure 35–25)

The PR interval is constant but characteristically prolonged greater than 0.2 s.

Second-Degree Atrioventricular Block (Mobitz Type I) (Figure 35–26)

There is progressive lengthening of the PR interval followed by a nonconducted P wave leading to a dropped QRS complex. Classically, the PP interval remains constant. The RR interval that includes the blocked P wave is the longest in duration.

Second-Degree Atrioventricular Block (Figure 35–27)

When every other P wave is blocked, one cannot distinguish between Mobitz type I or Mobitz type II AV block. This is described as 2:1 AV conduction.

Second-Degree Atrioventricular Block (Mobitz Type II) (Figure 35–28)

The PR interval is regular and can be either normal or prolonged. Periodically, a P wave is not conducted, leading to a dropped QRS complex.

Third-Degree Atrioventricular Block (Complete Heart Block) (Figures 35–29 through 35–31)

The PP interval (atrial rate) is usually shorter (faster) than the RR interval (ventricular rate). Because no atrial impulses are conducted through the AV node, no relationship exists between the atrial and ventricular activity.

Single-Chamber Ventricular Pacing (Figures 35–32 & 35–33)

When the intrinsic heart rate is faster than the programmed pacemaker rate, the pacemaker is inhibited from firing. When the intrinsic rate is slower, the pace-

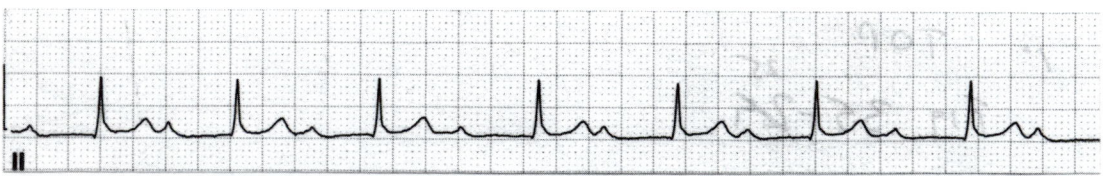

Figure 35–25. Sinus rhythm with first-degree AV block. The PR interval is 0.44 s.

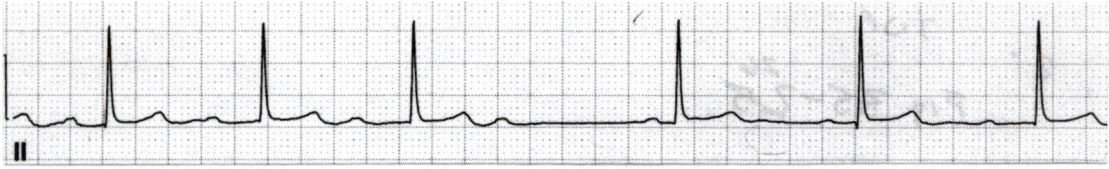

Figure 35–26. Sinus bradycardia with second-degree Mobitz type I AV block. Note the progressive lengthening of the PR interval until a QRS complex is dropped.

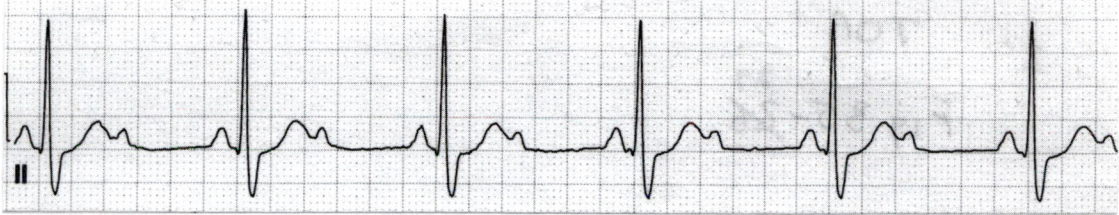

Figure 35–27. Sinus rhythm with second-degree AV block.

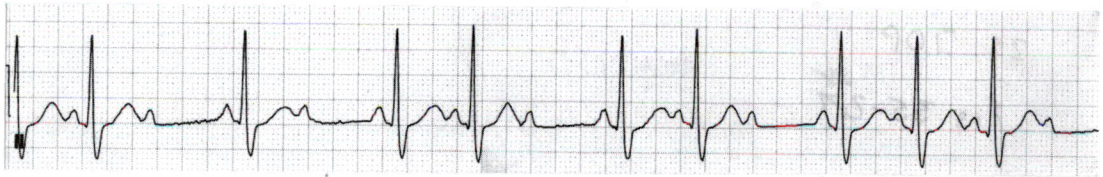

Figure 35–28. Sinus rhythm with second-degree Mobitz type II AV block. Note the variable AV conduction.

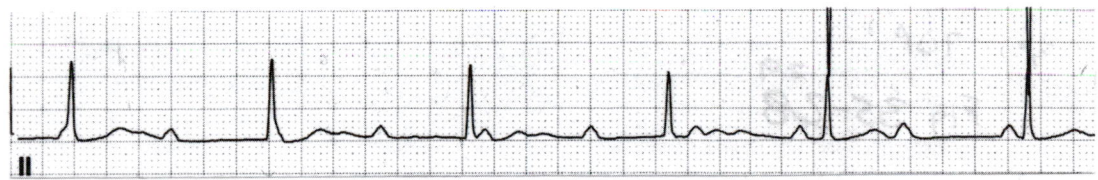

Figure 35–29. Third-degree AV block. The atrial rate is 92 beats/min, and the ventricular rate is 50 beats/min.

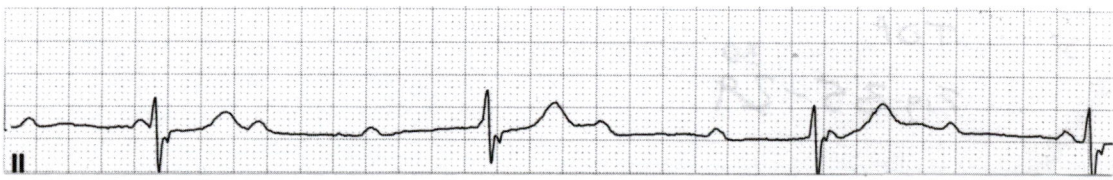

Figure 35–30. Third-degree AV block. The atrial rate is 88 beats/min, and the ventricular rate is 30 beats/min.

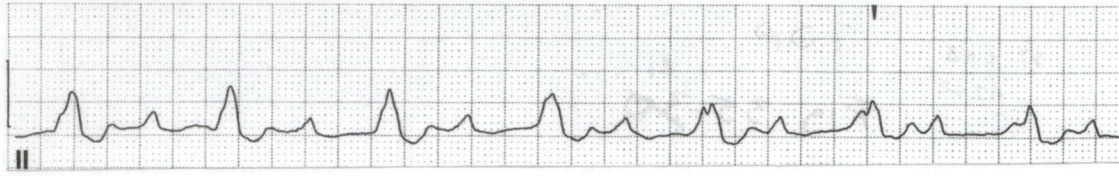

Figure 35–31. Third-degree AV block with an accelerated idioventricular escape rhythm with a ventricular rate of 60 beats/min.

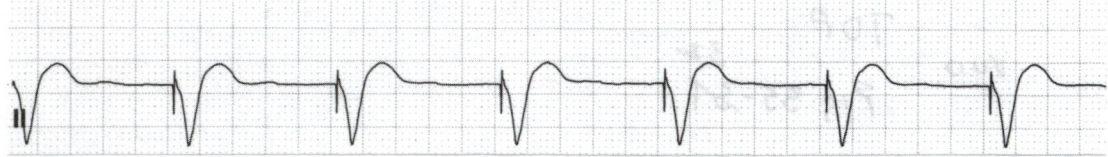

Figure 35–32. Asynchronous ventricular pacing. In this case, the intrinsic heart rate is slower than the programmed pacemaker rate. When this occurs, the pacemaker is triggered, taking over as the dominant pacemaker of the heart.

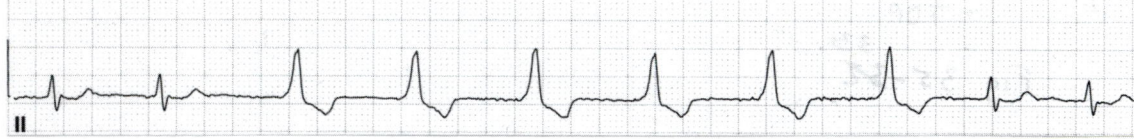

Figure 35–33. VVI pacing. Although the pacemaker spikes are difficult to appreciate, beats 3–8 are ventricular paced beats. When the intrinsic heart rate is faster than the programmed rate, the pacemaker is inhibited from firing.

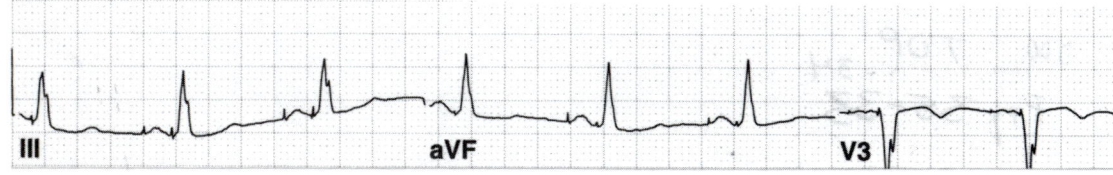

Figure 35–34. AV sequential pacing in a dual-chamber pacemaker. In this case, the pacemaker will pace both the atria and ventricles when no intrinsic cardiac activity is sensed.

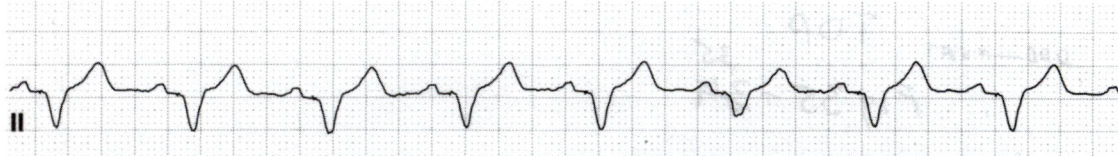

Figure 35–35. Dual-chamber pacemaker functioning in the VAT mode. The pacemaker paces the ventricles and senses the atria. If intrinsic atrial depolarizations are sensed, a ventricular pacing spike is triggered. This is evident on the ECG by the presence of atrial tracking.

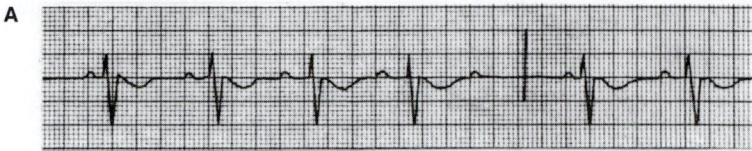

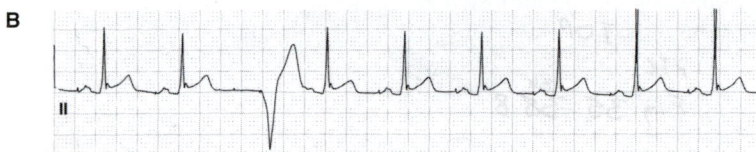

Figure 35–36. **A:** Single-chamber ventricular pacemaker showing failure to capture. The underlying rhythm is second-degree Mobitz type I AV block. A ventricular pacing spike occurs after the 5th atrial complex (P wave). This pacing spike fails to depolarize the ventricular myocardium. **B:** Dual-chamber pacemaker showing failure to capture. Beat 3 shows an atrial pacing spike that fails to depolarize the atrial myocardium. The pacemaker then proceeds to pace the ventricle. Beats 1, 2, and 4–9 show an atrial pacing spike with capture followed by normal AV conduction. (Part A reproduced, with permission, from Garson A: Stepwise approach to the unknown pacemaker ECG. Am Heart J 1990;119:924.)

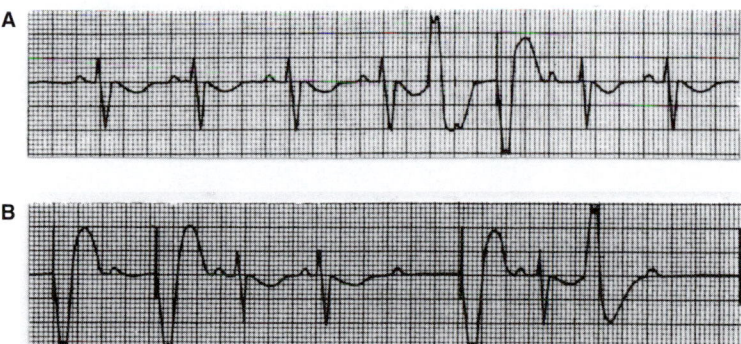

Figure 35–37. **A:** Undersensing. The 5th beat is a premature ventricular contraction (PVC). The next beat is a ventricular paced beat. Note that the paced beat occurs soon after the PVC, indicating a failure to sense the preceding complex. **B:** The 1st and 2nd beats are paced, the 3rd and 4th beats show normal AV conduction. There is a longer than expected pause between the 4th and 5th beats. This occurs secondary to ventricular oversensing. (Reproduced, with permission, from Garson A: Stepwise approach to the unknown pacemaker ECG. Am Heart J 1990;119:924.)

maker is triggered, taking over as the dominant pacemaker of the heart.

Dual-Chamber Atrioventricular Pacing (Figures 35–34 & 35–35)

The pacemaker is capable of pacing and sensing the atria and ventricles. Depending on the intrinsic rate, the pacemaker can either be triggered or inhibited.

Failure to Capture (Figure 35–36)

Failure to capture occurs when an appropriate pacemaker discharge fails to depolarize the myocardium. Physiologic failure to capture can occur if the pacing

stimulus occurs during the ventricular refractory period.

Failure to Sense (Undersensing) (Figure 35–37A)

Undersensing occurs when the pacemaker fails to detect intrinsic electrical cardiac activity. On the ECG, a P wave or QRS complex is inappropriately followed by a pacing spike.

Oversensing (Figure 35–37B)

Oversensing is the inappropriate inhibition of a pacing stimulus. On the ECG, it is evident by a pause that is longer than the programmed pacemaker rate.

Obstetric & Gynecologic Emergencies & Rape

36

Melissa Platt, MD, & Mary Nan Mallory, MD, RDMS[1]

Immediate Management of Life-Threatening Problems
    Abnormal Vaginal Bleeding
    Pelvic Pain with or without Bleeding
Emergency Management of Gynecologic Disorders
    Ectopic Pregnancy
    Spontaneous Abortion
    Septic Abortion
    Carcinoma & Other Tumors
    Genital Trauma
    Ruptured Ovarian Cyst
    Torsion of Ovarian Tumor
    Endometriosis
    Dysmenorrhea
    Mittelschmerz
    Uterine Prolapse
    Salpingitis & Tubo-ovarian Abscess
    Rape (Men & Women)

    1. Management of the Female Rape Victim
    2. Management of the Male Rape Victim
    Intrauterine Devices
    Postcoital Emergency Contraception
    Disorders of the Vulva & Vagina
    A Warning about Discontinuing Contraception
Emergency Management of Obstetric Disorders
    Pregnancy
    Discomforts of Pregnancy
    Hyperemesis Gravidarum
    Third-Trimester Bleeding
    Toxemia of Pregnancy (Preeclampsia-Eclampsia)
    Trauma in Pregnancy
    Labor & Delivery
    Postpartum Hemorrhage
    Puerperal Sepsis & Endometritis
    Puerperal Mastitis

■ IMMEDIATE MANAGEMENT OF LIFE-THREATENING PROBLEMS

ABNORMAL VAGINAL BLEEDING (See Table 36–1.)

Patients with active vaginal bleeding are at risk of exsanguination and require immediate evaluation and treatment.

Emergency Evaluation & Treatment

A. OBTAIN VITAL SIGNS

Examine the patient for hypotension or tachycardia due to depletion of intravascular volume.

1. Hypotension—If blood pressure and pulse are normal in the supine position, measure them in the sitting position. If they are still normal, measure them in the standing position to detect more subtle volume depletion. Supine or postural hypotension indicates life-threatening hemorrhage.

2. Tachycardia—Tachycardia while the patient is resting or when she assumes the upright posture also may indicate vascular depletion.

B. TREAT SHOCK, IF PRESENT

(See Chapter 9.) Briefly,

1. Insert at least 1 large-bore (≥ 16-gauge) intravenous catheter. A central venous catheter may be preferable if peripheral venous access is not readily obtainable (Chapter 6).

2. Determine the amount of blood loss, and draw blood for (a) typing and cross-matching (reserve 4 units of fresh-frozen plasma and 2–4 units of

---

[1]This chapter is a revision of the chapter by Phillip J. Goldstein, MD, from the 4th edition.

Table 36–1. Causes of abnormal vaginal bleeding.

Premenarcheal vaginal bleeding
  Menarche
  Tumor (vaginal, uterine)
  Genital trauma
  Foreign body
  Precocious puberty
  Hematuria
  Miscellaneous
Reproductive age bleeding
  Variations in normal cycle
    Hypermenorrhea (excessive bleeding at time of period)
    Polymenorrhea (menstrual periods < 21 days apart)
  Metrorrhagia (including ectopic)
    Abortion
    Pregnancy (including ectopic)
    Endocrine abnormality (idiopathic, estrogens, thyroid)
    Salpingitis
    Cervicitis
    Coagulopathy (factor VIII deficiency)
    Malignant neoplasm or polyps (cervical, vaginal, uterine)
    Ovarian cyst
    Myoma of uterus
    Trophoblastic tumor
  Miscellaneous (mittelschmerz)
Postmenopausal bleeding
  Carcinoma (cervical, uterine)
  Estrogen excess
  Atrophic vaginitis
  Cervical polyps
  Trauma
  Miscellaneous

---

packed red cells), (b) platelet count, prothrombin time, and partial thromboplastin time to uncover any bleeding abnormality, (c) complete blood count (CBC), (d) renal function tests and measurement of serum electrolytes, and (e) arterial blood gas measurements and pH (useful in assessing adequacy of ventilation and perfusion).

3. Insert a Foley catheter.

4. If the patient is of child-bearing age, obtain a serum or urinary pregnancy test.

5. Begin rapid infusion of crystalloid solution (Ringer's injection or normal saline), the rate depending on vital signs (eg, 200–1000 mL/h), to restore intravascular volume and maintain blood pressure until compatible blood becomes available for transfusion.

6. Infuse cross-matched blood as soon as possible. If the patient is unstable and cross-matched blood is

unavailable, transfuse O-negative blood. Give 2 or more units depending on vital signs.

C. DETERMINE THE CAUSE OF BLEEDING, AND STOP IT

The measures described here should not be used in third-trimester pregnancy.

1. Compression of uterus—Insert one hand in the vagina, elevate the uterus, and compress it against the abdominal wall and the other hand.

2. Pelvic ultrasonography—In the evaluation of a pregnant patient with vaginal bleeding, ultrasound can be used to rapidly identify fluid in the pelvis or abdomen (presumed to be blood in the setting of shock), which is highly suggestive of ruptured ectopic pregnancy. In the setting of symptomatic vaginal hemorrhage in the first trimester of pregnancy, ultrasound may show retained intrauterine products of conception, indicative of an incomplete spontaneous abortion. For the nonpregnant patient, an ultrasound showing significant pelvic or intraabdominal fluid may be representative of a hemorrhagic ruptured ovarian cyst, which occasionally requires surgical intervention.

D. TREAT FOR TRAUMA

If trauma has occurred, determine the extent of injury, and apply pressure to the bleeding site.

E. OBTAIN CONSULTATION

Obtain urgent gynecologic or surgical consultation for possible emergent dilation and curettage, laparoscopy, or laparotomy.

Disposition

Patients with vaginal bleeding resulting in abnormal hemodynamics or anemia should be hospitalized.

PELVIC PAIN WITH OR WITHOUT BLEEDING (See Table 36–2.)

Clinical Findings

A. HISTORY

Obtain information about the following points:

- Possible pregnancy (recent amenorrhea or abnormal period, intercourse without contraception, morning sickness, or tenderness of breasts of recent onset)
- History of trauma, including rape or nontherapeutic abortion
- History of salpingitis
- History of ectopic pregnancy
- Duration of symptoms and relation to menses

Table 36–2. Differential diagnosis of pelvic pain.

	History and Symptoms				Signs					Laboratory Findings	
	Relationship to Menstrual Period	Quality of Pain	Prior Salpingitis	Type of Vaginal Discharge	Fever	Cervix	Uterus	Adnexal Mass	Adnexal Tenderness	Urine Immunologic Pregnancy Test	Leukocytosis
Salpingitis	Accompanying or just after period	Constant and severe	+	Scant to purulent	+	Tender with motion	Tender	None	Usually bilateral	Indicated	++
Salpingitis plus tubo-ovarian abscess								+			Also, elevated erythrocyte sedimentation rate
Incomplete abortion	Period of amenorrhea with recent spotting	Cramping and suprapubic	±	Heavy blood clots	–	Dilated	Enlarged, tender	None	None	±	±
Septic abortion	Period of amenorrhea with recent spotting or frank blood		±	Thick and bloody; foul-smelling	+	Dilated, tender	Enlarged, tender	±	Bilateral	±	++
Ectopic pregnancy	Amenorrhea with recent spotting	Intermittent; variable severity	±	Scant but rarely none	±	Slightly tender	Normal to slightly enlarged	+	Unilateral	±	±
Ruptured ovarian cyst	Precedes period	Sudden and severe	–	None	±	Normal	Normal	±	Unilateral	Indicated.	±
Mittelschmerz	Midcycle	Sudden	–	Spotting	–	Normal	Normal	None	Unilateral	–	–
Torsion of ovarian tumor	None	Intermittent; radiates to thigh	–	None	±	Slightly tender	Slightly tender	None	Unilateral	±	–
Endometritis with or without IUD	Variable	Cramping	±	Scant or none	+	Variable	Slightly tender	+ if tubal abscess	Variable	±	±
Dysmenorrhea	Accompanies period	Cramping	±	Normal menses	–	Normal	Variable tenderness	Negative	Seldom	–	–
Appendicitis	None	Periumbilical; cramping; progressing to constant right lower quadrant	–	None	±	Normal	Normal	None	Unilateral	±	±

- Type of pain (cramping or constant)
- Type and amount of vaginal bleeding or discharge
- Use of intrauterine device (IUD)

B. Symptoms and Signs

Fever is often the first sign of infection, and pelvic warmth (from local inflammation) may be noted on bimanual examination. Pelvic organs are tender and engorged.

C. Laboratory Tests and Special Examinations

1. Blood tests—The white cell count, differential, and erythrocyte sedimentation rate may reflect inflammation.

2. Pregnancy test—A pregnancy test is important if pain or bleeding is present (Table 36–3). Qualitative tests of blood or urine are sensitive and may provide positive test results within 7 days of conception. They are also relatively inexpensive, easy to do, and can be performed in 5 minutes. Quantitative blood tests are more sensitive and may assist in the evaluation of gestational age. If the tests are performed using urine samples, false-positive results may rarely occur in the presence of psychotropic drugs, methadone, sperm, or proteinuria.

3. Cultures—Obtain cervical swab cultures for gonococci and *Chlamydia trachomatis* if infection is a possible diagnosis.

4. Ultrasound—Ultrasound may show an ectopic pregnancy, intrauterine pregnancy, inflamed fallopian tubes, ovarian cysts, or pelvic abscesses (Figures 36–1 and 36–2).

5. Laparoscopy—Laparoscopy may be helpful when the diagnosis is uncertain.

Treatment & Disposition

If the diagnosis is uncertain but either ectopic pregnancy or septic abortion is a possibility, consultation with a gynecologist for hospitalization or daily follow-up on an outpatient basis is mandatory.

■ EMERGENCY MANAGEMENT OF GYNECOLOGIC DISORDERS

ECTOPIC PREGNANCY

 ESSENTIALS OF DIAGNOSIS

- *Unilateral pelvic pain in early pregnancy.*
- *Vaginal bleeding present or absent.*
- *Risk factor assessment.*
- *Unilateral adnexal tenderness or mass.*
- *Uterine size less than dates.*
- *Quantitative hCG and pelvic ultrasound.*

General Considerations

Ectopic pregnancy is the leading cause of pregnancy-related death in the first trimester. Patients with ectopic pregnancy are often encountered in the emergency department, and the disorder may be difficult to identify given the varied presentations that occur. Overall, of the pregnant patients who present with vaginal bleeding or abdominal pain, 60% will have normally developing pregnancies, 30% will experience a miscarriage,

---

Table 36–3. Clinical manifestations of common pelvic disorders.

Clinical Findings	Possible Causes
Bleeding	Trauma Postpartum hemorrhage Dysfunctional uterine bleeding Carcinoma
Pain	Salpingitis and tubo-ovarian abscess Ruptured ovarian cyst Torsion of tube and ovary Mittelschmerz Abdominal disorders (appendicitis, etc.)
Pain and bleeding	Dysmenorrhea Endometriosis Endometritis
Pregnancy and bleeding	Placenta previa Ectopic pregnancy Spontaneous abortion Abruptio placentae
Pregnancy and pain	Ectopic pregnancy Degenerating fibroid (leiomyoma) Normal labor
Pregnancy with pain and bleeding	Labor with placenta previa Abruptio placentae Septic abortion Puerperal sepsis Ectopic pregnancy

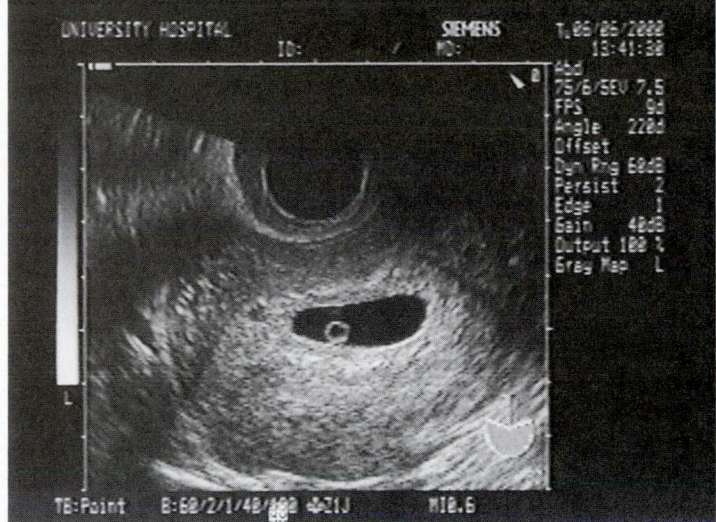

Figure 36–1. Bedside endovaginal ultrasound of an intrauterine pregnancy. An intrauterine gestational sac with a yolk sac is clearly visualized.

and 10% will have an ectopic pregnancy. Because ectopic pregnancy can be life threatening, it should be suspected in any patient presenting with menstrual irregularities, vaginal bleeding, and pelvic or lower abdominal pain. For some women, the initial presenting symptom of an ectopic pregnancy is syncope. The most common presenting complaint is vaginal bleeding, often scant at first, with cramping lower abdominal pain.

The incidence of ectopic pregnancy is increased in women using an IUD and in those with a history of pelvic infection (eg, salpingitis), tubal surgery, infertil-

ity treatments, or previous tubal pregnancies. About 98% of ectopic pregnancies are tubal.

The clinical presentation of ectopic pregnancy is variable, ranging from the asymptomatic patient to the patient with hemorrhagic shock. Rupture of the fallopian tube followed by free intraperitoneal bleeding from tubal vessels is the principal cause of illness and death.

With improved resolution of ultrasound and rapidly available quantitative β–human chorionic gonadotropin (β-hCG) assays, the diagnosis of ectopic pregnancy can be made more accurately and earlier than in the past (Figure 36–3).

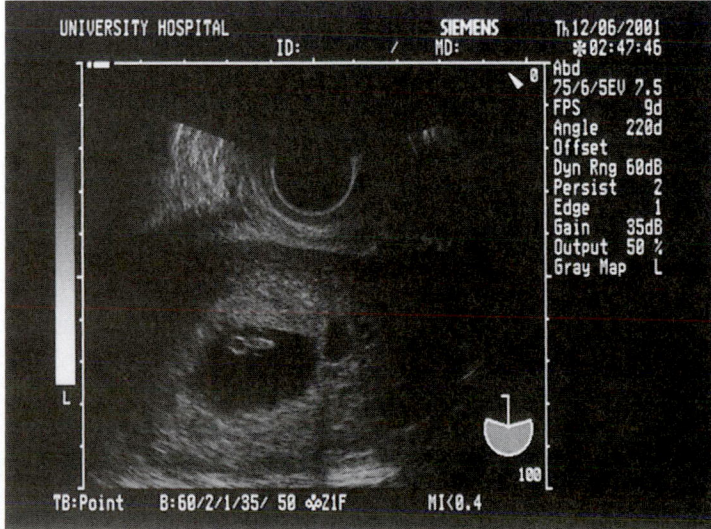

Figure 36–2. Bedside endovaginal ultrasound of an intrauterine pregnancy. An intrauterine gestational sac containing both a yolk sac and fetal pole is noted

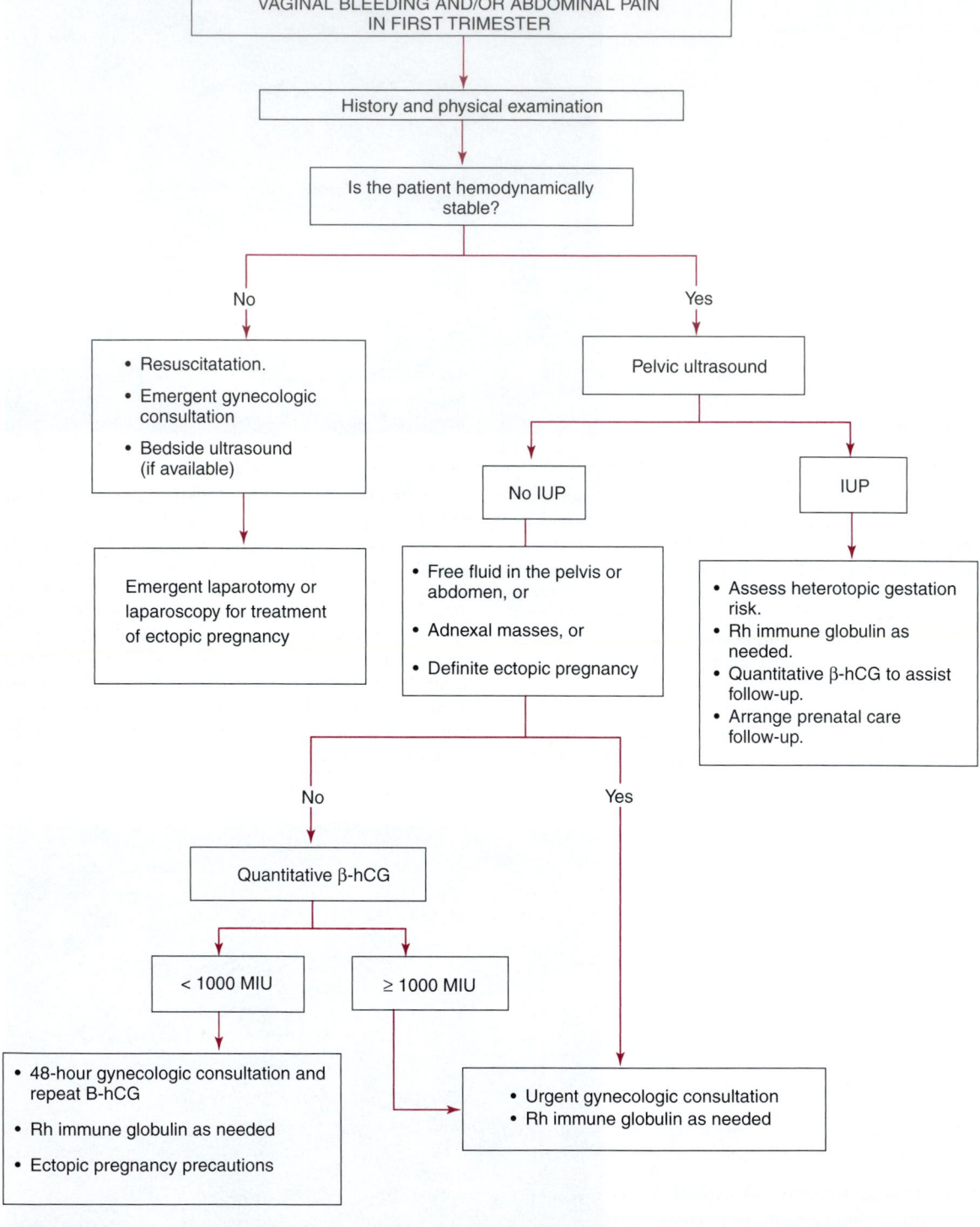

Figure 36–3. Diagnostic algorithm for the patient with possible ectopic pregnancy. IUP = intrauterine pregnancy.

Clinical Findings

A. SYMPTOMS AND SIGNS

Patients have a history of the following: (1) missed or abnormal menses or vaginal bleeding; however, 30% of patients with ectopic pregnancy have no vaginal bleeding; (2) pelvic pain, which may be unilateral, following amenorrhea; and (3) intermittent pain (occasionally). Rupture of the fallopian tube may bring temporary relief of pain.

Symptoms of early pregnancy (eg, breast tenderness, nausea) may be present. Peritoneal pain may develop after tubal rupture with bleeding into the peritoneum. Unilateral abdominal or pelvic pain may persist or improve. Referred shoulder pain is occasionally present. Syncope or lightheadedness may occur.

In the early stages of ectopic pregnancy, the results of pelvic examination may be normal. Symptoms, if present, may be completely nonspecific initially, because the tubal pregnancy producing them may be in the early stages of development. In advanced cases, a tender adnexal mass, enlarged uterus, or blood in the peritoneal cavity (eg, doughy cul-de-sac) may occur.

Obtain complete vital signs, including supine, sitting, and standing pulse and blood pressure measurements if these measures are normal in the supine position, to look for supine or orthostatic hypotension.

B. LABORATORY TESTS AND SPECIAL EXAMINATIONS

1. Pregnancy test—The qualitative urine and serum pregnancy test may be positive at levels as low as 10 mIU/mL. Check with the laboratory. The most specific and sensitive test is the serum quantitative β-hCG. It may detect levels as low as 5 mIU/mL depending on laboratory assay. Quantitative β-hCG values are invaluable in the interpretation of pelvic ultrasound in this setting. In a normal intrauterine first-trimester pregnancy, the β subunit of hCG should double about every 1.5 days.

2. Ultrasound—Endovaginal and transabdominal sonography have become key diagnostic tools in the differentiation of normal (see Figures 36–1 and 36–2) from abnormal early pregnancy (Figure 36–4). Occasionally, a mass can be seen in the adnexa or cul-de-sac, or products of conception can be visualized outside the uterine cavity, and ectopic pregnancy can be readily diagnosed (see Figure 36–4).

Ultrasound is often useful in excluding an ectopic pregnancy by ruling-in an intrauterine pregnancy. If the patient reports a history of infertility treatments, avoid making premature conclusions because the possibility of a heterotopic pregnancy (ie, simultaneous intrauterine and ectopic) has been reported to be as low as 1 in 5000. With a β-hCG of 6000–6500 mIU/mL, an intrauterine pregnancy can be visualized transabdominally 94% of the time. Likewise, a yolk sac can be identified at the

discriminatory β-hCG values of 1000–1500 mIU/mL. With endovaginal scanning, a small intrauterine collection of blood, or pseudosac, may be seen associated with an ectopic pregnancy. In very early pregnancy, at levels below the discriminatory values, the uterus may appear empty. Fluid in Morison's pouch on transabdominal scanning strongly suggests ruptured ectopic pregnancy in this clinical setting (Figure 36–5).

3. Laparoscopy or laparotomy—Laparoscopy or laparotomy may be necessary to make a definitive diagnosis of ectopic pregnancy.

Treatment & Disposition

Treatment of possible ectopic pregnancy is determined by the patient's risk factors for ectopic pregnancy (ie, infertility treatments, history of tubal ligation or pelvic inflammatory disease), hemodynamic stability, and physical examination findings. In addition, sonography is important in the evaluation of pregnant patients with either abdominal pain or vaginal bleeding (see Figure 36–3). Quantitative β-hCG results may help in the interpretation of ultrasound findings.

A. HIGH PROBABILITY OF ECTOPIC PREGNANCY

Obtain emergent pelvic sonography if hemodynamic stability allows. If the quantitative β-hCG value is greater than 1500–2000 mIU/mL in a patient with an empty uterine cavity on endovaginal ultrasound, ectopic pregnancy should be strongly suspected. An adnexal mass or extrauterine products of conception may or may not be readily identified. A large amount of pelvic or intraperitoneal fluid is highly suggestive of ectopic pregnancy (Figures 36–4C and 36–5). If ultrasound is unavailable for evaluation of a patient with a positive pregnancy test, physical findings worrisome for ectopic pregnancy include severe adnexal tenderness or an adnexal mass.

Prevent or correct hemorrhagic shock by inserting a large-bore ($\geq$ 16-gauge) intravenous catheter and infusing crystalloid solution for volume replacement. Type and cross-match for 2–3 units of packed red blood cells. Insert a Foley catheter, and send urine for analysis.

Obtain emergency obstetric consultation, and prepare the patient for surgery. Obtain CBC; serum electrolyte, blood urea nitrogen, and creatinine determinations; coagulation profile; and other studies as required.

B. ECTOPIC PREGNANCY EQUIVOCAL

Vaginal bleeding, pelvic pain, and tenderness without explanation may be present in a patient with a positive pregnancy test.

Insert an intravenous catheter, and send blood for CBC and typing and cross-matching. Obtain pelvic sonogram. A transvaginal sonogram may not show definite evidence of an ectopic pregnancy, but worrisome

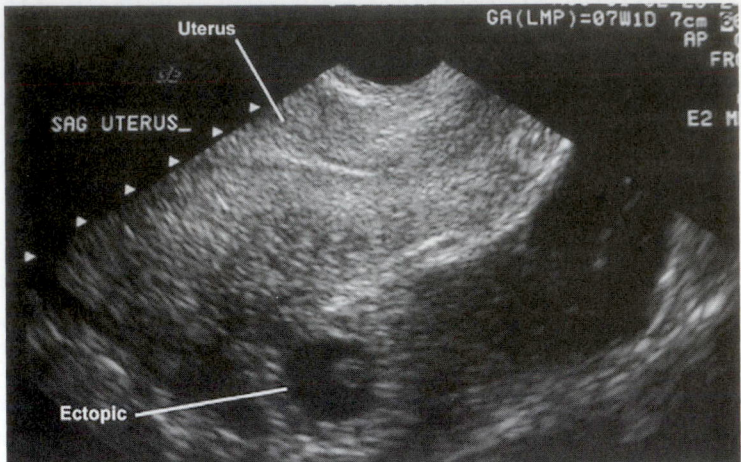

A

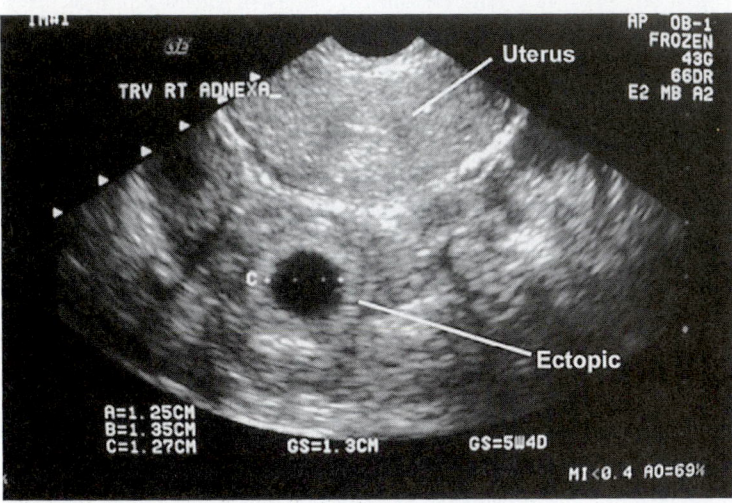

B

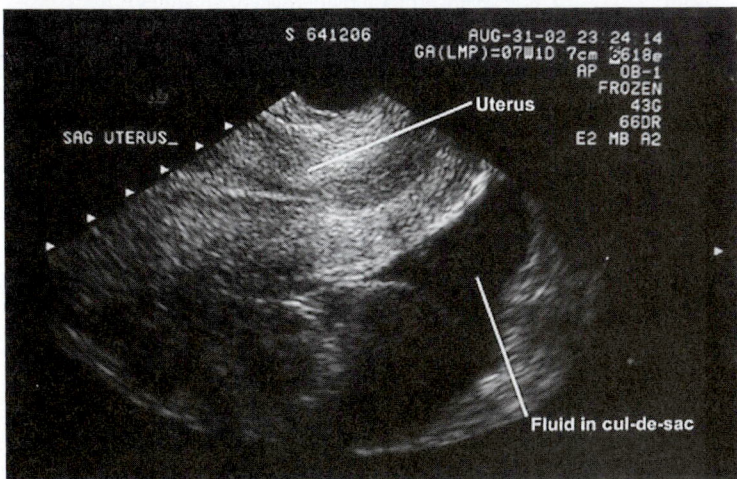

C

Figure 36–4. Endovaginal ultrasound clearly demonstrating an ectopic pregnancy. **A:** Longitudinal view of the uterus with a well-defined endometrial stripe and no intrauterine gestational sac. A gestational sac is noted posterior to the uterus. **B:** Transverse view of the uterus and right adnexa also demonstrating an extrauterine gestational sac. **C:** Longitudinal view demonstrating free fluid in the cul-de-sac.

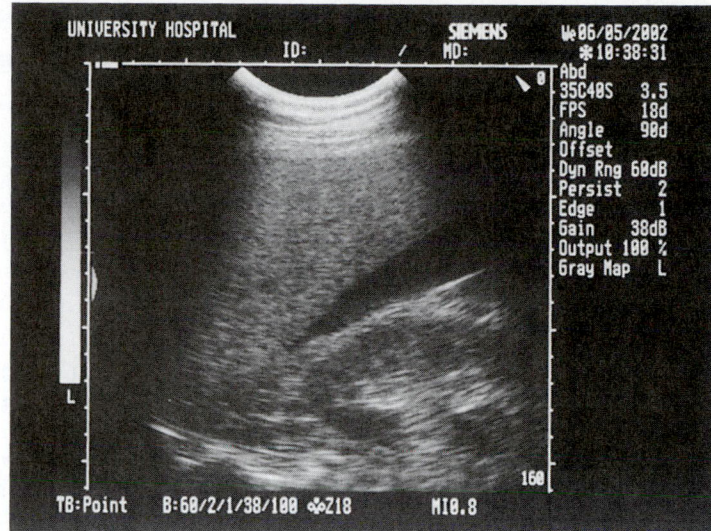

Figure 36–5. Bedside transabdominal ultrasound of free fluid in Morison's pouch (hepatorenal space) secondary to a ruptured ectopic pregnancy.

signs include fluid in the cul-de-sac or an empty uterus with a quantitative β-hCG at or above the discriminatory zone. Gynecologic consultation is recommended in these situations.

C. LOW PROBABILITY OF ECTOPIC PREGNANCY

Vaginal bleeding or pelvic pain is present. The results of physical examination and laboratory studies are normal. Some authors have developed clinical criteria for prediction of ectopic pregnancy. Suggested low-risk clinical criteria (ectopic pregnancy risk < 1%) for patients with pain or bleeding include absence of signs of peritoneal irritation on palpation, no cervical motion, no adnexal or uterine tenderness, and no abdominal or pelvic pain other than in the midline.

Send blood for quantitative β-hCG. If a pelvic sonogram demonstrates an intrauterine pregnancy, and the patient is at low risk for a heterotopic pregnancy (ie, no fertility medications or procedures), discharge the patient with 48-hour follow-up. Other patients who can be managed as outpatients with close gynecologic follow-up include those with quantitative β-hCG below the discriminatory zone (1000 mIU/mL) with an empty uterus and no abnormalities on endovaginal ultrasound suggestive of ectopic pregnancy. Patients with an isolated quantitative β-hCG below 1000 are not necessarily low risk because nearly one third of patients with ectopic pregnancies have a quantitative β-hCG level below 1000 mIU/mL.

Discharge the patient from the emergency department to outpatient care with a definite follow-up appointment for reevaluation within 1–2 days. Give the patient *written* instructions explaining that ectopic pregnancy is a possible diagnosis and that she must be

alert to the following symptoms, which would require that she return to the hospital immediately: (1) increased vaginal bleeding, (2) increased pelvic or abdominal pain, or (3) syncope.

SPONTANEOUS ABORTION

 ESSENTIALS OF DIAGNOSIS

- *Vaginal bleeding in early pregnancy.*
- *Pelvic and back pain common.*
- *Variable pelvic exam findings.*
- *Quantitative hCG and pelvic ultrasound.*
- *Exclude ectopic pregnancy.*

General Considerations

At least 20% of all pregnancies terminate in abortion, usually because of serious defects in the ovum. Half of abortions occur before the 8th week of gestation and another quarter before the 16th week. Many of these early spontaneous abortions go unnoticed as a delayed menstrual period. Nevertheless, early spontaneous abortions are also a common cause of visits to the emergency department.

If the fetus dies but is not expelled, a missed abortion occurs. If this state persists for longer than 4–6 weeks, disseminated intravascular coagulation may occur. Table 36–4 describes the various types of spontaneous abortion.

Table 36–4. Classification of spontaneous abortion.

Type	Symptoms and Signs
Threatened abortion	Mild, transient uterine cramps with minimal transient vaginal bleeding. The cervix is long and closed. Uterine size is compatible with the presumed length of pregnancy.[1] Symptoms of pregnancy continue, and the conceptus remains viable.
Inevitable abortion	Persistent uterine cramps and moderate vaginal bleeding. The cervical os is open (ie, a 0.5-cm [3/16-in] diameter sponge stick passes easily). Passage of some or all of the products of conception is inevitable or is about to occur; ie, fetal or placental tissue is found in the vagina or protrudes through the cervical os, or the patient gives a history of passage of tissue. Symptoms and signs of pregnancy disappear.
Incomplete abortion	Uterine cramps and vaginal bleeding are persistent and excessive. Symptoms of pregnancy may disappear. Products of conception are noted in the vagina, or the patient gives a history of passage of tissue.
Complete abortion	Uterine cramps markedly diminish or stop. Vaginal bleeding ceases. The entire conceptus is expelled. Symptoms of pregnancy disappear.
Missed abortion	The products of conception are retained. Symptoms and signs of pregnancy abate, and results of pregnancy tests change to negative. Brownish vaginal discharge (rarely, frank bleeding) occurs. Uterine cramps are rare. Examination shows a small and irregularly softened uterus. Ultrasonography fails to demonstrate a live fetus; ie, fetal heart motion is absent.

[1]Uterine size in centimeters measured from the top of the symphysis pubica to the top of the uterine fundus is a useful approximation of gestational age in weeks from 15–16 weeks through 32–33 weeks. A normal 20-week gestational age uterine size should be at the level of the umbilicus.

Clinical Findings

A. SYMPTOMS AND SIGNS

Almost all patients have a history suggesting possible pregnancy:

- Sexual intercourse
- Period of amenorrhea (absence of menses for a duration of 3 cycles or 6 months in women previously menstruating)
- Nausea and vomiting; breast tenderness
- Uterine cramps and vaginal bleeding
- Passage of fetal or placental tissue (in inevitable, incomplete, or complete abortion)

Caution: Pelvic examination should be performed on all patients with suspected abortion and on all pregnant patients with vaginal bleeding who have reached less than 20 weeks' gestation. Extreme care, however, must be exercised in examining patients in the second trimester; instruments should not be introduced into the cervical os. Beyond 20 weeks' gestation, pelvic examination should be done by an obstetrician because of the increasing risk of placenta previa.

B. LABORATORY TESTS AND SPECIAL EXAMINATIONS

In the first trimester of pregnancy, a β-hCG level that does not double in 48 hours suggests fetal demise. Real-time ultrasonography, using abdominal or vaginal probes, can be diagnostic, for example, demonstrating a fetus without heartbeat or movement. Pathologic examination of tissue expelled by the uterus confirms passage of the products of conception.

Treatment & Disposition

Blood typing and antibody screening are required in all patients with abortion of any type. If patients are Rh-negative, give $Rh_o(D)$ immune globulin (RhoGAM, many others), 1 vial, within 72 hours after any event in which fetal-maternal transfusion may occur, including abortion.

A. THREATENED ABORTION

Advise the patient to rest. Do not use hormones, douches, or tampons. The patient should not engage in coitus. Ultrasound scan may reveal a gestational sac or evidence of fetal cardiac activity. Discharge instructions must include follow-up instructions and indications for return to the emergency department, including passage of fetal tissue, severe vaginal bleeding greater than one pad per hour, significant abdominal or pelvic pain, or fever. The patient should also be given adequate narcotic analgesia for pain management.

B. INCOMPLETE OR INEVITABLE ABORTION

Hospitalize the patient if hypovolemia or anemia is present or if the pregnancy is past the first trimester. Treat hypovolemia if present. An obstetrical or gynecological consult should be obtained to perform suction curettage or dilation and curettage as the treatment of choice.

C. COMPLETE ABORTION

The patient may be discharged to home care if vital signs and hematocrit are stable and if vaginal bleeding is clearly decreasing. Pain must also be clearly decreasing and the cervical os closed. A physician must differentiate a complete abortion from an incomplete abortion. Several clues can help the physician determine that a complete abortion has occurred:

- A reliable history.
- Ultrasound revealing a clean uterine stripe.
- The products of conception are brought to the physician and confirmed by pathology. If pathology is not readily available, a physician can rub the specimen between a gauze pad; if the specimen is a blood clot it will dissolve. However, if the specimen is true products of conception, the specimen will not dissolve. A physician may also run the specimen under water; a blood clot will dissolve, whereas products of conception will not.

D. MISSED ABORTION (RETAINED CONCEPTUS)

Obtain CBC, differential, and coagulation panel (platelet count, prothrombin time, and partial thromboplastin time). Obtain disseminated intravascular coagulation screening tests if abnormal values are found. Hospitalize the patient, and prepare to perform dilation and curettage if evidence indicates infection or disseminated intravascular coagulation or if the products of conception have been retained more than 4 weeks.

Outpatient management of early missed abortion is possible if the patient is closely monitored for possible spontaneous abortion and if fibrinogen levels are measured weekly. Levels below 150 mg/dL call for evacuation of the uterine contents.

SEPTIC ABORTION

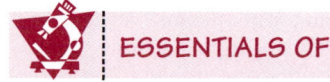

ESSENTIALS OF DIAGNOSIS

- *History of gynecologic procedure or abortion.*
- *Pelvic pain.*
- *Systemic signs of infection.*

- *Tender uterus.*
- *Profuse, malodorous vaginal discharge.*

General Considerations

Septic abortion is a rare complication after some obstetric-gynecologic procedures. Septic abortion may also arise as a result of nonsterile nontherapeutic abortion. The usual cause of sepsis is incomplete evacuation of the products of conception. Infection is usually due to mixed aerobic and anaerobic bacteria (bacteroides, *Prevotella,* group B streptococci, Enterobacteriaceae, and *C trachomatis*) and is rapidly progressive, extending quickly through the myometrium and involving the adnexa and pelvic peritoneum. Septic pelvic thrombophlebitis with or without septic pulmonary embolization is an uncommon but devastating complication.

Clinical Findings

A. SYMPTOMS AND SIGNS

Symptoms and signs are consistent with a history of recent pregnancy and induced abortion followed by pelvic pain and symptoms of infection. Nonjudgmental questioning in a private setting by a physician may be necessary to elicit a history of nontherapeutic abortion; in some cases, such a history is never obtained. Clinical findings include signs of infection (eg, fever, leukocytosis); diffuse pelvic tenderness; and profuse, foul vaginal discharge in most cases. Frank septic shock may be present.

B. IMAGING

Ultrasound or other imaging techniques (computed tomography [CT], magnetic resonance imaging) may show retained intrauterine material, uterine emphysema, or intraperitoneal air from uterine perforation.

Treatment & Disposition

Evacuation of the uterine contents is crucial and is the mainstay of treatment. It should be preceded by broad-spectrum antibiotic therapy (see below).

Note: Although antibiotic therapy alone is effective in the earliest stage of infection, many patients require emergency hysterectomy. Death may occur despite the best treatment.

A. IMMEDIATE MEASURES

Hospitalize the patient at once, and start general measures for septic shock (Chapters 9 and 40). Obtain emergency surgical obstetric and gynecologic consultation.

B. Laboratory Tests

Obtain samples of blood and uterine discharge for culture. Draw blood for CBC, tests of hepatic and renal function, serum electrolyte determination, prothrombin time, partial thromboplastin time, platelet count, and disseminated intravascular coagulation screening tests if initial findings are abnormal.

C. Antibiotics

After taking specimens for culture of aerobic and anaerobic organisms, give antibiotics (eg, doxycycline, 100 mg every 12 hours intravenously and one of the following: cefoxitin, 2.0 g every 6–8 hours intravenously, ticarcillin-clavulanate, 3.1 g every 6 hours intravenously, or imipenem cilastatin, 0.5 g every 6 hours intravenously).

CARCINOMA & OTHER TUMORS

Although gynecologic cancers seldom present as emergency situations, the emergency physician should be aware of the various presenting symptoms and risk factors associated with gynecologic cancers.

Carcinoma of the Vulva

Vulvar cancers are rarely sudden in onset and usually occur in women over age 50 years. They are more common in women with a history of cervical dysplasia or cancer.

Patients seeking treatment for vulvar lesions in the emergency department should be advised to seek gynecologic consultation if any lesion initially thought to be due to infection or trauma fails to heal in a short time. Persistent unremitting vaginal pruritus is the single most common symptom of vulvar cancer and should never be dismissed as a frivolous complaint in the postmenopausal patient.

Carcinoma of the vulva is not commonly seen in the emergency department.

Carcinoma of the Vagina

Vaginal cancers are rare. Bleeding is typically the presenting complaint. The patient is usually age 50 years or older, but even teenagers have developed clear cell carcinoma (eg, girls whose mothers were given diethylstilbestrol during pregnancy).

The source of the vaginal bleeding must be identified, and a speculum should be used to carefully inspect the vaginal walls. Careful digital examination of the vaginal mucosa is critical to detect submucosal infiltration by the tumor.

Carcinoma of the Cervix

Vaginal bleeding is the most common symptom in cervical cancer. Patients may be in their late 20s to (most commonly) early 40s. Patients often complain of persistent watery discharge. Speculum examination reveals a necrotic friable lesion on the cervix.

Uncontrollable bleeding from the cervix may be treated with applications of ferric subsulfate solution or vaginal packing. Manipulation should be kept to a minimum. Biopsy of the lesion at its margin with normal tissue usually confirms the diagnosis, but this procedure should be performed only in an operating room.

Carcinoma of the Endometrium

Postmenopausal bleeding is the most common symptom of endometrial carcinoma. Risk factors associated with endometrial carcinoma include ingestion of exogenous estrogens, obesity, infertility, polycystic ovarian syndrome, and age over 50 years.

The physician should not try to stop postmenopausal bleeding with administration of hormones (eg, estrogens or progesterone) without confirming the diagnosis beforehand. Consultation with a gynecologist should be obtained prior to discharge for further input.

Carcinoma of the Ovaries

Patients with ovarian cancer may have abdominal distention from ascites, intestinal obstruction, or rarely, acute abdominal pain. The possibility of ovarian cancer should be considered in any woman with abdominal or pelvic symptoms. Definitive diagnosis requires surgical or gynecologic consultation for laparotomy or laparoscopy.

Other Tumors

Patients with gestational trophoblastic disease may present with heavy vaginal bleeding and symptoms similar to those of early miscarriage, but the following symptoms and signs suggest trophoblastic disease: (1) heavy vaginal bleeding with or without passage of tissue, or great clusters of tissue aborted from the cervical os, (2) uterine size inappropriately large for dates, (3) profound anemia, (4) history of molar pregnancy, (5) first-trimester hypertension or preeclampsia, or (6) β-hCG remarkably elevated over the expected values. The diagnosis can be confirmed by ultrasound examination.

Any patient presenting with neurologic signs and with a recent history of molar pregnancy or trophoblastic disease may have cerebral metastasis. Central nervous system metastasis of trophoblastic disease represents a true oncologic emergency, because cerebral metastasis has the potential for cure as long as rapid growth or hemorrhage does not occur.

Patients with trophoblastic disease should be hospitalized for gynecologic consultation and possible referral to a regional trophoblastic disease center, where help is readily available.

GENITAL TRAUMA

Genital trauma in women almost always occurs as a result of sexual activity, either forced (rape) or voluntary (foreign bodies introduced into the vagina in sexual play). Penile thrusts rarely produce trauma unless it is the first sexual experience.

Clinical Findings

The most common presenting complaints are vaginal bleeding and pain or dyspareunia. Examination usually reveals bleeding from a tear in the genital mucosa or skin. Bleeding is rarely brisk enough to produce signs of hypovolemia, but if these are present, replace volume losses, and provide supportive care (Chapter 9). In prepubertal patients, general anesthesia may be required for adequate examination.

Treatment & Disposition

Determine whether rape has occurred, and proceed accordingly. Provide sedation or analgesia if necessary.

Treat hypovolemia if present. Control vaginal bleeding temporarily with a vaginal pack or, if bleeding is from the external genitalia, with direct firm pressure (combined with an indwelling urinary catheter).

Hospitalize the patient if bleeding cannot be easily and definitively controlled, and obtain gynecologic consultation. Small lesions at the introitus may be repaired in the emergency department under local anesthesia. However, small and seemingly minor vaginal tears may communicate with either the rectum or the peritoneum; consequently, such repairs are best performed by a gynecologist in an operating room with adequate anesthesia and good exposure.

RUPTURED OVARIAN CYST

ESSENTIALS OF DIAGNOSIS

- *Sudden, moderate to severe unilateral pelvic pain.*
- *Possible history of initial nausea, diaphoresis, near-syncope.*
- *Lack of systemic signs of infection.*
- *Negative pregnancy test.*

- *Unilateral adnexal tenderness without mass.*
- *Pelvic ultrasound excludes significant hemorrhage.*

Clinical Findings

Ruptured ovarian cyst is associated with sudden, moderately severe pelvic or lower abdominal pain. There are no gastrointestinal symptoms. The patient is afebrile, and leukocytosis is variable. Tenderness is found over the affected ovary, and there are no masses. A pregnancy test should be obtained, because ectopic pregnancy is a possible diagnosis. Ultrasonography may show the presence of an ovarian cyst or free pelvic fluid and is useful to detect ectopic pregnancy.

Treatment & Disposition

The physician should provide adequate analgesics, including narcotics if needed. The patient should be observed and may require hospitalization if the diagnosis is uncertain or if relief is required for severe pain not relieved by narcotics. Surgery is rarely required unless there is a significant hemoperitoneum from the rupture of a hemorrhagic corpus luteum cyst with hemodynamic instability.

TORSION OF OVARIAN TUMOR

ESSENTIALS OF DIAGNOSIS

- *Extremes of age.*
- *Single or recurrent moderate unilateral pelvic pain.*
- *Negative pregnancy test.*
- *Pelvic mass.*
- *Pelvic ultrasound.*

Clinical Findings

Torsion of ovarian tumor is associated with a history of attacks of cramps and pains, usually unilateral, in the lower abdomen and possibly in the flank. The symptoms, such as nausea, may be gradual, or they may occur suddenly if there is accompanying intraovarian bleeding. Discomfort is characterized by symptoms of pelvic mass (eg, painful defecation and dyspareunia). Ultrasonography may delineate the mass. Doppler studies may detect decreased or absent blood flow to the torsed ovary.

Treatment & Disposition

Hospitalize the patient, and obtain urgent gynecologic consultation. Pelvic ultrasonography may be a useful diagnostic tool, but laparoscopy is frequently required. Laparotomy is indicated if the diagnosis is confirmed or if the patient's condition deteriorates.

ENDOMETRIOSIS

 ESSENTIALS OF DIAGNOSIS

- *Recurrent pelvic, flank, or abdominal pain with menses.*
- *Negative pregnancy test.*

Clinical Findings

The patient with endometriosis gives a history of attacks of cramps and pains in the lower abdomen and possibly in the flank that are associated with menstruation. Symptoms may be gradual, or sudden if bleeding is present. Acquired dysmenorrhea is most commonly due to endometriosis. Other symptoms include painful defecation and dyspareunia.

Treatment & Disposition

Refer the patient for further gynecologic evaluation. Definitive diagnosis usually requires laparoscopy. Provide oral analgesia as needed.

DYSMENORRHEA

 ESSENTIALS OF DIAGNOSIS

- *Painful menstruation.*
- *Negative pregnancy test.*
- *Exclude pelvic infection.*

Clinical Findings

Many women experience painful menstruation (dysmenorrhea). The pain is cramping in nature, may be debilitating, and is usually relieved by release of menstrual contents from the uterus. The pain occurs because of elaboration of excessive quantities of prostaglandins by the endometrium with subsequent increased uterine tone. It is not psychological in origin.

Idiopathic dysmenorrhea usually begins at menarche and is probably more common than the acquired form. Acquired dysmenorrhea, occurring in the late teens and early 20s, may suggest endometriosis and is common in chronic pelvic inflammatory disease.

Treatment & Disposition

Both types of dysmenorrhea may be seen by the emergency physician and may be treated by prostaglandin inhibitors (eg, ibuprofen, 400 mg orally every 6 hours; naproxen, 250–500 mg twice daily, or controlled release, 750–1000 mg every day). Local application of heat to the lower abdomen may be helpful.

MITTELSCHMERZ

Midcycle pain (mittelschmerz) is common in women with regular menstrual periods who are not taking birth control pills. These patients may commonly have midcycle spotting caused by an estrogen surge. There is no fever and no other abnormal bleeding such as that resulting from trauma to the cervix (eg, coitus, douching). Pain usually occurs over several cycles. There is no history of intermittent lower abdominal pain. Examination at the time of mittelschmerz may reveal some lower quadrant tenderness with or without rebound. Bimanual examination may show localized tenderness. A palpable ovary may be present, but a history of regular menses, lack of fever, and negative pregnancy tests confirm the diagnosis.

Mild analgesics and reassurance are usually adequate for these patients.

UTERINE PROLAPSE

 ESSENTIALS OF DIAGNOSIS

- *Prior vaginal deliveries.*
- *History of pelvic heaviness, low back pain.*
- *Patient may present with urinary retention.*
- *Firm, muscular mass in or protruding from vagina.*

Clinical Findings

Uterine prolapse typically occurs because of muscular defects in the pelvic floor arising from childbirth. Prolapse is characterized by variable symptoms of pelvic heaviness or a dragging sensation and lower back pain.

Urinary retention of sudden onset may be a presenting complaint. Examination reveals a firm, muscular mass in the vagina or protruding from the vagina (procidentia) and having the shape and size of the uterus and cervix. Cystocele, rectocele, and enterocele are commonly associated with procidentia.

Treatment & Disposition

Acute postpartum prolapse is an emergency that requires immediate obstetric and gynecologic consultation. Patients with acute urinary retention or procidentia should have urgent gynecologic consultation. Patients with mild prolapse should be referred within 5–7 days for gynecologic evaluation and possible surgery.

SALPINGITIS & TUBO-OVARIAN ABSCESS (See Chapter 40.)

RAPE (MEN & WOMEN)

Proper care of the alleged rape victim requires concern for the social and emotional consequences of the event as well as for the medical sequelae. The best care fulfills the requirements of the law while providing proper support and reassurance to the patient. Every state has its own laws and regulations concerning rape; however, some general principles apply. The physician's responsibilities include the following:

- Recognizing and managing life-threatening trauma (eg, hemorrhagic shock).
- Obtaining informed written consent for physical examination, collection of evidence, photographic documentation, and treatment.
- Shielding the alleged rape victim from other patients, bystanders, and visitors.
- Accurately diagnosing and treating all physical injuries, both genital and nongenital.
- Recording a detailed and explicit history of the event in the patient's own words.
- Carefully collecting specimens for evidence, with accurate documentation and protection of the chain of evidence.
- Providing psychological support and follow-up.
- Offering prophylaxis against pregnancy and sexually transmitted disease.
- Avoiding a "diagnosis" of rape (it is not a medical diagnosis but a matter of jurisprudence). The physician should also avoid judgmental or conclusive language.
- Being willing to testify in court.

- Ensuring that discharge from the emergency department is to a safe place.
- Encouraging a physical examination even if the patient declines forensic examination.

Unless required to do so by statute, the emergency physician does not have a legal obligation to notify the police when providing treatment to a victim of alleged rape. Notifying the police is appropriate when the patient has consented (preferably in writing) to such notification. The physician may wish to refer the patient to a counseling organization that aids rape victims.

The responsibilities described above are often best fulfilled by having teams experienced in working with rape victims perform the evaluation. Such teams should follow an established written protocol and document all findings in writing.

1. Management of the Female Rape Victim

Evaluation

A. INITIAL STEPS

If required by law or with the patient's consent, inform the police (see below). Obtain written informed consent for examination.

B. HISTORY

Obtain and record the history in the patient's own words. Obtain answers to other specific questions (if they have not already been answered). Record the victim's general appearance and demeanor, and note whether clothing is torn or stained.

C. EVIDENCE

Collect and label relevant evidence, and protect the chain of evidence:

1. Scrape under the fingernails, and also take trimmings from them.
2. Comb pubic hair, and look for loose hairs from the assailant.
3. Pull a few pubic hairs and save them.
4. Collect any other loose hairs or dried blood.
5. Examine the perineum and other suspect areas with a Woods light (prostatic secretions are fluorescent even when dry).
6. Prepare 4 dried slides of vaginal contents (wash the vagina with saline if it is dry), and fix them with ether-alcohol.
7. Collect vaginal aspirate or washings into a screw-topped specimen tube for acid phosphatase determination (a positive reaction indicates the presence of prostatic fluid ejaculate).

8. Place a cotton swab of vaginal contents into a specimen tube (for typing of the blood group antigen in semen).

9. Obtain material from the cervix for culture for gonococci and *C trachomatis.*

10. Obtain urine for urinalysis (look for hematuria indicating genitourinary trauma). Perform a urine pregnancy test.

11. Photograph all external lesions, but only with the patient's written consent.

12. If oral or rectal penetration has occurred, steps 5–9 should be repeated with specimens from those sites.

D. PHYSICAL EXAMINATION

Thoroughly examine the patient for signs of trauma, discharge, or bleeding; record the results of the examination; and photograph all lesions (the last only with the patient's written consent).

E. PELVIC EXAMINATION

Look carefully for signs of trauma to the external genitalia. Note and record whether the hymen is intact and whether any hymenal tags are fresh (indicating trauma) or healed.

Using a warm, water-moistened speculum, carefully examine the vagina for lacerations. Topical application of toluidine blue may enhance identification of genital skin tears. Colposcopy enhances the identification of traumatic injury. Rarely, peritoneal perforation may occur.

Evaluate the cervix for signs of preexisting pregnancy and trauma. Examine the rectal area. If penetration has occurred, proctoscopy may be advisable.

F. LABORATORY TESTS

Obtain blood for blood chemistry studies (if indicated), a serologic test for syphilis, and blood typing (to compare the alleged assailant's type with that of the victim). Blood sampling may also be used for hepatitis B and human immunodeficiency virus (HIV) serologic testing.

Treatment

The physician should be empathic and concerned, never skeptical or judgmental.

A. PREVENT SEXUALLY TRANSMITTED DISEASE

Treatment for gonorrhea, *C trachomatis,* and syphilis (Chapter 40) should be offered but not forced on the patient. Only about 3% of rapes result in gonorrhea,

and only about 0.1% result in syphilis. Follow-up cultures for *N. gonorrhoeae* are essential. Perform follow-up serologic tests for syphilis 1 and 3 months after the rape.

B. PREVENT INFECTIOUS DISEASES

Offer the hepatitis B vaccine as well as follow-up in 3–4 weeks for repeat hepatitis vaccination and testing. HIV is also of concern. Start prophylactic medications based on risk factors with a follow-up for repeat HIV testing.

C. PREVENT PREGNANCY

Treatment for the prevention of pregnancy should be offered but not forced on the patient. Only about 1% of rapes result in pregnancy; the chances are much less if the victim is using an effective method of contraception. Give ethinyl estradiol, 200 µg, and norgestrel, 2 mg, orally over 12 hours in 2 divided doses (eg, norgestrel [Ovral], 2 tablets orally, repeating in 12 hours), to prevent implantation if it is certain that the patient is not already pregnant. Advise the patient that nausea and vomiting may occur. Give an antiemetic 40 minutes prior to the oral contraceptives.

Caution: Existing pregnancy is an absolute contraindication to the use of oral contraceptives. Warn the patient that this regimen may not be effective, and explain that a return visit within 1–2 weeks is essential for another pregnancy test.

D. REPORT THE INCIDENT

If required by law or if the patient consents, report the incident to the proper authorities before the patient leaves the emergency department, because the police will want to question her. If the alleged victim is a child, the incident may be child abuse and should be reported to the appropriate child welfare authorities (Chapter 48).

E. START RAPE COUNSELING IMMEDIATELY

Preferably, counseling should be directed by experienced personnel who are part of an established rape counseling program.

F. ARRANGE FOLLOW-UP

A definite appointment (time, place, and physician or clinic) should be made.

2. Management of the Male Rape Victim

Clinical Findings & Evaluation

A. INITIAL STEPS

If required by law or with the patient's consent, inform the police (see below). Obtain written informed consent for examination.

B. HISTORY

Obtain and record the history as described above.

C. EVIDENCE

Collect and label relevant evidence, and protect the chain of evidence:

1. Scrape under the fingernails, and also take trimmings from them.
2. Collect any loose hairs or dried blood.
3. Using the techniques and preparations described in steps 5–9 under Management of the Female Rape Victim, examine samples of material from the mouth and rectum.

D. PHYSICAL EXAMINATION

Thoroughly examine the patient for signs of trauma, discharge, or bleeding; record the results of the examination. Photograph all lesions, but only with the patient's consent.

Examine the mouth and the rectum for injuries. Proctoscopy may be advisable if penetration has occurred and if foreign objects were used, because peritoneal perforation may occur from rectal trauma.

E. LABORATORY TESTS

Obtain blood for blood chemistry studies (if indicated), a serologic test for syphilis, and blood typing (to compare the alleged assailant's type with that of the victim).

Treatment

A. PREVENT SEXUALLY TRANSMITTED DISEASE

Offer treatment and preventive therapy for sexually transmitted disease, as described above and in Chapter 40.

B. REPORT THE INCIDENT

If required by law or if the patient consents, report the incident to the proper authorities before the patient leaves the emergency department, because the police will want to question him. If the alleged victim is a child, the incident may represent child abuse and should be reported to the appropriate child welfare authorities (Chapter 48).

C. START RAPE COUNSELING IMMEDIATELY

Preferably, counseling should be directed by experienced personnel who are part of an established rape counseling program. Male victims of rape need counseling just as much as female victims.

INTRAUTERINE DEVICES

Problems with IUDs

A. "LOST" IUD

In the emergency department, the most common problem relating to these devices is the "lost" IUD. Check to see if the IUD is still properly placed by looking for the removal string protruding from the cervix (most women soon learn to feel for it with a finger). If no string can be found, the IUD may be located by uterine sonography or abdominal x-ray (for metallic IUDs). The IUD may be in an extrauterine position, in which case it should be removed surgically by laparoscopy or laparotomy, although this is usually not an emergency.

B. EMERGENCY REMOVAL OF IUD

1. Infection—The principal indication for removal of an IUD in the emergency department is infection (salpingitis, endometritis, pyosalpinx, or pelvic peritonitis). The incidence of endometritis, salpingitis, and tubal abscess is increased in women using IUDs. Any of these conditions requires removal of the IUD so that infection can be completely cleared. If possible, the patient should be started on appropriate antibiotics before the device is removed in order to ensure adequate blood levels of the drug (see "Salpingitis" section in Chapter 40).

2. Bleeding and pain—Persistent vaginal bleeding or pelvic pain usually requires removal of an IUD but not often on an emergency basis. Referral to the physician who inserted the device is preferable.

If referral is impractical, grasp the string of the IUD with a Kelly clamp or other long grasping forceps, and pull with gentle but increasing force until the IUD emerges from the uterus. Do not jerk the string, because it may detach from the device and make removal more difficult. If the string is not easily seen after manipulation with a speculum, use a special IUD remover to locate and grasp the string. Alternatively, explore the endocervix with a crochet hook; this generally frees the string so that it can be easily grasped and the device removed.

C. SERIOUS BUT RARE PROBLEMS

1. Perforation of the uterus—Perforation of the uterus is a probable diagnosis in patients with IUDs who have symptoms of endometritis, salpingitis, or peritonitis. Physical examination, an abdominal x-ray, and sonography show that the IUD is embedded in the uterine wall or free in the peritoneum. Emergency hospitalization is required.

2. Pregnancy with IUD in place—If pregnancy is confirmed by a positive pregnancy test, and an IUD is still in place, seek emergency obstetric consultation. Ectopic pregnancy is a distinct possibility in the pregnant patient with an IUD still in place.

POSTCOITAL EMERGENCY CONTRACEPTION

Postcoital emergency contraception, also known as the morning-after pill, can be given to prevent implantation. The U.S. Food and Drug Administration has approved 2 tablets, each containing 0.5 mg ethinyl estradiol and 0.5 mg DL-norgestrel, within 72 hours of intercourse and repeated again 12 hours later. Norgestrel [Ovral] has this combination; however, several prescriptive equivalents are available. Nausea and emesis frequently occur, and an antiemetic should be prescribed. Although the morning-after pill is reported to be 98% effective, a pregnancy test should be performed if menstruation does not occur within 21 days of treatment.

DISORDERS OF THE VULVA & VAGINA

Vaginal and vulvar cancers and other lesions are discussed earlier in this chapter. Vaginitis, gonorrhea, genital herpes virus infection, and genital abscesses are discussed in Chapter 40.

A WARNING ABOUT DISCONTINUING CONTRACEPTION

Treatment of gynecologic problems in the emergency department may require discontinuing the patient's current form of contraception. The emergency physician advising this course of action must warn the patient of the possibility of pregnancy and offer appropriate contraceptive advice. Discontinuation of oral contraceptives or IUD use because of treatment in the emergency department should not result in an unwanted pregnancy.

American College of Emergency Physicians: ACEP emergency ultrasound guidelines—2001. Ann Emerg Med 2001;38:470. [PMID: 11574810]

Ankum WM: Diagnosing suspected ectopic pregnancy: HCG monitoring and transvaginal ultrasound lead the way. [Editorial]. Br Med J 2000;321:1235. [PMID: 1182067]

Buckley RG et al: History and physical examination to estimate the risk of ectopic pregnancy: validation of a clinical prediction model. Ann Emerg Med 1999;34(5):589. [PMID: 10533005]

Ciancone AC et al: Sexual assault nurse examiner programs in the United States. Ann Emerg Med 2000;35(4):353. [PMID: 10736121]

Counselman FL et al: Quantitative B-HCG levels less than 1000 mIU/ML in patients with ectopic pregnancy: pelvic ultrasound still useful. J Emerg Med 1998;16:699. [PMID: 9754920]

Dart R et al: Normal intrauterine pregnancy is unlikely in emergency department patients with either menstrual days > 38 days or beta-HCG > 3,000 mIU/ml, but without a gestational sac on ultrasonography. Acad Emerg Med 1997;4:967. [PMID: 9332628]

Dart R, Dart L, Mitchell P: Normal intrauterine pregnancy is unlikely in patients who have echogenic material identified within the endometrial cavity at transvaginal ultrasonography. Acad Emerg Med 1999;6:116. [PMID: 10051902]

Dart RG: Role of pelvic ultrasonography in evaluation of symptomatic first-trimester pregnancy. Ann Emerg Med 1999;33 (3):310. [PMID: 10036346]

Durham B et al: Pelvic ultrasound performed by emergency physicians for the detection of ectopic pregnancy in complicated first-trimester pregnancies. Ann Emerg Med 1997;29(3):338. [PMID: 9055772]

Mateer JR et al: Outcome analysis of a protocol including bedside endovaginal sonography in patients at risk for ectopic pregnancy. Ann Emerg Med 1996;27(3):283. [PMID: 8599484]

Rodrigues I, Grou F, Joly J: Effectiveness of emergency contraceptive pills between 72 and 120 hours after unprotected sexual intercourse. Am J Obstet Gynecol 2001;184:531. [PMID: 11262449]

Shih CHY: Effect of emergency physician–performed pelvic sonography on length of stay in the emergency department. Ann Emerg Med 1997;29:348. [PMID: 9055773]

Wilcox AJ et al: Natural limits of pregnancy testing in relation to the expected menstrual period. JAMA 2001;286:1759. [PMID: 11594902]

■ EMERGENCY MANAGEMENT OF OBSTETRIC DISORDERS

PREGNANCY

Clinical Findings

The diagnosis and differential diagnosis of pregnancy are a critical skill in the emergency department, where many serious obstetric disorders (eg, abortion or ectopic implantation) may be seen.

A. EARLY SYMPTOMS AND SIGNS

Amenorrhea, nausea and vomiting, syncopal attacks, breast tenderness or tingling, and urinary symptoms (especially frequency) are early symptoms of pregnancy. Early signs of pregnancy include cervical cyanosis and softening, vaginal cyanosis, softening and enlargement of the uterus, and breast enlargement and tenderness.

B. LABORATORY TESTS

Urinary tests for pregnancy may occasionally be negative early in the pregnancy. False-positive results are rare at any time, unless trophoblastic tumors are present.

Patients with trophoblastic tumors ranging from benign hydatidiform mole to choriocarcinoma can present with incomplete abortion or bleeding during the second trimester of pregnancy without evidence of fetal activity. Serum hCG is often high (false-positive pregnancy test).

Ectopic pregnancies and spontaneous abortions may rarely cause false-negative results on urine immunologic pregnancy tests.

Differential Diagnosis of Pregnancy

The differential diagnosis of pregnancy includes disorders producing secondary amenorrhea (endocrinopathies, emotional stress, drugs, malnutrition, and menopause) and those producing abdominal or uterine enlargement (obesity, tumors, pseudopregnancy [pseudocyesis]).

DISCOMFORTS OF PREGNANCY

Pregnant women are subject to many discomforts, any of which may cause a visit to the emergency department. If drug therapy of these complaints is contemplated, only drugs generally recognized as safe in pregnancy should be used, and the patient should be informed of potential benefits and risks. Common problems include vomiting, backache, syncopal attacks, urinary symptoms (with and without demonstrable urinary tract infection), heartburn, constipation, hemorrhoids, varicose veins, leg swelling, and cramps.

Rarely, pregnant women may have severe abdominal pain localized to one or another quadrant. Patients with round ligament pain may present in this manner. The pain tends to be fairly constant, not cramping. Temperature and white blood cell count are usually normal. Treatment consists of oral analgesics and bed rest.

Nausea and vomiting are common in the first trimester and usually occur in the morning. Patients with persistent vomiting (hyperemesis gravidarum) with dehydration, elevated specific gravity of urine, ketonuria, and hemoconcentration may require hospitalization for parenteral hydration and nutrition. Symptomatic treatment of nausea and vomiting is preferred, for example, eating soda crackers immediately on arising in the morning, or consuming small, frequent, low-fat meals.

HYPEREMESIS GRAVIDARUM

Clinical Findings

Hyperemesis gravidarum is usually easily diagnosed. However, other causes of vomiting, such as infection, diabetes mellitus, or abdominal disorders, must be excluded.

A. SYMPTOMS AND SIGNS

Patients who are known to be pregnant or have symptoms and signs of pregnancy (see above) complain of persistent vomiting, often with postural dizziness, pre-syncope, weight loss, or other signs of dehydration. Hyperemesis gravidarum usually resolves early in the second trimester. Physical examination reveals signs of dehydration: hypotension or postural hypotension, tachycardia, dry mucous membranes, and collapsed neck veins. Patients are rarely in severe shock.

B. LABORATORY TESTS

The test for pregnancy usually is positive, although rarely urinary tests may be negative early in pregnancy. Blood tests may show hemoconcentration, elevated blood urea nitrogen or creatinine, hypokalemia, or metabolic alkalosis. The urine usually appears concentrated with high specific gravity and ketonuria.

Treatment

A. INITIAL STEPS

Insert an 18-gauge intravenous catheter (a larger bore is rarely needed). Draw blood for CBC, electrolytes, and renal function. Infuse crystalloid solution containing glucose (eg, 0.9% saline with 5% dextrose) to correct hypovolemia. (Glucose administration will inhibit ketogenesis.) The amount and rate of administration depends on the severity of dehydration. Replace potassium as needed.

B. ANTIEMETICS

If emesis persists, administer an antiemetic. Use prochlorperazine, 5–10 mg intravenously (or intramuscularly); promethazine, 25 mg intravenously (or intramuscularly); or ondansetron, 8 mg orally twice daily.

Medications should be avoided during the first 10 weeks of pregnancy because of fetal organogenesis, but a risk-to-benefit ratio must be weighed on a case-by-case basis. The patient should be made aware of such risks before being given antiemetics.

Disposition

Hospitalize patients who have persistent vomiting or ketonuria. Patients whose emesis is controlled and whose ketonuria resolves may be discharged with telephone follow-up in 1–2 days. Antiemetic tablets or suppositories may be prescribed for the patient to use only as needed.

THIRD-TRIMESTER BLEEDING

General Considerations

The most common causes of third-trimester bleeding are abruptio placentae, placenta previa, lower genital tract bleeding, or systemic coagulopathy. The least severe cause, lower genital tract bleeding, should be diagnosed only after the more severe conditions have been excluded systematically.

Third-trimester bleeding must be treated as a grave emergency threatening the life of both mother and fetus. Vaginal, rectal, or speculum examination must never be done in the emergency department, because it may initiate hemorrhage.

Clinical Findings

A. PLACENTAL DISORDERS

1. Abruptio placentae—Premature separation of the placenta from the endometrium is characterized by severe abdominal and pelvic pain and tenderness. The separation is associated with hemorrhage into the subplacental space (between the uterus and the placenta). In most cases, patients present with vaginal bleeding. Several risk factors are associated with abruptio placentae, including advanced maternal age, multiparity, smoking, hypertension, external abdominal trauma, cocaine use, or a history of previous abruption. Signs and symptoms include uterine tenderness, vaginal bleeding, back or abdominal pain, and an increase in contractions. In some cases, however, the subplacental hemorrhage may be concealed (occult abruption). Preeclampsia-eclampsia is common, and disseminated intravascular coagulation may occur.

2. Placenta previa—A placenta implanted in the lower uterine wall usually causes painless bleeding in small volumes that occurs regularly over a short period of observation. Such seemingly small blood loss may produce a false sense of security, because sudden massive hemorrhage can occur at any time. Risk factors for placenta previa include increased age, increased parity, multiple gestations, and previous cesarean sections or abortions.

B. SYSTEMIC COAGULOPATHIES

Coagulation disorders are uncommon as the sole cause of third-trimester bleeding. Diagnosis is confirmed by routine coagulation studies.

Treatment

A. INITIAL STEPS

Obtain emergency obstetric consultation. Evaluate the patient for hypovolemia (as shown by supine or postural hypotension), and if present, correct it with intravenous infusion of crystalloid solution or whole blood.

B. LABORATORY TESTS

Insert a large-bore (≥ 16-gauge) intravenous catheter. Draw blood for CBC, coagulation studies (prothrombin time, partial thromboplastin time, fibrinogen, and platelet count), and measurement of blood urea nitrogen and serum creatinine. Type and cross-match for 4 units of whole blood, preferably fresh.

Monitor fetal heart tones and toxicology especially looking for the presence of cocaine. Obtain urine for urinalysis, and monitor urine output with an indwelling urinary catheter.

C. OTHER CONSIDERATIONS

Ultrasound should be used to determine the placental location, but this should not delay delivery if the fetus is in distress.

The pregnant patient should never be maintained for any length of time in the supine, recumbent position (see Trauma in Pregnancy, below).

Disposition

Hospitalize the patient immediately, and move her to a delivery unit as soon as possible. Fetal bradycardia increases the urgency of the need for cesarean section.

TOXEMIA OF PREGNANCY (Preeclampsia-Eclampsia)

Clinical Findings

Preeclampsia-eclampsia describes a condition that covers a spectrum of symptoms and a continuum of severity. The condition is characterized by pregnancy-induced hypertension, by proteinuria, and when severe (eclampsia), by seizures. Symptoms of preeclampsia and eclampsia are so variable that whenever a woman in the third trimester of pregnancy or early postpartum period comes to the emergency department with *any* complaint, her blood pressure should be checked and urinalysis performed to detect early signs of preeclampsia-eclampsia.

A. SYMPTOMS AND SIGNS

Symptoms and signs are variable and may include headache, various visual symptoms, and vertigo. Nausea and vomiting, hyperreflexia, and abdominal pain may occur. Especially alarming is pain in the upper right quadrant and epigastrium (so-called hepatic pain), which is due to compression of the swelling liver by its capsule. Nervousness, irritability, and even frank seizures may occur.

Hypertension or rising blood pressure relative to the patient's normal blood pressure is a significant sign. Note that blood pressure may not be sufficiently elevated to be considered abnormal because of the physiologic decline in blood pressure usually associated with pregnancy.

Peripheral edema is usually present. Spasm of retinal arterioles and hemorrhage may occur. Hepatomegaly or hepatic tenderness (or both) may be present.

B. Laboratory Findings

Critical laboratory findings confirming the diagnosis of preeclampsia-eclampsia are decreased urine output, elevated blood urea nitrogen and serum creatinine levels, decreased creatine clearance, proteinuria, and evidence of disseminated intravascular coagulation.

Treatment & Disposition

Patients with suspected preeclampsia-eclampsia should be evaluated by an obstetrician before they are discharged from the emergency department.

A. Mild Preeclampsia

Mild preeclampsia is characterized by diastolic blood pressure under 105 mm Hg, trace to 1+ proteinuria, good urinary output, and absence of other symptoms. The patient should rest in bed at home and must be closely monitored (eg, twice weekly).

B. Moderate to Severe Eclampsia

Moderate to severe eclampsia is characterized by proteinuria greater than 2+, diastolic blood pressure greater than 105 mm Hg, seizures, anuria, or severe edema. Hospitalize patients who are more than mildly ill or who worsen on bed rest at home. It is better to err on the side of hospitalization, because eclampsia occurring out of the hospital greatly increases the chances of maternal or fetal death.

Treat hyperreflexia with magnesium sulfate, 2–6 g in 50 mL half-normal or normal saline given over 30 minutes as an intravenous loading dose, followed by 2 g/h.

Treat hypertension with intravenous hydralazine (Alazine, Apresoline), 20 mg in 50 mL of lactated Ringer's injection or 5% dextrose in water, infused at a rate of 1 mg every 2 minutes. An infusion pump should be used if possible. When blood pressure falls below 160/110 mm Hg, slow the infusion to a rate of about 1 mg/h, and adjust to maintain desired blood pressure. Do not reduce blood pressure to "normal" levels (120/80 mm Hg), because renal shutdown may result. Hypertension may also be controlled using nitroprusside or labetalol. Continued seizure activity raises the possibility of intracranial pathology such as a cerebral hemorrhage, and a CT scan of the head may be in order.

Insert a Foley catheter. Monitor fluid intake and urinary output closely, and test urine for specific gravity and hematuria.

When neurologic and cardiovascular status is stable, transfer the patient to a hospital equipped to manage high-risk obstetric patients.

TRAUMA IN PREGNANCY

Trauma due to gunshot wounds, assault, or automobile accident may cause abruptio placentae, ruptured fetal membranes, or direct fetal trauma.

A. Normal Physiologic Changes

An awareness of the normal physiologic changes in pregnancy is important in evaluating and providing treatment to the mother and fetus.

- Systolic and diastolic blood pressure decreases approximately 10 mm Hg by the middle of the second trimester.
- Resting heart rate increases by 10–15 beats.
- Uterine blood flow increases to 17% of the cardiac output.
- Hematocrit decreases to a range of 30–36%.
- Tidal volume increases by 30–40%.
- Residual volume and functional residual capacity decrease.
- Leukocytosis is common by the second trimester.
- PCO_2 decreases to approximately 35 mm Hg (mild respiratory alkalosis).

B. Injuries

1. Blunt abdominal trauma—Motor vehicle accidents account for most trauma. Be aware of abruptio placentae or uterine rupture.

2. Penetrating abdominal injuries—During pregnancy, the physical response to intraperitoneal irritation may be decreased. A cephalad and lateral displacement of maternal intraabdominal viscera occurs.

C. Laboratory Findings

The Kleihauer-Betke test detects fetal blood cells in the maternal circulation and is a helpful means of quantifying fetal bleeding; it may help identify fetal hypovolemia before obvious fetal distress occurs.

Treatment

A. Blunt Abdominal Trauma

Beyond 24 weeks' gestation the patient should be placed in the left lateral decubitus position unless potential spinal injury is a concern. For the patient who is unable to have her spines cleared clinically, maintain spinal immobilization on a long, rigid spine board tilted slightly to the left. Ensure that ventilation and resuscitative measures are adequate. Anticipate rapid oxygen desaturation and aggressively treat any acidosis. A complete physical examination including a bimanual exam for evaluation of the cervical os should be completed. Maternal vital signs, vaginal bleeding, and any abdominal tenderness should be the focus of examination.

For a pregnancy greater than 20 weeks' gestation, use a standard fetal monitor to monitor fetal heart tones and contractions. Fetal distress may precede maternal hemodynamic instability as an indicator of inadequately resuscitated shock. The need for aggressive resuscitation measures cannot be overemphasized because blood loss is easily underestimated. Early notification of surgical and obstetrical consultants is important. Radiologic studies should proceed as indicated.

B. PENETRATING TRAUMA

Most gunshot wounds to the abdomen should be explored surgically. In a pregnant patient, unstable vital signs with any penetrating abdominal wound is an indication for a laparotomy. However, not all penetrating trauma requires surgery. For instance, stab wounds to the lower abdomen are less likely to cause visceral injuries than upper abdominal wounds and may not need exploratory laparotomy. Although generally considered contraindicated in pregnancy, diagnostic peritoneal lavage (Chapter 6) may help diagnose hemoperitoneum and the need for surgery.

The decision to perform surgery with or without delivery should be made in conjunction with a surgeon and an obstetrician. Several factors are used to make interventional decision, including gestational age, penetration of amniotic cavity, and fetal injury.

Perimortem Cesarean Delivery

A. INDICATIONS

A fetus may survive up to 30 minutes after maternal cardiac arrest, but the greatest likelihood for fetal survival is if delivery occurs within 4–5 minutes after maternal cardiac arrest. Another indication for a perimortem cesarean section is to improve the ability to complete maternal cardiopulmonary resuscitation.

B. TECHNIQUE

1. Cardiopulmonary resuscitation should continue throughout the procedure.
2. Make an abdominal incision approximately 4–5 cm below the xiphoid to 2–3 cm above the pubis.
3. Separate the rectus muscles bluntly in the midline and enter the peritoneum with a midline incision usually below the umbilicus.
4. Make a vertical incision from the top of the uterine fundus to above the opaque insertion of the bladder.
5. Remove the fetus.
6. Remove the placenta.
7. Close the uterus in one or two layers using large sutures.

LABOR & DELIVERY

In many hospitals, patients in active labor are seen initially in the emergency department. A calm and orderly approach to evaluation of these patients—as well as established policies for transfer of responsibility from emergency department staff to obstetric staff—is essential for proper management.

Evaluation

A. HISTORY

If records from prenatal visits are not available, ask the patient about recent or intercurrent illness and risk factors such as diabetes mellitus, valvular heart disease, or previous cesarean section delivery. Ask whether the membranes have ruptured. Determine parity. Estimate the due date and gestational age of the fetus.

B. PHYSICAL EXAMINATION

Record complete maternal vital signs. Perform brief physical examination of the mother. Determine frequency and intensity of uterine contractions.

Check for vaginal discharge by speculum examination (blood or meconium). The presence of amniotic fluid may be detected by an alkaline reaction (yellow turning to blue) with Nitrazine paper.

Determine fetal position, and sketch it on an outline of the female figure. Determine the fetal heart rate during and between uterine contractions.

Perform vaginal examination. **Note:** Do not perform digital examination if vaginal bleeding is present. Determine the presenting part and the degree of dilation and effacement of the cervix by speculum.

Clinical Findings

Progressive labor is characterized by uterine contractions occurring every 3 minutes and dilation of the cervical os. Abnormal signs requiring emergency obstetric consultation include fetal bradycardia (< 100 beats/min during or after uterine contractions, vaginal bleeding (on history or examination), transverse or breech presentations, and maternal illness (eg, eclampsia, coma, major trauma).

Treatment

A. PREMATURE BIRTH

Infants under 36 weeks' gestational age are likely to require neonatal intensive care. If there is no such nursery in the facility where the mother has sought treatment, consider transferring her to another facility unless she is in active labor and delivery is imminent or likely during transport (ie, baby is crowning or very low station). See Chapter 5 for further discussion. Children are better off being born at the site where the nursery exists than being transferred to the site after birth.

Give crystalloid solution, 1000 mL over 3–4 hours, and monitor cardiovascular status carefully. In consultation with an obstetrician, decisions can be made about the use of tocolysis, administration of maternal betamethasone for fetal lung maturity, and prophylaxis against group B streptococci by administration of penicillin G.

B. Routine Labor

When delivery is imminent, give nothing (or sips of clear fluids only) by mouth. Maintain or reinstate adequate hydration with intravenous fluids. Give analgesia if there are no contraindications. Obtain a baby warmer, if available, and try to have a labor and delivery nurse present. Notify the patient's obstetric care provider that she is in the hospital and in active labor.

C. Emergency Department Delivery

If the examiner determines that the presenting part is in vertex position and is near the vulva, it is probably better to allow the patient to deliver in the emergency department than to rush her into elevators and through corridors to the delivery unit.

1. Delivery—Analgesia may be given as needed to the mother with an uncomplicated term pregnancy. Delivery may be accomplished in either the lithotomy or the Sims position. Try to prepare a clean field (wash the vulva and perineum). Prevent sudden uncontrolled delivery of the fetal head.

Clear the infant's nasal passages and airway. If thick meconium staining of the amniotic fluid is present, be prepared to clear the newborn's airway carefully and immediately, that is, clear the nostrils with a suction bulb (or DeLee suction trap, if available) after the head is delivered but before the body is delivered. Check for the umbilical cord. The physician may need to intubate the infant immediately, before spontaneous respirations occur, and apply suction to the trachea.

Cut the umbilical cord after ligating it about 2–3 in (5–7.5 cm) from the infant's abdomen.

Deliver the placenta with gentle traction on the cord if it comes out easily. Massage the fundus to help obtain hemostasis and uterine tone. If the patient is not bleeding vigorously, the placenta may be left in place while the patient is sent to the delivery room for further measures (eg, suture of lacerations).

2. Postpartum measures—Dry and examine the infant, and resuscitate if necessary. *Keep the baby warm.*

Monitor the mother's blood pressure every 5 minutes for 15 minutes and then every 15 minutes for 1 hour. A sample of the infant's clotted cord blood should be sent for ABO and Rh typing and a serologic test for syphilis.

Disposition

Hospitalize the newborn infant and mother for evaluation and supportive care.

POSTPARTUM HEMORRHAGE

 ESSENTIALS OF DIAGNOSIS

- *History of recent delivery.*
- *Painless, sudden, brisk vaginal bleeding.*

Clinical Findings

Rarely, a patient returns to the hospital a few days after delivery with brisk vaginal bleeding that may or may not be associated with hemorrhagic shock. The usual causes of postpartum hemorrhage are uterine atony, retention of products of conception, or uterine rupture following cesarean section. Other possible causes are subinvolution of the placental site, vaginal tears, or bleeding from an episiotomy. Signs of postpartum hemorrhage may include an enlarged uterus suggestive of atony, a vaginal mass suggestive of an inverted uterus, or uterine bleeding with good uterine tone and a normal size suggestive of retained products of conception.

Treatment & Disposition

A. Initial Steps

Treat hemorrhagic shock, if present (Chapter 9). If bleeding is brisk, insert the fingers of one hand into the vagina, and compress the uterus against the abdominal wall. Insert a large-bore (≥ 16-gauge) intravenous catheter, and start infusion of crystalloid solution, followed by whole blood if the hematocrit falls. Monitor vital signs and urinary output.

B. Laboratory Tests

Draw blood for CBC, coagulation studies (prothrombin time, partial thromboplastin time, and platelet count), blood urea nitrogen, and serum creatinine. Type and cross-match for 4 units of blood.

C. Consultation

Obtain emergency obstetric and gynecologic consultation.

D. Medications

Oxytocin, 20–30 mIU in 1 L of fluid given at 200 mL/h may be used for uterine atony. After an obstetrical consult is obtained, methylergonovine (Methergine) by mouth may be recommended prior to discharge.

E. Definitive Treatment

The definitive treatment is dilation and curettage, which should be performed by an obstetrician, because postpartum surgery may result in uterine perforation.

Disposition

If the cause of bleeding is definitively treated and the patient is otherwise stable, she can be discharged with close follow-up in 2–3 days. All other patients should be hospitalized and obstetric consultation obtained as needed.

PUERPERAL SEPSIS & ENDOMETRITIS

ESSENTIALS OF DIAGNOSIS

- *History of recent delivery.*
- *Systemic signs of infection.*
- *Abdominal pain, vaginal discharge.*
- *Peritoneal signs.*
- *Boggy, tender uterus and purulent lochia.*

Clinical Findings

Symptoms of puerperal sepsis in the early postpartum period are fever, peritoneal pain, and vaginal discharge. Examination reveals abdominal tenderness, exquisite uterine tenderness, and purulent lochia with leukocytes and bacteria on Gram stain.

Treatment & Disposition

If signs of sepsis are present, obtain obstetric and gynecologic consultation, and hospitalize the patient immediately. Patients with minimal symptoms may be managed as outpatients. Obtain samples of blood and discharge for diagnostic culture and sensitivity testing.

Start antibiotics in accordance with the following recommendations:

A. Severely Ill Patients

Give cefotaxime, 1–2 g intravenously every 6–8 hours; or a combination of ampicillin, 1 g intravenously every 6 hours, and gentamicin, 1.5 mg/kg intravenously every 8 hours. Before beginning treatment with gentamicin, obtain baseline serum creatinine levels; during treatment, obtain serum creatinine levels 1–2 times per week, and follow gentamicin peaks and troughs weekly.

B. Mildly Ill Patients

Doxycycline, 100 mg orally twice daily (or tetracycline, 500 mg orally 4 times daily), or ampicillin, 500 mg orally 4 times daily for 10–14 days, may be used for outpatients. ***Caution:*** Do not use doxycycline or tetracycline if the patient is breast feeding.

PUERPERAL MASTITIS

ESSENTIALS OF DIAGNOSIS

- *Postpartum breast infection.*
- *Increased localized breast pain.*
- *Variable systemic signs of infection.*
- *Localized tenderness, redness, induration, or warmth.*

Clinical Findings

Postpartum infection of the breast is almost always due to infection with *Staphylococcus aureus.* Pain, induration, redness, and warmth in the affected breast characterizes mastitis. Fever, chills, malaise, and axillary adenopathy may be present.

The diagnosis of puerperal mastitis is based on systemic signs of infection, pain, and tenderness of the involved breast. Abscess formation may occur, and blood cultures are occasionally positive.

Treatment & Disposition

A. Mild Cases (Afebrile)

Apply warm compresses to the affected breast. The patient may continue to breast feed. The patient should be given dicloxacillin, 500 mg by mouth twice daily, or cephalexin, 500 mg by mouth twice daily. Consultation with a lactation expert may be in order. Close follow-up with the obstetrician is recommended.

B. Severe Cases (Suspected Abscess)

Hospitalize the patient, and obtain surgical consultation. Give nafcillin or equivalent, 150 mg/kg/d intravenously. Penicillin-allergic patients may be given clindamycin, 450 mg intravenously every 8 hours, or erythromycin, 0.5 g intravenously every 6 hours.

American College of Obstetricians and Gynecologists: *Trauma During Pregnancy.* ACOG Technical Bulletin No. 161. American College of Obstetricians and Gynecologists, 1991.

Chames MC et al: Late postpartum eclampsia: a preventable disease? Am J Obstet Gynecol 2002;186:1174. [PMID: 12066093]

Coleman MT, Trianfo VA, Rund DA: Nonobstetric emergencies in pregnancy: trauma and surgical conditions. Am J Obstet Gynecol 1997;177:497. [PMID: 9322613]

Genitourinary Emergencies

37

Susan J. Letterle, MD[1]

Immediate Management of Serious & Life-Threatening Conditions
    Oliguria or Anuria
    Scrotal Pain
    Painless Scrotal Mass Lesions
    Dysuria
    Atraumatic Hematuria
Emergency Treatment of Specific Disorders
    Urolithiasis (Renal Colic)

Diseases of the Male Genitourinary System
    1. Torsion of the Testicle
    2. Orchitis
    3. Priapism
    4. Fournier Gangrene
    5. Phimosis & Paraphimosis

■ IMMEDIATE MANAGEMENT OF SERIOUS & LIFE-THREATENING CONDITIONS

OLIGURIA OR ANURIA

General Considerations

Decreased or absent urine output can occur from widely diverse disease states such as intravascular volume depletion or bladder outflow obstruction. In attempting to determine the cause of decreased urine output, it is helpful to categorize the mechanism as prerenal (eg, resulting from decreased or abnormal renal perfusion), renal (eg, resulting from intrinsic renal disease), or postrenal (eg, disease of the urinary collecting system distal to the renal parenchyma).

A. PRERENAL CAUSES

Prerenal causes include hypovolemia, sepsis, and heart failure.

B. RENAL CAUSES

Renal causes include tubular, glomerular, vascular, or interstitial disease.

C. POSTRENAL CAUSES

1. Supravesical obstruction—Supravesical obstruction rarely causes oliguria or anuria, because bilateral disease is required to reduce decreased urine flow. There are two types of supravesical obstruction: (1) ureteral obstruction (usually tumor) and (2) ureteropelvic or ureterovesical obstruction.

2. Intravesical or infravesical obstruction—Intravesical or infravesical obstruction is more common than supravesical obstruction (Table 37–1). Causes include prostatic hypertrophy or carcinoma, drugs with atropinic or adrenergic effects, neurologic diseases, bladder stones or tumors, and urethral strictures or valves.

Clinical Findings

A. HISTORY

1. Obstruction—Differentiate between reduced urine output (with normal or nearly normal voiding patterns) and oliguria associated with difficult in voiding, feeling of incomplete voiding, diminished urinary stream, and the like. The latter findings suggest obstruction.

2. Associated medical conditions—Ask about coexisting cardiac, pulmonary, renal, or other underlying disease that might contribute to renal or prerenal oliguria.

3. Drugs—The patient's medications might cause problems with urination or be nephrotoxic. Anticholinergics and sympathomimetics are most often the culprits of urinary retention.

---

[1]This chapter is a revision of the chapter by John Mills, MD, & Jack W. McAninch, MD, from the 4th edition.

Table 37–1. Diagnostic clues to the cause of bladder outlet obstruction.

Cause	Frequency of Occurrence	Results of History and Physical Examination	Laboratory Tests and Other Studies
Prostatic hypertrophy	Common.	Gradually increasing difficulty in voiding, often with abrupt worsening. Enlarged prostate on rectal examination is common.	Urethral catheterization may be difficult. Large amount of residual urine in bladder.
Urethral strictures or valves	Uncommon.	Often previous attacks of urethritis or urethral trauma. Onset may be gradual or abrupt.	Urethral catheterization often difficult. Large amounts of residual urine. Urethrogram or urethroscopy is diagnostic.
Bladder stones or tumor	Uncommon.	Hematuria is common. Obstruction may be intermittent.	Urethral catheter is passed without difficulty. Cystogram or cystoscopy is diagnostic.
Neuropathic bladder	Very uncommon.	Onset may be gradual and painless or abrupt and painful. Look for associated neurologic abnormalities (sacral dermatomal hypesthesia, poor rectal sphincter tone, neuralgic pain).	Urethral catheter passed without difficulty. Cystometrogram is diagnostic.
Traumatic urethral injury	Uncommon.	Male; history of trauma, prostatic dislocation, urthral bleeding.	*Do not pass catheter.* Retrograde urethrogram and percutaneous cystogram are diagnostic.

B. Physical Examination

1. Vital signs—Obtain a complete set of vital signs and orthostatic vitals to determine if volume depletion is an issue. Correct volume depletion, if present (Chapter 9).

2. General examination—Focus on signs of cardiac, pulmonary, renal, or hepatic disease that might contribute to oliguria of a prerenal or renal origin. Look for signs of volume depletion, such as dry mucous membranes or poor skin turgor.

3. Distended bladder—Palpate the lower abdomen to determine whether a suprapubic mass, consistent with a distended bladder, is present. A distended bladder is manifested as a firm (but not hard) mass that is adjacent to the symphysis pubica and is dull to percussion. The diagnosis may be confirmed by passage of a Foley catheter; ultrasonography; radiologic studies (computed tomography [CT] scan, abdominal x-ray); or, if necessary, percutaneous needle aspiration in the event of a urethral stricture, stenosis, or injury.

4. Prostate examination—Examine the prostate. Perform a rectal examination, looking especially for masses, prostatic hypertrophy, prostatic tenderness, or prostatic dislocation (associated with trauma).

C. Detection of Bladder Outlet Obstruction

Bladder outlet obstruction (complete or partial) is strongly suggested by a palpable bladder in a patient who is unable to void or who has a weak urinary stream or feeling of incomplete voiding. Whether lower abdominal pain is present depends on the rapidity of obstruction; acute obstruction causes rapid bladder distention and severe pain if sensation is intact.

Diagnostic features of some of the common causes of bladder outlet obstruction are set forth in Table 37–1.

Treatment

A. Serious Underlying Disease

If the patient is acutely ill or obviously in shock, is septic, or has heart failure or other serious coexisting conditions that might cause prerenal oliguria, these disorders must be evaluated and treated before those of the urinary tract.

B. Distended Bladder (Presumed Bladder Outlet Obstruction)

1. Gain intravenous access—Draw blood for complete blood count (CBC), electrolyte determination, and blood urea nitrogen and serum creatinine measurements.

2. Drain the bladder—

   a. Urethral catheter—Try to pass an indwelling urethral (Foley) catheter. If this maneuver is successful, drain the bladder, record the volume of urine obtained, and send a specimen for urinalysis and culture. Monitor the patient for postobstructive diuresis. Gradual bladder draining is not a proven method of decreasing bladder atony or mucosal hemorrhage. If bladder outlet obstruction is relieved by passage of a Foley catheter and is apparently due to a transient cause (eg, drugs), the catheter may be removed and the patient observed for ability to void after the effects of any drugs are presumed to have dissipated. In patients with fixed bladder outlet obstruction (eg, benign prostatic hypertrophy), leave the catheter in place, and obtain urologic consultation within 1 week.

b. Suprapubic catheter—If a standard Foley catheter cannot be passed secondary to prostatic hypertrophy, reattempt passage using a coudé catheter (which has a curved tip that usually allows passage beyond the enlarged prostate). If the coudé catheter is unsuccessful and a urologist is not available, insert a suprapubic catheter for temporary drainage (Chapter 6). A large (16-gauge) needle-clad catheter (eg, Intracath) will provide satisfactory emergency bladder drainage.

3. Treat cystitis and prostatitis, if present—See "Dysuria" section, below.

4. Hospitalize patients as needed—Hospitalize patients who have systemic symptoms (fever, rigors, intractable emesis) and those who need additional diagnosis and treatment (eg, for management of postobstructive diuresis, azotemia, sepsis, or electrolyte abnormalities).

C. Bladder Not Palpable; Patient Able to Void

If the patient can void on command but continues to have subjective or objective evidence of a weak urinary stream or if the patient experiences a feeling of incomplete voiding, partial bladder outlet obstruction is likely.

Draw blood for CBC, electrolyte, blood urea nitrogen, and serum creatinine measurements. Send a urine specimen for urinalysis and culture. Treat cystitis or prostatitis, if present.

If blood chemistry results and urinalysis are normal, refer the patient to a urologist. The presence of azotemia or electrolyte abnormalities indicates severe or longstanding obstructive uropathy, and the patient likely requires hospitalization.

D. Bladder Not Palpable; Patient Unable to Void

Consider the following in the differential diagnosis (1) intrinsic renal disease, (2) occult prerenal disease (unlikely, because most causes would be obvious on brief physical examination), (3) occult bladder outlet obstruction, or (4) supravesical obstructive uropathy (rare).

Draw blood for CBC; serum glucose, electrolyte, calcium, and phosphorus; and tests of renal and hepatic function. Obtain chest and abdominal x-rays to help evaluate the size of the kidneys and bladder. Ultrasonography is the best noninvasive test for evaluating kidney and bladder size.

Ensure adequate hydration. In an adult without obvious volume overload (eg, pulmonary or peripheral edema), give 1–2 L of fluid orally or intravenously, and observe the patient for 1–2 hours. In an individual with normal kidneys, this amount should produce a brisk flow of urine.

If anuria persists despite adequate hydration and if the bladder is not distended, the cause of the anuria is likely to be proximal to the bladder (prerenal, renal, or, rarely, bilateral ureteral obstruction). Bladder catheterization, with strict adherence to sterile technique, should be performed to confirm the lack of urine output. Hospitalize the patient for further evaluation.

Disposition

Hospitalization is required for patients with persistent unexplained anuria or severe oliguria (< 500 mL/d), those with systemic symptoms, and those with markedly abnormal electrolytes or renal function.

Patients with partial bladder outlet obstruction (ie, weak urinary stream, with or without palpable bladder) should be referred to a urologist if renal function is normal or nearly normal.

Asymptomatic patients with an indwelling urethral catheter should be reexamined or referred to a urologist within 1 week.

SCROTAL PAIN
(See Table 37–2.)

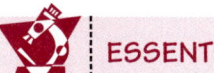 **ESSENTIALS OF DIAGNOSIS**

- *Trauma is a common cause.*
- *Infection accounts for orchitis and epididymitis.*
- *Flank pain, hematuria, and scrotal pain usually indicate urolithiasis.*
- *Incarcerated hernias cause scrotal pain.*
- *Testicular torsion requires urgent diagnosis to salvage the testicle. A torsed testis may be high riding or horizontally lying; ultrasound will show diminished blood flow to the torsed testis.*

Clinical Findings

A. Trauma

(See also Chapter 26.) Trauma commonly causes testicular or scrotal pain. Careful questioning may be required to elicit the circumstances under which the trauma occurred.

Table 37–2. Diagnostic clues to the cause of acute scrotal pain.

	History	Physical Examination	Urinalysis Results	Other Laboratory Studies	Treatment and Disposition
Trauma	History of injury.	Scrotal hematoma often present.	Variable; may have hematuria.	Sonogram.	Obtain urologic consultation (Chapter 26).
Urolithiasis	Antecedent flank or back pain; occasionally abdominal pain.	Testicle minimally tender or non-tender.	Hematuria.	Stones on excretory urogram.	Obtain urologic consultation.
Viral (eg, mumps) orchitis	Gradual onset, coexisting mumps parotitis common.	Tender testicles (unilateral or bilateral); epididymis rarely involved.	Normal.	Viral cultures (throat, stool) if available; characteristic 4-fold rise in serum antibody titer.	Elevate and immobilize testicle (eg, with atheletic supporter), give analgesics, and discharge for follow-up care.
Incarcerated hernia	Gradual onset; crampy pain.	Fluid rushes heard in scrotum (early); abdominal tenderness consistent with intestinal obstruction.	Normal.	Characteristically abnormal results on ultrasound studies; abdominal x-ray results often abnormal (intestinal obstruction).	Obtain general surgical consultation; hospitalize.
Epididymitis	Gradual onset; history of urethritis or urinary tract infection common; older men (> age 25 years).	Tender epididymis (often unilateral) with normal testicle early in course; pain relieved by elevating scrotum. If needed, use spermatic cord block (see text) to facilitate examination.	Leukocytes; bacteriuria in some cases (coexisting urinary tract infection).	Normal results on Doppler and ultrasound studies; radionuclide scan shows uptake in epididymis.	1. Prescribe bed rest and elevation and scrotum, with analgesics as needed. 2. Treat underlying urethritis or urinary-tract infection with antimicrobials (Chapter 40). 3. Discharge all patients for follow-up care.
Testicular torsion	Abrupt onset (minutes to hours); history of testicular pain in some; boys and young men (< age 25 years).	Tender testicle, often elevated and horizontally displaced; normal epididymis (if palpable). Use spermatic cord block to facilitate examination.	Normal.	Characteristically abnormal results on Doppler examination and radionuclide scan.	Obtain emergency urologic consultation; hospitalize for surgery. Attempt manual detorsion (see text).
Torsion of testicular appendage	Abrupt onset.	Firm nodule with point tenderness on upper anterior pole of testis; testical normal.	Normal.	Transillumination may reveal affected appendage as "blue dot," normal results on Doppler ultrasound and radionuclide studies.	1. Prescribed bed rest and elevation, with analgesics as needed. 2. Surgery is often needed to relieve pain. 3. Obtain urologic follow-up care.

B. VIRAL ORCHITIS

Mumps virus and the enteroviruses may cause acute unilateral or bilateral orchitis. In orchitis due to mumps virus, associated parotitis is usually present.

C. UROLITHIASIS

Rarely, patients with urolithiasis present with pain localized mainly in the scrotum; however, in most cases, back or flank pain has preceded the scrotal pain, or a history of nephrolithiasis is present. In such cases, the testicle and epididymis are normal to palpation. Hematuria is an important diagnostic clue. The diagnosis may be confirmed by unenhanced helical CT, intravenous pyelogram, or KUB (radiograph of the kidneys, urethras, and bladder).

D. INCARCERATED HERNIA

Inguinal hernias incarcerated in the scrotum may cause scrotal pain that may be confused with testicular pain. Bowel sounds are heard in the scrotum early in incarceration; if the hernia strangulates, bowel sounds are no longer audible. Intestinal hernia is almost always associated with clinical findings of intestinal obstruction (Chapter 13). Ultrasonography is diagnostic.

E. TESTICULAR TORSION, EPIDIDYMITIS, AND TORSION OF THE TESTICULAR APPENDAGES

(See Table 37–2.) Torsion of a testicular appendage, epididymitis, and testicular torsion are the 3 most common causes of acute scrotal pain and account for approximately 85–90% of cases. Because of the urgency to diagnose and treat testicular torsion within 6 hours to prevent loss of the testis, testicular torsion must be promptly ruled out in all patients with scrotal pain. It may be difficult to distinguish from epididymitis or torsion of testicular appendages as edema and inflammation progress to involve the entire scrotal sac and contents.

1. Testicular torsion—Testicular torsion tends to occur in young men and is rare in men over age 30 years; however, it can and does occur at all ages. There is often a history of episodes of similar scrotal pain, representing torsion with spontaneous repositioning of the testicle. The pain is abrupt in onset, severe, unilateral, and often associated with nausea and vomiting. Tenderness is initially noted only in the testicle; however, with persistent torsion and the resulting testicular hypoxia, pain and tenderness spread to involve contiguous intrascrotal structures.

Examination early in the illness shows an elevated testicle that is apt to have a horizontal lie (Bell clapper deformity). The epididymis may be felt in an abnormal position (eg, anteriorly) in the early stages. Later, the entire scrotal contents become swollen and tender, making the examination extremely difficult and less informative because the epididymis becomes indistinguishable from the testis on palpation.

2. Epididymitis—Epididymitis tends to occur in sexually active men over age 20 years and is the most common misdiagnosis for testicular torsion. There may be a history of urinary tract infection or urethritis. Pain begins gradually and is less severe than in testicular torsion. The Prehn sign is present if the pain is reduced when the scrotum is elevated. This finding is not specific to epididymitis nor is it a reliable discriminating clinical sign. Physical examination reveals a tender epididymis, often unilateral and often with erythema and edema of the scrotal skin. Early on, the testicle may be normal or minimally tender. However, as edema worsens, the epididymis becomes indistinguishable from the testicle on palpation, and a reactive hydrocele may develop, making it difficult to differentiate epididymitis from testicular torsion. Urinalysis frequently shows pyuria and possibly bacteriuria if a concomitant urethritis or urinary tract infection is present. Doppler ultrasound shows increased blood flow to the affected testis, in contrast to the decreased blood flow seen in testicular torsion.

3. Torsion of testicular or epididymal appendages—Of the 4 appendages, the appendix testis, located on the anterosuperior pole of the testis, is the most frequently (92%) torsed appendage followed by the appendix epididymis (7%), located on the head of the epididymis. Pain is usually sudden in onset and can be severe, with nausea and vomiting. Physical examination occasionally (21%) reveals a small, tender, firm nodule ("blue dot" sign), representing the infarcted appendage in the anterosuperior pole of the testis. The scrotal skin and testicle are usually normal and minimally tender. In advanced cases, marked edema and appearance of a reactive hydrocele may obscure the diagnosis of testicular torsion.

4. Specialized diagnostic tests for differentiating torsion from epididymitis—These tests should not delay emergent urologic consultation and surgical treatment of patients with high probability of testicular torsion (ie, patients under age 18 years with acute unilateral testicular pain and no signs or recent history of urinary tract infection).

a. Spermatic cord block—Anesthetizing the scrotal contents may facilitate accurate examination but should be attempted only by the consulting urologist. Inject lidocaine without epinephrine (2%), 5–10 mL, around the spermatic cord at the external inguinal ring.

b. Color-flow Doppler ultrasonography—Color-flow Doppler ultrasonography is the diagnostic study of choice at most institutions. It is widely available and has a sensitivity of 86–100% and a specificity of 100% as compared with a sensitivity of 80–100% and a specificity of 86–100% for radionucleotide imaging. The most frequent sonographic finding is absent or diminished blood flow to the affected testis, compared with the unaffected side. If the diagnosis is still unclear, then a nuclear study should be pursued. Ultrasound is more advantageous than nuclear scanning for elucidating other scrotal pathology including varicoceles, hydroceles, hernias, and masses.

   c. Radionuclide scan—In epididymitis, scanning of the scrotum after intravenous injection of technetium-^{99}m sodium pertechnetate reveals increased scrotal uptake on the affected side, whereas torsion shows decreased uptake.

Treatment & Disposition

(See Table 37–2.) If testicular torsion is present, obtain urgent urologic consultation, and prepare the patient for immediate surgery. Manual detorsion should be attempted if the urologist is not immediately available but should not delay definitive treatment. Detorsion of the testicle (either manual or surgical) must be accomplished within 6 hours to prevent testicular infarction. Torsion causes the patient's left testicle to rotate counterclockwise and the right to rotate clockwise (Figure 37–1); the affected testicle should be twisted in the opposite direction when detorsion is attempted. Because the testis affected by torsion is usually rotated a minimum of 360 degrees (one turn), the physician should initially attempt to untwist the testicle by counter-rotating it one turn. The testis will usually return to normal position on its own after this maneuver, even if it was originally twisted more than one complete revolution. The urologist may choose to infiltrate the spermatic cord near the inguinal ring with lidocaine without epinephrine (2%), 5–10 mL, to facilitate the maneuver, and give analgesics as needed. *Regardless of the result of manual detorsion, emergency surgery is indicated* to perform detorsion—if necessary—and to secure the testicle. Without surgery, torsion may occur again at any time.

   In patients with suspected epididymitis or orchitis, urologic consultation should be sought if the diagnosis is in doubt. If epididymitis is present, see Chapter 40 for treatment.

   Torsion of the testicular appendage (after testicular torsion is excluded) is managed with bed rest, scrotal elevation, analgesics, and follow-up care within 1–2 days. Surgical excision is often needed for adequate pain control.

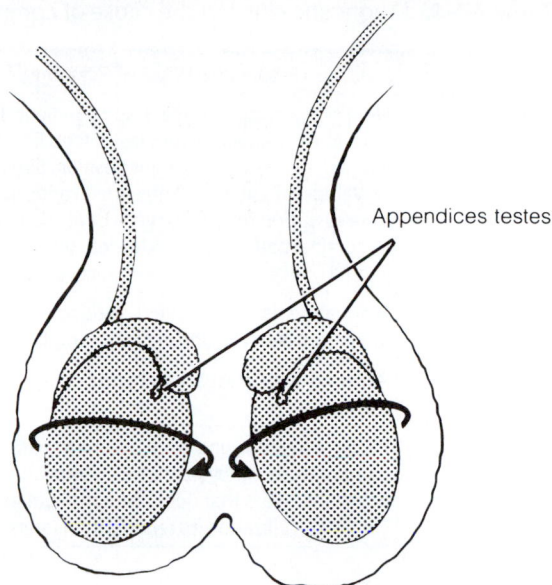

Figure 37–1. Torsion of the testicle. View of the testicles, epididymides, testicular appendages, and scrotum, showing direction of rotation of the testicles during torsion (as seen by the physician standing at the foot of the patient's bed and looking down at the patient). Manual detorsion should rotate the testicles in the opposite direction.

PAINLESS SCROTAL MASS LESIONS
(See Table 37–3.)

 ESSENTIALS OF DIAGNOSIS

- *Malignancy is often painless.*
- *A tense hydrocele or a firm spermatocele must be differentiated from a tumor. Ultrasound is the diagnostic study of choice.*
- *Sudden onset of a varicocele in an older male may be a late sign of a renal tumor.*

General Considerations

Conditions causing painless (relatively painless) scrotal swelling are not true emergencies, although testicular tumors are life threatening and require urgent evaluation (within a few days).

Table 37–3. Diagnostic clues to the cause of common painless scrotal masses.

	History and Physical Examination	**Other Diagnostic Studies**
Varicocele	Usually asymptomatic mass; some patients have mild pain. Mass is separate from testis; feels like "bag of worms," especially in upright position. Size increased by Valsalva maneuver. Right-sided variocele should raise suspicion for inferior vena cava and intra-abdominal pathology. Sudden left-sided variocele should raise suspicion for left renal vein obstruction.	Not usually required, physical examination is diagnostic. Ultrasonography also helpful in diagnosis of enigmatic cases.
Hydrocele	Gradually enlarging painless cystic mass that transilluminates. ***Note:*** Hydrocele may complicate tumor.	Aspiration yields clear fluid. Ultrasonography helpful in diagnosis.
Spermatocele	Asymptomatic mass separate from and superior to the testicle.	Aspiration reveals white cloudy fluid with immotile sperm. Ultrasonography also helpful in diagnosis.
Testicular tumor	Patient often a young adult. Asymptomatic enlargement of testis, rarely painful. Examination shows firm, nontender mass that does not transilluminate. Gynecomastia, virilization, or feminization rarely occur.	Ultrasonography helpful in confirming mass lesion. Surgical exploration required for exact diagnosis of all testicular mass lesions.

Table 37–3 sets forth helpful diagnostic features of conditions associated with painless scrotal swelling. Patients with newly diagnosed testicular enlargement or mass lesions should be referred to a urologist.

DYSURIA

 ESSENTIALS OF DIAGNOSIS

- *Painful urination that represents acute inflammation of the urethra, bladder, or prostate.*
- *Frequency and urgency may also be present.*
- *Workup should be guided by other associated symptoms, ie, hematuria or discharge.*
- *Urinalysis or sexually transmitted disease testing usually confirms the diagnosis.*

General Considerations

Common causes of dysuria and their associated clinical findings are given in Table 37–4. Urethral diverticula, urolithiasis, endocervical gonorrhea, balanitis, and urethral warts are uncommon causes of dysuria.

Clinical Findings

A. DYSURIA IN MALES

1. Urethritis—In males, urethritis is a much more common cause of dysuria than is urinary tract infection. Attempt to express urethral discharge by milking the ure-

thra, and send the material for culture and smear. If no discharge can be obtained, sample the anterior 2–3 cm (3/4–1 3/16 in) of the urethra with a calcium alginate, Dacron, or cotton swab, or wire loop; smear some of the urethral section obtained on a slide; and send the swab for culture for *Neisseria gonorrhoeae.* If facilities are available, also send a urethral swab in *Chlamydia* culture medium for culture and fluorescent antibody testing for *Chlamydia* infection. *Do not use a wood-handled cotton swab, because wood is toxic to the* Chlamydia *organism.* Smears should be stained with methylene blue or Gram stain and examined microscopically. The presence of more than 5 leukocytes per × 400 field indicates urethritis; the presence of intracellular diplococci (gram-negative if a Gram stain was done)—especially without other bacteria—indicates gonococcal urethritis. See Chapter 40 for treatment of gonorrhea and nongonococcal urethritis.

Dysuria without evidence of urethral or urinary tract inflammation (< 5 white blood cells per × 100 field, negative culture) is rare in men and may represent low-grade infection. Treatment for urethritis is usually indicated.

2. Prostatitis—If no evidence of urethritis is found, obtain a midstream clean-voided urine specimen (supervise the patient so that the sample is collected properly). Polymorphonuclear neutrophils in the urine in the absence of urethritis are diagnostic of urinary tract inflammation. Prostatitis (either alone or associated with urinary tract infection) may be excluded by rectal examination. For further information on treatment, see Chapter 40.

3. Urinary tract infection—Leukocytes, usually with bacteria, are found on microscopic examination of a midstream urine specimen. Urine dip reagent strips that test for the presence of leukocyte esterase and ni-

Table 37–4. Diagnostic clues to common causes of dysuria.

Condition	Sex More Commonly Affected	History and Physical Examination	Diagnostic Studies
Urethritis	Men.	Dysuria, usually severe. Clear or purulent urethral discharge.	Leukocytes in urethral discharge or on urethral swab. Tests for gonococcal or chlamydial infection are often positive.
Prostatitis	Men only.	Pelvic pain and dysuria. Fever common. Tender, boggy prostate on examination.	Prostatic massage produces leukocytes and bacteria in urethral discharge or urine ("3-glass test").
Urethral stricture	Men.	Dysuria, may have split or reduced urinary stream.	Urethroscopy or urethrogram.
Urethral caruncle	Women (usually postmenopausal).	Mild dysuria; examination may show lesion.	Urethroscopy.
Dysuria-frequency syndrome (urethral syndrome)	Women only.	Dysuria and urgency. May have urethral discharge.	Pyuria; leukocytes in urethral discharge or on urethral swab.
Vaginitis	Women only.	External dysuria, vaginal discharge dyspareunia.	Vaginal smear or culture shows *Candida*, *Gardnerella vaginalis*, or *Trichomonas vaginalis*.
Genital herpes	Women.	History of herpes (if recurrent); vesicles and ulcers on external genitalia.	Positive results on tests for herpes simplex.
Urinary tract infection	Mainly women.	Dysuria, urgency, frequency; cloudy or foul-smelling urine. May have fever, flank or supra-pubic tenderness.	Pyuria and bacteriuria, urine culture shows more then 10^3 bacteria/mL (often $> 10^5$/mL).
Urethral trauma	Either (mainly children).	History or evidence of genital manipulation or trauma.	Hematuria occasionally.
Psychogenic	Either.	No logical pattern to symptoms. Examination normal.	Normal results on urinalysis. No leukocytes on urethral swab. Tests for gonococcal and chlamydial infection negative.

trite are equivalent to the urine sediment analysis at detecting pyuria when both are positive. They are increasingly being used as a screening tool and often eliminate the need for microscopic examination. Culture usually shows bacteria of a single species (usually $> 10^5$ colony-forming units per milliliter but occasionally only 10^2–10^4, especially with certain organisms [eg, *Candida* species or enterococci]). **Note:** Urinary tract infection is unusual in men under age 60 years unless associated urinary tract abnormalities are present or the patient engages in homosexual sexual activity.

4. Local causes—Inspect the penis and urethral meatus for balanitis and intrameatal pathologic structures (warts, herpetic ulcers) that are commonly associated with dysuria. Urethral strictures often cause dysuria, and patients may describe a split or intermittent urinary stream.

B. Dysuria in Females

1. Collection of urine—Obtain an uncontaminated urine specimen for microscopic analysis. Contamination of the specimen is usually indicated by the presence of squamous (vaginal) epithelial cells visible microscopically (eg, ≥5 cells per × 100 field); if these are seen, discard the specimen and obtain another, uncontaminated specimen. Proper collection techniques for adults are as follows:

a. Midstream clean-voided urine—This method of collection is satisfactory in most cases but requires a cooperative patient and some coordination.

b. Catheterization—A small, straight (9F) catheter should be used for quick "in and out" catheterization, because it is more comfortable than the 14–19F Foley-type catheter. Contamination may occur.

c. Suprapubic aspiration—(See Chapter 6.) Suprapubic aspiration is useful in special situations (eg, for infants) and is associated with a very low contamination rate.

2. Clinical differentiation of causes of dysuria in women—

a. Dysuria-frequency syndrome (urethral syndrome) and urinary tract infection—These conditions are characterized by dysuria without vaginal symptoms (eg, discharge) and by pyuria (< 5 white cells per × 400 field). If bacteria are seen in the urinary sediment, urinary tract infection is a more likely diagnosis than urethral syndrome. Occasionally women with dysuria-frequency syndrome may have no pyuria.

b. Local causes—If results on urinalysis are normal, if vaginal symptoms associated with dysuria are present, or if pain is felt outside the urinary tract (external dysuria), perform a pelvic examination to look for vaginitis, genital herpes, or a urethral caruncle. Urethral caruncle is found in postmenopausal woman and is a small, nontender red lesion resembling a strawberry on the dorsal aspect of the urethral meatus. In addition, it is helpful to culture endocervical mucus for gonococci, because gonococcal infection in women may be associated with dysuria.

C. Dysuria Associated with Hematuria in Either Sex

The presence of large numbers of erythrocytes in the urine in either sex should suggest hemorrhagic cystitis, concomitant urolithiasis, or urethral manipulation (see "Hematuria" section, below).

Treatment & Disposition

Treat the various causes of dysuria as follows:

A. Urinary Tract Infections

For treatment of cystitis, pyelonephritis, and urethral syndrome, see Chapter 40.

B. Gonorrhea

See Chapter 40.

C. Vaginitis

See Chapter 40.

D. Prostatitis

See Chapter 40.

E. Other Conditions

Patients with other conditions (eg, urethral stricture or diverticulum) should be referred to a urologist or gynecologist for evaluation.

ATRAUMATIC HEMATURIA

ESSENTIALS OF DIAGNOSIS

- *Hematuria is often an early sign of genitourinary cancer.*
- *Hematuria with associated flank or groin pain is suggestive of urolithiasis.*
- *Dysuria and frequency may accompany hematuria of an infectious cause.*

General Considerations

Common causes of hematuria (microscopic defined as > 3 red blood cells per high-power field) and their associated clinical findings are set forth in Table 37–5. See Chapter 26 for management of hematuria associated with trauma or genitourinary manipulation. In all cases of atraumatic hematuria, nonglomerular diseases including infection account for 25% of cases, stones account for 20% of cases, and 10% of cases have an unknown cause.

Renal vein thrombosis, renal arterial embolization, drug-induced (cyclophosphamide, penicillins) interstitial cystitis, glomerular diseases, abdominal aortic aneurysm, and malignancy are less common causes of hematuria. In the elderly, painless gross hematuria is malignancy until proven otherwise.

Clinical Findings

A. History

Hematuria associated with abdominal or flank pain and tenderness suggests urolithiasis or, less commonly, renovascular disease. Diagnostic clues may come from timing of the hematuria. Initial, terminal, or total stream hematuria suggests bleeding from the following respective areas: anterior urethral, posterior urethra to trigone, or bladder sources or beyond.

Hematuria associated with dysuria and urinary urgency and frequency suggests hemorrhagic cystitis (drug-induced, infectious, or idiopathic).

Systemic conditions associated with hematuria include thrombotic thrombocytopenic purpura, Henoch-Schönlein purpura, sickling hemoglobinopathies, excessive anticoagulation therapy, or coagulopathies.

Bleeding from other perineal areas, especially menstrual flow, may be mistaken for hematuria.

Table 37–5. Diagnostic clues to common causes of hematuria.

	History and Physical Findings	Diagnostic Studies
Trauma	History or evidence of local genital, abdominal (renal), or pelvic trauma or recent genitourinary instrumentation.	See Chapter 26.
Tumor	Often long-standing painless hematuria.	Intravenous pyelogram reveals upper urinary tract tumors; cystogram or cystoscopy shows bladder tumor.
Urolithiasis	Intermittent hematuria usually associated with pain. Bladder stones may be painless but may be associated with intermittent urinary obstruction.	Intravenous pyelogram reveals ureteral stone, obstruction, or postobstructive hydroureter; cystoscopy or cystography shows bladder stones.
Infection (including tuberculosis)	Dysuria common.	Pyuria often present. Urine culture shows bacteria (usually $\geq 10^5$ colonies/mL).
Glomerulonephritis	May follow streptococcal infection; often associated with autoimmune diseases (eg, systemic lupus erythematosus). Gradual onset. Hypertension common.	Urinalysis shows leukocytes, red cell casts, and frequently proteinuria; blood urea nitrogen and serum creatinine elevated.
Prostatitis	Dysuria often present. Abnormal (large or tender) prostate.	Pyuria often present.
Urethral stricture, foreign body, or manipulation	Often painful. Local abnormality may be obvious on examination.	Urethroscopy reveals stricture or foreign body.
Sickling hemoglobinopathy or sickle cell trait	Intermittent hematuria that may be painless (trait) or painful (disease).	Urinalysis shows red blood cells and isosthenuria. Hemoglobin electrophoresis abnormal.
Bleeding diathesis	Painless hematuria. History of coagulation defect. Evidence of bleeding elsewhere (eg, purpura). Anticoagulant use.	Coagulation tests show thrombocytopenia, prolonged prothrombin time, etc (Chapter 39).

B. Physical Examination

Examine the external genitalia for local causes of hematuria (eg, intraurethral trauma). Examine the abdomen, back, and pelvis for tenderness and evidence of trauma.

In males, perform a rectal examination for evaluation of the prostate after a urine specimen has been obtained, because prostatic manipulation can induce pyuria.

C. Laboratory Examination

1. Urinalysis—Perform urinalysis to confirm the diagnosis of hematuria. Carefully performed microscopic examination of a freshly voided midstream urine specimen is essential to the evaluation of hematuria; look especially for erythrocyte casts, which suggest glomerulonephritis. In men, fractionate urinalysis (initial, midstream, and terminal specimens) is also helpful in localizing the source of hematuria.

2. Other laboratory tests—Further laboratory testing (except possibly urine culture) is not usually needed for bacterial hemorrhagic cystitis. Patients with urolithiasis should have baseline serum electrolyte determinations and renal function tests, especially prior to obtaining an intravenous pyelogram. Patients in whom a bleeding disorder is suspected or the cause of hematuria is unknown should have the following laboratory examinations: CBC with differential; prothrombin time, partial thromboplastin time, and international normalization ratio; serum electrolytes; and renal function.

D. Special Studies

An intravenous pyelogram may be necessary for the evaluation of urolithiasis, trauma, tumors, and other causes. However, compared with ultrasound, CT scanning is a better diagnostic study for evaluation of intraabdominal pathology and tumors, especially those that are less than 3 cm in size. In pregnant females, ultrasound is the test of choice for evaluating hematuria.

Cytoscopy is essential for evaluation of bladder or urethral hematuria due to tumors and other causes. It may also be helpful for localizing hematuria of the upper genitourinary tract to one side or the other. The need for cytoscopy should be determined by the consulting urologist.

Other studies such as radionuclide scans or angiograms may be needed in special situations, but urologic consultation should be obtained before these studies are requested.

Treatment & Disposition

Treat the various causes of hematuria as follows:

A. TRAUMA

See Chapter 26.

B. URINARY TRACT INFECTION

See Chapter 40.

C. SUSPECTED TUMOR

Refer the patient to a urologist for evaluation. Consider hospitalization in order to expedite diagnostic procedures.

D. UROLITHIASIS

See below.

E. GLOMERULONEPHRITIS

Hospitalize the patient, and obtain consultation with a nephrologist.

F. PROSTATITIS

See Chapter 40.

G. URETHRAL STRICTURES AND FOREIGN BODIES

Refer the patient to a urologist.

H. UNKNOWN CAUSE

Patients with hematuria of an unknown cause need urgent urologic consultation.

Agrawal M et al: Acute renal failure. Am Fam Physician 2000; 61:2077. [PMID: 10779250]

Anderson RU: Management of lower urinary tract infections and cystitis. Urol Clin North Am 1999;26:729. [PMID: 10584614]

Curtis LA et al: Acute urinary retention and urinary incontinence. Emerg Med Clin North Am 2001;19:591. [PMID: 11554277]

Farhat W et al: Urethral syndromes in children. Pediatr Rev 2001; 22:17. [PMID: 11139643]

Grossfeld GD et al: Evaluation of asymptomatic microscopic hematuria in adults: the American Urological Association best practice policy—part I: definition, detection, prevalence, and etiology. Urology 2001;57:599. [PMID: 11306356]

Grossfeld GD et al: Evaluation of asymptomatic microscopic hematuria in adults: the American Urological Association best practice policy—part II: patient evaluation, cytology, voided markers, imaging, cystoscopy, nephrology evaluation, and follow-up. Urology 2001;57:604. [PMID: 11306357]

Grossfeld GD et al: Evaluation of asymptomatic microscopic hematuria. Urol Clin North Am 1998;25:661. [PMID: 10026773]

Kass EJ: The acute scrotum. Pediatr Clin North Am 1997; 44:1251. [PMID: 97467752]

Lummus WE et al: Prostatitis. Emerg Med Clin North Am 2001; 19:691. [PMID: 11554282]

Miller O et al: Urinary tract infection and pyelonephritis. Emerg Med Clin North Am 2001;19:655. [PMID: 11554280]

Sokolosky MC: Hematuria. Emerg Med Clin North Am 2001; 19:621. [PMID: 11554278]

Strauss S et al: Torsion of the testicular appendages: sonographic appearance. J Ultrasound Med 1997;16:189. [PMID: 9166815]

■ EMERGENCY TREATMENT OF SPECIFIC DISORDERS

UROLITHIASIS (Renal Colic)

 ESSENTIALS OF DIAGNOSIS

- *Patients usually present with sudden onset of unilateral flank pain that may radiate to the ipsilateral lower quadrant, groin, scrotum, or labia.*

- *Hematuria is present in approximately 90% of cases.*

- *Spiral CT scan is the diagnostic study of choice at most institutions, but KUB, intravenous pyelogram, and ultrasound may also be used.*

General Considerations

Patients with stones in the urinary tract commonly present to the emergency department. Stones usually form in the renal pelvis, and symptoms occur with passage of the stone into the ureter, as the result of infection, or both. The incidence of stones is highest amongst whites with a peak incidence between ages 20 and 50 years, and the male to female ratio is 3:1. Bladder stones are less common, and patients may present with hematuria or intermittent urinary obstruction.

Clinical Findings

A. Symptoms and Signs

The initial symptom is usually acute, unilateral flank pain (stones near kidney) that rapidly becomes excruciating, radiating to the ipsilateral lower quadrant and often referred to the ipsilateral groin, testicle, or labia (stones near ureterovesicular). The pain may cause vasovagal syncope; occasionally patients are asymptomatic except for hematuria. Eliciting a history of pain that shifts anteriorly and inferiorly from the flank as the stone moves distally in the urinary tract may be helpful in differentiating renal colic from other types of abdominal pain.

Some patients note gross hematuria. Nausea and vomiting are frequent. If complicating infection is present, signs and symptoms of pyelonephritis also may be present. Inquire about a history of similar attacks or a predisposing condition (eg, previous documented urolithiasis, gout, hypercalcemia).

Vital signs are usually normal in the absence of infection, although bradycardia from vagal hypertonicity or tachycardia from pain may be seen. Some degree of ileus is usually present. Tenderness over the affected kidney (costovertebral angle tenderness) and ureter can be elicited.

B. Laboratory Findings

Obtain a urinalysis. Hematuria (gross or microscopic) is present in approximately 90% of cases. Occasionally a patient presents with pain and no hematuria.

A urine or serum human chorionic gonadotropin level should be obtained in all females of child-bearing age. Urine culture should be sent if an infected stone is suspected by bacteriuria and fever.

Blood urea nitrogen and serum creatinine levels are usually normal. Although they will not change the emergency department management, calcium, magnesium, phosphorus, and uric acid levels may be helpful to the urologist in assessing for metabolic causes of stone formation.

C. Imaging

Imaging studies should be performed during the first episode of suspected renal colic or if the diagnosis is uncertain (see Figures 37–2 and 37–3). Patients with recurrent stones with typical historical and physical examination consistent with urolithiasis may be managed symptomatically without any diagnostic studies unless obstruction or infection is of concern.

1. KUB—KUB, a study of the kidneys, urethras, and bladder, is useful because 90% of calculi are radiopaque. The sensitivity of this study is less than 70%.

2. Ultrasound—Renal ultrasound may be useful to detect stones or hydronephrosis but is not as sensitive (64%) as helical CT or intravenous pyelogram, particularly for detection of small stones. It may be of value in patients with a history of hypersensitivity to intravenous contrast, with radiolucent stones, and especially in pregnant women. Pediatric and geriatric patients should also be evaluated with ultrasound as the first screening modality.

3. Intravenous pyelogram—An intravenous pyelogram has a 90% sensitivity for detecting urolithiasis or the related obstruction as well as for assessing functional status and visualization of the entire urinary tract. *Caution:* This method is relatively contraindicated in the following settings: (1) patients with creatinine above 1.4 mg/dl, (2) elderly patients with proteinuria and elevated creatinine, and (3) patients with documented allergy to contrast media unless they are premedicated with antihistamines and steroids.

4. Unenhanced helical (spiral) CT—Helical CT scan is widely used and currently the study of choice at many institutions for the diagnosis of renal colic. Not only is it accurate, but it is less time consuming, no contrast is required, and additional intra-abdominal information may be obtained. It has a sensitivity of 98%, a specificity of 97%, and positive and negative predictive values of 100% and 97%, respectively. It does not provide information regarding the functional status of the kidney.

Treatment

About 90% of renal stones are passed spontaneously. Basic treatment is as follows:

A. Provide Analgesia

Begin analgesics as soon as the diagnosis has been established with reasonable certainty. Opioids and antiemetics are mainstays of therapy. Ketorolac, the only injectable nonsteroidal anti-inflammatory agent, is as equipotent as mild narcotic analgesics. Ketorolac provides analgesia, and given its antiprostaglandin effects, it can decrease the inflammatory response, promote relaxation of the ureteral spasm, and alleviate capsular distention. For patients who are not hospitalized, an antiemetic, an anti-inflammatory agent, and a narcotic may be required for control of pain and emesis.

B. Ensure Adequate Hydration

Although authorities usually recommend drinking 2–3 L of fluid per day, this is probably of more value in preventing the formation of more stones than in facilitating passage of an existing stone.

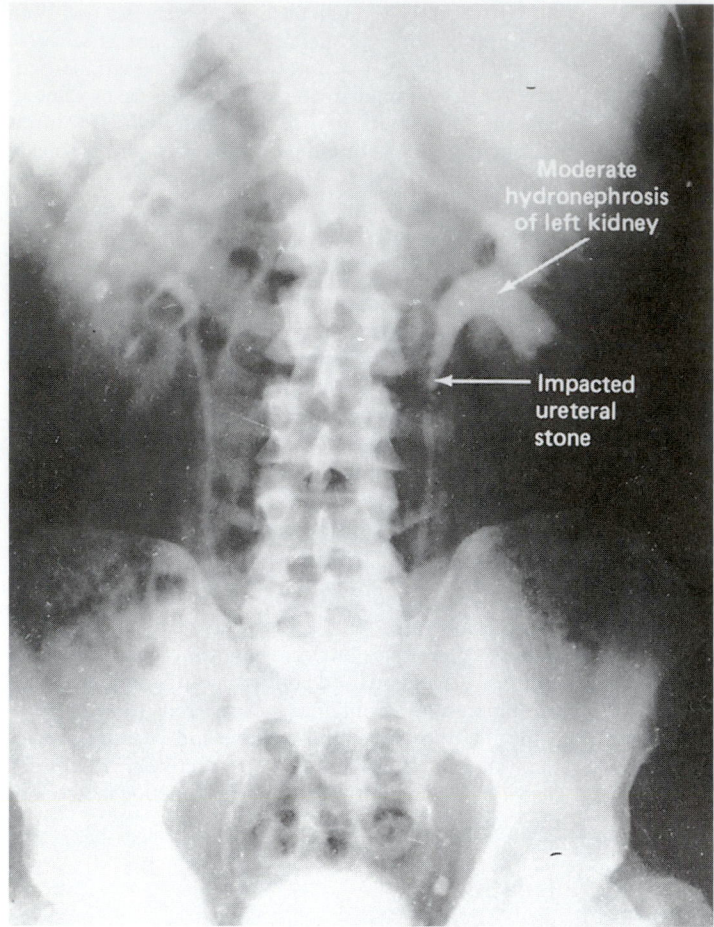

Figure 37–2. Stone in left upper ureter causing moderate obstruction. (Reproduced, with permission, from Tanagho EA, McAninch JW: *Smith's General Urology,* 13th ed. Appleton & Lange, 1992.)

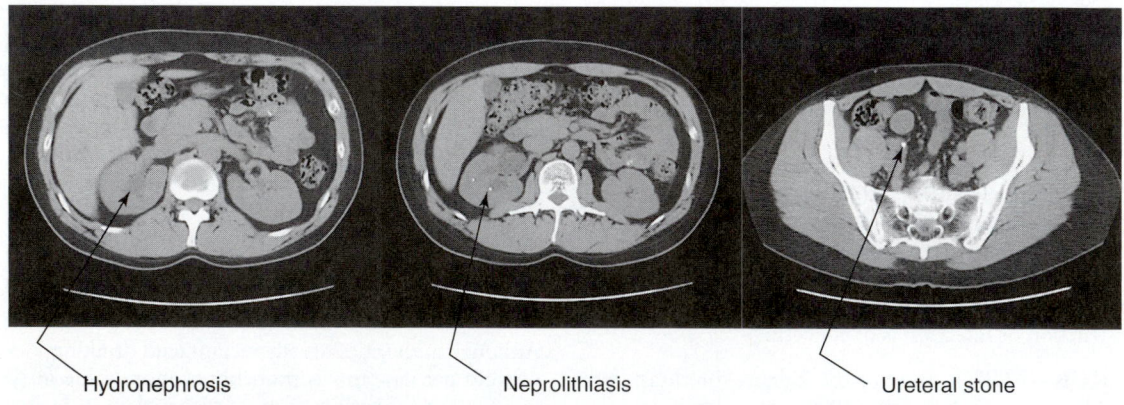

Figure 37–3. Unenhanced helical CT scan demonstrating right-sided hydronephrosis (**A**), right nephrolithiasis (**B**), and stone in right ureter (**C**).

C. Strain Urine

Patients with their first episode of urolithiasis or those who pass stones of unknown composition should strain their urine through a urine strainer or a coffee filter and submit the stone for chemical analysis.

Prevention

Specific preventive therapy can be recommended after the composition of the stone has been determined by chemical analysis.

Disposition

Patients with any of the following conditions require hospitalization:

- Pain requiring parenteral analgesics
- Intractable emesis
- Coexisting pyelonephritis
- Documented or suspected renal dysfunction (elevated blood urea nitrogen or serum creatinine levels, bilateral ureteral stones, oliguria or anuria, hydronephrosis)
- Pain that persists for more than 2–3 days, suggesting persistent urinary obstruction

Patients who do not require hospitalization should be referred to a urologist within 24–48 hours for further evaluation and treatment.

DISEASES OF THE MALE GENITOURINARY SYSTEM

1. Torsion of the Testicle

ESSENTIALS OF DIAGNOSIS

- *Testicular torsion, torsion of the testicular appendage, and epididymitis account for 85–90% of all cases of scrotal pain.*
- *Rare in males over age 30 years but occurs at all ages.*
- *The testicle may be high riding with "bell clapper" deformity.*
- *Detorsion must occur within 6 hours for testicular salvage.*
- *Attempt manual detorsion.*
- *Color-flow Doppler ultrasound demonstrates diminished blood flow to affected testis.*

Clinical Findings

Testicular torsion has a bimodal incidence with peaks occurring in neonates and pubescent males; however, it can occur in all age groups. Torsion of the testicular or epididymal appendages can also present as acute unilateral scrotal pain. Of the 4 appendages, the appendix testis becomes torsed the most often (99%) and usually requires only supportive care.

The history for testicular torsion is most often sudden onset of moderate to severe, unilateral scrotal pain. Patients may recount similar episodes that resolved spontaneously in the past. On physical examination, the testis can be high-riding with a transverse rather than vertical lie, slightly larger than the unaffected testis, and diffusely tender and erythematous. An absent cremasteric reflex on the affected side is the most sensitive physical finding. Nausea, vomiting, and abdominal pain may occur as a result of the ischemia.

Epididymitis, orchitis, neoplasms, peritonitis, hernia, abdominal aortic aneurysm, Fournier gangrene, and other scrotal diseases need to be considered in the differential diagnosis (see Table 37–2). Urinalysis is usually normal. Color-flow Doppler ultrasonography or radionucleotide scanning may confirm the diagnosis.

Epididymitis and orchitis may be confused with torsion of the testicle; helpful differentiating features are discussed in the section on scrotal pain and in Table 37–2. The diagnosis may be confirmed by Doppler ultrasound examination or radionuclide scanning.

Treatment & Disposition

A. Provide Analgesia

Parenteral narcotic analgesics usually are required.

B. Prepare for Surgery

Give nothing orally, obtain blood for CBC and renal function tests, and begin an intravenous infusion.

C. Obtain Immediate Urologic Surgical Consultation

If a delay in urologic consultation is anticipated, attempt manual detorsion as discussed earlier in this chapter. Testicular salvage approaches 100% if detorsion (manual or surgical) is performed within 6 hours.

2. Orchitis

Orchitis is commonly associated with epididymitis. It usually has an infectious cause, for example, from viral, bacterial, or mycobacterial agents. Viral orchitis is most often due to mumps. The orchitis commonly presents 5 days after the parotitis. Mumps orchitis may result in atrophy. If the diagnosis is in doubt or specific treatment appears warranted, obtain urologic consultation.

Symptomatic relief may be achieved with recumbency and analgesics.

3. Priapism

Clinical Findings

Priapism is a persistent involuntary, painful erection, unrelated to sexual stimulation and unrelieved by ejaculation. About 25% of cases are associated with leukemia, metastatic carcinoma, or sickling hemoglobinopathies. If the medical history is unclear, consider a CBC and sickling test. Alcohol, marijuana, cocaine, and now MDMA (Ecstasy) are among some of the recreational drugs known to induce priapism, but many prescriptions drugs are culprits as well. Regardless of treatment, there is a high incidence of corporal fibrosis and erectile dysfunction.

Treatment

Management is mainly to provide analgesia and hydration and to abort the erection to prevent permanent damage. Several modalities can be attempted, but success is often limited. Ice packs have limited success. Hydration, oxygenation, and sometimes exchange transfusion is necessary for sickle cell patients. Terbutaline has had some favorable results. Corporal aspiration and irrigation with a phenylephrine solution can be used but should be done in conjunction with urologic consultation.

Disposition

Hospitalize all patients with persistent priapism or those with serious underlying disease (sickling hemoglobinopathy, leukemia). Obtain urgent urologic consultation.

4. Fournier Gangrene

 ESSENTIALS OF DIAGNOSIS

- *Necrotizing fasciitis of the perineum.*
- *Fever, pain, edema, and erythema of the scrotum are typically present.*
- *Wide surgical debridement is crucial.*
- *Mortality is approximately 60–70%.*

Fournier gangrene is a necrotizing fasciitis of the perineum that primarily affects diabetic males aged 20–50 years. Patients typically present with fever, pain, edema, and erythema of the scrotum or penis. The most com-

mon causes are infection and trauma. Aerobes or anaerobes may be the causative infectious agents. Treatment includes antibiotic therapy, wide surgical incision, and drainage. Mortality is approximately 60–70%.

5. Phimosis & Paraphimosis

 ESSENTIALS OF DIAGNOSIS

- *Chronic balanoposthitis, due to a bacterial or fungal infection, is a risk factor for phimosis (inability to retract the foreskin).*
- *Physiologic phimosis is normal in the first few years of life.*
- *Paraphimosis (retracted, constricted foreskin proximal to the glans) may cause necrosis to the glans and urethra if not treated.*

Phimosis is a fibrous constriction of the foreskin preventing retraction; it is often associated with balanitis and may cause urinary retention. Phimosis or paraphimosis rarely results from chronic balanoposthitis, which is categorized as either irritant or infectious. Bal-

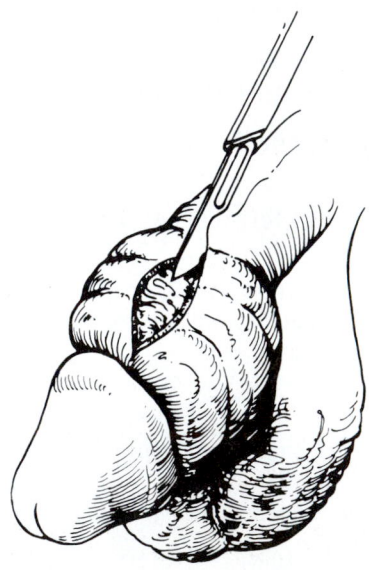

Figure 37–4. Method of performing a dorsal slit of the foreskin for balanitis and paraphimosis. An incision made through the tight band of skin as shown will relieve the paraphimosis.

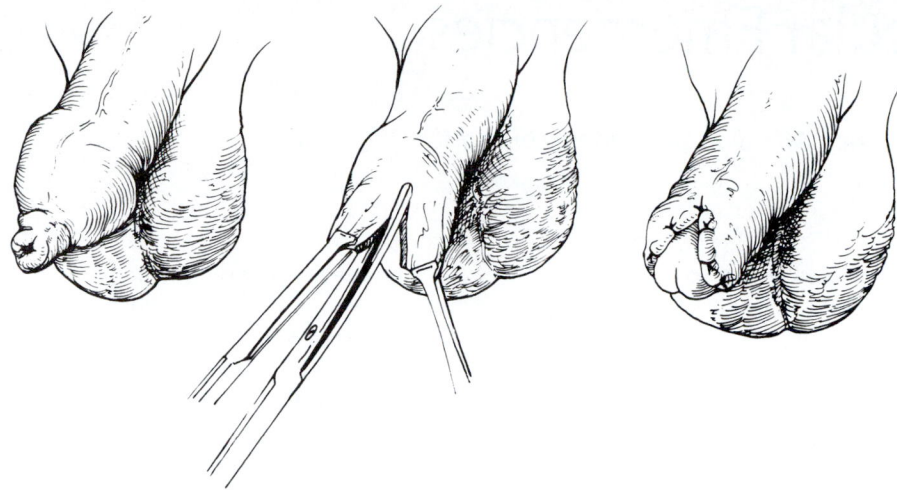

Figure 37–5. Method of performing a dorsal slit of the foreskin for phimosis.

anoposthitis is inflammation of the glans penis and the prepuce. Treatment for acute irritant balanoposthitis is sitz baths, cleansing with the foreskin retracted, and 0.5% hydrocortisone cream. Candidal infections are the most common infectious cause and are treated with good hygiene and topical antifungal cream. Phimosis without balanitis may be an indication for elective circumcision, but it is not an emergency. Surgical correction should not be attempted in the emergency department.

Paraphimosis occurs when the retracted foreskin develops a fixed constriction proximal to the glans. The penis distal to the constricting foreskin may become swollen and painful, or even gangrenous, and urinary retention may result. Attempt manual reduction: Squeeze the glans firmly for 5–10 minutes to reduce its size. Then move the prepuce distally while the glans is pushed proximally. If manual reduction is unsuccessful, a dorsal slit of the foreskin is necessary (Figures 37–4 and 37–5). Refer the patient to a urologist for elective circumcision to reduce risk of recurrence. In addition, a complication of the Plastibell device for pediatric circumcision occurs if the ring inadvertently slips behind the glans, creating a paraphimosis and causing penile ischemia. The ring should be removed immediately.

Abramson S et al: Impact in the emergency department of unenhanced CT on diagnostic confidence and therapeutic efficacy in patients with suspected renal colic: a prospective survey. 2000 ARRS President's Award. American Roentgen Ray Society. Am J Roentgenol 2000;175:1689. [PMID: 11090405]

Altman AL et al: Cocaine associated priapism. J Urol 1999;161:1817. [PMID: 10332443]

Burgher SW: Acute scrotal pain. Emerg Med Clin North Am 1998;16:781. [PMID: 9889740]

Choe JM: Paraphimosis: current treatment options. Am Fam Physician 2000;62:2623. [PMID: 11142469]

Dubin N et al: Priapism: Ecstasy related? Urology 2000;56:1057. [PMID: 11113767]

Herbener TE: Ultrasound in the assessment of the acute scrotum. J Clin Ultrasound 1996;24:405. [PMID: 8884519]

Kassim AA et al: Acute priapism associated with the use of sildenafil in a patient with sickle cell trait. Blood 2000;95:1878. [PMID: 10744389]

Langer JC et al: Circumcision and pediatric disorders of the penis. Pediatr Clin North Am 1998;45:801. [PMID: 9728187]

Larkin GL et al: Efficacy of ketorolac tromethamine versus meperidine in the ED treatment of acute renal colic. Am J Emerg Med 1999;17:6. [PMID: 9928687]

Lunquist ST et al: Diseases of the foreskin, penis, and urethra. Emerg Med Clin North Am 2001;19:529. [PMID: 11554274]

Majeed S et al: Refractory priapism of unknown etiology in a pediatric patient. Pediatr Emerg Care 2000;16:347. [PMID: 11063367]

Manthey DE et al: Nephrolithiasis. Emerg Med Clin North Am 2001;19:633. [PMID: 11554279]

Marcozzi D et al: The nontraumatic, acute scrotum. Emerg Med Clin North Am 2001;19:547. [PMID: 11554275]

Mulhall JP et al: Priapism: etiology and management. Acad Emerg Med 1996;3:810. [PMID: 8853679]

Rekant EM et al: Emergency department time for evaluation of patients discharged with a diagnosis of renal colic: unenhanced helical computed tomography versus intravenous urography. J Emerg Med 2001;21:371. [PMID: 11728762]

Siegel MJ: The acute scrotum. Radiol Clin North Am 1997;35:959. [PMID: 9216633]

Waugh MA: Balanitis. Dermatol Clin 1998;16:757. [PMID: 9891676]

Vascular Emergencies

Scott W. Hines, MD, & James J. Mensching, MD, DO, FACEP[1]

I. Vascular Emergencies Due to Trauma

Immediate Management of Life-Threatening Vascular Injuries

Emergency Management of Specific Vascular Injuries

Neck Injuries

Chest Injuries

Pulmonary Vascular Injuries

Abdominal Injuries

Injuries to the Extremities

Major Venous Trauma

II. Vascular Emergencies Not Due to Trauma

Acute Ischemia

Acute Peripheral Ischemia Due to Major Arterial Occlusion

Acute Peripheral Ischemia Due to Small-Vessel Occlusion ("Blue Toe Syndrome")

Acute Peripheral Ischemia Due to Venous Occlusion

Acute Visceral (Intestinal) Ischemia

Acute Cerebral Ischemia Due to Emboli

Arterial Aneurysms

Ruptured Abdominal Aortic Aneurysm

Visceral & Hypogastric Artery Aneurysms

Thoracic Aortic Aneurysm (Aortic Dissection)

Popliteal & Femoral Peripheral Aneurysms

Venous Disease

Lower-Extremity Deep Venous Thrombosis

Superficial Thrombophlebitis

Upper-Extremity Venous Thrombosis

Ruptured Venous Varicosities (Varicose Veins)

Pulmonary Embolism

Arteriovenous Fistula

Other Vascular Syndromes

Thoracic Outlet Syndrome

Complications of Percutaneous Transluminal Angioplasty & Retrograde Angiography

Ergotism

Intra-arterial Injection of Drugs

Frostbite

Most vascular emergencies are due either to disruption of the blood vessel wall with bleeding (eg, from penetrating trauma) or to occlusion of the blood vessel lumen (eg, by an embolus or thrombus). The major consequences of these events are blood loss or acute distal ischemia. If vascular injury is untreated, hypotension or tissue necrosis may occur.

■ I. VASCULAR EMERGENCIES DUE TO TRAUMA

IMMEDIATE MANAGEMENT OF LIFE-THREATENING VASCULAR INJURIES

Maintain Airway & Treat Associated Injuries

(See Chapters 7 and 11.) Treat associated life-threatening head, thoracic, and abdominal injuries (Chapters 10, 22, 24, and 25).

---

[1]This chapter is a revision of the chapter by Carol A. Raviola, MD, & Donald D. Trunkey, MD, from the 4th edition.

Stop Hemorrhage

1. Stop active bleeding from arterial or venous hemorrhage by gentle manual compression.
2. Avoid clamping the bleeding vessel, because this will cause further injury.
3. Avoid the use of tourniquets.
4. Do not remove embedded objects, because they may be preventing further bleeding.

Treat or Prevent Shock

(See also Chapter 9.) Insert 2 or more large-bore (≥ 16-gauge) intravenous catheters or perform venous cutdowns. Two intravenous access sites are preferable if the patient is already in shock or is bleeding profusely.

While intravenous catheters are being inserted, draw blood for complete blood count (CBC), serum electrolytes, glucose and creatinine measurements, prothrombin time (PT), partial thromboplastin time (PTT), and typing and cross-matching (reserve 6–8 units of packed red blood cells or whole blood).

Begin intravenous infusion of crystalloid solutions (eg, normal saline or lactated Ringer's) to support blood pressure. Up to 2–3 L of crystalloid solution may be given before blood products must be administered.

Replace blood. The number of units administered depends on the severity of existing blood loss and on anticipated loss from projected surgery. Use fresh whole blood whenever possible.

Prevent Further Vascular & Nerve Injury

All fractures and joint dislocations associated with abnormal pulses should be carefully reduced and splinted to reduce further neurovascular damage. Control hemorrhage by pressure; avoid clamping vessels to stop hemorrhage. Consider adjunctive studies for further evaluation as appropriate (eg, computed tomography [CT] scan, angiography).

Minimize Ischemia

Keep ischemic limbs horizontal. Do not use tourniquets.

Relieve Pain

Provide adequate analgesia; if necessary, give narcotic analgesics.

Obtain Surgical Consultation

All documented or suspected vascular injuries should be examined promptly by a general or vascular surgeon before the patient is transferred from the emergency department.

Hospitalize Patients as Required

Hospitalize all patients with arterial or major venous injuries.

General Considerations

Acute vascular injury may result in either hemorrhage or tissue ischemia.

A. ARTERIAL INJURY

1. Hemorrhage—Obvious external hemorrhage is present in many patients. Occult bleeding into soft tissue, the retroperitoneum, the pelvis, or body cavities may also occur.

2. Ischemia—Ischemia from arterial injury must be recognized and treated promptly, because increased tissue pressure and swelling from ischemia further compromise arterial perfusion, and prolonged ischemia results in irreversible tissue damage.

B. VENOUS INJURY

1. Hemorrhage—Obvious or occult bleeding usually occurs following venous injury. It is rarely life threatening except in the case of injuries to central veins (eg, vena cava) or their immediate branches (eg, femoral vein).

2. Ischemia—Tissue ischemia from venous trauma alone is rare, although venous obstruction and resultant tissue congestion may worsen preexisting tissue ischemia resulting from arterial injury.

C. CAUSES OF VASCULAR INJURY

1. Penetrating trauma—Penetrating trauma is the most common cause of peripheral vascular injury and ranges in severity from innocuous simple puncture wounds to extensive wounds caused by high-velocity missiles. Penetrating injuries to the central vessels may lead to massive hemorrhage and death.

2. Blunt trauma—Blunt trauma may also cause vascular injury. Contusions or crushing injuries of an artery may cause either transmural disruption with hemorrhage, or partial disruption of the artery and elevation of the intima from an intramural hematoma (ie, dissection). Thrombosis of a segment of artery may also occur. Blunt trauma with dislocation of a joint may result in disruption of the arteries crossing that joint line, leading to ischemia distal to the site of injury (eg, disruption of the popliteal artery with posterior dislocation of the knee). Blunt trauma may also contribute indirectly to vascular occlusion by creating large hematomas near a blood vessel. Hematoma formation may lead to arterial spasm, distortion, or compartment syndromes, all of which may interfere with arterial flow.

3. Chemicals—Chemical injury to blood vessels is increasing in frequency. It is generally iatrogenic or associated with parenteral drug abuse. Intra-arterial injection of drugs that are chemically irritating to tissues (eg, barbiturates) causes occlusion of small peripheral vessels. If occlusion is severe, all or part of the limb may be lost. Extravasation of an intravenously administered chemical may also cause associated arterial spasm or tissue necrosis. Barbiturates, phenytoin, vasopressors, and chemotherapeutic agents (eg, doxorubicin) are notable examples. High doses of certain intravenously administered vasopressors (eg, dopamine) can cause intense peripheral vasoconstriction with ultimate digital ischemic necrosis.

D. SEQUELAE

Late sequelae associated with major vascular injuries include the development of false aneurysms and arteriovenous fistulas.

1. False aneurysms—False aneurysms do not contain all three layers of the vessel wall (intima, media, and adventitia). They result from walled-off disruptions of vessel walls. They enlarge over time, may compress adjacent veins or nerves, and may rupture without warning.

2. Fistulas—Fistulas may occur after adjacent arteries and veins are injured simultaneously, usually as a result of stab wounds or missile injury. The fistula may enlarge over time and cause increased cardiac output if a large left-to-right shunting of blood is present. If the fistula involves the blood supply to an extremity, dilated veins may be observed in that extremity. Turbulent blood flow through the fistula results in an obvious thrill or bruit. Fistulas may also compress adjacent nerves or impede collateral circulation, or they may rupture, causing a severe hemorrhage.

Principles of Diagnosis

A. PHYSICAL EXAMINATION

If there is a wound in the vicinity of a major blood vessel, assume that vascular injury has occurred. The findings listed below may not appear for hours to days following a significant vascular injury, and absence of these findings does not rule out the possibility of vascular injury.

1. Signs—Clinical manifestations of vascular injury include an expanding or pulsating hematoma, to-and-fro or continuous murmurs of arteriovenous fistulas, a false aneurysm, loss of pulses, progressive swelling of the injured part, unexplained ischemia or dysfunction, and unilateral cool or pale extremities.

2. Pulses—Perform a complete vascular examination unless treatment of other life-threatening injuries precludes it.

a. Palpation—Palpate all peripheral pulses: carotid, axillary, brachial, radial, femoral, popliteal, dorsalis pedis, and posterior tibial.

b. Doppler ultrasound examination—The presence of blood flow in a peripheral vessel can be detected using a standard pocket Doppler apparatus. Any assessment of the normality of this flow requires concomitant pressure measurements or waveform analysis.

3. Murmurs and bruits—Auscultate over injured areas to detect bruits or murmurs.

4. Neurologic function—Assess neurologic function. Paresthesia may be an early sign of developing vascular problems (eg, compartment syndrome).

B. DIAGNOSTIC IMAGING

Arteriography is the single best method of confirming suspected peripheral, mesenterial, and cervical vascular injury. In addition, arteriography defines the nature and extent of injury and is essential to the surgeon contemplating corrective surgery. CT scan with contrast has emerged as the diagnostic study of choice to evaluate central vascular injuries (eg, aortic injury or rupture) due to its ready availability. Ultrasonography and arteriography are also useful in specific circumstances (discussed below).

Caution: Diagnostic imaging should not be performed in a patient whose condition is unstable and who needs emergency laparotomy or thoracotomy. The procedure should be delayed until after resuscitation and treatment of the life-threatening emergency, either in the emergency department or in the operating room.

EMERGENCY MANAGEMENT OF SPECIFIC VASCULAR INJURIES

NECK INJURIES
(See also Chapter 23.)

 ESSENTIALS OF DIAGNOSIS

- *History of blunt or penetrating trauma.*
- *Consider concomitant injury to nonvascular structures.*
- *Arteriography, ultrasound, or CT scan confirm diagnosis.*

General Considerations

Vascular injury to the neck is most often due to penetrating injuries; however, blunt trauma to the cervical vessels can result in intimal disruption, dissection, and thrombosis. Concomitant injury to nonvascular structures of the neck (eg, trachea, esophagus, and spinal cord) may also occur. The cervical spine must be protected until injury is excluded.

Penetrating Trauma

In penetrating trauma to the neck, two immediate concerns are massive hemorrhage and airway compromise secondary to a rapidly expanding hematoma.

A. EMERGENCY TREATMENT

Control hemorrhage, preferably with direct pressure. If this fails, balloon tamponade with a Foley catheter may act as a temporizing measure along with ongoing fluid resuscitation; neither of these measures should delay transport to the operating room for definitive repair. If a rapidly expanding hematoma is suspected, tracheal intubation via direct laryngoscopy or intubating bronchoscope should be conducted before compression of the trachea makes this procedure more difficult or impossible. Transtracheal jet insufflation and cricothyrotomy are methods of last resort; in this setting, emergent tracheostomy is preferable.

B. FURTHER TREATMENT

Further management is a function of the patient's hemodynamic stability and the location of the wound. All actively bleeding, hemodynamically unstable patients are taken immediately to the operating room for surgical exploration. For stable patients with wounds that penetrate the platysma muscle, management is a function of the zone of the neck affected (Figure 38–1). Wounds should never be probed beyond the level of the platysma muscle in the emergency department.

1. Zone I injuries—These wounds are frequently associated with injury to the great vessels and require imaging to exclude major arterial injury.

2. Zone II injuries—These injuries may be further evaluated by surgical exploration or imaging of the vessels and nonvascular structures at the discretion of the attending surgeon.

3. Zone III injuries—Because the relationship of the blood vessels to the base of the skull makes surgical exploration and distal control of hemorrhage difficult, preoperative imaging should be conducted to define the injury and help plan the surgical approach.

Blunt Trauma

Blunt trauma to the carotid artery can result in intimal disruption, dissection, and thrombosis leading to acute cerebral ischemia manifest as a gross hemispheric neurologic deficit not explained by intracranial trauma. Conduct emergent imaging of the neck arteries.

Diagnostic Imaging

The gold standard for detecting vascular injury in the neck remains arteriography. However, both ultrasonography and helical CT scan can be used.

Disposition

Asymptomatic patients with mild neck injuries due to blunt trauma or penetrating injuries that do not cross the platysma muscle may be discharged from the emergency department. Hospitalize all other patients with neck injuries, and consult with a general or vascular surgeon.

CHEST INJURIES
(See also Chapter 24.)

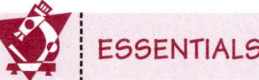

ESSENTIALS OF DIAGNOSIS

- *Significant mechanism of thoracic trauma.*
- *Tearing retrosternal or interscapular pain, dysphagia, hoarseness, or dyspnea.*
- *In blunt trauma, less than half of patients will have visible signs of chest wall injury.*
- *CT scan confirms diagnosis.*

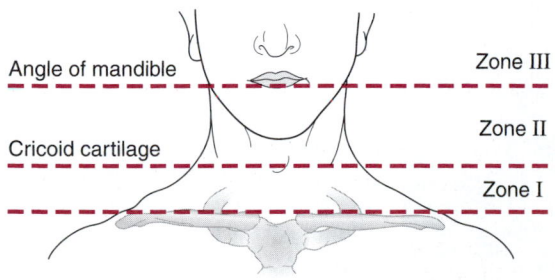

Figure 38–1. Zones of vascular injury in the neck.

General Considerations

Vascular injury to the chest occurs secondary to both penetrating and blunt trauma. If bleeding is not contained within fascial planes, these injuries can lead to exsanguination and death, often before the patient arrives in the emergency department. A high degree of suspicion for this type of injury must be maintained in any patient with a significant mechanism of thoracic trauma. With the evolution of helical (spiral) CT scan, CT with contrast has become the diagnostic study of choice in evaluating vascular injury in a hemodynamically stable patient with chest trauma.

Thoracic Aortic Injury

Penetrating and blunt trauma may cause thoracic aortic injury (TAI). Though penetrating TAI may be caused by any variety of objects or weapons, blunt TAI involves large, violent deceleration forces (eg, falls, motor vehicle collisions including occupant ejection or auto-pedestrian). The greatest risk of TAI in a motor vehicle collision exists when the impact occurs on the same side of the vehicle as the occupant, when there is greater than 15 inches of intrusion into the passenger compartment, and when the overall change in velocity experienced by the vehicle and its occupants is greater than 20 miles per hour. A significant mechanism of injury should heighten suspicion of blunt TAI, because less than half of these patients will have visible signs of chest wall injury.

Clinical Findings

A. SYMPTOMS AND SIGNS

Patients may complain of tearing retrosternal or interscapular pain. Less frequently, dysphagia, hoarseness, stridor, or shortness of breath is present. The physical examination often reveals no external evidence of chest wall injury. Classically, a difference in upper-extremity pulses and a harsh systolic murmur across the precordium and in the interscapular area are noted. Signs and symptoms of shock may be present.

B. IMAGING

The chest x-ray is frequently the first imaging study obtained (Figure 38–2); the classic chest x-ray findings associated with TAI are listed in Table 38–1. However, 7% of patients with TAI can have a normal chest x-ray and further imaging studies may be warranted, based on clinical suspicion and mechanism of injury. In the past, aortography had been the study of choice in evaluating TAIs. However, helical CT scan has emerged as the study of choice after initial chest x-ray. It is more readily available than aortography and less invasive, and prospective clinical trials have shown spiral CT scan to be 100% sensitive and 99.7% specific in diagnosing TAI following blunt trauma. In centers where transesophageal echocardiography (TEE) is readily available, it is a highly sensitive (98%) and specific (100%) modality for diagnosing TAI. TEE can be done at the bedside, requires no contrast dye, and evaluates real-time cardiac function.

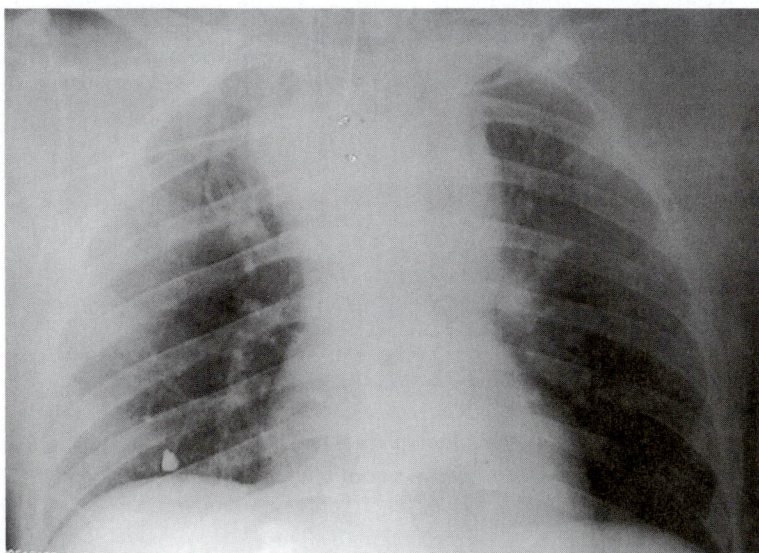

Figure 38–2. Chest x-ray from a patient with a traumatic aortic injury demonstrating a wide mediastinum, blurring of the aortic arch, left apical cap, and deviation of the nasogastric tube.

Table 38–1. X-ray findings associated with traumatic rupture of the thoracic aorta.

Left apical "cap" (fluid in the apical pleural space)
Widened mediastinum
Deviation of trachea to the right
Depression of left main-stem bronchus
Obscuration of the aortic arch
Hemothorax

Treatment & Disposition

Patients with TAI will require emergent consultation with a vascular or thoracic surgeon. In the emergency department it is important to maintain intravascular volume with crystalloid solutions and blood products. Systolic blood pressure should be lowered to less than 120 mm Hg. Exsanguinating hemorrhage may require emergency thoracotomy for the control of bleeding.

PULMONARY VASCULAR INJURIES

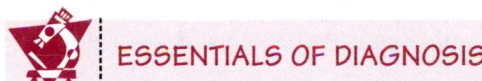 ESSENTIALS OF DIAGNOSIS

- *Usually due to penetrating thoracic or abdominal injury.*
- *Rapidly expanding hemothorax on chest x-ray.*

Clinical Findings

General Considerations

Most patients present with penetrating chest or abdominal trauma and rapidly expanding hemothorax, visible on chest x-ray. Rarely, blunt chest trauma is associated with pulmonary vascular injury.

Treatment & Disposition

Most patients can be managed with a chest tube that uses suction and allows the lung to reexpand and block the bleeding vessel. Continued massive bleeding requires prompt surgery. Consider the use of autotransfusion. Prompt consultation with a general, vascular, or thoracic surgeon is required, because exsanguination can occur rapidly. Hospitalization is indicated for all patients.

ABDOMINAL INJURIES
(See also Chapter 25.)

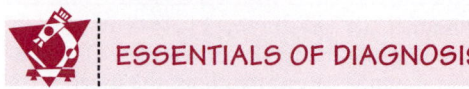 ESSENTIALS OF DIAGNOSIS

- *History of abdominal trauma.*
- *Signs and symptoms of shock that fail to respond to resuscitation efforts.*

Clinical Findings

Patients with injuries to major vessels within the abdominal cavity present mainly with hemorrhagic shock that fails to respond to resuscitative efforts. Although arteriography is rarely required to diagnose vessel injury in the abdomen, it is useful both diagnostically and therapeutically in patients with severe pelvic trauma who have ongoing bleeding, because angiographic embolization can be effective treatment in certain injuries. Aortography is also useful in establishing the diagnosis of renovascular pedicle injury in trauma patients with nonvisualization of a kidney on urography. CT scan may also be helpful.

Treatment & Disposition

Immediate operation is the only effective treatment for abdominal vascular injuries. Support blood pressure with infusion of intravenous fluids (colloid or crystalloid solutions) until surgery can be performed. Packed red blood cells or whole blood should be used as soon as available (Chapter 9).

A portable chest x-ray (upright, if possible) should be obtained before laparotomy, to rule out unsuspected thoracic injuries.

INJURIES TO THE EXTREMITIES

 ESSENTIALS OF DIAGNOSIS

- *History of blunt or penetrating trauma.*
- *Presence of a pulse does not rule out vessel injury.*
- *Use arteriography to evaluate.*

Clinical Findings

A. PENETRATING TRAUMA

Vascular injuries are present in 25–35% of patients with penetrating trauma to the extremities. Occasionally vascular trauma is present without the usual physical findings, and the presence of a pulse does not rule out injury to the vessel. Arteriography should be considered whenever the weapon's trajectory has passed close to major blood vessels.

B. BLUNT TRAUMA

Vascular injury may also occur after blunt trauma, especially if fractures and joint dislocations are present. Even if the pulse is restored with splinting and traction, an arteriogram is necessary to rule out significant injury to the intima.

C. POSTERIOR DISLOCATION OF THE KNEE

Posterior dislocation of the knee is associated with popliteal artery injury in half of cases, and arteriography is therefore mandatory.

Treatment

Stabilize the patient, and stop hemorrhage as outlined above. Splint fractures. Do not clamp vessels or use a tourniquet unless injury is exsanguinating the patient and compression fails to control the hemorrhage.

Disposition

All patients with suspected vascular injury should be hospitalized for arteriography. Obtain general or vascular surgical consultation.

MAJOR VENOUS TRAUMA

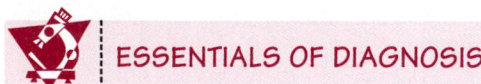

ESSENTIALS OF DIAGNOSIS

- *History of trauma.*
- *Injuries to major venous structures manifested by progressive hemorrhagic shock (not ischemia).*
- *Venography may aid diagnosis.*

General Considerations

Trauma to peripheral veins without associated arterial injury usually does not require operative correction; however, disruption of the central large veins (vena cava or its immediate branches, subclavian or iliac veins)—especially where they are not enclosed by dense fascia or muscles—requires prompt operation.

Clinical Findings

Venous injury is usually manifested by hemorrhage, not ischemia. Patients with bleeding from the central veins present with progressive hemorrhagic shock (Chapter 9). Superior vena cava and subclavian vein hemorrhage is usually associated with hemothorax visible on chest x-ray.

In contrast, hemorrhage from the inferior vena cava and iliac vein is more difficult to detect. The only common finding is progressive hemorrhagic shock, and many of these injuries are not suspected before they are discovered at surgery.

Diagnosis depends on venography (occasionally the lesion may be visible on the venous phase of an arteriogram) and on discovery at surgery, because most patients are too unstable to allow detailed radiologic evaluation.

Treatment & Disposition

Surgical correction in the operating room is indicated.

American College of Emergency Physicians: Clinical policy for the initial approach to patients presenting with penetrating extremity trauma. Ann Emerg Med 1999;33:612. [PMID: 10216346]

Asensio JA et al: Multiinstitutional experience with the management of superior mesenteric artery injuries. Am Coll Surg 2001;193:354. [PMID: 11584962]

Chen MY et al: Role of angiography in the detection of aortic branch vessel injury after blunt thoracic trauma. J Trauma 2001;51:1166. [PMID: 11740270]

Cook AD et al: Chest radiographs of limited utility in the diagnosis of blunt traumatic aortic laceration. J Trauma 2001;50:843. [PMID: 11371839]

Dyer DS et al: Thoracic aortic injury: how predictive is mechanism and is chest computed tomography a reliable screening tool? A prospective study of 1,561 patients. J Trauma 2000;48:673. [PMID: 10780601]

Exadaktylos AK et al: Do we really need routine computed tomographic scanning in the primary evaluation of blunt chest trauma in patients with "normal" chest radiograph? J Trauma 2001;51(6):1173. [PMID: 11740271]

Fishman JE et al: Direct versus indirect signs of traumatic aortic injury revealed by helical CT: performance characteristics and interobserver agreement. Am J Roentgenol 1999;172:1027. [PMID: 10587141]

Goarin JP et al: Evaluation of transesophageal echocardiography for diagnosis of traumatic aortic injury. Anesthesiology 2000;93:1373. [PMID: 11149428]

Horton TG et al: Identification of trauma patients at risk of thoracic aortic tear by mechanism of injury. J Trauma 2000;48:1008. [PMID: 10866244]

Ledbetter S et al: Helical (spiral) CT in the evaluation of emergent thoracic aortic syndromes: traumatic aortic rupture, aortic aneurysm, aortic dissection, intramural hematoma, and penetrating atherosclerotic ulcer. Radiol Clin North Am 1999; 37:575. [PMID: 10361547]

Malhotra AK et al: Minimal aortic injury: a lesion associated with advancing diagnostic techniques. J Trauma 2001;51:1042. [PMID: 11740248]

Mirvis SE et al: Use of spiral computed tomography for the assessment of blunt trauma patients with potential aortic injury. J Trauma 1998;45:922. [PMID: 9820704]

Munera F et al: Diagnosis of arterial injuries caused by penetrating trauma to the neck: comparison of helical CT angiography and conventional angiography. Radiology 2000;216:356. [PMID: 10924553]

Novelline RA et al: Helical CT in emergency radiology. Radiology 1999;213:321. [PMID: 10551209]

Simon BJ et al: Factors predicting early in-hospital death in blunt thoracic aortic injury. J Trauma 2001;51:906. [PMID: 11706338]

Thompson EC et al: Penetrating neck trauma: an overview of management. J Oral Maxillofac Surg 2002;60:918. [PMID: 12149739]

■ II. VASCULAR EMERGENCIES NOT DUE TO TRAUMA

Acute Ischemia

ACUTE PERIPHERAL ISCHEMIA DUE TO MAJOR ARTERIAL OCCLUSION

 ESSENTIALS OF DIAGNOSIS

- *History of arrhythmia, myocardial infarction, valvular disease, or atherosclerosis may be present.*
- *Pain, paresthesias, and coolness of affected extremity.*
- *Pale, mottled, cyanotic limb with decreased or absent pulses.*
- *Angiography confirms diagnosis.*

Clinical Findings

Acute arterial occlusion may be caused by an embolus, thrombosis, or trauma to an artery. Occlusion leads to distal ischemia, which if not corrected can progress to irreversible tissue damage and necrosis.

A. EMBOLIC OCCLUSION

Embolic occlusion is caused by the dislodgment of an intravascular thrombus which travels distally and occludes a smaller artery. The majority of thrombi originate in the heart, but they may come from anywhere within the vascular system. A history of arrhythmia, myocardial infarction, or valvular heart disease suggests an embolic cause for acute peripheral ischemia.

1. Cardiac emboli—Cardiac emboli generally originate in the left atrium in patients with atrial fibrillation or mitral valve disease and in the left ventricle in patients with recent myocardial infarction or ventricular aneurysm.

2. Vascular emboli—Vascular emboli originate on irregular luminal surfaces of atherosclerotic vessels (eg, ulcerative plaques or aneurysms). These emboli may contain cholesterol in the clot.

3. Tumor emboli—Tumor emboli are rare, the most common sources are atrial myxomas.

B. THROMBOTIC OCCLUSION

Thrombosis of an atherosclerotic artery resulting in acute ischemia is uncommon but may occur secondary to plaque disruption and resultant clot formation. A history of peripheral vascular disease, claudication, progressive rest pain, or nonhealing wounds of the distal extremities is suggestive of occlusion secondary to thrombosis, because these patients often lack sufficient collateral flow that can minimize ischemia.

C. CONSEQUENCES OF OCCLUSION

Acute occlusion of a previously patent major artery results in ischemia of the nerves, muscles, and skin distal to the occluded site. The severity of symptoms is a function of the adequacy of flow through collateral vascular channels. Within a few hours after persistent and severe occlusion, irreversible anesthesia, paralysis, and tissue infarction occur. During this time, the developing thrombus progressively occludes the distal vessels, reducing the likelihood of restoration of blood flow to distal parts. For these reasons, early recognition and appropriate treatment, before irreversible damage occurs, is critical.

Clinical Findings

A. SYMPTOMS AND SIGNS

Patients typically present with extremity pain but may also complain of paresthesias and even paralysis of the affected limb. Physical examination may reveal a pale, mottled, cool, or cyanotic limb. Pulses will be reduced or absent, and there may be tenderness to palpation of affected muscle groups.

B. IMAGING STUDIES

A Doppler ultrasound may be useful in evaluating a suspected acute arterial occlusion. Angiography of the affected limb confirms the diagnosis and is useful for planning surgical intervention.

Treatment

Obtain an immediate general or vascular surgery consultation.

Insert a large-bore (≥ 16-gauge) intravenous catheter. Obtain baseline laboratory studies, including CBC, PT, PTT, and blood chemistries. Also send a blood sample for typing and cross-matching. Begin intravenous heparin at full anticoagulation dosage as soon as possible.

Definitive treatment involves surgical thrombectomy or clot lysis through the use of localized intravascular thrombolytics.

Disposition

All patients with acute arterial insufficiency should be hospitalized for management.

ACUTE PERIPHERAL ISCHEMIA DUE TO SMALL-VESSEL OCCLUSION ("Blue Toe Syndrome")

 ESSENTIALS OF DIAGNOSIS

- Abrupt onset of small painful area on affected digit.
- Affected area is tender, cool, and cyanotic.
- Asymmetric distribution.
- Livedo reticularis may be present.

General Considerations

Acute occlusion of a digital artery by microemboli results in ischemia of the affected digit. The most common sources of these microemboli are proximal atherosclerotic plaques or aneurysms. Debris consisting of cholesterol, calcium, and platelet aggregates breaks off from these areas, travels distally through the vasculature, and lodges in the small digital arteries. Other sources of microemboli are clots on prosthetic heart valves and septic emboli from infected heart valves.

Clinical Findings

The diagnosis is based on clinical findings. Patients typically report the abrupt onset of a small painful area on the affected digit that is tender, cool, and cyanotic. If multiple areas are affected, the distribution of lesions is asymmetric. Pulses in the affected extremity are intact. A fine, lacelike rash (livedo reticularis) may be noted. If the patient presents late, gangrene may be present.

Treatment

Treatment is directed at identifying and treating the proximal source of the emboli because recurrence is likely if the source is not removed. Consult a vascular surgeon.

Disposition

Hospitalize the patient for evaluation and treatment of the source of the microemboli.

ACUTE PERIPHERAL ISCHEMIA DUE TO VENOUS OCCLUSION

 ESSENTIALS OF DIAGNOSIS

- Massive acute swelling of affected leg.
- Leg has doughy consistency.
- Cyanosis and gangrene may occur.
- Color-flow Doppler ultrasound or contrast venography confirms diagnosis.

General Considerations

Phlegmasia cerulea dolens (venous gangrene) is a severe form of iliofemoral thrombosis characterized by massive venous occlusion. Rapidly progressive venous hypertension results in diffuse limb swelling to the level of the groin. Distal ischemia occurs secondary to increased venous and tissue pressure. Cyanosis develops, and gangrene can occur.

Clinical Findings

Massive acute swelling of the entire leg and cutaneous cyanosis occur early. Distal pulses are diminished or absent. The leg has a doughy consistency, and bullae may be present. Gangrene is a late finding. The diagnosis is confirmed by color-flow Doppler ultrasound or contrast venography.

Treatment

Obtain immediate general or vascular surgery consultation. Begin intravenous heparin at full anticoagulant dosage. The first step in definitive treatment is catheter-directed intrathrombus thrombolysis. If this approach fails, or if the use of thrombolytics is contraindicated, the treatment is thrombectomy.

Disposition

Hospitalize all patients for definitive management.

ACUTE VISCERAL (INTESTINAL) ISCHEMIA

 ESSENTIALS OF DIAGNOSIS

- *Severe, poorly localized abdominal pain.*
- *May have history of intestinal angina.*
- *Pain out of proportion to physical exam findings.*
- *Gross or occult intestinal bleeding.*
- *Mesenteric arteriography confirms diagnosis.*

General Considerations

Significant arterial insufficiency can cause ischemia that results in necrosis of the bowel mucosa. This may progress to full-thickness involvement in 6–48 hours. The extent of necrosis depends on the vessel involved, the adequacy of collateral perfusion, and the degree of hypoperfusion. Untreated severe intestinal ischemia results in intestinal gangrene, diffuse peritonitis, cardiovascular collapse, and death.

Causes

A. Acute Mesenteric Vascular Occlusion

Acute mesenteric vascular occlusion is the cause of acute visceral ischemia in two thirds of patients. Occlusion may be due to an embolus from a cardiac mural thrombus or to arterial thrombosis that is the end result of atherosclerotic stenosis of the involved vessel. Some patients give a history of intestinal angina (pain after eating, often relieved by vomiting). Rarely, arterial thrombosis is due to a dissecting aneurysm (aortic or mesenteric artery), connective tissue disease (eg, polyarteritis), or other conditions.

Venous thrombosis occurs occasionally and is associated with portal hypertension, abdominal sepsis, hypercoagulable state, trauma, or use of oral contraceptives.

B. Nonocclusive Arteriolar Intestinal Ischemia

Nonocclusive arteriolar intestinal ischemia is the cause of acute visceral ischemia in one third of patients and can occur with cardiac arrhythmia, sepsis, or any prolonged hypotensive state. Splanchnic vasoconstriction causes ischemia secondary to a low-flow state.

Clinical Findings

Obscure abdominal pain and intestinal bleeding in elderly patients should suggest the diagnosis of intestinal ischemia.

A. Symptoms and Signs

Severe, poorly localized diffuse abdominal pain is invariable in intestinal ischemia. Classically the pain is out of proportion to that expected based on physical examination findings. See Chapter 13 for differential diagnosis of disorders causing acute abdominal pain. With major acute occlusion, the onset of pain is sudden. With nonocclusive ischemia, pain may develop more insidiously.

Usually, few abdominal findings occur early in the disease; later, abdominal distention and tenderness generally occur. Gross or occult intestinal bleeding may be present. Systemic toxicity may precede abdominal findings. Shock and generalized peritonitis occur late.

B. Laboratory and Other Findings

1. Laboratory tests—Laboratory tests show leukocytosis, metabolic acidosis, and elevated serum lactate.

2. X-ray findings—Upright plain films show ileus, absence of intestinal gas, or diffuse distention with an air-fluid level. Ischemia and intestinal necrosis are late findings. Abdominal plain films are abnormal in only 20% of cases. A barium enema (not recommended if vascular disease is strongly suspected) may show "thumbprinting" of the colonic mucosa.

3. Mesenteric arteriography—When performed early in the course of the disease, mesenteric arteriography is the definitive diagnostic procedure, because it demonstrates major vascular occlusion, if present. If it is done later, it merely delays necessary surgery and permits development of more extensive bowel necrosis and peritonitis. The catheter inserted in the superior mesenteric artery may be used to infuse vasodilating agents when the cause of disease is nonocclusive arteriolar intestinal ischemia and after the primary occlusive lesion is corrected.

Treatment

Treat hypotension and shock with infusion of intravenous crystalloid solutions and blood, if bleeding is present. Notify a vascular or general surgeon immediately to prepare for surgery. Prompt operation is required to resect necrotic bowel. In some cases, the embolus can be removed or the arterial obstruction bypassed.

Vasodilator drugs may be used as an adjunct to management of the vascular disease in selected cases of nonocclusive ischemia; however, operation is usually required to resect necrotic bowel. Begin parenteral administration of broad-spectrum antimicrobials.

Disposition

All patients with suspected or proved acute visceral ischemia should be hospitalized.

ACUTE CEREBRAL ISCHEMIA DUE TO EMBOLI

 ESSENTIALS OF DIAGNOSIS

- Unilateral motor or sensory deficits, dysarthria, aphasia, ataxia, visual disturbance, or vertigo.
- Noncontrast CT scan distinguishes between thrombotic or embolic etiologies and hemorrhagic etiologies.

General Considerations

Cerebrovascular accident (CVA) (stroke) due to infarction is in many cases the result of embolization of thrombotic or atheromatous debris from an extracranial vascular source. The advent of thrombolytic therapy for ischemic CVA or stroke has dramatically changed emergency department evaluation and management of cerebral embolic events.

Clinical Findings

A. Symptoms and Signs

Patients with CVA or transient ischemic attack (TIA) may present with unilateral motor or sensory deficits, dysarthria, aphasia, ataxia, visual disturbances, or vertigo, depending on the location of the insult. TIAs are classically defined as neurologic deficits spontaneously resolving within 24 hours.

B. Imaging

1. Emergent noncontrast cranial CT scanning— This diagnostic tool is vital to the evaluation of a patient presenting with a CVA within 3 hours of symptom onset; determining whether a CVA is ischemic or hemorrhagic may allow tissue plasminogen activator administration (provided no other contraindications are present and the hospital has a "brain attack" program involving emergency medical services, the emergency department, radiology, neurology, and neurosurgery).

2. Noncontrast CT scanning—This imaging method may be helpful for patients with TIA; duplex scanning of the carotid arteries may reveal atherosclerotic lesions responsible for the TIA.

Treatment & Disposition

For treatment and disposition of CVAs, see Chapter 18. Patients with TIAs should be started on antiplatelet therapy and referred to a neurologist. Certain patient characteristics (age > 60 years, diabetes, symptoms > 10 minutes, weakness, and speech impairment) are associated with a higher short-term risk of stroke and may warrant admission for an expeditious evaluation.

American Heart Association: Guidelines 2000 for cardiopulmonary resuscitation and emergency cardiovascular care. Circulation 2000;102:I204. [PMID: 11001640]

Centeno RF et al: An alternative approach: antegrade catheter-directed thrombolysis in a case of phlegmasia cerulea dolens. Am Surg 1999;65:229. [PMID 10075298]

Choucair MM et al: Leg ulcer diagnosis and management. Dermatol Clin 2001;19:659. [PMID: 11705353]

Eklof B et al: Indications for surgical treatment of iliofemoral vein thrombosis. Hematol Oncol Clin North Am 2000;14:471. [PMID: 10806568]

Greenwald DA et al: Ischemic bowel disease in the elderly. Gastroenterol Clin North Am 2001;30:445. [PMID: 11432300]

Johnston SC et al: Short-term prognosis after emergency department diagnosis of TIA. JAMA 2000;284:2901. [PMID: 11147987]

Novelline RA et al: Helical CT in emergency radiology. Radiology 1999;213:321. [PMID:10551209]

Verstraete M et al: Thrombolysis in the management of lower limb peripheral arterial occlusion—a consensus document. Am J Cardiol 1998;81:207. [PMID: 9591906]

Arterial Aneurysms

RUPTURED ABDOMINAL AORTIC ANEURYSM

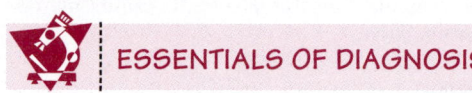 **ESSENTIALS OF DIAGNOSIS**

- *Sudden onset of abdominal or flank pain, pulsatile abdominal mass, and hypotension.*
- *CT scan with contrast confirms diagnosis.*

General Considerations

An artery is described as aneurysmal once it reaches more than twice its normal diameter. The exact mechanism behind the formation of an abdominal aortic aneurysm (AAA) is unknown and is likely multifactorial. The belief that aneurysms are due to atherosclerosis alone has undergone serious challenge in the past several years. Risk factors include a family history of AAA, male gender, age greater than 70 years, long-term smoking, and systemic hypertension. This condition is fairly common, affecting 2–5% of the population over age 60 years. The primary complication of AAA is spontaneous rupture, which carries a high mortality rate. The chance of rupture increases exponentially as the diameter of the aneurysm increases (Table 38–2).

If the aneurysm ruptures into the peritoneal space, exsanguination and death occur rapidly, usually prior to arrival in the emergency department. When rupture occurs into the retroperitoneal space, a tamponade effect may temporarily control hemorrhage and allow time for diagnosis and treatment.

Clinical Findings

A. Symptoms and Signs

The classic symptoms of AAA rupture include sudden-onset abdominal or flank pain, pulsatile abdominal mass, and hypotension. However, because this triad is seen in only 50% of patients presenting with AAA rupture, a high level of suspicion must be maintained. This diagnosis must be considered in patients with hypotension and shock of uncertain cause and in patients presenting with myocardial ischemia or infarction. Additionally, patients who have undergone previous aortic bypass grafting can present with gastrointestinal bleeding caused by erosion of the graft into the duodenum and subsequent rupture.

B. Laboratory Findings

The hematocrit may be normal or low.

C. Electrocardiogram

The electrocardiogram (ECG) may show signs of myocardial ischemia.

D. Imaging

CT scan with contrast is the diagnostic test of choice in evaluating symptomatic AAAs in normotensive, hemodynamically stable patients. Abdominal x-ray may reveal the presence of an AAA due to calcification of the wall of the aneurysm (70% of AAAs). Ultrasound is used to diagnose and follow progression of asymptomatic AAAs. Aortography is used to investigate the vascular anatomy in the workup for elective (nonemergent) AAA repair.

Treatment

Act quickly. Even if the patient appears hemodynamically stable at the time of initial evaluation, the contained rupture may progress rapidly to exsanguinating hemorrhage at any time.

Treat hypotension and shock (see Chapter 9 for more detail):

1. Begin oxygen, 4 L/min, by nasal cannula or mask.
2. Insert 2 large-bore (≥ 16-gauge) intravenous catheters by venous cutdown.
3. Obtain blood for CBC, electrolyte determinations, and renal function tests; and type and cross-match for 10 units of packed red blood cells or whole blood. Measure the hematocrit immediately and at frequent intervals thereafter. Remember that the delay in equilibration of blood volume may keep the hematocrit falsely elevated for 12–18 hours.
4. Give 1–3 L of crystalloid solution intravenously to restore adequate blood pressure, and follow with cross-matched blood. If the initial hematocrit is below 20%, either "universal donor" blood or type-specific blood may be necessary.
5. Insert a urinary catheter, send urine for analysis, and monitor urine output.

Table 38–2. Annual risk of rupture of an abdominal aortic aneurysm as a function of the size of the aneurysm.

Aneurysm Diameter	Annual Risk of Rupture
Less than 4 cm	Rare
4–5 cm	1–3% per year
5–6 cm	5–10% per year
Greater than 7 cm	Greater than 20% per year

Request urgent consultation with a general or vascular surgeon, because immediate surgery is the only definitive treatment.

Disposition

Hospitalize all patients with suspected or documented ruptured abdominal aortic aneurysm.

VISCERAL & HYPOGASTRIC ARTERY ANEURYSMS

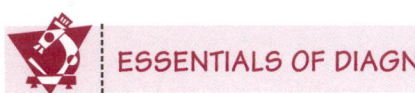 **ESSENTIALS OF DIAGNOSIS**

- *Abrupt onset of diffuse abdominal pain.*
- *Signs and symptoms of shock may be present.*
- *CT scan with contrast or visceral angiography confirms diagnosis.*

General Considerations

Congenital aneurysm occurs in younger patients, whereas atherosclerotic aneurysm occurs more commonly in older patients. The splenic artery is the most commonly involved vessel. Bleeding may be confined to the lesser sac of the peritoneal cavity for the first 24–48 hours. However, free rupture into the general peritoneal cavity invariably causes exsanguination. Rupture is most common during pregnancy. Hypogastric artery aneurysms may rupture into the retroperitoneum or erode into contiguous organs, in which case gastrointestinal bleeding or hematuria occurs.

Clinical Findings

There is abrupt onset of diffuse abdominal pain. Hypotension occurs secondary to blood loss. The hematocrit is low if the bleeding is more than a few hours old. CT scan with contrast is an excellent tool for diagnosis in the hemodynamically stable patient. Peritoneal lavage may reveal gross blood. A plain film of the abdomen may show an aneurysm if it has calcified.

The only definitive diagnostic procedure is selective visceral angiography, which should be performed in the hemodynamically stable patient in whom an aneurysm is not present on a plain film.

Treatment

Start resuscitative measures, including insertion of a large-bore (≥ 16-gauge) intravenous catheter, nasogastric tube, Foley catheter, and the like (see Treatment

section for ruptured abdominal aortic aneurysm, above, and Chapter 9). Draw blood for CBC, and type and cross-match for 8 units of packed red blood cells or whole blood.

Notify a vascular surgeon at once, because early operation is imperative.

Disposition

Immediately hospitalize all patients with suspected or documented visceral and hypogastric artery aneurysms.

THORACIC AORTIC ANEURYSM (Aortic Dissection)

 ESSENTIALS OF DIAGNOSIS

- *Sudden, severe, tearing chest pain radiating to the back or neck.*
- *Chest x-ray may show widened mediastinum.*
- *CT scan with contrast confirms diagnosis.*

General Considerations

Aortic dissection is defined as extraluminal blood entering and dissecting between the intima and media of the aortic wall. Aortic dissection is the most common aortic surgical emergency with an annual incidence of 5–10 cases per 100,000 population. Several classifications of aortic dissections have been described (Table 38–3). Approximately 65% of tears occur in the ascending aorta. Less frequently they occur in the aortic arch (10%) or descending thoracic aorta (20%). Nearly 5% of aortic dissections occur in the abdominal aorta. Untreated aortic dissections are associated with an overall mortality rate of 21% in the first 24 hours, 60% within

Table 38–3. Aortic dissection classification systems.

DeBakey System	
Type I	Involves both the ascending and descending thoracic aorta
Type II	Involves only the ascending thoracic aorta
Type IIIa	Involves only the descending thoracic aorta
Type IIIb	Involves the descending thoracic and abdominal aorta
Stanford System	
Type A	Involves the ascending aorta
Type B	All others

the first 2 weeks, and over 90% in the first 3 months. For dissection of the ascending aorta, the 24-hour mortality rate is 60% and the 2-week mortality rate is nearly 80%.

Aortic dissection typically occurs in men who are middle-aged or older. It is associated with hypertension in nearly 90% of cases. Other predisposing conditions include connective tissue disorders (Marfan syndrome, Ehlers-Danlos syndrome, Turner syndrome, tuberous sclerosis), congenital aortic anomalies including the valve, cocaine use, pregnancy, and weightlifting.

Clinical Findings

A. Symptoms and Signs

The classic symptoms of acute aortic dissection are a sudden, severe, sharp or tearing chest pain. Most patients are either normotensive or hypertensive; a murmur of aortic insufficiency is auscultated less than half the time. The pain may migrate and include the back, neck, and jaw as the dissection progresses. As the dissection advances it may occlude any of the branches of the involved section of the aorta, leading to coronary insufficiency, strokes, mesenteric ischemia, acute renal insufficiency, and neurologic deficits secondary to spinal cord ischemia. Patients may also present with cardiac tamponade, congestive heart failure, or Horner syndrome.

Depending on which vessels have been compromised, there may be signs of CVA, acute myocardial infarction, clinical findings associated with arterial occlusion of an extremity (ischemia, absent pulses), abdominal or back pain with or without hematuria or ileus, or wide difference in blood pressure measurements in the 2 arms or in an arm and a leg on the same side.

If the base of the aortic valve is involved, varying degrees of aortic insufficiency occur. The dissection may leak into the pleura or pericardium, causing a pericardial or pleural friction rub with effusion.

When rupture starts, shock of sudden and catastrophic onset may occur as a result of cardiac tamponade, massive hemothorax, or hemomediastinum. The patient may have a history of one or more of the conditions listed above.

B. Laboratory Findings

Hematuria may be present; the hematocrit may be normal or low.

C. Electrocardiogram

Approximately 40% of patients with aortic dissection will have ST-segment or T-wave changes on their ECG. Only 30% of patients will have a normal ECG (Table 38–4).

D. Imaging

Although the chest x-ray may show a widened mediastinum, abnormal aortic contour, or pleural effusion, these findings are inconsistent. According to the International Registry of Acute Aortic Dissection study, over 12% of patients presenting with an aortic dissection will have a normal chest x-ray (see Table 32–4). In recent years, CT scan with contrast has replaced aortography as the imaging mode of choice to diagnose aortic dissection. Although each method has a sensitivity and specificity approaching 100%, CT scan is noninvasive and is generally more available than arteriography. TEE has also been found to be highly reliable in the investigation of the thoracic aorta. Many authorities recommend TEE as the modality of choice when readily available, because of its expediency and accuracy.

Goals of Treatment

There are 3 main goals of treatment:

A. Reduce Hypertension

Hypertension must be controlled. The forces contributing to the development of dissection are a function of increased systolic blood pressure and the force generated with each systolic contraction of the left ventricle. Accordingly, once dissection is suspected, the essential first step is to reduce systolic pressure and the rate of rise of the left ventricular pressure wave (dp/dt) if the patient is not hypotensive. If the patient is hypotensive, treat for hypovolemic shock (Chapter 9).

B. Manage Pain

Use titrated narcotic analgesia to control the patient's pain.

C. Obtain Surgical Consultation

Obtain immediate vascular or thoracic surgery consultation for consideration of operative repair.

Treatment

A. All Patients

1. Insert 2 or more large-bore ($\geq$ 16-gauge) intravenous catheters or perform venous cutdowns.
2. Draw blood for CBC, electrolyte measurements, tests of renal function, PT, PTT, and typing and cross-matching (reserve 10 units of packed red blood cells of whole blood).
3. Insert a Foley catheter, send urine for urinalysis, and monitor urine output on an hourly basis.
4. Give oxygen, 5 L/min, by mask or nasal cannula.

Table 38–4. Chest radiography and electrocardiogram results for patients with acute aortic dissection.[1]

Category	Present, No. Reported (%)	Stanford Type A, No. (%)	Classification[2] Type B, No. (%)
Radiography findings (n = 427)	427 (100)	256 (88.6)	171 (97.7)
No abnormalities noted	53 (12.4)	26 (11.3)	27 (15.8)
Absence of widened mediastinum or abnormal aortic contour	91 (21.3)	44 (17.2)	47 (27.5)
Widened mediastinum	263 (61.6)	169 (62.6)	94 (56)
Abnormal aortic contour	212 (49.6)	124 (46.6)	88 (53)
Abnormal cardiac contour	110 (25.8)	69 (26.9)	41 (24.0)
Displacement/calcification of aorta	60 (14.1)	29 (11.3)	31 (18.1)
Pleural effusion	82 (19.2)	46 (17.3)	36 (21.8)
Electrocardiogram findings (n = 444)			
No abnormalities noted	139 (31.3)	85 (30.8)	54 (32.1)
Nonspecific ST-segment or T-wave changes	184 (41.4)	116 (42.6)	68 (42.8)
Left ventricular hypertrophy	116 (26.1)	67 (25)	498 (32.2)
Ischemia	67 (15.1)	47 (17.3)	20 (13.2)
Myocardial infarction, old Q waves	34 (7.7)	19 (7.1)	15 (9.9)
Myocardial infarction, new Q waves or ST segments	14 (3.2)	13 (4.8)	1 (0.7)
Initial modality (n = 453)			
Computed tomography	277 (61.1)	145 (50.2)	132 (75.4)
Echocardiogram (TEE and/or TTE)	148 (32.7)	122 (42.2)	26 (14.9)
Aortography	20 (4.4)	12 (4.2)	8 (4.6)
Magnetic resonance imaging	8 (1.8)	2 (0.7)	6 (3.4)
Images performed per patient, mean (*SD*)	1.83 (0.82)	1.64 (0.69)	2.15 (0.91)

SD = standard deviation; TEE = transesophageal echocardiography; TTE = transthoracic echocardiography.
[1]Reprinted, with permission. Copyright 2000, American Medical Association.
[2]Type A involves ascending aorta; Type B involves all others (see Table 38–3).

5. Obtain immediate vascular or thoracic surgical consultation.

B. Patients with Normotension, Hypotension, or Shock

1. Assume that free rupture or cardiac tamponade has occurred.

2. Begin intravenous infusion of crystalloid solutions to support blood pressure; give packed red blood cells or whole blood as soon as available.

3. Obtain chest x-ray (if possible) to confirm the diagnosis.

4. Consult with the surgeon, who will decide whether immediate operation or confirmatory studies are necessary.

5. Perform immediate surgery if cardiac tamponade or gross aortic insufficiency is present.

C. Patients with Hypertension

Institute emergency control of blood pressure with an intravenous infusion of nitroprusside and a β-blocker. Nitroprusside reduces both preload and afterload by causing arterial and venous dilation. The β-blocker counters the reflex tachycardia and increased contractility expected with preload and afterload reduction.

1. Start an infusion of Esmolol (short-acting, intravenous β-blocker). Give a loading dose of 500 μg/kg followed by an infusion of 25–200 μg/kg/min. Titrate the infusion to a goal heart rate of 60–70 beats/min.

2. Start an infusion of nitroprusside at a rate of 0.5–10 μg/kg/min. Titrate the infusion to the lowest blood pressure compatible with adequate organ perfusion, typically a mean arterial pressure of 60–70 mm Hg.

3. If intensive blood pressure monitoring is not available, labetalol hydrochloride, an α- and β-adrenergic receptor-blocking agent, may be used effectively by itself to reduce blood pressure and left ventricular dp/dt. Give 20 mg over 2 minutes by intravenous injection. Additional doses of 40–80 mg can be given every 10 minutes (maximum dose 300 mg) until the desired blood pressure has been reached. (Alternatively, 2 mg/min may be given by intravenous infusion, titrated to desired effect.)

Disposition

Hospitalize all patients without delay. Obtain urgent cardiothoracic surgical consultation for all patients, even those already receiving medical treatment.

POPLITEAL & FEMORAL PERIPHERAL ANEURYSMS

 ESSENTIALS OF DIAGNOSIS

- Symptoms are due to thrombus, embolization, or pressure from an expanding aneurysm.
- Pulsatile mass on physical examination (if not thrombosed).
- Ultrasound confirms diagnosis.
- Arteriography defines distal arterial circulation.

General Considerations

Occlusion or distal embolization of the friable lining of peripheral aneurysms results in symptoms of distal ischemia. Unlike AAA or visceral aneurysm, rupture is rare. The most common locations of peripheral aneurysms are the popliteal artery and, secondarily, the femoral artery. Popliteal aneurysms are often bilateral and are often associated with AAAs.

Acute occlusion can result in severe distal ischemia. Distal embolization can also result in severe distal ischemia; however, it is often associated with episodes of moderate ischemia that decrease as collateral circulation improves.

Clinical Findings

A. SYMPTOMS AND SIGNS

Symptoms are due to thrombosis, embolization, pressure from an expanding aneurysm, or (rarely) rupture. There may be an arterial mass in the popliteal fossa or the groin. The aneurysm is pulsatile unless it is thrombosed. Signs of acute arterial occlusion often coexist.

Popliteal aneurysms can cause symptoms (eg, signs of venous obstruction, weakness, sensory defects) when they compress the popliteal vein or tibial nerve. Rupture of the aneurysm is rare.

B. IMAGING

1. Plain x-ray—A rim of calcification may be apparent in the wall of the aneurysm.

2. Arteriography—Arteriography may not demonstrate the aneurysm if it is thrombosed, but this procedure is generally advised to define the status of the arterial circulation distal to the aneurysm.

3. Ultrasonography—Ultrasonography is helpful in identifying the presence of an aneurysm.

Treatment

Notify a vascular surgeon, because immediate operation is required when severe distal ischemia has occurred secondary either to acute thrombosis or to distal embolization.

Elective operation is recommended for any aneurysm producing compression of adjacent structures as well as for most documented popliteal aneurysms, because the rate of complication is high if these are left untreated.

Disposition

All symptomatic patients should be hospitalized immediately.

Dmowski AT et al: Aortic dissection. Am J Emerg Med 17;372. [PMID: 10452437]

Fikar CR et al: Etiologic factors of acute aortic dissection in children and young adults. Clin Pediatr 2000;39:71. [PMID: 10696543]

Hagan PG et al: The international registry of acute aortic dissection (IRAD): new insight into an old disease. JAMA 2000; 283:897. [PMID: 10685714]

Hallett JW: Management of abdominal aortic aneurysms. Mayo Clin Proc 2000;75:395 [PMID: 10761495]

Ledbetter S et al: Helical (spiral) CT in the evaluation of emergent thoracic aortic syndromes: traumatic aortic rupture, aortic aneurysm, aortic dissection, intramural hematoma, and penetrating atherosclerotic ulcer. Radiol Clin North Am 1999; 37:575. [PMID: 10361547]

Novelline RA et al: Helical CT in emergency radiology. Radiology 1999;213:321. [PMID: 10551209]

Sternbergh WC III et al: Abdominal and thoracoabdominal aortic aneurysm. Surg Clin North Am 1998;78:827. [PMID: 9891579]

VENOUS DISEASE

Lower-Extremity Deep Venous Thrombosis

 ESSENTIALS OF DIAGNOSIS

- *Unilateral swelling, warmth, and redness of affected limb.*
- *Physical examination is unreliable in diagnosing deep venous thrombosis.*
- *Contrast venography or ultrasound confirms diagnosis.*

Table 38–5. Factors predisposing to deep venous thrombosis.

Stasis of blood flow
  Recent travel
  Bedrest
  Immobilization (casting)
  Sedentary lifestyle
Hypercoagulopathy
  Malignancy
  Smoking[1]
  Exogenous estrogen[1]
  Intrinsic coagulopathies:
    Factor V Leyden
    Protein C deficiency
    Protein S deficiency
    Antithrombin III deficiency
    Homocysteinemia
Trauma
Surgery, particularly orthopedic surgery hip or lower
  extremity

[1]Causes secondary protein S deficiency.

General Considerations

Deep venous thrombosis (DVT) results in 600,000 hospitalizations each year in the United States. If untreated, DVT commonly results in pulmonary embolism, thus making it a significant source of morbidity and mortality.

As described by Virchow in 1856, venous thrombosis is predisposed by stasis of blood flow, hypercoagulopathy, and vascular endothelial injury. Specific conditions associated with development of DVT are shown in Table 38–5.

Clinical Findings

A. SYMPTOMS AND SIGNS

Patients with symptomatic DVT typically complain of unilateral lower-extremity pain and swelling that begins gradually and progresses over days. The described sense of fullness may worsen with standing or walking. Physical examination is of little help in diagnosing DVT and should not be used to exclude diagnosis. Possible findings include unilateral lower-extremity edema, warmth, or erythema. There may be tenderness along the course of the affected vessel, and rarely the clot will be palpable. The time-honored Homans sign (pain in posterior calf with passive dorsiflexion of the foot) has been shown to be unreliable in diagnosing DVT. Because the DVT results in a systemic inflammatory response, the patient may be febrile. Adjunctive testing is required because physical examination is unreliable in diagnosing DVT.

B. IMAGING AND LABORATORY FINDINGS

1. Contrast venography—Although contrast venography remains the gold standard for diagnosing DVT, it has been largely replaced by ultrasonography in most institutions. The advantages of contrast venography include a sensitivity and specificity of nearly 100% and the ability to detect DVTs of the calf, iliac vessels, and inferior vena cava that can be missed by ultrasound. Its primary disadvantages include its invasive nature, use of contrast material, and availability. Additionally, 5–15% of studies performed are technically inadequate.

2. Ultrasonography—Ultrasonography is the most accurate noninvasive study for diagnosing lower-extremity DVT, with a sensitivity of 93–100% and a specificity of 97–100% in detecting proximal DVTs. The limitations of ultrasonography are its ability to detect pelvic and calf DVTs (20% of which will extend into the popliteal vein and thigh).

3. D-Dimer assay—D-dimer is formed when fibrin is degraded by plasmin. The testing for the presence of D-dimer is by latex agglutination (least sensitive), whole blood agglutination (bedside, qualitative), and enzyme-linked immunoassay (ELISA) (most accurate). When combined with ultrasound, the whole blood agglutination and ELISA have an almost 100% negative predictive value.

Treatment

For DVT of proximal veins of the thigh, put the patient on bed rest and elevate the limb. Catheter-directed thrombolytic therapy with streptokinase or urokinase is effective in treating acute DVT less than 7 days old and may prevent postphlebitic complications. Alternatively, start anticoagulation with intravenous heparin or SC low-molecular-weight heparin. Obtain consultation with a vascular surgeon in cases of massive iliofemoral thrombosis. Surgery may be required for certain patients.

Management of calf DVT and the need for hospitalization are controversial. Isolated calf thrombi do not commonly produce pulmonary emboli, although they may propagate into proximal vessels. Traditional treatment has been low-dose heparin (eg, 5000 units subcutaneously twice a day), although some authors advocate serial noninvasive studies (eg, ultrasound) and treatment only if propagation occurs.

Disposition

All patients with proximal DVT should be hospitalized. Because of the association between DVT and malignancy, patients with a new diagnosis of DVT should be referred to a primary care provider for further evaluation.

SUPERFICIAL THROMBOPHLEBITIS

 ESSENTIALS OF DIAGNOSIS

- *Pain, tenderness, induration, and erythema along course of affected vein.*
- *Affected extremity shows only slight to no edema (no other signs of impaired venous return).*

General Considerations

Superficial venous thrombosis of the upper extremity is usually iatrogenic, occurring secondary to intravenous catheterization. Lower-extremity superficial venous thromboses may be associated with varicose veins, bacterial infection of surrounding tissues, trauma, or thromboangiitis obliterans. Trauma may play a part in the development of thrombi or may cause recurrences.

Clinical Findings

Pain, tenderness, induration, and erythema are noted along the course of the involved vein, which may feel like a cord. The extremity shows only slight or no swelling, and there are no other signs of impaired venous return.

Septic thrombophlebitis usually occurs following intravenous injections (especially among intravenous drug abusers) and at venous catheter sites. It should be suspected in the presence of the above symptoms or fluctuance along a superficial vein. Fever and rigors may be present. The diagnosis is confirmed if pus can be aspirated from the vein.

Treatment

A. CASES WITH NO COMPLICATIONS

For uncomplicated superficial venous thrombosis, only symptomatic treatment is required. Neither bed rest nor anticoagulation is indicated. An elastic bandage at and above the level of thrombosis helps to speed remission. Elevation of the leg when the patient is sitting and nonsteroidal anti-inflammatory drugs are also helpful.

B. CASES WITH COMPLICATIONS

Obtain general or vascular surgical consultation for all complications. If clinical examination suggests that the thrombosis is approaching the saphenofemoral junction, ligation and division of the saphenous vein are indicated, because pulmonary embolization can result from deep venous involvement.

If septic thrombophlebitis occurs, parenteral antimicrobials are required, and the involved segment of vein must be excised or ligated and drained to prevent persistent bacteremia.

Disposition

Patients with mild, localized superficial thrombosis may be discharged. Patients with more serious disease, including suspected or documented septic thrombophlebitis, should be hospitalized.

UPPER-EXTREMITY VENOUS THROMBOSIS

 ESSENTIALS OF DIAGNOSIS

- *Pain and swelling of affected limb.*
- *Occurs in 3% of patients with a central venous catheter.*
- *Examination reveals nonpitting edema, normal skin color, and intact distal pulses.*

• *Contrast venography or ultrasonography confirms diagnosis.*

General Considerations

Upper-extremity deep venous thrombosis (UEDVT) is much less common than lower-extremity DVT but remains an important cause of morbidity because of its association with pulmonary embolism and postphlebitic sequelae (persistent upper-extremity pain and swelling). Nearly 12% of cases of UEDVT will be complicated by pulmonary embolism. Mortality from UEDVT is approximately 1%.

The most common risk factor for UEDVT is central venous catheter placement, with clinically significant thrombus formation in 3% of patients with a central line. The second most common category of UEDVT is spontaneous (effort-related) thrombosis. Risk factors include repetitive activities involving hyperabduction of the shoulder and aberrant anatomy of the costoclavicular space. Other causes include intravenous drug use, thoracic tumors, and radiation. The most commonly affected site of thrombosis is the axillary-subclavian venous system.

Clinical Findings

A. SYMPTOMS AND SIGNS

Patients typically present with pain and swelling of the affected limb. The risk factors discussed above may be present. Physical examination may reveal nonpitting edema of the affected side forearm (occasionally the whole arm), normal skin color, and intact distal pulses. Venous cords may be palpable.

B. IMAGING

As with lower-extremity DVT, contrast venography remains the gold standard for diagnosis of UEDVT. However, it is slowly being replaced by ultrasonography, which has been shown to have a high degree of sensitivity and specificity for diagnosing UEDVT.

Treatment

Initial treatment involves immobilization, elevation, and the application of heat to the affected limb. This is followed by systemic anticoagulation with intravenous heparin or SC low-molecular-weight heparin. Other options include catheter-directed thrombolysis and surgical thrombectomy. Frequently surgery is required to correct underlying anatomic defects to prevent recurrence. Consult a vascular surgeon.

Disposition

Hospitalize all patients for definitive management.

RUPTURED VENOUS VARICOSITIES (Varicose Veins)

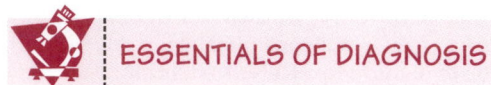

ESSENTIALS OF DIAGNOSIS

• *Bleeding from varicose veins, usually due to minor trauma.*

General Considerations

Rupture is an uncommon complication of varicose veins. The skin overlying varices can become thin, and erosion can occur spontaneously or with minor trauma.

Clinical Findings

Bleeding from varicose veins is present and may be brisk.

Treatment

Gentle digital pressure over the bleeding site and elevation of the leg control the initial bleeding. Suture ligature of the ruptured vein may be necessary to definitively stop the bleeding. When the initial bleeding has been controlled, the leg should be wrapped in an elastic bandage or Unna's paste boot. Consult a vascular or general surgeon about elective stripping of varicose veins.

Disposition

Brief hospitalization may be advisable.

PULMONARY EMBOLISM

Pulmonary embolism is an occasional complication of venous thrombosis. It is discussed in Chapter 33.

ARTERIOVENOUS FISTULA

ESSENTIALS OF DIAGNOSIS

- *Abnormal connection between arteries and veins.*
- *Constant systolic and diastolic (to-and-fro) murmur and palpable thrill at site.*
- *Arteriography confirms diagnosis.*

General Considerations

Arteriovenus fistulas are abnormal connections between arteries and veins. They may be congenital or acquired. Congenital lesions tend to have more diffuse connections and may involve an extremity. Acquired arteriovenous fistulas—other than those constructed to gain access for dialysis—generally occur secondary to trauma and result from erosion of the artery into a contiguous vein. Other causes include malignancy, infection, and arterial aneurysm. The physiologic effect depends on the size of the communication.

Clinical Findings

A constant systolic and diastolic (to-and-fro) murmur is heard, and a thrill is palpable over most arteriovenous fistulas. Cardiac output may be high if significant left-to-right shunting of blood exists. Patients with congenital arteriovenous fistulas may show increased muscle mass, increased bone length, clubbing, and cyanosis of the involved limb. Polycythemia may also be present.

Complications

Complications include cosmetic deformity due to limb disproportion, congestive heart failure, severe arterial insufficiency, expanding false aneurysm, and hemorrhage. Arteriography delineates the precise outlines of the lesion and may be used for therapeutic embolization.

Treatment & Disposition

Patients with pain, expanding mass, heart failure, or obvious high cardiac output require hospitalization. Others may be discharged from the emergency department and referred to a vascular surgeon or general surgeon.

Centeno RF et al: An alternative approach: antegrade catheter-directed thrombolysis in a case of phlegmasia cerulea dolens. Am Surg 1999;65:229. [PMID: 11705353}

Choucair MM et al: Leg ulcer diagnosis and management. Dermatol Clin 2001;19:659. [PMID: 10075298]

Dauzat M et al: Diagnosis of acute lower limb deep vein thrombosis with ultrasound: trends and controversies. J Clin Ultrasound 1997;25:343. [PMID: 9282799]

Eklof B et al: Indications for surgical treatment of iliofemoral vein thrombosis. Hematol Oncol Clin North Am 2000;14:471. [PMID: 10806568]

Heron E et al: Long-term sequelae of spontaneous axillary-subclavian venous thrombosis. Ann Int Med 1999;131:510. [PMID: 10507960]

Kennedy D et al: Physical examination findings in deep vein thrombosis. Emerg Med Clin North Am 2001;19:869. [PMID: 11762276]

Novelline RA et al: Helical CT in emergency radiology. Radiology 1999;213:321. [PMID: 10551209]

Rosen CL et al: The diagnosis of lower extremity deep vein thrombosis. Emerg Med Clin North Am 2001;19:895. [PMID: 11762272]

Stephens MB: Deep venous thrombosis of the upper extremity. Am Fam Physician 1997;55:533. [PMID: 9054222]

OTHER VASCULAR SYNDROMES

THORACIC OUTLET SYNDROME

ESSENTIALS OF DIAGNOSIS

- *Signs and symptoms caused by compression of the neural, arterial, or venous structures at the thoracic outlet.*
- *Hand or arm fatigue with use, especially with abduction of the arm.*
- *Elevated arm stress test may elicit symptoms.*

General Considerations

Thoracic outlet syndrome comprises a variety of disorders caused by abnormal compression of the neural, arterial, or venous structures at the superior aperture of the thorax (thoracic outlet); the most common is compression of nerve structures against the first rib. Symptoms of dysfunction of branches of the brachial plexus are far more common than symptoms secondary to compression of the axillary-subclavian artery or vein, accounting for approximately 95% of cases. Compression of the 8th cervical and 1st thoracic nerve roots (C8 and T1) is most common. The second most common pattern is involvement of the 3 uppermost nerve roots of the brachial plexus, the 5th through 7th cervical nerve roots (C5–C7). Thoracic outlet syndrome is rarely an emergency.

Clinical Findings

A. Symptoms

The diagnosis is typically made on clinical grounds with patients complaining of hand or arm fatigue with use, especially with activities involving abduction of the arm. More subtly, patients may note wasting of the muscles of the hand.

If symptoms are due to nerve compression, patients may complain of positional paresthesias in the distribution of one or more trunks of the brachial plexus. Compression of C8–T1 nerve roots results in paresthesias in the ulnar nerve distribution, whereas symptoms referable to C5–C7 compression may involve the ear, neck, upper thorax, or lateral aspect of the shoulder. Raynaud symptoms, secondary to compression of sympathetic nerve fibers may also be reported.

Symptoms of venous compression and thrombosis include pain and swelling of the affected limb. Patients with arterial thoracic outlet syndrome with resultant subclavian-axillary artery stenosis or aneurysm formation may present with symptoms of acute arterial occlusion or embolization.

B. Signs

Physical examination should include the elevated arm stress test (EAST test) in an attempt to provoke symptoms. In this test the patient externally rotates and abducts both arms to 90 degrees with elbows flexed 90 degrees and shoulders braced posteriorly. The patient then opens and closes both hands for a 3-minute period. Patients with thoracic outlet syndrome will complain of the rapid onset of fatigue and heaviness of the arms and are often unable to complete the entire test. Paresthesias may also be reproduced.

In neurologic thoracic outlet syndrome, wasting of the lateral thenar muscles of the hand, weakness of the intrinsic muscles of the hand, and patchy sensory deficits in the distribution of the involved nerve roots may be seen. Reproducible paresthesias during the EAST test may be elicited.

Findings in arterial thoracic outlet syndrome include a blood pressure differential in the upper extremities, a bruit with auscultation over the subclavian or axillary artery, and radial pulse deficit on the affected side during the EAST test. Findings of acute arterial occlusion or embolization may be found. Thoracic outlet syndrome secondary to venous occlusion or thrombosis may be associated with swelling of the affected extremity and normal pulses.

C. Imaging

1. X-rays—Plain film radiographs of the cervical spine or chest may reveal skeletal abnormalities predisposing to thoracic outlet syndrome (cervical rib, first rib, or clavicle deformity).

2. Angiography—Angiography may be indicated for evaluation of acute arterial occlusion or embolization.

3. Ultrasonography—Ultrasonography may be indicated for evaluation of arterial aneurysms or venous thrombosis.

4. Venography—Venography may be indicated for evaluation of venous thrombosis.

Treatment & Disposition

Patients with neurologic thoracic outlet syndrome can be discharged with a referral to a neurologist or thoracic surgeon. Patients with evidence of a venous or arterial abnormality and stable symptoms should be referred to a vascular or thoracic surgeon. If venous thrombosis or arterial occlusion or embolization is present, the patient should be hospitalized with immediate surgical consultation.

COMPLICATIONS OF PERCUTANEOUS TRANSLUMINAL ANGIOPLASTY & RETROGRADE ANGIOGRAPHY

 ESSENTIALS OF DIAGNOSIS

- *History of recent percutaneous procedure.*
- *May see complications at puncture site or signs and symptoms due to thrombosis or embolization.*

An increasing number of patients are undergoing percutaneous transluminal angioplasty (balloon dilatation of the arteries) and angiography via the femoral artery. These patients are observed for the development of immediate complications but are usually discharged from the hospital within 24–48 hours and may subsequently present to the emergency department with complications (Table 38–6).

Hospitalize the patient, and obtain prompt vascular or cardiothoracic surgical consultation, because many of these complications require surgical treatment.

Table 38–6. Complications of percutaneous transluminal angioplasty.

Puncture site complications
  Bleeding: massive, expanding, or pulsatile hematoma
  False aneurysm: pulsatile mass at puncture site
  Femoral artery occlusion: loss of pulse at or proximal to
    puncture site, due to thrombosis at catheter site or arter-
    ial injury (eg, luminal flap)
  Infection: superficial or deep, with or without arterial in-
    volvement
Dilatation site complications
  Thrombosis of dilated vessel (most commonly coronary,
    iliac, femoral, or renal artery)
Complications distal to insertion site
  Embolization (usually occurs before patient leaves the
    hospital)

ERGOTISM

 ESSENTIALS OF DIAGNOSIS

- *History of ergotamine use or exposure.*
- *Mottled cyanosis of the thighs and lower legs with intense cyanosis of the feet.*

General Considerations

Ergotism is caused by ergotamine tartrate or other ergot derivatives or by consumption of rye contaminated by ergot fungus. The disease is characterized by profound vasoconstriction that is almost always limited to the lower extremities.

Clinical Findings

There is mottled cyanosis of the thighs and lower legs, with intense cyanosis of the feet. Prolonged vasospasm may result in distal thrombosis. Secondary tissue loss may occur. Other findings include vomiting, diarrhea, cramps, and various central nervous system symptoms.

Treatment & Disposition

Hospitalize the patient, and maintain adequate blood pressure and intravascular volume. Withdraw ergota-mine medication. Vasodilators and heparin anticoagu-lation may be indicated. Hyperbaric oxygen therapy may be tried, although there is no evidence of benefit. Consult a general surgeon or vascular surgeon. Lumbar sympathectomy may be required.

INTRA-ARTERIAL INJECTION OF DRUGS

 ESSENTIALS OF DIAGNOSIS

- *History of parenteral drug injection.*
- *Severe burning pain distal to injection site.*

General Considerations

Inadvertent or intentional intra-arterial injection of drugs can cause intense vasospasm followed by arterial occlusion, with distal gangrene as a possible result. This is commonly known as a "hand trip" by intravenous drug abusers. Vasospasm may occur while the drug is being given, or the reaction may be delayed. Unfortu-nately, many patients with delayed reactions fail to seek medical attention until ischemia is advanced.

Clinical Findings

There is a history of therapeutic or illicit drug injection by the parenteral route. Severe burning pain in distal arterial distribution is followed by intense vasospasm. If the vasospasm has been prolonged, gangrene of the fin-gers or entire hand may occur even though the arterial vasoconstriction subsequently resolves.

Treatment & Disposition

Hospitalize the patient, and obtain vascular surgical consultation. If the needle is still in place, irrigate dis-tally with heparinized saline. Start systemic anticoagula-tion with heparin. Systemic vasodilating agents may be necessary to treat the intense vasospasm. Intra-arterial injection of vasodilators (eg, reserpine) is not usually beneficial. If sympathetic nerve block is indicated be-cause of persistent severe peripheral ischemia, consult an anesthesiologist or vascular surgeon.

FROSTBITE

Arterial injury is a major pathogenetic factor in frost-bite injury. See Chapter 44 for details of diagnosis and treatment.

Gelabert HA et al: Diagnosis and management of arterial com-
    pression at the thoracic outlet. Ann Vasc Surg 1997;11:359.
    [PMID: 9236991]
Wilbourn AJ: Thoracic outlet syndromes. Neurol Clin 1999;17:
    477. [PMID: 10393750]

Hematologic Emergencies

39

J. Stephan Stapczynski, MD, & Geoffrey A. Martin, MD

I. Hemostatic Disorders: General Considerations

II. Hemostatic Disorders: Platelet Disorders

Disorders of Decreased Platelet Production

Immune Thrombocytopenia

1. Idiopathic Thrombocytopenic Purpura
2. Drug-Induced Immune-Mediated Thrombocytopenia

Thrombotic Thrombocytopenic Purpura & Hemolytic Uremic Syndrome

1. Thrombotic Thrombocytopenic Purpura
2. Hemolytic Uremic Syndrome

Thrombocytopenia Due to Platelet Sequestration

Qualitative Platelet Abnormalities

Thrombocytosis

III. Hemostatic Disorders: Coagulation Factor Disorders

Hemophilia

von Willebrand Disease

Liver Disease

Renal Disease

Warfarin & Vitamin K Deficiency

Diffuse Intravascular Coagulation

IV. Anemia

Iron-Deficiency Anemia

Acute Hemolytic Anemia

Autoimmune Hemolytic Anemia

1. Warm-Type AIHA
2. Cold-Type AIHA: General Considerations
3. Cold-Type AIHA: Cold Agglutinin Syndrome
4. Cold-Type AIHA: Paroxysmal Cold Hemoglobinuria
5. Mixed-Type AIHA

Alloimmune Hemolytic Anemia

Drug-Related AIHA

Sickle Cell Anemia

Thalassemias

α-Thalassemia Carrier & Trait

Hemoglobin H Disease

β-Thalassemia Minor (β-Thalassemia Trait)

β-Thalassemia Major (Cooley Anemia)

Glucose-6-Phosphate Dehydrogenase Deficiency

Hereditary Spherocytosis

V. Polycythemia

Primary Polycythemia (Polycythemia Vera)

Secondary Polycythemia

VI. White Cell Disorders

Neutropenia

Leukocytosis

Acute Leukemia

Chronic Leukemia

1. Chronic Lymphocytic Leukemia
2. Chronic Myelocytic Leukemia

Infectious Mononucleosis

Multiple Myeloma

Waldenström Macroglobulinemia

VII. Transfusion Therapy

Packed Red Blood Cells

Platelets

Fresh Frozen Plasma

Cryoprecipitate

Other Plasma-Derived Products

Massive Transfusion

Complications of Transfusion Therapy

■ I. HEMOSTATIC DISORDERS: GENERAL CONSIDERATIONS

Most bleeding seen in the emergency department is due to trauma—the result of local wounds, lacerations, or other structural lesions—occurring in patients with normal hemostasis. Conversely, bleeding from multiple sites, bleeding from untraumatized sites, delayed bleeding several hours after trauma, and bleeding into deep tissues or joints suggests the possibility of a bleeding disorder. Historical data for the presence of a congenital bleeding disorder include the presence or absence of unusual or abnormal bleeding in the patient and other family members and the possible occurrence of excessive bleeding after dental extractions, surgical procedures, or trauma. Many patients with abnormal bleeding have an acquired disorder, commonly due to liver disease or drug use (particularly ethanol, aspirin, nonsteroidal anti-inflammatory drugs [NSAIDs], warfarin, and antibiotics).

The site of bleeding may provide an indication of the hemostatic abnormality. Mucocutaneous bleeding—including petechiae; ecchymoses; epistaxis; or gastrointestinal, genitourinary, or heavy menstrual bleeding—is characteristic of qualitative or quantitative platelet disorders. Purpura is often associated with thrombocytopenia and commonly indicates a systemic illness. Bleeding into joints and potential spaces, such as between fascial planes and into the retroperitoneum, as well as delayed bleeding, is most commonly associated with coagulation factor deficiencies (Figure 39–1). Patients who demonstrate both mucocutaneous bleeding and bleeding in deep spaces may have disorders such as disseminated intravascular coagulation (DIC), in which both platelet abnormalities and coagulation factor abnormalities are present. Basic hemostatic tests and clinical evaluation are generally adequate for diagnosis (Table 39–1). Additional hemostatic studies are ordered as indicated (Table 39–2).

■ II. HEMOSTATIC DISORDERS: PLATELET DISORDERS

DISORDERS OF DECREASED PLATELET PRODUCTION

Neonatal infections, such as cytomegalovirus (CMV) or rubella, may cause isolated thrombocytopenia. Many medications impair platelet production and produce

thrombocytopenia (Table 39–3). Chronic alcohol use is a common cause of thrombocytopenia and will generally resolve if the patient abstains from drinking for longer than 7 days. If multiple cell lines are affected, the differential diagnosis includes aplastic anemia, marrow infiltration from lymphoma or leukemia, or myelofibrosis. Usually the history and physical examination determines the most likely source of thrombocytopenia; however, bone marrow biopsy is sometimes needed.

IMMUNE THROMBOCYTOPENIA

Antibody-mediated platelet destruction can be related to medications, infections, or autoimmune diseases. Two of the more common antibody-mediated thrombocytopenic disorders are idiopathic thrombocytopenic purpura (ITP) and drug-induced immune thrombocytopenia.

1. Idiopathic Thrombocytopenic Purpura

General Considerations

ITP is an acquired autoimmune disease characterized by thrombocytopenia, the presence of purpura or petechiae, normal bone marrow, and no other identifiable cause for the thrombocytopenia. Platelet destruction is mediated by the production of autoantibodies that attach to circulating platelets, and the antibody-coated platelets are removed by the reticuloendothelial system. The bone marrow usually responds by increasing platelet production, but sometimes the same antibodies that bind to the platelets also bind to the megakaryocytes, limiting the bone marrow response. Despite the presence of antibodies, the circulating platelets function properly, and many people with ITP may not have significant bleeding despite low platelet counts.

ITP occurs in all age groups and may have an acute or chronic course. Acute ITP is more common among younger children, affects males and females equally, and typically resolves in 1–2 months. Chronic ITP lasts more than 3 months, is more common in adults, has a female predilection, and rarely remits spontaneously. Additionally, patients with chronic ITP are more likely to exhibit an underlying disease or autoimmune disorder, such as HIV infection, systemic lupus, Graves disease, Hashimoto thyroiditis, or antiphospholipid antibody syndrome.

Clinical Findings

The most common symptom of ITP is petechiae; mild bleeding may also be seen at mucosal surfaces, including epistaxis, gingival bleeding, and menorrhagia in women of child-bearing age. The physical examination is otherwise normal; the presence of lymphadenopathy,

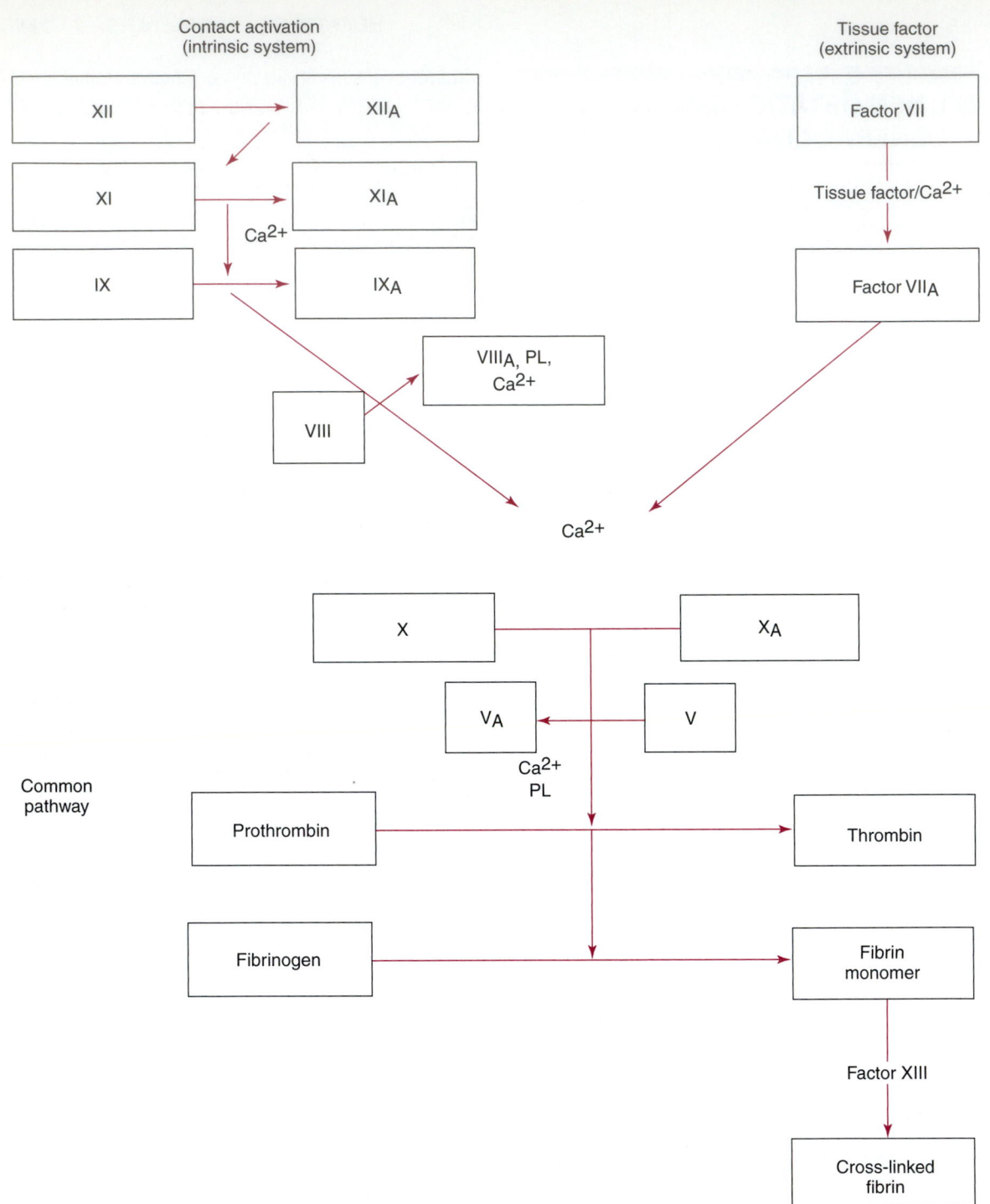

Figure 39–1. Coagulation cascade. Ca^{2+} = calcium; fibrinogen is factor I; PL, phospholipid surface (often platelets); prothrombin is factor II. (Reprinted, with permission, from Eberst ME: Evaluation of anemia and the bleeding patient. Page 1368 in Tintinalli JE, Kelen GD, Stapczynski JS (eds.): *Emergency Medicine. A Comprehensive Study Guide,* 5th edition. McGraw-Hill, 2000.

Table 39–1. Standard tests of hemostasis.

Test	Normal Value	Comments
Platelet count	150,000–400,000 platelets/µL	Traumatic bleeding not a serious concern unless platelet count < 50,000/µL, and spontaneous bleeding unlikely unless platelet count < 10,000/µL.
Prothrombin time and international normalized ratio (INR)	11–13 seconds, depending on reagent; INR 1.0	Tests extrinsic and common pathways: factors VII, X, V, prothrombin, and fibrinogen.
Activated partial thromboplastin time	22–34 seconds, depending on reagent	Tests intrinsic and common pathways: factors XII, XI, IX, VIII, V, prothrombin, and fibrinogen.
Fibrinogen level	150–450 mg/dL	Fibrinogen is cleaved by thrombin into fibrin monomer, which then polymerizes into cross-linked fibrin clot.
Fibrin degradation products by latex agglutination	< 2.5 mg/L, depending on assay methodology	Breakdown products of fibrinogen and fibrin monomer.
D-dimer by enzyme-linked immunoassay	< 500 µg/L, depending on assay methodology	Breakdown products of cross-linked fibrin.

hepatosplenomegaly, anemia, or hyperbilirubinemia should suggest an alternative diagnosis, such as leukemia, lymphoma, systemic lupus erythematosus, infectious mononucleosis, or hemolytic anemia. The complete blood count (CBC) should be normal in all cell lines except for the platelets. In some patients with bleeding, a mild anemia may be present. The peripheral blood smear should show large, well-granulated platelets that are few in number. The diagnosis of ITP is based primarily on the history, physical examination, CBC, and peripheral smear.

Treatment

Minimize bleeding risks in patients with ITP, for example, by avoiding the use of antiplatelet medications (eg, aspirin and NSAIDs), avoiding unnecessary invasive procedures, maintaining good blood pressure control, treating exacerbating comorbid conditions (eg, liver disease, renal disease), and addressing fall risks. Treatment of ITP depends on severity, comorbid conditions, and presence of bleeding. Asymptomatic patients, who are otherwise healthy, with platelet counts greater than 50,000/µL require no treatment. Treatment is indicated for (1) nonbleeding patients with platelet counts less than 20,000/µL and (2) patients with bleeding or significant risk factors for bleeding and platelet counts less than 50,000/µL. Initial therapy in adults is prednisone started at 60–100 mg/d (children, 1–2 mg/d) and tapered after the platelet count reaches normal (usually requires 4–8 weeks). For patients who do not respond to steroids, the main alternative therapy is splenectomy. For life-threatening bleeding, the current recommendation is high-dose steroid therapy (methylprednisolone

Table 39–2. Specialized tests of hemostasis.

Test	Normal Value	Comments
Bleeding time	2.5–10 minutes	Tests interaction between platelets and subendothelium.
Thrombin clotting time	10–12 seconds	Tests conversion of fibrinogen to fibrin monomer.
Mixing test	Variable	1:1 mixing of abnormal plasma with normal plasma will correct any single coagulation factor deficiency and normalize PT or PTT. If mixing does not normalize the PT or PTT, a coagulation inhibitor is present.
Specific factor assays	60–130% (0.6–1.3 units/mL)	Used to identify specific factor deficiencies.
Inhibitor screens	Variable	Used to detect inhibitors to coagulation factors (eg, lupus-anticoagulant).

PT = prothrombin time; PTT = partial thromboplastin time.

Table 39–3. Drugs that impair platelet production or function.

Impair Platelet Production (Thrombocytopenia)[1]	Impair Platelet Function (Prolonged Bleeding Time)
Heparin 4+	Aspirin
Gold salts 4+	Nonsteroidal anti-inflammatory drugs
Sulfa-containing antibiotics 4+	Antiplatelet agents: ticlopidine and clopidogrel
Quinine and quinidine 4+	Penicillins and cephalosporins
Ethanol (chronic use) 4+	Calcium channel blockers
Aspirin 3+	Propranolol
Indomethacin 3+	Nitroglycerin
Valproic acid 3+	Antihistamines
Heroin 3+	Phenothiazines
Thiazides 2+	Tricyclic antidepressants
Furosemide 2+	
Procainamide 2+	
Digoxin 2+	
Cimetidine and ranitidine 2+	
Phenytoin 1+	
Penicillins/cephalosporins 1+	

[1]The numerals following each drug indicate relative incidence based on case reports.

1–2 g/d intravenously for 2–3 days) with or without intravenous immunoglobulin. Transfuse platelets as needed following the first dose of methylprednisolone or immunoglobulin; holding the platelet transfusion until the first dose of either is completed results in a better response. Conjugated estrogen, 25 mg intravenously one time, can be given for severe uterine bleeding.

Disposition

Hospitalization is required for ITP-related bleeding. Hospitalization is generally not required for asymptomatic patients with platelet counts greater than 20,000/μL. At counts below 20,000/μL, hospitalization may not be required if patients are asymptomatic or have only mild purpura. Hospitalization is prudent when arranging patient follow-up is difficult, when compliance is in doubt, or when significant additional bleeding risk factors are present.

2. Drug-Induced Immune-Mediated Thrombocytopenia

Heparin is the drug most commonly associated with drug-induced immune-mediated thrombocytopenia. Platelet counts typically fall after the 5th day of therapy, usually to below 100,000/μL; less than 10% of patients develop profound thrombocytopenia with counts less than 20,000/μL. Paradoxically, the complications from heparin-induced thrombocytopenia are usually thromboembolic (deep venous thrombosis, pulmonary embolism, stroke), the conditions heparin is used to treat.

Immediate cessation of heparin therapy is indicated when the platelet count falls to below 100,000/μL or more than 50% from baseline. Substitute alternative agents (eg, danaparoid, hirudin, argatroban) for heparin. Avoid future exposure to either unfractionated heparin or the low-molecular-weight heparins.

The platelet glycoprotein IIb/IIIa receptor antagonists are associated with a 3–7% incidence of modest thrombocytopenia (platelet counts of 50,000– 100,000/μL), typically occurring within the first 24 hours of treatment. Severe thrombocytopenia (below 20,000/μL) occurs in less than 1% of patients. Petechiae, wound hematomas, mucosal bleeding, and hematuria are the most common hemorrhage complications. Platelet counts return to normal within 2–3 days after drug discontinuation.

Other drugs rarely cause immune-mediated thrombocytopenia; the sulfonamide, penicillin, and cephalosporin antibiotics have been most commonly reported. In this circumstance, thrombocytopenia typically develops 7–10 days after start of the medications, platelet counts typically fall to below 20,000/μL, and the most common symptoms are petechiae and oral mucosal hemorrhagic blisters.

THROMBOTIC THROMBOCYTOPENIC PURPURA & HEMOLYTIC UREMIC SYNDROME

Thrombotic thrombocytopenic purpura (TTP) and hemolytic uremic syndrome (HUS) involve platelet aggregation in the microvascular circulation via the mediation of von Willebrand factor (vWF), leading to consumption thrombocytopenia and microangiopathic hemolytic anemia (MAHA) or schistocyte-forming hemolysis as red blood cells (RBCs) are fragmented during travel through these occluded arterioles and capillaries. TTP and HUS are clinical syndromes with characteristic features, but overlap between the syndromes makes differentiation sometimes difficult. TTP is traditionally more common in adults, whereas HUS is more common in children. TTP typically induces more prominent neurologic deficits with deposition of platelet aggregates in a broader, systemic distribution; HUS more specifically impairs the renal system. In general, adults presenting with clinical and laboratory evidence of MAHA accompanied by thrombocytopenia should receive treatment for TTP once other diagnoses have been excluded (eg, sepsis, metastatic cancer, systemic vasculitis, preeclampsia-eclampsia, Evans syndrome, heparin-induced thrombocytopenia with thrombosis, and malignant hypertension). Untreated TTP has an 80–90% mortality rate.

Pallor, jaundice or scleral icterus, fatigue, and dyspnea on exertion are common because of the hemolytic anemia. With significant thrombocytopenia, purpura or mucosal bleeding may be evident. Focal neurologic deficits (often vacillating), aphasia, seizure, coma, visual disturbance, chest pain, cardiac conduction disorders, abdominal pain, oliguria, and hypertension indicate end-organ involvement.

1. Thrombotic Thrombocytopenic Purpura

Clinical Findings

A. SYMPTOMS AND SIGNS

TTP classically comprises the following pentad of symptoms and signs: (1) thrombocytopenia, (2) MAHA, (3) fever, (4) renal impairment, and (5) neurologic impairment. It is uncommon for all 5 features to occur in any one patient, but if they are, severe end-organ ischemia or damage has likely taken place. Thrombocytopenia and MAHA are the most common features, and fever is the least frequent finding.

A common feature of acquired TTP is the development of autoantibodies to a vWF-cleaving metalloprotease termed ADAMTS-13. Pregnancy is the most common precipitating event for TTP. Preeclampsia has some features similar to TTP, but TTP usually presents earlier during pregnancy, around 23–24 weeks, and delivery does not affect the course of TTP. By contrast, preeclampsia more commonly occurs in the third trimester, and delivery is the treatment of preeclampsia. Other triggers of TTP include infection (particularly HIV), vaccination, and autoimmune disorders such as systemic lupus erythematosus. Several drugs have been associated with TTP, including quinidine, cyclosporine, tacrolimus, and the antiplatelet agents ticlopidine and clopidogrel. A particularly refractory form of TTP has been seen in post–bone marrow transplant patients after treatment with the cancer chemotherapeutic agents mitomycin, cisplatin, gemcitabine, and bleomycin.

B. LABORATORY FINDINGS

TTP is still a clinical diagnosis, but characteristic laboratory findings include severe anemia, thrombocytopenia (μL), schistocytes or helmet cells on peripheral smear, decreased haptoglobin, elevated reticulocyte count, and elevated unconjugated (indirect) bilirubin seen with intravascular hemolysis. The direct Coombs test (DAT) is characteristically negative, because the hemolysis seen in TTP does not involve anti-RBC autoantibodies. Because TTP thrombi do not involve fibrin, TTP is distinguished from DIC based on normal coagulation studies. Compared with TTP, preeclampsia is associated with a reduced plasma antithrombin III level.

Treatment

Acquired TTP is treated with daily plasma exchange consisting of (1) plasmapheresis to remove large vWF multimers and autoantibodies and (2) plasma infusion to give the patient back one calculated daily volume of fresh frozen plasma (FFP) or cryoprecipitate-poor plasma (cryosupernatant). The use of plasma exchange has decreased TTP mortality rates from 90% to 10–20%. If plasmapheresis cannot be performed immediately, initial FFP infusion should be started but infusion should never replace exchange. Plasma exchange is performed daily until several days after remission is achieved. Remission usually occurs within 1 week but may require up to 4 weeks. Remission is defined by normalization of the platelet count and lactate dehydrogenase (LDH) combined with clinical resolution of tissue ischemia and thrombosis. Corticosteroids (usually prednisone, 1–2 mg/kg/d) may be helpful in the presence of a high autoantibody titer and if plasma exchange does not provide the desired response. Splenectomy can induce long-term remission or cure in cases of plasma exchange failure by removing a site of autoantibody production and by removing a site of microvascular occlusion, which mitigates MAHA.

Supportive measures may be needed to address systemic complications associated with TTP, including RBC transfusion for anemia, anticonvulsants for seizures, antihypertensives for hypertension, and hemodialysis for severe renal insufficiency. Avoid platelet transfusions, unless life-threatening bleeding or intracranial hemorrhage is present, because thrombosis may worsen acutely, leading to rapid renal failure and potentially death. Aspirin can worsen hemorrhagic complications in the setting of severe thrombocytopenia and also should be avoided. Heparin is not beneficial in TTP or HUS. Relapse rates after appropriate treatment may be as high as 30%, and maintenance therapies have not been shown to prevent relapse.

2. Hemolytic Uremic Syndrome

Clinical Findings

HUS is a disease primarily of early childhood, with a peak incidence between ages 6 months and 4 years. The adult form of HUS may be very difficult to distinguish from TTP. The overall mortality rate is 5–15%; the prognosis is worse in older children and adults. HUS is characterized by acute renal failure, MAHA, fever, and moderate thrombocytopenia. HUS often follows a viral or bacterial illness. Although several infectious agents have been implicated, *Escherichia coli* serotype O157:H7 is a well-recognized factor. Between 20% and 40% of patients with *E coli* O157:H7 infection have bloody diarrhea; 15% of children and 5% of adults go on to develop HUS. Onset of HUS is typically 2–14 days after diarrhea develops. Other organisms implicated in HUS include *Shigella, Yersinia, Campylobacter, Salmonella, Streptococcus pneumoniae,* varicella, echovirus, and coxsackievirus A and B.

In HUS the microthrombi are confined mostly to the kidneys, whereas in TTP they occur throughout the microcirculation. Laboratory studies reflect the presence of MAHA, and thrombocytopenia may be present but generally not to the degree seen in TTP. The serum creatinine may be markedly elevated, and urine, if present, contains protein and RBCs (although the urine can be normal).

Treatment

Patients with mild HUS with less than 24 hours of urinary symptoms require only fluid and electrolyte correction and supportive care. Steroid therapy may be beneficial. In the setting of more severe disease, plasma exchange or infusion have been performed with equivocal results. Patients whose disease resembles TTP may respond to plasma exchange, but the overall low mortality of HUS makes use routine use of plasma exchange questionable. Hemodialysis may be required in the setting of acute renal failure, especially in adults, because acute renal failure tends to be more severe. A shorter duration of dialysis therapy is associated with increased likelihood of recovery from HUS. Do not treat infection with *E coli* O157:H7 with antimotility drugs because these agents appear to increase the risk of developing HUS. Antibiotic treatment of *E coli* O157:H7 dysentery is controversial, but meta-analysis has found no evidence that antibiotic treatment increases or decreases the risk of developing HUS.

THROMBOCYTOPENIA DUE TO PLATELET SEQUESTRATION

In patients with marked splenomegaly, splenic sequestration may commonly produce platelet counts as low as 40,000/μL. However, isolated splenomegaly rarely results in clinically significant hemorrhage without the presence of another concomitant hemorrhagic disorder, and splenectomy is rarely indicated.

QUALITATIVE PLATELET ABNORMALITIES

Several disease processes can cause acquired qualitative or functional platelet abnormalities (Table 39–4). In the myeloproliferative diseases, despite frequently elevated platelet counts, the platelets are often dysfunctional and patients can develop mucosal hemorrhages or clinically significant bleeding. To control acute bleeding, consider transfusion to raise the level of normal platelets to 50,000/μL. In macroglobulinemia and related disorders, the elevated serum proteins interfere with platelet function and patients with clinically significant bleeding may require plasmapheresis to reduce the protein level and correct hemostatic function.

Many commonly used drugs can influence platelet function (see Table 39–3). Of these, the most commonly used are aspirin, the NSAIDs, and clopidogrel. Aspirin inhibits platelet function by acetylating and irreversibly inactivating platelet cyclooxygenase, which inhibits platelet aggregation. This antithrombotic effect can be seen in doses as small as 30 mg, occurs within 1 hour after ingestion, and continues for the lifespan of the platelets. Because the NSAIDs reversibly inhibit platelet cyclooxygenase, the impairment of platelet ag-

Table 39–4. Conditions associated with functional platelet disorders.

Renal failure
Liver disease
Myeloproliferative disorders: polycythemia vera, chronic myelogenous leukemia
Paraproteinemias: multiple myeloma, Waldenström macroglobulinemia
Antiplatelet antibodies: autoimmune disorders such as systemic lupus
von Willebrand syndrome

gregation lasts only as long as the active drug is present in the circulation, usually less than 24 hours. An exception is the drug piroxicam, which has a 2-day half-life. Ticlopidine and clopidogrel are related substances that inhibit platelet function by impairing fibrinogen binding to glycoprotein IIb/IIIa receptors and by inhibiting platelet binding. Platelet inhibition occurs within 24–48 hours after ingestion and continues for approximately 4–10 days after discontinuation of therapy.

THROMBOCYTOSIS

Thrombocytosis, a platelet count above 500,000/μL, can be seen in many disorders, including inflammatory reactions, malignancy, polycythemia vera, and postsplenectomy. Platelet function can be normal or abnormal depending on the underlying condition. With abnormal platelet function, thrombocytosis can be associated with bleeding (eg, mucosal or gastrointestinal bleeding or ecchymoses) or thromboembolism (eg, deep venous thrombosis, portal or mesenteric thrombosis, splenic vein thrombosis). However, these events are unusual, even with platelet counts in excess of 1 million/μL.

■ III. HEMOSTATIC DISORDERS: COAGULATION FACTOR DISORDERS

HEMOPHILIA

General Considerations

Hemophilia is a disorder of coagulation caused primarily by a deficiency or defect in one of two circulating plasma proteins. Hemophilia A, or classic hemophilia, is caused by a deficiency of factor VIII and is the most common cause of hemophilia in the United States, affecting 1 in 10,000 males. Hemophilia B, or Christmas disease, is caused by a deficiency of factor IX. This form of hemophilia is less common, affecting approximately 1 in 25,000 to 35,000 males. Together these forms of hemophilia account for about 99% of patients with inherited coagulation factor deficiencies; the remaining individuals have rare forms of factor deficiencies. Hemophilia A and B are clinically indistinguishable from each other, and specific factor testing is required for diagnosis. Both hemophilia A and B are X-linked recessive disorders; therefore, hemophilia is a disease overwhelmingly of men, and women are asymptomatic carriers. Approximately one third of new cases of hemophilia A and one fifth of new cases of hemophilia B arise from a spontaneous gene mutation.

Clinical Findings

A. SYMPTOMS AND SIGNS

Bleeding manifestations in patients with all forms of hemophilia are directly attributable to the decreased plasma levels of either factor VIII or IX (Table 39–5). Individuals with factor levels below 1% of normal are classified as having severe disease, and these people will experience severe spontaneous bleeding episodes and difficult-to-control bleeding related to traumatic events. Patients with factor levels of 1–5% of normal are classified as having moderate disease; although they may bleed spontaneously, more commonly their bleeding is related to a traumatic event. Patients with factor levels of 5–25% of normal are classified as having mild disease and usually bleed only after trauma. Those with factor levels of 25–50% may never be aware that they have hemophilia, or they might manifest unusual bleeding only after major surgery or severe trauma. Patients with hemophilia do not have problems with minor cuts and abrasions. As a result of exposure to blood products, many hemophiliacs have chronic viral hepatitis or are infected with HIV. Fortunately, as a result of newer viral inactivation procedures and recombinant technology, few seroconversions have resulted from the use of currently available factor replacement products.

B. LABORATORY FINDINGS

Routine coagulation studies (prothrombin time [PT] or activated partial thromboplastin time [aPTT]) require only 30% of normal factor VIII or IX level to be normal; therefore, patients with mild disease may have normal values. Coagulation studies are unlikely to yield new information in the known hemophiliac and are not routinely indicated when the patient presents with mild to moderate bleeding episodes.

Treatment

A general principle in managing major or life-threatening bleeding in a hemophilic patient is early and complete factor replacement, before or at the same time as other resuscitative and diagnostic maneuvers. Spontaneous or traumatic bleeding into the neck, tongue, retropharynx, or pharynx has a high potential for airway compromise. Any patient with hemophilia who complains of a new headache, localizing neurologic symptoms, or a blunt head injury requires immediate factor replacement therapy followed by urgent computed tomography scanning of the head. Hemophilic patients with complaints of back, thigh, groin, or abdominal pain may have bleeding into the retroperitoneum. At times the initial manifestations of bleeding can be subtle. Simple injuries such as ankle and wrist

Table 39–5. Common bleeding locations in hemophilia patients.

Location	Comments
Joint (hemarthrosis)	Common, can lead to joint destruction and chronic arthropathy
Soft tissue (hematomas)	Can occur in any location, dangerous in the neck (asphyxia), limb (compartment syndrome), and retroperitoneum (hemorrhagic shock)
Mucosa	Epistaxis, bleeding after dental extractions, gastrointestinal bleeding
Central nervous system	Can occur with minimal trauma, common cause of death
Kidney (hematuria)	Common, rarely serious

sprains may at first appear benign but can be complicated by bleeding. Compartment syndromes result from muscle bleeds within the fascial compartments of the extremities, both spontaneously and after minimal trauma to an extremity.

One of the most common manifestations of hemophilia is hemarthrosis. Clinical evidence of an acute problem with the joint may or may not present, but these patients can reliably report when bleeding is occurring. Prompt treatment of hemarthroses can prevent or reduce the long-term sequelae of hemophilic arthropathy. Many patients and their families have a sophisticated understanding of the disease. These patients will know to seek treatment at the first sign of a problem, and as stated earlier, little outward evidence of pathology may be present initially. Despite minimal findings, take seriously the concerns of these patients. Additionally, many known hemophiliacs will have in their medical records a detailed treatment plan for how to manage acute bleeding episodes. Consult these records when they are available.

Do not place central lines, including femoral lines and external jugular lines, in patients with hemophilia without giving factor replacement therapy. Similar rules apply to arterial blood gases or lumbar puncture. Patients with hemophilia should never receive intramuscular injections unless factor replacement is given and maintained for several days. Do not give compounds that contain aspirin for pain relief.

Two different factor replacement types exist: recombinant or plasma derived (Table 39–6). The highest level of purity comes from the recombinant factors, but these products cost 2–3 times more than plasma-derived products, and they are not available everywhere. Another concern with the plasma-derived factors is that some of the preparations may contain other coagulation factors, some partially activated. Prolonged use of the less pure concentrates may increase the risk of DIC or, in some cases, cause paradoxical clotting. Safety, cost, and availability must be considered when choosing the product to use in replacement therapy, but because the

recombinant forms are perceived to be safer, approximately 60% of patients with severe hemophilia in the United States receive these preparations.

The dosing regimen used in the hemophilic patient is based on the clotting factor's volume of distribution, the factor's half-life, and the hemostatic level of factor required to control the bleeding (Table 39–7). Clotting factor is dosed in units (U) of activity; 1 unit of factor represents the amount of factor present in 1 mL of normal plasma. For hemophilia A, 1 unit of factor VIII per kilogram of body weight raises the plasma level by approximately 0.02 U/mL (2%) with a half-life of approximately 8–12 hours. For hemophilia B, 1 unit of factor IX per kilogram of body weight will raise the plasma level by approximately 0.01 U/mL (1%) with a half-life of approximately 16 hours. The amount of factor needed can be calculated using the patient's weight and the desired increase in factor activity (to avoid wasting factor, round off all doses to the closest vial):

Factor VIII required = weight in kg × 0.5
× (% change in factor activity needed)

Factor IX required = weight in kg × 1.0
× (% change in factor activity needed)

Bleeding from the mouth is common in hemophiliacs, particularly children. If an oral bleed is present, identify the area, clean it of inadequate clot, and place a dry topical thrombin on the bleeding site. In addition to factor replacement, antifibrinolytic agents such as epsilon-aminocaproic acid (EACA) and tranexamic acid are useful to prevent bleeding when the clot falls off. For superficial mucosal injuries, it may be possible to manage the bleeding with antifibrinolytic therapy alone. The dose of EACA is 75–100 mg/kg for children (6 g for adults) every 6 hours, given orally or intravenously. Topical hemostatic agents used to help control oral or nasal bleeding include microfibrillar collagen hemostats, thrombin, and absorbable gelatin sponges.

Table 39–6. Available products for hemophilia treatment.

Hemophilia Type	Available Products	Comments

Hemophilia A	Human-plasma-derived factor VIII products:
	    Koate-HP
	    Humate-P
	    Alphanate
		All have a low risk of HIV and hepatitis transmission.

	Human-plasma-derived factor VIII with immunoaffinity purification:
	    Hemofil M
	    Monoclate-P
		Both products have reduced amounts of von Willebrand factor. Monoclate-P is highly purified source of factor VIII.

	Recombinant factor VIII products:
	    Recombinate
	    Gelixate
	    Bioclate
	    Kogenate
		Low to no risk of hepatitis or HIV.

	Porcine factor VIII products:
	    Antihemophilic Factor
	    Hyate C
		No evidence of porcine viral transmission to humans.

Hemophilia B	Factor IX complex products:
	    Koyne-80 factor IX complex
	    Proplex T factor IX complex
	    Profilnine SD
	    Bebulin VH
		Proplex T: HIV seroconversion has occurred. Other products have low risk of HIV and hepatitis transmission.

	Activated factor IX complex products:
	    Autoplex T
	    Feiba VH
		Low risk of HIV and hepatitis transmission.

	Purified factor IX products:
	    Alpha Nine SD
	    Mononine
		Low risk of HIV and hepatitis.

	Recombinant factor IX: BeneFIX	No known risk of viral transmission.

Patients with mild hemophilia A (factor levels of 5% or greater) who have mild bleeding may not always require factor replacement. Rather, these patients may be given desmopressin, which causes endothelial storage sites to release vWF that is capable of carrying additional amounts of factor VIII in the plasma. This medication is well tolerated, and patients can administer it at home by subcutaneous injection or intranasal spray. The dose of intravenous desmopressin is 0.3 μg/kg (maximum dose, 20 μg) over 30 minutes. The concentrated intranasal form of desmopressin is an antidiuretic agent, and fluid restriction may be needed during use. For children older than age 5 years, a single spray in a single nostril (150 μg total dose) is adequate. For adolescents and adults, a single spray in each nostril is used (300 μg total dose). This dose of intranasal desmopressin increases the factor VIII level by 2–3 times. This treatment can be repeated in 8–12 hours, but the patient's stores of factor VIII will be depleted, and subsequent effect will be less.

In response to the clotting factors used to treat bleeding episodes, some people will develop inhibitors, or antibodies against the replacement factor. Inhibitors tend to occur most commonly in patients with severe hemophilia because of frequent factor replacement. These inhibitors not only interfere with the effectiveness of factor replacement therapy but also cause anaphylaxis to factor administration in patients with hemophilia B. Inhibitors occur in 10–25% of those with hemophilia A and in 1–2% of those with hemophilia B. The use of factor replacement in hemophilic patients with inhibitors is guided by the concentration of inhibitor (measured in Bethesda Inhibitor Assay [BIA] units) and by the type of response the patient has to factor concentrates. Bleeding episodes are more difficult to treat in these patients, but options do exist. Given

Table 39–7. Initial factor replacement guidelines.

Site	Minimum Initial Factor Level	Hemophilia A Initial Dose	Hemophilia B Initial Dose	Details
Deep muscle	40–50%	20–40 U/kg	40–60 U/kg	Monitor total blood loss, watch for compartment syndrome. Duration of replacement: 1–3 days
Joint	30–50%	20–40 U/kg	30–40 U/kg	Orthopedic consult for splinting, physical therapy, and follow-up. Duration of replacement: 1–3 days
Epistaxis	80–100%	40–50 U/kg	80–100 U/kg	Local measures should be used. Replacement is given until bleeding resolves.
Oral mucosa	50%	25 U/kg	50 U/kg	Local measures and antifibrinolytic therapy will decrease need for additional factor replacement. Duration of replacement: 1–2 days
Gastrointestinal bleeding	100%	40–50 U/kg	80–100 U/kg	Consultation with gastroenterologist is appropriate to identify a lesion. Duration of replacement: 7–10 days
Central nervous system	100%	50 U/kg	100 U/kg	Early neurosurgical consultation. Lumbar puncture requires factor replacement.

the complexity of these patients, consultation or transfer to a center with hematology is recommended.

Disposition

Many patients with hemophilic bleeding episodes can receive factor replacement in the emergency department or clinic and then be discharged home with follow-up in 12–24 hours. Hemophilic patients with bleeding episodes that require hospital admission include (1) those with bleeding involving the central nervous system, neck, pharynx, retropharynx, or retroperitoneum, (2) those with potential compartment syndrome, (3) those for whom treatment requires more than 3 doses (relative indication), (4) those unable to use, or lacking access to, factor replacement, or (5) those in whom pain cannot be controlled with oral analgesics.

VON WILLEBRAND DISEASE

General Considerations

Von Willebrand disease is the most common congenital bleeding disorder; it is present in 1% of the population. This disease is a group of disorders caused by abnormalities of vWF. The disease is heterogeneously inherited and expressed, and although multiple subtypes exist, these can be classified into 3 major groups (Table 39–8). Type I is the most common and is a partial quantitative disease, type II is a qualitative (abnormal

function) disease, and type III is a severe and almost complete deficiency of vWF (this type is a rare autosomal recessive form). vWF is a glycoprotein that, as opposed to most other coagulation factors, is synthesized, stored, and then secreted by the vascular endothelial cells. It is a cofactor for platelet adhesion and the carrier protein for factor VIII.

Clinical Findings

A. SYMPTOMS AND SIGNS

Bleeding symptoms are common in people with von Willebrand disease, particularly in children and adoles-

Table 39–8. Classification of von Willebrand disease.

Type	Occurrence in Patients with von Willebrand Disease	von Willebrand Factor (vWF) Defect
I	70–80% of patients	All multimeric forms are present, but their quantity is diminished.
II	10–15% of patients	vWF is abnormal, missing some of the multimers.
III	< 10%	Essentially no vWF is present.

cents. Symptoms includes recurrent epistaxis, gingival bleeding, unusual bruising, gastrointestinal bleeding, and menorrhagia in young women. Hemarthrosis is not typical unless severe disease is present. In mild cases of von Willebrand disease, patients may be unaware of the disease until they undergo a surgical procedure or experience a traumatic event. Von Willebrand disease is relatively common, and its presence influences the treatment of other medical problems, because patients with this disease should not take medications with known antiplatelet effects, including aspirin, NSAIDs, antiplatelet agents, heparin, and some antibiotics.

B. LABORATORY FINDINGS

Common abnormalities on hemostatic testing include a prolonged bleeding time, low or normal vWF antigen, and low vWF activity. The PT is usually normal, but this can be variable, as can the factor VIII level. This variability sometimes makes von Willebrand disease difficult to differentiate from mild hemophilia A. The patient's blood type affects the vWF level; blood type O has as much as a 30% reduction in vWF levels compared to the other blood types.

Treatment

Desmopressin has become a mainstay of therapy for many patients with type I von Willebrand disease and may work in conjunction with other plasma products that contain vWF for types II and III. In responsive individuals, desmopressin causes a transient 2- to 4-fold increase in vWF. It also seems to have an effect on the endothelium that promotes hemostasis. The dose is 0.3 μg/kg (maximum dose, 20 μg) administered subcutaneously or intravenously every 12 hours for a total of 3–4 doses; after 4 doses, tachyphylaxis develops. Desmopressin can also be used as an intranasal spray. For children older than age 5 years, a single spray in a single nostril is adequate (150 μg total dose). For adolescents and adults, administer a single spray in each nostril (300 μg total dose).

Plasma derivatives that contain vWF are used for patients with type I disease that does not or no longer responds to desmopressin and for patients with type II or III disease. To be effective the chosen product must have vWF in the high molecular weight form. Cryoprecipitate meets this objective (contains factor VIII and vWF), but the potential for viral transmission is a concern. If cryoprecipitate is used, 10 bags every 12–24 hours will usually control bleeding. Humate-P is an intermediate-purity factor VIII concentrate that has significant amounts of vWF and can be used to treat bleeding episodes. Platelet transfusions may benefit patients with certain types of von Willebrand disease (es-

pecially type III) that do not respond to vWF-containing concentrates of cryoprecipitate.

Local measures to control bleeding in von Willebrand disease include (1) intranasal application of porcine strips (e.g., Surgicel), porcine strips sprinkled with microfibrillar collagen (e.g., Avitene), or cauterization for epistaxis, (2) birth control pills to help raise vWF levels and limit the degree of menstrual bleeding, and (3) EACA for dental injury or planned intraoral procedures.

LIVER DISEASE

Clinical Findings

Acute and chronic diseases of the liver can be associated with many hemostatic abnormalities. Hepatocytes synthesize all of the coagulation factors and related regulatory proteins, with the exception of factor VIII. Malabsorption of vitamin K can occur with processes that interfere with the absorption of fat-soluble vitamins, including impaired bile acid metabolism (ie, primary biliary cirrhosis), intrahepatic or extrahepatic cholestasis, and treatment with bile acid binders. Thrombocytopenia in severe liver disease is most often due to portal hypertension, which leads to congestive hypersplenism and splenic sequestration. Patients with significant liver disease have increased fibrinolysis due to decreased synthesis of α_2-plasmin inhibitor. In some patients with liver disease, abnormal fibrinogen molecules are synthesized that, when cleaved to fibrin monomers, do not polymerize correctly.

Patients with mild to moderate hepatic dysfunction frequently have subclinical hemostatic abnormalities. Patients with severe liver disease may have life-threatening bleeding. Laboratory studies should include a PT, aPTT, and platelet count. Also consider obtaining fibrinogen levels and measurement of fibrin degradation products (FDP) or D-dimer. In general, prolongation of the PT and a plasma fibrinogen level of less than 100 mg/dL is a poor prognostic sign in patients with liver disease.

Treatment & Disposition

Patients who have liver disease and laboratory abnormalities without clinically significant bleeding usually require only close observation. If clinically significant bleeding is present or an invasive procedure or surgery is pending, the coagulopathic state will need to be treated. Transfuse packed RBCs to maintain an adequate hemoglobin level and to maintain hemodynamic stability. Give oral or intravenous vitamin K to all patients. FFP can be used to replace coagulation factors temporarily, but the volume needed to completely replenish the coagulation factors may limit the amount given. Cryoprecipitate may be used to replace fibrinogen in patients with fibrinogen levels less than 100 mg/dL. Platelet transfusions may be appropriate if platelet counts are low. Desmopressin (either 0.3 μg/kg subcutaneously or intravenously [maximus dose, 20 μg], or 300 μg intranasal spray) shortens the prolonged bleeding time in some patients with liver disease. Although controlled trials are lacking, there are few side effects.

RENAL DISEASE

Hemostatic abnormalities commonly occurring in patients with renal disease include quantitative and qualitative platelet abnormalities and clotting factor abnormalities. Platelet counts are frequently normal, although mild thrombocytopenia may occur. Clinically significant bleeding may occasionally occur with dialysis-induced thrombocytopenia. Retention of uremic toxins causes inhibition of platelet aggregation.

Preventive measures include optimizing nutrition with folate, vitamin B_{12}, and iron repletion; optimizing dialysis; and correcting anemia with recombinant human erythropoietin. Acute bleeding can be treated with dialysis, transfusion of RBCs, desmopressin, and conjugated estrogens; cryoprecipitate transfusion and platelet transfusion are rarely used. Dialysis improves platelet function transiently, lasting for 1–2 days. Platelet function is optimized when the hematocrit (percentage of RBC mass to blood volume) is maintained at 26–30% because anemia contributes to bleeding. In uremic patients with prolonged bleeding times, 50–75% will have shortening or normalization of the bleeding time when given desmopressin. Conjugated estrogen, 25 mg intravenously, also improves both bleeding time and clinical bleeding in more than 80% of uremic patients. Cryoprecipitate carries the risk of viral transmission, and platelet transfusions are relatively ineffective because the infused platelets quickly acquire the uremic defect. Restrict the use of cryoprecipitate and platelet transfusions to life-threatening bleeding when used in combination with packed RBCs, desmopressin, and conjugated estrogens.

WARFARIN & VITAMIN K DEFICIENCY

General Considerations

The vitamin K–dependent coagulation factors produced in the liver are prothrombin (factor II), factor VII, IX, and X, as well as the anticoagulant proteins C and S. Nutritional deficiency of vitamin K is rare in adults. However, patients with liver disease can have vitamin K deficiency due to a combination of poor nutrition and malabsorption. Additionally, deficiency of the vitamin K–dependent factors can occur in patients receiving antibiotics, particularly the third-generation cephalosporins that contain the *N*-methylthiotetrazole side chain (ie, moxalactam, cefamandole, cefotaxime, cefoperazone).

Warfarin, the major oral anticoagulant used in the United States, inhibits the production of the vitamin K–dependent coagulation factors. The half-life of warfarin is approximately 36 hours with normal hepatic function. The standard starting dosage is usually 5 mg/d with subsequent dose adjustment guided by the international normalized ratio (INR). Observable anticoagulation effect is expected in 2–7 days. The goal INR is 2.0–3.0 for all indications except in patients with prosthetic mechanical valves and with antiphospholipid antibody syndrome; these patients require a higher INR of 2.5–3.5. Maintenance dosage can be influenced by different variables, including the patient's vitamin K stores, malnutrition, liver function, concurrent medical disorders, and numerous drug interactions.

Clinical Findings

The major adverse effects associated with warfarin treatment include warfarin embryopathy, warfarin-induced skin necrosis, and bleeding. Warfarin interferes with a vitamin K–dependent protein used to build the bone matrix, resulting in fetal bone abnormalities. This toxicity occurs with warfarin exposure during the 6th to 12th weeks of gestation, but warfarin should be avoided during the entire pregnancy. Warfarin-induced skin necrosis is an uncommon complication occurring during the first week after initiating therapy. Some patients who develop this complication have a hereditary heterozygous protein C deficiency or protein S deficiency.

Treatment

Treatment of warfarin complications includes discontinuation of warfarin, heparinization if anticoagulation is required, vitamin K administration, and screening for protein C and protein S deficiencies. The fear of creating a hypercoagulable state in persons with undiagnosed protein C deficiency is unfounded, but persons with a known hypercoagulable state should receive anticoagulation therapy with heparin before starting warfarin.

Bleeding is the most common complication of warfarin treatment; the risk of bleeding is related directly to the degree of anticoagulation. Additionally, individual risk factors for bleeding include age greater than 65 years, hypertension, anemia, prior cerebrovascular disease, gastrointestinal lesions, and renal disease. Medications that increase warfarin activity and antiplatelet medications can also increase bleeding risks. Management of bleeding depends on the type of bleeding and the INR value. The anticoagulated state can be reduced in 3 ways: withhold warfarin, administer vitamin K, or transfuse FFP (Table 39–9).

Table 39–9. Warfarin reversal guidelines.

International Normalized Ratio (INR) Value	Bleeding	Recommendations
Any elevation	Major to life threatening	Withhold warfarin. Replace coagulation factors with FFP or factor complex concentrates. Vitamin K, 5–10 mg IV (dose dependent on INR)
Any elevation	Mild to moderate	Withhold warfarin. Vitamin K, 2–4 mg PO (dose dependent on INR)
< 5	None	Withhold warfarin until INR therapeutic and then restart at same or lower dose.
5–9	None	Withhold warfarin until INR therapeutic and then restart at same or lower dose. Vitamin K, 1–2 mg PO
> 9	None	Withhold warfarin until INR therapeutic and then restart at same or lower dose. Vitamin K, 2–4 mg PO

Recent studies suggest that subcutaneous administration of vitamin K has an unpredictable and delayed response, whereas oral vitamin K is convenient to administer, is effective, and produces less resistance to subsequent warfarin use. Additionally, hypersensitivity reactions and anaphylaxis are uncommon with the oral administration of vitamin K. Intravenous administration of vitamin K results in the rapid reversal of hypercoagulation but is associated with anaphylaxis or hypersensitivity reactions, including flushing, diaphoresis, hypotension, dyspnea, and chest pain. Doses of vitamin K above 10 mg are associated with overcorrection of hypercoagulation and warfarin resistance for up to 1 week upon reinstitution of anticoagulation. In general, restrict the intravenous use of vitamin K to patients with life-threatening bleeding or to those with an INR greater than 20.

Superwarfarins with a prolonged duration of action are used as rodenticides; brodifacoum is the most widely available of these agents. Patients presenting with an overdose may develop severe coagulopathy with major mucosal bleeding and internal bleeding. Treatment with high doses of vitamin K, up to 100–125 mg/d for several weeks, may be required because of the long half-life of these products.

DISSEMINATED INTRAVASCULAR COAGULATION

General Considerations

DIC is an acquired syndrome characterized by both widespread activation of the coagulation system (resulting in fibrin formation and consumption of hemostatic factors) and activation of the fibrinolytic system (resulting in the breakdown of fibrin clots, consumption of coagulation factors, and bleeding). DIC is associated with a variety of disorders such as infection (usually bacterial and occasionally viral), malignancy (adenocarcinoma, acute leukemia, lymphoma), trauma (burns, fat embolism), liver disease, and environmental disorders (hyperthermia, envenomation). DIC may be acute and life threatening or chronic and compensated.

Clinical Findings

A. Symptoms and Signs

Clinical features of DIC vary with the underlying precipitating medical illness. The clinical complications of DIC are bleeding, thrombosis, purpura fulminans, and multiple organ failure. Although hemorrhage and thrombosis may occur simultaneously, in an individual patient, one manifestation usually predominates and the most common one is bleeding. Bleeding can range from petechiae and ecchymoses to bleeding from the gastrointestinal tract, genitourinary tract, surgical wounds, mucocutaneous sites, and venipuncture sites. Intravascular coagulation and fibrin deposition can cause multiple organ failure. Clinical signs include mental status changes, focal ischemia or gangrene, oliguria, renal cortical necrosis, and adult respiratory distress syndrome. Purpura fulminans results when widespread arterial and venous thromboses occur and is most commonly seen with significant bacteremia. In chronic DIC, the pathophysiology of disease is essentially the same, but the destruction of coagulation factors and platelets is balanced by hepatic and bone marrow production.

B. Laboratory Findings

The typical laboratory results in acute DIC include prolonged PT, low platelet count, and low fibrinogen level. The most commonly observed abnormality is thrombocytopenia. Fibrinogen levels may remain normal because fibrinogen is an acute-phase reactant. FDP and D-dimer may help differentiate DIC from other causes of prolonged coagulation times and low platelets; the D-dimer may be more specific than FDP in diagnosing DIC. Additional laboratory findings include increased LDH, decreased haptoglobin levels, and a peripheral smear with schistocytes. Patients with chronic DIC will have minor abnormalities on the screening assays, reflecting the limited consumption of coagulation factors that are being replaced by hepatic synthesis.

Treatment

Treatment of acute DIC rests on supportive measures and management of the underlying illness. Circulatory stabilization requires fluid, RBCs, and sometimes inotropic agents. If possible, the underlying cause of the DIC needs to be treated. Secondary treatment involves replacement therapy with platelets, fibrinogen, and coagulation factors. Many patients with DIC require no specific therapy if evidence of bleeding or thrombosis is lacking and laboratory study results are not deteriorating. Replacement therapy should be given only to patients with bleeding or an impending invasive procedure and should use specific replacement products: fibrinogen repletion with cryoprecipitate to raise the plasma fibrinogen level to 100–150 mg/dL, platelet concentrates to raise platelet count above 50,000/μL, and FFP to replace coagulation factors. Patients with DIC also should be given vitamin K and folate.

Heparin administration usually has a limited role in the treatment of acute DIC. It is usually considered in patients with documented DIC in whom thromboembolic complications predominant the clinical picture (ie, purpura fulminans). Consider heparin for patients with chronic DIC and thrombosis (ie, solid tumors). Antifibrinolytic agents, including EACA, are used with great caution in treating DIC. Although these drugs may reduce bleeding, their use is associated with serious or fatal thromboembolic complications. Restrict antifibrinolytic agents to patients who have documented hypofibrinogenemia and fibrinolysis; these agents should be given with heparin to minimize the potential for thrombosis.

Amitrano L et al: Coagulation disorders in liver disease. Semin Liver Dis 2002;22:83. [PMID: 11928081]

Cines DB, Blanchette VS: Immune thrombocytopenic purpura. N Engl J Med 2002;346:995. [PMID: 11919310]

Levi M, Ten Cate H: Disseminated intravascular coagulation. N Engl J Med 1999;341:586. [PMID: 10451465]

Levine MN et al: Hemorrhagic complications of anticoagulant treatment. Chest 2001;119(1 Suppl):108S. [PMID: 1157645]

Mannucci PM, Federici AB: Management of inherited von Willebrand disease. Best Pract Res Clin Haemtol 2001;14:455. [PMID: 11686109]

McCrae KR et al: Platelets: an update on diagnosis and management of thrombocytopenic disorders. Hematology (Am Soc Hematol Educ Program) 2001:282. [PMID: 11722989]

Moake JL: Thrombotic microangiopathies. N Engl J Med 2002; 347:589. [PMID: 12192020]

Opatrny K: Hemostasis disorders in chronic renal failure. Kidney Int Suppl 1997;62:S87. [PMID: 9350690]

Petrini P: Treatment strategies in children with hemophilia. Paediatr Drugs 2002;4:427. [PMID: 12083971]

Sallah S, Kato G: Evaluation of bleeding disorders. A detailed history and laboratory tests provide clues. Postgrad Med 1998; 103:209. [PMID: 9553596]

■ IV. ANEMIA

Anemia is a common problem, affecting an estimated one third of the world's population. Worldwide, the most common causes of anemia include iron deficiency, thalassemia, hemoglobinopathies, and folate deficiencies. Within the United States, the most common causes are iron deficiency, thalassemia, and anemia of chronic disease. Not only is anemia common in the general population, but also the prevalence of anemia increases with age. Given the ubiquity of this entity, some patients who present to the emergency department with anemia will be symptomatic, whereas anemia will be an incidental finding in other patients.

Anemia is defined as a reduced concentration of RBCs. Erythropoiesis ensures that the number of RBCs present is adequate to meet the body's demand for oxygen and that RBC destruction equals production with an average lifespan of 120 days for circulating erythrocytes. Any process or condition that impairs the production, increases the rate of destruction, or increases the loss of erythrocytes will result in anemia if the body cannot produce enough new RBCs to keep up with the loss.

Quantification of the RBC concentration is reflected in the RBC count per microliter, hemoglobin concentration, or hematocrit. Normal RBC values for adults vary slightly between males and females (Table 39–10). Based on RBC values, there are three categories of anemia (Table 39–11).

Regardless of the cause of anemia, many of the clinical manifestations are the same. The severity of symptoms and signs related to anemia depends on several

Table 39–10. Normal red blood cell (RBC) values for adults.[1]

Measure	Male	Female
RBC count (million/μL)	4.5–6.0	4.0–5.5
Hemoglobin (g/dL)	14–17	12–15
Hematocrit (%)	42–52	36–48
Mean corpuscular volume (fL)	78–100	78–102
Mean cellular hemoglobin (pg/cell)	25–35	25–35
Mean corpuscular hemoglobin concentration (g/dL)	32–36	32–36
Red cell distribution width (%)	11.5–14.5	11.5–14.5
Reticulocyte count (%)	0.5–2.5	0.5–2.5

[1]Normal values may vary depending upon the equipment used, patient's age, and altitude.

factors: the rate of development of anemia, the extent of anemia present, the patient's age, the patient's general physical condition, and other existing comorbid illnesses. Patients with chronic and slowly developing anemia may have almost no complaints even with hemoglobin levels as low as 5–6 g/dL. More typically, most people will begin to be symptomatic with hemoglobin levels at about 7 g/dL. Patients with chronic anemia may complain of weakness, fatigue, lethargy, dyspnea with minimal exertion, palpitations, and orthostatic symptoms. Physical examination findings in patients with significant chronic anemia may include orthostatic hypotension; tachycardia; skin, nail bed, and mucosal pallor; systolic ejection murmur; bounding pulse; or widened pulse pressure. Patients who develop anemia in a rapid fashion frequently have more pronounced symptoms. Additionally, these patients may have hypotension, resting and exertional dyspnea, palpitations, diaphoresis, anxiety, severe weakness that may progress to lethargy, and altered mental status. Loss of more than 40% of blood volume leads to severe symptoms that are due more to intravascular volume depletion than to anemia.

The diagnosis of anemia is established by the finding of a decreased RBC count, hemoglobin, or hematocrit on the routine CBC. A specific cause of anemia need not be established in the emergency department; however, appropriate workup should be initiated to help expedite a diagnosis and initial studies should be started before the transfusion of packed red blood cells. The basic evaluation of a patient newly diagnosed with anemia includes the following: RBC indices provided with the CBC, reticulocyte count, and peripheral blood smear. The mean cellular volume (MCV) is the most useful guide to the possible cause of an anemia. The

Table 39–11. Classification of anemias.

Type	Mean Corpuscular Volume (fL)	Mean Corpuscular Hemoglobin Concentration (g/dL)	Cause	Other Hematologic Findings
Microcytic	< 80	< 32	Iron deficiency	Low reticulocytes, low serum ferritin and iron, high total iron-binding capacity
	< 80	Variable, but usually < 32	Thalassemias	Elevated reticulocytes, target cells, normal or elevated serum ferritin and iron
	< 80	< 32	Chronic lead poisoning	Basophilic red blood cell stippling
	< 80	Variable, but usually < 32	Sideroblastic anemia	Elevated serum iron; ring sideroblasts in bone marrow
Normocytic	80–100	32–36	Acute blood loss	Elevated platelets
	80–100	32–36	Hemolytic anemia	Elevated reticulocytes, low haptoglobin, elevated LDH and indirect bilirubin
	80–100	32–36	Chronic disease	Low reticulocytes; low serum iron and total iron-binding capacity
Macrocytic	> 101 (usually > 130)	> 36	Vitamin B$_{12}$ or folate deficiency	Macroelliptocytes, hypersegmented neutrophils
	> 101–120	> 36	Liver disease	Decreased platelets

reticulocyte count reflects activity in the bone marrow. The red cell distribution width (RDW) measures the size variability of the RBC population, and in early nutritional deficiency anemias (iron, vitamin B_{12}, or folate) the RDW may be increased before the MCV becomes abnormal. As part of the general evaluation, the two most common sources of blood loss should be investigated: gastrointestinal (eg, checking the stool for occult blood) and uterine bleeding(eg, history).

IRON-DEFICIENCY ANEMIA

Iron-deficiency anemia occurs when body iron content is insufficient for erythropoiesis; it manifests as a microcytic, hypochromic anemia. Iron deficiency is seen with either inadequate iron intake (usually in undeveloped countries with little meat in the diet) or from a combination of iron loss (hemorrhage) and inadequate intake (in developed countries). Heme iron (as found in meat) is absorbed more efficiently than is nonheme iron (found in vegetables) and accounts for the higher incidence of iron deficiency in vegetarians. Total body iron content varies with age and gender at 35–60 mg/kg of body weight. Each gram of hemoglobin contains 3.47 mg of iron. The recommended daily intake of iron is about 7 mg in a man, 12–16 mg in a menstruating woman, and 5–7 mg in a postmenopausal woman.

Clinical Findings

A. Symptoms and Signs

The symptoms of iron-deficiency anemia (fatigue and weakness) are generally due to the anemia. Occasionally patients may describe a desire to chew ice or cold food (termed pagophagia) or leg cramps on climbing stairs. Gastrointestinal epithelial (angular stomatitis, glossitis, esophageal webs, and gastric atrophy) and nail (koilonychia) abnormalities have been described in iron deficiency, although their frequency varies and these findings are uncommon in the United States.

B. Laboratory Findings

Patients with iron-deficiency anemia have both microcytic (low MCV) and hypochromic (low MCHC) erythrocytes. The platelet count is often elevated. Examination of the peripheral smear is useful to exclude thalassemia; target cells are not seen in iron-deficiency anemia. Combined iron deficiency and folate deficiency produces variation in red cell size, some macrocytic and others microcytic, such that the measured MCV can be within the normal range. Iron-deficiency anemia produces a low serum ferritin, low serum iron, and elevated total iron-binding capacity. The absence of stainable iron on bone marrow aspirate establishes the diagnosis without other tests. Possible blood loss should be investigated in a patient with iron-deficiency anemia and often requires testing for occult blood loss from either the gastrointestinal tract (stool for occult blood) or the kidneys (hemoglobinuria or hemosiderinuria).

Treatment

Iron-deficiency anemia is treated effectively and economically with oral iron therapy using ferrous sulfate, 325 mg (children, 1–2 mg/kg) with each meal three times daily. A response with increased reticulocytes is seen within 3–4 days and peaks in 7–10 days, with the hemoglobin level increasing about 1 g/dL per week. Once normal hemoglobin levels are achieved, oral iron therapy should continue to replenish total body iron stores. Parenteral iron therapy is reserved for the rare patient who cannot absorb oral iron, but parenteral preparations are expensive and associated with adverse effects, including fatal anaphylactic reactions. The dose of parenteral iron preparations is calculated according to hemoglobin level and ideal body weight; the formula varies by specific product. Red cell transfusion is used for the patient with ongoing blood loss or acute symptoms of inadequate oxygen delivery to the brain or heart.

ACUTE HEMOLYTIC ANEMIA

The immune-mediated hemolytic anemias traditionally have been divided into 3 categories: autoimmune, alloimmune, and drug related.

AUTOIMMUNE HEMOLYTIC ANEMIA
General Considerations

Individuals with autoimmune hemolytic anemia (AIHA) make antibodies against their own RBCs or against the body's higher-incidence antigens. The overall incidence of AIHA is approximately 1–3 cases per 100,000 population per year. The incidence of AIHA in infants and children is less, approximately 0.2 cases per 100,000 population per year in those under age 20 years. AIHA in children is commonly associated with viral or respiratory infections; is mediated by immunoglobulin G (IgG); and causes acute, fulminant hemolysis. Pregnant women have a 5 times greater risk of developing autoantibodies, but significant RBC destruction is not common.

Diagnosis of AIHA requires evidence of an autoantibody against RBCs in the form of (1) detection of the autoantibody on the patient's red cells (positive DAT) *and* (2) identification of an autoantibody, after either eluting (washing off) the antibodies from a patient's red cells or detecting the autoantibodies in the patient's serum (indirect Coombs test). To make the diagnosis of AIHA, serologic evidence of autoantibodies should be correlated with clinical and other routine laboratory evidence of hemolytic anemia, including decreased hemoglobin, decreased haptoglobin, elevated reticulocyte count, elevated unconjugated (indirect) bilirubin, elevated LDH, or hemoglobinuria.

AIHA can be divided into primary and secondary varieties. Primary AIHA refers to cases without an underlying cause (idiopathic), and secondary AIHA refers to cases seen with an underlying disorder (Table 39–12). Primary AIHA is more common in women, with peak incidence during the 4th and 5th decades. The hemolytic process in AIHA can take place within the vascular space or in the liver or spleen. AIHA is also categorized according to autoantibody type: warm type, cold type, and mixed type.

1. Warm-Type AIHA

Clinical Findings

Warm-type AIHA comprises 70% of AIHA cases and is usually mediated by an IgG antibody directed against surface antigens of the RhD-erythrocyte system. Autoantibodies of the warm type react most strongly near 37 °C. These autoantibodies are usually pan-reactive and produce hemolysis both in the patient's RBCs and in transfused RBCs. Warm-type autoantibody-mediated hemolysis is predominantly extravascular, occurring in the spleen. Warm-type AIHA carries a 2:1 female preference but has no racial predilection. About half of warm-type AIHA cases can be labeled as primary or idiopathic. Secondary cases are most often associated with lymphoproliferative disorders (in about half) or a

Table 39–12. Causes of secondary autoimmune hemolytic anemia.

Lymphoproliferative disease: chronic lymphocytic leukemia, lymphoma, Hodgkin disease, Waldenström macroglobulinemia, multiple myeloma
Autoimmune disease: systemic lupus, rheumatoid arthritis, polyarteritis nodosa, pernicious anemia, autoimmune thyroid disease, scleroderma, ulcerative colitis, Crohn disease
Infection: infectious mononucleosis, cytomegalovirus infection, viral hepatitis, malaria, pediatric viral respiratory illness
Immunodeficiency syndrome: HIV, X-linked agammaglobulinemia, common variable immunodeficiency, IgA deficiency, Wiskott-Aldrich syndrome, dysglobulinemia
Non-lymphoid tumors: ovarian carcinoma and dermoid cysts, teratomas, Kaposi sarcoma, thymoma

systemic autoimmune disease. Viral-induced or HIV-associated warm-type AIHA is often mild and self-limited.

Treatment

Warm-type AIHA is initially treated with oral prednisone, 1–1.5 mg/kg/d for 1–3 weeks. Improvement is usually noted within 1 week, and 70–80% of patients are better within 3 weeks. Once the patient's hemoglobin level stabilizes, the steroids can be tapered. Complete remission is achieved in 15–20% of new-onset cases of warm-type AIHA, but half of patients will need low-dose prednisone for several months.

Between 10% and 20% of steroid-treated patients will fail to respond adequately or will require unacceptably high doses to maintain the desired response. In such patients the AIHA is treated with either splenectomy or cytotoxic drugs. Splenectomy removes both the main site of extravascular hemolysis and a major site of general autoantibody production. Splenectomy produces a 65–70% response rate and has the potential for long-term remission or a complete cure.

Cytotoxic drugs produce a 40–60% response rate and have been used for patients who have not responded to steroids or splenectomy. Severe hemolysis in cases of warm-type AIHA may be treated with plasma exchange as a transient stabilizing measure while waiting for steroids or cytotoxic agents to take effect. Intravenous immunoglobulin may be used as adjunctive treatment in children who cannot tolerate the side effects of chronic high-dose steroids or cytotoxic agents. Danazol, an attenuated androgen with fewer side effects than glucocorticoids, can produce remission in occasional patients.

For patients with life-threatening anemia, RBC transfusion of the least incompatible units may be transfused slowly with close monitoring. Transfusion may precipitate further production of autoantibodies as well as introduce a source for the production of allogeneic antibodies.

2. Cold-Type AIHA: General Considerations

Cold-type AIHA autoantibodies are usually immunoglobulin M (IgM) and are most strongly hemolytic at 0–4 °C. The presence of cold-type autoantibodies leads to clumping or agglutination of RBCs on peripheral smear at cooler temperatures. Hemolysis occurs in both the extravascular and intravascular spaces, and Kupffer cells in the liver are responsible for most of the extravascular RBC destruction. The two common cold-type AIHA disorders are cold agglutinin syndrome (CAS) and paroxysmal cold hemoglobinuria (PCH).

Fifty percent of secondary cold-type AIHA cases are associated with lymphoproliferative disorders.

3. Cold-Type AIHA: Cold Agglutinin Syndrome

CAS accounts for up to one third of all AIHA cases and is typically IgM mediated and directed against the I/i blood group antigens. Primary CAS is seen in older adults, particularly females, with a peak incidence at age 70 years. The hemolysis associated with the primary and chronic secondary forms of CAS tends to be mild and stable with hemoglobin levels of 9–12 g/dL. Secondary CAS can also occur as an acute attack, such as that seen in patients who have preceding infectious illnesses, including from *Mycoplasma pneumoniae,* Epstein-Barr virus (EBV), adenovirus, CMV, influenza, varicella zoster virus (VZV), HIV, *E coli, Listeria monocytogenes,* and *Treponema pallidum.*

Clinical Findings

Symptom onset corresponds with the peak antibody response to infection, usually 2–3 weeks after the onset of illness. The triggered cold-type AIHA resolves approximately 2–3 weeks later. Chronic cold-type AIHA associated with lymphoproliferative diseases, such as chronic lymphocytic leukemia, lymphomas, and Waldenström macroglobulinemia, produces high autoantibody levels with the potential for significant hemolysis. Cold weather exacerbates CAS; more episodes of acute hemolysis are seen during winter. Patients are apt to develop acrocyanosis because the peripheral circulation is typically cooler than the central circulation. Raynaud phenomenon, vascular occlusion, and tissue necrosis may complicate CAS. Clumping of cold agglutinins will elevate the MCV and decrease the RBC count. Peripheral smear findings include the spherocytosis caused by RBC membrane destruction, as well as anisocytosis, poikilocytosis, polychromasia, and agglutination. As with other forms of hemolytic anemia, patients will have elevated LDH and unconjugated bilirubin with moderate disease, and decreased haptoglobin, hemoglobinemia, and hemoglobinuria with severe, intravascular hemolysis.

Treatment

In primary and chronic CAS with mild anemia, treatment is symptomatic and involves simply keeping extremities, noses, and ears warm in cold weather. Patients with CAS should take daily folate supplements. Treatment for severe hemolysis has been successful with immunosuppressive or cytotoxic agents, such as chlorambucil, cyclophosphamide, α-interferon, or fludara-

bine. As in warm-type AIHA, plasmapheresis may prove helpful as a temporizing measure by removing autoantibodies, particularly as auto-IgM has an intravascular distribution, but such therapy should be combined with immunosuppressive agents. Unlike warm-type AIHA, CAS rarely responds to steroids though such treatment may be considered in atypical cases. Because splenic macrophages play a lesser role in IgM-mediated cold-antibody disease, splenectomy is not as helpful for cold-antibody mediated extravascular hemolysis. RBC transfusion can be performed for patients at risk for significant cardiac or cerebrovascular ischemia, but transfused blood should be kept at 37 °C using a blood warmer. Transfusions should be limited because they may worsen ongoing hemolysis. In addition to the risk of producing alloantibodies to transfused RBCs, most cold antibodies act against the I group antigens, which are found on most donor RBCs.

4. Cold-Type AIHA: Paroxysmal Cold Hemoglobinuria

PCH is caused by a biphasic IgG autoantibody called the Donath-Landsteiner antibody. The PCH autoantibody is directed against the P antigen system found on most RBCs. Despite the name, hemolysis may occur at both cold and normal temperatures.

Clinical Findings

Symptoms include high fever, chills, headache, abdominal cramps, nausea and vomiting, diarrhea, and leg and back pain that develops with cold exposure. Cold urticaria, extremity paresthesias, and Raynaud phenomenon may also develop. Primary PCH and PCH secondary to congenital or late-stage syphilis are characterized by chronic disease with cold-induced relapses. Secondary PCH caused by other infectious agents is most common in children and is one of the more common causes of childhood hemolytic anemia. Postinfection PCH is usually associated with measles, mumps, EBV, CMV, VZV, adenovirus, influenza A, *M pneumoniae, Haemophilus influenzae,* and *E coli.* Most cases of postinfectious PCH are self-limited, but severe cases may take weeks to resolve. With severe hemolysis, hemoglobinuria is common and methemoglobinuria may be seen. Acute renal failure may develop as a complication of PCH.

Treatment

Keep patients with PCH warm. Consider steroids in children with severe hemolytic anemia, but because infection-related PCH tends to be self-limited, the benefit is uncertain. PCH secondary to syphilis responds to effective antibiotic treatment. Splenectomy is not helpful, and plasmapheresis should be used only as a temporizing measure in life-threatening cases. RBC transfusion using a blood warmer should be limited to patients with severe hemolysis, because most donor units are P antigen positive and may stimulate further production of PCH autoantibodies.

5. Mixed-Type AIHA

Mixed-type AIHA occurs as primary or secondary disease (usually lymphoproliferative or autoimmune diseases). The course of illness is usually chronic with severe exacerbations. Like warm-type AIHA, mixed-type AIHA is steroid responsive, can be treated with splenectomy, and responds to cytotoxic therapy. Because relapses are not triggered by cold exposure, acrocyanosis and the Raynaud phenomenon are not characteristically seen. As with any secondary AIHA, treatment of the underlying disorder will reduce hemolytic activity.

ALLOIMMUNE HEMOLYTIC ANEMIA

Alloimmune hemolytic anemia requires exposure to allogeneic RBCs with subsequent formation of alloantibodies that react specifically with the allogenic RBCs that triggered their production; these antibodies do not react against a patient's own RBCs. A well-known example of alloimmune hemolytic anemia is when the RhD-negative maternal immune system develops IgG alloantibodies on exposure to RhD-positive fetal RBCs. The maternal alloantibodies can then cross the placenta to inflict fetal RBC destruction in a condition termed hemolytic disease of the newborn. Anemia can range from mild to potentially fatal producing intrauterine fetal death. By still uncertain mechanisms, administration of anti-D IgG with any fetomaternal hemorrhage event and soon after delivery will suppress maternal alloantibody formation and prevent hemolytic disease of the newborn. Treatment of established disease employs intrauterine and intravascular fetal transfusion and may include plasma exchange or intravenous immunoglobulin therapy.

Most adults who develop alloimmune hemolytic anemia have a history of RBC transfusion, which sensitizes patients to allogeneic RBC antigens. A subsequent transfusion can result in immediate alloantibody production, resulting in the fever, chest and flank pain, tachypnea, tachycardia, hypotension, hemoglobinuria, and oliguria seen in the hemolytic transfusion reaction. In patients with high alloantibody titers, the hemolytic reaction can be immediate, whereas patients with lower alloantibody levels develop delayed hemolysis occurring 3–7 days posttransfusion.

DRUG-RELATED AIHA

Drug-related AIHA can be divided into 3 types: autoimmune, drug adsorption, and neoantigen. Steroids can be used in cases of drug-related severe hemolysis. RBC transfusion will aggravate hemolysis if the recipient's serum contains antibodies against antigens found on the transfused RBCs.

Autoimmune Drug-Related AIHA

Autoimmune drug-related AIHA results when the offending drug triggers formation of autoantibodies that bind with RBC self-antigens, leading to a hemolytic process serologically indistinct from that seen in warm-type AIHA. The diagnosis is proved when the hemolytic process abates on withdrawal of the offending drug. Drugs implicated include α-methyldopa, levodopa, mefenamic acid, procainamide, diclofenac, quinidine, phenacetin, and the second- and third-generation cephalosporins (particularly cefotetan and ceftriaxone). Up to 71 drugs have been associated with development of a positive DAT; however, significant hemolysis is seen only occasionally. An extended drug exposure is usually required for autoantibodies to form. A positive DAT does not indicate that hemolysis will occur or that a drug must be discontinued. Within days of stopping the offending drug, hemolysis usually stops, though it may take months to see full resolution of the process.

Drug Adsorption–Type AIHA

Drug adsorption–type AIHA requires that the drug incite the formation of antidrug antibodies and that the drug bind to the RBCs with significant affinity. Antibodies formed against the drug will react against the drug bound to the RBC surface, producing hemolysis. This type of hemolysis has also been called drug-requiring because the absence of the offending drug eliminates the hemolytic reaction completely.

Neoantigen-Type Drug-Related AIHA

Neoantigen-type drug-related AIHA involves weak binding of the offending drug to normal RBCs. The body's immune system, seeing the formed immune complexes as foreign, will generate an immune response, which then produces hemolytic disease. The classic causative agent is penicillin, and isolated cases of diphtheria-tetanus-pertussis vaccination in children have been associated with hemolysis, possibly via this neoantigen mechanism.

SICKLE CELL ANEMIA

General Considerations

Sickle cell anemia is caused by the substitution of the amino acid valine for glutamine at position 6 in the β-globin chain producing an abnormal hemoglobin tetramer termed hemoglobin S (HbS). As a result of this mutation, deoxygenated HbS polymerizes, deforming the RBC and producing the characteristic sickled appearance. The distorted cell results in premature RBC destruction and also increases the viscosity of blood, leading to obstruction within the microvasculature. The overall effect is chronic ongoing hemolysis and episodic periods of vascular occlusion resulting in tissue ischemia affecting most organ systems.

This defect is inherited as an autosomal recessive trait, and disease is seen in patients who are homozygous for the sickle gene (HbSS). People with sickle cell trait (HbAS; heterozygous with one gene for normal β-globin chain and one gene for a β-globin chain with the sickle mutation) have a normal lifespan and are usually asymptomatic except in rare cases of severe physiologic stress when they may have an acute pain crisis, splenic infarction, or cerebrovascular complications. Approximately 8% of the African American population carries sickle cell trait (heterozygous for the sickle cell gene), and approximately 0.15–0.2% of African American newborns have sickle cell disease (homozygous for the sickle gene). A lesser percentage of individuals of Middle Eastern, eastern Mediterranean, and Indian descent may have the HbS gene.

Clinical Findings

A. SYMPTOMS AND SIGNS

Patients with sickle cell disease typically present to the emergency department because of complications (Table 39–13). Acute painful (vasoocclusive) sickle cell crisis is a common problem, and the average patient with sickle cell disease has 1–4 severe attacks per year. The initiating event may not be identifiable, but stressors such as infection, cold, dehydration, and altitude have been implicated. As a result of intravascular sickling and small vessel occlusion, infarction of bone, viscera, and soft tissue occurs. Infarction manifests as diffuse bone, muscle, and joint pain and, in some cases, symptoms related to a specific affected organ. Initial management includes

Table 39–13. Emergencies in sickle cell disease.

Type	Specific Emergencies
Vasoocclusive crises	Musculoskeletal pain (typical painful crisis) Dactylitis (hand-foot syndrome) Acute chest pain syndrome Stroke Priapism
Hematologic crises	Splenic sequestration Aplastic crisis Hemolytic crisis
Infections	Pneumonia Meningitis Sepsis Osteomyelitis Urinary tract infections

aggressive pain management and hydration, an assessment of the cause of the current crisis, and a search for additional complications.

B. LABORATORY FINDINGS

Generally a CBC and reticulocyte count help assess the degree of anemia and ensure that the marrow is still producing red cells. If the reticulocyte count is not available, the presence of polychromasia in the peripheral blood smear can indicate continued red cell production. Patients with sickle cell disease sometimes have a low-grade fever and an elevated white blood cell (WBC) count. This combination can make it difficult to determine whether an infection is present during a crisis. Consider infection if the WBC count has a left shift and is elevated above 20,000/μL. Because of the chronic hemolysis, mild elevations in bilirubin and serum LDH are common.

Treatment

Supplemental oxygen is commonly used for painful crises, but unless the patient is systemically hypoxemic, it has not proved to be of routine benefit. Treatment of acute pain requires opioids, and patients with severe pain should receive parenteral agents (commonly intravenously in the United States and subcutaneously in the United Kingdom). A potent opioid, such as morphine or diamorphine, is recommended, whereas meperidine, with the potential for neurotoxicity from the metabolite normeperidine, is not recommended. Some patients may be tolerant because of prior opioid treatment, and large doses may be required. Regular doses of analgesics for a few hours to several days are typically required. Patient-controlled analgesia can be used in selected patients. NSAIDs can be used for their additive effect in pain management of sickle cell crisis. Because patients with sickle cell disease with a painful crisis have an absolute or relative hypovolemia due to their disease (deficient renal concentrating ability) or crisis (anorexia, vomiting, fever), aggressive oral or intravenous rehydration is commonly carried out. Induced hyponatremia and purified poloxamer 188 shorten the duration and severity of an acute crisis but the effect is small, and no approach to shortening the duration and severity of a painful sickle cell crisis has proved reliable, safe, and appropriate for routine use. A common and recommended practice is to develop an individualized assessment and treatment protocol for specific patients who frequently present to the emergency department with painful crises.

Simple or exchange transfusion to reduce the concentration of HbS-containing red cells to below 30% can prevent or reverse the vasoocclusive process. Transfusion should not raise the hematocrit above 36% in sickle cell patients. Transfusion carries significant expense, risk of blood-borne disease transmission, and the potential for iron-overload, and it exposes the patient to the minor red cell antigens with the potential to induce antibodies that prevent or complicate future transfusions. Transfusion for sickle cell crisis or complications is reserved for specific indications such as aplastic crisis, pregnancy, stroke, respiratory failure, general surgery, and priapism. Hydroxyurea has been used to reduce the frequency and severity of painful crises. The major side effect is bone marrow, hepatic, and renal toxicity, and hydroxyurea has not been approved for use in children. Daily prophylactic penicillin V reduces the incidence of infections and reduces mortality from sepsis in children.

Sickle Cell Complications

A. Bone Pain

Bone pain is common during a sickle cell crisis and may include the back and the extremities. Usually the pain is diffuse, and no physical findings are present. However, redness, warmth, or swelling suggest infection (cellulitis or osteomyelitis). The complaint of localized pain to the hip with difficulty ambulating suggests the possibility of aseptic necrosis of the femoral head, and approximately 30% of those with sickle cell disease develop hip pathology by age 30 years. Bone infarctions may cause symptoms similar to osteomyelitis. Plain radiographs may show evidence of aseptic necrosis or osteomyelitis,

whereas bone infarcts are not usually visible on radiographs. Joint effusions are occasionally seen as a complication of sickle cell crisis, but arthrocentesis is often necessary to determine if the joint is infected.

B. Dactylitis

In young children an early manifestation of sickle cell disease is dactylitis (hand-foot syndrome). The syndrome is thought to be due to infarction of the red marrow with associated periosteal inflammation. The syndrome manifests as fever and painful swelling of the hands, feet, or both, and some redness and warmth may be present. As the child grows, the hematopoietic tissue in the metacarpal and phalangeal marrow is replaced by fatty tissue, making this entity less likely.

C. Chest Syndrome

The acute chest syndrome is used to describe a sickle cell crisis with pulmonary symptoms and a new pulmonary infiltrate found on radiograph. The patient might have pleuritic chest pain, shortness of breath, fever, nonproductive cough, and tachypnea. The exact cause of the chest syndrome is unclear, but infection, infarction (ribs or lung), and pulmonary fat embolism (from ischemic marrow fat necrosis) have all been implicated. Although a chest radiograph is not routinely required in all patients with painful sickle cell crisis, it is indicated in those with pulmonary symptoms or signs of fever. The onset of acute chest syndrome may be associated with a fall in hemoglobin level from the normal baseline. Pulmonary infiltrates may be present in one lobe or be diffuse and bilateral, and pleural effusions may be present. Severe cases may progress rapidly to respiratory failure. Treatment involves close monitoring of fluid status, oxygen, and pain control. Broad-spectrum antibiotics to cover S pneumoniae and M pneumoniae are recommended. In severe cases, simple transfusion or exchange transfusion can be done. Acute chest syndrome is currently the leading cause of death from sickle cell disease in the United States.

D. Abdominal Pain

Generalized and constant abdominal pain is a common complaint during an acute sickle cell crisis, and it may be difficult to distinguish between infarction of the abdominal and retroperitoneal organs associated with a sickle cell crisis and a focal abdominal problem such as cholecystitis or appendicitis. Frequently the patient can determine that the pain is similar to or different from prior episodes. Patients with a typical vasoocclusive episode should not have evidence of peritonitis (rebound). Hepatic infarction may cause the acute onset of jaundice and abdominal pain and can be difficult to distinguish from hepatitis or cholecystitis. Biliary disease is common because pigment-related cholelithiasis is seen in 30–70% of patients with sickle cell disease. Severe right upper quadrant pain and marked elevations of bilirubin may be due to intrahepatic cholestasis.

E. GENITOURINARY SYSTEM

Vasoocclusive events involving the kidneys are common but often asymptomatic. Infarction in the renal medulla may cause flank pain, renal colic-type pain, and costovertebral angle tenderness, mimicking pyelonephritis. Papillary necrosis may result in either gross or microscopic hematuria, but red cell casts are uncommon. Renal imaging studies are generally necessary for correct diagnosis. Priapism occurs in up to 30% of males with sickle cell disease. Initial treatment is fluid hydration, pain control, and transfusion. Urinary tract infections are more common in patients with sickle cell disease, and urinalysis is recommended.

F. SPLENIC INFARCTION

The spleen is particularly susceptible to the effects of sickled cells. During childhood, microinfarctions result in a nonfunctional spleen (in 14% of patients by age 6 months and 94% by age 5 years). Immunizations, prophylactic penicillin therapy, and parental education are critical to minimize the risk of infection and prompt early evaluation of fever in these patients. As sickle cell patients age, their risk of overwhelming sepsis decreases, but they remain predisposed to infection.

G. SPLENIC SEQUESTRATION

Splenic sequestration is more common in children than in adults, and it is a potential cause of death that can be averted with treatment. This syndrome is manifest by sudden enlargement of the spleen with an acute fall in the hemoglobin level due to sequestration of the blood volume within the spleen. Symptoms include tachycardia, hypotension, pallor, lethargy, and abdominal fullness. Left upper quadrant pain may or may not be present. The spleen is usually enlarged and firm. Platelets may also be sequestered, resulting in moderate thrombocytopenia. Therapy includes volume resuscitation, which may mobilize some of the red cells trapped within the spleen. Transfusion or exchange transfusion may be necessary; rarely, splenectomy is necessary. Unfortunately, recurrence of this syndrome is common.

H. HEMOLYTIC ANEMIA

Patients with sickle cell disease have a chronic hemolytic process with a baseline hemoglobin level usually between 6 and 9 g/dL; the reticulocyte count is 5–15%. With infections the hemolytic process may worsen and hemoglobin may drop from previous baseline. Typically, reticulo-cytosis will increase in response to the increased red cell destruction but may not be enough to compensate for the increased hemolysis. Acutely, the patient may notice symptoms of worsening fatigue, shortness of breath, dyspnea on exertion, and scleral icterus. The hemolysis is rarely severe enough to require transfusion.

I. APLASTIC CRISIS

Aplastic crisis results when the production of red cells declines significantly, producing a rapid decrease in the hemoglobin level with reticulocytopenia. The most common cause of aplastic crisis appears to be infection, specifically from parvovirus. Folate deficiency and bone marrow necrosis also may play a role. Aplastic crisis is more common in pediatric patients than in adults. The hemoglobin level will be unusually low, and few or no reticulocytes will be present (reticulocyte count typically < 0.5%. The WBC and platelet levels are usually normal. Generally this syndrome is self-limiting, and the marrow will begin producing red cells spontaneously within a week. Transfusion may be required in the interim.

J. NEUROLOGIC COMPLICATIONS

Complications of sickle cell disease include stroke and subarachnoid hemorrhage. The cause of strokes in most patients is cerebral infarction due to occlusion or narrowing of large cerebral vessels. Approximately 10% of patients with sickle cell disease experience a stroke before age 20 years. Acute treatment is emergent simple or partial exchange transfusion. Unfortunately, children who suffer a stroke are at 70–90% risk for recurrence. Chronic transfusion therapy is indicated to prevent recurrent stoke after the initial event. Cerebral aneurysms are also more common in sickle cell patients, perhaps due to local vessel occlusion or ischemia.

K. INFECTIONS

Patients with sickle cell disease are functionally asplenic after early childhood, making them susceptible to infections from encapsulated organisms, such as *H influenzae* and *S pneumoniae*. Other common infections associated with sickle cell disease include pneumonia caused by these organisms as well as *M pneumoniae*, meningitis, and osteomyelitis due to *Salmonella typhimurium*, *Staphylococcus aureus*, and *E coli*. Although low-grade fever sometimes occurs during an acute crisis, unexplained fevers of 38 °C (101 °F) or higher require evaluation for bacterial infection and consideration for early treatment with broad-spectrum antibiotics.

L. CARDIAC COMPLICATIONS

Cardiomegaly is common and correlates with the degree of chronic anemia. Additionally, cardiac dysfunction may occur from microinfarcts and hemosiderin deposition from hemolysis and blood transfusion. Because of the chronic anemia, enhanced cardiac contractility is present to maintain adequate systemic oxygen delivery producing a widely radiating systolic ejection murmur.

M. DERMATOLOGIC COMPLICATIONS

Chronic, poorly healing leg ulcers around the malleoli are common in older patients with sickle cell disease. Minor injury, impaired microcirculation due to repeated sickling episodes and microinfarcts, and infections all contribute to the development and persistence of these ulcers.

Disposition

Most sickle cell pain crises last 2–3 days. Patients with adequate clinical response and no indications for hospital admission can be discharged with oral pain medications and referred for follow-up with their primary care physician in the next 24–48 hours. The following are guidelines for hospital admission for sickle cell patients: (1) pulmonary or neurologic complications, (2) significant bacterial infection, (3) splenic sequestration or aplastic crisis, or (4) pain that remains poorly controlled or patients unable to maintain adequate hydration.

THALASSEMIAS

The thalassemias are a diverse group of disorders characterized by defective synthesis of globin chains that results in the inability to produce normal adult hemoglobin. The hallmark of these disorders is a microcytic, hypochromic, hemolytic anemia. These disorders are most common in individuals of Mediterranean, Middle Eastern, African, or Southeast Asian descent. Patients with the β-thalassemias have diminished production of the β-globin chain, which allows unmatched α-globin chains to accumulate as α_4 tetramers in the immature red cell. These tetramers are insoluble, and their precipitation damages the developing erythroid precursor cells, resulting in early death. Patients with α-thalassemia develop an excess of β-globin chains that accumulate as β_4 tetramers called hemoglobin H (HbH). HbH is more soluble and stable so that, in the severe α-thalassemia, ineffective erythropoiesis is less of a problem and increased destruction of the cells due to structural abnormality is more prominent. Thalassemia red cells contain decreased hemoglobin, which accounts for the hypochromia and target cell formation. Individuals with either α- or β-thalassemia can be minimally to severely affected due to the specific genotype and whether the mutation produces complete or partial reduction in globin chains.

α-THALASSEMIA CARRIER & TRAIT

α-Thalassemia carriers have normal RBC size, shape, and number and have no clinical consequences from this inherited gene. Those with a-thalassemia trait are detected by the finding of microcytic RBCs and a normal hemoglobin level.

HEMOGLOBIN H DISEASE

Hemoglobin H disease is a disorder in which 1 out of 4 α-globin chain genes is functional. Patients with hemoglobin H disease usually present in the neonatal period with a severe hypochromic anemia. Later in life the clinical picture includes a hypochromic, microcytic anemia with jaundice and hepatosplenomegaly. These patients may not require regular transfusions, but a transfusion may be necessary in conditions of increased oxidative stress (which may cause precipitation of the unstable hemoglobin H resulting in hemolysis) or infection. Most of these patients will know their diagnosis, and the emergency physician need provide only supportive care and blood transfusion when necessary. Medications that may precipitate hemolysis should be avoided in this population (Table 39–14).

Table 39–14. Drugs that produce oxidative stress on red blood cells and may induce hemolysis.

Class	Drug
Sulfonamides	Sulfacetamide Sulfamethoxazole Sulfanilamide Sulfapyridine
Antimalarials	Primaquine Chloroquine Pamaquine Pentaquine
Urinary agents	Nitrofurantoin Nalidixic acid Phenazopyridine
Miscellaneous antibiotics	Ciprofloxacin niridazole Norfloxacin Chloramphenicol
Mothballs	Naphthalene
Miscellaneous	Vitamin K analogs Methylene blue Acetanilid Doxorubicin Isobutyl nitrite Phenylhydrazine

β-THALASSEMIA MINOR (β-Thalassemia Trait)

Patients with β-thalassemia minor are heterozygous for the β-globin mutation and have only mild microcystic anemia. Splenomegaly may be present. These patients may exhibit microcytosis, hypochromia, and basophilic stippling on blood smear. An elevated hemoglobin A_2 level, typically 4–6%, confirms the diagnosis. These patients will generally not have clinical manifestations, and this form of thalassemia may come to the clinician's attention only during an evaluation for a mild anemia.

β-THALASSEMIA MAJOR (Cooley Anemia)

In patients with β-thalassemia major, both β-globin genes are defective and production of β-globin chains is severely impaired. β-Thalassemia major is characterized by a severe anemia that begins within the first year of life. These children develop hepatosplenomegaly, jaundice, expansion of the erythroid marrow (causing bone changes and osteoporosis), and increased susceptibility to infection. The anemia is severe and requires regular and lifelong blood transfusions. These transfusions and enhanced iron absorption eventually cause iron overload, which, if untreated, results in hemochromatosis with cardiac, hepatic, and endocrine dysfunction. The RBCs of these children show a low MCV with microcytic and hypochromic cells. Variation in size and shape of the RBCs will be notable (increased RDW) as will the presence of nucleated cells. Consider this diagnosis in any child with a severe microcytic anemia and the appropriate ethnic background. For those with a known diagnosis who present to the emergency department with significant symptoms related to anemia or hemolysis, consider transfusion and search for precipitating events.

GLUCOSE-6-PHOSPHATE DEHYDROGENASE DEFICIENCY

Glucose-6-phosphate dehydrogenase (G6PD) is an enzyme responsible for preventing oxidative damage to intraerythrocytic hemoglobin. Over 300 variant mutations are described for G6PD; the highest prevalence is in individuals of African, Asian, or Mediterranean descent. Because the gene for G6PD is carried on the X chromosome, males are affected when they are hemizygous. Females must carry two defective genes to be severely affected, but because expression of this gene is variable, women with one dysfunctional gene may show some symptoms. The severity of G6PD disease is related to the magnitude of enzyme deficiency; patients with severe deficiencies have less than 10% of normal enzyme activity and patients with moderate deficiencies have 10–60% of normal activity. G6PD deficiency is seen in approximately 10–15% of black males in the United States.

Oxidization of the hemoglobin sulfhydryl groups causes hemoglobin to precipitate within the cell; it is recognized by the presence of Heinz bodies on the peripheral blood smear. The affected RBC is removed from the circulation by the spleen. Oxidant damage also occurs at the RBC membrane, producing both extravascular and intravascular hemolysis.

A history of neonatal jaundice 1–4 days after birth is common. Patients with severe variants may have a severe chronic hemolytic anemia. In the more common variants of G6PD deficiency, the patient is usually asymptomatic except for acute hemolytic crises that occur due to bacterial and viral infections, exposure to oxidant drugs (most commonly sulfonamides, antimalarials, and nitrofurantoin), metabolic acidosis (such as diabetic ketoacidosis), renal failure, and in some patients, ingestion of fava beans (see Table 39–14). These episodes are usually self-limited and well tolerated because only the older RBCs will hemolyze. The incidence of pigmented gallstones and splenomegaly is increased in patients with G6PD deficiency. Treatment for this disease is supportive and preventative.

HEREDITARY SPHEROCYTOSIS

Hereditary spherocytosis is the result of an erythrocyte membrane defect and is the most prevalent hereditary hemolytic anemia among people of northern European descent. The disease is typically inherited in an autosomal dominant pattern, although a less common autosomal recessive variant exists; in up to 20% of patients the disease is the result of an apparent spontaneous mutation. The abnormal shape of the RBC results from molecular abnormalities in the cytoskeleton of the cell membrane, resulting in red cells with a microspherocytic shape, which is not pliable enough to pass through the spleen, leading to an increased rate of destruction and a compensatory increase in RBC production. The clinical spectrum of hereditary spherocytosis includes (1) mild disease, occurring in 20–30% of cases, with an autosomal dominant inheritance, (2) moderate disease, occurring in 60–75% of cases, with primarily autosomal dominant inheritance, and (3) severe disease, in about 5% of cases, occurring with autosomal recessive inheritance.

Neonatal jaundice during the first week of life occurs in 30–50% of hereditary spherocytosis patients.

After the neonatal period, the symptoms and signs depend on the severity of ongoing hemolysis. Patients with mild disease usually have a normal hemoglobin level and little or no splenomegaly but are susceptible to hemolytic or aplastic episodes triggered by infection. Patients with moderate disease have mild to moderate anemia, modest splenomegaly, periodic episodes of hemolysis with jaundice, and an increased incidence of pigmented gallstones. The rare patient with severe hereditary spherocytosis has chronic jaundice, an enlarged spleen, and significant hemolytic anemia requiring episodic blood transfusions.

The peripheral blood smear shows spherocytes with a normal to low MCV and increased MCHC (> 36%). The diagnosis of hereditary spherocytosis is established by the osmotic fragility test. In severe cases, splenectomy will generally reverse the anemia except in the unusual cases of autosomal recessive variants. After splenectomy, spherocytes are still present.

Ballas SK: Sickle anaemia: progress in pathogenesis and treatment. Drugs 2002;62:1143. [PMID: 12010077]

Bolton-Maggs PH: The diagnosis and management of hereditary spherocytosis. Baillieres Best Pract Clin Haemtol 2000;13:327. [PMID: 11030038]

Gehrs BC, Friedberg RC: Autoimmune hemolytic anemia. Am J Hematol 2002;69:258. [PMID: 11921020]

Hermiston ML, Mentzer WC: A practical approach to the evaluation of the anemic child. Pediatr Clin North Am 2002;49:877. [PMID: 12430617]

Mehta A, Mason PJ, Vulliamy TJ: Glucose-6-phosphatase dehydrogenase deficiency. Baillieres Best Pract Clin Haemtol 2000;13:21. [PMID: 10916676]

Scjroer SL: Pathophysiology of thalassemia. Curr Opin Hematol 2002;9:123. [PMID: 11844995]

Telen MJ: Principles and problems of transfusion in sickle cell disease. Semin Hematol 2001;38:315. [PMID: 11605166]

Vichinsky EP et al: Causes and outcomes of the acute chest syndrome in sickle cell disease. N Engl J Med 2000;342:1855. [Erratum in N Engl J Med 2000;343:824.] [PMID: 10861320]

Wonke B: Clinical management of beta-thalassemia major. Semin Hematol 2001;38:350. [PMID: 11605170]

Wright MS: Drug-induced hemolytic anemias: increasing complications to therapeutic interventions. Clin Lab Sci 1999;12:115. [PMID: 10387489]

■ V. POLYCYTHEMIA

The term *polycythemia* means increased cellular components in peripheral blood—RBCs, WBCs, and platelets—but in common practice is used to describe increased red cells or erythrocythemia. Polycythemia can be a primary disorder due to malignant transformation of a hematopoietic stem cell (called polycythemia vera) or can be secondary to overstimulation of red cell production. Polycythemia is characterized by an increased red cell mass. In relative or false polycythemia, the red cell mass is normal but decreased plasma volume results in elevated hemoglobin and hematocrit values.

PRIMARY POLYCYTHEMIA (Polycythemia Vera)

Polycythemia vera is an unregulated neoplastic proliferation of red cells, usually accompanied by increased WBC and platelet production. Peak age at onset is 50–70 years, although it can occur in young adults.

Clinical Findings

A. SYMPTOMS AND SIGNS

Onset is gradual, and symptoms are usually due to hyperviscosity and impaired circulation in the brain (headache, dizziness), eyes (impaired vision), heart (chest pain), or peripheral circulation (claudication). Increased production of basophils and mast cells can lead to pruritus after a hot shower from histamine release. Hemorrhagic or thrombotic complications are rare. Physical findings include hypertension (common), plethora or ruddy complexion, splenomegaly (in about 75% of cases), and hepatomegaly (in about 30% of cases).

B. LABORATORY FINDINGS

Determination of red cell mass with a radionuclide technique will show an elevated value (> 36 mL/kg in males or > 32 mL/kg in females) but is unnecessary when the hemoglobin value is above 20 g/dL or hematocrit is above 60% in males or above 56% in females; these values are always associated with an elevated red cell mass. The WBC and platelet counts are commonly elevated.

Treatment & Disposition

Standard treatment for polycythemia vera is periodic phlebotomy to remove excess red cells, reduce blood viscosity, and improve microcirculation. Polycythemia vera patients with altered mentation should have emergent phlebotomy with 500 mL of blood removed. Myelosuppressive agents are occasionally used, generally when excessive platelet production causes thrombotic or hemorrhagic complications.

SECONDARY POLYCYTHEMIA

Secondary polycythemia is produced by erythropoietin stimulation of bone marrow red cell production. Systemic hypoxia (eg, from chronic obstructive pulmonary disease, right-to-left cardiac shunts) or local renal hypoxia (eg, atherosclerotic renal vascular disease) can lead to stimulation of erythropoietin production by the kidney. Because of the widespread use of cigarettes, chronic obstructive pulmonary disease is the most common cause of secondary polycythemia. Less common causes include chronic carbon monoxide exposure, renal tumors that secrete erythropoietin, use of androgenic steroids, and familial hemoglobinopathies associated with high oxygen affinity.

Clinical Findings

Polycythemia should be suspected when the hematocrit is greater than 52% in males or 47% in females. Confirmation of red cell mass and plasma volume requires measurement via radionuclide techniques. Systemic hypoxia (arterial oxygen saturation < 92%) or chronic carbon monoxide exposure (carboxyhemoglobin levels > 8%) should be considered. Blood viscosity increases and impairs microcirculation with hematocrit values above 60–65%.

Treatment & Disposition

Symptomatic patients should undergo phlebotomy to reduce blood viscosity and improve microcirculation, and emergent phlebotomy may be necessary in the emergency department for patients with acute symptoms. Long-term management of secondary polycythemia depends on the primary disorder.

Prchal JT: Molecular biology of polycythemias. Intern Med 2001;40:681. [PMID: 11518102]

Tefferi A: Polycythemia vera: a comprehensive review and clinical recommendations. Mayo Clin Proc 2003;78:174. [PMID: 12583529]

■ VI. WHITE CELL DISORDERS

NEUTROPENIA

General Considerations

Neutropenia is defined as a decrease in circulating neutrophils as detected by measuring the absolute neutrophil count (ANC) in the peripheral blood. The ANC is determined by multiplying the total WBC count by the percentage of neutrophils and bands from the WBC differential. The ANC is normally greater than 1500 cells/μL in individuals of European descent and greater than 1000 cells/μL in African Americans. Neutropenia produces an increased susceptibility to bacterial infec-

tions inversely related to the ANC. Severe neutropenia is defined as an ANC less than 500 cells/μL.

Clinical Findings

Neutropenia can be congenital, associated with inherited immune defects and phenotypic abnormalities. A form of congenital neutropenia is chronic benign neutropenia, either familial with an autosomal dominant inheritance pattern, or nonfamilial. Patients with chronic benign neutropenia do not have significantly increased susceptibility to bacterial infections. Acquired neutropenia can be due to drugs, toxins, nutritional deficiencies, autoimmune disorders, or diseases that impair bone marrow granulocyte cell production. The list of drugs that can produce neutropenia is extensive, but the most likely agents are the cytotoxic chemotherapeutic agents used to treat malignancies.

Neutropenia should be suspected when a cancer patient receiving chemotherapy presents with fever or when an otherwise healthy patient presents with an infection that has not responded as expected to antibiotic treatment. The evaluation of the febrile neutropenic patient requires a careful evaluation for clinically occult infection. Because of the neutropenia, the patient may not be able to generate pus in a local site or wound, an infiltrate on chest radiograph, or pyuria on urinalysis in response to infection. Carefully examine the mouth, sinuses, and rectal area for evidence of local infection. Obtain blood cultures, urine culture, and a chest radiograph. When present, culture other body secretions such as diarrhea, wound exudate, or sputum.

Treatment & Disposition

The decision to initiate empiric antibiotic therapy is based on the estimated risk of serious bacterial infection as judged by the cause, severity, and expected duration of neutropenia and on the patient's clinical condition. The severely ill cancer patient with severe neutropenia (ANC ANC < 500 cells/μL) due to recent chemotherapy clearly requires broad-spectrum empiric antibiotic therapy and hospital admission. Conversely, a mildly ill cancer patient with mild neutropenia (ANC of 1000–1500 cells/μL) who has not received recent chemotherapy can likely be discharged home with symptomatic therapy and no antibiotic treatment as long as the evaluation does not find a specific bacterial infection requiring treatment. Consult with the hematologist-oncologist regarding treatment and admission decisions. If indicated, initiate empiric antibiotics in the emergency department after obtaining appropriate cultures. Multiple antibiotic regimens are used, typically a broad-spectrum agent such as a third-generation cephalosporin (ceftazidime), or a fluoroquinolone (levofloxacin), or a carbapenem (imipenem and cilastatin) with or without a specific antistaphylococcal agent such as vancomycin.

LEUKOCYTOSIS

Elevated WBC counts may represent an appropriate response to infection or may constitute an autonomous proliferation of cells due to a primary hematologic disorder. Elevated WBC count is not a problem by itself except in the unusual case of leukemia associated with hyperleukocytosis, when WBC counts exceed 100,000–300,000 cells/μL, causing increased blood viscosity and circulatory compromise. This can lead to central nervous system impairment and respiratory insufficiency; urgent treatment with leukocytapheresis is indicated. As a temporizing measure, intravenous hydration and exchange transfusion can be performed.

ACUTE LEUKEMIA

General Considerations

Acute leukemia is a malignancy of hematopoietic stem cells in which the leukemic cell population replaces and suppresses normal bone marrow cells, resulting in bone marrow failure with anemia, functional or absolute neutropenia, and thrombocytopenia. The usual causes of illness and death are infection (related to neutropenia) or hemorrhage (related to thrombocytopenia). These rapidly progressive disorders are uniformly fatal without treatment. Fortunately, effective treatment is available for most patients with acute leukemia, and depending on cell type, 20–40% of adult patients and 50–70% of pediatric patients with acute leukemia survive longer than 5 years with current therapy. Acute leukemias have historically been classified according to neoplastic cell morphology (acute lymphocytic leukemia, or ALL, and acute myelocytic leukemia, or AML), but immunologic analysis has found a wide diversity in neoplastic cell origin.

Clinical Findings

Patients with acute leukemia typically develop symptoms over a few weeks and present with fatigue (due to anemia), fever (due to neutropenia), or bleeding problems (due to thrombocytopenia or DIC). Leukemic organ infiltration accounts for symptoms such as bone pain (ALL), swollen gums (AML), and abdominal pain due to splenomegaly (ALL and AML)

The diagnosis of acute leukemia is suspected when the WBC count is elevated and the peripheral blood smear shows a large number of immature white cells (blast cells), along with anemia and thrombocytopenia. Uncommonly, blast cells may be absent from the peripheral blood (termed aleukemic leukemia) and the he

moglobin value and platelet count may be normal. Definitive diagnosis of acute leukemia is based on bone marrow examination showing more than 30% immature blast cells. Differentiation between the types of acute leukemia is made using morphologic, histochemical, and immunochemical staining.

Disposition

Hospitalize patients with suspected acute leukemia. Evaluate fever, if present, and initiation of empiric antibiotic treatment in the neutropenic patient is prudent. Patients with hyperleukocytosis (> 300,000 cells/μL) may develop symptoms of impaired microcirculation and require emergent treatment.

CHRONIC LEUKEMIA

Chronic leukemias are indolent diseases, typically found in older adults and producing nonspecific systemic symptoms (malaise, fatigue, weight loss, low grade fever) and signs of leukemic organ infiltration (splenomegaly, lymphadenopathy). Chronic leukemias have historically been classified according to neoplastic cell morphology (chronic lymphocytic leukemia, or CLL, and chronic myelocytic leukemia, or CML), but immunologic analysis has found a wide diversity in neoplastic cell origin.

1. Chronic Lymphocytic Leukemia

CLL is the most common leukemia seen in the adult population of Western countries. Most cases of CLL are seen in patients older than 55 years, and the majority of cases have a slow progression lasting up to 10 years before they enter a final terminal stage. These patients commonly experience repeated infections such as pneumonia, herpes simplex, and herpes zoster because the lymphocytes are functionally incompetent. Patients often have fatigue, lymphadenopathy, mucosal surface bleeding, or hepatosplenomegaly. Diagnosis is suggested by a peripheral blood smear with absolute lymphocyte count exceeding 5000 cells/μL and confirmed with bone marrow examination. Patients with an initial diagnosis of CLL and without any of the complications can be followed up with a hematologist. Patients with any of the above-mentioned complications (bleeding, fever, symptoms of hyperviscosity, bone marrow failure) need hospitalization and prompt consultation with a hematologist.

2. Chronic Myelocytic Leukemia

CML is a clonal disorder of hematopoietic stem cells most commonly due to a reciprocal translocation between the long arms of chromosomes 22 and 9, resulting in a shortened chromosome 22, termed the Philadelphia chromosome.

Patients typically present with fatigue, malaise, and weight loss. Often findings of leukocytosis and splenomegaly with or without hepatomegaly are found incidentally on routine examination. The CBC often shows a moderate leukocytosis of 20,000–60,000 cells/μL, a mild anemia, and variable platelet counts. The peripheral blood smear shows a predominance of myeloid progenitor cells (myeloblasts, myelocytes, metamyelocytes) and nucleated red blood cells.

Most patients are clinically stable and responsive to therapy for 3–5 years, then develop an acute blastic crisis (generally myeloid but occasionally lymphoid) that is refractory to treatment and progresses to death. A small subset of CML patients bypass the initial chronic phase and enter a rapidly progressive leukemic phase wherein they have profound leukocytosis and thrombocytopenia as evidenced by bleeding, petechiae, and ecchymoses. A serious complication is the hyperviscosity syndrome in which WBC counts exceed 300,000 cells/μL or with a leukocrit greater than 10%. This is evidenced by neurologic and ophthalmologic manifestations and respiratory failure.

Exchange transfusion can be a useful temporizing measure in the acute setting with severe stupor or seizure, but urgent leukocytapheresis is the most effective treatment.

INFECTIOUS MONONUCLEOSIS

General Considerations

Infectious mononucleosis is a primary infection with EBV characterized by fever, pharyngitis, adenopathy, and greater than 10% atypical lymphocytes in the peripheral smear. Only a minority of primary EBV infections come to medical attention; population studies indicate as many as 90% of young adults have serologic evidence of prior EBV infection, but only a minority of individuals describe a prior episode of infectious mononucleosis, supporting the concept that most primary EBV infections are mild or asymptomatic.

Clinical Findings

A. Symptoms and Signs

The incubation period of infectious mononucleosis is 1–2 months. Initial symptoms are fatigue, malaise, and sore throat. Fever is usually low grade, and chills are uncommon. The pharyngitis of infectious mononucleosis may be exudative or nonexudative, and tonsillar enlargement is common. The lymphadenopathy is usually bilateral and in the posterior cervical nodes, although other lymph nodes may be affected and generalized lymphadenopathy is possible. Splenic tenderness is common early in the disease, whereas splenomegaly is a later finding. A variety of other symptoms or signs are well described in infectious mononucleosis: (1) an early, faint, evanescent generalized maculopapular rash, (2) early bilateral periorbital edema, (3) hepatitis with liver tenderness and jaundice, (4) uvular edema, and (5) neurologic disorders such as Bell palsy, optic neuritis, other cranial nerve mononeuropathies, aseptic meningitis, encephalitis, Guillain-Barré syndrome, and transverse myelitis.

B. Laboratory Findings

Common laboratory findings of infectious mononucleosis include (1) leukocytosis (usually 12,000–20,000 cells/μL), (2) lymphocytosis (usually > 60% on the white cell differential), (3) atypical lymphocytosis (> 10% and frequently > 30%), (4) mild elevations in serum transaminases, and (5) elevated erythrocyte sedimentation rate. EBV infection induces the production of host antibodies that form the basis for serologic diagnosis of infectious mononucleosis. Specific antibody testing in clinical use for infectious mononucleosis includes both IgM and IgG antibodies to either the viral capsid antigen found on the viral surface or the Epstein-Barr nuclear antigen found in the viral core. The most commonly used antibody test is the Monospot, which detects an IgM antibody to the viral capsid antigen (historically named heterophile antibody) that produces agglutination of horse red blood cells. The Monospot is considered to have approximately 85% sensitivity and almost 100% specificity. However, the sensitivity of this test is lower early in the clinical disease (up to 6 weeks is required for maximal sensitivity) and in children under age 2 years, who are frequently Monospot negative. False-positive Monospot tests have been seen in patients with CMV, rubella, systemic lupus erythematosus, rheumatoid arthritis, HIV, and herpes simplex infections.

Differential Diagnosis

The differential diagnosis of infectious mononucleosis includes (1) streptococcal pharyngitis (complicated by the observation that up to 30% of infectious mononucleosis patients have detectable group A streptococci in the oropharynx), (2) primary CMV infection (the closest clinical mimic of infectious mononucleosis), (3) acute toxoplasmosis (usually with unilateral lymphadenopathy), and (4) viral hepatitis.

Treatment

There is no effective antiviral therapy for infectious mononucleosis. For the patient with excessive tonsillar enlargement, a 5- to 7-day course of oral prednisone, 1 mg/kg/d, provides symptomatic benefit. Steroids are also used for rare patients with central nervous system involvement or hemolytic anemia. Antibiotic treatment of coexistent group A streptococci is controversial. Some clinicians recommend withholding antibiotic treatment because a positive throat culture or streptococcal antigen test represents colonization rather than infection and antibiotic treatment may induce a rash that, though due to the infectious mononucleosis and not the drug, may be judged as a drug allergy and complicate future antibiotic therapy. Patients should be instructed to refrain from strenuous physical activity and especially contact sports for 3 weeks.

MULTIPLE MYELOMA

Clinical Findings

A. SYMPTOMS AND SIGNS

Multiple myeloma is a disease of malignant plasma cell proliferation and excessive secretion of monoclonal paraproteins. Multiple myeloma usually presents during the 6th to 7th decades of life. The most common initial symptoms are bone pain (in up to 70% of patients; involving the lumbar region) sometimes with pathologic fractures; constipation, nausea, confusion, and somnolence from hypercalcemia; fatigue and pallor from anemia; infection with impaired immunity; bleeding from thrombocytopenia or hyperviscosity; and paresthesias from peripheral neuropathies. Complications of multiple myeloma include renal impairment, amyloidosis from paraproteinemia, hypercalcemia, and spinal cord compression from extradural compression. Physical examination findings include bony tenderness, soft tissue plasmacytoma masses, pallor from anemia, ecchymoses or petechiae, epistaxis, or findings of spinal cord compression (lower extremity weakness or dysesthesias with incontinence of bowel or bladder with associated decreased rectal tone or saddle anesthesia).

B. LABORATORY FINDINGS

The diagnosis is suspected when the serum globulin protein level is elevated and is confirmed with serum protein immunoelectrophoresis demonstrating a monoclonal spike. Evaluate the patient's hematologic (CBC), hemostatic (PT, PTT), renal (blood urea nitrogen and creatinine), and metabolic (electrolytes, calcium, uric acid) status. Quantification of urinary protein excretion (Bence-Jones proteinuria; ie, lambda light chains) is sometimes useful for diagnosis and determining response to therapy. A skeletal series looking for sites of lytic lesions (commonly in the skull and long bones) can be helpful to identify potential pathologic fracture sites and to differentiate multiple myeloma from Waldenström macroglobulinemia (which does not typically have lytic bone lesions). Bone marrow examination typically finds sheets or clumps of plasma cells replacing normal marrow contents.

Treatment & Disposition

Many patients with multiple myeloma are asymptomatic, and specific treatment can be delayed until the patient shows signs of disease progression without affecting efficacy of treatment. Treatment is usually with the chemotherapeutic agents melphalan and prednisone. In occasional patients, multiple myeloma is treated with irradiation and chemotherapy followed by autologous bone marrow or peripheral blood stem cell transplantation. Adjunctive therapy may include bisphosphonates to prevent hypercalcemia and pathologic fractures, erythropoietin to treat anemia, and radiation to lytic lesions to prevent pathologic fractures. Complications of hypercalcemia, hyperviscosity, pathologic fracture, or spinal cord compression necessitate admission and specific therapy.

WALDENSTRÖM MACROGLOBULINEMIA

General Considerations

Waldenström macroglobulinemia is a rare malignancy of B lymphocytes characterized by excessive production of monoclonal IgM. Symptoms and signs are due to the elevated serum viscosity (from the IgM) and infiltration of organs (bone marrow, spleen, liver, lymph nodes) from the neoplastic lymphocytes. The disease most commonly occurs in the elderly; median age at onset is approximately 60 years.

Clinical Findings

The onset is typically gradual, and common symptoms are weakness, anorexia, and weight loss. Symptoms due to hyperviscosity include mental status changes, Raynaud phenomenon, peripheral neuropathy, and visual changes. Ocular signs of hyperviscosity include papilledema, enlarged retinal veins, and retinal hemorrhage. Hepatosplenomegaly and lymphadenopathy are common. Purpura can occur due to thrombocytopenia, and functional platelet impairment from the IgM paraproteinemia. The laboratory diagnosis of Waldenström macroglobulinemia is supported by (1) an IgM level above 3 g/dL and (2) hematologic abnormalities of anemia and thrombocytopenia and occasionally leukopenia. The malignant nature is identified with high-resolution serum protein immunoelectrophoresis or bone marrow biopsy with immunochemical staining.

Treatment & Disposition

Consider hyperviscosity for any Waldenström macroglobulinemia patient who presents with mental status or visual changes. Measure the serum viscosity; if elevated, start urgent plasmapheresis. Chemotherapy with alkylating agents (chlorambucil, melphalan, or cyclophosphamide) is used to reduce production of the IgM paraprotein and control symptoms of neoplastic organ infiltration. Prednisone is used to control autoimmune symptoms such as digital ischemia from cryoglobulinemia or immune hemolysis from agglutination. Other chemotherapeutic agents are sometimes used, but no combination is superior or changes median survival. Stable, asymptomatic patients typically do not receive treatment.

Aquino VM: Acute myelogenous leukemia. Curr Probl Pediatr Adolesc Health Care 2002;32:50. [PMID: 11951090]

Chan KW: Acute lymphoblastic leukemia. Curr Probl Pediatr Adolesc Health Care 2002;32:40. [PMID: 11951089]

Garcia-Sanz R et al: Waldenström macroglobulinaemia: presenting features and outcome in a series with 217 cases. Br J Haematol 2001;115:575. [PMID: 11736938]

Kalidas M, Kantarjian H, Talpaz M: Chronic myelogenous leukemia. JAMA 2001;286:895. [PMID: 11509034]

Oscier D: Chronic lymphocytic leukemia. Br J Haematol 1999; 105(Suppl 1):1. [PMID: 10330924]

Papesch M, Watkins R: Epstein-Barr virus infectious mononucleosis. Clin Otolaryngol 2001;26:3. [PMID: 11298158]

Porcu P et al: Leukocytoreduction for acute leukemia. Ther Apher 2002;6:15. [PMID: 11886572]

Rajkumar SV et al: Current therapy for multiple myeloma. Mayo Clin Proc 2002;77:813. [PMID: 12173715]

Viscoli C, Castagnola E: Treatment of febrile neutropenia: what is new? Curr Opin Infect Dis 2002;15:377. [PMID: 12130933]

Wendtner CM et al: New aspects on the pathogenesis, diagnostic procedures, and therapeutic management of chronic lymphocytic leukemia. Int J Hematol 2001;73:32. [PMID: 11372752]

■ VII. TRANSFUSION THERAPY

Transfusion in the emergency department is typically used for acute blood loss and circulatory shock. As medical care is moved to outpatient settings and emergency departments become more crowded, emergency physicians may be responsible for transfusion therapy that was once relegated to inpatient settings. An understanding of the available blood products, their indications, and potential complications of transfusions is important for safe and effective transfusion practice.

PACKED RED BLOOD CELLS

An adult's total blood volume is estimated to be 2.5 L/m^2, 75 mL/kg, or approximately 5 L in a 70-kg person. Fresh whole blood transfusion would be ideal to replace acute blood loss; however, during the storage of whole blood, platelets and other factors become inactive. In addition, the storage life of whole blood is less than that of individual components. Therefore, by necessity and convenience, whole blood is fractionated to its components for storage and transfusion.

PRBCs are prepared by the centrifugation of whole blood to remove about 80% of the plasma. Then a preservative solution is added, most commonly citrate-phosphate-dextrose, with additional nutrients adenosine, glucose, and mannitol. Each unit of PRBCs has a hematocrit of 65–80% and a volume of approximately 250–350 mL (Table 39–15). Transfusion of 1 unit of PRBCs into a typical adult will increase the hematocrit by 3% or the hemoglobin by 1 g/dL.

The primary reason for emergency transfusion of PRBCs is acute blood loss or profound anemia with impaired oxygen delivery. Based on animal and human studies, lactic acid production increases, oxygen extraction ratio exceeds 50%, and the mortality rate starts to increase in otherwise stable patients with hemoglobin levels of 3.5–4.0 g/dL. In an animal model of coronary stenosis, adverse cardiac effects are seen with hemoglobin levels of 6.0 g/dL. However, there are reports of Jehovah's Witnesses, who generally refuse blood products, tolerating surgery with hemoglobin levels below 6.0 g/dL as long as intravascular volume is maintained. Patients with chronic anemia have developed compensation mechanisms so that chronic anemia is better tolerated than acute anemia. Various consensus panels have recommended transfusion for hemoglobin less than 7 g/dL, whereas patients with hemoglobin greater than 10 g/dL rarely will benefit from transfusion. Some patients with cardiac or vascular disease may benefit from transfusion when hemoglobin levels are 7–10 g/dL. Transfusion thresholds for children may be higher and depend on the cause of their anemia.

Depending on the urgency of transfusion, most patients can be typed (ABO and RhD blood group type) and cross-matched against the blood intended for transfusion. The blood type can be determined in about 15 minutes, whereas typing and cross-matching takes approximately an hour. In critically ill patients, type O RhD negative (universal donor) may be transfused because it does not contain blood group antigens. Type O RhD-positive blood may also be used if type O RhD-negative blood is not available, but it is not the blood of choice for women of child-bearing potential. If an RhD-negative patient is transfused with 1 unit of RhD-positive PRBCs, approximately 80% will develop anti-D antibodies. Because the effect of 1 unit of PRBCs is small and clinically inconsequential, it is standard practice to transfuse a minimum of 2 units and raise the hematocrit by 6% and hemoglobin level by 2 g/dL.

Table 39–15. Characteristics of blood products and doses.

Component	Shelf Life	Volume/Unit	Approximate Content/Unit[1]	Typical Dose	Typical Dosage Effect
Packed red blood cells	21–42 days	250–350 mL	Red cells, 65–80% Plasma, 20–35%	2 units or 15 ml/kg	Raises hemoglobin concentration about 2g/dL.
Platelets (random-donor platelet concentrate)	5 days	50–60 mL	Platelets, 7.5×10^{10}	6 units or 5 mL/kg	Raises platelet count about 50,000/µL.
Platelets (apheresis-collected single-donor platelet concentrate)	5 days	250–300 mL	Platelets, $3–6 \times 10^{11}$	1 unit	Raises platelet count about 50,000/µL.
Fresh frozen plasma	1 year frozen and 24 hours thawed	200–250 mL	Each coagulation factor, 200–250 units; and fibrinogen, 400–500 mg	4 units or 15 mL/kg	Raises most coagulation factor levels about 20%.
Cryoprecipitate	1 year frozen	20–50 mL	Factor VIII, 80 units; fibrinogen, 225 mg; von Willebrand factor, variable amounts	10 units or 1 unit/5kg	Raises fibrinogen about 75 mg/dL.

[1]Blood-derived components often contain white blood cells, red blood cells, platelets, and plasma unless they have been specially prepared.

PRBCs may be further treated to meet specific uses, for example, leukocyte-reduced PRBCs, irradiated PRBCs, washed PRBCs, and frozen PRBCs. Leukocyte-reduced PRBCs have had 70–85% of the leukocytes removed. The advantages of leukocyte-reduced PRBCs is (1) to prevent or avoid nonhemolytic febrile reactions due to antibodies to WBC and platelets, if the patient has been exposed to previous transfusions or pregnancies, (2) to prevent sensitization in patients who may be eligible for bone marrow transplantation, and (3) to minimize the risk of virus transmission such as HIV and CMV. The leukocytes can be reduced by filtration or other methods before storage of the PRBCs or during transfusion. Irradiation of PRBCs eliminates the capacity of T cells to proliferate, therefore preventing the donor's T cells from reacting to the recipient's cells and causing graft-versus-host disease. Consider using irradiated cells in transplant patients, neonates, and immunocompromised patients. Washed PRBCs are indicated in patients who have a hypersensitivity to plasma, such as IgA deficiency. For rare blood types, PRBCs may be frozen and saved for up to 10 years for later use. This process is more expensive than normal storage, and once thawed the blood must be washed and transfused within 24 hours.

One unit of PRBCs, about 250–350 mL in volume, is generally transfused over 1–2 hours. However, blood may be transfused more rapidly in patients with hemodynamic instability. During standard transfusions the initial rate is slower over the first 30 minutes, so that if there is incompatibility, the transfusion may be stopped.

PLATELETS

Platelet transfusions may be used either prophylactically to prevent bleeding, or therapeutically when patients with thrombocytopenia are actively bleeding. Platelets are collected from whole blood donation or from single donors using apheresis techniques. One random-donor platelet concentrate prepared from 500 mL of donated whole blood contains an average of 7.5×10^{10} platelets (see Table 39–15). One apheresis-collected single-donor platelet concentrate generally contains $3–6 \times 10^{11}$ platelets, depending on local collection practice. Platelets should be given according to ABO compatibility, if available. A dose of 1 random-donor platelet concentrate per 10 kilograms (approximately 6–8 random-donor platelet concentrates for an adult) or 1 apheresis-collected single-donor platelet concentrate in an adult will increase the platelet count by about 50,000/µL. Response to platelet transfusions is variable; therefore, platelet levels should be checked at 1 hour and 24 hours. Failure of platelets to rise appropriately may be due to increased consumption of platelets from an underlying process, destruction due to platelet antibodies, or sequestration due to hypersplenism. Transfused platelets should survive 3–5 days, unless a consumptive process is present.

The cause of thrombocytopenia is important in the decision to transfuse platelets. With ITP, an antiplatelet antibody-mediated consumptive process, the platelets are larger, younger, and more functional; therefore, prophylactic transfusion is rarely indicated despite very low platelet counts. However, with platelet hypoplasia, platelet function is impaired, making the risk of bleeding greater. Patients with comorbid diseases such as infection, fever, medications, and central nervous system involvement may be more likely to bleed or may be at higher risk if they bleed; therefore, the threshold for platelet transfusion is higher.

The dose of platelets should reflect the indication. In general, spontaneous bleeding is possible, and prophylactic transfusion is indicated with platelet counts less than 10,000/μL. Platelet counts of greater than 50,000/μL rarely cause significant bleeding. Indications for platelet transfusion include the following:

- Platelet count 10,000 μL in asymptomatic patients
- Platelet count 15,000 μL and coagulation disorder or minor bleeding
- Platelet count 20,000 μL and major bleeding
- Platelet count 50,000 μL and invasive procedure (thoracentesis, paracentesis) or general surgery required, or during massive transfusion (1–2 blood volumes)
- Platelet count 100,000 μL and neurologic or cardiac surgery required

Like PRBCs, platelets can be leukocyte-reduced or washed. Patients who have had repeated transfusions may become alloimmunized and refractory to platelet transfusion, noted by the lack of expected rise of platelet count after transfusion. Such patients need HLA- or cross-matched platelets. Other disorders may affect the efficacy of platelet transfusion including duration of platelet storage, bacterial sepsis, antibiotics, graft-versus-host disease, DIC, and splenomegaly.

Relative contraindications to platelet transfusion are consumptive processes such as TTP or heparin-induced thrombocytopenia, in which transfusion may worsen thrombosis. In these diseases, platelet transfusion should be performed in consultation with a hematologist.

FRESH FROZEN PLASMA

FFP is plasma obtained after the separation of whole blood from RBCs and platelets, and then frozen within 6 hours. Each unit of FFP is 200–250 mL and contains

about 1 unit of each coagulation factor and 2 mg of fibrinogen per mL (see Table 39–15). FFP is appropriate for rapid replacement of multiple coagulation deficiencies such as in liver failure, warfarin overdose, DIC, and massive transfusion in bleeding patients. Administration of FFP prophylactically to nonbleeding patients is not indicated, and prophylaxis is not always needed for some procedures in patients with a coagulopathy. For example, patients undergoing paracentesis and thoracentesis are not at increased risk of bleeding until the INR is greater than 2 times control. During massive transfusion with replacement of an entire blood volume, coagulation factor levels are about one third of normal, and although PT and PTT may be abnormal, clinical coagulopathy does not always occur. Indications for FFP transfusion include the following:

- Rapid reversal of warfarin therapy
- Bleeding and multiple coagulation defects as evidenced by prolonged PT, INR, and aPTT greater than 1.5 control (eg, liver disease, DIC)
- Correction of coagulation defects for which no specific factor is available (specific factor replacement is safer and better but may not always be available)
- Transfusion of more than one total blood volume with evidence of active bleeding and prolonged PT or PTT

Other possible indications for FFP in consultation with an appropriate specialist include TTP, antithrombin III deficiency, and hereditary angioedema (FFP contains C1 esterase).

Because the efficacy of transfused coagulation factors varies, the increase in specific coagulation factors seen after FFP infusion also varies. In general, 1 unit of FFP will increase most coagulation factors by 3–5% in a 70-kg adult. The common adult dose of 7–8 mL/kg (or 2 units of FFP in a 70-kg individual) will increase coagulation factors by only 10%, a clinically inconsequential benefit in most circumstances. For clinically relevant correction of coagulation factor deficiencies, a dose of 15 mL/kg (or 4 units in a 70-kg adult) is required (see Table 39–15). As indicated by the name, FFP is stored frozen and there may be a delay while it is thawed. FFP should be ABO compatible. After transfusion, reevaluate bleeding and coagulation studies. If consumption is present, repeated FFP transfusion should be guided by the PT, INR, and aPTT response.

CRYOPRECIPITATE

Cryoprecipitate is the cold-insoluble protein fraction of FFP. Each unit of cryoprecipitate is about 20–50 mL and contains about 225 mg of fibrinogen, 80 units of factor VIII, and variable amounts of von Willebrand factor (vWF) (see Table 39–15). It also contains some factor XIII and fibronectin. With the development of recombinant factor VIII products for use in hemophilia, the primary role of cryoprecipitate is now replacement of fibrinogen or vWF. Bleeding patients with fibrinogen levels below 100 mg/dL due to severe liver disease, DIC, and dilutional coagulopathy may benefit from cryoprecipitate. The dose of cryoprecipitate is 1 unit/5 kg (or 10 units in an adult), which will raise fibrinogen by about 75 mg/dL.

OTHER PLASMA-DERIVED PRODUCTS

Immunoglobulin for Intravenous Administration

Immunoglobulin for intravenous administration is a pooled IgG product that has been virally attenuated. Labeled indications for its use are ITP, pediatric HIV infection, and primary humoral immunodeficiency; it is also indicated for several new and off-label treatments such as for Kawasaki disease and autoimmune disorders. Dose and administration varies by the indication. Adverse reactions include anaphylaxis especially in IgA deficiency (rare), febrile reactions, headache, and renal failure. Some patients develop transient positive serology to hepatitis C and CMV.

Albumin

Albumin is a virally inactivated purified plasma protein that usually accounts for 50% of circulating protein and 75% of plasma oncotic pressure. Albumin transfusion in patients with decreased oncotic pressures may transiently increase oncotic pressure; however, the albumin rapidly distributes to extravascular spaces. Therefore, because of its cost and the lack of proved efficacy over crystalloid, there is no advantage to using albumin.

Antithrombin III

Antithrombin III is a serum coagulation inhibitory protein. Deficiency can be acquired or congenital and is usually associated with difficult-to-treat thrombosis. Antithrombin III replacement is indicated in antithrombin III deficiency–related thrombosis and for thrombosis prophylaxis. This product should be considered in antithrombin III–deficient patients when difficulty is encountered in achieving adequate heparinization or when recurrent thrombosis is observed despite adequate anticoagulation. It is also reasonable to give concentrate to antithrombin III–deficient subjects before major surgeries or in obstetric situations where the risks of bleeding from anticoagulation are unacceptable. Currently, antithrombin III therapy is under investigation in sepsis, DIC, and other thrombotic diseases. The dose depends on the indication. An infusion of 50 units

(1 unit is the amount in 1 mL of pooled plasma) of antithrombin III concentrate per kilogram will usually raise the plasma antithrombin III level to about 120% of normal in a congenitally deficient individual. Monitor plasma antithrombin III levels to ensure that they remain above 80%. Subsequent administration of antithrombin III at 60% of the initial dose at 24-hour intervals is recommended to maintain antithrombin III levels in the normal range.

MASSIVE TRANSFUSION

Massive transfusion is defined as the replacement of one blood volume or about 10 units of PRBCs within a 24-hour period. Patients receiving less than one blood volume rarely need hemostatic factor (ie, FFP, platelets) replacement. In patients receiving two blood volumes or more than 20 units of PRBCs, transfusion of coagulation factors and platelets may be empirically helpful. For patients who receive 1–2 times total blood volume, hemostatic factor replacement should be guided by considerations noted above: (1) If the platelet count is less than 50,000/µL, platelet transfusion is warranted; (2) if the INR is greater than 1.5, FFP may be given; and (3) if fibrinogen levels are below 100 mg/dL, it may be replaced with cryoprecipitate. In massive transfusion, hypothermia is a risk and blood and crystalloid as well as the patient should be warmed. Hypocalcemia from the preservative citrate-chelating calcium is rare but should be considered in massive transfusion if symptoms or signs of hypocalcemia are present.

COMPLICATIONS OF TRANSFUSION THERAPY

Up to 20% of all transfusions may lead to some type of adverse reaction. Although most of these reactions are minor, some are life threatening (Table 39–16). In critically ill patients, transfusion reactions may be difficult to identify; therefore, attention should be paid to unexpected changes in patient status during a transfusion.

Infectious Complications of Blood Transfusion

Improved blood donor screening, serologic testing, safer handling of blood products, and viral inactivation of many blood products has reduced the risk of infection from blood transfusion (Table 39–17). Most cases of viral transmission are thought to occur during the window period between infection and antibody production in the donor. This window is reduced but not eliminated by the use of antigen testing. The prevalence of CMV-positive antibodies in the general population is 50–80%. Therefore, blood is not routinely tested for CMV unless the recipient is seronegative and is

Table 39–16. Acute transfusion reactions.

Reaction Type	Symptoms and Signs	Management	Evaluation
Acute intravascular hemolytic reaction	Fever, chills, low back pain, dyspnea, tachycardia, shock	Immediately stop transfusion. Intravenous hydration to maintain diuresis.	Retype and cross-match. Direct and in-direct Coombs tests. Serum haptoglobin, free hemoglobin, and indirect bilirubin. Urine hemoglobin.
Acute extravascular hemolytic reaction	Low grade fever, but may be asymptomatic	Stop transfusion. Rarely causes hemodynamic instability.	Retype and cross-match. Direct and in-direct Coombs tests. Serum haptoglobin, free hemoglobin, and indirect bilirubin. Urine hemglobin.
Febrile transfusion reaction	Fever, chills	Stop transfusion. Treat fever with acetaminophen.	Evaluate for intravascular hemolysis and infection.
Allergic reaction	Mild: urticaria, pruritus Severe: dyspnea, wheezing, hypotension, tachycardia, shock	Stop infusion. Treat urticaria and pruritus with antihistamines; bronchospasm with inhaled β-adrenergic agonists; and shock with intravenous fluids and epinephrine.	For mild symptoms that resolve with antihistamines: no further evaluation. For severe symptoms: evaluate for intravascular hemolysis.

(1) pregnant, (2) a potential or present transplant candidate, (3) immunocompromised, or (4) a premature infant. Use of leukocyte-reduced blood components further decreases the risk of CMV transmission to susceptible populations because most of the virus resides in the leukocytes. Bacterial sepsis resulting from RBC transfusion is most commonly due to *Yersinia enterocolitica,* which is able to grow easily in refrigerated blood. The risk of bacterial sepsis is highest with random-donor platelet concentrates.

Table 39–17. Risk of infection from transfusion of blood products.

Cause	Estimated Frequency[1]
HIV-1	1:1,000,000 (200,000–2,000,000)
HIV-2	Unknown
HTLV-I/II	1:500,000 (250,000–2,000,000)
Hepatitis B	1:40,000 (30,000–250,000)
Hepatitis C	1:40,000 (30,000–150,000)
Parvovirus B19	1:10,000
Bacterial contamination	1:12,000 random donor platelet concentrates 1:500,000 packed red blood cells

[1]One infection per number of units transfused (95% confidence interval where available).

Acute Hemolytic Transfusion Reactions

Hemolytic transfusion reactions occur when the recipient's antibodies recognize and induce hemolysis in the donor's RBCs. The reaction is usually acute when antibodies already exist in sufficient levels but can be delayed when an amnestic response occurs to a transfused RBC antigen to which the recipient is already sensitized. Acute transfusion reactions are most commonly caused by ABO incompatibility and are usually the result of technical errors made during the collection of blood, during pretransfusion testing, or in patient identification. The majority of transfusion-related fatalities are due to acute hemolytic reactions.

The risk of acute hemolytic transfusion reaction due to incompatible blood is 1–4 per million units transfused; the fatality rate is approximately 50%. With acute hemolytic reaction, most of the transfused cells are destroyed, which may result in activation of the coagulation system with DIC and release of anaphylotoxins and other vasoactive amines. Evidence of this type of reaction includes back pain, pain at the site of the transfusion, headache, alteration of vital signs (fever, hypotension, dyspnea, tachycardia), chills, bronchospasm, pulmonary edema, bleeding due to developing coagulopathy, and evidence of new or worsening renal failure. Recognition of transfusion reactions in critically ill patients who may already be hypotensive and tachycardic is difficult and requires a high degree of suspicion. Ongoing transfusion should be stopped immediately on first indication of potential problems. While laboratory confirmation is being performed, treat the sequelae of hemolysis supportively. Check renal function (serum creatinine, urinalysis), electrolytes, and coagulation status (PT, INR, aPTT). Maintain renal blood flow and urine output with fluids, mannitol, and furosemide as needed. Treat shock with volume and vasopressors to support blood pressure. Treat coagulopathy with FFP. Send the remaining donor blood, along with a posttransfusion blood specimen from the recipient, to the blood bank. Diagnosis is made by evidence of hemolysis (hemoglobinuria or hemoglobinemia) and by blood incompatibility. The blood bank will be able to test the blood, review records, confirm blood types, and determine if the patient's syndrome is from a transfusion reaction.

Risk of morbidity and mortality is proportional to the amount of blood received prior to recognition of the transfusion reaction. Therefore, in nonemergent blood transfusions, the initial rate of blood transfusion is low for the first 30 minutes to allow for the identification of a transfusion reaction while minimizing the volume of blood transfused. The best medicine is prevention by strict adherence to detail in obtaining blood for cross-match and initiating transfusion.

Extravascular Hemolytic Reactions

Extravascular hemolytic reactions occur in about 1 per 1000 PRBC units transfused. Hemolysis most commonly occurs in the spleen and occasionally in liver and bone marrow. This type of reaction is less serious than acute hemolytic transfusion reactions and is rarely fatal. It may be confirmed by a positive DAT, elevated unconjugated bilirubin, and poor response to transfusion. Treatment is supportive.

Febrile Transfusion Reactions

Febrile transfusion reactions are characterized by onset of fever during or within a few hours of a blood transfusion. This type of reaction is one of the more common transfusion-related complications and is more common in multiparous women or multiply transfused patients. The clinical presentation can range from a mild elevation in temperature to fever along with rigors, headache, myalgias, tachycardia, dyspnea, and chest pain. Initially it may be difficult to differentiate a febrile reaction from the more serious hemolytic transfusion reaction or sepsis. Febrile transfusions result from a combination of recipient antibody against donor leukocytes and the release of cytokines produced during storage. For non-leukocyte-reduced platelets the risk of fever during transfusion is about 20%, and with leukocyte reduction, the incidence of febrile reactions is about 2%. For the first-time febrile reaction, or in any severe reaction, the transfusion should be stopped and the product returned to the blood bank. Laboratory investigation similar to that done for possible hemolytic transfusion reaction should be done and blood cultures should be obtained. Febrile transfusion reactions are usually self-limited and respond to antipyretics. Premedication with diphenhydramine and acetaminophen may help prevent these reactions. For patients with recurrent febrile reactions, the use of leukocyte-reduced blood products and pretreatment with antipyretics may be helpful.

Allergic Transfusion Reactions

Allergic transfusion reactions are associated with onset of urticaria and pruritus during the transfusion and occur in approximately 1% of transfusions. Fortunately, only a small percentage of patients will have more severe reactions such as bronchospasm, wheezing, and anaphylaxis. These reactions are caused by an immune response to plasma proteins. Conservative therapy with an antihistamine usually controls the symptoms. The transfusion does not typically have to be stopped. For more severe symptoms the transfusion may need to be stopped and more aggressive management initiated. In patients with IgA deficiency, more severe anaphylactoid reactions can occur in response to exposure to the IgA in donor products. Washing the plasma from the cells minimizes this type of reaction.

Alderson P et al: Human albumin solution for resuscitation and volume expansion in critically ill patients. Cochrane Database Syst Rev 2002;(1):CD001208. [PMID: 11869596]

Bianco C: Choice of human plasma preparations for transfusion. Transfus Med Rev 1999;13:84. [PMID: 10218231]

Carson JL et al: Transfusion triggers: a systematic review of the literature. Transfus Med Rev 2002;16:187. [PMID: 12075558]

Dodd RY: Current viral risks of blood and blood products. Ann Med 2000;32:469. [PMID: 11087167]

Goodnough LT et al: Transfusion medicine. First of two parts—blood transfusion. N Engl J Med 1999;340:438. [PMID: 9971869]

Goodnough LT et al: Transfusion medicine. Second of two parts—blood conservation. N Engl J Med 1999;340:525. [PMID: 10021474]

Heddle NM: Pathophysiology of febrile nonhemolytic transfusion reactions. Curr Opin Hematol 1999;6:420. [PMID: 10546797]

Kopko PM, Holland PV: Mechanisms for severe transfusion reactions. Transfus Clin Biol 2001;8:278. [PMID: 11499977]

Rebulla P: Platelet transfusion trigger in difficult patients. Transfus Clin Biol 2001;8:249. [Erratum in Transfus Clin Biol 2002; 9:109.] [PMID: 11499971]

Rebulla P: Revisitation of the clinical indications for the transfusion of platelet concentrates. Rev Clin Exp Hematol 2001; 5:228. [PMID: 11703819]

Wilkes MM, Navickis RJ: Patient survival after human albumin administration. A meta-analysis of randomized, controlled trials: Ann Intern Med 2001;135:149. [PMID: 11487482]

Infectious Disease Emergencies

Brian Hawkins, MD, & Daniel F. Danzl, MD

I. Immediate Management of Life-Threatening Problems
Septic Shock
Evaluation of the Immunocompromised Patient with Suspected Infection

II. Emergency Management of Specific Disorders
Meningitis & Meningoencephalitis
Pneumonia
1. Pneumonia in Neonates (Aged < 2 months)
2. Pneumonia in Infants & Children (Aged 2 Months to 5 Years)
3. Pneumonia in Older Children (Aged 5–14 Years)
4. Pneumonia in Teenagers & Adults (Aged 15 Years & Older)
Bronchiolitis
Septic Arthritis
Osteomyelitis
Pharyngitis
Urinary Tract Infections
Acute Lower Urinary Tract Infection (Uncomplicated Cystitis)
Upper Urinary Tract Infection (Pyelonephritis)
Dysuria-Frequency Syndrome
Diseases of the Female Genitourinary Tract
Pelvic Inflammatory Disease
Vaginitis
Genital Abscesses
Mucopurulent Cervicitis
Diseases of the Male Genitourinary Tract
Acute Bacterial Prostatitis
Acute Epididymitis

Sexually Transmitted Diseases
Gonorrhea
Nongonococcal Urethritis (Nonspecific Urethritis)
Genital Herpes Simplex Virus Infection
Syphilis
Chancroid
Trichomoniasis
Skin & Soft Tissue Infections
Superficial Soft Tissue Infections
Deep Soft Tissue Infections
1. Infected Vascular Gangrene & Cellulitis
2. Clostridial Anaerobic Cellulitis
3. Nonclostridial Anaerobic Cellulitis
4. Synergistic Necrotizing Cellulitis
5. Necrotizing Fasciitis
6. Clostridial Myonecrosis

III. Management of Infections Caused by Specific Organisms
Acute Meningococcemia
Rocky Mountain Spotted Fever
Infective Endocarditis
Disseminated Gonococcemia
Toxic Shock Syndrome
Group A Streptococcal Infections Associated with a Toxic Shock–Like Syndrome
Lyme Borreliosis

IV. AIDS & HIV Infection

■ I. IMMEDIATE MANAGEMENT OF LIFE-THREATENING PROBLEMS

SEPTIC SHOCK

 ESSENTIALS OF DIAGNOSIS

- *Fever.*
- *Tachycardia, tachypnea.*
- *Leukocytosis, leukopenia, elevated or low white blood cell count.*
- *Left shift or bandemia.*
- *Hypotension.*
- *Clinical suspicion of infection.*

General Considerations

Sepsis results from a complicated interplay between the immune system and an infectious source, leading to a release of inflammatory cytokines in a cascade that affects every organ system in the body. Response to endotoxin and other immune modulators leads to a release of prostaglandins, histamine, and bradykinins that leads to arterial and venous dilation and increased endothelial permeability. Systemic inflammatory response syndrome (SIRS) is a nonspecific term describing the inflammatory processes seen after trauma, infection, burns, and medical disease such as pancreatitis. Sepsis is a systemic response (a form of SIRS) to infection. Sepsis syndrome is defined by (1) clinical evidence of infection, (2) fever or hypothermia, (3) tachypnea, (4) tachycardia, and (5) impaired organ system function or perfusion (such as altered mentation, hypoxemia, elevated plasma lactate level, or oliguria). Septic shock is sepsis-associated hypotension. Sepsis is the 13th leading cause of death in the United States; more than 700,000 cases of severe sepsis occur each year. Excluding fungal sepsis (which has a mortality rate of 83%), the mortality rate for sepsis is 28–50%.

Patients especially susceptible to infections include immunocompromised individuals and those whose natural mechanical barriers of defense have been breached or manipulated through injury or surgery. The incidence of bacteremia and sepsis is increased in patients who are receiving corticosteroids, immunosuppressive agents, cancer chemotherapy, or radiation as well as in those with diabetes, leukemia, severe granulocytopenia, genitourinary tract diseases, and cirrhosis. The age extremes are at risk.

Clinical Findings

The classical clinical pattern of abrupt onset of chills followed by fever and hypotension is present in only 30–40% of patients in septic shock. Other presenting symptoms include hypothermia, oliguria, alteration of mental function, unexplained hypotension, or metabolic acidosis.

Immediate Measures

A. MAINTAIN AIRWAY AND VENTILATION

Initiate continuous pulse oximetry and oxygenate by nasal cannula or face mask. Listen for stridor or other evidence of upper airway obstruction. Ensure that equipment necessary for definitive airway management is readily available because a patient with altered mental status or hypoxemia may require intubation.

Measure arterial blood gases (uncorrected for core temperature) and pH. Respiratory alkalosis may be present early in septic shock but usually progresses to a metabolic acidosis. The use of pulse oximetry can help as an overall indicator of perfusion and oxygenation but may be misleading if vasoconstriction is present.

B. ESTABLISH ADEQUACY OF CIRCULATION

Insert a large-bore catheter and obtain blood samples for laboratory studies. Two catheter sites will be necessary because of the large volumes of infusion and multiple medications necessary.

A flotation tip catheter (PAC) may be necessary for hemodynamic monitoring, but the role of a PAC is controversial in adults because studies have shown limited benefit. In children the role of the PAC appears to be more clearly defined. Insertion of a PAC is usually an intensive care unit procedure.

A central venous catheter will allow for infusion of inotropic agents as well as measurement of central venous pressure (CVP) and possibly central venous oxygen concentration (CVO_2), which may help guide patient management.

Place the patient on a continuous blood pressure monitor and consider placing an arterial line because of the inaccuracies associated with traditional blood pressure measurements in shock. The presence of an arterial line will also make it easier to obtain blood and measure arterial blood gases.

Monitor cardiac rhythm and obtain a 12-lead electrocardiogram because of the risk of precipitating ischemia in patients with preexisting coronary artery disease. Shock may also lead to arrhythmias secondary to electrolyte and acid-base abnormalities.

Begin volume replacement with crystalloid (studies have shown no difference between crystalloid and colloid with respect to mortality or development of pulmonary edema). In an adult, 1–2 L of crystalloid will typically improve blood pressure and urine output. The use of early goal-directed therapy in the emergency department (ie, monitoring central venous oxygen saturation, lactate, base deficit, and pH and having clearly set goals for improvement in these parameters during a set period of resuscitation) is beneficial to patients in septic shock. Significant impact on the final outcome of sepsis can be made in the emergency department prior to intensive care unit admission. This is partially based on the failure of traditional methods such as mean arterial pressure and urinary output in assessing tissue hypoperfusion and hypoxia and increased utility of other methods such as CVO_2. If a CVP catheter is available, a CVP of 15 suggests adequate volume unless the patient has acute respiratory distress syndrome, in which case the CVP should be maintained between 8 and 10. Large volumes of crystalloid (6–10 L) are usually required during the initial resuscitation, and in approximately 50% of patients, hypotension will reverse with fluid resuscitation alone.

Insert an indwelling urinary catheter.

C. Obtain Complete Vital Signs

1. Signs of septic shock—Hypotension in sepsis is the endpoint of a vicious cycle of inflammation that, if left untreated, will lead to multiorgan failure. Cardiovascular effects of sepsis include vasculature changes due to vasodilation and capillary leak, and direct myocardial depressant effects on the myocardium. Patients in sepsis who are deteriorating have worsening cellular function due to sepsis-induced mitochondrial dysfunction. This leads to a process termed cytopathic hypoxia, which is diminished adenosine triphosphate production despite a normal PO_2. Early in sepsis the extremities may be warm and dry and then progressively cool and clammy. Hypotension, tachycardia, tachypnea or hyperventilation, altered sensorium, and oliguria may be present.

2. Fever or hypothermia—A core temperature is indicated with seriously ill patients. Use a low-reading probe in hypothermic patients.

D. Regulate Blood Pressure

Give inotropic agents and vasopressors to patients unresponsive to fluids. The goal mean arterial pressure is 60 mm Hg.

1. Dopamine—Dopamine is the most commonly used initial agent for septic shock. It has dose-related α,

β, and dopaminergic sympathetic effects. The major side effects are increased heart rate, increased pulmonary artery wedge pressure, and decreased gastric pH. Acidosis is the most common cause of failure of this agent.

2. Dobutamine—Dobutamine may be warranted after volume replacement and vasoconstrictor therapy have begun for low cardiac output states. This agent is mainly a β agonist but has α activity as well and can cause peripheral vasodilation, pulmonary vasodilation, decreased pulmonary hypoxic vasoconstriction, and tachycardia.

3. Epinephrine—Epinephrine acts as an α and β agonist and increases cardiac output, blood pressure, heart rate, and blood lactate levels but decreases splanchnic blood flow and gastric pH. Consider using this agent if others fail.

4. Norepinephrine—Norepinephrine acts as an α and β agonist and has potent peripheral vasoconstrictor and inotropic effects. Its administration can lead to severe systemic, pulmonary, renal, and splanchnic vasoconstriction. Norepinephrine is useful in patients who respond to dopamine with excessive tachycardia or in patients who remain hypotensive. *Note:* Norepinephrine is gaining support in the management of sepsis without serious organ dysfunction and may eventually replace dopamine as the initial agent of choice.

5. Phenylephrine—Phenylephrine is a selective α-adrenergic agonist that lacks direct myocardial effects and may be indicated for patients with tachyarrhythmias.

E. Correct Acidosis

Correct acidosis by improving oxygen delivery and hemodynamic parameters. Patients with severe acidosis have a decreased response to catecholamines; nevertheless, bicarbonate therapy is recommended only for severe acidosis (eg, pH < 7.1) because bicarbonate may lead to diffusion of CO_2 into the cells, leading to intracellular acidosis.

F. Correct Coagulopathy

If the patient is coagulopathic or actively bleeding, administer fresh frozen plasma or packed red blood cells. The hemoglobin should be maintained between 8 and 10.

G. Select Therapy

Because sepsis is a heterogeneous entity, a one-therapy-for-all approach is not suitable. Therapy should be directed by specific metabolic or biochemical derangements that are present.

1. Corticosteroids—Because the efficacy of steroids in treating sepsis is unclear, they are not recommended for acute sepsis.

2. RhAPC (recombinant human activated protein C; drotrecogin α [Xigris])—RhAPC is approved for treatment of severe sepsis. Studies show 40% relative risk reduction in mortality at 28 days in patients given Xigris. In vitro studies have shown this drug to have anti-inflammatory action.

3. Vasopressin—Vasopressin infusions can cause a pressor response and decrease the required doses of conventional catecholamines.

4. Dopexamine—Dopexamine is a synthetic catecholamine, with β-adrenergic and dopaminergic effects without α stimulation, that may be beneficial in septic shock.

5. Other agents—Numerous studies have concluded that agents such as interleukin antagonists, monoclonal antibody against tumor necrosis factor α, and platelet-activating factor antagonists have no proven benefit.

H. Search for Source of Infection

Thoroughly but rapidly examine the patient for an obvious source of infection. Examine skin and nails, looking carefully for a rash, petechiae, purpura, abscesses, ulcers, an infected intravenous catheter insertion site, needle marks, and splinter hemorrhages. Examine the patient's scalp, back, perineum, mucosal surfaces, palms, and soles. Check for signs of meningeal irritation. Listen for heart murmurs or abnormal lung sounds. Examine the abdomen and perform a rectal examination because rectal abscesses are frequently overlooked on physical examination. Percuss and palpate all joints and vertebrae. Perform a bimanual pelvic examination on all female patients.

I. Perform Diagnostic Tests

1. Blood cultures—Obtain 2 sets of blood cultures (aerobic and anaerobic) from separate sites on all seriously ill patients.

2. Gram staining and culture—Obtain Gram-stained smears and cultures of all accessible body fluids, purulent material, and other potentially infected tissue. Typical sources of infection include urine, pulmonary secretions, cerebrospinal fluid (CSF), surgical wounds and drains, intravenous catheter sites, ascitic fluid, and decubiti. Microscopic examination of the buffy coat of a centrifuged blood sample may identify the organism, particularly in meningococcemia.

3. Other laboratory studies—A complete blood count may display leukocytosis, leukopenia, or left shift as well as thrombocytopenia. Increased consumption

and decreased hepatic production of clotting factors, as well as the possible development of disseminated intravascular coagulation, may lead to coagulation abnormalities. Hypotension and acute tubular necrosis may lead to acute renal failure. Elevated liver function tests may be seen in hepatic dysfunction. Electrolyte abnormalities include hypokalemia, hyponatremia, hypomagnesemia, and hypophosphatemia. A patient can present with either hyperglycemia (secondary to stress response) or hypoglycemia.

4. Radiologic studies—Obtain chest x-ray, bone and soft tissue x-rays, and other studies as needed.

J. Start Antibiotic Treatment

Early antibiotic therapy is associated with decreased mortality. Ideally antibiotic treatment should be targeted at a specific organism, but the causative agent is frequently unknown. Empiric therapy must be used until the infectious agent is identified (Table 40–1). The most common route of entry for organisms is the genitourinary tract, followed by the respiratory tract, wounds, and the gastrointestinal tract. Gram-negative organisms are currently the most common organisms and include *Escherichia coli, Klebsiella* spp., *Proteus* spp., *Enterobacter* spp., and *Pseudomonas* spp. Gram-positive organisms include *Staphylococcus aureus,* pneumococci, enterococci, and *Streptococcus viridans.* Anaerobic organisms such as *Bacteroides fragilis* are increasingly common as causative organisms.

Provide surgical treatment as needed: antibiotics and volume replacement will not provide much aid in the face of a surgical cause of sepsis that requires further surgery. Examples include intra-abdominal abscess, biliary obstruction with cholangitis, perirectal abscess, or septic abortion.

Disposition

Intensive care is required for all patients in septic shock and for those seriously ill with infection.

Annane D: Corticosteroids for septic shock. Crit Care Med 2001;29:S117. [PMID: 11445691]

Anonymous: Practice parameters for hemodynamic support of sepsis in adult patients in sepsis. Task Force of the American College of Critical Care Medicine, Society of Critical Care Medicine. Crit Care Med 1999;27(3):639. [PMID: 10199548] (Review.)

Balk RA: Severe sepsis and septic shock: definitions, epidemiology and clinical manifestations. Crit Care Clin 2000;16(2):179. [PMID: 10768078] (Review.)

Butt W: Pediatric critical care: a new millennium: septic shock. Pediatr Clin North Am 2001;48(3):601. [PMID: 11411296] (Review.)

Table 40–1. Organisms and empiric therapy for sepsis.

Suspected Source of Sepsis	Major Community–Acquired Pathogens	Empiric Antibiotic Therapy	Major Nosocomial Pathogens	Empiric Antibiotic Therapy
Lung	*Streptococcus pneumoniae* *Haemophilus influenzae* *Legionella* spp. *Chlamydia pneumoniae* *Pneumocystis carinii*	Macrolide and third-generation cephalosporin OR levofloxacin	Aerobic gram-negative bacilli	Cefepime OR imipenem-cilastatin + aminoglycoside
Abdomen	*Escherichia coli* *Bacteroides fragilis*	Imipenem-cilastatin OR piperacillin-tazobactam ± aminoglycoside	Aerobic gram-negative rods Anaerobes *Candida* spp.	Imipenem-cilastatin ± aminoglycoside OR piperacillin-tazobactam ± amphotericin B
Skin and Soft Tissue	Group A streptococci *Staphylococcus aureus* *Clostridium* spp. Polymicrobial enteric gram-negative rods *Pseudomonas aeruginosa* Anaerobes Staphylococci	Vancomycin ± imipenem-cilastatin OR piperacillin-tazobactam	*Staphylococcus aureus* Aerobic gram-negative rods	Vancomycin +cefepime
Urinary Tract	*Escherichia coli* *Klebsiella* spp. Enterobacteria *Proteus* spp.	Ciprofloxacin + aminoglycoside	Aerobic gram-negative enterococci	Vancomycin + cefepime

Choi PT et al: Crystalloids vs. colloids in fluid resuscitation: a systematic review. Crit Care Med 1999;27(1):200. [PMID: 9934917]

Cohen JC et al: UK Medical Research Council International Working Party. New strategies for clinical trials in patients with sepsis and septic shock. Crit Care Med 2001;29(4):880. [PMID: 11373487] (Review.)

Dellinger RP: Bacterial sepsis and septic shock: current therapy for sepsis. Infect Dis Clin North Am 1999;13(2):495. [PMID: 10340180] (Review.)

Friedman G, Silva E, Vincent JL: Has the mortality of septic shock changed with time? Crit Care Med 1998;26:2078. [PMID: 9875924]

Glauser MP: Pathophysiologic basis of sepsis: considerations for future strategies of intervention. Crit Care Med 2000;28 (9)(Suppl):S4. [PMID: 11007189]

Holmes C et al: Physiology of vasopressin relevant to management of septic shock. Chest 2001;120(3):989. [PMID: 11555538] (Review.)

Jindal NJ, Hollenberg SM, Dellinger RP: Pharmacologic issues in the management of septic shock. Crit Care Clin 2000;16 (2):233. [PMID: 10768081] (Review.)

Lerosa SP: Sepsis: menu of new approaches replaces one therapy for all. Cleve Clin J Med 2002;69(1):65. [PMID: 11811722]

Martin C et al: Effects of norepinephrine plus dobutamine alone on left ventricular performance of septic shock patients. Crit Care Med 1999;27(9):1708. [PMID: 10507587]

Mizock BA: Metabolic derangements in sepsis and septic shock. Crit Care Clin 2000;16(2):319. [PMID: 10768084] (Review.)

Opal S: Therapeutic rationale for antithrombin III in sepsis. Crit Care Med 2000;28(9):1681. [PMID: 11007195]

Opal S, Cross A: Bacterial sepsis and septic shock: clinical trials for severe sepsis; past failures and future hopes. 1999;13(2):285. [PMID: 10340167] (Review.)

Rivers E et al: Early goal-directed therapy in the treatment of severe sepsis and septic shock. N Engl J Med 2001;345:1368. [PMID: 11794169]

Schexnayder SM: Pediatric septic shock. Pediatr Rev 1999;20 (9):303. [PMID: 10473659]

Simon D, Trenholme G: Sepsis and septic shock: antibiotic selection for patients with septic shock. Crit Care Clin 2000; 16(2):215. [PMID: 10768080] (Review.)

Sriskandan S, Cohen J: Bacterial sepsis and septic shock: gram-positive sepsis; mechanisms and differences from gram-negative sepsis. Infect Dis Clin North Am 1999;13(2):397. [PMID: 10340174]

Turner A, Tsamitros M, Bellomo R: Myocardial cell injury in septic shock. Crit Care Med 1999;27(9):1775. [PMID: 10507416]

EVALUATION OF THE IMMUNOCOMPROMISED PATIENT WITH SUSPECTED INFECTION

Classification of Immune Dysfunction

Identification of the type of immune dysfunction will often enable the physician to predict the agent causing infection, so that the differential diagnosis and, in some cases, treatment may be started in the emergency department. Types of immune dysfunction include the following:

1. Granulocytopenia—Patients with circulating granulocyte counts below 500 are especially susceptible to infections caused by gram-negative bacilli (including *Pseudomonas aeruginosa*) and staphylococci. Profound granulocytopenia is usually due to myelosuppressive therapy or irradiation, which in addition to causing toxic effects on the bone marrow, damages the mucosa of the alimentary canal. Bowel flora may thereby enter the bloodstream and cause septicemia and secondary pneumonia. Perirectal and perineal infections are also common.

2. Cellular immune dysfunction—Defects in cell-mediated immunity may be due to underlying disease (eg, congenital defects in cell-mediated immunity, Hodgkin disease, AIDS) or may occur as a result of antineoplastic or immunosuppressive treatment (eg, treatment of lymphoma or transplant rejection). Patients with this type of immune dysfunction are especially susceptible to infections caused by intracellular pathogens such as *Listeria monocytogenes*, *Mycobacterium* spp., *Cryptococcus neoformans* and other fungi, and herpes viruses (herpes simplex virus [HSV], cytomegalovirus [CMV]), as well as *Pneumocystis carinii*.

3. Humoral immune dysfunction—Defects in opsonizing antibody production occur in patients with untreated multiple myeloma and in patients who have undergone splenectomy. These patients are susceptible to infections caused by encapsulated organisms, particularly *Streptococcus pneumonia* and *Haemophilus influenzae*. Patients with multiple myeloma usually develop pneumonia; splenectomized patients may develop overwhelming sepsis.

Clinical Findings

A. SYMPTOMS AND SIGNS

Fever is the most reliable sign of infection in immunocompromised patients and must never be ascribed to an underlying disease until infection has been excluded. Localized collections of pus (abscesses or fluctuant areas) are generally absent in neutropenic patients, and the only sign of serious infection may be a localized area of redness or tenderness in a febrile patient. In all immunocompromised patients, careful examination of the lungs, skin, and mucous membranes for signs of infection is important. The lungs may show signs of pneumonia, and signs of disseminated infection may be found in the skin and mucous membranes (eg, the ulcerated pustules characteristic of ecthyma gangrenosum in patients with sepsis caused by *P aeruginosa,* and perirectal cellulitis in patients with neutropenia).

B. LABORATORY AND X-RAY FINDINGS

Determination of the absolute number of circulating granulocytes is mandatory in the evaluation of immunocompromised patients. For example, if the patient's white cell count is 1500 with a total of 10% mature and immature polymorphonuclear neutrophil leukocytes (PMNs), then the granulocyte count is 150. For all immunocompromised patients, samples of blood, urine, and sputum should be sent for Gram stain and culture. A chest x-ray will often show signs of pneumonia, even in patients with very low white blood cell counts. Other studies (eg, sinus x-rays) should be obtained, depending on localized symptoms and signs.

Treatment

A. ANTIBIOTICS

In febrile patients with granulocyte counts under 1000, antibiotic therapy should be started immediately after material for routine culture has been obtained. Circumstances that strengthen the directive for urgent empiric therapy include (1) a rapidly falling granulocyte count, (2) a very low granulocyte count (< 500 further increases the risk of infection; < 100 is frequently associated with fulminant infection), and (3) other clinical findings suggesting infection.

(Current therapy for neutropenic fever involves monotherapy using ceftazidime, imipenem, and cefepime or dual therapy with an aminoglycoside plus an antipseudomonal penicillin, ticarcillin-clavulanic acid, piperacillin-tazobactam, or ceftazidime.

B. ISOLATION

Neutropenic patients should be hospitalized in private rooms, and strict hand-washing precautions observed. Protective isolation as usually practiced (ie, masks and gowns) does not appear to be effective. Patients should be prescribed a diet free of fresh fruits and vegetables, which are often heavily contaminated with gram-negative bacilli.

Disposition

All immunocompromised patients with new findings of fever or other signs of infection should be hospitalized.

Sumaraju V, Smith LG, Smith SM: Infectious complications in asplenic hosts. Infect Dis Clin North Am 2001;15(2):551. [PMID: 11447709] (Review.)

■ II. EMERGENCY MANAGEMENT OF SPECIFIC DISORDERS

MENINGITIS & MENINGOENCEPHALITIS

 ESSENTIALS OF DIAGNOSIS

- Fever.
- Nuchal rigidity.
- Mental status change.
- Photophobia.
- Headache.
- Cerebrospinal fluid findings.

General Considerations

Meningitis is defined as inflammation of the meninges; it is the major infectious syndrome affecting the central nervous system (CNS). When meningitis is accompanied by parenchymal involvement, it is referred to as meningoencephalitis. The epidemiology of meningitis has changed drastically since *H. influenzae* immunizations became available. The incidence of meningitis caused by the agent has decreased by 94%. The average age of a meningitis patient has risen from 15 months to 25 years, and there is an increasing trend for adult meningitis to be nosocomial rather than community acquired (with a corresponding increase in gram-negative organisms). Acute bacterial meningitis is a life-threatening medical emergency. The current mortality rate is 25%, the morbidity rate is 60%, and survival depends on prompt recognition and early treatment.

Clinical Findings

A. SYMPTOMS AND SIGNS

Patients with meningitis present with fever, headache, nuchal rigidity, and mental dysfunction. Seizures and cranial nerve deficits are also common. Infants with meningitis may present with only vomiting, lethargy, irritability, and poor feeding. Elderly patients may present with only low-grade fever and delirium. The headache associated with meningitis is continuous and throbbing and, although generalized, is usually most prominent over the occiput. The pain is increased by jugular vein compression or any other maneuver that increases intracranial pressure (eg, coughing, sneezing, straining at stool). Neck stiffness and other signs of

Table 40–2. Contraindications to lumbar puncture.

Impending or established septic shock
Glasgow Coma Scale score of less than 13 or deteriorating
  score
Other signs of raised intracranial pressure (marked instability
  of blood pressure or heart rate)
Focal neurologic signs
Confident diagnosis of meningococcal infection
Infection at the planned lumbar puncture site
Bleeding disorder

---

meningeal irritation must be sought with care, because they may not be obvious early and may disappear during coma. (For contraindications to lumbar puncture, see Table 40–2). Patients with meningitis may be divided into 2 groups on the basis of the presentation of the disorder.

1. Acute presentation (septic meningitis)—Symptoms and signs have been present for less than 24 hours and are rapidly progressive. The causative organisms are usually pyogenic bacteria, and the mortality rate is approximately 50%.

2. Subacute presentation—Symptoms and signs have been present for 1–7 days. Meningitis is due to bacteria, viruses, or fungi, and the death rate due to bacterial infection is much lower than in patients with acute presentation of disease. Aseptic meningitis is typically caused by viruses (enteroviruses, HSV, or Epstein-Barr virus identified by polymerase chain reaction [PCR] in 95% of patients). Suggestive features such as respiratory tract syndrome and hand-foot-mouth syndrome

strengthen the diagnosis. Chronic meningitis is defined as meningitis present for more than 4 weeks; the major infectious causes are tuberculous meningitis and cryptococci.

B. LABORATORY FINDINGS

Perform lumbar puncture immediately in the absence of papilledema and focal neurologic findings (see Table 40–2). Interpretation of CSF findings is shown in Table 40–3. Draw blood for serum glucose measurement and for culture. Gram staining of CSF will allow presumptive identification of the causative agent. Even if no organisms are seen on Gram-stained smears of CSF, bacterial meningitis is a likely diagnosis and warrants empiric antimicrobial therapy if total CSF leukocytes number more than 1000, if PMNs make up at least 85% of the white cells in CSF, or if the CSF glucose is less than 50% of the serum glucose level in a simultaneously drawn blood sample. The differential diagnosis in patients in whom PMNs are less than 85% of the CSF white count must include several possible causes of acute lymphocytic meningitis (Table 40–4). Prior treatment with antibiotics could result in sterile cultures of CSF.

Treatment

A. ANTIMICROBIAL THERAPY

1. Acute presentation—When bacterial meningitis is suspected, begin administration of appropriate empiric antibiotics immediately (Table 40–5). Give the first dose as soon as samples of CSF and blood have been collected for tests; the goal is to begin intravenous administration of antimicrobials within 30 minutes after a patient with acute presentation of meningitis has

Table 40–3. Cerebrospinal fluid (CSF) findings in meningitis.

Measure	Normal	Bacterial Meningitis	Viral Meningitis	Fungal Meningitis	Tuberculous Meningitis	Abscess
WBC/mL	0–5	> 1000	< 1000	100–500	100–500	10–1000
PMNs (%)	0–15	> 80	< 50	< 50	< 50	< 50
Lymphocytes (%)	> 50	< 50	> 50	> 80	Increased monocytes	Variable
Glucose	45–65	< 40	45–65	30–45	30–45	45–60
CSF/blood glucose ratio	0.6	< 0.4	0.6	< 0.4	< 0.4	0.6
Protein	20–45	> 150	50–100	100–500	100–500	> 50
Pressure	6–20	> 25–30	Variable	> 20	> 20	Variable

PMN = polymorphonuclear leukocytes; WBC = white blood cells.

Table 40–4. Some causes of acute lymphocytic meningitis.

Early or partially treated bacterial meningitis
Viral meningitis and meningoencephalitis (including HIV)
Tuberculous or fungal meningitis
Syphilis
Parameningeal infection (eg, brain abscess)
Central nervous system collagen vascular disease
Central nervous system tumor, leukemia, lymphoma, or carcinomatosis
Intracranial injury (eg, subdural hematoma)
Subarachnoid hemorrhage

---

sought treatment. If lumbar puncture must be delayed for computed tomography (CT) scan, obtain 2 blood samples for culture and begin appropriate antimicrobials. Perform lumbar puncture after mass lesion has been excluded and obtain CSF for microscopic examination as soon as possible. For pathogen-specific antibiotic therapy for bacterial meningitis, see Table 40–6.

2. Subacute presentation—Treatment is based on results of Gram staining of CSF and other tests. If meningitis is likely but gram staining is negative, begin empiric treatment based on the patient's clinical characteristics pending the results of CSF studies.

3. Suspected brain abscess—In patients thought to have a brain abscess, begin intravenous therapy with a combination of penicillin and metronidazole or a third-generation cephalosporin. Obtain an emergency CT scan.

B. SUPPORTIVE CARE

General supportive care measures should be started in the emergency department. Protect the patient's airway, and provide padded rails or restraints for agitated or delirious patients. If seizures occur, begin anticonvulsant therapy. Avoid overhydration, which may worsen cerebral edema. In children older than age 2 months who have bacterial meningitis, dexamethasone reduces neurologic sequelae and hearing loss. Dexamethasone should preferably be given prior to antibiotic therapy.

Disposition

Immediate hospitalization is warranted for all patients, except those with aseptic (viral) meningitis who appear well and can be observed at home.

Cartwright KAV: Early management of meningococcal disease. Infect Dis Clin North Am 1999;13(3):661. [PMID: 10470561] (Review.)

Coyle PK: Overview of acute and chronic meningitis. *Neurol Clin* 1999;17(4):691. [PMID: 10517924] (Review.)

Kaplan SL: Clinical presentations, diagnosis, and prognostic factors of bacterial meningitis. Infect Dis Clin North Am 1999;13(3):579. [PMID: 10470556] (Review.)

Saez-Llorens X, McCracken GH: Antimicrobial and anti-inflammatory treatment of bacterial meningitis. Infect Dis Clin North Am 1999;13(3):619. [PMID: 10470558] (Review.)

Spach DH, Jackson LA: Bacterial meningitis. Neurol Clin 1999;177(4):711. [PMID: 10517925] (Review.)

Wubbel LW, McCracken GH: Management of bacterial meningitis: 1998. Pediatr Rev 1998;19(3):78. [PMID: 9509854] (Review.)

PNEUMONIA

1. Pneumonia in Neonates (Aged < 2 Months)

 ESSENTIALS OF DIAGNOSIS

- *Fever, cough, dyspnea.*
- *Tachypnea.*
- *Focal lung exam.*
- *Sputum findings.*

Clinical Findings

A. SYMPTOMS AND SIGNS

Neonates with pneumonia often have widely disseminated infection caused by group B streptococci, gram-negative bacilli, viruses, or other pathogens. Patients present with fever or labile temperature, poor feeding, irritability, jaundice, and apneic spells. Concurrent meningitis is frequent in bacterial infections.

B. LABORATORY AND X-RAY FINDINGS

Draw samples of blood, urine, and CSF for culture for bacteria and viruses. Order routine blood tests and a chest x-ray.

Treatment & Disposition

See "Treatment" and "Disposition" sections after discussion of pneumonia in teenagers and adults.

2. Pneumonia in Infants & Children (Aged 2 Months to 5 Years)

Clinical Findings

A. SYMPTOMS AND SIGNS

In infants, tachypnea out of proportion to fever is the most common sign of lower respiratory tract infection.

Table 40–5. Recommended empiric antimicrobial therapy for bacterial meningitis based on age.

Age	Major Pathogens	Antibiotic Regimen	Alternative Regimens	Comment
Less than 3 months	Group B streptococci, Listeria monocytogenes, Escherichia coli, Streptococcus pneumoniae	Ampicillin plus ceftriaxone (or cefotaxime)	Chloramphenicol plus gentamicin	Cerebrospinal fluid levels are not reliable in low-brith-weight infants and should be monitored.
3 months–18 years	Neisseria meningitidis, Streptococcus pneumoniae, Haemophilus influenzae	Ceftriaxone (or cefotaxime)	Meropenem or chloramphenicol	Add vancomycin in areas with greater than 2% incidence of highly drug resistant Streptococcus pneumoniae.
18–50 years	Streptococcus pneumoniae, Neisseria meningitides, Haemophilus influenzae	Ceftriaxone (or cefotaxime)	Meropenem or chloramphenicol	Add vancomycin in areas with greater than 2% incidence of highly drug resistant Streptococcus pneumoniae.
50 years and older	Streptococcus pneumoniae, Listeria monocytogenes, gram-negative bacilli	Ampicillin plus ceftraxone (or cefotaxime)	Ampicillin plus fluoroquinolone (ciprofloxacin, levofloxacin)	Add vancomycin in areas with greater than 2% incidence of highly drug resistant Streptococcus pneumoniae; for patients who have major penicillin allergy, trimethoprim–sulfamethoxazole can substitute for ampicillin to treat Listeria monocytogenes infection.

Table 40–6. Pathogen-specific therapy for patients who have bacterial meningitis.

Organism	Preferred Regimen	Alternative Choices	Duration
Group B streptococci	Penicillin G (or ampicillin)	Vancomycin	14–21 days
Haemophilus influenzae	Ceftriaxone (or cefotaxime)	Chloramphenicol	7–10 days
Listeria monocytogenes	Ampicillin plus gentamicin	Trimethoprim-sulfamethoxazole	14–21 days
Neisseria meningitidis	Penicillin G (or ampicillin)	Ceftriaxone (or cefotaxime); chloramphenicol	7–10 days
Streptococcus pneumoniae (MIC < 0.1)	Ceftriaxone (or cefotaxime)	Penicillin; meropenem	10–14 days
Streptococcus pneumoniae (MIC < 0.1)	Vancomycin plus ceftriaxone (or cefotaxime)	Substitute rifampin for vancomycin; use vancomycin monotherapy if patient is highly allergic to cephalosporins	10–14 days

MIC = minimum inhibitory concentration.

Grunting respirations secondary to air trapping and expiratory obstruction suggest pneumonia. Localized findings (rales, decreased breath sounds) are more common in children over age 1 year.

B. LABORATORY AND X-RAY FINDINGS

A peripheral leukocyte count over 15,000 suggests bacterial pneumonia, although lower blood counts do not exclude the diagnosis. Arterial blood gas analysis may be obtained to assess the adequacy of ventilation. Electrolyte levels and blood urea nitrogen are useful in assessing the degree of dehydration, the most frequent complication seen in this age group. When obtainable, Gram-stained smears of sputum may be diagnostic. Lobar consolidation, pneumatoceles, and pleural effusions suggest pneumonia. Blood cultures are frequently positive in pneumonia due to *H. influenzae.* Severely ill or immunocompromised patients may benefit from pneumocentesis.

Treatment & Disposition

See "Treatment" and "Disposition" sections after discussion of pneumonia in teenagers and adults.

3. Pneumonia in Older Children (Aged 5–14 Years)

Clinical Findings

A. SYMPTOMS AND SIGNS

Infection with *Mycoplasma pneumoniae* is the most common cause of pneumonia in this age group and usually develops insidiously with fever and malaise followed in 3–5 days by nonproductive cough, hoarseness, and sore throat, with or without chest pain. Physical examination may disclose pharyngeal erythema and areas of fine rales, wheezes, or dullness, especially in the lower lobes. Myringitis occurs in approximately 15% of patients, occasionally with the development of tympanic bulla, and maculopapular rashes are common. Pneumonia due to *S. pneumoniae, H. influenzae,* and *S. aureus* usually follows a viral upper respiratory infection and is characterized by abrupt onset of fever, chills, tachypnea, and cough accompanied by signs of lobar consolidation or bronchopneumonia.

B. LABORATORY AND X-RAY FINDINGS

In pneumonia due to *M. pneumoniae,* the white cell count is usually normal or slightly elevated, and chest x-ray reveals scattered segmental infiltrates, atelectasis, interstitial disease, or, less frequently, lobar consolidation.

In pneumonia due to bacteria other than *M. pneumoniae,* the white cell count usually exceeds 15,000. Chest x-ray abnormalities include patchy infiltrates, increased bronchovascular markings, lobar consolidation, cavitary infiltrates, and pleural effusions or empyema. Gram-stained smears of sputum may allow for a presumptive diagnosis if numerous PMNs, few epithelial cells, and a predominant microorganism are found. Pleural fluid should be examined if present.

Treatment & Disposition

See "Treatment" and "Disposition" sections after discussion of pneumonia in teenagers and adults.

4. Pneumonia in Teenagers & Adults (Aged 15 Years & Older)

General Considerations

In teenagers and young adults, *M. pneumoniae* and *S. pneumoniae* are the most common causative agents of pneumonia. In older adults, *S. pneumoniae* is the most common cause, although many other pathogens may also cause disease. Aspiration pneumonia due to mixed anaerobic and aerobic flora is common in patients with depressed consciousness. Alcoholic patients are predisposed to severe pneumonia due to *Klebsiella pneumoniae* and other gram-negative bacilli. Patients with chronic lung disease may develop pneumonia due to *H. influenzae. Legionella* spp. are an uncommon but important cause of community-acquired pneumonia in middle-aged adults; special diagnostic tests (sputum for direct fluorescent antibody) and treatment with erythromycin or azithromycin is required for successful management.

Clinical Findings

A. SYMPTOMS AND SIGNS

The clinical signs of pneumonia due to *M. pneumoniae* are similar to those in younger patients. In pneumonia due to other bacteria, there is often abrupt onset of malaise, fever with or without rigors, productive cough, and pleuritic chest pain. Rales and signs of consolidation are noted on physical examination. Elderly or debilitated patients may manifest only fever and obtundation. In Legionnaire disease, high, spiking fevers, diarrhea, and delirium are especially common. Foul-smelling sputum and involvement of dependent parts of the lung suggest aspiration pneumonia due to mixed anaerobic and aerobic flora.

B. LABORATORY AND X-RAY FINDINGS

Chest x-ray findings are similar to those described for mycoplasma and other bacterial pneumonias in older children, except that pneumatoceles are rare in adults. Bilateral pneumonia indicates severe or atypical disease (eg, septic emboli due to endocarditis). In pneumonia due to *M. pneumoniae,* the white cell count is usually normal or only slightly elevated. In pneumonia due to other bacteria, leukocytosis commonly exceeds 15,000. In elderly or critically ill patients, however, leukopenia with a shift to the left sometimes occurs and is a poor prognostic sign. Gram-stained smear of a good sputum sample (showing many PMNs, few epithelial cells) is the most important diagnostic test in acute pneumonia. In general, all but the smallest pleural effusions should be aspirated to rule out empyema. Send fluid to the laboratory for Gram staining and culture and for measurement of protein, lactate dehydrogenase, glucose, and pH. Blood cultures and arterial blood gas measurements should be obtained for all patients severely ill with pneumonia. Results of other laboratory tests are less specific: prerenal azotemia is common in elderly patients; in Legionnaire disease, hyponatremia, hypophosphatemia, and elevated liver enzyme levels are common enough to be important diagnostic clues.

Treatment

The correct choice of treatment for pneumonia is essential. The initial antibiotic choices given in the emergency department influence patient outcome and should be based on the patient's age and the probable causative organism (Table 40–7). Patients with nosocomial pneumonia who receive the appropriate antibiotic therapy are more than twice as likely to survive compared with patients who had inappropriate therapy selected.

Disposition

Neonates should be hospitalized. Severely ill infants (ie, with respiratory distress, hyperthermia, or $PO_2 < 70$) should be hospitalized. Hospitalization is indicated for most older patients with pneumonia, especially for patients with preexisting pulmonary disease, and is required for all patients with bilateral bacterial pneumonia.

BRONCHIOLITIS

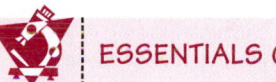 **ESSENTIALS OF DIAGNOSIS**

- *Wheezing, cough, low-grade fever.*
- *Tachypnea.*

General Considerations

Bronchiolitis is an acute inflammation of the bronchioles, most commonly resulting from a viral infection. It typically affects children from birth to age 2 years and occurs mostly during the winter months (November to March). Respiratory syncytial virus (RSV) is the cause in 60–90% of cases; the remaining cases are caused by parainfluenza, adenovirus, rhinovirus, and influenza.

Clinical Findings

A. SYMPTOMS AND SIGNS

The child with bronchiolitis typically has a 4-day history of clear profuse rhinorrhea and congestion, usually accompanied by low grade fever followed by the development of a cough, tachypnea, and wheezing. Signs of respiratory distress including cyanosis and accessory muscle use may be evident, and inspiratory wheezing and crackles are typically heard on auscultation of the patient's lungs. Apnea can occur, and approximately 2–7% of children ill enough to require hospitalization develop respiratory failure and require intubation.

Table 40–7. Treatment of pneumonia.

Age Group	Cause	Primary Treatment	Alternative Treatment

Neonates	**Viruses**
	    Cytomegalovirus, rubella,
	    herpes simplex virus
	Bacteria
	    Group B streptococci
	Listeria spp.
	Coliforms
	Staphylococcus aureus
	Pseudomonas aeruginosa
	Other
	    Chlamydia trachomatis
		Ampicillin (or nafcillin) plus
		    gentamicin (or cefotaxime)
		Use vancomycin plus gentamycin if
		    methicillin-resistent *S aureus* is a
		    concern.
			For chlamydial
			    infection, use
			    erythromycin

Infants (1–3 months;
    pneumonitis syndrome)
	Chlamydia trachomatis
	RSV and other respiratory
	    viruses
	Bordetella spp.
		Erythromycin	Clarithromycin

Children (1–24 months)	RSV and other respiratory
	    viruses
	Streptococcus pneumoniae
	Haemophilus influenzae
	Chlamydia spp.
	Mycoplasma spp.
	Staphylococcus aureus
		Hospitalization
		Cefuroxime
			**Intensive care unit
			    admission**
			Cefotaxime or
			    ceftriaxone plus
			    cloxacillin

Children (3 months –5 years)	Respiratory viruses *Streptococcus pneumoniae* *Mycoplasma* spp. *Chlamydia* spp.	**Outpatient** Erythromycin Clarithromycin or azithromycin	**Hospitalization** Cefuroxime plus azithromycin

Children (5–18 years)	*Mycoplasma* spp. and
	    respiratory viruses are
	    most common
		Clarithromycin or azithromycin	Doxycycline or
			    azithromycin

Adults (community
    acquired, nonhospitalized)
		Azithromycin or clarithromycin	Fluoroquinolone or
			    Augmentin or
			    doxycycline

Adults (community
    acquired, hospitalized)
		Third-generation cephalosporin plus
		    erythromycin or azithromycin or a
		    fluoroquinolone	

Adults (hospital acquired)		Imipenem or meropenem or antipseu-
		    domonal penicillin, plus amino-
		    glycoside or third-generation
		    cephalosporin plus aminoglycoside
		    or ticarcillin-clavulanate or pipera-
		    cillin-tazobactam plus ciprofloxacin
		    or fourth-generation cephalosporin
		    ± clindamycin	

Aspiration pneumonia		Clindamycin	Cefoxitin or ticarcillin-
			    clavulanate or pipera-
			    cillin tazobactam

RSV = respiratory syncytial virus.

B. LABORATORY AND X-RAY FINDINGS

A nasopharyngeal swab can be sent for viral culture and is the gold standard for diagnosis but is rarely indicated clinically. A chest x-ray is recommended for all patients and may show findings characteristic of bronchiolitis: hyperinflation, atelectasis, peribronchial thickening, and diffuse interstitial infiltrates.

Treatment

Oxygen rapidly relieves hypoxemia and is the most important therapeutic agent for bronchiolitis. The use of bronchodilators is controversial and does not decrease hospitalization rates. Racemic epinephrine is a potential agent for bronchiolitis; its use is associated with improvement in clinical scores and increase in oxygen saturations. Studies evaluating the use of glucocorticoids show no improvement in outcome. Ribavirin is a synthetic nucleoside analogue that has virostatic activity against RSV and is recommended for use in patients with a history of congenital heart disease or chronic lung disease, preterm infants, infants younger than age 6 weeks, and infants ventilated for RSV infection.

Disposition

Criteria suggestive of severe disease include the following: ill or toxic appearing, oxygen saturation less than 95%, gestational age less than 34 weeks, respiratory rate greater than 70 breaths/min, atelectasis on x-ray, and age less than 3 months. The infant's oxygen saturation while feeding is the single best objective measure of severe disease.

Cross JT, Campbell GD: Drug-resistant pathogens in community and hospital-acquired pneumonia. Clin Chest Med 1999;20(3):499. [PMID: 10516899] (Review.)

Cunha BA: Community-acquired pneumonia: diagnostic and therapeutic approach. Med Clin North Am 2001;85(1):43. [PMID: 11190352] (Review.)

Fiel S: Guidelines and pathways for hospital-acquired pneumonia. Chest 2001;119(2):412S. [PMID: 11171778] (Review.)

Mandell LA: Antibiotic therapy for community-acquired pneumonia. Clin Chest Med 1999;20(3):589. [PMID: 10516906] (Review.)

Wright RB, Pomerantz WJ, Luria JW: New approaches to respiratory infections in children: bronchiolitis and croup. Emerg Med Clin North Am 2002;20(1):93. [PMID: 11826639] (Review.)

SEPTIC ARTHRITIS

 ESSENTIALS OF DIAGNOSIS

- *Fever.*
- *Painful joint.*
- *Joint effusions.*
- *Arthrocentesis findings.*

General Considerations

Left untreated, septic arthritis rapidly destroys articular cartilage, causing permanent joint damage. Delay between the onset of symptoms and treatment is the major determining factor for prognosis. Joint infection may occur by hematogenous route, direct inoculation, or spread of contiguous infections. The peak incidence occurs in children under age 3 years, and boys are affected twice as often as girls. Septic arthritis typically affects only one or a few asymmetrically distributed joints. Because joint infection superimposed on rheumatoid arthritis sometimes occurs, any joint that develops inflammation out of proportion to that in other affected joints should be aspirated to rule out the possibility of infection in patients with rheumatoid arthritis. Some studies have shown that up to 50% of cases of septic arthritis occur in patients with rheumatoid arthritis. Other groups at high risk include intravenous drug abusers and patients on hemodialysis. Rarely, acute arthritis is caused by fungi, mumps, or hepatitis B virus or, in women, may be due to wild or vaccine strains of rubella virus. Aspiration of the affected joint in the emergency department is often necessary to differentiate septic arthritis from other causes of synovitis, such as gout or pseudogout.

Clinical Findings

A. SYMPTOMS AND SIGNS

Patients with septic arthritis usually have acute or subacute onset of pain, erythema, swelling, and limitation of motion in the affected joints. The arthritis more commonly affects the large joints, especially the knee. Systemic symptoms and signs of infection (malaise, fever, and leukocytosis) are common but not always present. In infants or neonates, failure to feed or pseudoparalysis of the extremity may be present.

B. LABORATORY FINDINGS

Definitive diagnosis is established by demonstration of the infecting organism in synovial tissue or joint fluid. Blood cultures may be positive even though cultures of joint fluid are negative and should be obtained for all patients thought to have septic arthritis.

1. Joint fluid analysis—Joint fluid typically shows high leukocyte counts, usually over 50,000, although the count may not be strikingly elevated in early disease. Synovial fluid should be considered inflammatory and possibly infectious if the count is above 7500. The higher the white cell count in joint fluid, the greater the likelihood of bacterial or fungal arthritis. The glucose content of synovial fluid is usually lower than normal but occasionally may be normal. If no antimicrobial therapy has been given, smears and cultures often reveal the causative organism. The most common organisms are gram positive; *S. aureus* is the most common pathogen of this group. A synovial fluid lactic acid test may be useful in excluding septic arthritis; the test has a negative predictive value of 97%. Results of other laboratory tests are variable, and plain x-rays of affected joints are usually negative early in the disease.

2. Gonococcal arthritis—In gonococcal arthritis, Gram-stained smears and cultures of joint fluid are negative in 50–75% of cases, although in 86% of patients, cultures of exudates from the cervix, urethra, pharynx, or rectum demonstrate gonococci. Because the gonococcus is a fastidious organism, demonstration of its growth in cultures depends on prompt processing of specimens by the laboratory. Because special handling is also required, all specimens submitted should bear the instruction "Rule out gonorrhea." Prompt response to antimicrobial therapy helps confirm the diagnosis of gonococcal arthritis.

Treatment

A. ASPIRATION

Aspirate affected joints, and repeat aspiration as often as necessary to evacuate accumulating joint fluid. Aspiration is necessary except for infections in inaccessible joints, such as the hip. Open drainage is almost never required in gonococcal arthritis.

B. ANTIBIOTICS

High doses of intravenous antibiotics should be given (Table 40–8). Intra-articular instillation of antibiotics is unnecessary, because high antibiotic levels are attained in synovial fluid when drugs are given intravenously. If no organisms are seen on Gram-stained smears of synovial fluid, but other findings suggest septic arthritis, empiric antibiotic therapy based on the type of patient and clinical findings should be started pending results of culture and sensitivity.

Disposition

Hospitalize all patients with suspected or documented septic arthritis.

OSTEOMYELITIS

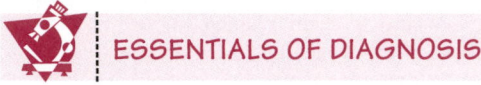 ESSENTIALS OF DIAGNOSIS

- *Pain, fever.*
- *Increased erythrocyte sedimentation rate.*
- *Biopsy findings.*

General Considerations

Osteomylitis is an infection of bone that affects all age groups. The infecting organisms are bacteria, mycobacteria, or fungi. For purposes of discussion, osteomyelitis

Table 40–8. Treatment of septic arthritis.

Age Group	Cause	Primary Treatment	Alternative Treatment
Infant (< 3 months)	*Staphylococcus aureus* Enterobacteriaceae Group B streptococci *Neisseria gonorrhoeae*	Antistaphylococcal penicillin + third-generation cephalosporin	Antistaphylococcal penicillin + aminoglycoside
Children (3 months–14 years)	*Staphylococcus aureus* *Streptococcus pyogenes* *Streptococcus pneumoniae* *Haemophilus influenzae*	Antistaphylococcal penicillin + third-generation cephalosporin	Vancomycin + third-generation cephalosporin
Adults (acute monoarticular; sexually active)	*Neisseria gonorrhoeae*	Ceftriaxone or cefotaxime or ceftizoxime	Nafcillin if gram-positive organisms are found
Adults (acute monoarticular; not sexually active)	*Staphylococcus aureus* Streptococci Gram-negative bacilli	Antistaphylococcal penicillin + third-generation cephalosporin	Antistaphylococcal penicillin + ciprofloxacin
Adult (polyarticular)	*Neisseria gonorrhoeae*	Ceftriaxone	

can be classified according to the pathogenic mechanism: (1) hematogenous osteomyelitis, (2) osteomyelitis secondary to contiguous focus of infection, and (3) osteomyelitis associated with peripheral vascular disease. Hematogenous osteomyelitis is common in children, although its incidence is increasing in older age groups. Hematogenous osteomyelitis in adults usually involves the vertebral bodies. Spread of disease from a contiguous focus of infection is the most common pathogenic mechanism in adults. Osteomyelitis associated with vascular insufficiency occurs almost exclusively in adults who have diabetes mellitus or severe peripheral vascular disease.

In both children and adults, the most commonly involved bones are the long bones, especially those of the lower extremities; this is particularly true in children. Orthopedic procedures or traumatic wounds predispose to osteomyelitis of the extremities.

Clinical Findings

A. SYMPTOMS AND SIGNS

1. Hematogenous osteomyelitis—In children, abrupt onset of high fever, systemic toxicity, and physical findings of local suppuration surrounding the involved bone (local pain, swelling, and tenderness) are typical. The child is often unwilling to move the affected extremity. The most common location is the metaphysis of long bones.

In adults, the disease may be more indolent, particularly in patients with vertebral osteomyelitis. About half of patients may have pain, swelling, chills, and fever. Patients with vertebral osteomyelitis may have low-grade or intermittent fever or back pain that may be either severe or only nagging and may not cause extreme discomfort or immobility until late in the disease. Focal tenderness over the dorsal spines of the involved vertebral bodies may be the only physical finding.

2. Osteomyelitis secondary to contiguous infection—The most common predisposing factor is postoperative infection, such as that following open reduction of fractures. Extension of soft tissue infections to bone from infected fingers and toes, infected teeth, or infected sinuses also occurs. Most patients are over age 50 years and may present with fever, swelling, and erythema in the initial episode. During recurrences, sinus formation and drainage are the major presenting signs.

3. Osteomyelitis associated with vascular insufficiency—Patients with osteomyelitis associated with vascular insufficiency invariably have diabetes mellitus or severe peripheral vascular disease. The toes and small bones of the feet are usually affected. Local signs and symptoms such as pain, swelling, redness, or frank cellulitis with deep ulcers in the soft tissue are prominent. Pain is often absent because of diabetic neuropathy.

B. LABORATORY FINDINGS

Routine laboratory tests are of limited value in the diagnosis of osteomyelitis. The leukocyte count is often elevated in acute disease but may be normal in more chronic infection. The erythrocyte sedimentation rate is elevated in most patients. Radiographic procedures are the primary diagnostic tool, although plain x-rays may not show signs of disease until 10–14 days after symptom onset. The earliest visible x-ray changes are adjacent soft tissue swelling and periosteal reaction. Lytic lesions and areas of sclerosis may then develop. If osteomyelitis is suspected and plain x-rays fail to reveal signs of disease, CT scan or technetium bone scan should be performed. The diagnosis is confirmed by culture and histologic examination of bone. Bacteriologic findings vary, and cultures should be obtained from bone (via needle aspiration or surgical biopsy) or blood (results are positive in 50% of cases in patients with acute hematogenous osteomyelitis). Magnetic resonance imaging (MRI) is an important imaging modality for detecting vertebral osteomyelitis.

Treatment

The most important therapeutic measures are systemic antibiotics and surgery to drain abscesses or for debridement of necrotic tissue. The selection of an antibiotic depends on identification of the causative organism. If the disease is uncomplicated (ie, involves a long bone in a patient without underlying medical problems), if the patient is a child, or if the patient is critically ill, then antistaphylococcal therapy should be initiated, because *S. aureus* is the most common infective organism.

Surgery in acute osteomyelitis should be limited to biopsy for diagnosis, drainage of suppurative areas, and debridement of necrotic bone. Surgical drainage is also indicated if neurologic abnormalities are present or develop in patients with vertebral or cranial osteomyelitis or if infection spreads to the hip joint in a child.

Disposition

Patients with acute osteomyelitis should be hospitalized for intravenous antimicrobial therapy.

Carek PC, Dickerson LM, Sack JL: Diagnosis and management of osteomyelitis. Am Fam Physician 2001;63(12):2413. [PMID: 11430456]

Pioro MH, Mandell BF: Septic arthritis. Rheum Dis Clin North Am 1997;23(2):239. [PMID: 9156391] (Review.)

Shitty AK, Gedalia AG: Septic arthritis in children. Rheum Dis Clin North Am 1998;24(2):287. [PMID: 9606760] (Review.)

PHARYNGITIS

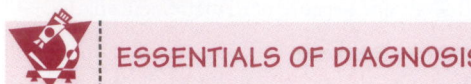

ESSENTIALS OF DIAGNOSIS

- Sore throat, fever.
- Cervical lymphadenopathy.
- Odynophagia.
- Erythematous pharynx.

General Considerations

Acute pharyngitis is inflammation of the pharynx. It is often caused by viral or bacterial infections. The most important task in the evaluation of pharyngitis is to identify and treat group A streptococcal infection and to recognize less common causes of pharyngitis associated with more serious systemic illness. Viral infections (rhinovirus, adenovirus, and many others) are responsible for 90–95% of sore throats.

Clinical Findings

A. SYMPTOMS AND SIGNS

1. Group A streptococcal infection—The most common cause of bacterial pharyngitis, presentations of group A streptococci vary and include fever, sore throat, anterior cervical lymphadenopathy, headache, beefy red pharynx, tonsillar exudates, lymphatic hyperplasia, and scarlatiniform rash. The so-called classic findings of high fever, pharyngeal exudates, and anterior cervical lymphadenopathy only suggest streptococcal pharyngitis and do not confirm the diagnosis. The three clinical features that are most helpful in differentiating streptococcal from viral pharyngitis are fever of 38.9 °C or higher, painful cervical adenitis, and absence of flulike symptoms such as cough and coryza.

2. Infectious mononucleosis—Acute infection by Epstein-Barr virus (the causative agent of infectious mononucleosis), by adenovirus, or by the human immunodeficiency virus (HIV) may produce an exudative pharyngitis with fever, posterior cervical adenopathy, malaise, and enlarged spleen. Patients with acute CMV infection may have pharyngeal soreness, but examination shows a few findings of note.

3. Diphtheria—Diphtheria should be considered in patients with exudative or membranous pharyngitis in whom the status of immunization for diphtheria is either incomplete or in question. The characteristic tonsillar or pharyngeal membrane varies from light to dark gray and is firmly attached to the tonsillar and pharyngeal mucosa. Toxemia and tachycardia out of proportion to the degree of fever are other clues.

4. Vincent angina—Vincent angina is a membranous pharyngitis caused by a mixture of aerobic and microaerophilic bacteria and spirochetes. It is generally encountered in children and young adults and is characterized by foul breath, cervical lymphadenitis, and low-grade fever in association with membranous pharyngitis. Removal of the necrotic gray pseudomembrane usually results in bleeding.

5. Other causes—Other causes of bacterial pharyngitis include *M. pneumoniae, N. gonorrhoeae, Chlamydia trachomatis, Arcanobacterium haemolyticus,* groups C and G streptococci, and secondary syphilis.

B. LABORATORY FINDINGS

Definitive diagnosis of group A streptococcal pharyngitis can be made by results on culture of exudates from the throat and demonstration of a rise in titers to antistreptolysin-O or other streptococcal products, because many people are asymptomatic carriers of group A streptococci. Rapid streptococcal antigen tests are highly specific but not as sensitive as culture. The American Heart Association has revised its recommendation for throat cultures before antibiotic therapy. Throat cultures are considered "valuable" for children and adolescents and "not as essential" for adults. They are indicated primarily to avoid the unnecessary use of antibiotics for the 70–80% of adult patients with pharyngitis due to virus. In the patient with culture-proved streptococcal pharyngitis, follow-up test-of-cure throat cultures are not indicated unless the patient remains symptomatic. Cultures of asymptomatic family members and contacts should be reserved for special circumstances—for example, if the patient has a history of rheumatic fever or if there is an epidemic of group A streptococcal pharyngitis. An elevated white cell count (> 12,000) suggests bacterial pharyngitis. Obtain a heterophil agglutination test or mononucleosis spot test for patients thought to have infectious mononucleosis. A complete blood count with differential may also reveal a lymphocytosis with atypical lymphocytes.

Treatment

Begin empiric treatment in children and young adults if the classic signs and symptoms of streptococcal pharyngitis, scarlatiniform rash, or a history of rheumatic fever or valvular heart disease are present, or if illness occurs during an epidemic of group A streptococcal infection.

A throat culture is not necessary in most cases because its results would not influence the management strategy. Effective antibiotic regimens are penicillin V, 250 mg orally 4 times a day for 10 days, or benzathine penicillin G, 1.2 million units intramuscularly (children < age 10 years, 600,000 units; children aged 10–15 years, 900,000 units). For penicillin-allergic patients, erythromycin, 250 mg orally 4 times a day for 10 days, is suggested. For both penicillin and erythromycin, a full 10 days of therapy is necessary to eradicate infection and prevent rheumatic fever.

Patients with a sore throat but no other features of streptococcal pharyngitis should receive symptomatic therapy (throat lozenges, saline gargles). A throat culture is not necessary. Patients with sore throat or one or two features (fever, exudates, or adenopathy) have an intermediate chance of having streptococcal pharyngitis. A throat culture may be useful to avoid unnecessary use of antibiotics and to reassure the patient. Antibiotic treatment should be withheld until the results of the culture are known.

Disposition

Patients with pharyngitis without complications may receive treatment on an outpatient basis. Patients thought to have diphtheria, Vincent angina, epiglottitis, or possible localized abscess should be hospitalized.

Hayes CS, Williamson HW: Management of group A beta-hemolytic streptococcal pharyngitis. Am Fam Physician 2001;63(8):1557. [PMID: 1132743] (Review.)

Richardson MA: Sore throat, tonsillitis, and adenoiditis. Med Clin North Am 1999;83(1):75. [PMID: 9927961] (Review.)

URINARY TRACT INFECTIONS

ACUTE LOWER URINARY TRACT INFECTION (Uncomplicated Cystitis)

 ESSENTIALS OF DIAGNOSIS

- Dysuria.
- Frequency, urgency, resistancy.
- Suprapubic pain.
- Hematuria.
- Pyuria.

General Considerations

Uncomplicated bacterial cystitis is defined as a urinary tract infection confined to the bladder. It affects women more commonly than men and tends to recur even in the absence of anatomic abnormalities. Many patients with apparent lower urinary tract infection also have asymptomatic involvement of the upper urinary tract (absence of fever, chills, or flank pain). Children present with cystitis without the complaint of dysuria much more commonly than do adults. Conditions such as vesicoureteral reflux may predispose children to infections, and an aggressive workup to evaluate for these possibilities is required. Prior to age 1 year, the incidence is nearly equal in males and females, but after age 1 year, females are 30 times as likely to develop a urinary tract infection until age 50 years, when men begin developing an increased incidence of these infections.

Most cystitis is caused by bacterial infection, usually *E coli* (80%) and other enteric gram-negative bacilli such as *Proteus mirabilis, Klebsiella pneumonia,* and *P aeruginosa.* Gram-positive bacteria such as *Streptococcus faecalis, S. epidermis,* and *S. viridans* are less common causes. Adenovirus is a common cause of hemorrhagic cystitis in children (typically males) and occasionally young adults.

Clinical Findings

A. SYMPTOMS AND SIGNS

A history of urinary tract infections is frequently elicited. Dysuria and urinary frequency and urgency are the most common symptoms in adults, although they may be absent in children. Patients may report that their urine is cloudy, smelly, or dark.

Suprapubic discomfort and tenderness are common. Patient are usually afebrile or have a low-grade fever. The presence of high fever (> 38.3 °C [101 °F]) or rigors is inconsistent with a diagnosis of uncomplicated cystitis and suggests pyelonephritis. Nausea and vomiting, though uncommon in adults, are not unusual in children with uncomplicated cystitis.

Neonates may present with poor feeding, vomiting, jaundice, or irritability and may not always have fever. Young children may present with new bed-wetting or loss of bladder training.

B. LABORATORY FINDINGS

1. Urinalysis—Accurate diagnosis of urinary tract infection depends on obtaining a urine specimen uncontaminated by perineal secretions. The presence of squamous epithelial cells or of mixed flora on Gram-stained smears suggests contamination, and the specimen should be discarded and a better one obtained. Urine should be examined while it is fresh (within 1 hour) or should be refrigerated if delay is expected. Urine should be obtained by catheter or clean-catch specimens only because bagged specimens are usually contaminated.

a. Chemistry—Mild degrees of proteinuria and hematuria are common on dipstick tests of urine. If the infection is caused by a urea-splitting bacterium (eg, *P. mirabilis*), urinary pH may be abnormally high (eg, 6–8). The leukocyte esterase dipstick test is a reliable indicator of infection. Chemical tests for the presence of bacteria in urine (eg, nitrate reduction) are not sensitive and specific enough to be generally recommended.

b. Sediment—Many leukocytes and often some erythrocytes are present. Clumps of leukocytes must be differentiated from white blood cell casts, which signify upper urinary tract involvement. In most cases, numerous bacteria are visible.

c. Gram-stained smears—Microscopic examination of Gram-stained specimens of urinary sediment from centrifuged urine usually shows bacteria of a single morphologic type. If uncentrifuged urine is examined, and an average of one bacterium is found per oil-immersion field, there is about an 80% probability that there are 10^5 organisms per milliliter of urine (strongly indicative of infection).

2. Urine culture—In women of child-bearing age with a history of recurrent cystitis (2–3 times per year) who are otherwise healthy, treatment may be started on the basis of urinalysis results alone, and urine culture may be postponed until 1 week after treatment (test-of-cure culture) or may be omitted in patients who respond well to treatment. In all other patients, quantitative urine cultures should be obtained. Growth of at least 10^5 organisms of a single species per milliliter of urine indicates a high probability of active urinary tract infection. A urine culture should be ordered for all febrile infants under age 2 years, for children with a history of urinary tract infection, for children who are taking suppressive antibiotic therapy, and for children in whom antibiotic therapy is started regardless of urinalysis results. Smaller numbers (10^2–10^4/mL) of bacteria (especially of a single species) are significant and indicate the need for therapy (see "Dysuria-Frequency Syndrome" section, below).

Treatment

A. Antimicrobials

Nonpregnant women of child-bearing age who have a history of recurrent cystitis and findings compatible with uncomplicated cystitis may be given a short course (3 days) of therapy. Single-dose therapy has fallen into disfavor because of the frequency of relapse and because it requires that the patient be seen 2–4 days later for a test-of-cure urine culture. All other patients should receive multidose therapy for at least 7–10 days. Because men often harbor occult infection in the prostate or kidney, some authorities recommend that treatment be extended for at least 3 weeks in an effort to prevent relapse of infection. Current American Academy of Pediatrics guidelines recommend treatment for children for 7–14 days with coverage by antibiotics until radiologic studies are completed and urologic referral conducted.

Select an antimicrobial from those listed in Table 40–9. Trimethoprim-sulfamethoxazole (TMP-SMZ) and ciprofloxacin, because of their good penetration into the prostate and high level of activity against uropathogens, are recommended for men with urinary tract infection who have normal serum creatinine levels.

There is an increasing trend of bacterial resistance in urinary tract pathogens; 40% are resistant to ampicillin

Table 40–9. Empiric antibiotic therapy for urinary tract infection.

Type of Infection	First-Line Therapy	Alternative Regimens	Comments
Urinary tract infection with mild pyelonephritis (outpatient therapy)	Fluoroquinolone	Amoxicillin-clavulanate, oral cephalosporin, or Bactrim DS	
Urinary tract infection with pyelonephritis (inpatient therapy)	Intravenous fluoroquinolone, ampicillin + gentamicin, third-generation cephalosporin, or antipseudomonal penicillin	Ticarcillin-clavulanate, ampicillin-sulbactam, or piperacillin-tazobactam	
Complicated urinary tract infection (obstruction, reflux, indwelling catheter)	Ampicillin + gentamicin, piperacillin-tazobactam Ticarcillin-clavulanate, imipenem, or meropenem	Intravenous fluoroquinolone	Rule out obstruction

or amoxicillin, 5% are resistant to TMP-SMZ, and 17% are resistant to cephalexin.

B. ADJUNCTIVE MEASURES

Phenazopyridine (Pyridium, many others), 200 mg orally 3 times a day, may help relieve severe dysuria. The drug should be taken for only 2–3 days. Warn patients that their urine will turn orange.

C. FOLLOW-UP

In uncomplicated cystitis, follow-up urine cultures are optional in patients who respond to therapy. Patients given single-dose or 3-day therapy and whose symptoms recur should have urine culture and be given a 10-day course of therapy.

Disposition

Infants, children, and men with diagnosed urinary tract infection should receive treatment and be referred to a urologist. Hospitalization is indicated for children younger than age 3 months and for children with dehydration, toxicity, vomiting, or failure of outpatient regimen. Urologic referral is also recommended for women with frequent recurrences of cystitis (monthly) and probably also for those who have had 3 or more infections in 1 year, although the latter recommendation is controversial. Hospitalization is not indicated for patients with uncomplicated cystitis.

UPPER URINARY TRACT INFECTION (Pyelonephritis)

General Considerations

Acute pyelonephritis is symptomatic inflammatory bacterial infection of the kidney. Because it most commonly results from spread of infection up the ureters from the bladder, it is usually caused by the same organisms that cause cystitis (ie, *E. coli*, *P. mirabilis*). In elderly men, pyelonephritis may be caused by *S. faecalis*. In patients who have received prior antimicrobial therapy (eg, during recent hospitalization, because of chronic indwelling Foley catheter), the infecting organisms may be resistant to commonly used antimicrobials. *Note:* Pregnant patients are especially prone to upper urinary tract infection. Because pyelonephritis in pregnancy is associated with an increased risk of premature delivery, pregnant patients with urinary tract infection should always receive multidose antimicrobial therapy.

Between 15% and 25% of children and young adults with endstage renal failure have chronic pyelo-nephritis that results in renal scarring and decreased renal function, termed reflux nephropathy. This renal scarring can be prevented by avoiding urinary tract infection. Emphysematous pyelonephritis is acute pyelonephritis associated with gas in the collecting system; it typically occurs in patients with diabetes. This disease has a 75% mortality rate, and emergency nephrectomy is required.

Clinical Findings

A. SYMPTOMS AND SIGNS

Pyelonephritis is characterized by symptoms of cystitis (dysuria, urgency, and frequency) accompanied by flank pain and tenderness. Fever, rigors, and, in patients with complicating bacteremia or endotoxemia, systemic signs of sepsis (eg, hypotension, delirium) may be present. In young children, fever is the predominant symptom; only 32% of boys and 40% of girls display dysuria as a symptom, and flank pain is an even less common symptom. In pyelonephritis occurring as a complication of nephrolithiasis, severe flank pain radiating to the groin may be the most prominent symptom. In patients with sickle cell disease, diabetes, or nephropathy caused by analgesic abuse, necrosis of the renal papillae with sloughing into the ureters occurs as a complication of renal infection, and the patient may present with symptoms of ureteral obstruction that mimic nephrolithiasis.

B. LABORATORY FINDINGS

1. Urine—The findings on urinalysis, microscopic examination, and culture are the same as in cystitis (see above), except that leukocyte casts (granular casts) occur only with pyelonephritis. Gross hematuria and pain suggest pyelonephritis complicating urolithiasis. For all patients with suspected pyelonephritis, send urine for culture and susceptibility testing.

2. Other laboratory studies—Serum electrolyte, blood urea nitrogen, and creatinine measurements should be obtained, because azotemia may be present. The white cell count is usually elevated. A normal or low white cell count with a shift to the left in a patient with suspected pyelonephritis is often a sign of sepsis, indicating the need for hospitalization.

C. X-RAY AND OTHER FINDINGS

Some authorities suggest that excretory urography be performed in all nonpregnant women with pyelonephritis after the infection has cleared. In patients with pyelonephritis in whom urinary obstruction is suspected, radiologic and other examinations should be performed as soon as possible. Ultrasonography is a safe and sensitive means of assessing hydronephrosis and may reveal intrarenal and perinephric abscesses. Remember that in pregnancy some degree of ureteral dilatation (usually greater in the right ureter than the left) is normal.

Treatment

A. ANTIMICROBIALS

(See Table 40–9.) Patients with anatomic abnormalities of the urinary tract or concomitant prostatitis may require up to 6 weeks of therapy. In patients with suspected bacteremia or suspected infection due to antibiotic-resistant organisms, an aminoglycoside should be added.

B. GENERAL MEASURES

If vomiting or dehydration is present, begin intravenous fluid replacement with crystalloid solutions. Provide analgesia for flank pain if needed. Give antipyretics for high fever regularly (rather than as needed) until the patient is afebrile.

Disposition

Patients who meet the criteria listed below or who have any of the following conditions should be hospitalized:

- Inability to maintain oral hydration or take medications
- Concern about compliance or follow-up
- Diagnostic uncertainty
- Severe illness with high fevers, severe pain, and marked debility
- Comorbid illness (eg, diabetes, renal failure, immunosuppression)
- Failure of outpatient therapy

Patients who are not hospitalized should have a follow-up appointment within 1–2 days to assess their response to therapy.

Some patients with pyelonephritis, especially young women, may not be sick enough for hospitalization but do not appear well enough to go home. For these patients, a 12- to 24-hour period of intravenous antimicrobial therapy, intravenous hydration, and observation in the emergency department may be indicated. If rapid resolution of signs and symptoms occurs, the patient may be discharged with a prescription for oral antimicrobials and a follow-up appointment in 1–2 days.

DYSURIA-FREQUENCY SYNDROME

General Considerations

The dysuria-frequency syndrome (urethral syndrome) occurs by definition only in women, usually young women. These patients have symptoms of lower urinary tract infection but have urine cultures that are sterile or contain fewer than 10^5 organisms per milliliter of urine. Patients with dysuria-frequency syndrome may be divided into 2 groups: those with accompanying pyuria (> 10 leukocytes per high power field) and those without. In women with pyuria, symptoms are usually due either to a low-grade bacterial cystitis (bacteriuria with < 100,000 organisms per milliliter of urine) or to chlamydial urethritis with or without accompanying chlamydial cervicitis. *N. gonorrhoeae* also causes urethritis. HSV causes urethritis during primary infection and, on occasion, during recurrent infection. In some patients with pyuria and in most patients who lack pyuria, no causative agent can be identified.

Clinical Findings

A. SYMPTOMS AND SIGNS

The principal symptoms are those of cystitis: dysuria, urgency, and frequency. The dysuria is "internal" dysuria as opposed to the "external" dysuria occurring in vaginitis or genital HSV infection and results from urine coming into contact with denuded skin. Findings on physical examination are normal except that there may be urethral inflammation or mucopurulent cervical discharge and cervical edema in patients whose symptoms are due to gonococcal or chlamydial infection. Pelvic examination is important to diagnose vaginitis, which may also cause dysuria.

B. LABORATORY FINDINGS

The urine may be normal or may contain PMNs with few or no bacteria. Swabs of urethral discharge should be obtained for smear and culture for *N. gonorrhoeae* in patients with a history of gonorrhea, in those with multiple sexual partners, and in those whose recent sexual partner has had urethritis. Urine culture shows scant growth or no growth of organisms. A cervical swab for *Chlamydia* antigen (fluorescent or ELISA slide test) is indicated in sexually active women with cervicitis accompanying this syndrome, because this organism causes concurrent cervicitis and urethritis.

Treatment

Antimicrobial therapy is usually reserved for patients with pyuria. Tetracyclines and erythromycin are the most effective drugs for suspected chlamydial infection; other bacterial pathogens may be resistant to these drugs. Optimal treatment of chlamydial infection requires 7 days of therapy. Short-course, 3-day therapy may be tried initially in patients with low-grade bacteriuria. None of the single-dose regimens provides reliable empiric therapy for both chlamydial and bacterial infection.

Disposition

Because of the difficulties of empiric therapy in the urethral syndrome, a follow-up visit to a primary care physician should be arranged. If ordinary bacterial cultures of urine are sterile in patients with pyuria, the patient's sexual partners should be screened for urethritis and *Chlamydia* infection.

Miller O, Hemphill RR: Urinary tract infection and pyelonephritis. Emerg Med Clin North Am 2001;19(3):655. [PMID: 11554280] (Review.)

Orenstein R, Wong ES: Management of urinary tract infections in adults. Am Fam Physician 1999;59(5):1225. [PMID: 10088877] (Review.)

Roberts JA: Management of pyelonephritis and upper urinary tract infections. Urol Clin North Am 1999;26(4):753. [PMID: 10584616] (Review.)

Roberts KB: The AAP practice parameter on urinary tract infections in febrile infants and young children. Am Fam Physician 2000;62(8):1815. [PMID: 11057838] (Review.)

Santen SA, Altieri MF: Pediatric urinary tract infection. Emerg Med Clin North Am 2001;19(3):675. [PMID: 11554281] (Review.)

DISEASES OF THE FEMALE GENITOURINARY TRACT (See also "Sexually Transmitted Diseases" section.)

PELVIC INFLAMMATORY DISEASE

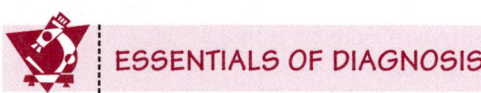

ESSENTIALS OF DIAGNOSIS

- Lower abdominal pain.
- Vaginal discharge.
- Fever.
- Cervical motion tenderness.
- Bilateral lower adnexal tenderness.

General Considerations

Infection of the uterine tubes may be acute or chronic and unilateral or bilateral. It may lead to pyosalpinx or tuboovarian abscess. Pelvic peritonitis is frequently present. Causative agents include *C. trachomatis, N. gonorrhoeae,* anaerobic bacteria (which include *Bacteroides* and gram-positive cocci), facultative gram-negative bacilli (such as *E. coli*), *Mycoplasma hominis,* and rarely *Actinomyces israelii.* Because it is often impossible to differentiate among these agents in individual patients, treatment regimens that are active against the broadest possible range of these pathogens should be used. Risk factors for pelvic inflammatory disease (PID) include young age, multiple sexual partners, intrauterine device insertion, vaginal douching, tobacco smoking, chlamydial or gonococcal infection, and bacterial vaginosis.

Clinical Findings

A. SYMPTOMS AND SIGNS

Patients are usually young (< age 30 years) and sexually active. Symptoms include fever (sometimes with rigors), severe pelvic pain that may be either continuous or crampy (pelvic pain is usually bilateral and is the most common presenting symptom), dyspareunia, menstrual disturbances, vaginal discharge, and gastrointestinal disturbances (anorexia, nausea and vomiting, constipation).Patients usually are menstruating or just finished their periods (risk of ascending infection is increased secondary to the loss of the cervical mucus plug during menses).

Physical examination in acute cases discloses marked tenderness on manipulation of the cervix and palpation of the adnexa. There is a unilateral tender adnexal mass if tuboovarian abscess or pyosalpinx is present. The clinical spectrum in PID includes a gradual progression from subclinical endometritis to salpingitis to pyosalpinx to tuboovarian abscess to pelvic peritonitis to perihepatitis. A ruptured tuboovarian abscess carries with it a mortality rate of 7% and may require emergency surgery. Table 40–10 presents physical examination criteria.

B. LABORATORY TESTS AND SPECIAL EXAMINATIONS

There is usually leukocytosis or an elevated erythrocyte sedimentation rate or C reactive protein. Obtain a serum pregnancy test. Purulent fluid should be cultured for aerobic and anaerobic pathogens, specifically for *N.*

Table 40–10. Criteria for diagnosis of pelvic inflammatory disease.

Minimum criteria
   Lower abdominal tenderness
   Adnexal tenderness
   Cervical motion tenderness
Additional criteria
   Oral temperature > 101°F
   Abnormal cervical or vaginal discharge
   Elevated erythrocyte sedimentation rate
   Elevated C-reactive protein
   Laboratory documentation of cervical infection with
     N. gonorrhoeae or *C trachomatis*
Elaborate criteria
   Histopathologic evidence of endometritis on endometrial
     biopsy
   Transvaginal sonography or other imaging techniques
     showing thickened, fluid-filled tubes with or without free
     pelvic fluid or tuboovarian complex
   Laparoscopic abnormalities consistent with pelvic in-
     flammatory disease

gonorrhoeae and *Chlamydia.* Ultrasonography may be helpful in detecting or assessing the size of tuboovarian abscess.

Treatment

A. ANTIBIOTIC THERAPY

Table 40–11 presents treatment options. No single agent is active against the entire spectrum of pathogens. Several antibiotic combinations provide a broad spectrum of activity against the major pathogens, but none

Table 40–11. Antimicrobial therapy for pelvic inflammatory disease.

Outpatient Treatment	Inpatient Treatment
Ceftriaxone IM + doxycycline PO	Cefoxitin IV + doxycycline IV
Ceftriaxone IM + ofloxacin PO and clindamycin PO or metronidazole PO	Cefotetan IV + doxycycline IV
Cefoxitin IM + probenecid PO + doxycycline PO	Clindamycin IV + gentamicin IV + doxycycline IV
Cefoxitin IM + probenecid PO + ofloxacin PO and clindamycin PO or metroidazole PO	

have been adequately evaluated. Treatment with penicillin, ampicillin, amoxicillin, or a cephalosporin alone is not recommended.

B. REEVALUATION

Patients who are not hospitalized should be reevaluated in 2–4 days and hospitalized if their condition has not improved markedly.

C. ADJUNCTIVE MEASURES

Relieve pain. Narcotics are frequently required. If present, an intrauterine device should be removed as soon as adequate antibiotic levels are achieved in the blood. Surgery should be delayed at least 2–3 days, until the effect of antibiotic therapy can be assessed, even if pyosalpinx or tuboovarian abscess is present. Pelvic abscesses often regress with antibiotic therapy alone or may drain externally via the vagina or rectum. Repeated ultrasound examinations help to determine the patient's progress.

Disposition

There is an increasing trend toward the outpatient management of PID. Indications for admission include uncertain diagnosis, pelvic abscess, pregnancy, adolescence, severe illness, failure of outpatient management, an inability to arrange follow-up, and HIV-positive status.

VAGINITIS

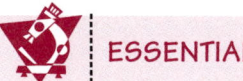 **ESSENTIALS OF DIAGNOSIS**

- *Abnormal vaginal discharge.*
- *Pruritus, irritation, odor.*
- *Inflamed cervix.*

General Considerations

Vaginitis is a common and annoying disorder that in the absence of other symptoms or signs rarely indicates serious disease. Common pathogens include *Candida albicans, Trichomonas vaginalis, Gardnerella vaginalis* with anaerobic bacteria (bacterial vaginosis), and gonococci (in prepubertal girls). Other common causes are estrogen deficiency (atrophic vaginitis) and vaginal foreign body. Systemic antibiotics (especially tetracyclines), oral contraceptives, diabetes mellitus, primary genital HSV infection, and pregnancy predispose to the development of candidiasis. Less common causes include allergy, cervicitis, polyps, tumors, vaginal ulcer, shigellosis, irradiation for cancer, and certain bubble bath preparations.

Clinical Findings

A. SYMPTOMS AND SIGNS

Vaginal discharge and pruritus are the chief symptoms. Vaginal discharge with varying degrees of inflammation of the vaginal wall (minimal in atrophic vaginitis) is usually found. Search for foreign bodies in the vagina, particularly in young girls, and examine for associated disorders (eg, salpingitis).

B. LABORATORY FINDINGS

1. Examination of smears—

a. Gram stain—Look for *Candida* and *G. vaginitis* (small gram-negative rods usually adherent to epithelial cells; "clue cells"). Methylene blue stain also demonstrates clue cells. Vaginitis due to *Candida* or *Trichomonas* is usually associated with a polymorphonuclear exudate, whereas inflammatory cells are absent in bacterial vaginosis caused by *G. vaginalis*. In prepubertal girls with gonococcal vulvovaginitis, Gram stain of smears usually shows typical gram-negative intracellular diplococci, but cultures should be performed to confirm the diagnosis.

b. Saline wet mount—Look for motile trichomonads. *Candida* and clue cells of *G. vaginalis* may also be seen.

c. Potassium hydroxide wet mount—Addition of a few drops of potassium hydroxide to a sample of vaginal secretions releases a typical amine odor (fishy) in cases of bacterial vaginosis due to *G. vaginalis*. Microscopic examination reveals *Candida* in cases of *Candida* vaginitis, but Gram staining is more sensitive and specific.

2. Urinalysis—Obtain a clean-catch urine specimen for analysis and culture if dysuria is present.

3. Other tests—Obtain fasting blood glucose measurement in cases of recurrent candidiasis, to rule out diabetes mellitus.

Treatment

A. GENERAL MEASURES

Avoid systemic antibiotic therapy, if possible. Advise patients regarding adequate perineal ventilation. Patients should wear loose-fitting cotton underpants with skirts and avoid tight-fitting constrictive clothing. Sitz baths may give relief. Occasional douches with white vinegar (2 tablespoons per quart of warm water) may provide symptomatic relief but seldom influence recovery. Advise patients to avoid intercourse for a few days after treatment. Partners also should receive treatment, as described below.

B. SPECIFIC MEASURES

1. *C albicans* vaginitis—

a. Imidazole regimens—(1) Miconazole nitrate (vaginal suppositories, 200 mg) or clotrimazole (vaginal suppositories, 200 mg), intravaginally at bedtime for 3 days, or (2) butoconazole (2% cream, 5 g), intravaginally at bedtime for 3 days, or (3) terconazole, 80 mg suppository or 0.4% cream, intravaginally at bedtime for 3 days.

b. Reinfection—The male partner should wear a condom, or both partners should abstain from intercourse for 2–3 days. Balanitis due to *Candida* occurs almost exclusively in uncircumcised men. Occasionally the patient's gastrointestinal tract is a reservoir for *Candida*, in which case oral nonabsorbable antifungal preparations (eg, nystatin), are necessary.

2. *T. vaginalis* vaginitis—Give the patient and her sexual partner metronidazole, 2 g orally in a single dose (eight 250-mg tablets). This regimen is curative in about 95% of cases. An alternative regimen involves metronidazole, 250 mg orally 3 times daily for 7 days. Resistance of *T. vaginalis* to metronidazole has been observed but is rare. If treatment fails, the patient should receive the same treatment regimen again. Address persistent treatment failure in consultation with an expert.

3. Bacterial vaginosis—Several species of vaginal bacteria (including *G. vaginalis*) interact to produce this syndrome. Metronidazole, 500 mg orally 2 times daily for 7 days, is an effective treatment. Warn the patient about side effects. Clindamycin, 300 mg orally 2 times daily for 7 days, may be used in pregnant patients. Because bacterial vaginosis may be a factor in premature rupture of membranes and premature delivery, close clinical follow-up of pregnant women is essential. Treatment for male sexual partners does not reduce the risk of recurrence of bacterial vaginosis in the index case.

4. Atrophic vaginitis—Prescribe estrogen suppositories or creams. Diethylstilbestrol, one 0.5-mg vaginal suppository every 3 days for 3 weeks, followed by 1 week without treatment, may be tried.

5. Gonococcal vaginitis—See "Gonorrhea" section, below.

Disposition

Patients should have a follow-up appointment with a gynecologist or primary care physician in 7–10 days so that the results of treatment can be assessed and follow-up cultures obtained.

GENITAL ABSCESSES

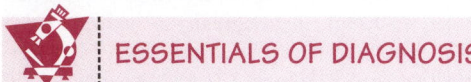 ESSENTIALS OF DIAGNOSIS

- *Labial pain, swelling.*
- *Fluctuant lesion.*

General Considerations

Vulvar abscesses may rise in a sebaceous gland or Bartholin gland (Bartholin cyst). Skene glands, adjacent to the urethra, may also be the site of abscess formation. *N. gonorrhoeae* is responsible for some vulvar abscesses: the remainder are caused by a variety of bacteria, often in mixed culture.

Clinical Findings

The patient complains of tender swelling of the labia majora that is confirmed by examination. Gram stain and culture of pus from the abscess help to identify the causative organism. Endocervical culture for *N. gonorrhoeae* should be performed, if possible.

Treatment

A. Nonfluctuant Lesions

If lesions are not fluctuant, incision and drainage is not indicated. If gonorrhea is suspected, give ceftriaxone, 250 mg intramuscularly. In addition, give a broad-spectrum antibiotic such as amoxicillin clavulanate, 500 mg 3 times daily. Prescribe sitz baths and application of warm compresses. Ask the patient to return in 1–2 days for reevaluation of the need for incision and drainage.

B. Fluctuant Lesions

When drainage is performed, pack the abscess. Administer antimicrobials as described above. Have the patient return in 2–3 days.

Disposition

Gynecologic follow-up is mandatory, because surgery may be necessary. Occasionally marsupialization may be performed at the time of diagnosis of acute bartholinitis.

MUCOPURULENT CERVICITIS

 ESSENTIALS OF DIAGNOSIS

- *Vaginal discharge.*
- *Pruritus.*
- *Cervical exudate.*

General Considerations

The presence of mucopurulent endocervical exudates strongly suggests cervicitis due to chlamydial or gonococcal infection.

Clinical Findings

A. Symptoms and Signs

Vaginal discharge and pruritus may be present. Mucopurulent endocervical exudate may be observed.

B. Laboratory Findings

1. Swab test—Mucopurulent secretion from the endocervix may appear yellow or green when viewed on a white cotton-tipped swab. Cervicitis is present if bleeding occurs when the first swab culture for gonococci is taken or if erythema or edema is present within a zone of cervical ectopy.

2. Slide test—Fluorescent antibody or ELISA slide test should be used to diagnose *Chlamydia*.

3. Gram stain—Gram-stained smears of endocervical secretions show greater than 10 PMNs per microscopic oil-immersion field. The presence of gram-negative, diplococci suggest infection with *N. gonorrhoeae* but is not diagnostic. Culture is necessary to confirm infection with *N. gonorrhoeae*.

Treatment

If *N. gonorrhoeae* is suspected or found on Gram stain of endocervical or urethral discharge, treatment should be given as recommended for uncomplicated gonorrhea in adults. If *N. gonorrhoeae* is not suspected, treatment should be as recommended for chlamydial infection in adults.

DISEASES OF THE MALE GENITOURINARY TRACT

ACUTE BACTERIAL PROSTATITIS

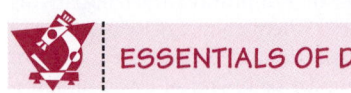

ESSENTIALS OF DIAGNOSIS

- *Fever.*
- *Low back pain.*
- *Dysuria.*
- *Urgency.*
- *Prostatic tenderness.*

Clinical Findings

A. SYMPTOMS AND SIGNS

Patients with acute bacterial prostatitis often have chills, fever, low back and perineal pain or pressure, malaise, dysuria, urgency, and difficulty voiding or decreased urinary stream. Recurring attacks of acute prostatitis are common. Urethral discharge may be present if prostatitis is secondary to urethritis (uncommon). The prostate is tender and enlarged. Prostatic abscess should be suspected when localized prostatic tenderness, swelling, or fluctuance is present. Prostatic massage is contraindicated in severe, acute prostatitis because it may induce bacteremia. A simple rectal examination may be performed, however. Prostatitis is the most common urologic diagnosis in men over age 50 years; as many as 50% of men are affected in their lifetime.

B. LABORATORY FINDINGS

When acute bacterial prostatitis is suspected based on the patient's symptoms and on physical examination, presumptive diagnosis may be made based on the results of urinalysis and urine Gram stain and culture. The bacterial pathogen found in the urine will usually be the same as that infecting the prostate. The presence of bacteria should be confirmed by culture and susceptibility testing. Leukocytosis is common. Azotemia suggests obstructive uropathy. Obtain blood cultures for all patients who have high fever or rigors.

Treatment

A. ANTIMICROBIALS

Enterococcal prostatitis may require inpatient treatment with intravenous ampicillin and gentamicin. Fluoroquinolones are the first-line agents of choice for outpatient therapy. Other inpatient regimens include TMP-SMZ intravenously in 2 divided doses or an aminoglycoside. Gonococcal prostatitis is uncommon and should be managed in consultation with a urologist.

B. ADJUNCTIVE MEASURES

Analgesics (often including a narcotic) should be provided. Hot sitz baths may provide relief. Bed rest is usually helpful. α-1-Blockers may be useful to decrease pain and recurrence rates.

Disposition

Patients with acute bacterial prostatitis causing systemic symptoms (high fever, rigors) or with suspected prostatic abscess should be hospitalized for treatment with parenteral antibiotics and consultation with a urologist.

Patients who are not hospitalized should return for follow-up in 3–4 days to ensure that recovery is progressing and again 7–10 days after stopping antimicrobial therapy for a test-of-cure culture of expressed prostatic secretions or of urine. Refer the patient to a urologist or to a source of regular medical care.

ACUTE EPIDIDYMITIS

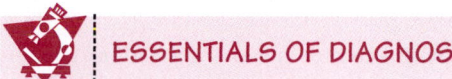

ESSENTIALS OF DIAGNOSIS

- *Testicular pain.*
- *Epididymal tenderness.*

General Conditions

Epididymitis usually results from retrograde spread of urethral or urinary tract infection into the epididymis. Epididymitis is therefore usually caused by the same pathogens causing urethritis (eg, gonococci, *Chlamydia*) or urinary tract infection (eg, *E. coli*). The former pathogens are found more commonly in men younger than age 35 years, and *E. coli* is seen more often in men over age 35 years.

Clinical Findings

A. SYMPTOMS AND SIGNS

Pain and tenderness of the epididymis is present on one or both sides. Epididymitis must be differentiated from testicular torsion and from torsion of the testicular appendage. In orchitis the testicle is diffusely and tensely swollen, warm, firm, and tender.

Urethritis or urinary tract infection usually coexists with epididymitis, and evidence of these conditions must be sought with appropriate laboratory tests. At a minimum, Gram or methylene blue stain of urethral exudates (or swab of material in the anterior urethra if no exudates can be obtained) and a clean-voided midstream urine specimen should be obtained for analysis.

Treatment

A. ANTIMICROBIALS

1. Epididymitis with urinary tract infection—Give TMP-SMZ for 10 days.

2. Epididymitis in sexually active heterosexual men younger than age 35 years—Regardless of whether *N. gonorrhoeae* is demonstrated, the Centers for Disease Control (CDC) recommends treatment for gonorrhea and *Chlamydia*. Administer ceftriaxone intramuscularly followed by doxycycline or tetracycline for 10 days.

B. ADJUNCTIVE MEASURES

Prescribe analgesics as needed. Hot sitz baths may be helpful. Bed rest and scrotal elevation for 1–2 days will provide symptomatic relief. If the patient must be ambulatory, an athletic supporter may be helpful.

Disposition

Refer the patient to a urologist or primary care physician within a few days. Hospitalization is indicated for orchitis that does not respond within 48 hours to oral therapy and adjunctive measures.

SEXUALLY TRANSMITTED DISEASES

The management of all sexually transmitted diseases should include counseling regarding safe sex practices and the performance of HIV antibody test in consenting patients.

GONORRHEA

N. gonorrhoeae causes primary genitourinary tract infections, localized infections, and the disseminated arthritis-dermatitis syndrome. Approximately 600,000 new cases are diagnosed each year.

Clinical Findings

A. SYMPTOMS AND SIGNS

In men, gonococcal urethritis is characterized by acute onset of dysuria, sometimes with hematuria, and a copious creamy urethral discharge. Less profuse urethral discharge requiring milking of the penile urethra may

also occur. Local extension of infection may produce inflammation of preputial glands, epididymitis, seminal vasculitis, and prostatitis. In women, gonococcal cervicitis may be asymptomatic or patients may present with vaginal discharge or symptoms of accompanying urethritis (eg, dysuria, frequency). Occasionally a Bartholin gland abscess is the initial complaint. Patients with gonococcal salpingitis complain of lower abdominal pain (unilateral or bilateral), vaginal discharge, and metromenorrhagia. Pain on cervical motion and adnexal tenderness is usual; nausea and vomiting and marked abdominal tenderness or rebound suggest pelvic peritonitis.

Rectal infection with *N. gonorrhoeae* is usually asymptomatic, although patients occasionally present with proctitis (rectal pain, discharge, tenesmus, and constipation). Pharyngeal infection is almost always asymptomatic.

Patients with gonococcal conjunctivitis present with marked conjunctival erythema and purulent discharge, often unilateral. In adults, it usually follows contact between contaminated fingers and the eye.

B. LABORATORY FINDINGS

In men, obtain a Gram-stained smear of urethral discharge, examine it microscopically, and obtain culture and antimicrobial susceptibility testing. The presence of leukocytes (usually PMNs) and intracellular gram-negative diplococci on the smear is more than 99% specific for gonorrhea. A smear showing only PMNs with no gram-negative diplococci is a predictor of a negative gonococcal culture in over 90% of patients, although culture for gonorrhea is generally recommended. These patients should receive treatment for nongonococcal urethritis. Culture of the pharynx and rectum is necessary if there is a history of oral or receptive rectal intercourse, because negative results on Gram-stained smears from these areas do not rule out gonorrhea.

In women, findings on Gram-stained smears of cervical secretions may suggest gonorrhea (PMNs with intracellular gram-negative diplococci), but culture should be performed to confirm the diagnosis. Culture of rectal secretions is recommended in all women, because sometimes it is the only site yielding positive cultures. Culture of pharyngeal secretions is necessary in patients with a history of oral sexual intercourse.

Express the exudates in purulent conjunctivitis, and examine a Gram-stained smear. Gram-negative diplococci confirm a diagnosis of gonococcal conjunctivitis. Send a sample of the exudates for culture.

Culture on Thayer-Martin media remains the gold standard for diagnosis. The PCR is 97–99% sensitive, with specificity of 99%. A serologic test for syphilis (eg, VDRL) should be ordered for all patients.

Treatment

Because there has been worldwide spread of strains of *N. gonorrhoeae* that are resistant to penicillin, amoxicillin, and tetracycline, these agents are no longer recommended for empiric treatment of gonococcal infections. Use ceftriaxone, 150 mg intramuscularly, an oral fluoroquinolone (eg, ciprofloxacin, 500 mg, or ofloxacin, 400 mg, single dose), or azithromycin (2 g single dose). Because of the high frequency of coexisting chlamydial infection (up to 45%), a tetracycline, doxycycline, or azithromycin regimen should follow the treatment of gonococcal infections.

Patients with gonococcal conjunctivitis must be hospitalized and should receive ophthalmologic consultation. Therapy consists of ceftriaxone, 1 g intramuscularly or intravenously once daily for at least 5 days, combined with immediate and at least hourly irrigation of the eye with saline or buffered ophthalmic solutions. Simultaneous ophthalmic infection with *C. trachomatis* can also occur. Careful ophthalmic follow-up is necessary to prevent ocular complications.

Disposition

Hospitalization is not required for patients with localized gonococcal infection, except for gonococcal conjunctivitis. Sexual partners with gonorrhea must be notified and receive treatment. Cases of gonorrhea must be reported to the local public health department.

NONGONOCOCCAL URETHRITIS (Nonspecific Urethritis)

Nongonococcal urethritis, or nonspecific urethritis, is due to infection with *C. trachomatis* in over half the cases. Genital *Mycoplasmas* (*Ureaplasma*), HSV, and *Trichomonas* are occasional causes.

Clinical Findings

A. SYMPTOMS AND SIGNS

Most male patients have urethral discharge and dysuria. Symptoms are often insidious in onset, with urethral discharge that is scanty, mucoid, watery, and most prominent in the morning. Women may be asymptomatic or may complain of dysuria or frequency. Infection may involve the cervix as well and extend to the oviducts, producing low-grade fever.

B. LABORATORY FINDINGS

Urethral discharge should be stained with Gram stain and examined microscopically. The presence of more than 4 leukocytes per high-power field confirms the diagnosis of urethritis. If no organisms morphologically consistent with gonococci are found, then presumptive diagnosis of nongonococcal urethritis can be made. A Gram-stained smear with findings diagnostic of gonorrhea does not exclude nongonococcal urethritis, because dual infection with *Chlamydia* and the gonococcus is common, particularly in a heterosexual population. The specimen should be sent for culture but because of difficulties in culturing this organism, culture is 80% sensitive. PCR testing is the most sensitive (93–99%), with specificity of 99–100%. A serologic test for syphilis should also be obtained.

Treatment

First-line agents recommended by the CDC include single-dose azithromycin or a 7-day course of doxycycline. If nongonococcal urethritis is suspected (negative or equivocal findings on Gram-stained smear with culture results pending) or documented (culture negative for nongonococcal urethritis), sexual partners should also receive treatment.

Disposition

Patients with nongonococcal urethritis can receive treatment on an outpatient basis.

GENITAL HERPES SIMPLEX VIRUS INFECTION

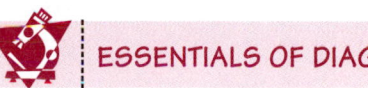

ESSENTIALS OF DIAGNOSIS

- *Fever, adenopathy.*
- *Vesicles on an erythematous base.*
- *Pain.*

General Considerations

HSV is a major cause of recurrent genital lesions. The initial (primary) infection is the most severe, although it is sometimes asymptomatic. After the primary lesion has healed, the virus remains latent in the paraspinous ganglia, where it periodically causes reactivation of infection. Genital infection is usually caused by HSV type 2, and about 99% of patients with recurrent disease will be infected by type 2 virus. Spread of infection is almost exclusively by sexual intercourse.

Clinical Findings

Obtain a serologic test for syphilis (eg, VDRL) to rule out coexisting syphilis.

A. Symptoms and Signs

1. First clinical episode of genital HSV—The first clinical attack of HSV is usually the most severe. Patients may present with fever, malaise, myalgias, and arthralgias. Aseptic meningitis occurs in 10–20% of cases, particularly in women. Associated symptoms may include dysuria, dyspareunia, and urinary retention. Successive crops of grouped vesicles on an erythematous base denude, form ulcers, and heal by secondary intention, usually in 2–3 weeks but sometimes not until after 6 weeks. Genital edema is common. Local pain and regional adenopathy are usually marked. In men, the glans and penile shaft are involved. In women, the vulva, vagina, and cervix are the usual sites of involvement. Male or female patients with herpetic proctitis present with fever, tenesmus, constipation, and rectal pain.

2. Recurrent HSV episodes—Recurrent infection is common and may be triggered by a variety of stimuli (eg, friction, menstruation, sexual intercourse, pregnancy, or stress). Recurrent attacks are frequently heralded by a prodrome consisting of local itching, pain, or aching in the buttocks or leg. Initially, a papule develops that rapidly vesiculates, breaks down into an ulcer, and then heals, usually within 7–10 days. The virus may be recovered as long as lesions are moist. Patients should avoid direct skin-to-skin contact until the area is completely dried and healed.

The presence of HSV may be confirmed by the Tzanck test (about 60% sensitivity and 80% specificity) or virus culture. Virus culture is recommended in most cases.

Treatment

Antipyretics and analgesics may help to relieve systemic symptoms. Antiviral regimens (Table 40–12) accelerate resolution of the signs and symptoms of herpetic eruptions but do not affect the subsequent risk, frequency, or severity of recurrences after the drug is discontinued. Immunocompromised patients (especially AIDS patients) with extensive, ulcerative, or progressive mucocutaneous herpes should receive oral therapy. Continuous therapy is necessary in some patients. Hospitalization for intravenous therapy may be warranted if the patient is unable to take medications orally or if the lesions are extensive. Antibiotics are not necessary unless Gram-stained smears suggest bacterial superinfection. Women with primary genital herpes frequently have associated *Candida* vaginitis, which should be treated as described above. The patient should bathe the exposed affected areas with warm tap water, or apply warm compresses every 4 hours. Because lesions shed infectious virus, patients should avoid manipulating lesions with their bare hands and should wash their hands after exposure (autoinoculation of the eye or other sites may occur). Any

Table 40–12. Outpatient treatment for herpes infections.

Type of Therapy	Agent and Dosing
Primary outbreak	Acyclovir, 200 mg PO 5 times a day for 10 days Valacyclovir, 1000 mg PO bid for 10 days Famciclovir, 250 mg PO tid for 5–10 days
Recurrent	Acyclovir, 200 mg PO 5 times a day for 5 days Famciclovir, 125 mg PO bid for 5 days Valacyclovir, 500 mg PO bid for 5 days
Suppression therapy	Acyclovir, 400 mg PO bid Famciclovir, 250 mg PO bid Valacyclovir, 1000 mg PO qd

other contact with the lesions (eg, sexual) should be avoided until they have healed.

Disposition

Hospitalization is occasionally indicated for patients with primary HSV infection because of severe pain, systemic symptoms, and other complications (urinary retention, obstipation, aseptic meningitis, dehydration). Hospitalization is also required for patients with extensive, large, or rapidly progressive lesions.

Patients with genital HSV infection are often frightened and confused about the nature and transmission of the disease and may suffer both physically and psychologically. Counseling should be initiated and provided in the emergency department, if possible, and patients should be referred to a gynecologist or primary care provider who is experienced in treating HSV infection and who can explain the disease, answer any questions, and provide information on various methods of treatment, so that the patient can make an informed evaluation of the associated efficacy, risks, and side effects.

Obtain obstetric consultation for pregnant patients with HSV infection.

SYPHILIS

 ESSENTIALS OF DIAGNOSIS

- *Chancre (painless).*
- *Rash.*
- *Positive VDRL, RPR, FTA-ABS.*

General Considerations

Disease following infection due to *Treponema pallidum* may be divided into primary, secondary, latent, and tertiary stages. Infection with *T. pallidum* has been identified as an important risk factor for HIV infection. An HIV antibody test should be obtained for all consenting patients with syphilis.

Clinical Findings

A. SYMPTOMS AND SIGNS

1. Primary stage—A chancre develops at the site of entry of the spirochete between 10 days and 6 weeks after exposure. The ulcer, located on the genitals or occasionally on extragenital sites (finger, mouth), is nontender and has a depressed center and rolled, pearly edges. Associated inguinal adenopathy, if present, is usually firm, hard, and nontender.

2. Secondary stage—Secondary disease develops about 4 weeks after the appearance of the chancre. Clinical manifestations reflect the presence of spirochetes in the bloodstream. Most common is a rash that ranges from macular to maculopapular to plaques (condyloma lata). The rash is generally distributed over the thorax, abdomen, and extremities; it may involve the palms and soles; and it is nonpruritic. Associated findings may include low-grade fever, generalized lymphadenopathy, hepatitis, meningitis, alopecia, and weight loss.

3. Latent stage—A positive serologic test is the only sign, and this stage may last from 1 to 2 months up to more than 20 years.

4. Tertiary stage—This stage is characterized by destructive lesions of the aorta, CNS, skeletal structures, and skin.

B. LABORATORY FINDINGS

The diagnosis of infectious syphilis is confirmed by serologic testing or by positive results on microscopic darkfield examination of scrapings from the chancre or lesions of secondary disease. Obtain blood for serologic testing (eg, VDRL or RPR); if results are positive, perform a treponemal antibody test (eg, FTA-ABS or MHA-TP).

Treatment

A. INFECTIOUS SYPHILIS

1. Benzathine penicillin G—The treatment of choice is benzathine penicillin G (2.4 million units intramuscularly). Patients who claim to be allergic to penicillin should be tested (ie, skin testing) and desensitized, if necessary.

2. Doxycycline—An alternative regimen for penicillin-allergic patients is doxycycline, 100 mg orally twice daily, or tetracycline, 500 mg 4 times daily for 14 days.

3. Erythromycin—Patients who cannot take penicillin, doxycycline, or tetracycline and who are reliable and can be followed closely can take erythromycin, 500 mg orally 4 times daily for 14 days.

B. JARISCH-HERXHEIMER REACTION

Asprin or acetaminophen may be prescribed for the Jarisch-Herxheimer reaction that commonly occurs within a few hours after treatment for secondary syphilis has been started. The reaction is characterized by malaise, fever, faintness, and intensification of the rash. Patients with secondary syphilis who are released from the emergency department following penicillin therapy should be warned about the symptoms of the reaction and should be told that it is not due to penicillin allergy.

C. SYPHILIS IN HIV-INFECTED PATIENTS

A lumbar puncture should be performed in HIV-infected patients with early syphilis because of increased risk of treatment failure and CNS relapse. If the CSF cell count is normal and the VDRL test nonreactive, give 1–3 doses of benzathine penicillin G therapy. Serum VDRL testing must be repeated at monthly intervals for at least 3 months. Tetracyclines are probably inadequate therapy for HIV-infected patients with syphilis. Ceftriaxone, 250 mg intramuscularly once daily for 10 days, can be tried.

Disposition

Patients may receive treatment on an outpatient basis. Cases of syphilis must be reported to the local public health department. Sexual partners of patients should be notified and receive treatment. Arrangements must be made for follow-up serologic testing.

CHANCROID

General Considerations

Chancroid is an ulcerating genital infection caused by *Haemophilus ducreyi*. It is common in tropical and subtropical regions and is believed to be underdiagnosed in the United States.

Clinical Findings

Chancroid is manifested by the appearance of a small pustule that rapidly ulcerates with an irregular and purulent exudative base that is painful. It is associated with tender inguinal lymphadenopathy in 50% of cases.

Definitive diagnosis requires growth on culture media, and the diagnosis should be considered for any patient who has painful genital ulceration and for whom darkfield fluoroscopy and HSV testing are negative.

Treatment

Recommended treatments include azithromycin orally or ceftriaxone intramuscularly; ciprofloxacin and erythromycin are alternatives.

TRICHOMONIASIS

 ESSENTIALS OF DIAGNOSIS

- *Erythematous pustule.*
- *Adenopathy.*
- *Pain.*
- *Gram stain or culture.*

Clinical Findings

A. SYMPTOMS AND SIGNS

Most men with *T. vaginalis* infections develop nongonococcal urethritis, but women typically develop malodorous yellow-green frothy discharge, dysuria, dyspareunia, vulvar irritation, and pruritus.

B. LABORATORY FINDINGS

Motile parasites are seen on a wet-mount smear.

Treatment

Single-dose metronidazole or metronidazole therapy for 7 days is the only treatment option. No effective alternatives are available.

Lawson MA, Blythe MJ: Pelvic inflammatory disease in adolescents. Pediatr Clin North Am 1999;46(4):767. [PMID: 10494256]

Lummus WE, Thompson I: Prostatitis. Emerg Med Clin North Am 2001;19(3):691. [PMID: 11554282]

McKininzie J: Sexually transmitted diseases. Emerg Med Clin North Am 2001;19(3):723. [PMID: 11554284]

SKIN & SOFT TISSUE INFECTIONS

SUPERFICIAL SOFT TISSUE INFECTIONS

 ESSENTIALS OF DIAGNOSIS

- *Erythema, pain, edema.*
- *Fever.*
- *Elevated white blood cell count.*

General Considerations

Superficial soft tissue infections (eg, impetigo, erysipelas, cellulitis) are rarely emergencies. However, these infections may be potentially life- or limb-threatening in 3 situations: (1) when infection is near the face or hand, (2) when cellulitis occurs in the presence of diabetes, peripheral vascular disease, or venous or lymphatic insufficiency, or (3) when local infection occurs in the presence of immunodeficiency, particularly leukopenia, leukemia, or AIDS.

Clinical Findings

A. SYMPTOMS AND SIGNS

1. Impetigo—Impetigo is a superficial skin infection seen mainly in children. It is usually due to group A streptococci. Less commonly, staphylococci alone or in conjunction with streptococci may cause the disease. It has 2 forms: bullous (impetigo bullosa) and nonbullous (impetigo contagiosa). Nonbullous impetigo begins with small vesicles that rapidly pustulate and rupture easily. The purulent discharge dries, forming the characteristic thick, golden yellow (honey-crusted) appearance. Bullous impetigo is related to toxin formation and initially appears as a vesicle that rapidly enlarges to form a bulla, which then forms a dark brown crust. Exposed areas are the most common sites of lesions. Mild regional lymphadenopathy is common. The lesions are painless and often pruritic; systemic symptoms are minimal.

2. Ecthyma—Ecthyma is a deeper form of impetigo that is associated with ulceration and scarring. It occurs frequently on the legs, often as a complication of debility or infestation with ectoparasites.

3. Staphylococcal scalded skin syndrome—This is the most severe manifestation of skin disease caused by widespread bullae and exfoliation. It usually occurs in young children but may rarely develop in adults. It begins abruptly with fever, skin tenderness, and scarlatiniform rash. Large, flaccid, clear bullae form and promptly rupture, resulting in separation of sheets of skin.

4. Erysipelas—Erysipelas is a distinctive superficial cellulitis characterized by prominent lymphatic involvement. It is almost always due to group A streptococci and is more common in infants, young children, and older adults than in younger adults. The face is most often involved. The lesion is painful and has a bright red, edematous, indurated appearance and an advancing raised border that is sharply demarcated from adjacent normal skin. A common form of the disease affects the bridge of the nose and cheeks. Fever is common. Erysipelas is usually limited to the dermis and lymphatics but can occasionally extend more deeply to produce cellulitis and bacteremia.

5. Cellulitis—Cellulitis is an acute spreading infection of the skin that extends deeper than erysipelas. Group A streptococci and *S. aureus* are the most common causative agents. Previous trauma or underlying skin lesions (eg, furuncle, ulcer) predispose to the development of cellulitis. Local tenderness, pain, and erythema develop within several days and intensify rapidly. The lesion has poorly demarcated borders, and the skin is red, hot, and edematous. Malaise, fever, and chills may develop. In older patients, cellulitis in the lower extremity may be complicated with thrombophlebitis. In patients with diabetes or peripheral vascular disease, cellulitis in the lower extremity may be caused by gram-negative bacilli and anaerobes, in addition to streptococci and staphylococci.

B. Laboratory Findings

Leukocytosis with a shift to the left may be present. Obtain a Gram-stained smear and culture of material from vesicles, bullae, or exudates. Examination of material aspirated at the leading edge of cellulitis may reveal the causative organism. Obtain blood cultures from patients with high fever, chills, or rapid progression of infection.

Treatment

A. Impetigo and Ecthyma

Penicillin is the treatment of choice and is administered either as a single intramuscular injection of benzathine penicillin G (children, 300,000–600,00 units; adults, 1,200,000 units) or as oral penicillin, 125–500 mg every 6 hours for 10 days. Erythromycin (children, 30–50 mg/kg/d orally in divided doses every 6 hours for 10 days; adults, 250–500 mg orally every 6 hours). Erythromycin is an alternative for penicillin-allergic patients. Topical mupirocin can also be used for impetigo. It is helpful to remove the crust by soaking it in soap and water.

Bullous impetigo responds to treatment with a penicillinase-resistant penicillin (eg, dicloxacillin); erythromycin may be substituted in penicillin-allergic patients.

B. Staphylococcal Scalded Skin Syndrome

Staphylococcal scalded skin syndrome is treated with a penicillinase-resistant penicillin (eg, nafcillin, 50–100 mg/kg/d intravenously in newborns; 100–200 mg/kg/d intravenously in older children). Topical treatment consists of application of cool saline compresses. Corticosteroids should not be used.

C. Erysipelas

Mild cases in adults may be treated with procaine penicillin G (600,000 units intramuscularly once or twice daily) or with oral penicillin, 250–500 mg orally every 6 hours for 2 weeks. Erythromycin, 250–500 mg orally every 6 hours, is a suitable alternative. For more extensive erysipelas, hospitalization for treatment with parenterally administered aqueous penicillin G, 600,000–2,000,000 units intramuscularly every 6 hours, is required.

D. Cellulitis

Mild, early cellulitis may be treated with oral antibiotics. Because *S. aureus* may be involved, empiric therapy is with a penicillinase-resistant penicillin or first-generation cephalosporin. For more severe infection thought to be caused by streptococci or staphylococci, give penicillinase-resistant penicillin intravenously with or without penicillin G. A first-generation cephalosporin equivalent to cefazolin (1–2 g/d intravenously) is an alternative for patients who are not critically ill. Vancomycin (1–2 g/d intravenously) is an alternative for penicillin-allergic patients. If superinfection with gram-negative bacteria is present or suspected, add an aminoglycoside such as gentamycin or amikacin. Local care includes immobilization and elevation of the involved limb.

Disposition

Patients with lymphangitis and patients with cellulitis that has progressed rapidly over the preceding 12 hours can be given parenteral antibiotic therapy in the emergency department if they are reliable for follow-up within 12–24 hours. Hospitalize patients who worsen despite parenteral antibiotic therapy, those who are unreliable, and those who cannot be closely followed in an outpatient setting. Cellulitis involving the face or hand usually requires hospitalization for parenteral antibiotic therapy. The presence of diabetes, venous or lymphatic insufficiency, or systemic symptoms usually requires inpatient or outpatient parenteral therapy.

DEEP SOFT TISSUE INFECTIONS

Deep soft tissue infections involve subcutaneous tissues and may also involve muscles and fascial planes. Classification of these infections is complicated by use of varied nomenclature. Most of these infections are due to anaerobic and aerobic gram-positive and gram-negative organisms.

1. Infected Vascular Gangrene & Cellulitis

Infected vascular gangrene and cellulitis is a mixed infection occurring mostly in the lower extremities in patients with peripheral vascular disease or diabetes. Anaerobic organisms, aerobic gram-negative bacilli, and staphylococci may be involved.

Clinical Findings

An underlying ulcer is often the source of infection that may spread to involve not only superficial and deep soft tissue but also muscles or an entire limb. Gas formation may occur. Edema and foul-smelling pus are noticeable. Pain and tenderness may be present.

Treatment & Disposition

Hospitalization is required for surgical debridement and intravenous therapy with a combination of antibiotics (eg, cefoxitin alone, or clindamycin plus gentamicin). Underlying osteomyelitis is common if an ulcer is present. Amputation is sometimes necessary.

2. Clostridial Anaerobic Cellulitis

Clinical Findings

Clostridial anaerobic cellulitis is a necrotizing clostridial infection of devitalized subcutaneous tissue. The deep fascia is not appreciably involved, and there is ordinarily no associated myositis. Gas formation is common and often extensive. Onset of infection is gradual after an incubation period of several days. Local pain, swelling, and systemic toxicity are not prominent. A thick, dark, sometimes foul-smelling drainage is characteristic. Frank crepitus is present. Gram-stained smears of drainage material show numerous blunt-ended, thick, gram-positive bacilli. Soft tissue x-rays show abundant gas. Obtain cultures for aerobic and anaerobic organisms.

Treatment & Disposition

Hospitalize patients for treatment with high doses of intravenous penicillin (chloramphenicol for penicillin-allergic patients) and surgery.

3. Nonclostridial Anaerobic Cellulitis

Clinical Findings

A clinical picture similar to clostridial cellulitis can be produced by nonclostridial anaerobic bacteria alone or in mixed infection with aerobic gram-negative and gram-positive organisms.

Treatment & Disposition

Antimicrobial therapy is based on the findings on Gram-stained smears of drainage material. Because these are frequently mixed infections, several antibiotics may be needed (eg, cefoxitin, clindamycin, or penicillin plus an aminoglycoside). Surgical incision and drainage is necessary.

4. Synergistic Necrotizing Cellulitis

Clinical Findings

Synergistic necrotizing cellulitis is a rapidly progressive infection with high fever and systemic manifestations caused by infection with anaerobes and anaerobic gram-negative bacilli. It occurs most commonly on the perineum and lower extremities and is associated with a high mortality rate. The disease is first manifested as skin ulcers from which drains foul-smelling, reddish-brown ("dishwater") pus. Circumscribed areas of blue-gray gangrene surround these drainage sites, but intervening skin appears normal. Local pain and tenderness are marked. Tissue gas is noted in about one fourth of patients.

Treatment & Disposition

Hospitalization for prompt surgical incision and drainage of necrotic tissue must be combined with antimicrobial therapy (eg, clindamycin plus gentamicin).

5. Necrotizing Fasciitis

Clinical Findings

Necrotizing fasciitis is a mixed anaerobic and aerobic infection that rapidly dissects deep fascial planes and produces severe toxicity associated with a high mortality rate. It most commonly occurs on the extremities but may occur on the abdomen in patients with diabetes mellitus, especially after abdominal surgery, or on the perineum or scrotum (Fournier gangrene) in patients with diabetes mellitus, especially after urinary tract manipulation. The affected area is initially erythematous, swollen, and painful. Bullae containing serosanguineous material appear, and subcutaneous gas is common. Systemic toxicity with high fever is prominent. When a lesion is probed with a hemostat through a limited incision, the instrument passes easily along a plane just superficial to the deep fascia, a distinguishing feature that does not occur with ordinary cellulitis. Leukocytosis is present. About half the cases are due to group A streptococci alone; the remainder are due to mixtures of gram-positive and gram-negative bacteria, both aerobic and anaerobic.

Treatment & Disposition

Hospitalization for prompt surgical therapy with extensive incision and excision of necrotic tissue is of paramount importance. The initial empiric antimicrobial therapy (eg, cefoxitin alone, or clindamycin and gentamicin) should be altered based on the results of Gram-stained smears and cultures of tissue biopsies.

6. Clostridial Myonecrosis

Clostridal myonecrosis (gas gangrene) is a necrotizing infection of fascia and muscle. Infection most commonly occurs following surgical procedures or as a result of contaminated wounds. Patients with peripheral vascular disease, diabetes, and neoplastic diseases are especially at risk for this infection.

Clinical Findings

The incubation period is usually less than 3 days. Severe pain is the earliest symptom, followed by intense swelling and edema. A thin hemorrhagic exudate may be seen. The skin is exquisitely tender to touch and has a bronze to dusky discoloration that darkens with time. Bullae may appear and are filled with serosanguineous fluid. Crepitus is uncommon early in the disease. There may be a watery brown discharge with a peculiar sweet smell. Systemic symptoms of tachycardia and low-grade fever are usually present. Gram-stained smears may demonstrate *Clostridium perfringens,* but surgical exploration is necessary for confirmation of the diagnosis.

Treatment & Disposition

Hospitalization for prompt, complete excision of necrotic muscle is mandatory. Penicillin G or chloramphenicol is recommended for the penicillin-allergic patient. Because some species of *Clostridium* are resistant to clindamycin and cefoxitin, these agents should not be used as initial empiric drugs in suspected cases of clostridial myonecrosis. General supportive measures include administration of oxygen and adequate volume replacement to counteract shock. Hyperbaric oxygen, though useful, is not a substitute for immediate surgery.

Callahan EF et al: Cutaneous infections. Dermatol Clin 2000;18 (3):497. [PMID: 10943544] (Review.)

Dong SL et al: ED management of cellulites: a review of five urban centers. Am J Emerg Med 2001;19(7):535. [PMID: 11698996]

Rhody CR: Bacterial infections of the skin. Primary Care Clinics in Office Practice 2000;27(2):459.

Sadick NS: Current aspects of bacterial infections of the skin. Dermatol Clin 1997;15(2):341. [PMID: 9098643] (Review.)

Stone DR, Gorbach SL: Necrotizing fasciitis. Dermatol Clin 1997;15(12):213. [PMID: 9098631] (Review.)

■ III. MANAGEMENT OF INFECTIONS CAUSED BY SPECIFIC ORGANISMS

ACUTE MENINGOCOCCEMIA

 ESSENTIALS OF DIAGNOSIS

- *Fever.*
- *Petechial rash.*
- *Hypotension, shock.*
- *Positive blood culture.*

Clinical Findings

A. SYMPTOMS AND SIGNS

Meningococcemia often follows a mild upper respiratory infection. Onset may be acute or subacute, with fever and malaise, with or without symptoms and signs of meningitis or septic shock. A petechial rash appears early in the course of the illness, usually on the trunk and lower portion of the body and over pressure points (eg, under elastic underwear or stockings). The petechiae are small (1–2 mm), irregular, gunmetal gray, and often palpable. Petechiae may become confluent (purpura) or may progress to form vasculitic ulcers. Mucosal petechiae (eg, on the palpebral conjunctiva) also occur. Early in the disease, the number of petechiae correlates with the degree of thrombocytopenia and with the probability of disseminated intravascular coagulation. A majority of patients with meningococcal disease (80–85%) present with meningitis and most of the remaining (15–20%) present with septicemia without meningitis.

B. Laboratory Findings

Results of routine laboratory studies are consistent with the findings of bacteremia with or without sepsis. All patients should be evaluated for disseminated intravascular coagulation (prothrombin time, international normalized ratio, partial thromboplastin time, fibrinogen level, and fibrin degradation products). Always obtain blood cultures. The likelihood of a positive culture is 50% in patients prior to antibiotic treatment and only 5% after receiving antibiotics. Other special laboratory tests that may be helpful include the following:

1. *Bacteria on stained smear.* Meningococci (gram-negative kidney bean–shaped diplococci) may be found on the stained smears of the buffy coat of a centrifuged blood sample or in material taken from petechial skin lesions. If meningitis has developed, meningococci and PMNs may often be seen on careful examination of gram-stained smears of CSF.

2. *Blood sample for PCR.*

3. *CSF for microscopy, culture, PCR, and antigen detection.* Contraindications to lumbar puncture include a Glasgow Coma Scale score of less than 13 or deteriorating scores, other signs of raised intracranial pressure, focal neurologic signs, impending or established septic shock, infection at the planned puncture site, or bleeding disorder.

4. *Throat (nasopharyngeal) swab culture.* Throat culture is typically useful only in infants and young children. Results are not likely to be significant in an adult because of the high nasal carriage rate.

Differential Diagnosis

Rickettsial infections, septicemia caused by organisms other than meningococci (eg, *H. influenzae, S. pneumonia, S. aureus*), and atypical measles may resemble meningococcemia. Bleeding diatheses (eg, idiopathic thrombocytopenia purpura) and cutaneous vasculitides (eg, Henoch-Schönlein purpura) may also be confused with meningococcemia.

Complications

A. Septic Shock

Septic shock is a common complication of meningococcemia. Myocarditis is often found at autopsy and may contribute to vascular collapse.

B. Disseminated Intravascular Coagulation

Disseminated intravascular coagulation is frequently diagnosed in meningococcemia. Therapy is directed mainly at treating the underlying sepsis while giving supportive care.

C. Adrenal Hemorrhage

Waterhouse-Friderichsen syndrome is characterized by shock and vascular collapse caused by glucocorticoid deficiency due to adrenal hemorrhage.

D. Metastatic Infection

Meningitis, arthritis, and pericarditis are common complications.

Treatment

A. Antibiotics

Empiric treatment with ceftriaxone or cefotaxime is appropriate with a change to aqueous penicillin G when meningococcal disease is verified. Chloramphenicol may be used if the patient has a history of serious allergy to penicillin.

B. Steroids

Treat suspected adrenal insufficiency with doses of injectable hydrocortisone (Solu-Cortef) or methylprednisolone (Solu-Medrol). Dexamethasone should be used to treat meningococcal meningitis but not meningococcal septicemia without meningitis.

Disposition

Patients with meningitis should be hospitalized in an intensive care unit.

Prophylaxis of Exposed Contacts

Current recommendations include rifampin orally in 4 divided doses, a single dose of oral ciprofloxacin, or a single intramuscular dose of ceftriaxone.

Cartwright KAV: Early management of meningococcal disease. Infect Dis Clin North Am 1999;13(3):661. [PMID: 10470561]

Cohen J: Meningococcal disease as a model to evaluate novel antisepsis strategies. Crit Care Med 2000;28:S64. [PMID: 11007201]

ROCKY MOUNTAIN SPOTTED FEVER

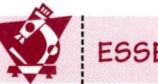 ESSENTIALS OF DIAGNOSIS

- *Fever.*
- *Headache.*
- *Petechial rash (palms or soles).*

General Considerations

Rocky mountain spotted fever is an acute febrile tick-borne illness caused by *Rickettsia rickettsii*. Although it has been reported in most states in the United States, it is most common in the southern Atlantic and south central states and in Oklahoma. Most cases occur in warm months, when ticks are most active. Eighty percent of patients have a history of tick bite.

Clinical Findings

A. SYMPTOMS AND SIGNS

Following an incubation period of about 1 week, there is sudden onset of fever, chills, malaise, myalgias, and severe frontal headache. On the 2nd to 5th day of illness, a pink macular rash 1–4 mm in diameter appears on the palms, soles, hands, feet, wrists, and ankles. Over the next 24–48 hours, the rash becomes petechial, purpuric, and even gangrenous and spreads centripetally to involve the rest of the body. (At this stage the rash may mimic the lesions of fulminant meningococcemia, although in meningococcemia, the skin eruption appears earlier in the disease.) There may be diffuse edema due to capillary leakage; hypotension, splenomegaly, and delirium may be seen. A common treatment error is to give the patient penicillin for streptococcal disease.

B. LABORATORY FINDINGS

Results on ordinary laboratory testing are not exceptional. The white cell count is usually not elevated. Hyponatremia, hypochloremia, and hypoalbuminemia may be present. Thrombocytopenia may occur as an isolated finding or in association with disseminated intravascular coagulation, which is common in Rocky Mountain spotted fever. The CSF is usually normal, but protein levels may be elevated and a few mononuclear cells may be present. No specific laboratory test is available for the diagnosis of Rocky Mountain spotted fever during the acute stage; therefore, the diagnosis must be made on clinical grounds.

Treatment

Give tetracycline or doxycycline to adults and older children. Give chloramphenicol to children younger than age 8 years.

Disposition

Hospitalization is required for all patients except those with the mildest symptoms. Severely ill patients should be in an intensive care unit.

INFECTIVE ENDOCARDITIS

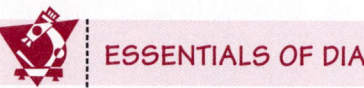

ESSENTIALS OF DIAGNOSIS

- *Fever, chills.*
- *New or changing murmur.*
- *Cutaneous lesions.*

General Consideration

Infective endocarditis denotes infection of the endothelial surface of the heart, most often the cardiac valves. The disease may either be acute or subacute and may affect normal valves, previously damaged cardiac valves, or prosthetic valves. It is usually caused by bacteria, but fungi are also common pathogens in intravenous drug abusers with acute endocarditis. Seeding of bacterial emboli or deposition of immune complexes in the skin may cause characteristic skin lesions that can alert the physician to the correct diagnosis before progressive damage to the heart leads to circulatory collapse. Common pathogenic organisms include *S. viridans, Streptococcus bovis,* and the HACEK group of gram-negative organisms (*Haemophilus, Actinobacillus, Cardiobacterium, Eikenella,* and *Kingella*). *S. aureus* is particularly virulent, and infection is associated with a high mortality rate. *Staphylococcus epidermis* and coagulase-negative staphylococci are the leading causes of infective endocarditis in patients with prosthetic valves.

Clinical Findings

A. SYMPTOMS AND SIGNS

Patients usually present with fever and malaise. In subacute endocarditis, there may be a history of anorexia, night sweats, and weight loss. Patients may also present in cardiac failure, with a stroke due to cerebral embolism, or with a cold extremity due to arterial emboli. Patients with infective endocarditis of the tricuspid valve (usually seen in intravenous drug abusers) commonly present with acute, often bilateral, embolic pneumonia. Examination of the heart often reveals a murmur, although heart murmurs are commonly absent in right-sided endocarditis.

Characteristic (but not specific) cutaneous and mucosal lesions in bacterial endocarditis include conjunctival and palatal petechiae, subungual (splinter) hemorrhages, Osler nodes, and Janeway lesions. Osler nodes are tender erythematous nodules with opaque centers that appear on the pulp of the fingertips and toes. Janeway lesions are nontender red or maroon macules or nodules that develop on the palms and soles. Careful ophthalmologic examination may also reveal Roth spots (pale oval areas surrounded by hemorrhage) near the optic disk.

The Duke criteria were developed in 1994 to aid in the diagnosis of endocarditis. The diagnosis requires 2 major criteria or 1 major and 3 minor criteria or 5 minor criteria (Table 40–13).

B. LABORATORY FINDINGS

Laboratory findings are variable and nonspecific for infective endocarditis. A normochromic normocytic anemia may be present, especially for patients with subacute disease. The white cell count may be elevated, especially in acute disease. The erythrocyte sedimentation rate is usually elevated. Microscopic hematuria is present in 30–50% of patients. Immune complex glomerulonephritis with renal failure may occur. Transthoracic echocardiography is 98% specific for endocarditis, but sensitivity may be less than 60%. Transesophageal echocardiography is close to 100% sensitive for examination of native valves and 84–94% sensitive for prosthetic valves.

Definitive diagnosis depends on isolating the causative organisms in blood cultures; however, 5–20% of patients with clinical endocarditis have persistently negative blood cultures (termed culture-negative endocarditis). Gram-stained smears of aspirates from skin lesions (usually Janeway lesions) occasionally permit

Table 40–13. Duke criteria for diagnosis of infective endocarditis.

Major criteria
Positive blood cultures:
   Typical microorganisms for endocarditis on 2 separate
      blood cultures
   Persistently positive blood cultures
Evidence of endocardial involvement: positive echocardiogram (oscillating intracardiac mass on valve or supporting structures; in the path of regurgitant jets; or on implanted material, abscess, or new partial dehiscence of a prosthetic valve)
New valvular regurgitation (increase or change in preexisting murmur not sufficient)

Minor criteria
Fever > 38 ˚C
Predisposing heart conditions or intravenous drug abuse
Vascular phenomenon: major arterial emboli, septic pulmonary infarcts, mycotic aneurysms, intracranial hemorrhage, conjunctival hemorrhages, Janeway lesions
Immunologic phenomena: glomerulonephritis, Osler nodes, Roth spots, rheumatoid factor
Microbiological evidence: positive blood culture but not meeting major criteria
Echocardiogram: consistent with endocarditis but not meeting major criterion

rapid diagnosis. In patients with embolic pneumonia, Gram-stained smears of sputum may demonstrate the causative agent (usually *S. aureus*); however, in intravenous drug abusers, possible concurrent infection with other organisms (streptococci, gram-negative bacilli) must be treated pending blood culture results.

Treatment

In patients who are not acutely ill and in whom symptoms and signs of cardiac failure or major emboli are absent, antibiotic therapy may be withheld pending blood culture results. In all other patients, empiric antibiotic therapy should be initiated after samples of blood, urine, and (when present) sputum and aspirates from skin lesions have been obtained for culture.

A. ABNORMAL CARDIAC VALVE OR CONGENITAL HEART DISEASE

Usual pathogens in patients with abnormal cardiac valves or congenital heart disease are *S. viridans* and group D streptococci. Aqueous penicillin G intravenously is an acceptable empiric regimen. Vancomycin intravenously may be substituted for penicillin.

B. PROSTHETIC CARDIAC VALVES

Many pathogens cause prosthetic cardiac valve endocarditis. Infection occurring less than 6 months postoperatively may be caused by *S. aureus, S. epidermidis*, gram-negative aerobic bacilli, diphtheroids, or fungi. Infection occurring more than 6 months after prosthetic valve insertion is usually caused by *S. viridans*, aerobic gram-negative bacilli, enterococci, or staphylococci. Because growth of some of these organisms requires multiple blood cultures using special techniques, it is best to avoid early empiric therapy whenever possible. In a patient who requires immediate surgery because of hemodynamic decompensation, empiric therapy may be started with vancomycin and gentamycin.

C. PARENTERAL DRUG ABUSE

The usual pathogens in intravenous drug abusers are *S. aureus, Pseudomonas* spp., and streptococci, including group D streptococci. Empiric treatment should include vancomycin and gentamicin with substitution for vancomycin with penicillin and nafcillin, oxacillin, or methicillin in patients with compromised renal function.

Disposition

Patients with suspected bacterial endocarditis should be hospitalized. Obtain cardiothoracic surgical consultation for patients with infected prosthetic heart valves, new onset of cardiac failure, or emboli in major vessels, because emergency valve replacement is often necessary.

Brook MM: Pediatric bacterial endocarditis: treatment and prophylaxis. Pediatr Clin North Am 1999;46(2):275. [PMID: 10218075]

Giessel BE et al: Management of bacterial endocarditis. Am Fam Physician 2000;61(6):1725. [PMID: 10750879]

Ryan EW, Bolger AF: Transesophageal echocardiography (TEE) in the evaluation of infective endocarditis. Cardiol Clin 2000;18(4):773. [PMID: 11236165]

DISSEMINATED GONOCOCCEMIA

 ESSENTIALS OF DIAGNOSIS

- *Fever.*
- *Skin lesions.*
- *Septic arthritis.*
- *Positive culture results.*

General Considerations

Gononoccal bacteremia occurs in 1–3% of patients with infections and is the leading cause of acute septic arthritis in adults. A presumptive diagnosis based on the characteristic clinical picture is usually possible in sexually active patients.

Clinical Findings

A. SYMPTOMS AND SIGNS

Disseminated gonococcemia begins as a subacute febrile illness with migratory polyarthralgia. Typically, in the first week of illness, 5–40 discrete lesions develop on the extremities; the face and trunk are spared. Lesions vary and range from petechiae and erythematous, palpable purpura to vesiculopustules with an erythematous halo, and they often have necrotic centers. About one fourth of patients have tenosynovitis, usually affecting the wrist or ankle. Acute septic arthritis, affecting one or more large joints, may follow disseminated gonococcemia or may occur in its absence.

B. LABORATORY FINDINGS

The white cell count may be elevated. Blood cultures are often positive in disseminated gonococcemia. Although Gram stains and culture of skin lesions are generally negative, cultures of all sites are negative in as many as 50% of patients, and a presumptive diagnosis is based instead on the prompt response to ceftriaxone therapy.

Treatment

A. ANTIMICROBIAL THERAPY

Give ceftriaxone (1 g intravenously or intramuscularly every 24 hours).

B. ARTHROCENTESIS

Arthrocentesis should be performed as often as necessary to prevent accumulation of fluid in an infected joint. Open drainage is usually not necessary in gonococcal arthritis.

Disposition

Most patients with septic arthritis should be hospitalized, but outpatient treatment with daily visits for joint aspiration is an acceptable alternative for reliable patients. Many patients with only dermatitis or tenosynovitis may receive outpatient treatment with close follow-up.

TOXIC SHOCK SYNDROME

General Considerations

Toxic shock syndrome results from absorption of toxin from localized *S. aureus* colonization or infection. In the past, most cases occurred in young women who had vaginal colonization with *S aureus* that produce toxic shock syndrome toxin-1 (TSST-1); however, nonmenstrual-related cases currently outnumber menstrual-related cases. Most of the nonmenstrual cases occur in the postoperative setting. The toxin functions as a superantigen that allows the antigen to bind directly to the MHC-II (major histocompatibility complex) receptor in a nonspecific fashion. This may result in activation of 5–30% of the total T cell population, leading to massive cytokine production. Streptococcal toxic shock syndrome (STSS) is similar in appearance to toxic shock syndrome but is associated with invasive streptococci infection. A majority of cases of STSS have occurred in young, otherwise healthy individuals aged 20–50 years. The initial presentation in STSS is localized pain in an extremity with cutaneous signs of a soft tissue infection. Toxic shock syndrome rarely shows the signs of cutaneous skin involvement commonly seen in STSS.

The mortality rate in STSS is 5 times higher than in toxic shock syndrome.

Clinical Findings

Menstrual-related toxic shock syndrome usually starts abruptly during menses. It occurs most commonly in women using tampons or contraceptive sponges. In nonmenstrual cases associated with postoperative infection, signs of localized infection in the wound may be absent.

A. SYMPTOMS AND SIGNS

There is a short prodrome consisting of various combinations of the following symptoms and signs: fever, myalgias, vomiting, diarrhea, and pharyngitis. Patients then develop shock (systolic blood pressure < 80 mm Hg) with fever (> 39 °C) and signs of multiple organ dysfunction. At the time of presentation to the emergency department or within 24 hours of admission to the hospital, a diffuse, blanching, macular erythema appears, accompanied by signs of mucous membrane inflammation (pharyngitis, conjunctivitis, vaginitis, and strawberry tongue). The rash fades in about 3 days, but desquamation of the hands and feet occurs in all patients 5–12 days after the rash disappears. Patients typically prefer to remain motionless in bed because of intense myalgias. Confusion and agitation occur in about half of patients. Pedal edema is common.

B. LABORATORY FINDINGS

Laboratory findings reflect dysfunction of several organ systems. There may be leukocytosis and thrombocytopenia, elevated blood urea nitrogen and creatinine levels, hyperbilirubinemia, elevated hepatic enzymes, or sterile pyuria. The prothrombin, INR, and partial thromboplastin times may be elevated, with or without thrombocytopenia. Other laboratory abnormalities include acidosis, elevated creatine kinase levels (indicating rhabdomyolysis), hypocalcemia, decreased serum albumin and total protein due to capillary leakage, and elevated liver enzyme levels. Cultures of material from the vagina or cervix are usually positive for *S. aureus*. Blood cultures are negative in 85% of patients with toxic shock syndrome and in 50% of patients with STSS.

Treatment & Disposition

Remove the vaginal tampon or nasal or wound packing if present. Begin volume replacement with saline or colloid solutions and with vasopressors, if necessary. Admit the patient to an intensive care unit, and monitor hemodynamic status. Start treatment with a first-generation cephalosporin, penicillinase-resistant synthetic penicillin, or vancomycin intravenously. Some studies have shown intravenous immunoglobulin to be useful in treating STSS.

GROUP A STREPTOCOCCAL INFECTIONS ASSOCIATED WITH A TOXIC SHOCK–LIKE SYNDROME

An infection with group A streptococci that is remarkable for severity of local tissue destruction, life-threatening systemic toxicity, and toxic shock–like syndrome has been described in adults. Clinical isolates frequently produce pyrogenic exotoxin A. The portal of entry may be the skin or the mucous membranes, or infection may occur subsequent to a surgical procedure, but many patients do not have obvious evidence of a portal of entry.

Clinical Findings

A. SYMPTOMS AND SIGNS

Pain is the most common initial symptom and is frequently severe and abrupt in onset. The pain usually involves the extremity but may be intra-abdominal. Before symptom onset, some patients complain of an influenza-like syndrome characterized by fever, chills, myalgia, vomiting, and diarrhea. Patients often have oral temperatures above 37 °C, may have confusion that rapidly deteriorates into coma, or may be combative. Shock is apparent at the time of presentation or within hours with evidence of hypotension, renal dysfunction, and respiratory failure. Most patients present with soft tissue infection, such as cellulitis or necrotizing fasciitis. Deeper infections may be present, including osteomyelitis, myometritis, peritonitis, suppurative phlebitis, or endophthalmitis. A major difference between these patients and patients with STSS is that the former have extensive soft tissue infection and bacteremia. The mortality rate is approximately 30%.

B. LABORATORY FINDINGS

Laboratory findings reflect dysfunction of several organ systems. There may be leukocytosis and thrombocytopenia. The hematocrit is initially normal but may drop within 48–72 hours. Serum creatinine and creatine kinase levels are elevated, but calcium and albumin levels are low. Microscopic hematuria is often present and correlates with the presence of renal impairment. Group A streptococci are cultured from the blood, body fluid, or tissues of all patients who have not received antibiotic therapy.

Treatment & Disposition

Intensive fluid replacement, central venous or pulmonary capillary wedge pressure monitoring, and timely surgical debridement are essential. Start antibiotic therapy with intravenous penicillin or a cephalosporin. Admit patients to the intensive care unit.

Manders SM: Toxin-mediated streptococcal and staphylococcal disease. J Am Acad Dermatol 1998;39(3):1725. [PMID: 10750879] (Review.)

LYME BORRELIOSIS

Lyme borreliosis (Lyme disease, Lyme arthritis) is a chronic disease caused by the spirochete *Borrelia burgdorferi*. Transmission is by several tick vectors (*Ixodes, Amblyomma, Rhipicephalus*) and occurs throughout the United States; the highest prevalence is in the Northeast and Midwest. It has been recognized in Europe, Asia, and Australia. In stage 1, a rash is present, sometimes accompanied by fever. Timely treatment at this stage may prevent disease progression.

Clinical Findings

A. Symptoms and Signs

Between 3 and 32 days following the tick bite, which the patient may not notice, a gradually expanding area of redness with clearing (erythema migrans) occurs at the bite site. The involved skin is warm but not particularly tender to touch. About half of affected patients will develop smaller lesions of similar morphology at areas remote from the bite site over ensuing days to weeks.

In stage 1 disease (erythema migrans), often there are fever, chills, malaise, and regional lymphadenopathy. In stage 2 (days to weeks after infection), symptoms related to the multisystemic nature of Lyme borreliosis often appear, such as meningitis, hepatitis, sore throat, dry cough, heart block and other cardiac abnormalities, musculoskeletal pain, and neuropathy. Fatigue and lethargy are prominent and may persist for months after the skin lesions have disappeared.

A persistent illness (stage 3) may linger for months to years and usually involves the musculoskeletal system (chronic arthritis), neurologic system (both central and peripheral), and skin (acrodermatitis chronica atrophicans). Stage 3 illness responds more slowly to treatment, and treatment at this stage has higher failure rates compared to stages 1 and 2.

B. Laboratory Findings

Laboratory testing is currently not reliable or standardized. Diagnosis depends on recognition of the pathognomonic rash. Serodiagnosis by either indirect immunofluorescence or ELISA may be negative in early infection. Nonspecific laboratory abnormalities include an elevated erythrocyte sedimentation rate, mild anemia, and transient elevations in SGOT (AST), SGPT (ALT), and lactate dehydrogenase enzyme levels.

Treatment & Disposition

The treatment of choice for early Lyme borreliosis is tetracycline for at least 10 days, or for 20 or 30 days if symptoms persist or recur. For children under age 12 years, give amoxicillin or penicillin V. In pediatric patients with penicillin allergy, give erythromycin for 15–30 days. For more serious disease (eg, Lyme carditis or meningitis), use intravenous therapy with ceftriaxone or penicillin G for 14–21 days.

Edlow JA: Lyme disease and related tick-borne illnesses. Ann Emerg Med 1999;33(6):680. [PMID: 10339684] (Review.)

Gayle A: Tick-borne diseases. Am Fam Physician 64(3):1461. [PMID: 11515835] (Review.)

■ IV. AIDS & HIV INFECTION (See Table 40–14.)

General Considerations

AIDS patients can present in extremis, with shock, acute respiratory distress syndrome, or multiple organ failure secondary to overwhelming infection. Acute adrenal failure can occur secondary to CMV and tuberculosis affecting the adrenals. AIDS and HIV can complicate virtually any organ system, and a detailed history and physical examination are necessary. AIDS is the end stage of chronic infection by HIV, a lymphotrophic retrovirus. Transmission occurs by sexual contact, perinatally, and by contact with infected blood. The virus causes slow destruction of the helper T cell subset and in most affected individuals leads to fatal immunosuppression.

Clinical Findings

Assess mental status carefully because mental status changes may be early signs of CNS infection or neuropsychiatric problems such as HIV dementia. Examine the eyes carefully for retinal lesions such as yellowish exudates and large hemorrhages seen in CMV or toxoplasma retinitis. The presence of nuchal rigidity may not be a presenting symptom of meningitis in an HIV-positive patient but should be assessed. Examine the mouth for evidence of oral candida (thrush) or leukoplakia, herpes, and Kaposi sarcoma. Pulmonary examination could reveal tachypnea or unequal breath sounds. A cardiac examination is essential in evaluating for murmurs that could be secondary to an infectious endocarditis (especially in intravenous drug abusers).

Table 40–14. Common HIV emergencies.

Findings	Common Causes	Helpful Diagnostic Tests
Pulmonary Cough, dyspnea, pulmonary infiltrates	*Pneumocystis carinii* *Mycobacterium tuberculosis* Pneumococci *Haemophilus influenzae*	Arterial blood gas measurements Chest x-ray Giemsa, acid-fast, and gram-staining of sputum; culture Bronchoscopy with lavage with biopsy
Neurologic Seizures; focal neurologic deficit; encephalopathy, hydrocephalus	*Toxoplasma gondii* Crytococcal or tuberculous meningitis Cerebral lymphoma Encephalitis (HIV, herpes virus)	CT scan, MRI Lumbar puncture (after CT scan) Brain biopsy
Systemic Fever, rigors, night sweats	Neutropenia with sepsis Cryptococcal infection Disseminated mycobacterial infection (several species) Sinusitis *Pneumocystis carinii* Cytomegalovirus *Salmonella* spp.	Complete blood count Blood cultures (viruses, bacterial, fungi, mycobacteria) Lumbar puncture and CSF examination Chest x-ray
Gastrointestinal Diarrhea, dehydration	*Cryptosporidium* spp. *Shigella* spp. *Salmonella* spp. *Campylobacter jejuni* *Entamoeba histolytica*	Culture of stool and microscopic examination for parasites
Hematologic Bleeding, purpura	Thrombocytopenia Intestinal or pulmonary Kaposi sarcoma (rare)	Complete blood count and platelet count Endoscopy

Examine genitalia for lesions such as the chancre of syphilis. An anorectal examination can reveal fissures or fistulas, perianal abscesses, or prostatitis. A careful neurologic examination can disclose a CNS lesion that could be either infectious or neoplastic in origin.

Organ System–Specific Presentations

A. PULMONARY

The most common presenting complaint for an HIV-positive patient is pulmonary in origin. *P. carinii* pneumonia (PCP) is the most common identifiable cause of death in AIDS patients and remains common (70% of HIV-positive patients will get it, and 70% of those will get reinfected). PCP is typically associated with fever and nonproductive cough, in contrast to bacterial pneumonia, in which the cough tends to be productive. Other causes of pulmonary pathology include tuberculosis, CMV, *Cryptococcus, Histoplasma,* and neoplasms (Kaposi sarcoma, lymphoma).

B. NEUROLOGIC

Ninety percent of patients with AIDS and 10–20% of HIV-positive patients will present with neurologic symptoms at some point (eg, seizure, mental status change, headache). It is crucial to rule out infectious causes (*Cryptococcus,* bacterial meningitis, *Histoplasma,* CMV, progressive multifocal leukoencephalopathy, HSV, neurosyphillis, tuberculosis) but also to consider HIV encephalopathy (also known as AIDS dementia or subacute encephalitis; occurring in up to 15% of AIDS patients), lymphoma, cerebrovascular accident, and metabolic encephalopathy.

C. GASTROINTESTINAL

Fifty percent of HIV-positive patients will have a gastrointestinal complication, presenting with complaints such as odynophagia, abdominal pain, bleeding, or diarrhea. Common infections include *Shigella, Salmonella, E. coli, Campylobacter, Cryptosporidium, Isospora,* CMV, or *Mycobacterium avium* complex (MAV). Bacterial infection is typically fulminant. If bacterial infection is suspected, give a fluoroquinolone empirically. Hepatitis is commonly seen secondary to high rates of coinfection with hepatitis B and C but can also be due to CMV, *Cryptosporidium,* or MAV. Proctocolitis is common in HIV-positive patients, and unless a careful examination is carried out, this diagnosis is easily overlooked (common causative organisms include *Campylobacter, Shigella, Salmonella,* gonococcus, and *Chlamydia*).

D. SYSTEMIC

Acute HIV infection causes an acute flulike illness in 50–90% of patients. Patients may present with fever, weight loss, adenopathy, or fatigue. MAV causes disseminated disease in up to 50% of AIDS patients (with fever, weight loss, and diarrhea). Fever is a common symptom and, in the absence of organ-specific clues, needs to be evaluated carefully. It may be due to HIV infection itself or another infectious cause. Patients with PCP may present with fever in the absence of respiratory symptoms. Cryptococcal meningitis can begin as fever without headache. Also consider *Mycobacterium* tuberculosis, MAV, endocarditis (especially if the patient is an intravenous drug abuser), and fever associated with neoplasm (lymphoma).

E. OPHTHALMOLOGIC

The most common ocular finding is retinal microvasculopathy ("cotton wool spots"). CMV retinitis is common, and patients with this disorder present with visual loss, blindness, photophobia, scotomata, and floaters. On examination, CMV retinitis appears as fluffy white perivascular lesions with hemorrhage. HSV ophthalmicus is a worrisome complication; patients present with conjunctivitis, episcleritis, iritis, and keratitis.

F. RENAL

HIV-positive patients commonly display prerenal azotemia secondary to volume depletion but also must deal with the consequences of drug nephrotoxicity, HIV nephropathy (focal segmental glomerulosclerosis), and renal tubular acidosis (hyperchloremic metabolic acidosis non-anion-gap acidosis), which are common in HIV infection and AIDS.

G. SKIN

Patients can display a multitude of symptomology related to the skin. Infections are common (eg, *Staphylococcus, Pseudomonas,* HSV, herpes zoster, syphilis, intertriginous *Candida*), as are xerosis or pruritus associated with HIV infection.

H. DRUG REACTIONS

See Table 40–15.

Table 40–15. Side effects of HIV antiviral therapy.

Drug	Side Effects
Abacavir	Nausea, vomiting, fever, rash, dizziness
Adefovir	Elevated LFTs, diarrhea, nausea
Amprenavir	Rash, nausea, headache, vomiting
Delavirdine	Rash, headache, fatigue
Didanosine	Diarrhea, pancreatitis, neuropathy, elevated LFTs
Efavirenz	Central nervous system effects, rash, elevated LFTs
Hydroxyurea	Nausea, headache, stomatitis, white blood cells, platelets, hemoglobin
Indinavir	Nephrolithiasis, elevated bilirubin, nausea, abdominal pain
Lamivudine	Headache, fatigue, nausea
Nelfinavir	Diarrhea, nausea
Nevirapine	Rash, nausea, headache, elevated LFTs
Ritonavir	Nausea, headache, diarrhea, elevated LFTs
Saquinavir	Diarrhea, nausea, elevated LFTs
Stavudine	Neuropathy, elevated LFTs
Zalcitabine	Neuropathy, rash
Zidovudine	Headache, neutropenia, nausea, myalgias

LFT = liver function tests.

Laboratory Data

Obtain an arterial blood gas measurement to aid in investigating pulmonary complaints ($PaO_2 < 60$ or oxygen saturation < 90 is suggestive of pneumonitis). A fall in oxygen saturation of greater than 3% with activity is 80% sensitive for PCP. A chest x-ray can be useful in narrowing the differential diagnosis of pulmonary complaints based on appearance, but these findings are often nonspecific. Chest x-rays are read as negative in 15–20% of patients with documented PCP. Obtain blood and urine cultures (remember fungal and mycobacterial studies) as needed to evaluate systemic complaints or for focal complaints related to possible infection. Sputum culture and Gram stain are particularly useful for pulmonary complaints.

A complete blood count is helpful as a general index to evaluate for infection and for hematologic complications of HIV infection. In the absence of a CD4 count, an absolute lymphocyte count can be helpful. If the total lymphocyte count is less than 1000, then the CD4 is likely less than 200. CMV or MAC usually do not occur unless CD4 is less than 50. CSF should be sent for typical studies such as opening-closing pressures, cell count, glucose, protein, Gram stain, and culture, as well as other studies in selected cases: India ink, viral culture, fungal culture, *Toxoplasma* and cryptococci antigens, and coccidioidomycosis titer.

Evaluation of gastrointestinal complaints should proceed by sending stool for Wright stain, ova and parasite testing, acid-fast stain, and culture. Send standard stool cultures, Thayer-Martin culture, *Chlamydia* culture or immunoassay, and viral culture for HSV if proctocolitis is suspected on clinical examination.

HIV-positive patients should receive a head CT scan prior to lumbar puncture if mental status changes are present. MRI scans are superior to CT scan for detection of cerebral toxoplasmosis and other lesions.

Treatment

Manifestations of HIV infection can range from asymptomatic to life-threatening and can affect any organ system. Because of the complexity of opportunistic infections and malignancies occurring in HIV-positive patients, the diagnosis often cannot be made in the emergency department. In general, admit patients if a fever of unknown source or CNS findings are present or in the event of seizure, suspected PCP, hypoxia worse than baseline, intractable diarrhea, disseminated Herpes zoster, marrow suppression, extreme weakness, or inability to care for self or obtain follow-up.

Disposition

Disposition depends on the organ system in question. Ensure that the patient is adequately resuscitated. Final diagnoses may require biopsy or complicated studies to obtain a final diagnosis.

Aftergut K, Cockerell CJ: Update on the cutaneous manifestations of HIV infection. Dermatol Clin 1999;17(3):445. [PMID: 10410852] (Review.)

Barbaro G et al: HIV-associated cardiovascular complications: a new challenge for emergency physicians. Am J Emerg Med 2001;19(7):566. [PMID: 11699002] (Review.)

Patton LL, van der Horst C: Oral infections and other manifestations of HIV disease. Infect Dis Clin North Am 1999;13(4)445. [PMID: 10410852] (Review.)

Stone VE: Primary care of the patient with HIV/AIDS. Infect Dis Clin North Am 2000;14(4):967. [PMID: 11144647] (Review.)

Metabolic & Endocrine Emergencies 41

Micheal D. Rush, MD, & Wason W. S. Louie, MD

Emergency Management of Disorders of Carbohydrate Metabolism

    Diabetic Ketoacidosis

    Hyperglycemic Hyperosmolar Nonketotic Syndrome

    Hyperglycemia without Ketoacidosis or Unrecognized Type 2 Diabetes

    Hypoglycemia

    Lactic Acidosis

    Alcoholic Ketoacidosis

Emergency Management of Other Metabolic & Endocrine Abnormalities

    Thyroid Disorders

      1. Thyroid Storm

      2. Myxedema Coma

    Acute Adrenal Insufficiency/Addisonian Crisis

    Pheochromocytoma

    Pituitary Apoplexy

    Inappropriate Secretion of Antidiuretic Hormone

    Central Diabetes Insipidus

■ EMERGENCY MANAGEMENT OF DISORDERS OF CARBOHYDRATE METABOLISM

Disorders of carbohydrate metabolism represent a broad category of emergent and potentially emergent conditions. Most are related to diabetes and associated complications. They may also occur as a result of or be mimicked by drug or alcohol toxicity, multisystem trauma, head injury, cardiovascular disease, cerebrovascular disease, and infection. Patients may present with coma or altered mental status or look remarkably well clinically yet be on the brink of metabolic decompensation. These disorders may be a challenge not only to diagnose early but also to treat in the most severe cases. Often they are precipitated by underlying illness or injury. Early diagnosis and effective treatment of these underlying entities is a crucial element in resolving the metabolic decompensation.

DIABETIC KETOACIDOSIS

ESSENTIALS OF DIAGNOSIS

• *Signs and symptoms include fatigue, tachypnea (Kussmaul respiration), tachycardia, altered men-*

tal status, abdominal pain, vomiting, polyuria, and polydipsia.

• *Arterial pH < 7.3, serum glucose ≥ 250 mg/dL, and serum bicarbonate ≤ 15 mEq/L.*

General Considerations

Diabetic ketoacidosis (DKA) is the most common acute life-threatening complication of diabetes. It is more commonly seen in type 1 diabetes but may occur rarely in type 2 diabetes. It is a result of insulin-producing β cell failure in the islets of Langerhans located in the pancreas. This results in insulin deficiency, which then shifts the normal metabolic processes from using glucose for fuel to using lipids for fuel. Metabolic stress, most commonly from trauma or infection, may accelerate this process. The result is osmotic diuresis from severe hyperglycemia leading to dehydration, electrolyte loss, and metabolic acidosis, which results from a combination of dehydration and the overproduction of ketone bodies from fat metabolism, primarily β-hydroxybutyrate and acetoacetate, which further acidify the blood. Eventually, hypovolemia leads to inadequate blood flow to the kidneys and limits renal excretion of glucose. As serum osmolality rises above 320 mOsm/L, lethargy and coma may ensue. If left untreated, severe metabolic acidosis from DKA can lead to depression of cardiovascular function, severe hyperkalemia, and potentially lethal cardiac dysrhythmias.

Clinical Findings

A. History

Determine if the patient has diabetes. Direct the history to ascertain potential precipitating causes of DKA:

- Recent or current infection of any type (most common)
- Injury or trauma
- Acute coronary syndrome or myocardial infarction
- Transient ischemic attack or stroke
- Medications (corticosteroids, thiazides, or sympathomimetics)
- Acute or acute-on-chronic pancreatitis
- Alcohol or drug abuse
- Psychosocial factors, such as depression or inability to afford medications, limiting compliance
- Noncompliance with insulin regimen

B. Symptoms and Signs

Symptoms and signs include general fatigue and weakness, abdominal pain (be aware of precipitating causes such as appendicitis, cholecystitis, pancreatitis, and pregnancy), and Kussmaul respirations (rapid deep respirations attempting to compensate for acidosis). Patients may have a fruity or acetone-like smell to the breath. Other findings include polyuria, polydipsia, and polyphagia (the body's attempt to compensate for inefficient use of fuel and water loss in excreting glucose); nausea and vomiting (hemorrhagic gastritis occurs in 25% of patients); altered mental status ranging from agitation to coma; hypothermia (may be fever equivalent; if present, prognosis is poor).

C. Laboratory Findings

1. Key findings—Key laboratory features include serum glucose ≥ 250 mg/dL, ketonuria (ketonemia is unreliable unless β-hydroxybutyrate is measured), serum bicarbonate ≤ 15 mEq/L, and arterial pH < 7.3 (venous pH has been shown to be a consistent, acceptable substitute for arterial pH). Limit arterial blood gas analysis to patients in whom oxygenation or ventilation is a concern or when diagnosis may be uncertain.

2. Serum potassium—Serum potassium is often elevated initially despite total body deficits estimated at 3–5 mEq/kg body weight. Additionally, potassium may be lost through vomiting or urinary losses. Metabolic acidosis shifts potassium out of the cells and into the extracellular fluid space. Because insulin therapy drives potassium back into the cells, serum potassium should be monitored every 2 hours during the first 8 hours of treatment. Low initial serum potassium (< 3.2 mEq/L) represents a severe total body potassium deficit, and

emergent repletion of potassium is essential to prevent life-threatening cardiac dysrhythmias.

3. Serum sodium—Serum sodium is usually low from losses in the urine and vomitus coupled with dilution effects of water being drawn out of the cells into the extracellular compartment by hyperglycemia. This effect can be corrected by adding 1.8 mEq/L to the serum sodium concentration for each 100 mg/dL the serum glucose concentration is above normal. Serum sodium may also be artificially lowered by severe hypertriglyceridemia. Although sodium deficits may approach 7–10 mEq/kg, sodium repletion must proceed gradually to avoid cerebral edema, especially in children.

4. Serum phosphate—Serum phosphate is usually normal or elevated despite deficits approaching 1 mmol/kg body weight. Routine phosphate repletion has not been shown to improve clinical outcomes in DKA and is not indicated. There is significant potential to cause severe hypocalcemia, which may manifest without the typical finding of tetany. Severe hypophosphatemia (< 1 mg/dL) may cause skeletal, cardiac, and respiratory muscle depression; phosphate should be replaced in this circumstance.

5. Other important laboratory findings—

a. Anion gap—Anion gap is useful to assess severity of acidosis and to follow progress of therapy. The anion gap is obtained from the following formula:

$$\text{Anion gap} - [\text{Na}] \ (\text{in mg}/\text{dL}) - [\text{Cl}^-] \ (\text{in mg}/\text{dL})$$
$$+ [\text{HCO}_3^-] \ (\text{in mEq}/\text{L})$$

Normal values are ≤ 10. Effective serum osmolality may be estimated from the following formula:

$$\text{Effective serum osmolality} - 2 \, [\text{Na}] \ (\text{in mg}/\text{dL})$$
$$+ (\text{glucose})/18 \ (\text{in mg}/\text{dL})$$
$$+ [\text{blood urea nitrogen}/2.8] \ (\text{in mg}/\text{dL})$$

Values of at least 320 mOsm/kg are associated with central nervous system involvement, usually lethargy or coma. Below this value, other causes for lethargy or coma such as head injury, subarachnoid hemorrhage, or cerebrovascular accident should be investigated. This value may also be used to diagnose hyperglycemic hyperosmolar nonketotic syndrome (HHNS) or ingestions of ethanol or other osmotically active substances such as ethylene glycol or other alcohols.

b. Serum ketones—Standard laboratory tests measure only acetoacetate. The primary ketone body formed in DKA initially is β-hydroxybutyrate, which is broken down into acetoacetate in the presence of insulin. Serum ketones are not reliable as a diagnostic test because initially they may be reassuringly negative even in a severely ill DKA patient. They are not useful to track therapy because in most cases they will increase as the patient improves.

c. Blood urea nitrogen (BUN) and creatinine—These levels may be elevated because of severe dehydration, even to the point at which acute tubular necrosis and renal failure occur. If these levels are elevated on initial chemistries, be sure to establish urine output prior to initiating potassium repletion.

d. Electrocardiogram—The electrocardiogram (ECG) may reveal severe electrolyte disturbances or diagnose cardiac ischemia or myocardial infarction, a common precipitating cause of DKA or HHNS in older patients. History and physical examination should dictate whether to order cardiac enzymes.

Treatment & Disposition

Given the similar nature of treatment for DKA and HHNS, treatment and patient disposition for these two entities are presented together in the discussion of HHNS, below.

HYPERGLYCEMIC HYPEROSMOLAR NONKETOTIC SYNDROME

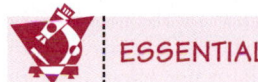 **ESSENTIALS OF DIAGNOSIS**

- *Most symptoms relate to severe dehydration.*
- *Kussmaul respirations and abdominal pain are unusual findings.*
- *Absence of acidosis, small or absent serum ketones, and hyperglycemia usually ≥ 600 mg/dL.*

General Considerations

HHNS, formerly called hyperglycemic hyperosmolar nonketotic coma or hyperosmolar coma, is differentiated from DKA in that patients with HHNS have enough insulin activity to prevent lipolysis and ketogenesis. DKA often manifests suddenly over hours to a few days, whereas HHNS is more insidious, developing over several days to weeks. Also, in mild or early DKA, mental status is normal, whereas in HHNS, mental status is nearly always abnormal, ranging from confusion to stupor or coma. HHNS occurs most commonly in older (> 65 years) patients who may or may not have diagnosed diabetes and who are often residents in chronic care facilities. Symptoms of hyperglycemia such

as frequent urination may be attributed to aging, and the thirst response may be depressed as normal physiology of aging or unrecognized secondary to dementia. Patients also may not have or be given proper access to fluids.

Usually, a severe physiologic stressor, most commonly infection, is a precipitating cause. Myocardial infarction, cerebrovascular accident, trauma, and drug effects or interactions may also precipitate HHNS. Electrolyte deficits are similar in DKA and HHNS, and the free water loss is on the order of 9 L in HHNS compared with an average water loss of 6 L in DKA.

Clinical Findings

A. History

Risk factors for HHNS include age of 65 years or older, residence in a chronic care facility or nursing home, change in diabetes regimen, addition of medications that may elevate glucose levels (eg, corticosteroids, thiazides, anticonvulsants, sympathomimetics), recent or current infection, and dementia.

B. Symptoms and Signs

Symptoms and signs include polydipsia, polyuria, or polyphagia; generalized weakness; altered mental status (clouded thinking to confusion to lethargy or coma); dry mucous membranes; poor skin turgor; and delayed capillary refill. Kussmaul respiration is usually not present unless metabolic acidosis from sepsis or hypoperfusion occurs.

Abdominal pain is not a typical finding in HHNS (in contrast to DKA); its presence merits aggressive investigation for precipitating causes. Acute cholecystitis and appendicitis may be insidious and occur atypically in elderly patients.

C. Laboratory Findings

1. Key laboratory findings—Key findings to diagnose HHNS and differentiate it from DKA include the following:

- Serum glucose is usually ≥ 600 mg/dL.
- Urine or serum ketones are small or absent (a small amount of ketone may be detected secondary to starvation). Glucosuria is prominent.
- Serum bicarbonate is usually > 15 mEq/L.
- pH is usually > 7.30.
- The anion gap may be variable depending on precipitating cause but is usually ≤ 10
- Effective serum osmolality is ≥ 320 mOsm/kg.

2. Serum sodium—In the early stages of HHNS, serum sodium findings are similar to those in patients with DKA. Urinary losses and fluid shifts out of the cell and into the extracellular compartment create hyponatremia usually in the 125–130 mg/dL range (remember to correct by adding 1.8 mg/dL for every 100 mg/dL glucose above normal). As water losses worsen, hypernatremia ensues and osmolality rises, leading to progressive lethargy and coma.

3. Serum potassium—Potassium levels will most commonly be normal or low, unless renal failure is present. An associated metabolic acidosis driving potassium out of the cells is usually not present in HHNS.

4. Blood urea nitrogen and creatinine—BUN is often markedly elevated. Gastrointestinal bleeding may also elevate BUN, and this is a possible precipitating cause of HHNS in elderly patients.

5. Other studies—Other studies should be dictated by the history and physical examination findings, but have a low threshold to obtain serial ECGs and cardiac enzymes to rule out cardiac ischemia or myocardial infarction, computed tomography (CT) scan of the head to rule out cerebrovascular accident or subdural hematoma, and rectal exam and nasogastric tube to look for gastrointestinal hemorrhage. Order an abdominal CT scan or ultrasound to work up abdominal pain if the patient is stable enough to leave the emergency department.

Treatment

Initial treatment for DKA and HHNS is similar. The various aspects of therapy should be initiated concurrently whenever possible. Differences in therapy of DKA and HHNS are noted when appropriate. Frequent reassessment of vital signs, mental status, and laboratory parameters are essential to successful therapy of DKA and HHNS.

A. Resuscitation Issues

Assess the airway and consider obtaining arterial blood gases for any patient who appears not to be oxygenating or ventilating properly or who is obtunded or comatose. Consider proceeding directly to rapid-sequence intubation in patients who are unresponsive or who have depressed gag or swallow reflexes. Avoid succinylcholine if hyperkalemia is suspected based on peaked T waves on ECG or rhythm strip.

Oxygen therapy is indicated for all DKA or HHNS patients at flow rates adequate to maintain oxygen saturation above 96% or $P_{O_2} \geq 70$ mm Hg. Hypoxia should trigger an investigation for aspiration, pneumonia, or pulmonary edema in the differential diagnosis of precipitating causes.

B. Fluid Therapy

Fluid therapy is dictated by 3 parameters: vital signs, corrected serum sodium, and serum glucose. Overall fluid deficits approach 6–10 L in most patients, and daily maintenance fluid requirements must also be considered. Multiple, preferably large-bore ($\geq$ 18-gauge), intravenous lines are essential. Central venous access should be strongly considered.

Hypotension should prompt a bolus of 1 L of 0.9% NaCl solution to restore blood pressure to at least 90 mm Hg.

Caution: Assess patients for cardiogenic shock and renal failure before giving large volumes of intravenous fluids. Reassess patients frequently for adequate urine output and absence of pulmonary edema or congestive heart failure. Hemodynamic monitoring (Swan-Ganz) is indicated to facilitate fluid management if cardiogenic shock is present. In the absence of hypotension, administer 1–1.5 L (~ 15–20 mL/kg) normal saline in the first hour of therapy.

Using the serum sodium corrected for excess glucose:

- If serum sodium is high or normal, give 0.45% NaCl or half normal saline at a rate of 5–15 mL/kg for the next liter of fluids.
- If serum sodium is low, give 0.9% NaCl or normal saline for next liter of fluids at a rate of 5–15 mL/kg.
- Once serum glucose reaches approximately 250 mg/dL, 5% dextrose in 0.45% NaCl is the fluid of choice at a rate of 250 mL/h; or use 5% dextrose in normal saline if the corrected serum sodium remains low.

Follow serum electrolytes, venous pH, BUN and creatinine, and glucose, and calculate the osmolality frequently (every 2 hours in the first 8 hours) as measures of progress in therapy. The aim is a decrease in serum osmolality of no more than ~ 3 mOsm/kg/h. Urine output may be unreliable while glucose levels remain high secondary to osmotic diuresis. Once glucose levels approach normal, urine output may be used to guide therapy; 30–50 cc/h is considered adequate.

C. Electrolyte Replacement

1. Potassium—Potassium repletion may commence once urine output is confirmed and should be accomplished according to the following algorithm, with target levels of 4.0–5.0 mEq/L:

- If serum potassium is 3.3 mEq/L or less, hold insulin therapy and give 40 mEq/h intravenously as potassium chloride or as a mixture of two-thirds potassium chloride and one-third potassium phosphate (~ 5 mmol) if serum phosphate is less than 1 mmol/L. If patient is not vomiting, potassium chloride, 20–40 mEq, may also be given orally or by nasogastric tube. Assume a deficit of about 100 mEq potassium for each 1 mEq/L below normal.

- If serum potassium is 3.3–5.0 mEq/L, give 20–30 mEq potassium chloride in each liter of intravenous fluid.
- If serum potassium is 5.0 mEq/L or more, hold potassium repletion and recheck serum potassium in 2 hours.
- Follow serum potassium every 2 hours during the first 8 hours of therapy.

D. INSULIN THERAPY

Insulin therapy for DKA and HHNS is generally accomplished intravenously using regular human insulin. Subcutaneous insulin may be absorbed erratically in severely volume-depleted patients. Begin therapy with a bolus of 0.1–0.15 U/kg body weight. In DKA this dose rapidly halts lipolysis and further ketogenesis. In HHNS it helps in rapidly lowering very high serum glucose and halting further water loss to osmotic diuresis. Start a continuous infusion at 0.1 U/kg body weight per hour, and monitor capillary blood glucose hourly. If glucose is not decreasing at least 50–70 mg/dL/h, insulin dosage may be doubled hourly until this rate of decline is achieved. Hold insulin therapy for any potassium level less than 3.3 mEq/L until repletion is undertaken and the level has risen on recheck in 2 hours.

E. SODIUM BICARBONATE THERAPY

Sodium bicarbonate therapy is generally indicated only for severe cases of DKA (arterial pH < 6.9). Bicarbonate therapy will seldom if ever be indicated for HHNS. At pH higher than 6.9, no benefit has been proved in controlled trials on DKA outcomes, whereas studies have shown aggressive bicarbonate therapy leading to increased rates of cerebral edema, especially in children. No controlled data exist on bicarbonate therapy when pH is less than 6.9. Given the catastrophic potential of such severe acidosis on cellular metabolism, bicarbonate therapy is indicated in these patients and is accomplished by giving 100 mmol of $NaHCO_3$ diluted in a 500-cc bag of 5% dextrose in water given over 2 hours. This may be repeated every 2 hours until venous pH is greater than 7.0

F. TREATMENT OF SUSPECTED OR KNOWN PRECIPITATING CAUSES

Infection is the most common precipitating cause of DKA and HHNS. Be sure to examine the patient's entire skin surface for wounds and cellulitis. Obtain a urine pregnancy test and conduct a pelvic examination in women of child-bearing age who have DKA to rule out pelvic inflammatory disease or pregnancy as sources

of physiologic stress. Analysis and cultures of all appropriate body fluids (blood, sputum, urine, cerebrospinal fluid) should be obtained as dictated by the history and physical examination or broadly in obtunded or comatose patients. Consider empiric administration of broad-spectrum antibiotics until culture results are available. Treat other precipitating causes as they become known, for example, cardiac catheterization and percutaneous transluminal coronary angioplasty for myocardial infarction.

G. FLOW SHEET

It is a good idea to organize vital signs, mental status findings, monitored laboratory values, intravenous fluid therapy types and rates, insulin dosages, electrolyte repletion, urine output, and bicarbonate administration (if any) into a flow sheet that can be included in the patient's chart.

Disposition

Patients with all but the mildest cases of DKA and all patients with HHNS should have cardiac monitoring and a higher level of nursing care for at least 24 hours. Whether the patient goes to an intermediate care or telemetry unit or the intensive care unit is based on severity of the case and response to initial therapy as judged by the treating physician.

Kitabchi AE et al: Management of hyperglycemic crises in patients with diabetes mellitus. (Technical Review). Diabetes Care 2001;24:131. [PMID: 11194218] (Definitive and extremely comprehensive review on diagnosis and therapy of DKA and HHNS by the foremost authorities in these aspects of endocrinology and diabetes care. Contains helpful therapeutic algorithms.)

Hyperglycemia without Ketoacidosis or Unrecognized Type 2 Diabetes

Hyperglycemia in the absence of metabolic decompensation (DKA or HHNS) is an increasingly common finding in the emergency department. Obesity, pre-diabetes, and diabetes are epidemic in the United States. Sedentary lifestyles and high-carbohydrate and high-fat diets have contributed to the epidemic. Patients with diabetes may present with hyperglycemia from self-monitored blood glucose, or they may have no history of diabetes. Patients without diabetes may present with symptoms of hyperglycemia, most typically polydipsia, polyuria, fatigue, and blurred vision, or they may present with one or more complications of unrecognized diabetes, such as ischemic heart disease, cerebral or peripheral vascular disease, nonhealing wounds, or persistent or recurrent infections (especially of the skin and genitourinary tract). Some patients present with unrelated complaints, and diabetes and hyperglycemia are found incidentally. The astute emergency clinician should know the risk factors for type 2 diabetes and recognize any of these symptomatic presentations as an indication to investigate the possibility of hyperglycemia or unrecognized diabetes.

Clinical Findings

A. History

Risk factors for hyperglycemia and unrecognized type 2 diabetes are listed in Table 41–1.

B. Symptoms and Signs

Symptoms of hyperglycemia may include polydipsia, polyuria, polyphagia, weakness, fatigue, headache, blurred vision, lightheadedness, or dizziness. When present, symptoms are generally mild to moderate.

Superficial skin and skin structure infections (cellulitis, furuncles, abscesses, nonhealing wounds or ulcers), urinary tract infections, candidal genital infections, malignant otitis externa, and rhinocerebral mucormycosis all have epidemiologic associations to hyperglycemia and diabetes. Chronic hyperglycemia impairs neutrophil function and other cellular immune responses. Glycosuria is thought to contribute directly to urine bacterial colonization.

To excrete excess glucose, large volumes of water are lost, and the patient rapidly becomes dehydrated if fluid intake is not keeping up. Symptoms may include weakness, dizziness, near-syncope, and headache. Signs

Table 41–1. Risk factors for hyperglycemia and unrecognized diabetes mellitus.

Age 45 years or older
Obesity (body mass index ≥ 25 kg/m²)
Family history in first-degree relative
Habitual physical inactivity
Ethnicity (African Americans, Hispanic Americans, Asian Americans, Native Americans, and Pacific Islanders are all at greater risk for diabetes than are whites.)
History of gestational diabetes or delivering an infant weighing ≥ 9 lb
Hypertension (≥ 140/90 mm Hg)
Dyslipidemia (high-density lipoproteins ≤ 35 mg/dL or triglycerides ≥ 250 mg/dL)
Polycystic ovary disease
History of impaired fasting glucose or impaired glucose tolerance
Vascular disease, peripheral or cerebral

are sunken eyes, poor skin turgor, and poor capillary refill.

C. Laboratory Findings

Random serum glucose of greater than 200 mg/dL in the setting of symptoms of hyperglycemia or metabolic decompensation (DKA or HHNS) or fasting serum glucose of greater than 126 mg/dL on repeat occasions are both diagnostic of diabetes. Impaired fasting glucose is defined as a fasting plasma glucose of 110–126 mg/dL.

Glycosylated hemoglobin, or A1C, is increasingly available as a rapid assay, and the role of A1C in diagnosing diabetes is evolving. Levels of 6.1% or more are about 80% sensitive in diagnosing diabetes; levels of 7.0% or more are nearly always consistent with diabetes.

It is always prudent to assume that severe hyperglycemia (≥ 400 mg/dL) represents impending decompensation. An underlying cause should be sought aggressively, most commonly infection, but cardiac ischemia or myocardial infarction sometimes occur and an ECG plus cardiac enzymes may be helpful. Lack of compliance with antidiabetic regimen or diet should always be exclusionary. Have a low threshold in this setting to check electrolytes and BUN and creatinine to screen for metabolic decompensation, severe electrolyte imbalance, and renal insufficiency.

Treatment

A growing body of literature suggests that hyperglycemia is a risk factor for adverse outcomes and that tight glucose control is a strong component of therapy for nearly every acute illness or injury experienced by diabetes patients. If hyperglycemia is mild (< 300 mg/dL), patients are not significantly volume-depleted, no specific cause is identified, and medical follow-up is readily available, no specific treatment is required other than to refer patients to primary care for diabetes testing (fasting plasma glucose is preferred over oral glucose tolerance test) or for adjustment of antidiabetic regimen in patients with known diabetes. When serum glucose is greater than 300 mg/dL, treatment is as follows:

A. Fluids

Normal saline or lactated Ringer's solution, 1 L given over 1 hour, may be adequate monotherapy for hyperglycemia.

B. Insulin

Mildly volume-depleted patients may be given 0.1 U/kg regular human insulin or insulin lispro (Humalog) or insulin aspart (Novolog) subcutaneously. Regular insulin at a dose of 0.1–0.15 U/kg should be given intravenously to dehydrated patients because subcutaneous insulin absorption may be erratic in these patients. Insulin may be rebolused intravenously if glucose does not decline by 50–75 mg/dL in the first hour.

C. Oral Hypoglycemic Agents

Oral hypoglycemic agents are generally not indicated for acute therapy of severe hyperglycemia, but if a patient is newly diagnosed with diabetes, the emergency physician may wish to prescribe an oral agent on discharge. Metformin, which inhibits fasting hepatic glucose production and promotes weight loss, is the oral agent least likely to cause hypoglycemia. Metformin can be safely started at 500 mg orally once per day; the dosage can be increased by 500 mg/d each week until 500 mg 4 times a day is reached. Metformin therapy may be initiated if serum creatinine levels are 1.4 mg/dL or lower. Above this level, the patient is at risk for developing lactic acidosis. Sulfonylurea or insulin therapy is best undertaken after the patient has received diabetes education and knows the symptoms of hypoglycemia, how to treat them, and when to call for help. If adjusting an existing oral agent or insulin dosage, it is a good rule of thumb not to increase insulin dosages by more than 10% or sulfonylurea dosage by more than about 20%. Patients may also be taking insulin resistance–reduction agents such as thiazolidinediones or agents that inhibit breakdown of complex carbohydrates in the small intestine, such as α glucosidase inhibitors.

D. Treatment of Underlying Causes

Treat any underlying causes for hyperglycemia appropriately as they are discovered (eg, antibiotics for urinary tract infection).

Disposition

Most patients with hyperglycemia in the absence of metabolic decompensation can be safely discharged after thorough evaluation for underlying causes and therapy has reduced blood glucose to less than 250–300 mg/dL. Patients with serious underlying causes or in whom hyperglycemia is resistant to treatment should be hospitalized for further workup and treatment.

Expert Committee on the Diagnosis and Classification of Diabetes Mellitus: Report of the Expert Committee on the Diagnosis and Classification of Diabetes Mellitus. Diabetes Care 2003;26(Suppl. 1):S5. [PMID:12502614] (Defines the various types of diabetes, their presentation, and diagnostic criteria.)

Montori VM, Bistrian BR, McMahon MM: Hyperglycemia in acutely ill patients. JAMA 2002;288:2167. [PMID: 12413377] (Outstanding brief review of the pathophysiology of hyperglycemia, its causes, and the rationale and literature supporting aggressive blood glucose control in acutely ill patients.)

HYPOGLYCEMIA

 ESSENTIALS OF DIAGNOSIS

- *Common signs and symptoms include irritability, diaphoresis, and tachycardia related to increased circulating catecholamines.*
- *As hypoglycemia progresses, neuroglycopenic effects range from focal neurologic deficits such as diplopia and paresthesias to coma.*
- *Always remember to check the fingerstick blood glucose on every patient presenting with altered mental status or who appears to be acutely ill.*

Causes

Hypoglycemia may occur for many reasons. Most commonly hypoglycemia results from an excess of endogenous or exogenous insulin or oral hypoglycemic agents, such as sulfonylureas. Failure of other organs that either produce glucose or mediate the production of glucose and glucose homeostasis may also precipitate hypoglycemia.

A. Exogenous Insulin

In patients with known diabetes, hypoglycemia may occur as a result of the following:

- Delay in eating after taking insulin, or general malnutrition or inadequate caloric intake from acute nausea and vomiting or gastroparesis
- Increased or unusual physical exertion
- Increased physiologic stress resulting from illness (most commonly infection or sepsis), injury, or emotional upset
- Excessive dose of exogenous insulin (**Note:** Remember to check the patient's vision and confirm that he or she can read the syringe appropriately.)
- Variable absorption from injection site
- Impaired counter-regulatory hormone axis (glucagon and epinephrine) secondary to autonomic failure caused by iatrogenic (insulin therapy–related) hypoglycemia
- Excessive insulin release produced by sulfonylurea drugs, especially in the presence of renal insufficiency
- Alterations in therapeutic regimen, particularly increases in insulin or oral agent dosages or the addition of new oral agents such as thiazolidinediones, which may reduce insulin resistance and improve therapeutic action of endogenous or exogenous insulin

Rarely, insulin or sulfonylurea drugs have been given to nondiabetics with the intent to harm. Comprehensive toxicology, insulin, and C-peptide levels can help diagnose these problems. C-peptide is not present in manufactured insulin; therefore, a high insulin level without a correspondingly high C-peptide level is diagnostic of insulin overdose.

B. PANCREATIC β CELL TUMOR

Tumor of the insulin-secreting β cells in the islets of Langerhans may cause refractory hypoglycemia and even coma. C-peptide levels will elevate concurrently with insulin levels.

C. ALCOHOL

Excessive ethanol intake, especially without adequate caloric intake, may cause severe hypoglycemia. Alcohol abuse depletes hepatic glycogen production and storage and also reduces NADH-mediated gluconeogenesis. *Caution:* Administer thiamine, 100 mg, prior to giving large amounts of glucose to alcoholic patients with hypoglycemia to avoid Wernicke encephalopathy.

D. POSTPRANDIAL OR REACTIVE HYPOGLYCEMIA

The intake of large amounts of calories in nondiabetics may produce enough excess insulin to induce mildly symptomatic hypoglycemia. Seldom is the hypoglycemia severe enough or persistent enough to cause decreased level of consciousness or coma.

Clinical Findings

A. HISTORY

Try to obtain history of diabetes from emergency medical services; family; or Medic Alert bracelet, necklace, or wallet card. Emergency medical services or family may also be helpful in disclosing alcohol use, recent caloric intake, alterations of medication regimen, and recent illness or injury.

B. SYMPTOMS AND SIGNS

Most early symptoms and signs are the result of increased catecholamine release (glucose usually 30–50 mg/dL): tachycardia, irritability, diaphoresis, paresthesias, hunger, decreased concentration. Later or more severe symptoms and signs of neuroglycopenia (glucose usually < 30 mg/dL) include confusion or bizarre behavior; visual disturbances (blurred vision, diplopia, hallucinations); hypothermia; seizurelike activity (myoclonus, tremor) and even seizures; focal neurologic deficits similar to Todd paralysis that resolve with glucose administration or remain transiently; and lethargy, syncope, or coma.

C. LABORATORY FINDINGS

The capillary or fingerstick glucose test is the most rapid diagnostic method to test blood glucose levels. Because glucometers can become unreliable at readings less than 40 mg/dL, always try to draw a serum or plasma sample for glucose before administration of glucose.

Search for ancillary causes of hypoglycemia such as infection or sepsis, myocardial infarction, cerebrovascular accident, alcohol use, pregnancy, drug use (particularly stimulants), occult trauma, depression (poor caloric intake or insulin or oral agent overdose), other endocrinopathies (Addison disease, myxedema, thyrotoxicosis, pituitary insufficiency) as dictated by history and physical examination, and, when appropriate or if history is not available, laboratory studies.

Treatment

A. AIRWAY

Make sure the patient's tongue is not obstructing the airway and that the gag reflex and preferably the ability to phonate and swallow are present.

B. EMERGENCY THERAPEUTIC MEASURES

1. Intravenous glucose—If intravenous access is readily obtainable, administer 50 cc of 50% dextrose in water (containing approximately 25 g of glucose, which is enough to resolve most hypoglycemic episodes). *Caution:* Remember to give thiamine, 100 mg intravenously or intramuscularly, to alcoholic patients prior to administration of glucose to prevent Wernicke encephalopathy. Monitor the patient's mental status and recheck capillary blood glucose 30 minutes after glucose administration. Repeat dosages of 50% glucose or even infusion of glucose glucose-containing intravenous fluids (5–10%) may be necessary to maintain adequate blood glucose levels. Neuroglycopenia (altered level of consciousness, seizurelike activity, focal neurologic deficits) may take time to resolve completely; however, if abnormalities persist longer than 30 minutes after glucose administration and hypoglycemia has not recurred, other causes should be investigated with a head CT scan and appropriate laboratory studies.

2. Oral feeding—As soon as the patient regains consciousness, clear fruit juice (eg, apple, grape; 6 oz = ~ 15 g glucose) is a good choice to maintain glucose levels, and if the patient has not eaten, a snack or meal is appropriate.

3. Glucagon—If intravenous access is not readily available, 1 mg of glucagon may be given intramuscularly. The response time is typically 10–15 minutes, and nausea and vomiting along with overcorrection of glucose levels are common. Given that glucagon can be given intramuscularly, all patients with insulin-treated diabetes (or their families) should carry and be familiar with the use of glucagon emergency kits, which come with syringe, lyophilized glucagon, and diluent.

4. Monitoring—Consider the duration of action of the insulin and/or oral agents taken by the patient. Hourly capillary glucose checks should be taken until glucose levels are stable. Generally the patient should be observed through the peak time of the longest-acting insulin, typically 30 minutes to 1 hour after the dose with insulin lispro or insulin aspart, 2 hours with regular insulin, or 6 hours with NPH. Insulin glargine has no peak activity and does not generally cause hypoglycemia by itself. Patients taking long-acting insulins with peak activity, such as lente or ultralente, and patients taking sulfonylurea oral agents should generally be observed for a day in the hospital.

Disposition

Indications for admission include persistent or recurrent hypoglycemia despite appropriate therapy, hypoglycemia related to an oral agent or long-acting insulin, or serious ancillary cause (eg, severe infection, persistent nausea and vomiting).

Conditions for discharge include availability of responsible adult to be with the patient for next 8–12 hours; ability to take oral fluids and food; medical follow-up available within 24–48 hours; and ability to (and understanding of the need to) perform blood glucose checks, especially if changes are made in the therapeutic regimen.

American Diabetes Association: Position Statement: Hospital admission guidelines for diabetes mellitus. Diabetes Care 2003;26(Suppl. 1):S118. [PMID: 12502634] (American Diabetes Association recommendations on when to admit patients with hypoglycemia.)

Cryer PE: Hypoglycaemia: the limiting factor in the glycaemic management of type I and type II diabetes. Diabetologia 2002;45:937. [PMID: 12136392] (An excellent review of therapeutic hypoglycemia and the counter-regulatory response, both normal and pathologic.)

McAulay V, Deary IJ, Frier BM: Symptoms of hypoglycaemia in people with diabetes. Diabet Med 2001;18:690. [PMID: 11606166] (Extensive review of literature on clinical presentation and symptomatology in diabetes-related hypoglycemia.)

LACTIC ACIDOSIS

General Considerations

Lactic acidosis is a common complication of critical illness. It is defined as serum lactic acid concentration greater than 5 mmol/L and arterial pH less than 7.35. Typically lactic acidosis results from the metabolism of glucose in the presence of inadequate tissue oxygenation or inadequate disposal of lactic acid by the liver. Severe acidosis can lead to impairment of cardiac contractility, increased pulmonary vascular resistance, sensitization of the myocardium to dysrhythmias, hyperkalemia, and inhibition of metabolism at the cellular or molecular level. The mortality rate is high, approaching 40–60%.

Causes

Lactic acidosis may occur in any severe illness in which the combination of inadequate tissue oxygenation, inadequate tissue perfusion, and inadequate lactic acid disposal is present. Common underlying causes include the following:

- Respiratory, hepatic, renal, or heart failure
- Sepsis
- Shock
- Cancer, especially leukemias
- Acute infarction of lung, bowel, or extremities
- Severe abdominal or multisystem trauma
- Alcohol, methanol, or ethylene glycol poisoning
- Drugs: cocaine, metformin, isoniazid

Clinical Findings

Diagnostic efforts should focus on finding the underlying cause of the lactic acidosis. Treatment of the underlying cause is crucial to recovery.

A. SYMPTOMS AND SIGNS

The clinical presentation varies according to the underlying illness or injury. Symptoms may include hyperventilation, generalized weakness, abdominal pain, or hypotension. Often there is a general lack of symptoms, especially in the early stages of the underlying pathology. As a result, diagnosis is frequently difficult in the period when the underlying illness and the acidosis itself are most treatable. A high index of suspicion is essential in older patients and in patients with the underlying illnesses identified above.

B. LABORATORY FINDINGS

Laboratory findings include pH less than 7.35 and often less than 7.2; anion gap greater than 15 mEq/L; and lack of explanation of acidosis by other causes—such as salicylates; alcohol, methanol, or ethylene glycol poisoning; or diabetic or alcoholic ketoacidosis. Hyperphosphatemia is a common finding secondary to anaerobic glycolysis or cellular disruption. Samples collected for lactate should be chilled immediately and centrifuged promptly to avoid continued lactic acid production by red and white blood cells, which can distort results.

Treatment

Detailed attention to resuscitation issues is essential in improving outcome. Improving tissue oxygenation through delivery of adequate oxygen through the lungs and adequate perfusion to carry the oxygen to the tissues via the circulatory system is critical.

A. Oxygen

High flow rates are indicated. Consider rapid-sequence intubation, mechanical ventilation, or noninvasive ventilation (eg, bilevel positive airway pressure) when arterial blood gas analysis indicates that oxygenation or ventilation is inadequate.

B. Fluids

Rapid infusion of 1 L of 0.9% saline is indicated to restore intravascular volume. Reassess the patient frequently to avoid volume overload in the setting of acute renal failure or cardiogenic shock and circulatory failure.

C. Pressors

Avoid vasoconstrictive pressors such as norepinephrine and higher doses of β active pressors such as dopamine and dobutamine because they tend only to worsen tissue hypoxia. Low doses of dopamine and dobutamine may improve cardiac output and renal blood flow and are worth trying.

D. Sodium Bicarbonate

The use of sodium bicarbonate is one of the most controversial issues in the treatment of metabolic acidosis. The majority of data available suggest that at pH levels greater than 6.9, no benefit has been shown supporting the administration of sodium bicarbonate, at least in the clinical settings of severe metabolic acidosis resulting from DKA and sepsis. Significant risks of administering bicarbonate include hypernatremia and hyperosmolality, volume overload, paradoxical increase of intracellular acidosis secondary to excess carbon dioxide as a result of bicarbonate metabolism, and cerebral edema. If pH is less than 6.9, especially if the patient is exhibiting one or more complications of severe acidosis as listed above, consider administering 1–2 amps (~ 44 mEq/amp) diluted in 1 L of 5% dextrose in water or 0.2% saline infused over 2 hours. Reassess pH after allowing at least 2 hours for equilibration.

E. Treatment of Underlying Causes

Treatment of underlying causes may include revascularization therapy or balloon pump support in patients with cardiogenic shock, antibiotics for suspected sepsis after appropriate culture material is obtained, amputation or revascularization of ischemic extremities, removal or revascularization of ischemic bowel, hemodialysis for renal failure, or removal of toxic components such as ethylene glycol or methanol.

Disposition

The prognosis is grim, and mortality is high. Prompt identification and treatment of the underlying root cause of lactic acidosis remains the best hope for a positive outcome.

Adrogue HJ, Madias NE: Management of life-threatening acid-base disorders. N Engl J Med 1998;338:26. [PMID: 9414329] (Excellent overview of pathophysiology of severe acidosis and the management of several common causes.)

Forsythe SM, Schmidt GA: Sodium bicarbonate for the treatment of lactic acidosis. Chest 2000;117:260. [PMID: 10631227] (An intelligent debate on the rationale, or more accurately lack thereof, for giving sodium bicarbonate as therapy for severe metabolic acidosis.)

ALCOHOLIC KETOACIDOSIS

 ESSENTIALS OF DIAGNOSIS

- Signs include tachypnea (Kussmaul respirations are common), tachycardia, abdominal tenderness, poor skin turgor, and delayed capillary refill.
- In general, serum glucose < 250 mg/dL distinguishes alcoholic ketoacidosis from DKA.

General Considerations

Alcoholic ketoacidosis (AKA) typically occurs in the alcoholic patient who is on a long drinking binge and either is unwilling or unable to take in food calories secondary to nausea and vomiting, gastritis, or pancreatitis. Lipolysis is driven by the lack of caloric intake and catecholamine release from alcohol intoxication or withdrawal. Acid-base disturbances are frequently mixed in these patients because volume depletion alkalosis and respiratory alkalosis frequently coincide. As in DKA, underlying causes and contributors such as infection, trauma, gastrointestinal hemorrhage, hepatic or renal failure, concurrent cocaine or methamphetamine use, and rhabdomyolysis must be investigated and treated as part of the overall diagnostic and therapeutic plan.

Clinical Findings

A. History

The patient's history most often includes a recent or ongoing alcohol binge with poor food intake, nausea and vomiting, and abdominal pain.

B. Symptoms and Signs

The physical examination most often shows tachypnea (Kussmaul respirations are common), tachycardia, and abdominal tenderness to palpation. Poor skin turgor and delayed capillary refill are also common. Fever is not generally part of the syndrome, and causes of fever should be sought aggressively.

C. Laboratory Findings

1. Metabolic acidosis—Low pH (often < 7.2) and low serum bicarbonate are common.

2. Plasma or urine ketones—Most of the ketone bodies produced in AKA are β-hydroxybutyrate, which does not show up on the standard test for ketones in serum or urine. Negative initial ketone test does not rule out AKA.

3. Electrolyte disorders—Hyponatremia, hyperkalemia, hypokalemia, hypophosphatemia, hypomagnesemia, and hypocalcemia are common findings in patients with AKA.

4. Glucose—Glucose levels range from hypoglycemia to moderately elevated (up to 250 mg/dL) in the absence of diabetes.

5. Alcohol levels—Alcohol levels may not be elevated by time of presentation because the patient may not have been able to maintain oral intake of even alcohol for some time. Be alert for signs and symptoms of alcohol withdrawal or delirium tremens.

Treatment

A. Glucose

After giving thiamine, 100 mg intravenously or intramuscularly, give 5% dextrose solution in 0.9% normal saline, 1 L/h for the first 1–2 hours; 5% dextrose in 0.45% normal saline is then appropriate at 250 cc/h.

B. Potassium

Total body potassium levels are generally low secondary to losses from vomiting, but severe acidosis may elevate serum potassium levels and AKA patients may present with hyperkalemia. If urine output is established, up to 20 mEq/L of potassium chloride may be given per hour. If vomiting is controlled, consider supplementing with oral potassium chloride at up to 40 mEq every 2 hours. Assume a total body deficit of at least 100 mEq of potassium for each 1 mEq/L below normal. Potassium levels should be reevaluated every 2 hours for the first 4–8 hours of therapy.

C. Insulin

Generally, mild hyperglycemia will resolve with intravenous fluid therapy. Intravenous insulin, 0.1 units regular insulin/kg, may be required along with glucose to treat severe hyperkalemia (> 6.0 mEq/L) if changes such as peaked T waves, prolonged QRS interval, or loss of P waves are evident on the ECG.

D. Magnesium

Consider giving magnesium sulfate, 1–2 g, empirically in the first liter of fluid because magnesium deficiency is extremely common in alcoholic patients. This therapy makes the myocardium less susceptible to dysrhythmias and also helps restore calcium homeostasis.

E. Bicarbonate

Bicarbonate is indicated only as therapy for acute hyperkalemia; acidosis generally responds rapidly to volume repletion.

F. Treatment of Underlying Causes

Do not assume that severe abdominal pain is due to AKA alone; pancreatitis or upper gastrointestinal bleeding are often concurrent illnesses contributing to AKA.

Disposition

Although metabolic problems tend to correct reasonably rapidly with intravenous fluids and glucose administration, most AKA patients are extremely unreliable and would have difficulty complying with outpatient treatment and follow-up. Alcohol withdrawal may also complicate the course as the ketoacidosis improves. Hospitalization for observation is a prudent choice for patients with AKA.

Fulop M: Alcoholic ketoacidosis. Endocrinol Metab Clin North Am 1993;22:209. [PMID: 8325283] (Most recent comprehensive review on the topic in English.)

Wrenn KD et al: The syndrome of alcoholic ketoacidosis. Am J Med 1991;91:119. [PMID: 1867237] (Presents the only existing data on emergency department patients (retrospective) with AKA regarding clinical presentation, underlying illnesses, and laboratory findings.)

EMERGENCY MANAGEMENT OF OTHER METABOLIC & ENDOCRINE ABNORMALITIES

THYROID DISORDERS

1. Thyroid Storm

 ESSENTIALS OF DIAGNOSIS

- Typical stigmata of hyperthyroidism, thyromegaly, ophthalmopathy, tremor, stare, diaphoresis, and agitation.
- Fever (usually).
- Tachycardia (out of proportion to fever) often with associated atrial arrhythmias.
- Mental status changes ranging from confusion to coma.

General Considerations

Thyroid storm represents a disorder of extreme thyrotoxicosis, or the overproduction of thyroid hormone. Thyroid storm, if not diagnosed and treated promptly, is a life-threatening emergency. The diagnosis is made clinically, and although laboratory testing may suggest the diagnosis, interpretation of thyroid function tests in the setting of acute illness may be difficult. No laboratory test is available that will confirm the diagnosis. The classic findings of thyroid storm include fever (> 38.5 °C [101.5 °F]); tachycardia out of proportion to fever; gastrointestinal symptoms; cardiovascular symptoms; and central nervous system abnormalities, most commonly confusion, agitation, or delirium rather than lethargy, obtundation, or coma.

Causes

Thyroid storm is frequently associated with serious concurrent illness or injury. Common factors that may trigger thyroid storm include infection, recent surgery, trauma, pregnancy, stroke, metabolic disorders such as diabetic ketoacidosis, radioiodine therapy, drug abuse (stimulants most commonly), alcohol abuse, iodinated contrast material, and discontinuation of antithyroid medications.

Clinical Findings

The diagnosis of thyroid storm is made clinically. Laboratory results may be of little help because thyroid hormone secretion and metabolism may be altered by acute stress or illness and may not be significantly abnormal. Most patients who present with thyroid storm have had a history of partially treated hyperthyroidism or have signs and symptoms of antecedent thyroid disease, such as thyromegaly, proptosis, stare, myopathy, or myxedema. The diagnosis should be made empirically and treatment initiated when a patient with prior or current thyroid disease decompensates rapidly in the setting of fever, tachycardia, central nervous system hyperactivity, and unexplained cardiac or gastrointestinal symptomatology.

A. Symptoms and Signs

Fever is characteristic and may exceed 40 °C (104 °F). The fever may be primarily from thyrotoxicosis or may be secondary to a precipitating infection. Always assume infection is the primary cause, obtain appropriate cultures, and treat accordingly with empiric broad-spectrum antibiotics.

Cardiac findings include sinus tachycardia, supraventricular tachycardia, atrial arrhythmias, and congestive heart failure. The tachycardia seen with a thyroid storm is usually out of proportion to the fever. Gastrointestinal symptoms include nausea, vomiting, diarrhea, abdominal pain, and in rare cases jaundice. Mental status changes are commonly seen. Patients may present with delirium, confusion, psychosis, or coma. Neuromuscular findings include agitation, tremor, generalized weakness (especially in the proximal muscles), and periodic paralysis.

Findings consistent with prior thyroid disease include thyromegaly, orbitopathy, tremor, stare, pretibial myxedema and other integumentary changes such as coarse hair and thick, dry skin. Death may occur from hypovolemic shock, coma, congestive heart failure, tachydysrhythmias, or any combination of these.

Apathetic hyperthyroidism is important to consider in the elderly population. Because of advanced age and other comorbid conditions, the classic signs and symptoms of thyroid storm and thyrotoxicosis may be subtle or absent. This may make diagnosis of thyrotoxicosis especially difficult in the elderly population.

B. Laboratory Findings

Thyroid function tests are frequently not helpful in diagnosing acute thyroid storm. Previous abnormal thyroid test may inform the clinician of a preexisting thyrotoxicosis but will not confirm the diagnosis of a thyroid storm. The most helpful thyroid function tests are thyroid-stimulating hormone (TSH), which will be markedly low in most patients with thyroid storm, and free thyroxine (T_4), which will be elevated. These studies may not be readily available in a timely manner to all emergency department clinicians. Electrolyte and glucose abnormalities may be present, most commonly resulting from gastrointestinal losses, dehydration, physiologic stress, and fever.

Laboratory and imaging studies should be directed toward findings in the history and physical examination. Blood cultures, urine cultures, chest X-ray, complete blood count (CBC) with differential, chemistry panel, and ECG and cardiac enzymes are generally indicated to look for precipitating causes. Head CT scan is indicated for delirious or comatose patients.

C. ELECTROCARDIOGRAPHIC FINDINGS

The ECG is usually abnormal; common findings are sinus tachycardia, increased QRS interval and P wave voltage, nonspecific ST-T wave changes and atrial dysrhythmias, usually atrial fibrillation or flutter. Conduction defects, most commonly first-degree AV block and nonspecific interventricular conduction delay, may occur. Ischemic findings or myocardial infarction may be present, especially in older patients with concurrent illness such as diabetes or hypertension.

Treatment

A. EMERGENCY MEASURES

Maintain an airway. Consider rapid-sequence intubation for severely agitated or comatose patients, and give supplemental oxygen. Ensure adequate intravenous access, preferably with a large-bore ($\geq$ 18-gauge) catheter. Draw blood samples for free T_4 and TSH radioimmunoassay, CBC, serum electrolytes and glucose measurements, renal and hepatic function tests, and arterial blood gas determination. Electrocardiographic monitoring is indicated.

Initiate intravascular volume replacement with isotonic fluids, at least 1 L normal saline or lactated Ringer's in the first hour, and vasopressors as needed if the patient is hypotensive. Frequent reassessment is necessary to prevent fluid overload, especially in patients exhibiting signs of high output cardiac failure (tachycardia, dyspnea, wide pulse pressure).

B. HORMONE SYNTHESIS BLOCKERS

Thionamides block thyroid hormone synthesis. They are not available in parenteral forms and should be administered orally or by nasogastric tube. Propylthiouracil, 200–300 mg every 6 hours, is the drug of choice.

In addition to blocking thyroid hormone synthesis, propylthiouracil has the ability to block peripheral conversion of T_4 to the more physiologically active triiodothyronine (T_3).

C. HORMONE RELEASE BLOCKERS

Iodine therapy is a therapeutic adjunct to propylthiouracil. Iodide compounds should be given 2–4 hours after initial propylthiouracil dose. Potassium iodide (SSKI, 35 mg iodide/drop), 5 drops 3–4 times daily given orally or by nasogastric tube, will inhibit thyroid hormone release.

Alternatively, Lugol's iodine solution (8 mg iodide/drop), 10 drops every 8 hours given orally or by nasogastric tube, may be used. Seriously ill patients may be given iodinated radiographic contrast agents such as sodium ipodate (Oragrafin) or sodium iopanoate (Telepaque). The dose for either is 1 g by mouth daily as a single dose or 500 mg twice daily. These medications can only be given orally.

D. HORMONE ACTION BLOCKERS

β-Adrenergic antagonists such as propanolol block the peripheral effects or excess thyroid hormone and decrease conversion of T_4 to T_3. A typical dose is 0.5–1.0 mg intravenously every 10–15 minutes until pulse reduction is achieved. In patients with bronchospastic disease, cautious use of esmolol, 0.05–0.1 mg/kg/min intravenously, or calcium channel blockers such as diltiazem, 5–15 mg/h intravenously, may be considered.

E. CORTICOSTEROIDS

Corticosteroids inhibit peripheral conversion of T_4 to T_3. In addition, they also treat the relative adrenal insufficiency that may be present. Intravenous hydrocortisone, 100 mg every 8 hours, may be used; if concurrent adrenal insufficiency is in the differential diagnosis, dexamethasone, 0.1 mg/kg intravenously every 8 hours, may be given and an adrenocorticotropic hormone (ACTH) stimulation test of the adrenocortical axis may still be undertaken.

Disposition

Hospitalization in an intensive care unit is indicated for all patients with thyroid storm. A Swan-Ganz catheter may be necessary to facilitate fluid management and assess progress of therapy in cases complicated by cardiac failure.

Dabon-Almirante CL, Surks MI: Clinical and laboratory diagnosis of thyrotoxicosis. Endocrinol Metab Clin North Am 1998;

27:25. [PMID: 9534025] (Good overview of thyrotoxicosis, outlining the clinical manifestations by organ systems.)

Ringel MD: Management of hypothyroidism and hyperthyroidism in the intensive care unit. Crit Care Clin 2001;17:59. [PMID: 11219235] (Complete coverage of hyperthyroid treatments, detailing both medical and surgical options.)

2. Myxedema Coma

ESSENTIALS OF DIAGNOSIS

- *A potentially lethal complication of severe hypothyroidism.*
- *Look for typical stigmata: dry skin, delayed reflex relaxation, generalized weakness, edema, or a transverse scar across the low anterior neck.*
- *Alteration in mental status (although coma is rare).*
- *Often hypothermic (< 35.5 °C [95.9 °F]).*

General Considerations

Myxedema coma is a rare complication of hypothyroidism related to severe deficiency of thyroid hormone production resulting in encephalopathy. The most common causes for hypothyroidism include autoimmune disorders (Hashimoto thyroiditis), prior thyroidectomy, and radioactive iodine ablation of the thyroid. Myxedema coma typically occurs in the winter months often after cold exposure. Other predisposing factors include cerebrovascular accident, anesthesia or surgery, trauma, medications, and infections. Cardinal features include hypothermia, hyporeflexia, central nervous system depression, coma, bradycardia, and slow verbal responses. Oxygenation and ventilation may be impaired because of decreased respiratory drive and respiratory muscle weakness. Onset may be rapid or may be insidious, especially in the elderly. Mortality is estimated at up to 60–70%; the elderly population is at highest risk. When myxedema coma is recognized and treated appropriately, mortality drops to 15–20%.

Clinical Findings

The presumptive diagnosis of myxedema coma should be made when clinical manifestations of hypothyroidism are accompanied by disturbances of consciousness, hypothermia, hypoventilation, and hypotension.

A. HISTORY

The history, if available, is usually that of classic hypothyroidism and may include discontinuation of thy-

roid medication, previous radioactive iodine treatment, thyroidectomy, or drug administration (sedatives, iodides, or amiodarone).

B. SYMPTOMS AND SIGNS

Symptoms and signs of hypothyroidism include cold intolerance, dry skin, constipation, weight gain, irregular or absent menses, muscle cramps, paresthesias, angina, or seizures. Neurologic complaints such as generalized weakness, slow speech, disorientation, apathy, ataxia, inappropriate humor (myxedema wit), or psychosis are also common. As hypothyroidism worsens, neurologic symptoms progress to lethargy, disorientation, grand mal seizures, and myxedema coma.

Hypothermia is found in approximately 80% of patients with myxedema coma. Hypoventilation often occurs secondary to decreased respiratory drive and generalized muscle weakness. Hypotension may be present. Gastrointestinal ileus or urinary retention are common.

In comatose patients, the only data the clinician may have are physical findings: bradycardia; generalized puffiness; periorbital edema; ptosis; cutaneous myxedema; coarse, dry skin; macroglossia; delayed deep tendon reflexes; thyroidectomy scar or a goiter; or coarse, sparse hair.

C. LABORATORY FINDINGS

Thyroid studies typically reveal low serum free T_4 and T_3 levels. The serum TSH level is high in primary hypothyroidism and low or undetectable in secondary hypothyroidism. Secondary hypothyroidism represents a failure of the hypothalamus to secrete adequate thyrotropin-releasing hormone (TRH) or failure of the anterior pituitary to secrete TSH.

Obtain routine blood cultures, urine cultures, chest radiography, and ECG in the search for a precipitating cause. Arterial blood gases may reveal hypoxemia, hypercapnia, and a respiratory or mixed respiratory-metabolic acidosis. Hyponatremia and hypoglycemia may be signs of concurrent adrenal insufficiency. These are also potential contributors to central nervous system depression. Serum creatine kinase may be elevated. Myocardial pathology or rhabdomyolysis must be excluded as causes.

D. IMAGING

Chest radiography may show an enlarged heart from a pericardial effusion or other precipitating cause for the myxedema coma, such as pneumonia. A bedside echocardiogram can confirm a pericardial effusion.

E. ELECTROCARDIOGRAPHIC FINDINGS

The ECG shows bradycardia, low voltage of the QRS complex in all leads, flattening or inversion of the T waves, and conduction abnormalities.

Treatment

A. GENERAL AND SUPPORTIVE MEASURES

1. ABCs—Assess airway. Patients with myxedema coma may need rapid-sequence intubation and mechanical ventilation for hypoxemia and hypoventilation. Patients may need assistance with bag-valve-mask ventilation to achieve adequate preoxygenation. Electrocardiographic monitoring is indicated.

2. Venous access—Establish large-bore ($\geq$ 18-gauge) intravenous access. Draw blood samples for free T_4, free T_3, TSH, cortisol, CBC, renal and hepatic function tests, arterial blood gases, and electrolyte and glucose levels.

3. Fluid replacement—Isotonic crystalloid solution (normal saline or lactated Ringer's) should be given for hypotension. Avoid hypotonic solutions because hyponatremia may be present. Avoid giving vasopressors because they may provoke dysrhythmias, especially when used with intravenous thyroid replacement therapy. In addition, vasopressors are not likely to be effective because of a reduced adrenergic receptor response.

4. Treatment for hypothermia—Hypothermia is usually corrected by administration of thyroid hormone; however, passive rewarming methods may be used. Avoid external warming blankets. Active methods of rewarming may cause vasodilation and cardiovascular collapse.

5. Treatment for hypoglycemia—Treat hypoglycemia with 50% dextrose initially, then by 5% dextrose infusion (in normal saline or lactated Ringer's). Treat gastrointestinal ileus and urinary retention with a nasogastric tube and Foley catheter, respectively.

6. Other medications—Avoid unnecessary medications that may further exacerbate a myxedema coma such as central nervous system depressants. Treat severe hyponatremia ($\leq$ 120 mEq/L) with isotonic intravenous fluids (normal saline); be careful not to correct too rapidly to avoid fluid overload. Thyroid replacement therapy and corticosteroids will generally correct mild hyponatremia.

Intravenous corticosteroids (hydrocortisone sodium phosphate or sodium succinate), 100 mg every 8 hours, are indicated as treatment for frequently concurrent adrenal insufficiency.

7. Treatment of precipitating causes—Treat appropriately any identified precipitating cause for myxedema coma. Recovery from myxedema coma is slow because reversal of severe metabolic abnormalities is required.

B. SPECIFIC THERAPY

Although thyroid replacement therapy is indicated for myxedema coma, the method of replacement is controversial. T_3 has the advantage of being more physiologically active than T_4; however, it carries the increased risk of dysrhythmia and ischemic heart disease in susceptible populations such as the elderly. T_4 in low doses has not proved effective. A frequently used and generally safe method appears to be high-dose intravenous T_4 therapy, 200–500 μg as an initial intravenous loading dose over the first hour, followed with 50–100 μg/d intravenously until oral intake is tolerated and the patient can begin taking an initial oral replacement dose of 50–100 μg/d. In younger comatose patients without comorbid coronary artery disease, T_3 at low intravenous doses of 10 μg every 8 hours may be given in addition to T_4 until the patient is conscious. All patients receiving any form of intravenous thyroid hormone therapy should have continuous cardiac monitoring.

Disposition

Hospitalization in an intensive care unit is indicated for all patients with myxedema coma.

Ringel MD: Management of hypothyroidism and hyperthyroidism in the intensive care unit. Crit Care Clin 2001;17:59. [PMID: 11219235] (Good overview of thyroid pathology, diagnosis, and treatment. Details the rationale and various methods of thyroid hormone replacement.)

Wall CR: Myxedema coma: diagnosis and treatment. Am Fam Physician 2000;11:2485. [PMID: 11130234] (Highlights the variable presentations of myxedema coma and emphasizes the need for a high index of suspicion.)

ACUTE ADRENAL INSUFFICIENCY (Addisonian Crisis)

 ESSENTIALS OF DIAGNOSIS

- *Consider addisonian crisis in patients with hypotension refractory to intravenous fluids or in acutely ill patients with typical stigmata of chronic glucocorticoid use such as moon facies and buffalo hump.*
- *Common symptoms include orthostasis, weight loss, anorexia, lethargy, abdominal cramps, nausea, vomiting, diarrhea, and mental depression.*
- *Classic electrolyte abnormalities include hyponatremia associated with hyperkalemia.*

General Considerations

The adrenal glands produce four different groups of hormones: glucocorticoids, mineralocorticoids, catecholamines, and sex hormones. Failure to produce all but the sex hormones may induce a life-threatening emergency because cardiovascular stability, extracellular fluid and electrolyte balance, glucose homeostasis, and the body's ability to deal with metabolic stress all depend on the other three classes of adrenal hormones. Recognizing the clinical manifestations of adrenal insufficiency requires a high index of suspicion because signs and symptoms are often nonspecific.

Classification

A. PRIMARY ADRENOCORTICAL INSUFFICIENCY

Primary adrenocortical insufficiency (Addison disease) results from primary destruction of the adrenal glands. Causes include autoimmune insults (most common), infection, systemic inflammatory response, thrombosis, hemorrhage, malignant metastatic carcinoma (most commonly lung, breast, hematogenous), and medications (most commonly warfarin, antifungals, and corticosteroids). Etomidate, a medication used with increasing frequency in emergency medicine for rapid- sequence intubation and for procedural sedation, may also cause transient and occasionally serious primary adrenal insufficiency. Whereas tuberculosis was the most common infectious cause in the past, HIV and related opportunistic complications are now responsible for most infectious insults to the adrenal glands. The infection may be primary or secondary via an opportunistic infection, most commonly systemic fungal, protozoal, or herpes simplex or cytomegalovirus infections. Patients with coagulopathy or thromboembolic disease are at higher risk for bilateral adrenal hemorrhage. Waterhouse-Friderichsen syndrome related to *Neisseria meningitidis* or pneumococcal septicemia consists of bilateral adrenal hemorrhage and abrupt circulatory collapse.

B. SECONDARY ADRENOCORTICAL INSUFFICIENCY

Secondary adrenocortical insufficiency results from pathology of the hypothalamus and pituitary. Corticotropin-releasing hormone (CRH) and ACTH release are impaired causing dysfunction along the entire hypothalamus-pituitary-adrenal axis. Common causes include corticosteroid withdrawal and systemic inflammatory states such as sepsis. A primary pituitary or hypothalamic mass must also be considered.

Clinical Findings

A. SYMPTOMS AND SIGNS

As with other endocrine disorders, signs and symptoms are typically nonspecific because a number of different organ symptoms are involved. Clinical findings are typically secondary to low glucocorticoid and mineralocorticoid levels.

1. Glucocorticoid deficiency—Symptoms and signs include hypotension (particularly hypotension refractory to fluids), orthostasis, weight loss, anorexia, lethargy, abdominal cramps, nausea, vomiting, diarrhea, and mental depression.

2. Mineralocorticoid deficiency (primary deficiency only)—Symptoms and signs include hypovolemia, orthostasis, hypotension, and salt craving.

Acute bilateral adrenal hemorrhage is not accompanied by the above chronic manifestations but should be suspected in the following situations:

- Patients with sepsis who have rapid or unexplained deterioration
- Adults with major medical illnesses who have abdominal, flank, or chest pain; dehydration; hypotension; shock; or fever (especially if anticoagulants have been used)

Patients with secondary adrenal insufficiency may present with acute adrenal insufficiency; in these patients it is preceded by one of the following:

- History of or physical features characteristic of chronic glucocorticoid administration (eg, moon facies, buffalo hump)
- Symptoms of hypopituitarism (hypogonadism, hypothyroidism) and manifestations of a hypothalamic or pituitary tumor (including headache, bitemporal visual field defects, or enlargement of the sella turcica) in patients with hypothalamic or pituitary disorders

3. Symptoms and signs of acute crisis—Rapid worsening of glucocorticoid-deficiency symptoms is associated with severe weakness. Symptoms of mineralocorticoid deficiency occur only with primary adrenal insufficiency:

- Fever
- Increased nausea and vomiting with nonspecific abdominal pain
- Rapid dehydration and hypovolemia
- Hypotension and shock
- Altered mental status ranging from lethargy to obtundation and coma

B. LABORATORY FINDINGS

Mineralocorticoid deficiency causes a classic hyponatremia and hyperkalemia. The finding of the two together should suggest the diagnosis of primary adrenal insufficiency.

Other findings may include anemia of chronic disease, elevated blood urea nitrogen, hypoglycemia, hypocalcemia, lymphocytosis, and eosinophilia. Hyperkalemia is typically not seen in secondary adrenal insufficiency because aldosterone production is usually preserved.

C. IMAGING

Calcification of the adrenals may be present as a result of tuberculosis, histoplasmosis, or other disseminated fungal disease. Magnetic resonance imaging (MRI) of the head is usually the test of choice for secondary adrenal insufficiency to reveal sellar and hypothalamic-pituitary tumors, and CT scan of the abdomen is the test of choice in primary adrenal insufficiency to image the adrenal glands. Enlarged adrenal glands suggest tuberculosis, fungal disease, cancer, hemorrhage, or AIDS. Small adrenal glands suggest autoimmune disease, chronic infection, or chronic vascular abnormalities.

D. ELECTROCARDIOGRAPHIC FINDINGS

The ECG may reveal low voltage in all leads and changes characteristic of electrolyte abnormalities, most commonly hyperkalemia with peaked T waves, prolongation of QRS interval, and loss of P waves in severe cases.

Diagnosis

Draw blood for serum cortisol level. A serum cortisol exceeding 20 µg/dL at any time of the day makes the diagnosis of adrenal insufficiency unlikely. Ideally the blood is drawn when the patient is under duress.

An ACTH stimulation test, however, is the study of choice. After the initial serum cortisol is drawn, 250 µg of synthetic ACTH (Cosyntropin) is given. Serum cortisol levels are drawn 30 and 60 minutes later. Failure of the adrenals to produce cortisol to levels of 25–30 µg/dL suggests primary adrenal insufficiency. A normal response to the test does not rule out adrenal insufficiency because partial adrenal insufficiency may be present. **Note:** An ACTH stimulation test cannot be undertaken if hydrocortisone was given as initial therapy. Dexamethasone is a reasonable and effective alternative to hydrocortisone that will not disrupt the results.

In addition, the 250 µg of Cosyntropin is thought to be supratherapeutic, being many times the normal physiologic levels seen in a stress situation. A low-dose ACTH test has been suggested that uses only 1–2 µg of the drug. The rest of the parameters of the test—including timing of cortisol levels and the cortisol levels

of 25–30 µg/dL needed to suggest adequate adrenal function—remain the same, and the test is thought to be more sensitive with the lower dose of cosyntropin.

Treatment

A. GENERAL AND SUPPORTIVE MEASURES

Assess the airway, intubate as necessary for decreased mental status, and provide supplemental oxygen as needed. Establish large-bore intravenous access. Draw blood for CBC, electrolytes, glucose level, renal and hepatic function tests, and serum cortisol. Perform an ACTH stimulation test.

Monitor body weight, fluid intake, and urine output. Check serum electrolytes, glucose, and renal function every 4–6 hours, then once or twice daily until these measures are stable. Monitor potassium levels carefully. Even though potassium levels may be high initially, total body deficits often exist and will appear in conjunction with hydrocortisone therapy. Replace fluid volume and correct electrolyte abnormalities as appropriate.

B. SPECIFIC THERAPY

Hydrocortisone, 100 mg intravenously every 8 hours, is the mainstay for treating adrenal insufficiency. Alternatively, dexamethasone, 0.1 mg/kg every 8 hours, may be used without disruption of diagnostic testing although it supports only glucocorticoid function. Once diagnostic testing has been done, hydrocortisone is the drug of choice because it has both glucocorticoid and mineralocorticoid functions. Once patients are stable, the dose may be tapered gradually over 1–2 weeks.

Patients receiving less than 50 mg/d of hydrocortisone will likely need mineralocorticoid support as well. Fludrocortisone, 0.05–0.2 mg/d, is the drug of choice. Fludrocortisone therapy is necessary as transition to oral therapy begins.

Disposition

Admission to the hospital is indicated if an addisonian crisis is suspected or confirmed. Intensive care unit admission is warranted for hemodynamically unstable patients.

Marik PE, Zaloga GP: Adrenal insufficiency in the critically ill. A new look at an old problem. Chest 2002;5:1784. [PMID: 12426284] (Reviews adrenal insufficiency in light of modern causes.)

Zolga GP, Marik P: Hypothalamic-pituitary-adrenal insufficiency. Crit Care Clin 2001;17:25. [PMID: 11219233] (Comprehensive review of the pathophysiology and management of adrenal insufficiency emphasizing the need for a high index of suspicion.)

PHEOCHROMOCYTOMA
(Catecholamine Crisis)

 ESSENTIALS OF DIAGNOSIS

- Catecholamine crisis symptoms are headache, palpitations, flushing, or diaphoresis associated with hypertension.
- Symptoms associated with pheochromocytoma are often intermittent (with asymptomatic periods in between episodes), whereas those of a monoamine oxidase inhibitor (MAOI) crisis or of sympathomimetic intoxication are not.

General Considerations

A catecholamine crisis is typically caused by one of three entities (1) a pheochromocytoma, (2) a MAOI crisis, or (3) intoxication from cocaine or other similar sympathomimetics. Occasionally a catecholamine crisis may be induced by sudden cessation of clonidine therapy. Catecholamines bind to α-1 and β receptors and in excess may cause various signs and symptoms such as headache, palpitations, diaphoresis, and often severe hypertension. A thorough history will usually lead to the cause of catecholamine crisis, except in the case of pheochromocytoma, which often remains an elusive cause because the symptoms are nonspecific and often intermittent. This section focuses on diagnosis and treatment of pheochromocytoma.

Clinical Findings

A. SYMPTOMS AND SIGNS

Classic manifestations include headache, diaphoresis, pallor, palpitations, nervousness, apprehension, nausea, vomiting, and abdominal pain. Hypertension, often severe ($\geq$ 120 mm Hg diastolic), is a striking sign that usually prompts the clinician to include catecholamine crisis in the differential diagnosis.

Hypertension is frequently intermittent and may not always be present at the time of examination. Labile hypertension is the hallmark of a pheochromocytoma. Recent reviews have placed the frequency of hypertension at 72.4% and sustained hypertension at only 47.9%.

Complications that occur late in the course of the disease may cloud the diagnosis because they can be dramatic and distracting. Presentations in severe cases may include abdominal or chest pain, aortic dissection, encephalopathy, cardiomyopathy, pulmonary edema, fever, and anion gap metabolic acidosis.

Neurocutaneous syndromes such as neurofibromatosis, von Hippel-Lindau disease, ataxia-telangiectasia, tuberous sclerosis, and Sturge-Weber syndrome are sometimes associated with pheochromocytoma. Cutaneous findings (ie, café-au-lait spots, telangiectasias) may provide clues to a diagnosis.

Mucosal neuromas and a marfanoid appearance suggest multiple endocrine neoplasia type IIB. Other findings include weight loss, heat intolerance, hyperglycemia, and tachycardia.

B. LABORATORY FINDINGS AND SPECIAL TESTS

The diagnosis of pheochromocytoma is made along two pathways. First, a biochemical diagnosis must be made. Second, the tumor must be defined by radiologic studies for possible surgical excision.

The initial test of choice is a 24-hour urine collection for catecholamine and catecholamine metabolites (norepinephrine, epinephrine, dopamine, vanillylmandelic acid [VMA], and metanephrine). In the absence of grossly positive results, plasma catecholamine levels have been unreliable for diagnosis; however, new research has shown free plasma metanephrine to be useful as a diagnostic marker.

Although 90% of pheochromocytomas arise from the adrenal glands, 10% are found in extra-adrenal sites. Localization of the tumor is performed by CT scan, MRI, and isotope scanning with metaiodobenzylguanidine.

C. CARDIAC EFFECTS OF A CATECHOLAMINE CRISIS

In addition to tachydysrhythmias, a prolonged QT interval, which can predispose the patient to more lethal arrhythmias, may be present on the ECG. Findings of cardiac ischemia and coronary artery disease (ST elevation or depression and T wave inversion) also complicate the diagnostic picture because many of these findings resolve after tumor removal.

Treatment

A. GENERAL AND SUPPORTIVE MEASURES

Assess airway, and provide supplemental oxygen as needed (5–10 L by nasal cannula or mask). Establish large-bore intravenous access. Draw blood for routine studies (CBC, serum electrolytes, glucose, hepatic and renal function). Replace volume deficits, and correct electrolyte abnormalities. Avoid drugs or procedures that may exacerbate a catecholamine crisis. Begin 24-hour urine collection for fractionated catecholamines, metanephrine, and VMA.

B. SPECIFIC THERAPY

1. Phentolamine—The α-adrenergic blockade of phentolamine has been the traditional cornerstone of acute therapy for pheochromocytoma. The dose is 1–2 mg intravenously every 5 minutes. ***Caution:*** Higher initial doses may cause sudden severe hypotension. If no response is seen, increase the dose to 5 mg intravenously every 5 minutes until adequate blood pressure control occurs. Orthostatic hypotension is a common side effect and can be managed by ensuring adequate hydration and keeping the patient recumbent.

2. Nitroprusside—Intravenous sodium nitroprusside infusion, 0.5–10 μg/kg/min, may be useful in a hypertensive crisis. Risks of cyanide toxicity with prolonged therapy and the need for careful continuous cardiovascular monitoring have prompted clinicians to switch to newer agents such as fenoldopam and labetalol to control blood pressure in hypertensive crisis.

3. Fenoldopam—Fenoldopam, a dopamine-1 receptor agonist, is a promising alternative to nitroprusside. An intravenous infusion beginning at 0.1 μg/kg/min vasodilates renal, splanchnic, and coronary circulation. Improved renal blood flow, lack of a toxic metabolite, and a short half-life of 7–9 minutes are its major advantages.

4. β-Blockers—β-Adrenergic blockade is usually reserved for patients with severe tachydysrhythmias. Propranolol, 1–2 mg intravenously at a rate of 1 mg/min repeated every 5 minutes to a total of 10 mg, may be used. β-Blockade should begin only after α-blockade has been established to avoid unopposed peripheral α-receptor vasoconstriction. Mixed α-β receptor antagonists are an excellent alternative to simple β-blockade and significantly lessen the risk of unopposed α effects. Labetalol may be given in 10–20 mg intravenous boluses every 10 minutes until the desired blood pressure is achieved with maintenance intravenous infusion of 0.5–2.0 mg/min.

5. Benzodiazepines—Benzodiazepines may also be useful in blunting the body's sympathetic response to excess catecholamines. Lorazepam, 1–2 mg intravenously, or diazepam, 5–10 mg intravenously, are common starting doses. Administer these drugs judiciously to avoid oversedation and hypotension, particularly if the patient is volume depleted.

Disposition

Hospitalization in an intensive care unit is indicated in all patients with pheochromocytoma.

Elliott WJ: Hypertensive emergencies. Crit Care Clin 2001;17:435. [PMID: 11450325] (An excellent review of the literature on diagnosis and treatment of all causes of hypertensive emergency, including pheochromocytoma.)

Liao WB et al: Cardiovascular manifestations of pheochromocytoma. Am J Emerg Med 2000;18:622. [PMID: 10999582] (Focuses on the presentation and treatment of cardiovascular problems associated with pheochromocytoma.)

Young WY: Pheochromocytoma and primary aldosteronism: diagnostic approaches. Endocrinol Metab Clin North Am 1997;26:801. [PMID: 9429861] (Emphasis of this article is on the diagnostic approach to pheochromocytoma.)

PITUITARY APOPLEXY

 ESSENTIALS OF DIAGNOSIS

- *Rare disease with variable presentation.*
- *Patients often have headache.*
- *Neurologic deficits including hemiparesis; cranial nerve defects including ophthalmoplegia and bitemporal hemianopsia.*

General Considerations

Pituitary apoplexy is a massive hemorrhagic infarction of the pituitary gland. Clinically the condition almost always occurs in the setting of a preexisting pituitary tumor or tumor in structures adjacent to the sella turcica. Pituitary adenomas are particularly prone to hemorrhage and necrosis. The symptoms seen in pituitary apoplexy result from (1) leakage of blood and necrotic material into the subarachnoid space, (2) development of a rapidly expanding hemorrhagic intrasellar mass lesion compressing the optic chiasm, cavernous sinuses, cranial nerves, and adjacent structures (hypothalamus and internal carotid arteries), and (3) acute hypopituitarism.

Risk factors for pituitary apoplexy include head trauma, irradiation, estrogen, anticoagulation use, DKA, hypertension, diuretics, use of bromocriptine, and pregnancy (Sheehan syndrome, which occurs when massive intrapartum hemorrhage and shock occur, leading to vasospastic necrosis of the pituitary).

Clinical Findings

A. SYMPTOMS AND SIGNS

Diagnosis is challenging, because pituitary apoplexy is a rare disease with variable presentation. Onset may be acute and dramatic or subacute, developing over days to weeks. Neurologic symptoms are most prominent and are usually the most striking features seen when a patient with pituitary apoplexy is examined.

Headache is a common feature. Pituitary apoplexy should enter the differential whenever a pathologic headache is suspected. The quality of the headache has been described as subacute and worsening, as retroorbital, and as a sudden thunderclap. Meningeal irritation may be prominent feature. Nausea and vomiting may be present. Fever often is present from blood in the subarachnoid space or hypothalamic compression disturbing normal temperature regulation. Neurologic symptoms range from paresthesias to ataxia to unilateral weakness mimicking cerebrovascular accident.

Ophthalmologic symptoms are also common. Compression of the optic chiasm from an expanding mass can cause visual disturbances, particularly bitemporal hemianopsia. Cranial nerve III compression can cause ophthalmoplegia. Further encroachment on the cavernous sinus can lead to dysfunction in cranial nerves IV, V, and VI (cavernous sinus syndrome). Compression of the internal carotid artery can lead to mental status changes ranging from mild lethargy to delirium to coma. Internal carotid artery compression can also cause hemispheric ischemia.

With pituitary apoplexy, numerous endocrinopathies may be present. A history of pituitary hormone dysfunction may be helpful in making the diagnosis of pituitary apoplexy; however, adrenal insufficiency is the most life-threatening complication and requires immediate attention in the emergency department. Respiratory failure may occur because of hypothalamic compression or increased intracranial pressure.

B. LABORATORY FINDINGS

Hypernatremia and hyponatremia may occur as a result of diabetes insipidus or inappropriate secretion of antidiuretic hormone. Obtain thyroid function tests, cortisol levels, growth hormone levels, and prolactin levels to assess global pituitary function. Cerebrospinal fluid will often be xanthochromic or grossly bloody, with elevated opening pressure. Analysis reveals elevated protein concentrations and increased numbers of red and white cells. Do not perform lumbar puncture if an intracranial mass is suspected.

C. IMAGING

CT scan and MRI are the imaging studies of choice for diagnosis of pituitary apoplexy. Acute hemorrhage appears hyperdense on CT scan. Blood appears hypodense on T2-weighted MRI scans. MRI is helpful in detecting hemorrhage in the subacute setting. Because these patients are often unstable, exercise care in deciding to send the patient out of the emergency department for a prolonged period of time for an MRI. CT may miss small pituitary tumors, but CT scans are rapid and will pick up most clinically significant lesions in the sella turcica and surrounding structures. A negative CT scan does not necessarily exclude the diagnosis of pituitary apoplexy.

Treatment

Assess for a patent airway, consider rapid-sequence intubation and mechanical ventilation in obtunded or comatose patients, and provide supplemental oxygen as needed. Cardiac monitoring is indicated.

Hydrocortisone sodium succinate or phosphate, 100 mg intravenously, should be given to all patients suspected of having pituitary apoplexy to treat frequently concurrent and potentially lethal acute adrenal insufficiency.

Definitive treatment for pituitary apoplexy is neurosurgical decompression, generally accomplished by transsphenoidal approach. Indications for surgery are decreasing consciousness, progressive vision loss, or increasing extraocular motor palsy indicating cavernous sinus compression.

Disposition

Hospitalization and immediate neurosurgical consultation are indicated. Surgery is the definitive treatment, but not every patient will require an operation. Some patients recover without sequelae with conservative management alone.

Inamasu J et al: Pituitary apoplexy without ocular/visual symptoms. Am J Emerg Med 2001;19:88. [PMID: 11146033] (Covers the classic clinical presentation of pituitary apoplexy along with an unusual presentation.)

Laws ER, Kamal T: Pituitary surgery. Endocrinol Metab Clin North Am 1999;28:119. [PMID: 10207687] (Good information on the medical management of pituitary apoplexy prior to surgery. Also covers general surgical approaches.)

Lee CC et al: Emergency department presentation of pituitary apoplexy. Am J Emerg Med 2000;18:328. [PMID: 10830692] (Good review on the presentation, diagnosis, and management of pituitary apoplexy.)

INAPPROPRIATE SECRETION OF ANTIDIURETIC HORMONE

 ESSENTIALS OF DIAGNOSIS

- *Hyponatremia in the setting of a reduced plasma osmolality, persistent urinary secretion of sodium (> 20 mEq/L), and urine osmolality that is inappropriately high for the degree of hyponatremia and hypoosmolality found.*

- *Mental status changes ranging from mild to severe dependent on the degree of hyponatremia.*

General Considerations

Antidiuretic hormone (ADH), also known as arginine vasopressin (AVP), is secreted from the posterior pituitary and acts on the collecting ducts in the nephron to induce water reabsorption. Inappropriate secretion of antidiuretic hormone (SIADH) is a state of pathological hormone excess. Classic diagnostic criteria include (1) hyponatremia with lower than normal plasma osmolality in the absence of dehydration or volume depletion, (2) failure of the kidney to dilute the urine in the presence of reduced serum osmolality (urine osmolality is frequently > 300 mOsm/kg), (3) continued sodium excretion (usually > 20 mEq/L) despite hyponatremia, and (4) absence of hyponatremia producing states such as hypothyroidism, adrenal insufficiency, congestive heart failure, cirrhosis, or renal disease.

Causes

Numerous diseases and drugs can cause SIADH. Of particular note are malignancies (small cell carcinoma of the lung, pancreatic carcinoma, thymoma, Hodgkin disease), central nervous system disorders, surgery, pulmonary disorders (tuberculosis, pneumonia, lung abscess, bronchiectasis). Several medications have been implicated in SIADH, most commonly antidepressants, antipsychotics, anticonvulsants, sulfonylureas, angiotensin-converting enzyme inhibitors, narcotics, and MDMA (Ecstasy).

The elderly are at higher risk for SIADH because several physiologic effects of aging contribute to its pathogenesis, including an increased ADH response to osmotic stimulation; declining renal function; and decreased renin, angiotensin, and aldosterone production.

Clinical Findings

A. SYMPTOMS AND SIGNS

The clinical presentation of SIADH depends on the level of hyponatremia and water intoxication:

- In mild cases (serum sodium ≥ 120 mEq/L), patients are usually asymptomatic.
- When serum sodium reaches 105–120 mEq/L, patients begin to experience neurologic manifestations such as anorexia, nausea, vomiting, personality changes, depressed tendon reflexes, and muscle weakness.
- With severe hyponatremia (≤ 105 mEq/L), coma, seizures, delirium, cranial nerve palsies, hypothermia, and altered patterns of respiration (Cheyne-Stokes) may be evident.

Because SIADH can be caused by various pathologic conditions, patients will also present with signs or symptoms of their underlying disease (eg, malignancy, pulmonary disease). Edema and other signs of volume overload are highly unusual even with severe hyponatremia and water intoxication. Signs of volume overload indicate an alternative diagnosis.

B. LABORATORY FINDINGS

Hyponatremia is the classic feature of SIADH. Other findings include a reduced plasma osmolality, persistent urinary secretion of sodium (> 20 mEq/L), and urine osmolality that is inappropriately high for the degree of hyponatremia and hypoosmolality found.

Treatment

A. GENERAL AND SUPPORTIVE MEASURES

Assess airway, protect the airway with endotracheal intubation in obtunded or comatose patients and initiate mechanical ventilation, and provide supplemental oxygen as needed. Establish large-bore intravenous access. Draw blood for measurement of serum sodium and other electrolytes, creatinine, blood urea nitrogen, osmolality, cortisol levels, and thyroid function studies (TSH and free T_4). Send urine for urinalysis and measurement of urinary osmolality, electrolytes, and specific gravity.

Monitor carefully the patient's body weight, intravenous and oral intake, and urine output. Measure serum and urine electrolytes and osmolality every 4–6 hours during the acute phase and then once or twice daily until the patient's condition has stabilized.

Assess the patient for evidence of renal, hepatic, or cardiac dysfunction. Obtain a history of drugs and medications used by the patient. Evaluate for manifestations of cancer, central nervous system disease, or pulmonary disease.

B. SPECIFIC THERAPY

Fluid restriction is the treatment of choice for the correction of hyponatremia.

1. Mild SIADH (serum sodium ≥ 120 mEq/L)— Restrict fluids to 800–1000 mL per 24 hours.

2. Moderate SIADH (serum sodium 105–120 mEq/L)—Restrict fluids to 500 mL per 24 hour.

3. Severe SIADH (serum sodium < 105 mEq/L or at any level if the patient develops neurologic complications such as coma or seizures)—This is a medical emergency. Treatment is as follows:

- Administer hypertonic saline, 3% solution, at 1–2 mL/kg/h for the first 3–4 hours.
- Use intravenous furosemide, 1 mg/kg, to counteract volume overload.
- Monitor sodium and potassium every 1–2 hours and adjust fluids and replace as needed.
- Correct to a serum sodium level of 125 mEq/L or until central nervous system involvement resolves, then resume fluid restriction therapy as described previously.

Serum sodium correction should average 0.5–2 mEq/L/h and no more than 12 mEq/L in the first 24 hours. Faster rates of sodium correction increase the risk for central pontine myelinolysis. Symptoms of tetraparesis and bulbar palsy are seen. Once central pontine myelinolysis occurs as a complication, there are no proved methods of treatment.

Disposition

Responsible patients with mild SIADH without any neurologic symptoms may be managed on an outpatient basis with fluid restriction and close follow-up. Patients with more severe symptoms of SIADH and those who may not follow proposed treatment recommendations should be hospitalized. Patients receiving hypertonic saline should be admitted to the intensive care unit.

Miller M: Syndromes of excess antidiuretic hormone release. Crit Care Clin 2001;17:11. [PMID: 11219224] (Discusses the various causes, pathophysiology, and management options of SIADH.)

Robertson GL: Antidiuretic hormone. Normal and disordered function. Endocrinol Metab Clin North Am 2001;30:671. [PMID: 11571936] (Covers antidiuretic hormone physiology in both normal and disease states.)

CENTRAL DIABETES INSIPIDUS

 **ESSENTIALS OF DIAGNOSIS**

- *Signs and symptoms include lethargy, altered mental status, irritability, hyperreflexia, and spasticity.*
- *Urine osmolality of < 150 mOsm/kg in the setting of serum hypertonicity and polyuria is generally diagnostic of diabetes insipidus.*

General Considerations

Central diabetes insipidus can be defined by the abnormal excretion of large amounts of solute-free water in the urine. Urine volumes in patients with central diabetes insipidus have exceeded 45 mL/kg per 24 hours. The pathology behind central diabetes insipidus is ADH deficiency, usually resulting from an insult to the hypothalamic-posterior-pituitary axis. Most patients will have an intact thirst mechanism, and polydipsia (fluid intake > 3.5 L/d) occurs in an attempt to maintain adequate hydration. If water intake does not keep up with urinary losses, extracellular volume depletion and hypernatremia soon develop.

Causes

Central diabetes insipidus can be acquired or caused by congenital factors. Acquired causes include head trauma, surgery, tumors (craniopharyngiomas, primary or metastatic hypothalamic tumors), infection (tuberculosis, syphilis, basilar meningitis, fungal infections), cerebrovascular events (cerebral aneurysms, cavernous sinus thrombosis, postpartum pituitary infarction, cerebrovascular accidents), granulomatous diseases (sarcoidosis, histiocytosis X, Wegener granulomatosis). Congenital forms of both central and nephrogenic diabetes insipidus exist.

Clinical Findings

A. SYMPTOMS AND SIGNS

1. ADH deficiency—Profound polydipsia and polyuria are present. Polyuria may lead to associated nocturia, incontinence, or enuresis. Urine osmolality is typically less than 300 mOsm/kg.

2. Hypernatremia and hyperosmolality—Hypernatremia causes intracellular dehydration as water shifts to the more hypertonic extracellular fluid space. The organ most susceptible to these effects is the brain. Signs and symptoms include lethargy, altered mental status, irritability, hyperreflexia, and spasticity.

Intracranial hemorrhage may occur as the brain shrinks and mechanical tension is placed on dural veins and venous sinuses. Patients with marked volume deficits typically have hypotension, tachypnea, tachycardia, and decreased level of consciousness. Fever may be present. With severe dehydration, hypovolemic shock and coma are common. Patients whose diabetes insipidus is caused by intracranial neoplasms may also have visual field defects and anterior pituitary insufficiency.

Symptoms are milder in chronic hypernatremia because the brain has had a chance to produce its own osmotic components. In the patient presenting with polydipsia and polyuria, a number of pathologic processes can be present and the differential diagnosis is broad. As a general rule, a urine osmolality of less than 150 mOsm/kg in the setting of hypertonicity and polyuria is diagnostic of diabetes insipidus. A good history can identify drug-induced diabetes insipidus caused by lithium or demeclocycline. A trial of DDAVP (exogenous ADH) can also distinguish neurogenic from nephrogenic diabetes insipidus. Urine osmolality will increase and volume will decrease with DDAVP administration in central but not nephrogenic diabetes insipidus.

B. Laboratory Findings

Hypernatremia and hyperosmolality are found in uncompensated patients. Serum sodium may be greater than 160 mEq/L in severe cases, and prerenal azotemia is common in these patients. Specific gravity and osmolality of urine are low in proportion to serum osmolality.

C. Imaging

Urgent MRI of the brain is indicated to rule out tumor, mass, or hemorrhage in the region of the hypothalamus or pituitary gland. CT scanning may help exclude other central nervous system lesions.

Treatment

A. General and Supportive Measures

Assess airway, consider rapid-sequence intubation and mechanical ventilation in obtunded or comatose patients, and provide supplemental oxygen as needed. Establish large-bore intravenous access. Draw blood samples for measurement of electrolytes, osmolality, glucose, calcium, serum cortisol levels, and renal and thyroid function tests. Measure plasma ADH; if very low, this may be diagnostic.

Obtain urine specimens for routine urinalysis and specific gravity and osmolality measurements. Monitor volume status, body weight, fluid intake, and urine output and specific gravity.

B. Volume and Electrolyte Deficits

Water administration—whether orally, by nasogastric tube, or intravenously—is the treatment for hypernatremia. Whenever possible, the oral or nasogastric route is preferred because water absorption and resultant decline in serum sodium concentrations are more gradual.

Free water deficit can be calculated by the following equation:

$$\text{Free water deficit} = 0.6 \times \text{premorbid body weight (in kg)}$$
$$\times [1 - (140 / \text{plasma sodium in mmol/L})]$$

Hypotonic saline (0.45% normal saline) or 5% dextrose in water may be given. The latter is given to patients who show severe signs of neurologic compromise from hypernatremia. Be wary of hyperglycemia when using dextrose-containing solutions; it may cause an osmotic diuresis and worsen the hypernatremia.

Replace half the volume deficit within the first 12–24 hours. When serum sodium decreases to less than 150 mEq/L, 0.45% or 0.9% saline should be used. Decreasing the serum sodium greater than 1–2 mEq/L/h can cause fluid shifts back into the intracellular compartment causing cerebral edema. Neurologic deterioration after hydration therapy should raise serious concern and prompt action.

C. Specific Therapy

Desmopressin acetate or DDAVP, 1–2 µg every 12–24 hours subcutaneously or intravenously or 5–20 µg every 12 hours intranasally, is a synthetic AVP analogue that is the drug of choice when treating central diabetes insipidus. It is preferred over other AVP preparations because it has a longer half-life and has almost no pressor effect.

Disposition

Patients with diabetes insipidus should be hospitalized for definitive diagnosis and initiation of treatment. Patients who are severely hypernatremic or who present in hypovolemic shock merit intensive care unit admission for at least the first 24 hours of treatment.

Robertson GL: Antidiuretic hormone. Normal and disordered function. Endocrinol Metab Clin North Am 2001;30:671. [PMID: 11571936] (Excellent review of normal and pathologic antidiuretic hormone physiology.)

Singer I, James OR, Fishman LM: The management of diabetes insipidus in adults. Arch Intern Med 1997;157:1293. [PMID: 9201003] (Discusses the various causes of diabetes insipidus, gives two case studies, and gives a comprehensive overview of initial and chronic treatment.)

Fluid, Electrolyte, & Acid-Base Emergencies

Michael E. Chansky, MD, FACEP, Andrew Nyce, MD, & Jason Friedman, MD[1]

I. Diagnosis of Fluid & Electrolyte Disorders
    Electrolyte Abnormalities
    Approach to the Patient
II. Management of Specific Disorders
    Disorders of Serum Sodium Concentration
    Hyponatremia
        1. Hyponatremia with Hypovolemia
        2. Hyponatremia with Fluid Overload
        3. Hyponatremia with Isovolemia
    Hypernatremia
    Disorders of Serum Potassium Concentration
    Hypokalemia
    Hyperkalemia
    Disorders of Serum Calcium Concentration
    Hypocalcemia
    Hypercalcemia
    Disorders of Serum Phosphorus Concentration

    Hypophosphatemia
    Hyperphosphatemia
    Disorders of Serum Magnesium Concentration
    Hypomagnesemia
    Hypermagnesemia
    Acid-Base Disorders
    Definitions
    Classification of Acid-Base Disorders
    Compensation
    Clinical Acid-Base Disorders
        1. Respiratory Acidosis
        2. Metabolic Acidosis
        3. Respiratory Alkalosis
        4. Metabolic Alkalosis
        5. Mixed Acid-Base Disorders
Appendix: Useful Equations & Formulas

■ I. DIAGNOSIS OF FLUID & ELECTROLYTE DISORDERS

Variations in Total Body Water

Variations in total body water can usually be detected on the basis of the history and physical examination. Intravascular volume and serum osmolarity are regulated by homeostatic mechanisms involving thirst, antidiuretic hormone (ADH), and renal sodium excretion and absorption.

A. VOLUME EXCESS

Volume excess is manifested as peripheral edema or circulatory overload (jugular venous distention, pleural effusion, ascites, cardiac gallop).

B. VOLUME DEPLETION

Volume depletion is shown by poor skin turgor, dry mucous membranes, or thirst.

C. CIRCULATORY COMPROMISE AND DECREASED INTRAVASCULAR VOLUME

Compromised circulation and decreased intravascular volume are manifested by resting tachycardia, narrowed pressure, orthostatic hypotension, or shock.

ELECTROLYTE ABNORMALITIES

Disordered electrolyte concentrations produce vague symptoms that are referable primarily to the neuromuscular system and are often mistaken for primary neurologic or metabolic abnormalities.

Detection of electrolyte abnormalities requires a high index of suspicion in the proper clinical setting and laboratory measurement of blood constituents (sodium, potassium, chloride, bicarbonate [HCO_3^-], calcium, magnesium, and phosphorus). Serum glucose,

---

[1]This chapter is a revision of the chapter by Michael H. Humphreys, MD, from the 4th edition.

blood urea nitrogen, and creatinine are also helpful. These tests are indicated for any patient with even vague neuromuscular symptoms and a pertinent history, examination, or medications.

APPROACH TO THE PATIENT

A. NORMAL VALUES

Evaluation and treatment are based on (1) assessment of total body water and its distribution and (2) electrolyte concentrations.

1. Body water—Table 42–1 lists the normal volumes of various body fluid compartments both as fractions of body weight and as amounts in liters in a hypothetical man or woman.

2. Electrolytes—Table 42–2 presents the normal ranges of serum electrolyte concentrations.

3. Osmolality—The osmolality of fluid in any one compartment is identical to that in all other compartments; normally, it is about 290 mOsm/kg.

B. HISTORY

The history should include information about the following:

- Salt and water retention
  - Symptoms of congestive heart failure
  - Recent weight gain
  - Peripheral edema or ascites
  - History of congestive heart failure or liver or renal disease
- Volume depletion
  - Gastrointestinal losses from vomiting, diarrhea, or nasogastric tube
  - Urinary losses associated with renal disease, diuretics, or diabetes insipidus
  - Excessive insensible loss from skin associated with fever or sweating

Table 42–1. Volume of body fluid compartments.

	Fraction of Body Weight	Typical Volume Woman (120 lb [55 kg])	Typical Volume Man (154 lg [70 kg])
Total body water	0.5–0.6	28 L	42 L
Intracellular fluid	0.35–0.4	20 L	28 L
Extracellular fluid	0.15–0.2	8 L	14 L
Plasma volume	0.05–0.07	3 L	5 L

Table 42–2. Normal serum electrolyte concentrations.

Sodium (Na^+)	136–146 mEq/L
Potassium (K^+)	3.5–5 mEq/L
Chloride (Cl^-)	96–106 mEq/L
Bicarbonate (HCO_3^-)	24–28 mEq/L
Calcium (Ca^{2+})	8.5–10.5 mg/dL (4.2–5.2 mEq/L)
Magnesium (Mg^{2+})	1.8–3 mg/dL (1.5–2.5 mEq/L)
Phosphate (PO_4^{3-})	3–4.5 mg/dL (1–1.5 mmol/L)

C. PHYSICAL EXAMINATION

The physical examination supports the historical data. Particularly helpful are any documented changes in body weight, skin turgor, mucous membranes, or vital signs that have occurred over a short time. A decrease in blood pressure and an increase in pulse rate when the patient changes from the supine to an upright (sitting or standing) position is a relatively sensitive measure of intravascular hypovolemia.

D. LABORATORY FINDINGS

Laboratory measurements provide corroboration and quantification of abnormalities.

■ II. MANAGEMENT OF SPECIFIC DISORDERS

DISORDERS OF SERUM SODIUM CONCENTRATION

HYPONATREMIA (See Figure 42–1.)

 ESSENTIALS OF DIAGNOSIS

- *Hyponatremia is a disorder of impaired water excretion.*
- *Assess volume status, measure urine osmolality, and review all medications and thyroid and adrenal function.*
- *Symptoms relate to the rate of change.*
- *Therapy is geared toward replacing volume and treating the underlying condition.*

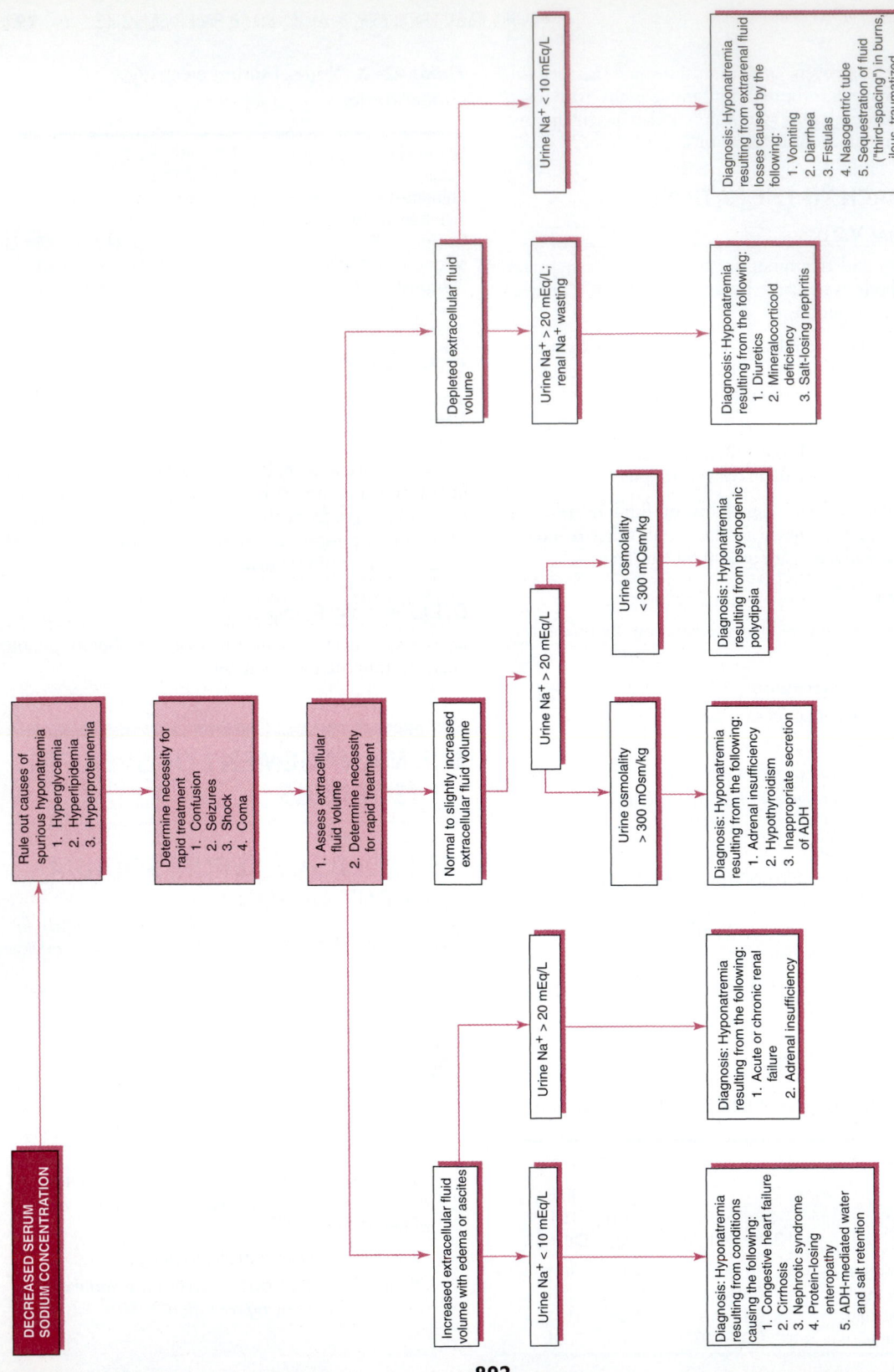

Figure 42–1. Emergency evaluation of hyponatremia.

General Considerations

Hyponatremia is commonly associated with many disease processes (Table 42–3) and use of certain drugs (Table 42–4). It is characterized by a serum sodium concentration under 130 mEq/L. Hyponatremia is a manifestation of decreased water excretion. Appropriate water excretion occurs only when the kidneys are adequately perfused, chloride is transported in the ascending loop, and ADH secretion is inhibited. Symptoms of hyponatremia vary but relate primarily to the rate of serum sodium change. Alterations in central nervous system function dominate the clinical presentation and include delirium, drowsiness, and lethargy progressing to coma and seizures. These symptoms may coexist with those caused by concurrent volume depletion: faintness and dizziness, orthostatic hypotension, tachycardia, dry mucous membranes, poor skin turgor, oliguria, and thirst.

Rule out spurious hyponatremia arising from erroneous sampling, especially when the serum sodium concentration fails to correlate with the clinical scenario, (ie, sample drawn above an intravenous line of hypotonic fluid). In the following conditions, the measurement is accurate but does not represent a true hypoosmolar state (pseudohyponatremia):

A. HYPERLIPIDEMIA AND HYPERPROTEINEMIA

In hyperlipidemia and hyperproteinemia, markedly increased amounts of lipid or protein occupy an increased

Table 42–3. Conditions causing hyponatremia.

True hyponatremia
  Hypervolemic:
    Heart failure
    Liver failure
    Kidney failure
    Nephrotic syndrome
  Normovolemic:
    Adrenal corticosteroid insufficiency
    Inappropriate secretion of antidiuretic hormone
    Hypothyroidism
    Drugs (see Table 36–4)
    Poisons (methanol, ethylene glycol)
    Psychogenic polydipsia
  Hypovolemic:
    Renal salt loss (diuretics, mineralocorticoid deficiency)
    Extrarenal salt loss (sweating, vomiting, diarrhea, peritonitis, burns, muscle trauma)
Spurious hyponatremia
  Hyperglycemia
  Hyperlipidemia
  Hyperproteinemia

Table 42–4. Drugs implicated in the development of hyponatremia.

Hypoglycemic agents
  Phenformin
  Sulfonylureas (chlorpropamide, tolbutamide)
Antineoplastic compounds
  Vincristine
  Cyclophosphamide
Tricyclic compounds
  Carbamazepine
  Amitriptyline
  Thioridazine
Thiazide diuretics
Others
  Acetaminophen
  Clofibrate
  Indomethacin
  Morphine

portion of the plasma volume, resulting in decreased volume of water for electrolytes and other solutes. The sodium concentration in total plasma volume is decreased; however, if sodium concentration in plasma water is measured, it is normal.

The plasma is turbid and milky if hyperlipidemia is present. Excess plasma proteins can be detected quickly in the laboratory using a protein refractometer. In each of these cases, a normal sodium concentration can be expected if serum osmolality is normal despite the measured hyponatremia.

B. HYPERGLYCEMIA

The increase in extracellular fluid osmolality produced by excess glucose molecules causes the transfer of water from the intracellular to the extracellular compartment, thereby increasing the volume of water there. Because sodium is confined principally in the extracellular space, serum sodium concentration falls. Correction of hyperglycemia usually corrects hyponatremia by approximately 1.6 mEq/L of sodium for every 100-mg/dL fall in glucose concentration. Correction of hyperglycemia only shifts water between the intracellular and the extracellular spaces, so that the total body sodium does not change.

Preliminary Evaluation

A. ASSESS URGENCY OF TREATMENT

1. Serious symptoms—Prompt therapy is indicated if muscle cramps, weakness, myoclonus, confusion, delirium, lethargy, seizures, coma, or increased deep tendon reflexes are associated with reliable laboratory evidence of severe hyponatremia (serum sodium < 120 mEq/L).

Hyponatremia should be presumed to be the cause of symptoms until proved otherwise.

2. Rapidity and intensity of treatment—These factors depend on the rate of development of hyponatremia, its severity, and any life-threatening complications (eg, seizures, altered mental status). Slowly developing chronic hyponatremia is well tolerated even to a serum sodium concentration as low as 120 mEq/L. An abrupt fall in serum sodium concentration, even though it is of lesser degree, may be poorly tolerated.

B. Assess Extracellular Fluid Volume

The history and physical examination may suggest increased or decreased extracellular fluid volume. This finding—as well as determination of the sodium concentration in a urine specimen obtained before treatment has been started—provides a basis for diagnosis.

1. Hyponatremia with Hypovolemia

Clinical Findings

Hyponatremia with hypovolemia occur because losses of water and salt have been partially replaced with water, via appropriate ADH secretion. Patients show signs of hypovolemia (postural hypotension or tachycardia; oliguria) and (occasionally) frank shock.

A. With Renal Sodium Conservation

(Urine sodium < 10 mEq/L unless diuretics have been given.) Hyponatremia is due to extrarenal losses of sodium with continued intake of water. Usual causes include gastrointestinal losses (vomiting, nasogastric tube, or diarrhea), severe sweating, or increase in volume of fluid sequestered from extracellular fluid ("third-spacing") (eg, from burns, pancreatitis, intestinal obstruction, or crush injuries).

B. With Renal Sodium Wasting

(Urine sodium > 20 mEq/L.) Hyponatremia is due at least in part to renal sodium wasting such as occurs with diuretic therapy or in patients with adrenal insufficiency. Patients with chronic renal disease may also present with this clinical picture.

Treatment

Restore depleted extracellular fluid volume with infusions of isotonic saline solutions (eg, normal saline or lactated Ringer's injection). Hypertonic saline is rarely necessary to treat this form of hyponatremia.

Disposition

The need for hospitalization depends on the underlying cause and the need for prolonged treatment.

2. Hyponatremia with Fluid Overload

Clinical Findings

Hyponatremia with fluid overload occurs because of a relative decreased intravascular volume and ADH secretion. This results in an impaired ability to excrete water. Total body sodium is greater than normal. Signs of fluid overload (jugular venous distention, sacral or peripheral edema, pulmonary edema or pleural effusions, ascites, or anasarca) are present. Evidence of the underlying disease (eg, heart failure, cirrhosis) is usually apparent. The urine sodium concentration is characteristically less than 10 mEq/L unless the patient has been taking diuretics.

Treatment

A. Water Restriction

Restrict salt and water intake (eg, 2 g of sodium; 1–2 L of water daily). Water restriction is necessary so that insensible water losses will produce slow correction of hyponatremia.

B. Diuretics

Loss of water may need to be accelerated in some patients (eg, those with pulmonary edema) by giving diuretics (eg, furosemide [Lasix], 0.5–1.0 mg/kg intravenously). If diuretics aggravate renal hypoperfusion, hyponatremia may worsen.

C. Hypertonic Saline

It may be advisable to administer small amounts of hypertonic saline (100–200 mL of 3% sodium chloride solution) to patients who already have expanded extracellular fluid volume if they have profound hyponatremia (serum sodium < 110 mEq/L) with serious manifestations (eg, coma or seizures). In such cases, monitoring of central venous pressure or pulmonary capillary wedge pressure in an intensive care unit setting is advisable, and concomitant administration of furosemide (as above) is usually necessary.

D. Dialysis

In patients with concurrent renal failure, emergency dialysis may be necessary to help correct hyponatremia.

Disposition

Hospitalization is required in most cases.

3. Hyponatremia with Isovolemia

Clinical Findings

Occasionally, hyponatremia develops in euvolemic patients. In this setting, evaluation of urine osmolality in addition to determination of urine sodium may be helpful. Hyponatremic patients should have a urine osmolarity significantly less than serum osmolarity (ie, indicating appropriate excretion of water).

A. DEFICIENCY OF POTASSIUM

The uncommon occurrence of hyponatremia resulting from a deficiency in total body potassium has been reported in patients who have taken diuretics without potassium supplementation.

B. INAPPROPRIATE ANTIDIURETIC HORMONE SECRETION

In the syndrome of inappropriate secretion of ADH, mild hyponatremia is universal, and urine osmolality is usually over 300 mOsm/kg. Drugs other than diuretics have also been associated with hyponatremia (see Table 42–4). The mechanisms by which these drugs cause hyponatremia are not firmly established but may include inappropriate secretion or enhanced effect of ADH.

C. HYPOTHYROIDISM

Hypothyroidism may also be associated with isovolemic hyponatremia.

D. PSYCHOGENIC POLYDIPSIA

Psychogenic polydipsia may produce mild to moderate hyponatremia caused by excess free-water intake. Euvolemia is maintained through the renal excretion of sodium. Urine sodium is typically elevated (> 20 mEq/L), and urine osmolality is low (< 300 mOsm/kg).

Treatment

Treatment depends entirely on the underlying cause. In patients with precarious hemodynamic status, monitoring of central venous pressure in an intensive care unit is essential.

Inappropriate secretion of ADH is treated primarily by water restriction (eg, 1–2 L/d).

Hypokalemic hyponatremia is corrected by restoring body potassium stores. Replace potassium by intravenous infusion at a rate not to exceed 10–15 mEq/h, via a central line in a monitored setting. Concentrations of solutions should seldom exceed 40 mEq/L. Oral therapy is preferable to parenteral administration, if the patient's condition permits it. The usual dose for an adult is 40–120 mEq/d.

Drugs associated with hyponatremia should be stopped.

Severe hyponatremia (serum sodium < 120 mEq/L) without life-threatening symptoms may be treated by administration of isotonic saline with concomitant administration of potent diuretics (eg, furosemide, 0.5–1.0 mg/kg intravenously). Profound hyponatremia

(serum sodium < 110 mEq/L) or severe hyponatremia with life-threatening manifestations (eg, coma, seizures) should be corrected more rapidly by the infusion of 100–200 mL of hypertonic (3%) sodium chloride solution (adult dose) along with a diuretic in an intensive care unit.

Disposition

Most patients with isovolemic hyponatremia and all patients with abrupt hyponatremia require hospitalization. Abrupt hyponatremia may be associated with permanent neurologic damage, as may rapid or overcorrection.

HYPERNATREMIA

 ESSENTIALS OF DIAGNOSIS

- *Hypernatremia is related to pure water loss, hypotonic fluid, or rarely salt gain.*
- *Most common in infants and the elderly.*
- *Symptoms are primarily neurologic and related to severe hypovolemia.*
- *Measure urine osmolality.*
- *Therapy is emergent and aimed toward restoring volume and water deficits.*
- *Address the underlying condition.*

General Considerations

Hypernatremia is characterized by a serum sodium concentration over 150 mEq/L. Hypernatremia is much less common than hyponatremia but may also cause serious neuromuscular symptoms and signs. Hypertonicity normally stimulates ADH release and thirst. Hypernatremia arises from an inability either to concentrate the urine or to drink water. Excessive salt intake may rarely play a role. Thus, hypernatremia may arise from excessive water loss, decreased water intake, or salt gain.

A. EXCESSIVE WATER LOSS

Excessive water loss often occurs when the thirst mechanism is deficient (eg, in infants or when coma, intubation, or dementia are present). Causes can be classified as nonrenal or renal.

1. Nonrenal—Nonrenal causes of excessive water loss include protracted fever, burns, and thyrotoxicosis.

2. Renal—There are 5 main renal causes:

- Tube feeding syndrome (ie, more water than sodium is lost in relation to intake of water and sodium, producing osmotic diuresis)
- Diabetes insipidus
- Hypercalcemia
- Renal failure
- Drugs (eg, demeclocycline, lithium)

B. INADEQUATE WATER INTAKE

Inadequate water intake may occur when coma is present or when the thirst mechanism is lost.

C. EXCESSIVE SODIUM INTAKE: MASSIVE SALT INGESTION

Excessive sodium intake may result from ingestion of salt pills, from ocean drowning, or from iatrogenic causes (eg, inadvertent hypertonic solution administration).

Clinical Findings

A. SYMPTOMS AND SIGNS

Symptoms and signs of hypernatremia relate to the severity and rate of development. These include thirst, lethargy, and dehydrated appearance (eg, dry mucous membranes, poor skin turgor). Tachycardia, low blood pressure, and oliguria may be present. Fever, confusion, delirium, seizures, and coma are manifestations of severe hypernatremia. Intracerebral hemorrhage may occur in severe cases, perhaps secondary to tearing of bridging veins stretched by shrinking brain tissue. Elevated blood urea nitrogen level and hematocrit may also occur.

B. RENAL CONSERVATION OF WATER

The approach to the patient with hypernatremia depends primarily on urine osmolality.

1. Urine osmolality greater than 400 mOsm/kg— If urine osmolality is greater than 400 mOsm/kg, renal water-conserving mechanisms are operating.

a. Nonrenal losses—Hypernatremia is due to nonrenal losses of water from skin, lungs, gut, or burn areas, with attendant failure of water intake to keep pace with water losses. In this situation, total body sodium deficits may also be present despite the hypernatremia.

b. Tube feedings—Hypernatremia with concentrated urine also occurs with high-protein tube feedings with limited water intake. The increased urine urea concentration results in osmotic diuresis, with loss of more water than sodium.

c. Diabetes mellitus—Osmotic diuresis from glycosuria in patients with diabetes mellitus may also result in hypernatremia (after correction for the elevated glucose concentration).

2. Urine osmolality less than 250 mOsm/kg—

a. Diabetes insipidus—Hypernatremia accompanied by a urine osmolality of less than 250 mOsm/kg is characteristic of diabetes insipidus.

b. Central diabetes insipidus—Impaired secretion of ADH from the pituitary may occur following damage to or disease of the pituitary gland or the hypothalamus.

c. Nephrogenic diabetes insipidus—Nephrogenic diabetes insipidus results from insensitivity of the renal distal tubule and collecting duct to ADH. Acquired nephrogenic diabetes insipidus may occur in patients taking lithium or demeclocycline or after relief of prolonged urinary tract obstruction.

3. Urine osmolality approximately equal to plasma osmolality—Hypernatremia may also develop when urine osmolality is about the same as plasma osmolality. In this case, hypernatremia results from impaired renal water conservation, which may occur (1) in the diuretic phase of acute renal failure, (2) in certain cases of postobstructive diuresis, with severe potassium depletion, (3) in prolonged hypercalcemia, or (4) in some cases of chronic renal disease.

Treatment

Acute hypernatremia is a medical emergency because of the risk of brain damage and impaired ability to regulate water intake.

A. HYPOVOLEMIA

Hypernatremia in the presence of severe hypovolemia should be treated initially with isotonic saline to correct the volume deficit, followed by 5% dextrose in water to replace the free-water deficit. A mild volume deficit may be treated initially with 0.45% saline in 5% dextrose in water.

B. WATER DEFICIT

Replace water with intravenous dextrose solutions (eg, 5% dextrose in water). The amount of sodium excess and the amount of water required to restore serum sodium concentration to normal can be estimated from equations 6 and 7 (Appendix). For example, a 70-kg man with a serum sodium concentration of 155 mEq/L has an estimated total body water of 35 L and excess sodium of 525 mEq (15 mEq/L × 35). It would take 3.75 L of water to restore serum sodium to 140 mEq/L. In general, the rate of correction of hypernatremia should not exceed 1–2 mEq/L/h.

C. Body Deficit of Sodium

Because total body sodium deficits frequently exist with hypernatremia, fluid therapy often must include sodium in hypotonic replacement solutions.

D. Correction of the Underlying Disorder

After initiating therapy, it is important to address the cause of water loss, inadequate water intake, or salt intoxication.

Disposition

Patients with serum sodium over 150 mEq/L require hospitalization. Patients with lesser degrees of hypernatremia may be discharged from the emergency department with close follow-up.

DISORDERS OF SERUM POTASSIUM CONCENTRATION

Potassium is the principal intracellular electrolyte; over 95% of the body's potassium is stored within cells. The body's potassium content is given in Table 42–5. Disorders of serum potassium concentration may not reflect accurately the condition of body potassium stores for the following reasons:

- Serum pH alters the distribution of potassium between cells and plasma: acidosis promotes transfer of potassium from intracellular to extracellular fluid, causing hyperkalemia; alkalosis does the reverse, causing potassium to enter the cells.

Table 42–5. Potassium content of the body.[1]

Body Compartment	Body Potassium (%)
Plasma	0.4
Interstitial fluid and lymph	1
Cartilage and dense connective tissue	0.4
Bone	7.6
Transcellular	1
Intracellular	89.6

[1]Modified and reproduced, with permission, from Ganong WF: *Review of Medical Physiology*, 13th ed. Appleton & Lange, 1987.

- Extensive cell injury (eg, from burns or crush injuries) may release large amounts of potassium into the extracellular fluid and cause hyperkalemia, because tissue cells contain most of the body's potassium.

- Body potassium content and serum concentrations of potassium are regulated by the kidney; however, the kidneys adjust to alterations in serum potassium more slowly and with less efficiency than is the case with sodium.

- Diuretic-induced potassium loss is one of the major causes of hypokalemia. Diminished food intake alone is rarely a cause of hypokalemia, because most foods contain large amounts of potassium.

- Potassium distribution may be affected by circulating levels of hormones such as insulin (which causes potassium influx into cells) and catecholamines (which cause potassium influx via their β-adrenergic effects).

HYPOKALEMIA

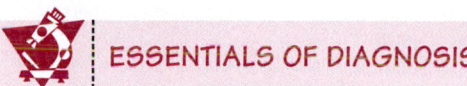 ESSENTIALS OF DIAGNOSIS

- *Most commonly occurs in diuretic therapy and metabolic alkalosis.*
- *Symptoms are primarily neuromuscular and cardiac.*
- *Serum potassium represents only 2% of total body potassium.*
- *Whenever possible, utilize oral replacement; never give more than 15 mEq/h intravenously.*

General Considerations

Hypokalemia is defined as a serum potassium concentration of less than 3.5 mEq/L. It is a common complication of diuretic therapy. Other causes are listed in Table 42–6. Most cases of hypokalemia result from excessive potassium wasting.

Clinical Findings

A. Symptoms and Signs

Clinical signs and symptoms suggestive of hypokalemia include varying degrees of weakness, including muscular paralysis; paralytic ileus; rhabdomyolysis; and cardiac dysrhythmias, including A-V dissociation, ventricular tachycardia, and ventricular fibrillation.

Table 42–6. Causes of hypokalemia.[1]

Poor intake
  Starvation, alcoholism
  Prolonged use of intravenous fluids lacking potassium
Reduced absorption
  Malabsorption
  Small bowel bypass; short bowel
Increased loss
  Gastrointestinal: Vomiting, gastrointestinal suction, obstruction, small bowel fistula, diarrhea, villous adenoma, laxative abuse
  Renal: Diuresis (diuretics, osmolar); congenital tubular defects (renal tubular acidosis, Franconi's syndrome); renal failure; acidosis (especially diabetes); metabolic alkalosis; corticotropin or glucocorticoid excess (Cushing's syndrome); mineralocorticoid excess (aldosterone-renin); licorice abuse; Bartter's syndrome; some antibiotics (amphotericin B, aminoglycosides, sodium load with carbenicillin or ticarcillin); magnesium depletion
  Skin: Burns; excessive sweating
Hypokalemia with no deficit (shift into cells)
  Insulin; β-adrenergic agonists
  Athletic training; testosterone (anabolic agent) therapy
  Respiratory alkalosis
  Familial periodic paralysis
  Treatment of megaloblastic anemia

---

[1]Modified and reproduced, with permission, from Schroeder SA et al (editors): *Current Medical Diagnosis & Treatment 1991.* Appleton & Lange, 1991.

B. Laboratory Findings

The most important laboratory tests to obtain are a basic chemistry panel and consider a venous pH. Hypokalemia can be seen in both acidosis and alkalosis. Determining whether a metabolic derangement exists, and what that derangement is, remains the key to correcting the electrolyte abnormality (Figure 42–2) .

C. Electrocardiographic Findings

Typical electrocardiogram (ECG) changes seen with hypokalemia include ST depression, T wave flattening, and the appearance of U waves (Figure 42–3).

Treatment

A. Hypokalemia Due to Alkalosis

If hypokalemia is not associated with depletion of body stores of potassium and is due solely to metabolic alkalosis, the initial goal of treatment is to correct the alkalosis or the condition causing it. Hypokalemia, however, may cause or exacerbate metabolic alkalosis (eg, prolonged gastric suction), thus necessitating potassium repletion.

B. Hypokalemia Associated with Depletion of Body Potassium Stores

Treat hypokalemia arising from depleted body potassium stores with oral or intravenous potassium salts, depending on severity and associated symptoms.

Intravenous emergency replenishment of potassium stores is indicated for patients with severe hypokalemia (serum potassium < 2.5 mEq/L), especially if neuromuscular or ECG manifestations are present.

If intravenous replenishment is necessary, the solution should be no more concentrated than 60 mEq/L and is generally infused at a rate of 10–15 mEq/h. The solution should be mixed in normal saline or other dextrose-free solutions, because the addition of dextrose will stimulate insulin release and lead to intracellular uptake of the cation. Potassium should always be infused as a drip, never pushed rapidly. Although there is some debate over the use of central versus peripheral venous access for the infusion, it appears that either is acceptable. However, peripheral infusion may be complicated by painful irritation, especially at faster infusion rates.

If patients are able to take fluids orally, they can be given oral potassium, which is safe and rapidly absorbed. Give K^+ solution, 40 mEq orally every 3–4 hours, until hypokalemia is corrected. Avoid giving high doses of potassium-containing tablets or capsules for rapid potassium repletion, because esophageal injury has been reported if stricture is present.

A good estimate for potassium repletion is that the administration of 20 mEq will cause a 0.25 mEq/L rise in concentration. Therefore, a serum potassium of 2.5 mEq/L, or a potassium deficit of 1.0 mEq/L, will require approximately 80 mEq of oral or intravenous replacement. In general, the overall rate of intravenous potassium replacement should not exceed 5 mEq/kg/ 24 h (0.2 mEq/kg/h).

Occasionally patients may have hypokalemia and potassium depletion that are refractory to administration of potassium salts. Magnesium deficiency may contribute to this abnormality, and repletion of magnesium will be necessary to bring about full correction of the potassium depletion and hypokalemia.

Disposition

Patients with severe hypokalemia (serum potassium < 2.5 mEq/L) require hospitalization in a monitored setting for proper diagnosis and correction. Patients with lesser degrees of hypokalemia may be discharged from the emergency department but should have close follow-up and repeat testing within 1 week.

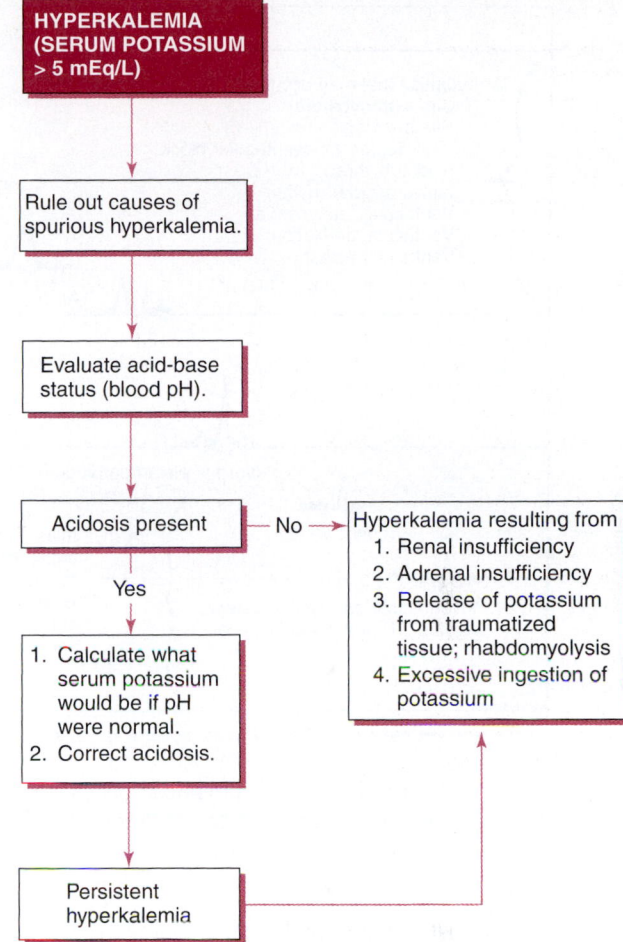

Figure 42–2. Emergency evaluation of hyperkalemia.

HYPERKALEMIA
(See Figure 42–2.)

 **ESSENTIALS OF DIAGNOSIS**

- *A true life-threatening medical emergency.*
- *Suspect in patients with renal disease, diabetic patients, or those taking potassium supplements.*
- *Symptoms are primarily neuromuscular and cardiac.*
- *ECG progression from hyperacute T waves to ventricular fibrillation may be rapid.*
- *Beware of spurious hyperkalemia.*
- *Therapy stabilizes cardiac membranes, shifts potassium into cells, and causes potassium elimination.*

- *Always admit patients to monitored setting and address the underlying condition.*

General Considerations

Hyperkalemia is generally defined as a serum potassium concentration greater than 5.0. It is less common (Table 42–7), but more immediately life threatening, than hypokalemia.

Clinical Findings

A. SYMPTOMS AND SIGNS

Clinical symptoms and signs of hyperkalemia include generalized weakness or paresthesias, diarrhea, and cardiac dysrhythmias.

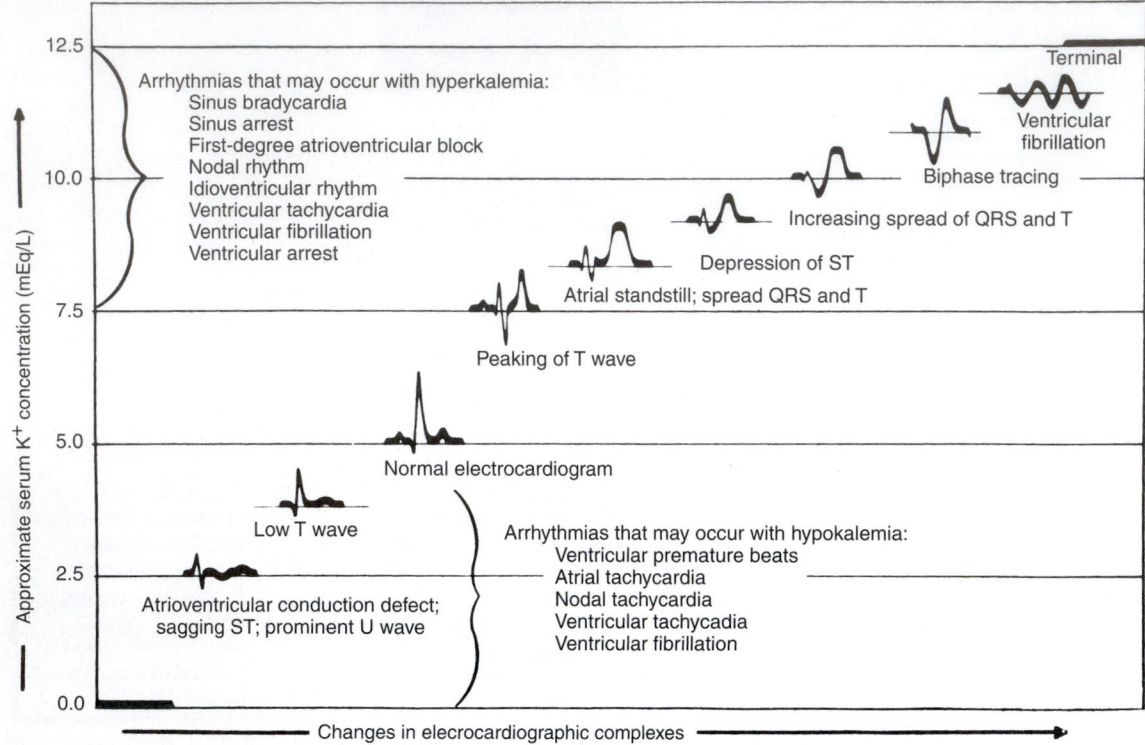

Figure 42–3. Correlation between serum potassium concentration and ECG findings. The correlation is approximate and depends on serum pH and concentrations of other ions (Na⁺, Ca²⁺). (Reproduced, with permission, from Schroeder SA [editor]: *Current Medical Diagnosis & Treatment 1992.* Appleton & Lange, 1992.)

Table 42–7. Causes of hyperkalemia.

True hyperkalemia
Acidosis (movement of potassium from cells into extracellular fluid)
Impaired renal potassium excretion:
Renal disease; oliguria due to severe dehydration
Mineralocorticoid deficiency
Drugs (triamterene, spironolactone, amiloride)
Increased potassium load:
Tissue death (eg, crush injury), burns, severe infections
Potassium ingestion (eg, salt substitutes)
Spurious hyperkalemia (true serum potassium concentration is normal)
Thrombocytosis (potassium release from platelets during clotting)
Hemolysis during clotting
Delayed separation of serum from clot (diffusion of potassium from erythrocytes)
Fist clenching during phlebotomy (loss of potassium from exercising muscle)

B. ELECTROCARDIOGRAPHIC FINDINGS

The ECG changes seen in hyperkalemia are varied and well-documented (see Figure 42–3). A thorough understanding of these changes is crucial to the emergency physician, because they are often the first clinical indication of an abnormality. Tall, hyperacute, or "peaked" T waves are most often associated with mild hyperkalemia. As hyperkalemia worsens, prolongation of the PR interval and the QRS duration can be seen. Severe hyperkalemia can be manifest in many ways, including loss of P waves, intraventricular conduction delays, bundle branch blocks, bizarre QRS morphologies, ventricular fibrillation, and asystole.

In addition to these changes, ECG findings consistent with ischemia or infarction, including ST-segment changes and (less frequently) Q waves, can be seen in hyperkalemia. These changes will resolve with treatment of the underlying disorder. Because of the wide variety of possible ECG manifestations, hyperkalemia should be suspected in any high-risk patient (eg, with renal insufficiency or taking potassium-sparing diuretics) who has ECG abnormalities.

C. SPURIOUS HYPERKALEMIA

Rule out spurious hyperkalemia caused by the following conditions:

1. Hemolysis—If serum in the sample appears hemolyzed (pink), draw a new blood sample. Hemolysis is also associated with markedly elevated serum lactate dehydrogenase concentrations.

2. Marked thrombocytosis—Platelet counts over 1 million/μL may result in liberation of significant amounts of potassium as clotting occurs. This effect may be avoided by measuring potassium concentrations or heparinized plasma rather than serum.

3. Fist clenching during antecubital phlebotomy—This action can raise serum potassium concentration in the sample (but not in the body) by releasing potassium from the exercising forearm muscles.

D. TRUE HYPERKALEMIA

If hyperkalemia is still present after acidosis has been corrected, the cause of hyperkalemia must be determined and treatment instituted accordingly.

1. Renal disease—Renal disease associated with hyperkalemia is always manifested by decreased creatinine clearance and elevated serum creatinine.

2. Mineralocorticoid deficiency—Mineralocorticoid deficiency (eg, Addison disease, acute adrenal insufficiency) may be manifested by hyperkalemia and hyponatremia. In severe cases, orthostatic hypotension or shock may also be present.

In certain cases of renal insufficiency and type 4 renal tubular acidosis, hyporeninemic hypoaldosteronism may also be associated with hyperkalemia. In either case, serum sodium is usually low, which is unusual in other causes of hyperkalemia.

3. Drug-induced hyperkalemia—Drug-induced hyperkalemia (eg, ingestion of aldosterone antagonists or large amounts of potassium) may be diagnosed from the history. Penicillin G, administered as a potassium salt in high doses, may be an iatrogenic cause of hyperkalemia. The use of potassium-containing salt substitutes in patients with sodium-retaining disorders may also predispose to hyperkalemia. Other medications that may cause hyperkalemia include potassium-sparing diuretics, nonsteroidal anti-inflammatory drugs, and digoxin.

4. Crush injuries or burns—Rhabdomyolysis or burns sufficient to produce hyperkalemia are grossly apparent in most cases.

Treatment

The speed with which treatment must be initiated depends on the degree of hyperkalemia and on symptoms, signs, and ECG abnormalities. Any unstable patient (serum potassium > 7.0 mEq/L, or with any degree of hyperkalemia and concurrent ECG changes) requires emergency stabilizing measures before further treatment, such as potassium elimination, is initiated.

A. EMERGENT STABILIZATION

Emergent stabilization is indicated for patients discussed above. Two amps of calcium gluconate, or 1 amp of calcium chloride, administered as an intravenous push, helps to decrease the irritability of cardiac myositic membranes. This can be repeated after 2–5 minutes and followed by an infusion of 5 amps mixed in 500 mL of 5% dextrose in water, because the stabilizing effect of calcium is transient. Although calcium chloride provides a larger and more rapidly bioavailable source of calcium, it also carries a theoretical risk of worsening acidosis and should be used with caution in cases of hyperkalemia caused by acidosis.

Insulin (10 units regular, intravenous push) can be administered to force a temporary influx of potassium into the cells. This should be given in concert with glucose to prevent iatrogenic hypoglycemia. Adding β-2 agonists, either intravenously or via nebulization, can also enhance potassium influx.

In patients with acidosis, sodium bicarbonate can be administered; however, this approach is not indicated in diabetic ketoacidosis (see "Acid-Base Disorders" section, below).

B. POTASSIUM ELIMINATION

Potassium elimination can be accomplished in one of two ways. Kayexalate (sodium polystyrene sulfate) is a potassium exchange resin that will bind the cation and enhance its elimination in the gastrointestinal tract. Hemodialysis is the definitive treatment and should be considered in patients with renal failure or following the above emergent measures in a severely unstable patient.

C. CORRECTION OF THE UNDERLYING DISORDER

In almost all cases, correction of the underlying acidosis, or other secondary cause of the hyperkalemia, will resolve the electrolyte abnormality. This should be noted when undertaking corrective measures, because treatment of the underlying cause combined with emergent treatment of hyperkalemia may result in a hypokalemia. This is especially true in diabetic ketoacidosis, where patients often have depleted their total-body potassium stores, despite an apparent serum hyperkalemia. For this reason, treatment should be aimed at the underlying disorder, and chemistry panels should be checked every 1–2 hours until the patient has been stabilized. Serial blood gases may also be warranted.

Disposition

Patients with hyperkalemia require hospitalization in a monitored setting.

DISORDERS OF SERUM CALCIUM CONCENTRATION

Calcium, the most abundant cation, is 99% bound to bone and 1% extracellular. Serum calcium is composed of 2 major fractions. About 55% of total serum calcium is bound to serum proteins (chiefly albumin) or complexed to organic anions such as citrate; the other 45% exists as free, or ionized, calcium. Symptoms and signs of disordered serum calcium concentration are due to changes in the ionized fraction. Proper interpretation of serum calcium concentration requires measure of serum albumin concentration. Serum calcium is usually reported in mg/dL; this unit is easily converted to mEq/L by dividing by 2. The ionized calcium level in plasma is controlled chiefly by the action of parathyroid hormone, calcitonin, and vitamin D metabolites and is related to the patient's acid-base status. Acidosis increases the fraction of total calcium in the ionized form by displacing it from albumin, whereas alkalosis decreases it. As a result, symptomatic hypocalcemia may develop in patients who hyperventilate (acute respiratory alkalosis) or in those in whom metabolic acidosis has been rapidly corrected with infusion of sodium bicarbonate.

HYPOCALCEMIA

 ESSENTIALS OF DIAGNOSIS

- *May accompany shock, sepsis, or massive transfusion of blood products.*
- *Neuromuscular and respiratory symptoms predominate.*
- *Rarely life-threatening by itself and may be associated with disorders of magnesium and phosphate.*
- *A prolonged QT interval may be only ECG manifestation.*
- *Address the underlying cause.*

General Considerations

Hypocalcemia is defined as an ionized calcium concentration of less than 2.0 mEq/L. It may result from decreased intake or decreased absorption of calcium (eg, vitamin D deficiency, malabsorption syndromes), increased renal loss (eg, renal failure, diuretic therapy), endocrine disease (hypoparathyroidism), hypomagnesemia, or hyperphosphatemia. Hypocalcemia may accompany shock, hemorrhagic pancreatitis, sepsis, or massive transfusion of blood products (Table 42–8).

Clinical Findings

A. SYMPTOMS AND SIGNS

Many patients with mild hypocalcemia are asymptomatic. Symptoms and signs of more severe hypocalcemia include tetany, weakness, fatigue, cramps, carpopedal spasm, convulsions, diplopia, and stridor and dyspnea due to laryngospasm. Positive Trousseau and Chvostek signs and fasciculations of skeletal muscle also occur. Cataracts may also occur with long-standing hypocalcemia.

B. LABORATORY FINDINGS

An arterial or venous blood gas may be useful to identify (1) respiratory or metabolic alkalosis as a cause of transient tetany and (2) hypercapnia secondary to severe hypocalcemia. It is important to determine renal

Table 42–8. Causes of hypocalcemia.[1]

Decreased intake or absorption
    Malabsorption
    Small bowel bypass, short bowel
    Vitamin D deficit (decreased absorption, decreased production of 25-hydroxyvitamin D or 1,25-dihydroxyvitamin D)
Increased loss
    Chronic renal insufficiency
    Diuretic therapy
Endocrine disease
    Hypoparathyroidism (genetic, acquired)
    Pseudohypoparathyroidism
    Calcitonin secretion with medullary carcinoma of the thyroid
Physiologic causes
    Associated with decreased serum albumin
    Decreased end organ response to vitamin D
    Hyperphosphatemia
    Induced by aminoglycoside antibiotics, mithramycin, loop diuretics

[1]Reproduced, with permission, from Schroeder SA et al (editors): *Current Medical Diagnosis & Treatment 1991.* Appleton & Lange, 1991.

function and serum potassium and magnesium concentrations (coexisting abnormalities are common and may require treatment).

C. Electrocardiographic Findings

A prolonged QT interval may be noted on the ECG without U waves (Figure 42–4).

Treatment

Hypocalcemia is rarely life threatening but must be addressed in conjunction with treating the primary disorder. Severe hypocalcemia can cause laryngeal stridor and grand mal seizures. Because of the potential for severe symptoms, even mild symptoms attributable to hypocalcemia should be treated. Asymptomatic patients require close outpatient follow-up and an appropriate workup.

For initial treatment in a symptomatic adult, give calcium chloride (5%) or calcium gluconate (10%), one to two 10-mL ampules by intravenous infusion. Then give 1 ampule in 500 mL of normal saline intravenously over 8 hours to provide 100–500 mg of calcium and maintain the serum calcium concentration at 7–8 mg/dL, the level at which symptoms are usually alleviated. During massive transfusions, 10 cc of calcium chloride should be given for every 4–6 units of blood. Long-term treatment of chronic hypocalcemia requires oral calcium supplements and vitamin D. Treat hypomagnesemia, if present (see below).

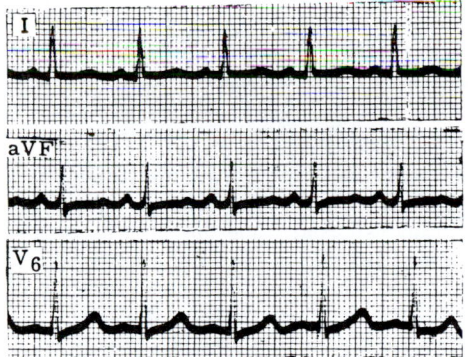

Figure 42–4. The ECG in hypocalcemia. T waves are upright, but the QT interval is prolonged at 0.4 s (corrected for RR of 0.66 s, $QT_c = 0.48$ s). The lengthening of the QT interval is due to a lengthening of the ST segment and not to any abnormality in the T wave itself. Blood calcium at the time the above recording was made was 6.8 mg/dL. (Reproduced, with permission, from Goldman MJ: *Principles of Clinical Electrocardiography*, 12th ed. Lange, 1986.)

Caution: Rarely, hypocalcemia requiring treatment is accompanied by markedly elevated phosphorus concentration (> 6 mg/dL). To prevent metastatic calcification, correct hyperphosphatemia before or while giving calcium. Give intravenous glucose and insulin (see "Hyperphosphatemia" section, below).

Disposition

Patients with acute symptomatic hypocalcemia require hospitalization in a closely monitored setting. Patients with less severe disease may be discharged from the emergency department but should have close follow-up.

HYPERCALCEMIA

 ## ESSENTIALS OF DIAGNOSIS

- *Usually caused by a malignancy or hyperparathyroidism.*
- *Symptoms are primarily neuromuscular and renal.*
- *Serum calcium above 12 mg/dL requires acute diagnosis and therapy.*
- *Therapy is primarily volume repletion because natriuresis promotes renal calcium excretion.*
- *Bisphosphonates are effective osteoclast inhibitors.*
- *Always admit symptomatic patients.*

General Considerations

Hypercalcemia is characterized by a serum calcium concentration over 11 mg/dL. It is commonly associated with numerous conditions (Table 42–9) and may have life-threatening consequences. The majority of patients with symptomatic hypercalcemia have either hyperparathyroidism or a malignancy.

Clinical Findings

A. Symptoms and Signs

Symptoms of hypercalcemia usually begin at levels over 12 mg/dL and are nonspecific. The diagnosis may be missed unless it is suspected and serum calcium measured. Central nervous system depression, stupor, somnolence, weakness, psychosis, and coma may occur. Anorexia, vomiting, constipation, and abdominal pain may also be seen. Symptoms become severe at serum concentrations greater than 15 mg/dL.

Table 42–9. Causes of hypercalcemia.[1]

Increased intake or absorption
Milk-alkali syndrome
Vitamin D or vitamin A excess
Endocrine disorders
Primary hyperparathyroidism (adenoma, hyperplasia, carcinoma)
Secondary hyperparathyroidism (renal insufficiency, malabsorption)
Acromegaly
Adrenal insufficiency
Neoplastic disease
Tumors producing PTH-like peptides (ovary, kidney, lung)
Metastases to bone
Lymphoproliferative disease, including multiple myeloma
Secretion of prostaglandins and osteolytic factors
Miscellaneous causes
Thiazide diuretic-induced
Sarcoidosis
Paget's disease of bone
Hypophosphatasia
Immobilization
Familial hypocalciuric hypercalcemia
Complications of renal transplantation
Iatrogenic

[1]Reproduced, with permission, from Schroeder SA et al (editors): *Current Medical Diagnosis & Treatment 1991.* Appleton & Lange, 1991.

Renal damage may occur in chronic cases, for example, when impaired concentration ability of the kidney leads to polyuria, dehydration, hypernatremia, thirst, and finally azotemia. Band keratopathy may occur in long-standing hypercalcemia.

Hypercalcemia reflects an increase in the concentration of the ionized fraction of calcium, because elevated levels of calcium-binding serum proteins (chiefly albumin) do not occur except in cases of extreme dehydration.

B. ELECTROCARDIOGRAPHIC FINDINGS

ECG abnormalities include prolonged PR interval, shortened QT interval, and flattened T waves.

Treatment

Any serum calcium concentration above 12 mg/dL requires prompt treatment, especially if symptoms are present. The goal of treatment is to lower serum calcium by general measures and by measures appropriate to the specific cause of hypercalcemia. Avoid immobilization if at all possible.

A. PROMOTE EXCRETION OF CALCIUM BY THE KIDNEY

1. Fluids—Volume expansion with isotonic saline promotes a natriuresis and calcium excretion, and is the first step in treating hypercalcemia in patients with normal renal function. The vast majority of these patients are initially dehydrated. Infuse saline until the patient is clinically euvolemic and producing adequate urine. Rarely patients may require monitoring of central venous pressure.

2. Diuretics—Furosemide is also effective in increasing excretion of calcium in patients in whom volume expansion with isotonic saline has been achieved. Do not use thiazide diuretics, because they may aggravate hypercalcemia. Give furosemide, 0.5–1.0 mg/kg intravenously, and monitor fluid status closely, because hypovolemia induced by furosemide will diminish calcium excretion and prolong hypercalcemia.

B. INCREASE DEPOSITION OF CALCIUM IN BONE

Another treatment approach is to promote deposition of calcium into bone or decrease the rate of resorption of calcium from bone.

1. Bisphosphonates—These analogues of pyrophosphate are concentrated in areas of boney turnover and inhibit osteoclast activity. The first-generation bisphosphonate etidronate is poorly absorbed orally and is most effective intravenously (7.5 mg/kg intravenously each day for 3 days). It may cause hypophosphatemia through a renal mechanism. Second-generation pamidronate, 60–90 mg intravenously, infused over 24 hours, has higher potency and prolonged duration of action. Fever is common and thought to be secondary to cytokine release from osteoclasts and macrophages. Pamidronate is the agent of choice in severe hypercalcemia associated with malignancy and is used with forced diuresis.

2. Mithramycin—Given in an intravenous dose of 25 µg/kg, mithramycin lowers serum calcium concentration within 8–12 hours, and this effect may last several days. Close monitoring of serum calcium is necessary because toxicity is related to frequency and dose administered. Toxicity is unusual with only 1 or 2 doses. Mithramycin use has been displaced by the second-generation bisphosphonates in the treatment of malignancy-induced hypercalcemia.

3. Calcitonin—Calcitonin may be effective in some cases of hypercalcemia; it should be reserved as adjunctive rather than primary therapy. Action is immediate, inhibiting calcium and phosphorus release at the osteoclast level. Therapy is short lived, most likely due to tachyphylaxis. The starting dose is 4 IU/kg intramuscularly or subcutaneously every 12 hours. Calcitonin should be reserved as a rapid modality in life-threatening hypercalcemia while waiting for more sustained therapies (eg, pamidronate) to work. Glucocorticoids may prolong the hypocalcemic effect of calcitonin.

4. Phosphate—*Caution:* Hypercalcemia complicated by hypophosphatemia (common in primary hyperparathyroidism) will respond to slowly raising the patient's serum phosphate concentration to near normal. Although intravenous phosphate can dramatically lower serum calcium, there is significant risk of toxicity, including potentially fatal metastatic calcification. Use intravenous phosphate only in consultation with a nephrologist in a critical care setting.

C. Decrease Absorption of Calcium by the Intestine

Corticosteriods reduce any increase in gastrointestinal absorption of calcium, such as occurs in vitamin D intoxication and sarcoidosis. Steroids are also effective in hypercalcemia secondary to lymphoproliferative malignancies, due to antitumor effects. Hydrocortisone, 3–4 mg/kg/d orally or intravenously, should cause a fall in serum calcium concentration within 1–2 days.

D. Perform Hemodialysis

In patients with renal insufficiency or in whom the above measures are ineffective, hemodialysis with calcium-free dialysate effectively removes calcium from the extracellular fluid.

Disposition

Patients with a serum calcium concentration over 12 mg/dL should be hospitalized. Those with lower levels may be discharged from the emergency department but require close follow-up and outpatient workup.

DISORDERS OF SERUM PHOSPHORUS CONCENTRATION

HYPOPHOSPHATEMIA

General Considerations

Hypophosphatemia is characterized by a serum phosphorus concentration under 2 mg/dL. It is a common condition with diverse causes (Table 42–10). An isolated serum phosphate level may not reflect total body stores, because phosphate is prone to shifting intracellularly. Phosphate is critical to many cellular functions,

Table 42–10. Causes of hypophosphatemia.

Alcoholism
Primary hyperparathyroidism
Phosphorus-deficient parenteral nutrition
Treatment with phosphate-binding antacids
Metabolic or respiratory alkalosis
Severe burns
Recovery from diabetic ketoacidosis
Starvation

and severe hypophosphatemia has profound effects on multiple organ systems.

Clinical Findings

Diagnosis of hypophosphatemia depends on laboratory measurement of serum phosphorus concentration, because clinical symptoms are usually vague and nonspecific. Acute respiratory alkalosis or a recent glucose load may lead to hypophosphatemia. Fatigue, neuromuscular weakness, irritability, paresthesias, dysarthria, confusion, convulsion, and coma may occur. At serum levels below 1 mg/dL, hemolysis and impaired neutrophil phagocytosis become evident. Erythrocyte 2,3-disphosphoglycerate is lowered, resulting in decreased delivery of oxygen to the tissues. Rhabdomyolysis may occur.

Treatment

Treatment consists of replacing phosphorus by intravenous or oral phosphate supplements. All patients with a serum phosphorus concentration under 2 mg/dL should receive supplements. Milk is an excellent source of phosphate. Aluminum phosphate gel (Phosphaljel) or neutral phosphate salts (adults, 0.5–1.0 g/d of phosphate orally) can be given.

Sodium or potassium phosphate may be carefully given intravenously in severe symptomatic hypophosphatemia, (usually phosphate < 1.0 mg/dL). Serum phosphate, calcium, potassium, and magnesium must be carefully monitored during therapy, because hypocalcemia and metastatic calcifications may occur during therapy. Intravenous therapy of severe hypophosphatemia should be given by experienced physicians in a monitored, critical care setting. Oral therapy is safer and should be used whenever possible.

Disposition

Hospitalization is invariably necessary for patients with a serum phosphorus concentration under 1 mg/dL and is strongly advised for those whose serum phosphorus is under 2 mg/dL. Patients for whom hospitalization is not indicated require close follow-up.

HYPERPHOSPHATEMIA

General Considerations

Hyperphosphatemia is characterized by a serum phosphorus concentration over 7 mg/dL. It may result from chronic or acute renal disease; hypoparathyroidism; growth hormone excess; cytolysis (rhabdomyolysis or chemotherapy of lymphoproliferative tumors); excessive enemas with phosphate-containing solutions; or ingestion of large amounts of phosphate, vitamin D, or laxatives.

Clinical Findings

No signs are directly referable to hyperphosphatemia. However, hypocalcemia or hypomagnesemia may develop because of tissue deposition of calcium phosphate.

Treatment

A. GLUCOSE AND INSULIN

Administer 50% glucose and regular insulin as described above (see "Hyperkalemia" section) to produce an initial fall in serum phosphorus.

B. VOLUME EXPANSION

Infuse isotonic saline to achieve volume expansion and promote excretion of phosphate by the kidneys in patients with normal renal function. Acetazolamide (Diamox) will also facilitate urinary phosphate excretion. Give 500 mg every 6 hours, but monitor fluid balance closely.

C. PHOSPHATE-BINDING ANTACIDS

Oral phosphate-binding antacids such as aluminum hydroxide will cause binding of phosphate in the gut and reduce phosphate absorption.

D. DIALYSIS

Dialysis is required to lower serum phosphorus concentration in patients with renal failure.

Disposition

Indications for hospitalization usually depend on factors other than hyperphosphatemia itself (eg, renal insufficiency, rhabdomyolysis).

DISORDERS OF SERUM MAGNESIUM CONCENTRATION

Magnesium, the most abundant intracellular divalent cation, is distributed approximately 1% extracellularly, 30% intracellularly, and 69% in bone. Serum concentration may not reflect total body stores. Magnesium is essential to life and plays an important role in regulating cellular adenosine triphosphate and maintaining intracellular potassium concentration. Green vegetables, nuts, peas, and beans are rich in magnesium. Excretion is via the kidneys and depends on glomerular filtration. Magnesium deficiency is usually caused by decreased intake (nutritional deficiency) or enhanced excretion (endocrine or renal disorders).

HYPOMAGNESEMIA

 ESSENTIALS OF DIAGNOSIS

- *Frequently associated with disorders of calcium, potassium, and phosphate.*
- *Common in malnourished patients and in those with renal disease.*
- *Symptoms are primarily neuromuscular and similar to those of hypocalcemia.*
- *Utilize oral replacement whenever possible.*
- *Symptomatic patients require admission.*
- *Identify and treat the underlying cause.*

General Considerations

Hypomagnesemia is characterized by a serum magnesium concentration under 1 mEq/L (< 1.2 mg/dL). It is commonly associated with several conditions (Table 42–11). It is frequently associated with hypocalcemia and disorders of potassium and phosphate, and should be suspected in high-risk patients and those with other electrolyte and elemental deficiencies.

Clinical Findings

Carpopedal spasm, tetany, athetoid movements, jerking, coarse and flapping tremors, and hyperexcitability may occur. A positive Babinski sign, seizures, and weakness are seen. Hypertension and vasomotor changes as well as confusion, disorientation, and psychotic behavior can occur. Severe hypomagnesemia and hypokalemia may lead to significant prolongation of the QT interval and subsequent ventricular tachycardia and fibrillation.

Table 42–11. Causes of hypomagnesemia.[1]

Diminished absorption or intake
   Malabsorption, chronic diarrhea, laxative abuse
   Prolonged gastrointestinal suction
   Small bowel bypass
   Malnutrition
   Alcoholism
   Parenteral alimentation with inadequate Mg^{2+} content
Increased loss
   Diabetic ketoacidosis
   Diuretic therapy
   Diarrhea
   Hyperaldosteronism, Bartter's syndrome
   Associated with hypercalciuria
   Renal magnesium wasting
Unexplained
   Hyperparathyroidism
   Postparathyroidectomy
   Vitamin D therapy
   Induced by aminoglycoside antibiotics, cisplatin

---

[1]Reproduced, with permission, from Schroeder SA et al (editors): *Current Medical Diagnosis & Treatment 1991.* Appleton & Lange, 1991.

Treatment

Hypocalcemia and hypokalemia associated with hypomagnesemia are characteristically resistant to calcium supplementation but respond quickly to magnesium replacement. Great caution must be used in patients with renal insufficiency. Monitor and correct associated electrolyte abnormalities.

A. Oral Replacement

The oral route is preferred in patients with long-standing magnesium deficiency. For adults, give magnesium oxide, 400 mg 4 times daily.

B. Parenteral Replacement

Reserve parenteral administration of magnesium for patients with severe hypomagnesemia, usually those who have evidence of neuromuscular or cardiac dysfunction.

1. Intramuscular route—Give magnesium sulfate, 1.0 g intramuscularly every 4–6 hours. This route is painful.

2. Intravenous route—Intravenous therapy is reserved for severe hypomagnesemia (usually in alcoholic patients). One cc of 50% magnesium sulfate contains 50 mg of magnesium. The usual recommended dose of intravenous magnesium is 1 g of magnesium sulfate every 6 hours. In the presence of ventricular tachycardia (torsade de pointes), 4 cc of 50% magnesium sulfate should be infused over 1–2 minutes.

Disposition

Patients with symptomatic hypomagnesemia require hospitalization. Patients with less severe magnesium depletion may require hospitalization because of associated conditions.

HYPERMAGNESEMIA

General Considerations

Hypermagnesemia is characterized by a serum magnesium concentration over 3 mEq/L (3.6 mg/dL). It is usually due to renal failure (acute or chronic) that is often associated with excessive magnesium intake (eg, from magnesium-containing antacids or magnesium sulfate).

Clinical Findings

A. Symptoms and Signs

Symptoms and signs are uncommon and vary depending on the severity of hypermagnesemia.

1. Serum concentration of 3–4 mEq/L—Peripheral vasodilatation may result in hypotension. Nausea and vomiting may also occur.

2. Serum concentration of 5–7 mEq/L—Drowsiness, confusion, and lethargy develop, and deep tendon reflexes are depressed or absent.

3. Serum concentration above 10 mEq/L—Coma and death occur, preceded by progressive weakness and skeletal muscle paralysis, with depression of the respiratory centers.

B. Electrocardiographic Findings

ECG changes include a prolonged PR interval, widened QRS complexes, and elevated T waves.

Treatment

A. Patients with Renal Insufficiency

In patients with severe renal insufficiency, significant hypermagnesemia must be treated by dialysis using a magnesium-free dialysate.

B. Patients with Normal Renal Function

Infusion of isotonic saline solution for volume expansion promotes urinary excretion of magnesium. Potent diuretics such as furosemide, 0.5–1.0 mg/kg intravenously, may also be effective. Intravenous infusion of calcium will temporarily neutralize the neuromuscular effects of hypermagnesemia.

Disposition

All patients with hypermagnesemia require hospitalization.

Adrogue HJ et al: Hypernatremia. N Engl J Med 2000;342 (20):1493. [PMID: 10816188] (A thorough review of hypernatremia, with an emphasis on, and examples of, recommended therapy.)

Adrogue HJ et al: Hyponatremia. N Engl J Med 2000;342 (21):1581. [PMID: 10824078] (A thorough review of hyponatremia, with an emphasis on, and examples of, recommended therapy.)

Agus ZS: Hypomagnesemia. J Am Soc Nephrol 1999;10:1616. [PMID: 10405219] (Signs and symptoms of hypomagnesemia are reviewed, as are the causes, approach to diagnosis, and therapy.)

Carlstedt F, Lind L: Hypocalcemic syndromes. Crit Care Clin 2001;17:139. [PMID: 11219226] (A review of calcium metabolism, hypocalcemia, and benefits of calcium replacement in the critically ill.)

Dacey MJ: Hypomagnesemic disorders. Crit Care Clin 2001;17 (1):155. [PMID: 11219227] (A review of the causes of hypomagnesemia as well as pathophysiology and therapeutics in critically ill patients.)

Davidson T: Conventional treatment of hypercalcemia of malignancy. Am J Health Syst Pharm 2001;58(Suppl 3):S8. [PMID: 11757206] (A review of the pathophysiology of hypercalcemia of malignancy, comparing available treatments and suggesting treatment guidelines. An excellent review of all FDA-approved therapies.)

Fulop M: Algorithms for diagnosing some electrolyte disorders. Am J Emerg Med 1998;16:76. [PMID: 9451320] (Presents an algorithmic approach to differentiating the causes of abnormalities in serum sodium, potassium, and calcium.)

Halperin ML et al: Potassium. Lancet 1998;352:135. [PMID: 9672294] (An overview of the pathophysiology of potassium disorders as well as a stepwise approach to the diagnosis and treatment of potassium disturbances.)

Kapoor et al: Fluid and electrolyte abnormalities. Crit Care Clin 2001;17:503. [PMID: 11525047] (A comprehensive review of electrolyte abnormalities with a focus on critical care.)

Mandal AK: Hypokalemia and hyperkalemia. Med Clin North Am 1997;81:611. [PMID: 9167648] (A thorough review of the causes and effects of disturbances in potassium homeostasis.)

Mattu A et al: Electrocardiographic manifestations of hyperkalemia. Am J Emerg Med 2000;18:721. [PMID: 11043630] (A case-based review of the common ECG changes seen in hyperkalemia.)

Singer FR: Medical management of nonparathyroid hypercalcemia and hypocalcemia. Otolaryngol Clin North Am 1996;29:701. [PMID: 8844739] (A comprehensive review of the medical management of both hypocalcemia and hypercalcemia.)

Ziegler R: Hypercalcemic crisis. J Am Soc Nephrol 2001;12(Suppl 17):S3. [PMID: 11251025] (A comprehensive review of the pathophysiology, diagnosis, and treatment of hypercalcemia.)

ACID-BASE DISORDERS

An understanding of acid-base disorders is paramount to the emergency physician. These disorders are encountered on a daily basis, and command of this complex topic guides appropriate management in the emergency department.

DEFINITIONS

Although the hydrogen ion concentration [H+] in humans is extremely low (normal level is 40 nmol/L), its regulation is vital to the function of many proteins and enzyme systems. Acid-base disorders are generally not characterized by [H+], but rather by the pH of the disturbance. Normal pH in humans is 7.4 (range 7.36–7.44). Acidemia is a state in which the blood pH is less than 7.36, and alkalemia is a state in which the blood pH is greater than 7.44. The pH of any solution is determined by the Henderson-Hesselbach equation:

$$pH = pK_a + \log \frac{[base]}{[acid]}$$

According to this equation, pH equals the pK_a (the pH at which one half of the compound is ionized) added to the ratio of the log of the concentration of base to its related acid.

In humans the most important acid base buffer is the bicarbonate-carbonic acid system.

CLASSIFICATION OF ACID-BASE DISORDERS

An arterial blood gas and an electrolyte panel are essential tests needed to determine the nature of the disorder(s) in patients with potential acid-base disorders. Acidosis is a process that tends to produce an acidemia, whereas alkalosis is a process that tends to produce an alkalemia. A metabolic or respiratory process alone (primary acid-base disorder) or a combination of the two processes (mixed acid-base disorder) may result in an alteration of blood pH. Metabolic processes involve a primary alteration in the HCO_3^- concentration, whereas respiratory disorders involve a primary alteration in the $PaCO_2$.

Primary processes that change pH from normal are generally only partially compensated; therefore, the primary acidosis or alkalosis is always evident by the acidemic (< 7.36) or alkalemic (> 7.44) pH. Patients with a primary respiratory alkalosis always have PCO_2 less than 35 mm Hg, whereas patients with a primary respiratory acidosis always have PCO_2 greater than 45 mm Hg. Patients with a primary metabolic alkalosis always have a HCO_3^- concentration greater than 28 mEq/L, whereas patients with a primary metabolic acidosis always have a HCO_3^- concentration less than 22 mEq/L.

COMPENSATION

Many metabolic and respiratory processes can cause swings in pH, but pH homeostasis is maintained by the combination of physiologic buffers, the lungs, and the kidneys. The bicarbonate-carbonic anhydrase buffer system is the most important buffering system in the blood and interstitial fluid. Cell metabolism produces carbon dioxide that combines with water to form carbonic acid. Carbonic acid then dissociates to form HCO_3^- and H^+:

$$H_2O + CO_2 \rightarrow H_2CO_3$$

$$H_2CO_3 \rightarrow H^+ + HCO_3^-$$

The normal concentration of carbonic acid is 1.2 mmol/L compared to the plasma HCO_3^- concentration of 24 mmol/L.

Under physiologic stress, the lungs and kidneys play a vital role in maintaining near-normal pH by altering the concentrations of this buffer system. The respiratory system provides compensation for primary metabolic processes, whereas the kidneys compensate for primary respiratory processes.

An alteration in blood pH secondary to a metabolic disturbance is sensed by chemoreceptors, which in turn signal the respiratory center. The generation of a metabolic acidosis (decrease in pH and HCO_3^-) will stimulate the respiratory center, causing a decrease in the $PaCO_2$ and consequently increasing the blood pH. The generation of a metabolic alkalosis (increase in pH and HCO_3^-) will inhibit the respiratory center, causing an increase in the $PaCO_2$ and consequently decreasing the blood pH.

In contrast to the almost immediate compensation provided by the respiratory system, the kidneys provide little compensation until after 6–12 hours of sustained alteration in blood pH. The kidneys maintain normal pH by excreting acids produced by normal metabolism in addition to adjusting HCO_3^- reabsorption in the proximal tubule. The kidneys respond to acidosis by stimulating renal synthesis and retention of HCO_3^- and actively excreting H^+ while retaining HCO_3^-. More than 6–12 hours of alkalemia stimulates the kidney to excrete HCO_3^- and retain H^+.

Table 42–12 displays the compensatory responses in primary acid-base disturbances. One should recognize the pattern in primary disturbances: the compensatory response of elevation versus lowering of the HCO_3^- or $PaCO_2$ is in the same direction as the primary abnormality. Discordance between the direction of compensation and the primary abnormality indicates two pri-

Table 42–12. Primary disorders and compensatory responses.

Disorder	Primary Abnormality	Compensation
Respiratory acidosis	Increased $PaCO_2$	Increased bicarbonate
Metabolic acidosis	Decreased bicarbonate	Decreased $PaCO_2$
Respiratory alkalosis	Decreased $PaCO_2$	Decreased bicarbonate
Metabolic alkalosis	Increased bicarbonate	Increased $PaCO_2$

mary disorders (see below). Generally, primary processes that change pH from normal are only partially compensated (the exception is chronic respiratory alkalosis); therefore, compensation does not approach total correction, nor can one overcompensate.

CLINICAL ACID-BASE DISORDERS

1. Respiratory Acidosis

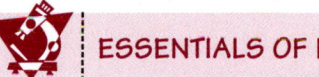

ESSENTIALS OF DIAGNOSIS

- *Impairment in rate of alveolar ventilation generates a hypercapnic state.*
- *Clinical feature is alteration of consciousness.*
- *Treat the underlying disorder.*

General Considerations

Respiratory acidosis is defined as an elevated $PaCO_2$ (> 45 mm Hg) and a subsequent drop in serum pH below 7.35. This results from an impairment of the rate of alveolar ventilation. Respiratory acidosis can be caused by central nervous system disorders, diseases affecting the respiratory muscles directly, airway obstruction, or primary pulmonic processes (Table 42–13).

Clinical Findings

The hallmark clinical finding of respiratory acidosis is an alteration in level of consciousness. The characteristic features of hypercapnia range from fatigue, irritability, headache, confusion, stupor, or obtundation to coma and depend on the severity and chronicity of this process. A $PaCO_2$ of 70mm Hg secondary to acute respiratory acidosis may result in a coma, whereas a person

Table 42–13. Causes of respiratory acidosis.

Acute
Respiratory center depression
Narcotic/sedative overdose
Cardiac arrest
Paralysis of respiratory muscles
Anticholinesterases, anesthetics
Cerebral, brainstem, or high spinal cord infarct
Primary neuromuscular diseases: Guillain-Barré, myasthenia gravis, amyotrophic lateral sclerosis, poliomyelitis, botulism, tetanus
Myopathy of respiratory muscles: muscular dystrophy, hypokalmemic myopathy, electrolyte imbalance (decreased phosphorus, magnesium), familial periodic paralysis
Primary hypoventilation
Diaphragmatic paralysis
Airway obstruction
Upper: laryngeal edema/spasm, tracheal edema/stenosis, obstructive sleep apnea
Lower: mechanical (foreign body, aspirated fluid, neoplasm, bronchospasm)
Pulmonic/musculoskeletal abnormalities
Pneumonia, pulmonary edema, acute respiratory disease syndrome, restrictive lung disease, pulmonary embolism
Pneumothorax, hemothorax, chest wall trauma, flail chest, smoke inhalation
Iatrogenic (mechanical ventilation)
Chronic
Chronic airway disease (chronic obstructive pulmonary disease, emphysema)
Extreme kyphoscoliosis
Extreme obesity (Pickwickian syndrome)

with a chronic respiratory acidosis may not progress into a coma until the $PaCO_2$ exceeds 100 mm Hg. Prolonged states of hypercapnia may result in elevated intracranial pressure from cerebral vasodilatation.

Physiology

A. ACUTE RESPIRATORY ACIDOSIS

An acute increase in the $PaCO_2$ results in a rise of $[H^+]$ and subsequent drop in the serum pH. Within 10–15 minutes of an acute rise in $PaCO_2$, intracellular proteins begin the buffering process, resulting in a 3- to 4-mEq/L increase in the HCO_3^- concentration. This immediate buffering will elevate the pH only slightly (0.05–0.10 units), and no further compensation occurs until the kidney responds to the sustained acidosis. In the acute setting, a 10 mm Hg increase in the $PaCO_2$ will decrease the pH by 0.08 and increase the HCO_3^- concentration by 1.0 mEq/L.

B. CHRONIC RESPIRATORY ACIDOSIS

Chronic obstructive pulmonary disease and extreme obesity are two common conditions that may produce chronic respiratory acidosis secondary to inadequate alveolar ventilation. With sustained acidosis from an elevated $PaCO_2$, the kidneys begin compensation within the first 6–12 hours but may not reach a steady state for 2–3 days. The kidneys buffer the acidosis by increasing acid secretion in addition to excreting chloride in preference to HCO_3^-. This buffering results in the characteristic elevated HCO_3^- (usually not greater than 38 mEq/L), hypochloremia, and near normal pH of chronic respiratory acidosis. A 10 mm Hg increase in $PaCO_2$ will decrease the pH by 0.03 and increase the HCO_3^- concentration by 3.5 mEq/L.

Treatment & Disposition

The primary treatment goal must be focused on reversing or stabilizing the underlying process that generated the respiratory acidosis. Depending on the clinical scenario, naloxone, oxygen, or β agonists may be needed to improve the patient's respiratory status. Additionally, a trial of bilevel positive airway pressure (BiPAP) or tracheal intubation may be required to improve alveolar ventilation, but avoid decreasing the $PaCO_2$ faster than 5 mm Hg/h in patients with chronic respiratory acidosis. Rapid correction of the pH can cause acute hypocalcemia and subsequent dysrhythmias and seizures.

Patients with acute respiratory acidosis should be admitted, whereas patients with chronic respiratory acidosis may require hospitalization depending on the patient's clinical status (ie, hypoxemia).

2. Metabolic Acidosis

 ESSENTIALS OF DIAGNOSIS

- Anion gap acidosis caused by ketones, lactate, toxins, uremia.
- Non-anion-gap acidosis rarely life-threatening.
- Use Winter's formula to identify respiratory compensation.
- Treat the underlying cause.

General Considerations

Metabolic acidosis occurs due to an imbalance between the plasma concentration of H^+ and HCO_3^-. This imbalance is caused by an overproduction of organic acids such as ketones or lactate, loss of HCO_3^- through intestinal or renal wasting, or by the inability to excrete normal acid production. These mechanisms result in a decrease in the plasma concentration of HCO_3^- to less than 22 mmol/L and a pH less than 7.35.

Clinical Findings

The identification of a metabolic acidosis is made by laboratory values, but the diagnosis of the process generating the metabolic acidosis depends on the clinical situation and the anion gap (AG).

The AG is a measure of the difference between the predominant cation, sodium, and the combination of the predominant anions, chloride and HCO_3^-.

$$AG = [NA^+] - ([Cl^-] + [HCO_3^-])$$

The normal AG is 8–14 mEq/L. The calculation of an increased versus normal AG is the key step in determining the cause of metabolic acidosis.

A. Increased Anion Gap

An elevated AG is synonymous with the presence of a metabolic acidosis and implies an overproduction of acids or a decrease in acid clearance by the kidney. The accumulation of acidic anions that are not measured by routine laboratory testing lowers the serum HCO_3^- via buffering, hence generating an increased AG. An increased AG is associated with the following conditions:

- Ketoacidosis: in diabetic or alcoholic patients; starvation
- Renal failure
- Lactic acidosis
- Exogenous toxins leading to lactic acidosis: cyanide, carbon monoxide, ibuprofen, isoniazid, iron, strychnine, toluene
- Exogenous toxins metabolized to acids: aspirin, methanol, ethylene glycol, paraldehyde

B. Normal Anion Gap

A metabolic acidosis with a normal AG is generated by the loss of bicarbonate with a reciprocal increase in the chloride concentration. Causes of normal AG (hyperchloremic) metabolic acidosis can be classified according to serum potassium concentration. Causes associated with hypokalemia include diarrhea, small bowel or pancreatic fistula, ureteral diversion, ileal loop (obstruction verus too long), type 1 renal tubular acidosis, and carbonic anhydrase inhibitors. Normal and hyperkalemic sources include type 4 renal tubular acidosis, early renal failure, hydronephrosis, tubulointerstitial renal disease, and hypoaldosteronism. Other causes of a normal AG metabolic acidosis include rapid normal saline hydration and posttreatment of diabetic ketoacidosis.

The urinary anion gap (UAG) is calculated as follows:

$$UAG = ([NA^+] + [K^+]) - [Cl^-]$$

The UAG grossly reflects urine ammonium excretion and can help differentiate the source of the normal AG metabolic acidosis. A negative value for the UAG indicates the acidosis and hypokalemia are generated from gastrointestinal sources (ie, diarrhea), whereas a near neutral or positive value for the UAG points toward a renal cause for the acidosis.

Physiology

The body buffers an acute metabolic acidosis by utilizing intracellular and extracellular proteins, increasing H^+ elimination by the kidney, and stimulating the respiratory drive. A decreased pH stimulates the chemoreceptors in the brain to increase the alveolar ventilation, which decreases the $PaCO_2$. If appropriate compensation is occurring in response to the metabolic acidosis (gap or nongap), then the $PaCO_2$ should equal the value calculated by Winter's formula, or $PaCO_2 = 1.5([HCO_3^-]) + 8 \pm 2$. If the $PaCO_2$ via arterial blood gas is higher than the calculated value, then the patient has a superimposed primary respiratory acidosis (hypoventilation). If the $PaCO_2$ via arterial blood gas is below the calculated range, the patient has a superimposed primary respiratory alkalosis (hyperventilation). Respiratory compensation will not decrease the $PaCO_2$ below 10–15 mm Hg, and it may take 12–24 hours of respiratory compensation to reach a steady state.

Treatment

Metabolic acidosis requires treatment of the underlying cause that generated the acidosis. The appropriate treatment depends on the underlying illness. For example, diabetic ketoacidosis is treated with hydration, insulin, and electrolyte supplementation as needed. The restoration of tissue perfusion by supporting the patient's respiratory and cardiovascular state is essential in the treatment of metabolic acidosis. These two measures will help correct the acidosis, but sometimes intravenous sodium bicarbonate is needed to correct the metabolic derangement. This is generally withheld from treatment unless the pH falls below 7.1. The estimation of the HCO_3^- dose is as follows:

$$0.5 \ (weight \ [kg]) \times (desired \ [HCO_3^-]$$
$$- \ measured \ [HCO_3^-])$$

As a general rule, initially correct the deficit with one half of the calculated HCO_3^- dose, followed by a recheck of the serum HCO_3^- and pH to guide further therapy. The dose of HCO_3^- should not exceed 0.5–1.0 mEq/kg at a time. Be careful with the administration of intravenous HCO_3^- because of potential complications of volume overload, hypokalemia, decreased ionized calcium, paradoxical cerebrospinal fluid acidosis, and serum alkalosis.

3. Respiratory Alkalosis

ESSENTIALS OF DIAGNOSIS

- Hypocapnia generated by many common causes.
- Chronic state may result in near normal compensation.
- Treat the underlying cause.

General Considerations

Respiratory alkalosis is defined as a $PaCO_2$ concentration below 35 mm Hg and subsequent elevation in serum pH above 7.45. An acute respiratory alkalosis is caused by hyperventilation secondary to other causes. Common causes include early shock, early sepsis, trauma, fear, anxiety, pulmonary disease (congestive heart failure, asthma, pneumonia, pulmonary embolism), central nervous system infection, cerebrovascular accident, pregnancy, liver disease, hyperthyroidism, and acute salicylate ingestion. These causes generally decrease the $PaCO_2$ to 25–35 mm Hg, but further hypocapnia can result from metabolic acidosis or hypoxia.

Clinical Findings

The clinical findings of respiratory alkalosis vary depending on the severity and acuity of the process. An acute respiratory alkalosis can produce circumoral and digital paresthesias in addition to carpopedal spasm and possibly tetany. These symptoms may be caused partly by a modest hypocalcemia secondary to the acute respiratory alkalosis. Severe hypocapnia causes cerebral vasoconstriction that in part produces the clinical symptoms of lightheadedness, dizziness, confusion, and possibly loss of consciousness. Chronic respiratory alkalosis may produce hypophosphatemia and lower the seizure threshold.

Physiology

A. Acute Respiratory Alkalosis

Acute hyperventilation lowers the $PaCO_2$ concentration, and within minutes compensation begins. H^+ ions attempt to buffer the hypocapnic state by moving from inside the cell to the extracellular space. A 10 mm Hg decrease in the $PaCO_2$ will lower the HCO_3^- concentration by 2.5 mEq/L and increase the pH by 0.8. There is no significant renal loss of HCO_3^- in the acute setting.

B. Chronic Respiratory Alkalosis

In response to chronic hypocapnia, the kidney decreases the H^+ secretion while retaining chloride in exchange for HCO_3^-. In chronic states, a 10 mm Hg decrease in $PaCO_2$ will increase the pH by 0.03 and decrease the HCO_3^- concentration by 5 mmol/L. Additionally, mild hypokalemia is produced by potassium shifting into cells in exchange for H^+. After 2 weeks, this compensation will bring the pH to normal levels.

Treatment & Disposition

Treatment for respiratory alkalosis focuses on treating the underlying disorder. Symptomatic patients with respiratory alkalosis caused by anxiety or psychogenic hyperventilation may require a rebreathing device such as a paper bag in an attempt to increase the $PaCO_2$ concentration. Appropriate disposition of patients with respiratory alkalosis depends on the underlying process.

4. Metabolic Alkalosis

ESSENTIALS OF DIAGNOSIS

- Commonly results from vomiting or volume depletion secondary to diuretics.
- Evaluate urine chloride concentration to help guide therapy.

General Considerations

Metabolic alkalosis is defined as a primary elevation of plasma HCO_3^- above 28 mmol/L, with a subsequent elevation of pH above 7.45. A primary metabolic alkalosis usually results from the loss of gastric acid contents (via vomiting or nasogastric tube) or from volume depletion secondary to diuretics. Although the majority of metabolic alkaloses are generated from volume depletion, various medical conditions can generate hyperbicarbonatemia (Table 42–14). The diagnosis of the process generating the metabolic alkalosis depends on the clinical situation and measurement of the urinary chloride.

Table 42–14. Causes of metabolic alkalosis.

Saline Responsive (Urine [Cl⁻] < 10 mEq/L)	Saline Resistant (Urine [Cl⁻] > 20 mEq/L)	Other Causes
Gastrointestinal: vomiting, nasogastric suction, Cl⁻ diarrhea, villous adenoma Diuretic therapy Cystic fibrosis Posthypercapnia Alkali syndrome	Mineralocorticoid excess: Primary aldosteronism Secondary causes: congestive heart failure, cirrhosis, Bartter syndrome, licorice, renin tumor, tobacco Cushing syndrome, severe K⁺ depletion Congenital adrenal hyperplasia	Refeeding alkalosis Massive blood transfusion Hypercalcemia (bone metastases)

Clinical Findings

Metabolic alkalosis produces hypokalemia, hypocalcemia, and hypomagnesemia. Depending on the degree of alkalosis (usually pH > 7.55), increased neuromuscular activity can occur and become clinically apparent via positive Chvostek and Trousseau signs, twitching, and tetany. Metabolic alkalosis can also produce cardiac tachyarrhythmias and reduce oxygen availability.

Physiology

The generation of a metabolic alkalosis is compensated in part by hypoventilation. A 1.0 mEq/L increase in the HCO_3^- concentration will increase the pH by 0.015 and the $PaCO_2$ by 0.7 mm Hg. This compensatory increase in $PaCO_2$ from hypoventilation is usually limited to 55 mm Hg because the chemoreceptors will not allow the associated hypoxemia below a PaO_2 of 60 mm Hg.

Many different physiologic processes can generate a metabolic alkalosis. Hyperbicarbonatemia can result from diuretics secondary to an excessive loss of chloride relative to HCO_3^-, resulting in a so-called contraction alkalosis. The loss of H^+ from excessive vomiting or from the enhanced renal excretion in a mineralocorticoid excess state can also generate a metabolic alkalosis. Additionally, massive blood transfusions can cause a metabolic alkalosis from the metabolism of sodium citrate into sodium bicarbonate. Hypokalemia causes hyperbicarbonatemia by causing a shift of H^+ into cells, and the kidney maintains the alkalosis by secreting H^+ while reabsorbing HCO_3^-.

The kidneys compensate for a metabolic alkalosis initially by excreting some of the excess HCO_3^- in the urine. Under circumstances of severe volume depletion, the kidney actually maintains the alkalosis by reabsorbing HCO_3^- in an attempt to maintain plasma volume regardless of the acid-base status. As the kidney responds to the metabolic alkalosis, the urine chloride concentration can be evaluated. A level below 10 mEq/L indicates tubular reabsorption of chloride, signifying

volume depletion. This urine chloride concentration can help guide subsequent therapy.

Treatment

Patients with a urine chloride concentration below 10 mEq/L require volume expansion. Normal saline infusion should correct the alkalosis by suppressing renal acid excretion and enhancing renal HCO_3^- excretion. The kidneys can correct for a metabolic alkalosis only if sufficient volume is replaced. Additionally, potassium replacement in the form of potassium chloride may be needed to correct the alkalosis. Depending on the clinical situation, generally 100–500 mEq of K^+ may be needed to correct the hypokalemia associated with the alkalosis.

Patients with a urine chloride concentration above 20 mEq/L are not as responsive to volume expansion. Specific therapy should be guided toward the underlying processes generating the alkalosis. Patients with a mineralocorticoid excess state require potassium replacement. Patients with significant edema may require acetazolamide to enhance HCO_3^- secretion.

5. Mixed Acid-Base Disorders

 ESSENTIALS OF DIAGNOSIS

- *Up to 3 disorders can coexist.*
- *Approach in a stepwise fashion.*
- *Metabolic acidosis and respiratory alkalosis commonly coexist.*
- *Accurate evaluation of data will guide treatment.*

General Considerations

Whenever a primary disturbance exists, the lungs and kidneys begin to adjust their physiologic parameters in an attempt to bring the pH toward normal. If the degree of compensation is inadequate, or if an acid-base disorder causes no shift in arterial pH (except in chronic respiratory alkalosis), or if the clinical picture does not fit with a primary disturbance alone, then consider the presence of a second primary process. The presence of 2 or more primary processes occurring simultaneously is referred to as a mixed acid-base disorder. Respiratory acidosis and respiratory alkalosis can never be present simultaneously, but any other combination of processes can occur.

Approach the patient with a mixed acid-base disorder in a stepwise fashion:

1. A thorough history and physical examination can provide clues about the disorders.
2. The predominant disorder (acidosis versus alkalosis) is reflected by the acidemic or alkalemic pH. Confirm the accuracy of the laboratory data via the Henderson-Hesselbach equation.
3. Determine the predominant process altering the pH by interpreting the HCO_3^- concentration and $PaCO_2$ (see above).
4. *Always* calculate the serum AG.
5. Determine the degree of compensation (described below).
6. Calculate the delta gap (described below).
7. Interpret urine and serum electrolytes.

Combined Metabolic Acidosis & Respiratory Acidosis

Upon identification of a metabolic acidosis from the blood gas and electrolyte panel, determine whether the respiratory compensation to the metabolic acidosis is appropriate (see "Primary Metabolic Acidosis" section, above). If the $PaCO_2$ is higher than expected, then the patient has a superimposed primary respiratory acidosis. This is an ominous mixed disorder and is found in patients in cardiopulmonary arrest. In patients with a chronic respiratory acidosis, HCO_3^- should be increased by 3.5 mEq/L for every 10 mm Hg increase in PCO_2. A smaller increase in HCO_3^- implies a superimposed primary metabolic acidosis or a compensation that is not complete.

Combined Metabolic Acidosis & Respiratory Alkalosis

If the respiratory compensation results in a lower PCO_2 than expected in response to a metabolic acidosis, the patient has a superimposed primary respiratory alkalosis. This mixed disorder is commonly encountered in the emergency department. Causes include congestive heart failure, early sepsis, early shock, liver disease, and salicylate ingestion. In patients with chronic respiratory alkalosis, HCO_3^- should be decreased by 5 mEq/L for every 10 mm Hg decrease in PCO_2. A greater decrease in HCO_3^- implies a superimposed primary metabolic acidosis.

Combined Metabolic Alkalosis & Respiratory Acidosis

Once an acute metabolic alkalosis is identified, the appropriate respiratory compensation should be an increase in the PCO_2 of 0.6 mm Hg for each 1 mEq/L increase in HCO_3^- concentration. A greater increase in PCO_2 implies a superimposed primary respiratory acidosis. In patients with chronic respiratory acidosis, HCO_3^- concentration should be increased by 3.5 mEq/L for every 10 mm Hg increase in the PCO_2. A greater increase in HCO_3^- implies a superimposed primary metabolic alkalosis. This mixed disorder can occur in patients with chronic respiratory acidosis who develop a metabolic alkalosis from diuretics for cor pulmonale.

Combined Metabolic Alkalosis & Respiratory Alkalosis

A smaller increase in the PCO_2 of 0.6 mm Hg for each 1 mEq/L increase in HCO_3^- secondary to an acute metabolic alkalosis implies a superimposed respiratory alkalosis. In patients with chronic respiratory alkalosis, HCO_3^- should be decreased by 5 mEq/L for every 10 mm Hg decrease in PCO_2. A smaller decrease in HCO_3^- implies a superimposed primary metabolic alkalosis or a compensation that is not complete. This mixed disorder is present in patients with hepatic failure who are taking diuretics and in patients who require mechanical ventilation and are taking diuretics or given nasogastric suction.

Triple Disturbances

Patients may present with a maximum of three primary disturbances. For example, a 55-year-old man with alcoholic liver disease presents to the emergency department with protracted vomiting and a blood pressure of 70/40. Laboratory values reveal an AG of 25 (metabolic acidosis from lactate) and a HCO_3^- concentration of 22 mEq/L. The calculated $PaCO_2$ for appropriate respiratory compensation is 39–43 mm Hg [1.5(22) + 8 ± 2]. The patient's $PaCO_2$ is 25 mm Hg, which clearly reflects a respiratory alkalosis (hyperventilation) from liver disease. A third disturbance (metabolic alkalosis) should be suspected if laboratory values reveal a high AG with a HCO_3^- concentration close to normal.

Determine the presence of a triple disturbance by calculating the delta gap. The delta gap is defined as the deviation of the AG from normal minus the deviation of the HCO_3^- from normal. Prior to calculating the delta gap, assume a normal AG of 10 mmol/L, and in a high AG acidosis every unit rise in the AG above 10 lowers the patient's HCO_3^- concentration by 1 unit via buffering. This patient's deviation in the AG is 15 (25 − 10), and the deviation in the HCO_3^- concentration is 2 (24 − 22). This difference of 13 (15 − 2) represents an elevated delta gap (normal range 0 ± 6). In this example, the presence of an elevated delta gap represents a higher than expected HCO_3^- level, hence a simultaneous third disorder: metabolic alkalosis from the protracted vomiting.

Adrogue HJ, Madias NE: Management of life-threatening acid-base disorders. First of two parts. N Engl J Med 1998;338(1):26. [PMID: 9414329] (Discussion of the complications and management of severe metabolic and respiratory acidosis.)

Adrogue HJ, Madias NE: Management of life-threatening acid-base disorders. Second of two parts. N Engl J Med 1998;338(2):107. [PMID: 9420343] (Discussion of the complications and management of severe metabolic and respiratory alkalosis.)

Bia M, Their SO: Mixed acid base disturbances: a clinical approach. Med Clin North Am 1981;65:347. [PMID: 7230962] (Classic article for the approach to mixed acid-base disturbances.)

Fall PJ: A stepwise approach to acid-base disorders. Practical patient evaluation for metabolic acidosis and other conditions. Postgrad Med 2000;107(3):249. [PMID: 10728149] (Stepwise approach to evaluation of acid-base disorders using a clinical example to guide discussion.)

Fulop M: Flow diagrams for the diagnosis of acid-base disorders. J Emerg Med 1998;16(1):97. [PMID: 9472767] (Approach to acid-base disorders using flow diagrams.)

Gluck SL: Acid-base. Lancet 1998;352:474. [PMID: 9708769] (Discussion of acid-base disorders focused on metabolic processes.)

Kraut JA, Madias NE: Approach to patients with acid-base disorders. Resp Care 2001;46(4):392. [PMID: 11262558] (Practical approach to acid-base disturbances with case examples.)

Laski ME, Kurtzman NA: Acid-base disorders in medicine. Disease-A-Month 1996;42(2):51. [PMID: 8631223] (In-depth discussion of acid-base disorders.)

Rutecki GW, Whittier FC: An approach to clinical acid-base problem solving. Compr Ther 1998;24(11–12):553. [PMID: 9847971] (Five-step approach to acid-base disorders including algorithms for metabolic acidosis.)

■ APPENDIX: USEFUL EQUATIONS & FORMULAS

Osmolality

$$P_{osm} = 2[Na^+]_{serum} + \frac{[Glucose]}{18} + \frac{[Blood\ urea\ nitrogen]}{2.8}$$

P_{osm} is in mOsm/L, $[Na^+]$ in mEq/L, and [glucose] and [blood urea nitrogen] in mg/dL.

When measured osmolality exceeds calculated osmolality by more than 10 mOsm/L, an osmolal gap exists owing to the presence of significant quantities of unmeasured solute:

$$Osmolal\ gap = P_{osm\ (measured)} - P_{osm(calc)}$$

If the solute is alcohol, the blood alcohol concentration can be estimated:

$$Blood\ alcohol\ above\ concentration\ (mg/dL)$$
$$= 4.6 \times Osmolal\ gap$$

Hyponatremia

To determine whether the cause of the serum sodium concentration ($[Na^+]_{serum}$) abnormality is due to total body sodium, potassium, or water abnormality, equation 4 may be helpful.

$$[Na^+]_{serum} = \frac{[Na_e^+] + [K_e^+]}{TBW}$$

where TBW = total body water (in L), $[Na_e^+]$ = total body Na^+ (in mEq), and $[K_e^+]$ = total body K^+ (in mEq). TBW may be estimated using equation 5. (See also Table 42–1.) For example, if $[Na^+]_{serum}$ is low and TBW is estimated to be normal, total body sodium or potassium must be decreased, and sodium or potassium replacement is the necessary treatment. However, if TBW is increased and $[Na^+]_{serum}$ is low, diuresis is the necessary treatment.

$$TBW\ in\ L = 0.6\ Body\ weight\ in\ kg$$

$$Na^+\ deficit\ above\ in\ mEq$$
$$= 0.6 \times (Body\ weight\ in\ kg)\ (140 - [Na^+]_{serum})$$

$$Water\ excess\ in\ L$$
$$= \frac{0.6 \times (Body\ weight\ in\ kg)\ (140 - [Na^+]_{serum})}{140}$$

The relationship between serum sodium concentration and serum glucose concentration is as follows: For each increase in serum glucose concentration of 100 mg/dL, there will be a reciprocal decrease of 1.6 mEq/dL in serum sodium concentration.

Hypernatremia

$$Na^+ \text{ excess in mEq} = ([Na^+]_{serum} - 140)\,(TBW)$$

Water deficit in L

$$= \frac{0.6 \times (\text{Body weight in kg})\,([Na^+]_{serum} - 140)}{140}$$

Plasma Calcium Concentration & Plasma Albumin Concentration

For every fall in serum albumin of 1 g/dL, plasma calcium will fall about 0.8 mg/dL. This reduction does not reflect a change in free Ca^{2+} (ionized) concentration and therefore does not represent true hypocalcemia.

Burns & Smoke Inhalation

43

Melissa M. Cheeseman, MD, & Harriet L. Boozer, MD[1]

Immediate Management of Life-Threatening Problems

Further Evaluation of Patient with Burns or Inhalation Injury

Emergency Treatment of Specific Types of Burns

    Smoke Inhalation

    Chemical Burns

    Tar Burns

Sunburn

Electrical Burns

Ocular Burns

Circumferential Burns of Neck, Chest, & Extremities

Burns Due to Child Abuse

Outpatient Management of Minor Burns

■ IMMEDIATE MANAGEMENT OF LIFE-THREATENING PROBLEMS (See Figure 43–1.)

Begin CPR If Needed

See Chapter 7.

Establish an Adequate Airway

Severe burns to the lower face and neck may be associated with upper airway and laryngeal edema that cause airway obstruction. Inhalation of superheated air or steam in a confined space may also cause significant upper airway edema. Full-thickness chest wall burns, especially if they are circumferential, may limit chest wall movement and cause respiratory failure. Consider early endotracheal intubation in all patients with such injuries. When the burn size exceeds 60% total body surface area, including the face, early endotracheal intubation is advisable. If endotracheal intubation is impossible, cricothyrotomy may be necessary.

Support Ventilation & Oxygenation

Give oxygen, 2–12 L/min, by nasal cannula or face mask. If smoke inhalation might have occurred, give 100% oxygen by tight-fitting reservoir face mask or endotracheal tube. Monitor oxygen saturation by pulse oximetry. (Note that the actual oxygen saturation can be obtained by subtracting the percent of carboxyhemoglobin from the measured value.) Burn patients with inhalation injuries require frequent reevaluation because of possible progressive respiratory compromise.

Gain Intravenous Access

Patients with deep burns covering more than 15% of body surface area (Figure 43–2) require intravenous fluid resuscitation. Insert 1 or 2 large-bore (≥16-gauge) peripheral intravenous catheters, preferably inserted through nonburned skin. Central venous access is needed only if large-bore peripheral access is impossible.

Obtain Laboratory Data

Arterial blood gas analysis is helpful if respiratory involvement is present. In addition, for assistance in overall patient management and resuscitation, submit blood for carboxyhemoglobin level, complete blood count, and electrolytes and urine for myoglobin. Obtain chest x-ray and electrocardiogram (ECG).

Begin Fluid Resuscitation

Burns are associated with the loss of large volumes of intravascular fluid, electrolytes, and protein through capillaries with increased permeability. Loss begins soon after injury and is maximal during the first 6–8 hours. Several formulas may be used as guidelines to fluid resuscitation (Table 43–1). Most burn centers use

---

[1]This chapter is a revision of the chapter by Anthony A. Meyer, MD, PhD, & Patricia R. Salver, MD, FACEP, FACP, from the 4th edition.

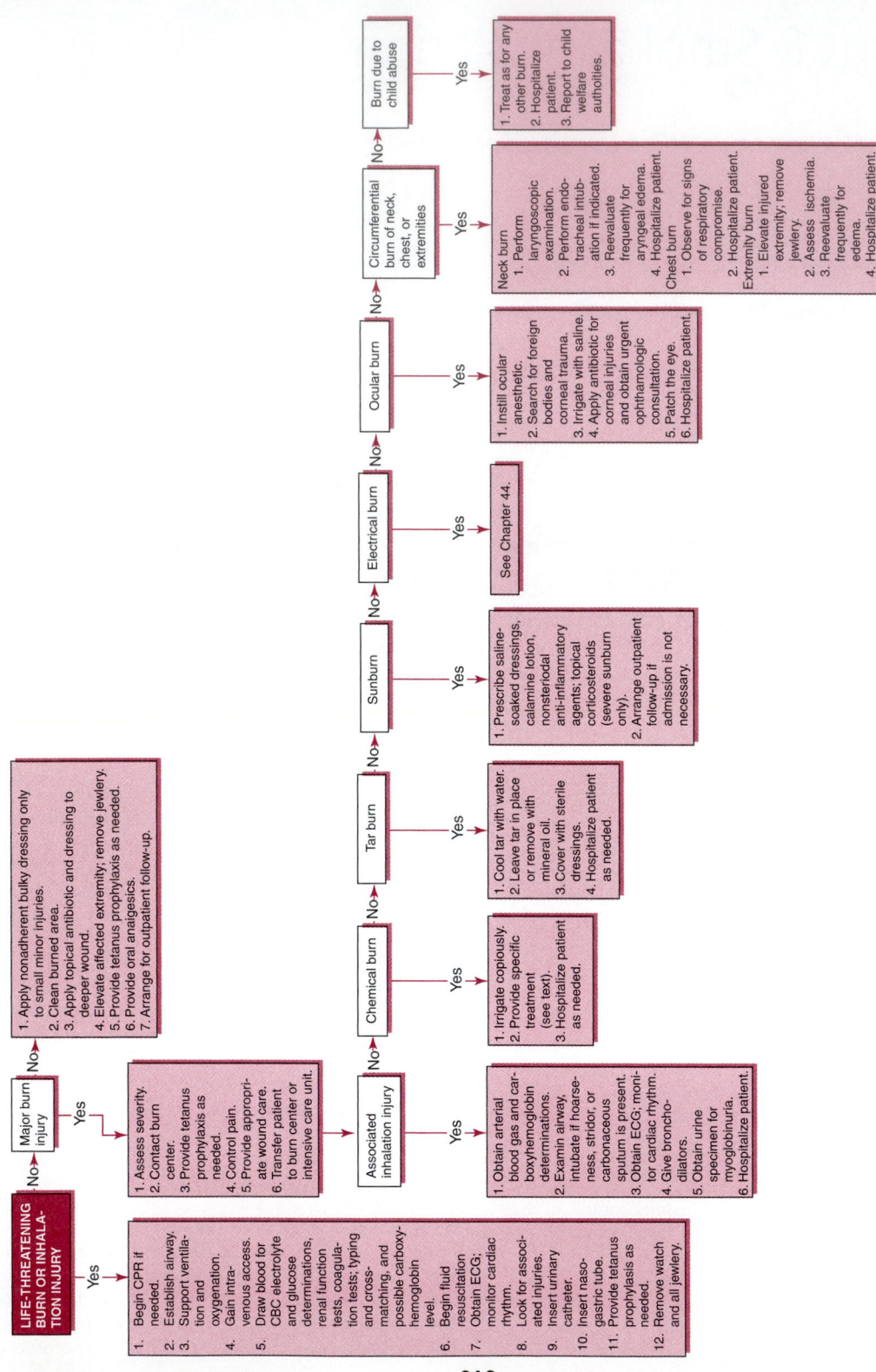

Figure 43–1. Management of life-threatening burn or inhalation injury.

918

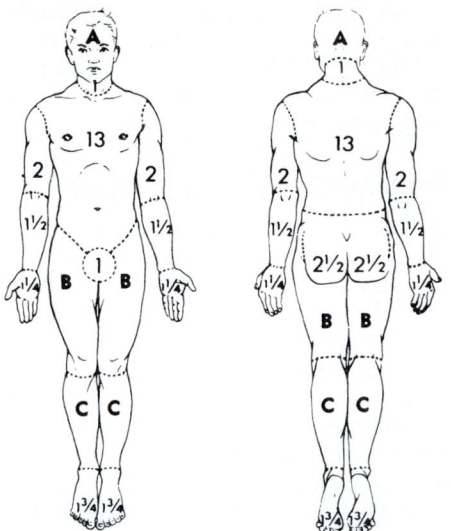
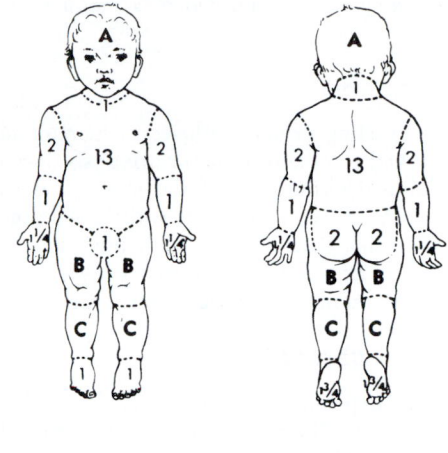

Relative Percentages of Areas Affected by Growth

Area	Age		
	10	15	Adult
A = half of head	5½	4½	3½
B = half of one thigh	4¼	4½	4¾
C = half of one leg	3	3¼	3½

Relative Percentages of Areas Affected by Growth

Area	Age		
	0	1	5
A = half of head	9½	8½	6½
B = half of one thigh	2¾	3¼	4
C = half of one leg	2½	2½	2¾

Figure 43–2. Burn size may be estimated using an age-adjusted burn chart. (Reproduced, with permission, from Way LW, [editor]: *Current Surgical Diagnosis & Treatment*, 9th ed. Appleton & Lange, 1991.)

Table 43–1. Formulas for fluid resuscitation in burn patients.

Formula	Day 1[1]
	Crystalloid
Parkland (Baxter)	Lactated Ringer's injection, 4 mL/kg per percentage of body surface area burned
Modified Brooke	Lactated Ringer's injection **Adult:** 2 mL/kg per percentage of body surface area burned **Child:** 3 mL/kg per percentage of body surface area burned

[1]One-half of the calculated volume is given in the first 8 hours; the remainder is given over the next 16 hours.

only crystalloid for the first 18–24 hours and use either the Parkland or the modified Brook formula. These formulas should be individualized for each patient on the basis of the patient's response to therapy. In general, infusion rates should be adjusted to maintain urine output at 0.5–1.0 mL/kg/h for adults and 1.0 mL/kg/h for children under 10 kg.

Obtain 12-Lead ECG & Monitor Cardiac Rhythm

Hypoxemia, shock, electrolyte disturbances, or carbon monoxide poisoning in a burn patient may predispose to development of myocardial ischemia or cardiac arrhythmias.

Evaluate for Possible Associated Injuries

Burn patients frequently have other injuries in addition to the burn. Patients who have been burned in motor vehicle accidents or explosions should be evaluated as described in Chapter 10. Search for fractures and injuries of the hand, cervical spine, chest, and abdomen in patients who may have jumped or fallen from a burning building or been burned in a motor vehicle crash.

Insert a Urinary Catheter

Insert an indwelling urinary catheter to monitor urinary output and to obtain urine for urinalysis (including myoglobin determination if the patient has sustained an electrical burn). Patients with full-thickness burns of the penile glans or shaft may require suprapubic cystostomy. An indwelling urinary catheter is the most important monitoring device in burn patients.

Insert a Nasogastric Tube

Patients with deep burns covering more than 20% of their body surface will develop ileus. A nasogastric tube will decrease the risk of emesis and possible aspiration. If the patient is to be transported by air to a burn facility, a nasogastric tube is mandatory, because decreased cabin pressure may cause gastric distention and vomiting. The tube should be on suction or open to air and not clamped during transport.

Provide Tetanus Prophylaxis

See Chapter 30.

Remove Jewelry

Remove all rings, watches, and other jewelry, which could act as a tourniquet when edema develops.

Gueugniaud PY et al: Current advances in the initial management of major thermal burns. Intensive Care Med 2000;26:848. [PMID: 10990098]

Ramzy PI et al: Thermal injury. Crit Care Clin 1999;15:333. [PMID: 10331132]

Rose JK, Herndon DN: Advances in the treatment of burn patients. Burns 1997;23:S19. [PMID: 9177897]

Yowler CJ, Fratianne RB: Current status of burn resuscitation. Clin Plast Surg 2000;27:1. [PMID: 10665352]

■ FURTHER EVALUATION OF THE PATIENT WITH BURNS OR INHALATION INJURY

Obtain a History

Ask the patient, witnesses, and family about the mechanism of injury (eg, explosion, spilled liquid, house fire) and about the possible presence of combustibles known to be toxic. Find out whether the patient was burned in an open space or in an enclosed space; the latter increases the risk of inhalation injury. Also ask about underlying medical problems, tetanus immunization status, and medication allergies.

Determine the Severity of Injury

An accurate estimate of the severity of injury is crucial in determining the need for hospital admission or referral to a burn center and in guiding initial fluid resuscitation and establishing a prognosis. Table 43–2 lists several important determinants of burn severity. Table 43–3 is the American Burn Association's classification of burns according to severity. In general, patients with minor burns may be managed as outpatients, patients with moderate uncomplicated burns should be hospitalized, and patients with major burns should be transferred to a burn center. If local personnel or facilities do not have experience in caring for burn patients, then patients with moderate or major burns should be referred to a burn center.

A. BURN SIZE

Accurate measurement of the burned area, expressed as a percentage of body surface area, should be performed in all burn patients. Burn size may be estimated by using an age-adjusted surface area chart (see Figure 43–2) or by using the "rule of nines" for adults or the "rules of fives" for infants and children (Table 43–4). The size of scattered small burns can be estimated by comparing them with the size of the patient's hand, which constitutes about 1¼% of body surface area. The extent of all burns should be recorded on a drawing (front and back views) on the patient's chart.

B. BURN DEPTH

Burns are typically described as first, second, third, or fourth degree. A more useful description, based on the wound's ability to heal, is partial-thickness (heals spontaneously) and full-thickness (requires skin grafting). Deep partial-thickness burns usually require grafting to

Table 43–2. Determinants of burn severity.

Burn size
Burn depth
Burn site
Presence of circumferential burns
Inhalation injury
Electrical injury
Age of patient
Associated injuries
Major underlying medical problems

Table 43–3. Summary of American Burn Association burn severity categorization.

Major burn injury
Second-degree burn of > 25% body surface area in adults
Second-degree burn of > 20% body surface area in children
Third-degree burn of > 10% body surface area
Most burns involving hands, face, eyes, ears, feet, or perineum
Most patients with the following:
    Inhalation injury
    Electrical injury
    Burn injury complicated by other major trauma
Poor-risk patients with burns
Moderate uncomplicated burn injury
Second-degree burn of 15–25% body surface area in adults
Second-degree burn of 10–20% body surface area in children
Third-degree burn of < 10% body surface area
Minor burn injury
Second-degree burn of < 15% body surface area in adults
Second-degree burn of < 10% body surface area in children
Third-degree burn of < 2% body surface area

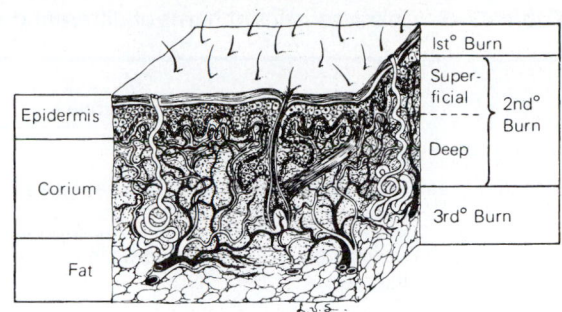

Figure 43–3. Layers of the skin, showing depth of first-, second-, and third-degree burns. (Reproduced, with permission, from Way LW [editor]: *Current Surgical Diagnosis & Treatment*, 9th ed. Appleton & Lange, 1991.)

expedite healing and decrease contractures and hypertrophic scar. Figure 43–3 shows the level of skin involved with each type of burn. Table 43–5 outlines the physical findings usually associated with each type of burn. The depth of burn should be recorded accurately on a drawing (front and back views) on the patient's chart.

Table 43–4. Rule of nines (rapid means of estimating body surface area burned in adult patients) and rule of lives (rapid means of estimating body surface area burned in infants and children.

Area	Percentage		
	Adult	Infant	Child
Head and neck	9	20	15
Arm			
Right	9	10	10
Left	9	10	10
Torso			
Front	18	20	20
Back	18	20	20
Leg			
Right	18	10	15
Left	18	10	15
Genitalia and perineum	1	. . .	. . .
Total	100	100	= 100

Several principles must be kept in mind when considering burn depth. First, because it is difficult to distinguish deep partial-thickness burns from full-thickness burns, these burns should be assumed to be full-thickness injuries and should be treated accordingly. Second, burn wounds change over 48–72 hours, and what may appear to be superficial injury on initial examination may progress to a deeper-level injury, especially if the patient has poor perfusion or the wound becomes desiccated or infected.

C. BURN SITE

Burns in the following areas are considered major injuries:

1. Hands and feet—Deep burns of the hands or feet cause scarring and may produce permanent disability.

2. Face—Partial- or full-thickness facial burns may cause severe scarring, with profound physical and emotional impact. They are also often associated with inhalation injury and compromised airway.

3. Eyes—Burns of the eyes may cause corneal scarring and eyelid dysfunction that may ultimately lead to blindness. ***Note:*** Patients with possible eye burns should be examined as quickly as possible, preferably in the emergency department, because massive periorbital edema often develops and hinders later examination.

4. Ears—Deep burns of the ears predispose to development of pressure deformity and infection. Examine the tympanic membrane in patients with external ear injuries caused by hot liquids or chemicals.

5. Perineum—Burns of the perineum are difficult to manage on an outpatient basis and are more susceptible to infection than are other types of burns.

Table 43–5. Characteristics of burns of different depth.

	Depth of Burn	Color and Appearance	Skin Texture	Capillary Refill	Pinprick Sensation	Healing
First-degree	Superficial epidermis	Red	Normal	Yes	Yes	5–10 days; no scar
Second-degree	Superficial partial-thickness	Red; may be blistered	Edematous	Yes	Yes	10–21 days; no or minimal scar
	Deep partial-thickness	Pink to white	Thick	Possibly	Possibly	25–60 days; dense scar
Third-degree	Full-thickness	White, black, or brown	Leathery	No	No	No spontaneous healing
Fourth-degree	Involves underlying subcutaneous tissue, tendon, or bone	Variable	Variable	No	No	No spontaneous healing

D. PRESENCE OF CIRCUMFERENTIAL BURNS

Any deep circumferential burn is a potential major injury. Circumferential deep burns of the neck may cause lymphatic and venous obstruction that leads to laryngeal edema and airway obstruction. Circumferential burns of the extremities may restrict blood flow, causing an increase in tissue pressure and ischemia. Circumferential chest wall injuries may impede chest wall movement and lead to respiratory failure.

E. INHALATION INJURY

Inhalation injury (burn sustained in a confined space, singed nasal nares, soot around the nares, carbonaceous sputum, hoarseness, stridor, symptoms of respiratory distress, carboxyhemoglobin level > 10%) signifies a major burn. Diagnosis and management of inhalation injuries are discussed below.

F. ELECTRICAL INJURY

Damage from electrical injury may be extensive, even though the outward signs of injury are minimal. Cardiac arrhythmias and renal failure from myoglobinuria are possible complications. All electrical injuries should be considered major injuries.

G. AGE OF PATIENT

The mortality rate from burn injury is increased in very young or very old patients; these are also the age groups in which burns most commonly occur. Burns in a child under age 5 years or in an adult over age 55 years are more likely to be serious than are burns in other age groups.

H. ASSOCIATED INJURIES

Burns may occur in patients with other injuries, such as fractures or internal injuries due to vehicular accidents, falls, or explosions. The associated injuries often place the patient at increased risk of serious complications or death, even though the burns themselves are small.

I. MAJOR UNDERLYING MEDICAL PROBLEMS

Major preexisting medical problems in a burn patient are associated with an increased rate of serious complications and death. Patients with a history of myocardial infarction, angina, significant pulmonary disease, diabetes mellitus, or renal failure are considered poor-risk patients even if their burns are not serious. Burned patients with a history of alcohol or other drug abuse are also at higher risk for complications following burn injury.

Control Pain

Patients with minor burns, especially of the extremities, may relieve pain by immersing the burned part in cool water; do not use this method in patients with larger burns, because of the risks of inducing hypothermia. Oral, subcutaneous, or intramuscular administration of narcotic analgesics may provide adequate pain relief for outpatients; however, intravenous morphine (in increments of 1–3 mg for adults or 0.1–0.2 mg/kg for children) should be used to control pain in patients with moderate or major burn injuries. Take care to avoid precipitating respiratory failure in a burn patient with compromised respiration. Ventilator support may be required in some patients to permit administration of adequate amounts of analgesics safely.

Provide Appropriate Wound Care

Gently remove clothing, dirt, and other foreign material adhering to the burn; irrigation with sterile saline (at room temperature) may be helpful. Do not scrub wounds or use harsh detergents or chemical disinfectants (eg, benzalkonium chloride, povidone-iodine). Little or no debridement of moderate or major wounds should be performed in the emergency department. Redundant skin from ruptured blisters of minor superficial partial-thickness burns may be removed. The wounds of patients with moderate or major burns, especially those who will be transferred to a burn facility, should not be treated with topical ointments or complex dressings in the emergency department, because these will have to be removed for evaluation upon arrival at the receiving facility. A simple nonadherent dressing such as petrolatum-impregnated gauze or sterile saline-soaked dressings should be applied instead. Outpatient management of minor burns is discussed in the "Emergency Treatment of Specific Types of Burns" section, below.

Transfer the Patient to a Burn Center

All major burns and many moderate burn injuries are best treated in a burn center, which has the personnel, equipment, and experience needed to treat major burns effectively. When a patient with a serious burn is first evaluated, the closest burn center should be contacted immediately, so that recommendations for care can be obtained and plans made for transfer, if indicated. Transfer should be coordinated with the physician at the burn center, and unnecessary delays should be avoided. If transfer can be carried out quickly, escharotomy may be performed at the receiving facility in patients with circumferential burns of the extremities, chest, or neck who do not have signs of respiratory compromise or tissue ischemia. Fluid resuscitation and all other supportive measures should be continued during transport, and the patient should be kept warm. Complete medical records should be sent with the patient.

Kao CC, Garner WL: Acute burns. Plast Reconstr Surg 2000; 105:2482. [PMID: 10845306]

Sheridan RL: Comprehensive treatment of burns. Curr Probl Surg 2001;38:641. [PMID: 11568825]

■ EMERGENCY TREATMENT OF SPECIFIC TYPES OF BURNS

SMOKE INHALATION

ESSENTIALS OF DIAGNOSIS

- Look for evidence of thermal injury (airway edema).

- Consider signs of chemical injury including cyanide.
- Evaluate for carbon monoxide intoxication.

Mechanisms of Injury

The mechanisms of injury in smoke inhalation may be divided into 3 categories: (1) thermal injury of the airways, (2) chemical injury of airways and lung parenchyma, and (3) systemic chemical poisoning. Although one type of injury may predominate in some patients, most patients have a combination of injuries. All victims of smoke inhalation should be examined carefully for the presence of any of these injuries.

A. THERMAL INJURY

Patients who have been trapped in a fire in a confined space inhale superheated gases and may also have direct flame injury of the face and neck, which is associated with development of marked upper airway edema and possible airway obstruction. Because of the efficient thermal exchange system of the upper airway, direct thermal injury to the lower respiratory tract is unusual; rarely, exposure to water or steam in the heated gas mixture may produce thermal damage in the lower trachea and bronchi.

B. CHEMICAL INJURY

Chemical injury to the airways and lung parenchyma may be caused by noxious products of combustion of flammable materials (Table 43–6). Some of these products are directly toxic to the airways and lung parenchyma. Only the most commonly produced toxins are discussed below.

Table 43–6. Common toxic products of combustion.

Material Burned	Toxic Product
Wood, paper, cotton	Acrolein, acetaldehyde, formaldehyde, acetic acid, formic acid, nitrogen dioxide, carbon monoxide
Polyvinyl chloride	Hydrochloric acid, phosgene, chlorine
Polyurethane	Hydrocyanic acid, isocyanates (eg, toluene diisocyanate), carbon monoxide
Petroleum products	Acrolein, acetic acid, formic acid
Agricultural wastes, automobile exhaust	Nitrogen dioxide and other oxides of nitrogen; acetic acid; formic acid; carbon monoxide

1. Acrolein—Acrolein is a highly reactive aldehyde that results from combustion of wood and petroleum products. It rapidly reacts with lung and airway tissues, causing injury by protein denaturation. Prolonged inhalation or exposure to high concentrations (> 150 parts per million) for short periods of time (minutes) can be fatal. Lesser exposure causes pulmonary edema due to alveolar capillary leakage; bronchorrhea and bronchospasm, which may be severe; and ventilation-perfusion disturbances that cause hypoxemia that may persist even after the person is no longer exposed to smoke. Acrolein also causes conjunctivitis and ocular tearing even at low concentrations.

2. Hydrochloric acid—Hydrochloric acid is one of the main products of combustion of polyvinyl chloride, a material commonly found in the structural components of houses and high-rise buildings as well as in furnishings and plastics. Hydrolysis occurs when hydrochloric acid comes in contact with the mucosa of the upper airway and tracheobronchial tree, causing protein denaturation and cell death. Even limited exposure may cause marked ocular irritation and tearing, although individuals with repeated or prolonged exposure may become desensitized to this effect. More severe exposure is associated with dyspnea, chest pain, and irritation of mucous membranes. Onset of pulmonary edema may be delayed for 2–12 hours after exposure, and the patient may appear asymptomatic in the interim. Toxic levels of hydrochloric acid gas may persist for as long as 1 hour after a fire has been extinguished. Patients exposed to products of combustion of polyvinyl chloride may also demonstrate premature ventricular contractions and may be at risk for development of lethal cardiac arrhythmias.

3. Toluene diisocyanate—Toulene diisocyanate is a product of combustion of polyurethane, a synthetic material found in almost all homes and offices, where it is used in seat cushions, mattresses, and carpet backing. Toluene diisocyanate is also found in insulation material. Toluene diisocyanate may cause severe bronchospasm, especially in persons with underlying obstructive lung disease, and is also an ocular irritant.

4. Nitrogen dioxide—Nitrogen dioxide is produced in fires involving automobiles or agricultural wastes. It is an uncommon though important toxin, because even brief exposures to high concentrations may cause severe bronchospasm, laryngospasm, and pulmonary edema. If the patient survives, late development of bronchiolitis fibrosa obliterans and chronic interstitial lung disease may occur.

5. Other noxious products—Particulate matter in smoke may stimulate irritant receptors in the large airways and cause bronchoconstriction.

C. Systemic Chemical Poisoning

1. Carbon monoxide—(See Chapter 45.) The most widely recognized and most common complication of smoke inhalation is carbon monoxide poisoning. Carbon monoxide is a product of incomplete combustion and is produced in varying amounts in all fires. Carbon monoxide binds to hemoglobin with an affinity that is 260 times greater than that of oxygen, forming carboxyhemoglobin. The presence of even small amounts of carboxyhemoglobin drastically alters the affinity of the remaining unbound hemoglobin. Thus, even small concentrations of carbon monoxide may markedly reduce the binding of oxygen to hemoglobin, and the carbon monoxide that is bound is not easily displaced by oxygen. The presence of carboxyhemoglobin shifts the oxyhemoglobin dissociation curve to the left, making it more difficult for hemoglobin to release bound oxygen to the tissues. The net result is tissue hypoxia and lactic acidosis due to cellular anaerobic metabolism. Carbon monoxide also binds to the cytochromes, interfering with intracellular energy production, but this binding is 9 times weaker than that to oxygen. In high concentrations, carbon monoxide is also bound to myoglobin; rhabdomyolysis with myoglobinuria and renal failure may occur. The half-life of carboxyhemoglobin is about 4 hours, which can be reduced to 40–50 minutes by administration of 100% oxygen.

2. Cyanide—(See Chapter 45.) Reports have documented the presence of cyanide in the smoke of residential fires. Because of the difficulties in measuring cyanide levels in patients and because of the difficulty in recognizing smoke-related cyanide poisoning, the clinical relevance of cyanide poisoning in smoke inhalation is uncertain. Because there are risks associated with treating cyanide poisoning—which involves the production of methemoglobin by infusion of sodium nitrite—in a patient who also demonstrates carboxyhemoglobinemia, empiric therapy for cyanide poisoning is not recommended. The diagnosis and treatment of cyanide poisoning are discussed in Chapter 45.

Clinical Findings

A. Thermal Injury

Thermal injury to the upper airway should be suspected in any patient who has been in a fire occurring in a confined space, in patients with obvious face or neck burns, and in patients with soot around the nares and soot-tinged sputum or burned nasal or facial hairs. Patients may complain of dyspnea; there may be stridor, drooling, or dysphonia. The diagnosis is confirmed by direct visualization of the larynx by laryngoscopy or in some cases bronchoscopy.

B. CHEMICAL INJURY

Chemical injury to the airways and lung parenchyma is difficult to diagnose in the emergency department. Direct laryngoscopy or flexible fiberoptic bronchoscopy may reveal mucosal friability and edema of the airways. Initially the chest x-ray is often normal; noncardiogenic pulmonary edema may develop hours after exposure. Xenon lung scans, pulmonary function tests, and nitrogen washout studies have all been used to document the extent of pulmonary involvement, but they seldom provide more information than is obtainable by bronchoscopy.

C. CARBON MONOXIDE POISONING

Systemic chemical poisoning due to carbon monoxide should be suspected in every victim of fire and may be confirmed by measuring the serum carboxyhemoglobin level. The often-described cherry-red skin color is not a frequent or reliable finding in patients with carbon monoxide poisoning. Similarly, arterial blood gas measurements are not reliable determinants of carbon monoxide poisoning, because PO_2 and the calculated percentage of oxygen saturation of hemoglobin (the value that is routinely reported by clinical laboratories) are not affected by carboxyhemoglobin. The oxygen saturation measured by pulse oximetry does not distinguish oxyhemoglobin from carboxyhemoglobin. Hence, the actual saturation is obtained by subtracting the percent of carboxyhemoglobin from the measured saturation obtained from the pulse oximeter.

Typical nonexposed, nonsmoking individuals may have serum carboxyhemoglobin levels of up to 1%; smokers usually have levels of 4–6%. Levels above 10% signify significant exposure and may be associated with symptoms as outlined in Table 45–11. Patients may be asymptomatic when carboxyhemoglobin levels are below 10–15%. Levels higher than 50–60% are associated with a high incidence of coma and seizures, and levels higher than 70% are frequently fatal. Myocardial ischemia or infarction and cardiac arrhythmias occur frequently, especially in patients with underlying atherosclerotic heart disease. Some patients who initially appear to have recovered may experience delayed onset of a neurologic syndrome characterized by dementia, ataxia, and other sensory and motor abnormalities. This syndrome may be due to infarcts in the globus pallidus.

Treatment

For the critically ill patient, proceed as outlined earlier in this chapter. If there are signs of thermal injury to the airway, endotracheal intubation is necessary. In patients with major burns, even if the airway is patent initially, edema frequently occurs minutes or hours later. Prophylactic intubation prevents later urgent, difficult intubation.

Obtain arterial blood gas and carboxyhemoglobin determinations in all patients with possible smoke inhalation. While waiting for the results, give 100% oxygen by tight-fitting reservoir mask or, if indicated, by endotracheal tube. Avoid alkalosis and hypothermia, which decrease the dissociation of carbon monoxide from hemoglobin. Indications for hyperbaric oxygen therapy have been described as a carboxyhemoglobin level greater than 25%, neurologic symptoms, seizures, or depressed consciousness. The efficacy of hyperbaric oxygen in clinical management remains unproved. Although therapy shortens the half-life of carboxyhemoglobin to less than 30 minutes, the hazards and the length of time involved in transporting a critically ill patient to the nearest hyperbaric oxygen facility and the limits of resuscitating the patient in the chamber may outweigh the benefits of treatment. Hyperbaric oxygenation may be useful, however, in the severely poisoned patient who fails to respond to therapy with 100% oxygen. If carboxyhemoglobin levels are under 2% and if oxygenation is adequate, the inspired oxygen content can be decreased.

In stable patients with suspected thermal or chemical injury of the airway, evaluate mucosa injury using direct laryngoscopy.

Obtain an ECG, and monitor cardiac rhythm. Carbon monoxide poisoning is associated with myocardial ischemia and cardiac arrhythmias.

Obtain a chest x-ray to look for signs of lung injury if smoke inhalation has occurred and to serve as a baseline for further changes.

Give inhaled and parenteral bronchodilators to patients with clinical evidence of bronchospasm.

Obtain a urine specimen for assessment of myoglobinuria. If present, treat as described in Chapter 18.

No evidence supports the use of prophylactic antibiotics or systemic corticosteroids in the treatment of inhalation injuries.

Disposition

Because victims of smoke inhalation may develop late respiratory failure, these patients should be hospitalized for 24 hours for observation. All patients with carboxyhemoglobin levels higher than 25% should be hospitalized. Patients who present to the emergency department with respiratory compromise or respiratory failure should be hospitalized in an intensive care unit.

CHEMICAL BURNS

General Considerations

Most chemical burns result from exposure of the skin to strong acids or alkalis. Other chemicals that may cause skin damage include phosphorus and phenol. Because full development of chemical burns is slower than that of other types, the size of chemical burns is usually underestimated during initial evaluation.

Clinical Findings

Definitive diagnosis of chemical burns depends on the history. The physician should try to ascertain both the type of chemical involved and its concentration. Physical examination of a patient unable to give a history may aid in diagnosis. Alkali burns are frequently full-thickness injuries, appear pale, and feel leathery and slippery. Acid burns are usually partial-thickness injuries and are accompanied by erythema and erosion. Skin is stained black by hydrochloric acid, yellow by nitric acid, and brown by sulfuric acid.

Treatment

The mainstay of treatment of any chemical burn is copious irrigation with large amounts of tap water. To be most effective, treatment should be started immediately after exposure, preferably before arrival in the emergency department.

Remove any contaminated clothing. Do not attempt to neutralize the burn with weak reciprocal chemicals (acids for alkali burns and alkali for acid burns), because the heat generated from the chemical reaction may cause severe thermal injury. Occasionally the leathery skin of an alkali burn may make it difficult to completely wash off the alkali, and injury may continue; further irrigation and emergency excision of burned tissue by a surgeon experienced in this procedure may be indicated.

After copious irrigation *with water,* the following treatment for specific types of chemical burns may be used:

A. Hydrofluoric Acid

Cover burns with calcium gluconate (2.5%) gel prepared by mixing 3.5 g of calcium gluconate powder in 150 cc of water-soluble lubricant, secured by an occlusive cover. In fingertip burns, the fluoride ion often penetrates under the nail bed and matrix, so that it is usually wise to remove the nail or make a large wedge. For persistent pain or more severe burns, the treatment of choice is subcutaneous and intradermal injections of calcium gluconate (10%), 0.5 mL/cm^2 of burned area by a 30-gauge needle. Larger volumes should not be used, especially in the fingers, because further damage may occur from compartment pressure or the intrinsic toxicity of calcium. For extremely severe burns, some authors recommend intra-arterial perfusion of calcium.

B. Phenol

After copious irrigation with water, enhance the removal of phenol by applying polyethylene glycol, which increases the solubility of phenol. Follow with additional water irrigation.

C. Phosphorus

Phosphorus, a potent oxidizing agent, ignites and melts on air contact and often leaves embedded deposits on the skin. Immersion in cool water is recommended, followed by attempts to remove embedded material. Some authors recommend applying a solution of copper sulfate (1–3%) in hydroxycellulose (1%) to inactivate the phosphorus and aid in its removal, but few studies of this treatment have been made, and systemic toxicity from copper absorption may occur if copper is used repeatedly or over large areas.

Fluid resuscitation in the patient with large chemical burns is the same as that for patients with similar-size thermal burns. Because the size of chemical burns may be underestimated initially, reevaluate the patient after 24–48 hours.

Disposition

The choice between hospitalization or outpatient management of chemical burns should be made using the same criteria as for thermal burns. However, remember that the full extent of skin injury may not be readily apparent during the initial emergency department evaluation.

TAR BURNS

General Considerations

Roofing tar usually varies in temperature from 51.1 to 80 °C (124–176 °F). The hands, arms, head, and neck are the most commonly burned areas.

Treatment

Cool the tar immediately with water, which often separates the tar from the skin. If the tar continues to adhere, either leave it in place or apply one of the commercially available cream- or oil-based solvents specially made for this purpose. If these are not available, use mayonnaise or mineral oil. Do not use hydrocarbon solvents, such as paint thinner, because they may further injure burned skin. Cover the wound with sterile dressings. When dressings are changed after 12–24 hours, much of the tar will have separated and will be removed with the dressings.

Initial stabilization of the patient with large tar burns should follow the procedures outlined for thermal burns.

Disposition

The criteria for admission or transfer to a burn center for patients with tar burns are the same as for patients with thermal burns.

SUNBURN

General Considerations

Most sunburn is a first-degree (erythema) or superficial partial-thickness (blisters) burn. Skin changes from sunburn are maximal about 12–24 hours after exposure. Patients usually present to the emergency department for pain relief. Occasionally a patient with extensive superficial partial-thickness burns will require fluid resuscitation and parenteral analgesics for pain control.

Clinical Findings

Diagnosis is based on a history of exposure to the sun (or to ultraviolet light in tanning booths) and physical findings of erythema and blistering.

Treatment

Sunburn can be difficult to treat. Saline-soaked dressings or calamine lotion may provide some relief from pain and itching. Aspirin or other nonsteroidal anti-inflammatory agents (eg, indomethacin, 25–50 mg orally 3–4 times a day) work by blocking the production of prostaglandins that are thought to be important mediators of pain in sunburned skin. More severe burns may benefit from the application of topical corticosteroid preparations such as triamcinolone acetonide, 0.1%, or a short course of systemic corticosteroids (prednisone, 40 mg orally to start, with the dose tapered over 3–5 days). Patients with extensive partial-thickness sunburn should receive treatment according to the guidelines described for other thermal burns.

Disposition

Almost all patients with sunburn may receive treatment on an outpatient basis. If there are large blisters, the patient should be seen again in 2–3 days to make sure that secondary infection has not developed. Patients should be advised to avoid prolonged exposure to the sun in the future and to use a sunscreen (eg, over-the-counter preparations containing PABA [p-aminobenzoic acid] or dioxybenzone) before exposure. Patients requiring fluid resuscitation or parenteral analgesics should be hospitalized.

ELECTRICAL BURNS
(See Chapter 44.)

OCULAR BURNS
(See also Chapter 31.)

 ESSENTIALS OF DIAGNOSIS

- *High level of suspicion in patients with facial burns.*
- *Evaluate for foreign bodies.*
- *Examine eyes with fluorescein.*

General Considerations

Patients with facial burns may also have burns to the eyelid and the eye itself. Such burns are associated with the development of massive periorbital edema that makes delayed examination difficult. It is therefore important that patients with suspected ocular burns be examined promptly, preferably in the emergency department and by an ophthalmologist.

Clinical Findings

Instill tetracaine, 0.5%, or proparacaine, 0.5%, in the conjunctival sac to decrease pain during examination. Retract the eyelids, and look for foreign bodies. Remove contact lenses to prevent injury to the cornea due to pressure from edematous lids. Corneal abrasions and thermal injury may be detected by instilling fluorescein in the conjunctival sac and examining the eye using the blue light on an ophthalmoscope or, if the patient's condition permits, a slit lamp.

Treatment

Irrigate any suspected chemical burn of the eye with large amounts (2 L) of sterile normal saline using a Morgan lens. Treat corneal abrasions and thermal injuries by instilling an ophthalmic antibiotic in the conjunctival sac. Alkali burns may require larger amounts of irrigating fluid, and irrigation should continue until the effluent pH is normal. Alkali burns require emergent ophthalmologic consultation.

Disposition

Burns of the eyes are major injuries. Hospitalize the patient, and obtain urgent ophthalmologic consultation.

CIRCUMFERENTIAL BURNS OF NECK, CHEST, & EXTREMITIES

General Considerations

Circumferential deep burns of the neck may cause lymphatic and venous obstruction leading to laryngeal edema and airway obstruction. Circumferential chest wall injuries may impede chest wall movement and lead to respiratory failure. Circumferential burns of the extremities may restrict blood flow, causing increased tissue pressure with resultant ischemia.

Clinical Findings

Patients with deep circumferential neck wounds should undergo direct visualization of the larynx by laryngoscopy. Because laryngeal edema may develop hours after initial examination, frequent reevaluation may be necessary.

Monitor patients with circumferential chest wounds for signs of respiratory compromise (tachypnea, dyspnea, deteriorating arterial blood gas levels); measurement of forced vital capacity or peak airway pressure may be useful.

Carefully examine the extremity distal to the wound in patients with circumferential burns of the extremities. Look for evidence of ischemia (diminished pulses, poor capillary refill, anesthesia); loss of vibratory sense is an early sign. If available, a Doppler ultrasound device is useful to assess distal blood flow. Because edema continues to develop during the first 6–8 hours after burn injury of the extremities, frequent reevaluation is important.

Treatment

Patients with deep circumferential burns of the neck are candidates for early endotracheal intubation.

Elevate the injured extremity of patients with circumferential wounds of the extremities in order to minimize development of edema. Remove rings or other jewelry that could act as a tourniquet when edema develops. If evidence of distal ischemia develops, escharotomy is indicated. Ideally this should be performed in a burn center by a surgeon experienced in this procedure. Occasionally escharotomy must be performed in the emergency department before the patient is transported to a burn center for definitive care. Sterilize the overlying skin (Chapter 6), and make medial and lateral incisions through the eschar using a No. 20 scalpel or electrocautery. Incise deeply enough to cut entirely through the burned skin and release the constricting eschar (typically this occurs at the level of the subcutaneous fat). No anesthesia is required. Blood loss is seldom significant but can be controlled by cautery or suture if necessary.

Patients with a circumferential chest wall burn may require escharotomy in the emergency department. Using sterile technique, incise the eschar along the anterior axillary line bilaterally to the costal margins, and then join these incisions with incisions along the costal margins and just below the clavicles. This releases a segment of chest wall eschar that can move with respiratory excursion.

Disposition

All patients with deep circumferential burns of the neck, extremities, or chest wall should be hospitalized, preferably in a burn center.

BURNS DUE TO CHILD ABUSE

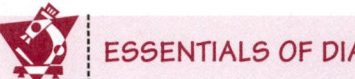 **ESSENTIALS OF DIAGNOSIS**

- *High index of suspicion.*
- *Discrepancy between the history and physical findings.*
- *Err on the side of protecting the child.*

General Considerations

Burns represent 8–14% of child abuse injuries seen in the United States; about 15% of abused children have been intentionally burned at some time.

Clinical Findings

Suspect child abuse if there is a delay in seeking medical care, if there is a history of other injuries, or if there is a discrepancy between the history and the physical findings. The injuries most commonly encountered in the emergency department are burns of the perineum caused by immersion in hot water in children who are being toilet-trained, and cigarette burns in children of any age.

Treatment & Disposition

The treatment of burns in children is the same as that of a burn of comparable size in any other patient, but if there is any suspicion that the injury was due to abuse, *the child must be hospitalized and the attending physician informed of the emergency physician's suspicions.* By law, suspected child abuse must be reported to the appropriate child welfare authorities (Chapters 5 and 48). Obtain consultation with appropriate personnel as soon as possible (eg, social worker, nurse, psychologist, pediatrician).

OUTPATIENT MANAGEMENT OF MINOR BURNS

General Considerations

Burns that meet the criteria for outpatient management (described above) may be treated initially in the emergency department, after which arrangements should be made for close follow-up on an outpatient basis.

Treatment

First-degree burns (erythema only) are best treated with application of nonadherent dressings (eg, petrolatum-impregnated gauze). Clean deeper burns by gently irrigating them with sterile normal saline solution. Leave blisters intact, and perform only minimal debridement. Wounds may be covered with a topical antibiotic such as silver sulfadiazine cream or triple antibiotic ointment and wrapped in a bulky dressing. Instruct the patient to keep the wound clean and to change dressings and apply topical antibiotic cream twice a day at home. A nonadherent, semipermeable, polyurethane dressing (eg, Epi-Lock), which is left in place for 5–7 days, may be an acceptable alternative for some patients. Such dressings should be covered with roll gauze, which is changed daily. Have the patient elevate affected extremities to minimize development of edema. All patients should receive tetanus prophylaxis as outlined in Chapter 30. Prophylactic systemic antibiotics are not indicated. Control pain with oral analgesics (eg, codeine, oxycodone).

Disposition

Patients should be seen on an outpatient basis in 1–2 days. Ruptured blisters or dead tissue may be debrided at that time. Promptly treat any minor infection with oral antistaphylococcal drugs (eg, dicloxacillin, 250– 500 mg orally 4 times a day [children < 40 kg, 25–50 mg/kg/d orally divided into 4 equal doses]; or a first-generation cephalosporin such as cephalexin, 250–500 mg orally 4 times a day [children, 25–50 mg/kg/d orally divided into 2 or 4 equal doses]). Patients who develop infections (fever, extensive cellulite, lymphadenitis), poor-risk patients (diabetics), and unreliable patients must be hospitalized for administration of parenteral antibiotics and continued wound care.

Heimbach D: What's new in general surgery: burns and metabolism. J Am Coll Surg 2002;194:156. [PMID: 11848634]

Lee-Chiong TL Jr: Smoke inhalation injury. Postgrad Med 1999; 105:55. [PMID: 10026703]

Reilly DA, Garner WL: Management of chemical injuries to the upper extremity. Hand Clin 2000;16:215. [PMID: 10791168] (Review.)

Schrage NF et al: Eye burns: an emergency and continuing problem. Burns 2000;26:689. [PMID: 11024601]

Smith ML: Pediatric burns: management of thermal, electrical, and chemical burns and burn-like dermatologic conditions. Pediatr Ann 2000;29:367. [PMID: 10868433]

Wong L, Spence RJ: Escharotomy and fasciotomy of the burned upper extremity. Hand Clin 2000;16:165. [PMID: 10791164]

Disorders Due to Physical & Environmental Agents

44

D. Shannon Waters, MD, & Rebecca C. Bowers, MD[1]

Emergency Treatment of Disorders Due to Cold
- Systemic Hypothermia
- Cold Injury of the Extremities
  1. Chilblains (Pernio)
  2. Frostbite
  3. Immersion Syndrome (Immersion Foot; Trench Foot)

Emergency Treatment of Disorders Due to Heat
- Heat Edema
- Heat Syncope
- Heat Cramps
- Heat Exhaustion
- Heat Stroke

Emergency Treatment of Electrical Injuries
- Lightning Injuries
- Electric Shock & Burns

Emergency Treatment of Radiation Injuries

Emergency Treatment of Near-Drowning

Emergency Treatment of Disorders Due to Atmospheric Pressure Changes
- Decompression Sickness (Caisson Disease, "Bends")
- Arterial Gas Embolism

High-Altitude Sickness (Mountain Sickness)
  1. Acute Mountain Sickness
  2. Acute High-Altitude Pulmonary Edema
  3. High-Altitude Cerebral Edema

Emergency Treatment of Disorders Due to Venomous Animals
- Snake Bites
- Bees & Wasp Stings
- Black Widow Spider Bites
- Brown Recluse Spider Bites
- Scorpion Stings
- Hazardous Marine Life
  1. Stingrays
  2. Sea Snakes
  3. Jellyfish
  4. Scorpion Fish
  5. Sea Urchins

Ingestion of Poisonous Fish
  1. Ciguatera Toxin Poisoning
  2. Scombroid Poisoning
  3. Puffer Fish (Tetrodotoxin) Poisoning
  4. Paralytic Shellfish Poisoning

■ EMERGENCY TREATMENT OF DISORDERS DUE TO COLD

Individuals vary considerably in their response to environmental cold. Factors that increase the possibility of injury due to cold include poor general physical condition, nonacclimatization, childhood or advanced age, systemic illness, anoxia, and the use of alcohol and other sedative drugs. High wind velocity (windchill factor) and moisture may markedly increase the propensity for cold injury at low temperatures.

SYSTEMIC HYPOTHERMIA

 ESSENTIALS OF DIAGNOSIS

- *Signs and symptoms depend on degree of hypothermia.*

---

[1]This chapter is a revision of the chapter by Paul S. Auerbach, MD, from the 4th edition.

• *Rewarming methods include passive external active, external, and active internal rewarming.*

General Considerations

A. HEALTHY PERSONS

Accidental hypothermia occurs when an external cold challenge overwhelms an individual's capacity to produce or conserve heat. Hypothermia may occur in otherwise healthy individuals during occupational or recreational exposure to cold or as a result of accidents or other misfortunes. Alcohol abuse is a common predisposing cause.

B. PERSONS WITH PREDISPOSING FACTORS

Systemic hypothermia may follow exposure to even slightly lowered temperatures when preexisting altered homeostasis exists as a result of debility or disease. Accidental hypothermia is more likely to occur in elderly or inactive people and those with cardiovascular, dermatologic, or cerebrovascular disease; mental retardation; myxedema; hypopituitarism; or alcoholism. The use of sedative-hypnotic or antidepressant drugs may be a contributing factor.

Clinical Findings

Because lowered body temperature is the sole finding in some patients brought to the emergency department, making the diagnosis often depends on awareness of the possibility of hypothermia.

A. TEMPERATURE

In the hypothermic patient, oral and axillary temperatures are not accurate. Infrared tympanic thermometers or rectal probes should be used. The temperature varies widely in hypothermia, and accurate monitoring is essential.

B. SYMPTOMS AND SIGNS

At rectal temperatures of 35 °C (95 °F), hypothermia is classified as mild. Shivering is at a maximum and consciousness is normal. At 34 °C (93.2 °F), the victim develops apathy, drowsiness, slurred speech, and poor judgment. At 32 °C (89.6 °F), the hypothermia is profound with marked alteration in mental status, lethargy, and ataxia. At 31 °C (87.8 °F), shivering stops and failure of the thermoregulatory mechanism is imminent. The patient soon becomes unresponsive; profound bradycardia, hypotension, and hypoventilation can occur; and fixed pupils may develop. The patient may appear to be in a state of rigor mortis. Ventricular

fibrillation and asystole may occur spontaneously at core temperatures below 28 °C (82.4 °F). *Note:* For this reason, a hypothermic patient should not be considered dead until all reasonable resuscitative measures have failed. No one is dead until he or she is "warm and dead."

C. LABORATORY FINDINGS

Several laboratory findings are unique to hypothermia. The electrocardiogram (ECG) may demonstrate prolongation of any conduction interval; atrial fibrillation is common. A pathognomonic positive deflection in the RT segment is known as a J, or Osborne, wave (Figure 44–1).

Hypoglycemia, hypomagnesemia, and hypophosphatemia are common in hypothermia, particularly in alcoholic individuals. Hyperglycemia may be seen as a result of hemorrhagic pancreatitis in patients with long-lasting exposure to the cold. Sodium and potassium levels may be elevated or depressed. Arterial blood gas samples drawn at cold temperatures are generally analyzed at 37 °C (98.6 °F), which causes lowering of pH and elevation of PO_2 and PCO_2 readings. However, clinical therapy is based on the uncorrected determinations recorded at 37 °C.

D. COMPLICATIONS

Metabolic acidosis, pneumonia, pancreatitis, renal failure, sepsis, and ventricular fibrillation may occur. Death due to systemic hypothermia usually results from cardiac arrest associated with ventricular fibrillation, which may occur during rewarming.

E. UNDERLYING CONDITIONS

Obtain a brief history from witnesses or relatives of a patient with hypothermia, and perform a general physical and laboratory examination to detect underlying conditions that might predispose to hypothermia. Examination should include an evaluation of renal function (uremia), thyroid function (myxedema), and adrenal function (Addison disease). If sepsis is a diagnostic possibility, obtain blood for culture.

Treatment

Bundle the victim of suspected hypothermia in dry, warm blankets at the scene of discovery, and transport the person to the nearest hospital as soon as possible. *Note:* Transport should be as gentle as possible because of the risk of cardiac arrhythmias due to increased myocardial irritability. Hospitalization and monitoring in an intensive care unit are required for all victims with initial core temperatures below 32 °C (89.6 °F) or for those with complications of hypothermia.

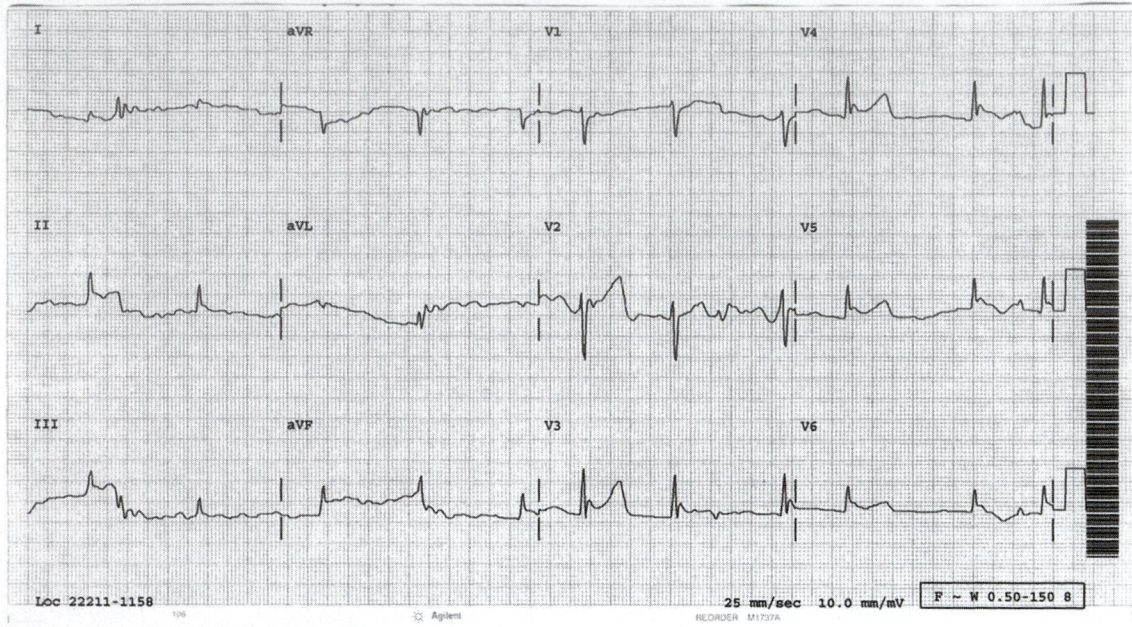

Figure 44–1. Hypothermia. The patient is in atrial fibrillation with a slow ventricular response. The QRS complexes are narrow, and there is an additional positive slurred deflection, the J wave (Osborne wave), just prior to the ST segment.

A. CARDIOPULMONARY RESUSCITATION

Adequacy of ventilation and circulation must be ensured by careful clinical observation, continuous electrocardiographic monitoring, and serial determinations of arterial blood gases. If cardiac arrest occurs, start cardiopulmonary resuscitation (CPR) (Chapter 7). If the victim has any detectable pulse or breathing, no matter how slow, do not initiate CPR; unnecessary brisk closed chest compression may induce ventricular fibrillation. Because of the protective effects of hypothermia, bradycardia and hypotension are generally well tolerated.

1. Establish an airway—Intubation of the unprotected airway and frequent suctioning may be required.

2. Give warm, humidified oxygen—Depression of the respiratory center in hypothermia causes hypoxemia or hypercapnia, requiring controlled ventilation and supplemental oxygen. Avoid hyperventilation, because a rapid fall in PCO_2 may trigger ventricular fibrillation.

3. If arterial blood pH is below 7.1, cautiously give bicarbonate—(See Chapter 42). Do not try to attain neutral pH, because sudden changes in acid-base equilibrium may cause cardiac arrhythmias. Mild acidosis (pH 7.25–7.35) due to hypothermia in the absence of

sepsis is generally well tolerated. Management should be based on arterial blood gas measurements recorded at 37 °C (98.6 °F).

4. Correct ventricular fibrillation—Electrical defibrillation is rarely successful at core temperatures below 30 °C (86 °F). Bretylium tosylate is the drug of choice in ventricular fibrillation; lidocaine and other class Ib agents are generally ineffective. Other pharmacologic measures to correct bradycardia and hypotension should generally be avoided.

5. Correct fluid, electrolyte, and glucose abnormalities—Give thiamine, 100 mg intravenously; naloxone, 2.0 mg intravenously; and dextrose, 25 g intravenously, to all patients with altered mental status who are thought to be hypothermic. Volume expansion with warmed fluid generally helps the rewarming process. Avoid lactated Ringer's solution because the lactate is not metabolized efficiently by a cold liver.

B. TREATMENT OF UNDERLYING CONDITIONS

Treat underlying and predisposing conditions as necessary (eg, heart disease, hypoglycemia, malnutrition, adrenocortical insufficiency [hydrocortisone, 200 mg intravenously], hypothyroidism [levothyroxine, 400 µg intravenously; plus hydrocortisone, 100 mg intravenously]).

C. Rewarming

Rewarming is essential but potentially harmful, because peripheral vasodilatation may divert blood flow from internal organs to the skin and shunt cooled blood to the central circulation, causing a brief drop in core temperature. *Note:* Rapid rewarming may be hazardous, because hypothermic patients are particularly vulnerable to lethal cardiac arrhythmias. Core rewarming should be undertaken only if hypothermia is severe and the patient shows cardiovascular instability (eg, cardiac arrest, ventricular fibrillation).

1. Mild hypothermia (core temperature ≥ 33 °C [91.4 °F])—Passive rewarming to prevent further heat loss is sufficient for most patients with mild hypothermia, because their thermoregulatory mechanism is intact, and many of these patients are able to generate heat by shivering. Most patients should be wrapped in dry, heated blankets and carefully monitored. Patients with mild hypothermia who are otherwise healthy usually respond well to heated blankets and the administration of heated (45 °C [113 °F]) intravenous solutions. Another conservative approach—often used with elderly or debilitated patients—is to wrap the patient in an electric blanket kept at 37 °C (98.6 °F). Patients must be carefully monitored when any of these rewarming methods are used.

2. Moderate to severe hypothermia (core temperature < 33 °C [91.4 °F])—Moderate to severe hypothermia often requires additional rewarming measures, because thermoregulation is altered or absent. Individualized supportive care is mandatory, because active rewarming is hazardous. As mentioned previously, active core rewarming is necessary only for patients with cardiovascular instability.

 a. Active external rewarming methods—Heated blankets, forced-air blankets (Bair Hugger), or warm baths have been used, with a rate of rewarming of about 1–3 °C/h (up to 600 kcal/h using hydraulic pads at 45 °C). Because it is easier to monitor the patient and to carry out diagnostic and therapeutic procedures when heated blankets rather than warm baths are used for active rewarming, heated baths are not widely recommended. There is some potential risk with active external rewarming, because marked vasodilation may occur. Combining active external rewarming with active core rewarming may prevent the resultant hypotension and core temperature after-drop sometimes seen during rewarming. If active external rewarming is used, the patient should be carefully monitored and supported hemodynamically. The application of commercial heat packs directly to hypothermic skin may cause serious burns.

 b. Active internal (core) rewarming methods—Internal rewarming is suggested for patients with profound hypothermia of long duration in which there is suspected underlying debilitation, for patients with complications of cardiovascular or respiratory insufficiency, and for patients in cardiac arrest.

 Repeated peritoneal dialysis may be performed using warm (45 °C [113 °F]) potassium-free dialysate solution or normal saline. The usual exchange rate is 6 L/h, which can increase the core temperature 1–3 °C/h.

 Warm fluids (crystalloid solutions) administered by gastrointestinal, colonic, or bladder lavage may be employed. Placement of a nasogastric tube is less invasive but may run the risk of stimulating ventricular dysrhythmias owing to the irritability of the hypothermic heart.

 Administration of heated intravenous fluids contributes only 17 kcal/h, which accounts for an increase in body temperature of less than $\frac{1}{3}$ °C/L. Microwave rewarming of crystalloid solutions to 40–42 °C (104–107.6 °F) may be safely accomplished in about 2–3 minutes. This technique causes some hemolysis of erythrocytes, and if blood products are used they should be administered through a high-flow countercurrent fluid infuser or reconstituted with warmed normal saline.

 Heated humidified oxygen, either via a tight-fitting mask or by endotracheal tube, will raise the core temperature 1 °C/h or 1.5–2 °C/h, respectively.

 Thoracic cavity lavage may achieve rapid rewarming with the added advantage of warming the heart more quickly. Insert 2 thoracostomy tubes, and continuously infuse fluid warmed to 41 °C (105.8 °F) through one tube and drain it through the other.

 Extracorporeal blood rewarming methods including arteriovenous and venovenous rewarming as well as hemodialysis have been reported as treatment options but are limited to medical centers with the available resources.

 Negative pressure rewarming is a new technique based on the principle that thermoregulatory blood flow to certain skin areas is regulated by arteriovenous anastomosis. Negative pressure and a thermal device are used to increase local subcutaneous blood flow, allowing heat to be transferred directly from the skin to the critical body core despite the central drive for vasoconstriction. The devices have reported good rewarming rates, although more studies are needed.

D. Antimicrobials

Patients with severe hypothermia—especially those who are comatose—are at high risk for development of aspiration pneumonia; subsequent pulmonary, urinary tract, or intraperitoneal infections; and sepsis. If severe infection is suspected, obtain a chest x-ray and samples of blood and urine for culture, and take material for culture from any other appropriate sites (eg, cerebrospinal fluid). If sepsis is likely, administer broad-spectrum antibiotics. Prophylactic antimicrobial drugs are unnecessary if infection is unlikely. Many hypothermic alcoholic, debilitated, or elderly patients will have an underlying infection, and the cause should be aggressively sought and treatment initiated.

E. COMPLICATIONS OF REWARMING

Observe the patient for signs of metabolic acidosis, cardiac arrhythmias, acute respiratory distress syndrome, pancreatitis, ischemic bowel, pneumonia, myoglobinuria with renal failure, or clotting abnormalities.

Disposition

Hospitalize all patients who present with core temperatures below 33 °C (91.4 °F), especially if the sensorium is altered. Patients with coexisting illness and core temperatures under 35 °C (95 °F) should be hospitalized. The mortality rates in hypothermia are variable and depend on the cause of hypothermia and the patient's underlying condition.

COLD INJURY OF THE EXTREMITIES

 ESSENTIALS OF DIAGNOSIS

- Tissue injury or death is caused by ischemia and thrombosis in capillaries or by formation of ice in the tissues.
- Treatment of frostbite or chilblains depends on the severity of skin injury and includes rewarming by both passive and active measures.

In the normal person, exposure of the extremities to cold produces immediate intense localized vasoconstriction followed by reflex generalized vasoconstriction. When skin temperature falls to 25 °C (77 °F), tissue metabolism is slowed but the relative demand for oxygen exceeds the supply from diminished circulation; thus, the area becomes cyanotic. At 15 °C (59 °F), tissue metabolism is markedly decreased and the dissociation of oxyhemoglobin is reduced, which may give the skin a pink, well-oxygenated appearance. Tissue damage occurs at this temperature. Tissue death may be caused either by ischemia and thrombosis in capillaries or by actual freezing. Freezing (frostbite) does not occur until the skin temperature drops to −10 to −4 °C

(14–24.8 °F). The body's "hunting reaction," or alternating vasoconstriction and vasodilation of vessels in the frozen area, results in repetitive cycles of partial thawing with refreezing. This process causes the most damage. The incidence of frostbite depends on factors such as wind, moisture, mobility, venous stasis, trauma, malnutrition, and occlusive arterial disease.

1. Chilblains (Pernio)

Clinical Findings

Chilblains, a less severe form of cold injury than frostbite, is more common in children and women as well as people with any form of peripheral vascular disease. Chilblains are red or violaceous pruritic skin lesions, usually on the face or extremities, caused by exposure to cold and humidity without actual freezing of tissues. Lymphocytic vasculitis is common. Chilblains may be associated with edema or blistering and are subsequently aggravated by excessive warmth. With continued exposure, ulcerative or hemorrhagic lesions may appear and progress to scarring, fibrosis, and atrophy.

Treatment & Disposition

Elevate the affected part on pillows or sheepskin, and allow it to warm gradually at room temperature.

Do not rub or massage injured tissues or apply ice or heat. Protect the area from trauma and secondary infection. Refer the patient to a primary care physician or clinic for follow-up.

2. Frostbite

Clinical Findings

A. CLASSIFICATION

Frostbite is injury of the tissues due to freezing. The classification of injury is applied after rewarming because most frostbite appears similar initially.

1. First-degree—Freezing without blistering; peeling is occasionally present.

2. Second-degree—Freezing with clear blistering.

3. Third-degree—Freezing with death of skin, hemorrhagic blisters, and subcutaneous involvement.

4. Fourth-degree—Freezing with full-thickness involvement (including bone); ultimate loss or deformity of body part.

This classification scheme neither accurately predicts clinical outcome nor aids in initial management because a discrepancy exists between skin lesions and the extent of deep tissue injury, and demarcation is not complete for 3–5 weeks.

B. Symptoms and Signs

Frostbitten tissue appears white or blue-white, is firm or hard (frozen), cool to the touch, and generally insensitive. Because cold injury produces anesthesia, many symptoms are not apparent until rewarming begins or the part is closely inspected. In patients with mild frostbite, the symptoms are numbness, paresthesias, pruritus, and lack of fine motor control. With increasing severity, decreased range of motion, blister formation, and prominent swelling are noted. Thawing unmasks local tenderness and throbbing pain. The tissue becomes discolored, loses its elasticity, and becomes immobile. Profound edema, hemorrhagic blisters, necrosis, and gangrene may occur. Long-term sequelae include cold sensitivity, loss of sensation, and hyperhidrosis.

Treatment

A. Systemic Hypothermia

Treat moderate to severe associated systemic hypothermia before managing frostbite.

B. Rewarming

1. Superficial frostbite—Rewarm extremities affected by superficial frostbite (frostnip) by removing wet clothing and applying constant warmth, which can be accomplished by exerting gentle pressure with a warm hand.

2. Full-thickness frostbite—Rapid rewarming is the most important aspect of management. It should not be attempted, however, until the risk of refreezing is gone. Once rewarming can begin, it should be performed with a waterbath containing an antimicrobial agent. Strict adherence to a narrow water temperature window of 40–42 °C (104–107.6 °F) is necessary. When a red-purple color appears and the skin becomes pliable, the rewarming may cease.

C. Resuscitation

Unless concomitant hypothermia exists, intravenous hydration is not usually necessary. Severe cases of frostbite have led to subsequent rhabdomyolysis with renal failure, which then requires aggressive hydration. Intravenous narcotics are almost always necessary secondary to the severe pain associated with rewarming.

D. Protection of the Injured Part

In the prehospital setting, padding, splinting, and avoidance of rewarming are all that is necessary. Once in the secure hospital setting and after rewarming has been achieved, avoidance of further trauma is important. Affected body parts should be elevated and padded, uncovered or loosely dressed, and left at room temperature. Debride clear blisters because prostaglandins and thromboxane are present in the exudate. Leave hemorrhagic blisters intact. Apply aloe vera cream every 6 hours. Administer ibuprofen, 400–600 mg every 8–12 hours for 72 hours.

E. Anti-infective Measures

Infection prevention is important after rewarming. Maintain a sterile environment. Protect skin blebs from physical contact. Whirlpool therapy at temperatures of 32–38 °C (89.6–100.4 °F) twice daily for 30 minutes for a period of 3 or more weeks helps to cleanse the skin and debride superficial dead tissue. Penicillin prophylaxis is highly recommended for severe cases.

F. Adjunctive Therapies

1. Anticoagulation—Consistent benefit from anticoagulation has not been demonstrated.

2. Dextran—Animal experiments have shown promise, but human clinical trials have not been attempted.

3. Vasodilators—Intra-arterial injections of reserpine reduce vasospasm but have not prevented tissue loss.

4. Thrombolysis—Thrombolytics have been extremely successful in aiding tissue survival in the animal model. Small clinical studies with tissue plasminogen activator are also showing success in humans, but the results of larger, multicenter trials are needed.

5. Surgery—Amputation or debridement should not be considered until it is definitely established that tissues are dead. Although rare, the development of a compartment syndrome necessitates fasciotomy. The line of demarcation between injured and normal tissue may not appear until 3–5 weeks after injury; mummification of the injured extremity may require the same length of time. Technetium-^{99} pyrophosphate scanning accurately predicts the level of ultimate amputation. Magnetic resonance imaging and magnetic resonance angiography are under investigation as possible techniques for assessing demarcation lines much earlier.

Regional sympathectomy performed 24–48 hours after injury has reportedly ameliorated the early sequelae of frostbite, including a reduction in edema and decreased subsequent tissue loss. Appropriate clinical studies have yet to be performed to support the use of this therapy.

6. Hyperbaric oxygen—Considerable disagreement exists as to the effectiveness of hyperbaric oxygen therapy. In animal models, early institution after rewarming, with subsequent daily therapy, decreased tissue loss.

Disposition

Hospitalize all patients with second- or third-degree frostbite and patients with extensive areas of first-degree frostbite.

3. Immersion Syndrome (Immersion Foot; Trench Foot)

 ESSENTIALS OF DIAGNOSIS

- *Caused by prolonged immersion in cold water.*
- *Alternating vasospasm and vasodilatation results in initial cold and anesthetic feet followed by blistering and ulceration.*
- *Treatment includes rewarming and wound care.*

Clinical Findings

Immersion foot (or hand) is caused by prolonged immersion in cool or cold water or mud that causes alternating arterial vasospasm and vasodilatation. The affected parts are first cold and anesthetic. Hyperemia follows after 24–48 hours, and the parts become warm, with intense burning and tingling pain. Blistering, swelling, redness, ecchymoses, and ulceration are noted. The posthyperemic phase occurs after 2–6 weeks and causes the limbs to become cyanotic, with increased sensitivity to cold. Complications include lymphangitis, cellulitis, thrombophlebitis, and wet gangrene.

Prevention

Changing out of wet socks and shoes as soon as possible is paramount to the prevention of immersion syndrome. In the military, individuals at risk for immersion foot apply silicone ointment to the bottoms of their feet twice daily as a preventive measure.

Treatment & Disposition

Treatment is best started during or before the stage of reactive hyperemia.

Immediate treatment consists of protecting the extremities from trauma and secondary infection. Rewarm the injured areas gradually by exposing them to air (not to ice or extreme heat). Do not soak or massage the skin. The patient should remain at bed rest until all ulcers have healed. Keep the affected parts elevated to aid in removal of edema fluid, and protect pressure sites (eg, heels) with pillows or booties lined with cotton batting. Give antimicrobials only if infection occurs.

Hospitalize all patients with immersion syndrome.

Giesbrecht GG: Cold stress, near drowning and accidental hypothermia: a review. Aviat Space Environ Med 2000;71:733. [PMID: 10902937] (Review of therapy and new techniques in the treatment of hypothermia.)

Humphrey W et al: Warm water immersion: still a threat to the soldier. Mil Med 1997;162:610. [PMID: 9290296] (Case reports of soldiers with immersion foot syndrome.)

Kulkarni RD et al: Severe accidental hypothermia: the need for prolonged aggressive resuscitative efforts. Prehosp Emerg Care 1999;3:254. [PMID: 10424866] (Case report and review of the treatment of hypothermia.)

Lazar HL: The treatment of hypothermia. N Engl J Med 1997;337:1545. [PMID: 9366589] (Review of the treatment of hypothermia and discussion about the findings of the Walpoth et al article [see below].)

Murphy JV et al: Frostbite: pathogenesis and treatment. J Trauma 2000;48:171. [PMID: 10647591] (Review article on frostbite.)

Soreide E et al: A non-invasive means to effectively restore normothermia in cold stressed individuals: a preliminary report. J Emerg Med 1999;17:725. [PMID: 10431966] (A prospective study to evaluate the use of subatmospheric pressure and heat to restore normothermia.)

Stavem K et al: Accuracy of infrared ear thermometry in adult patients. Intensive Care Med 1997;23:100. [PMID: 9037647] (Prospective comparison of infrared ear thermometry vs. core reference [pulmonary artery] temperature.)

Vassal T et al: Severe accidental hypothermia treated in an ICU: prognosis and outcome. Chest 2001;120:1998. [PMID: 11742934] (A retrospective analysis of the characteristics and outcome of patients admitted to an intensive care unit with severe accidental hypothermia.)

Walpoth BH et al: Outcome of survivors of accidental deep hypothermia and circulatory arrest treated with extracorporeal blood warming. N Engl J Med 1997;337:1500. [PMID: 9366581] (An analysis and testing of survivors of severe hypothermia for residual deficits. Cardiopulmonary bypass is recommended as the rewarming method of choice.)

Walsh S: More red toes. J Pediatr Health Care 2000;14:205. [PMID: 10900417] (Discussion of cold-induced skin disorders.)

■ EMERGENCY TREATMENT OF DISORDERS DUE TO HEAT

The 5 main disorders due to environmental heat stress are (1) heat edema, (2) heat syncope, (3) heat cramps, (4) heat exhaustion, and (5) heat stroke.

Acclimatization usually results after 8–10 days of exposure to high temperatures, but even a fully acclimatized person may suffer a heat disorder when heat exposure is combined with excessive fatigue; severe infection; alcohol intoxication; use of anticholinergic drugs; or failure to maintain hydration, salt intake, or caloric intake. Elderly or obese persons and those with chronic debilitating diseases are most susceptible to heat disorders due to circulatory failure or failure of the sweating mechanism.

HEAT EDEMA

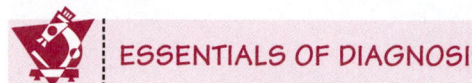

ESSENTIALS OF DIAGNOSIS

- *Swelling of feet and ankles due to vasodilatation and venous stasis.*
- *Treatment is elevation of the limbs.*

Nonacclimatized individuals, particularly the elderly, may develop swelling of the feet and ankles that is generally associated with periods of prolonged sitting or standing. The edema is not complicated by manifestations of congestive heart failure or lymphatic disease. The cause of heat edema is muscular and cutaneous vasodilation combined with venous stasis. Interstitial fluid then accumulates in the lower extremities. Because the problem is self-limited, treatment involves use of support hose and simple elevation of the lower limbs. Diuretics are not indicated.

HEAT SYNCOPE

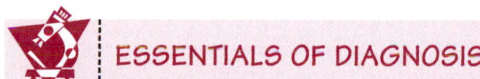

ESSENTIALS OF DIAGNOSIS

- *Caused by peripheral pooling of the intravascular volume.*
- *Patient responds promptly to rest, cooling, and rehydration.*

Simple fainting may occur suddenly after exertion in the heat. Cutaneous and muscular vasodilation redistributes intravascular volume to the periphery of the body. Volume loss and prolonged standing (pooling in the lower extremities) also contribute to the development of inadequate central venous return and insufficient cerebral perfusion. The patient's skin is cool and moist, the pulse is weak, and transient hypotension occurs. In general, core temperature is normal or mildly elevated. The patient usually responds promptly to rest in a recumbent position, cooling, and oral rehydration. Evaluate elderly people who experience syncopal episodes for hypoglycemia, arrhythmias, and fixed myocardial or cerebrovascular lesions.

HEAT CRAMPS

ESSENTIALS OF DIAGNOSIS

- *Spasms of the voluntary muscles of the abdomen and extremities.*
- *Caused by salt depletion.*
- *Treatment consists of fluid and salt replacement.*

Clinical Findings

Heat cramps are due primarily to salt depletion and are manifested by painful spasms of the voluntary muscles of the abdomen and extremities. The skin may be moist or dry, and cool or warm. Muscle fasciculations may be present. The core temperature is normal or only slightly elevated. Laboratory studies (rarely indicated) may reveal hemoconcentration and low serum sodium levels, although this is variable, and normal serum sodium levels are frequently noted. Hypokalemia occurs occasionally.

Treatment & Disposition

Treatment includes oral fluid and salt replacement with 0.1–0.2% salt solution (¼–½ teaspoon table salt in 1 cup water) or, in severe cases, intravenous normal saline solution. Give supplementary potassium as dictated by measured serum levels. Replace glucose if needed. An alternative therapy for mild symptoms is a commercial electrolyte solution (eg, Gatorade). Place the patient in a cool place, and massage sore muscles gently.

The patient should rest for 1–3 days, depending on the severity of the attack. Hospitalization is usually not required.

HEAT EXHAUSTION

ESSENTIALS OF DIAGNOSIS

- *Caused by either primary water loss or primary sodium loss due to prolonged heat exposure.*
- *Rapidly leads to heat stroke.*
- *Symptoms of dehydration are present, but central nervous system symptoms are not seen.*
- *Treatment includes rehydration and cooling.*

General Considerations

Heat exhaustion is a systemic reaction to prolonged heat exposure (hours to days) and is due to sodium depletion, dehydration, accumulation of metabolites, or a combination of these factors. It is a premonitory syndrome that rapidly evolves to heat stroke. Central nervous system symptoms are generally not present, and the core body temperature is usually less than 40 °C (104 °F).

Clinical Findings

Two types of heat exhaustion have been described: hypernatremic (primary water loss) and hyponatremic (primary sodium loss). The hypernatremic form is seen in persons without access to free water and results from inadequate water replacement. The hyponatremic form results from excessive thermal sweating with pure water replacement. It differs from heat cramps in that systemic symptoms are present. Pure forms of either type are rare, and most cases have a mixed salt and water depletion. The signs and symptoms of heat exhaustion are nonspecific and include headache, nausea, vomiting, malaise, muscle cramps, and dizziness. Dehydration is manifested by tachycardia, hypotension, and diaphoresis. In a hypernatremic patient, the water deficit can be calculated using the following formula:

$$\text{Water deficit in liters} = TBW - (TBW \times \text{desired}$$
$$[Na^+] / \text{measured } [Na^+]),$$

where TBW = total body water, calculated as follows:

$$\text{TBW for men} = \text{wt in kg} \times 0.6$$
$$\text{TBW for women} = \text{wt in kg} \times 0.5$$

Measurement of serum electrolytes and renal function is advisable in most patients, because serum sodium concentration may be markedly low in patients with heat exhaustion. Myoglobinuria indicates subclinical rhabdomyolysis.

Treatment & Disposition

Initial treatment includes placing the patient in a cool place and giving adequate cool water and salted (< 200 mOsm/L) fruit drinks or salt tablets according to the estimated amount of water and salt depletion. If the patient is unable to drink fluids, give normal saline or lactated Ringer's injection with 5% glucose supplementation intravenously in accordance with clinical and laboratory findings. If marked hyponatremia with water intoxication is present, administration of intravenous hypertonic saline may be required (Chapter 42).

Hospitalize patients with moderate to severe symptoms and those who are elderly or have comorbid illnesses.

HEAT STROKE

 ESSENTIALS OF DIAGNOSIS

- Extremely high body temperatures causing altered mental status and multiorgan dysfunction.
- Rhabdomyolysis and severe hepatic damage occur.
- Treatment is rapid reduction in body temperature.

General Considerations

Heat stroke is characterized by dysfunction of the heat-regulating mechanism, with altered mental status (ranging from confusion to coma) and elevated core body temperature in excess of 41 °C (105.8 °F). Sweating is variable. The extremely high body temperature rapidly causes widespread damage to body tissues, with significant rhabdomyolysis and multiorgan dysfunction. Illness and death result from destruction of cerebral, cardiovascular, hepatic, and renal tissue.

Heat stroke usually follows excessive exposure to heat or strenuous physical activity under exceptionally hot environmental conditions, although it may develop in elderly, infirm, or otherwise susceptible individuals in the absence of unusual exposure to heat. Cardiovascular disease, diabetes, cystic fibrosis, alcoholism, obesity, recent febrile illness, and debility are predisposing factors. Anesthetics, paralyzing agents, diuretics, sedatives, antidepressants, and anticholinergic drugs may also be contributing factors.

Clinical Findings

A. SYMPTOMS AND SIGNS

Premonitory findings include headache, dizziness, nausea, diarrhea, and visual disturbances. Most patients have profound central nervous system dysfunction including seizures, delirium, and coma. The skin is hot, flushed (cyanosis may be present), and usually dry (although sweating may be present). Prior to cardiovascular collapse, the pulse may be strong and rapid. Blood pressure is initially elevated, and hypotension is a late finding that signals circulatory collapse. Hyperventilation may cause initial respiratory alkalosis, which is generally followed by metabolic acidosis. Stigmas of coagulopathy may be present and include hematuria, hematemesis, bruising, petechiae, and oozing at sites of venipuncture. Core body temperatures as high as 46 °C (114.8 ° F) have been reported in some patients who have achieved full recovery.

B. Laboratory Findings

Laboratory findings include hemoconcentration, decreased blood coagulation, and evidence of disseminated intravascular coagulation. Hypoprothrombinemia, hypofibrinogenemia, or thrombocytopenia may be present. The white blood cell count is routinely elevated. Hypophosphatemia and hypokalemia sometimes occur. Hyperkalemia is associated with acute renal failure due to rhabdomyolysis. The patient has scantly concentrated urine ("machine oil urine") containing protein, tubular casts, and myoglobin. A consistent finding in patients with heatstroke is severe hepatic injury. Serum transaminase levels rise to tens of thousands, although complete recovery usually ensues if treatment is initiated quickly.

Treatment

Act quickly to prevent further inquiry.

A. Airway and Ventilation

Maintain an adequate airway and ventilation; monitor arterial blood gas levels. Give supplemental oxygen, 6–10 L/min, by mask or nasal cannula.

B. Temperature Reduction

Reduce body temperature promptly. As a first-aid measure, place the patient in a shady, cool place and remove his or her clothing. Sprinkle the patient's entire body with water, and cool by fanning. Alcohol sponge baths are contraindicated and can result in alcohol toxicity. If the victim is near a cold stream, it may be helpful to immerse the patient in the water to facilitate cooling.

In the emergency department, place the patient on a cooling blanket, and place ice packs on the axilla, posterior neck, and inguinal areas (do not apply ice directly to the skin). Water should be sprayed on the patient with a fan blowing on him or her to maximize evaporative cooling. If the temperature cannot be rapidly lowered, or if the victim is unresponsive and the initial core temperature exceeds 42 °C (107.6 °F), begin peritoneal lavage with cold potassium-free dialysate, 2 L every 10–15 minutes. When the rectal temperature drops to 39 °C (102.2 °F), discontinue active measures to lower temperature to avoid hypothermia, but continue temperature monitoring. Hyperthermia may recur due to thermoregulatory instability, and additional cooling may be required.

Benzodiazepines may be given as needed to control shivering. Because the hypothalamic set point is not elevated as it is in fever, aspirin and acetaminophen are ineffective and should not be given. They may even worsen coagulopathy and liver damage.

C. Maintenance of Urine Output

Maintain adequate urinary output (30–50 mL/h). Insert an indwelling urinary catheter to monitor urine output. If myoglobinuria is present, alkalize the urine with intravenous administration of bicarbonate, and consider the use of mannitol, 0.25 g/kg intravenously, to promote diuresis. Maintain blood pressure and urine output with intravenous infusion of crystalloid solutions and inotropic agents as necessary (monitoring of central venous pressure or pulmonary capillary wedge pressure may be required). α-Adrenergic drugs are contraindicated because they produce vasoconstriction and decrease heat exchange. Dobutamine may be preferable to dopamine as an inotropic agent, because it does not have the α-adrenergic renal effects associated with dopamine at rapid rates of infusion.

Disposition

Hospitalize all patients whose core temperature has exceeded 41 °C (105.8 °F) for treatment of possible complications (disseminated intravascular coagulation, renal failure, hepatic failure, rhabdomyolysis, cardiac arrhythmias, myocardial infarction, and coma).

With early diagnosis and proper care, 80–90% of previously healthy patients should survive. Extreme hyperpyrexia (rectal temperature > 42 °C [107.6 °F]), persistent coma after cooling, markedly elevated alanine aminotransferase (serum glutamic pyruvic transaminase) and aspartate aminotransferase (serum glutamic oxalacetic transaminase) levels, and hyperkalemia associated with extensive rhabdomyolysis are unfavorable prognostic signs.

Backer HD et al: Exertional heat illness and hyponatremia in hikers. Am J Emerg Med 1999;17:532. [PMID: 10530529] Retrospective analysis of the presentation of exercise-associated hyponatremia and heat disorders in hikers.

Khosla R et al: Heat-related illnesses. Crit Care Clin 1999;15:251. [PMID: 10331127] (Review of minor and major heat illnesses and temperature regulation.)

Waters TA: Heat illness: tips for recognition and treatment. Cleve Clin J Med 2001;68:685. [PMID: 11510526] (Review of heat exhaustion versus heat stroke.)

■ EMERGENCY TREATMENT OF ELECTRICAL INJURIES

LIGHTNING INJURIES

 ESSENTIALS OF DIAGNOSIS

- *Lightning injuries can result not only in burns but also in multiorgan dysfunction.*
- *Respiratory arrest is the most common cause of death; ventricular fibrillation and asystole are also seen in severe cases.*
- *Management is the same as that for a person with blunt trauma.*

General Considerations

Lightning associated with thunderstorms strikes the earth more than 120 times per second. Although the number of lightning strikes in human beings is low, at least 200–400 people are killed each year as a result of injuries caused by lightning.

A stroke of lightning travels from a thundercloud to the ground at a speed of 10,000 km/s (10^7 m/s), and it briefly attains voltages over 100 million V and temperatures of up to 3000 °C (5432 °F). Lightning is direct current (DC). The most common form of lightning is streak lightning. Injuries are caused by a direct strike, splash (eg, from trees, building, fences), step voltage, or blunt trauma. In step voltage, ground surface current is transmitted through a circuit created by the victim's legs (pathway of least resistance).

Clinical Findings

Suspect lightning injury in a person found dazed, unconscious, or injured in the vicinity of a thunderstorm. Certain pathognomonic clinical signs help to establish the diagnosis.

A. Burns

Although enormous levels of electrical energy are generated in a lightning strike, burns are frequently superficial. The flashover phenomenon channels most of the current along the outside of the body (over the skin) rather than through the victim, as occurs in other types of electrical injury. As the current races over the body, it vaporizes moisture on the skin and may destroy clothing in an explosive manner. Burns of unusual patterns may be noted.

1. Linear burns—Linear burns are first- and second-degree burns that begin at the head and neck and course in a branching pattern down the chest and legs. They tend to follow areas with a heavy concentration of sweat.

2. Punctate burns—Punctate burns are clusters of discrete, circular, partial- or full-thickness burns that form starburst patterns on the skin.

3. Feathering burns—Feathering burns are not true burns but rather cutaneous imprints from electron showers that track through the skin. They create a fernlike pattern with delicate branching. These patterns are also called ferning, keraunographic markings, and Lichtenberg flowers or figures.

4. Thermal burns—Thermal burns from clothing or heated metal are typical second- and third-degree burns. Cranial burns (direct or indirect head strike) and leg burns (ground current) are associated with increased death rates.

B. Altered Mental Status

Victims of lightning strikes are usually disoriented, combative, or comatose. Rarely they are alert, but they typically have amnesia for the event.

C. Cardiac Arrest

Cardiac arrest is a result of sudden cardiac standstill induced by the massive DC countershock of the lightning strike. Spontaneous resumption of normal cardiac function is the rule if cardiac standstill is not complicated by simultaneous respiratory arrest (brain-stem shock or contusion). Both asystole and ventricular fibrillation have been associated with lightning strike. Myocardial infarction is a potential acute complication.

D. Neurologic Injuries

Central nervous system injuries include epidural and subdural hematomas (due to associated falls), subarachnoid hemorrhage, coagulation burn injuries of brain, intraventricular hemorrhage, and respiratory paralysis. Seizures, loss of consciousness, and peripheral neurovascular instability are common. Anterograde amnesia and confusion are noted in most patients. Paraplegia and quadriplegia have also been described.

E. Musculoskeletal Injuries

Victims of lightning strikes are frequently thrown to the ground by tetanic muscle contractions, or they may be injured by falls from heights. Fractures of the skull, spine, ribs, and extremities may occur. Intrathoracic and abdominal injuries result from blunt trauma.

F. Eye and Ear Injuries

Eye injuries associated with lightning strikes include cataracts, corneal abrasions, hyphema, uveitis, vitreous hemorrhage, and iridocyclitis. ***Note:*** Dilated pupils should never be the sole criterion for termination of resuscitative efforts, because they may merely reflect transient autonomic sympathetic discharge or parasympathetic inhibition.

Temporary sensorineural hearing loss with or without rupture of the tympanic membrane may result from the loud noise and physical shock wave.

Treatment

A. Maintain the Airway, and Begin Cardiopulmonary Resuscitation

Respiratory arrest is the most common cause of death in persons who have been struck by lightning. Artificial respiration should be continued until spontaneous respiration resumes or the rescuer cannot continue because of exhaustion. Begin closed chest compression if no pulse (carotid or femoral) is present (Chapter 7). Victims struck by lightning and apparently dead have been successfully resuscitated after prolonged efforts.

B. Anticipate Traumatic Injury

Management of the victim of lightning strike is the same as that for a person who has sustained severe blunt trauma. Examine the entire body for evidence of significant skeletal, muscular, or internal injury. Immobilize the spine. Obtain x-rays of the cervical spine and chest, an ECG, and appropriate laboratory tests (urinalysis; complete blood count; blood urea nitrogen and serum electrolyte and creatinine measurements; and CK-MB, lactic dehydrogenase, and aspartate aminotransferase enzyme determinations). If the patient's level of consciousness deteriorates, if focal neurologic signs are present, or if coma is prolonged, obtain a computed tomography (CT) scan of the brain. Fasciotomy of paralyzed or pulseless extremities should be guided by measurement of intracompartmental tissue pressures to avoid unnecessary surgery on limbs that are pulseless and cyanotic as the result of transient sympathetic overactivity with intense vasospasm.

C. Begin Burn Therapy and Fluid Replacement

Management of burn wounds follows standard procedures (Chapter 43). Rhabdomyolysis and myoglobinuria are rarely caused by lightning strike unless severe thermal injury or blunt trauma to muscle has occurred. Administration of intravenous fluids should be adjusted according to blood pressure readings and urine output. Alkalization of the urine and administration of mannitol are not necessary unless myoglobinuria is present. If significant brain injury is present, intracranial and pulmonary artery pressure monitoring may be necessary for proper evaluation of fluid replacement. Tetanus should be updated appropriately (Chapter 30).

Disposition

Prolonged cardiac monitoring and serial cardiac enzymes are required only if the patient has a history of cardiac arrest, loss of consciousness, cardiac arrhythmia, or abnormal ECG or if admission is considered for other reasons (burns, trauma). Screen the urine regularly for evidence of myoglobinuria. Record results of visual acuity and hearing tests to establish a baseline measurement.

If the victim has experienced cardiopulmonary arrest and resuscitation efforts have been successful (resumption of spontaneous cardiac activity), allow a minimum of 12–24 hours before weaning the patient from the ventilator to see if spontaneous respiratory activity resumes. If electroencephalographic abnormalities are present, they may clear over 24–72 hours. Dilated pupils cannot be used as an early diagnostic criterion for brain death.

ELECTRIC SHOCK & BURNS

 ESSENTIALS OF DIAGNOSIS

- *Direct current is less dangerous than alternating current.*
- *Alternating current (most house current) can cause ventricular fibrillation and respiratory arrest.*
- *Burns can result from the electrical current and, although they may look mild, can indicate significant internal damage.*
- *Treatment includes cardiopulmonary resuscitation, wound care, and possibly fasciotomy.*

General Considerations

Electric shock may result from carelessness or ignorance in working with electricity, faulty appliances and equipment, or severed electric power lines, or it may be an accident of nature (lightning). Dry skin offers high resistance to passage of ordinary levels of electric current. However, skin moistened with water, ointment, sweat, saline solution, or urine offers greatly reduced resistance to electric current. The amount and type of current, the duration and area of exposure, and the pathway of the current through the body determine the degree of damage. If current passes through the heart or the brain, death may be rapid.

Direct current is much less dangerous than alternating current (AC) and is generally tolerated at much higher strengths. High-voltage AC current with a high number of cycles per second (hertz, Hz) may be less dangerous than low-voltage current with fewer cycles per second.

Alternating current of 25–300 Hz and 25–200 V, a range that includes house current in most locales, tends to cause ventricular fibrillation if the pathway includes the heart. With voltages over 1000 V, respiratory paralysis often occurs. With intermediate voltages (220–1000 V), a mixed picture of respiratory insufficiency and arrhythmias is noted.

Clinical Findings

A. ELECTRIC SHOCK

Electric shock may produce momentary or prolonged loss of consciousness. Ventricular fibrillation is the most serious immediate arrhythmia, although ectopic beats, sinus tachycardia or bradycardia, atrial fibrillation, and asystole can occur. Respiration may continue for a few minutes after injury or be absent, with immediate respiratory paralysis. When respiratory failure occurs, the patient becomes unconscious. Although a pulse can be felt, the patient is cyanotic and has cool, clammy skin and marked hypotension. Seizures, deafness, blindness, aphasia, and neuropathy can also result from electric shock. Multiple orthopedic injuries may be seen, including posterior shoulder dislocations and femoral neck fractures.

After recovery from mild to moderate electric shock, muscular pain, fatigue, headache, and generalized or focal nervous irritability occur. Physical signs vary according to the sites of action of the current.

B. ELECTRICAL BURNS

There are 3 distinct types of electrical burns: (1) flash (arc) burns, (2) flame burns, and (3) direct burning of the tissues by electric current. Direct burns cause entry wounds that are usually sharply demarcated, round or oval, painless gray areas with a surrounding inflammatory reaction. The exit wounds are more ragged looking, with an "exploded" appearance. Initial examination of the surface wound is often misleading, because the injury may appear relatively innocuous despite extensive deep tissue destruction. Little destruction may be evident for the first 7–10 days; ischemia and sloughing then occur slowly in severely affected areas. The temperature generated in an arc burn from household electric current (110–220 V) may reach 3000 °C (5432 °F).

Common complications include cardiac arrhythmias or cardiac failure, circulatory shock, hemorrhage, and myoglobinuria.

Treatment

A. ELECTRIC SHOCK

Free the victim from the current at once. This may be done in many ways, but the rescuer must be protected. Turn off the power, sever the wire with a dry wooden-handled ax, make a proper ground to divert the current, or drag the victim carefully away using dry clothing, a leather belt, rubber or other dry nonconductive materials.

Check cardiac and ventilatory function. If the patient is apneic or pulseless, begin artificial ventilation or CPR (Chapter 7).

B. ELECTRICAL BURNS

Treat tissue burns conservatively. The direction and extent of tissue injury may not be apparent for 7–10 days. Treat circulatory shock, if present, with intravenous infusion of crystalloid solutions. Locate entrance and exit wounds to help determine the pathway of the current. If current has passed through the chest, obtain an ECG. Serum CK-MB isoenzyme levels may be falsely elevated immediately after high-voltage electrical injuries and should not be considered a reliable indicator of myocardial damage. Monitor cardiac rhythm to detect rhythm disturbances in unconscious victims, those who have presented with cardiac arrhythmias, or those with an abnormal ECG. If myoglobinuria is present, monitor arterial blood pH at regular intervals to detect acidosis, which requires intravenous bicarbonate therapy to alkalize the urine and maintain blood pH above 7.45. Use intravenous mannitol, 2.5 g initially, to promote moderate diuresis.

Assess the need for fasciotomy by measurement of intracompartmental tissue pressures. In children who have bitten electrical cords, be alert for delayed (up to 3 weeks) erosion of the labial artery.

Disposition

Hospitalize all small children and patients who have lost consciousness or experienced cardiac or respiratory arrest, as well as those with ischemic chest pain, myoglobinuria, or significant burn wounds.

Fahmy FS et al: Lightning: the multisystem group injuries. J Trauma 1999;46:937. [PMID: 10338416] (Case presentation of a group lightning injury with description of clinical features.)

Fish RM: Electric injury, part II: specific injuries. J Emerg Med 2000;18:27. [PMID: 10645833] (Review of the diagnostic and treatment considerations for electric injuries.)

Fish RM: Electric injury, part III: cardiac monitoring indications, the pregnant patient, and lightning. J Emerg Med 2000;18:181. [PMID: 10699519] (Review and analysis of publications about cardiac monitoring indications, pregnancy and electric injury, and lightning injury.

Jain S et al: Electrical and lightning injuries. Crit Care Clin 1999;15:319. [PMID: 10331131] (Review of pathophysiology and management of electrical and lightning injuries.)

Lederer W et al: Electricity-associated injuries I: outdoor management of current-induced casualties. J Emerg Med 1999;43:69. [PMID: 10636320] (Review article of epidemiology, clinical manifestations, and resuscitation in electric shock injuries.)

EMERGENCY TREATMENT OF RADIATION INJURIES

RADIATION INJURIES

 ESSENTIALS OF DIAGNOSIS

- *Radiation exposure can cause damage to multiple organ systems.*
- *Organ system damage depends on the dose of radiation delivered.*
- *Treatment is supportive regardless of radiation dose.*

General Considerations

The effects of radiation have been observed in the clinical use of x-rays and radioactive agents, after occupational or accidental exposure, and following the use of atomic weapons. The harm derived depends on the quantity of radiation delivered to the body, the type of radiation (x-rays, neutrons, gamma rays, or alpha or beta particles), the site of exposure, and the duration of exposure.

Tolerance to radiation is difficult to define, and there are no absolute standards for all types and levels of radiation. In the United States, the National Committee on Radiation Protection has set the maximum permissible limits of radiation exposure for occupationally exposed workers over age 18 years at 0.1 rem per week for the whole body (not to exceed 5 rems per

year) and 1.5 rems per week for the hands.[2] (For purposes of comparison, routine chest x-rays deliver 0.1–0.2 rem). If recommended limits are exceeded, radiation injury may occur.

Death after acute lethal radiation exposure is usually due to destruction of hematopoietic organs, gastrointestinal mucosal damage, central nervous system damage, or widespread vascular injury. Vomiting within 1 hour after radiation exposure is often a sign of lethal exposure.

A. 4–6 Gy (400–600 Rads)

Doses of 4–6 Gy (400–600 rads) of x-ray or gamma radiation applied to the entire body at one time will kill more than half of exposed persons within 60 days; death is usually due to hemorrhage, anemia, and infection secondary to injured hematopoietic cells.

B. 10–30 Gy (1000–3000 Rads)

Doses of 10–30 Gy (1000–3000 rads) to the entire body are associated with a death rate of 100%. Destruction of gastrointestinal mucosa and bone marrow leads to death within 2 weeks. Bloody diarrhea begins within 4–5 days and is followed by hemorrhage and sepsis.

C. 30 Gy (3000 Rads) and Above

Doses above 30 Gy (3000 rads) to the entire body cause widespread vascular damage, cerebral anoxia with seizures, ataxia, coma, hypotensive shock, and death within a few days.

Clinical Findings

A. Injury to Skin and Mucous Membranes

Irradiation causes erythema, epilation, destruction of fingernails, or epidermolysis, depending on the dose.

B. Injury to Deep Structures

1. Hematopoietic tissues—Injury to bone marrow may cause a decrease in production of blood elements. Lymphocytes are most sensitive, polymorphonuclear neutrophils next most sensitive, and erythrocytes least sensitive. Damage to blood-forming organs may vary from transient depression of one or more blood elements to pancytopenia. The degree of lymphocyte depression within the first 24–48 hours can be used to estimate the dose received.

2. Cardiovascular system—Pericarditis with effusion or constrictive pericarditis may occur many months after exposure to ionizing radiation. Myocarditis is less common than pericarditis. Smaller vessels (capillaries and arterioles) are more readily damaged than larger blood vessels. If injury is mild, recovery of function occurs.

3. Gonads—In males, small single doses of radiation (2–3 Gy; 200–300 rads) cause transient aspermatogenesis, and larger doses (6–8 Gy; 600–800 rads) may cause sterility. In females, single doses of 2 Gy (200 rads)

[2] In radiation terminology, a rad is the unit of absorbed dose and a rem is the unit of dose of any radiation to body tissue in terms of its estimated biologic effect. The gray (Gy) is a unit of measure for the dose of ionizing radiation equal to 1 J/kg of tissue. One gray is equal to 100 rad.

may produce sterility. Moderate to heavy irradiation of the embryo in utero results in injury to the fetus or causes embryonic death and abortion.

4. Respiratory tract—High or repeated moderate doses of radiation may cause delayed pneumonitis (weeks or months).

5. Mouth, pharynx, esophagus, and stomach—Mucositis with edema and painful swallowing of food may occur within hours to days after exposure to radiation. The salivary glands are relatively radioresistant. Gastric secretion may be temporarily (occasionally permanently) inhibited by moderately high doses of radiation.

6. Intestines—Loss of mucosa with ulceration and inflammation may follow moderately large doses of radiation.

7. Viscera and endocrine glands—Hepatitis and nephritis may be delayed complications of therapeutic irradiation. Normal thyroid, pituitary, pancreas, adrenals, and bladder are relatively resistant to low to moderate doses of radiation.

8. Nervous system—High doses of radiation may damage the brain and spinal cord by impairing their blood supply. Peripheral and autonomic nerves are highly resistant to radiation.

C. SYSTEMIC REACTION (RADIATION SICKNESS)

Symptoms vary with type and amount of exposure. Each phase will be shortened for increasing dosages. The prodromal phase consists of incapacitating vomiting and malaise. An asymptomatic latent phase then follows. A third phase then occurs with dose-dependent symptoms and findings. Bone marrow suppression may occur as early as 24 hours. A gastrointestinal syndrome involving massive fluid losses and bloody diarrhea will begin a few days to a week after exposure to higher doses. The neurovascular syndrome will occur with extremely high doses within a few hours to 1–3 days. This syndrome includes seizures, coma, and eventual death.

Treatment

There is no specific treatment for the biologic effects of ionizing radiation. Safe and effective radioprotective drugs are not available.

A. DECONTAMINATION

Decontamination in most instances will occur prior to arrival at a medical facility. If it does not, simple removal of clothing with placement in marked containers will achieve 90% reduction in contamination. Bare skin and hair should be washed thoroughly and the effluent secured for disposal. Radioactive particles will not cause acute injury to medical personnel and should not interfere with emergency management.

B. LOCAL TREATMENT

The success of treatment of local radiation injury depends on the extent, degree, and location of tissue injury. A victim exposed to more than 0.25–0.5 Gy (25–50 rads) of radioactive iodine should receive potassium iodide, 130 mg (65 mg for children) orally every day for 10 days, to prevent uptake in the thyroid gland. The drug should be given in the first hour after exposure, because it is only 50% effective after a delay of 3 hours.

C. SYSTEMIC TREATMENT

Treatment of the systemic reaction following irradiation is symptomatic and supportive. No truly effective antiemetic is available for the distressing nausea that frequently occurs. Granisetron and ondansetron are the most effective. Massive fluid replacement will be necessary, as will nutrition replacement. Isolation and neutropenic precautions must be implemented. Blood products will be needed, and cytokines may be of benefit. Consider bone marrow transplantation for all victims with exposures exceeding 3 Gy (300 rads). Patients with neurovascular syndrome usually receive expectant treatment.

Disposition

All patients with signs or symptoms of radiation exposure must be hospitalized. Advice may be obtained from the Radiation Emergency Assistance Center/Training Site (REAC/TS) in Oak Ridge, Tennessee ([865] 576-3131). The 24-hour emergency network telephone number is (865) 481-1000.

Armed Forces Radiobiology Research Institute, Military Medical Operations Office: Military Manual of Medical Management of Radiological Casualties. http://www.afrri.usuhs.mil/www/outreach/pdf/radiologicalhandbooksp99-2.pdf

Goans RE: Early dose assessment following severe radiation accidents. Health Phys 1997;72:513. [PMID: 9119674] (Early approximation of radiation exposure to guide initial medical management.)

Goans RE: Early dose assessment in criticality accidents. Health Phys 2001;81:446. [PMID: 11569639] (Early approximation of radiation exposure to guide initial medical management.)

■ EMERGENCY TREATMENT OF NEAR-DROWNING

General Considerations

The asphyxia associated with drowning is usually due to aspiration of fluid, but it may result from airway obstruction caused by laryngeal spasm that occurs while the victim is gasping under water. About 10% of victims develop laryngospasm after the first gulp and never aspirate water ("dry drowning"). The rapid sequence of events after submersion—hypoxemia, laryngospasm, fluid aspiration, ineffective circulation, brain injury, and brain death—may occur within 5–10 minutes. This sequence may be delayed for longer periods if the victim, especially a child, has been submerged in very cold water or if the victim has ingested significant amounts of barbiturates.

The differences in the pathophysiology of aspiration of fresh water (hypotonic) and seawater (hypertonic) usually have little clinical significance in humans, because the amount of fluid aspirated in most patients is small. The primary effect in both instances is disruption of the vascular endothelium and dilution of pulmonary surfactant, with resulting atelectasis and perfusion of poorly ventilated alveoli (large physiologic shunt). Foreign materials such as sand, algae, microorganisms, oil, or chemicals in the aspirated fluid may cause additional pulmonary injury. Fresh water, when absorbed, may produce hemodilution and intravascular hemolysis. Aspiration of large amounts of seawater may result in hypovolemia and hemoconcentration. Clinical features in both types of drowning are similar, and prompt ventilatory management is mandatory.

A number of initial factors may precede near-drowning and may need to be considered in management: (1) use of alcohol or other drugs (a contributing factor in an estimated 25% of adult drownings), (2) extreme fatigue, (3) intentional hyperventilation just prior to diving or swimming under water ("shallow water blackout"), (4) sudden acute illness (eg, epilepsy, myocardial infarction), (5) head or spinal cord injury sustained in diving or surfing accidents, (6) venomous stings by aquatic animals, and (7) decompression illness or air embolism associated with scuba diving.

Hypoxemia, acidosis, and hypoperfusion of vital organs are common factors accounting for the high incidence of illness and death associated with drowning. Other problems include variations in vascular volume, cardiac failure, renal insufficiency, electrolyte abnormalities, hematologic disturbances, and infection.

Clinical Findings

The victim of near-drowning may present with a wide range of clinical manifestations. Spontaneous return of consciousness often occurs in otherwise healthy individuals when submersion is brief. Other patients respond promptly to immediate artificial ventilation. Vomiting is common. Patients with more severe near-drowning may experience frank pulmonary failure, pul-

monary edema, shock, anoxic encephalopathy, cerebral edema, or cardiac arrest. A few patients may be deceptively asymptomatic during the recovery period, only to deteriorate as a result of acute respiratory failure in the ensuing 6–24 hours.

A. SYMPTOMS AND SIGNS

The patient may be unconscious, semiconscious, or awake and apprehensive. Cyanosis, trismus, apnea, tachypnea, and wheezing may be present. A pink froth from the mouth and nose indicates pulmonary edema. Cardiovascular manifestations may include tachycardia, arrhythmias, hypotension, shock, and cardiac arrest.

B. LABORATORY FINDINGS

Urinalysis may show proteinuria, hemoglobinuria, and ketonuria. The white blood cell count is elevated because of leukocyte demargination induced by stress. The P_{O_2} is usually decreased and the P_{CO_2} increased or decreased. Metabolic acidosis is always present.

C. X-RAY FINDINGS

Chest x-rays may show pneumonitis or pulmonary edema. Preliminary x-rays may appear normal in patients with mild symptoms.

Treatment

Begin resuscitation immediately. Do not waste time attempting to drain water from the victim's lungs or stomach. (If, however, a tense, water-filled stomach prevents adequate lung expansion, place the victim supine, perform the Heimlich maneuver [Chapter 7], clear the victim's mouth with a finger sweep, and resume artificial ventilation.) Place the patient in a slightly head-down position (15 degrees) to allow fluid to drain from the mouth.

A. OPEN AIRWAY AND MAINTAIN VENTILATION

Open the airway, and ventilate the patient. If the victim is not breathing, clear the mouth and pharynx with the finger, open the victim's airway, and institute immediate mouth-to-mouth or mouth-to-nose breathing. Give oxygen in high concentrations by continuous positive airway pressure.

Perform endotracheal intubation for assisted ventilation as soon as possible, and begin positive end-expiratory pressure breathing. Consider the possibility of cervical spine injury, particularly in a diving or surfing accident.

B. ESTABLISH CIRCULATION

Check for a carotid or femoral pulse. If a pulse cannot be detected, start CPR without delay (Chapter 7). External chest compression cannot be performed effectively in the water; therefore, bring the victim ashore or out of the water as quickly as possible in order to attempt resuscitation. In the hospital setting, monitor the effectiveness of CPR with arterial blood gas measurements.

C. Treat Hypothermia

Measure the patient's core temperature and treat systemic hypothermia. Hypothermia improves the chances for survival. If the patient is in full cardiac arrest (ventricular fibrillation or pulseless ventricular tachycardia, asystole, or mechanical dissociation), use core rewarming techniques (see Systemic Hypothermia, above) to attain a core temperature of 33–35 °C (91.4–95 °F) before discontinuing CPR. If the patient shows signs of life (spontaneous respirations, detectable pulse), core rewarming techniques may not be necessary. Complete recovery has been reported after prolonged resuscitative efforts, even when victims have had dilated, fixed pupils. This is particularly true of infants and children, in whom the brain is protected by hypothermia. Studies have also shown that children involved in warm water near-drowning with initial signs and symptoms that portend a bad outcome can ultimately have a near or total recovery. Therefore, aggressive resuscitation efforts should be attempted after warm water incidents as well.

Disposition

Near-drowning victims who are initially asymptomatic must be monitored for "secondary drowning" or respiratory distress that develops later. Studies have shown that signs and symptoms of secondary drowning occur within 6–8 hours. If the patient has a normal physical examination and respiratory effort, a Glasgow Coma Scale score of 13 or greater, and a room air oxygen saturation of 95% or greater on presentation, he or she may be safely discharged home after 6–8 hours.

Causey AL: Predicting discharge in uncomplicated near-drowning. Am J Emerg Med 2000;18:9. [PMID: 10674523] (Retrospective cohort study to determine if routine, noninvasive parameters could be used to predict early discharge.)

Spack L: Failure of aggressive therapy to alter outcome in pediatric near-drowning. Pediatr Emerg Care 1997;13:98. [PMID: 9127416] (Retrospective chart analysis of pediatric drowning victims and their outcome.)

Zuckerman GB: Predictors of death and neurologic impairment in pediatric submersion injuries. The pediatric risk of mortality score. Arch Pediatr Adolesc Med 1998;152:134. [PMID: 9491038] (Retrospective chart review of pediatric drowning victims and their outcome.)

■ EMERGENCY TREATMENT OF DISORDERS DUE TO ATMOSPHERIC PRESSURE CHANGES

DECOMPRESSION SICKNESS (Caisson Disease, "Bends")

 ESSENTIALS OF DIAGNOSIS

- Caused by release of nitrogen bubbles from plasma and tissues during ascent.
- Type 1: joint pain; Type 2: cardiorespiratory or neurologic involvement.
- Treatment is immediate recompression in a hyperbaric chamber.

General Considerations

Decompression sickness has long been recognized as an occupational hazard for professional divers. In recent years, the popular sport of scuba diving has exposed a large number of variably trained individuals to the hazards of decompression sickness.

Divers using conventional diving gear (scuba; self-contained underwater breathing apparatus) breathe air or other oxygen-containing gas mixtures that are at the same pressure as that of the surrounding water. Water pressure increases by 1 atmosphere for every 10 m (33 ft) below the surface. The increased pressure increases the amount of gas dissolved in plasma and tissues. During ascent, as external pressure decreases, the dissolved gases (predominantly nitrogen) escape from tissues as gas bubbles. A similar disorder occurs in persons who rapidly ascend to altitudes above 2000 m (6600 ft) in unpressurized aircraft. The size and number of gas bubbles escaping from the tissues are functions of the depth and duration of the dive, the degree of physical exertion (exercise increases the amount of dissolved nitrogen), and the speed of ascent. The quantity and site of release of nitrogen bubbles determines the symptoms.

Clinical Findings

Symptoms begin to appear within 6 hours but may be delayed up to 24 hours. The clinical picture varies and can be divided into 2 types of decompression sickness. Type 1, or the minor symptom complex, includes deep, aching pain in the large joints of the extremities. This has been termed the bends. Type 2 involves any cardiorespiratory or focal neurologic symptoms. Neurologic symptoms include ataxia, paralysis, vertigo, visual or speech disturbance, and cognitive deficits. A propensity for the spinal cord seems to be prevalent in many cases. Chest pain and shortness of breath occur with involvement of pulmonary artery circulation.

Treatment

A. EARLY MEASURES

Give oxygen, 6–10 L/min, by mask. Give mild analgesics as needed. In the absence of congestive heart failure, give intravenous fluids (5% dextrose in normal saline or lactated Ringer's injection) to correct dehydration and maintain normal hydration.

B. RECOMPRESSION

Immediate recompression is the only effective treatment. Rapid transport to a treatment facility for immediate recompression is necessary not only to relieve symptoms but also to prevent permanent impairment. Persistent symptoms may be treated successfully with hyperbaric oxygen up to 7 days after the onset of serious decompression sickness. All emergency department physicians should know the location of the nearest hyperbaric chamber. The local public health department or nearest naval facility may be able to provide such information. In the United States, clinical advice may be obtained rapidly by telephoning the National Diving Alert Network (DAN) at Duke University ([919] 684-8111, or [919] 684-4326 after hours). A patient who is transported to a hyperbaric chamber by aircraft must not be exposed to a cabin altitude higher than 300 m (1000 ft).

C. COMPLICATIONS

Further measures may be necessary to relieve some of the complications associated with the bends (eg, shock, spinal cord injury, bladder paralysis, hemoconcentration, and disseminated intravascular coagulation).

Disposition

Transport the patient immediately to the nearest recompression center (hyperbaric chamber) for evaluation and treatment. ***Caution:*** Never attempt recompression in the water.

ARTERIAL GAS EMBOLISM

 ESSENTIALS OF DIAGNOSIS

- *Increased pressure in the lungs causing air to escape from alveoli.*
- *Results in air in the interstitial space or in the pulmonary venous circulation.*
- *Can result in pneumothorax or occlusion of the coronary or cerebrovascular systems.*
- *Treatment is immediate recompression in a hyperbaric chamber.*

General Considerations

Diving regulators maintain the pressure of the gas being breathed and thereby enable the diver to descend and maintain lung expansion against the pressure of the surrounding water. Because of the pressure-volume relationship (Boyle's law: $P_1V_1 - P_2V_2$), greater volume changes for a given change in depth occur near the surface than at a greater depth.

If the breath is held on ascent (by closure of the glottis) or if air is trapped in the lung by bronchospasm during ascent, the volume of gas in the lung expands. When a pressure differential of about 80 mm Hg is reached, air will be forced from the alveoli through the pulmonary alveolocapillary membrane. The result will be air in the interstitial space (creating pneumothorax or mediastinal emphysema) or formation of bubbles in the pulmonary venous circulation. These bubbles travel through the left side of the heart into the systemic arterial circulation, where they may be trapped in smaller arteries and cause coronary artery or cerebrovascular occlusion. Larger bubbles may occlude the large vessels of the central circulation and become lodged in the heart, causing complete circulatory collapse. One study has found that this process may be the cause of death in most fatal cases of arterial gas embolism.

Clinical Findings

A. ARTERIAL EMBOLISM

Patients usually present with dramatic symptoms. If the symptoms occur more than 10 minutes after the diver has surfaced, they are not due to air embolism. Many victims of arterial gas embolism die immediately upon surfacing.

If air bubbles enter the cerebral circulation, the victim becomes unconscious or has a seizure during ascent or immediately upon surfacing. Other symptoms include blindness, confusion, or an apparent acute stroke.

If the bubbles have entered the coronary arteries, the person presents with symptoms similar to those of acute myocardial infarction, with chest pain, arrhythmias, and collapse. Complete, sudden circulatory collapse occurs with occlusion of the central circulation.

B. PNEUMOTHORAX

Signs of pneumothorax or mediastinal emphysema develop more slowly and are not as life threatening; signs include shortness of breath, hyperresonance of the chest to percussion and decreased breath sounds on the affected side, and subcutaneous crepitus that may extend into the neck.

Treatment

A. EARLY MEASURES

Give oxygen, 6–10 L/min, by mask. Position the victim head down (15–30 degrees) on the left side in the Trendelenburg position. Give 5% dextrose in normal saline or lactated Ringer's injection intravenously to maintain urine output at 1–2 mL/kg/h.

B. RECOMPRESSION

Immediate recompression is the only effective treatment; the patient should be transported to a hyperbaric chamber immediately (see Decompression Sickness, above).

Disposition

Transport the patient immediately to the nearest recompression center (hyperbaric chamber) for evaluation and treatment. ***Caution:*** Never attempt recompression in the water.

Certain anatomic risk factors predispose divers to pulmonary barotrauma. A history of obstructive lung disease or an anatomic abnormality such as lung cysts may increase the likelihood of pulmonary barotrauma. A helical (spiral) CT scan of the chest may help assess future fitness to dive in survivors of pulmonary barotrauma by revealing previously undiagnosed lung pathology.

HIGH-ALTITUDE SICKNESS (Mountain Sickness)

General Considerations

Rapid means of modern transportation have increased the number of unacclimatized people who are exposed to the effects of high altitude. Lack of sufficient time for acclimatization, increased physical activity, and varying degrees of ill health may be responsible for the acute and chronic disturbances that result from hypoxemia at altitudes greater than 2000 m (6600 ft). Marked individual differences in tolerance to hypoxemia exist. Acclimatization involves a variety of changes that affect the respiratory, circulatory, hematopoietic, renal, and pulmonary systems.

1. Acute Mountain Sickness

 ESSENTIALS OF DIAGNOSIS

- Flulike symptoms due to lack of acclimatization to higher altitudes.
- Treatment is descent, oxygen, and antiemetics.
- If descent is not possible, dexamethasone or acetazolamide can be used to aid acclimatization.

Clinical Findings

Symptoms and signs include headache (the most common and usually the most prominent symptom), lassitude, difficulty in concentrating, sleep disturbances, drowsiness, dizziness, insomnia, anorexia, nausea and vomiting, dyspnea on exertion, and palpitations.

Symptoms are often worse on the second and third day after ascent but usually clear completely within 5–7 days. Serious illness is rare; deaths from mountain sickness do not occur, by definition.

Treatment

The most effective treatments are descent to lower altitude and administration of oxygen. Headache responds to analgesics. Use narcotics judiciously to avoid distorting sleep patterns or masking signs of altered mental status, which accompany impending high-altitude encephalopathy. Antiemetics are indicated for nausea and vomiting. By decreasing periodic breathing, acetazolamide has been useful in treating insomnia. Studies show that severe or rapidly progressive mountain sickness may respond favorably to dexamethasone, 4–6 mg orally every 6 hours, until signs of improvement occur; the dose is then tapered over 3–5 days.

Prevention

Preventive measures include gradual ascent, adequate rest, avoidance of alcohol and tobacco, and avoidance of strenuous exercise until acclimatization has been achieved. Acetazolamide, 125 mg twice a day before and during ascent, is the preferred drug for prophylaxis; dexamethasone is an alternative. Studies have also found Ginkgo biloba to reduce acute mountain sickness dramatically in both gradual and rapid ascent.

Disposition

If symptoms persist, returning to lower altitude is curative.

2. Acute High-Altitude Pulmonary Edema

ESSENTIALS OF DIAGNOSIS

- Pulmonary edema due to rapid ascent to altitudes above 2400 m (8000 ft).
- Cough and dyspnea on exertion lead to pink, frothy sputum and dyspnea at rest.
- Chest x-ray findings show patchy infiltrates but normal heart size.
- Treatment is rapid descent, continuous positive-pressure ventilation, oxygen, and nifedipine.

Clinical Findings

Acute high-altitude pulmonary edema is a serious disorder usually occurring at levels above 2400 m (8000 ft). High-altitude pulmonary edema is associated with exercise and rapid ascent and is commonly noted in young, previously healthy individuals who have not become properly acclimatized. Known risk factors for development of high-altitude pulmonary edema are previous episodes of the disease, congenital absence of one pulmonary artery, and brief sojourn at low altitude by persons acclimatized to living at high altitudes.

A. SYMPTOMS AND SIGNS

Early symptoms of high-altitude pulmonary edema generally appear on the second night at a new altitude. Early symptoms include dry cough and dyspnea on exertion. As illness progresses, cough productive of pink, frothy sputum occurs as does dyspnea at rest. Orthopnea is uncommon. Extreme weakness and drowsiness ensue.

Physical signs include tachycardia, tachypnea, cyanosis, rales, rhonchi, and confusion that progresses to coma. Tachycardia begins with exertion and progresses to tachycardia at rest. Rales most often originate in the right axilla and become bilateral as illness progresses.

Death may occur in untreated high-altitude pulmonary edema.

B. LABORATORY FINDINGS

The white blood cell count and hematocrit are often slightly elevated. The erythrocyte sedimentation rate is usually normal. Fluid collected by bronchoalveolar lavage shows high protein and cellular content associated with the high-permeability vascular leak due to hypoxia and increased pulmonary vascular pressures.

C. X-RAY FINDINGS

Findings on chest x-ray are variable. In mild disease, patchy infiltrates in a solitary lung field (commonly the right middle lobe) are noted. The infiltrates rarely coalesce and generally do not involve the base of the lungs. The central pulmonary arteries are dilated, but the cardiac shadow is of normal size. In severe illness, infiltrates are more generalized, but no left atrial enlargement or Kerley lines are noted. Unilateral pulmonary edema is consistent with unilateral atresia of the pulmonary artery.

D. ELECTROCARDIOGRAPHIC FINDINGS

Transient, nonspecific electrocardiographic changes such as tachycardia, right axis deviation, right ventricular strain, and occasional right bundle branch block can occur.

Treatment

Early recognition of the disease is crucial. Persistent dry cough and dyspnea in a person who has recently arrived at high altitude should be considered high-altitude pulmonary edema until proved otherwise.

A. REST

Limit the patient's physical activity as much as possible. The sitting or semi-Fowler position is usually the most comfortable.

B. OXYGEN

Give oxygen, 4–6 L/min, by mask; otherwise, deliver the maximum amount possible with the equipment at hand.

C. CONTINUOUS POSITIVE-PRESSURE VENTILATION

Application of continuous positive pressure during spontaneous ventilation (which can be achieved with a portable apparatus) relieves symptoms and improves oxygenation in patients with high-altitude pulmonary edema and is a useful temporizing measure during descent. Portable hyperbaric chambers, or Gamow Bags, are also helpful if descent is impossible.

D. Descent

Development of high-altitude pulmonary edema is an automatic indication for descent to lower altitude as quickly as possible (a descent of 500–1000 m [1650–3300 ft] is usually sufficient), although it is best to descend below an altitude of 1500 m [5000 ft]). Supplemental oxygen and descent to a lower altitude should bring about marked improvement within 12–72 hours.

E. Drugs

Acetazolamide, 250 mg every 6 hours, has been used, but its usefulness is still debated in acute illness. Nifedipine, 10 mg orally initially and then 30 mg of extended-release preparation every 12–24 hours, has been shown to be beneficial by lowering pulmonary artery pressures.

Prevention

Preventive measures include (1) education of prospective mountaineers about the possibility of serious pulmonary edema, (2) gradual ascent to permit acclimatization, and (3) rest and avoidance of strenuous exercise for 1–2 days after arrival at high altitudes. Medical attention should be sought promptly if respiratory symptoms develop.

Patients with a history of high-altitude pulmonary edema have a 60% chance of the illness recurring with repeat ascents. Prophylaxis with nifedipine, 20–30 mg of the extended release form every 12–24 hours, is helpful.

Mountaineering parties climbing at 2400 m (8000 ft) or higher should carry a supply of oxygen and equipment sufficient for several days if hospital facilities are not available.

People with symptomatic cardiac or pulmonary disease should avoid high altitudes. Detection of a heart murmur and recurrent episodes of high-altitude pulmonary edema should prompt investigation for a previously existing valvular, shunt, or pulmonary hypertension problem.

Disposition

Hospitalization is generally recommended if symptoms persist for more than a few hours after return to lower altitudes.

3. High-Altitude Cerebral Edema

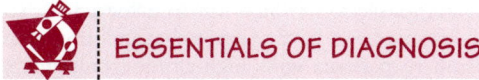

ESSENTIALS OF DIAGNOSIS

- *Cerebral edema due to rapid ascent to altitudes above 2400 m (8000 ft).*

- *Signs and symptoms include headache, ataxia, papilledema, and global encephalopathy.*

- *Treatment is immediate descent, oxygen, and dexamethasone.*

Clinical Findings

Acute high-altitude cerebral edema, a syndrome related to hypoxemia, occurs at elevations above 2400 m (8000 ft). Like its counterpart high-altitude pulmonary edema, it is more common in unacclimatized individuals and is the end-stage form of acute mountain sickness. Death occurs from brain-stem herniation.

Early symptoms include severe headache, ataxia, confusion, incoordination, and drunken behavior. Ataxia is usually the first sign of advancement to high-altitude cerebral edema in someone with acute mountain sickness. The physical examination may reveal papilledema, retinal hemorrhages, and occasionally a cranial nerve palsy. Patients with high-altitude cerebral edema typically present with global encephalopathy. Focal neurologic deficits are present only in the most severe forms of high-altitude cerebral edema and should prompt investigation into other causes of headache and mental status changes. Seizures are uncommon. Because high-altitude pulmonary edema commonly accompanies high-altitude cerebral edema, the patient may be lethargic and short of breath and may demonstrate tachycardia.

Treatment

It is crucial to recognize early manifestations. Because the symptoms of early high-altitude cerebral edema are similar to those of acute mountain sickness, anyone with headache and fatigue at high altitude must be watched closely for signs of deterioration. Inability to walk a straight line is a fairly sensitive test for incipient high-altitude cerebral edema.

A. Oxygen

Give oxygen, 6–10 L/min, by mask, or give 100% oxygen if possible. Keep the patient in a sitting position, with the head elevated.

B. Descent

Development of high-altitude cerebral edema is an automatic indication for descent to lower altitude as quickly as possible (a descent of 500–1000 m [1650–3300 ft] is usually sufficient, although it is best to descend below an altitude of 1500 m [5000 ft]). Dexamethasone, 8 mg orally or intramuscularly initially followed by 4–6 mg orally every 6 hours, is recommended. Nifedipine for high-altitude pulmonary edema is contraindicated in patients with concomitant severe high-altitude cerebral edema.

Disposition

Hospitalization is generally recommended if symptoms persist for more than a few hours after return to lower altitudes.

Cheshire WP Jr et al: Headache in divers. Headache 2001;41:235. [PMID: 11264683] (Review of decompression illness.)

Erdmann J: Effects of exposure to altitude on men with coronary artery disease and impaired left ventricular function. Am J Cardiol 1998;81:266. [PMID: 9468065] (Prospective study evaluating the effect of exposure to high altitude in men with coronary artery disease.)

Hackett PH et al: High altitude illness. N Engl J Med 2001;345:107. [PMID: 11450659] (Review of acute mountain sickness, high-altitude pulmonary edema, and high-altitude cerebral edema.)

Levine BD et al: Effect of high-altitude exposure in the elderly: the Tenth Mountain Division Study. Circulation 1997;96:1224. [PMID: 9286953] (Prospective study to evaluate the impact of high altitude on elderly patients.)

Neuman TS: Arterial gas embolism and decompression sickness. News Physiol Sci 2002;17:77. [PMID: 11909997]

Neuman TS et al: Fatal pulmonary barotrauma due to obstruction of the central circulation with air. J Emerg Med 1998;16:413. [PMID: 9610969] (Case studies of patients with severe barotrauma and discussion of the treatment.)

Reuter M et al: Computer tomography of the chest in diving-related pulmonary barotraumas. Br J Radiol 1997;70:440. [PMID: 9227223] (Retrospective chart analysis of patients diagnosed with pulmonary barotrauma who underwent a CT scan of the chest.)

Tetzlaff K et al: Risk factors for pulmonary barotrauma in divers. Chest 1997;112:654. [PMID: 9315797] (Retrospective chart analysis of patients with pulmonary barotrauma to determine potential risk factors for the development of barotraumas.)

Yarnell PR et al: High-altitude cerebral edema (HACE): the Denver/Front Range experience. Semin Neurol 2000;20:209. [PMID: 10946741] (Retrospective case analysis and discussion of patients with high-altitude illness.)

■ EMERGENCY TREATMENT OF DISORDERS DUE TO VENOMOUS ANIMALS

SNAKE BITES

ESSENTIALS OF DIAGNOSIS

- *Venomous bites can result from either pit vipers or elapids.*

- *Pit viper envenomation results in symptoms related to cytolysis, whereas elapid bites can result in neurotoxic symptoms.*

- *Antivenin is available for both pit viper and elapid bites and should be administered for symptomatic envenomations.*

General Considerations

Snakes bite at least 50,000 humans each year in the United States. Most snake bites are from nonpoisonous snakes. There are 2 main types of poisonous snakes: crotalids, or pit vipers (rattlesnakes, cottonmouths [water moccasins]), and elapids (coral snakes, cobras). Among venomous bites in the United States, 95% are from pit vipers (mostly rattlesnakes). Envenomation occurs in only 15–20% of venomous bites.

Snake venom is a complex mixture of proteolytic enzymes and toxic proteins. In general, crotalid venom is mainly cytolytic, whereas elapid venom is mainly neurotoxic. Cytolytic venom lyses cells; enhances local spread of venom; and causes hemolysis, increased capillary permeability, and altered hemostasis. Neurotoxic venom can disrupt neuromuscular activity, causing paresthesias, weakness, and respiratory paralysis.

Clinical Findings

Identify the snake if at all possible. Pit vipers have large triangular heads with pits between the eyes and the nose. Coral snakes have black and red circumferential bands separated by narrower yellow bands ("red on yellow, kill a fellow; red on black, venom lack"). If the identity of a snake is not obvious, obtain help from a herpetologist or a poison control center.

Collect the snake, if possible, for positive identification; take care to avoid being bitten. Remember that the head of a decapitated snake may exhibit reflex actions for as long as 1 hour after it has been severed from the body. The predominantly cytolytic venom of crotalids can cause edema, hemorrhage, and necrosis around the bite site as well as distant from the site in severe envenomations. Systemic signs and symptoms consist of hemolysis, thrombocytopenia, disseminated intravascular coagulopathy, vomiting, and, rarely, respiratory failure with cardiovascular instability or collapse.

The predominantly neurotoxic venom of elapids and the Mojave green rattlesnake may produce few or no early local signs of envenomation, but neurologic symptoms (paresthesias, blurred vision, dysphagia, hypersalivation, ptosis, and respiratory depression) may appear after a delay of 2–6 hours.

Treatment

A. EMERGENCY FIRST-AID MEASURES

Many of the most well-known first-aid measures are no longer recommended. Cryotherapy, tourniquets, and incision and suction have not been shown to be helpful and in many cases cause more harm. The best management is to transport the patient to the nearest hospital. Immobilize the bitten part as if it were a fracture, and hold it below the level of the heart. Keep the patient on strict bed rest, if possible. If the patient has a severe envenomation with progression of symptoms, emergency medical service providers may place a constriction band over the site of the bite. A constriction band is a broad, flat band exerting 20 mm Hg of pressure that still permits 1–2 fingers under the band. However, if the patient is stable, application of a constriction band is not recommended, even if transport time is long. If a constriction band or suction device has been placed prior to the arrival of emergency medical services, it should be left in place for transport. Suction devices have been shown to cause injury themselves, however, and can be removed if no liquid is being extracted.

B. HOSPITAL MEASURES

Assess the patient's respiratory and cardiovascular status. Determine if airway management or cardiovascular resuscitation with crystalloid or vasopressors is needed.

Obtain intravenous access. Assess bite site for local progression. Determine species of snake if possible. Check complete blood count, electrolytes, coagulation profile, and urine myoglobin. Type and cross-match blood.

Antivenin is warranted if abnormalities are found in any of the above measures. Crotalidae polyvalent immune Fab, also known as CroFab or FabAV, has been approved by the U.S. Food and Drug Administration (FDA) and should be used as needed (Table 44–1). Antivenin must be reconstituted and then administered slowly intravenously for 10 minutes. If no signs or symptoms of anaphylaxis occur, then the infusion rate may be increased to be complete in 1 hour. No reports of anaphylaxis have occurred thus far with the use of FabAV, but vigilant monitoring must continue throughout infusion. For coral snake (Eastern or Texas variety) bites, give 3–6 vials of Eastern coral snake antivenin. Coral snake antivenin is not effective against the bites of the Arizona or Sonoran coral snake.

Tetanus should be updated and antibiotics administered in severe bites.

Surgical management of a snake bite is not needed in the acute phase unless evidence of compartment syndrome is present. Many of the signs and symptoms of compartment syndrome are present with snake bite, but it is extremely rare for intracompartmental pressures to be elevated. Fasciotomy should be reserved for patients with elevated pressure measurements. Delayed debridement of necrotic tissue may ultimately be necessary.

Disposition

Place patients requiring antivenin in the intensive care unit for monitoring. Asymptomatic patients with no local progression and normal laboratory values may be discharged after 8 hours with close wound follow-up.

Boyer LV: Recurrence phenomena after immunoglobin therapy for snake envenomations: part 2. Guidelines for clinical management with crotaline Fab antivenom. Ann Emerg Med 2001;37:196. [PMID: 11174239] (Review of the use of crotaline Fab antivenom at the time of presentation and with symptom recurrence.)

Bush SP: Immediate removal of extractor is recommended. Ann Emerg Med 2001;38:607. [PMID: 11679882] (Comment on the use of the extractor in snake bites and its complications.)

Dart RC: Efficacy, safety, and use of snake antivenoms in the United States. Ann Emerg Med 2001;37:181. [PMID: 11174237] (Review of the use of Crotalidae and CroFab in snake envenomation.)

Hall EL: Role of surgical intervention in the management of crotaline snake envenomation. Ann Emerg Med 2001;37:175. [PMID: 11174236] (Review of surgical techniques in the treatment of snake bites.)

Table 44–1. Indications and dosages of Crotalidae Polyvalent Immune Fab (FabAV).

Symptoms	Dosing	Goal
None	No FabAV required.	
Local progression, systemic symptoms, or clinically significant coagulopathy	The patient should be given enough vials to achieve the goal. This generally ranges from 3 to 12 vials, although up to 25 vials have been used.	Achieve control of local progression, resolution of systemic symptoms, or reversal of the coagulopathy.
Stabilization of signs and symptoms and no progression of signs and symptoms after FabAV given.	Administer 2 vials at 6, 12, and 18 hours.	Prevent recurrence.

McKinney PE: Out-of-hospital and interhospital management of crotaline snakebite. Ann Emerg Med 2001;37:168. [PMID: 11174235] (Review of out-of-hospital management including constriction bands in the treatment of snake bites.)

Seifert SA: Recurrence phenomena after immunoglobulin therapy for snake envenomations: part I. Pharmacokinetics and pharmacodynamics of immunoglobulin antivenoms and related antibodies. Ann Emerg Med 2001;37:198. [PMID: 11174238] (Review of the use of antivenins and the recurrence of symptoms after their use.)

BEES & WASP STINGS

 ESSENTIALS OF DIAGNOSIS

- *Most people who experience a Hymenoptera envenomation have only a painful and urticarial lesion at the site of the sting; more severe reactions can occur and result in anaphylaxis and multiorgan dysfunction.*
- *Oral pain control, tetanus prophylaxis, and diphenhydramine are generally the only treatment needed. In severe reactions, airway management, vasopressors, and even dialysis may be needed.*

General Considerations

Bees, wasps, and ants are members of the order Hymenoptera. In the United States, domesticated honey bees, feral bumblebees, paper wasps, yellow jackets, and fire ants are the most common attackers, although the aggressive, swarming Africanized bees have been present in the United States since the early 1990s. These insects inject venom through a stinger connected to a venom reservoir supplied by venom glands. The venom causes hemolysis and destruction of platelets and leukocytes. It is also capable of destroying vascular endothelium and necrosing skeletal muscle.

Clinical Findings

Patients with Hymenoptera envenomation can present with a wide array of signs and symptoms. The most common effect of a sting is a small pruritic and urticarial-type lesion that also causes pain. Ten percent of people have a large local reaction greater than 5 cm in diameter. These reactions may last longer than the smaller lesions. Less than 1% of patients experience a systemic reaction. Some have a milder reaction with only nausea, vomiting, and diarrhea as well as pruritic urticarial lesions distant from the sting site. Rarely a victim will experience anaphylaxis. Persons who experience multiple stings or who are taking β-adrenergic blocking drugs may experience more severe reactions. Immediate and delayed toxic reactions may occur with envenomation by 50 or more stings. These reactions include hemolysis and rhabdomyolysis with subsequent renal failure, thrombocytopenia, disseminated intravascular coagulopathy, and liver dysfunction.

Treatment

Remove stings or fragments by scraping, not with forceps. Apply topical ice packs. Oral pain control, diphenhydramine, and tetanus prophylaxis are usually all that is necessary for small or large local reaction. Mild systemic reactions may require intravenous diphenhydramine as well as intravenous corticosteroids and a short period of monitoring to allow early intervention for progression to anaphylaxis. Anaphylaxis requires intubation, intravenous access, aggressive fluid resuscitation, aerosolized β-agonists for bronchospasm, subcutaneous or intravenous epinephrine, and possibly pressor agents. Toxic reactions will require the above measures with possible blood products, dialysis, and extensive hospital care.

Disposition

Patients with local reactions may be discharged home. Patients with severe systemic reactions require admission. The Phoenix Poison Control Center recommends mandatory 24-hour admission for children, the elderly, and patients with underlying medical problems or if 50 or more stings are sustained. Otherwise, young healthy individuals with massive envenomation require 6 hours of monitoring with initial and discharge laboratory evaluations of renal and liver function, coagulation studies, and red blood cell count; if no abnormalities are found, patients may be discharged to home. Studies of sensitized individuals have found that the vast majority never experience escalating symptoms with future stings; many have less severe reactions. Victims with less severe systemic reactions should undergo immunotherapy and carry an emergency epinephrine pen.

BLACK WIDOW SPIDER BITES

 ESSENTIALS OF DIAGNOSIS

- *Symptoms of envenomation include severe pain in the bitten extremity and muscle spasms of the abdomen and trunk.*
- *Abdominal muscle spasms can mimic a surgical abdomen.*

- *Severe hypertension and tachycardia can occur.*
- *Treatment includes narcotic analgesics, intravenous calcium gluconate, and antivenin in the seriously ill.*

Clinical Findings

The female black widow spider (Latrodectus mactans) is shiny black, with a red hourglass marking on its abdomen. Only the female is dangerous. This spider is common in California and other parts of the United States. Other Latrodectus species may be found in other countries. The venom is a neurotoxin that acts on the myoneural junction.

The bite itself is minor and often unnoticed at first. Characteristic symptoms of envenomation occur within 10–60 minutes, including severe pain in the bitten extremity and muscle spasms of the abdomen and trunk. Diffuse paresthesias are noted as well as muscle fasciculation, piloerection, and diaphoresis. Headache, nausea and vomiting, hyperactive deep tendon reflexes, and ptosis may be noted. Victims are in agonizing pain; the rigidity of abdominal muscles may mimic a surgical emergency. Severe hypertension and tachycardia may occur. Deaths are rare; at greatest risk are small infants or older patients with preexisting cardiovascular disease. Symptoms peak at 2–3 hours after the bite and may last up to 24 hours.

Treatment

Most patients respond to narcotic analgesics. Calcium gluconate, 0.1–0.2 mL/kg slowly intravenously, is often effective in alleviating muscle spasm. Methocarbamol, 1 g intravenously, infused at a rate no faster than 100 mg/min, is less effective. Local applications of ice should be used judiciously. Antivenin should be reserved for use in seriously ill infants and older patients and should be preceded by horse serum sensitivity testing. One vial of antivenin is sufficient for most patients; give 1 ampule (2.5 mL) in 10–50 mL of normal saline by slow intravenous infusion.

Disposition

All patients who have been bitten by a black widow spider should be observed for 12–24 hours, because hypertension and muscle spasm commonly recur. Hospitalization is necessary for all patients under age 14 years, those older than age 65 years, those with a history of hypertension, and those who present with severe symptoms.

BROWN RECLUSE SPIDER BITES

 ESSENTIALS OF DIAGNOSIS

- *The venom of the brown recluse spider is cytotoxic and causes local tissue destruction.*
- *The bite progresses from an initial pustule to a bull's eye–like lesion to a larger craterlike ulcer (severe cases).*
- *Most bites require only tetanus prophylaxis and local wound care; more symptomatic patients may require more aggressive wound care including dapsone, antivenin, and excision.*

Clinical Findings

The brown recluse spider (*Loxosceles reclusa;* other *Loxosceles* spp.) has a dark, violin-shaped area on its back. It is found in old wood piles, attics, closets, and clothes piles and prefers dark, undisturbed places. The venom, which contains sphingomyelinase D, is chiefly cytotoxic, causing local tissue destruction by destroying endothelial cells; it also has a hemolytic component, which on rare occasions may cause massive hemolysis. The enzyme may also disrupt nerve impulses, thus causing skin anesthesia at the bite site.

The bite initially seems mild and often goes unnoticed. Pain at the site begins 1–4 hours later, and an erythematous area with a central pustule or hemorrhagic vesicle may be seen. The typical bull's-eye lesion is created when the red blister is encircled by a pale, irregularly shaped and ischemic halo, which in turn is surrounded by extravasated blood. The pustule may gradually grow to form a craterlike lesion over 3–4 days, with associated lymphadenopathy and low-grade fever. Healing is slow, and large lesions may occasionally require skin grafting. Rarely, ulcerating skin lesions may appear years after a bite. A generalized systemic reaction termed loxoscelism may occur 24–48 hours after the bite, with fever, malaise, arthralgias, rash, and hemolysis. Rare fatalities have occurred in small children, who have shown massive intravascular hemolysis, accompanied by hemoglobinuria, jaundice, hypotension, renal failure, pulmonary edema, and disseminated intravascular coagulation. There appears to be little correlation between the development of a systemic reaction and the severity of the skin lesion.

The bites of many other insects may be mistaken for brown recluse spider bites and lead to unnecessary treatment. One helpful clue (although not absolutely reliable) is that spiders tend to bite only once, whereas other insects leave multiple bites.

Treatment

Because of the progressive necrosis associated with many brown recluse bites, early surgical excision is not recommended. Excision of a necrotic area should occur only after the area has stabilized. Many recent studies have failed to show any significant benefit to corticosteroid therapy. Dapsone has been one of the more effective treatments if administered within 36 hours of the bite. The drug has severe side effects, however, and is not recommended for children. It should be reserved for rapidly progressing lesions and systemic illness. Hyperbaric oxygen therapy and wound coverage with nitroglycerin patches have failed to produce consistent effective reduction in progression of the necrosis. Brown recluse antivenin, if given within 24 hours, has been shown to be the most effective approach to limiting dermonecrosis. Many brown recluse spider bites are minor and heal without specific treatment other than tetanus prophylaxis (Chapter 30) and local wound care.

Disposition

Most brown recluse spider bites can be treated on an outpatient basis. Patients with large or infected wounds or those who have signs of a systemic reaction should be hospitalized.

SCORPION STINGS

ESSENTIALS OF DIAGNOSIS

- *Most bites produce only local reactions including a painful sting site with or without erythema.*
- *The bite of the* Centruroides exilicauda *scorpion can produce severe systemic symptoms including extreme restlessness, diaphoresis, seizures, and hypertension.*
- *Severe reactions should be treated in the intensive care unit with neuroleptics, antihypertensives, and atropine; antivenin is available for treatment failures.*

General Considerations

Most scorpions are relatively harmless, producing only local envenomation reactions. However, *C. exilicauda* [*sculpturatus*] may produce severe systemic toxicity.

This arthropod is small and yellowish, has a small tubercle (telson) at the base of its stinger, and is 2.5–7.5 cm (1–3 in) long. It is found mostly in the southwestern United States (Arizona, New Mexico, Texas, and along the Colorado River) but may rarely be transported in freight to distant states. Related arthropods are found in many other parts of the world.

The venom of *C. exilicauda* contains a neurotoxin that may produce severe systemic symptoms. Other scorpion stings generally produce only local reactions.

Clinical Findings

The initial sting is intensely painful with little or no erythema or swelling. Light percussion of the wound causes intense pain. Although pain and paresthesias generally resolve within 4 hours, local symptoms may persist for several days.

Generalized reactions may occur within 60 minutes and include extreme restlessness, uncontrollable jerking, nystagmus, diaphoresis, diplopia, incontinence, hypersalivation, confusion, seizures, hypertension, and occasionally wheezing or stridor.

Children under age 10 years are more likely to have severe or prolonged reactions; older children and adults usually recover in 10–12 hours.

Treatment

Periodic applications of ice may relieve local pain; avoid intense cooling. Immobilize the affected part. Do not apply a tourniquet.

Most children recover with supportive care alone but should be observed in an intensive care unit. Strong depressants or tranquilizers do not appear to shorten the duration of symptoms and may produce respiratory depression; specifically, opiate analgesics seem to potentiate the toxicity of the venom. Diazepam or phenobarbital may be used to control seizures; sympatholytic antihypertensive agents may be required to control hypertension. Secondary to the adrenergic effects of most foreign scorpion stings, atropine has not been recommended for treatment of excessive oral secretion. Centruroides venom, however, has predominantly cholinergic-mediated neuromuscular effects and little to no adrenergic effect. Therefore, atropine use to dry oral secretions and prevent the necessity of intubation is becoming much more popular.

Goat serum antivenin is available in Arizona (Arizona Poison and Drug Information Center [800] 222-1222 or [602] 495-6360) but has not been approved by the FDA. It is effective only for stings from *C. exilicauda* and is not of benefit for stings from scorpions from South America, Asia, or the Middle East. It is recommended only for use in severe envenomations with respiratory compromise unresolved by symptomatic treatment.

Disposition

Hospitalize all patients with *C. exilicauda* stings for supportive care.

Curtis J: Insect sting anaphylaxis. Pediatr Rev 2000;21:256. [PMID: 10922021] (Review of insect stings and their complications.)

Forks TP: Brown recluse spider bites. J Am Board Fam Prac 2000;13:415. [PMID: 11117338] (Review of the presentation and treatment of brown recluse spider bites.)

Graudins A et al: Red-back spider (*Latrodectus hasselti*) antivenom prevents the toxicity of widow spider venoms. Ann Emerg Med 2001;37:154. [PMID: 11174232] (Study assessing the efficacy of the antivenin in preventing in vitro and in vivo toxicity of widow spider bites.)

Jelinek GA: Widow spider envenomation (latrodectism): a worldwide problem. Wilderness Environ Med 1997;8:226. [PMID: 11990169] (Review of the problem of black widow spider envenomation.)

Kolecki P: Delayed toxic reaction following massive bee envenomation. Ann Emerg Med 1999;33:114. [PMID: 9867899] (Case report and review of massive bee envenomation.)

Lowry BP et al: A controlled trial of topical nitroglycerin in a New Zealand white rabbit model of brown recluse spider envenomation. Ann Emerg Med 2001;37:161. [PMID: 11174233] (Randomized, blinded controlled study assessing topical nitroglycerin treatment in brown recluse spider bites.)

Suchard JR et al: Atropine use in Centruroides scorpion envenomation. J Toxicol Clin Toxicol 2001;39:595. [PMID: 11762667] (Case study series of the use of atropine in the scorpion bite.)

Vetter RS et al: Mass envenomations by honey bees and wasps. West J Med 1999;170:223. [PMID: 10344177] (Review of the literature on mass stinging events.)

HAZARDOUS MARINE LIFE

Many ocean-dwelling animals are potentially harmful to humans because of their ability to traumatize, envenom, or otherwise poison their victims with bites or stings. Most human injuries result from envenomation.

1. Stingrays

ESSENTIALS OF DIAGNOSIS

- *Evenomation occurs when the tail of the stingray releases venom into its victim.*

- *The sting causes intense local pain as well as nausea and vomiting, weakness, tachycardia, and muscle cramps.*

- *Removal of any foreign material and irrigation with hot water are the mainstays of treatment.*

General Considerations

Stingrays are the fish most commonly responsible for human envenomations; at least 2000 stings occur annually in the United States. Stingrays are usually encountered in the waters off coastal regions, where they lie partially submerged in the sand. When disturbed, they splash upward with a muscular tail, which carries 1–4 venomous stings. Each sting is a retroserrate vasodentin spine containing multiple venom glands surrounded by an integumentary sheath. Injury due to stingrays therefore involves both a traumatic wound (which can be quite severe) and envenomation. The most common sites of injury are the lower extremities, followed by the upper extremities, abdomen, and chest. Wound necrosis is not uncommon.

Clinical Findings

The sting is followed by immediate intense local pain and moderate swelling with bleeding. The pain radiates centrally and can be so severe that it causes disorientation. Systemic symptoms occur within 30 minutes of the sting and include nausea and vomiting, weakness, diaphoresis, vertigo, tachycardia, and muscle cramps. If envenomation has been severe, syncope, paralysis, hypotension, cardiac arrhythmias, and death may occur.

Treatment

A. IRRIGATE THE WOUND

Irrigate the wound with whatever diluent is at hand (preferably sterile saline or water). Remove any obvious pieces of foreign matter. Immediate basic first aid is necessary to help prevent eventual necrosis, ulceration, and infection.

B. ANESTHETIZE THE WOUND

Soak the wound in hot water to tolerance (45–50 °C [113–122 °F]) for 30–60 minutes. Stingray venom is heat labile and may be denatured in hot water. If heat fails to relieve the pain, infiltrate the wound with lidocaine, 1–2% without epinephrine; or perform regional nerve block. Do not apply ice to the wound.

C. EXPLORE THE WOUND

Wound exploration and an x-ray should be performed so that all tissue fragments may be removed. Close the wound loosely around drains, or pack it open.

D. GIVE ANTIBIOTICS

Administer standard tetanus prophylaxis (Chapter 30), and start treatment with trimethoprim-sulfamethoxazole (160 mg and 800 mg, respectively, twice a day), ciprofloxacin (500 mg twice a day), or tetracycline (500 mg 4 times a day) for 7 days.

E. SURGICAL DEBRIDEMENT

If necrosis develops, early surgical debridement is recommended. Serial debridement may be necessary to stop any progression.

F. HYPERBARIC OXYGEN

Hyperbaric oxygen has been used successfully in the setting of myonecrosis when serial debridement is required. If used, it should be instituted immediately after debridement takes place.

Disposition

Any patient with significant envenomation from a stingray sting should be observed for 4–6 hours for appearance of systemic side effects. Patients who are discharged should have close outpatient follow-up for wound care.

2. Sea Snakes

ESSENTIALS OF DIAGNOSIS

- The initial bite is painless, but limb and respiratory paralysis as well as myolysis can occur with envenomation.
- Treatment is the same as for land snake envenomation and includes sea snake antivenin if paralysis or myolysis is present.

General Considerations

Sea snakes are present in all oceans except the Atlantic and are very similar to terrestrial snakes except for the shape of their tail. Although 90% of sea snake bites are dry, the venom is highly toxic to the nervous system and can cause significant myolysis. The sea snake is not aggressive, and some type of provocation is necessary to be bitten.

Clinical Findings

The initial bite is relatively painless, but with significant envenomation comes rapid limb and respiratory muscle paralysis, ptosis, ophthalmoplegia, and myolysis. Renal failure can occur if myolysis is severe. The hemolysis and coagulopathy associated with U.S. snake bites is not seen.

Treatment

The same basic first-aid principles used for terrestrial envenomation still apply. Monitor respiratory status and prepare for intubation. Screen for signs of myolysis with CK, urine myoglobin, and renal function panel. Signs should be present by 6 hours. If paralysis or myolysis is present, administer sea snake antivenin. Between 1 and 3 ampules should be given initially, although more may be necessary. Tiger snake antivenin may be used if sea snake antivenin is not available. Polyvalent snake venin is the third-line choice.

3. Jellyfish

ESSENTIALS OF DIAGNOSIS

- Jellyfish envenomations are associated with extreme pain both locally and distant from the sting site.
- Extensive skin changes may be seen shortly after envenomation.
- Systemic signs and symptoms include nausea and vomiting, autonomic changes, and paralysis.
- Death is usually caused by respiratory paralysis or drowning secondary to limb paralysis.

General Considerations

There are 3 types of jellyfish that cause the vast majority of the morbidity and mortality associated with jellyfish envenomation of humans: box jellyfish, Irukandji jellyfish, and Portuguese man-o-war. Jellyfish envenomate by touching prey or unsuspecting bathers with long tentacles containing hundreds of stinging cells called nematocysts. The jellyfish sting can cause a wide array of symptoms ranging from skin irritation to death.

Clinical Findings

Most jellyfish stings cause only a localized inflammatory skin reaction and require only symptomatic care. A few jellyfish, however, can cause severe systemic envenomation syndromes.

A. Box Jellyfish

Severe incapacitating localized pain occurs immediately with the development of wide, erythematous bands on the skin. Confusion progressing to unconsciousness as well as respiratory failure and cardiac arrest can occur within 5 minutes. If the patient lives, skin changes occur over the next few hours with the development of blistering and necrosis that may cause permanent scarring.

B. Irukandji Jellyfish

The initial sting is hardly felt. Approximately 30 minutes later, the Irukandji syndrome begins. Unbearable pain generally begins in the sacral area and rapidly progresses to the rest of the body. The pain is always present but worsens in waves. Other symptoms include profuse diaphoresis, restlessness, headache, nausea and vomiting, severe hypertension, and tachycardia. Later complications include pulmonary edema, transient cardiomyopathy, and left ventricular dysfunction.

C. Portuguese Man-o-War

Portuguese man-o-war stings are very painful and leave a "string of beads" appearance. Shortly afterward, an Irukandji-like syndrome can occur, which consists of nausea and vomiting, and muscle cramps, particularly in the abdomen and chest. Pain may be so severe in the chest as to cause hypoxia. Death can occur.

Treatment

A. Box Jellyfish

Due to the rapidity of possible fatality, basic life support on the scene and advanced cardiac life support once in medical hands must be a priority. Vinegar application to the sting sites will inactivate venom. Compression bandages should be applied next. An antivenin exists and should be used if available. Intramuscular injection above the sting sites should be performed with 3 ampules. Intravenous pain control is always necessary in all but the most trivial stings.

B. Irukandji Jellyfish

Initial first aid is not usually necessary. The role of vinegar is uncertain because it is not known whether vinegar inactivates the nematocysts. Intravenous pain medication will be needed. Control of blood pressure with an α-adrenergic blocking agent will also be necessary.

Monitoring for early signs of heart failure with echocardiography within the first 24 hours is recommended. Respiratory and cardiovascular support may ultimately be needed. Development of an antivenin is under way.

C. Portuguese Man-o-War

First aid consists of removing tentacles. Vinegar is not indicated. Rinsing with seawater, not fresh water, is the treatment of choice. Cold packs and intravenous pain medicine will ease pain. Rarely, respiratory support may be needed.

Disposition

Victims of envenomation should be monitored for 6–8 hours for systemic effects. The elderly or the very young should be monitored for 24 hours.

4. Scorpion Fish

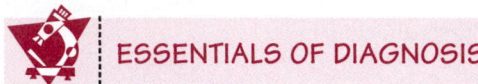 ESSENTIALS OF DIAGNOSIS

- *Extreme pain at sting site.*
- *Wound sites commonly become ischemic or secondarily infected.*
- *Systemic signs and symptoms include neurologic changes, respiratory failure, and autonomic dysfunction.*

General Considerations

Scorpion fish are divided into 3 groups on the basis of appearance and structure of the venom organ: zebra fish, scorpion fish, and stonefish. The venom apparatus consists of 12 or 13 dorsal spines, 3 anal spines, and 3 pelvic spines, all of which can be erected upon stimulation. The venom can be highly toxic (stonefish) and contains chemical fractions analogous to those contained in stingray venom.

Clinical Findings

Scorpion fish stings vary in intensity depending on the species. Most cause immediate pain, with central radiation of discomfort. Local ischemia at the wound site progresses over days to marked swelling, erythema, and cellulitis. Prolonged indolent wound infections sometimes result. Systemic symptoms occur within the first few hours and include vomiting, weakness, diarrhea, delirium, seizures, paresthesias, fever, arthritis, hypertension, cardiac arrhythmias, respiratory failure, hypotension, and death.

Treatment

Manage systemic symptoms and dysfunctions supportively. An antivenin is available in Australia for management of stings by the Indo-Pacific stonefish. It is manufactured by Commonwealth Serum Laboratories, Melbourne, Australia. For scorpion fish stings occurring in coastal waters surrounding the United States, institute the following regimen:

A. PROVIDE PAIN RELIEF

Immerse the wound in hot water to tolerance (45–50 °C [113–122 °F]) for 30–60 minutes. If heat fails to relieve the pain, infiltrate the wound with lidocaine, 1–2% without epinephrine; or perform regional nerve block. Pain from a stonefish sting may be so severe that it causes delirium requiring parenteral narcotic analgesics for relief.

B. MANAGE THE WOUND

Debride and explore the wound, and remove all foreign material. If there is a chance that a spine may have entered a joint, these procedures should be performed in the operating room, and the surgeon should use magnifying loupes to explore the joint. Do not suture wounds tightly; allow adequate drainage.

C. GIVE ANTIBIOTICS

Administer standard tetanus prophylaxis (Chapter 30), and start treatment with trimethoprim-sulfamethoxazole (160 mg and 800 mg, respectively, twice a day), ciprofloxacin (500 mg twice a day), or tetracycline (500 mg 4 times a day) for 7 days.

Disposition

Patients who have sustained significant envenomation from a scorpion fish sting should be observed for 4–6 hours for development of systemic symptoms. All patients should be seen frequently on an outpatient basis for wound care after discharged.

5. Sea Urchins

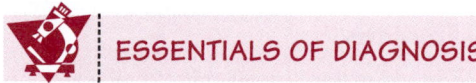

ESSENTIALS OF DIAGNOSIS

- *Extreme pain at sting site.*
- *Skin changes at site.*
- *May have retained spines.*

- *Systemic signs and symptoms include neurologic changes and respiratory failure.*

General Considerations

Sea urchins are egg-shaped, globular, or flattened echinoderms found in areas ranging from the shallow intertidal zone to great oceanic depths. Some species are covered with sharp, brittle, venom-filled spines that readily break off. Most sea urchin venom contains several toxic fractions that may include cholinergic compounds and potent neurotoxins. Envenomation occurs when a victim inadvertently handles or falls on a sea urchin and the spines penetrate the skin.

Clinical Findings

Injuries caused by sea urchin spines are associated with immediate intense burning pain, followed by erythema, edema, and aching. One or more spines typically break off in the skin. A purplish discoloration indicates penetration of the skin but does not necessarily mean that a spine remains. Multiple wounds may cause a systemic reaction, including nausea and vomiting, intense pain, paralysis, aphonia, respiratory distress, and death. Pain may subside within the first 2 hours, but paralysis may remain for 6–8 hours.

Treatment

Systemic symptoms and dysfunctions are managed supportively. No antivenin is available for sea urchin venom.

A. RELIEVE PAIN

Immerse the wound in hot water to tolerance (45–50 °C [113–122 °F]) for 30–60 minutes. If heat fails to relieve the pain, infiltrate the wound with lidocaine, 1–2% without epinephrine; or perform regional nerve block.

B. REMOVE EMBEDDED SPINES

Halt the envenomation process by carefully removing the spines (avoid fragmentation). Although some thin spines may be absorbed over 2–3 weeks, remove as many as possible. Remove all thick spines, because of the potential for foreign body reactions and infections. Many spines are radiopaque and can be visualized using soft tissue x-ray techniques. Obtain surgical consultation if there is a chance a spine may have entered a joint, if a spine is near a significant neurovascular structure, or if a spine has been lost in a closed space in the hand. In these cases, the spine should be removed in the operating room with the aid of magnifying loupes.

Do not suture the wounds tightly; allow adequate drainage.

Disposition

Patients with significant sea urchin envenomation should be observed for 4–6 hours for appearance of systemic effects. Patients who are discharged should have frequent outpatient follow-up for wound care.

INGESTION OF POISONOUS FISH

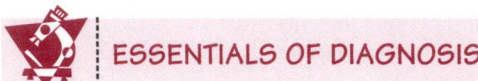

ESSENTIALS OF DIAGNOSIS

- Consider ingestion of poisonous fish in anyone with gastroenteritis, neurologic symptoms, and respiratory compromise.

The more intensive harvesting of marine plants and animals for food has increased the number of poisoning episodes due to ingestion of such items. Emergency physicians should obtain a dietary history from any patient who presents with gastroenteritis, respiratory compromise, confusing neurologic signs, or sudden unexplained systemic illness.

1. Ciguatera Toxin Poisoning

General Considerations

Ciguatera fish poisoning is caused by tropical and semi-tropical marine coral reef fish whose tissues accumulate toxins that originate in the toxic dinoflagellate *Gambierdiscus toxicus*. The toxin is ingested by small herbivorous fishes, which are eaten by larger carnivorous fishes. Humans are then the final consumer. Larger and older fish are more toxic in ciguatera-endemic areas. The most frequently implicated fishes in the United States include barracuda, jack, snapper, and grouper.

Clinical Findings

Symptoms usually occur within 15–60 minutes of ingestion—almost always within 12 hours—and increase in severity over the next 4–6 hours. Symptoms include abdominal pain, nausea and vomiting, diarrhea, chills, paresthesias, pruritus, dysphagia, odontalgia, pathognomonic reversal of the sensation of hot and cold, fatigue, athetosis, ataxia, vertigo, headache, myalgias, bradycardia, hypotension, central respiratory failure, and coma, with an overall death rate of 0.1–12%. More severe reactions often occur in persons previously poisoned by the toxin. Untreated, the gastroenteritis usually resolves

in 24–48 hours, whereas the neurologic syndrome may last for weeks. The diagnosis is made on the basis of clinical findings; there is currently no test that indicates the presence of ciguatoxin in human blood.

Treatment & Disposition

Treatment is largely supportive and symptomatic. Gastric emptying (via gastric lavage or emesis), catharsis, and instillation of activated charcoal may be of limited value if performed within 3 hours after ingestion. Avoid magnesium-based cathartics. Treat hypotension with intravenous infusion of crystalloid solutions and vasopressors. Mannitol infusion, 1 g/kg intravenously, has been reported to reverse cardiac depression and severe neurologic symptoms. Bradyarrhythmias generally respond well to atropine. Treat persistent myocardial failure with judicious administration of calcium gluconate, 1–2 intravenously over 24 hours; the rationale is that the toxin occupies calcium receptor sites that affect the permeability to sodium of the pores in neural and myocardial membranes. Although many other drugs have been recommended, none have proven benefit.

Admit patients with cardiovascular symptoms for observation.

2. Scombroid Poisoning

General Considerations

Scombroid poisoning follows the ingestion of toxic fish of the families Scomberesocidae and Scombroidei, which include albacore, tuna, mackerel, bonito, kingfish, and wahoo. Scombroid poisoning can also be caused by nonscombroid fish such as dolphin, sardine, anchovy, amberjack, and ocean salmon. This pseudoallergic syndrome results from the improper preservation or refrigeration of dark-fleshed fish. These fish contain certain bacteria, most commonly *Vibrio* spp. Muscle tissue undergoes degradation induced by these bacteria that transforms histidine to histamine if not stored below 0 °C (32 °F). Histamine levels higher than 20–50 mg/100 mL are noted in toxic fish. It has been suggested that histamine alone is unlikely to be the sole toxin, because oral histamine is converted in the bowel to *N*-acetyl histamine. Cooking does not prevent the toxic effects.

Clinical Findings

Symptoms occur within 15–90 minutes of ingestion and are the same as those caused by histamine (eg, flushing of the face, neck, and upper torso; sensation of warmth; urticaria; pruritus; angioneurotic edema; epigastric pain; abdominal cramps; diarrhea; nausea and vomiting; headache; thirst; pharyngitis; tachycardia; palpitations; bronchospasm; and hypotension). Untreated mild to moderate scombroid poisoning resolves within 6–12 hours.

Treatment & Disposition

Treatment is directed at reversing the effects of histamine. Patients with minor poisoning without respiratory distress should receive diphenhydramine, 25–75 mg orally. If the reaction is severe, give epinephrine, 0.3–0.5 mL of 1:1000 solution subcutaneously. Nausea and vomiting are usually controlled by the antihistamine. In refractory cases, the histamine antagonists cimetidine, 300 mg intravenously, or ranitidine, 50 mg intravenously, may be given. Oral cimetidine, 300 mg every 6 hours, may be used to combat persistent headache. If the patient presents in the emergency department within 1 hour of consuming a large amount of scombroid fish, it may be helpful to empty the stomach (via gastric lavage or emesis) and administer activated charcoal, 50–100 g in sorbitol.

Admit patients with serious illness for observation.

3. Puffer Fish (Tetrodotoxin) Poisoning

General Considerations

Tetrodotoxin is one of the most potent nonprotein poisons found in nature and is characteristic of the order Tetraodontiformes. The poison is found in puffer fish, also known as toadfish, blowfish, blowfish, swellfish, balloonfish, and porcupine fish. The microbial flora of the fish produces the toxin. Some of these tropical and subtropical fish are prepared as delicacies (*fugu*) in Japan by trained and licensed chefs. The toxin is distributed throughout the entire fish, with the greatest concentrations in the liver, gonads, intestine, and skin. The poison interferes with central and peripheral neuromuscular transmission, causing depression of the medullary respiratory mechanism, intracardiac conduction, and myocardial and skeletal muscle contractility. The toxin is water soluble but very difficult to remove from the fish by cooking.

Clinical Findings

The onset of symptoms can be as rapid as 10 minutes or can be delayed for up to 5 hours. Victims initially develop paresthesias, followed by hypersalivation, diaphoresis, lethargy, headache, nausea, vomiting, abdominal pain, diarrhea, weakness, ataxia, tremor, paralysis, respiratory failure, coma, and hypotension. Sixty percent of victims die, most within the first 6 hours.

Treatment

A. MANAGE THE AIRWAY

If the victim is obtunded or evidence of dysphagia or respiratory insufficiency is present, endotracheal intubation should be performed and supplemental oxygen administered, guided by serial arterial blood gas measurements. Prompt ventilatory support in the setting of rapid paralysis is the most important intervention to prevent anoxic brain damage.

B. GIVE ACTIVATED CHARCOAL

If treatment is within 3 hours of ingestion, perform intragastric placement of 50–100 g of activated charcoal in 70% sorbitol solution. In the paralyzed or obtunded patient, protect the airway before giving charcoal.

C. PROVIDE SYMPTOM-BASED LIFE SUPPORT

Hypotension may necessitate administration of crystalloid solutions or, rarely, the addition of a pressor agent. Bradyarrhythmias generally respond to atropine; heart block may necessitate temporary placement of a transvenous or transcutaneous pacemaker.

Disposition

Patients with respiratory difficulties, cardiovascular symptoms, or paralysis should be hospitalized in an intensive care unit. Patients with symptoms of a minor intoxication, which may be limited to paresthesias and mild dysphagia, should be observed in the emergency department or intensive care unit for at least 8 hours to detect deterioration.

4. Paralytic Shellfish Poisoning

General Considerations

Bivalve mollusks filter large quantities of water unselectively to gather plankton and extract oxygen. This action leads to concentration of bacteria, viruses, biologic toxins, and other substances in the tissues of such shellfish. Paralytic shellfish poisoning is induced by ingesting any of a variety of clams, oysters, scallops, mussels, chitons, limpets, murex, starfish, and sand crabs. The source of toxicity is the toxin elaborated by various planktonic dinoflagellates and protozoan organisms. The most common dinoflagellates are *Protogonyaulax* (or *Alexandrium*) and *Ptychodiscus* spp, which are responsible for colored tides and enormous mortality in bird and marine populations. Saxitoxin, elaborated by *Protogonyaulax,* is found in greatest concentrations in the digestive organs, gills, and siphon. No physical characteristic distinguishes the carrier animal. A toxin concentration of greater than 75–80 μg/100 g of shell-fish tissue is considered hazardous. The toxin blocks sodium conductance, inhibiting neuromuscular transmission at the axonal and muscle membrane levels. In humans, a lethal dose of purified saxitoxin is 0.1 mg.

Clinical Findings

Within minutes to a few hours of ingestion of contaminated shellfish, intraoral and perioral paresthesias ensue. These rapidly involve the neck and distal extremities. Other symptoms include dizziness, incoordination, weakness, incoherence, dysarthria, sialorrhea, dysphagia, diarrhea, nausea, vomiting, dysmetria, headache, loss of vision, and tachycardia. Flaccid paralysis and respiratory insufficiency may follow. Unless a period of anoxia occurs, the victim will often remain awake and alert, although paralyzed. Death due to respiratory arrest occurs in up to 25% of victims within the first 12 hours.

Treatment

A. MANAGE THE AIRWAY

If the victim is obtunded or evidence of dysphagia or respiratory insufficiency is present, endotracheal intubation should be performed and supplemental oxygen administered, guided by serial arterial blood gas measurements. Prompt ventilatory support in the setting of rapid paralysis is the most important intervention to prevent anoxic brain damage.

B. PERFORM GASTRIC EMPTYING

If the victim shows any neurologic signs that indicate impending paralysis or respiratory difficulty, gastric emptying should be preceded by endotracheal intubation. The toxin is gastric acid stable and partially inactivated in alkaline solutions. If treatment is within 3 hours of ingestion, perform gastric lavage with at least 2 L of 2% sodium bicarbonate solution in 200-mL aliquots, followed by intragastric placement of 50–100 g of activated charcoal in 70% sorbitol solution.

C. PROVIDE SYMPTOM-BASED LIFE SUPPORT

Hypotension may necessitate administration of crystalloid solutions or, rarely, the addition of a pressor agent. Bradyarrhythmias generally respond to atropine; heart block may necessitate temporary placement of a transvenous or transcutaneous pacemaker.

Disposition

Patients with respiratory difficulties, cardiovascular symptoms, or paralysis should be hospitalized in an intensive care unit. Patients with symptoms of a minor intoxication, which may be limited to paresthesias and mild dysphagia, should be observed in the emergency department or intensive care unit for at least 8 hours to detect deterioration

Australian Venomous Research Unit at the University of Melbourne: Australian CSL Antivenom Handbook. http://www.wch.sa.gov.au/paedm/clintox/cslb_index.html

Centers for Disease Control and Prevention: Scombroid fish poisoning—Pennsylvania 1998. JAMA 2000;283:2927. [PMID: 10896527] (Morbidity and mortality weekly report on puffer fish poisoning.)

Fenner PJ: Dangers in the ocean: the traveler and marine envenomation. I. Jellyfish. J Travel Med 1998;5:135. [PMID: 9772332] (Review of venomous jellyfish and treatment of envenomations.)

Fenner PJ: Dangers in the ocean: the traveler and marine envenomation. II. Marine vertebrates. J Travel Med 1998:5:213. (PMID: 9876198) (Review of venomous marine vertebrates and treatment of envenomations.)

Field J: Puffer fish poisoning. J Accid Emerg Med 1998;15:334. [PMID: 9785165] (Case report of puffer fish poisoning and review of the literature.)

Hawdon GM et al: Venomous marine creatures. Aust Fam Physician 1997;26:1369. [PMID: 9470289] (Review of the features of envenomation by venomous marine creatures.)

Lipp EK et al: The role of seafood in foodborne diseases in the United States of America. Rev Sci Tech 1997;16:620. [PMID: 9501377] (Review of seafood poisoning.)

Rocca AF et al: Hyperbaric oxygen therapy in the treatment of soft tissue necrosis resulting from a stingray puncture. Foot Ankle Int 2001;22:318. [PMID: 11354445] (Case study of stingray puncture with resultant complications and treatments.)

Poisoning

D. Shannon Waters, MD, Darren Waters, MD, & Travis Sewalls, MD[1]

Immediate Management of Life-Threatening Conditions

Further Management of Victims of Poisoning

Management of Conditions Associated with Poisoning

Emergency Treatment of Specific Poisonings

Acetaminophen

Amphetamines & Other Related Stimulants

Anticholinergics

β-Adrenergic Blocking Agents

Calcium-Channel Blocking Agents

Carbon Monoxide

Cardiac Glycosides

Caustics & Corrosives

Cocaine & Local Anesthetics

Cyanide

Drug-Induced Methemoglobinemia

Ethanol & Other Alcohols

1. Ethanol
2. Methanol
3. Ethylene Glycol
4. Isopropanol

Heavy Metals

1. Iron
2. Lead
3. Arsenic
4. Mercury

Hydrocarbons

Inhalants (Toxic Gases & Vapors)

Isoniazid

Lithium

Opiates

Organophosphates & Other Cholinesterase Inhibitors

Phencyclidine

Phenothiazines & Other Antipsychotics

Poisonous Mushrooms

Poisonous Plants

Salicylates

Sedative-Hypnotics

Theophylline & Methylxanthines

Tricyclic Antidepressants

Warfarin & Other Anticoagulants

■ IMMEDIATE MANAGEMENT OF LIFE-THREATENING CONDITIONS

Victims of Poisoning with Coma, Seizures, or Marked Obtundation

A. KEEP AIRWAY OPEN

Establish and maintain an adequate airway and ventilation. Begin supplemental oxygen, 12 L/min, by nonrebreathing mask. If the patient has no gag reflex, intubate for airway protection, to facilitate oxygenation, and to remove airway secretions.

B. OBTAIN ARTERIAL BLOOD GAS AND pH MEASUREMENTS

Obtain arterial blood for blood gas and pH measurements to determine adequacy of ventilation and perfusion.

C. GAIN INTRAVENOUS ACCESS

Insert a large-bore (≥ 18-gauge) peripheral or central intravenous catheter, and draw blood for complete blood count, serum electrolyte and blood glucose measurements, and tests of renal and hepatic function.

D. TREAT COMA PROMPTLY

(See Chapter 16.) Give glucose, 50 mL of a 50% solution (25 g of glucose) intravenously over 3–4 minutes.

[1]This chapter is a revision of the chapter by Kent R. Olson, MD, FACEP, & Charles E. Becker, MD, from the 4th edition.

Give naloxone (Narcan, others), 0.4–2 mg intravenously. If the patient's response is weak or if narcotic overdose is suspected, give repeated doses of 2 mg every 1–2 minutes up to a total dosage of 10–20 mg. *Note:* The duration of action of naloxone (2–3 hours) is shorter than that of many of the narcotics it reverses. Patients responding to naloxone must be observed for at least 3 hours after the last dose.

If alcoholism or malnutrition is suspected, give thiamine, 100 mg intramuscularly or in intravenous solution with or prior to glucose administration.

E. Maintain Circulation

Maintain circulation, and treat shock by restoring intravascular volume with intravenous infusion of crystalloid solutions (Chapter 9). *Caution:* Fluid overload and pulmonary edema may occur with overly vigorous hydration. If administration of more than 20–30 mL/kg of crystalloid solution and usual doses of dopamine (ie, 5–15 µg/kg/min intravenously) fail to restore blood pressure, insert a pulmonary artery catheter to obtain pressure readings and help guide further therapy with fluids or pressor agents.

F. Treat Seizures

(See Chapter 17.) If the patient is experiencing seizures, give diazepam, 0.1–0.2 mg/kg intravenously over 1–2 minutes. If this is not effective, give phenytoin, 15–20 mg/kg, or fosphenytoin, 15–20 phenytoin equivalents per kilogram, at a rate no faster than 100–150 mg/min.

G. Start Electrocardiographic Monitoring

Start cardiac monitoring. Obtain a 12-lead electrocardiogram (ECG), and note especially the rate; rhythm; presence of arrhythmias; and PR, QRS, and QT intervals. If overdose of tricyclic antidepressants is suspected, obtain serial ECGs.

H. Perform Gastric Lavage

Perform gastric lavage with a large-bore orogastric or nasogastric tube (Ewald tube) for any potentially lethal ingestion and in any patient with altered mental status who might have ingested a toxic substance within 1 hour prior to arrival (see section on decontamination, below).

I. Search for Associated Illness

Look for other causes of coma or seizures (Chapters 16 and 17). In particular, look for (1) head trauma (focal neurologic deficits or asymmetric seizures), (2) other trauma causing hemorrhage or shock, (3) infection (generalized or central nervous system), (4) metabolic disorders (hyponatremia, hypoglycemia, hyperglycemia), (5) hypothermia (use a rectal thermometer that can measure temperatures lower than 32 °C [89.6 °F]), or (6) hyperthermia.

Victims of Poisoning with Intact Gag Reflex & Lethargy

Management is the same as that outlined above for patients with absent gag reflex, except that endotracheal intubation may not be necessary before gastric lavage. The airway may be adequately protected by placing the patient in the lateral decubitus position with the head and trunk slightly lower than the feet (Trendelenburg position).

■ FURTHER MANAGEMENT OF VICTIMS OF POISONING

For assistance in identifying drugs and poisons and access to expert toxicologic consultation, refer to www.aapcc.com for appropriate poison center listings. Experts at the poison center can (1) provide immediate assistance in selecting appropriate laboratory or toxicity tests and in recommending preferred methods of gut decontamination or the use of antidotes and (2) advise on patient disposition.

Obtain Brief History

Obtain as much information as possible from paramedics, bystanders, police, family, and friends. Ask about recent use of drugs or medications, and find out whether any empty pill bottles, medications, or drug paraphernalia were found at the scene. If several patients present with similar symptoms of poisoning, consider carbon monoxide poisoning, food poisoning, or other toxins that can affect multiple victims simultaneously. Correlate the history with physical findings and results of laboratory tests, but do not be misled by the history. What the patient or friends say was ingested may differ from what was actually swallowed, especially in suicide attempts.

Decontaminate as Soon as Possible

A. Inhaled Poisons

Remove the patient from the source of poison, and give oxygen by mask. Inhalation of a water aerosol may help to dilute inhaled irritants in the nasopharynx. Check for hoarseness and singed nasal hairs (eg, after smoke inhalation), and be alert for delayed development of upper airway obstruction or pulmonary edema.

B. Contaminated Eyes

(See Chapter 31.) Wash the eyes immediately with copious amounts of plain water or normal saline; *do not* use neutralizing solutions. Hang a bottle containing

500–100 mL of normal saline above the patient, and dribble the solution slowly into the corner of the injured eye through the intravenous tubing.

If the contaminating material was acidic or basic, tears may be checked with pH paper after the eyes have been washed to make sure that all toxic material has been removed. A careful eye examination is indicated following irrigation (Chapter 31).

C. Contaminated Skin

Wash the skin immediately with plenty of water and dilute soap solution. Discard contaminated clothes in a marked plastic bag. Certain toxins, such as organophosphates, are well absorbed through the skin and are difficult to remove. Remove all particulate matter prior to irrigation.

Hydrofluoric acid burns are particularly penetrating and corrosive. Prompt immersion of the burn into quaternary ammonium salt solution or 10% calcium gluconate solution or 2.5% gel, or subcutaneous injection of calcium gluconate deep to the burn (0.5 mL of 10% solution per square centimeter of burn area) may be helpful. A plastic surgeon (or hand surgeon) should be consulted for injuries involving the fingers.

D. Ingested Poisons

The traditional approach has been to remove ingested toxins by emesis or gastric lavage, followed by activated charcoal and catharsis. However, recent evidence suggests that gastric emptying (particularly emesis) may have limited efficiency, especially if initiated more than 1 hour after the ingestion, and may delay the administration of charcoal. Gastric lavage is the preferred method of gastric emptying, particularly in patients who have taken a rapid-acting convulsant or those with a rapidly declining level of consciousness.

1. Ipecac—Induced emesis is no longer recommended in the emergency department. Although controversial, ipecac may still have a role in the domestic setting (eg, mushroom poisoning).

2. Gastric lavage—Use gastric lavage in patients with suspected serious poisonings who present to the emergency department within 1 hour of ingestion. Unless a patient is intubated, gastric lavage is contraindicated if airway protective reflexes are absent.

Gastric lavage is performed with a large-bore (at least 36F for adults) orogastric or nasogastric tube. (Pill fragments cannot be removed through standard-sized nasogastric tubes.) Use tap water or saline at body temperature in 250-mL increments, and continue lavage until fluid returns clear or free of pill fragments.

3. Activated charcoal—Activated charcoal, 50–100 g as a slurry, can be given if a patient has ingested a potentially toxic amount of a poison. Unless a patient has an intact or protected airway, the administration of activated charcoal is contraindicated. For oral administration, charcoal can be made more palatable by adding a small amount of cherry, licorice, or chocolate flavoring just before administration. Mixing the charcoal with 1 mL/kg of 70% sorbitol improves taste and also provides cathartic action. Although routine use of a cathartic with activated charcoal is not endorsed, if used, it should be limited to a single dose in order to minimize adverse effects. As with gastric lavage, the effectiveness of activated charcoal decreases with time.

Charcoal has great adsorptive properties and can bind most poisons (exceptions include alcohols, potassium, lithium, and iron). If the ingested dose of poison is known, attempt to give at least 10 times that weight of charcoal, in divided doses if necessary.

4. Whole bowel irrigation—Whole bowel irrigation has been used successfully for removal of iron tablets and sustained-release and enteric-coated preparations. This technique utilizes a balanced electrolyte–polyethylene glycol solution (Colyte, GoLYTELY) to flush out the entire intestinal tract. It is given by nasogastric tube, 1–2 L/h (400–500 mL/min in children), until the rectal effluent is clear (3–5 hours or more).

Perform Complete Physical Examination

Look for characteristic physical signs of various kinds of poisoning while immediate treatment measures are being started. Physical signs associated with specific poisons are listed in Tables 45–1 and 45–2.

Order Other Laboratory & X-ray Studies as Needed

Appropriate laboratory evaluation of the patient is determined, in part, by the patient's clinical condition.

A. Blood Tests

Obtain arterial blood gas and pH measurements to determine adequacy of ventilation and circulation. Draw blood for measurement of serum electrolytes, blood urea nitrogen, blood glucose, and serum osmolality. Calculate anion and osmolar gaps (Tables 45–3 and 45–4).

B. Electrocardiogram

Obtain an ECG, and look for widened QRS complexes or QT intervals, atrioventricular block, ventricular tachyarrhythmias, or evidence of ischemia (Table 45–5).

C. X-ray Studies

Obtain a chest x-ray to look for pulmonary edema (caused by narcotics, barbiturates, salicylates, ethchlorvynol, or corrosive chemicals) or infiltrates (due to

Table 45–1. Physical findings associated with various types of poisons.

Altered vital signs
> Hypertension: amphetamines, phencyclidine, phenyl propanolamine, anticholinergics, cocaine, nicotine
> Hypotension: sedative-hyponotics, narcotics, antihypertensives, theophylline, cloridine, β-blockers, tricyclic antidepressants
> Hyperthermia: salicyates, amphetamines, cocaine, phencyclidine, anticholinergics, seizures due to any cause
> Hypothermia: narcotics, barbiturates, ethanol, other sedative-hypnotics, clonidine, phenothiazines
> Hyperpnea: salicylates or other agents causing metabolic acidosis

Ocluular signs
> Miosis (pinpoint pupils): narcotics, clonidine, organophosphates, phenothiazines, severe sedative-hypnotic overdose, pilocarpine
> Mydriasis (dilated pupils): anticholinergics, amphetamines, cocaine, LSD, glutethimide
> Nystagmus: phenytoin, phencyclidine (especially vertical nystagmus), alcohol, many sedative-hypnotics
> Ophthalmoplegia: botulism, sedative-hypnotics
> Oculogyric crisis: haloperidol, other antipsychotics
> Optic neuritis: methanol

Breath odors
> Smoke: fire-associated toxins (see sectin on inhalants)
> Garlic: arsenic, arsine gas, organophosphates
> Bitter almond or silver polish; cyanide
> Wintergreen: methyl salicylate
> Pearlike: chloral hydrate
> Rotten eggs: hydrogen sulfide
> Acetone: diabetic ketoacidosis, isopropanol
> Typical odors of ethanol, ammonia, tobacco, disinfectants, camphor, glue, paraldehyde

Skin signs
> Cyanosis: ergotamine, agents causing hypoxemia, hypotension, or methemoglobinemia
> Flushed, red: carbon monoxide (rare), cyanide (rare), anticholinergics, boric acid
> Acneiform rash: bromides, chlorinated aromatic hydrocarbons
> Bullae: nonspecific for sedative-hypnotic overdose, carbon monoxide, and other causes of coma

Altered muscle tone
> Increased: amphetamines, phencyclidine, antipsychotics
> Flaccid: sedative-hypnotics, narcotics, cloridine
> Fasciculations: organophosphates, lithium
> Rigidity: haloperidol, phencyclidine, strychnine
> Dystonic posturing: antipsychotics, phencyclidine
> Tremor: lithium, nicotine, or stimulant overdose; alcohol or sedative-hypnonotic withdrawal
> Asterixis (flapping tremor): agents causing hepatic encephalopathy
> Seizures: tricyclic antidepressants, theophylline, amphetamines, cocaine, phencyclidine, phenothiazines isoniazid, lindane, other chlorinated hydrocarbons and pesticides

---

aspiration of gastric contents, inhalation of certain metal fumes, or hydrocarbon aspiration). Obtain an abdominal x-ray to look for radiopaque pills or toxins (Table 45–6).

D. URINE STUDIES

Obtain urine for toxicologic screening and routine analysis, and look for calcium oxalate crystals (ethylene glycol poisoning); positive test for occult blood (myoglobinuria, hemolysis); or positive test for phenylpyruvic acid (eg, Phenistix) in phenothiazine or salicylate overdose (may be negative in patients with acid urine).

E. TOXICOLOGIC STUDIES

Request toxicologic studies. Results of toxicologic studies may be useful in later confirmation of the diagnosis but are rarely helpful in the emergency department. It is more cost-effective to save serum and urine samples in the laboratory and analyze them later only if necessary. For certain types of poisoning, however, obtaining estimates of drug concentration quickly is valuable in determining the need for specific therapy. These drugs and their antidotes are discussed later in this chapter, under each specific poisoning.

Accelerate Elimination of Poisons

A. TOXICOKINETICS

The rational management of drug overdose requires an understanding of the absorption, distribution, and elimination of the toxin. Most published kinetic parameters have been determined at normal doses, whereas pharmacokinetics in victims of poisoning are often more complex.

Dissolution and absorption of toxin or gastric-emptying time may be altered in poisoned patients, so that the peak effects may be delayed (as occurs with anticholinergics). The gastrointestinal tract may be injured, allowing increased absorption of certain materials (eg, iron). If the finite capacity of the liver to metabolize a drug is exceeded, an increased amount of the drug may be delivered to the systemic circulation. If the concentration of the toxin in the bloodstream increases dramatically, protein binding may be saturated (eg, in salicylate poisoning), so that the fraction of free toxin increases. Circulatory insufficiency, hypothermia, and electrolyte and acid-base imbalance influence the metabolism and excretion of ingested drugs. Any of these factors may drastically alter normal kinetics and confuse calculations. Despite these limitations, pharmacokinetic principles may be useful in the management of drug overdose. Some terms commonly used in toxicology are defined below.

Table 45–2. Toxidromes.[1]

Toxidrome	Representative Agent(s)	Most Common Findings	Additional Signs and Symptoms	Potential Interventions
Opioid	Heroin Morphine	CNS depression, miosis, respiratory depression	Hypothermia, bradycardia. Death may result from respiratory arrest, pulmonary edema	Ventilation or naloxone
Sympathomimetic	Cocaine Amphetamine	Psychomotor agitation, mydriasis, diaphoresis, tachycardia, hypertension, hyperthermia	Seizures, rhabdomylosis, myocardial infarction Death may result from seizures, cardiac arrest, hyperthermia	Cooling, sedation with benzodiazepines, hydration
Cholinergic	Organophosphate insecticides Carbamate insecticides	Salivation, lacrimation, diaphoresis, nausea, vomiting, urination, defecation, muscle fasciculations, weakness, bronchorrhea	Bradycardia, moisis/mydriasis, seizures, respiratory failure, paralysis Death may result from respiratory arrest 2° to paralysis and/or bronchorrhea, seizures	Airway protection and ventilation, atropine, pralidoxime
Anticholinergic	Scopolamine Atropine	Altered mental status, mydriasis, dry/flushed skin, urinary retention, decreased bowel sounds, hyperthermia, dry mucous membranes	Seizures, dysrhythmias, rhabdomyolysis Death may result from hyperthermia and dysrhythmias	Physostigmine (if appropriate) sedation with benzodiazepines, cooling supportive management
Salicylates	Aspirin Oil of wintergreen	Altered mental status, respiratory alkalosis, metabolic acidosis, tinnitus hyperpnea, tachycardia, diaphoresis, nausea, vomiting	Low-grade fever, ketonuria Death may result from pulmonary edema, cardiorespiratory arrest	MDAC, alkalinization of the urine with potassium repletion, hemodialysis, hydration
Hypoglycemia	Sulfonylureas Insulin	Altered mental status, diaphoresis, tachycardia, hypertension	Paralysis, slurring of speech, bizarre behavior, seizures Death may result from seizures, altered behavior	Glucose, containing solution intravenously, and oral feedings if able, frequent capillary blood for glucose measurement
Serotinin syndrome	Meperidine/dextromethorphan + MAOI, SSRI + TCA, SSRI/ TCA/MAOI + amphetamine, SSRI overdose	Altered mental status, increased muscle tone, hyeprreflexia, hyperthermia	"Wet dog shakes" (intermittent whole body tremor) Death may result from hyperthermia	Cooling, sedation with benzodiazepines, supportive management, theoretical benefit—cyproheptadine

CNS = central nervous system; MDAC = multidose activated charcoal; MAOI = monoamine oxidase inhibitor; SSRI = selective serotonin reuptake inhibitor; TCA = tricyclic antidepressant.
[1]Reproduced, with permission, from Tintinalli JE, Kelen GD, Stapczynski S: *Emergency Medicine: A Comprehensive Study Guide* 5th ed. McGraw-Hill, 2000.

Table 45–3. Drugs causing metabolic acidosis associated with an elevated anion gap.[1]

Direct causes of acidosis
Alcohols: methanol, ethanol, ethylene glycol
Salicylates
Paraldehyde
Phenformin
Indirect causes of acidosis
Seizures (eg, isoniazid)
Hypotension (eg, barbiturates)
Hypoxemia (eg, carbon monoxide, cyanide)

[1]Anion gap = $(Na^+ + K^+) - (HCO_3^- + Cl^-)$ = 12–16 mEq/L.

Table 45–4. Calculation of the osmolar gap in toxicology.

The osmolar gap (ΔOsm) is determined by subtracting the calculated serum osmolality from the measured serum osmolality. Calculated osmolality:

$$Osm = 2(Na^+) + \frac{Glucose}{18} + \frac{BUN}{2.8}$$

Osmolar gap:

$$\Delta Osm = measured\ Osm - Calculated\ Osm$$

Serum osmolality may be increased by contributions of circulating alcohols and other low-molecular-weight substances. Because these substances are not included in the calculated osmolality, there will be a gap proportionate to their serum concentration and inversely proprotional to their molecular weight:

$$Serum\ concentration\ (mg/dL) = \Delta Osm \times \frac{Molecular\ weight}{10}$$

For ethanol (the most common cause of ΔOsm), a gap of 30 mOsm/L indicates an ethanol level of

$$30 \times 46/10 = 138\ mg/dL$$

	Molecular Weight	Lethal Concentration (mg/dL)	Corresponding ΔOsm (mOsm/L)
Ethanol	46	350	75
Methanol	32	80	25
Ethylene glycol	62	200	35
Isopropanol	60	350	60

Note: Most laboratories use the freezing point method for calculating osmolality. If the vaporization point method is used, alcohols are driven off and their contribution to osmolality is lost.

Table 45–5. Electrocardiographic manifestations of poisoning.

Sign	Examples of Causes
Prolonged QT interval	Hypocalcemia (ethylene glycol) Tricyclic antidepressants Type I antiarrhythmic agents
Prolonged QRS interval	Phenothiazines (selected) Tricyclic antidepressants Type I antiarrhythmic agents
Atrioventricular block	Beta-adrenergic blockers Calcium-channel blocking agents Digitalis glycosides Tricyclic antidepressants Type I antiarrhythmic agents
Ventricular tachyarrhythmias	Amphetamines, cocaine Digitalis glycosides Theophylline Tricyclic antidepressants Type I antiarrhythmic agents
Ischemic pattern or current of injury	Cellular, asphyxiants (cyanide, carbon monoxide) Hypoxemia (pneumonia) Hypotension

1. Half-life—The half-life of a toxin is the time required to eliminate one half of the toxin from the body. This parameter is most meaningful for the many drugs (eg, barbiturates, theophylline) that exhibit first-order kinetics, in which a fixed percentage of the toxin is removed per unit of time. Other drugs (eg, alcohol) have zero-order kinetics, in which a fixed amount of toxin is removed per unit of time. In an overdose, pathways of elimination are often saturated, and first-order kinetics are replaced by fixed-rate, or zero-order, elimination.

Table 45–6. Drugs and toxins that may be radiopaque.[1]

Chloral hydrate Heavy metals (iron, arsenic) Iodide Psychotropics (phenothiazines, tricyclic antidepressants) Sodium Enteric-coated tablets	Mnemonic is CHIPS

[1]**Caution:** Recent studies suggest that these drugs are *not* routinely visible on x-ray. If tablets have dissolved, false-negative x-ray results may occur. Abdominal x-rays are therefore useful only if positive findings are seen.

2. Volume of distribution—The volume of distribution (V_d) is the volume into which the toxin is distributed after absorption. If a drug is sequestered outside the blood and is highly tissue bound, it will have a large volume of distribution. Table 45–7 gives the volumes of distribution for several common drugs.

3. Clearance—Clearance is the volume of plasma that can be cleared of toxin per unit of time. Clearance includes both renal and metabolic components, and the proportion that each contributes to total clearance is important. For example, a toxin may be 95% metabolized and 5% renally excreted, in which case doubling the renal clearance of the toxin will not significantly enhance its total elimination from the body.

Knowledge of these parameters is helpful when measures to increase drug elimination (eg, forced alkaline diuresis, hemodialysis, or hemoperfusion) are under consideration. For example, toxins with large volumes of distribution are present in only minute quantities in plasma and are not effectively removed by dialysis or diuresis. Measures to enhance elimination of drugs with rapid intrinsic clearance rates will not contribute significantly to the overall elimination rate.

B. Methods to Enhance Drug Elimination

The decision to use measures to improve drug elimination should be based on a rational understanding of the drug's properties and the patient's clinical condition. Most patients respond satisfactorily to appropriate supportive care. The risks, time, and expense involved in hemodialysis or hemoperfusion must be weighed against the possible benefits. In some patients, the severe potential toxicity of the poison warrants immediate hemodialysis (Table 45–8). With other poisons, dialysis is of no theoretic or proved benefit.

1. Diuresis and pH manipulations—Because many toxins are weak acids or bases, they can be ionized in solutions of varying pH. In the ionized state, they are less

Table 45–7. Volumes of distribution for some common drugs.

Drugs with Large Volumes of Distribution		Drugs with Small Volumes of Distribution	
Chlorpromazine	10–20 L/kg	Acetaminophen	0.8 L/kg
Haloperidol	20–30 L/kg	Digitoxin	0.5 L/kg
Amitriptyline	> 40 L/kg	Ethanol	0.6 L/kg
Imipramine	10–20 L/kg	Isoniazid	0.6 L/kg
Digoxin	6–10 L/kg	Lithium	1.1 L/kg
Meperidine	4 L/kg	Phenytoin	0.6 L/kg
Methadone	5 L/kg	Salicylate	0.2 L/kg
		Theophylline	0.5 L/kg

Table 45–8. Indications for hemodialysis (HD) or hemoperfusion (HP) in the management of poisoned patients unresponsive to antidotal or supportive therapy.

Indicated immediately if intoxication is significant
Methanol (HD)
Ethylene glycol (HD)
Lithium (HD)
Paraquat (HP)
Salicylate (HD)
Theophylline (HP preferred over HD)
Indicated if supportive measures are unsuccessful or if prolonged coma is expected
Phenobarbital (HP preferred over HD)
Ethchlorvynol (HP)
Digitoxin (HP)
Tricyclic antidepressants (HP)
Not indicated
Digoxin
Benzodiazepines (diazepam, chlordiazepoxide)
Glutethimide
Narcotics
Short-acting barbiturates
Amphetamines, phencyclidine, cocaine
Quinidine, procainamide
Chlorpromazine, haloperidol, and other antipsychotics

likely to cross cell membranes, and their reabsorption to the renal tubular epithelium is decreased. The clinical significance of these measures depends on the contribution of renal elimination to total body clearance. It is also important to consider the possible adverse effects of overhydration, alkalemia, or acidemia. **Note:** Most studies have failed to show a significant effect of forced diuresis or pH manipulation on the outcome of poisoning.

Weak acids such as salicylate and phenobarbital are more fully ionized in basic solutions, so that alkalizing the urine may serve to trap them in the tubular lumen, thus increasing excretion of the drug in the urine.

Weak bases such as amphetamines, strychnine, and phencyclidine are more ionized in an acid medium; acidification of the urine has been proposed to enhance their removal. However, acidification may promote myoglobinuric renal failure in patients with rhabdomyolysis, a common complication of poisoning by these agents, and is no longer recommended.

2. Hemodialysis—During hemodialysis, toxin is removed from the blood into a dialysate solution across a semipermeable membrane. The toxin must be relatively water soluble and not highly protein bound. It should have a small volume of distribution and slow rate of intrinsic elimination (ie, a long half-life). Hemodialysis is effective in removing methanol, ethylene glycol, salicylates, and lithium, among other drugs (see Table 45–8). It is also of value in correcting pH and electrolyte imbalances, especially in anuric patients.

3. Peritoneal dialysis—This method is much less efficient than hemodialysis in removing most drugs.

4. Hemoperfusion—In hemoperfusion, blood is pumped through a column of adsorbent material (charcoal or resin) and returned to the patient's circulation. Vascular access similar to that for hemodialysis is required. The kinetic conditions required are the same as in hemodialysis; that is, the drug should have a small volume of distribution and a slow rate of intrinsic clearance. Hemoperfusion has the advantage that the drug or toxin is in direct contact with the adsorbent material; therefore, high molecular weight, poor water solubility, and even plasma protein binding are not limiting factors as they are in hemodialysis. Hemoperfusion is commonly associated with thrombocytopenia. Hemoperfusion will not correct pH or electrolyte imbalances.

5. Repeated doses of activated charcoal—Repeated doses of charcoal given orally or via gastric tube (20–30 g every 3–4 hours without a cathartic) may enhance elimination of some drugs and toxins from the bloodstream by a type of so-called gut dialysis. Drugs for which this may be useful can be recalled by the mnemonic ABCD: **a**ntimalarials (quinine) and **a**minophylline, **b**arbiturates (phenobarbital), **b**-blockers (nadolol), **c**arbamazepine, and **d**apsone.

C. ANTIDOTES

Table 45–9 sets forth several common useful antidotes. Their indications and dosages are discussed below in the sections on specific toxins. The half-life of the antidote relative to that of the toxin must be considered. Most important, antidotes should not be used indiscriminately and without regard for the patient's clinical condition. They may have serious side effects and in some cases may be more toxic than the poison. *Note:* Always treat the specific symptoms manifested by the patient, not those known to be associated with a certain poison.

■ MANAGEMENT OF CONDITIONS ASSOCIATED WITH POISONING

Airway Management

It is essential to protect the lungs from aspiration and maintain adequate ventilation and oxygenation. In the patient with a depressed gag reflex, gastric lavage and

Table 45–9. Some poisons for which there are specific antidotes.

Poison	Specific Antidote
Acetaminophen	Acetylcysteine
Anticholinergics	Physostigmine
Anticholinesterases (organophosphates, carbamates, physostigmine)	Atropine Pralidoxime (2-PAM)
Benzodiazepines	Flumazenil
β-Blockers	Glucagon
Calcium-channel blockers	Calcium
Carbon monoxide	100% Oxygen
Cyanide	Sodium nitrite Sodium thiosulfate Vitamin B_{12} (not yet approved for use in the United States)
Digoxin	Digoxin-specific antibodies
Heavy metals	Chelating agents
Isoniazid	Pyridoxine (vitamin B_6)
Methanol, ethylene glycol	Ethanol, folate, 4-methyl pyrazole (not approved for use in the United States)
Narcotics	Naloxone
Tricyclic antidepressants	Sodium bicarbonate

administration of activated charcoal may result in significant aspiration.

A. PATIENTS IN COMA OR WITH MARKEDLY DEPRESSED GAG REFLEX

Endotracheal intubation should always be performed in these patients, especially before gastric lavage.

B. AWAKE PATIENT WITH NORMAL GAG REFLEX

Gastric intubation and lavage may be performed without special precautions.

C. LETHARGIC PATIENT

The lethargic patient with fluctuating mental status and a variable gag reflex poses a more difficult problem in management. If the gag reflex is intact, cautious gastric lavage may be performed with the patient in the left lateral decubitus position and with the head of the bed or stretcher tilted down at an angle of 10–20 degrees. *Note:* If there is any doubt about the patient's ability to protect the airway with a gag or cough reflex, gastric lavage must be preceded by intubation with a cuffed endotracheal tube.

If intubation is not immediately performed, it is critical to monitor the status of the airway closely and to position the patient so as to preserve aspiration. An initially responsive patient may rapidly become more obtunded. Significant swelling and upper airway obstruction may be late developments after thermal, chemical, or caustic burns.

Seizures

See Chapter 17.

A. General Management

Management of drug-induced seizures is generally the same as that for seizures due to other causes, that is, protection of the airway; use of anticonvulsants; and correction of acidosis, hypoxemia, electrolyte abnormalities, and hyperthermia. Seizures unrelated to poisoning may also occur as a result of intracranial bleeding from trauma, hypoglycemia, or hyponatremia. Seizures caused by poisoning are rarely focal, nor are they associated with asymmetric neurologic findings. Meningitis may mimic metabolic or toxic encephalopathy and must be ruled out by lumbar puncture (Chapter 40).

B. Specific Therapy

In certain types of poisoning, refractory seizures may require specific therapy:

1. Seizures occurring as a result of theophylline, lithium, or salicylate overdose usually require hemodialysis or hemoperfusion to accelerate removal of the drug.

2. In isoniazid poisoning with seizures refractory to diazepam, administer pyridoxine, 5 g (or 1 g per gram of isoniazid ingested) intravenously.

3. Seizures due to organophosphate poisoning may respond to atropine and pralidoxime. (See "Organophosphates & Other Cholinesterase Inhibitors" section, below.)

Hypotension

(See Chapter 9.) Hypotension is a common associated condition in victims of poisoning. The mechanism of hypotension may be direct cardiac depression, peripheral vasodilation, or fluid defects or shifts that result in hypovolemia. Concurrent hypothermia may aggravate hypotension. Be alert for possible concurrent trauma with occult internal bleeding or concurrent infection with septic shock.

In the absence of associated pulmonary edema, a fluid challenge should be given with intravenous bo-luses of 1 L of normal saline. A central venous or pulmonary artery catheter may need to be inserted to monitor fluid needs and response to therapy in cases of refractory hypotension. Monitoring of urine output with an indwelling catheter is recommended. If hypotension and hypoperfusion are severe and unresponsive to administration of fluids and temperature correction, vasopressors may be of benefit.

Thermodysregulation

See Chapter 44 for further details of the management of hypothermia and hyperthermia.

A. Hyperthermia

1. Causes—Many drugs cause hyperthermia, either by direct toxic effects on temperature-regulating mechanisms or through associated hyperactivity or seizures.

a. Salicylates—Salicylate intoxication causes hyperthermia by uncoupling of oxidative phosphorylation, resulting in inefficient (and therefore heat-generating) production of ATP.

b. Phenothiazines—Phenothiazines inhibit the autoregulatory ability of the central nervous system, leading to environmentally induced hypothermia or hyperthermia.

c. Seizures or hyperactivity—Hyperthermia may result from seizures or extreme hyperactivity (particularly if the patient has to be forcibly restrained) following poisoning by phencyclidine or amphetamines.

d. Anticholinergic properties—The anticholinergic properties of many drugs (eg, antihistamines, tricyclic antidepressants) can aggravate hyperthermia by inhibiting sweating.

2. Treatment—For dangerous core temperatures above 41 °C (105.8 °F), cool the patient rapidly by sponge bathing with evaporation accelerated by fanning and ice packs; treat seizures. Muscular hyperactivity is most effectively treated with benzodiazepines or neuromuscular paralysis and assisted ventilation.

B. Hypothermia

Hypothermia may be caused by certain drugs, exposure to cold, hypoglycemia, sepsis, or hypothyroidism. The diagnosis may be missed if a rectal thermometer capable of reading temperatures in the range of 24–32 °C (75.2–89.6 °F) is not used.

For severe hypothermia, rapidly restore normal body temperature with warm intravenous fluids, warm gastric or peritoneal lavage, or ventilation with warmed, humidified air. Slow passive rewarming by external means is usually sufficient in milder cases.

Delayed Severe Toxicity

Initial evaluation may fail to reveal the seriousness of poisoning with some drugs. Severe, potentially preventable hepatic damage may occur after acetaminophen overdose unless the physician determines acetaminophen levels and administers the antidote acetylcysteine, when appropriate, early in treatment. Other poisons with characteristically delayed severe toxicity are listed in Table 45–10.

The development of sustained-release preparations has increased the chances of nearly normal results on initial evaluation. The possibility that a sustained-release preparation has been used must be considered in theophylline or salicylate poisoning, because with these drugs, serum or blood concentrations are used to evaluate the severity of intoxication. Under these circumstances, it is prudent to observe the patient longer and obtain a second blood-level reading before deciding on further treatment and disposition.

Barceloux D, McGuigan M, Hartigan-Go K: Position statement: cathartics. American Academy of Clinical Toxicology; European Association of Poisons Centres and Clinical Toxicologists. J Toxicol Clin Toxicol 1997;35:743. [PMID: 9482428] (Guidelines on the use of cathartics in overdose.)

Bowden CA et al: Clinical applications of commonly used contemporary antidotes. Drug Saf 1997;16:9. [PMID: 9010641] (Review of commonly used antidotes in poisoning.)

Chyka PA et al: Position statement: single-dose activated charcoal. American Academy of Clinical Toxicology; European Association of Poisons Centres and Clinical Toxicologists. J Toxicol Clin Toxicol 1997;35:721. [PMID: 9482427] (Guidelines on the use of charcoal in overdose.)

Krenzelok EP et al: Position statement: ipecac syrup. American Academy of Clinical Toxicology; European Association of Poisons Centres and Clinical Toxicologists. J Toxicol Clin Toxicol 1997;35:699. [PMID: 9482425] (Guidelines on the use of ipecac syrup in overdose.)

Table 45–10. Selected examples of poisons with delayed severe toxicity.

Poison	Delayed Effect
Acetaminophen	Hepatic necrosis
Amanita mushrooms	Hepatic necrosis
Carbon tetrachloride	Hepatic and renal damage
Methanol	Blindness
Paraquat	Pulmonary fibrosis
Super-warfarins	Bleeding
Thallium	Peripheral neuropathy, hair loss
Ethylene glycol	Renal failure

Larsen LC et al: Oral poisoning: guidelines for initial evaluation and treatment. Am Fam Physician 1998;57:85. [PMID: 9447216] (Practical review of the evaluation and treatment of the poisoned patient.)

Poisindex. http://www.micromedex.com/products/poisindex (Web site containing information on individual drugs and treatment for poisoning.)

Proudfoot A: Practical management of the poisoned patient. Ther Drug Monit 1998;20:498. [PMID: 9780125] (Review of the management of the poisoned patient.)

Tenenbein M: Position statement: whole bowel irrigation. American Academy of Clinical Toxicology; European Association of Poisons Centres and Clinical Toxicologists. J Toxicol Clin Toxicol 1997;35:753. [PMID: 9482429] (Guidelines on the use of whole bowel irrigation in overdose.)

Vale JA: Position statement: gastric lavage. American Academy of Clinical Toxicology; European Association of Poisons Centres and Clinical Toxicologists. J Toxicol Clin Toxicol 1997;35:711. [PMID: 9482426] (Guidelines on the use of gastric lavage in overdose.)

Watson ID: Laboratory support for the poisoned patient. Ther Drug Monit 1998;20:490. [PMID: 9780124] (Discussion of the types of laboratory analysis available in the evaluation of the poisoned patient.)

■ EMERGENCY TREATMENT OF SPECIFIC POISONINGS

ACETAMINOPHEN

ESSENTIALS OF DIAGNOSIS

- *Patient may be asymptomatic early after ingestion or present with anorexia, nausea, and right upper quadrant pain.*
- *Draw 4-hour postingestion levels, and use the nomogram (Figure 45–1) to predict severity.*
- *Acetylcysteine therapy is antidote if level of acetaminophen is above the possible toxicity line.*

General Considerations

Acetaminophen is a widely used ingredient in numerous over-the-counter and prescription preparations. One of the products of the normal metabolism of acetaminophen is hepatotoxic; at toxic levels, it saturates the glutathione detoxification system in the liver and accumulates, causing delayed hepatic injury (24–72 hours after ingestion). The toxic dose of acetaminophen is considered to be over 140 mg/kg. The margin of safety

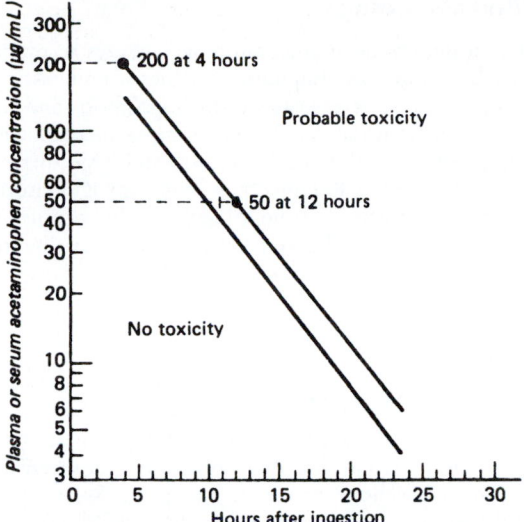

Figure 45–1. Nomogram for prediction of aceta-minophen hepatotoxicity following acute overdosage. The upper line defines serum acetaminophen concentrations known to be associated with hepatotoxicity. The lower line defines serum levels 25% below those expected to cause hepatotoxicity. To give a margin for error, the lower line should be used as a guide to treatment. (Modified and reproduced, with permission, from Rumack BM, Matthew M: Acetaminophen poisoning and toxicity. Pediatrics 1975;55:871.)

is probably lower in patients who are chronic alcohol abusers, those with liver disease who have been fasting, and those with induced microsomal enzymes (most commonly from other drugs).

Clinical Findings

Caution: Shortly after ingestion of acetaminophen, there may be no symptoms or only anorexia or nausea; hepatic necrosis may not become clinically apparent until 24–48 hours later, when nausea, jaundice, and markedly elevated results on liver function tests may appear. Hepatic failure may follow.

Treatment

A. GENERAL MANAGEMENT

Provide intensive supportive care and gastrointestinal decontamination as described previously. Administer activated charcoal regardless of the possibility that acetylcysteine may be administered (see below).

B. ESTIMATION OF SEVERITY

Obtain a 4-hour postingestion acetaminophen serum concentration measurement, and use the nomogram (see Figure 45–1) to predict the range of severity. If the 4-hour level is over 150 µg/mL, or if a toxic dose (7.5 g) is suspected to have been ingested, begin treatment with acetylcysteine. Because acetaminophen and salicylate are often ingested simultaneously, a measurement of serum salicylate concentration should also be obtained immediately.

The Rumack-Matthew nomogram (see Figure 45–1) is not helpful in determining the need for *N*-acetylcysteine (NAC) in chronic or enteric-coated ingestions. In these cases, 2 serum acetaminophen levels should be obtained 4–6 hours apart and treatment given if either level is above the possible toxicity line.

C. ACETYLCYSTEINE THERAPY

Acetylcysteine (Mucomyst) substitutes for glutathione and binds the toxic metabolite of acetaminophen, thus inactivating and detoxifying it. Give 140 mg/kg orally of a 10% or 20% solution diluted to 5% with citrus juice or soda. Follow with 70 mg/kg orally every 4 hours for 18 doses. If the patient vomits a dose within 1 hour, it should be repeated; slow drip by nasogastric tube and administration of an antiemetic (eg, metoclopramide, 10–20 mg intravenously) may be helpful. The intravenous dosing of NAC is used extensively in the United Kingdom and in Canada and is beginning to be used in the United States, although it has not been approved by the U.S. Food and Drug Administration (FDA). Intravenous NAC, 0.2 g/mL, is given after a 1:5 dilution in 5% dextrose in water over 1 hour. The initial dose is 140 mg/kg followed by 70 mg/kg every 4 hours for an additional 12 doses. Anaphylactoid reactions have been reported with the use of intravenous NAC. Both the oral and intravenous routes have been demonstrated in multiple studies to be effective.

The effectiveness of acetylcysteine depends on its use early in treatment; it must be given within 12–16 hours of ingestion of acetaminophen and preferably within 8–10 hours. Do not delay treatment if a serum acetaminophen level is not readily available and a toxic dose may have been taken. Treat with NAC empirically and reevaluate treatment after the acetaminophen level has returned. NAC can be given in conjunction with activated charcoal without any change in dosing. NAC can also be safely given in pregnancy.

Disposition

Use serum concentration of acetaminophen as a guide to the severity of poisoning, and hospitalize all patients requiring acetylcysteine therapy and those with evidence of hepatotoxicity.

Bailey B et al: Management of anaphylactoid reactions to intravenous N-acetylcysteine. Ann Emerg Med 1998;31:710. [PMID: 9624310] (Retrospective case study and literature review of patients who developed anaphylactoid reactions to intravenous NAC.)

Cetaruk EW et al: Tylenol Extended Relief overdose. Ann Emerg Med 1997;30:104. [PMID: 9209234] (Retrospective case analysis of the evaluation and management of overdose with Tylenol Extended Relief.)

Kozer E et al: Management of paracetamol overdose: current controversies. Drug Saf 2001;24:503. [PMID: 11444723] (Review of both oral and intravenous NAC in acetaminophen overdose.)

Woo OF et al: Shorter duration of oral N-acetylcysteine therapy for acute acetaminophen overdose. Ann Emergency Med 2000;35:363. [PMID: 10736123] (Retrospective case series evaluating the safety and efficacy of a shorter NAC regimen.)

AMPHETAMINES & OTHER RELATED STIMULANTS

 ESSENTIALS OF DIAGNOSIS

- *All drugs in this class are central nervous system stimulants.*
- *Predominant symptom is sympathetic hyperactivity.*
- *Treatment is supportive; no specific antidote is available.*

General Considerations

Amphetamines and other stimulants are easily abused because of their wide availability, primarily through street sales of illicit drugs but also in the so-called legal-high diet preparations. These drug combinations may contain varying amounts of methamphetamine, methylene-dioxyamphetamine (MDA), caffeine, ephedrine, and phenylpropanolamine. Illicitly obtained stimulants may also contain phencyclidine. Cocaine is discussed later in this chapter.

All of these drugs are central nervous system stimulants and cause sympathetic hyperactivity. Some may produce significant vasoconstriction, causing hypertension and bradycardia. Most of these drugs have short half-lives, and their peak effect and toxicity occur within 30 minutes after intravenous or intramuscular administration and 2–3 hours after oral ingestion. As a result, serum drug level measurements are of little value, and measures to enhance elimination generally do not alter the outcome.

Clinical Findings

Significant amphetamine poisoning is always accompanied by symptoms. Euphoria, mydriasis, and restlessness progress in severe cases to toxic psychosis and seizures. Hypertension can be severe and associated with palpitations or arrhythmias. Seizures and hyperthermia may produce rhabdomyolysis and myoglobinuria. Phenylpropanolamine is no longer available because of documented cases of severe toxic encephalopathy and even cerebrovascular accidents.

Treatment

A. GENERAL MANAGEMENT

Provide intensive supportive care and gastrointestinal decontamination as described previously. For severe agitation or psychotic behavior, diazepam, 5–10 mg in adults (0.2–0.5 mg/kg intravenously in children), may be helpful; repeat every 5–10 minutes until sedation has been achieved. Lorazepam, 4–8 mg intravenously in adults (0.05–0.1 mg/kg in children), or haloperidol, 0.1–0.2 mg/kg intramuscularly, is also effective.

B. TREATMENT OF SEIZURES

Treat seizures with diazepam, followed by phenobarbital, phenytoin, or both if seizures are uncontrollable or recur (Chapter 17.)

C. TREATMENT OF HYPERTENSION

Hypertension is generally transient and, unless severe, does not require treatment. Often the hypertension responds to benzodiazepine administration, but in severe cases (eg, diastolic blood pressure > 120 mm Hg, encephalopathy), intravenous nitroprusside, 0.5–1.0 μg/kg/min, is effective and easily titratable. Phentolamine, 0.1 mg/kg slowly intravenously, is an alternative drug.

D. TREATMENT OF ARRHYTHMIAS

Tachycardia and ventricular tachyarrhythmias may respond to administration of propranolol, 0.05–0.1 mg/kg intravenously.

E. OTHER MEASURES

Monitor temperature, and start cooling measures if hyperthermia occurs. Check the urine for myoglobin. Acidification of the urine is not recommended.

If chest pain is present, perform an ECG and cardiac enzymes, and consider hospitalization to rule out myocardial ischemia or infarction.

Patients with seizures may require computed tomography (CT) scanning to rule out intracranial hemorrhage.

Disposition

Hospitalize patients with complications (psychotic behavior, hypertension, hyperthermia, chest pain, arrhythmias) or those with prolonged symptoms.

Albertson TE et al: Methamphetamine and the expanding complications of amphetamines. West J Med 1999;170:214. [PMID: 10344175] (Review of the toxicity of methamphetamine use.)

Chan TC et al: Drug-induced hyperthermia. Crit Care Clin 1997;13:785. [PMID: 9330841] (Review of the pathophysiology, presentation, and treatment of sympathomimetic poisoning.)

Mersfelder TL: Phenylpropanolamine and stroke: the study, the FDA ruling, the implications. Cleve Clin J Med 2001;68: 208. [PMID: 11263849] (Review of phenylpropanolamine side effects and toxicity.)

Richards JR et al: Methamphetamine abuse and rhabdomyolysis in the ED: a 5-year study. Am J Emerg Med 1999;17:681. [PMID: 10597089] (Retrospective case review of patients with rhabdomyolysis and methamphetamine use.)

ANTICHOLINERGICS

 ## ESSENTIALS OF DIAGNOSIS

- *Ingestion produces many symptoms prompting the phrase "blind as a bat, hot as Hades, red as a beet, dry as a bone, and mad as a hatter."*
- *Treatment is primarily supportive, although physostigmine can be used in life-threatening situations.*

General Considerations

Atropine, scopolamine, belladonna, many antihistamines, and tricyclic antidepressants are anticholinergics. Many plants (eg, jimsonweed [*Datura stramonium*], nightshade, *Amanita muscaria* mushrooms) also contain anticholinergic compounds.

Clinical Findings

These drugs block cholinergic receptors both centrally and peripherally. Ingestion of a significant amount of an anticholinergic drug can produce many clinical effects. The popular phrase "blind as a bat, hot as Hades, red as a beet, dry as a bone, mad as a hatter" describes many of the manifestations of anticholinergic toxicity. Other signs and symptoms include tachycardia, gastrointestinal ileus, urinary retention, delirium, and hallucinations. Seizures can also occur.

Treatment

Provide intensive supportive care and gastrointestinal decontamination as described previously. Most patients can be managed with supportive measures alone, including sedation with benzodiazepines, cooling, and bladder emptying. If a patient develops life-threatening complications of anticholinergic toxicity (hemodynamically significant tachycardia, hyperthermia, or seizures resistant to benzodiazepines), physostigmine, 1–2 mg intravenously over 2 minutes, can be given. Physostigmine works within minutes, and the duration of effect is 30–60 minutes. It has been associated with severe complications, including bradycardia, heart block, and seizures. Atropine should be readily available if the antidote is used, and ECG monitoring is necessary. ***Note:*** Physostigmine should never be used as a diagnostic test for patients with an altered mental status or hallucinations. Physostigmine is contraindicated in patients with an overdose of any drug that could delay intraventricular conduction (tricyclic antidepressants), asthma, or mechanical bowel or bladder obstruction.

Disposition

Hospitalize patients who have incapacitating signs or symptoms of anticholinergic poisoning.

Chan TC et al: Drug-induced hyperthermia. Crit Care Clin 1997;13:785. [PMID: 9330841] (Review of the pathophysiology, presentation, and treatment of anticholinergic poisoning.)

Dewitt MS et al: The dangers of jimson weed and its abuse by teenagers in the Kanawha Valley of West Virginia. WV Med J 1997;93:182. [PMID: 9274142] (Case review of jimson weed ingestion evaluation and treatment.)

Grace RF: Benztropine abuse and overdose—case report and review. Adverse Drug React Toxicol Rev 1997;16:103. [PMID: 9359932] (Case report and review of the management of anticholinergic overdose.)

Weiner AL et al: Anticholinergic poisoning with adulterated intranasal cocaine. Am J Emerg Med 1998;16:517. [PMID: 9725971] (Case report of the presentation of cocaine and anticholinergic toxicity.)

β-ADRENERGIC BLOCKING AGENTS

 ## ESSENTIALS OF DIAGNOSIS

- *Ingestion of a large amount of β-blockers primarily affects the cardiac system.*
- *Symptoms of ingestion include hypotension, bradycardia, and bronchoconstriction.*
- *Plasma levels are not useful.*
- *Glucagon can be used to treat hypotension if fluids are unsuccessful; glucagon can also be used to*

treat arrhythmias, but cardiac pacing may be required in severe cases.

General Considerations

β-Adrenergic blocking agents are widely used in clinical medicine to treat hypertension, arrhythmias, angina pectoris, migraine headache, and thyrotoxicosis. β-Blockers act by competing with catecholamines for a finite number of β_1 and β_2 receptor sites. The β_1 receptors are responsible for increasing the force and rate of cardiac contraction. The β_2 receptors mediate vasodilatation; bronchial smooth muscle dilation; and a number of metabolic effects, including glycogenolysis. Excessive β blockade can therefore cause hypoglycemia, bradycardia, bronchoconstriction, and hypoglycemia. In overdose, β_1 and β_2 selectivity is lost, and generalized β blockade is seen. Some agents (eg, pindolol) have partial intrinsic sympathomimetic activity and may cause hypertension and tachycardia in overdose.

Clinical Findings

The main features of massive β-blocker overdose are hypotension and bradycardia. Pulmonary edema or bronchospasm may also occur, especially in patients with preexisting congestive heart failure or asthma. Hypoglycemia and hyperkalemia are sometimes seen. Convulsions are common with propranolol and other agents (eg, oxprenolol) with high lipid solubility and marked membrane-depressant effects. Seizures have not been reported with atenolol, pindolol, or practolol. The ECG may show sinus bradycardia, atrioventricular blocks, or a prolonged QRS interval. In rare cases ventricular tachyarrhythmias may occur, especially with sotalol overdose. Death is usually due to profound myocardial depression, with advanced atrioventricular block or asystole. The heart may not respond to attempts at pacing, even with high currents.

Plasma levels of β-blockers are not clinically useful and are not routinely available.

Treatment

A. GENERAL MANAGEMENT

General management of overdose, including airway protection, treatment of hypoglycemia, and gastrointestinal decontamination should be undertaken as outlined earlier.

B. TREATMENT OF HYPOTENSION

Treat hypotension initially with fluids. If this is unsuccessful, use glucagon, 5–10 mg (100–150 μg/kg) as an intravenous bolus, followed by an infusion of 2–5 mg/h.

Glucagon increases intracellular cyclic AMP by a mechanism different from that of β receptors. If the initial bolus is unsuccessful, a second bolus may be tried up to a maximum dosage of 10 mg.

C. TREATMENT OF ARRHYTHMIAS

Advanced atrioventricular block or bradycardia resulting in hypotension can also be treated initially with glucagon; atropine, 0.01–0.03 mg/kg intravenously, or isoproterenol, 0.05–0.3 μg/kg/min by intravenous infusion, may also be used. If these are unsuccessful, cardiac pacing may be necessary.

D. OTHER MEASURES

Enhance elimination. Because of the relatively large volume of distribution and extensive protein binding, dialysis is not likely to be of value for propranolol overdose. Less lipophilic agents (eg, atenolol, nadolol) have much smaller volumes of distribution and may be eliminated by dialysis or hemoperfusion, but they are less likely to cause profound toxicity.

Disposition

Patients should remain under observation for at least 6–8 hours after ingestion. Patients with significant β-blocker intoxication (eg, profound bradycardia, conduction abnormalities, hypotension, shock) should be hospitalized.

Love JN et al: Characterization of fatal beta blocker ingestion: a review of the American Association of Poison Control Centers data from 1985–1995. J Toxicol Clin Toxicol 1997;354:353. [PMID: 9204094] (Retrospective review of β-blocker-related fatalities.)

White CM: A review of potential cardiovascular uses of intravenous glucagon administration. J Clin Pharmacol 1999;39:442. [PMID: 10234590] (Review of the use of glucagon in the treatment of β-blocker overdose.)

CALCIUM-CHANNEL BLOCKING AGENTS

 ESSENTIALS OF DIAGNOSIS

- *Ingestion of a large amount of calcium-channel blockers can cause hypotension, bradycardia, and central nervous system depression.*
- *Treatment is primarily supportive, although both calcium and glucagon can be used to treat hypotension and bradycardia.*
- *Levels of calcium-channel blockers are not useful.*

General Considerations

Calcium-channel blockers are being used with increasing frequency for supraventricular tachycardia, hypertension, rate control in atrial fibrillation or atrial flutter, angina, and vasospasm. These agents block the slow calcium channels and have the following cardiovascular effects: they depress sinus node activity, slow atrioventricular nodal conduction, cause coronary and peripheral vasodilatation, and depress myocardial contractility. Verapamil and diltiazem have the most marked myocardial effects and are especially dangerous in patients with sinus or atrioventricular nodal disease, Wolff-Parkinson-White syndrome, on digitalis therapy or in patients receiving β-blockers, quinidine, disopyramide, or other myocardial depressant drugs. Nifedipine is especially dangerous in patients receiving nitrates or β-blockers and in patients with obstructive valvular heart disease. Nifedipine is more likely than verapamil or diltiazem to be associated with increased heart rate and vasodilatation. Calcium-channel blockers may also block insulin release, resulting in hyperglycemia.

Clinical Findings

The main manifestations of calcium-channel blocker overdose are hypotension, bradycardia, and depressed mental function. Bradydysrhythmias result from sinoatrial and atrioventricular nodal conduction dissociation. If the ingestion is a sustained-release preparation, toxicity and symptoms may be delayed for 6–8 hours. With regular-release preparations, toxicity is generally seen in 2–3 hours. Hyperkalemia and seizures, which are sometimes observed in overdoses of β-blockers, are not prominent in overdoses of calcium-channel blockers. The ECG shows evidence of bradyarrhythmia with atrioventricular block. Death results from severe myocardial depression leading to asystole.

Treatment

A. GENERAL MANAGEMENT

General management includes airway protection and gastrointestinal decontamination. Give multidose activated charcoal and initiate whole bowel irrigation in a patient who may have ingested sustained-release preparations.

B. CARDIAC CARE

Constant cardiac monitoring is essential. Appropriate pharmacologic management in seriously ill patients may require placement of central intravenous lines.

Leg elevation, Trendelenburg positioning, and fluid management may be required.

Advanced atrioventricular block and bradycardia resulting in hypotension may be treated initially with atropine, 0.01–0.03 mg/kg intravenously. Cardiac pacing may be required.

C. OTHER MEASURES

In hypotensive patients not responding to the therapy outlined above, calcium solutions have sometimes been successful. Administer 10% calcium chloride, 10–20 mL for adults (10–30 mg/kg for children) intravenously, or 10% calcium gluconate, 10–20 mL for adults (0.2–0.4 mL/kg for children), followed by repeated boluses or continuous intravenous infusion as necessary. Calcium administration improves the blood pressure more than the heart rate. As in β-blocker overdose, glucagon may improve both heart rate and blood pressure. An initial bolus of 2–5 mg intravenously may be given and followed by up to a total of 10 mg if no response is seen. If glucagon improves the patient's hemodynamics, then an infusion should be started. Isoproterenol, epinephrine, phenylephrine, or amrinone may be required for severe, unresponsive hypotension.

Disposition

Asymptomatic patients should be observed for at least 8–10 hours. Patients with significant calcium-channel blocker overdose should be hospitalized for monitoring and observation.

Adams BD et al: Amlodipine overdose causes prolonged calcium channel blocker toxicity. Am J Emerg Medi 1998;16:527. [PMID: 9725975] (Case report of amlodipine overdose with treatment overview.)

Papadopoulos J et al: Utilization of a glucagon infusion in the management of a massive nifedipine overdose. J Emerg Med 2000;18:453. [PMID: 10802424] (Case report of nifedipine overdose with glucagon as the treatment.)

White CM: A review of potential cardiovascular uses of intravenous glucagon administration. J Clin Pharmacol 1999;39:442. [PMID: 10234590]. (Review of the use of glucagon in the treatment of calcium-channel blocker overdose.)

CARBON MONOXIDE

 ESSENTIALS OF DIAGNOSIS

- *Carbon monoxide is a colorless and odorless gas that binds with great affinity to hemoglobin.*
- *Severe tissue hypoxia results.*
- *Carbon monoxide levels correlate with severity of symptoms and should be used to guide treatment.*

• *Treatment is with 100% oxygen; hyperbaric oxygen can also be used in certain circumstances.*

General Considerations

Carbon monoxide, a colorless, odorless, and tasteless gas, is produced by incomplete combustion of organic materials and is found in engine exhaust, gas heaters, burning charcoal briquettes, and solid alcohol (Sterno Canned Heat, many others). Any fire may also produce large quantities of carbon monoxide.

Carbon monoxide binds to hemoglobin with an affinity about 200 times greater than that of oxygen. The resulting carboxyhemoglobin complex cannot transport oxygen, causing tissue hypoxia that can lead to death or permanent neurologic damage if untreated. Hemoglobin saturation and blood oxygen content are dangerously low despite adequate (or elevated) arterial PO_2 levels.

Clinical Findings

The severity of symptoms usually correlates with carboxyhemoglobin levels (Table 45–11). The carboxyhemoglobin level can be from either venous or arterial blood. The earliest reliable diagnostic symptom is headache. Usually, PO_2 is normal, although metabolic acidosis due to tissue hypoxia may be present. Using oxygen saturation calculated from PO_2 (based on assumption of normal hemoglobin) or measured by pulse oximetry will provide an incorrect estimate of oxygen-carrying capacity. Blood may be cherry-red, but the patient rarely appears pink. The ECG may show ischemia or infarction in a person with coronary disease. Delayed central nervous system effects such as parkinsonism, memory loss, and personality changes can occur after recovery.

Treatment

Note: Act quickly. Delay in treatment may worsen neurologic damage.

A. GENERAL MANAGEMENT

Administer 100% oxygen by nonrebreathing face mask or endotracheal tube, *not* by nasal cannula or loose-fitting face mask. Oxygen competes with carbon monoxide for hemoglobin-binding sites. The half-life of carboxyhemoglobin in a person breathing room air is 5–6 hours; in 100% oxygen, it is only 1 hour. Hyperbaric 100% oxygen lowers the carboxyhemoglobin level even more rapidly (23 minutes), but it is seldom readily available and no studies have demonstrated a reduction in post–carbon monoxide poisoning neurologic deficits in patients receiving hyperbaric oxygen versus 100% oxygen. Consider hyperbaric oxygen for patients with major symptoms of carbon monoxide intoxication such as loss of consciousness or myocardial ischemia or if the patient is pregnant.

B. BLOOD TESTS

Obtain arterial blood for measurement of carboxyhemoglobin content and arterial blood gases.

C. CHEST X-RAY

If carbon monoxide poisoning is associated with smoke inhalation, obtain a chest x-ray and consider hospitalization and monitoring for development of noncardiogenic pulmonary edema.

Table 45–11. Clinical findings in carbon monoxide poisoning.

Estimated Carbon Monoxide Concentration (parts per million)	Carboxyhemoglobin (% of Total Hemoglobin)	Symptoms
Less than 35 ppm (cigarette smoking)	5	None, or mild headache
0.005% (50 ppm)	10	Slight headache, dyspnea on vigorous exertion
0.01% (100 ppm)	20	Throbbing headache, dyspnea with moderate exertion
0.02% (200 ppm)	30	Severe headache, irritability, fatigue, dimness of vision
0.03–0.05% (300–500 ppm)	40–50	Headache, tachycardia, confusion, lethargy, collapse
0.08–0.12% (800–1200 ppm)	60–70	Coma, convulsions
0.19% (1900 ppm)	80	Rapidly fatal

D. OTHER MEASURES

The use of corticosteroids and mannitol for cerebral edema has been recommended, but their value in preventing late neurologic sequelae remains unproved.

Disposition

All patients with significant carbon monoxide poisoning (ie, with chest pain or other evidence of cardiac ischemia, neurologic signs, or carboxyhemoglobin concentrations above 25%) and pregnant patients must be hospitalized and given oxygen. Oxygen may be administered in a hyperbaric chamber, in the circumstances described earlier in this section.

Gilmer B et al: Hyperbaric oxygen does not prevent neurologic sequelae after carbon monoxide poisoning. Acad Emerg Med 2002;9:1. [PMID: 11772662] (An animal model study evaluating the efficacy of hyperbaric oxygen to treat carbon monoxide poisoning.)

Greingor JL et al: Acute carbon monoxide intoxication during pregnancy. One case report and review of the literature. Emerg Med J 2001;18:399. [PMID: 11559621] (Case report of carbon monoxide poisoning in pregnancy and review of the literature.)

Juurlink DN et al: Hyperbaric oxygen for carbon monoxide poisoning. Cochrane Database System Review 2000;(2): CD002041. [PMID: 10796853] (Meta-analysis of hyperbaric oxygen for carbon monoxide poisoning.)

Sheridan RL et al: Hyperbaric oxygen treatment: a brief overview of a controversial topic. J Trauma 1999;47:426. [PMID: 10452491] (Review of the use of hyperbaric oxygen in carbon monoxide poisoning.)

CARDIAC GLYCOSIDES

ESSENTIALS OF DIAGNOSIS

- *These cardiotoxic drugs result in rhythm and conduction disturbances in the heart and occasionally severe hyperkalemia.*
- *Digoxin levels are indicative of the degree of poisoning in the acute overdose.*
- *Patients with severe arrhythmias or hyperkalemia may benefit from digitalis antibodies to reverse toxicity.*
- *All patients with poisoning require hospitalization.*

General Considerations

Digoxin; digitoxin; and several plant digitalis derivatives including oleander, foxglove, and lily of the valley are the sources of digitalis and the cardiac glycosides.

They are used therapeutically primarily for their ability to slow conduction through the atrioventricular node in disease states such as atrial fibrillation. They also increase the force of myocardial contractility and enhance automaticity. These therapeutic effects also mediate the severity of toxicity.

Digoxin has a large volume of distribution (6–10 L/kg) and a half-life of about 40 hours; for the most part, it is excreted unchanged in the urine. Digitoxin, by contrast, has a small volume of distribution, is highly protein bound, and undergoes extensive enterohepatic recirculation; its half-life is 7 days. In the elderly, the half-life may be increased owing to decreased creatinine clearance.

Clinical Findings

Blurred vision, color vision disturbance (especially with green or yellow vision), and neurologic symptoms may occur. The most serious toxic effects are those that cause rhythm and conduction disturbances in the heart, for example, third-degree atrioventricular block, bradycardia, ventricular ectopy, bidirectional ventricular tachycardia, and paroxysmal atrial tachycardia with atrioventricular block. In patients with chronic atrial fibrillation, digitalis toxicity may cause nonparoxysmal junctional tachycardia, which is characterized by a regular rhythm with narrow QRS complexes and a heart rate of 90–120 beats/min (Chapter 35). Although hypokalemia may aggravate digitalis toxicity in the patient receiving chronic therapy, acute ingestion of an overdose is often associated with hyperkalemia. The plasma potassium level in digoxin overdose is indicative of the degree of poisoning of the Na^+-K^+-ATPase pump; if the potassium is elevated, the toxicity is severe. Therapeutic serum levels of digoxin are 0.5–2 ng/mL; for digitoxin, they are 18–22 ng/mL.

Treatment

A. GENERAL MANAGEMENT

Provide intensive supportive care and gastrointestinal decontamination as described previously. Gastric lavage may worsen bradycardia by enhancing vagal tone.

B. ELECTROLYTE ABNORMALITIES

If hypokalemia is present, replace potassium (Chapter 42). For severe hyperkalemia, measures to reduce the potassium level may be necessary (Chapter 42) in order to reduce the cardiotoxic effects of digitalis. Because the total body potassium is not high, potassium-binding resins (ie, Kayexalate) should not be used. Other measures such as insulin, glucose, and sodium bicarbonate can be attempted in addition to specific antidotal therapy. Avoid the use of calcium, which may potentiate the cardiac toxicity of digitalis. Magnesium replacement may be beneficial.

C. ARRHYTHMIAS

(See also Chapter 35.) For symptomatic bradycardia or second- or third-degree atrioventricular block, atropine, 0.5–1.0 mg intravenously, repeated every 5 minutes if there is no response, may be helpful. The total dose should not exceed 2 mg. A transcutaneous pacemaker may be used.

For ventricular ectopic beats, both lidocaine and phenytoin are effective, although lidocaine is easier to use. Give 1 mg/kg as an intravenous bolus, followed by 1–4 mg/min by continuous infusion. Phenytoin and the new prodrug fosphenytoin are also effective at suppressing atrial and ventricular ectopy.

Avoid direct current (DC) countershock, because it may cause serious conduction and rhythm disturbances including asystole or ventricular fibrillation in patients with digitalis toxicity. If countershock is unavoidable, use the lowest voltage that is effective.

D. DRUG REMOVAL

Dialysis or hemoperfusion is of no value for digoxin because of its large volume of distribution. Digitoxin may be effectively removed by hemoperfusion and by repeated doses of activated charcoal or cholestyramine, which interrupt enterohepatic recirculation.

E. DIGITALIS ANTIBODIES

Digitalis-specific Fab fragment antibodies are extremely effective and are indicated for patients with serious arrhythmias or severe hyperkalemia. Each vial of Digibind binds 0.6 mg of digoxin. Toxicity usually is reversed within 5–10 minutes, and the digoxin-antibody complex is excreted in the urine. After Digibind administration, serum digoxin levels are elevated owing to cross-reaction of the complex in the assay. For information on Digibind use and how to calculate the dosage,

see Table 45–12. When the ingested amount is unknown, 5–10 vials may be given initially.

Disposition

All patients with digitalis and other cardiac glycoside poisoning require hospitalization in a cardiac-monitored unit for observation and treatment. Onset of cardiac toxicity may be delayed for 6–12 hours after acute ingestion.

Barron SW et al: Advances in the management of digoxin toxicity in the older patient. Drugs Aging 1997;10:18. [PMID: 9111705] (Review of digoxin toxicity and treatment in the elderly.)

DiDomenico RJ et al: Analysis of the use of digoxin immune Fab for the treatment of non-life-threatening digoxin toxicity. J Cardiovasc Pharmacol Ther 2000;5:77. [PMID: 11150387] (Analysis of the use of digoxin immune Fab in the treatment of digoxin toxicity.)

Gupta A et al: A case of nondigitalis cardiac glycoside toxicity. Ther Drug Monit 1997;19:711. [PMID: 9421116] (Case study of cardiac glycoside poisoning from oleander.)

Ma G et al: Electrocardiographic manifestations: digitalis toxicity. J Emerg Med 2001;20:145. [PMID: 11207409] (Review of the electrocardiographic manifestations of digitalis toxicity.)

CAUSTICS & CORROSIVES

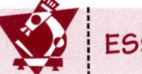 ESSENTIALS OF DIAGNOSIS

- *Includes both acids and alkalis.*
- *Ingestion can result in coagulative (acids) or liquefactive (alkalis) necrosis of tissue.*
- *Treatment is supportive and includes dilution of the material with water, milk, or normal saline.*
- *Endoscopy is recommended to assess degree of damage.*

Table 45–12. Digoxin immune Fab dosing.

To calculate the body load of digoxin:
  Dose ingested (if known) × 0.8
    or

$$\frac{\text{Serum digoxin concentration (ng/mL)} \times 5.6 \text{ L/kg} (V_D) \times \text{wt (kg)}}{1000}$$

$$\text{Digibind dose (number of vials)} = \frac{\text{Body load (mg)}}{0.5 \text{ mg/vial}}$$

$$\textit{Quick estimation: Number of vials} = \frac{\text{Serum digoxin concentration} \times \text{wt (kg)}}{1000}$$

General Considerations

Corrosive agents include strong agents, alkalis (caustics), oxidizing agents, and other chemicals. They are commonly used in household cleaners (Table 45–13).

A. Acids

Toilet bowl cleaners, bleaches, battery acid, soldering flux (zinc chloride), and many industrial sources contain acids.

B. Alkalis

Lye (drain cleaners, reagent tablets used to detect glucose in urine [Clinitest, many others]), ammonia, and industrial-grade detergents contain caustic alkalis.

The mechanism of toxicity is tissue destruction resulting from coagulative (acids) and liquefactive (alkali) necrosis and heat injury during neutralization of the chemical by water in body tissues. Most household bleaches and detergents are dilute and do not cause severe corrosive burns. Concentrated alkalis are common in the household, especially in granular form or strongly concentrated liquids (pH > 12.5), and these cause severe tissue damage. Corrosive burns may lead to airway or intestinal edema and obstruction, mucosal perforation, and (later) stricture formation.

Clinical Findings

Symptoms are almost always present with significant ingestion and include mouth and throat pain, dysphagia, drooling, and substernal or abdominal pain. However, significant gastric or esophageal burns may be present without oral lesions. Skin and eye burns may also occur (Chapters 31 and 43).

Table 45–13. Common corrosive agents.

Type	Examples	Injury
Concentrated alkali	Clinitest tablets Drain cleaners Ammonia Lye Oven cleaners Denture cleaners	Penetrating liquefaction necrosis
Concentrated acids	Pool disinfectants Toilet bowl cleaners	Coagulation necrosis
Weaker cleaning agents	Cationic detergents (dishwasher detergents) Household bleach	Superficial burns and irritation; deep burns (rare)

Treatment

A. General Management

Dilute the corrosive material with water, normal saline, or milk (8 ounces for adults, 4 ounces for children). *Do not* give neutralizers, because they may increase the heat of hydration and worsen subsequent tissue destruction.

Do not induce vomiting, because this may produce further tissue damage. Activated charcoal is contraindicated because it can interfere with endoscopy.

After liquid corrosive ingestion, careful insertion of a nasogastric tube and gastric lavage is recommended by some gastroenterologists.

B. Endoscopy

Diagnostic endoscopy should be performed in any symptomatic patient with or without oral burns. Endoscopy may not be necessary in asymptomatic patients, although this remains controversial.

C. Pharmacologic Treatment

No studies support the efficacy of corticosteroids in preventing stricture formation, and the authors do not recommend them. Esophageal or gastric perforation is a contraindication to their use. Antibiotics are indicated for suspected perforation or infection.

Disposition

Hospitalize all patients known or thought to have ingested or inhaled (aspirated) caustic or corrosive agents with a potential for tissue damage. Skin burns may be managed on an outpatient basis if they are of mild to moderate severity (Chapter 43). Eye injuries should be copiously irrigated and evaluated by an ophthalmologist (Chapter 31).

Gupta SK et al: Is esophagogastroduodenoscopy necessary in all caustic ingestions? J Pediatr Gastroenterol Nutr 2001;32:50. [PMID: 11176325] (Chart review of caustic ingestions evaluating the need for esophagogastroduodenoscopy depending on the initial presentation.)

Millar AJ et al: Detection of caustic esophageal injury with technetium 99m-labelled sucralfate. J Pediatr Surg 2001;36:262. [PMID: 11172412] (Prospective study evaluating radiolabeled sucralfate in the evaluation of caustic injury.)

COCAINE & LOCAL ANESTHETICS

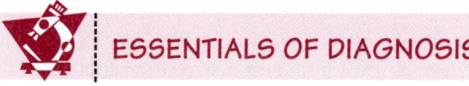

ESSENTIALS OF DIAGNOSIS

- *Overdose of local anesthetics causes initial central nervous system excitement and seizures, followed by central nervous system depression.*

- *Cocaine intoxication causes sympathetic hyperactivity and can result in severe hypertension, myocardial ischemia, and even aortic dissection.*
- *Treatment is supportive and should address any resulting cardiac or central nervous system symptoms.*

General Considerations

Cocaine is a natural extract from coca leaves. It is a local anesthetic that also has sympathomimetic effects. Overdoses of all local anesthetics are manifested by initial excitement and seizures, followed by central nervous system depression. Peak effects occur rapidly, usually in less than 1 hour.

A. COCAINE

All significant overdoses are associated with symptoms. Intravenous injection of cocaine and inhalation (smoking) of freebase, or crack, cocaine may result in very high levels. Cocaine causes euphoria, excitement, and restlessness; toxic psychosis, seizures, hypertension, tachycardia, dysrhythmias, and hyperthermia may follow absorption of toxic amounts. Chest pain, myocardial ischemia and infarction, and aortic dissection have occurred. Blood cocaine and metabolite concentrations vary widely and do not predict the development of clinical findings.

B. LOCAL ANESTHETICS

Common local anesthetics such as lidocaine, mepivacaine, and procaine have no toxic effects in usual doses. With excessive doses, they cause tremors, anxiety, and restlessness, followed by seizures and then cardiorespiratory depression. Toxic doses for these drugs vary and depend on the route and duration of administration. Maximum recommended doses for infiltration anesthesia in adults are lidocaine, 4.5 mg/kg; bupivacaine, 2 mg/kg; and procaine, 7 mg/kg. Larger doses may be tolerated if epinephrine has been included in the preparation.

Treatment

A. GENERAL MANAGEMENT

Provide intensive supportive care and gastrointestinal decontamination as described previously.

B. TREATMENT OF COCAINE OVERDOSE

Treat manifestations of sympathetic hyperactivity in the same way as for amphetamine overdose. Because effects peak rapidly, measures to enhance elimination of the drug from the body are unnecessary.

If a patient is thought to have ingested packets of cocaine (body packers), whole bowel irrigation should be instituted immediately and a surgical consult obtained for removal of the packets.

Patients with chest pain suggestive of ischemia should be evaluated with a 12-lead ECG and considered for admission to rule out myocardial infarction. Myocardial infarction may be present even with a normal ECG. Patients with a new onset of seizures may need CT scanning to rule out intracranial hemorrhage.

C. TREATMENT OF OVERDOSE WITH COMMON LOCAL ANESTHETICS

Treatment consists of supportive measures with particular attention to respiratory depression and hypotension. Seizures are usually brief and easily treatable with benzodiazepines and usually do not require other anticonvulsant therapy.

Disposition

Hospitalize patients with cocaine or local anesthetic poisoning manifested by multiple seizures, hyperthermia, ischemic chest pain, or severe hypertension.

Blaho K et al: Blood cocaine and metabolite concentrations, clinical findings, and outcome of patients presenting to an ED. Am J Emerg Med 2000;18:593. [PMID: 10999576] (Prospective study of cocaine and its metabolites correlated with clinical findings and outcome.)

Dribben WH et al: A pilot study to assess the safety of dobutamine stress echocardiography in the emergency department evaluation of cocaine-associated chest pain. Ann Emerg Med 2001;38:42. [PMID: 11423811] (Prospective case series of patients with cocaine-associated chest pain, evaluating the efficacy of dobutamine stress echocardiography.)

Naguib M et al: Adverse effects and drug interactions associated with local and regional anaesthesia. Drug Saf 1998;18:221. [PMID: 9565736] (Review of the adverse effects with the use of local and regional anesthesia.)

Olmedo R et al: Is surgical decontamination definitive treatment of "body-packers"? Am J Emerg Med 2001;19:593. [PMID: 11699007] (Case reports of body packers and their medical management.)

Singh R et al: Local anaesthetics: an overview of current drugs. Hosp Med 1998;59:880. [PMID: 10197123] (Review of the pharmacology and side effects of local anesthetics.)

Steinhauer JR et al: Spontaneous coronary artery dissection associated with cocaine use: a case report and brief review. Cardiovasc Pathol 2001;10:141. [PMID: 11485859] (Case report and literature review of coronary artery dissection associated with cocaine use.)

CYANIDE

 ESSENTIALS OF DIAGNOSIS

- *Cyanide acts as a cellular asphyxiant that inhibits the use of oxygen by the body's tissues.*

- *Symptom onset is rapid and ultimately results in hypotension.*
- *In mild cases, supportive care including 100% oxygen is adequate.*
- *If poisoning is severe, a cyanide antidote kit of sodium nitrite, amyl nitrite, and sodium thiosulfate should be used.*
- *Cyanide levels are not readily available and should not be used to determine treatment.*
- *All patients with cyanide intoxication should be hospitalized.*

General Considerations

Fumigants, hydrocyanic acid gas used in industry, amygdalin (Laetrile) in fruit pits (eg, apricot, cherry, peach), and burning plastics and fabrics are sources of cyanide. Sodium nitroprusside used to treat severe hypertension undergoes a biotransformation to methemoglobin and cyanide and can be a source of poisoning. Cyanide poisoning has also resulted from metabolism of ingested acetonitrile in an artificial nail-removing solution.

Cyanide is a rapidly absorbed cellular asphyxiant that inhibits the cytochrome oxidase system for oxygen utilization in cells. The inability of the body's tissues to use oxygen leads to anaerobic metabolism and a profound metabolic acidosis. Death may occur within minutes after a dose of 200 mg. In fatal poisoning, blood levels usually exceed $1–2\ \mu g/mL$. Cyanide gas is much more toxic than salt forms because of its rapid absorption, and its effects are usually immediate.

Clinical Findings

Significant poisoning is associated with rapidly developing symptoms, including headache, nausea and vomiting, anxiety, confusion, and collapse. Initial hypertension and tachycardia progress to hypotension, bradycardia, and apnea. The smell of bitter almonds is present occasionally. The skin may appear pink. The measured oxygen saturation of venous blood may be elevated as a result of failure of oxygen uptake by the tissues.

Treatment

Note: Act quickly. To be successful, treatment must be started within 5–10 minutes in cases of severe poisoning. In witnessed cases of cyanide poisoning, begin therapy without waiting for symptoms.

A. GENERAL MANAGEMENT

Supportive care only, including 100% oxygen, may be given to patients with mild to moderate symptoms.

Close observation is needed because the antidote may need to be administered if the patient deteriorates. If activated charcoal is available, administer it at once. Although its binding affinity for cyanide is low, it can adsorb a lethal dose.

B. ANTIDOTE ADMINISTRATION

Every emergency department should have a prepackaged cyanide antidote kit containing sodium nitrite, 300 mg in 10-mL ampules (2); sodium thiosulfate, 12.5 g in 50-mL ampules (2); amyl nitrite inhalant, 0.3 mL (12 Aspirols); and syringes and stomach tube (Table 45–14).

1. Nitrites—Nitrites produce methemoglobin, which binds free cyanide.

1. Break a capsule of amyl nitrite under the patient's nose for deep inhalation while starting an intravenous infusion of sodium nitrite and thiosulfate. A new ampule should be used every 3 minutes until intravenous medication has begun.

2. Give sodium nitrite, 300 mg (10-mL ampule) intravenously for adults; for children, 0.12–0.33 mL/kg up to 10 mL with a normal hemoglobin concentration (for alternate dosing in a child with abnormal hemoglobin, consult Poisindex). ***Caution:*** Do not overtreat; fatal methemoglobinemia has resulted from overzealous use of nitrites. After initial therapy, guide subsequent treatment by monitoring symptoms and signs. The goal of nitrite therapy is a methemoglobin level of 25–30%.

2. Thiosulfate—Sodium thiosulfate is a cofactor in the rhodanese enzyme conversion of cyanide to thiocyanate, which is less toxic and readily excreted. Give thiosulfate, 50 mL of a 25% solution in adults and 1.65 mL/kg of a 25% solution in children, intravenously.

C. VITAMIN B$_{12A}$

Vitamin B$_{12A}$ (hydroxocobalamin) has been successfully used in Europe. Hydroxocobalamin reverses cyanide

Table 45–14. Prepackaged cyanide antidote kit.[1]

Antidote	How Supplied	Dose
Amyl nitrite	0.3 mL (aspirol inhalant)	Break 1–2 aspirols under patient's nose
Sodium nitrite	3 g/dL (300 mg in 10 mL [vials])	300 mg intravenously
Sodium thiosulfate	25 g/dL (12.5 g in 50 mL [vials])	500 mg intravenously

[1]In the United States, manufactured by Taylor Pharmaceuticals.

toxicity by combining with cyanide to form cyano-cobalamin (Vitamin B_{12A}). The usual dose is 50 mg/kg; a single dose of 5 g is usually sufficient.

D. HYPERBARIC OXYGEN

Hyperbaric oxygen may be considered in cases that are refractory to standard care, including use of the antidote kit. It has not been proven, however, to have any significant clinical advantage over 100% oxygen.

E. TREATMENT FOR PERSISTENT SYMPTOMS

If symptoms of cyanide poisoning persist, the sodium nitrite and sodium thiosulfate can be repeated at half of the original dose.

Disposition

All patients with suspected or documented cyanide poisoning should be hospitalized.

Chin RG et al: Acute cyanide poisoning: a case report. J Emerg Med 2000;18:441. [PMID: 10802422] (Case report and review of the treatment of cyanide poisoning.)

Mueller M et al: Delayed cyanide poisoning following acetonitrile ingestion. Postgrad Med J 1997;73:299. [PMID: 9196706] (Case report of cyanide toxicity from acetonitrile ingestion.)

Sauer SW et al: Hydroxocobalamin: improved public health readiness for cyanide disasters. Ann Emerg Med 2001;37:635. [PMID: 11385334] (Review of the use of hydroxocobalamin to treat cyanide poisoning.)

Suchard JR et al: Acute cyanide toxicity caused by apricot kernel ingestion. Ann Emerg Med 1998;32:742. [PMID: 9832674] (Case report of cyanide toxicity from ingestion of an apricot kernel.)

DRUG-INDUCED METHEMOGLOBINEMIA

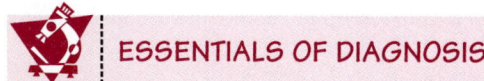 ESSENTIALS OF DIAGNOSIS

- *Methemoglobinemia cannot bind oxygen or carbon dioxide.*
- *Symptoms correlate with the degree of methemoglobinemia and can include asymptomatic cyanosis, dyspnea, and severe central nervous system depression.*
- *Treatment includes methylene blue, which can reduce methemoglobin levels in less than 1 hour.*

General Considerations

Hemoglobin becomes methemoglobin when iron is oxidized from the ferrous to the ferric form. Methemoglobin is a dark chocolate color and can no longer bind oxygen or carbon dioxide. Conversion of hemoglobin to methemoglobin decreases both delivery of oxygen to the tissues and removal of carbon dioxide, and tissue hypoxia may result.

Methemoglobin is produced endogenously in small quantities and is reduced by methemoglobin reductase; normally, less than 1–2% of hemoglobin is methemoglobin. Methemoglobinemia is caused by various oxidant drugs and poisons, including nitrites (food preservatives, some well water), nitrous gases, chloroquine and primaquine, phenazopyridine (Pyridium, others), sulfonamides, sulfones, aniline dye derivatives, phenacetin, dapsone, local anesthetics, and nitrobenzenes.

Clinical Findings

Symptoms correlate with the degree of methemoglobinemia. At concentrations of 1.5 g/dL (about 10% of the total hemoglobin), patients may seek care for cyanosis without any shortness of breath. When the level of methemoglobin exceeds 15% of total hemoglobin, blood appears chocolate brown when it is dripped onto filter paper. The exact concentration of methemoglobin in the blood may be determined spectrophotometrically. However, the Po_2 and calculated oxyhemoglobin on routine arterial blood gases are falsely normal, and the measured saturation by pulse oximetry is unreliable.

Conversion of up to 25% of normal hemoglobin to methemoglobin is usually not associated with clinical findings other than peripheral and perioral cyanosis, although anxiety, headache, weakness, and lightheadedness can develop. At conversion levels of 35–40%, patients experience lassitude, fatigue, and dyspnea. At conversion levels exceeding 60%, coma and death may occur as a result of severe central nervous system depression. Anemia, acidosis, respiratory compromise (eg, chronic obstructive pulmonary disease), and cardiac disease may make patients more symptomatic than expected for a given methemoglobin level.

Treatment

A. GENERAL MANAGEMENT

Provide intensive supportive care and gastrointestinal decontamination as described previously.

B. OXYGEN

Oxygen per se does not affect the methemoglobin level, but it should be given to improve tissue oxygenation pending the start of specific therapy. Give oxygen, 5–10 L/min, by mask or nasal cannula; in comatose or severely acidotic patients, give 100% oxygen by rebreathing mask or endotracheal tube. Continue oxygen therapy for 1–2 hours after giving methylene blue (see below). Always give oxygen if the percentage of methemoglobin is higher than 40% or if the patient has severe symptoms.

C. METHYLENE BLUE

Methylene blue is a specific antidote for methemoglobinemia. The dose is 1–2 mg/kg, or 0.1 mL/kg of a 1% solution, given intravenously over 5 minutes. The dose may be repeated at 1 mL/kg once after 1 hour, but the amount specified should not be exceeded, because an overdose of methylene blue can also cause methemoglobinemia. Methylene blue should reduce methemoglobin levels significantly in less than 1 hour. Patients with glucose-6-phosphate dehydrogenase deficiency may not respond to methylene blue and may experience hemolysis. Exchange transfusions may be required in these patients. **Note:** Methylene blue is contraindicated in patients with methemoglobinemia associated with nitrite treatment of cyanide poisoning because it may cause release of cyanide, resulting in toxic concentrations.

D. REMOVAL OF SOURCE

Discontinue the offending drug or chemical.

Disposition

Symptomatic patients with methemoglobinemia should be hospitalized for treatment. Some agents (eg, dapsone) may produce prolonged or recurrent methemoglobinemia over several days.

Griffey RT et al: Cyanosis. J Emerg Med 2000;18:369. [PMID: 10729678] (Discussion of the diagnosis, evaluation, and management of methemoglobinemia.)

Khan NA et al: Methemoglobinemia induced by topical anesthesia: a case report and review. Am J Med 1999;318:415. [PMID: 10616167] (Case report and overview of the treatment of methemoglobinemia caused by topical anesthesia.)

Wright RO et al: Methemoglobinemia: etiology, pharmacology, and clinical management. Ann Emerg Med 1999;34:646. [PMID: 10533013] (Review of methemoglobinemia and its cause, pharmacology, and clinical management.)

ETHANOL & OTHER ALCOHOLS

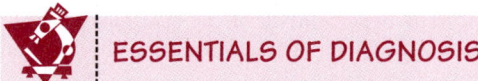

ESSENTIALS OF DIAGNOSIS

- *Ethanol, methanol, ethylene glycol, and isopropanol are all central nervous system depressants. Levels of all alcohols should be obtained, although the level may not predict the severity of the intoxication.*

- *Treatment of ethanol intoxication is supportive and includes glucose and thiamine.*

- *Treatment of methanol and ethylene glycol ingestions includes either fomepizole or an ethanol drip to inhibit the formation of toxic metabolites.*

- *Treatment of isopropanol ingestion is supportive and may include dialysis if the level is greater than 400 mg/dL.*

General Considerations

Methanol, ethylene glycol, and even isopropanol have been used as cheap substitutes for ethanol, although this practice is less common now than formerly. These alcohols may also be ingested accidentally or in suicide attempts. All are capable of causing intoxication similar to that produced by ethanol, and all can widen the osmolar gap (see Table 45–4). Additional toxic effects can occur as a result of the metabolism of ethylene glycol and methanol.

1. Ethanol

Ethanol is a central nervous system depressant. It is metabolized by alcohol dehydrogenase (in most cases by fixed-rate, zero-order kinetics) at a rate of about 7–10 g/h, resulting in a decrease in blood alcohol concentration of 20–30 mg/dL/h. The rate of elimination among individuals varies, as does tolerance. In the United States, legal impairment for purposes of driving is generally defined as blood (or breath) ethanol concentrations above 80–100 mg/dL; coma usually occurs with levels exceeding 300 mg/dL, except in chronic ethanol abusers who have developed tolerance.

Clinical Findings

Symptoms of alcohol intoxication include ataxia, dysarthria, depressed sensorium, and nystagmus. The breath may smell of alcohol, but this finding is neither sensitive nor specific. Alcohol intoxication is frequently seen with trauma and can contribute significantly to morbidity and mortality. Coma and respiratory depression with subsequent pulmonary aspiration due to intoxication is also a common cause of illness and death. Laboratory diagnosis may be aided by direct determination of the blood ethanol concentration or by its estimation from the calculated osmolar gap (see Table 45–4).

Treatment

A. GENERAL MANAGEMENT

Provide intensive supportive care and gastrointestinal decontamination as described previously. Supportive care is the primary mode of therapy. Special care should be taken to prevent aspiration.

B. THIAMINE AND GLUCOSE

Give thiamine and glucose as needed. Give thiamine, 100 mg intramuscularly or intravenously, to prevent Wernicke syndrome. Check for hypoglycemia, because ethanol inhibits gluconeogenesis, and give glucose, 50 mL of a 50% solution (25 g of glucose) intravenously over 3–4 minutes, if needed.

C. OTHER MEASURES

Diagnose and correct disorders such as hypovolemia, hypothermia, infection, trauma, or gastrointestinal tract bleeding. Do not use fructose therapy or forced diuresis.

Disposition

Hospitalize patients with ethanol poisoning if ethanol intoxication has caused abnormalities that would by themselves require hospitalization (eg, obtundation, seizures, refractory hypoglycemia).

2. Methanol

Methanol is a highly toxic alcohol found in a variety of commercial products, including paint stripper, antifreeze, automobile windshield washer fluid, and solid alcohols (Sterno Canned Heat, many others). It is metabolized by alcohol dehydrogenase to formaldehyde and formic acid. An osmolar gap and metabolic acidosis with an anion gap result. Optic neuritis (caused by formate) that results in blindness has been described after overdose. Early diagnosis is essential, because permanent blindness or death may result if methanol intoxication is left untreated.

Clinical Findings

The major clinical effect of methanol before it is metabolized is central nervous system depression. As the methanol is metabolized to formic acid (this may be delayed 6–18 hours if ethanol has also been ingested), visual disturbances invariably occur (blurred vision or hazy, snowlike patterns), along with hyperemia of the optic disk, headache, dizziness, and breathlessness. In severe toxicity, seizures and coma may occur.

Examination shows variable degrees of central nervous system dysfunction (agitation and intoxication to coma). Pupillary dysfunction has been shown to be a strong predictor of mortality. The retinas may appear suffused and bright red. Early after ingestion, the only finding may be inebriation with an elevated osmolar gap. Later, severe metabolic acidosis occurs.

Treatment

If serious intoxication is suspected, begin therapy even before receiving the results of blood methanol concentration determination.

A. GENERAL MANAGEMENT

Provide intensive supportive care and gastrointestinal decontamination as described previously. The main objective of treatment is to limit the accumulation of formate by blocking the metabolism of methanol by alcohol dehydrogenase. Two drugs have been shown to be effective, fomepizole (Antizol) and ethanol.

1. Fomepizole—Fomepizole is approved by the FDA for the treatment of ethylene glycol poisoning and is also effective in methanol intoxication. Fomepizole, like ethanol, inhibits alcohol dehydrogenase and the formation of toxic metabolites. Give a loading dose of 15 mg/kg intravenously, followed by 10 mg/kg every 12 hours for 48 hours. After 48 hours the dose is increased to 15 mg/kg every 12 hours until the level of methanol is undetectable or both symptoms and acidosis resolve and the level is less than 20 mg/dL. Fomepizole has several advantages over ethanol infusion, including ease of dosing, lack of central nervous system depression, and no requirement for constant serum monitoring because of its reliable therapeutic concentration. Ethanol infusion can also be used if fomepizole is unavailable.

2. Ethanol—Ethanol is metabolized in preference to methanol by alcohol dehydrogenase, thus blocking further metabolism of methanol. The loading dose of ethanol for an average 70-kg adult is 0.7 g/kg (2 mL/kg of 100-proof [50%] ethanol orally; or 7 mL/kg of 10% ethanol intravenously). Maintain continuous infusion of 0.07–0.1 g/kg/h to keep blood concentration of ethanol between 100 and 200 mg/dL. These levels are sufficient to produce clinically evident intoxication. Ethanol may be given intravenously or orally, but intravenous solutions must be at concentrations of 10% or less to prevent hypertonicity of the solution. Monitor and maintain adequate ventilation during the infusion of ethanol.

B. OTHER MEASURES

Correct metabolic acidosis with sodium bicarbonate; keep the pH at 7.2 or higher. Because folate deficiency increases the toxicity of methanol (in animals), folate replacement may be helpful. It can be given as a 50-mg intravenous dose every 4 hours for 5 doses, then once a day.

C. HEMODIALYSIS

Hemodialysis is indicated for methanol blood concentrations higher than 50 mg/dL and in patients with severe acidosis, high formate levels, seizures, optic changes, or mental status changes; it should be started as soon as possible. The ethanol infusion must be adjusted to replace ethanol lost in dialysis (increase ethanol to 0.15–0.2 g/kg/h). Fomepizole is also dialyzed, and dosing should be increased to every 4 hours during dialysis.

Disposition

Hospitalize all patients with suspected or documented methanol poisoning. If the osmolar gap and anion gap are both normal 1 hour after suspected injection, serious intoxication is unlikely.

3. Ethylene Glycol

Ethylene glycol is a common ingredient of deicers and antifreeze products. It is sweet tasting, and some preparations are attractively colored. Following ingestion, it is metabolized by alcohol dehydrogenase to glycolate and ultimately to oxalate, which precipitates with calcium to form calcium oxalate crystals. Symptoms may occur within 30 minutes or after a delay of several hours.

Clinical Findings

The clinical course of ethylene glycol intoxication can be divided into 3 phases. The first phase occurs less than 1 hour after ingestion and is characterized by central nervous system depression. The second phase affects the cardiopulmonary system, and heart failure or pulmonary edema can occur approximately 12 hours after ingestion. The final phase occurs 24–72 hours after ingestion and is characterized by renal tubule necrosis, flank pain, hematuria, and renal failure. Visual symptoms are usually not present, and the ocular fundi appear normal (as distinguished from their appearance in methanol poisoning). An osmolar gap is present, and after metabolism to toxic products, a severe acidosis usually occurs, and crystals of calcium oxalate may be seen in the urine. The urine may be fluorescent under an ultraviolet lamp owing to the fluorescent often added to commercial antifreeze products.

Treatment

Fomepizole is the treatment of choice, although ethanol can be used if fomepizole is unavailable. The dosing is the same as in methanol poisoning. Hemodialysis is now indicated only in patients with severe acidosis or abnormal renal function; the ethylene glycol level by itself does not determine the need for dialysis.

Disposition

Hospitalize all patients with suspected or documented ethylene glycol intoxication.

4. Isopropanol

Isopropanol is a common ingredient in many household products, especially rubbing alcohol. It causes intoxication with central nervous system and cardiac depression; blood concentrations of 150 mg/dL are frequently associated with deep coma. It is metabolized by alcohol dehydrogenase to acetone, although most of the clinical effects of isopropanol intoxication are due to the parent compound. Both the alcohol and its metabolite cause an elevated osmolar gap, but acidosis is rare. The odor—and acetonemia without acidosis—is characteristic of isopropanol intoxication.

Treatment

Treatment is primarily supportive and similar to that for ethanol intoxication. Hemodialysis is indicated for patients with an isopropanol level greater than 400 mg/dL and significant central nervous system depression.

Disposition

Hospitalize patients with isopropanol intoxication who have significant signs (eg, stupor, coma, or hypotension).

Abramson S et al: Treatment of the alcohol intoxications: ethylene glycol, methanol and isopropanol. Curr Opin Nephrol Hypertens 2000;9:695. [PMID: 11128434] (Review of diagnosis and treatment of intoxication with ethylene glycol, methanol, and isopropanol.)

Barceloux DG et al: American Academy of Clinical Toxicology practice guidelines on the treatment of ethylene glycol poisoning. Ad Hoc Committee. J Toxicol Clin Toxicol 1999; 37:537. [PMID: 10497633]

Brent J: Current management of ethylene glycol poisoning. Drugs 2001;61:979. [PMID: 11434452] (Review of the treatment of ethylene glycol poisoning.)

Sivilotti ML et al: Toxicokinetics of ethylene glycol during fomepizole therapy: implications for management. For the Methylpyrazole for Toxic Alcohols Study Group. Ann Emerg Med 2000;36:114. [PMID: 10918102] (Evaluation of drug concentration data obtained in the ethylene glycol arm of the Methylpyrazole for Toxic Alcohols trial.)

HEAVY METALS

ESSENTIALS OF DIAGNOSIS

- *Signs and symptoms of heavy metal ingestion can vary widely and include all major organ systems.*
- *Levels can be obtained and in many cases guide treatment.*
- *Chelation therapy is available for iron, lead, arsenic, and mercury poisoning.*

1. Iron

General Considerations

Iron poisoning results primarily from ingestion of mineral supplements containing divalent iron: ferrous sulfate (20% elemental iron), ferrous fumarate (33%), and ferrous gluconate (12%).

Absorption of iron is dose related and may increase dramatically with overdose levels, especially when the corrosive action of iron has damaged the intestinal mucosal barrier. Iron also causes vasodilatation and disruption of cellular electron transport. The elemental iron equivalent should be used when toxic doses are being estimated; an amount higher than 20–30 mg/kg causes toxicity, and amounts over 60 mg/kg are potentially lethal. Blood concentrations of iron may assist in the diagnosis of acute toxicity but may be unreliable owing to concurrent absorption of iron and distribution in the tissues. A peak concentration in serum often occurs 4–5 hours after ingestion. Serum concentrations over 400 µg/dL are potentially serious, and levels over 1000 µg/dL are associated with severe poisoning.

Clinical Findings

Four stages of intoxication are commonly described:

1. Severe nausea and vomiting and abdominal pain occur within 1–4 hours. Hyperglycemia and leukocytosis are common. In severe cases, hemorrhagic gastroenteritis, shock, acidosis, and coma may follow. A plain film of the abdomen may show radiopaque iron tablets.
2. During the next period, which lasts 6–12 hours and sometimes up to 24 hours, the patient may appear relatively well or may even improve. Patients with significant ingestions, however, can still have progressive, silent systemic deterioration.
3. A stage of shock, acidosis, coagulopathy, and hypoglycemia may occur 12–24 hours after ingestion of significant amounts of iron and reflects a severe course and poor outlook. Serum iron concentration at this stage may be deceptively low, because most absorbed iron has been taken up by tissues.
4. The last stage is characterized by hepatic poisoning with possible progression to hepatic failure.

Treatment

A. General Management

Provide intensive supportive care and gastrointestinal decontamination as described previously. Empty the stomach by induced emesis with syrup of ipecac or gastric lavage. For serious or massive ingestion, enhance removal or iron from the gastrointestinal tract with whole bowel irrigation. Activated charcoal is not effective.

B. Chelation Therapy

Intravenous chelation with deferoxamine is the treatment of choice when symptoms of iron poisoning are evident or when the serum iron level is over 400 µg/dL (Table 45–15). The iron-deferoxamine complex is excreted in the urine and has a pink color. If urinary output is inadequate, the complex may be removed by peritoneal dialysis or hemodialysis. The deferoxamine intramuscular challenge is no longer recommended, and any patient with a significant ingestion who appears toxic or has a serum iron level greater than 400 mg/dL should receive treatment.

Observe the patient for several hours when ingestion of significant amounts of iron is suspected, because symptoms in the initial phase may be deceptively mild.

Disposition

Hospitalize all patients with suspected or documented cases of iron poisoning. If patients remain asymptomatic, with a negative abdominal x-ray and no elevation of white blood cell count or blood glucose 6 hours after ingestion, they may be discharged to home care.

2. Lead

General Considerations

Inorganic lead is found in paint in older homes; pottery glazes containing lead (not used commercially in the United States); and fumes from welding, smelting, and battery manufacturing. Gasoline may contain organic lead (tetraethyl lead). Most adult cases of lead poisoning are due to inhalation exposure; chronic ingestion is the most common cause of lead poisoning in children.

Table 45–15. Chelating agents.

Metal	Chelating Agent	Dose	Side Effects
Iron	Deferoxamine	10–15 mg/kg h until serum iron levels fall to less than 400 µg/dL or until urine no longer has characteristic pink color. Higher doses have been used in massive overdose. Consult a poison control center.	Hypotension with rapid intravenous route of administration.
Lead	Edetate calcium disodium (EDTA)	50–75 mg/kg/d IM divided q 6–8 h × 5 d. Should be started *after* first dose of BAL. May also be given by slow IV drip at concentrations no greater than 0.5% (5 mg/mL).	Reversible acute tubular necrosis; zinc and vitamin B_6 depletion. Do not give orally. If urinary output inadequate with administration, initiate hemodialysis.
Lead, arsenic, and mercury	2,3-Dimercaptosuccinic acid (DMSA) (Succimer)	Children: 10 mg/kg q 8 h PO × 5 d, then q 12 h for the next 14 d. Adults: 30 mg/kg q 8 h × 5 d, then 20 mg/kg/d q 12 h × 14 d.	Nausea, vomiting, diarrhea, transient liver function enzyme elevation.
	Dimercaprol (BAL)	3–5 mg/kg/dose IM q 4 h × 5 d	Hypertension, lacrimation, burning lips, nausea and vomiting.
	Penicillamine	100 mg/kg/d (maximum dose 1 g) orally in 4 divided doses on an empty stomach.	Nephrotic syndrome, loss of sense of taste.

Lead is well absorbed from the respiratory tract and usually poorly absorbed from the gastrointestinal tract; target organs are bone, kidney, bone marrow, and the nervous system. Lead toxicity usually occurs with chronic absorption of more than 0.4–0.5 mg/dL; a single chip of lead-based paint may contain 50–100 mg of lead. Most lead poisoning results from chronic, subacute exposure rather than acute exposure to large amounts.

Clinical Findings

Early symptoms of lead poisoning are nonspecific, for example, listlessness, irritability, headache, abdominal pain, and constipation. Subtle behavioral changes and intellectual impairment may occur in children. With severe toxicity, lethargy, clumsiness, ataxia, seizures, and coma occur. Peripheral neuropathy (lead palsy)—characterized chiefly by extensor muscle weakness with minimal sensory loss—occurs after prolonged chronic exposure and occurs more frequently in adults than in children. Exposure to organic lead compounds produces a more dramatic acute encephalopathy than does exposure to inorganic lead. Delirium and hallucinations are associated symptoms.

The best standard diagnostic tool is the concentration of lead in the blood. (The concentration in the hair is not useful.) Up to 25 µg/dL is considered normal but may in fact be toxic over long periods, especially in children. Over 70 µg/dL is serious and usually

requires hospitalization. Plain films of the abdomen may show radiopaque (ingested) lead in the gastrointestinal tract. Microcytic anemia may be present, and when it is associated with basophilic stippling of red blood cells on the peripheral blood smear, it strongly suggests lead poisoning. In children, so-called lead lines can be visualized radiographically as opacities at the metaphyseal plate; these lines represent toxic effects of lead on bone growth rather than lead deposition in bone.

Treatment

A. GENERAL MANAGEMENT

Provide intensive supportive care and gastrointestinal decontamination as described previously. Consider whole bowel irrigation if a lead foreign body has been ingested.

B. CHELATION THERAPY

(See Tables 45–15 and 45–16.) Treatment depends on blood lead concentration; if the hematocrit is less than 20%, adjust the lead level as shown in the following equation:

$$\frac{\text{Normal hematocrit}}{\text{Patient's hematocrit}} \times \text{Blood lead level} = \frac{\text{Corrected blood}}{\text{lead level}}$$

Proceed with treatment as outlined in Table 45–16. Because of concerns that lead may be redistributed to the brain with an edetate calcium disodium (EDTA) chal-

Table 45–16. Recommended treatment for lead poisoning by blood concentration.

Blood Lead Concentration	Treatment
< 25 μg/dL	None.
25–45 μg/dL	Stop further exposure to lead and monitor blood levels monthly.
45–70 μg/dL	Children: Give DMSA (Succimer) in the absence of encephalopathy or protracted vomiting. BAL and EDTA can also be used. Adults: Give EDTA and BAL. Although not FDA-approved for adults, consider use of DMSA.
> 70 μg/dL	Considered a medical emergency. Institute chelation with BAL, EDTA, and possibly DMSA immediately.

BAL = dimercaprol; DMSA = 2,3-dimercaptosuccinic acid; EDTA = edetate calcium disodium.

lenge, toxicologists no longer recommend this practice. Several chelating agents can be used to treat lead poisoning. 2,3-Dimercaptosuccinic acid (DMSA) (Succimer) is now FDA approved for oral chelation in children with lead levels greater than 45 mg/dL and can also be used in adults. Dimercaprol (BAL) and EDTA are still used as well; penicillamine is a less effective chelating agent, but is also less expensive.

Disposition

Hospitalize patients with symptoms of severe lead poisoning or blood lead concentrations higher than 70 μg/dL.

3. Arsenic

General Considerations

Many insecticides, rodenticides, and wood preservatives are sources of trivalent arsenic. The much less toxic pentavalent organic arsenic found in shellfish and other foods produces positive urine screens for arsenic but is not associated with clinical toxicity. Highly toxic arsine gas is produced by burning arsenic-containing ores and is used in the electronics industry.

Arsenic is absorbed mainly through the gastrointestinal tract but may be absorbed through intact skin or after inhalation, binds avidly to tissue proteins, and

accumulates in tissue. The lethal dose of trivalent arsenic is about 100–300 mg in an adult; the pentavalent form is rapidly excreted and less toxic.

Clinical Findings

A. Symptoms and Signs

1. Arsenic salt ingestion—

a. Acute poisoning—Symptoms and signs include crampy abdominal pain, vomiting, profuse watery diarrhea, a burning sensation in mucous membranes, conjunctivitis, tremor, hypotension, tachycardia, and seizures. A garlic odor is sometimes noted on the breath. Abdominal plain films may show radiopaque material in the gut. Periorbital edema may occur after 1–2 days.

b. Chronic poisoning—Symptoms include stocking-glove peripheral sensory and motor neuropathy, malaise, anorexia, alopecia, anemia, and stomatitis. These symptoms are also noted during recovery from an episode of acute poisoning.

2. Arsine gas inhalation—Arsine gas is highly toxic and causes rapid intravascular hemolysis and renal failure. Other characteristics of arsenic toxicity are often not seen.

B. Laboratory Findings

Measurement of 24-hour urinary arsenic excretion levels is useful but can be misleading, because ingestion of shellfish containing nontoxic forms of arsenic may cause transient elevation of arsenic levels. The chief usefulness of this measurement lies in monitoring the response to chelation therapy. In chronic poisoning, arsenic concentrations are elevated in the hair and nails.

Treatment

A. Acute Poisoning

Provide intensive supportive care and gastrointestinal decontamination as described previously. Perform gastric lavage. Give DMSA (if the patient can tolerate oral medications) or BAL (see Table 45–15), and continue until the urine arsenic level is less than 50 μg/24 h.

B. Chronic Poisoning

Management usually consists of prevention of further arsenic absorption and gastrointestinal decontamination. Penicillamine is no longer recommended.

C. Arsine Gas Inhalation

Blood transfusion may be necessary for severe hemolysis. Give adequate fluids to prevent renal hemoglobin deposition. Chelation therapy is of no value for acute exposure to arsine gas.

Disposition

Hospitalize all patients with suspected or documented arsenic poisoning.

4. Mercury

General Considerations

Elemental mercury vapor is produced in the course of various manufacturing procedures, during repair of mercury-containing instruments, and when the liquid metal is heated (eg, home ore processing). Inorganic mercury salts are present in disinfectants and older cathartics and diuretics. Organic mercury is found in fungicides used in seed grain and in environmentally contaminated seafood.

Mercury poisoning can result from ingestion (mercury salts), inhalation (elemental mercury), injection, and dermal absorption. Mercury is avidly bound to sulfhydryl groups and disrupts cellular enzyme and membrane function.

Clinical Findings

A. SYMPTOMS AND SIGNS

1. Elemental mercury poisoning—Liquid mercury is nontoxic if swallowed, but mercury vapor is well absorbed by inhalation and rapidly enters the central nervous system. With large exposure, encephalopathy, gingivitis, and pneumonitis may occur. The predominant manifestations of chronic mercury poisoning are various neuropsychiatric symptoms (erethism): tremor, anxiety, incapacitating shyness, and irritability.

2. Inorganic mercury poisoning—Salts of inorganic mercury are corrosive and irritating to the gastrointestinal tract. Mercurous salts (eg, calomel) are poorly absorbed and generally less toxic than mercuric salts, which cause gastroenteritis with bloody emesis and diarrhea. The target organ is the kidney; acute tubular necrosis is common. Chronic intoxication may cause gingivitis, salivation, dysarthria, intention tremor (mainly of the fingers, eyes, and tongue), nervousness, emotional outbursts, and memory loss.

3. Organic mercury poisoning—Organic mercury (methyl mercury, ethyl mercury) has been implicated in epidemic poisonings resulting from ingestion of seed grain fumigated with mercury compounds or from consumption of heavily contaminated seafood. These compounds are well absorbed and reach high levels in the nervous system with devastating effects. They can also cross the placenta.

Tremor and neuropsychiatric symptoms are similar to those occurring with exposure to the vapor of elemental mercury, but the development of peculiar sensory deficits is unique to this type of mercury poisoning. These distinctive symptoms include paresthesias; constriction of visual fields; loss of hearing, smell, and taste; incoordination; choreoathetosis; stupor; and incontinence. Uncontrollable crying and laughter are also seen. The developing fetus may concentrate mercury in the central nervous system, with resulting congenital cerebral palsy, mental retardation, and other birth defects.

B. LABORATORY FINDINGS

Blood levels are not always reliable indicators of excessive mercury burdens because of its wide distribution; levels may even be elevated 2–3 days after a seafood meal. Whole blood levels are recommended for acute intoxications; normal levels are less than 5 µg/dL. A 24-hour urine collection can be more helpful than a blood level, and a level greater than 20 µg/dL indicates meaningful exposure.

Treatment

A. GENERAL MANAGEMENT

Provide intensive supportive care and gastrointestinal decontamination as described previously. A kidney-ureter-bladder x-ray may be helpful in elemental mercury ingestion to document its presence and passage through the gastrointestinal tract.

B. CHELATION THERAPY

DMSA has been shown to lower mercury levels, although it is not FDA approved for this indication (see Table 45–15). BAL can also be used, although it is contraindicated in methyl mercury poisoning because it can exacerbate central nervous system symptoms. Penicillamine is rarely used.

C. SUPPORTIVE TREATMENT

Renal failure, a common occurrence after poisoning with inorganic mercuric salts, is treated with general supportive measures, which may include dialysis.

Disposition

Hospitalize all patients with suspected or documented mercury poisoning.

Gordon RA et al: Aggressive approach in the treatment of acute lead encephalopathy with an extraordinarily high concentration of lead. Arch Pediatr Adolesc Med 1998;152:1100.

[PMID: 9811288] (Case report and review of literature on the treatment of lead toxicity.)

Graeme KA et al: Heavy metal toxicity, part I: arsenic and mercury. J Emerg Med 1998;16:45. [PMID: 9472760] (Review of the toxicity of arsenic and mercury and the diagnosis and treatment of arsenic and mercury poisoning.)

Graeme KA et al: Heavy metal toxicity, part II: lead and metal fume fever. J Emerg Med 1998;16:171. [PMID: 9543397] (Review of the toxicity of lead and the diagnosis and treatment of lead poisoning.)

Ioannides AS et al: Acute respiratory distress syndrome in children with acute iron poisoning: the role of intravenous desferrioxamine. Eur J Pediatr 2000;159:158. [PMID: 10664227] (Case report of severe acute respiratory decompensation in a child given intravenous desferrioxamine.)

Levin SM et al: Clinical evaluation and management of lead-exposed construction workers. Am J Ind Med 2000;37:23. [PMID: 10573595] (Review of the adverse effects and treatment of lead exposure in industry and treatment guidelines.)

Muckter H et al: Are we ready to replace dimercaprol (BAL) as an arsenic antidote? Hum Exp Toxicol 1997;16:460. [PMID: 9292286] (Animal model of the treatment of arsenic poisoning with BAL, DMSA, and 2,3-dimercaptopropane-1-sulfate.)

Siff JE et al: Usefulness of the total iron binding capacity in the evaluation and treatment of acute iron overdose. Ann Emerg Med 1999;33:73. [PMID: 9867890] (Review of reported cases of iron overdose using total iron-binding capacity as part of the laboratory analysis.)

Staudinger KC et al: Occupational lead poisoning. Am Fam Physician 1998;57:719. [PMID: 9490995] (Diagnosis and management of occupational lead exposure.)

HYDROCARBONS

 ESSENTIALS OF DIAGNOSIS

- *Choking, gagging, or gasping following ingestion.*
- *Hypoxia.*
- *Delayed (4–6 hours) physical findings.*
- *Infiltrates on chest x-ray (chemical pneumonitis).*

General Considerations

Hydrocarbons—a large group of compounds that includes petroleum distillates—exert various toxic effects. They are classified by 2 characteristics: viscosity (low-viscosity products are more likely to cause chemical aspiration pneumonia) and their potential for systemic toxicity (central nervous system or cardiac toxicity). These properties are summarized in Table 45–17.

The major complication following ingestion of petroleum distillates is aspiration pneumonitis, which may occur with poisoning caused by any of the low-viscosity compounds.

Most cases of poisoning are accidental, and exposure is rarely more than a taste (5–10 mL). As little as 1–2 mL of low-viscosity compounds may produce severe chemical pneumonitis if aspirated into the tracheobronchial tree.

Accidental or intentional inhalation of hydrocarbon vapors may produce irritation, nausea, and headache. Exposure to volatile vapors in an enclosed area may result in hypoxia owing to displacement of oxygen from the atmosphere. Inhalation of aromatic (eg, toluene) or halogenated (eg, freon, trichloroethylene) hydrocarbon solvents may cause euphoria, confusion, hallucinations, coma, and cardiac arrhythmias. Chronic exposure to toluene may cause myopathy, hypokalemia, renal tubular acidosis, and neuropathy.

Clinical Findings

Symptoms suggesting aspiration are choking, coughing, or gasping immediately following ingestion of a toxic compound. Physical signs of aspiration are often present but may be delayed for up to 4–6 hours. For example, chest x-ray may reveal infiltrates before physical signs appear. Systemic signs of toxicity include narcosis, delirium, and for certain compounds, seizures. Some of these effects may result from hypoxemia due to pneumonitis. Hydrocarbons may sensitize the myocardium to the arrhythmogenic effects of endogenous catecholamines.

Treatment

Although gastric aspiration of any ingested hydrocarbon may increase the chances of aspiration, ingestion of even small amounts of low-viscosity compounds with known significant systemic toxicity requires gastric aspiration and administration of activated charcoal. For example, the camphor contained in 10 mL of Campho-Phenique is sufficient to cause seizures in a child. The toxic dose of benzene or toluene is unknown but may be less than 10 mL.

A. HIGH-VISCOSITY LUBRICANTS

No treatment is required.

B. LOW-VISCOSITY COMPOUNDS WITH NO KNOWN SYSTEMIC TOXICITY

If there are unequivocal signs of aspiration pneumonitis, protect the airway if necessary to prevent further aspiration, and give oxygen. However, there are case reports of pulse corticosteroid therapy used successfully in the treatment of late acute respiratory distress syndrome following hydrocarbon ingestion.

Table 45–17. Clinical features of hydrocarbon poisoning.

Type	Examples	Risk of Phenumonia	Risk of Systemic Toxicity	Treatment
High-viscosity	Vaseline, motor oil, gasoline	Low	Low	None.
Low-viscosity, nontoxic	Furniture polish, mineral spirits, kerosene, lighter fluid	High	Low	Observe for pneumonia. *Do not* induce emesis.
Low-viscosity, unknown systemic toxicity	Turpentine, pine oil	High	Variable	Observe for penumonia. *Do not* induce emesis if less than 1–2 mL/kg was ingested.
Low-viscosity, known systemic toxicity	CHAMP: **C**amphor, **H**alogenated or **A**romatic hydrocarbons (benezene, toluene), **M**etals, **P**esticides	High	High	Gastric aspiration followed by activated charcoal.

If the patient is asymptomatic and has no history of coughing or choking after ingestion, aspiration is unlikely. Do not induce emesis, because it may increase the risk of aspiration. Observe the patient closely for 4–6 hours to detect signs of possible aspiration. Obtain a chest x-ray even in asymptomatic patients.

C. LOW-VISCOSITY COMPOUNDS WITH UNKNOWN OR UNPROVED TOXICITY

It is unclear whether these compounds have inherent systemic toxic effects apart from chemical pneumonitis, and controversy exists regarding the use of lavage to clear a compound of this group from the body. Evaluate the patient, and give treatment for possible pulmonary aspiration, as described above.

D. LOW-VISCOSITY COMPOUNDS WITH KNOWN SYSTEMIC TOXICITY

Consider gastric emptying for ingestions of more than 30 mL of hydrocarbons with systemic toxicity, intentional overdoses, and mixed overdoses with other toxins. In the absence of the above scenarios, avoid gastric emptying. Activated charcoal should also be initiated under the same pretenses. Activated charcoal is especially useful if the toxin (eg, camphor) is known to produce coma or seizures abruptly. If lethargy, coma, or seizures are present, intubate the patient with a cuffed endotracheal tube, and perform gastric aspiration. Evaluate the patient for possible pulmonary aspiration.

Disposition

Hospitalize patients who have ingested low-viscosity petroleum distillates if symptoms or signs of systemic toxicity (lethargy, seizures) or pneumonitis (coughing, choking, abnormal findings on chest x-ray) are present.

Because delayed onset of pulmonary complications may occur after hydrocarbon poisoning, it is prudent to observe patients for 4–6 hours before discharging them from the emergency department.

Kamijo Y et al: Pulse steroid therapy in adult respiratory distress syndrome following petroleum naphtha ingestion. J Toxicol Clin Toxicol 2000;38:59. [PMID: 10696927] (Case report and discussion of the treatment of hydrocarbon ingestion.)

Mickiewicz M et al: Hydrocarbon toxicity: general review and management guidelines. Air Med J 2001;20:8. [PMID: 11331818] (Review of hydrocarbon toxicity and management guidelines.)

INHALANTS (Toxic Gases & Vapors)

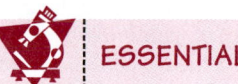 ESSENTIALS OF DIAGNOSIS

- *Hypoxia.*
- *Irritation of upper airway and conjunctiva.*
- *Chemical pneumonitis and pulmonary edema.*

General Considerations

Many toxic inhalants (eg, carbon monoxide, phosgene) are produced by combustion of household or industrial products in accidental fires or as byproducts of work activity (eg, welding). Many toxic chemicals exist in gaseous form (eg, chlorine, arsine), and exposure occurs during an accidental spill or leak. Toxic gases can be classified as (1) simple asphyxiants, (2) chemical asphyxiants and systemic poisons, and (3) irritants or corrosives (Table 45–18).

A. SIMPLE ASPHYXIANTS

Methane, propane, and inert gases cause toxicity by lowering the ambient oxygen concentration.

B. CHEMICAL ASPHYXIANTS AND SYSTEMIC POISONS

Examples include carbon monoxide, cyanide, and hydrogen sulfide. These substances possess intrinsic systemic toxicity manifested after absorption into the circulation.

C. IRRITANTS OR CORROSIVES

These substances cause cellular destruction and inflammation when they come in contact with the tracheobronchial tree, usually by producing acids or alkali upon contact with moisture. Gases that are highly water soluble (eg, chlorine, ammonia) cause immediate irritation, mainly of the upper airway and conjunctiva, whereas gases that are poorly soluble in water (eg, nitrogen dioxide) may be more deeply inhaled, producing delayed lower airway destruction with chemical pneumonitis and pulmonary edema.

Clinical Findings

Symptoms and signs vary depending on the toxin. In an accidental fire, combinations of all classes of toxic inhalants may be responsible for symptoms of toxicity, for example, a burning sensation in the eyes and mouth, sore throat, brassy cough, dyspnea, and headache. Look for singed nasal hairs, carbonaceous deposits on the nose and face, upper airway swelling or obstruction, wheezing or signs of pulmonary edema, and manifestations of systemic toxicity. Obtain arterial blood gas determinations, carboxyhemoglobin level measurements, and chest x-ray.

Treatment

Remove the patient from the source of toxic gases, and begin supplemental oxygen, 10 L/min, by mask. For victims of smoke inhalation or carbon monoxide poisoning, give 100% oxygen.

Treatment of poisoning caused by chemical asphyxiants and systemic toxins depends on the specific toxin. For cyanide, see previous discussion; for hydrogen sulfide poisoning, use sodium nitrate and hyperbaric oxygen, as outlined in the "Cyanide" section. Although unproved, nitrite therapy may decrease sulfide toxicity by binding it with methemoglobin. Do not give thiosulfate for hydrogen sulfide intoxication, because the enzyme rhodanese is not involved in elimination of sulfide.

For upper airway irritation, humidified oxygen is often effective. Carefully observe the patient for stridor and other signs of progressive airway obstruction that would require endotracheal intubation.

For bronchospasm, give nebulized bronchodilators (Chapter 33).

Disposition

Hospitalize for observation and treatment all patients with significant symptoms or signs of poisoning caused by inhalation of toxic gases. Patients exposed briefly to high-solubility irritant gases whose symptoms have resolved can be safely discharged; however, those exposed to low-solubility irritants such as nitrogen oxides or phosgene may experience delayed-onset pulmonary edema or chemical pneumonitis and should be admitted for 16–24 hours' observation.

Brouette T et al: Clinical review of inhalants. Am J Addict 2001;10:79. [PMID: 11268830] (Epidemiology, pharmacology, and sequelae of inhalant abuse.)

Lau FL et al: A fatal laboratory accident with toxic gases inhalation. Eur J Emerg Med 1998;5:265. [PMID: 9486258] (Case reports and discussion of exposure of toxic gases.)

Meng Y et al: Inhalation studies with drugs of abuse. NIDA Res Monogr 1997;173:201. [PMID: 9260190] (Review of inhalants and their pharmacology.)

ISONIAZID

 ESSENTIALS OF DIAGNOSIS

- *Seizures, metabolic acidosis, and coma.*
- *Seizures may be refractory to standard management (benzodiazepines).*
- *Estimated acute toxic dose is 80–100 mg/kg.*

General Considerations

Isoniazid is a common antituberculosis drug often prescribed as a 3- to 6-month supply. The principal manifestations of isoniazid overdose are seizures, metabolic acidosis, and coma. Seizures may be due to depression of γ-aminobutyric acid levels in the central nervous system. Severe metabolic acidosis accompanies recurrent

Table 45–18. Clinical features of toxic gases and fumes.

Class of Toxin	Toxin	Source	Clinical Features	Treatment
Simple asphyxiants	Propane	Cooking gas	All displace normal air and lower F_{IO_2}. Symptoms of hypoxemia, without airway irritation.	Remove patient from source; give oxygen.
	Methane	Cooking gas		
	Carbon dioxide	All fires		
	Inert gases (nitrogen, argon)	Industry (especially welding)		
Chemical asphyxiants	Carbon monoxide	Fires	Forms carboxyhemoglobin; inhibits oxygen transport. Headache is earliest symptom.	100% oxygen.
	Hydrocyanic acid	Industry; burning plastics, furniture, fabrics	Highly toxic cellular asphyxiant (see section on cyanide).	Use cyanide antidote (Table 45–14)
	Hydrogen sulfide	Liquid manure pits, decaying organic materials	Highly toxic cellular asphyxiant similar to cyanide; sudden collapses; ability to smell characteristic odor of rotten eggs is rapidly fatigued.	Use sodium nitrite as for cyanide (makes sulmethemoglobin). **Do not** use thiosulfate.
Irritants High solubility in water	Chlorine gas Hydrochloric acid	Industry; swimming pool chemical; bleach mixed with acid at home	Early onset of lacrimation, sore throat, stridor, tracheobronchitis; with heavy exposure, may progress to pulmonary edema in 2–6 hours.	Humidified oxygen; bronchodilators; airway management.
	Ammonia	Industry; burning fabrics		
Low solubility in water	Nitrogen dioxide	Burning cellulose; fabrics. Grain silos (acid red gas)	Has sweet "electric" smell. Delayed onset (12–24 hours) of tracheobronchitis, pneumonitis, and pulmonary edema. Late chronic bronchitis.	Oxygen; observation for 24–48 hours; steroids (controversial).
	Ozone	Inert gas arc welding industry		
	Phosgene	Burning of chlorinated organic material		
Allergenic	Toluene diisocyanate	Manufacture of polyurethanes	Reactive bronchoconstriction; may have long-term effects (chronic obstructive pulmonary disease) in susceptible persons.	Bronchodilators.
Metal fumes	Zinc Copper Tin Teflon	Welding (especially galvanized metal welding)	"Metal fumes fever." Chills, fever, myalgias, headache, nonproductive cough, leukocytosis (4–8 hours after exposure).	Self-limited (12–24 hours).
	Arsine	Burning arsenic-containing ores; electronics industry	Highly toxic. Hemolysis, pulmonary edema, renal failure; chronic arsenic toxicity.	Exchange transfusion; use dimercaprol (BAL) for chronic arsenic toxicity only.
	Mecury Lead	Industry, welding	See specific metals.	

seizure activity. The estimated acute toxic dose is 80–100 mg/kg, although this range may be lower in patients with preexisting seizure disorders, vitamin B₆ deficiency, or chronic alcoholism.

Clinical Findings

Symptoms occur 30 minutes to 3 hours following ingestion and include nausea and vomiting, slurred speech, dizziness, lethargy progressing to stupor, hyperreflexia, seizures, metabolic acidosis, hyperglycemia, and cardiovascular and respiratory depression. Symptoms and signs occur promptly after significant poisoning.

Treatment

A. GENERAL MANAGEMENT

Provide intensive supportive care and gastrointestinal decontamination as described previously.

B. TREATMENT OF SEIZURES

Treat seizures with lorazepam or diazepam, as described in Chapter 17. If these medications are not effective, give pyridoxine (vitamin B₆) in doses equivalent to the amount ingested (gram for gram). If the amount ingested is unknown, start with 5 g (0.1 g/kg) intravenously given over 3–5 minute, and repeat every 10–15 minutes until seizures are controlled. If the intravenous form of pyridoxine is not available, pyridoxine can be given as a slurry in a similar dose via a nasogastric tube. Unfortunately, many hospitals are ill-equipped and do not have the recommended 5-g aliquot available.

C. ENHANCED ELIMINATION

Consider hemodialysis for patients unresponsive to conventional therapy.

Disposition

Hospitalize all patients who have ingested more than 80 mg/kg of isoniazid and those who have signs or symptoms suggesting isoniazid poisoning.

Ramero JA et al: Isoniazid overdose: recognition and management. Am Fam Physician 1998;57:749. [PMID: 9490997] (Case study and discussion of the treatment of isoniazid overdose.)

Santucci KA et al: Acute isoniazid exposures and antidote availability. Pediatr Emerg Care 1999;15:99. [PMID: 10220077] (Prospective study to determine the availability of pyridoxine in emergency departments.)

LITHIUM

ESSENTIALS OF DIAGNOSIS

- *Apathy, lethargy, tremor, slurred speech, and ataxia.*
- *In severe overdose, choreoathetosis, seizures, and coma.*
- *Toxicity often accidental and seen with diuretic therapy and dehydration.*
- *Lithium levels > 2 mEq/L are usually toxic.*

General Considerations

Lithium is frequently used to treat bipolar disorder and other psychiatric disorders. It is a monovalent cation like sodium and potassium; unlike these cations, however, it has only a small gradient of distribution across cell membranes and cannot maintain membrane potentials. It is rapidly absorbed into extracellular fluid, with an initial volume of distribution of 0.1–0.2 L/kg. Its distribution into selected tissues then occurs slowly over several hours. Its final volume of distribution is about 1 L/kg. It is excreted unchanged in the urine and actively reabsorbed, with a half-life of approximately 22 hours (with normal renal function). Sodium and water depletion lead to marked increases in the reabsorption of lithium and to elevation of blood concentrations of lithium.

Clinical Findings

Symptoms of lithium overdose include apathy, lethargy, tremor, slurred speech, ataxia, and fasciculations, which may progress in severe overdose to choreoathetosis, seizures, coma, and death. Persistent neurologic sequelae may occur. Toxicity is frequently accidental and occurs secondary to chronic sodium depletion, diuretic therapy, and dehydration. In these cases, the serum lithium level is a more reliable index to the severity of overdose, because adequate time has passed for distribution into the central nervous system. In such circumstances, blood concentrations of lithium higher than 2 mEq/L are usually associated with toxicity.

In acute overdose, in contrast, initially elevated serum lithium concentrations may be misleading, because distribution into tissues occurs over several hours. For example, an initial toxic level of 4 mEq/L may easily fall to 1 mEq/L with final distribution. Thus, in acute overdose, repeated measurements of serum lithium levels and assessment of mental status (eg, every 4 hours) are more helpful than a single assessment in evaluating toxicity.

Treatment

A. GENERAL MANAGEMENT AND PREVENTION OF ABSORPTION

Provide intensive supportive care and gastrointestinal decontamination as described previously. Whole bowel irrigation is an effective means of increasing lithium removal. Sodium polystyrene sulfonate is also effective in decreasing the lithium concentration, but the dose and effect on the potassium level have not been determined.

B. ENHANCED ELIMINATION

The treatment of choice for serious intoxication is hemodialysis. Specific indications for hemodialysis have not been well defined by careful studies, but dialysis should be considered for any patient with obtundation, seizures, or coma, or when serum levels at equilibrium exceed 4 mEq/L. However, many patients with high levels do not have serious clinical toxicity. Dialysis is the only route of elimination in patients with renal failure. Hemoperfusion is not effective.

Because lithium is reabsorbed in the kidney when sodium and fluids are depleted, administration of intravenous saline may promote lithium excretion. Normal urine flow rates are adequate. The value of forced saline diuresis using large fluid volumes is unclear, and the authors do not recommend it.

Activated charcoal does not adsorb lithium and is of no value.

C. PREVENTION OF ACCIDENTAL TOXICITY

To prevent chronic (accidental) toxicity, frequent assessment of fluid and sodium balance and lithium levels is recommended for patients taking lithium.

Disposition

Hospitalize all patients with serum lithium concentrations above 2–3 mEq/L and those who show objective signs of lithium intoxication.

Linakis JG et al: Use of sodium polystyrene sulfonate for reduction of plasma lithium concentrations after chronic lithium dosing in mice. J Toxicol Clin Toxicol 1998;36:309. [PMID: 9711196] (Placebo-controlled animal study to determine whether multiple oral doses of sodium polystyrene sulfonate are effective in reducing chronic lithium toxicity.)

Micheli F et al: Blepharospasm and apraxia of eyelid opening in lithium intoxication. Clin Neuropharmacol 1999;22:176. [PMID: 10367183] (Case study and discussion of lithium overdose.)

Newland KD: Hemodialysis reversal of lithium overdose cardiotoxicity. Am J Emerg Med 2002;20:67. [PMID: 11781927]

(Case study and discussion of the use of hemodialysis in lithium overdose.)

Scharman EJ: Methods used to decrease lithium absorption or enhance elimination. J Toxicol Clin Toxicol 1997;35:601. [PMID: 9365427] (Meta-analysis of the methods used to decrease lithium absorption or enhance elimination.)

OPIATES

 ESSENTIALS OF DIAGNOSIS

- *Sedation, hypotension, bradycardia, hypothermia, and respiratory depression.*
- *Diagnosis is confirmed if patient regains consciousness after naloxone.*

General Considerations

Codeine, propoxyphene, and other opiates with varying potencies and durations of action are found in a wide range of prescription analgesic preparations. Some opiates, such as dextromethorphan, are found in nonprescription drugs.

The opiates act on central nervous system receptors and cause sedation, hypotension, bradycardia, hypothermia, and respiratory depression. Most opiates have a half-life of 3–6 hours; the major exceptions are methadone (15–20 hours) and propoxyphene (12–15 hours).

Clinical Findings

Consider opiate intoxication in any comatose or lethargic patient, especially when the clinical findings listed above are present. Pinpoint pupils are a typical sign, although in mixed overdoses, pupils may be in mid position. Signs of parenteral drug abuse may or may not be apparent. Pulmonary edema may occur. The diagnosis is confirmed if toxic concentrations of opiates are found in blood or urine or if the patient regains consciousness after administration of naloxone.

Treatment

A. GENERAL MANAGEMENT

Provide intensive supportive care and gastrointestinal decontamination as described previously. Maintain adequate airway and ventilation.

B. NALOXONE OR NALMEFENE

1. Naloxone—Give naloxone (a specific narcotic antagonist) to all patients with suspected opiate overdose. Start with 0.4–2 mg intravenously. Repeat 3 or 4 times if no response occurs and narcotic overdose is suspected. Some authorities recommend up to 10–20 mg to treat suspected narcotic overdose. Propoxyphene poisoning seems to be particularly resistant to the usual doses of naloxone. Because naloxone has a half-life of 1 hour and effects lasting only 2–3 hours (shorter than many opiates), its effects may wear off before those of the narcotic, permitting the patient to lapse into coma again. If relapse occurs after the first response to naloxone, a naloxone continuous infusion may be started, using approximately two thirds the dose required to initially awaken the patient given over each hour.

2. Nalmefene—Another option in the busy emergency department is a long-acting opioid antagonist such as nalmefene. Nalmefene, 2 mg, has been shown to last for as long as 8 hours, thereby reducing the need for any drips or repeated doses of naloxone. Naloxone is still the preferred initial antidote for comatose patients when the cause is uncertain because it will produce a shorter period of withdrawal in the chronically opioid-dependent patient.

C. Prevention of Narcotic Withdrawal Symptom

Watch carefully for withdrawal symptoms caused by naloxone or nalmefene. Chronic narcotic abusers who have developed tolerance to opiates may develop acute narcotic withdrawal when these agents are given. Although this syndrome is not life threatening, it is a management problem in the emergency department if the patient becomes combative or uncooperative or signs out of the hospital before adequate treatment can be given. Careful titration of the naloxone dose may help to prevent narcotic withdrawal syndrome. Some authors have even recommended the use of home-based supplies of naloxone to prevent opiate overdose death among misusers.

Disposition

Hospitalize and observe all patients thought or known to have ingested significant amounts of opiates and those who relapse after the initial response to naloxone. Patients with heroin overdose who respond to naloxone may be safely discharged if they are asymptomatic 3 hours after the last dose.

Rice EK et al: Heroin overdose and myoglobinuric acute renal failure. Clin Nephrol 2000;54:449. [PMID: 11140805] (Retrospective case analysis evaluating the use of heroin and the development of renal failure.)

Sporer KA: Acute heroin overdose. Ann Intern Med 1999;130:584. [PMID: 10189329] (Literature review of the use and toxicity of heroin.)

Stang J et al: Preventing opiate overdose fatalities with take-home naloxone: pre-launch study of possible impact and acceptability. Addiction 1999;94:199. [PMID: 10396785] (Structured interviews of a community and treatment sample of opiate-addicted individuals regarding the possible home use of naloxone.)

Wang DS et al: Nalmefene: a long-acting opioid antagonist. Clinical applications in emergency medicine. J Emerg Med 1998;16:471. [PMID: 9610980] (Review of the pharmacology and clinical use of nalmefene.)

Watson WA et al: Opioid toxicity recurrence after an initial response to naloxone. J Toxicol Clin Toxicol 1998;36:11. [PMID: 9541035] (Retrospective case-control study to determine the frequency and potential predictors of opioid toxicity recurrence after a response to naloxone.)

ORGANOPHOSPHATES & OTHER CHOLINESTERASE INHIBITORS

ESSENTIALS OF DIAGNOSIS

- Toxicity and potency vary widely.
- DUMBELS (**d**iarrhea; **u**rination; **m**iosis; **b**ronchorrhea; **e**xcitation with muscle fasciculation, anxiety, and seizures; **l**acrimation; and **s**eizures). Death is usually from respiratory depression.
- Diagnosis usually confirmed with low plasma or red blood cell cholinesterase level.

General Considerations

Cholinesterase inhibitors are found in a variety of insecticides (organophosphates and carbamates) available for home and commercial use (eg, crop sprays, bug bombs, flea collars). Some chemical warfare agents (nerve gases) are also cholinesterase inhibitors.

These compounds inhibit acetylcholinesterase and therefore allow accumulation of acetylcholine at muscarinic and nicotinic receptors in nerve endings. Organophosphates bind irreversibly with the enzyme, whereas carbamates are considered reversible inhibitors. All are rapidly absorbed from the skin, gastrointestinal tract, and respiratory tract. Toxicity and potency vary widely. Workers constantly exposed to organophosphates and infants with underdeveloped cholinesterase activity are at greater risk for intoxication.

Clinical Findings

Miosis, excessive salivation, bronchospasm, hyperactive bowel sounds, and lethargy typically occur shortly after exposure. Either bradycardia (muscarinic effect) or tachycardia (nicotinic effect) may be observed. QT-interval prolongation and pleomorphic ventricular tachyarrhythmias are a late consequence of poisoning. Symptoms of toxicity are easily remembered with the mnemonic DUMBELS (**d**iarrhea; **u**rination; **m**iosis; **b**ronchorrhea; **e**xcitation with muscle fasciculation, anxiety, and seizures; **l**acrimation; and **s**alivation). Death is usually caused by respiratory depression.

Measurement of the plasma or red blood cell cholinesterase level is helpful in confirming acute toxicity; cholinesterase levels become low soon after exposure.

Treatment

A. GENERAL MANAGEMENT

Provide intensive supportive care and gastrointestinal decontamination as described previously. Careful management of the airway is important, because significant bronchial secretions, bronchospasm, and hypoventilation may occur. Position the patient so as to avoid aspiration, and provide suction and oxygen as required. Early recognition of respiratory distress and subsequent intubation may decrease the mortality among these patients.

Remove and isolate the patient's clothing, and carefully wash the skin with soap and water. Medical personnel should be careful to avoid cross-contamination.

B. PHARMACOLOGIC TREATMENT

Atropine is a symptomatic treatment for muscarinic signs (salivation, bronchorrhea, bronchospasm, sweating). Large doses may be required. Start with 1–2 mg intravenously (0.5 mg in children), followed by repeated doses of 2–4 mg every 5–10 minutes until signs of atropinization occur (ie, flushing, mydriasis, drying of secretions, and tachycardia). The use of up to 50 mg in 24 hours is not unusual.

Pralidoxime (Protopam, 2-PAM) competitively inhibits binding of organophosphates to acetylcholinesterase and should be given to all patients with significant intoxication. It is not required for carbamate poisoning, because carbamate toxicity is transient. The dose is 1–2 g (25–50 mg/kg in children) in saline intravenously over 5–10 minutes. Continuous pralidoxime infusion has also been shown to improve the outcome in organophosphate poisoning. Adequate renal function is a prerequisite for use of pralidoxime, because it is excreted in the urine.

C. NEUROLOGIC SEQUELAE

Patients who receive prompt treatment usually recover from acute toxicity. However, 2 neurologic sequelae of severe intoxication—organophosphate-induced delayed neuropathy and intermediate syndrome—may occur after significant exposure.

Disposition

Hospitalize all patients with suspected or documented serious organophosphate poisoning. Carbamate poisoning is usually transient, and patients who recover rapidly may be discharged.

Kwong TC: Organophosphate pesticides: biochemistry and clinical toxicology. Ther Drug Monit 2002;24:144. [PMID: 11805735] (Review of the biochemistry and clinical toxicology of organophosphates.)

Singh S et al: Aggressive atropinisation and continuous pralidoxime (2-PAM) infusion in patients with severe organophosphate poisoning: experience of a northwest Indian hospital. Hum Exp Toxicol 2001;20:15. [PMID: 11339619] (Noncontrolled study to determine if continuous pralidoxime infusion and atropine improved the outcome in patients with severe organophosphate poisoning.)

Sungur M et al: Intensive care management of organophosphate insecticide poisoning. Crit Care 2001;5:211. [PMID: 11511334] (Retrospective case study analysis to evaluate the clinical course of organophosphate poisoning.)

Wang MH et al: Q-T interval prolongation and pleomorphic ventricular tachyarrhythmia ('Torsade de pointes') in organophosphate poisoning: a report of a case. Hum Exp Toxicol 1998;17:587. [PMID: 9821023] (Case report and discussion of organophosphate poisoning.)

PHENCYCLIDINE

 ESSENTIALS OF DIAGNOSIS

- *Rapid onset of action.*
- *Vertical and horizontal nystagmus are common.*
- *Symptoms may fluctuate, unpredictably, from severe agitation to quiet stupor.*
- *Hyperthermia and rhabdomyolysis may lead to myoglobinuria and renal failure.*

General Considerations

Phencyclidine (PCP)—a common adulterant of marijuana, amphetamines, and street hallucinogens—is also called angel dust, crystal, supergrass, ozone, whack, rocket fuel, and peace pill by its users. It may be smoked, snorted, ingested, or injected.

PCP is a sympathomimetic, hallucinogenic, dissociative agent originally used as a veterinary anesthetic. It has a rapid onset of action when smoked or snorted, causing euphoria and hallucinations. Serious overdose does not usually occur with smoking, because users can titrate the dose to achieve the desired effect. Ingestion of 20–25 mg of PCP can cause severe intoxication. PCP has a large volume of distribution (2–4 L/kg) and a half-life of several hours to days. As a weak base, it is ionized in acidic media such as the stomach and acidic urine. It is eliminated primarily by metabolism. Because only about 10% is excreted into the urine, increasing urinary output or urinary acidification (to cause ion trapping) is unlikely to increase elimination of the drug significantly.

Clinical Findings

Symptoms typically fluctuate, with patients alternating unpredictably from severe agitation to quiet stupor. Bizarre, paranoid behavior and extreme violence may occur unexpectedly. Both vertical and horizontal nystagmus are common. The pupils may be large or small. Hypertension, tachycardia, and hyperthermia are common. Marked muscle rigidity, dystonias, and seizures may occur. Hyperthermia and rhabdomyolysis resulting in myoglobinuria and renal failure are a major cause of subsequent illness. The diagnosis is made primarily on clinical grounds but may be confirmed by demonstrating PCP in urine or gastric aspirate. Serum PCP concentrations are not of value in emergency management.

Treatment

A. General Management

Provide intensive supportive care and gastrointestinal decontamination as described previously. Most instances of PCP intoxication are mild and self-limited, and patients need no specific treatment other than to be in a quiet and supportive environment.

B. Treatment of Moderate to Severe Poisoning

Diazepam, 2–5 mg intravenously every 30 minutes until sedation is achieved, is effective in controlling moderate agitation or anxiety.

Haloperidol, 5–10 mg intravenously, may also be effective in controlling toxic psychosis. The goal of treatment is to prevent complications stemming from muscular hyperactivity and subsequent hyperthermia and rhabdomyolysis.

C. Treatment of Rhabdomyolysis or Myoglobinuria

If the patient has rhabdomyolysis or myoglobinuria, maintain urine output with intravenous fluids and mannitol. Alkalization of urine is recommended in order to minimize renal deposition of myoglobin.

D. Enhanced Elimination

Because PCP has a large volume of distribution, dialysis procedures are not useful. Acidification of the urine with ammonium chloride or hydrogen chloride has been used, but it does not significantly increase the total elimination rate, and it is not recommended. Evidence indicates that aciduria may worsen myoglobinuric renal toxicity. It is no longer recommended.

Disposition

Hospitalize patients who have moderate to severe PCP poisoning, particularly if hyperthermia, severe muscular rigidity, or evidence of rhabdomyolysis is an accompanying manifestation.

Cruz R et al: Pulmonary manifestations of inhaled street drugs. Heart & Lung: The Journal of Acute and Critical Care 1998;27:297. [PMID: 9777375] (Review of the pulmonary manifestations of snorting or smoking PCP.)

Piecuch S et al: Acute dystonic reactions that fail to respond to diphenhydramine: think of PCP. J Emerg Med 1999;17:527. [PMID: 10338254] (Case report of a presentation of PCP use initially thought to be due to phenothiazines.)

PHENOTHIAZINES & OTHER ANTIPSYCHOTICS

 ESSENTIALS OF DIAGNOSIS

- *Extrapyramidal side effects (eg, dystonia, orofacial spasms)*
- *Sedation, miosis, and hypotension are common.*
- *Coma, seizures, and ventricular arrhythmias may occur with large doses.*

General Considerations

Antipsychotic drugs include chlorpromazine (Thorazine, many others), prochlorperazine (Compazine), haloperidol (Haldol, others), and many other phenothiazines and butyrophenones.

The mechanism of toxicity of the antipsychotics is complex. Antiadrenergic properties cause sedation and hypotension, anticholinergic effects are manifested by dry mouth and tachycardia, and antidopaminergic properties may produce extrapyramidal side effects (most commonly seen with haloperidol). The contribution of each of these effects in drug overdose depends on the specific drug and on the individual patient.

Most of these compounds have large volumes of distribution (10–30 L/kg) and long half-lives (12–30 hours); dialysis is not effective.

Clinical Findings

Extrapyramidal side effects may occur even at therapeutic doses and include dystonic posturing, spasm of orofacial muscles, cogwheel rigidity, and spasticity. With acute overdose, sedation, miosis, and hypotension are common. Coma and seizures may occur with very large ingestions. Prolongation of the QT interval and ventricular arrhythmias may occur. Disruption of the temperature-regulating mechanism may lead to hyperthermia or hypothermia. Abdominal x-rays may show radiopaque tablets in the gut.

Treatment

A. GENERAL MANAGEMENT

Provide intensive supportive care and gastrointestinal decontamination as described previously. Treat hypotension with intravenous crystalloid solution; if a vasopressor is needed, norepinephrine is preferable.

B. TREATMENT OF EXTRAPYRAMIDAL REACTIONS

Diphenhydramine (Benadryl, many others), 0.5–1 mg/kg intravenously slowly; or benztropine (Cogentin), 1–2 mg intramuscularly for adults, is recommended for extrapyramidal reactions. Relapse may occur; dispense oral anticholinergics for 2–3 days. Sophisticated drug-seeking patients have been known to simulate dystonias in order to receive these medicines.

C. TREATMENT OF ATYPICAL ANTIPSYCHOTIC OVERDOSE

Patients who overdose on atypical antipsychotics (eg, risperidone, olanzapine) present in a manner similar to patients who overdose on the high-potency antipsychotics and should be managed similarly.

Disposition

Hospitalize patients with suspected or documented poisoning due to antipsychotics. In the acute period, close cardiac monitoring for arrhythmias and hypotension is warranted. Indications of significant poisoning include (1) a large number of pill fragments found in the stomach or intestines by means of lavage, emesis, or abdominal plain film, (2) rapidly worsening clinical findings, and (3) obtundation. Patients with extrapyramidal reactions who respond to anticholinergic therapy may be discharged.

Catalano G et al: Atypical antipsychotic overdose in the pediatric population. J Child Adolesc Psychopharmacol 2001;11:425.

[PMID: 11838825] (Case report and literature review of the treatment of risperidone overdose.)

Chan-Tack KM: Neuroleptic malignant syndrome due to promethazine. South Med J 1999;92:1017. [PMID: 10548178] (Case report and discussion of promethazine as a cause of neuroleptic malignant syndrome.)

James LP et al: Phenothiazine, butyrophenone, and other psychotropic medication poisonings in children and adolescents. J Toxicol Clin Toxicol 2000;38:615. [PMID: 11185968] (Retrospective case analysis of phenothiazine and butyrophenone ingestions in children.)

POISONOUS MUSHROOMS

 ESSENTIALS OF DIAGNOSIS

- *Delayed onset of symptoms (gastrointestinal irritation) of 6–12 hours suggests a toxic mushroom ingestion.*
- *Mushrooms containing amatoxin may produce fatal hepatic necrosis.*

General Considerations

Of the over 5000 varieties of mushrooms found in the United States, about 100 can be toxic. Most poisonous mushrooms act as gastrointestinal irritants. Table 45–19 lists several types of poisonous mushrooms, symptoms, and treatment. The most significant are *Amanita phalloides* and other mushrooms containing amatoxin, which may produce fatal hepatic necrosis.

Assistance with identification of specimens can often be obtained from a university biology department or mycology society. Poisindex and regional poison control centers may also help with identification. However, because accurate identification of mushrooms is difficult without an experienced mycologist and impractical because many types of mushrooms are often ingested at one time, the best approach to mushroom ingestion is to assume that the most toxic types have been consumed. Delayed onset (6–12 hours) of gastrointestinal symptoms suggests amatoxin or monomethylhydrazine poisoning.

Treatment

Provide intensive supportive care and gastrointestinal decontamination as described previously.

If the identity of the ingested mushrooms is not known, induce emesis at home or perform gastric lavage in the emergency department. This should be followed by activated charcoal every 2–4 hours.

Table 45–19. Mushrooms: symptoms, toxicity, and treatment.

Symptoms	Mushrooms	Toxicity	Treatment
Gastrointestinal symptoms Onset < 2 h	*Chlorophyllum molybdites* *Omphalotus illudens* *Cantharellus cibarius* *Amanita caesarea*	Nausea, vomiting, diarrhea (occasional bloody) Initial: nausea, vomiting, diarrhea	IV hydration Antiemetics IV hydration, glucose, monitor, AST, ALT, PT, PTT, bilirubin, BUN, creatinine
Onset 6–24 h	*Gyromitra esculenta:* fall season *Amanita phalloides, Amanita verna,* and *Amanita virosa:* spring season	Day 2: rise in AST, ALT Day 3: hepatic failure	For *Amanita:* activated charcoal Penicillin G, 300,000–1,000,000 U/kg/d Silymarin, 20–40 mg/kg/d Consider cimetidine, 4–10 g/d Hyperbaric oxygen
Muscarinic (SLUDGE) syndrome Onset < 30 min	*Inocybe* *Clitocybe*	Salivation, lacrimation, diarrhea, gastrointestinal distress, emesis	Supportive atropine, 0.01 mg/kg, repeated as needed for severe secretions.
CNS excitement Onset < 30 min	*Amanita muscaria* *Amanita pantherina*	Intoxication, dizziness, ataxia, visual disturbances, sei- zures, tachycardia, hyper- tension, warm dry skin, dry mouth, mydriasis (anti- cholinergic effects)	Supportive sedation with pheno- barbital, 30 mg IV, or diazepam, 2–5 mg IV, as needed for adults
Hallucinations Onset < 30 min	*Psilocybe* *Gymnopilus*	Visual hallucinations, ataxia	Supportive sedation with pheno- barbital, 0.5 mg/kg, or, for adults, 30–60 mg IV, or diaze- pam, 0.1 mg/kg or 5 mg IV, for adults
Disulfiram 2–72 h after mushroom, and < 30 min after alcohol	*Coprinus*	Headache, flushing, tachycar- dia, hyperventilation, short- ness of breath, palpitations	Supportive IV hydration Propranolol for supraventricular tachycardia Norepinephrine for refractory hypotension

ALT = alanine amino transferase; AST = aspartate amino transferase; BUN = blood urea nitrogen; CNS = central nervous system; PT = prothrombin time; PTT = partial thromboplastin time; SLUDGE syndrome = salivation, lacrimation, urination, defecation, gastrointestinal
hypermotility, and emesis.
Reproduced, with permission, from Tintinalli JE, Keten GD, Stapczynski S: *Emergency Medicine: A Comprehensive Study Guide,* 5th ed.
McGraw-Hill, 2000.

If poisoning with amatoxin is suspected, hospitalize
the patient for observation and obtain baseline hepatic
and renal function measurements. A variety of potential
antidotes have been recommended, including corticosteroids, penicillin G, thioctic acid, silymarin, and NAC.
No well-designed controlled human studies have addressed the efficacy of these antidotes. More important
than specific antidotes is supportive care, including aggressive fluid replacement for massive gastroenteritis,
supplemental glucose, and supportive treatment for hepatic encephalopathy. Early charcoal hemoperfusion or
dialysis may be beneficial. Liver transplant has been successful in several patients with massive hepatic necrosis.

Table 45–19 describes specific treatment for various
kinds of mushroom poisoning.

Disposition

Hospitalize patients thought or known to have ingested
mushrooms known to cause serious poisoning (see
Table 45–19).

Broussard CN et al: Mushroom poisoning—from diarrhea to liver
transplantation. Am J Gastroenterol 2001;96:3195. [PMID:
11721773] (Case study series and discussion of the toxicity of
mushrooms.)

Wellington K et al: Silymarin: a review of its clinical properties in the management of hepatic disorders. BioDrugs 2001;15: 465. [PMID: 11520257] (Literature review and discussion of the potential for silymarin use in hepatic disorders.)

POISONOUS PLANTS

 **ESSENTIALS OF DIAGNOSIS**

- *Identification of plant is often difficult but essential to diagnosis of toxicity.*
- *Symptoms are dependent on plant toxin ingested (eg, cyanide, cardiac glycosides, anticholinergics).*

General Considerations

Several hundred species of plants in the United States contain toxic compounds. Tables 45–20 and 45–21 give examples of nontoxic and toxic plants. Details about identification, mechanism of toxicity, and treatment are best obtained from a local poison control center or from Poisindex. If the identity of a plant is unknown, it is helpful to take along a sample to a local nursery or to a botanist. Gardening books are also useful sources of identification. Despite the potential for plants to cause serious toxicity, physicians have a general lack of knowledge about plant poisoning.

Treat the specific symptoms manifested by the patient, not those thought to be associated with the type of poisonous plant believed to have been ingested. Many similar species of plants have widely varying potencies and combinations of toxins; the plant's age, the

Table 45–20. Some nontoxic plants.

African violet (*Saintpaulia ionantha*)
Baby tears (*Helxine soleirolii*)
Bridal veil (*Genista monosperma pendula*)
Coleus species
Fuchsia species
Gardenia (*Gardenia radicans*)
Jade plant (*Crassula argentea*)
Piggyback *Begonia* (*Begonia hispida cucullifera*)
Piggyback plant (*Tolmiea menziesii*)
Rubber plant (*Ficus elastica "Decora"*)
Spider plant (*Chlorophytum comosum*)
Swedish ivy (*Plectranthus australis*)
Wandering Jew (*Tradescantia albiflora, T fluminensis, Zebrina pendula*)
Zebra plant (*Calathea zebrina*)

soil conditions, and other factors influence the severity of toxic symptoms.

Classes of Toxins

Some of the more common plant toxins are described below. The list is not complete.

A. OXALATES

Insoluble calcium oxalate crystals in the leaves and stems of some plants irritate the mucous membranes and can cause edema of the mouth, throat, and tongue. In rare severe reactions, drooling, dysphagia, and airway obstruction may occur. Renal failure may occur if sufficient amounts of oxalates are absorbed.

B. AMYGDALIN AND CYANOGENIC GLYCOSIDES

Cyanide is produced by the gastrointestinal hydrolysis of chewed-up fruit pits or seeds. (*Prunus* species: cherry, apricot, peach) or leaves and stems (*Hydrangea*, elderberry). Severe poisoning is uncommon. See "Cyanide" section for symptoms and therapy.

C. CARDIAC GLYCOSIDES

Digitalis and similar compounds are present in varying amounts in certain plants. Death after consumption of only one oleander leaf has been reported (see "Cardiac Glycosides" section).

D. ANTICHOLINERGICS

The typical anticholinergic syndrome of dry mouth, tachycardia, delirium, urinary retention, and mydriasis is seen. Most poisonings are mild, and supportive treatment is sufficient (see "Anticholinergics" section).

E. NICOTINELIKE TOXINS

These toxins include nicotine and aconitine. Symptoms include nausea and vomiting, salivation, diarrhea, restlessness, and seizures. Mydriasis may also occur. Following an initial phase of excitement, respiratory depression and hypotension may occur.

F. SOLANINE

Solanine has effects similar to those of nicotine. In addition, plants containing solanine often have significant amounts of atropinic alkaloids, so that the net effect is unpredictable. Onset of symptoms may be delayed several hours.

G. TOXALBUMINS

These highly toxic compounds (eg, abrin, ricin, phallin) can cause acute gastroenteritis, dehydration, and shock. Convulsions, hemolysis, and renal and hepatic injury can also occur. Oral and esophageal irritation or burns may be seen.

Table 45–21. Some poisonous plants.[1]

Plant name	Type of Toxin
Azalea (*Rhododendron* species)	Andromedotoxin (nicotinelike and cardiotoxic)
Black nightshade (*Solanum nigrum*)	Solanine
Caladium	Oxalates
Castor bean (*Ricinus communis*)	Toxalbumin (ricin)
Deadly nightshade (*Atropa belladonna*)	Anticholinergic
Delphinium	Nicotinelike
Dumb cane (*Dieffenbachia*)	Oxalates
Elderberry (*Sambucus*)	Cyanogenic (ripe berries nontoxic)
Foxglove (*Digitalis purpurea*)	Cardiac glycosides
Hydrangea	Cyanogenic
Jequirity bean, rosary bean (*Abrus precatorius*)	Toxalbumin (a lectin)
Jerusalem cherry (*Solanum pseudocapsicum*)	Solanine
Jimsonweed (*Datura stramonium*)	Anticholinergic
Lantana	Anticholinergic
Lily of the valley (*Convallaria majalis*)	Cardiac glycosides
Lobelia	Nicotinelike
Mistletoe (*Viscum album, Phoradendron flavescens*)	Tyramine (hypertension; gastroenteritis)
Mountain laurel (*Kalmia latifolia*)	Andromedotoxin (nicotinelike and cardiotoxic)
Oleander (*Nerium oleander*)	Cardiac glycosides
Philodendron	Oxalates
Pits (of cherry, apricot, peach)	Cyanogenic (amygdalin)
Poison hemlock (*Conium maculatum*)	Nicotinelike
Poinsettia (*Euphorbia pulcherrima*)	Oxalatelike
Tobacco (*Nicotiana tabacum*)	Nicotine
Water hemlock (*Cicuta maculata*)	Cicutoxin (seizures)
Yew (*Taxus* species)	Taxine (gastrointeritis, cardiac toxicity)

[1]This short list is for illustrative purposes only. Consult other sources (eg, regional poison control center) for information on specific plants.

Treatment

In general, emesis is recommended after ingestion of any unidentified plants or those with known potentially serious toxic effects. Follow emesis with activated charcoal, a cathartic, and symptomatic treatment as needed. Keep the patient under observation. Begin specific treatment as indicated for the specific toxins involved.

Disposition

Disposition depends on the plant ingested and the symptoms experienced.

Lawrence RA: Poisonous plants: when they are a threat to children. Pediatr Rev 1997;18:162. [PMID: 9114716]

Manriquez O et al: Analysis of 156 cases of plant intoxication received in the Toxicologic Information Center at Catholic University of Chile. Vet Hum Toxicol 2002;44:31. [PMID: 11824773] (Retrospective analysis of plant and mushroom ingestions.)

SALICYLATES

 ESSENTIALS OF DIAGNOSIS

- *Toxicity generally occurs at levels > 150 mg/kg.*
- *Early manifestations include nausea, vomiting, and hyperventilation.*
- *Initial respiratory alkalosis is often followed by a severe metabolic acidosis, creating a mixed acid-base status.*
- *Hypoglycemia is prominent in children.*

General Considerations

Salicylates are present in numerous prescription and nonprescription medications, for example, analgesics, bismuth subsalicylate (Pepto-Bismol, many others), or oil of wintergreen (methyl salicylate).

The mechanism of toxicity with salicylate poisoning is complex and includes direct central nervous system stimulation, uncoupling of oxidative phosphorylation, inhibition of Krebs cycle enzymes, and interference with hemostatic mechanisms. The volume of distribution is dose dependent and usually small; with significant ingestion, however, the drug is redistributed into the central nervous system. Because salicylate is a weak acid, acidemia increases its penetration of the central nervous system. The half-life may increase from 2 to 20 hours at overdose levels as a result of saturation of liver metabolism. The elimination of salicylate is increased in alkaline urine. The minimum acute toxic dose is 150 mg/kg, with severe toxicity occurring at doses over 300–500 mg/kg. However, many cases of toxicity are a result of prolonged excessive treatment of minor illnesses (subacute or accidental overdose). The chronically ill and the elderly are at greater risk for subacute toxicity because of relative hypoalbuminemia and renal insufficiency.

Clinical Findings

Early manifestations of overdose include nausea and vomiting, tinnitus, listlessness, and hyperventilation. Loss of fluid and electrolytes is common. Initial respiratory alkalosis is followed by severe metabolic acidosis, hypokalemia, and hypoglycemia. Seizures, hyperpyrexia, and coma occur as toxicity becomes more severe. Measurement of the blood salicylate concentration is essential for effective management, although it is not as reliable an indicator of the severity of illness if subacute toxicity is present. In cases of acute salicylate ingestion, the Done nomogram has been shown to have a poor predictive value and the prognosis and patient management should not be based solely on an aspirin level. Consider the patient's clinical presentation, age, aspirin level, and acid-base status in making treatment decisions. In the presence of acidosis, toxicity occurs with considerably lower levels. Salicylate determinations should be repeated every 4–5 hours. Repeated measurements are especially important for ingestion of sustained-release or enteric-coated preparations, which are absorbed slowly and may result in delayed peak levels.

With subacute (accidental) toxicity, severity of poisoning does not correlate well with serum salicylate concentration, but levels above 30 mg/dL (300 mg/L) are significant. Patients with subacute toxicity are frequently very young or very old, and they usually present with dehydration, obtundation, and acidosis. The diagnosis is often missed while the physician concentrates on the more prominent secondary complications. Cerebral and pulmonary edema and death are more common in patients with subacute toxicity.

A Phenistix test of urine may be positive (purple or purple-brown) with salicylate toxicity, but false-negative results have been reported in patients with acid urine.

Treatment

A. GENERAL MANAGEMENT

Provide intensive supportive care and gastrointestinal decontamination as described previously. After acute overdose, give adequate charcoal to bind ingested salicylate. Multidose activated charcoal may be beneficial. For enteric-coated aspirin, toxicologists recommend lavage followed by activated charcoal, with further doses of activated charcoal and possibly even whole bowel irrigation if the salicylate level is rising.

B. CORRECTION OF ACID-BASE STATUS

Correct dehydration, hypoglycemia, hypokalemia, and acidosis. For significant dehydration, start with 20 mL/kg of an intravenous crystalloid solution given over 1–2 hours, and then give 3–5 mL/kg/h to maintain the urine output at 2–3 mL/kg/h. To correct acidosis and promote excretion of salicylate in the urine, give sodium bicarbonate, 1 mEq/kg/h. Concurrent correction of potassium deficit is mandatory. Urine pH should be maintained at 7–7.5. Alkalization of the urine is often unsuccessful in critically ill patients (especially the elderly), and it may aggravate pulmonary and cerebral edema.

C. Enhanced Elimination

Hemodialysis is recommended for critically ill patients with persistent seizures, acidosis that fails to respond to treatment, or cerebral or pulmonary edema. Although high salicylate concentrations (eg, > 120 mg/dL [1200 mg/L] at 6 hours) generally represent severe toxicity, hemodialysis should be based on the patient's complications and not the drug level. Hemodialysis is efficient in removing salicylate and can help to correct pH and electrolyte abnormalities. Consider early hemodialysis in ill patients with subacute overdose. Although there are no proved guidelines, elderly patients with serum salicylate levels over 60 mg/dL, and those with significant neurologic toxicity, should probably receive immediate hemodialysis. If the patient is hemodynamically unstable or hemodialysis is unavailable, continuous hemodiafiltration has been reported to be a viable alternative.

D. Other Measures

Obtain measurements of serum salicylate every 4–6 hours to monitor adequacy of treatment. If evidence of salicylate-induced hypoprothrombinemia is present, give vitamin K, 10 mg intramuscularly.

Rehydration and rapid correction of acidemia are essential. Give glucose, and replace potassium deficits.

Disposition

Hospitalize all patients with known or suspected severe salicylate poisoning. Patients who have ingested enteric-coated tablets (eg, Ecotrin) may remain asymptomatic for several hours or even days; repeated blood levels and abdominal x-rays or even endoscopy may be necessary if a massive ingestion is suspected.

Higgins RM et al: Alkalinization and hemodialysis in severe salicylate poisoning: comparison of elimination techniques in the same patient. Clin Nephrol 1998;50:178. [PMID: 9776422]

Juurlink D et al: Gastrointestinal decontamination for the enteric-coated aspirin overdose: what to do depends on who you ask. J Toxicol Clin Toxicol 2000;38:465. [PMID: 10981955] (Survey of poison control centers and their individual recommendations for gastrointestinal decontamination in overdose with enteric-coated aspirin.)

Wrathall G et al: Three case reports of the use of haemodiafiltration in the treatment of salicylate overdose. Hum Exp Toxicol 2001;20:491. [PMID: 11776412] (Case reports and discussion of the use of hemodiafiltration in the treatment of salicylate overdose.)

SEDATIVE-HYPNOTICS

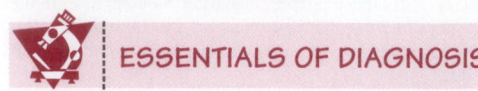

ESSENTIALS OF DIAGNOSIS

- *Symptoms include nystagmus, atonia, lethargy, somnolence, respiratory depression, hypotension, and hypothermia.*
- *Sedative-hypnotics such as γ-hydroxybutyric acid may be associated with symptoms ranging from respiratory depression and coma to seizurelike activity with aggressive behavior.*

General Considerations

Sedative-hypnotics include a broad range of drugs used to treat anxiety or insomnia. They can induce tolerance and can cause a withdrawal syndrome similar to that associated with ethanol withdrawal (except for the time of onset and duration). These agents are found singly and in various drug combinations. Of note, one sedative-hypnotic, γ-hydroxybutyric acid (GHB), has become a relatively new drug of abuse. Effects range from respiratory depression, apnea, and coma to seizurelike activity along with aggressive behavior.

Absorption, distribution, and elimination of sedative-hypnotics vary. In general, the mechanism of toxicity of these drugs is central nervous system depression similar to that caused by ethanol.

Clinical Findings

Clinical manifestations of overdose include nystagmus, ophthalmoplegia, ataxia, dysarthria, lethargy, somnolence, respiratory depression, hypotension, and hypothermia. With the onset of deep coma, oculocephalic reflexes are lost, and the pupils become nonreactive to light. The initial electroencephalogram may be flat, although the patient may subsequently recover completely. Serum drug levels may be misleading, because levels of intoxication and rates of elimination vary enormously from person to person, depending on prior drug use and the patient's physical state.

Treatment

A. General Management

Provide intensive supportive care and gastrointestinal decontamination as described previously. Treat shock and hypotension with an initial bolus of 200–1000 mL of intravenous crystalloid solution (Chapter 9). Restore the patient's core temperature to normal levels, because hypothermia will worsen hypotension. Monitoring the pulmonary capillary wedge pressure is helpful in avoiding fluid overload and determining the need for pressor agents. Vasopressors should be used only if adequate fluid replacement is ineffective (as determined by pulmonary capillary wedge pressure measurements).

B. Enhanced Elimination

Reserve hemodialysis or hemoperfusion for patients who remain hypotensive or otherwise unstable despite aggressive supportive care. These measures successfully remove only a few sedative-hypnotics (eg, phenobarbital, meprobamate, ethchlorvynol).

C. Other Measures

The benzodiazepine antagonist flumazenil (Mazicon) should be used with extreme caution, if at all. The dose is 0.2 mg intravenously slowly repeated every 5–10 minutes as needed, up to a maximum 3–5 mg. Effects wear off in 1–3 hours, and repeated sedation is common. Contraindications include known seizure disorder, benzodiazepine addiction, and tricyclic antidepressant overdose. General supportive care usually suffices.

Treatment of GHB toxicity is similar to the treatment of toxicity from all other sedative-hypnotics in that supportive care will usually suffice. However, flumazenil has no effect on GHB toxicity, but intravenous physostigmine (slowly over 2–3 minutes) has been found in some case studies to reverse the respiratory depression of GHB toxicity and obvert the need for intubation. The use of physostigmine should be discouraged, however, because of the potential for the development of life-threatening cardiac complications.

Disposition

Hospitalize patients with sedative-hypnotic drug poisoning resulting in depression of vital reflexes (eg, respiration, gag reflex).

James L et al: A tale of novel intoxication: a review of the effects of gamma-hydroxybutyric acid with recommendations for management. Ann Emerg Med 1998;31:729. [PMID: 9624313] (Literature review of the effects and management of GHB intoxication.)

Rachel LC et al: Clinical course of gamma-hydroxybutyrate overdose. Ann Emerg Med 1998;31:716. [PMID: 9624311] (Retrospective case analysis of patients with GHB overdose.)

Yates SW et al: Physostigmine in the treatment of gamma-hydroxybutyric acid overdose. Mayo Clin Proc 200;75:401. [PMID: 10761496] (Case report of the use of physostigmine in the treatment of GHB overdose.)

THEOPHYLLINE & METHYLXANTHINES

 ESSENTIALS OF DIAGNOSIS

- *Minimum acute toxic dose is 10 mg/kg.*
- *Mild symptoms include nausea and vomiting, tremor, anxiety, and abdominal cramping.*
- *Severe symptoms include arrhythmias and seizures.*

General Considerations

Theophylline causes bronchodilatation; gastric, central nervous system, and cardiac stimulation; and vasodilatation. The half-life is 4–8 hours and is shortened in chronic smokers and prolonged in patients with congestive heart failure or cirrhosis. In acute overdose, the half-life may be markedly prolonged (up to 50 hours).

The minimum acute toxic dose is over 10 mg/kg, or 700 mg, in the average adult. Because drug metabolism varies markedly depending on the patient's clinical status, careful monitoring of patients receiving therapeutic doses is necessary to avoid iatrogenic toxicity.

Clinical Findings

Mild symptoms of toxicity are nausea and vomiting, abdominal cramps, tremor, and anxiety. Arrhythmias and seizures occur with more serious intoxication. Seizures are often refractory to treatment with standard anticonvulsants. The characteristics of acute single overdose differ from those of chronic, subacute overmedication. Acute overdose is characterized by hypotension, tachycardia, and hypokalemia. Seizures and serious arrhythmias are common with levels over 100 mg/L but rare with levels under 90 mg/L. By contrast, chronic intoxication more commonly results in seizures and arrhythmias with much lower serum levels (ie, 20–70 mg/L). Hypotension and hypokalemia are uncommon. The elderly are at highest risk for fatal outcome.

Sustained-release theophylline preparations are now commonly used, so that after acute overdose, early blood concentrations of the drug may be low and gastrointestinal symptoms absent. Obtain serial blood levels until the theophylline level begins to fall.

Treatment

A. General Management

Provide intensive supportive care and gastrointestinal decontamination as described previously.

B. Gastrointestinal Decontamination

Consider gastric lavage if a significant dose has been ingested within 1 hour of arrival at the emergency department. Administer multidose activated charcoal; consider whole bowel irrigation for sustained-release preparations.

C. Treatment of Seizures

Seizures (Chapter 17) are usually difficult to control with standard drugs. Start with diazepam, 0.1–0.2 mg/kg as an intravenous bolus, followed by phenobarbital, 15 mg/kg, intravenously over 20–30 minutes. Perform hemoperfusion immediately if seizures are not controlled.

D. Treatment of Hypotension

Treat hypotension with intravenous fluids. Propranolol, 0.02–0.05 mg/kg, or esmolol, 25–50 μg/kg/min, intravenously, may reverse hypotension associated with tachycardia, both of which are mediated by excessive β-adrenergic stimulation.

E. Treatment of Arrhythmias

Ventricular tachyarrhythmias and rapid atrial fibrillation may be controlled with propranolol or esmolol intravenously (see above) or with standard antiarrhythmics.

F. Enhanced Elimination

Charcoal hemoperfusion, hemofiltration, or hemodialysis are the treatments of choice for severe poisoning. Hemoperfusion is the treatment of choice for severe poisoning (intractable seizures, acute overdose with serum level over 80–100 mg/L, and hemodynamic instability). Repeated doses of activated charcoal may be effective at lowering theophylline levels, obviating extracorporeal treatment.

Disposition

Hospitalize patients with significant theophylline poisoning (serum concentrations above 30 μg/mL or signs or symptoms of toxicity).

Henderson JH et al: Continuous venovenous haemofiltration for the treatment of theophylline toxicity. Thorax 2001;56:242. [PMID: 11182020] (Case study and discussion of the use of venovenous hemofiltration in theophylline toxicity.)

Seiko O et al: Recovery from theophylline toxicity by continuous hemodialysis with filtration. Ann Intern Med 2000;133:922. [PMID: 11103070] (Case report of the use of hemodialysis with filtration to treat theophylline toxicity.)

Shannon M: Life-threatening events after theophylline overdose. Arch Intern Med 1999;159:989. [PMID: 10326941] (Prospective longitudinal cohort study of patients with theophylline overdose.)

TRICYCLIC ANTIDEPRESSANTS

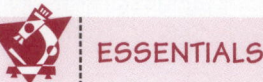

ESSENTIALS OF DIAGNOSIS

- *Average toxic dose is 5 mg/kg.*
- *Anticholinergic symptoms range from mydriasis, agitation, and tachycardia to seizures and coma.*
- *Cardiovascular manifestations are often life threatening and include QRS widening, profound hypotension, atrioventricular blocks, and ventricular arrhythmias.*

General Considerations

Major tricyclic antidepressants include amitriptyline (Elavil, many others), imipramine (Tofranil, many others), and doxepin (Adapin, Sinequan). Maprotiline (Ludiomil) is a tetracyclic antidepressant with similar properties.

The antidepressants are analogs of phenothiazines, with complex effects, including anticholinergic, α-adrenergic-receptor blocking, and quinidinelike activity on the heart. They are well absorbed and highly tissue bound, with volumes of distribution of 10–40 L/kg. These drugs are eliminated primarily by metabolism in the liver, and the half-lives are 10–30 hours. The average toxic dose is more than 5 mg/kg, with severe poisoning occurring at doses of 10–20 mg/kg.

Clinical Findings

Many symptoms are the result of the anticholinergic activity of these drugs, for example, mydriasis, dry mouth, tachycardia, agitation, and hallucinations. The onset of coma may be rapid, even precipitous. Twitching and myoclonic jerking have been noted, and seizures occur frequently and may be difficult to treat.

Cardiovascular manifestations are the most dramatic and life threatening (Figure 45–2). Quinidinelike slowing of conduction is reflected by widening of the QRS complex (> 100 ms) and prolonged QT and PR intervals. Varying degrees of atrioventricular block and ventricular tachycardia are common. Atypical (torsades de pointes) ventricular tachycardia may occur. Profound hypotension resulting from decreased contractility and

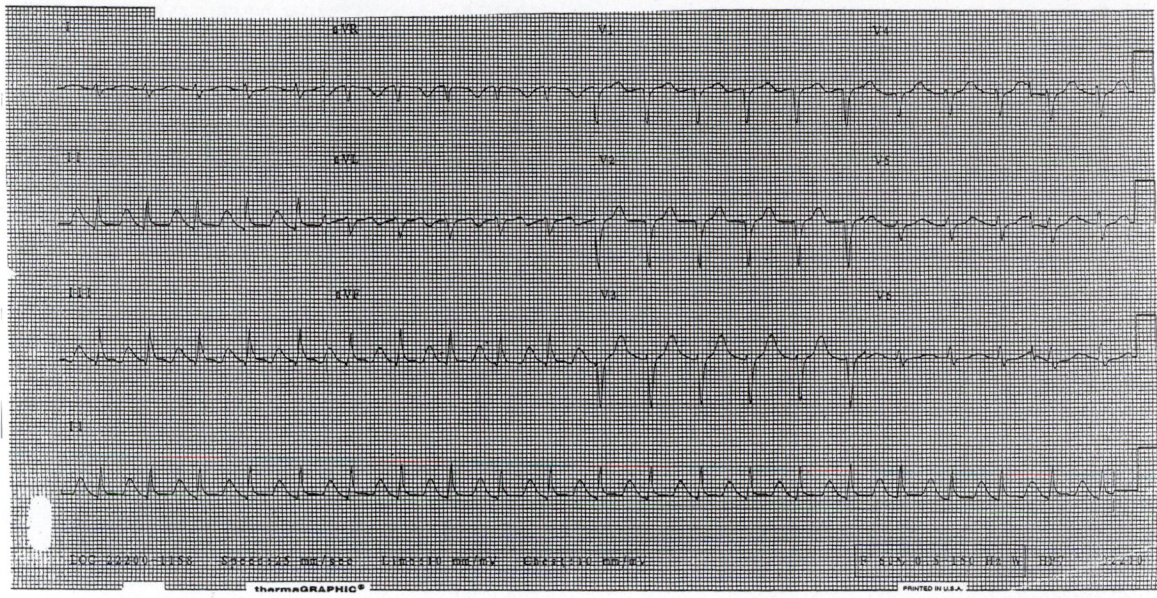

Figure 45–2. Supraventricular tachycardia with prolonged QT$_c$ and terminal right axis resulting from tricyclic antidepressant overdose.

vasodilatation may occur and is a frequent cause of death. Hypoxemia and acidosis aggravate the cardiovascular toxicity of tricyclic antidepressants.

Diagnosis is generally based on history, relevant physical findings, widened QRS complexes, and prolonged QT intervals (3 C's: **c**ardiac abnormalities, **c**onvulsions, and **c**oma). The diagnosis may be confirmed by qualitative or quantitative tests for these drugs in the blood or urine. Plasma concentrations are rarely available and often lack sensitivity in detecting active metabolites. Prolongation of the QRS complex or the terminal axis in lead aVR is a better predictor of severity of poisoning than is the drug concentration.

Note: Some newer cyclic antidepressants (amoxapine) and antipsychotics (loxapine) can cause seizures and coma without associated cardiovascular toxicity or electrocardiographic changes.

Treatment

A. GENERAL MANAGEMENT

Provide intensive supportive care and gastrointestinal decontamination as described previously. Do not induce emesis because of the well-established risk of seizures and coma. Perform gastric lavage if the patient has ingested a toxic amount and is seen within 1 hour.

Also, administer activated charcoal at the beginning and again at the end of the procedure.

B. CARDIAC MONITORING

Constant monitoring of the ECG for at least 6 hours is mandatory. Progressive widening of the QRS complex indicates worsening toxicity.

C. TREATMENT OF SEIZURES

Treat seizures with diazepam and phenytoin (Chapter 17). Do not use physostigmine to treat seizures, because it may cause seizures and other complications as described below.

D. TREATMENT OF ARRHYTHMIAS

Sinus tachycardia is benign and usually does not require treatment. Physostigmine and propranolol may aggravate conduction abnormalities and should not be used.

Ventricular arrhythmias and conduction defects may respond to sodium bicarbonate, 50–100 mEq (1–2 mEq/kg) as an intravenous bolus. It is not clear whether the improvement is merely a result of correction of acidosis, a result of transient hypernatremia, or a result of a shift in the protein binding of the drug with alkalosis. Lidocaine, 1–2 mg/kg as an intravenous bolus (Chapter 35), is frequently effective. Phenytoin, 15–18 mg/kg intravenously over 20–30 minutes, is the logical drug of choice because it enhances conduction while decreasing automaticity, but there is no proof that it is more effective. Quinidinelike drugs (eg, quinidine, procainamide, disopyramide) are contraindicated, because they worsen cardiotoxicity.

E. TREATMENT OF HYPOTENSION

Treat hypotension initially with intravenous infusion of sodium bicarbonate, 50–100 mEq (1–2 mEq/kg), and crystalloid solutions. If the patient fails to respond after 1–2 L have been infused, further therapy should be guided by measurement of pulmonary artery wedge pressures and cardiac output. Norepinephrine and epinephrine have been found to be more effective than dopamine in refractory hypotension.

F. OTHER MEASURES

Hemoperfusion has no role in tricyclic antidepressant poisoning. However, several new antidotes, including α-1 acid glycoprotein and hypertonic saline, are under investigation.

Disposition

Hospitalize all symptomatic patients with overdose of tricyclic antidepressants. Use serial ECGs along with the patient's clinical appearance to predict impending toxicity. Observe asymptomatic patients for a minimum of 6–8 hours, taking repeated measurements of the vital signs and QRS interval.

Kerr GW et al: Tricyclic antidepressant overdose: a review. Emerg Med J 2001;18:236. [PMID: 11435353] (Review of the pharmacokinetics, clinical presentation, and treatment of tricyclic antidepressant overdose.)

Ma Y et al: The antidotal effect of alpha(1)-acid glycoprotein on amitriptyline toxicity in cardiac myocytes. Toxicology 2001;169:133. [PMID: 11718954] (Animal model study to evaluate the use of α-1 acid glycoprotein in the treatment of QRS prolongation caused by amitriptyline.)

McCabe J et al: Experimental tricyclic antidepressant toxicity—a randomized, controlled comparison of hypertonic saline solution, sodium bicarbonate, and hyperventilation. Ann Emerg Med 1998;32:329. [PMID: 9737495] (Randomized, controlled animal-model comparison of hypertonic saline solution, sodium bicarbonate, and hyperventilation in severe tricyclic antidepressant overdose.)

Mehta NJ et al: Tricyclic antidepressant overdose and electrocardiographic changes. J Emerg Med 2000;18:463. [PMID: 10802426] (Case report and discussion of ECG changes in tricyclic antidepressant overdose.)

Singh N et al: Serial electrocardiographic changes as a predictor of cardiovascular toxicity in acute tricyclic antidepressant overdose. American Journal of Therapeutics 2002;9:75. [PMID: 11782822] (Case report and discussion of the predictive value of ECG changes in acute tricyclic antidepressant overdose.)

WARFARIN & OTHER ANTICOAGULANTS

ESSENTIALS OF DIAGNOSIS

- A single overdose with warfarin usually does not cause significant bleeding.
- May see ecchymosis, hematuria, melena, epistaxis, gingival bleeding, hematoma, and hematemesis.
- Life-threatening cardiac tamponade and intracranial hemorrhage may occur.

General Considerations

Dicumarol and other natural anticoagulants are found in sweet clover. Warfarin and other synthetic coumarinlike anticoagulants are used therapeutically and as rodenticides.

Warfarin and other coumarinlike compounds inhibit blood clotting by interfering with the synthesis of vitamin K–dependent clotting factors (II, VII, IX, X). Only the synthesis of new factors is affected, and the anticoagulation effect is delayed until currently circulating factors have degraded. Thus, effects may be seen within 8–12 hours after ingestion because factor II has only a 6-hour half-life, but peak effects are usually not observed until 1–2 days after ingestion because of the longer half-lives (24–60 hours) of the other clotting factors.

The potency and pharmacokinetics of the different coumarin anticoagulants vary. Warfarin is highly bound to albumin and has a half-life of 35 hours. It is metabolized by the liver. Multiple drug interactions are known to increase or decrease the anticoagulation effect (Table 45–22).

A single overdose with warfarin does not usually cause significant bleeding, because the half-life of warfarin is shorter than that of some of the clotting factors. Chronic warfarin administration carries a greater risk of excessive anticoagulation and bleeding. However, some newer, extremely potent and long-acting anticoagulants, also known as super-warfarins (brodifacoum, indanediones), may produce severe bleeding disturbance for several weeks to months following a single overdose.

Clinical Findings

Excessive anticoagulation may result in ecchymoses, hematuria, uterine bleeding, melena, epistaxis, gingival bleeding, hemoptysis, or hematemesis. Hematomas may result in compression neuropathy or compartment

Table 45–22. Interactions of warfarin and oral anticoagulants with selected drugs.

Increased Anticoagulation Effect	Decreased Anticoagulation Effect
Allopurinol	Barbiturates
Chloral hydrate	Carbamazepine
Cimetidine	Cholestyramine
Disulfiram	Glutethimide
Indomethacin	Oral contraceptives
Quinidine	Antibiotics (rifampin)
Salicylates	
Sulfonamides	
Antibiotics (erythromycin)	

syndrome. Life-threatening cardiac tamponade and intracranial hemorrhage have been reported. Such complications can be prevented if the international normalized ratio (INR) is carefully monitored and kept within the desired therapeutic range, if interacting drugs are avoided, and if antidotal therapy is begun promptly when necessary.

Treatment

A. GENERAL MANAGEMENT

Provide intensive supportive care and gastrointestinal decontamination as described previously. Gastric lavage and emesis are not recommended. Treatment is rarely required for acute single overdose of warfarin, because the dose involved (eg, from typical rodenticide) is small, and any anticoagulation effect is usually brief and mild. However, caution and careful follow-up are indicated after ingestion of the super-warfarins. Obtain a baseline prothrombin time, and repeat the measurement after 24 and 48 hours.

B. TREATMENT OF MAJOR HEMORRHAGE

For major hemorrhage (eg, intracranial hemorrhage, aortic dissection, shock), control bleeding with fluid resuscitation and withhold further doses of warfarin. Vitamin K, 5–10 mg intravenously, should be given along with fresh-frozen plasma, 15 mL/kg, or prothrombin complex concentrates. For patients with asymptomatic prolongation of the INR (> 10), give vitamin K, 2–5 mg orally, without fresh-frozen plasma. Recheck the INR in 6–12 hours. If the INR is between 6 and 10, give vitamin K, 2 mg, orally without fresh-frozen plasma and recheck the INR in 12–24 hours. In all the above cases, vitamin K should be given intravenously or orally, not intramuscularly, because of the risk of erratic absorption and hematoma formation.

Disposition

Hospitalize all patients with significantly prolonged prothrombin times, evidence of bleeding, or history of ingestion of massive amounts of anticoagulants. Patients who have documented anticoagulant effect after ingestion of the super-warfarin rodenticides will need close follow-up and repeated vitamin K dosing for up to several weeks.

Cruickshank J et al: Warfarin toxicity in the emergency department: recommendations for management. Emerg Med 2001;13:91. [PMID: 11476421] (Retrospective analysis of adult patients with warfarin toxicity and literature review of the treatment guidelines.)

Walter-Michael H: Rational, high quality laboratory monitoring before, during and after infusion of prothrombin complex concentrates. Thrombosis Research 1999;95:S25. [PMID: 10499906] (Review of the use of prothrombin complex concentrates to treat warfarin overdose.)

Weibert RT et al: Correction of excessive anticoagulation with low-dose oral vitamin K. Ann Intern Med 1997;126:959. [PMID: 9182473] (Case analysis of patients with excessive anticoagulation who received oral vitamin K.)

Dermatologic Emergencies

Joseph A. Salomone III, MD, FAAEM, & Martha Ann Pratt, MD

Immediate Recognition & Management of Life-Threatening Problems

    Angioedema & Urticaria

        1. Angioedema

        2. Urticaria

    Stevens-Johnson Syndrome & Toxic Epidermal Necrolysis

    Exfoliation & Erythroderma

    Staphylococcal Scalded Skin Syndrome

Recognition & Management of Potentially Life-Threatening Problems

    Cellulitis & Erysipelas

    Pustular Psoriasis

    Pemphigus vulgaris

Recognition & Management of Non-Life-Threatening Problems

    Contact Dermatitis & *Rhus* Dermatitis

    Impetigo

    Herpes zoster

    Herpes simplex

    Psoriasis

    Scabies

    Pediculosis

    Cutaneous Dermatophytes/Tinea

    Pityriasis rosea

    Molluscum contagiosum

■ IMMEDIATE RECOGNITION & MANAGEMENT OF LIFE-THREATENING PROBLEMS

To some observers, emergency medicine and dermatology may seem to be two of the most unrelated specialties in medicine, but the emergency physician will encounter many patients presenting with dermatologic complaints. The astute clinician will realize that, although rare, some of these problems can be life threatening. Some patients may even require emergent airway protection and vigorous resuscitation. This chapter reviews those special situations and discusses common and uncommon dermatologic complaints.

Initial Evaluation

The initial evaluation begins with the primary survey and vital signs. Always focus special attention on airway, breathing, and circulation (the ABCs). Note any abnormal vital signs and oxygen saturation, and be alert to subtle changes in mental status or behavior that may indicate impending airway or cardiovascular collapse. The ABCs apply to all clinical situations, and thorough histories and examinations are often the most helpful tools in arriving at any diagnosis. Early and appropriately aggressive airway management and fluid resuscitation may prevent morbidity or even death.

History

Parallel to the assessment of the ABCs is the beginning of a thorough history that includes potential recent exposures to foods, medications, plants, insects, and the like that may have triggered the condition. An AMPLE history, addressing the patient's allergies, medications, past medical and surgical history, last meal, and events leading up to the presentation may provide information necessary to begin appropriate management.

ANGIOEDEMA & URTICARIA

1. Angioedema

 ESSENTIALS OF DIAGNOSIS

- *Swelling of face, lips, tongue.*
- *May lead to airway compromise.*

General Considerations

Angioedema is edema that forms in the mucous membranes and subcutaneous tissues of the face and neck. Particularly dangerous is the involvement of the mouth, tongue, and lower airway, which can lead to severe airway compromise. Two subtypes exist, the rare hereditary form and the acquired form. The hereditary variant is usually due to C1-esterase deficiency. The acquired form is most commonly secondary to angiotensin-converting enzyme (ACE) inhibitors and has increased in prevalence because of widespread usage of these drugs.

Treatment

Emergent airway protection is mandated if airway compromise is impending or present. Treat shock if present. Discontinue any implicated medications or substances. Supply oxygen to maintain oxygen saturation at greater than 90%. In severe angioedema with airway compromise, administer epinephrine (0.3–0.5 mL of 1:1000 solution) subcutaneously or intramuscularly. This may be repeated every 10 minutes and is used to maintain a patent airway. Give antihistamines, such as diphenhydramine HCl, 1–2 mg/kg or 25–50 mg parenterally. Methylprednisolone sodium succinate, 125 mg intravenously, may be repeated every 6 hours. This drug is used to help blunt or block any late-phase response.

Disposition

Admit patients to an intensive care unit if airway compromise is present; otherwise, they may need observation in the emergency department. If a patient is thought to have experienced a reaction to a medication, instruct the patient to discontinue that medication and contact his or her primary care physician to discuss an alternative medication.

2. Urticaria

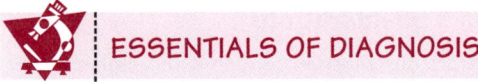

ESSENTIALS OF DIAGNOSIS

Urticaria

- *Localized areas of dermal edema.*
- *Intense itching.*

Anaphylaxis

- *May have urticaria.*

- *Bronchospasm.*
- *Angioedema.*
- *Shock.*

General Considerations

Urticaria (hives) may be either acute or chronic and may appear in any age group. The condition represents one end of a continuum, ranging from urticaria to anaphylactic shock. Because various medications and foods are most often implicated as causes, take a thorough history of possible exposures. The lesions themselves represent localized areas of edema in the dermis. They appear as intensely pruritic, sharply demarcated areas with either an erythematous or a blanched base and border. Their appearance may wax and wane, and individual lesions often resolve within an hour. With anaphylaxis, there may be an initial decrescendo of the presenting symptoms with early interventions. A late-phase response may occur hours later with a more severe presentation than the initial symptom complex.

Treatment

If airway compromise is not present, patients can be given H_1-receptor blockers (see diphenhydramine dosing, above), steroids, and even epinephrine. H_2-receptor blockers, such as ranitidine, may also be added. If airway compromise is present, treat emergently as for angioedema (see above).

Disposition

Disposition is the same as for angioedema (see above). Remember the sometimes-biphasic nature of anaphylactic reactions. Instruct patients to avoid any potentially responsible agents. Give any patient with a history of anaphylaxis a prescription for an auto-injector epinephrine device and instruct the patient on its proper use prior to discharge.

Chin AG et al: Angiotensin-converting enzyme inhibitor-induced angioedema: a multicenter review and an algorithm for airway management. Ann Otol Rhinol Laryngol 2001;110 (9):834. [PMID: 11558759] (A brief review with a focus on airway management and outcomes at two tertiary care centers.)

Rusznak C et al: Anaphylaxis and anaphylactoid reactions. A guide to prevention, recognition, and emergent treatment. Postgrad Med 2002;111(5):101. [PMID: 12040857] (A review of pathophysiology and emergent treatment of anaphylaxis with specific treatment recommendations.)

STEVENS-JOHNSON SYNDROME & TOXIC EPIDERMAL NECROLYSIS

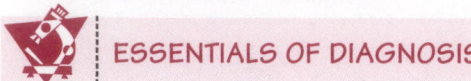 ESSENTIALS OF DIAGNOSIS

- Epidermal detachment.
- Drug-induced or post–viral illness.
- Patients may be critically ill.

General Considerations

A disorder of epidermal detachment was initially reported in 1922, when Stevens and Johnson published a description of two children with fever, erosive stomatitis, severe conjunctivitis, and a disseminated cutaneous eruption. It is now known to be a drug-induced state or one that follows a viral illness. Stevens-Johnson syndrome (SJS) and toxic epidermal necrolysis (TEN) are now thought to represent ends of a spectrum of reactions involving detachment of the epidermis. Both conditions share inciting factors. The range of disorders has been classified into three categories: SJS, involving less than 10% of body surface area (BSA); transitional cases, involving 10–30% of BSA; and TEN, with greater than 30% of BSA with detached epidermis. Mortality rates for SJS are approximately 5%; rates are much higher (30%) with TEN. Death is most commonly from sepsis secondary to infections from *S. aureus* and *P. aeruginosa*.

Clinical Findings

Patients with SJS present with severe, intensely painful bullae and mucosal ulcerations with a truncal distribution of target-like lesions. The skin lesions are typically purpuric macules. The Nikolsky sign may be elicited. This refers to easy separation of the upper layers of the epidermis from the lower layers with very minor trauma, such as lateral traction or gentle rubbing on the skin. Patients with TEN typically present with fever, pruritus, pharyngitis, and conjunctivitis. These symptoms and signs precede mucous membrane and skin involvement. Mucous membrane involvement usually occurs first, followed by skin involvement. The rash is painful and usually starts on the upper trunk or face. Affected skin may be erythematous or have bullae. There may be eroding of the bullae, or the affected skin may slough in large sheets. This may progress over hours to days. The sloughing may involve other organ systems, including the gastrointestinal tract and the respiratory tree.

Treatment

Discontinue any potentially responsible medications. This usually requires that all nonessential medicines be stopped, because no tests are available to identify culprit agents. Careful correction of electrolyte abnormalities and fluid replacement are critical, because significant fluid losses occur with loss of the protective skin barrier. In TEN, airway protection and mechanical ventilation may be necessary if the trachea and upper airway are involved. Sloughing and detachment of mucosa can lead to airway compromise. Antibiosis may be necessary to avoid sepsis-related complications. Pain control is essential.

Disposition

In severe cases, treatment in a burn center may be necessary. Guard carefully against infection. Avoid central lines if possible. Avoid steroids because they have not proved beneficial.

Becker DS: Toxic epidermal necrolysis. Lancet 1998;351(9113): 1417. [PMID: 9593426] (A review of TEN with a practical focus on treatment strategies.)

Revus J: New advances in severe adverse drug reactions. Dermatol Clin 2001;19(4):697. [PMID: 11705355] This is an extensive review of various drug-related reactions.

Wolkenstein P et al: Toxic epidermal necrolysis. Dermatol Clin 2000;18(3):485. [PMID: 10943543] (A thorough review of the diagnosis, cause, and treatment of TEN.)

Wolkenstein PE et al: Drug-induced toxic epidermal necrolysis. Clin Dermatol 1998;16(3):399. [PMID: 9642534] (A thorough review of TEN.)

EXFOLIATION & ERYTHRODERMA

 ESSENTIALS OF DIAGNOSIS

- A diffuse, generalized erythema and scaling.
- Occurs secondary to many disease states.

General Considerations

Many cutaneous diseases present with exfoliative erythroderma, or generalized redness and scaling. This condition is associated with a high risk for morbidity and mortality, independent of the inherent risks of the disease process it represents. Most commonly, this condition occurs secondary to psoriasis, atopic dermatitis, cutaneous T-cell lymphoma, or reactions to any of a wide range of inciting drugs. The erythrodermic state usually has a slow progression, but an acute onset may occur in patients who have cutaneous dermatoses or severe drug reactions.

Clinical Findings

Clues to the diagnosis may be from the underlying disease, such as psoriatic plaques or characteristic nail changes. Bullous pemphigoid typically exhibits tense bullae in addition to erythroderma. Long-standing erythroderma may be associated with keratoderma, alopecia, and ectropion. Peripheral edema occurs in 50% of patients. Patients with severe drug reactions may appear acutely ill with fever, malaise, and lymphadenopathy. A leukocytosis with eosinophilia, organomegaly, and hepatic or renal impairment may be present. In the most severe cases, high-output cardiac failure may occur. Severe alterations in fluid balance may occur, leading to shock. Sepsis may ensue, and hepatic necrosis may be fatal.

Treatment

Correction of derangements in fluid balance must begin early. Take care with the skin, applying moist dressings to weeping areas. Low-potency topical steroids may be used. Avoid high-potency preparations, because the large surface areas involved could lead to the absorption of large doses of steroids. Treat secondary infections.

Disposition

Hospital admission is often required, preferentially in an intensive care unit, depending on the needs of the patient.

Rothe MJ et al: Erythroderma. Dermatol Clin 2000;18(3):405. [PMID: 10943536] (A review of erythroderma with a focus on inciting agents, diagnosis, and treatment and includes excellent photographs of skin findings.)

STAPHYLOCOCCAL SCALDED SKIN SYNDROME

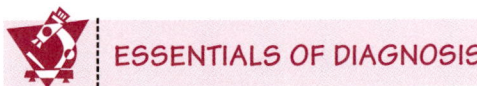 ESSENTIALS OF DIAGNOSIS

- *Skin appears scalded and blistered.*
- *Affects primarily children.*
- *Skin barrier is broken and leads to* S. aureus *infection.*

General Considerations

Primarily a disease of children, staphylococcal scalded skin syndrome (SSSS) refers to a series of toxin-induced blistering dermatoses. The exfoliative toxins are primarily attributed to *S. aureus,* and all phage groups of the bacterium have now been implicated. Mortality rates are low (2–3%) in children but can reach as high as 60% in adults who have comorbidities or preexisting conditions.

Clinical Findings

The clinical presentation ranges from a milder form with localized eruption of a few fragile fluid-filled bullae surrounded by normal skin, to a more involved state. The more widespread form is often associated with fever, generalized erythema, and poor feeding in infants. Subsequently, large bullae form with a predilection for sites of friction. Erosion can occur in large areas, resulting in open, painful lesions. The Nikolsky sign is present. Unlike in SJS or TEN, mucous membranes are spared in SSSS. This may be a helpful distinguishing factor. The process is thought to result from a break in the protective skin barrier, which leads to a *S. aureus* infection. Typical areas involved in the primary infection include the umbilicus in neonates, as well as the nasopharynx, urinary tract, and other sites.

Treatment

Cases of localized eruptions may be treated with oral antibiotics. The widespread form usually requires parenteral antibiotics to cover penicillin-resistant *S. aureus.* Treatment for adults is nafcillin, 1.5 g, or oxacillin, 2 g intravenously every 4 hours. For pediatric patients, treatment is nafcillin or oxacillin, 150 mg/kg/d intravenously in divided doses for 5–7 days. If superinfection is suspected, an aminoglycoside may be needed. Rehydration and thermoregulation are essential, as is adequate pain control.

Disposition

Severe cases require treatment in an intensive care unit or burn center. Because the cleavage of the epidermis and exfoliation are extremely superficial, the lesions typically heal with little or no residual scarring.

Callahan EF et al: Cutaneous (non-HIV) infections. Dermatol Clin 2000;18(3):497. [PMID: 10943544] (A concise and thorough review of major cutaneous infections.)

Ladhani S: Recent developments in staphylococcal scalded skin syndrome. Clin Microbiol Infect 2001;7(6):301. [PMID: 11442563] (A review of the latest knowledge regarding the pathophysiology and cause of SSSS, with a discussion of the diagnosis and treatment.)

■ RECOGNITION & MANAGEMENT OF POTENTIALLY LIFE-THREATENING PROBLEMS

CELLULITIS & ERYSIPELAS

 ESSENTIALS OF DIAGNOSIS

Cellulitis
• *Deeper infection.*
• *Affects skin and subcutaneous tissues.*

Erysipelas
• *Well-demarcated, superficial, erythematous infection.*
• *Often affects face and extremities.*

General Considerations

Cellulitis and erysipelas refer to infections of the subcutaneous tissues. Erysipelas involves the more superficial upper dermis, and cellulitis is deeper, with more extensive involvement of the subcutaneous tissues and fat. Both conditions are acute and are related to a breach in the skin's protective barrier function. This can be secondary to fissuring and maceration, burns, venous stasis, malnutrition, or any of a number of other factors. The primary causative agent is group A β-hemolytic streptococcus. Other causes include streptococci B, C, and G and, less commonly, staphylococci infection. Causative organisms associated with cellulitis include *S. aureus, H. influenzae, S. pneumoniae, Pseudomonas,* and several others. If untreated, both conditions can lead to devastating complications such as local abscesses and gangrene with severe cellulitis. Facial erysipelas may lead to cavernous sinus thrombosis. Both cellulitis and erysipelas may lead to septicemia.

Clinical Findings

Erysipelas is characterized by well-demarcated, erythematous, indurated plaques. The borders may be palpable. Primary sites include the face, scalp, and lower extremities. Patients are usually in the extremes of age. Cellulitis is usually associated with painful swelling and erythema of the involved area. The borders are usually less well defined, and the affected area is typically warm.

Treatment

Although many cases can be managed on an outpatient basis, patients may have constitutional symptoms, and those with comorbid conditions may be quite ill and require hospitalization. Antibiotics are used empirically to cover streptococci and *S. aureus.* Recommended therapies include penicillin G, 600,000 to 2 million units intravenously every 6 hours, for streptococci; and nafcillin, 1.5–2 g intravenously every 4 hours, for staphylococci. Treat methicillin-resistant cases with vancomycin. If *H. influenzae* is suspected, use ampicillin, 200–250 mg/kg intravenously divided into 6 doses. Trimethoprim-sulfamethoxazole may be used in penicillin-allergic patients. Patients who appear well and without constitutional symptoms may be given oral therapy. This includes oxacillin, 0.5–1 g orally 4 times daily, or erythromycin, 0.25–0.5 g orally 4 times daily, in the penicillin-allergic patient. Simple measures may be helpful in both conditions, including rest, cool compresses, elevation of the affected part, and antibacterial soaks. Debridement is used in secondary abscesses.

Callahan EF et al: Cutaneous (non-HIV) infections. Dermatol Clin 2000;18(3):497. [PMID: 10943544] (A concise and thorough review of major cutaneous infections.)

Sadick NS: Current aspects of bacterial infections of the skin. Dermatol Clin 1997;15(2):341. [PMID: 9098643] (A review of cutaneous infections with practical applications to diagnosis and treatment.)

PUSTULAR PSORIASIS

 ESSENTIALS OF DIAGNOSIS

• *Most patients have preexisting plaque psoriasis.*
• *Patients are systemically ill and febrile.*
• *Large areas of erythema with multiple pustules.*

General Considerations

This condition usually occurs in patients with the preexistent plaque variant of psoriasis (see later for a description). Patients typically appear ill or toxic. Constitutional symptoms are present, including fever and malaise. Patients are often bedridden. A thorough history often reveals a recent withdrawal from systemic corticosteroid therapy.

Clinical Findings

Psoriatic plaques may be seen in conjunction with large areas of erythema. These are usually covered with small pustules. The pustules enlarge and merge to form large purulent collections on the skin. Patients become extremely ill and are usually febrile and experience arthralgias and gastrointestinal symptoms. A more localized variant may be seen on the palms and soles, without concomitant plaque psoriasis.

Treatment & Disposition

The generalized form of pustular psoriasis can be difficult to treat. It usually mandates inpatient treatment with the close collaboration of a dermatologist.

Drew GS: Psoriasis. Prim Care 2000;27(2):385. [PMID: 10815050] (A thorough review of various types of psoriasis with a discussion of multiple treatment modalities.)

PEMPHIGUS VULGARIS

ESSENTIALS OF DIAGNOSIS

- *Blistering of skin and mucous membranes.*
- *Usually affects older adults.*

General Considerations

Pemphigus is one of several autoimmune diseases of the skin that present with blistering. The antibodies attack skin proteins and result in the inability of cells in the epidermis to hold together normally. Blisters form within the superficial epidermis. Although rare, pemphigus can be life threatening. Several subtypes exist, and pemphigus vulgaris is the most common and the most severe. Prior to newer developments in therapy, mortality rates were as high as 50% at 2 years and 100% at 5 years.

Clinical Findings

Pemphigus most often occurs in older adults. The skin and mucous membranes are usually affected, and oral lesions often appear first. All mucous membranes may eventually be affected. As described earlier, the blistering is superficial. This results in fragile, flaccid blisters. The underlying skin may be erythematous. In the oral cavity, the blisters often slough prior to presentation, and the clinician may find only ulcerations. Hoarseness may occur if the lower airway is involved. Oral involvement can be extremely painful, interfering with the patient's ability to tolerate oral intake. The blisters slough

easily, and the erosions enlarge by extending their borders. The Nikolsky sign is present. These erosions often crust over, but scarring is not usually a problem.

Treatment

Patients may have only isolated lesions, but more commonly there is widespread involvement. Patients may appear ill or toxic. Initial management involves fluid resuscitation, because fluid losses from the blistering are significant. Institute antibiotic therapy if secondary infection is present. Causative organisms are usually streptococci or staphylococci. This chronic disease usually mandates lifelong immunosuppressive therapy. The advent of glucocorticoids has decreased the mortality rates to approximately 5%. Start steroid therapy immediately. The suggested doses are 1–2.5 mg/kg/d of prednisone. Prednisone doses of 60 mg/d are recommended for treating isolated oral lesions. Topical high-potency steroids, such as clobetasol propionate 0.05%, can also be used in mild cases of skin involvement but should not be used on mucous membranes. Other immunosuppressive agents, such as azathioprine, are usually added to the oral steroid regimen later.

Disposition

Admit patients who appear ill to an intensive care unit for careful management of their fluid balance, with the close help of consultants to aid in the diagnosis.

Cotell S et al: Autoimmune blistering skin diseases. Am J Emerg Med 2000;18(3):288. [PMID: 10830686] (A discussion of pemphigus and pemphigoid disorders from the perspective of the emergency physician.)

Toth GG et al: Therapy of pemphigus. Clin Dermatol 2001; 19(6):761. [PMID: 11705686] This is a review of current methods of treating pemphigus.

■ RECOGNITION & MANAGEMENT OF NON-LIFE-THREATENING PROBLEMS

CONTACT DERMATITIS & *RHUS* DERMATITIS

ESSENTIALS OF DIAGNOSIS

Rhus dermatitis
- *Intense itching.*

- *Erythema with vesicles.*
- *Linear distribution.*
- *Lesions appear 8–48 hours after exposure to poison ivy, poison oak, or poison sumac.*

General Considerations

Contact dermatitis refers to a collection of disorders resulting from an inciting environmental agent that has contacted the skin. The usual manifestation is a papulosquamous eruption, but vesicles may also be present.

A classic example is *Rhus* dermatitis, which is induced by plants in the *Rhus* genus (Toxicodendron). This collection of plants includes poison ivy, poison oak, and poison sumac. The culprit agent is the plant oil urushiol, and 50–70% of the U.S. population is sensitive to this substance. Factors affecting the clinical significance of any contact include the extent of exposure, the patient's age and activity level, and the patient's immunocompetence. Poison ivy, poison oak, and poison sumac are native plants of North America, rarely found at elevations above 4000 feet. Their appearance is quite variable, and they do not always exhibit the classic three-leaf morphology. The oil urushiol is widely distributed in almost all parts of the plant. The resultant dermatitis is classically described as a form of delayed hypersensitivity (type IV) reaction.

Clinical Findings

After the first exposure, lesions can erupt within 8–48 hours, and they may persist for up to 3 weeks. The presence of an intensely pruritic, erythematous, papulovesicular eruption after an environmental exposure is highly suggestive of *Rhus* dermatitis. The lesions are usually linear. Transfer of the allergenic urushiol can continue and produce more lesions if it is not completely removed. It must be cleansed from the fingernails, skin, and clothing and from pets. Transfer of the oil, not the vesicles or the vesicular fluid, is responsible for the development of new lesions. Immediate eruption after exposure is not consistent with *Rhus* dermatitis, because it takes at least 8 hours for the cell-mediated response to develop. The most common sites for eruptions are the face and extremities. The lesions may range from erythematous papules to large bullae. Any of the commonly used rules for estimation of body surface area of burns, such as the "rule of nines" or preprinted estimation sheets, may be used to estimate the percentage of body surface area involved.

Treatment

The condition is self-limiting, with resolution within 3 weeks if all of the urushiol is removed. The most important therapy is prevention of exposure, but if exposure occurs, the individual should attempt to remove the oil within 10–30 minutes of exposure.

Treatment can decrease the severity of the symptoms, but it does not shorten the course. Oral antihistamines are effective symptomatic therapy for the intense pruritus. Topical preparations, including calamine, camphor, and cool compresses, are useful measures for comfort. Extreme caution must be used with topical antihistamines, zirconium, and benzocaine. These medications are no longer advocated, secondary to systemic absorption and sensitization. Over-the-counter steroid preparations are typically not helpful, because they contain too little steroid to be of benefit.

The backbone of therapy is usually a moderate-potency topical corticosteroid, such as triamcinolone 0.1% cream or betamethasone 0.1% cream. If the case is more severe or widespread, high-potency preparations such as clobetasol propionate 0.05% may be used. Extreme caution must be used with these creams, because systemic effects can occur secondary to steroid absorption. Steroid therapy can also be used orally, but to be effective it must begin within 18 hours of exposure. Therapy must be tapered for 2–3 weeks. If the dose is too low or the course is too brief, intense rebound flares will often occur. A single 40-mg intramuscular dose of triamcinolone will typically produce good results in adults. Superinfection of the lesions with staphylococci or streptococci is the most common complication.

Disposition

Outpatient therapy is sufficient in all but the most severe cases, which may require parenteral steroids. Systemic glucocorticoids may be used at doses starting with 1 mg/kg/d and continuing until the symptoms resolve.

Tanner TL: Rhus (Toxicodendron) dermatitis. Prim Care 2000; 27(2):493. [PMID: 10815057] (A thorough review of *Rhus* dermatitis with practical applications to diagnosis and treatment.)

IMPETIGO

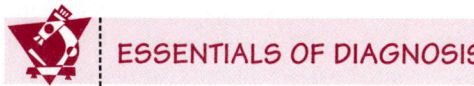 **ESSENTIALS OF DIAGNOSIS**

- *Infection due to* Staphylococcus *or* Streptococcus *species.*

- *Lesions appear honey-crusted.*
- *More common in children but may affect all ages.*

General Considerations

Impetigo is an infection of the skin primarily due to group A streptococci and, less commonly, *S. aureus.* The infection is classified into bullous and nonbullous forms; the nonbullous form comprises approximately 70% of cases. Young children are the predominant age group affected, but adults are not excluded. A break in the protective skin barrier is the inciting event. Conditions such as chickenpox, abrasions, and burns are typically associated with impetigo. Predisposing situations include crowded living conditions, poor hygiene, and contact sports.

Clinical Findings

Impetigo is associated with the classic history of the emergence of a small vesicle or pustule. This is often in the context of one of the above-mentioned conditions. The vesicle or pustule develops into the classic honey-crusted lesion. These lesions are usually less than 2 cm in diameter and may be mildly pruritic. The lesions are usually not painful. Although in healthy individuals the lesions will usually heal spontaneously with little scarring, the potential complications can be life threatening. Complications include septicemia, pneumonia, osteomyelitis, and glomerulonephritis.

Treatment

Correction of predisposing environmental conditions is important. The honey-colored crust must be removed. Cleansing with antibacterial soaps and solutions is helpful. The only topical antibiotic therapy currently indicated for the treatment of localized lesions is mupirocin (Bactroban) ointment. Patients should apply the ointment until the lesions resolve. Scalp and oral lesions typically require oral therapy, as do disseminated cases. Effective oral therapies include cloxacillin, amoxicillin/clavulanate, or clindamycin. Cephalosporins may be used, such as cephalexin, cefaclor, cefadroxil, cefprozil, or cefpodoxime proxetil. Seven days of therapy has been demonstrated as effective. If symptoms persist beyond 7 days, cultures should be taken and further treatment based on the results. Treat lesions suspected of being due to *S. aureus* with a β-lactamase-resistant penicillin such as oxacillin or nafcillin.

Sadick NS: Current aspects of bacterial infections of the skin. Dermatol Clin 1997;15(2):341. [PMID: 9098643] (A review of cutaneous infections with practical applications to diagnosis and treatment.)

HERPES ZOSTER

 ESSENTIALS OF DIAGNOSIS

- *Most cases are very painful.*
- *Prodrome of paresthesias may occur.*
- *Rash appears as a bandlike distribution of vesicles.*
- *Usually has a dermatomal distribution.*
- *Usually does not cross the patient's midline.*

General Considerations

Herpes zoster (HZ), or shingles, is a painful condition that results from reactivation of a latent infection with the varicella zoster virus (VZV). A patient who is naive to the virus develops chickenpox after an initial exposure. After resolution of this primary infection, the VZV remains dormant in the satellite cells of the dorsal root ganglion of the sensory nerves. It remains there for the rest of the patient's life. The triggers of subsequent reactivation in certain patients are not fully understood. Events such as trauma and exposure to ultraviolet radiation have been implicated in provoking eruptions of shingles. The incidence of HZ is increased in the elderly population. This is thought to result from diminishing immune function with increasing age. Although usually a localized process, disseminated HZ can develop in immunocompromised individuals.

Clinical Findings

The diagnosis is primarily clinical. Previous history of chickenpox and the progression of current symptoms are important points in the history.

Three phases of HZ have been described. During the prodrome phase, 80% of patients feel altered sensations in the affected dermatome. These are typically described as pain, burning, or paresthesias. These feelings may be intense and will often be present several days before the appearance of any lesions. This can often make the diagnosis difficult during this phase.

Patients in the acute phase present with the eruption of vesicles, usually in a band-like pattern, which follows a dermatomal distribution. Only rarely will the lesions cross the midline. The two most common sites are the trunk and face, respectively. The lesions will dry and form a crust within 7–10 days. The lesions usually resolve within 2–3 weeks.

An unfortunate subset of patients will go on to develop the chronic phase of HZ, known as postherpetic neuralgia (PHN). This is an extremely painful condition, which persists at least 30 days after the eruption resolves. PHN can be quite difficult to treat and is much more likely in the older patient. It may occur in up to 50% of elderly patients with HZ.

Several dangerous complications can develop from HZ, including ophthalmic HZ. This condition occurs when the ophthalmic branch of the trigeminal nerve is involved. Up to half of these patients will have ocular HZ. A clue to the presence of ocular HZ can be involvement of the tip of the patient's nose. Conjunctivitis, uveitis, and ulcerative keratitis can occur as a result of HZ. These serious conditions can lead to blindness if not managed properly. A complete ocular examination and urgent ophthalmologic referral are essential. Other potential complications of HZ include the Ramsay Hunt syndrome (an acute facial paralysis), meningitis, and encephalitis.

Treatment

It is important to educate patients who have HZ. They must understand that they are contagious to those who are not immune to VZV and to those who have not had chickenpox. This infective state lasts until the vesicles have dried and crusted, or approximately 1 week from the onset of the rash. During this time, patients should avoid pregnant women, those who are immunocompromised, and those who have never had chickenpox.

Pain relief is important and is usually achieved with short-term combinations of oral analgesics and narcotics. Antiviral drugs are of use in the treatment of HZ, if therapy is started within 72 hours of the eruption of the rash. Oral acyclovir, 800 mg 5 times daily, is effective in improving resolution of the rash and decreasing the incidence of PHN. Famciclovir and valacyclovir are other options, with similar efficacy to acyclovir. One study showed valacyclovir as having some superiority in pain control. Studies have shown that steroids do not prevent the development of PHN. Some authors suggest that steroids are beneficial in treating Ramsay Hunt syndrome. Treatment of ocular involvement requires the assistance of an ophthalmologist.

Morgan R: Shingles: a review of diagnosis and management. Hosp Med 1998;59(10):770. [PMID: 9850292] (A discussion of varicella zoster and herpes zoster with a good review of the diagnosis and treatment of shingles.)

HERPES SIMPLEX

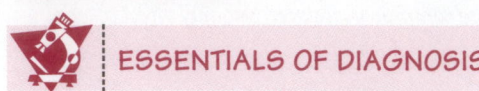

ESSENTIALS OF DIAGNOSIS

- *Vesicles on an erythematous base.*
- *HSV-1: usually oral; HSV-2: usually genital.*
- *Spread by direct contact.*

General Considerations

Herpes simplex virus (HSV) is a major cause of recurrent orofacial and genital lesions and causes other types of illness as well (eg, keratitis, encephalitis). Infection is spread by direct contact. Primary infection is often the most severe, although it may be asymptomatic. After the primary lesion has healed, the virus remains latent in sensory neurons in ganglion tissue, where it periodically reactivates in response to diverse stimuli.

HSV type 1 (HSV-1) tends to be associated with oral lesions and is spread through contact with saliva from an infected person, whereas HSV type 2 (HSV-2) causes mainly genital lesions and is spread primarily by sexual contact.

Clinical Findings

A. Primary Herpes Simplex Infection

The first clinical attack of HSV infection is usually the most severe. Patients may present with fever, malaise, and arthralgias. Infection is characterized at first by grouped vesicles and later by denudation, erosions, or punctate lesions on a swollen, tender, painful erythematous base. Local pain and regional adenopathy are usually marked. Gingivostomatitis is the most common manifestation of HSV-1 infection; patients with HSV-2 infection usually present with genital lesions (ie, of the vulva, vagina, penis, anus, or perineum). Patients (especially women) with genital herpes may have aseptic meningitis. The primary illness usually disappears in 2–3 weeks but may last as long as 6 weeks.

B. Recurrent HSV Infection

Recurrence of infection is common and may be triggered by fever, exposure to ultraviolet light, friction or trauma associated with sexual intercourse, menstruation, and possibly stress or fatigue. Focal itching, pain, or aching may precede the appearance of vesicles by hours to a few days in some patients. Vesicles usually rupture spontaneously within a few days and heal within a week without scarring. The virus may be recovered as long as lesions are moist; until the area is completely dry and healed, the patient should avoid direct skin-to-skin contact with others.

C. SPECIFIC DIAGNOSIS

For either primary or recurrent herpes simplex, especially genital herpes, confirm the diagnosis by culture or antigen detection.

Treatment

A. PRIMARY INFECTION

Antipyretics or analgesics may help to relieve systemic symptoms. Give oral acyclovir, valacyclovir, or famciclovir to all patients who have primary infection. Hospitalize severely ill patients for administration of intravenous acyclovir, 15 mg/kg/d in 2–3 divided doses. Give other patients oral acyclovir, 200 mg 5 times daily for 7–10 days; valacyclovir, 1 g twice a day for 7–10 days; or famciclovir, 250 mg 3 times daily for 5–10 days.

Antibiotics are not necessary unless local purulence or cultures or Gram-stained smears positive for bacteria suggest concomitant bacterial infection. *Candida* vaginitis occurs frequently in women with primary genital herpes.

B. RECURRENT INFECTION

Patients should not touch or manipulate lesions and should avoid physical contact with others around the area of moist or active lesions. Acyclovir, 200 mg orally twice daily for 5 days; valacyclovir, 500 mg twice daily for 5 days; or famciclovir, 125–250 mg 3 times daily for 5 days, will somewhat reduce healing time and the duration of virus shedding if started within a day of lesion onset.

Disposition

Hospitalization is often indicated for patients with primary genital herpes, who may have severe pain, systemic symptoms, and other complications (eg, aseptic meningitis, neuropathic bladder). Hospitalization is also required for patients with large or rapidly progressive lesions, especially if the patient is immunocompromised.

Refer pregnant patients with newly diagnosed genital herpes to an obstetrician. Order a serologic test for syphilis (eg, VDRL) for all patients to rule out coexisting syphilis. Consider testing for HIV if risk factors are present.

Taylor TJ et al: Herpes simplex virus. Front Biosci 2002;7:d752. [PMID: 11861220] (A review of herpes simplex virology.)

Whitley RJ, Roizman B: Herpes simplex virus infections. Lancet 2001;357:1513. [PMID: 11377626] (A comprehensive review of pathophysiology, diagnosis, and treatment of herpes simplex infections.)

PSORIASIS

 ESSENTIALS OF DIAGNOSIS

- *Common disorder.*
- *Well-circumscribed plaques.*
- *Erythematous base with silvery scale.*
- *Predilection for extensor surfaces.*

General Considerations

Psoriasis is a common skin condition affecting up to 2% of the U.S. population. It has been described among all age groups with a similar male-to-female ratio. Onset is usually in the third decade of life. The disease process is well described and understood, but its cause is still unknown. A family history is present in 30% of patients. Psoriasis significantly affects the patient's quality of life. It is chronic, and there is no known cure. The plaque variant of psoriasis, or psoriasis vulgaris, is the most common form.

Clinical Findings

Thorough examination reveals the characteristic erythematous, raised, scaly plaques. These are often described as having a salmon-colored base with tightly adherent silvery scales. They are typically found on the extensor surfaces of major joints, such as elbows and knees. Other sites of predilection include the scalp, ears, and umbilicus. Lesions are often found to be in various stages of plaque formation and healing. Potassium hydroxide preparations can be used to differentiate psoriasis from tinea. Classic nail findings, such as pitting and onycholysis, can also aid in the diagnosis. Cultures play no role in the diagnosis of psoriasis.

Treatment

Many remedies have been tried over the years, but no cure has been found for psoriasis. Therapies often merely decrease scaling and increase the patient's comfort. Tar preparations and shampoos are well-known effective keratolytics, which decrease scaling. Avoidance of skin trauma is helpful, because the Koebner phenomenon is associated with psoriasis. This phenomenon refers to a flare in symptoms and initiation of plaque formation after local skin trauma, including scratching and even surgical incisions. Judicious use of topical low-potency steroids may be helpful initially.

Calcipotriene is a newer preparation that is a topical vitamin D_3 analogue. Applied twice daily, effects are typically seen within 8 weeks. Oral and parenteral steroids play little or no role in the treatment of plaque psoriasis. Their use has been demonstrated as harmful in certain situations, such as the exacerbation of the more serious pustular psoriasis.

Disposition

Outpatient therapy is sufficient, except in the most severe cases. Referral should be made to a primary care physician or a dermatologist for more involved therapies, including topical preparations, ultraviolet phototherapy, and systemic agents such as methotrexate.

Drew GS: Psoriasis. Prim Care 2000;27(2):385. [PMID: 10815050] (A thorough review of various types of psoriasis with a discussion of multiple treatment modalities.)

Feldman SR et al: Psoriasis. Med Clin North Am 1998;82(5):1135. [PMID: 9769796] (A concise review of psoriasis and its treatment.)

SCABIES

 ESSENTIALS OF DIAGNOSIS

- *Human parasite.*
- *Causes intense itching.*
- *Spread by contact.*
- *May affect entire households.*

General Considerations

Scabies have been known to affect the human condition for thousands of years. The culprit organism in scabies is a mite, *Sarcoptes scabiei*. This mite is found in varying stages of development in the epidermis of the infested individual. There it makes tunnels, leaving behind eggs and feces. The mites are obligate parasites of humans and are spread by skin-to-skin contact between persons. This includes both sexual and nonsexual interactions.

Clinical Findings

The diagnosis of scabies is primarily a clinical one, with the usual history of intense pruritus that is especially worse at night. Consider scabies when entire households complain of the onset of pruritus. The classic physical findings are tiny burrows in the web spaces between the fingers, in intertriginous areas, and in flexural creases. Burrows may not always be seen. Only excoriations and impetiginization may be found. The lesions may be difficult to differentiate from atopic dermatitis. In the most extreme cases, heavy mite loads may result and lead to the crusted or Norwegian variant. This is usually limited to individuals with severe disabilities or in immunocompromised states. The diagnosis of scabies is confirmed by microscopic visualization of mites or eggs in skin scrapings.

Treatment

A. ADULTS

The treatment for adults (except pregnant or lactating women) and older children includes permethrin 5% cream (Elimite). It should be applied after a shower or bath over the entire body from the neck down. It should be left on for 8 hours, after which it should be carefully washed off. A 60-g tube is usually sufficient to treat one to two people. All clothing and bed linens should be laundered in hot water to kill all remaining mites. Alternative regimens include lindane cream or lotion. Used for many years, it is effective but some strains of lindane-resistant scabies exist. Also, dangerous central nervous system side effects have occurred in the elderly and in immunocompromised patients, or in normal hosts after repeated uses. Sulfur in petrolatum 6% is another treatment option. It should be applied to the entire body from the neck down for three consecutive nights. Patients should bathe between applications and 24 hours after the final treatment. Although it has no dangerous systemic effects, this remedy has an unpleasant odor. Crotamiton 10% cream may be applied for two consecutive nights and then washed off 24 hours after the last application.

B. CHILDREN

The treatment for infants, children younger than 10 years of age, and pregnant or lactating women is permethrin 5% cream, crotamiton 10% cream, or sulfur and petroleum as described above. The lindane preparation should not be used.

PEDICULOSIS

 ESSENTIALS OF DIAGNOSIS

- *Lice infestation.*
- *Different distributions: head, body, pubic area.*

• Spread by direct contact or sharing of personal items.

General Considerations

Pediculosis refers to infestation of the body with lice. Similar to scabies, pediculosis results from a parasite. These organisms feed on the blood of humans. Several variants exist, and the organisms are named in reference to the area of the body they inhabit. These include *P. humanus var. capitis* (head lice), *P. humanus var. corporis* (body lice), and *P. pubis* (pubic lice). Head lice are the most common, with the classic scenario of outbreaks in school children seen in all levels in society. The lice are transmitted by direct contact as well as by sharing of hats, brushes, and other personal items. Body lice predominantly affect adults of lower socioeconomic standing, such as the homeless and those in refugee situations. Pubic lice are spread by sexual contact, and they often occur in conjunction with other sexually transmitted diseases.

Clinical Findings

Recognition of the lice as described above is essential in the diagnosis. Pruritus may lead to excoriations that may become secondarily infected. Infestation of head lice is diagnosed by visualizing live lice or nits (eggs) attached to the proximal portion of the hair shaft. Body lice and eggs are found in the clothing of the affected individual, with excoriations over the body. Pubic lice are intensely pruritic, and the lice themselves may be transferred to other hair-bearing areas of the body. Remember to screen these patients for other sexually transmitted diseases. When pubic lice are found in children, they have often resulted from nonsexual contact; however, abuse should be considered in the differential.

Treatment

For the treatment of pediculosis capitis, corporis, and pubis, permethrin 1% cream rinse can be used. It can be applied to the groin, armpit, or scalp for 10 minutes and then washed off. Lindane 1% shampoo may be used as an alternative regimen. It is applied as above but is left on for 8 hours before washing off. For pediculosis capitis, it may be used as a shampoo, left on for 4 minutes, and then rinsed. Lindane should never be used on pregnant or lactating women, or on children younger than 10 years of age.

Chosidow O: Scabies and pediculosis. Lancet 2000;355(9206):819. [PMID: 10711939] (A thorough review of scabies and pediculosis with a discussion of treatment modalities.)

CUTANEOUS DERMATOPHYTES/TINEA

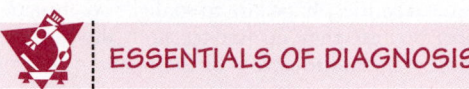

ESSENTIALS OF DIAGNOSIS

• *Superficial fungal infections.*
• *Flat, scaly patches.*

General Considerations

Dermatophytes include a group of fungi that infect the skin. The organisms themselves survive on the dead keratin found in the uppermost layer of the epidermis. The infections are limited to this superficial distribution in immunocompetent individuals. The dermatophytoses are classified by the distribution of the lesions.

Clinical Findings

A. TINEA CORPORIS

Tinea corporis refers to tinea of the body. Some authors and clinicians include the face in this category, but the American Academy of Dermatology refers to tinea of the face separately as tinea faciei. The most common causative organisms are *Trichophyton rubrum, Microsporum canis,* and *Trichophyton mentagrophytes.* Classic ringworm (tinea circinata) is the most common form of tinea corporis. It usually begins as a flat scaly patch with a raised, palpable border. It enlarges by advancing its border outward, leaving an area of central clearing.

B. TINEA PEDIS

Also known as athlete's foot, tinea pedis is a common condition. It affects up to 70% of adults. It is divided into three subtypes. The most prevalent is the interdigital type. It is chronic and occurs with fissuring and maceration between the toes. Moccasin-type tinea pedis has a plantar distribution. The plantar surface is tender and erythematous. It is usually covered with a silvery scale. The third type is the wet, vesicular type.

C. TINEA CRURIS

Tinea cruris, commonly called "jock itch," affects the groin area, sparing the genitalia. Men are affected more commonly than women, and the condition has a predilection for summer months.

D. TINEA VERSICOLOR

Tinea versicolor affects a deeper layer of the skin than the previously described tineas. It is caused by the yeast *Malassezia furfur.* It often is associated with multiple hypopigmented macular lesions distributed over the trunk and extremities. Exposure to sunlight accentuates the lesions, because they do not tan normally like the surrounding skin. A fine scale is often present.

Treatment

A. TINEA CORPORIS

Mild cases of tinea corporis can usually be treated with over-the-counter topical preparations, such as miconazole nitrate or clotrimazole. Prescription agents include ketoconazole 2% cream or econazole nitrate. All topical remedies should be used for 1–2 weeks after resolution of symptoms. Extensive disease or difficult cases may require oral therapy. Agents include griseofulvin, itraconazole, terbinafine, and fluconazole.

B. TINEA PEDIS

Most mild cases of tinea pedis can be treated successfully with 1–4 weeks of therapy with an over-the-counter preparation, in conjunction with the use of drying powders. Severe cases may require oral therapy. Drugs such as griseofulvin, fluconazole, and itraconazole are effective. Cases are often recurrent if concomitant nail disease is present.

C. TINEA CRURIS

Tinea cruris can often be treated with topical antifungal therapies used for 2–3 weeks (see as for tinea corporis). The area should be kept dry, because moisture and maceration are problems with this disease. Antifungal powders and loose-fitting clothing are often useful adjuncts. A mild topical corticosteroid may be used cautiously for a short time to help relieve the pruritus, which is often severe. Corticosteroids may be used only for 48–72 hours; longer use is contraindicated. As with tinea corporis, resistant disease may require oral therapy.

D. TINEA VERSICOLOR

Limited tinea versicolor can be treated with topical selenium sulfide 2.5%. Daily application of ketoconazole to the affected areas for 3 days is an alternative regimen. Recurrence of the disease may be prevented with the use of a once-monthly bedtime application of selenium sulfide 2.5%.

Goldstein AO et al: Mycotic infections. Effective management of conditions involving the skin, hair, and nails. Geriatrics 2000;55(5):40. [PMID: 10826264] (A thorough review with an extensive discussion of treatment modalities and pharmaceutical regimens.)

Rupke SJ: Fungal skin disorders. Prim Care 2000;27(2):407. [PMID: 10815051] (A review of various fungal disorders, including tinea, pityriasis, and candida.)

PITYRIASIS ROSEA

 **ESSENTIALS OF DIAGNOSIS**

- *Herald patch is initial lesion.*
- *Rash is usually truncal and has a "Christmas tree" distribution.*
- *May be pruritic.*

General Considerations

Pityriasis rosea is a common rash that may easily be confused with tinea corporis. It is a papulosquamous eruption that most commonly affects patients in the second to the fourth decades of life. Pityriasis rosea affects men and women equally. Although its cause is thought to be related to a viral process, the exact cause of pityriasis rosea is unknown.

Clinical Findings

The classic progression of the exanthem begins with the appearance of a herald patch. This is an isolated lesion usually found on the trunk. It is typically oval shaped and can be as large as 10 cm in diameter. It usually has an erythematous border, and there may be central clearing. The subsequent lesions usually develop within 1–2 weeks, and their distribution has been described as resembling the shape of a Christmas tree. The individual lesions are smaller than the herald patch, are usually a lighter shade, and have a scaly border.

Treatment

The lesions are self-limiting and usually disappear within 6–8 weeks. The initial lesions regress, and new lesions develop during this time. No effective treatment has been found for pityriasis rosea. If pruritus is present, it may be treated symptomatically with antihistamines or topical hydrocortisone 1% ointment. Patients should be reassured that recurrences are uncommon, occurring in only approximately 3% of cases.

Hsu S et al: Differential diagnosis of annular lesions. Am Fam Physician 2001;64(2):289. [PMID: 11476274] (A basic discussion comparing various skin lesions and their diagnoses.)

Wyndham M: Pityriasis. Practitioner 1997;241(1575):358. [PMID: 9254391] (A brief discussion of pityriasis and its diagnosis and treatment.)

MOLLUSCUM CONTAGIOSUM

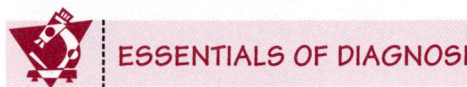

ESSENTIALS OF DIAGNOSIS

- *Viral infection.*
- *Pearly pink papules with central umbilication.*

General Considerations

Molluscum contagiosum is a viral infection of the skin. It is associated with multiple lesions, typically papules, spread over the skin. Molluscum contagiosum is present worldwide. In normal hosts, it is a self-limited disease and usually resolves within 8 weeks. Recently there has been increased prevalence in the immunocompromised population, especially in patients with HIV. In this population the disease presentation can be dramatic, with large, widespread lesions and a longer duration.

Clinical Findings

The diagnosis is made by the identification of the lesions. They are typically flesh-colored papules. The lesions may also appear pearly pink. The papules are rounded with a distinctive central umbilication and are firm to palpation. They usually are 1–5 mm in diameter, but in certain situations they may be quite large. The lesions may be distributed anywhere on the body, but they are rarely found on the palms or soles. They are usually found in groups, and usually fewer than 20 lesions are present. Molluscum contagiosum is spread by close contact with infected persons, by contact with contaminated surfaces, or by autoinoculation with scratching or shaving. It can also be spread by sexual contact.

Treatment

Most lesions resolve without treatment in immunocompetent patients. Lesions involving the perineum and genitalia should be treated to avoid spread via sexual contact. If lesions require treatment, the two most commonly used modalities are cryosurgery and curettage. Various topical therapies have had varying levels of success, including lactic acid, podophyllin, cantharidin, and silver nitrate. In pediatric patients, use of a topical anesthetic, such as lidocaine plus prilocaine, should be considered prior to curetting. Instruct patients to avoid contact sports, swimming pools, and other such activities until the lesions have resolved.

Lewis EJ et al: An update on molluscum contagiosum. Cutis 1997; 60(1):29. [PMID: 9252731] (A discussion of the latest information regarding the diagnosis and treatment of molluscum contagiosum, with a focus on the immunocompromised population.)

Psychiatric Emergencies

47

Gregory Hall, MD, & Denis J. Fitzgerald, MD

I. Introduction

II. The S.A.F.E.S.T. Approach to Violent or Agitated Patients

III. Emergency Department Screening Assessment

Targeted History

Focused Physical Examination

Mental Status Examination

Screening Laboratory Tests

Diagnostic Focus: Organic versus Functional Cause

Psychiatric Safety Check

IV. Organic Causes for Psychiatric Emergencies

Dementia

Delirium

Drug Intoxication & Withdrawal

Infection

Endocrine & Metabolic Disorders

Neurologic Disorders

Cardiopulmonary Disease

V. Functional Causes for Psychiatric Emergencies

Cognitive (Thought) Disorders: Schizophrenia

Affective (Mood) Disorders

Depression

Manic States

Borderline Personality Disorder

Other Functional Causes

Somatoform Disorders & Hysterical States

Dissociative States: Psychogenic Fugue

Developmental Disorders

VI. Psychopharmacotherapy

Traditional Antipsychotics

Neuroleptic Malignant Syndrome

Atypical Antipsychotics

Antidepressants

VII. Disposition

■ I. INTRODUCTION

Psychiatric emergencies are acute changes in behavior that negatively impact a patient's ability to function in his or her environment. Often such patients are in a state of crisis in which their baseline coping mechanisms have been overwhelmed by real or perceived circumstances. In dealing with such emergencies, the emergency physician faces many challenges and must prioritize his or her clinical efforts toward four main concerns.

First, the physician must ensure his or her own safety and the patient's well-being if violence or agitated behavior is present. Second, the physician must perform an effective screening assessment, probing for organic causes and completing a psychiatric safety check. The screening assessment ensures that there is no underlying medical cause for the patient's condition, ei-

ther initially inducing the aberrant behavior or evolving as a consequence of that behavior (eg, malnutrition or dehydration). The screening assessment also involves a psychiatric safety check to explore for suicidal ideation, homicidal ideation, or the patient's inability to care for him- or herself. Third, the physician must ensure that the patient receives appropriate psychological support and medical treatment, even if that treatment needs to be provided without the patient's consent. Fourth, the physician must determine the appropriate disposition for the patient.

The algorithm in Figure 47–1 provides a decision-making guide to the management of psychiatric emergencies. This algorithm reflects the four main priorities in patient care and provides a framework for this chapter.

Frumin M et al: Psychotic and behavioral problems. Neurol Clin 1998;16:521. [PMID: 9537973]

Richards CF, Gurr DE: Psychosis. Emerg Med Clin North Am 2000;18:253. [PMID: 10767882]

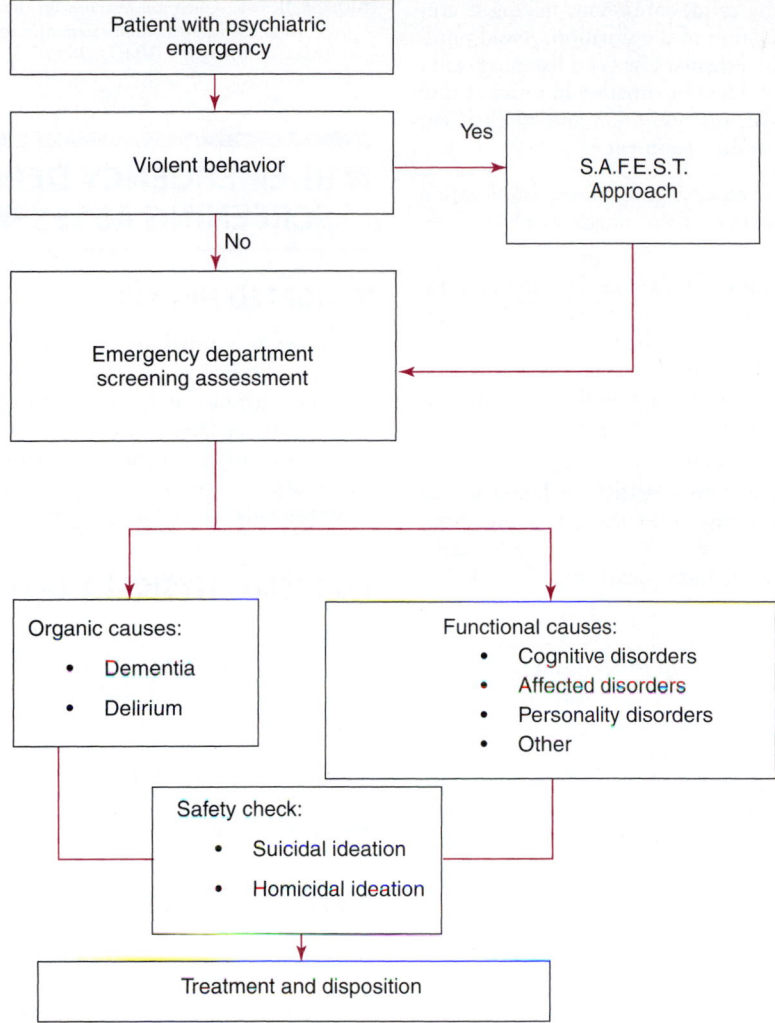

Figure 47–1. Decision-making algorithm for psychiatric emergencies.

▪ II. THE S.A.F.E.S.T. APPROACH TO VIOLENT OR AGITATED PATIENTS

The emergency physician may find him- or herself dealing with a patient who threatens or exhibits violent behavior toward staff. In these cases, it is important to recognize the early warning signs of impending violence and adopt an approach to management that reduces the likelihood of injury to staff and patient. Early warning signs of impending violence include threatening state-ments, clenched fists, loud vocalizations, shifting body position toward a fighting posture, agitated movements, and striking inanimate objects. If such behavior is detected, adopt the S.A.F.E.S.T. Approach:

Spacing—Maintain distance from the patient. Allow both the patient and you to have equal access to the door. Do not touch a violent person.

Appearance—Maintain empathetic professional detachment. Use one primary contact person to build rapport. Have security staff available as a show of strength.

Focus—Watch the patient's hands. Watch for potential weapons. Watch for escalating agitation.

Exchange—Delay by calm, continuous talking is crucial to permit deescalation of the situation. Avoid punitive or judgmental statements. Use good listening skills. Target the current problem or situation in order to find face-saving alternatives for resolution and to elicit the patient's cooperation with treatment.

Stabilization—If necessary, use three stabilization techniques to get control of the situation: physical restraint, sedation, and chemical restraint.

1. Physical restraint—Once the situation permits, it is advisable to restrain any violent or agitated patient to ensure safety. This activity is best done by trained security personnel who should also search the patient for weapons. Implement documentation that indicates the need for restraints and provides a record of safety checks on the restrained patient.

2. Sedation—If agitation persists, sedation is best achieved by administering lorazepam, 1–2 mg intramuscularly or intravenously. Dosing may be repeated every 30 minutes for 4 doses maximum, if needed to achieve effect.

3. Chemical restraint—Chemical restraint is best achieved with neuroleptics. For patients not responding to sedation, haloperidol may be administered (5 mg intramuscularly). In elderly patients, it is best to start with lower dosing and increase by 1- to 2-mg increments. Dosing may be repeated every 30 minutes until the patient is more in control. Be alert for the emergence of extrapyramidal symptoms, seizure activity, or neuroleptic malignant syndrome (see below, in discussion of psychopharmacotherapy).

Treatment—Once the patient is more manageable, initiate treatment based on the patient's symptoms. The patient may refuse treatment and may need to receive treatment involuntarily in order to ensure his or her safety.

American College of Emergency Physicians: Use of patient restraints. Ann Emerg Med 2001;38:619. [PMID: 11699510]

Annas GJ: The last resort—the use of physical restraints in medical emergencies. N Engl J Med 1999;341:1408. [PMID: 10536135]

Buckley PF: The role of typical and atypical antipsychotic medications in the management of agitation and aggression. J Clin Psychiatry 1999;60:52. [PMID: 10340688]

Citrome L, Volavka J: Violent patients in the emergency setting. Psychiatr Clin North Am 1999;22:789. [PMID: 10623971]

FitzGerlad D: S.A.F.E.S.T. Approach. In: TIGER Coursebook (in press).
http://www.ucemergencymedicine.com/pdfs/Tiger.pdf

Hill S, Petit J: The violent patient. Emerg Med Clin North Am 2000;18:301. [PMID: 10767886]

Hillard JR: Emergency treatment of acute psychosis. J Clin Psychiatry 1998;59:57. [PMID: 9448670]

Richards JR et al: Chemical restraint for the agitated patient in the emergency department: lorazepam versus droperidol. J Emerg Med 1998;16:567. [PMID: 9696171]

■ III. EMERGENCY DEPARTMENT SCREENING ASSESSMENT

TARGETED HISTORY

Focus on precipitating causes and circumstances that brought the patient to the emergency department. It may be necessary to elicit information from multiple sources such as family, friends, or ambulance personnel. Other key topics include previous psychiatric treatment, seizure disorders, polysubstance abuse, and any recent suicidal attempts including possible ingestions.

FOCUSED PHYSICAL EXAMINATION

Perform a thorough physical examination, including neurologic assessment. Complete vital signs are essential. Look for physical clues to the source of an altered mental status, such as evidence of head injury, drug use, or toxidromes (constellation of symptoms produced by a toxic ingestion or exposure). Assess the patient for adverse consequences of his or her behavior such as malnutrition or dehydration.

MENTAL STATUS EXAMINATION

It is important to document the mental status examination in patients presenting with psychiatric emergencies. The mental status assessment should probe for global functioning, thought disorders, mood disorders, and personality disorders.

A. GLOBAL FUNCTIONING

Assess the patient for general orientation (person, place, time, reason for visit), memory (short and long-term), judgment, and concentration.

B. THOUGHT DISORDERS

Assess the patient for abnormal thought content such as hearing voices, experiencing command hallucinations, or having paranoid thoughts.

C. MOOD DISORDERS

Assess the patient for evidence of depression or mania. Compare the appropriateness of the patient's stated mood with his or her overt affect. Look for clues such as emotional lability or unbalanced emotional extremes.

D. Personality Disorders

Try to assess whether the patient's current behavior is an acute psychiatric event that represents a decompensation in his or her normal functioning or a representative sample of a maladaptive pattern of behavior derived from an underlying socially inappropriate personality matrix.

SCREENING LABORATORY TESTS

The following studies are often helpful in the evaluation of patients presenting with psychiatric emergencies:

- Electrolyte panel with glucose
- Pulse oximetry
- Toxicology screen
- Liver function tests
- Computed tomography (CT) scan of the head
- Electrocardiogram (ECG)
- Thyroid function tests

DIAGNOSTIC FOCUS: ORGANIC VERSUS FUNCTIONAL CAUSE

The emergency department is the first stop, in many instances, for patients with many different types of acute, and sometimes chronic, complaints. Often a patient presents with an alteration in his or her mental state, behavior, level of functioning, mood, or personality. The emergency physician must distinguish between those patients needing medical treatment for an organic problem (eg, delirium or dementia) and those individuals who would benefit from psychiatric treatment for a functional problem (eg, thought disorder, mood disorder, personality disorder).

Functional disorders may be very difficult to differentiate from an acute mental status change caused by an organic condition. However, some factors may point to an organic cause of the behavioral change. Organic causes often are acute in onset, whereas functional disorders develop over time. Visual hallucinations are much more common with organic syndromes or medical illness than are auditory hallucinations. Age of onset may also be a clue. Patients presenting with functional etiologies are usually younger, typically 12–40 years of age. Exceptions are always possible, but older patients need special consideration when disease is being attributed to psychiatric origin, especially when no history of previous psychiatric disorder is present. Patients with organic disorders generally present with emotional lability, whereas patients with a flat affect

usually have functional disease. Finally, any abnormality in vital signs or features of a toxidrome should immediately point to an organic cause.

PSYCHIATRIC SAFETY CHECK

General Considerations

The emergency physician must directly assess for the presence of suicidal or homicidal ideation in all patients presenting with a psychiatric emergency. In general, the patient's ability to care for him- or herself is a cardinal component of the initial assessment.

Suicidal Patients

The management of suicidal ideation involves recognition of the problem, an assessment of risk, and development of a treatment plan.

A. Recognition of Suicidal Ideation

Patients with suicidal ideation may present with an obvious attempt to cause self-harm. However, such patients may present to the emergency department more indirectly, with suicidal ideation as the underlying cause behind other presentations, such as through an automobile accident. The best screening approach involves general questions about the patient's emotional state. Inappropriate, irrational, or dysphoric answers should prompt further investigation, culminating in direct questions about suicidal intent.

B. Assessment of Risk

Several factors increase the risk of suicide. Patients with prior suicide attempts are at increased risk. Patients who employ violent means are more serious about their intent. Existence of a detailed plan reflects significant commitment to following through with the suicide attempt, particularly when coupled with a depressed emotional state or altered mental status. Poor social support or inadequate coping mechanisms also puts patients at increased risk.

C. Treatment

Admit patients who have clear suicidal ideation, unless immediate psychiatric evaluation is an option. The admission may be directly to the psychiatry service or to the medical service with a psychiatry consult. It may be necessary to sign involuntary admission holds on patients who resist efforts to ensure their safety. Patients with suicidal ideation should be monitored closely at all times, ideally with a one-on-one sitter. They should be given emotional support throughout their stay, and their environment should be carefully screened for any potential means of suicide.

Homicidal Patients

Patients expressing homicidal intent require special measures to ensure staff safety and the safety of the third party threatened by the patient. The patient's threats should be believed, particularly if he or she has a specific plan. The third party, if specifically named, should be contacted through appropriate authorities to ensure his or her safety. The patient should be closely monitored by security personnel, with restraints, as indicated, in a setting devoid of potential weapons. Acute psychiatric consultation is mandatory.

■ IV. ORGANIC CAUSES FOR PSYCHIATRIC EMERGENCIES

Patients with acute behavior, mood, or thought disturbances must be medically evaluated for the presence of dementia or delirium. Dementia is a chronic, progressive alteration in memory associated with cognitive decline and agnosia, apraxia, and aphasia. Alzheimer disease is the classic type of dementia. However, infections, such as HIV, and other neurologic conditions, such as stroke, can also cause dementia. Delirium, by contrast, is an acute disturbance in consciousness. It may also involve cognitive decline, but the patient's level of consciousness is decreased, unlike in dementia. Delirium has a short onset and usually a fluctuating course.

DEMENTIA

Alzheimer disease is the most common type of dementia. It starts with memory loss affecting recent memory. Long-term memory is usually preserved. As the disease progresses, more cognitive deficits become apparent until the patient is no longer able to function. History and physical exam are the most important contributors to the diagnosis. Magnetic resonance imaging (MRI) is an important adjunct. Acetylcholinesterase inhibitors (eg, tacrine, donepezil) are used to increase central nervous system (CNS) levels of acetylcholine. This treatment helps to delay the progression of the disease in some patients. However, no agent is currently available that can prevent the ultimate progression of Alzheimer disease.

DELIRIUM

Multiple medical problems can cause a delirious state, which may be confused with psychosis. Drug intoxication or withdrawal; infection; and endocrine, metabolic, neurologic, and cardiopulmonary disturbances are most often implicated.

DRUG INTOXICATION & WITHDRAWAL

Stimulants

The stimulant drugs such as cocaine and amphetamines, including MDMA (Ecstasy), can cause symptoms of behavioral and personality disturbance. These drugs can also induce someone with a compensated psychiatric illness such as schizophrenia to decompensate. Therefore, when evaluating a patient with mental status changes and bizarre behavior, the physician should determine whether stimulant drugs are present. The diagnosis is based on history of substance abuse, characteristic signs, and a positive drug screen. Cocaine and amphetamines both cause a sympathetic rush. They cause hypertension, tachycardia, dilated pupils, and diaphoresis. MDMA causes less sympathetic hyperactivity and has more hallucinogenic properties.

Psychological manifestations of stimulants include dysphoria, paranoid psychosis, and potentially a delirious state. Stimulants also cause a disinhibition leading to poor impulse control. As a result, patients with acute ingestion are more likely to be violent, homicidal, or suicidal. This property is seen especially in patients taking amphetamines. Management of patients with acute toxicity is supportive. Benzodiazepines are the treatment of choice for the acutely agitated and violent person taking cocaine or amphetamines.

Withdrawal from stimulants initially involves anxiety, anhedonia, depression, fatigue, and severe craving for the drug of abuse. Withdrawal does not cause a significant risk for death from cardiac or pulmonary disturbances. The withdrawal state may be a risk factor, however, for suicide. Patients receive supportive measures, usually lasting 1–2 weeks until improvement in the anxiety and lethargy is seen. However, the anhedonia and cravings may continue for weeks.

Depressants

Alcohol and benzodiazepines are the classic depressants. The diagnosis is based on clinical findings coupled with a positive drug level. They cause a decrease in sensorium, lethargy, ataxic gait, nystagmus, and respiratory depression. Individuals presenting with symptoms of intoxication and lethargy warrant evaluation for depressant use. These chemicals, however, can inhibit impulse control, and some people have a paradoxical excitation when using depressants. Monitoring of airway and breathing status is crucial. Searching for any other cause of the behavior (eg, head injury) is also important.

Alcohol withdrawal is noteworthy due to the continued morbidity and even mortality that occurs from such a widely used substance. Delirium tremens can cause a clinical picture very similar to that of an acute psychotic break. Patients with delirium tremens have stopped drinking for as little as a few hours to days. Patients clinically show signs of sympathetic overload, including hypertension and tachycardia. They are usually diaphoretic and, by definition, tremulous. This delirious state can be differentiated from functional psychosis due to the history, autonomic dysfunction, and visual hallucinations. Treatment is with benzodiazepines. A titrated lorazepam infusion may be needed to decrease the hypertension, tachycardia, and CNS symptoms.

Opioids

All opioid medications, such as morphine and heroin, can cause the classic triad of respiratory depression, miosis, and decreased mental status. Diagnosis is based on the clinical picture, positive drug screen, or response to naloxone. Usually the patient abusing opiates presents with lethargy and not bizarre behavior. However, if these chemicals are mixed with stimulants (eg, cocaine, amphetamines), the result may be any type of delirium that can mimic functional psychosis or mood disorder.

Hallucinogens

Lysergic acid diethylamide (LSD) and phencyclidine (PCP) are the traditional hallucinogenic drugs. LSD is absorbed through the oral mucosa and binds to postsynaptic serotonergic receptors. The patient may report kaleidoscopic hallucinations. However, the drug may also cause violence, suicidal ideation, and bizarre memories or flashbacks. PCP is a dissociative anesthetic. Patients are awake but exhibit bizarre behavior that can become suddenly violent. Patients may be hypertensive and tachycardic. Patients may also experience a host of behavioral and neurologic changes such as loss of concentration or the presence of illogical speech, nystagmus, or ataxia. Diagnosis is based on the history of use, clinical findings, and drug screen results. Treatment for hallucinogens includes ruling out any other associated acute medical problem and providing supportive care in a calm, quiet environment. Benzodiazepines may be used in acutely agitated patients.

INFECTION
Systemic

Many patients, especially the elderly, with systemic infections present with delirium. Sometimes the delirious state involves behavioral changes. Any elderly patient with acute mental status changes should be evaluated for systemic infection. Diagnosis is based on the clinical picture coupled with the source of infection on urinalysis, chest x-ray, or cultures.

Central Nervous System

Encephalopathy is an infectious process that causes inflammation around the brain. The etiology often is viral (eg, herpes, HIV). Clinical manifestations usually involve fever and headache. If the infection affects the limbic area of the brain, personality and behavioral changes can occur, including floridly psychotic behavior and aggression. Meningitis, likewise, may cause delirium and altered mental status. Therefore, if an infectious cause is suspected, especially in a patient with fever, the patient should receive a head CT scan and lumbar puncture. Diagnosis is based on these two tests in the appropriate clinical setting. Treatment is aimed at the underlying infectious or inflammatory process. If infection is suspected, initiate acyclovir and antibiotics as soon as possible.

ENDOCRINE & METABOLIC DISORDERS
Hepatic Encephalopathy

Patients with stigmata of liver failure routinely present with altered mental status. These patients may be delirious. At times they may be violent or aggressive. Pathophysiology is debated, but there is a correlation with high ammonia levels. Therefore, in the context of liver failure, an ammonia level may be helpful in narrowing down the differential diagnosis to hepatic encephalopathy. Treatment is usually supportive along with lactulose to enterally clear toxins usually cleared by the liver.

Electrolyte Abnormalities

Hypercalcemia and alterations in sodium, either hyponatremia or hypernatremia, are the most common causes of altered mental status. Personality and behavioral changes are much less common than lethargy. Seizures, coma, and death are possible if the electrolyte abnormality is not corrected appropriately. Fortunately, the diagnosis is easily made with routine electrolyte chemistry panels.

Hypoglycemia

The brain requires glucose to function. A low blood glucose level can mimic any type of CNS event. Patients may present with decreased consciousness or focal neurologic findings similar to a stroke. Blood glucose level should be checked as soon as possible in any patient with behavioral changes. Rapid correction of hypoglycemia can itself cause behavioral changes. Violence and aggression from the rapid correction are usually short in duration. However, if a patient continues to have symptoms after the glucose level has been corrected, further investigation into the cause is warranted.

Thyroid Disease

Hyperthyroidism and hypothyroidism have been implicated in acute behavioral changes mimicking psychiatric disorders. Hyperthyroidism may cause anxiety and tremor. These patients usually present with mild to moderate hypertension and tachycardia along with weight loss and heat intolerance. Patients with hypothyroidism can present with symptoms of fatigue all the way to delirium or coma. Other symptoms include gastrointestinal complaints such as constipation, cold intolerance, weight gain, and menstrual irregularities. Diagnosis can be reliably made based on laboratory levels of thyroid hormones.

NEUROLOGIC DISORDERS

Seizure Disorder

Patients who have had a seizure may present with normal mental status or may have decreased consciousness from a postictal state. A history of seizure or witnessed seizure activity may guide the workup. Nonconvulsive status epilepticus is much more difficult to determine. These patients may present with decreased consciousness or may be awake and alert. Patients may even have behavioral changes from blank stare to aggression depending on the location of the seizure focus. Nonconvulsive status epilepticus should be considered in patients with behavioral or neurologic changes, especially if a history of epilepsy is present. If necessary, neurologic consultation and an electroencephalogram would be appropriate to confirm the diagnosis.

Cerebral Vascular Accident

Cerebral vascular accidents (CVAs) are usually associated with focal weakness and a variable level of consciousness. Depending on the area of the brain affected, patients may have significant cognitive deficits. Patients may present with bizarre behavior secondary to aphasia or neglect. Therefore, a CVA should be considered in patients with risk factors for vascular disease or cardioembolic phenomenon. CT scanning and MRI can be helpful in diagnosis.

Wernicke-Korsakoff Syndrome

A clinical diagnosis, Wernicke encephalopathy is secondary to thiamine deficiency and occurs mostly in alcoholic patients. The main features clinically are ataxia, ophthalmoplegia (either nystagmus or gaze palsy), and mental status changes. The mental status change involves anything from confusion to delirium or even coma. Thus, this entity should be considered in anyone with a history of alcohol abuse, eye changes, and mental status changes. The development of Korsakoff psychosis can accompany these findings. Patients with malnutrition and alcohol abuse should be given thiamine. Theoretically, anyone with this history who is given dextrose should receive a thiamine supplement first although there is little evidence in the dogma that it must be given before the glucose.

CARDIOPULMONARY DISEASE

Diseases of the cardiopulmonary system can cause significant behavioral changes. Myocardial infarction, pulmonary edema, and pulmonary embolism can cause anxiety secondary to pain, shortness of breath, and a possible sense of doom. These disorders may elicit significant fear in patients, which may manifest itself as panic attack or even aggression. Patients may also be hypoxic or hypotensive, which may cause decreased consciousness and cognitive dysfunction. Diagnosis is based on clinical suspicion coupled with basic cardiac function evaluation (ECG, cardiac enzymes, pulse oximetry, chest x-ray).

■ V. FUNCTIONAL CAUSES FOR PSYCHIATRIC EMERGENCIES

Patients with psychiatric illness present to the emergency department with a disorder of behavior secondary to abnormal thought process, mood, or personality traits. The changes that result in the visit to the emergency department usually occur over a period of weeks. Patients may present with depressed mood, labile affect, paranoid delusions, auditory hallucinations, and psychomotor retardation, or they may be in a manic state. The clinical picture is quite variable, and organic cause for the decompensation should be investigated.

COGNITIVE (THOUGHT) DISORDERS: SCHIZOPHRENIA

Diagnosed clinically, schizophrenia is a common disorder. Most patients with schizophrenia are not institutionalized and routinely present to the emergency department for acute medical care. The visit may be due to medication noncompliance, ineffective medication, or substance abuse. Onset of disease is usually in the late teens or early adult years. The cause of schizophrenia is not fully understood, but it is heralded by a disturbance in thought process. Current medications work on dopaminergic and serotonergic receptors.

Clinical Findings

Patients with schizophrenia present with positive symptoms (delusions, hallucinations, and bizarre behavior) and negative symptoms (withdrawal, blunted affect, catatonia). Organic causes of the behavior must be sought (eg, steroid toxicity, substance abuse or withdrawal, encephalitis, HIV encephalopathy). Common manifestations of disorganized thought include the following:

- Social withdrawal, often with poor personal hygiene
- Preoccupation with inner thoughts and auditory hallucinations, which are often violent, sexual, or religious in nature
- Labile affect, often presenting with flat emotionless affect but rapidly changing
- Poor ability to focus on a topic, making it difficult to follow the patient in conversation
- Flight of ideas
- Hallucinations, often derogatory to the patient
- Grandiose or persecutory delusions
- Catatonia
- Paranoia

Treatment

Provision of a safe and supportive environment is important, both for the patient and emergency department staff. Patients with aggression and grossly disruptive or dangerous behavior require antipsychotic agents such as haloperidol, 5–10 mg intramuscularly, for management. Patients who are unable to care for themselves or who pose a high risk of harm to themselves require psychiatric consultation and admission. Often patients present in a withdrawn state (catatonia). These patients are at high risk for dehydration, electrolyte imbalances, and malnutrition. Therefore, along with psychiatric consultation, evaluation for organic disease that results from the psychiatric condition is imperative.

AFFECTIVE (MOOD) DISORDERS

DEPRESSION

Diagnosed based on a constellation of symptoms, depression is the most common mood disorder. Patients have variable presentations ranging from an acute depressive state lasting days after an emotionally taxing event to chronic depression lasting years.

Clinical Findings

Depression is characterized by a change in mood. Patients commonly have intense feelings of sadness, guilt, and hopelessness. Patients are often anhedonic, with no interest in pleasurable activity. These patients also may have psychomotor retardation or agitation with variable sleeping patterns. Depressed patients routinely are evaluated in the emergency department for complaints of fatigue or decreased appetite, suicidal ideation or attempt, overdose, substance abuse, dehydration, or malnutrition.

Patients with depression may present with delusions or frank psychosis. These patients may or may not have a diagnosis of schizoaffective disorder, which is a disorder of both thought and mood. The delusions are usually persecutory or somatic in nature.

Treatment

Life-threatening medical conditions must be detected and treated. Dehydration, overdose, and illicit drug ingestion must be medically managed. Many general medical conditions may cause depression and must also be ruled out. Neurodegenerative disorders, stroke, thyroid disorders, epilepsy, metabolic disorders, and infection are just some of the conditions that may involve a depressed state. Once patients are medically stable, those at risk of harming themselves or others must receive psychiatric consultation and be admitted.

MANIC STATES

Mania is another type of mood disorder. Many patients with mania have bipolar affective disorder, alternating between episodes of mania and depression. Mania is diagnosed clinically and is characterized by variable degrees of heightened mood and activity. The symptoms may be mild, characterized by an overly friendly and talkative personality. This condition is called hypomania. Others may present with grandiose delusions, insomnia, and aggressive behavior. Caution must be used in the emergency department when dealing with a manic patient. The disorder can cause an increase in unpredictable behavior.

Clinical Findings

The predominance of an infectious, inappropriate euphoria coupled with hyperactivity and talkativeness suggests the diagnosis. Mania is also characterized by decreased need to eat or sleep. Patients routinely are awake all hours of the night and may go for extended periods of time without a significant amount of sleep. The disorder is also characterized by flight of ideas, decreased ability to concentrate on a task, inappropriate laughing and joking, increased uninterrupted speech, and grandiose delusions. Patients with bipolar affective disorder may be rapid cycling. In this state, patients, over hours to days, alternate between severely depressed mood and a state of euphoria. When disorganization of thought process is a prominent feature, a diagnosis of schizoaffective disorder should be considered.

Treatment

Initially, evaluate patients for an organic cause or signs of organic disease resulting from the manic state. Illicit drug use, especially stimulants, may cause a clinical picture of mania. In addition, patients with mania may be dehydrated or have an electrolyte or nutritional disorder secondary to decreased consumption of food and water while in a manic state.

Evaluate patients for toxicity from drugs used to treat mania, such as lithium or antiepileptics. Once patients are medically stable, evaluate them for risk of harming themselves or others. If a patient is found to be at risk, psychiatric consultation and admission are required. Treat acute hostile behavior medically as appropriate. Reducing the environmental stimuli in the emergency department is important. Place the patient in a safe and quiet room after ensuring that he or she has no objects that may be used to cause harm. If the patient continues to be agitated, medical management with lorazepam, 1–2 mg intravenously or intramuscularly, or haloperidol, 5–10 mg intramuscularly, is appropriate.

BORDERLINE PERSONALITY DISORDER

Borderline personality disorder presents a special situation in the emergency department. Patients with this disorder regularly present to the emergency department and are usually well known for their frequent visits. The diagnosis is clinical, based on patient behavior.

Clinical Findings

Patients with borderline personality disorder are characterized by their volatile interpersonal relationships. They can be very impulsive and have labile affect. Patients are usually very demanding, frequently presenting with suicide threats and other self-destructive behavior. They commonly experience paranoid thoughts and have other comorbid conditions such as substance abuse and affective disorders.

Treatment

Evaluation of the patient for medical illness is the first priority. Treat medical and surgical issues resulting from self-destructive behavior rapidly, and evaluate the patient for continued threat to self or others. If such a threat exists, seek psychiatric consultation for the patient and arrange for admission.

Additional techniques for dealing with patients with borderline personality disorder involve contacting the patient's support structure (eg, family, friend, or therapist) and ensuring adequate follow-up. The number of visits to the emergency department is inversely proportional to the amount of social support the patient receives outside the hospital. Furthermore, emergency department staff should treat the patient's abrasiveness as a symptom of the disorder and avoid being abrasive toward the patient in response. Addressing the patient's complaints promptly may prevent escalation of symptoms.

OTHER FUNCTIONAL CAUSES

SOMATOFORM DISORDERS & HYSTERICAL STATES

Somatoform disorders and hysterical states are psychiatric functional disorders diagnosed by exclusion of organic disorders. Patients present with physical complaints of different types. Patients perceive the complaints as real, even though no underlying physical organic cause is responsible. These disorders must be separated from malingering, which involves deliberate and conscious deception for secondary gain.

1. Conversion Disorder

Conversion disorder is characterized by motor or sensory dysfunction caused by psychological stress with no true physical dysfunction. These symptoms are not intentionally produced and frequently are seen in the emergency department after a traumatic event, especially if a loved one is injured or killed. Different types of conversion disorder involve motor symptoms, sensory symptoms, or seizures.

Clinical Findings

The most important factor for the emergency physician is to differentiate between somatic symptoms due solely to functional cause and true organic disease exacerbated by psychologic stress. Evaluate patients for disorders such as Guillain-Barré syndrome, botulism poisoning, herpes encephalitis, and CVAs. Obtain a thorough history, including history of psychiatric disease, and conduct a thorough physical exam. Pay close attention to discrepancies in the physical findings. A patient with hysterical blindness can be tested for nystagmus by running a strip of paper with multiple vertical lines on it (ECG paper) in front of the patient's eyes. Doing so will elicit tracking and nystagmus if the patient has vision (optokinetic reflex). The diagnosis of conversion disorder is strengthened by a fluctuating pattern of disability; a lack of concern about the disability; a pattern that does not follow known anatomic relationships; intact sphincter tone; and, when the complaint is paralysis, presence of the Hoover sign (in which counterpressure with the heel of the unaffected leg is absent when the patient is asked to lift the affected leg).

Treatment

Differentiating a conversion disorder from a true motor or sensory disorder is imperative. If the diagnosis is difficult, an elaborate workup may be initiated. If the diagnosis of conversion disorder is made, psychiatric consultation and counseling are appropriate.

2. Somatization Disorder

Somatization disorder is characterized by 4 or more different pain complaints along with at least 2 gastrointestinal complaints, a sexual complaint, and a neurologic complaint. Patients usually have a history of multiple surgeries, numerous emergency department visits, multiple medications, multiple reported allergies, and no relief from intractable chronic pain. The emergency physician must rule out significant medical disease and at the same time avoid elaborate workups. Evaluating available medical records and contacting the patient's other physicians or counselors is imperative.

3. Hypochondria

Hypochondria represents an anxious preoccupation with physical signs and symptoms. Patients have a fear of having a serious medical condition. Evaluation of the patient based on clinical reasoning is important, followed by reassurance and referral for psychiatric counseling.

DISSOCIATIVE STATES: PSYCHOGENIC FUGUE

Clinical Findings

Psychogenic fugue is the dissociative state most commonly encountered in the emergency department. The disorder is diagnosed clinically and characterized by the sudden loss of memory. It usually begins abruptly after a psychologically catastrophic event, such as the loss of a close family member. Patients are usually in good health and able to communicate, but they are unable to answer personal questions, for example, regarding their name and address. Patients may travel long distances without recall and are often found in bus or train stations. Recovery of memory can occur within a few hours or take several weeks. Afterward, the patient often has amnesia for the period of dissociation.

Treatment

The emergency physician must rule out organic disorders. Alcohol abuse is the most common cause of blackouts, which may mimic psychogenic fugue. Malingering must also be considered, especially if the patient is confronted with legal problems. Once other etiologies have been ruled out, it is important to reassure the patient that the disorder is not permanent. Social support is important to help the patient emotionally cope until the problem resolves.

DEVELOPMENTAL DISORDERS

Patients with developmental disorders such as autism and mental retardation require special attention. Patients are usually diagnosed by the age of 3 years due to poor functional development and failure to reach milestones. These patients may present to the emergency department with hostility or a change from baseline functioning. It is imperative that the physician discuss the changes with the patient's parents or caregivers and then evaluate the patient for recent trauma, signs of infection, and comorbid medical conditions. The inciting event often is organic in cause and must be treated before the patient's symptoms will improve.

Bair BD: Frequently missed diagnosis in geriatric psychiatry. Psychiatr Clin North Am 1998;21:941. [PMID: 9890132]

Broderick KB, et al: Emergency physician practices and requirements regarding the medical screening examination of psychiatric patients. Acad Emerg Med 2002;9:88. [PMID: 11772676]

Brust JC: Acute neurologic complications of drug and alcohol abuse. Neurol Clin 1998;16:503. [PMID: 9537972]

Goldman LS: Medical illness in patients with schizophrenia. J Clin Psychiatry 1999;60:10. [PMID: 10548136]

Korn CS, Currier GW, Henderson SO: "Medical clearance" of psychiatric patients without medical complaints in the emergency department. J Emerg Med 2000;18:173. [PMID: 10699517]

Perrone J, et al: Drug screening versus history in detection of substance use in ED psychiatric patients. Am J Emerg Med 2001;19:49. [PMID: 11146019]

Radomsky ED, et al: Suicidal behavior in patients with schizophrenia and other psychotic disorders. Am J Psychiatry 1999; 156:1590. [PMID: 10518171]

Reeves RR, Pendarvis EJ, Kimble R: Unrecognized medical emergencies admitted to psychiatric units. Am J Emerg Med 2000;18:390. [PMID: 10919525]

Richards CF, Gurr DE: Psychosis. Emerg Med Clin North Am 2000;18:253. [PMID: 10767882]

Tolbot-Stern JK, et al: Psychiatric manifestations of systemic illness. Emerg Med Clin North Am 2000:18:199. [PMID: 10767878]

Tse SK, et al: How good are accident and emergency doctors in the evaluation of psychiatric patients? Eur J Emerg Med 1999; 6,297. [PMID: 10646916]

Tueth MJ, Zuberi P: Life-threatening psychiatric emergencies in the elderly: overview. J Geriatr Psychiatry Neurol 1999;12:60. [PMID: 10483926]

Williams ER, Shepherd SM: Medical clearance of psychiatric patients. Emerg Med Clin North Am 2000;18:185. [PMID: 10767877]

■ VI. PSYCHOPHARMACO-THERAPY

Psychiatric medications have changed significantly in recent years. New atypical antipsychotics are being prescribed ever more frequently because of their more benign side-effect profiles. Psychiatrists and primary care providers are prescribing antidepressants to patients with symptoms of depression. Due to the rapid increase in the use of these medications, an understanding of their indications and potential toxicities is essential for an emergency physician faced with medically evaluating patients who are taking these drugs. Emergency physicians also need to be aware of potential uses for typical antipsychotic medications and the risks of using them.

TRADITIONAL ANTIPSYCHOTICS

Traditionally, high-potency antipsychotic agents such as haloperidol are used to treat agitation, violence, and acute psychosis in the emergency department. The high-potency agents are associated with less sedation, hypotension, and anticholinergic effects than are low-potency agents such as chlorpromazine or thioridazine. However, the high-potency agents are associated with a higher incidence of dystonic reactions and extrapyramidal side effects (EPS).

For an acutely agitated patient, the intravenous or intramuscular route of administration is preferred. Haloperidol is thought to have less potential for EPS or dystonic reaction when given intravenously. These agents may be used in combination with minor tranquilizers such as benzodiazepines, but prolonged sedation is a risk. Like its closely related cousin droperidol, haloperidol has the potential, like many other psychoactive agents, to cause a prolonged QTc. This factor should be considered before such drugs are used, and appropriate cardiac monitoring should be established. The potential for cardiac conduction delays should be of particular concern when giving haloperidol to patients with overdose or toxin exposure.

Any toxic overdose of typical antipsychotics should be treated with supportive care. Dyskinesias are treated with diphenhydramine, 25–50 mg intravenously or intramuscularly, or benztropine, 1–2 mg intravenously or intramuscularly. The usual dose of haloperidol for agitation in a patient whose appearance does not appear to be due to overdose or toxicologic origin is 5–10 mg intravenously or intramuscularly. Escalating doses of haloperidol are no longer considered appropriate. Effects should start within 30 minutes and peak at 1–2 hours.

NEUROLEPTIC MALIGNANT SYNDROME

Diagnosis

Neuroleptic malignant syndrome is an uncommon and potentially fatal reaction usually due to high-potency antipsychotic medications. The condition is characterized by hypertension, tachycardia, hyperthermia, and muscle rigidity. It may also occur in cases of acute delirium. Consider neuroleptic malignant syndrome in any patient who is known to have a psychiatric condition and who is taking neuroleptic medications.

Treatment

Treatment begins with management of airway, breathing, and circulation. Discontinue antipsychotic medication immediately. The patient should be cooled and rehydrated with crystalloid. Initiate muscle relaxation with intravenous benzodiazepines or dantrolene (1 mg/kg). Bromocriptine has also been used to help treat this condition because it is potentially caused by CNS depletion of dopamine. Further management includes supportive care and evaluation for rhabdomyolysis.

ATYPICAL ANTIPSYCHOTICS

In the 1990s, atypical antipsychotic medications (eg, risperidone, clozapine, quetiapine, olanzapine) started to replace the traditional antipsychotics in the treatment of schizophrenia. This trend is due to their improved efficacy for treating both positive and negative symptoms of schizophrenia. These agents have a much improved side-effect profile. EPS are minimal, if occurring at all. Tardive dyskinesia, likewise, is very rare even with long-term use. Overall, the medications have enhanced efficacy, fewer side effects, and greater patient compliance.

Atypical agents appear to be relatively safe. Most patients who overdose on these medications have few if any signs of toxicity. Death is especially rare but is more commonly associated with pediatric overdose and in adults not accustomed to taking the medications. Toxic signs and symptoms depend on age and dose ingested. The effects usually range from CNS depression, slurred speech, and ataxia to coma and, rarely, seizure. Respiratory depression, hypotension, and anticholinergic symptoms also occur. Sinus tachycardia is the most common cardiac disturbance. Prolongation of QTc and dysrhythmias happen infrequently. Treatment for overdose is largely supportive, paying attention to airway, breathing, and cardiac monitoring. Hemodialysis is unlikely to be of any benefit secondary to the large volume of distribution of these agents.

Some of the agents have more specific side effects. Clozapine has a higher risk of seizures as compared to the other agents. Risperidone is the one agent that can cause EPS when used in higher doses. Finally, clozapine has a risk of agranulocytosis that usually becomes evident in the first few months of therapy. Therefore, a complete blood count should be routinely obtained in patients taking this medication.

ANTIDEPRESSANTS

Antidepressants have been around for decades. The older antidepressants such as tricyclic antidepressants (TCAs) and monoamine oxidase inhibitors (MAOIs) were effective, but they had the potential for serious side effects or death. Selective serotonin reuptake inhibitors (SSRIs) are now the predominant antidepressant agents. However, even newer agents are increasingly becoming available that combat depression and other disorders such as anxiety and obsessive-compulsive disorder.

The SSRIs include fluoxetine, sertraline, paroxetine, and fluvoxamine. SSRIs are metabolized by cytochrome P450 enzymes. Of note, SSRIs can inhibit these enzymes, causing altered levels of other medications that are metabolized by the liver in the same way. Therefore, caution must be used when a patient is taking an SSRI and other medications such as theophylline or warfarin.

SSRI overdoses usually cause minor symptoms but rarely death. The serotonin syndrome, marked by tremulousness and delirium, is also a risk. However, it occurs much less frequently than with MAOIs. Symptoms of SSRI overdose can include nausea, vomiting, tachycardia, dizziness, and drowsiness. Seizures, coma, and death are possible but rare. Treatment includes supportive measures and observation. Base the decision to use charcoal and gastric lavage on the time since ingestion and the patient's level of consciousness.

Newer agents such as venlafaxine (Effexor) and mirtazapine (Remeron), like the SSRIs, are relatively safe agents. Common symptoms of overdose include drowsiness and sinus tachycardia. Patients who overdose on these agents usually require only observation and supportive care. However, two exceptions should be noted. Citalopram in doses greater than 600 mg has caused seizures and cardiac conduction abnormalities. A patient who has ingested a large quantity may require monitoring in an intensive care setting. Buproprion, likewise, has been associated with seizures in people with bulimia nervosa and in individuals who overdose on high doses.

Buckley PF: Broad therapeutic uses of atypical antipsychotic medications. Biol Psychiatry 2001;50:912. [PMID: 11743945]

Burns MJ: The pharmacology and toxicology of atypical antipsychotic agents. J Toxicol Clin Toxicol 2001;39:1. [PMID: 11327216]

Goldberg JF: New drugs in psychiatry. Emerg Med Clin North Am 2000;18:211. [PMID: 10767879]

Welch R, Chue P: Antipsychotic agents and QT changes. J Psychiatry Neurosci 2000;25:154. [PMID: 10740988]

■ VII. DISPOSITION

General Considerations

Disposition is critical in patients with psychiatric emergencies. Patients should be admitted to the hospital if they meet any of the following criteria, which constitute a psychiatric crisis:

- Unable to care for self
- Actively suicidal

- Actively homicidal
- Unresolved symptoms with an organic cause

Admit such patients to the psychiatric service or, alternatively, to the general medicine service with a psychiatry consult. Assign patients full-time sitters for their safety.

Involuntary Procedures & Admission

One of the unique aspects of managing patients with psychiatric disease is the potential need to initiate involuntary procedures or admission when such patients refuse life-saving intervention. Generally, patient care is conducted under the auspices of the patient's informed consent. However, care can be rendered without consent in four recognized situations: (1) if the patient is a minor, in which case consent must come from parents unless the treatment is immediately required to save the child's life, (2) if the patient lacks the current capacity to comprehend the choice or weigh the factors needed to make the decision, in which case the physician or significant other(s) may need to make the decision, (3) if the patient is unable to offer consent because of a life-threatening medical condition (such as a comatose state) that precludes the patient's ability to offer input into the decision, in which case consent is presumed for life-saving measures until the patient's wishes become known via advance directive or next of kin, or (4) if the patient is having an acute psychiatric crisis in which he or she is not exhibiting a rational pattern of behavior with regard to self-preservation and what reasonable individuals would consider to be consistent with the patient's best interests, in which case the physician is obligated by his or her oath to act to preserve the patient's life until the situation changes to permit the patient's consensual participation in the care.

Patients experiencing an acute psychiatric crisis may therefore need procedures and admission performed for their safety without their consent. Involuntary procedures include physical or chemical restraint. Such patients may also require involuntary admission or 72-hour holds to permit psychiatric assessment. In most venues, this type of involuntary care may be authorized by a practicing physician, police officer, or social service worker who has reason to believe that the patient is a safety risk to him- or herself or another because of psychiatric illness. This individual must document evidence to support the decision, and it is good practice to seek the independent corroboration of two physicians if available. Under such circumstances, the patient may then receive treatment and be held against his or her will for up to 72 hours until the psychiatric evaluation is completed to verify that the patient is no longer at risk of harming him- or herself or others due to psychiatric illness or other treatable cause.

Pediatric Emergencies

48

Roger L. Humphries, MD, Keith D. Bricking, MD, & Thomas M. Huhn, MD[1]

Cardiovascular Emergencies
  Dehydration
  Shock
  Congestive Heart Failure
  Cardiac Dysrhythmias
Respiratory Distress
  Apnea
  Upper Airway Obstruction
  Lower Airway Disorders
    1. Bronchiolitis
    2. Asthma
    3. Pneumonia
Neurologic Emergencies
  Seizures
Infectious Diseases
  Fever
    1. Fever in Infants
    2. Fever in Children
  Meningitis
  Acute Otitis Media

Pharyngitis
Periorbital Cellulitis
Urinary Tract Infection
Gastroenteritis
Septic Arthritis
Acute Osteomyelitis
Exanthems
Gastrointestinal Disorders
  Abdominal Pain
  Vomiting
  Bleeding
  Foreign Body
Hematologic Diseases
  Anemia
  Sickle Cell Disease
  Idiopathic Thrombocytopenic Purpura
Newborn Emergencies
Child Abuse
  Physical Abuse
  Sexual Abuse

General Considerations

A. EPIDEMIOLOGY

Children constitute the most diverse and challenging patient population facing the emergency physician. They represent approximately 10% of prehospital and 30% of emergency department patients. Critical illness and injury in children are less frequent than in the adult population and occur in only about 5% of emergency department pediatric patients.

The epidemiology of pediatric emergency medicine changes with the clinical setting. In the prehospital environment, the common presenting complaints are trauma, seizures, respiratory distress, and toxicologic emergencies. In the emergency department, the most common complaints are either infections, including upper respiratory infections, gastroenteritis, and otitis media, or trauma.

Injury is the leading cause of pediatric morbidity and mortality between the age of 1 year and adulthood. Illness also exacts a terrible toll on the childhood population, especially in the youngest age groups, even though many childhood maladies are preventable or their complications could be reduced through preventive measures or earlier recognition of distress.

B. ASSESSMENT

Assessment of the pediatric patient in the emergency department requires an age-specific approach. A calm, reassuring, and gentle manner on the physician's part will facilitate information collection and encourage patient cooperation in examination and testing.

---

[1]This chapter is a revision of the chapter by Ronald A. Dieckmann, MD, MPH, FAAP, FACEP, & Kevin Coulter, MD, FAAP, from the 4th edition.

Knowledge of the child's growth and development often is required for the diagnosis, management, and disposition of the pediatric emergency department patient. Assessment of growth is most accurate when considered in terms of prior growth in the same individual.

Severity of acute pediatric illness and injury is often difficult to discern. In contrast to the direct anatomic examination that underlies physical evaluation of the adult, observational methods of assessment may be more sensitive to illness and injury acuity in children (Table 48–1). Such observations appear to be more predictive of serious illness than anatomic physical examination using standard palpation, percussion, and auscultation techniques.

Assessment and management of the distressed pediatric patient require appropriately sized equipment. Table 48–2 itemizes emergency department equipment and supplies for children. Table 48–3 provides equipment sizes for invasive procedures in children of different age groups.

Vital signs vary by age (Table 48–4). A rapid formula for estimating systolic blood pressure is 80 + (2 × age [in years]). The maximum effective heart rate in infants is 200 beats/min; in young children, 150 beats/min; and in school-aged children, 120 beats/min. Respiratory rate decreases with advancing age, ranging from 50 breaths/min in the newborn period to 40 breaths/min at 1 year, 30 breaths/min at 2 years, 20 breaths/min at 3 years, and 16 breaths/min through-

out school ages. The use of vital signs to assess vital functions in pediatric patients, however, is hazardous. Appropriate-sized measuring equipment is imperative, techniques must be applied carefully, and interpretation must be age-related. Furthermore, even accurately obtained, age-adjusted vital signs may be insensitive. Instead, other objective measures of cardiopulmonary function—such as the pediatric observational scale (Table 48–1)—and simple physical signs—such as skin color, temperature, and capillary refill—are often better triage and assessment tools.

C. Concept of the Distressed Family

The emergency department physician must appreciate the intimate relationship of the child to the family. Acute pediatric illness and injury are inextricably part of the family environment and dynamics. The child as well as the entire nuclear and extended family may experience major psychological, emotional, and financial consequences of pediatric emergencies. Effective care requires appropriate consideration of the child within the distressed family, enlistment of parental assistance in evaluation and management, and provision of psychological support.

D. Pain and Sedation

Too often, the inexperienced physician neglects pain control or procedural sedation because of misunderstanding about the significance of pain in the young

Table 48–1. Predictive model: acute illness observational scale.[1]

Observation Item	1 Normal	2 Moderate Impairment	3 Severe Impairment
Quality of cry	Strong with normal tone, or content and not crying	Whimpering or sobbing	Weak or moaning or high pitched
Reaction to parent stimulation	Cries briefly then stops, or content and not crying	Cries off and on	Continual cry or hardly responds
State variation	If awake, stays awake, or if asleep and stimulated, wakes up quickly	Eyes close briefly, awake or wakes with prolonged stimulation	Falls to sleep or will not rouse
Color	Pink	Pale extremities or acrocyanosis	Pale or cyanotic or mottled or ashen
Hydration	Skin normal, eyes normal, and mucous membranes moist	Skin normal, eyes normal, and mouth slightly dry	Skin doughy or tented, and dry mucous membranes or sunken eyes
Response (talk, smile) to social overtures	Smiles or alerts (≤ 2 mo)	Brief smile or alerts briefly (≤ 2 mo)	No smile; face anxious, dull, expressionless; or no alerting (≤ 2 mo)

Score: < 10, only 2.7% had a serious illness; 11–15, 26.2% had a serious illness; > 16, 92.3% had a serious illness.

[1]Reproduced, with permission, from McCarthy PL et al: Observational scales for febrile children. Pediatrics 1982;70:806.

Table 48–2. Guidelines for equipment and supplies for use in pediatric patients in the emergency department.[1]

Monitoring equipment
   Cardiorespiratory monitor with strip recorder
   Defibrillator with pediatric and adult paddles (4.5 cm and 8 cm) or corresponding adhesive pads
   Pediatric and adult monitor electrodes
   Pulse oximeter with sensors and probe sizes for children
   Thermometer or rectal probe[2]
   Sphygmomanometer
   Doppler blood pressure device
   Blood pressure cuffs (neonatal, infant, child, and adult arm and thigh cuffs)
   Method to monitor endotracheal tube and placement[3]
   Stethoscope
Airway management
   Portable oxygen regulators and canisters
   Clear oxygen masks (standard and nonrebreathing—neonatal, infant, child, and adult)
   Oropharyngeal airways (sizes 0–5)
   Nasopharyngeal airways (12F through 30F)
   Bag-valve-mask resuscitator, self-inflating (450- and 1000-mL sizes)
   Nasal cannulae (child and adult)
   Endotracheal tubes: uncuffed (2.5, 3.0, 3.5, 4.0, 4.5, 5.0, 5.5, and 6.0 mm) and cuffed (6.5, 7.0, 7.5, 8.0, and 9.0 mm)
   Stylets (infants, pediatric, and adult)
   Laryngoscope handle (pediatric and adult)
   Laryngoscope blades: straight or Miller (0, 1, 2, and 3) and Macintosh (2 and 3)
   Magill forceps (pediatric and adult)
   Nasogastric/feeding tubes (5F through 18F)
   Suction catheters—flexible (6F, 8F, 10F, 12F, 14F, and 16F)
   Yankauer suction tip
   Bulb syringe
   Chest tubes (8F through 40F)[4]
   Laryngeal mask airway (sizes 1, 1.5, 2, 2.5, 3, 4, and 5)[5]
Vascular access
   Butterfly needles (19–25 gauge)
   Catheter-over-needle devices (14–24 gauge)
   Rate limiting infusion device and tubing[4,6]
   Intraosseous needles (may be satisfied by standard bone needle aspiration needles)
   Arm boards[5]
   Intravenous fluid and blood warmers[4]
   Umbilical vein catheters (size 5F feeding tube may be used)[4,7]
   Seldinger technique vascular access kit[4]
Miscellaneous
   Infant and standard scales
   Infant formula and oral rehydrating solutions[4]
   Heating source (may be met by infrared lamps or overhead warmer)[4]
   Towel rolls, blanket rolls, or equivalent
   Pediatric restraining devices
   Resuscitation board
   Sterile linen[8]
   Length-based resuscitation tape or precalculated drug or equipment list based on weight
Specialized pediatric trays
   Tube thoracotomy with water seal drainage capability[4]
   Lumbar puncture
   Pediatric urinary catheters
   Obstetric pack

(continued)

Table 48–2. Guidelines for equipment and supplies for use in pediatric patients in the emergency department.[1] (Continued)

Specialized pediatric trays (con't)
  Newborn kit[4]
  Umbilical vessel cannulation supplies[4]
  Venous cutdown[4]
  Needle cricothyrotomy tray
  Surgical airway kit (may include a tracheostomy tray or a surgical cricothyrotomy tray)[4]
Fracture management
  Cervical immobilization equipment[4,9]
  Extremity splints[4]
  Femur splints[4]
Medical photography capability

[1]Adapted from Committee on Pediatric Equipment and Supplies for Emergency Departments, National Emergency Medical Services for Children Resource Alliance. Reproduced, with permission, from ACEP policy statement. Care of children in the emergency department: guidelines for preparedness. American College of Emergency Physicians, 2001.
[2]Suitable for hypothermic and hyperthermic measurements with temperature capability from 25°C to 44°C.
[3]May be satisfied by a disposable CO_2 detector of appropriate size for infants and children. For children 5 years or older who are $\geq$ 20 kg in body weight, an esophageal detection bulb or syringe may be used additionally.
[4]Equipment that is essential but may be shared with the nursery, pediatric ward, or other inpatient service and is readily available to the emergency department.
[5]Equipment or supplies that are desirable but not essential.
[6]To regulate rate and volume.
[7]Ensure availability of pediatric sizes within the hospital.
[8]Available within hospital for burn care.
[9]Many types of cervical immobilization devices are available, including wedges and collars. The type of device chosen depends on local preferences and policies and procedures. Chosen device should be stocked in sizes to fit infants, children, adolescents, and adults. Use of sandbags to meet this requirement is discouraged, because they may cause injury if the patient has to be turned.

Table 48–3. Equipment and sizes available for invasive procedures.

Age	Inner Diameter Endotracheal Tube (mm)	Laryngoscope Blade	Chest Tube (F)	Nasogastric/Foley (F)
Newborn	2.5–3	0–1	8–12	5
1 month	3.5	1	12	8
6 months	3.5	1	16	8
1 year	4	1	20	8
2–3 years	4.5	1	24	8
4–5 years	5–6	2	28	10
6–8 years	6–6.5	2	32	10
10–12 years	7	2–3	32	12
14 years	7.5	3	40	12

Table 48–4. Age-related vital signs.

Age	Mean Weight (kg)	Minimum Systolic Blood Pressure	Normal Heart Rate	Normal Respiratory Rate
Premature	2.5	40	120–170	40–60
Term	3.5	50	100–170	40–60
3 months	6	50	100–170	30–50
6 months	8	60	100–170	30–50
1 year	10	65	100–170	30–40
2 years	13	65	100–160	20–30
4 years	15	70	80–130	20
6 years	20	75	70–115	16
8 years	25	80	70–110	16
10 years	30	85	60–105	16
12 years	40	90	60–100	16

child, unwarranted fear of addicting children to narcotic agents, or ignorance of appropriate agents. When a painful procedure is necessary, an effective approach integrates careful explanation directly to the child and enlistment of parental understanding and assistance. Whenever conscious or deep sedation procedures are performed, the emergency department physician must ensure the patient's safety by strict adherence to guidelines of monitoring. This includes preparation for any potential airway complications, such as aspiration or apnea. In general, only previously healthy or mildly chronically ill children should be considered as candidates for sedation procedures in the emergency department. Sometimes a restraint apparatus will facilitate the procedure.

The following are guidelines for a variety of clinical situations:

1. Topical anesthetics for wound repair—The formulation TAC (0.5% tetracaine, 1:2000 epinephrine or adrenaline, and 11.8% cocaine) has been associated with seizures after systemic absorption of the cocaine component. Another topical anesthetic, LET (2% lidocaine, 1:1000 epinephrine, and 2% tetracaine), has a more favorable safety profile. However, because the onset of action of LET is about 30 minutes, it should be applied early in the evaluation of wounds to avoid unnecessary treatment delays. Any anesthetic containing epinephrine (such as LET or TAC) should be avoided on end-arterial structures, such as the ears, nose, digits, or penis.

2. Sedation and analgesia for painful procedures—Use a combination of fentanyl, 1.0–1.5 µg/kg intravenously every 3 minutes, and midazolam, 0.05–0.075 mg/kg intravenously every 3–5 minutes. The reversal agents naloxone, 0.01–0.1 mg/kg intravenously, and flumazenil, 0.01 mg/kg to a maximum of 0.2 mg, should also be available at the bedside and can be administered for respiratory depression. Use pulse oximetry to monitor the child's respiratory status after administration.

3. Sedation for imaging studies—For individuals requiring imaging studies such as computed tomography (CT) scan or magnetic resonance imaging (MRI), use pentobarbital, 5 mg/kg intramuscularly, midazolam, 0.5 mg/kg orally (maximum dose, 20 mg), or methohexital, 1 mg/kg intravenously.

4. Other drugs used for painful procedures—

   a. Inhaled nitrous oxide—Administration of inhaled nitrous oxide requires a reliable scavenging system to avoid exposure to staff as well as a careful regulatory method for oxygen delivery in the oxygen-nitrous oxide mix.

   b. Ketamine—Ketamine, 3–4 mg/kg intramuscularly, or 1 mg/kg intravenously, may be used for procedural situations involving children under 10 years, especially burn debridement, foreign body removal, deep wound care, abscess incision and drainage, sexual abuse evaluation, and interventions such as lumbar puncture or orthopedic reductions. Use atropine, 0.01 mg/kg (maximum, 0.5 mg), or glycopyrrolate, 0.005 mg/kg (maximum 0.25 mg), as part of the same intramuscular injection to avoid hypersalivation. Intravenous administration is better for longer procedures. Ketamine may elevate intracranial and intraocular pressure, induce emesis, and occasionally precipitate laryngospasm; because ketamine use in older children may also cause an adverse behavioral reaction upon emergence from sedation, the concomitant use of midazolam, 0.025–0.05 mg/kg intravenously, is recommended in children over age 5 years. Nonetheless, it is an effective drug when used by trained personnel and with appropriate cardiopulmonary monitoring including vital signs and continuous pulse oximetry.

5. Outpatient analgesia—Outpatient analgesia should ordinarily include a nonsteroidal, anti-inflammatory drug such as ibuprofen, 4–10 mg/kg every 6–8 hours. This drug can also be used in combination with oral narcotic agents for treatment of severe pain. Acetaminophen, 10–15 mg/kg/dose every 4–6 hours, can also be used for treatment of mild pain on an outpatient basis.

E. Drug and Fluid Administration

All parenterally and orally administered agents must be given strictly on a per-kilogram basis, until maximum adult doses and volumes are reached. Overdosing and overhydration are dangerous errors in emergency pediatrics. Underdosing is also frequent, especially in infants and small children. Initial treatment of dehydration should include isotonic fluids (normal saline or lactated Ringer's). Deaths due to acute hyponatremic cerebral edema have been reported with administration of as little as 40 mg/kg intravenous 5% dextrose in water. Physicians and nurses must meticulously review drug and fluid orders to ensure that they are age- and weight-corrected.

Vascular access is often the rate-limiting step in provision of life-saving therapy to critically ill and injured children. The emergency department physician must be familiar with a variety of techniques for access into the cardiopulmonary system.

1. Endotracheal tube—In critically ill, intubated patients, the endotracheal route is an effective conduit for administration of a variety of life-saving drugs, including epinephrine, atropine, lidocaine, naloxone, and diazepam. Epinephrine is by far the most commonly used. When administered through the endotracheal tube, higher doses of epinephrine, up to 10 times the intravenous dose, must be used to achieve adequate serum concentrations. The pharmacokinetics of endotracheal epinephrine administration may be optimized by delivering the drug directly into the highly vascular trachea and proximal tracheobronchial tree instead of

directly into the endotracheal tube. The preferred technique requires insertion of a nasogastric tube or a size 5F umbilical catheter past the distal tip of the endotracheal tube with direct instillation of drugs through the tube. Because endotracheal drugs may be more effective if aerosolized, dilute the drug with normal saline to a maximum volume of 0.5–1 mL//kg, and then inject rapidly to achieve a partially aerosolized form.

2. Intravenous access—In infants, the scalp is an ideal site for cannulation; use a size 25 butterfly needle. In children past the neonatal period, the dorsal veins of the hand, antecubital fossa, or dorsum of the foot are usually accessible with a 24- or 22-gauge intravenous catheter. The external jugular vein is a large vein, usually easily visualized and readily cannulated with a 20-gauge catheter if the child is properly restrained and the head is held in a dependent position.

3. Intraosseous infusion—(See also Chapter 6.) For patients under age 5 years in extremis and requiring life-saving drug and fluid administration, intraosseous infusion is an alternative method of administration. A short, thick needle with trocar tip is inserted into the intramedullary space of the bone. The richly vascularized intramedullary space allows for direct entry of drugs and fluids into the central circulation through emissary veins. The easiest insertion sites are the medial proximal tibia or the distal midline femur. Intraosseous infusion is a rapid and effective technique of achieving therapeutic serum concentrations of almost all important drugs; moreover, a large fluid volume can be rapidly administered in injured or dehydrated patients. When necessary, insert multiple intraosseous lines. The most common complication of this procedure is osteomyelitis.

F. Medicolegal Considerations

Most exposure to legal liability derives from the patient's status as a minor. Although state laws protecting children vary significantly, some common legal principles apply.

Consent issues are frequent and often vexing problems in the emergency department. Consent may be difficult to obtain either because the legal guardian is absent or because the child's actual caregiver may be neither the legal guardian nor a legally authorized surrogate. If the child's legal guardian is unavailable, the health care provider must make and clearly document every effort to communicate directly with the child's legal representative.

If the child's condition allows, informed consent must be obtained from the legal representative. If the child's condition is life threatening, and permanent harm or physical disability will result from delay of appropriate medical interventions, treatment, including appropriate analgesia, must be implemented under the concept of implied consent. If the characteristics of this legal action are not clearly spelled out by emergency department policy, consultation with the hospital's legal authority is prudent. Whenever treatment is instituted without formal consent, the reasons for such action must be documented on the patient's medical record.

Another dilemma occurs when a child presents to the emergency department with acute serious injury or illness, and the legal representative refuses appropriate medical assistance. If the patient's condition is such that permanent impairment or death may result from failure to treat, emergency legal recourse through the local juvenile court system may be required, especially if the legal representative is incompetent owing to substance abuse or other debilitating mental conditions. The hospital administrator, legal counsel, and social services should also be notified.

In some circumstances, parental consent is not needed for emergency care. For example, "emancipated minors" are, by law, able to act as adults and consent to medical care, even though they have not obtained legal age of maturity. Emancipated minors include individuals who are married, pregnant, in active duty in the armed services, or declared emancipated by the Superior Court. Moreover, many states recognize "mature minors," a status whereby a minor also has the power to consent to medical care in situations involving substance abuse, mental disease, sexually transmitted disease, or pregnancy.

G. Death in the Emergency Department

The sudden and unexpected death of an infant or child in the emergency department constitutes one of the most difficult situations in emergency practice. Careful and compassionate dialogue between the physician and parents, and between the physician and emergency department staff, is essential to minimize chaos in the clinical setting and to reduce confusion and anger among bereaved families and department personnel. Debriefing for health care workers may also be appropriate within 48–72 hours to alleviate stress that may impair work performance or cause psychological disability.

■ CARDIOVASCULAR EMERGENCIES

Evaluation of cardiopulmonary function in children, especially in infants and younger children, requires special techniques. Vital signs are generally insensitive and

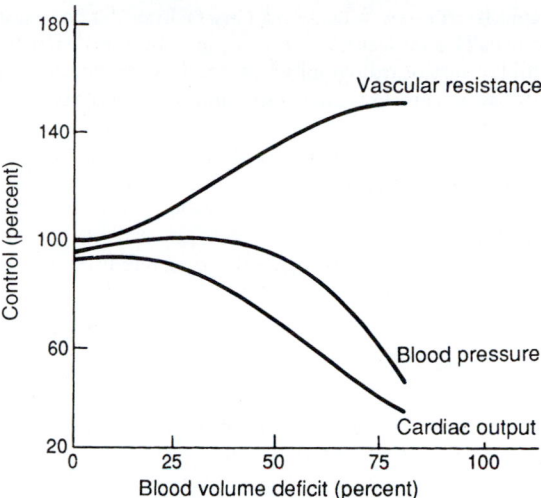

Figure 48–1. Relationship of blood volume to blood pressure in children during acute blood loss. (Reproduced, with permission, from Schwaitzberg SD, Bergman KS, Harris BH: A pediatric trauma model of continuous hemorrhage. J Pediatr Surg 1988;23:605.)

nonspecific. Blood pressure poorly reflects volume status. When perfusion is mistakenly equated with blood pressure, early signs of hypovolemia can be missed. Figure 48–1 demonstrates the relationship of a child's blood volume to blood pressure during acute blood loss. In children, hypovolemia triggers compensatory tachycardia and intense peripheral vasoconstriction, which effectively maintains blood pressure until volume loss exceeds about 50% of intravascular volume.

Tachycardia, while sensitive to cardiopulmonary duress, is nonspecific. Normal heart rate also varies with age, and tachycardia is a common response to many types of stress (eg, fever, anxiety, hypoxia, hypovolemia). In children, assessment of volume status should focus primarily on skin signs (temperature, color, capillary refill, turgor) in combination with heart rate. Feeling the skin at the knee is an excellent first maneuver to assess warmth and skin perfusion. Rate of urine output may be the next best measure of core perfusion. Adequate core blood flow results in 1–2 mL/kg/h of urine production. Therefore, in the unstable child with suspected perfusion abnormalities, a urinary bladder catheter is imperative to monitor output.

Cardiac rhythm disturbances in children are unusual. The most common disturbance is bradycardia, usually secondary to hypoxia. Properly applied pulse oximetry, at the triage desk or as part of initial clinical assessment, is an easy and useful method for rapid evaluation of oxygen saturation in patients with slow or rapid heart rates. When a primary tachycardia occurs, it is usually supraventricular in origin. In the distressed child, electrocardiographic monitoring will assist in evaluating cardiovascular status and in judging response to therapy.

DEHYDRATION

 ESSENTIALS OF DIAGNOSIS

- *Commonly occurs after severe or prolonged episodes of diarrhea and vomiting.*
- *Significant signs include acute weight loss, listlessness, sunken eyes, dry mucous membranes, poor capillary refill, and tachycardia.*

General Considerations

Acute dehydration is a common pediatric emergency. Diarrhea and vomiting are the most frequent causes. Other common causes are blood loss, burn wounds, open wounds, fever or hyperthermia, sweating, inadequate fluid intake, polyuria, and poisoning.

Clinical Findings

Clinical evaluation of the dehydrated child requires assessment of hydration status. Comparison of presenting weight with recent weights may be useful. Management is dictated by degree of acuity (mild, 3–5% weight loss; moderate, 10%; severe, 15%). Formulate initial treatment on the basis of clinical evaluation of degree of dehydration. Dry or pasty mucous membranes, sunken eyes, doughy and cool peripheral skin with poor capillary refill, and listlessness signal severe dehydration. Laboratory assessment of type of dehydration assists the physician in later strategies for specific electrolyte replacement. Serum sodium concentration is the most important laboratory parameter. Serum sodium concentration does not indicate degree of hydration but does provide a useful measure for titrating sodium repletion (see below).

Treatment

After rapid assessment of degree of dehydration, management must match severity of illness.

A. OXYGEN AND INTRAVENOUS ACCESS

For severely dehydrated patients, provide supplemental oxygen, attach pulse oximeter and cardiac monitor, and establish intravenous or intraosseous access with one or two secure catheters.

B. VOLUME RESUSCITATION

For a severely dehydrated infant or young child, rapidly infuse a balanced isotonic solution (eg, normal saline or lactated Ringer's injection). Infants and children have limited glycogen stores and are prone to hypoglycemia when stressed; rapid blood glucose analysis (eg, fingerstick blood sugar) should be performed, and glucose should be replaced if less than 60 mg/dL. Administer 5 mL/kg 10% dextrose in water for infants and young children and 2 mL/kg 25% dextrose in water for older children.

Administer a fluid bolus of 20 mL/kg, and then repeat boluses of 20 mL/kg until physical signs (heart rate, skin temperature, and capillary refill) indicate improved perfusion. After 60 mL/kg of isotonic fluid have been administered, if vital signs have not normalized, consider administration of packed red blood cells, 10–20 mL/kg, fresh-frozen plasma, or occasionally 5% albuminated saline.

C. OTHER MEASURES

After stabilizing the patient, slow the intravenous infusion to a maintenance rate (Table 48–5) and devise a therapeutic plan. Insert a urinary bladder catheter if the child has uncertain volume replacement requirements. Send blood for complete blood count (CBC); electrolytes; and glucose, blood urea nitrogen (BUN), and creatinine measurements. Arterial blood gas determination is indicated for the child who remains unstable after 60 mL/kg of volume administration.

When laboratory data are available, titrate sodium and water repletion accordingly. For hyponatremic and isotonic dehydration, replace the calculated volume deficit over 24 hours, giving 50% of the deficit in the first 8 hours and the remaining 50% over the following 16 hours. Ongoing losses and maintenance requirements must also be included. Control fever, because insensitive water losses are significantly increased by tem-

Table 48–5. Daily maintenance requirements for fluids and electrolytes.

Weight	Water Requirement[1]	Sodium Requirement	Potassium Requirement[2]
1–10 kg	100 mL/kg		
11–20 kg	50 mL/kg + 1000 mL	3 mEq/kg	2 mEq/kg
> 20 kg	20 mL/kg + 1500 mL		

[1]Assume child is normothermic. Fever significantly increases insensible water losses.
[2]Do not exceed 0.25 mEq/kg/h intravenously. Use oral route when possible. Add KCl to intravenous infusion after urination.

perature elevation. Add small amounts of potassium to the ongoing infusion, once urination is observed, and replace calculated potassium deficits over 48 hours. The minimum daily maintenance requirements for water, sodium, and potassium are noted in Table 48–5. For hypernatremic dehydration, divide fluid and electrolyte replacement evenly over 48 hours to avoid rapid osmolal shifts and central nervous system complications.

D. ORAL REHYDRATION THERAPY

Use oral rehydration therapy (ORT) in most dehydrated patients. Children can usually take fluids by mouth. Vomiting does not contraindicate use of ORT. Unless shock, altered mental status, or severe weakness is present, ORT may be used as part of early emergency department and inpatient management for most dehydrated patients. Other patients not requiring hospitalization can be easily rehydrated using this technique. The composition of ORT as set by the World Health Organization includes 90 mEq/L of sodium, 20 mEq/L of potassium, 30 mEq/L of citrate, and a 1–2% glucose concentration. Commercial preparations that provide approximately these electrolyte constituents include Pedialyte, Lytren, and Infalyte. Other commonly used clear liquids, such as colas, have too few electrolytes (Na^+, K^+, and Cl^-), and their high sugar content may contribute to worsening of osmotic diarrhea. If the child can be discharged, prescribe home fluid replacement that is appropriate for the age of the child, the calculated deficit, and ongoing losses.

SHOCK

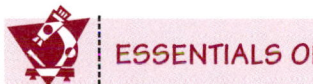

ESSENTIALS OF DIAGNOSIS

- Altered mental status.
- Tachypnea, tachycardia.
- Hypotension is a late sign in children.

Clinical Findings

Shock is inadequate oxygen delivery to tissues. Most causes of shock in children (eg, gastrointestinal fluid losses, burns, blood loss from acute injury) involve decreased stroke volume usually from hypovolemia (hypovolemic shock). Septic shock, a form of distributive shock, occurs usually in the patient under age 2 years and must always be considered in the sick-appearing, febrile child. Anaphylactic shock, another form of distributive shock, may develop after bee stings or after in-hospital use of parenteral drugs or contrast agents. Cardiogenic shock is extremely rare in children but may complicate congenital heart disease or toxicologic emergencies.

Shock is not hypotension. Successful management includes early recognition of the compensated, normotensive phase of shock. During the compensated phase of hypovolemic shock, vital signs in the supine patient are usually normal, except for mild tachycardia. Skin signs of hypoperfusion are usually evident, and laboratory testing may disclose metabolic acidosis. Intervention is usually successful during this phase. When the hypotensive, decompensated phase develops in the absence of recognition and effective treatment, irreversible shock and death may result.

Treatment

Rapid clinical assessment should disclose a shock category, so that focused treatment can be immediately instituted (Chapter 9). Failure to act expeditiously and aggressively is a common error and may significantly increase mortality risk. Figure 48–2 is an algorithm for treatment of uncompensated shock in children.

A. GENERAL MANAGEMENT

Consider immediate endotracheal intubation. In the ill-appearing child with signs of shock and sepsis or the frankly hypotensive child, intubation should be accomplished either immediately or after the patient fails to respond to first-line resuscitation with oxygen and fluids. After intubation, insert a nasogastric tube.

Apply supplemental oxygen, attach pulse oximeter and cardiac monitor, establish 2 secure intravenous catheters, check fingerstick blood sugar, and insert urinary bladder catheter.

B. VOLUME RESUSCITATION

Initiate volume resuscitation if indicated, or begin administration of an inotropic agent. When inotropic agents are used, the intravascular volume must be adequate. Inotropic infusions can then be titrated at the bedside, often using multiple infusions (dopamine, epinephrine, dobutamine), until perfusion is restored. Start with epinephrine at 0.1–1.0 µg/kg/min, and then add a second inotropic agent if cardiovascular response does not occur. If physical examination is equivocal for hydration status, a chest x-ray may help: dehydration or overhydration is reflected in the appearance of pulmonary vessels.

C. OTHER MEASURES

Obtain arterial blood gases, CBC, electrolytes, platelets, coagulation studies, blood cultures (if infection is suspected), and urinalysis, and consider a urine drug

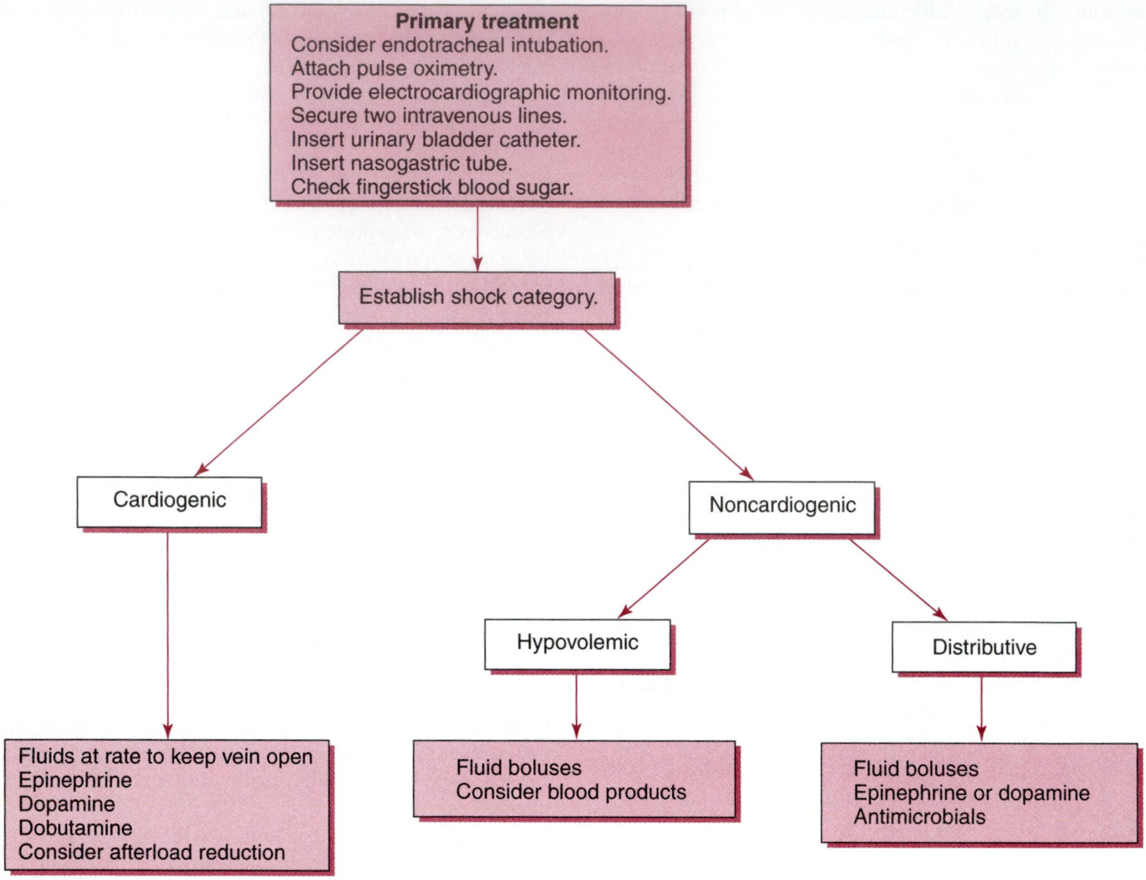

Primary treatment
Consider endotracheal intubation.
Attach pulse oximetry.
Provide electrocardiographic monitoring.
Secure two intravenous lines.
Insert urinary bladder catheter.
Insert nasogastric tube.
Check fingerstick blood sugar.

Establish shock category.

Cardiogenic

Noncardiogenic

Hypovolemic

Distributive

Fluids at rate to keep vein open
Epinephrine
Dopamine
Dobutamine
Consider afterload reduction

Fluid boluses
Consider blood products

Fluid boluses
Epinephrine or dopamine
Antimicrobials

Figure 48–2. Treatment algorithm for pediatric uncompensated shock.

screen to help guide secondary treatment after stabilization. A chest x-ray is also necessary in most cases.

Bardella IJ: Pediatric advanced life support: a review of the AHA recommendations. Am Fam Physician 1999;60:1743. [PMID: 10537389] (Review.)

CONGESTIVE HEART FAILURE

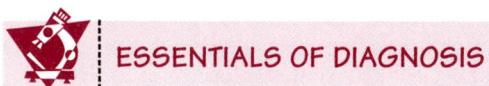

ESSENTIALS OF DIAGNOSIS

- *Sweating during feeding or crying; failure to thrive.*
- *Tachypnea, tachycardia.*
- *Hepatomegaly.*

Clinical Findings

Congestive heart failure (CHF) is unusual in childhood. It usually presents in the first year of life in patients with congenital heart disease. Table 48–6 lists the structural conditions causing CHF at different times during infancy. Myocarditis and other cardiomyopathies, toxicologic conditions, and coronary artery disease are also included in the differential diagnosis of new heart failure in childhood.

Treatment

When congestive heart failure has progressed to frank pulmonary edema, treat as follows:

A. GENERAL MANAGEMENT

Assess need for immediate endotracheal intubation in the severely distressed, hypotensive, or hypoxic patient (pulse oximetry < 85% on 100% oxygen).

Table 48–6. Structural causes of congestive heart failure during infancy.

Newborn period
Hypoplastic left heart
Arteriovenous fistula
Large placental-fetal transfusion
Regurgitation of the pulmonic or tricuspid valves
Third-degree atrioventricular block
Paroxysmal atrial tachycardia
First month
Aortic coarctation with patent ductus arteriosus
Ventricular septal defect
Total anomalous pulmonary venous return
Tricuspid atresia
Truncus arteriosus
First 6 months
Transposition of the great vessels
Ventricular septal defect
Patent ductus arteriosus
Truncus arteriosus with large left-to-right shunt
6–12 months
Ventricular septal defect
Endocardial fibroelastosis
Total anomalous pulmonary venous return

[1]Reproduced, with permission, from Hoffman JIE: Congestive heart failure, Page 54 in: *Pediatric Emergency Medicine: A Clinician's Reference.* Grossman M, Dieckmann RA (editors). Lippincott, 1991.

Apply 100% oxygen, sometimes with positive-pressure ventilation through an endotracheal tube, and attach pulse oximeter and cardiac monitor. Insert urinary bladder catheter and check fingerstick blood sugar.

Establish a secure intravenous line with 5% dextrose in water at a rate to keep the vein open.

B. Pharmacologic Treatment

Administer morphine sulfate, 0.1 mg/kg intravenously. Administer furosemide, 1–2 mg/kg intravenously.

C. Other Measures

Obtain arterial blood gas, CBC, electrolyte, BUN, creatinine, and digoxin levels if appropriate. Obtain an ECG. Order a chest x-ray in the room or with a nurse or physician in attendance in the radiology suite.

Administer digoxin. Digitalization doses are 10 μg/kg intravenous load, a second dose at 6 hours, and a third dose at 24 hours. Occasionally, patients with severe pulmonary edema unresponsive to initial therapy require dopamine, dobutamine, or both.

McCollough M, Shafieff G: Common complaints in the first thirty days of life. Emerg Med Clin North Am 2002;20:27. [PMID: 11826636] (Review.)

O'Laughlin MP: Congestive heart failure in children. Pediatr Clin North Am 1999;46:263. [PMID: 10218074] (Review.)

CARDIAC DYSRHYTHMIAS

Clinical Findings

Although uncommon, dysrhythmias sometimes occur in children with known congenital heart disease, acquired heart disease (eg, myocarditis), or secondary to other metabolic or toxicologic disorders. Therapy is aimed at the underlying condition. Evaluation of dysrhythmias includes clinical assessment of cardiopulmonary status and interpretation of the electrocardiogram (ECG). Key electrocardiographic features are heart rate and width of the QRS complex. These constituents must be evaluated against age-specific norms.

Treatment

See Table 48–7.

A. General Management

Apply supplemental oxygen; attach pulse oximeter and cardiac monitor. Establish a secure intravenous line with 5% dextrose in water at a rate to keep the vein open. Obtain an ECG if the patient is hemodynamically stable.

B. Cardioversion

Unstable patients with tachydysrhythmias require immediate electrical direct current countershock. Initial mode (synchronized or asynchronized) and exact energy levels are dictated by the nature of the dysrhythmia. (See Table 48–7.)

If electrical conversion does not occur with initial shock, double electrical doses until conversion occurs or until the maximum electrical dose is 8 J/kg. If synchronized countershock fails at 4 J/kg, switch to asynchronized mode (defibrillation). Ensure that paddles are held firmly against chest wall and that a good conductive agent is employed. Standard 4.5-cm pediatric paddles are used for infants up to age 1 year. If standard 4.5-cm pediatric paddles are unavailable for sternoapical placement, use adult paddles in an anteroposterior configuration.

Pretreat conscious patients requiring cardioversion with light anesthesia (diazepam, 0.1 mg/kg), and be prepared to perform endotracheal intubation and full cardiopulmonary resuscitation.

Fulton S, Jackimczyk KC: Antidysrhythmics. Emerg Med Clin North Am 2000;18:655. [PMID: 11130932] (Review.)

Table 48–7. Treatment of common pediatric dysrhythmias.

Rhythm	Rate/min	QRS	Initial Treatment	Drug Therapy
Narrow complex tachycardias Sinus tachycardia	100–250	< 0.10	Oxygen, fluids, warmth, calm manner.	Treatment of primary condition.
Atrial flutter	300–500	< 0.10	If unstable, synchronized electrical DC cardioversion, 0.25 J/kg. If stable, vagal maneuvers (rectal stimulation, ice water to face, Valsalva).	Digoxin, 10 µg/kg intravenously. Procainamide, 15 mg/kg intravenously, over 30 min.
Atrial fibrillation	60–190	< 0.10	As for atrial flutter.	As for atrial flutter.
Supraventricular	120–300	0.10	As for atrial flutter.	Adenosine, 0.1 mg/kg rapid intravenous push. Repeat at 0.2 mg/kg (Maximum single dose of 12 mg).
Wide complex tachycardias Ventricular tachycardia	150–260	> 0.10	If unstable with a pulse, synchronized electrical DC cardioversion, 0.5 J/kg, then double. If pulseless, treat like ventricular fibrillation. If stable, lidocaine, 1 mg/kg, then 20–50 µg/kg/min.	Lidocaine, 1.0–1.5 mg/kg, then 20–50 µg/kg/min.
Wolff-Parkinson-White syndrome	150–300	> 0.10	As for ventricular tachycardia.	As for ventricular tachycardia.
Ventricular fibrillation	300–500	Variable	DC cardioversion, 2 J/kg, then double.	Epinephrine, 0.01 mg/kg. Lidocaine, 1 mg/kg, then 20–50 µg/kg/min.
Bradycardia Sinus	Age-related	< 0.10	Oxygen, stimulation.	Epinephrine, 0.01 mg/kg. Atropine, 0.01–0.02 mg/kg (minimum, 0.1 mg).
Atrioventricular block	Age-related	Variable	Oxygen. If unstable, transcutaneous or transvenous pacing.	As for sinus bradycardia.

■ RESPIRATORY DISTRESS

In children, normal ventilation and oxygenation occurs with minimal visible effort. Evaluation of respiratory function includes assessment of rate, work of breathing, skin and mucous membrane color, and mental status. Respiratory rate alone is an insensitive indicator of respiratory distress, because rates vary significantly with age, excitement, anxiety, or fever. Tachypnea may be an early manifestation of respiratory distress, or it may re-sult from respiratory compensation for metabolic acidosis caused by shock, diabetic ketoacidosis, inborn errors of metabolism, salicylism, or chronic renal insufficiency. A slow respiratory rate may indicate impending respiratory failure.

Observation alone will usually disclose distress or increased work of breathing. A child with noisy breathing is especially worrisome, especially if inspiratory stridor is present. This denotes upper airway obstruction. Immediate therapy is indicated to relieve obstruction and improve oxygenation and ventilation. Increased work of breathing is also evidenced by nasal flaring and by suprasternal, intercostal, and subcostal retractions. Retractions become more pronounced cephalad to caudad with increasing hypoxia. Grunting is produced by premature glottic closure and usually represents alveolar collapse and loss of lung volume, which develop in patients with pulmonary edema, pneumonia, or atelectasis. Auscultation will provide further differentiation of disease possibilities. Wheezing, rales, or decreased breath sounds may be present. However, auscultation is often inaccurate in the busy, noisy emergency department setting. Cyanosis, when present, represents severe distress and is best seen on mucous membranes of the mouth and nail beds. Peripheral cyanosis is more likely due to circulatory failure than to pulmonary failure. Finally, mental status changes may be a clue to gas exchange abnormalities. Hypoxic patients are restless and agitated; hypercapnic patients are drowsy or even comatose.

Rapid evaluation of respiratory function is imperative in all distressed emergency department pediatric patients. Respiratory failure and respiratory arrest due to a wide spectrum of causes (eg, head trauma, coma, poisoning, pneumonia, asthma, foreign body aspiration) are the most common causes of cardiac arrest in childhood. Timely, aggressive intervention in early stages as well as meticulous respiratory monitoring by means of pulse oximetry and continuous observation will avert preventable adverse patient outcomes. Children with respiratory distress should not be sent for imaging studies without qualified personnel in attendance. Early hospital admission is usually warranted for such patients.

Pulse oximetry must be used liberally in the emergency department setting in order to disclose undetected oxygen desaturation states. Pulse oximetry is noninvasive, simple, and reasonably accurate. Use this assessment modality in all cases of suspected respiratory distress, cardiopulmonary disease, or serious trauma. In selected patients, especially those with significant tachypnea or work of breathing, pulse oximetry may underestimate degree of distress, and it provides no indication of adequacy of ventilation (ie, PCO_2). In such patients, obtain arterial blood gas levels to help measure the severity and nature of the ventilation or oxygenation disturbance.

APNEA

General Considerations

Apnea means cessation of ventilation for 20 seconds or for 10–20 seconds in patients who also manifest bradycardia, cyanosis, or pallor. Ordinary sleep will sometimes cause breathing irregularities easily confused with apnea. There are 2 classifications of apnea: central and obstructive. Central apnea is characterized by an absence of respiratory effort secondary to diminished muscular activation. It occurs in newborn infants, often in preterm infants. Infection, metabolic abnormalities, anemia, hypoxia, or central nervous system injury may be associated with newborn apnea. Obstructive apnea occurs in later infancy and childhood and is related to obstructive upper airway conditions. This results in cessation of airflow despite respiratory effort, as can be seen with chest and abdominal movement.

Treatment

A. APNEA IN INFANTS

Apnea in infants may be symptomatic of life-threatening illness. Such patients ordinarily require hospital admission for observation and full workup for infections and for central nervous system, metabolic, and feeding problems. Initial management in the emergency department is discussed here.

1. Oxygenation and ventilation—Place child on supplemental oxygen, and apply pulse oximeter and cardiac monitor or apnea monitor.

2. Volume resuscitation—If evidence of dehydration is present, establish intravenous access with lactated Ringer's solution or isotonic normal saline. Otherwise, if the patient is euvolemic, begin 5% dextrose in quarter-normal saline at maintenance rate for weight (see Table 48–5).

3. Laboratory and imaging studies—Obtain blood for CBC with differential, electrolytes, BUN, creatinine, ionized calcium and magnesium, and cultures. Obtain clean urine for urinalysis, culture, and toxicology studies. Consider spinal fluid analysis in most infants and any young child with meningeal signs, toxicity, or altered mental status. CT scan can usually precede spinal fluid analysis in the child who does not appear acutely infected.

Obtain a chest x-ray and respiratory syncytial virus (RSV) and pertussis studies. Consider an ECG. Consider an EEG if the patient has an altered mental status or if a seizure focus is suspected.

4. Other measures—Admit for observation and further evaluation on an apnea monitor.

B. APNEA IN CHILDREN

Obstructive apnea in slightly older patients may be serious. Focus evaluation on obstructive upper pharyngeal lesions such as tonsillitis and pharyngitis or laryngomalacia. Chest x-ray and lateral neck films, along with transnasal laryngoscopy, are often necessary. Emergency department evaluation may be insufficient to exclude a serious diagnosis, and hospital admission may be indicated.

UPPER AIRWAY OBSTRUCTION

ESSENTIALS OF DIAGNOSIS

- Inspiratory stridor.
- Suspect foreign body aspiration if symptoms develop rapidly without associated signs of infection.
- Anteroposterior and lateral neck x-rays are helpful to differentiate croup from epiglottitis.

Clinical Findings

Upper airway obstruction is usually readily apparent. Inspiratory stridor is the hallmark. The child is dyspneic and shows signs of respiratory distress, including tachypnea; flaring; and supraclavicular, intercostal, and subcostal retractions. Ventilation and sometimes oxygenation abnormalities are present. If obstruction is severe, hypercapnia will be present, usually along with depressed mental status, cyanosis, and decreased air movement. Arterial blood gases will demonstrate carbon dioxide retention and often hypoxemia. Pulse oximetry will be abnormal in most advanced cases but normal in typical cases.

Differential Diagnosis

In children, the common causes of stridor and upper airway obstruction are croup, epiglottitis, and foreign body aspiration. The epidemiologic and clinical characteristics of these entities are compared in Table 48–8. Other less common conditions producing stridor are bacterial tracheitis (usually *Staphylococcus aureus* or *Haemophilus influenzae*), retropharyngeal or peritonsillar abscess, trauma, caustic ingestions, neoplasm, or angioneurotic edema.

Treatment

(See Figure 48–3.) Clear the airway using procedures recommended in Table 48–9 for the patient with complete airway obstruction. Avoid airway clearance maneuvers in the patient with incomplete or partial airway obstruction, because this may worsen obstruction. Allow the child to adopt a position of comfort, usually on the parent's lap. Apply supplemental oxygen, and attach pulse oximeter and cardiac monitor.

A. Epiglottis

If a child presents with clinical findings suggestive of epiglottitis, immediately arrange to establish a definitive airway, preferably by orotracheal intubation in the operating room. In the rare case in which abrupt airway obstruction occurs, first attempt bag-valve-mask ventilation and prepare for orotracheal intubation. If bag-valve-mask and orotracheal intubation fails, perform needle cricothyrotomy or surgical tracheostomy. Minimize all invasive interventions in order to avert patient agitation and potential precipitous airway obstruction.

Once the airway is secured, obtain blood and throat cultures and begin antibiotic therapy. Intravenous cefuroxime, 50 mg/kg every 8 h; intravenous cefotaxime, 50 mg/kg every 8 h; or intravenous ceftriaxone, 50 mg/kg every 24 h, may be used. Alternatives include trimethoprim-sulfamethoxazole (TMP-SMZ), 4–6 mg/kg TMP and 20–30 mg/kg SMZ every 12 h, or ampicillin-sulbactam, 25–75 mg/kg every 6 h.

In a patient with a lower likelihood of epiglottitis, a soft tissue lateral film of the neck may be useful to help demonstrate the swollen epiglottis (Figure 48–4).

A physician should be at the patient's bedside at all times, including in the radiology suite, prepared to perform definitive airway maneuvers.

B. Croup (Laryngotracheobronchitis)

Croup is a clinical syndrome characterized by barking cough, inspiratory stridor, and hoarseness of voice. These symptoms are believed to be secondary to viral inflammation of the upper airway. If history and clinical assessment, sometimes in combination with lateral neck x-rays and chest x-rays, suggest croup, therapy includes the following:

1. Initial steps—Apply humidified oxygen, and attach pulse oximeter and cardiac monitor. Rarely is immediate endotracheal intubation necessary before attempts at medical management. Keep the child in a position of comfort, usually on the parent's lap.

2. Pharmacologic treatment—Give glucocorticoids to any child who presents with croup symptoms and demonstrates increased work of breathing. Give either nebulized budesonide, 2 mg, or oral or intramuscular dexamethasone, 0.15–0.6 mg/kg.

For children who are moderately or severely distressed, consider nebulized racemic epinephrine (0.5 mL of 2.25% racemic epinephrine) or nebulized L-epinephrine (5 mL of 1:1000). Previously all children who received epinephrine were hospitalized because of concerns over severe rebound airway swelling. Current recommendations allow for discharge if the patient remains comfortable without stridor or signs of respiratory distress for 2–3 hours after 1 epinephrine nebuliza-

Table 48–8. Differential diagnosis of upper airway obstruction.

	Croup	**Epiglottitis**	**Foreign Body**
Age	6 months to 3 years	2–5 years	Under 3 years
Cause	Parainfluenza	*S pyogenes, S pneumoniae, S aureus, H influenzae* (rare)	Foreign body
Season	Fall or winter	Any	Any
Time of day	Night or morning	Any	Daytime
Illness features			
Onset	Slow	Abrupt	Abrupt
Upper respiratory infection	Yes	No	No
Fever	Generally low grade	High	None
Toxic	Mild	Yes	No
Pharyngitis	Possible	Yes	No
Drooling	No	Yes	No
Stridor	Inspiratory + expiratory	Inspiratory	Inspiratory + expiratory
Position	Variable	Sitting	Variable
Hoarseness	Yes	Rare	No
Ancillary tests			
White blood count	Normal	High	Normal
Chest x-ray	Steeple sign	Normal	Hyperinflation
Lateral neck	Normal	Swollen epiglottis, "thumb-print sign"	May show radiopaque body

tion. Patients who require a second epinephrine nebulization should be hospitalized for further observation and treatment. Discharged patients must have reliable guardians and be able to return if their symptoms worsen.

3. Humidified oxygen with saline—For the minimally distressed child with no stridor at rest and pulse oximetry greater than 92% on room air, consider cool, humidified oxygen with nebulized saline. If this approach is effective in the emergency department at reducing upper airway obstruction, such patients may ordinarily be discharged and may use cool mist therapy at home.

C. Foreign Body Aspiration

The anatomic level and completeness of airway obstruction will dictate physical findings. The history is usually highly suggestive, with a brief asymptomatic interval followed by sudden dyspnea, coughing, and gagging, after the child has handled a small object such as

jewelry, a toy, a pin, a peanut, or candy. In 20% of cases, the object is in the upper airway; in 80%, it is in the main-stem or lobar bronchus. Stridor is present if the object is lodged high, at the level of the larynx; wheezing and decreased breath sounds occur if is it lodged below the larynx. Mild tachypnea may be the only finding. Lateral neck x-rays may be helpful for radiopaque foreign bodies in the neck. When lower airway occlusion is suspected, chest x-rays taken in decubitus positions bilaterally (preferentially in expiration) will often reveal hyperinflation in the affected lung area. This finding is most visible in the dependent lung, which will be more radiolucent when compared with the superior lung in the same decubitus view or with the contralateral dependent lung in the other decubitus view.

1. Complete obstruction—If obstruction is complete and airway clearance maneuvers (see Table 48–9) fail, perform laryngoscopy immediately, and attempt to remove the foreign body with Magill forceps under direct

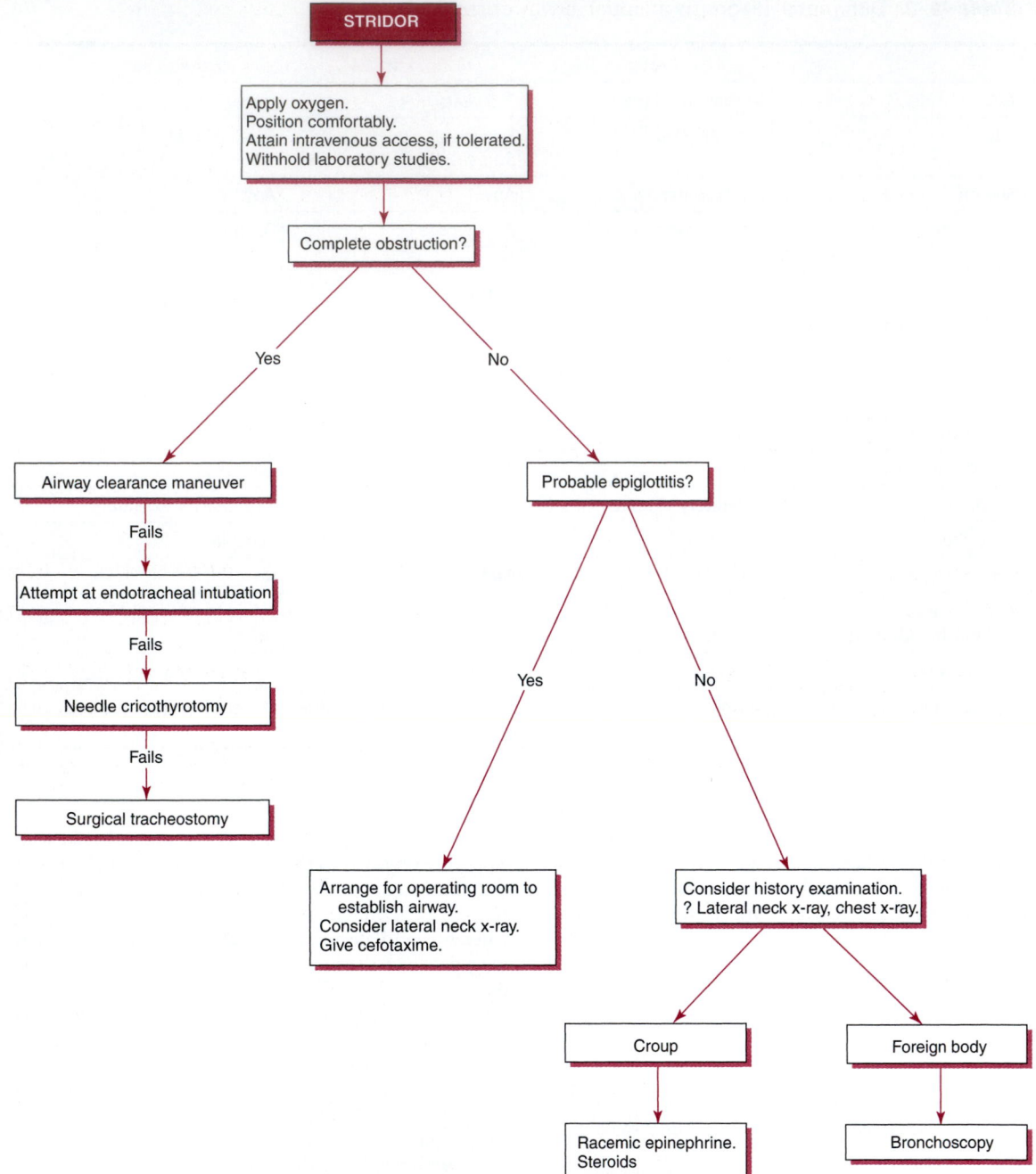

Figure 48–3. Treatment algorithm for pediatric stridor.

Table 48–9. Management of complete foreign body airway obstruction in infants and children.

Status	Infant (up to age 1 year)	Child (1–8 years)
Conscious	Patient unable to ventilate: 　5 back blows with infant in prone, head-down position, then 5 chest thrusts with infant supine, head-down position. 　Repeat as above until patient becomes unconscious.	Patient unable to ventilate: 　Perform Heimlich maneuver: abdominal thrusts above the umbilicus standing behind the victim. 　Continue thrusts until foreign body is expelled or victim becomes unconscious.
Unconscious	Open airway, perform tongue-jaw lift. If able to visual foreign body, remove it. If no spontaneous respirations, attempt rescue breathing. If unsuccessful . . . Reposition airway and try again, then . . . Start cycle again, repeat back blows, chest thrusts, open airway, attempt to ventilate. Emergency medical services activation after 1 minute. If spontaneous respirations resume, place in recovery position.	Lower victim to the ground. Open airway with tongue-jaw lift. Remove any visible foreign body. If no spontaneous respirations, attempt to ventilate. If unsuccessful . . . Straddle or kneel beside the victim. Begin abdominal thrusts with heel of hand positioned above umbilicus and below xiphoid process. Open airway and repeat steps until obstruction is relieved.

vision. After removal of the foreign body, insert a properly sized endotracheal tube to prevent later inflammatory obstruction.

2. Partial obstruction—In most patients, obstruction is partial. Apply supplemental oxygen, and attach pulse oximeter and cardiac monitor. Do not attempt endotracheal intubation.

Establish venous access and begin 5% dextrose in quarter-normal saline, at maintenance rate (see Table 48–5). Allow the patient to assume a position of comfort, usually on the parent's lap.

Obtain chest x-rays (see above). Maintain constant observation of the patient by nurse or physician. Arrange for rigid bronchoscopy, under general anesthesia, to remove the foreign object.

Wright RB, Pomerantz WJ, Luria JW: New approaches to respiratory infections in children. Bronchiolitis and Croup. Emerg Med Clin North Am 2002;20:93. [PMID: 11826639] (Review.)

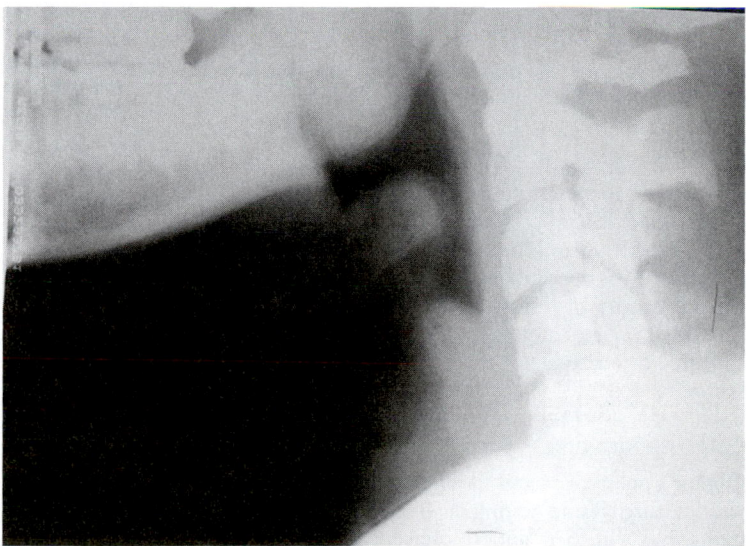

Figure 48–4. Lateral soft tissue x-ray of the neck, showing thumbprint sign of epiglottitis.

LOWER AIRWAY DISORDERS

Lower airway disorders are a disparate group of conditions with varying clinical presentations that may affect oxygenation and ventilation. Lower airway disease includes both obstructive conditions and parenchymal or alveolar disease. The clinical hallmarks are dyspnea and tachypnea, often with cough. Wheezing denotes an obstructive process.

In children, the most common causes of lower airway obstruction are bronchiolitis, asthma, and foreign body obstruction. In infants, congenital anomalies of the airway (tracheal web, cysts, vascular rings, lobar emphysema) must also be considered. Pneumonia is the most frequent pediatric alveolar disorder, although pulmonary edema, inhalation injury, and cystic fibrosis must also be excluded.

1. Bronchiolitis

Clinical Findings

Bronchiolitis is a wintertime acute lower airway respiratory disease, usually caused by RSV, that produces small airway obstruction. It primarily affects children under age 12 months. Cough, coryza, and upper respiratory symptoms, usually with fever, precede wheezing and dyspnea. Clinical signs of respiratory distress are variable. The white blood cell count is normal, and the chest x-ray shows shifting patterns of hyperaeration and atelectasis. Hypercapnia, hypoxemia, or both may be present.

Treatment

A. General Management

Apply supplemental humidified oxygen, and attach pulse oximeter. Keep child on parent's lap.

B. Bronchodilator Therapy

If wheezing is present, a trial of nebulized epinephrine or albuterol (0.15 mg/kg of 0.5% solution or 0.03 mL/kg by mask; maximum, 2.5 mg) is recommended. Albuterol can be repeated every 15–60 minutes depending on severity of disease and response to the medication. If bronchodilator therapy produces improvement, continue bronchodilator therapy as discussed below for asthma.

C. Other Measures

Obtain a chest x-ray and nasopharyngeal swab for RSV viral culture. Rapid testing such as enzyme-linked immunoassay (ELISA) and fluorescent antibody testing may also be available.

Disposition

Admission is required for children who appear ill or toxic. Admission is recommended if any of the following are present: oxygen saturation less than 95%, respiratory rate greater than 70 breaths/min, atelectasis on chest x-ray, gestational age less than 34 weeks, or age less than 3 months.

Klassen TP: Recent advances in the treatment of bronchiolitis and laryngitis. Pediatr Clin North Am 1997;44:249. [PMID: 9057793] (Review.)

2. Asthma

Clinical Findings

The most common pediatric respiratory disease is reactive airway disease, or asthma. Dyspnea, cough, and wheezing are part of the usual presentation. In infancy, wheezing is typically associated with bronchiolitis, caused by RSV. The relationship of bronchiolitis in infancy to childhood asthma is not clear, although approximately one half of infants with bronchiolitis later develop asthma. Bronchiolitis may respond to bronchodilator therapy with albuterol or subcutaneous epinephrine, which indicates reversible smooth muscle spasm. In both conditions, mucus plugging of small airways, edema, and bronchial constriction are key pathophysiologic features. Asthma appears to be increasing in prevalence, and morbidity and mortality rates associated with this condition are rising.

When a patient presents during an asthma exacerbation, important historical information includes recent steroid use, prior intensive care unit admissions, prior intubations secondary to asthma, preceding triggers, medications and frequency of their use, and baseline peak expiratory flow rates (PEFRs).

PEFR is extremely useful in asthma evaluation, and handheld pediatric-sized devices should be available in the emergency department. PEFR is more sensitive than auscultation, pulsus paradoxus, or other physical signs in gauging severity of obstruction and response to therapy. Children aged 4–5 years can successfully use handheld peak flow meters. Comparison of presenting PEFR with known baseline values is especially helpful. Arterial blood gas measurements and chest x-ray are necessary in severe cases. Physical exam findings also guide the management and treatment of asthma. Inability to speak, cyanosis, accessory muscle use, pulsus paradoxus, or signs of infection may indicate more serious disease.

Treatment

See Figure 48–5.

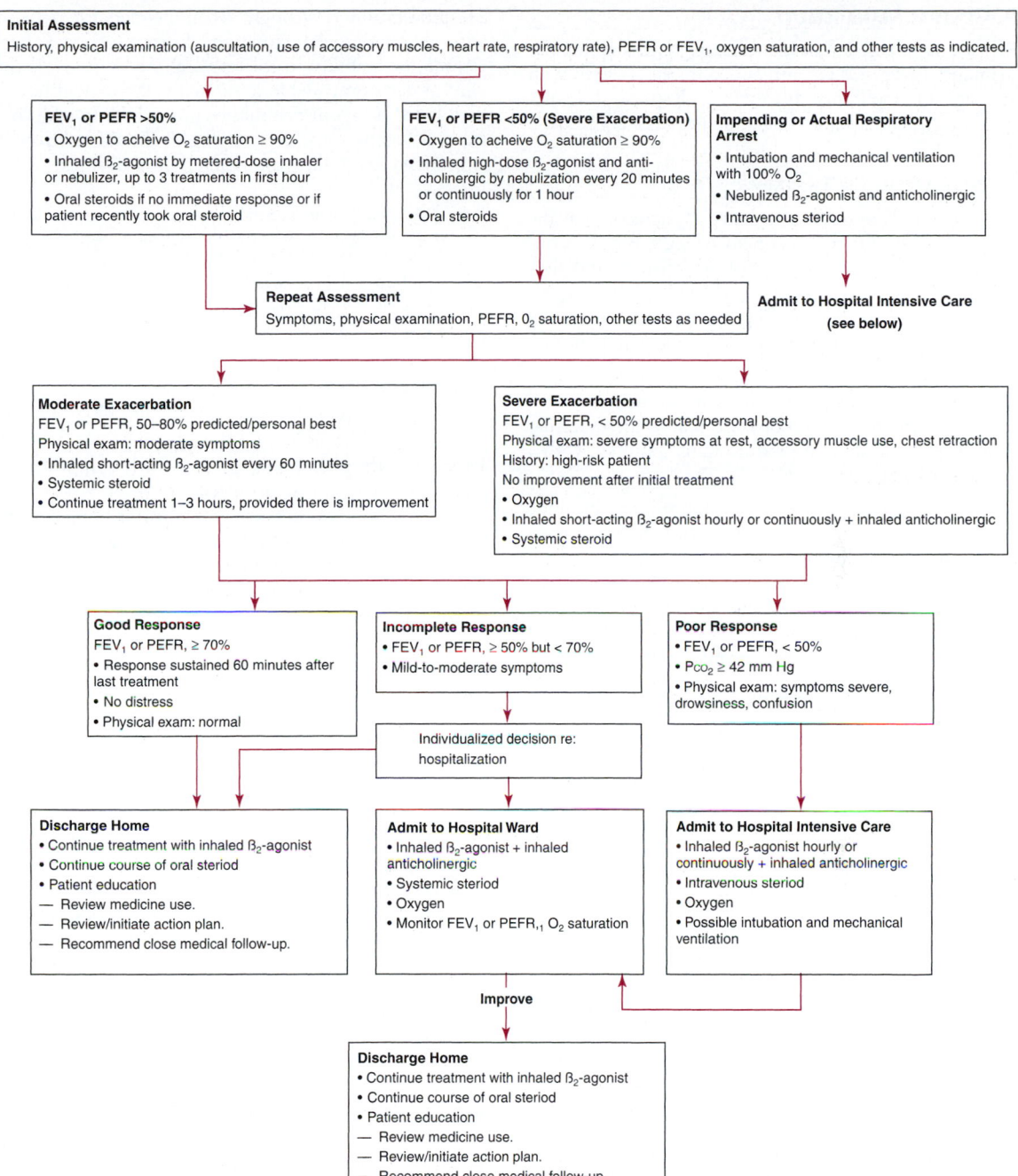

Figure 48–5. Management of asthma exacerbation: emergency department and hospital-based care. FEV$_1$ = forced expiratory volume in 1 second; PEFR = peak expiratory flow rate. (Reproduced from National Institutes of Health: *National Asthma Education and Prevention: Practical Guide for the Diagnosis and Management of Asthma,* p. 29. NIH Publication No. 97-4053. National Institutes of Health, 1997.)

A. GENERAL MANAGEMENT

Provide supplemental oxygen therapy, and attach pulse oximeter. Oxygen is recommended for all children with any sign of respiratory distress (eg, dyspnea, difficulty speaking, mental status changes, or accessory muscle use).

B. PHARMACOLOGIC THERAPY

1. Inhaled β_2-agonists—Inhaled β_2-agonists are the drugs of choice for the treatment of acute bronchoconstriction. Nebulizers, metered-dose inhalers, and dry-powder inhalers are equally effective. Nebulized albuterol treatment (0.15 mg/kg; maximum, 5 mg) may be preferred by children who cannot adequately inspire medications from other routes.

2. Glucocorticoids—Consider glucocorticoids for all children with asthma who present in an acute exacerbation. The initial dose of prednisone is 2 mg/kg, with a maximum of 80 mg.

3. Ipratropium bromide—Ipratropium bromide alone is not recommended and is not a first-line therapy. Although a dosing regimen has not been determined, when used as an adjunct with albuterol, ipratropium bromide has been shown to improve pulmonary function tests and to decrease emergency department time in an acute asthma exacerbation.

4. Epinephrine or terbutaline—In general, subcutaneous epinephrine, 0.01 mg/kg up to 0.3–0.5 mg, or terbutaline intravenously or subcutaneously offers no advantage over an inhaled β-agonist but should be considered in addition to inhaled albuterol for critically ill children with severe respiratory distress, poor air movement, or rapid decompensation. A terbutaline intravenous bolus of 2–10 μg/kg should be followed by an infusion starting at 0.4 μg/kg/min to a maximum of 5.0 μg/kg/min.

5. Magnesium—The benefit of intravenous magnesium, 25–50 mg/kg (maximum, 2 g), is unclear and may be considered for moderate to severely ill patients who have not responded to other therapies.

C. INTUBATION

Absolute indications for intubation include apnea, respiratory failure, and coma. Relative indications include marked hypoxia, rapidly rising hypercarbia with respiratory acidosis, inability to speak, mental status changes, and exhaustion.

Disposition

There are no absolute guidelines for admission or discharge of a pediatric asthma patient. Intensive care unit admission is required for patients with an altered level of consciousness, hypotension, or respiratory failure.

Hospitalization is strongly recommended for patients with a poor social situation, history of near fatal asthma, or inability to tolerate oral medications. If the clinical decision is made to discharge the patient home, an inhaled β_2-agonist should be prescribed. In addition, steroids (eg, prednisone, 2 mg/kg/d) should be strongly considered and follow-up within 3 days arranged.

Baren JM, Zorc JJ: Contemporary approach to emergency department management of pediatric asthma. Emerg Med Clin North Am 2002;20:115. [PMID: 11831222] (Review.)

Smith SR, Strunk RC: Acute asthma in the pediatric emergency department. Pediatr Clin North Am 1999;46:1145. [PMID: 10629678] (Review.)

3. Pneumonia

Clinical Findings

Patients with pneumonia present with symptoms of cough and dyspnea, with or without fever. Abdominal pain may be the presenting complaint. Nonspecific symptoms in a young child or infant may include irritability, poor feeding, decreased physical activity, vomiting, diarrhea, or apneic episodes. Signs of respiratory distress, including wheezing, rales, rhonchi, or focal absence of breath sounds, usually are present. Physical evaluation may be nonspecific. Tachypnea and respiratory distress may be present with a clear chest on auscultation or with discrete rales in affected lung segments. Chest x-rays show lobar or peribronchial perihilar patterns of infiltration, sometimes with pleural effusion.

Pediatric pneumonia can be caused by bacteria, viruses, *Mycoplasma*, mycobacteria, or *Chlamydia*. Age is an important consideration in determining possible pathogens in children with pneumonia (Table 48–10). Certain clinical or laboratory features suggest specific causes: high fever, appearance of illness, significant leukocytosis, and pleural effusion suggest bacteria; afebrile pneumonia with eosinophilia in infancy suggests *Chlamydia;* extreme lymphocytosis in an unimmunized infant with whooping cough suggests pertussis; hilar adenopathy and upper lobe infiltration suggest primary tuberculosis. In younger children, rapid diagnostic testing for RSV (by immunofluorescent and ELISA antigen techniques performed on nasal or conjunctival specimens) may provide the cause. In older children, sputum Gram staining may guide initial therapy.

Treatment

Rapid evaluation of respiratory status, in combination with pulse oximetry and occasionally arterial blood gas determination, will direct the immediate therapy.

Table 48–10. Causes of pneumonia by age.[1]

Age	Infecting Organism
2 weeks	Bacteria Group B streptococcus Gram-negative bacilli Viruses
2 weeks–2 months	Chlamydia Viruses Bacteria S pneumoniae S aureus H influenzae
2 months–3 years	Viruses Bacteria S pneumoniae S aureus H influenzae
3–12 years	Viruses Bacteria S pneumoniae M pneumoniae
13–19 years	Viruses Bacteria S pneumoniae M pneumoniae

[1]Reproduced, with permission, from Fleisher G: Infectious disease emergencies. Page 750 in: Fleisher G (editor): *Textbook of Pediatric Emergency Medicine*, 4th ed. Williams & Wilkins, 2000.

A. GENERAL MANAGEMENT

Provide supplemental oxygen, and attach pulse oximeter and cardiac monitor. Evaluate degree of respiratory distress. Significant respiratory distress is best defined as pulse oximetry less than 92% on room air.

B. LABORATORY AND IMAGING STUDIES

Obtain a chest x-ray (posteroanterior and lateral). Consider CBC with differential, absolute neutrophil count, C-reactive protein, RSV studies, and blood culture.

C. ANTIMICROBIAL THERAPY

Administer antimicrobial therapy based on age and clinical appearance. See Table 48–11 for guidelines.

D. TREATMENT OF SUSPECTED TUBERCULOSIS

Arrange for in-hospital multiple drug therapy with isoniazid, rifampin, and pyrazinamide for children with clinical and epidemiologic evidence of primary pulmonary tuberculosis. Consider applying an intradermal PPD test and arrange 48-hour follow-up for patients at risk of having tuberculosis.

E. OTHER MEASURES

Children with a parapneumonic pleural effusion require a thoracentesis and subsequent hospital admission for observation and intravenous antibiotics after the procedure. Analysis of the fluid should include Gram stain, culture, cell count and differential, total protein, pH, and glucose.

Disposition

Most children can be discharged home with appropriate follow-up on antibiotics. Hospitalization is required if the patient demonstrates signs of toxicity, dehydration, significant respiratory distress, hypoxemia, or pleural effusion or if the patient is less than 20–30 days old. Consider hospitalization for children younger than age 3 months and for patients with preexisting pulmonary disease. Twenty-four hour follow-up is required for all children diagnosed with pneumonia and discharged.

McCracken GH: Diagnosis and management of pneumonia in children. Pediatr Infect Dis J 2000;19:924. [PMID: 11001128] (Review.)

McIntosh K: Community-acquired pneumonia in children. N Engl J Med 2002;346:429. [PMID: 11832532] (Review.)

■ NEUROLOGIC EMERGENCIES

Objective neurologic evaluation of the emergency department patient involves recognition of age-appropriate differences in cognitive function. For patients with altered mental status, an objective scale, such as the pediatric Glasgow Coma Scale (Table 48–12) will help reduce interobserver differences in assessment and provide a measure for comparison during serial examinations.

SEIZURES

General Considerations

Seizures are common pediatric emergencies in both the prehospital environment and the emergency department. Approximately 5% of all children have one or more seizures before age 16 years. Epilepsy is a chronic condition of recurrent seizures that develops in only a small portion of patients who have single seizures. Most seizures in childhood are single, generalized tonic-clonic events lasting a few minutes. Seizures may be generalized or focal. Status epilepticus is defined as continuous seizure activity for 30 minutes or as recurrent seizures without intervening return of consciousness.

Table 48–11. Suggested drug treatment for community-acquired pneumonia in children, according to whether they are hospitalized.[1]

Age Grouping	Outpatient	Inpatient, without Lobar or Lobular Infiltrate, Pleural Effusion, or Both	Inpatient, with Signs of Sepsis, Alveolar Infiltrate, Large Pleural Effusion, or All Three
Birth–20 days	Admit patient.	Administer ampicillin and gentamicin, with or without cefotaxime.	Administer IV ampicillin and gentamicin, with or without IV cefotaxime.[2]
3 weeks–3 months	If patient is afebrile, give oral erythromycin, 30–40 mg/kg/d in 4 divided doses, or oral azithromycin, 1 dose of 10 mg/kg, then 5 mg/kg/d for 4 days. Admit patient if fever or hypoxia is present.	If patient is afebrile, administer IV erythromycin, 40 mg/kg/d in 4 divided doses given 6 hours apart.[3] If patient is febrile, add cefotaxime, 200 mg/kg/d in 3 divided doses given 8 hours apart.	Administer IV cefotaxime, 200 mg/kg/d in 3 divided dose given 8 hours apart[2,4]
4 months–4 years	Administer oral amoxicillin, 80–100 mg/kg/d in 3 or 4 divided doses).	In cases of apparent viral pneumonia, no antibiotics should be given. Otherwise, consider treatment with IV ampicillin, 200 mg/kg/d in 4 divided doses given 6 hours apart.	Administer IV cefotaxime, 200 mg/kg/d or IV cefuroxime, 150 mg/kg/d in 3 divided doses given 8 hours apart[2,4]
5–15 years	Administer oral erythromycin, 30–40 mg/kg/d in 4 divided doses, oral clarithromycin, 15 mg/kg/d in 2 divided doses), or oral azithromycin, 1 dose of 10 mg/kg, then 5 mg/kg/d for 4 days. In children older than 8 years of age, consider oral doxycycline, 4 mg/kg/d in 2 divided doses.	Administer IV erythromycin, 40 mg/kg/d in 4 divided doses given 6 hours apart or IV azithromycin, 5 mg/kg/d in 2 divided doses given 12 hours apart. In children older than 8 years of age, consider IV doxycycline 4 mg/kg/d in 2 divided doses given 12 hours apart. If there is strong evidence of a bacterial cause (eg, high white-cell count, chills, or no response to outpatient therapy with a macrolide), add ampicillin.	Administer IV cefotaxime, 200 mg/kg/d or IV cefuroxime, 150 mg/kg/d in 3 divided doses given 8 hours apart.[4] Consider adding IV azithromycin if patient is not doing well.[2]

[1]Reproduced, with permission, from McIntosh K: Community-acquired pneumonia in children. N Engl J Med 2002; 346:435.
[2]Staphylococcal pneumonia is unusual; however, if cultures of blood or pleural fluid grow *Staphylococcus aureus* or, in other exceptional circumstances, oxacillin or, in areas where methicillin-resistant *S aureus* is a reasonable possibility, vancomycin should be added.
[3]In infants younger than 6 weeks of age, treatment with azithromycin, 5 mg/kg/d in 2 divided doses given 12 hours apart, should be considered in view of reports of hypertrophic pyloric stenosis in infants who received erythromycin.
[4]Some experts suggest treatment with ampicillin, 200–300 mg/kg/d intravenously in 4 divided doses given 6 hours apart, in patients who have lobar, and therefore most likely pneumococcal, pneumonia.

Seizures may be generalized or focal, or focal with secondary generalization. Patients with focal status epilepticus may present with or without preserved consciousness. Status epilepticus is often the first presentation of seizures in childhood.

The causes of seizures and status epilepticus in children are multiple and age-dependent. Children under age 3 years presenting with status epilepticus are most likely to have serious conditions, for example, central nervous system infections or vascular disorders, anoxia, trauma, intoxications, or metabolic abnormalities. Many of these conditions are treatable. In older children, however, status epilepticus is usually the result of chronic epilepsy with noncompliance for anticonvulsive medications, chronic progressive encephalopathy, or idiopathic encephalopathy. The likelihood of serious underlying disease in a child presenting with status epilepticus is inversely correlated with age.

Febrile seizures are also common in childhood. The peak age is 8–20 months, although they may occur in

Table 48–12. Pediatric Glascow Coma Scale.[1]

Eyes Opening

	> 1 Year	< 1 Year
4	Spontaneously	Spontaneously
3	To verbal command	To shout
2	To pain	To pain
1	No response	No response

Best Motor Response

	> 1 Year	< 1 Year
6	Obeys	Spontaneous
5	Localizes pain	Localizes pain
4	Flexion-withdrawal	Flexion-withdrawal
3	Flexion-abnormal (decorticate rigidity)	Flexion-abnormal (decerebrate rigidity)
2	Extension (decerebrate rigidity)	Extension (decorticate rigidity)
1	No response	No response

Best Verbal Response

	> 5 years	2–5 Years	0–23 Months
5	Oriented and converses	Appropriate words and phrases	Smiles, coos appropriately
4	Disoriented and converses	Inappropriate words	Cries, consolable
3	Inappropriate words	Persistent cries and/or screams	Persistent, inappropriate crying and/or screaming
2	Incomprehensible sounds	Grunts	Grunts, agitated/restless
1	No response	No response	No response

Total: 3–15

[1]Reproduced, with permission, from Johnson LA: Altered mental status. Page 1148 in: The Clinical Practice of Emergency Medicine, 3rd Ed. Lippincott Williams & Wilkins, 2001.

children from approximately 6 months to 6 years of age. Often, underlying diseases are simply upper respiratory tract infections or gastroenteritis. Febrile seizures may be simple or complex. A simple febrile seizure typically occurs as a generalized self-limited tonic-clonic seizure of several minutes' duration. Complex febrile seizure denotes a seizure with high-risk features, including focal onset, postictal neurologic abnormalities, or duration greater than 15 minutes. Other high-risk features include prior neurologic or developmental abnormalities or a history of epilepsy in the nuclear family. The simple febrile seizure is usually benign and requires no therapy; however, children presenting with high-risk features are at greater risk for recurrent afebrile features.

Clinical Findings

Many children will present in the postictal state. In such patients, search for a specific cause. Obtain a history from the parents beginning with a precise description of the seizure itself, including the nature of onset (focal or generalized), duration, and quality of motor features. Exclude syncope, hysteria, breath-holding, and night terrors. Other confusional states that may be difficult to distinguish from seizures include migraine headache, hereditary chin trembling, familiar choreoathetosis, and narcolepsy. Also exclude head trauma and alcohol and drug intoxication. Several drugs are well associated with seizure activity: cyclic antidepressants, sympathomimetics (cocaine, amphetamine, phencyclidine), theophylline, isoniazid, phenothiazines, camphor, anticholinergics, antihistamines, and lindane. Physical examination should specifically exclude head trauma, bulging fontanelle, papilledema, meningeal irritation, focal neurologic signs, cutaneous lesions, and systemic disease.

Treatment

A well-organized approach to seizure management minimizes the complications of the acute electrical and metabolic derangements and averts iatrogenic complications. Ensure adequate ventilation and oxygenation in the patient with active seizures, and then address termination of the seizure and reversal of metabolic imbalances. Finally, attempt to establish the cause in order to implement specific therapy.

A. GENERAL MANAGEMENT

1. Initial steps—Open the airway, use suction to clear secretions or foreign bodies, and then administer oxygen. Ordinarily, reserve intubation for failure of medical management.

Protect the child from injury by manually holding the head. Remove tight-fitting clothing from the child.

2. Laboratory studies—Establish intravenous access, and draw blood for immediate bedside glucose determination and other appropriate laboratory investigations, including CBC; glucose, lead, calcium, and magnesium levels; liver and renal function; and electrolytes, ammonia, and pertinent drug levels. Send urine for toxicologic screening. Consider obtaining an arterial blood gas if significant acidosis is suspected. The best alternative to intravenous access in children younger than age 5 years with prolonged refractory status epilepticus may be the intraosseous route.

3. Volume resuscitation—If rapid bedside glucose determination is less than 90 mg/dL, administer 25% dextrose in water, 2 mL/kg/dose slowly intravenously. In children over age 3 years, give 50% dextrose in water at 1 mL/kg. If evidence of dehydration is present, provide lactated Ringer's solution or isotonic normal saline. Otherwise, if the patient is euvolemic, start 5% dextrose in quarter-normal saline at maintenance rate for weight (see Table 48–5).

4. Pharmacologic therapy—Consider naloxone, 0.1 mg/kg (max 2 mg) intravenously. If the child is febrile, administer rectal acetaminophen, 10–15 mg/kg. If fever fails to respond to acetaminophen, use tepid water baths to reduce temperature.

5. Other measures—After a febrile seizure, children who appear toxic or do not return to baseline mental status (after a brief postictal period) should undergo a full septic workup including a lumbar puncture.

B. SPECIFIC MANAGEMENT

If seizures continue after first-line supportive care, consider immediate anticonvulsant therapy (Figure 48–6). Duration of seizure activity may be related to ultimate neurologic outcome, particularly in patients with severe underlying disease.

Alternatives to intravenous lorazepam include rectal diazepam, 0.5 mg/kg administered by lubricated tuberculin syringe approximately 5 cm into the rectum, or intramuscular midazolam, 0.2 mg/kg. Phenytoin, barbiturates, and benzodiazepines may be given intraosseously.

Hanhan UA, Fiallos MR, Orlowski: Status epilepticus. Pediatr Clin North Am 2001;48:683. [PMID: 11411300] (Review.)

Reuter D, Brownstein D: Common emergent pediatric neurologic problems. Emerg Med Clin North Am 2002;20:155. [PMID: 11826632] (Review.)

■ INFECTIOUS DISEASES

FEVER

The evaluation of febrile children is a common problem for the emergency physician. Although most of these children will have benign, self-limited viral infections, a few will have invasive disease with bacterial pathogens that may cause significant illness and even death. No source of infection will be evident after history and physical examination in 20% of febrile children. The ability to identify those children at increased risk for serious disease is the key to management. Because young children are at increased risk for more serious disease, the child's age frequently determines the extent of the evaluation.

1. Fever in Infants

General Considerations

Management of fever in infants under age 3 months is complicated and controversial. Signs of disease at this age are frequently subtle and nonspecific, and there are multiple sources of infection. Relative to older infants, these infants uncommonly have febrile disease, and when present, it more likely reflects a serious invasive infection. Causes of fever at this age include (1) infections acquired in the household, (2) late onset of disease acquired in the nursery, at delivery, or in utero, and (3) infections secondary to anatomic or physiologic abnormalities.

Household-acquired infections are the most likely cause of fever in this age group, particularly with an uncomplicated prenatal and delivery history. Respiratory and gastrointestinal infections are most common. The incidence of invasive disease caused by *Streptococcus pneumoniae* is significant in the first 2 months of life. Other causes include the late onset of signs of congenital infection, such as rubella, cytomegalovirus, or syphilis. In addition, the delayed onset of infection acquired at delivery, for example, group B streptococci, *Escherichia coli,* and *Listeria,* are potentially life-threatening infections in this age group. Disease acquired in the nursery before discharge (eg, *S. aureus*) may also become manifest during this time. Additionally, infections associated with an underlying anatomic abnor-

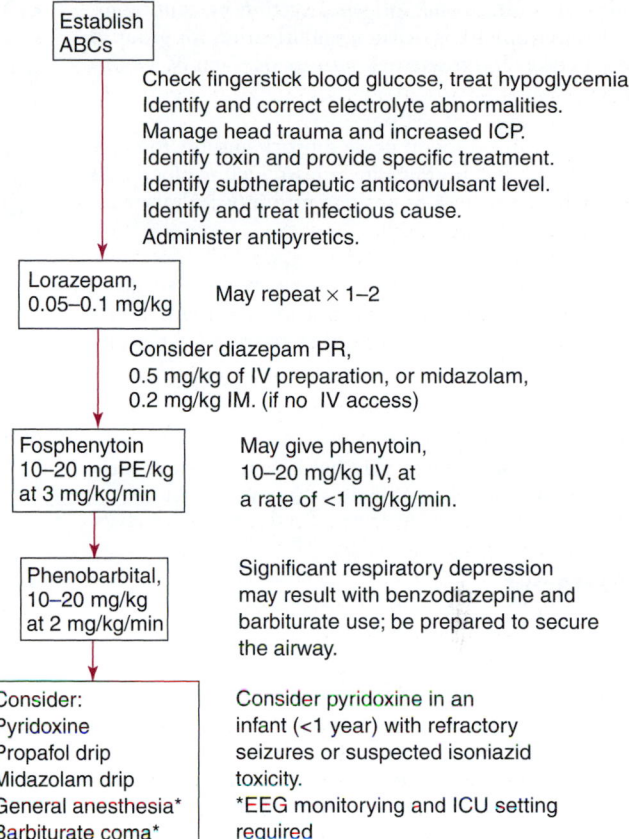

```
Establish
ABCs
```
Check fingerstick blood glucose, treat hypoglycemia.
Identify and correct electrolyte abnormalities.
Manage head trauma and increased ICP.
Identify toxin and provide specific treatment.
Identify subtherapeutic anticonvulsant level.
Identify and treat infectious cause.
Administer antipyretics.

```
Lorazepam,
0.05–0.1 mg/kg
```
May repeat × 1–2

Consider diazepam PR,
0.5 mg/kg of IV preparation, or midazolam,
0.2 mg/kg IM. (if no IV access)

```
Fosphenytoin
10–20 mg PE/kg
at 3 mg/kg/min
```
May give phenytoin,
10–20 mg/kg IV, at
a rate of <1 mg/kg/min.

```
Phenobarbital,
10–20 mg/kg
at 2 mg/kg/min
```
Significant respiratory depression
may result with benzodiazepine and
barbiturate use; be prepared to secure
the airway.

```
Consider:
Pyridoxine
Propafol drip
Midazolam drip
General anesthesia*
Barbiturate coma*
```
Consider pyridoxine in an
infant (<1 year) with refractory
seizures or suspected isoniazid
toxicity.
*EEG monitorying and ICU setting
required

Figure 48–6. Management of status epilepticus. ICP = intracranial pressure; ICU = intensive care unit; PE = phenytoin equivalent; PR = per rectum. (Reproduced, with permission, from Chiang VW: Seizures. Page 578 in: Fleisher G [editor]: *Pediatric Emergency Medicine,* 4th ed. Williams & Wilkins, 2000.)

mality, particularly those of the urinary tract, are potential sources of infection.

The younger the infant, the greater the risk of disease. The incidence of bacterial disease in febrile infants under age 1 month with a temperature of at least 38 °C (100.4 °F) is approximately 13%; in infants aged 1–2 months, the incidence is approximately 10%. In infants under age 3 months with temperatures over 40 °C (104 °F), the incidence of serious disease may be as high as 30–40%.

Clinical Findings

Evaluation includes a careful history of the pregnancy, delivery, and nursery course of the infant. Inquire about household infections. Look for general signs of illness, including lethargy and irritability. Otitis media can occur in infants under age 2 months. Other clues to the source of fever are (1) rash, jaundice, hepatosplenomegaly, macrocephaly (congenital infection), (2) direct hyperbilirubinemia (urinary tract infection),

(3) pseudoparalysis, cellulitis, meningitis (group B streptococci), and (4) meningitis (*Listeria*).

A. LABORATORY FINDINGS

The laboratory evaluation of febrile infants under age 3 months includes the following:

1. CBC with differential and blood culture—A white blood cell count less than 5000 or greater than 15,000; absolute neutrophil count greater than 10,000; or band count greater than 1500 increases the probability of sepsis.

2. Peripheral blood smear—Toxic granulation and vacuolization of white cells are sensitive indicators for invasive bacterial disease.

3. Lumbar puncture—Both bacterial and aseptic meningitis may be serious in febrile infants under age 3 months. Lumbar puncture is mandatory for infants under age 1 month and is strongly recommended for infants aged 1–3 months. Spinal fluid studies include cell count and differential, glucose, protein, Gram stain, and culture and antigen detection by counterimmunoelectrophoresis or latex agglutination for group B streptococci, *H. influenza, S. pneumoniae,* and *N. meningitidis.*

4. Urinalysis—Obtain urine dipstick and microscopic analysis. Positive findings are at least 5 white blood cells per high-power field or positive nitrite or leukocyte esterase.

5. Urine culture—A bagged specimen is not adequate because of the high incidence of contamination. Suprapubic aspiration or bladder catheterization are the preferred methods of obtaining urine.

B. X-ray Findings

Findings of pneumonia may be present on chest x-ray even in infants without cough, tachypnea, or rales.

Treatment

See Figure 48–7.

A. General Management

Management must be conservative. If evaluation discloses a local infection (eg, meningitis, pneumonia, or urinary tract infection), hospitalize the infant and promptly institute intravenous antibiotic therapy.

1. Antimicrobials for infants birth to age 4 weeks—If the suspected causative organism is group B streptococci, *Listeria,* or *E. coli,* give ampicillin, 50 mg/kg every 6–8 hours, and gentamicin, 2.5 mg/kg every 12 hours.

2. Antimicrobials for infants aged 4–8 weeks—If the suspected causative organism is group B streptococci, *Listeria, H. influenzae,* or *S. pneumoniae,* give ampicillin, 50 mg/kg every 6–8 hours, and either ceftriaxone, 100 mg/kg/d, or cefotaxime, 50 mg/kg every 6 hours.

3. Other antimicrobials—The cephalosporins are not active against *Listeria* and thus are not recommended as the sole treatment for presumed sepsis in infants under age 8 weeks. If *S. aureus* infection is possible, replace ampicillin with a penicillinase-resistant antibiotic such as nafcillin, 50–200 mg/kg/d, depending on the child's age.

B. Treatment of Otitis Media

The infant older than age 1 month with otitis media who clinically appears well may be discharged with antibiotics and careful follow-up.

C. Treatment for Fever without Clear Cause

Clinical and laboratory screening criteria have been developed for febrile infants under age 3 months without an evident source of infection after detailed history and physical examination. These criteria attempt to classify infants into high- and low-risk categories. Infants meeting low-risk criteria (Philadelphia criteria) are considered safe to discharge home provided the parents are reliable and follow-up is assured at 24 hours. The Philadelphia criteria have demonstrated excellent sensitivity (100%) for identifying those infants aged 1–2 months with serious bacterial infections. These criteria, however, were not adequate when applied to infants under age 1 month. Therefore, all infants less than age 1 month with fever of 38 °C (100.4 °F) or higher require a full septic workup, intravenous antibiotics, and hospitalization until culture results are negative (see Figure 48–7).

2. Fever in Children

General Considerations

Of emergency department visits for children aged 3–36 months, 8% are for fever. Differentiating serious illnesses such as bacterial diseases from self-limited viral infections can be difficult in febrile children in this age group. They are at increased risk for occult invasive bacterial diseases (eg, pneumonia, urinary tract infection, meningitis, occult bacteremia). Children with invasive bacterial disease may present with an undifferentiated febrile illness.

Clinical Findings

Young children with pneumonia may present without auscultatory findings in the chest; occasionally, the only clues to diagnosis are a history of cough with fever and tachypnea on physical examination. Urinary tract infections are occult infections in young children because dysuria and urinary frequency are not clinically apparent in this age group. Although children with meningitis may present with significant obtundation, initially children show only high fever and irritability.

Occult bacteremia is the presence of bacteremia in a young child who is only moderately ill-appearing. Risk factors appear to be the child's age and height of the fever at presentation. The incidence is greatest under age 3 years. Approximately 6% of children presenting to an emergency department with temperatures over 38.5 °C (101.3 °F) have bacteremia. The likelihood of bacteremia increases with increasing fever and may exceed 10% in children with temperatures over 40 °C (104 °F). *S. pneumoniae* is the most common pathogen.

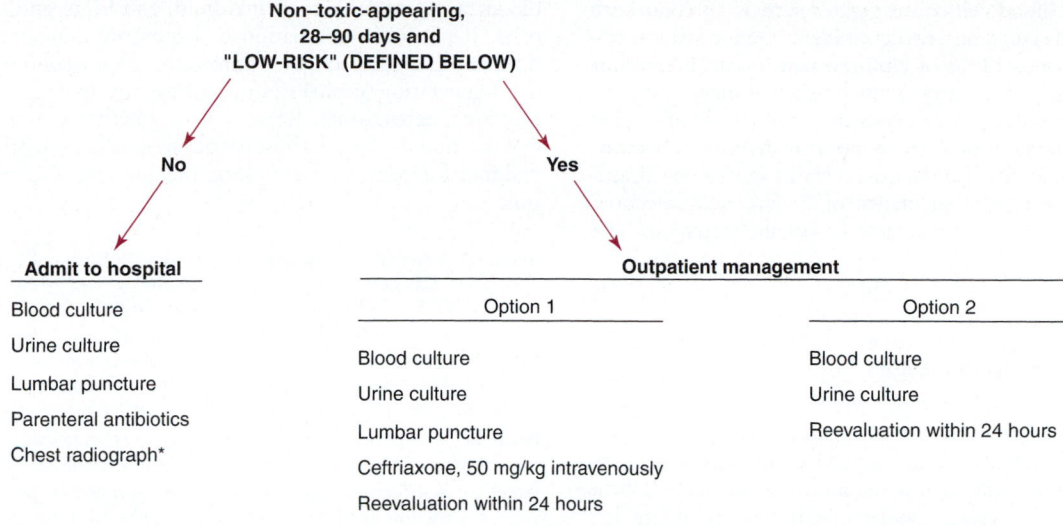

Non–toxic-appearing,
28–90 days and
"LOW-RISK" (DEFINED BELOW)

No

Yes

Admit to hospital

Blood culture

Urine culture

Lumbar puncture

Parenteral antibiotics

Chest radiograph*

Outpatient management

Option 1

Blood culture

Urine culture

Lumbar puncture

Ceftriaxone, 50 mg/kg intravenously

Reevaluation within 24 hours

Option 2

Blood culture

Urine culture

Reevaluation within 24 hours

*Chest radiograph if signs of pneumonia: respiratory distress, abnormal breath sounds, tachypnea, pulse oximetry < 95%.

Follow-up of low-risk infants treated as outpatients with positive culture results:

Blood culture positive (pathogen):   Admit for sepsis evaluation and parenteral antibiotic therapy pending results.

Urine culture positive (pathogen):   Persistent fever: admit for sepsis evaluation and parenteral antibiotic therapy pending results.

Outpatient antibiotics if afebrile and well.

Low-risk criteria for febrile infants:

Clinical criteria:

    Previously healthy, term infant with uncomplicated nursery stay

    Nontoxic clinical appearance

    No focal bacterial infaction on examination (except otitis media)

Laboratory criteria:

    WBC count 5–15,000/mm^3, <1500 bands/mm^3, or band-neutrophil ratio < 0.2.

    Negative Gram stain of unspun urine (preferred), or negative urine leukocyte esterase and nitrite, or < 5 WBCs/hpf.

    When diarrhea present: < 5 WBCs/hpf in stool.

    CSF: < 8 WBCs/mm^3 and negative Gram stain (option 1 only).

Figure 48–7. Algorithm for the management of a previously healthy infant (birth to 90 days) with fever without a source with a temperature of 38 °C (100.4 °F) or greater. CSF = cerebrospinal fluid; WBC = white blood cell. (Reproduced, with permission, from Baraff LJ: Management of fever without a source in infants and children. Ann Emerg Med 2000; 36:605.)

A white blood cell count greater than 15,000 has been used for screening febrile children, but it lacks specificity. Almost 90% of children with occult bacteremia recover spontaneously. Sequelae such as meningitis, cellulitis, pneumonia, or sepsis may develop. Studies have shown the rates of occult bacteremia have been decreasing. Use of the *H influenzae* b (Hib) vaccine has drastically reduced the incidence of *H influenza* infection, which is now a rare cause of occult bacteremia and meningitis.

Treatment

A. GENERAL MANAGEMENT

Evaluate the child before administering acetaminophen and then again after the temperature has been lowered. Acetaminophen is equally effective in lowering the temperature in both bacteremic and nonbacteremic febrile children. However, children with meningitis are less likely to be clinically improved after the use of antipyretics. If the examination discloses a source of infection, initiate appropriate laboratory studies and treatment.

B. FEVER WITH AN APPARENT SOURCE

A recognizable viral syndrome (eg, herpetic gingivostomatitis, hand-foot-and-mouth disease) can qualify as a source of a high fever in a child and may require no further ancillary studies. If a virus is suspected, treat the infection symptomatically with oral fluids and antipyretics, and follow up by telephone contact or reexamine the patient within 24 hours.

C. FEVER WITHOUT AN APPARENT SOURCE

The treatment of febrile children younger than age 36 months with fever greater than 39 °C (102.2 °F) and no apparent source of infection after appropriate laboratory screening (ie, urinalysis, stool studies, chest x-ray) remains controversial. In 1993, Baraff and others published guidelines recommending intramuscular antibiotics (ceftriaxone, 50 mg/kg/d) for febrile children (≥ 39 °C [102.2 °F]) aged 3–36 months without a source of infection and a white blood cell count greater than 15,000. Follow-up in 24 hours is required, at which time cultures are checked and a second dose of antibiotic is administered. In 2000, Baraff modified the widely adopted recommendations, taking into account the 90% efficacy of the pneumococcal conjugate vaccine in reducing pneumococcal disease (Figure 48–8).

D. MANAGEMENT OF THE CHILD APPEARING SERIOUSLY ILL

The young febrile child appearing seriously ill requires aggressive diagnostic evaluation and prompt institution of parenteral antibiotic therapy. Obtain cultures of blood, urine, and cerebrospinal fluid, and begin antibiotics. If physical examination or laboratory evaluation does not disclose a source of infection, use a second- or third-generation cephalosporin intravenously (eg, cefuroxime, ceftriaxone). Regardless of whether a source of infection is found, hospitalize seriously ill febrile children for continued antibiotic therapy and observation.

Avner JR, Baker MD: Management of fever in infants and children. Emerg Med Clin North Am 2002;20:49. [PMID: 11826637] (Review article of the evaluation and management of fever in young children.)

Baker MD, Bell LM, Avner JR: Outpatient management without antibiotics of fever in selected patients. N Engl J Med 1993;329:1437. [PMID: 8413453] (Controlled clinical trial.)

Baraff LJ: Management of a fever without a source in infants and children. Ann Emerg Med 2000;36:605. [PMID: 11097701]

Baraff LJ et al: Practice guideline for the management of infants and children 0 to 36 months of age without source. Ann Emerg Med 1993;22:1198. [PMID: 8517575] (Practice guidelines for evaluation and management of febrile infants and children based on meta-analysis.)

Kramer MS: The young febrile child: evidence-based diagnostic and therapeutic strategies. Emergency Medicine Practice 2000;2:7 (revised edition). (Comprehensive clinical discussion of the evaluation and management of previously healthy febrile children aged 3–36 months.)

Kuppermann N, Fleisher GR, Jaffe DM: Predictors of occult pneumococcal bacteremia in young febrile children. Ann Emerg Med 1998;31:679. [PMID: 9624306] (Prospective, multicenter, randomized trial of antibiotic use in young febrile children at risk for occult bacteremia.)

Lee GM, Harper MB: Risk of bacteremia for febrile young children in the post-Haemophilus influenzae type b era. Arch Pediatr Adolesc Med 1998;152:624. [PMID: 9667531] (Prospective clinical trial.)

MENINGITIS

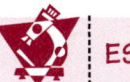

ESSENTIALS OF DIAGNOSIS

- *Fever, headache, stiff neck, mental status changes or excessive irritability.*
- *Cerebrospinal fluid Gram stain or culture may be diagnostic for a specific organism.*

General Considerations

Meningitis is an infection of the central nervous system characterized by fever, alteration in the level of consciousness, and in some instances a stiff neck. Acute bacterial meningitis is of particular concern to the

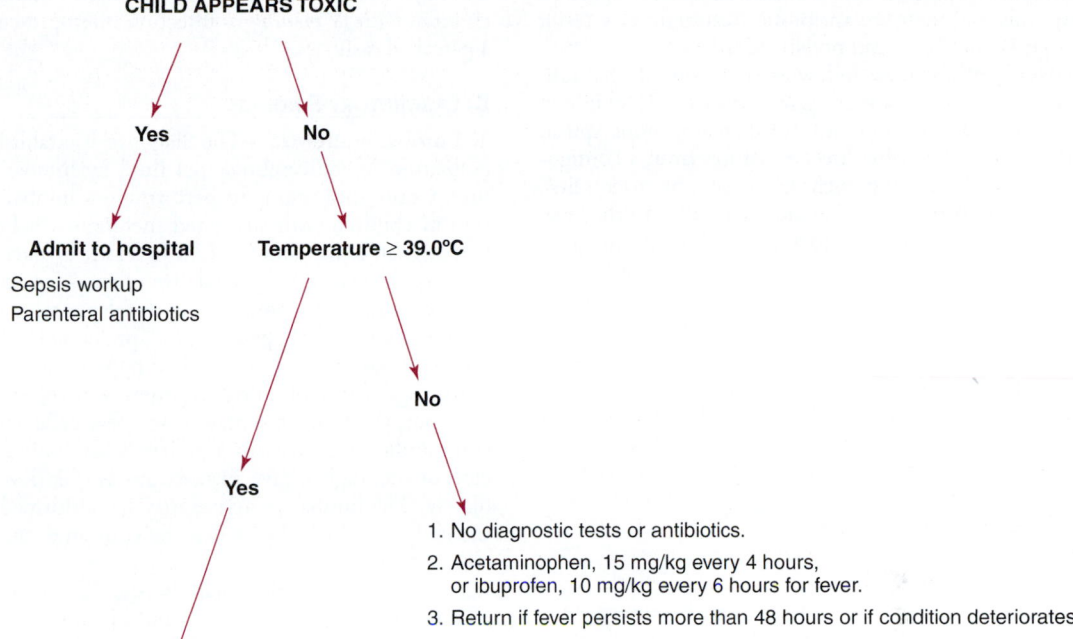

CHILD APPEARS TOXIC

Yes → **Admit to hospital**
Sepsis workup
Parenteral antibiotics

No → **Temperature ≥ 39.0°C**

No →
1. No diagnostic tests or antibiotics.
2. Acetaminophen, 15 mg/kg every 4 hours, or ibuprofen, 10 mg/kg every 6 hours for fever.
3. Return if fever persists more than 48 hours or if condition deteriorates.

Yes →

1a. Urine leukocyte esterase (LE) and nitrite or urinalysis and urine culture:

All males ≤ 6 months and uncircumcised males 6–12 months

All females < 12 months

If urine screening test positive: outpatient antibiotics (oral third-generation cephalosporin)

1b. Urine LE and nitrite or urinalysis and hold urine culture:

Circumcised males 6–12 months and all females 12–24 months

If urine screening test positive: send urine culture and outpatient antibiotics (oral third-generation cephalosporin)

2. For infants and children who have not received the conjugate *S pneumoniae* vaccine:

Temperature ≥ 39.5°C: obtain WBC count (or ANC) and hold blood culture

If WBC count ≥ 15,000 (for ANC ≥ 10,000):

Send blood culture

Ceftriaxone, 50 mg/kg up to 1 g

3. Chest radiograph: If O_2 saturation < 95%, respiratory distress, tachypnea, rales, or temperature ≥ 39.5°C and WBC count ≥ 20,000 (see below).

4. Acetaminophen: 15 mg/kg every 4 hours, or ibuprofen, 10 mg/kg every 6 hours for fever.

5. Return if fever persists more than 48 hours or condition deteriorates.

Follow-up of children treated as outpatients with positive culture results:

Blood culture positive (pathogen): Admit if febrile or ill-appearing
Outpatient antibiotics if afebrile and well

Urine culture positive (pathogen): Admit if febrile or ill-appearing
Outpatient antibiotics if afebrile and well

Figure 48–8. Algorithm for the management of a previously healthy child (3–36 months) with fever without a source. ANC = absolute neutrophil count; WBC = white blood cell. (Reproduced, with permission, from Baraff LJ: Management of fever without a source in infants and children. Ann Emerg Med 2000; 36:605.)

emergency physician because failure to make a prompt diagnosis and institute antibiotic treatment may result in significant illness and possibly death.

Meningitis occurs following invasion of the subarachnoid space by a pathogenic organism. In children, this occurs most commonly by hematogenous spread but may also occur by direct extension from a contiguous focus of infection such as sinusitis or mastoiditis. Disruption of the normal anatomic barriers to the cerebrospinal fluid secondary to a basilar skull fracture or a congenital sinus tract may also result in infection. Acute meningitis is usually of viral or bacterial origin (Table 48–13). The onset of meningitis in children usually follows one of 2 patterns: (1) The illness develops over several days as a nonspecific febrile illness, or (2) signs of central nervous infection develop over hours.

Clinical Findings

A. SYMPTOMS AND SIGNS

In infants, the clinical findings may be nonspecific: restlessness, irritability, poor feeding, emesis, diarrhea, lethargy, decreased tone, respiratory distress, full fontanelle (late finding), and seizures. Obvious neck stiffness or other signs of meningeal irritation (eg, Kernig or Brudzinski signs) are not reliably present in infants under age 18 months. In children over age 18 months, headache, nausea, vomiting, signs of increased intracranial pressure, focal neurologic signs, fever, lethargy, and photophobia are common. Infants and children with *N meningitis* infection often present with a petechial rash.

B. LABORATORY FINDINGS

1. Lumbar puncture—The diagnosis is established by evaluation of the cerebrospinal fluid by lumbar puncture. Contraindications to performing a lumbar puncture in children with suspected meningitis include (1) hemodynamic instability (child in shock or having respiratory difficulties), (2) evidence of mass lesion or increased intracranial pressure (eg, focal neurologic signs [hemiparesis, facial palsy, gaze preference], altered pupillary reactions, bradycardia, hypotension, apnea, posturing), (3) a bleeding disorder, and (4) infection overlying the lumbar puncture site (eg, cellulitis). If a contraindication exists in a patient with clinical suspicion of meningitis, give intravenous antibiotics immediately. The lumbar puncture may be performed when the child is stabilized or when the contraindication has resolved.

Cerebrospinal fluid analysis should include cell count, Gram staining, protein and glucose determinations, and culture (Table 48–14). The cell count in the cerebrospinal fluid should be performed quickly because delay over 90 minutes will result in lysis of white blood cells.

2. Other tests—Blood tests include peripheral white blood cell count and serum glucose determination. Ideally, these should be done before the lumbar puncture,

Table 48–13. Common causes of meningitis and empiric antibiotic therapy.

Age of patient	Common Bacterial Causes	Antibiotic	Dose	Other Causes
Preterm to < 1 month	Group B streptococcus E coli Listeria	Ampicillin plus cefotaxime or gentamicin	50 mg/kg, q 6–8 h 50 mg/kg q 8–12 h 2.5 mg/kg q 12 h	Enterovirus *Candida albicans*
1–3 months	Group B streptococcus E coli Listeria S pneumoniae N meningitidis H influenzae type B (*rare*)	Vancomycin plus cefotaxime or ceftriaxone	15 mg/kg q 6 h 50 mg/kg q 6 h 100 mg/kg q 24 h	Enterovirus
3 months–6 years	S pneumoniae N meningitidis H influenzae type B (*rare*)	Vancomycin plus cefotaxime or ceftriaxone	15 mg/kg q 6 h 50 mg/kg q 6 h 100 mg/kg q 24 h	Enterovirus Mumps M tuberculosis
> 6 years–adult	S pneumoniae N meningitidis	Vancomycin plus cefotaxime or ceftriaxone	15 mg/kg q 6 h 50 mg/kg q 6 h 100 mg/kg q 24 h	Enterovirus Mumps M tuberculosis

Table 48–14. Cerebrospinal fluid values in normal and disease states.[1]

Diagnosis	White Blood Cell Count (%PMN)	Glucose (% serum) (mg/dL)	Protein (mg/dL)	Gram Stain	Intracranial Pressure (mm H$_2$O)
Normal	< 6 (0)	> 40 (> 50)	< 35	Negative	< 180
Bacterial meningitis	200–10,000 (80–100)	< 40 (< 50)	100–500	Positive	> 200
Partially treated	200–10,000 (40–100)	< 40 (< 50)	100–500	Positive or negative	> 200
Viral	25–1000 (< 50)	> 40 (> 50)	50–100	Negative	< 180
Mycobacterial	50–1000 (< 50)	< 40	50–300	Negative	> 200

PMN = polymorphonuclear neutrophils.
[1]Adapted from Tureen J: Meningitis. In: *Pediatric Emergency Medicine: A Clinician's Reference.* Grossman M, Dieckmann RA (editors). Lippincott, 1991.

because both will increase during a lumbar puncture. It takes approximately 30 minutes for serum glucose to equilibrate with spinal fluid. Blood culture should also be performed and serum electrolytes obtained. The syndrome of inappropriate secretion of antidiuretic hormone (SIADH) may occur in acute meningitis, with resulting hyponatremia and volume overload. Urinalysis should be performed.

C. IMAGING

If a mass lesion or increased intracranial pressure is suspected, give antibiotics immediately and obtain an emergent CT scan.

Treatment

A. GENERAL MANAGEMENT

Assess the airway. In a child with significant central nervous system depression who has an impaired gag reflex or is hypoventilating, perform an elective orotracheal intubation.

Apply oxygen. Use 100% nonrebreathing reservoir bag-mask if the child is severely ill. Monitor with pulse oximetry. Attach an electrocardiographic monitor, and watch closely for bradycardia.

B. VOLUME RESUSCITATION

Assess the child's intravascular volume by means of blood pressure, heart rate, and capillary refill. Hypovolemia can compromise perfusion of the central nervous system. Aggressive rehydration is indicated if signs of hypovolemia are present. If the child is euvolemic, give fluids at two-thirds the normal maintenance rate until serum electrolyte results have been obtained. If evidence of SIADH is present, continue fluids at two-thirds the maintenance rate. If no SIADH is present,

increase intravenous fluids to the normal maintenance rate (see Table 48–5).

C. STEROID THERAPY

The administration of steroids (dexamethasone) in patients with bacterial meningitis is controversial. Studies have shown a benefit of steroids (although only statistically significant when the cause is *H. influenzae*) in reducing neurologic sequelae (sensorineural hearing loss) in patients with bacterial meningitis. In the post–Hib vaccine era, the current applicability of these results has been questioned because *H. influenzae* is now a rare cause of meningitis. Studies have suggested benefit for pneumococcal meningitis if steroids are commenced before or with antibiotics. Further complicating recommendations are concerns that steroids may decrease meningeal permeability, preventing adequate penetration of some antibiotics through the blood-brain barrier and resulting in subtherapeutic cerebrospinal fluid concentrations. Many authors still advocate steroids for children over age 2 months with bacterial meningitis. The recommended dose of dexamethasone is 0.15 mg/kg every 6 hours for 2–4 days, given before or concomitant with the initiation of antibiotic therapy.

D. ANTIMICROBIAL THERAPY

Administer antimicrobial therapy based on the child's age and the most likely pathogens (see Table 48–13). In critically ill children suspected of having meningitis, administer antibiotics rapidly without delay prior to lumbar puncture.

E. OTHER MEASURES

Treat seizures aggressively with anticonvulsants (see Figure 48–6).

Disposition

Children with proved or suspected bacterial meningitis require prompt hospitalization, ideally in an intensive care unit.

McIntyre PB et al: Dexamethasone as adjunctive therapy in bacterial meningitis. A meta-analysis of randomized clinical trials since 1988. JAMA 1997;278:925. [PMID: 9302246] (Meta-analysis.)

Quagliarello VJ, Scheld WM: Treatment of bacterial meningitis. N Engl J Med 1997;336:708. [PMID: 9041103] (Review.)

Wubbel L, McCracken GH: Management of bacterial meningitis: 1998. Pediatr Rev 1998;19:78. [PMID: 9509854] (Review.)

ACUTE OTITIS MEDIA

 ESSENTIALS OF DIAGNOSIS

- *Loss of light reflex or bulging tympanic membrane is suggestive of otitis media.*
- *Loss of mobility of the tympanic membrane with otitis media is sensitive and specific sign.*

General Considerations

After viral upper respiratory infection, otitis media is the next most common infectious pediatric disease. It accounts for up to one third of pediatric office visits and a high proportion of illness visits to the emergency department.

Acute otitis media results from auditory (eustachian) tube dysfunction, usually following an upper respiratory infection. In infants and children, *S. pneumoniae, H. influenzae,* and *Moraxella catarrhalis* are the most common pathogens.

Clinical Findings

The history is typically that of an infant or child who has had an upper respiratory infection for a few days and then presents with symptoms of ear pain. The pain of otitis media is typically acute in onset, severe, constant, and associated with hearing loss. Younger, preverbal children tend to have nonspecific symptoms of irritability, lethargy, gastrointestinal disturbances, and frequently poor sleeping. Children with acute otitis media may be afebrile or have only mild temperature elevation. High fever (> 40 °C [104 °F]) should alert the physician to the possibility of a more serious underlying infection, such as meningitis or pneumonia.

Older children can accurately describe the source of their pain. Pus may rupture through the tympanic membrane, producing a purulent discharge and a prompt decrease in pain. Otoscopy reveals an opaque white tympanic membrane bulging outward and loss of visible ossicles. Erythema of the tympanic membrane is a common finding but is not nearly as sensitive as loss of normal tympanic membrane landmarks. Decreased movement of the tympanic membrane, demonstrable by pneumatic otoscopy, is sensitive and specific.

Occasionally, facial nerve paralysis develops acutely. Vertigo and sensorineural hearing loss may occur if inflammation spreads to the inner ear and causes serous or purulent labyrinthitis. Mastoiditis occurs with infection of the bony structure of these air cells. The mastoid area becomes red, tender, and swollen. Typically the auricle is pushed laterally and downward.

No laboratory tests or x-rays are generally required. The bacteriology of otitis media has been clearly defined. Tympanocentesis is indicated only when unusual organisms may be present (eg, in neonates or immunosuppressed patients) or if acute otitis media is complicated by meningitis. If mastoiditis is a clinical concern, CT scan can detect small collections of fluid within the mastoid air cells as well as destruction of the bony septa.

Treatment

A. ANTIMICROBIAL THERAPY

Begin antimicrobial therapy (Figures 48–9 and 48–10, and Table 48–15). Consider alternative antibiotics if a child is less than age 24 months, attends daycare, has received multiple antibiotic courses, or has received antibiotics in the past 30 days. Treat uncomplicated otitis media for up to 10 days, and arrange for reevaluation.

B. TREATMENT OF PAIN AND FEVER

Treat associated pain and fever with acetaminophen or ibuprofen. A commercially available mixture of benzocaine, antipyrine, and oxyquinoline sulfate (Auralgan) applied topically into the ear canal may also provide pain relief.

C. TREATMENT FOR INFANTS UNDER AGE 4 WEEKS

Infants under age 4 weeks with acute otitis media require hospitalization because of the risk of associated hematogenous spread of disease. If fever is present or an infant appears ill, a full evaluation for meningitis and sepsis is required.

D. MANAGEMENT OF FACIAL NERVE PARALYSIS

If facial nerve paralysis accompanies acute otitis media, perform myringotomy, administer intravenous antibiotics, and hospitalize the patient.

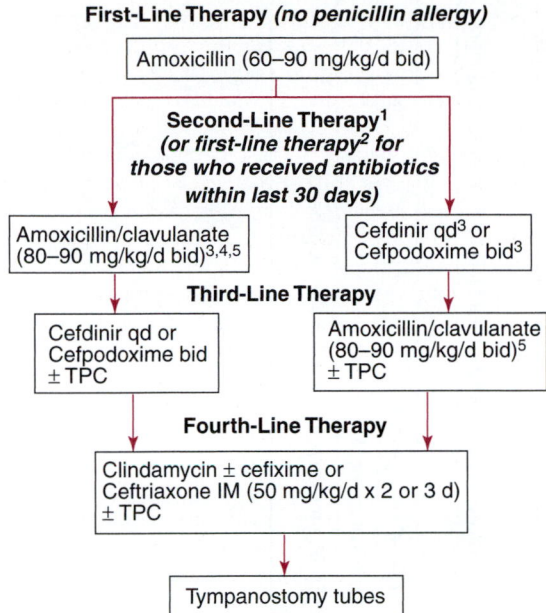

First-Line Therapy (no penicillin allergy)

Amoxicillin (60–90 mg/kg/d bid)

Second-Line Therapy[1]
(or first-line therapy[2] for
those who received antibiotics
within last 30 days)

Amoxicillin/clavulanate (80–90 mg/kg/d bid)[3,4,5]

Cefdinir qd[3] or Cefpodoxime bid[3]

Third-Line Therapy

Cefdinir qd or Cefpodoxime bid ± TPC

Amoxicillin/clavulanate (80–90 mg/kg/d bid)[5] ± TPC

Fourth-Line Therapy

Clindamycin ± cefixime or Ceftriaxone IM (50 mg/kg/d x 2 or 3 d) ± TPC

Tympanostomy tubes

Figure 48–9. Antibiotic choices for acute otitis media. TPC = tympanocentesis with culture and susceptibility testing. Recommendations are for children aged 3–36 months with acute otitis media (AOM).[1] If fully vaccinated with pneumococcal conjugated heptavalent vaccine, cefixime can be used as an alternative second-line antibiotic.[2] Azithromycin (5 days) may be an alternative for the older child with recurrent AOM who has (1) concomitant pneumonia suggestive of atypical pathogens or (2) significant gastroenteritis. Because azithromycin has limited coverage of *Haemophilus influenza* (~50%), some experts recommend adding trimethoprim-sulfamethoxazole.[3] Also AOM with concomitant conjunctivitis.[4] Also AOM with concomitant impetigo.[5] Augmentin ES-600 may be substituted. (Reproduced, with permission from Block SL, Harrison CJ: *Diagnosis and Management of Acute Otitis Media,* 1st ed. Professional Communications, 2001.)

E. Treatment of Mastoiditis

Treat mastoiditis like osteomyelitis. Perform myringotomy, culture, and Gram staining of middle ear fluid, and give antibiotics based on Gram-stain results. Drainage of the mastoid may be required.

Disposition

Modify risk factors for otitis media to improve resolution. For example, limit passive smoke exposure, control food and inhalant allergies, and treat sinusitis. The

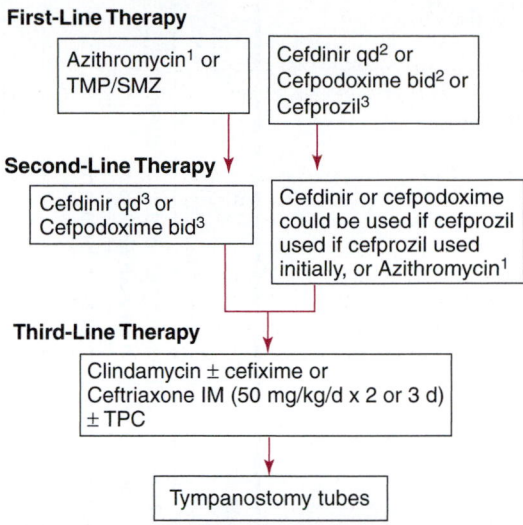

First-Line Therapy

Azithromycin[1] or TMP/SMZ

Cefdinir qd[2] or Cefpodoxime bid[2] or Cefprozil[3]

Second-Line Therapy

Cefdinir qd[3] or Cefpodoxime bid[3]

Cefdinir or cefpodoxime could be used if cefprozil used if cefprozil used initially, or Azithromycin[1]

Third-Line Therapy

Clindamycin ± cefixime or Ceftriaxone IM (50 mg/kg/d x 2 or 3 d) ± TPC

Tympanostomy tubes

Figure 48–10. Antibiotic choices for acute otitis media for the penicillin-allergic child. TMP-SMZ = trimethoprim-sulfamethoxazole; TPC = tympanocentesis with culture and susceptibility testing. Recommendations are for children aged 3–36 months with acute otitis media (AOM).[1] Because azithromycin has limited coverage of *Haemophilus influenza* (~50%), some experts recommend adding TMP-SMZ. Also AOM with concomitant pneumonia suggestive of atypical pathogens.[2] Also AOM with concomitant conjunctivitis.[3] With concomitant impetigo (*Staphylococcus aureus*). In AOM, coverage of β-lactamase-positive *H. influenza* is 10–25%. (Reproduced, with permission from Block SL, Harrison CJ: *Diagnosis and Management of Acute Otitis Media,* 1st ed. Professional Communications, 2001.)

primary benefit of antibiotics in treating acute otitis media is to decrease the incidence of suppurative complications (ie, mastoiditis) and to shorten the duration of symptoms.

A repeat ear examination should be performed at the end of therapy. Children should be reexamined if no clinical improvement occurs in 48 hours.

Dowell SF et al: Acute otitis media: management and surveillance in an era of pneumococcal resistance—a report from the Drug-Resistant *Streptococcus pneumoniae* Therapeutic Working Group. Pediatr Infect Dis J 1999;18:1. [PMID: 9951971] (Review.)

Hoberman A et al: Efficacy of Auralgan for treating ear pain in children with acute otitis media. Arch Pediatr Adolesc Med 1997;151:675. [PMID: 9232040] (Prospective randomized, controlled trial.)

Table 48–15. Drugs used for the treatment of acute otitis media.

Drug	Dosage	Comments
Amoxicillin (Amoxil)	40–60 mg/kg/d (bid) × 10 d	Standard dose for children without risk factors > age 24 months
Amoxicillin (Amoxil)	80–90 mg/kg/d (bid) × 10 d	Indicated for children > age 24 months with any risk factors (daycare attendance, multiple antibiotic courses, or antibiotics use in previous 30 days)
Amoxicillin-clavulanate (Augmentin)	80–90 mg/kg/d of amoxicillin 10 mg/kg/d of clavulanate (bid-tid) × 10 days	Alternative to high-dose amoxicillin, gastrointestinal intolerance common
Azithromycin (Zithromax)	10 mg/kg/d × 1 d then 5 mg/kg/d × 4 d	Alternative for penicillin-allergic patients
Cefdinir (Omnicef)	14 mg/kg/d (qd) × 10 d	Alternative to high-dose amoxicillin
Cefpodoxime (Vantin)	10 mg/kg/d (qd) × 10 d	Alternative to high-dose amoxicillin
Cefprozil (Cefzil)	30 mg/kg/d (bid) × 10 d	
Ceftriaxone (Rocephin)	50 mg/kg/d IM × 3 d	Documented efficacy in acute otitis media treatment failures from other antibiotics
Cefuroxime axetil (Ceftin)	30 mg/kg/d (bid) × 10 d	
Clarithromycin (Biaxin)	15 mg/kg/d (bid) × 10 d	Alternative for penicillin-allergic patients
Clindamycin (Cleocin)	25 mg/kg/d (tid)	No activity against *H influenzae* or *M catarrhalis*
Trimethoprim-sulfamethoxazole (TMP-SMZ; Septra, Bactrim)	8 mg/kg/d TMP 40 mg/kg/d SMZ (bid) × 10 d	No activity against DRSP, alternative for penicillin-allergic patients

DRSP = drug resistant *Streptococcus pneumoniae*.

Klein JO: Review of consensus reports on management of acute otitis media. Pediatr Infect Dis J 1999;18:1152. [PMID: 10608648] (Review.)

Louie JP, Bell LM: Appropriate use of antibiotics for common infections in an era of increasing resistance. Emerg Med Clin North Am 2002;20:69. [PMID: 11826638] (Review.)

Takata GS et al: Evidence assessment of management of acute otitis media: I. The role of antibiotics in treatment of uncomplicated acute otitis media. Pediatrics 2001;108:239. [PMID: 11483783] (Meta-analysis.)

PHARYNGITIS

General Considerations

Infections of the pharynx cause mucosal inflammation and ulceration, resulting in pain that is exacerbated by swallowing. The most common causes of pharyngitis in children are viruses and group A streptococci. Enteroviruses, particularly coxsackievirus, cause erythematous and vesicular lesions on the soft palate and pharynx. Other viruses associated with pharyngitis include adenovirus, influenza virus, parainfluenza virus, rhinovirus, Epstein-Barr virus, and RSV. Bacteria other than group A streptococci occasionally cause pharyngitis. *Corynebacterium diphtheriae* is now a rare cause of membranous pharyngitis in the United States. *Corynebacterium hemolyticum* has been associated with pharyngitis and erythematous rash in adolescents. Sexually active teenagers and victims of sexual abuse may have pharyngeal infection with *Neisseria gonorrhoeae*. *Mycoplasma pneumoniae* may also cause pharyngitis, but this is usually associated with more prominent lower respiratory tract infections. Acute uvulitis has been associated with *H. influenzae* type B.

Clinical Findings

Most cases of streptococcal pharyngitis are in school-aged children, but recent studies have suggested that disease can be found in all age groups including children younger than age 2 years. Common presenting signs and symptoms include fever, sore throat, pharyngeal hyperemia, exudate, or petechiae. The characteristic erythematous fine, raised, generalized "sandpaper" rash of scarlet fever supports the diagnosis of streptococcal infection (see Table 48–18). Abdominal pain and headache are frequent findings in children with streptococcal pharyngitis and may distract the physician from the diagnosis.

Throat cultures remain the most practical and reliable means of diagnosing streptococcal pharyngitis. Rapid detection of streptococcal antigen from throat swabs is possible, but because the sensitivity is only 76–87%, a negative test should be followed by a throat culture.

The white blood cell count may be elevated with streptococcal pharyngitis, but this is a nonspecific finding. White blood cell count may also be increased with Epstein-Barr virus infection, where the blood smear will show 10–20% atypical lymphocytes and a mononucleosis test (Monospot, many others) is positive. Children over age 4 years with infectious mononucleosis will develop heterophilic antibodies 1–2 weeks into the course of infection in 30% of cases. Heterophilic antibodies are less common in children under age 4 years.

Tonsillar infections with group A streptococci may extend into surrounding tissues and result in peritonsillar cellulitis or abscess; the child will usually present with fever, toxicity, muffled voice, tender superior cervical lymphadenopathy, trismus, and drooling. Peritonsillar abscess is commonly unilateral. Initially there is edema and erythema of the soft palate and tonsil and frequently but not invariably a whitish tonsillar exudate. Peritonsillar abscess is characterized by deviation of the tonsil and soft palate on the affected side medially, causing the uvula to point away from the side of the abscess. Retropharyngeal or lateral pharyngeal abscesses may also develop in concert with group A streptococcal pharyngitis and are often associated with stridor and signs similar to those of peritonsillar abscess.

Treatment

A. SYMPTOMATIC THERAPY

Use symptomatic therapy to decrease discomfort, including acetaminophen and saltwater gargles.

B. ANTIMICROBIAL THERAPY

If streptococcal pharyngitis is likely, begin antibiotic therapy at the time of the examination. The duration of symptoms can be decreased if treatment is begun before culture results are available.

Prescribe oral penicillin (or an alternative) for suspected streptococcal pharyngitis. If antibiotic therapy is initiated within 7–9 days of onset of illness, acute rheumatic fever can be prevented.

1. Penicillin V—Dosing of penicillin V for children under age 12 years is 250 mg 2 or 3 times daily for 10 days; dosing for adolescents is 500 mg 2 or 3 times daily for 10 days.

2. Benzathine penicillin G—If compliance is a problem, benzathine penicillin G, 25,000 units/kg intramuscularly (maximum, 1.2 million units), is a good alternative to the multiple-daily dosing of penicillin V. The pain may be lessened if it is used in a mixture with procaine penicillin G. The total dose is still based on the amount of benzathine penicillin G.

3. Alternatives for penicillin-allergic patients—For children allergic to penicillin, the macrolides are the drug of choice. Erythromycin estolate, 40 mg/kg/d divided 2–4 times daily for 10 days; erythromycin ethylsuccinate, 40 mg/kg/d divided 2–4 times daily for 10 days; clarithromycin, 15 mg/kg/d 2 times daily for 10 days; or azithromycin, 12 mg/kg/d for 5 days are all approved by the U.S. Food and Drug Administration.

C. RAPID ANTIGEN TEST

If the rapid antigen test is positive, begin treatment. A negative rapid antigen test should be followed up with a throat culture.

D. TREATMENT FOR PERITONSILLAR CELLULITIS

Treat early stages of peritonsillar cellulitis on an outpatient basis with penicillin and follow-up. If the disease has progressed to deviation of the soft palate and uvula, hospitalize the child and initiate intravenous antibiotics with aqueous penicillin G, 250,000 units/kg/d in divided doses every 4 hours, after needle aspiration. Consult an otorhinolaryngologist if the abscess cannot be aspirated easily and for consideration of definitive incision and drainage.

Disposition

A repeat examination is indicated if no improvement occurs in 48 hours. Particularly in older children and adolescents, a mononucleosis test should then be done. Children with early signs of peritonsillar abscess must be reexamined in 12–24 hours.

Berkovitch M et al: Group A streptococcal pharyngotonsillitis in children less than 2 years of age—more common than thought. Clin Pediatr 1999;38:361. [PMID: 10378094] (Prospective randomized, controlled trial.)

Hayes CS, Williamson H: Management of group A beta-hemolytic streptococcal pharyngitis. Am Fam Physician 2001;63:1557. [PMID: 11327431] (Review.)

Louie JP, Bell LM: Appropriate use of antibiotics for common infections in an era of increasing resistance. Emerg Med Clin North Am 2002;20:69. [PMID: 11826638] (Review.)

PERIORBITAL CELLULITIS

ESSENTIALS OF DIAGNOSIS

- *Erythema and swelling around the eye.*
- *No pain with range of motion of the extraocular muscles.*
- *No diplopia or proptosis.*

Clinical Findings

Periorbital swelling is a common problem in children. The primary task is to differentiate serious and life-threatening causes of this finding from those that are benign. Cellulitis restricted to the eyelid is preseptal or periorbital. Orbital cellulitis refers to infection involving orbital contents posterior to the septum. Differentiation of these 2 entities is essential to management. Table 48–16 lists the differential considerations of periorbital swelling. Periorbital cellulitis can be classified as secondary to sinusitis (group I), secondary to disruption of local skin integrity (group II), or secondary to bacteremia with no apparent predisposing focus (group III).

A. GROUP I

Periorbital swelling from sinusitis is usually subacute in onset, evolves over several days, and is neither tender nor indurated. Fever is typically absent or low grade. This condition can occur at any age, but it is rare in infancy. X-rays show sinus opacification. Blood cultures are almost always negative. This is the most common

Table 48–16. Differential diagnosis of periorbital swelling.[1]

Diagnosis	Onset	Appearance	Other Features
Periorbital and orbital cellulitis	Rapid	Reddish, violaceous	Usually unilateral Tender swelling with fever
Trauma	Variable	Reddish, blue	Tense or soft nontender Swelling not associated with fever
Insect bite	Variable	Red, no color	Bite may be visible
Allergic reaction	Rapid	No color	Bilateral, nontender, afebrile
Reactive edema	Days	No color	Unilateral or bilateral evidence of sinusitis

[1]Adapted, with permission, from Luten RC: Evaluation of periorbital swelling. In: *The Emergency Ill Child.* Barkin R (editor). Aspen Publishers, 1987.

form of periorbital cellulitis and is caused by organisms that commonly cause sinusitis (ie, nontypeable *H influenzae, S pneumoniae, M catarrhalis, S pyogenes,* and anaerobic bacteria).

B. Group II

Primary skin infection about the eye may result from secondary infection, prior trauma, or insect bite. There is rapid onset of tender and indurated preseptal swelling with fever. Blood cultures are typically negative. *S aureus* and group A streptococci are the most common pathogens. Human and animal bites may produce a polymicrobial infection.

C. Group III

Children with idiopathic periorbital cellulitis are generally younger than those in the previous 2 groups. These children have a history of a mild upper respiratory infection for 1–5 days followed by rapid onset of high fever and preseptal swelling. Swelling is often tender and indurated. Prior to the institution of the Hib vaccine, *H. influenzae* was a common organism causing periorbital cellulitis as a complication of bacteremia. Current cases are most likely to be from *S. pneumoniae.*

Orbital cellulitis can be distinguished clinically from periorbital cellulitis by the presence of proptosis, ophthalmoplegia, pain on eye movement, and loss of vision. Patients are usually febrile; blood cultures are usually negative. Orbital cellulitis is usually secondary to extension of pus from sinusitis (usually ethmoidal) into the orbit or due to penetrating orbital trauma. The most common bacterial organisms include *S. pneumoniae, M. catarrhalis, S. aureus, H. influenzae* (in nonimmunized patients), and anaerobes.

Management of orbital cellulitis should include blood cultures and CBC if the patient is febrile or appears bacteremic. Infants under age 3 months with these symptoms should be worked up as outlined in Figure 48–7. Obtain a CT scan without contrast for all patients suspected of having orbital cellulitis. Mild cases may be managed with daily ceftriaxone injections. More severe cases should receive inpatient intravenous antibiotics (second- or third-generation cephalosporins). A nasal decongestant and warm compresses may also be beneficial to patients.

Treatment

A. Afebrile Patients

Consider ambulatory therapy for children with early mild periorbital cellulitis who are afebrile and do not appear ill. Use ceftriaxone, 50–75 mg/kg/d intramuscularly for 5 days, or amoxicillin-clavulanate, 45 mg/kg/d divided twice daily for children weighing more than 40 kg, and perform a repeat evaluation in 24 hours. If contiguous skin infection is present, treat with dicloxacillin, 25 mg/kg/d divided 4 times daily.

B. Febrile Patients

Hospitalize any child with periorbital swelling who is febrile and appears ill. Begin intravenous antibiotic therapy. For young children whose periorbital cellulitis is not secondary to an external skin infection, give cefuroxime, 100 mg/kg/d divided 3 times daily, or ceftriaxone, 100 mg/kg/d divided twice daily. For children whose infection is secondary to an external skin source, use nafcillin, 50–200 mg/kg/d in divided doses every 6 hours.

Hospitalize children with orbital cellulitis secondary to direct extension from a contiguous sinus, or a subperiosteal abscess, for treatment with intravenous antibiotics. Coverage for *H. influenzae, S. pneumoniae, S. aureus,* and anaerobes must be included (ie, ceftriaxone, 50–100 mg/kg/d divided twice daily, and clindamycin, 15–40 mg/kg/d divided 3 or 4 times daily). Consult an ophthalmologist whenever orbital cellulitis is suspected.

Disposition

Children with acute onset of fever, toxicity, and periorbital swelling should be hospitalized promptly for intravenous antibiotic therapy. Children less acutely ill who receive outpatient treatment should be reexamined in 12–24 hours.

Donahue SP, Schwartz G: Preseptal and orbital cellulitis in childhood. Ophthalmology 1998;105:1902. [PMID: 9787362] (Retrospective chart review and discussion.)

Mawn LA et al: Preseptal and orbital cellulitis. Ophthalmol Clin North Am 2000;13:633. (Review.)

URINARY TRACT INFECTION

General Considerations

Urinary tract infections are relatively common in children. Risk in the first 10 years of life for boys and girls is 1.1% and 3.5%, respectively. About 40% of these children will have recurrent infections.

In children, *E. coli* is the predominant pathogen (approximately 95% of initial infections and 80% of all infections). Other organisms causing urinary tract infections are *Klebsiella, Proteus mirabilis* (particularly in males), coagulase-negative staphylococci (in adolescent females), adenovirus (hemorrhagic cystitis), *Chlamydia trachomatis* (frequency-dysuria syndrome), *Pseudomonas, Streptococcus faecalis, Streptococcus viridans, N. gonorrhoeae, Ureaplasma urealyticum,* herpes simplex virus, and *H. influenzae* (uncommon).

Children with congenital anomalies of the urinary tract are at increased risk for infection. Vesicoureteral reflux is present in over 30% of children with urinary tract infection. Other abnormalities include obstruction at the level of the urethra, bladder, or ureter and duplication of the urinary tract and ureteroceles. In male infants, increased susceptibility to infection may be related to an uncircumcised penis.

In the first months of life, urinary tract infections are most common in males. By age 4 months, however, urinary tract infections are 10 times more common in females, and this female predominance continues through childhood and adolescence. Approximately one third of newborns with urinary tract infection are bacteremic. By age 1–3 months, the incidence of bacteremia with urinary tract infection is decreased to 18%; and by age 3–8 months, the incidence is 6%.

Clinical Findings

In the neonate, nonspecific symptoms predominate. Poor feeding, irritability, fever, vomiting, diarrhea, and slow weight gain are common symptoms. The neonate may also develop a direct hyperbilirubinemia. In infants aged 1 month to 2 years, nonspecific symptoms still predominate. Alert parents may note urinary frequency, dribbling, weak stream, and abdominal distress during voiding. Many young infants with urinary tract infection are febrile. In preschool and school-aged children, dysuria is a frequent symptom and may be accompanied by abdominal and flank pain, frequency, urgency, enuresis, and fever. Dysuria is a nonspecific symptom in children, however. Dysuria in children often has causes other than urinary tract infection, such as chemical urethritis from strong soaps, diaper rash, herpes, or pinworm. In adolescent females, dysuria and frequency are common with urinary tract infection but may also be secondary to vaginitis or the acute urethral syndrome.

The key to diagnosis is demonstration of bacteria in the urine. Methods of collecting urine in children include a urine bag taped to the perineum, clean-catch specimens, bladder catheterization, and suprapubic aspiration. The urine specimen collected by bag is helpful only if it proves to be negative. Most positive cultures from urine bag specimens in infants and newborns represent contamination. Febrile infants under age 3 months who are likely to be admitted to the hospital should undergo either bladder catheterization (using an 8–10F pediatric feeding tube) or suprapubic aspiration. Older infants and children should undergo bladder catheterization if the bag urine specimen shows evidence of infection. Midstream clean-catch specimens are acceptable in children who can void on command.

Urine test strips using a nitrite and leukocyte esterase indicator are helpful. Most urinary pathogens will convert nitrite to nitrate, and false-positive reactions are uncommon. However, false-negative results can occur with urinary pathogens unable to convert nitrite to nitrate (eg, *Staphylococcus saprophyticus,* enterococci). Therefore, if the urine test strip is negative for nitrite and clinical findings or history suggest possible urinary infection, other tests are still indicated.

Urine collected by the clean-catch method is likely to be infected if more than 10^4 colonies of a single organism are found. If urine is collected by bladder catheterization or suprapubic aspiration, 10^3 colonies or more of a single organism represents infection. More than 5 white blood cells per high-power field of urine sediment in a child who is symptomatic for urinary tract infection is highly suggestive. However, pyuria alone is not a reliable guide for identification of a urinary tract infection. Any bacterium present on Gram staining of unspun urine, when viewed under oil immersion, is a sensitive indicator of urinary tract infection.

Obtain a blood culture in neonates, infants, and any child who is highly febrile. Assume that children with fever, back pain, and costovertebral angle tenderness have pyelonephritis. As many as 25% of children with urinary tract infections and no symptoms of pyelonephritis have upper tract disease. No effective noninvasive means exist to identify upper tract infections.

Treatment

A. OUTPATIENT TREATMENT

In children who are to receive outpatient treatment, use oral antibiotics effective against *E. coli.* Cystitis should be treated for 7 days, whereas pyelonephritis and febrile urinary tract infection should be treated for 10–14 days. Treatment options include the following: TMP-SMZ, 6–12 mg/kg/d TMP and 30–60 mg/kg/d SMZ; sulfisoxazole, 120–150 mg/kg/d; amoxicillin, 20–40 mg/kg/d; cephalexin, 50–100 mg/kg/d; or cefixime, 8 mg/kg/d. Phenazopyridine, 10 mg/kg/day divided every 8 hours, can be used for symptomatic relief.

Outpatient therapy can be instituted for febrile but nontoxic-appearing children older than age 3 months, provided they can tolerate fluids and medications by mouth. Follow-up should occur at 24–48 hours. It is advisable to administer a parenteral first dose of antibiotics (intravenous or intramuscular gentamicin or third-generation cephalosporin) in the emergency department, and start oral antibiotics at home. Any child, regardless of age, who appears toxic should be admitted for parenteral antibiotics.

B. Inpatient Treatment

Hospitalize neonates and young infants with urinary tract infections, and give intravenous antibiotics on the presumption of pyelonephritis. Use ampicillin, 100 mg/kg/d in divided doses every 12 hours, and gentamicin, 7.5 mg/kg/d in divided doses every 8 hours.

C. Evaluation for Urinary Tract Anomalies

Because of the frequency of urinary tract anomalies in children who have urinary tract infections, evaluation of the urinary tract by sonogram and voiding cystourethrogram are frequently indicated in boys of any age; girls aged 2 months to 2 years with their first culture-proven urinary tract infection; and children with febrile urinary tract infection or pyelonephritis. The sonogram can be done during the acute illness if necessary. Order a voiding cystourethrogram approximately 1 month after diagnosis. Postpubertal females with recurrent uncomplicated cystitis do not require imaging studies.

Disposition

Admit infants, febrile or not, under age 3 months with urinary tract infection for intravenous antibiotic administration. Nontoxic-appearing, febrile, older infants and children with urinary tract infection can receive treatment on an outpatient basis with follow-up at 24–48 hours.

Children receiving outpatient treatment will require a repeat urine culture to document cure in 1 week. At 24- to 48-hour follow-up, check the urine culture to ensure appropriate antibiotic selection. If clinical improvement is not evident, consider hospitalization for parenteral antibiotics. Discharge instructions should caution parents to return if persistent vomiting, lethargy, or other worsening symptoms occur.

Santen SA, Altieri MF: Pediatric urinary tract infections. Emerg Med Clin North Am 2001;19:675. [PMID: 11554281] (Review.)

Shaw K, Gorelick MH: Urinary tract infection in the pediatric patient. Pediatr Clin North Am 1999;46:1111. [PMID: 10629676] (Review.)

GASTROENTERITIS

General Considerations

Diarrhea is a common reason for bringing a child to medical attention. Dehydration frequently complicates diarrhea in children, particularly in young infants who experience a greater net fluid and electrolyte loss. Acute diarrhea in children most commonly results from infectious gastroenteritis. Keys to management include identification of children who will benefit from antimicrobial therapy, prevention or treatment of dehydration, and identification of children with diarrhea secondary to other processes (eg, intussusception, hemolytic uremic syndrome). In the United States, rotavirus is the most common cause of acute diarrhea, particularly in winter months.

Clinical Findings

A. Symptoms and Signs

Information regarding the duration of diarrhea, number of stools per day, frequency of urination, presence of tears when crying, and most recent weight of the child are helpful in assessing the risk of dehydration. A history of frequent vomiting, particularly early in the course of the disease, suggests a viral cause. High fever, lack of vomiting, abdominal pain with bowel movements, and the presence of gross blood and mucus in the stool suggest a bacterial cause. A history of recent antibiotic use suggests the possibility of pseudomembranous colitis. A history of recent travel suggests the possibility of a parasitic infection or traveler's diarrhea. Children in daycare are particularly susceptible to infections with *Giardia lamblia*. Inquire about a common outbreak of symptoms in family members that may suggest food poisoning. When more than one member of the family has symptoms of nausea, vomiting, or headache, explore the possibility of carbon monoxide poisoning. Assess the child's hydration status, and look for signs of appendicitis or intussusception. Serial abdominal examinations are recommended to rule out surgical conditions. Gastroenteritis is one of the most common diagnoses listed in cases of missed appendicitis.

B. Laboratory Findings

1. Stool culture—A stool culture is the most reliable means of identifying a bacterial cause. It is not cost effective, however, to culture the stool of every child with diarrhea. Obtain cultures from children at highest risk for bacterial disease. Stool cultures for *Shigella*, *Salmonella*, and *Campylobacter* should be obtained in the following circumstances:

- If the child presents with obvious symptoms of acute bacterial dysentery (ie, fever, watery stool, fecal leukocytes, and gross blood in the stool).
- If the child has abrupt onset of frequent stools without the initial vomiting common to viral gastroenteritis. Perform methylene blue slide examination for the presence of fecal leukocytes. A positive result

(> 5 white blood cells per high-power field) is a sensitive indicator of a bacterial pathogen. Trophozoites of *G. lamblia* may also be identified.

- If the child has hemoglobinopathies or immunodeficiencies.

2. Peripheral white blood cell count—A peripheral white blood cell count may be helpful, because *Salmonella* and *Shigella* can cause leukocytosis. Some patients with *Shigella* infection may have a low white blood cell count with a marked shift to the left.

3. Other laboratory tests—If the child appears dehydrated, check serum electrolytes, BUN, creatinine, and fingerstick blood sugar. Blood cultures are also indicated in young infants with bloody diarrhea and any child who appears significantly ill.

If the child is in daycare or has a history of recent travel, examine the stool examined for parasites.

Treatment

A. REHYDRATION

The use of oral rehydration solutions for children with mild to moderate dehydration and of intravenous fluids for children with more severe dehydration is critical to prevent severe morbidity and mortality. Breast-feeding infants should continue to breast feed while taking oral rehydration.

B. ANTIEMETICS AND ANTIDIARRHEAL AGENTS

Antiemetic and antidiarrheal drugs occasionally worsen symptoms in children with gastroenteritis.

C. ANTIMICROBIAL THERAPY

The empiric use of antibiotic therapy is indicated for obvious symptoms of bacterial dysentery. TMP-SMZ (TMP, 8–12 mg/kg/d, and SMZ, 30–60 mg/kg/d, in divided doses every 12 hours) can be given empirically until culture results are available.

Disposition

Hospitalize children with moderate to severe dehydration, particularly if vomiting prohibits oral rehydration, and young infants with fever and bloody diarrhea. Young infants are at increased risk for *Salmonella* bacteremia.

Instruct parents about the signs of dehydration and the proper use of oral rehydration solutions. Parents should encourage children to continue small but frequent amounts of liquids at home and to resume a normal diet as tolerated.

Infants under 6 months of age should be followed up by telephone or be seen in 24 hours. Reevaluate older children if diarrhea persists longer than 3 days. Children with bloody diarrhea should be reexamined in 24 hours.

SEPTIC ARTHRITIS

 ESSENTIALS OF DIAGNOSIS

- *Patient usually febrile.*
- *Involved joint is tender, swollen, erythematous with painful range of motion.*
- *Aspiration with fluid analysis is diagnostic.*

General Considerations

Septic arthritis is an acute bacterial infection of a joint. Delay in treatment may result in permanent damage and loss of function of the infected joint. Septic arthritis in children usually occurs through hematogenous seeding. It may also result from contiguous spread of osteomyelitis or through a penetrating injury. The bacterial cause is age related (Table 48–17). Special clinical

Table 48–17. Causes and antibiotic therapies for septic arthritis and osteomyelitis in infants and children.[1]

Age	Possible Pathogen	Therapy for Septic Arthritis	Therapy for Osteomyelitis
0–3 months	Gram negative rods, group B streptococcus	Ampicillin, 100 mg/kg/d, plus gentamicin, 7.5 mg/kg/d, or cefotaxime, 100–150 mg/kg/d	Ampicillin, 200 mg/kg/d, plus gentamicin, 7.5 mg/kg/d
3 months–5 years	S aureus, rarely H influenzae	Nafcillin, 100–200 mg/kg/d, plus cefotaxime, 100–150 mg/kg/d	Nafcillin, 100–200 mg/kg/d, plus cefotaxime, 150 mg/kg/d
> 5 years	S aureus, group A streptococcus	Nafcillin, 100–200 mg/kg/d	Nafcillin, 100–200 mg/kg/d

[1]Modified, with permission, from Nurico S, Walker WA: Acute diarrhea. In: Dersheurtz RA (editor): *Ambulatory Pediatric Care.* Lippincott, 1980.

situations include *N. gonorrhoeae* joint infections in young children who have been sexually abused and patients with sickle cell disease, who are at a high risk for joint infections with *Salmonella.*

Clinical Findings

A. SYMPTOMS AND SIGNS

Almost all patients have fever and malaise. Typically the infected joint is hot, painful, and swollen and has overlying erythema. Early in the disease, the child may present with an unexplained limp. In young infants with hip involvement, the obvious findings of swelling and erythema may be absent. More commonly the infant will not move the leg on the infected side and will keep the leg abducted and externally rotated. Movement of the hip causes pain. Patients with toxic synovitis may have similar complaints but in general have a lower-grade temperature and less pain on joint manipulation.

B. LABORATORY FINDINGS

1. Joint aspiration—Definitive diagnosis is established by joint aspiration. Examine joint fluid for cell count and differential, Gram staining and culture, protein and glucose determinations, and mucin clot. Synovial white blood cell count greater than 50,000 is considered positive for septic arthritis. Gram staining of joint fluid is important, because up to 33% of joint aspirates may be sterile.

2. Blood tests—CBC, C-reactive protein, and erythrocyte sedimentation rate are helpful, particularly when considering noninfectious diagnoses. Perform a blood culture, because it may produce a pathogen even with a negative joint aspirate culture.

C. IMAGING

Radiographic studies of the joint are of limited help in the older child with obvious joint infection. They usually demonstrate capsular swelling. Radiographic studies may be helpful in the evaluation of the hip, because the physical examination may not be definitive. Ultrasound may be able to identify small joint effusions.

Radionuclide studies may show diffuse uptake within the joint. MRI may be helpful in differentiating septic arthritis from transient or toxic synovitis.

Treatment

Successful management depends on prompt antibiotic therapy (see Table 48–17) and surgical drainage as indicated. Gram staining may be helpful in guiding choice of antibiotics.

Septic arthritis of the hip is a surgical emergency, and these patients should undergo prompt surgical drainage. Children with sickle cell disease should receive adequate therapy for *Salmonella* until culture results are known.

Disposition

Hospitalize children with suspected septic arthritis for intravenous antibiotic therapy. Obtain orthopedic consultation to evaluate the need for surgical drainage of the involved joint.

Leet AI, Skaggs DL: Evaluation of the acutely limping child. Am Fam Physician 2000;61:1011. [PMID: 10706154] (Review.)

ACUTE OSTEOMYELITIS

 ESSENTIALS OF DIAGNOSIS

- *Usually warm, tender, swollen area.*
- *Initially x-rays may be normal.*
- *Bone scan may be diagnostic.*

General Considerations

Acute osteomyelitis is a pyogenic infection of bone that occurs in about 1 in 5000 children before the age of 13 years. Although any bone may be involved, in children the long bones are more frequently infected. Infection usually is the result of seeding, although spread from a contiguous focus or through direct traumatic inoculation can also occur.

Over 90% of cases of acute hematogenous osteomyelitis are caused by *S. aureus.* Group A streptococci and *H. influenzae* are less common causes. In neonates, osteomyelitis may also be caused by group B streptococci and gram-negative enteric organisms. Children with sickle cell disease are at risk for *Salmonella* and *S. pneumoniae* osteomyelitis. Puncture wounds to the plantar surface of the foot may result in *Pseudomonas aeruginosa* osteomyelitis.

Clinical Findings

A. SYMPTOMS AND SIGNS

The clinical hallmarks are fever and well-localized bone tenderness. Chills, malaise, and appearance of illness are frequently present. Lower extremity disease will frequently result in a limp. Point tenderness is usually evident on careful examination. There may also be swelling, warmth, redness, and focal induration at the site of infection. The young infant is usually irritable when the affected extremity is touched or moved. Pseudoparalysis is common, and occasionally significant swelling of the extremity will occur.

B. LABORATORY FINDINGS

Draw blood for culture, CBC, C-reactive protein, and erythrocyte sedimentation rate. Blood cultures are positive in about 30–50% of patients with osteomyelitis. Obtain orthopedic consultation regarding aspiration of bone at the site of tenderness, because there may be some risk of epiphyseal damage.

C. IMAGING

Obtain plain x-rays of the affected extremity. Radiographic changes are usually not evident until 7–10 days after disease onset. However, soft tissue swelling and obliteration of the tissue planes may be the initial radiographic findings. Later findings include periosteal reaction and osteolysis.

After the child has been admitted to the hospital, technetium bone scans may be helpful.

Treatment

The mainstay of treatment of acute bacterial hematogenous osteomyelitis is parenteral antibiotics (see Table 48–17). Because culture results are usually not available when the diagnosis is first made, empiric therapy depends on the patient's age.

In children with puncture wound osteomyelitis of the foot, surgical debridement is an important part of therapy. Parenteral antibiotics active against *Pseudomonas* should be started.

Disposition

Hospitalize children in whom acute osteomyelitis is suspected.

Kothari NA, Pelchovitz DJ, Meyer JS: Imaging of musculoskeletal infections. Radiol Clin North Am 2001;39:653. [PMID: 11549164] (Review.)

EXANTHEMS
(See Table 48–18.)

Important considerations are the child's age, the time of year, knowledge of illnesses currently present in the community, history of exposure to individuals with rashes, medication history, prodromal symptoms such as fever, and initial appearance and progression of the rash. Note how ill the child appears, the morphology and distribution of the rash, mucous membrane involvement, associated lymphadenopathy, and presence of hepatosplenomegaly.

Gable EK, Liu G, Morrell DS: Pediatric exanthems. Prim Care 2000;27:353. [PMID: 10815048] (Review.)

■ GASTROINTESTINAL DISORDERS

ABDOMINAL PAIN

General Considerations

Abdominal pain is a common complaint. Causes are many and include both intra-abdominal and systemic illnesses. The child presenting with acute severe abdominal pain may have an acute abdomen requiring immediate surgical intervention. Recognition of the acute abdomen in children may be difficult but is critical in reducing morbidity and mortality.

Abdominal pain can originate from 3 neural pathways. Visceral pain originates from distention of a viscus, which stimulates nerves locally that send impulses to the central nervous system through autonomic parasympathetic fibers. Because these nerve fibers from different organs overlap, visceral pain is not specific to the site of the viscus involved. Somatic pain is generally intense and well localized. It arises from irritation of the parietal perineum. Frequently there is abdominal muscle reflex spasm over the site of pain. Referred pain is somatic or visceral in origin but is felt elsewhere.

Common causes of abdominal pain in infants are colic, constipation, gastroenteritis, intussusception, viral syndrome, and volvulus; in younger children, appendicitis, constipation, gastroenteritis, pneumonia, streptococcal pharyngitis, urinary tract infection, and viral syndrome; and in school-aged children, appendicitis, pregnancy, gastroenteritis, pneumonia, peptic ulcer, and pelvic inflammatory disease. Other more rare causes include pancreatitis, Henoch-Schönlein purpura, and hemolytic uremic syndrome.

Clinical Findings

See Table 48–19.

A. SYMPTOMS AND SIGNS

Note the nature of the pain, including time of onset, duration, severity, and location; associated gastrointestinal symptoms, including anorexia, vomiting, diarrhea, and constipation; associated systemic symptoms, including fever, cough, sore throat, dysuria, rash, and joint pain; and history of significant disease, particularly sickle cell disease, renal disease, and gynecologic disorders (for adolescents). Obtain a thorough menstrual, sexual, and medication history from the patient.

Obtain accurate vital signs. Observe the child over a period of time. Children with colicky pain may appear quiet and even lethargic and then suddenly develop crampy pain. Perform a complete physical examination, and assess the child's state of hydration and perfusion. Group A streptococcal pharyngitis and lower lobe pneumonia are 2 common sources of referred abdominal pain. Inspect the abdomen for signs of generalized distention or visible bowel loops. Auscultate the abdomen to evaluate the nature of the bowel sounds. Decreased or absent bowel sounds may signal an ileus, whereas sudden rushes of bowel sounds associated with crampy abdominal pain may indicate the presence of an intussusception. Gently seek out the areas of maximal tenderness. Careful percussion will determine areas of rebound pain. Perform a rectal examination. In boys, examine the testicles to rule out epididymitis or testicular torsion. In sexually active girls, rule out pelvic inflammatory disease. Appendicitis, which is the most common nontraumatic surgical emergency in the pediatric population, must be considered in all children who present with abdominal pain. Incidence peaks in adolescent years, but appendicitis has also been reported in neonates and infants. Perforation is nearly universal in children younger than age 3 years old compared to the less than 15% rate of perforation in adolescents. Common presenting symptoms in children younger than age 3 years include emesis, pain, diarrhea, and fever. Irritability, grunting respirations, cough, and right hip complaints may also be present. Localized tenderness to digital examination of the rectum may disclose a retrocecal appendix.

B. Laboratory Findings

1. Urinalysis—Look for evidence of a urinary tract infection. More than 5 white or red blood cells per high-power field are occasionally seen in patients with appendicitis.

2. Complete blood count with differential—CBC with differential may be useful in suggesting an infectious cause for abdominal pain. The white blood cell count is an insensitive and nonspecific test and cannot be used to rule out appendicitis.

3. Other laboratory studies—Electrolytes, BUN, and creatinine measurements should be obtained for children who appear dehydrated after protracted vomiting or diarrhea. Consider lipase, and hepatic function tests if biliary disease, pancreatitis, or hepatitis are possible causes. Obtain a serum pregnancy test in adolescent girls.

B. Imaging

Obtain a chest x-ray for children with abdominal pain and respiratory symptoms (ie, cough, tachypnea).

Lower lobe pneumonia in children may frequently result in referred pain to the abdomen that can mimic an acute abdomen. Obtain flat and upright, or decubitus, abdominal films for children with an acute abdomen to demonstrate obstruction, a radiopaque ureteral stone, an appendolith, or free air from a perforated viscus.

CT scanning with oral and intravenous contrast is a sensitive test in the workup of appendicitis. Abdominal ultrasound is another modality commonly used at some centers instead of CT for detecting inflammation of the appendix. Ultrasound may also aid in diagnosing cholecystitis, hydronephrosis, appendiceal abscess, and ovarian torsion. Testicular ultrasound is indicated to rule out torsion.

Barium or air-contrast enema may be used to look for intussusception in children with recurrent episodes of cramping abdominal pain, vomiting, and bloody stools. These tests are contraindicated if signs of peritonitis are present.

Disposition

Keep the patient on nothing-by-mouth status, and obtain surgical consultation. Broad-spectrum antibiotics should be started if obvious signs of perforation are present. If surgery is not immediately indicated, ensure close observation and follow-up. Admit the child to the hospital for frequent abdominal examinations.

Outpatient management is indicated only when an acute abdomen appears unlikely and the physician is certain that the child will be returned for an examination within 12–24 hours.

D'Agostino JD: Common abdominal emergencies in children. Emerg Med Clin North Am 2002;20:139. [PMID: 11826631] (Review.)

Irish MS et al: The approach to common diagnoses in infants and children. Pediatr Clin North Am 1998;45:729. [PMID: 9728184] (Review.)

Pearl RH et al: The approach to common diagnoses in infants and children, part II. Pediatr Clin North Am 1998;45:1287. [PMID: 9889755] (Review.)

Rothrock SG, Pagane J: Acute appendicitis in children: emergency department diagnosis and management. Ann Emerg Med 2000;36:39. [PMID: 10874234] (Review.)

VOMITING

General Considerations

Causes of vomiting in children may be categorized as due to direct irritation to the gastrointestinal tract, intestinal or gastric outlet obstruction, effect of a toxin or other noxious stimulus on the central nervous system, or elevated intracranial pressure.

Table 48–18. Exanthems.[1]

Disease (Etiology)	Usual Age	Season	Prodrome	Morphology
Measles (rubeola virus)	Infants to young adults	Winter/spring	High fever, symptoms of upper respiratory infection, conjunctivitis	Erythematous macules and papules, become confluent
Rubella (rubella virus)	Adolescents/young adults	Spring	Absent or low-grade fever, malaise, upper respiratory symptoms	Rose pink maculopapules, not confluent
Erythema infectiosum (parvovirus B19)	3–12 years	Winter/spring	Usually none	Slapped cheeks; reticular erythema or maculopapular
Enteroviral exanthems (coxsackie, echovirus, other enteroviruses)	Young children	Summer/fall	Fever (occasional)	Extremely variable; maculo-papular, petechial, purpuric, vesicular
Hand-foot-mouth syndrome (several coxsackieviruses)	Children	Summer/fall	Fever (occasional), sore mouth	Grey-white vesicles 3–7 mm on normal or erythematous base
Adenovirus exanthems (adenoviruses)	5 months to 5 years	Winter/spring	Fever, symptoms of upper respiratory infection	Rubellaform, morbilliform, roseola-like
Chickenpox (varicellazoster virus)	1–14 years	Late fall/winter/spring	Fever, headache, malaise 48 hours prior to exanthem	Macules, papules rapidly be-come vesicles on erythematous base, then crusts
Roseola (?herpesvirus 6)	Under 3 years	Spring/fall	High fever for 3–5 days prior to exanthem	Maculopapular rash in rosettes appears *after* fever declines
Lyme disease (Borrelia burgdorferi carried by ticks)	School age	Summer, geographical distribution	None	Erythema chronicum migrans
Rocky Mountain spotted fever (Rickettsia rickettsii carried by ticks)	Any age	Summer	Fever, malaise, headache, restlessness	Maculopapular and petechial rash that blanches
Kawasaki disease	Under 5 years	Winter/spring	High fever, irritability	Polymorphous—papular, vesicobullous, or morbilliform, erythema with desquamation
Gilanotti-Crosti syndrome (hepatitis B, cytomega-lovirus coxsackievirus, Epstein-Barr virus, etc.)	1–6 years	Any season	Upper respiratory symp-toms with generalized lymphadenopathy and hepatosplenomegaly	Papules or papulovesicles; may become confluent
Scarlet fever (group B streptococcus)	School age	Fall to spring	Acute onset with fever, sore throat	Diffuse erythema with sandpaper texture

Table 48–18. Exanthems.[1] (Continued)

Distribution	Associated Findings	Diagnosis	Special Management
Begins on face and moves centrifugally	Koplik's spots, "toxic" appearance, photophobia, cough, adenopathy, high fever	Usually clinical; acute/convalescent hemagglutinin (HAI) serologic test	Report to public health. Immunoglobulin within 6 days of exposure.
Begins on face and moves downward rapidly	Postauricular and occipital adenopathy, headache, malaise, mild pruritis	Rubella IgM or acute/convalescent HAI serologic test	Report to public health; check for exposure to pregnant women.
Usually arms/legs, may be generalized	Waxes and wanes for several weeks, occasional arthritis, headache, malaise	Usually clinical, acute/convalescent serologic test	Potential complication of aplastic crisis and hydrops fetalis.
Usually generalized, may be acral	Low-grade fever, occasional myocarditis, aseptic meningitis, pleurodynia	Usually clinical; viral culture from throat, rectal swabs in selected cases	If petechiae or purpura, *must consider* meningococcemia.
Hands/feet most common, diaper area, occasionally generalized	Oral ulcers, occasional fever, adenopathy	Same as for enteroviral exanthems	
Generalized	Fever, symptoms of upper respiratory infection, occasionally pneumonia	Viral isolation or acute/convalescent seroconversion	
Often begins on scalp or face, more profuse on trunk than extremities	Pruritus, fever, oral and genital lesions, occasional malaise	Usually clinical; Tzanch preparation or direct immunofluorescence	Antihistamines for itching; aspirin contraindicated (Reye syndrome). Varicella zoster virus vaccination.
Trunk, neck, may be generalized, lasts hour to days	Cervical and postauricular adenopathy	Clinical	
Trunk, extremities	Fever, later arthritis; cardiac, neurologic complications	Serologic test	Penicillin for children < 9 years of age, tetracycline for older children.
Wrists, ankles, plams, soles, later trunk	Central nervous system, pulmonary, cardiac lesions, nausea, vomiting, diarrhea	Serologic test	Treat on presumptive clinical grounds.
Generalized, often with perineal accentuation and desquamation	Conjunctivitis, cheilitis, glossitis, peripheral edema, adenopathy, and strawberry tongue	Clinical	Admit to hospital for intravenous gamma globulin, salicylates.
Face, arms, legs, buttocks, spares the torso	Occasional lymphadenopathy, hepatomegaly, splenomegaly fever, diarrhea, malaise	Clinical; hepatitis B and Epstein-Barr serologic test; elevated liver function tests	
Facial flushing with circumoral pallor, linear erythema in skin folds	Exudative pharyngitis, palatal petechiae, abdominal pain	Throat cultures	Intramuscular penicillin or oral erythromycin.

(continued)

Table 48–18. Exanthems.[1] (Continued)

Disease (Etiology)	Usual Age	Season	Prodrome	Morphology
Staphylococcal scalded skin syndrome (*S aureus* epidermolytic toxin)	Under 5 years	Any season	None	Abrupt onset, tender erythroderma
Toxic shock syndrome/ *Staphylococcus* toxin	Adolescents/young	Any season	None	Macular erythroderma
Meningococcemia/ meningococcus	< 2 years	Winter/spring	Malaise, fever, symptoms of upper respiratory infection	Papules, petechiae, purpura
Henöch-Schonlein Purpura	4–7 years	Spring	Possibly abdominal pain	Palpable, purpuric or petechial rash
Erythema multiforme (minor)	Any age	Any season	Malaise, fever, itching, burning	Erythematous macules, papules, vesicles or bullae; classic target lesions

Clinical Findings

Look for precipitating factors including trauma, medications, feeding techniques, and recent illness. It is helpful to know the nature of the vomitus (eg, bilious bloody, coffee ground, bright red, or feculent), the relationship to eating and position, and whether projectile vomiting occurs. The absence of passage of stool or gas implies obstruction. Inspect the abdomen for signs of obstruction, and look for evidence of a systemic illness (eg, otitis media, urinary tract infection).

A. VOMITING IN THE NEWBORN

Infants commonly regurgitate a portion of feedings. Nonforceful regurgitation is usually benign. Forceful vomiting, however, often indicates serious disease. Causes of gastrointestinal obstruction in newborns include the following:

1. Intestinal atresia—Vomiting begins shortly after birth. Abdominal x-rays reveal distention of the stomach and duodenum with an absence of colonic air. Early surgical intervention is necessary.

2. Meconium ileus—Antenatal perforation of the intestines secondary to obstruction with meconium results in vomiting shortly after birth; 90% of patients have cystic fibrosis.

3. Meconium plug syndrome—The distal colon becomes obstructed with a plug of meconium. A barium enema shows the plug and usually relieves the obstruction. This entity is suggestive of Hirschsprung disease.

4. Midgut volvulus—This abdominal emergency usually presents in the first month of life with bile-stained vomiting and abdominal distention. An upper gastrointestinal series usually demonstrates obstruction. Immediate surgical management is essential because many of these obstructions are associated with vascular compromise.

5. Hirschsprung disease—Delayed passage of meconium associated with abdominal distention and bilious vomiting is suggestive. A barium enema is helpful in diagnosis.

6. Pyloric stenosis—Patients with muscular hypertrophy of the pylorus typically present in the third week of life with nonbilious vomiting. Observe the infant during feeding to evaluate this event. Patients may present with altered consciousness if dehydrated. An olive-like mass may be palpable when examining the patient's mid-epigastrium. Ultrasound is the preferred diagnostic study. Pyloromyotomy is curative.

B. VOMITING IN INFANTS AND CHILDREN

Most infants and children who vomit have gastroenteritis. More serious causes of vomiting include the following:

• Gastrointestinal obstruction in the young child, particularly intussusception, should be considered. Ex-

Table 48–18. Exanthems.[1] (Continued)

Distribution	Associated Findings	Diagnosis	Special Management
Eruption with intensification in neck, face, axillae, and groin	Fever, conjunctivitis, rhinitis	Clinical: culture of *S aureus* from systemic site (not skin)	Neonate; if blistering present, hospitalize for intravenous nafcillin and fluid/electrolyte therapy.
Generalized	Hypotension; fever, myalgias, diarrhea/vomiting	Clinical case definition criteria, isolation, of *S aureus* from cervix, etc.	Treat hypotension, admit to hospital; antibiotics to eradicate *S aureus*.
Trunk, extremities, palms, soles	Temp > 40°C, meningism, circulatory collapse	Clinical, blood culture, spinal tap	Immediate intravenous penicillin, cefotaxime, or ceftriaxone in emergency department; treat for shock, if present.
Begins on malleoli and extends to buttocks	Arthralgia, nausea, vomiting, diarrhea, gastrointestinal bleeding	Clinical	Consider Rocky Mountain Spotted Fever or meningococcemia; steroids for severe cases.
Palms, soles, back of hands		Clinical	Hospitalization if severe; remove offending agent.

amine the abdomen for a sausage-shaped mass in the right upper quadrant and the rectum for "currant jelly stools" in the child presenting with intermittent crampy abdominal pain followed by vomiting. If a history of trauma is present, duodenal hematoma and traumatic pancreatitis should be considered.

- Appendicitis may begin with a history of nausea and vomiting prior to the appearance of right lower quadrant abdominal pain.
- Hepatitis in children is commonly associated with anorexia and vomiting.
- In children with protracted vomiting and increasing lethargy, consider the diagnosis of Reye syndrome. Obtain blood for liver function tests and ammonia and glucose measurements.
- Consider incarcerated inguinal hernia in a child with abdominal pain and vomiting.

Treatment

(See Figure 48–11.) Administer fluids if the child is dehydrated or if an obstruction is present. Insert a nasogastric tube if obstruction is suggested.

Obtain upright and supine x-rays if signs of obstruction are present. A barium or air-contrast enema is indicated when considering the diagnosis of intussusception. Perform an upper gastrointestinal series emergently in the infant with bilious emesis who may have a midgut volvulus.

Obtain urinalysis, CBC, platelet count, and electrolyte measurement as indicated by the child's clinical condition.

Irish MS et al: The approach to common diagnoses in infants and children. Pediatr Clin North Am 1998;45:729. [PMID: 9728184] (Review.)

BLEEDING

General Considerations

Gastrointestinal hemorrhage in children usually results from ulceration of the bowel mucosal lining secondary to infection or ischemia. Subsequent bleeding into the gastrointestinal tract can be manifest in a number of ways. Hematemesis (vomiting of blood) and melena (black stool) usually indicate that the site of bleeding is in the stomach or duodenum proximal to the ligament of Treitz. Hematochezia (red blood per rectum) usually indicates bleeding in the distal small bowel or colon. In children, however, rapid gastrointestinal transit may result in hematochezia following upper gastrointestinal bleeding.

Clinical Findings

The patient's age and the amount and type of bleeding help determine the most likely cause. Bleeding in neonates is usually benign and self-limited. Profuse,

Table 48–19. Common nontraumatic causes of abdominal pain.

Organ System	Clinical Entity and Demographics	History	Physical Examination and Laboratory Findings	Imaging Studies
Gastrointestinal	Appendicitis Peak: 10–12 years M:F 3:2	Periumbilical pain followed by right lower quadrant pain, anorexia, and emesis.	Temperature > 100.5°F, right lower quadrant pain, peritoneal signs (if perforated); often elevated white blood cell count	*X-rays:* concave curvature of the spine to the right; fecalith (5–10%) *Ultrasound:* pericolic or appendiceal fluid; edema *Abdominal CT scan with intravenous contrast:* enlarged appendix or right lower quadrant stranding or fluid
	Meckel diverticulitis Mean: 2 years	Typically painless gastro-intestinal bleeding; stool appears bright red or tarry.	Anemia, elevated blood urea nitrogen and creatinine	*X-rays:* typically normal, possible obstruction or perforation *Meckel's scan with technetium 99m* recommended
	Intussusception 5–9 months M:F 3:2	Paroxysmal crampy ab-dominal pain followed by periods of calmness, emesis, currant jelly stools.	Fever, distension (late), right-sided mass; dehydration, anemia, leukocytosis (late)	*X-rays:* obstructive pattern *Ultrasound:* intussusception "pseudokidney" and "target" signs *Contrast enema:* intussusception and failure of gas or contrast to reflux into the small bowel is diagnostic and often thera-peutic
	Pyloric stenosis	Nonbilious projectile vom-iting following feeds.	Scaphoid abdomen, peristaltic waves, palpable olive; hypo-chloremic, hypokalemic meta-bolic acidosis	*X-rays:* dilated stomach *Ultrasound:* hypertrophied pylorus "bulls-eye" and "sausage" sign
	Malrotation/ midgut volvulus < 1 month M:F 3:2	Sudden onset of bilious emesis, abdominal pain, and feeding intolerance.	Normal (early), tenderness, possi-ble distension, peritonitis (late); dehydration; anemia; leukocy-tosis (late)	*X-rays:* distended stomach, gasless abdomen (high obstruction) *Upper GI:* abnormal duodenal sweep *Lower GI:* cecum in the left abdomen or right lower quadrant
	Incarcerated inguinal hernia < 1 year F > M	Irritability; crampy, abdom-inal pain; nonbilious emesis (early); bilious emesis (late).	Firm, tender groin or scrotal mass; dehydration leukocytosis (late)	*X-rays:* obstructive pattern

	Hirschprung disease	Infant unable to pass meconium in 24 hours after birth, diarrhea ± emesis, no rectal stool.	Asymptomatic (early), lethargy, fever, obtunded, shock (late), abdominal distension, normal or hyperactive bowel sounds	*X-rays:* distended bowel loops, abrupt cutoff below pelvic brim; relatively airless rectum *Barium enema:* postevacuation films show transition zone
	Constipation	Two or fewer bowel movements per week with excessive straining.	Crampy abdominal pain without peritoneal signs; may have abdominal mass	*X-rays:* not required; may show large amount of stool in colon or rectum
Gynecologic	Ectopic pregnancy	Delayed menses, abdominal pain, vaginal bleeding.	Positive urine pregnancy test, lower quadrant pain and tenderness, amenorrhea, adnexal tenderness	*Ultrasound:* free fluid in pelvis, adnexal mass, gestational sac outside uterus, ectopic fetal heart beat activity
	Salpingitis	Increased vaginal discharge, pelvic pain, symptoms of urethritis.	Cervical motion tenderness, adnexal tenderness, possible fever	*Ultrasound:* free fluid in pelvis, adnexal mass
Pulmonary	Influenza	Signs and symptoms of viral illness.	Altered breath sounds, low grade fever	*X-rays:* viral pattern
	Pneumonia	Dyspnea, cough, ± chest pain.	Altered breath sounds, fever; elevated absolute neutrophil count, elevated C-reactive protein	*X-rays:* infiltrate, possible consolidation
Renal	Cystitis F > M	Urinary frequency, dysuria, nocturia, history of congenital abnormalities.	Suprapubic tenderness, pyuria, bacteruria, varying degrees of hematuria	None recommended
	Pyelonephritis F > M	Flank pain, possible frequency or dysuria, nausea and vomiting, history of congenital abnormalities.	Flank and occasionally lower quandrant tenderness, fever	*Ultrasound:* may show hydronephrosis in cases of chronic reflux *Abdominal CT scan with intravenous contrast:* decreased enhancement, enlargement of kidney

Modified and reproduced, with permission, from Irish MS, Pearl RH, Caty M, Glick P: The approach to common abdominal diagnoses in infants and children. Pediatr Clin North Am 1998;45[4]:730.

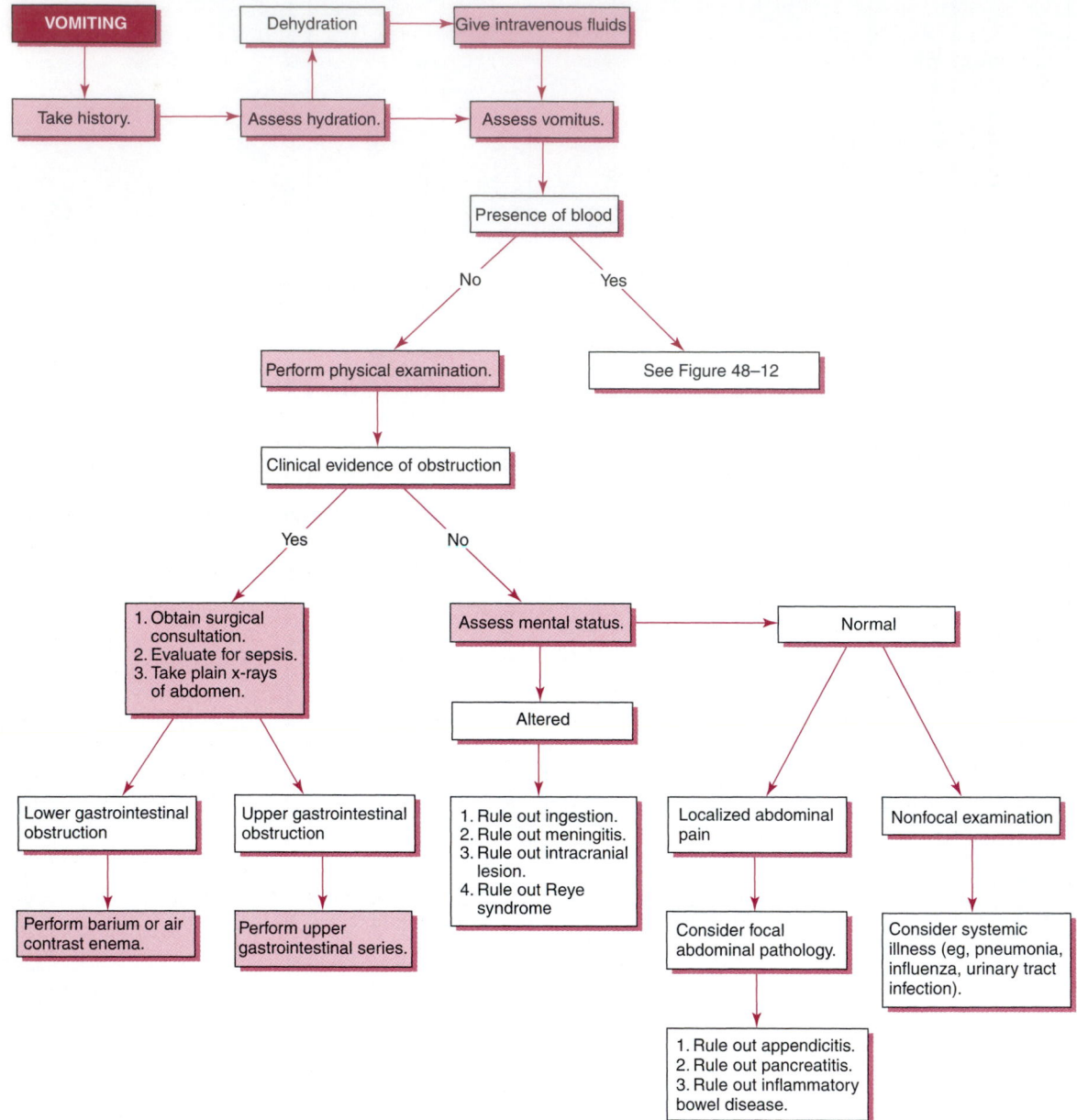

Figure 48–11. Algorithmic approach to vomiting in children.

painless bleeding may indicate Meckel diverticulum. Bleeding associated with pain may occur with intussusception. Diarrhea associated with bleeding per rectum usually indicates bacterial dysentery.

Obtain vital signs to detect cardiovascular compromise. Clinical signs of liver disease may indicate a coagulopathy or esophageal varices as a possible cause of

bleeding. Elicit a careful history for nonsteroidal antiinflammatory drug use or exposure to warfarin-containing drugs.

Occasionally what appears to be gastrointestinal hemorrhage is not truly from the gastrointestinal tract. Epistaxis, nasopharyngeal trauma, and hemoptysis may result in coffee-ground emesis. Some substances may color the emesis or stool red (eg, food colorings, beets, red gelatin, artificial fruit drinks, and antibiotic syrups). The stool should be routinely checked with a guaiac test for occult blood.

A. Bleeding in the Newborn

1. Swallowed maternal blood—Swallowed maternal blood at delivery or from a bleeding nipple can result in hematemesis or melena in the newborn. These infants usually appear otherwise healthy. An Apt-Downey test can differentiate infant from maternal blood by identifying fetal hemoglobin.

2. Hemorrhagic disease—Newborns with hemorrhagic disease may present with melena or hematochezia. However, other evidence of a generalized bleeding disorder usually is present. Maternal medications such as aspirin or anticoagulants may result in neonatal hemorrhage. Consider vitamin K deficiency if the neonate did not receive an intramuscular injection after birth.

3. Stress ulcers—In an infant with asphyxia or sepsis, stress ulcers may cause significant gastrointestinal bleeding. Stress ulcers can be secondary to sepsis, asphyxia, intracranial pathology, or heart disease.

4. Other causes—Consider necrotizing enterocolitis, anal fissures, malrotation with midgut volvulus, and Hirschsprung disease with enterocolitis.

B. Upper Gastrointestinal Bleeding in Infants and Children

The most common cause of upper gastrointestinal bleeding is esophagitis or gastric and duodenal ulceration. Esophageal varices are an uncommon cause of bleeding in young children that may develop with severe liver disease. With forceful vomiting, tears of the distal esophagus (Mallory-Weiss syndrome) can occur in the esophagus, causing upper gastrointestinal hemorrhage.

C. Lower Gastrointestinal Bleeding in Infants and Children

1. Anal fissures—Anal fissures are the most common cause of hematochezia in infants.

2. Cow's milk sensitivity—Sensitivity to cow's milk protein can result in severe colitis with bloody stools.

3. Intussusception—Always consider intussusception in a child who presents with colicky abdominal pain followed by vomiting. Typically these children may appear well between episodes of vomiting. Bloody stool helps establish the diagnosis.

4. Meckel diverticulum—Patients with Meckel diverticulum may present with the painless appearance of bright red blood per rectum. Sufficient blood may be lost to result in cardiovascular compromise. The gastric mucosa within the diverticulum can be identified on technetium scan.

5. Bacterial or viral infection—Fever and diarrhea associated with blood per rectum are usually secondary to an invasive bacterial infection of the colon. Culture stool for *Campylobacter, Shigella,* and *Salmonella.* Viral pathogens such as rotavirus and Norwalk virus must also be considered as possible causes.

6. Hemolytic uremic syndrome—Hemolytic uremic syndrome is characterized by acute renal failure with thrombocytopenia, hemolytic anemia, and bloody diarrhea. Children with this syndrome are usually quite ill and require hospitalization and close observation.

7. Intestinal polyps—Intestinal polyps are sometimes found in young children and may result in bright red blood per rectum. A diagnosis can be established by colonoscopy.

8. Henoch-Schönlein purpura—This disorder is characterized by small vessel vasculitis of the skin, gastrointestinal tract, and kidneys. Patients will at times have palpable purpura of the skin, joint swelling and pain, and colicky abdominal pain. Gastrointestinal bleeding may be secondary to submucosal hemorrhage. These children are also at an increased risk for intussusception.

9. Inflammatory bowel disease—Patients with inflammatory bowel disease may present with evidence of gastrointestinal bleeding associated with anemia, poor growth, abdominal pain, and diarrhea.

Treatment

(See Figures 48–12 and 48–13.) Evaluate cardiovascular status. Achieve intravenous access if significant blood loss has occurred. Send blood for CBC, platelet count, coagulation studies, and typing and crossmatching. Consider stool evaluation for fecal leukocytes, bacterial culture, ova and parasites.

Infuse saline or Ringer's lactated injection initially if the child is in shock. Alternatively, infuse type O, Rh-negative blood.

Place a nasogastric tube to determine if the site of bleeding is in the upper gastrointestinal tract. Lavage with saline (10 mL/kg) until active bleeding stops. Unstable patients are at risk for aspiration and may require intubation.

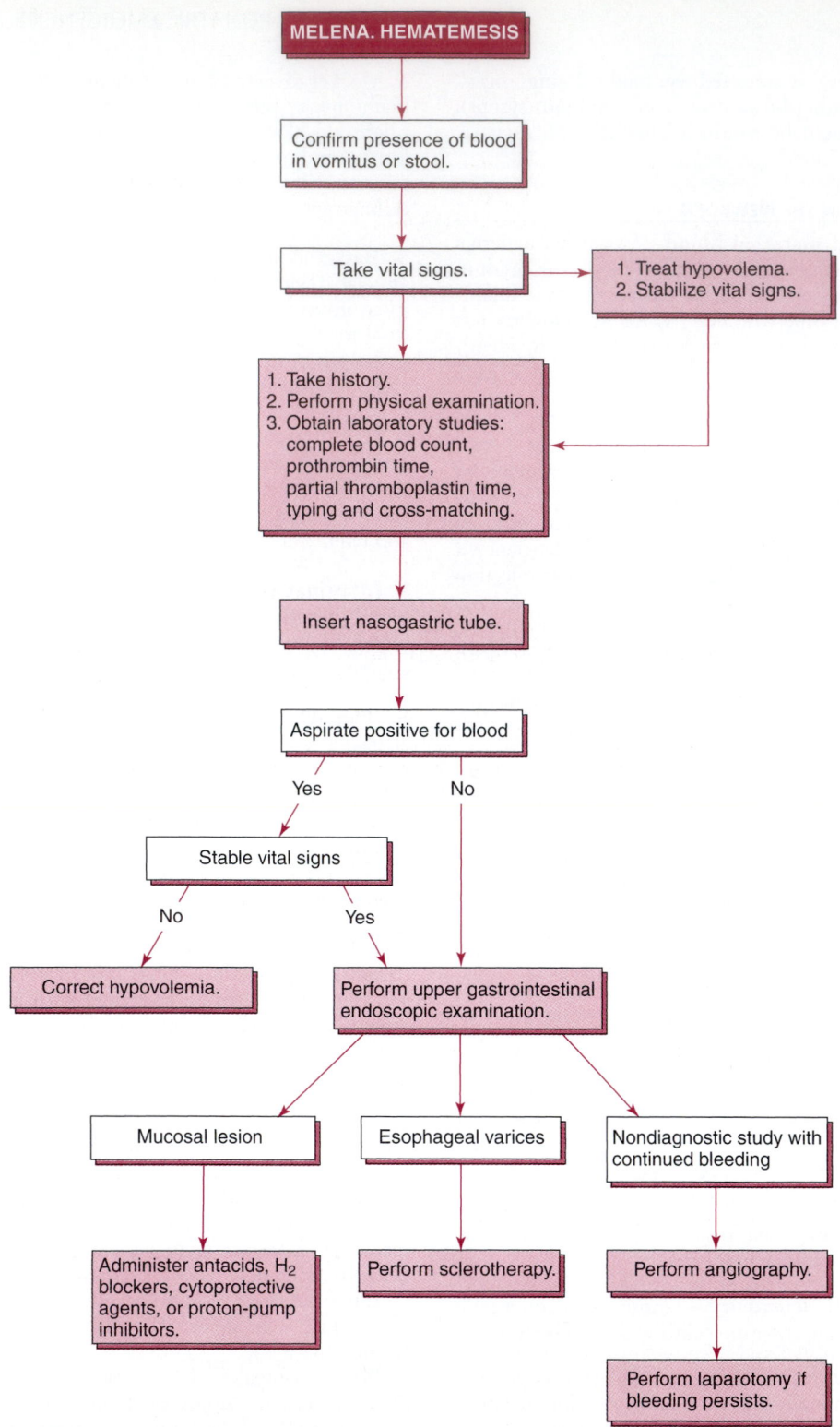

Figure 48–12. Treatment algorithm for melena and hematemesis.

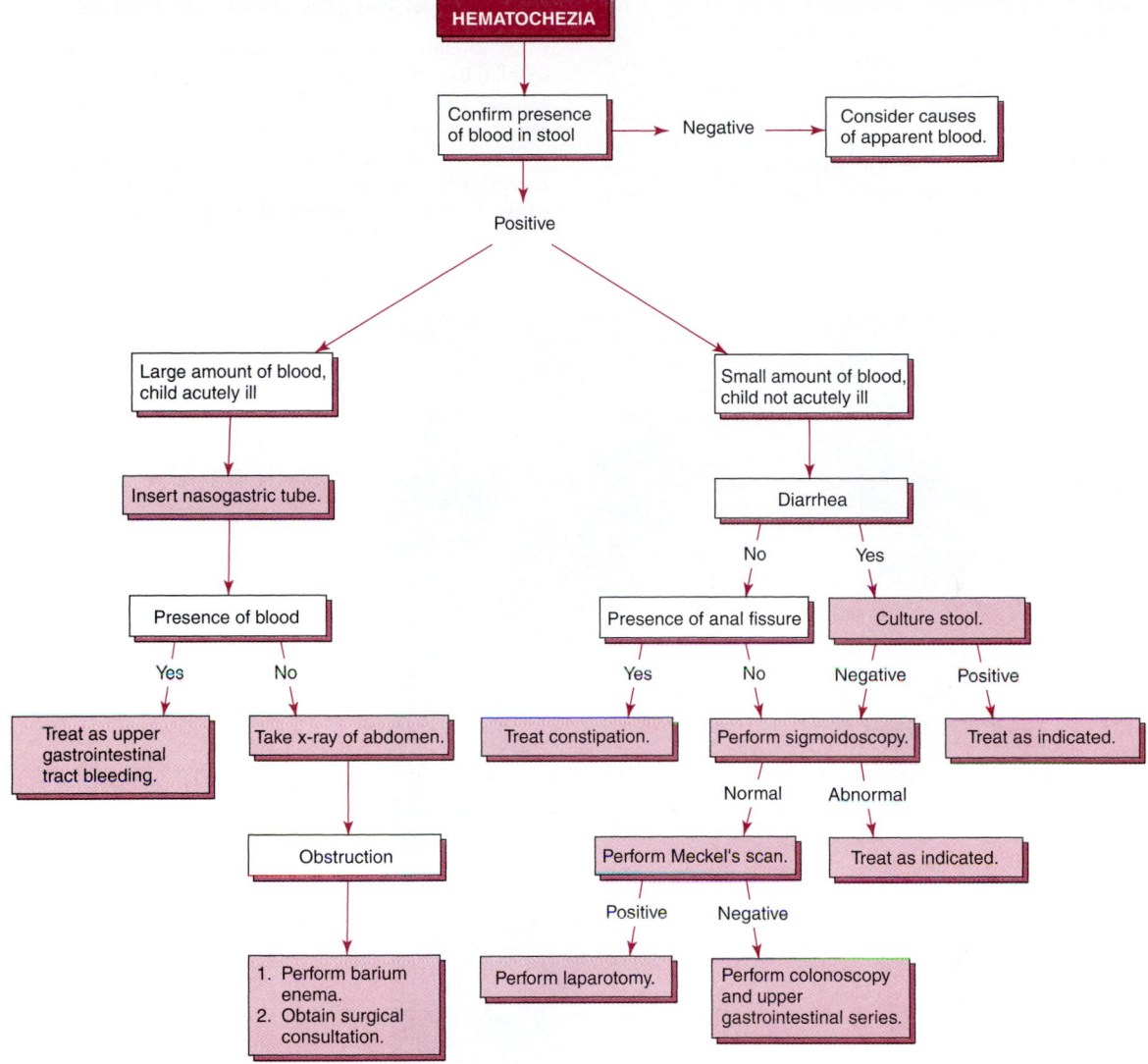

Figure 48–13. Treatment algorithm for hematochezia.

If blood loss is greater than 10 mL/kg/h, emergent surgical intervention may be necessary to control bleeding.

Disposition

Admit children with acute upper gastrointestinal bleeding to the hospital for stabilization and endoscopic evaluation. Children with lower gastrointestinal bleeding can be evaluated as outpatients as long as they appear well and are hemodynamically stable. Stabilize a hemodynamically unstable patient before performing diagnostic procedures. Emergent surgical intervention may be necessary to identify the site of bleeding.

Pearl RH et al: The approach to common diagnoses in infants and children, part II. Pediatr Clin North Am 1998;45:1287. [PMID: 9889755] (Review.)

FOREIGN BODY

Esophageal Foreign Bodies

Foreign bodies within the esophagus become lodged at the cervical esophagus, aortic arch, or lower esophageal sphincter. Esophageal obstruction secondary to a foreign body may result in substernal chest pain and increased salivation secondary to inability to swallow. The physical examination is usually normal unless perforation has occurred. X-ray examination of the chest will usually disclose the foreign body; in the esophagus it is best seen on an anteroposterior film (Figure 48–14). A radiolucent foreign body (eg, plastic) may not be visible on x-ray.

Gastric & Small Bowel Foreign Bodies

Most foreign bodies that successfully pass through the esophagus will navigate the remainder of the gastrointestinal tract without difficulty. The occasional object that is unable to pass through the stomach after a period of 3 days should be removed by endoscopy. Intestinal obstruction may occur if a foreign body becomes lodged in the region of the ileocecal valve.

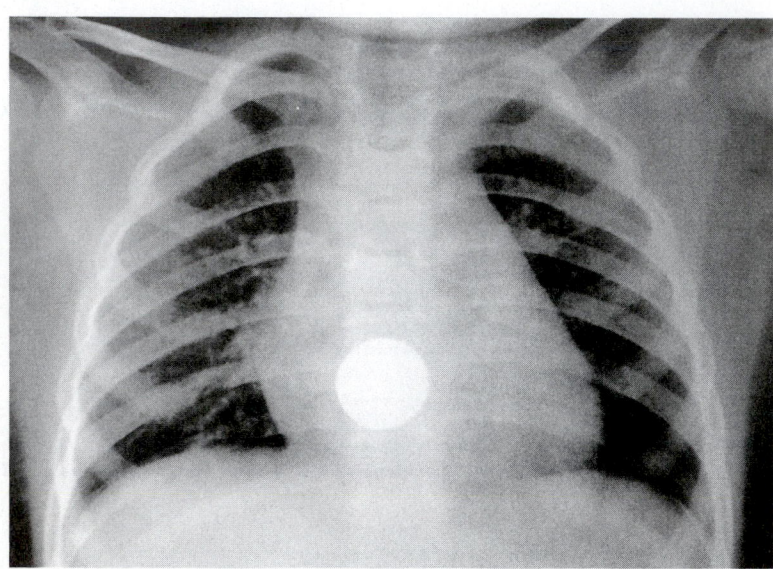

A

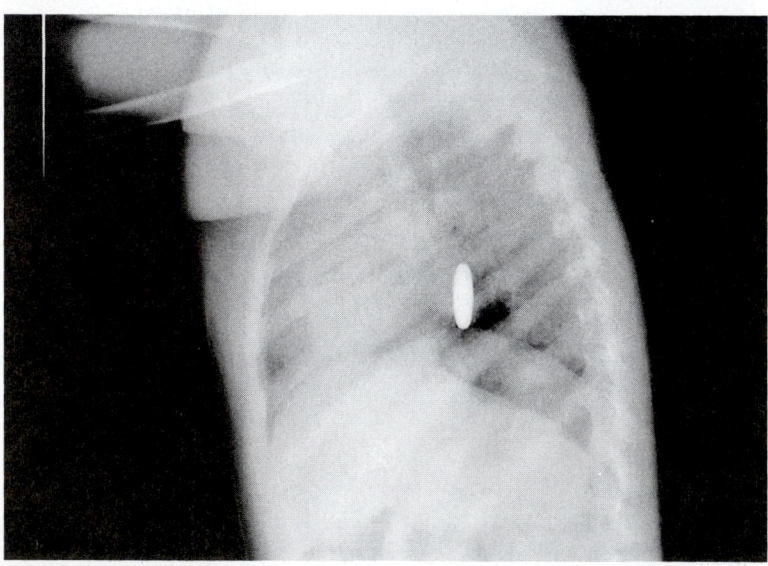

B

Figure 48–14. Posteroanterior (**A**) and lateral (**B**) chest x-rays, showing esophageal foreign body.

■ HEMATOLOGIC DISEASES

ANEMIA

General Considerations

In children, over 75% of anemias are due to iron deficiency or thalassemia minor, both of which are characterized by microcytosis. The most common cause of anemia in children aged 6 months to 2 years is nutritional iron deficiency. Typically this results from excessive cow's milk intake. Less commonly iron deficiency anemia will occur secondary to chronic blood loss, usually from the gastrointestinal tract (eg, duodenal ulcer, Meckel diverticulum, and polyps).

Anemias not due to iron deficiency are caused by one of 2 processes: (1) Decreased erythrocyte production or release from the bone marrow, for example, transient erythroblastopenia of childhood (TEC). TEC typically occurs in children aged 1–2 years. Severe anemia and reticulocytopenia spontaneously resolve in 1–2 months. (2) Increased destruction, sequestration, or acute loss of circulating red cells owing to sickle cell disease, autoimmune hemolytic anemia, or hemolytic uremic syndrome, or blood loss due to trauma, surgery, or peptic ulcer disease.

Clinical Findings

A. SYMPTOMS AND SIGNS

With rapid onset of anemia from blood loss or hemolysis, signs of cardiovascular compromise as well as impending cardiac failure may be present. With slow onset of anemia, children typically show pallor and decreased exercise tolerance but no evidence of cardiovascular compromise even with extremely low levels of hemoglobin. Hemolytic anemias may cause jaundice and splenomegaly. Petechiae may indicate hemolytic uremic syndrome.

B. LABORATORY FINDINGS

Laboratory evaluation should include a complete blood count with hemoglobin, red blood cell indices, white blood cell and platelet counts, peripheral smear, and reticulocyte counts. Anemia with microcytosis in a young child strongly suggests iron deficiency. If the stool is negative for occult blood, further tests are not necessary if the child is not severely anemic.

Treatment

A. IRON THERAPY

Treat iron deficiency with elemental iron at 3–6 mg/kg/d (ferrous sulfate, 75 mg/0.6 mL dropper, equivalent to 15 mg elemental iron/0.6 mL dropper) in 1–2 daily doses. Continue iron therapy for 2 months after the anemia is corrected. Restrict cow's milk intake.

If anemia has developed slowly, patients can often tolerate remarkably low hemoglobin levels, even to 4–5 g/dL, without the need for transfusion if other effective therapy is available.

B. TRANSFUSION

Transfuse children who experience a rapid decline in hemoglobin to less than 7, particularly if signs of cardiovascular compromise are present.

In patients with gradual onset of anemia who require transfusion, slow transfusion is recommended, because these children are at risk for congestive heart failure with rapid transfusion. Administer a diuretic prior to transfusion to prevent circulatory overload (eg, furosemide, 1 mg/kg intravenously).

Disposition

Obtain consultation with a hematologist for anemias requiring transfusion, anemias associated with hemolysis, and anemias without an obvious cause.

Recheck the hemoglobin level in children receiving iron therapy in 2–4 weeks to document response.

SICKLE CELL DISEASE

Clinical Findings

A. SYMPTOMS AND SIGNS

Vasoocclusive events are associated with severe local pain, fever, leukocytosis, and impaired organ function. Abdominal pain may be severe and suggest appendicitis or cholecystitis. In young children, a common initial vasoocclusive episode is manifested by hand-foot syndrome, or dactylitis, with fever, acute swelling, and pain in one or both hands or feet. Bone and joint pain may be quite severe, and differentiation from skeletal infection may be difficult.

Splenic infarcts may cause severe abdominal pain and lead to progressive atrophy of the spleen. Because of impaired splenic clearance of bacteria, children with sickle cell anemia are partially susceptible to infection by encapsulated organisms. Acute splenic sequestration, a severe vasoocclusive crisis, occurs in 10% of children aged 5 months to 2 years with sickle cell disease. Symptoms include left upper quadrant pain, massive splenomegaly, and hypovolemic shock.

Vasoocclusive crises may involve the central nervous system and produce neurologic symptoms of severe headache, visual disturbances, coma, and seizures. Also in 10% of patients with sickle cell disease, cerebral vessel thrombosis during these crises may result in stroke.

A combination of pulmonary infarcts and infection may lead to the acute chest syndrome manifested by chest pain, dyspnea, and tachypnea. These children may become severely hypoxic. Priapism is another complication of sickling and can be extremely uncomfortable to the child.

B. Laboratory Findings

Obtain a complete blood count and reticulocyte count. A decrease in hematocrit from baseline may indicate the need for transfusion. The absence of reticulocytosis indicates an aplastic crisis (often from parvovirus B19) and heralds an abrupt decrease in the hematocrit.

Obtain cultures of blood and urine if fever is present. Obtain blood for electrolytes if dehydration is a concern.

If bone pain is associated with high fever, chills, toxicity, and leukocytosis, bone aspiration is indicated to diagnose osteomyelitis.

B. Imaging

Obtain x-rays of the chest if hypoxemia, cough, tachypnea, or dyspnea is present. Infiltrates may be present in patients with acute chest syndrome.

Treatment

A. General Management

Administer oxygen only if the patient is hypoxemic or in respiratory distress. Intravenous fluid hydration is important in reversing the sickling process if dehydration is present.

B. Venous Access

Begin an intravenous line if fluids or parenteral pain medications are anticipated. For patients with acute splenic sequestration, bolus with intravenous fluids and perform exchange transfusion when available.

C. Antimicrobial Therapy

Children with sickle cell disease have an increased susceptibility to sepsis from encapsulated organisms. Figure 48–15 is an algorithm for the management of the febrile child with sickle cell disease without an obvious localizing source of infection.

D. Pain Management

Treatment of pain in a sickling crisis is important for the child's recovery. Ask the patient to use an objective scale (eg, 1–10) to grade pain severity. Use this scale to guide pain management. Do not hesitate to use parenteral narcotics for adequate pain control because of concerns about drug addiction. Acetaminophen with or without codeine can be used for mild pain. For severe pain, give intravenous morphine sulfate, 0.1 mg/kg every 2–4 hours, or meperidine, 1 mg/kg every 3–4 hours.

E. Treatment of Acute Chest Syndrome

Treatment of acute chest syndrome includes hospitalization, intravenous antibiotics, and supplemental oxygen to keep oxygen saturation above 95% on pulse oximetry. Administer intravenous fluids to maintain hydration. If hypoxemia worsens, exchange transfusion may be required. Consider vancomycin for patients not responding to initial antibiotics.

Disposition

Children who can maintain adequate oral fluid intake and whose pain is controlled with oral medication can be managed as outpatients with close follow-up.

Hospitalize children who require continued parenteral therapy for pain, those who cannot maintain adequate oral hydration, or those who have required more than 2 visits for treatment of the same painful crisis.

Freeman L: Sickle cell disease and other hemoglobinopathies: approach to emergency diagnosis and treatment. Emergency Medicine Practice 2001;3:11.

Sadowitz P, Amanullah S, Souid AK: Hematologic emergencies in pediatric emergency room. Emerg Med Clin North Am 2002;20:177. [PMID: 11826633] (Review.)

Wethers DL: Sickle cell disease in children: part II. Diagnosis and treatment of major complications and recent advances in treatment. Am Fam Physician 2000;62:1309. [PMID: 11011859] (Review.)

IDIOPATHIC THROMBOCYTOPENIC PURPURA

 ESSENTIALS OF DIAGNOSIS

- *Usually children present with petechia, purpura, or spontaneous bleeding involving the mucous membranes.*
- *Platelet counts usually less than 100,000.*

General Considerations

The differential diagnosis of thrombocytopenia involves one of 3 mechanisms: (1) increased destruction (idiopathic thrombocytopenia purpura [ITP], hemolytic uremic syndrome, or disseminated intravascular coagulopathy), (2) decreased production (aplastic crisis, marrow infiltrating neoplasms), and (3) splenic sequestration (sickle cell disease). ITP results from increased destruction of only platelets, causing severe isolated thrombocytopenia. It commonly follows a viral

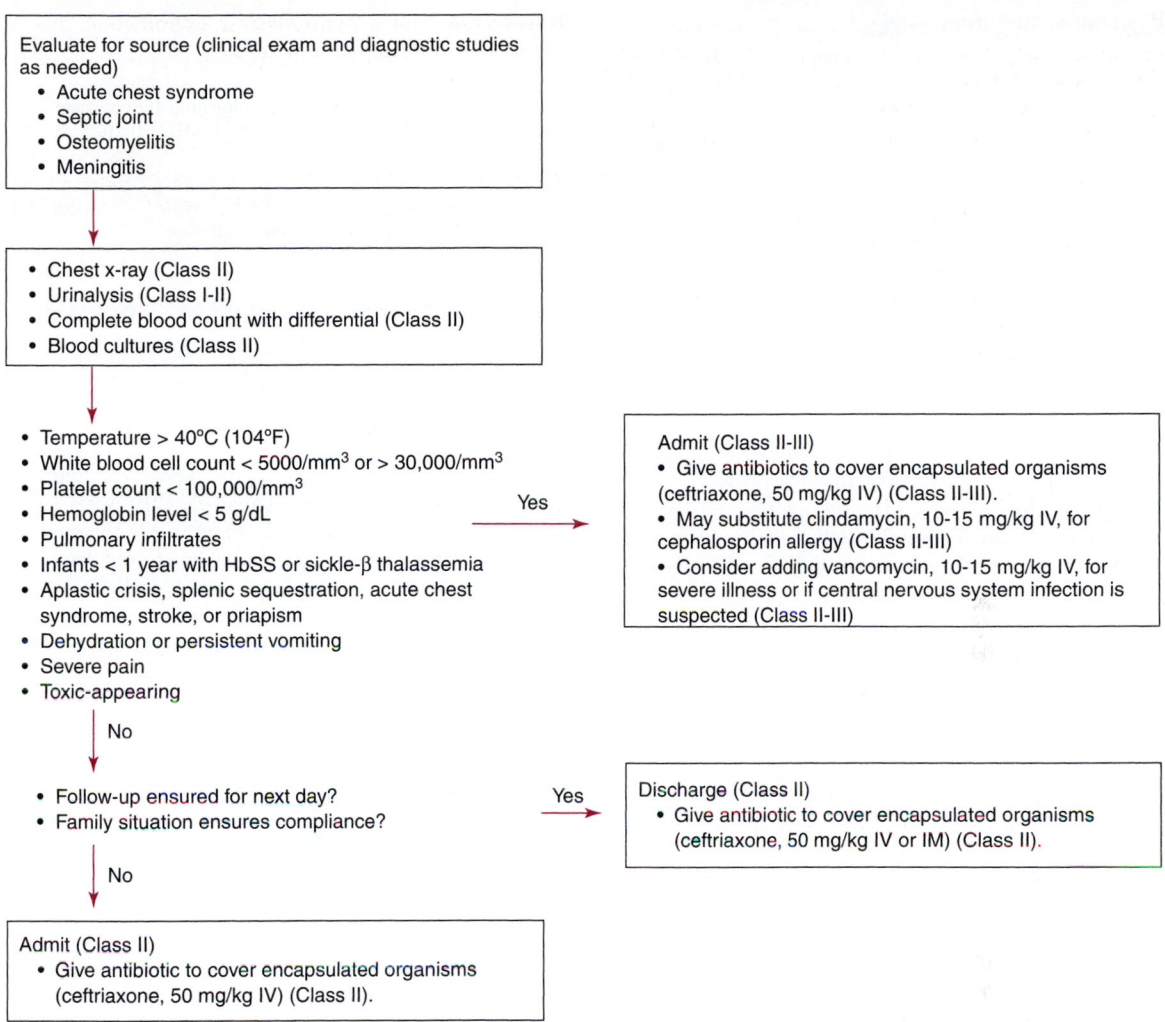

Figure 48–15. Clinical pathway: management of the febrile child with sickle cell disease. Give antibiotics emergently—before obtaining diagnostic studies—if signs of toxicity or sepsis are present. (May draw blood cultures if done expediently.) The evidence for recommendations is graded using the following scale: Class I = definitely recommended. Definitive, excellent evidence provides support. Class II = acceptable and useful. Good evidence provides support. Class III = may be acceptable, possibly useful. Fair-to-good evidence provides support. Indeterminate = continuing area of research. (Reproduced, with permission, from Freeman L: Sickle cell disease and other hemoglobinopathies: approaches to emergency diagnosis and treatment. Emerg Med Practice 2001;3[12]:14.)

illness. It is usually benign and self-limited; approximately 80–90% of cases resolve within 6 months.

Clinical Findings

A. SYMPTOMS AND SIGNS

Children usually present with the abrupt appearance of petechiae, purpura, and spontaneous bleeding of the skin and mucous membranes. They may also have epistaxis. Early in the disease, intracranial hemorrhage occurs in less than 1% of patients. These patients usually manifest severe headache or altered level of consciousness. Children with ITP typically appear in good health. They usually are not febrile and do not have splenomegaly. Children with platelet counts under 10,000/μL are at risk for life-threatening complications.

B. CLINICAL FINDINGS

Obtain a CBC, blood smear, and platelet count. Typically the platelet count is less than 100,000/μL and sometimes is less than 20,000/μL.

Bone marrow examination may be recommended by the hematologist if the presentation is atypical.

Treatment

A. GENERAL MANAGEMENT

Observation is adequate for children with only moderately severe thrombocytopenia.

B. CORTICOSTEROID THERAPY

If the platelet count is less than 10,000–20,000/μL or if extensive bleeding is present, consultation with a pediatric hematologist and corticosteroid therapy are recommended. Corticosteroids will usually cause the platelet count to increase to 20,000/μL within 48–72 hours.

C. EMERGENT INTERVENTIONS

Emergent intervention is needed for severe gastrointestinal bleeding, hematuria, or intracranial hemorrhage. Whole-blood transfusion may be required for severe anemia. Intravenous corticosteroids should be administered as methylprednisolone, 10–30 mg/kg/d for 3–5 days (maximum, 1 g over 30 minutes).

D. GAMMA GLOBULIN

Intravenous infusion of gamma globulin, 1 g/kg/d for 2 consecutive days, or a single dose of anti-Rh D, 40–80 mg/kg over 5 minutes in Rh-positive patients, will also result in a rapid rise in platelet count.

E. PLATELET TRANSFUSIONS

Platelet transfusions are indicated for refractory ITP and life-threatening hemorrhage, but the half-life of transfused platelets is brief. Splenectomy may be indicated if medical treatments fail.

Disposition

Hospitalize children with ITP if the platelet count is less than 10,000/μL or if significant bleeding is present, particularly young children for whom avoidance of traumatic play is difficult.

Advise older children to avoid all contact sports and vigorous playground activities during the acute phase of the disease.

Obtain emergent neurosurgical consultation for any signs of intracranial hemorrhage. Obtain hematologic consultation and a bone marrow examination before corticosteroid therapy is initiated.

Chu YW, Korb J, Sakamoto KM: Idiopathic thrombocytopenia purpura. Pediatr Rev 2000;21:95. [PMID: 10702324] (Review.)

Sadowitz P, Amanullah S, Souid AK: Hematologic emergencies in pediatric emergency room. Emerg Med Clin North Am 2002;20:177. [PMID: 11826633] (Review.)

■ NEWBORN EMERGENCIES

Clinical Findings

The need for resuscitation of the newborn infant is based on the Apgar score (Table 48–20). Vital signs should be recorded frequently to monitor the success of resuscitation. Physical examination should establish the degree of maturity of the infant as well as the integrity of the infant's respiratory and cardiovascular functions.

Treatment

A. GENERAL MANAGEMENT

The key to treatment in the newborn infant is to be prepared and use an organized team approach. A "code card" posted in the emergency department, or use of the Broselow tape, can help guide drug dosing and choice of equipment sizes.

If time permits, alert the obstetric service and nursery staff prior to the birth of the baby. Electronic fetal monitoring is helpful if time and equipment availability permit.

Table 48–20. Evaluation of the newborn infant using the APGAR score.

	Score		
	0	1	2
Appearance (color)	Pale or blue	Pink trunk and pale limbs	Pink trunk and limbs
Pulse (heart rate)	Absent	< 100	> 100
Grimace	Absent	Some response	Crying; withdraws
Activity	Absent	Some flexion	Extremities well flexed
Respiration	Absent	Weak cry	Active cry

An overhead radiant warmer should be present and turned on. If one is not available, use heating lamps or warm blankets. Proper equipment should be available and functioning (Table 48–21).

At birth the umbilical cord should be quickly clamped and then cut. The infant should be placed under the radiant warmer and immediately assessed, and an Apgar score should be assigned (see Table 48–20). The heart rate can be monitored by palpation of the umbilical arterial pulse. The oropharynx can be gently suctioned and the infant stimulated by rubbing its back. The infant should be towel-dried. Apgar scores should be assigned at 1 and 5 minutes.

B. Neonatal Resuscitation

Infants who are bradycardic, apneic, or significantly depressed require immediate resuscitative efforts (Figure 48–16).

Epinephrine, atropine, or naloxone can be administered endotracheally during resuscitative efforts prior to the establishment of vascular access. When this route is used, double the usual intravenous dosages of these medications.

Umbilical vein catheterization can also be used for emergent drug administration or volume expansion. Umbilical artery catheterization can be used for frequent arterial blood gas analysis and blood pressure readings.

Continue to assign Apgar scores at 5-minute intervals to determine the need for continued resuscitative efforts. Be alert to complications particular to the newborn when resuscitation does not result in expected improvement (eg, meconium aspiration, respiratory distress syndrome, shock, maternal substance abuse, pneumothorax, choanal atresia, diaphragmatic hernia, tracheoesophageal fistula). As the Apgar score improves, prepare the infant for transport to the nursery for close monitoring and care as indicated.

CHILD ABUSE

PHYSICAL ABUSE

General Considerations

In 2000, over 3 million referrals concerning child abuse or neglect were reported to child protective services in the United States. Almost 1 million children were found to be victims of maltreatment, which included neglect, medical neglect, physical abuse, sexual abuse, and psychological abuse. The rate of child maltreatment was 12.2 victims per 1000 children in the United States. Management of possible child abuse is one of the most difficult clinical problems facing the emer-

Table 48–21. Equipment required for neonatal resuscitation.[1]

	Prehospital/ Field	Emergency Department
Blankets (warm)	+	
Heat lamp or radiant warmer		+
Thermometer, temperature probe	±	+
Oxygen source (warm, humid)	+	+
Lighting	+	+
Infant stethoscope	+	+
Suction catheter with syringe	+	
Suction catheter with machine	±	+
Face masks (preterm, term)	+	+
Self-inflating bag, pop-off	+	
Anesthesia bag, manometer		+
Endotracheal tubes (2.5–4 mm)	+	+
Stylet	±	±
Sterile needles, syringes, stop cocks	+	+
Oral airways (000–0)	±	±
Laryngoscope (0 and 1 Miller blades)		+
Spare bulbs and batteries		+
Cord tie, clamps	+	
Hemostat, forceps, scissors, scalpel	+	+
Umbilical catheters (3.5 and 5F)		+
Resuscitation drugs	+	+
Sterile attire, drapes		+
ECG monitor		+
Blood pressure monitor		+
Blood gas machine		+
Glucose reagent sticks	+	+
Defibrillator	±	+
Umbilical catheter tray		+
Thoracostomy tray		+

[1]Reproduced, with permission, from Partridge JC: Neonatal resuscitation. In: *Pediatric Emergency Medicine: A Clinician's Reference.* Grossman M, Dieckmann RA (editors). Lippincott, 1991.

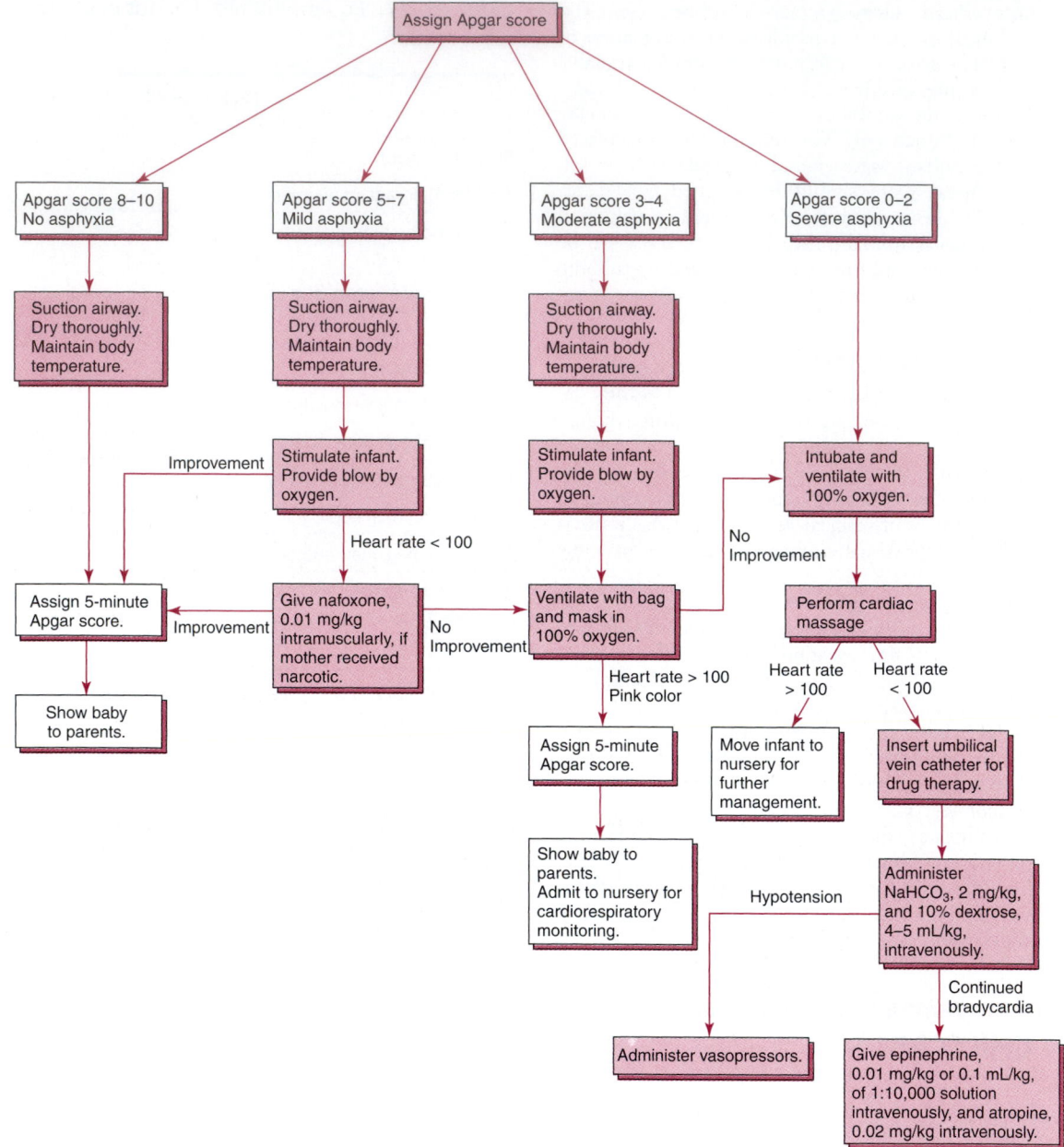

Figure 48–16. Algorithmic guide to neonatal resuscitation.

gency physician. The initial presentation of a physically abused child frequently occurs in the emergency department. The physician's responsibilities are to (1) acknowledge that a problem exists, (2) maintain a high index of suspicion, (3) discuss concerns with the parents in a sensitive and compassionate manner, (4) en-

sure protection of the child, (5) perform a complete medical evaluation of injuries or neglect, including documentation and radiologic imaging if indicated, and (6) report suspicions to child protective services.

The key to diagnosis of physical abuse is matching a carefully taken history with the extent of injury. Historical indicators of abuse include (1) a history that overestimates or underestimates the injury, (2) a history that suggests a lack of proper supervision, (3) inconsistencies or changes in the history, and (4) a delay in seeking medical care.

Note the quality of the parent-child interaction. Note whether the parents appear to be under the influence of drugs or alcohol.

Consider the child's motor skills and capabilities when evaluating the worthiness of the history. Injuries that could occur accidentally only in an older child with more advanced motor skills strongly suggest the possibility of nonaccidental injury.

Physical indicators of abuse include (1) injuries that do not match the history, (2) specific pathognomonic injuries (eg, looped wire marks or cigarette burns), (3) multiple injuries in various stages of healing, (4) different types of injuries or disease (eg, burns and fractures), (5) overall evidence of poor care, and (6) evidence of failure to thrive.

Clinical Findings

A. SYMPTOMS AND SIGNS

1. Bruises—The skin is the most commonly injured site. Injuries from physical abuse may be either nonspecific bruises or pathognomonic injuries that clearly reflect the instrument used to strike the child. The specific pattern of bruising may be indicative of nonaccidental trauma. Young children accidentally bruise themselves in predictable ways. A pattern of bruising significantly different from that of accidental bruises should raise suspicion of nonaccidental trauma. Locations of possible accidental cutaneous injuries in the young child are the shins and knees, hips (iliac crests), spinal prominences, chin, forehead, face (facial scratches in infants), lower arms, and elbows. Locations of injuries that probably are not accidental are the buttocks, inner thighs, genitalia, perineum, rectum, abdomen, chest, cheeks, neck, ears, and inner surface of upper arms. Be alert to specific abusive cutaneous injuries, for example, wire loop marks made by extension cords, belt marks, burns from hot objects such as silverware or heat vents, and belt buckle marks.

2. Skeletal trauma—Skeletal trauma occurs in one fifth to one third of abuse cases. More than half of these fractures occur in children under age 1 year. Suspicious fractures include femoral, epiphyseal metaphyseal, and rib fractures.

a. Femoral fractures—Femoral fractures (spiral or transverse) in children under age 3 years are suspicious. Minor falls, less than 30–60 cm, usually do not result in femoral fractures.

b. Epiphyseal metaphyseal fractures—Epiphyseal metaphyseal fractures in young infants and children are virtually diagnostic of abuse because they usually do not occur with accidental falls. These fractures usually occur as a result of severe pulling, twisting, or shaking of a child's limbs. These activities produce severe acceleration-deceleration forces on the limbs, resulting in metaphyseal chip fractures.

c. Rib fractures—Rib fractures in infants under age 2 years are extremely uncommon because the infant's rib cage is extremely pliant. Rib fractures in these children should always raise the possibility of nonaccidental trauma.

3. Burns—Burn injuries should raise the possibility of abuse in young children when they do not fit the normal accidental pattern. Children may be held down in scalding water as a means of discipline. These immersion burns typically cause injury to the buttocks and to the hands and feet in a stocking-glove distribution. The line of demarcation between burned and normal skin is usually quite abrupt. The flexion creases of the legs are usually spared. Children may also be burned by hot objects such as heater grates, curling irons, or cigarettes. Cigarette burns typically cause a deep circular burn about 5–10 mm in diameter. They may be difficult to differentiate from impetigo or insect bites.

4. Skin lesions—See Table 48–22.

5. Head injuries—Head injuries carry the highest incidence of morbidity and mortality. Abusive head injuries either are due to direct impact with a fist or other object or are secondary to severe rotational forces during vigorous shaking. Many children with abusive intracranial injury suffer a combination of impact and shaking injuries. Both shaking and impact can cause severe acceleration-deceleration forces to the brain, resulting in shearing injury to the bridging vessels that connect the brain to the dura. Subdural hematomas can then occur with resulting cerebral compression. In addition, these forces can cause direct neuronal injury within the brain. Infants who are severely shaken can present with sudden onset of seizure or coma but have no signs of head trauma. Typically infants who are severely shaken will have bilateral retinal hemorrhages and on CT scan may have bilateral subdural hemorrhages.

6. Abdominal injuries—Nonaccidental abdominal injury may produce severe injury to the viscera, including intramural hematomas of the small bowel, splenic or hepatic lacerations, traumatic pancreatitis, and renal contusions.

Table 48–22. Differential diagnosis of skin lesions in child abuse.

Skin Lesion	Diagnostic Procedure
Bruising Trauma	
Hemophilia	Prothrombin time, partial thromboplastin time
von Willebrand disease	Bleeding time, von Willebrand factor, antigen and ristocetin cofactor
Idiopathic thrombocyto-penic purpura	Complete blood count, platelet count
Periorbital ecchymoses secondary to neuroblastoma	CT scan
Mongolian spots	History, location
Coin rubbing	History, location, configuration
Self-inflicted	Depression, mental retardation
Local erythema, bullae Burn	
Impetigo	Culture, Gram staining
Photosensitivity reaction	History of sensitizing agent
Herpes simplex, herpes zoster	Culture, Tzanck smear
Car-seat burn	History
Hair loss Traumatic alopecia	History
Tinea capitis	Fungal culture, KOH slide
Alopecia areata	Clinical appearance
Seborrhea, eczema	Clinical appearance

B. Diagnostic Procedures

The following diagnostic studies should be ordered:

- CBC, platelet, and coagulation studies
- Urinalysis (recommend urine pregnancy test for adolescent females)
- A skeletal x-ray series, if indicated, of the skull, ribs, and long bones

Jain AM: Emergency department evaluation of child abuse. Emerg Med Clin North Am 1999;17:575. [PMID: 10516839] (Review.)

National Clearinghouse on Child Abuse and Neglect Information: http://www.calib.com/nccanch/pubs

SEXUAL ABUSE

General Considerations

Sexual abuse is involvement of children and adolescents in sexual activities they cannot comprehend because of their developmental level, activities to which they are unable to give informed consent, or activities that violate social taboos. These activities may physically injure the child and leave detectable patterns of trauma, but often sexual abuse may involve genital touching or fondling that does not cause detectable injury and may even be physically pleasurable to the child. Most victims of sexual abuse are female, and the mean age is approximately 7–8 years. Children are usually molested by males who are well known to them, either as a family member or trusted friend. Adolescents are more commonly molested by strangers.

Clinical Findings

Various behavioral reactions may ensue following sexual abuse. In preschool children, these can be fear states (eg, fear of adult males), nightmares, precocious sexual behavior, enuresis, encopresis, or behavior regression. In school-aged children, indicators may be precocious sexual behavior, sexual aggression toward other children, cross-dressing, school failure, truancy, running away, or depression. Adolescents may demonstrate behavioral problems with drugs, promiscuity, prostitution, running away, sexual aggression toward other children, depression, somatic complaints, or school failure.

Disclosures of sexual abuse often are incomplete and may later be retracted because the perpetrator is typically someone to whom the child feels great allegiance and on whom the child is dependent.

Some children who are sexually abused show signs of abuse, including genital and nongenital trauma as well as the presence of sexually transmitted diseases (STDs). An STD may be the only indication of molestation (Table 48–23). Direct injuries to hymenal tissue are rarely accidental. Hymenal lacerations should always raise the possibility of sexual abuse. Typical straddle injuries do not cause hymenal lacerations. Anal penetration may result in erythema and swelling of the perianal tissue as well as lacerations, abrasions, and bruising.

Children in whom sexual abuse is being considered should be evaluated at a center where health care providers accustomed to examining sexual abuse victims are located. The goals of the medical evaluation are to (1) treat any medical illness or injuries, (2) provide crisis counseling, (3) provide protection for the child if necessary, and (4) precisely document injuries and collect evidence for use by the legal system.

Table 48–23. Sexually transmitted diseases in children.[1]

Organism	Incubation Period	Clinical Features	Nonabusive Transmission	
			Perinatal Transmission	Nonsexual Contact
Neisseria gonorrhoeae	3–7 days	Vaginitis (prepubertal females); profuse discharge Cervicitis, pelvic inflammatory disease (postpubertal females) Pharyngitis, proctitis, urethritis Disseminated disease: rash, arthralgias, tenosynovitis, arthritis Asymptomatic carriage: vagina, cervix, pharynx, rectum	Yes, neonatal conjunctivitis	Not documented in children
Chlamydia trachomatis	7–21 days	Vaginitis (prepubertal females) Cervicitis, endometritis (postpubertal females) Urethritis, proctitis, epididymitis, prostatitis, Reiter syndrome, perihepatitis Asymptomatic carriage: vagina, cervix, rectum	Yes, may have asymptomatic vaginal, rectal carriage for up to 2 years	Not documented in children
Herpes simplex types 1 and 2	5–7 days	Painful vesicles on labia, vagina, anus, rectum	Yes	Documented with type 1: autoinoculation from oral to genital sites
Condyloma acuminatum, human papillomavirus	2–3 months average ? over 1 year	Mucosa: red, mulberry-type lesions Skin: verrucous warts common; may be pigmented papules	Yes	Possible
Trichomonas vaginalis	3–28 days	Vaginitis Asymptomatic carriage: urethra	Yes, neonate may carry in the vagina for 3–6 weeks after birth	Not documented in children
Syphilis	Primary: 10–90 days	Primary: chancre Secondary: rash, lymphadenitis, mucous patches, condyloma latum	Yes	Yes

[1]Reproduced, with permission, from Coulter K: Sexual abuse. In: *Pediatric Emergency Medicine: A Clinician's Reference.* Grossman M, Dieckmann RA (editors). Lippincott, 1991.

Approach the child in a compassionate, nonthreatening manner, and ask nonleading questions in an attempt to uncover whether sexual abuse has occurred. The physical examination should be performed immediately if sexual assault has occurred within 72 hours or the child has signs or symptoms of genital injury or infection. Look for both nongenital and genital injuries. Many examiners employ a colposcope with a camera attachment to provide photographic documentation of genital injuries. A speculum examination in a prepubertal child is indicated only when symptoms of vaginal injury (eg, vaginal bleeding) are present. This is best done under general anesthesia. Laboratory tests in the diagnosis of STDs should be obtained routinely, including wet mount and Gram staining of genital or rectal discharge; genital and rectal cultures for *N. gonorrhoeae* and *C. trachomatis;* pharyngeal culture for *N. gonorrhoeae;* culture of lesions suspicious for herpes simplex; and serologic studies for hepatitis B, syphilis, and human immunodeficiency virus, if indicated.

If the sexual assault has occurred within 72 hours of the examination, seminal fluid may be present on or within the child. The proper collection of this evidence is essential. Physicians who examine sexual abuse victims must be fully knowledgeable of the protocol for evidence collection in their locale.

Treatment

A. Treat Physical Injuries

Treat physical injuries as necessary. Inspect vaginal lacerations for possible extension into the abdominal cavity. Significant perineal or vaginal lacerations are best examined under general anesthesia in the operating room.

B. Treat Sexually Transmitted Diseases

Because STDs are relatively uncommon in prepubertal victims of sexual abuse, empiric therapy is recommended only if the child has a vaginal or rectal discharge that on Gram staining is suggestive of gonorrhea. Adolescent victims of sexual assault should routinely be given treatment for STDs at the time of the examination, because the incidence of STDs in this group is significant. Give empiric treatment for both *Chlamydia* (doxycycline, 100 mg twice a day for 10 days) and gonorrhea (ceftriaxone, 125 mg intramuscularly).

C. Offer Pregnancy Prevention

After documentation of a negative urine pregnancy test, adolescent girls should be offered prophylaxis against conception with norgestrel (Ovral), 2 pills at the time of examination and 2 pills 12 hours later orally.

D. Offer Counseling

Pediatric and adolescent victims of sexual abuse should be offered counseling following the initial evaluation. Many children will require extensive counseling, particularly those who are victims of long-term incestuous relationships.

Disposition

Children and adolescents may be discharged home if their medical condition permits and safety can be ensured. If the child is at risk for further sexual abuse, removal from parental custody and placement in shelter care is indicated.

Index

Page numbers in **bold face** type indicate a major discussion. Page numbers followed by *t* or *i* indicate tabular material or illustrations, respectively. Drugs are listed under generic names. When a drug trade name in listed, the reader is referred to the generic name.

Abacavir, side effects of, 865*t*
Abandonment, **67–68**
ABCs (airway, breathing, and circulation)
  in adult basic life support, 147–152
  in chest trauma, establishment of, 454
  in hemoptysis, 653–654
  in multiply injured patient, 210–211
  in shock, 194–195
  in spinal cord injury, 508
Abdomen. *See under Abdominal*
Abdominal aortic aneurysm, ruptured, **777–778**
  and abdominal pain, 261*t*, **277**
  and chest pain with hypovolemia, 242*t*
  diagnosis of, 271*t*
  and gastrointestinal bleeding, 292
  risk of, size of aneurysm and, 777, 777*t*
  and shock, 196
Abdominal bleeding, and shock, 200, 213
Abdominal emergencies. *See also specific type; Abdominal pain; Abdominal trauma*
  diarrhea and vomiting, **297**, 297*t*
Abdominal examination
  auscultation in, 264
  for diarrhea, 302
  for gastrointestinal bleeding, 285
  inspection in, 264
  palpation in, 264–265
  percussion in, 265
  for vomiting, 302
Abdominal fullness, 263
Abdominal infection, septic shock in, treatment of, 828*t*
Abdominal injuries. *See Abdominal trauma*
Abdominal pain, **257–282**
  abrupt, 262, 262*i*
  absence of, 263
  acute, not amenable to surgery, 282
  in acute intermittent porphyria, 361
  and anorexia, 263
  character of, 262–263
  and chest pain, 262
  in children, **1080–1081**, 1086*t*–1087*t*
  constipation and, 264, 1087*t*
  diarrhea and, 264, 297, 297*t*
  differential diagnosis, 260*t*, 271*t*
  dull, 262, 262*i*
  evaluation of patient with, **259–270**, 260*t*–261*t*
    history in, **259–264**
    laboratory examination in, **266–267**
    physical examination in, **264–266**, 264*t*
    radiologic examination in, **267–270**
  and fever, 263
  gastrointestinal bleeding and, 288
  gradual, 262, 262*i*
  gynecologic disorders and, **280–281**
  with hematuria, 758
  hepatobiliary disorders and, **275–277**
  intermittent with cramps, 262, 262*i*
  intestinal disorders and, **272–275**
  life-threatening problems, immediate management of, **257–259**, 258*i*
  localized, 263

  location of, 263
  management of, 258*i*, 270–272, **272–282**
  mode of onset, 262, 262*i*
  and nausea, 263
  pain management for, 270
  radiation of, 263
  and rigors, 263
  severe, 262, 262*i*
  shift in, 263
  shock and, 259
  in sickle cell anemia, 809–810
  surgery for, 272
  syncope with, 339
  urinary disorders and, **278–279**
  vascular disorders and, **277–278**
  in visceral (intestinal) ischemia, 775
  and vomiting, 263
Abdominal paracentesis, **121–122**, 122*i*
Abdominal tenderness
  gastrointestinal bleeding and, 288
  one-finger palpation in evaluation of, 264–265
Abdominal thrust, **152–153**, 153*i*, 154*i*
Abdominal trauma, **218–219**, **467–476**, 576
  airway management in, 467
  assessment of, 467–468
  blunt, 467, **469–470**
    in pregnancy, 745–746
  breathing in, 467
  child abuse and, 1099
  circulation in, 467
  computed tomography in, 468–469
  diagnostic peritoneal lavage in, 468
  diagnostic testing in, 468
  diaphragmatic hernia in, 460
  diaphragmatic injuries in, **470–472**
  disability in, 467
  emergency laparotomy in, 468
  emergency treatment of specific injuries in, **470–476**
  exposure of patient for examination in, 467–468
  flank injuries in, **476**
  fluid resuscitation in, 467, 468, 767
  intestinal injuries in, **473–476**
  laboratory evaluation of, 468
  laparoscopy in, 469
  life-threatening injuries in, immediate management of, **467–470**
  liver injuries in, **472**
  pancreatic injuries in, **472**
  penetrating, 467, **470**
    in pregnancy, 745–746
  plain radiography in, 468
  renal injuries in, **472–473**
  and shock, 195
  splenic injuries in, **470**
  surgical consultation in, 468
  treatment of, 468
  types of, 469–470
  ultrasound in, 468, 469, 469*i*
  vascular injuries in, **771**
  wound care in, 576
Abductor pollicis longus muscle, 552

ABO incompatibility, 822–823
Abortion
  complete, 734*t*, 735
  incomplete, 734*t*, 735, 742–743
    pelvic pain in, 727*t*
  inevitable, 734*t*, 735
  missed, 733, 734*t*, 735
  septic, **735–736**
    pelvic pain in, 727*t*
  spontaneous, **733–735**, 743
    classification of, 734*t*
  threatened, 734, 734*t*
"Abrasion tattooing," 580
Abrin, in poisonous plants, 1003
Abruptio placentae, 743–744
Abrus precatorius, toxins in, 1004*t*
Abscesses. *See also specific type or structure affected*
  superficial, incision and drainage of, **140–142**
Absolute neutrophil count (ANC), 814
Absorbable sutures, 582
Absorption dressings, for wounds, 588
Abuse
  alcohol (*See under Alcohol*)
  child, **1097–1102**
    burn injuries in, 928–929
    orthopedic injuries in, 515
    physical, **1097–1100**
    radial head subluxation in, 523
    reporting of, 68
    sexual, 740, 741, 1079, **1100–1102**, 1101*t*
Accelerated idioventricular rhythm (AIVR), 706
Accidents
  industrial, **45**
  nuclear, **45**
  radiation, **45**
  transportation, **45**
Acclimatization, 936–937
ACD CPR. *See* Active compression/decompression CPR
ACE inhibitors. *See* Angiotensin-converting enzyme inhibitors
ACEP. *See* American College of Emergency Physicians
Acetaminophen
  for chronic degenerative disk disease, 417
  with codeine, for corneal abrasion, 620
  for fever, in children, 1066
  and hyponatremia, 893*t*
  for Jarisch-Herxheimer reaction, 853
  for lumbosacral strain, 417
  for osteoarthritis, 410
  for otitis media, 1070
  pediatric dosing, 1044
  poisoning/overdose of, **972–973**, 973*i*
  for seizures, in children, 1062
  for sickle cell disease, in children, 1094
  for transfusion reaction prevention, 823
Acetazolamide
  for acute angle-closure glaucoma, 605
  for acute high-altitude pulmonary edema, 950
  for central retinal artery occlusion, 605
  for eye trauma, 619

Acetazolamide (*cont.*)
  for hyperphosphatemia, 906
  for hypokalemic periodic paralysis, 367
  for mountain sickness, 948–949
  for pseudotumor cerebri, 386
  for uveitis, 613
Acetylcholine esterase, nerve agents and, 37
Acetylcysteine, for acetaminophen poisoning/overdose, 973
Achilles tendon injuries, **541–542**
  in ankle sprains, 543
  testing for, 541–542, 542*i*
Acid burns, **925–926**
  ocular, **616**
Acid-base disorders, **908–915**. *See also* Acidosis; Alkalosis
  classification of, 908–909
  compensatory mechanisms in, 909, 909*t*
  definitions of, 908
  metabolic, **910–913**, 913*t*
  mixed acid-base disorders, **913–915**
  respiratory, **909–910**, 910*t*, **912**
  triple disturbances, **914–915**
Acid-base status, correction of, for salicylate overdose, 1005–1006
Acidosis, 908
  and alcoholic ketoacidosis, 876–877
  and cardiogenic shock, 202
  and diabetic ketoacidosis, 867–869
  and hyperkalemia, 901–902
  lactic, **875–876**
  metabolic, 231*t*, **238–239**, **910–912**
    drugs causing, 968*t*
    and respiratory acidosis, **914**
    and respiratory alkalosis, **914**
    and respiratory distress/dyspnea, 231*t*, **238–239**
    in septic shock, 825, 826
  respiratory, **909–910**, 910*t*
    acute, 910
    chronic, 910
      in chronic bronchitis and emphysema, 658
      and metabolic acidosis, **914**
      and metabolic alkalosis, **914**
    seizure activity causing, 334, 341
Acids, poisoning with, 981, 981*t*
Aconitine, in poisonous plants, 1003
Acoustic neuroma, 630
  peripheral vertigo with, 631*t*
Acquired immune deficiency syndrome (AIDS), **863–866**. *See also* Human immunodeficiency virus infection
  clinical findings in, 863–864
  disposition in cases of, 866
  drug reactions in, 866, 866*t*
  gastrointestinal presentation of, 864–865
  general considerations in, 863
  laboratory data in, 865–866
  neurologic presentations of, 864
  ophthalmologic presentations of, 865
  organ system-specific presentations of, 864–865
  pericardial effusions in, 687
  and pneumonia, 234
  pulmonary presentations of, 864
  renal presentations of, 865
  skin presentations of, 865
  systemic presentations of, 865
  treatment of, 866
Acrolein, and inhalation injury, 924
Acromioclavicular joint injuries, **517**
β-actam/β-lactamase inhibitors, for pneumonia, 661, 668

ACTH. *See* Adrenocorticotropic hormone
Actinic keratitis, 617
Activated charcoal, for poisoning/overdose, 970
  of acetaminophen, 973
  of cardiac glycosides, 980
  of hydrocarbons, 992, 993
  of ingested poisons, 965
  of paralytic shellfish, 962
  of poisonous mushrooms, 1001
  of puffer fish, 961
  of salicylates, 1005
  of theophylline, 1008
Active compression/decompression (ACD) CPR, 165
Acute abdomen. *See* Abdominal pain
Acute adrenal insufficiency (Addisonian crisis), **881–883**
Acute angle-closure glaucoma, 602, 604*i*, **604–605**
Acute chest syndrome, in sickle cell disease, 809, 1094
Acute coronary syndrome, **675–684**
Acute high-altitude pulmonary edema, **949–950**
Acute intermittent porphyria
  drugs therapy for, contraindicated and accepted, 361*t*
  weakness caused by, **361–362**
Acute lymphocytic leukemia (ALL), 815
Acute mountain sickness, **948–949**
Acute myelocytic leukemia (AML), 815
Acute osteomyelitis, in children, 1078*t*, **1079–1080**
Acute otitis media, in children, **1070–1072**
Acute respiratory distress syndrome (ARDS), **671–673**, 672*t*
Acute tubular necrosis, in septic shock, 827
Acyclovir
  for Bell palsy, 358
  for genital herpes infection, 852
  for herpes pharyngitis, 639*t*
  for herpes simplex, 1021
  for herpes zoster, 1020
  for herpetic whitlow, 563
  for zoster, 256
ADAMTS-13, in thrombotic thrombocytopenic purpura, 793
Adapin. *See* Doxepin
Addisonian crisis (acute adrenal insufficiency), **881–883**
Addison's disease, 882
  and abdominal pain, 271*t*
Adefovir, side effects of, 865*t*
Adenosine
  in advanced life support, 159*t*, 161
  drug interactions of, 696
  in EMS field treatment, 15
  in heart transplant patients, 696
  for paroxysmal supraventricular tachycardia, 696
  for preexcitation arrhythmias, 700
  side effects of, 696
Adenovirus infections
  and exanthems, 1082*t*–1083*t*
  and keratoconjunctivitis, 611–612
  and pharyngitis, in children, 1073
  and urinary tract infections, in children, 1075
ADH. *See* Antidiuretic hormone
Adhesives, tissue, for wound closure, 584
Adjunctive drugs, for intubated patient, 189
Admission, to hospital, 5
  involuntary, **1038**
  through emergency department, 70–71
Adnexa, blunt trauma of, **618–620**
Adolescent(s)
  Osgood-Schlatter disease in, 535–536

pneumonia in, **834–835**
  tuberculosis in, 670
Adrenal hemorrhage, in meningococcemia, 858
Adrenal insufficiency
  acute (Addisonian crisis), **881–883**
  in meningococcemia, 858
  treatment of, 858
Adrenaline, for wound care, in children, 1043
β-Adrenergic receptor agonists
  for asthma and COPD, 659–660
  for bronchitis, 668
  for complete heart block, 706
α-Adrenergic receptor antagonists
  for jellyfish stings, 958
  for prostatitis, 849
β-Adrenergic receptor antagonists
  in advanced life support, 161
  for angina, 683–684
  for atrial fibrillation, 698
  for atrial flutter, 699
  bee/wasp stings and, 953
  bradycardia caused by, 704
  for catecholamine crisis, 885
  for chest pain, 243
  for delirium tremens, 398
  for heart failure, 686
  for hypertension, in aortic dissection, 780
  for mitral valve prolapse, 251
  for multifocal atrial tachycardia, 699
  for myocardial infarction, 677
  for paroxysmal supraventricular tachycardia, 696
  poisoning/overdose of, **975–976**
  for preexcitation arrhythmias, 700
  for shock, 211
  for thyroid storm, 879
Adrenergic responses, in shock, 194
β-Adrenergic sympathomimetic bronchodilators
  for asthma, 227
  for COPD, 227
  for pulmonary fibrosis, 227
Adrenocortical insufficiency
  primary, 882
  secondary, 882
Adrenocorticotropic hormone (ACTH) stimulation test, for adrenal insufficiency, 883
Adrenocorticotropic hormone (ACTH) therapy
  contraindications to, in delirium tremens, 398
  for gouty arthritis, 409
Adult advanced life support, **156–163**
Adult basic life support, **147–156**, 148*i*
Adult respiratory distress syndrome. *See* Acute respiratory distress syndrome
Advanced life support
  adult, **156–163**
  airway management in, **157**
  cardiac rhythm correction in, **157–162**
  cardiopulmonary resuscitation in, for infants and children, **163–165**
  pediatric, **164–165**
  pharmacologic therapy for, **158–162**, 158*t*–160*t*
  pharmacologic therapy in, in EMS field treatment, 15
  postresuscitation stabilization, **162**
  termination of, **162–163**
AEDs. *See* Automated external defibrillators
Aeromonas hydrophila, and dysentery, 308*t*
Affective disorders, **1033–1034**
African American(s), sickle cell anemia in, 808–811
Age, and vital signs, 1040, 1043*t*
Agitated confusion, **402**
Agitated patients, S.A.F.E.S.T. approach to, 1027–1028

β-Agonists
  for anaphylactic shock, 207
  for asthma, 1058
Agraphesthesia, in stroke patients, 371
AHA. *See* American Heart Association
AIDS. *See* Acquired immune deficiency syndrome
AIDS-related dementia, 863–864
Air, in abnormal locations, in abdominal pain, 268, 269i–270i
Air embolism, systemic, in chest trauma, **464–465**
Air transport, in EMS system, 12, **18**, 53
Airborne precautions, 25t
Airplane crashes, 45
Airway
  assessment of, 167
  compromised (*See* Compromised airway)
  injuries to
    in facial trauma, 439
    laryngeal, **436**
    in neck trauma, 436, 438–439
    pharyngeal, **436**
    tracheal, **436**
  management of
    in abdominal trauma, 467
    in advanced life support, 157
    in anaphylactic shock, 206
    in angioedema, 1013
    in asthma and COPD, 660
    in basic life support, **147**, 149i, 150i
    in burn injuries, 917
    in cardiogenic shock, 201–202, 679
    in chest trauma, 454
    in children, **186–187**, 186t
    in congestive heart failure, 680
    in croup, 647
    in delirium or confusion, 391
    in EMS field treatment, **14**
    equipment for, 169t, 186t
    in esophageal varices, 291
    in gastrointestinal bleeding, 285
    in head injury, 421–422
    in heat stroke, 939
    in hemoptysis, 653–654
    in hypoglycemia, 874
    in laryngeal airway injury, 436
    in lightning injuries, 941
    in maxillary (Le Fort) fracture, 445
    in maxillofacial trauma, 435–436
    in multiply injured patient, 210–211
    in near-drowning, 945
    in neck trauma, 435–436, 437
    needle cricothyroidotomy for, **175–178**
    nonsurgical alternatives for, **174–175**
    in paralytic shellfish poisoning, 962
    in pediatric basic life support, 164
    in pharyngeal airway injury, 436
    in pneumothorax, 655–656
    in poisoning/overdose, 963, 970, 971
    in puffer fish poisoning, 961
    in pulmonary aspiration syndrome, 671
    in respiratory distress/dyspnea, 230t, **235–237**
    in seizures, 332–334
    in septic shock, 825
    in shock, 194
    in smoke inhalation, 917
    in sore throat, 634–635
    in spinal cord injury, 493–494, 508
    in status asthmaticus, 188
    in stroke, 369
    surgical, **178**
    techniques for, 98–102

  in trauma patients, 188–189
  universal precautions for, 173
  in vascular trauma, 766, 769
obstruction of
  in asthma and chronic obstructive pulmonary disease, 656–661, 659
  in chronic bronchitis, 656
  in emphysema, 656
  foreign body, **152–153**, 153i, 154i
    in children, 164, 187–188
    and respiratory distress/dyspnea, **224–225**
  upper, traumatic injury to, **214**
AKA. *See* Alcoholic ketoacidosis
Albumin
  for hypovolemic shock, 199
  plasma concentration, determination of, **916**
  transfusion of, **821**
Albuminocytologic dissociation, in Guillain-Barré syndrome, 360
Albuterol
  for anaphylactic shock, 207
  for asthma, 227, 659–660, 1058
  for bronchiolitis, 1056
  for bronchitis, 668
  for COPD, 227, 659–660
  in EMS field treatment, 15
  for pulmonary fibrosis, 227
Alcohol intoxication, and coma, **327**
Alcohol poisoning, 985–987
Alcohol use/abuse. *See also* Ethanol
  and cluster headache, 389
  and delirium, 1030–1031
  electrolyte abnormalities in, 367
  head injuries in, **434**
  hypoglycemia in, 874
  lactic acidosis in, 875
  pneumonia in, 835
  pulmonary aspiration syndrome in, 671
  syncope in, 346
  and thrombocytopenia, 789
  TMJ dislocation in, 652
Alcohol withdrawal, 1031
  clinical findings in, 397
  delirium or confusion in, **396–398**
  magnesium deficiency in, 399
  seizures in, 341, 396, **397**, 398
Alcoholic hepatitis, 276
Alcoholic ketoacidosis, **876–877**
Aldosterone, in heart failure, 684
Alertness level
  in spinal cord injury, 496
  in stroke patients, 371
Alexandrium, 961
Algorithms
  for abdominal pain, 258i
  for altered mental status, 17i
  for asthma, 1057i
  for automated external defibrillator, 157i
  for burns, 918i
  for burns/burn injuries, 918i
  for cardiac arrest, 148i
  for chest pain, 241i
  for compromised airway, 168i
  for confusion, 392i
  for delirium, 392i
  for diarrhea, 294i, 298i, 300i
  for fever
    in children, 1067i
    in infants, 1065i
  for gastrointestinal bleeding, 284i
    lower, 294i
    upper, 287i

  for genitourinary trauma, 478i, 479i, 480i
  for headache, 380i
  for hematemesis, 1090i
  for hematochezia, 1091i
  for hyperkalemia, 899i
  for hyponatremia, 892i
  for inhalation injury, 918i
  for loss of consciousness, 333i
  for melena, 1090i
  for multiply injured patient, 209i
  for neonatal resuscitation, 1098t
  for psychiatric emergencies, 1027i
  for respiratory distress/dyspnea, 223i
  for resuscitation, of children, 1098i
  for seizures, 333i
  for shock, 192i
    in children, 1048i
  for standing orders, 13i
  for stridor, in children, 1054i, 1054t
  for syncope, 333i
  for unconsious patient, 312i
  for vomiting, 294i, 298i, 300i
    in children, 1088i, 1088t
Alkali burns, **925–926**
  ocular, **616**, 616i, 927
Alkalis, poisoning with, 981, 981t
Alkalosis, 908
  and hypokalemia, 898
  metabolic, **912–913**, 913t
    and respiratory acidosis, **914**
    and respiratory alkalosis, **914**
  respiratory, **912**
    in hyperventilation, 346
    and metabolic acidosis, **914**
    and metabolic alkalosis, **914**
    in septic shock, 825
Allen test, **97**
Allergenics, 995t
Allergies
  anaphylactic shock with, 206–207
  conjunctivitis with, 610, 611i
  epistaxis (nosebleed) with, 632
  sore throat with, 638t
  to transfusion, 822t, 823
  and treatment of wounds, 575
Allis technique, for reduction of posterior hip dislocation, 532, 532i
Alloimmune hemolytic anemia, **807**
Almotriptan, for migraine, 389
Alpha particles, 21
Alprazolam, for psychogenic hyperventilation, 346
Alteplase, for myocardial infarction, 677–678
Altered mental status
  protocol for, 17i
  shallow breathing and, **225**
  shock and, 194
Altered states of consciousness, rare causes of, **346–347**
Alternative airway, establishing, in EMS field treatment, 14
Alternative basic life support techniques, 165
Altitude, high
  and cerebral edema, **950–951**
  disorders associated with, **948–951**
  and pulmonary edema, **949–950**
Aluminum phosphate, for hypophosphatemia, 905
Alveolar bone, 648–649
Alzheimer disease, and dementia, 1030
Amanita mushrooms, poisoning, 1002t
Amatoxin poisoning, 1001–1002
Amaurosis fugax, in transient ischemic attacks, 376

Ambulances
  air, 12
  in multicasualty incidents/disasters, 51–52
  surface, 12
American College of Emergency Physicians (ACEP)
  Core Content Task Force II, 3
  emergency medicine definition of, 1
  expert witness guidelines of, 71
American Heart Association (AHA), chain of survival, 147
Amikacin, for cellulitis, 855
Aminocaproic acid, for hyphema, 613
Aminoglycoside(s)
  for cellulitis, 855
  contraindications to
    in botulism, 364
    in myasthenia gravis, 366
  for hepatic abscess, 276
  for nonclostridial anaerobic cellulitis, 856
  for open fractures, 220
  for pneumonia, 836*t*
  for pulmonary infections in cystic fibrosis, 673
  for septic arthritis, 838*t*
  for septic shock, 828*t*
  for suppurative cholangitis, 276
Aminophylline, for complete heart block, 706
Amiodarone
  in advanced life support, 159*t*, 161
  for atrial fibrillation, 698, 700
  for atrial flutter, 699
  in EMS field treatment, 15
  for multifocal atrial tachycardia, 699
  for paroxysmal supraventricular tachycardia, 697
  for preexcitation arrhythmias, 700
  for ventricular fibrillation, 158, 703
  for ventricular tachycardia, 702
Amitriptyline
  for headache prophylaxis, 388
  and hyponatremia, 893*t*
  overdose of, 1008–1010
Ammonia poisoning, 994, 995*t*
Amnesia, **400–401**
  causes of, 401, 401*t*
  delirium or confusion in, 394*t*, **400–401**
  episodes of, **400–401**
  in head injuries, 430–431
  hysterical, 402–403
  transient global, **401**
Amobarbital, for status epilepticus, 336*t*
Amoxapine, poisoning/overdose of, 1009
Amoxicillin
  for nasal fracture, 448
  for otitis media, 628*t*, 1071*t*, 1072*t*
  resistance to, 842–843, 851
  for urinary tract infections, in children, 1076
  in zygomaticomaxillary complex fractures, 446
Amoxicillin-clavulanate
  for animal bites, 564–565, 596
  for dacryocystitis, 608
  for eyelid infections, 609
  for glanders, 24*t*
  for human bites, 565
  for impetigo, 1019
  for melioidosis, 24*t*
  with nasal packing for epistaxis, 633
  for otitis media, 628*t*, 1071*t*, 1072*t*
  for periorbital cellulitis, 1075
  for Q fever, 24*t*
  for sinusitis, 643
  for tooth pain, 649
  for urinary tract infections, 842*t*
Amoxicillin-sulbactam, in human bites, 565

Amoxil. *See* Amoxicillin
Amphetamine(s)
  delirium or confusion with, 399, 2030
  poisoning/overdose of, 967*t*, **974–975**
Amphotericin B, for septic shock, 828*t*
Ampicillin
  for cellulitis, 1016
  for encephalitis, 314
  for erysipelas, 1016
  for fever, in infants, 1064
  for meningitis, 314, 833*t*, 834*t*
    in children, 1068*t*
  for osteomyelitis, in children, 1078*t*
  for pneumonia, 836*t*, 1060*t*
  prophylactic, in wound care, 590*t*
  for prostatitis, 849
  for puerperal sepsis, 748
  for pyelonephritis, 279
  resistance to, 842–843
  for septic arthritis, in children, 1078*t*
  for urinary tract infections, in children, 1077
Ampicillin-sulbactam
  for acute abdomen, 259*t*
  for epiglottitis, 1052
  for suppurative cholangitis, 276
  for urinary tract infections, 842*t*
Amprenavir, side effects of, 865*t*
Amputation(s), **511–512**, **595–596**
  fingertip, **557–558**
  for frostbite, 935
  hand, **568–569**
  traumatic, **511–512**
Amrinone, for calcium-channel blocker poisoning, 977
Amygdalin, in poisonous plants, 1003
Amyl nitrite, for cyanide poisoning, 40, 983, 983*t*
Amylase
  in abdominal pain, 266
  in abdominal trauma, 468
Anal fissures, in children, 1089
Analgesia. *See also* Pain management/relief (analgesia)
  poisoning/overdose of, 1005–1006
  in rapid-sequence intubation, 181–182
Anaphylactic shock, 197, **206–207**
  bee/wasp stings and, 953
  in children, 1047
Andromedotoxin, in poisonous plants, 1004*t*
Anemia, **802–813**. *See also specific type*
  in children, **1093**
  of chronic disease, 802
  classification of, 802, 803*t*
  definition of, 802
  diagnosis of, 803–804
  hemolytic, **804–808**
    hereditary, 812–813
    microangiopathic, 792–794
    in sickle cell anemia, 810
  iron-deficiency, 802, **804**
  lower gastrointestinal bleeding and, 293
  macrocytic, 803*t*
  microcytic, 803*t*
  normocytic, 803*t*
  in pneumonia, 668
  red blood cell quantification in, 802, 803*t*
  respiratory distress/dyspnea in, **239**
  sickle cell, **808–811** (*See also* Sickle cell anemia/disease)
  in Waldenström macroglobulinemia, 817
Anesthesia
  in hand trauma, 549–550, 550*i*, 551*i*, 552*i*, 578, 578*i*, 579*i*
    avoidance of inflamed areas in, 550

  dosage of, 549
  local infiltration of, 549, 577*i*
  inhalation, 576
  initiation of, checklist for, 181*t*
  local, 576–578
    drugs used for, 577*t*
    for intubation, 179, 179*t*
    ophthalmic, 621, 622*t*, 624
    properties of, 179*t*
    for tooth pain, 649
  local infiltration, 576–578
    method of injection, 576–577, 577*i*
  for nasal fracture, 448
  regional, 578
    for facial surgery, 579, 579*i*
    for hand surgery, 578, 578*i*, 579*i*
  spinal, 578
  topical, 576
    for children, 1043
    and intubation, 99, 179, 180
  for wounds, 576–579
Aneurysms
  aortic, abdominal, ruptured, **777–778**
    abdominal pain in, 261*t*, **277**
    chest pain with hypovolemia in, 242*t*
    diagnosis of, 271*t*
    gastrointestinal bleeding in, 292
    leaking, 265
    shock in, 196
  arterial, **777–781**
    cerebral, in sickle cell anemia, 810
  false, 768
  femoral artery, **781**
  hypogastric artery, **778**
  peripheral, **781**
  popliteal artery, **781**
  stereotactic microsurgery for, 377
  in subarachnoid hemorrhage, 372
    rebleeding of, 373
  thoracic aortic, **778–781**
  visceral artery, **778**
Angel dust. *See* Phencyclidine
Angina, **682–684**
  atypical, 683
  diagnosis of, 247*t*
  of effort, 683
  Ludwig, 639*t*
  pectoris, **682–684**
  Prinzmetal (variant), 683–684
  stable, 683
  unstable, 683
  Vincent, 638*t*, 840, 841
Angiodysplasia, and gastrointestinal bleeding, **293**
Angioedema, **1012–1013**
  hereditary, 237
Angiography
  in abdominal pain, 270
  in angiodysplasia, 293
  in aortic injury, 462
  in arterial dissection, 376
  in diverticulitis, 293
  in headache, 379
  in intracerebral hemorrhage, 373
  in lower gastrointestinal bleeding, 289
  in penetrating chest trauma, 465
  in pulmonary embolism, 661, 663
  retrograde, complications of, **786**
  in stroke, 371
  in subarachnoid hemorrhage, 372
  in thoracic outlet syndrome, 786
  in upper gastrointestinal bleeding, 288

Angioplasty
  for angina, 684
  for cardiogenic shock, 680
  carotid artery, 377
  for myocardial infarction, 679, 680
  percutaneous transluminal, complications of, **786,** 787t
Angiotensin, in heart failure, 684
Angiotensin-converting enzyme (ACE) inhibitors
  and angioedema, 1013
  for central venous hypervolemia, 245
  for heart failure, 686
Animal bites, **596**
  antibiotics for, 564–565, 596
  cellulitis with, **564–565**
  to hand, 564–565, 572
  and rabies infection, 590–593, 591i
  reporting of, 69
  venomous, weakness with, **353–354**
Anion gap
  and diabetic ketoacidosis, 868
  and metabolic acidosis, 911
Anistreplase (APSAC), for myocardial infarction, 677–678
Ankle
  abscess of, incision and drainage of, 142
  anatomy of, 540
  arthrocentesis of, 136, 138, 139i
  dislocations of, **542–543**
  injuries of, **540–544**
    radiography in, criteria and rules of, 540, 543
Ankle ligaments, 540
  injuries to, 543–544
Ankle sprains, **543–544**
Ankylosing spondylitis, **412–413**
  back pain in, 412–413, 415
Anomia, 402
Anorexia, and abdominal pain, 263
Anoscopy, for lower gastrointestinal bleeding, 288
Anoxic spells, **692**
Antacids
  for gastritis, 291
  and gastrointestinal bleeding, 285
  phosphate-binding, for hyperphosphatemia, 906
Antecubital fossa venous cutdown, emergency, **76–78,** 78i, 79i
Antecubital veins, for venipuncture, 75
Anterior chamber
  blunt trauma to, 618
  depth of, estimation of, 604i, 624
Anterior chamber paracentesis, 605, 607
Anterior cord syndrome, 506
Anterior cruciate ligament
  injuries of, 537–538
    and hemorrhagic arthritis, 407
  stability of, assessment of, 537, 538i
Anterior drawer test, of cruciate ligaments, 537
Anterior horn cells, in poliomyelitis, 351, **357**
Anterior nasal packing, for epistaxis, **133–136,** 134i
Anthrax
  as biologic weapon, **22–25,** 46
  cutaneous, **22,** 23t
  gastrointestinal, **22,** 23t
  inhalational, **22,** 23t
Anthrax meningitis, **22**
Antibiotic prophylaxis
  in bite injuries, 564, 596, 597
  in blast injuries, 595
  in foreign body injuries, 567, 568
  for meningococcemia exposure, 858
  with nasal packing for epistaxis, 633
  in wound care, 564, 589, 590t, 597

Antibiotic resistance
  in gonorrhea, 851
  in urinary tract infection, 842–843
Antibiotic therapy. *See also specific agent and Antimicrobials*
  for abdominal trauma, 470
  for animal bites, 564–565, 596
  for anthrax, 25
  for aspiration, 225
  for asthma and COPD, 660–661
  for botulism, 364
  for brain abscess, 321
  for brucellosis, 28
  for bursitis, 414
  for cellulitis, 855–856
  for complex hand injuries, 568
  for conjunctivitis, 610
  for corneal and conjunctival foreign body injuries, 620
  for dacryoadenitis, 609
  for dacryocystitis, 608
  for disseminated gonococcemia, 861
  for dysuria-frequency syndrome, 845
  for ear pain, 627t–628t
  for encephalitis, 314
  for epiglottitis, 638t, 1052
  for esophageal injury, 461
  for eye trauma/disorders, 621, 622t
  for eyelid infections, 609
  for frontal nasal fracture, 449
  for glanders, 29
  for gonorrhea, 851
  for hand trauma, 557
  for herpes simplex, 1021
  for human bites, 565
  for impetigo, 1019
  for infected burns, 929
  for infected vascular gangrene and cellulitis, 856
  for infection in immunocompromised patients, 830
  for mandibular fracture, 443
  for mangling injuries, 572
  for melioidosis, 29
  for meningitis, 314, 381, 384, 831–832, 833t, 834t
  for meningococcemia, 858
  for mononucleosis, 816–817
  for nasal fracture, 448
  for necrotizing fasciitis, 857
  for neutropenia, 814–815
  for ocular burn injuries, 616
  for open fractures, 220
  for orbital cellulitis, 606
  for osteomyelitis, 839
  for pelvic inflammatory disease, 846, 846t
  for perforated duodenum, 254
  for perforated stomach, 254
  for peritonsillitis, 639t, 646
  for pharyngitis, 840–841
  for plague, 26
  for pneumonia, 234, 668, 835, 836t
  for prostatitis, 849
  for puerperal sepsis, 748
  for pulmonary infections in cystic fibrosis, 673
  for pyelonephritis, 844
  for Q fever, 28
  for septic abortion, 735–736
  for septic arthritis, 410, 838, 838t
    in children, 1078t, 1079
  for septic shock, 205, 827, 828t, 828t
  for sinusitis, 643
  for skull fractures, 425

  for soft tissue infections, 855
  for sore throat, 636, 638t–639t
  for spinal cord injury, 495
  for spinal epidural abscess, 356
  for spinal infection, 420
  for stingray wound, 957
  for subungual hematoma, 528, 558
  for sulfur mustard exposure, 39
  for suppurative tenosynovitis, 565
  for syphilis, 853
  for tendonitis, 414
  for tooth pain, 649, 650t–651t
  topical, for wounds, 589
  for toxic shock syndrome, 862
  for toxic shock-like syndrome, 862
  in traumatic amputation, 511
  for tularemia, 27
  for urinary tract infection, 842t, 842–843, 844
  for zygomaticomaxillary complex fractures, 446
Anticholinergic agents
  for asthma and COPD, 660–661
  centrally acting, 399, 399t
    delirium and confusion caused by, **399**
  poisoning/overdose of, 967t, **975**
  in poisonous plants, 1003, 1004t
  for vertigo, 632
Anticholinergic properites, and hyperthermia, 971
Anticoagulation therapy
  for angina, 684
  for arterial dissection, 376
  for atrial fibrillation, 698
  contraindicated in pericarditis, 682
  for deep venous thrombosis, 783
  drug interactions, 1010, 1011t
  for ergotism, 787
  for frostbite, 935
  poisoning/overdose of, **1010–1011**
  for pulmonary embolism, 664, 682
  for stroke prevention, 377
Anticonvulsant therapy, 338t
  for confused or delirious patient, 395
  for meningitis, 384
  for status epilepticus, 334, 335, 336t
  for stroke patients, 369
  for subarachnoid hemorrhage, 373
  for trigeminal neuralgia, 385
Antidepressants, **1037**
  for headache prophylaxis, 388
  tricyclic
    central anticholinergic syndrome caused by, 399t
    proarrhythmic activity of, 702
Antidiarrheal agents, for gastroenteritis, 274, 309
Antidiuretic hormone
  deficiency of, and central diabetes insipidus, 888
  inappropriate secretion of, **886–888**
    and hyponatremia, 895
Antidotes, for poisoning, 970, 970t
Antidysrhythmics
  in advanced life support, 161–162
  for ventricular fibrillation, 157–158
Antiemetics
  for hyperemesis gravidarum, 743
  for infectious gastroenteritis, 306–309
  for migraine, 388–389
  for urolithiasis, 761
Antifibrinolytic agents
  for disseminated intravascular coagulation, 802
  for hemophilia, 796
Antihistamines
  for allergic transfusion reaction, 823
  for angioedema, 1013

Antihistamines (*cont.*)
  central anticholinergic syndrome caused by, 399*t*
  for contact dermatitis, 1018
  poisoning/overdose of, 975
Antimicrobials. *See also* Antibiotic prophylaxis; Antibiotic therapy
  for acute abdomen, 259*t*, 270–272
  for fever, in infants, 1064
  for gastroenteritis, in children, 1078
  for hepatic abscess, 276
  for hypothermia, 933–934
  for meningitis, in children, 1068*t*, 1069
  for otitis media, 1070, 1071*i*, 1072*t*
  for pharyngitis, in children, 1073–1074
  for sickle cell disease, in children, 1094
  for skin and wound cleansing, 580
  for suppurative cholangitis, 276
Antiparkinsonism agents, central anticholinergic syndrome caused by, 399*t*
Antiplatelet therapy, 792*t*, 794
  for stroke prevention, 376–377, 776
Antipsychotic agents
  atypical, **1037**
  and neuroleptic malignant syndrome, **1036–1037**
  poisoning/overdose of, **1000–1001**, 1036
  for psychotic confusional states, 402
  traditional, **1036**
Antipyrine, for otitis media, 1070
Antiretroviral therapy, for HIV/AIDS, side effects of, 865, 865*t*
Antiseizure agents, for rapid-sequence intubation, 182
Antiseptics, in hand trauma, 556
Antispasmodic agents, central anticholinergic syndrome caused by, 399*t*
Antithrombin III replacement, **821**
Antivenin
  for black widow spider bites, 954
  for brown recluse spider bites, 955
  for jellyfish stings, 958
  for scorpion bites, 955–956
  for sea snake bites, 957
  for snake bites, 952, 952*t*
Antiviral therapy
  for genital herpes simplex virus infection, 852, 852*t*
  for HIV/AIDS, side effects of, 865, 865*t*
Antizol. *See* Fomeprizole
Anuria, **750–752**
Anus, abscesses around, incision and drainage of, 142
Anxiety
  and abdominal examination, 265
  and hyperventilation, 346
  and syncope, 346
  and tension headache, 388
Aorta
  injury of
    in chest trauma, **462**
    imaging of, 462, 463*i*
    thoracic, injury of, **770–771**
Aortic aneurysm
  abdominal, ruptured, **777–778**
    and abdominal pain, 261*t*, **277**
    diagnosis of, 271*t*
    and gastrointestinal bleeding, 292
    leaking, 265
      and chest pain with hypovolemia, 242*t*
  and shock, 196
  thoracic, **778–781**

Aortic coarctation, 691, 692, 693, **693**
Aortic dissection, **778–781**, 778*t*, 780*t*
  and chest pain with hypovolemia, 242*t*
  diagnosis of, 248*t*
  and shock, 196
  syncope in, 339
    treatment and disposition of, 344
Aortic murmurs, with heart failure in infants, 692
Aortic regurgitation
  and chest pain, **251–252**
  diagnosis of, 247*t*
Aortic rupture, traumatic, **217–218**, 462
Aortic stenosis, 691, 693
  and chest pain, **251–252**
  diagnosis of, 247*t*
  syncope caused by, **343–344**
Aortoenteric fistula, and gastrointestinal bleeding, 290*t*
Aortography, 767, 777, 779
Ape hand deformity, in median nerve injury, 570*i*
Apgar score, 1096, 1096*t*, 1097
Aphasia
  expressive, 401
  fluent, 394*t*, **401–402**
  nonfluent, 401
  receptive, 401
  in stroke patients, 371, 401–402
Aphthous stomatitis, diagnosis and treatment of, 650*t*
Aplastic crisis, in sickle cell anemia, 810
Apley tests, for meniscal tears, 538
Apnea
  and airway management, 167
  in bronchiolitis, 835
  central, 1051
  in children, **1051–1052**
  obstructive, 1051
  in spinal cord injury, 493, 494
Apneustic breathing, coma and, 316
Apoplexy, pituitary, **885–886**
Appendicitis, 269*i*–270*i*, **272**
  and abdominal pain, 260*t*, 263, 1086*t*
  in children, 1081
  diagnosis of, 271*t*
  pelvic pain in, 727*t*
  traumatic, 476
Apricot pits, toxins in, 1004*t*
ARDS. *See* Acute respiratory distress syndrome
Arenaviridae, 31*t*
Argentine hemorrhagic fever, 31*t*
Arginine vasopressin. *See* Antidiuretic hormone
Argon poisoning, 995*t*
Arm
  burns of, **928**
  cold injury to, **934–936**
Arm fatigue, in thoracic outlet syndrome, 786
Arm pain, in myocardial infarction, 676
Arm veins, for venipuncture, 75
Arrhythmias (dysrhythmias), **694–724**. *See also specific type*
  in asthma and COPD, 658
  atrial, 697–699
  in β-adrenergic blocker poisoning, 976
  bradyarrhythmias, **703–706**
  in cardiogenic shock, 202
  in children, **1049**, 1050*t*
  commonly encountered, **712–724**
  in digitalis poisoning, 980
  in myocardial contusion, 459–460
  in myocardial infarction, 676
  preexcitation, **699–700**
  proarrhythmic ventricular, **702**

  in septic shock, 825–826
  in stimulant overdose, 974
  in stroke patients, 371
  supraventricular, **695–700**
  syncope in, 339, 339*t*, 342, **343**
  tachyarrhythmias, **694–703**
  in theophylline overdose, 1008
  in tricyclic antidepressant overdose, 1008–1010
  ventricular, **700–703**, 711
Arsenic poisoning, 989*t*, **990–991**
  blindness in, 607
  neuropathy and weakness in, **360–361**
Arsenic salt ingestion, 990
Arsine gas inhalation, 990
Arsine poisoning, 995*t*
Arterial aneurysms, **777–781**
Arterial blood gases
  in acute lung injury, 672
  in air embolism, 465
  in asthma, 658
  in atelectasis, 667
  in botulism, 364
  in chronic bronchitis, 658
  in chronic obstructive pulmonary disease, 658
  in coma, 316
  in emphysema, 658
  in head injuries, 422
  in heart failure, 685
  in HIV/AIDS, 865
  in hyperventilation, 346
  in intubated patient, 190
  in metabolic disorders, 396
  in pleural effusion, 666
  in pneumonia, 668, 834
  in pneumothorax, 655
  in pulmonary aspiration syndrome, 671
  in pulmonary edema, 685
  in pulmonary embolism, 662
  in septic shock, 825
  in spinal cord injury, 493, 506
  in status epilepticus, 334
  in weak patient, 349
Arterial dissection, **376**
Arterial gas embolism, **947–948**
Arterial injury
  in blunt trauma, 767
  in frostbite, 787
  hemorrhage in, 767
  ischemia in, 767
Arterial lines
  for intubated patients, 190
  in septic shock, 825
Arterial occlusion, acute peripheral ischemia due to, **773–774**
Arterial puncture, inadvertent, in lumbar puncture, 132
Arteriogram
  in arteriovenous fistula, 785
  in distal femoral fractures, 535
  in hemoptysis, 654
  in knee dislocations, 536, 772
  mesenteric, in visceral (intestinal) ischemia, 775–776
  in peripheral aneurysms, 781
  in pulmonary embolism, 681
  in trauma, indications for, 215, 215*t*
  in vascular injuries, 768, 769, 771
Arteriolar visceral ischemia, nonocclusive, 775
Arteriovenous fistula, 574, **785**
Arteriovenous malformations, 370, 372, 377
Arthritis, **404–415**
  acute

evaluation of, **404–407,** 405*i*
  specific conditions causing, emergency management of, **408–414**
arthrocentesis in, **407,** 407*t*
back pain in, 415
classification of, **407,** 407*t*
in degenerative joint disease (osteoarthritis), **410–411**
gonococcal, 404, 409–410, 838
gouty, **408–409**
hemorrhagic (class IV), **407,** 407*t*
  in hemophilia, 796
  in von Willebrand disease, 799
inflammatory (class II), **407,** 407*t*
intestinal, **412**
joint examination in, 406
in Lyme disease, 863
monarticular, **408–410**
  versus nonarticular rheumatism, 406, 406*t*, **413–414**
noninflammatory (class I), **407,** 407*t*
oligoarticular, 406–407, **408–411**
polyarticular, 406–407, **410–413**
poststreptococcal reactive, **411**
in pseudogout, **409**
psoriatic, **412**
in Reiter syndrome, **412**
in rheumatic fever, **411**
rheumatoid, **411–412**
  infection in, 837
septic (class III), 407, 407*t*, **409–410, 837–838**
  in children, **1078–1079,** 1078*t*
  in disseminated gonococcemia, 861
  with puncture wounds, 597
systemic causes of, 404
in systemic lupus erythematosus, **413**
traumatic, **408**
viral, **413**
Arthrocentesis, **136–140,** 407, 407*t*, 861
of ankle, 138, 139*i*
of elbow, 138, 138*i*
of feet, 139
of hands, 139
of knee, 137, 137*i*
of shoulder, 137–138, 138*i*
and synovial fluid analysis, 139–140
of wrist, 138–139
Arthrogram, in rotator cuff injuries, 518
Arthroscopy
  in cruciate ligament injuries, 538
  in meniscal tears, 538
  in tibial spine fractures, 536
Ascites, in primary peritonitis, **281**
Asphyxia
  in near-drowning, 944–946
  traumatic, **465**
Asphyxiants
  chemical, 994, 995*t*
  simple, 994, 995*t*
Aspiration
  of gastric contents, 671
  of joint, in septic arthritis, 410, 837, 838
  massive, **225**
  of oropharyngeal secretions, 671
  positive-pressure ventilation and, 170
  and respiratory distress/dyspnea, 230*t*, **235**
Aspiration pneumonia, 671, 835
  hydrocarbon poisoning and, 992
  treatment of, 836*t*
Aspirin
  for angina, 684
  for basilar artery insufficiency, 345

for central venous hypervolemia, 245
for chest pain, with normal hemodynamics, 245
contraindications to, in thrombocytopenia, 794
in EMS field treatment, 15
for Jarisch-Herxheimer reaction, 853
for migraine, 388
for myocardial infarction, 677, 684
  platelet function impaired by, 794
for pleurisy, 252
for pleurodynia, 252
poisoning/overdose of, 967*t*
for rheumatoid arthritis, 411–412
for stroke prevention, 376
  combined with dipyridamole, 377
for sunburn, 927
Assessment, in triage, 50, 51*i*
Astereognosis, in stroke patients, 371
Asterixis, in metabolic disorders, 396, 403
Asthma, **656–661**
in adults, 659
and airway management, 188
cardiac, 226, 680
in children, 659, **1056–1058,** 1057*i*
clinical findings in, 657
conditions associated with, 656, 657*t*
differential diagnosis of, 659
disposition in cases of, 661
evaluation of, 658–659
history of, 657
impending respiratory failure in, 657
laboratory findings in, 658–659
life-threatening exacerbations, 660–661
medical history in, 658
mild exacerbations, 657, 659–660
moderate exacerbations, 657, 660
peak expiratory flow in, 657, 658
physical examination in, 657
precipitating factors in, 657, 657*t*
radiographic findings in, 658
and respiratory distress/dyspnea, 230*t*, **237**
severe, **227–228**
severe exacerbations, 657, 660
treatment of, 659–661
Asystole, 158
Ataxia
  cerebellar hemorrhage and, 373
  in stroke patients, 371, 375
  in Wernicke encephalopathy, 398
Ataxic hemiparesis, 375
Atelectasis, **666–667**
  intrinsic (resorption), 667
  and respiratory distress/dyspnea, 230*t*, **232–233**
Atenolol
  in advanced life support, 160*t*, 161
  poisoning/overdose of, 976
Atherosclerosis
  and arterial occlusion, 773
  and myocardial infarction, 675
  risk factors for, 375*t*
  and stroke, 374–377, 776
  surgical interventions for, 377
Athletes, concussions in, 430–431
Athlete's foot. *See* Tinea pedis
Ativan. *See* Lorazepam
Atmospheric pressure changes, disorders due to, **946–951**
Atopic dermatitis, and exfoliative erythroderma, 1014
Atrial fibrillation, **697–698**
  in children, 1050*t*
  electrocardiogram in, 697, 712, 716*i*
  in stable patients, 698

  thromboembolic complications of, 697–698
  treatment of, 698, 700
  in unstable patients, 698
  in Wolf-Parkinson-White syndrome, 700
Atrial filling pressure, resuscitation and, 199
Atrial flutter, **698–699**
  in children, 1050*t*
  electrocardiogram in, 698, 712, 717*i*
  in stable patients, 699
  thromboembolic complications of, 698–699
  in unstable patients, 699
Atrial myxoma, syncope with, 343
Atrial tachycardia, 695, 712, 713*i*
  multifocal, **699**
    electrocardiogram in, 699, 712, 717*i*
Atrioventricular block, **704–706**
  in children, 1050*t*
  first-degree, 705
    electrocardiogram in, 705, 720, 721*i*
  second-degree, Mobitz type I, 705
    electrocardiogram in, 705, 720, 721*i*
  second-degree, Mobitz type II, 705
    electrocardiogram in, 705, 720, 721*i*
  third-degree, 705–706
    electrocardiogram in, 705, 720, 721*i*, 722*i*
  treatment and disposition of, 707
Atrioventricular conduction disturbances, 703
Atrioventricular junctional rhythm, **707**
  electrocardiogram in, 707, 719*i*, 720
Atrioventricular nodal reentrant tachycardia (AVNRT), 695–697
  electrocardiogram in, 695, 712, 713*i*–715*i*
Atrioventricular reciprocating tachycardia (AVRT), 695–697
  antidromic, 699–700
  electrocardiogram in, 695, 712, 715*i*
  orthodromic, 699
  treatment of, 700
  in Wolf-Parkinson-White syndrome, 699–700
Atropa belladonna, toxins in, 1004*t*
Atrophic vaginitis, 846–848
Atropine
  in advanced life support, 159*t*, 161
  for arrhythmias, 976, 980
  in children, 187, 1043–1044
  for cholinesterase inhibitor poisoning, 314
  for ciguqtera toxin poisoning, 960
  for complete heart block, 705–706
  for drug-induced seizures, 971
  in EMS field treatment, 15
  endotracheal administration of, 189
  for eye trauma/disorders, 619, 620, 622*t*
    misuse of, 624
  for gastroenteritis, 309
  for nerve agent exposure, 37
  for organophosphate poisoning, 365, 998
  poisoning/overdose of, 967*t*, 975
  for rapid-sequence intubation, 180–181
  for scorpion bites, 955
  side effects of, 706
Auditory nerve injury, 440
Augmentin. *See* Amoxicillin-clavulanate
Aura
  epileptic, 340
  in migraine, 388
Auricle
  frostbite of, 642
  lacerations of, **451**
Auscultation
  of abdomen, 264
  for respiratory distress, in children, 1051
Austere medical care, 51

Autoimmune hemolytic anemia, **804–807**
  cold-type, 805–807
  drug-adsorption type, 807
  drug-related, 807, **807–808**
  mixed-type, 807
  neoantigen-type drug-related, 807–808
  primary, 805
  secondary, 805
    causes of, 805, 805*t*
  warm-type, 805
Automated external defibrillators (AEDs), 155,
  156*i*, 157*i*
  for children, 164
  in EMS field treatment, 14
Autonomy, of patient, and refusal to consent, 66
Autotransfusion
  for hemorrhagic shock, 214
  for hemothorax, 457
Avascular necrosis
  in carpal bone fractures, 526
  in hip injuries, 531, 532
AVPU mnemonic, for level of consciousness assess-
    ment, 219
Avulsion
  of fingernails, **558–559**
  of teeth, **450, 636–640,** 651*t*
Avulsion flaps, in wound care, 576
Avulsion fracture, 513
Axillary artery injury, in luxatio erecta, 519
Axillary nerve block, 578
Azalea, toxins in, 1004*t*
Azathioprine, for pemphigus vulgaris, 1017
Azithromycin
  for bullous myringitis, 627*t*
  for chancroid, 854
  for gonorrhea, 851
  for otitis media, 1071*t*, 1072*t*
  for pharyngitis, in children, 1074
  for pneumonia, 668, 835, 836*t*, 1060*t*
  for urethritis, 851
Aztreonam, for acute abdomen, 259*t*

Bacillus anthracis, 22, 23*t*
Bacillus cereus, and gastroenteritis, 304*t*
Bacitracin
  for burn injuries, 566
  for eye trauma/disorders, 621, 622*t*
Back, physical examination of, in headache patients,
    383
Back pain, **415–420**
  acute, evaluation of, **415–417,** 416*i*
  in ankylosing spondylitis, 412–413, 415
  in arthritis, 415
  baseline evaluation of, **415–417**
  and chest pain, 251
  in children, **419**
  in chronic degenerative disc disease, **417–418**
  in epidural compression syndrome, 415, **419**
  in facet syndrome, **419**
  history of, 415
  laboratory findings in, 415–417
  in lumbosacral strain, **417–418**
  neoplasm causing, **420**
  neurologic deficit with, 415
  nonorthopedic (visceral) causes of, 415, 417*t*
  physical examination in, 415
  radicular distribution of, 415
  radiographic findings in, 415–417
  red flags in evaluation of, 415
  in sciatica, **418–419**
  specific conditions causing, emergency treatment
    of, **417–420**
  in spinal cord injury, 496
  in spinal infections, **419–420**
  traumatic, 415, **417**
  in zoster infection, **420**
Bacteremia
  in children, 1064–1066
  and urinary tract infections, in children, 1076
Bacterial agents, as biologic weapons, **22–29,**
    23*t*–24*t*
Bacterial colonization, of wound, 581
Bacterial gastroenteritis, **303**
Bacterial peritonitis, 259
Bacteriodes fragilis, and suppurative cholangitis, 276
Bactrim. *See* Trimethoprim-sulfamethoxazole
Bactroban. *See* Mupirocin
Bag-mask ventilation, 150, 151
  in pediatric basic life support, 164
Bag-valve-mask ventilation
  and asthma, 188
  in children, 187
  for positive-pressure ventilation, 170
BAL. *See* Dimercaprol
Balanitis, 847
  dysuria in, 757
  phimosis in, 764–765
  treatment of, 764*i*
Balanoposthitis
  phimosis in, 764–765
  treatment of, 765
Balloon, nasal, for epistaxis, 633, 634*i*
Balloon occlusion, for epistaxis, 135
Balloon pump, intra-aortic
  for cardiogenic shock, 680
  for mitral regurgitation, 681
  for ventricular septal rupture, 681
Balloon tamponade, for esophageal varices, 292
Balloonfish poisoning, 961
Band ligation, for esophageal varices, 292
Bankart fracture, 519
Barbiturate(s)
  extravasation of, 768
  for seizures, in children, 1062
Barium enema
  and abdominal pain, 269
  for lower gastrointestinal bleeding, 289
  in visceral (intestinal) ischemia, 775
Barium swallow, in esophageal injury, 461
Bartholin gland cyst, **848,** 851
Barton bandage, for mandibular fracture, 443
Barton fracture, 524
Base station hospitals, for EMS systems, 9–10
Basic life support, **147–156,** 148*i*
  ABCs of, **147–152**
  airway in, **147,** 149*i*, 150*i*
  alternative techniques, 165
  breathing in, 149*i*, **150–151**
  chain of survival, 147
  circulation in, **151–152,** 152*i*
  complications of, **152**
  defibrillation, **153–156,** 155*i*
  early, 147
  pediatric, **163–164**
  techniques of, **147–152**
Basilar artery insufficiency, syncope in, **345**
Basilar artery thrombosis, and coma, **323**
Basilar skull fractures, 219, **425,** 449–450
Basilic vein, deep, identification of, 77
Battery, failure to obtain consent and, 64
Battle sign
  in basilar skull fractures, 425, 449
  in temporal bone fracture, 441

Beck triad, of cardiac tamponade, 216
Bed rest
  for chronic degenerative disk disease, 418
  for lumbosacral strain, 418
  for pulmonary agent exposure, 38
  for Wernicke encephalopathy, 399
Bee sting, **953**
Bell clapper deformity, in testicular torsion, 754
Bell palsy, **357–358**
Belladonna poisoning, 975
Benadryl. *See* Diphenhydramine
Bence-Jones proteinuria, 817
"Bends," **946–947**
Benign paroxysmal vertigo, 631*t*
Benign pericardiocentesis, 118, 118*i*
Bennett fracture, 526–527
Benzathine penicillin. *See* Penicillin G
Benzene, toxicity, 992
Benzocaine
  cautions for use, 1018
  for otitis media, 1070
Benzocaine-tetracaine, for drainage of peritonsillar
    abscess, 645
Benzodiazepine(s)
  for acute intermittent porphyria, 362
  for alcohol withdrawal, 1031
  for catecholamine crisis, 885
  and coma, 311
  and delirium, 1030–1031
  for delirium tremens, 397–398
  in EMS field treatment, 15
  for epistaxis, 633
  for hallucinogen withdrawal, 1031
  for head injuries, 423
  for heat stroke, 939
  for hypertension, 974
  for neuroleptic malignant syndrome, 1036
  for organophosphate poisoning, 365
  psychiatric uses, 1036
  for sedative-hypnotic drug withdrawal, 398
  for seizures, in children, 1062
  for status epilepticus, 334
  for stimulant intoxication, 1030
Benztropine, for antipsychotic overdose, 1001, 1036
Berry aneurysm, and subarachnoid hemorrhage,
    372
Beta blockers. *See* β-Adrenergic receptor antagonists
Beta particles, 21
Betamethasone
  for contact dermatitis, 1018
  for fetal lung maturity, 747
Biaxin. *See* Clarithromycin
Bicarbonate
  for acidosis, in septic shock, 826
  for alcoholic ketoacidosis, 877
  for anoxic spells, 692
  for arrhythmias, 1009
  for diabetic ketoacidosis, 871
  in EMS field treatment, 15
  for hyperglycemic hyperosmolar nonketonic syn-
    drome, 871
  for hyperkalemia, 901
  for hypotension, 1010
  for lactic acidosis, 876
  for proarrhythmic ventricular arrhythmias, 702
Bicarbonate retention, in chronic bronchitis and
    emphysema, 658
Bicarbonate studies, for coma, 316
Bilevel positive airway pressure (BiPAP)
  for asthma and COPD, 660
  for pulmonary edema, 226
  for respiratory acidosis, 910

Biliary colic
  and abdominal pain, 260t, **275**
  diagnosis of, 271t
Biliary disease, in sickle cell anemia, 810
Biologic toxins, as biologic weapons, **32–36**, 33t
Biologic weapons, **22–36**, 46
  bacterial agents, **22–29**, 23t–24t
  biologic toxins, **32–36**, 33t
  defense against, 46
  drug therapy for, 46
  viral agents, **29–32**
Biot breathing, coma and, 316
Bioterrorism
  and declaration of need by hospital, 46
  detection of, 46
BiPAP. See Bilevel positive airway pressure
Bipartite patella, 534
Biphasic defibrillation, 155, 156i
Bipolar affective disorder, 1034
Birth, **746–747**
  emergency room, 747
  premature, 746–747
Bismuth subsalicylate
  for gastroenteritis, 274, 309
  poisoning/overdose of, 1005–1006
Bisphosphonates
  for hypercalcemia, 904
  for multiple myeloma, 817
Bite(s), 575, **596–597**
  animal, **596**
    antibiotics for, 564–565, 596
    cellulitis with, **564–565**
    to hand, 564–565, 572
    and rabies infection, 590–593, 591i
    venomous, weakness with, **353–354**
  black widow spider, **953–954**
  human, **596–597**
    antibiotics for, 564, 565, 596, 597
    cellulitis with, **564–565**
    to clinician, in TMJ reduction, 652
    with metacarpal fractures, 527, 565
  intubation and, 173
  sea snake, **957**
  snake, **951–952**
Biventricular failure, in infants, 692
Black death. See Septicemic plague
Black eye, **619**
Black nightshade, toxins in, 1004t
Black widow spider bites, 354, **953–954**
Blackouts, 1035
Bladder
  distended, in oliguria or anuria, 751–752
  neuropathic, 750, 751t
Bladder catheterization. See Urinary catheterization
    (bladder catheterization)
Bladder dysfunction, in spinal cord injury, 495
Bladder infection, 752, 758, 759, **841–843**
Bladder injuries, 486i, **486–488**, 487i
  in abdominal trauma, **473**
  blunt, 486, 487i
  imaging of, 481, 486–488, 487i
  special examinations and procedures in, 477–481
  with urethral injuries, 488
Bladder outlet obstruction
  causes of, diagnostic clues to, 751t
  detection of, 751
  differential diagnosis of, 752
  drainage in, 751–752
  intravenous access in, 751
  oliguria or anuria in, 750–752
  partial, 752
  treatment of, 751–752

Bladder rupture, 486i; 486–488
Bladder stones, 750, 751t, 760
Bladder tumors, bladder outlet obstruction with,
    750, 751t
Blast injuries, **594–595**
Bleeding. See also specific site or structure affected and
    Hemorrhage
  in children, **1085–1091**
  gastrointestinal (See Gastrointestinal bleeding)
  in newborn, 1089
Bleeding diathesis, hematuria in, 759t
Bleeding disorders, **789–802**
Bleeding time, 791t
Blepharospasm, with corneal abrasion, 620
Blindness
  monocular
    in temporal arteritis, 381
    in transient ischemic attacks, 376
  snow, 617
  toxic causes of, **607–608**
Blisters, pemphigus vulgaris and, 1017
Blood
  in pleural space, and respiratory distress/dyspnea,
    231–232, 233i
  warming of, 214
Blood alcohol samples, consent for, 66–67
Blood count, for abdominal pain, 266
Blood cultures, in septic shock, 827
Blood gases
  in acute lung injury, 672
  in air embolism, 465
  in asthma, 658
  in atelectasis, 667
  in botulism, 364
  in chronic bronchitis, 658
  in chronic obstructive pulmonary disease, 658
  in coma, 313, 316
  in emphysema, 658
  in head injuries, 422
  in heart failure, 685
  in HIV/AIDS, 865
  in hyperventilation, 346
  in intubated patient, 190
  in metabolic disorders, 396
  in pleural effusion, 666
  in pneumonia, 668, 834
  in pneumothorax, 655
  in pulmonary aspiration syndrome, 671
  in pulmonary edema, 685
  in pulmonary embolism, 662
  radial artery puncture for analysis of, **96–98**, 97i
  in septic shock, 825
  in spinal cord injury, 493, 506
  in status epilepticus, 334
  in weak patient, 349
Blood loss
  in children, 1045, 1045i
  in closed fractures, 511, 512t
  in conscious patient with history of syncope,
    335–339
  and hemorrhagic shock, 213
  internal, hidden sources of, 213
  and shock, 195, 196, 200
Blood pressure
  in children, 1045, 1045i
  in conscious patient with history of syncope,
    335–337
  and diarrhea, 302
  elevated (See Hypertension)
  in head injuries, 423
  and headache, 382
  in intracerebral hemorrhage, 374

  in lacunar stroke, 376
  in septic shock, regulation of, 826
  in spinal cord injury, 495
  and vomiting, 302
Blood pressure cuff
  for hemostasis, in extremity wounds, 574
  as tourniquet, 211
Blood pressure support, in cardiac tamponade, 689
Blood products, refusal to consent to, 66
Blood supply, revascularization of, 377
Blood tests
  in cardiogenic shock, 202
  in diarrhea, 302
  in pelvic pain, 728
  in poisoning/overdose, 965, 968t
  in stroke, 371
  in vomiting, 302
Blood transfusions. See Transfusions
Blood urea nitrogen
  in coma, 316
  in diabetic ketoacidosis, 869
  in heart failure, 686
  in hyperglycemic hyperosmolar nonketonic syn-
    drome, 870
Blood volume, in children, 1045, 1045i
Blood warming, 214
Blowfish poisoning, 961
Blowout fractures, **447, 619–620**
  computed tomography of, 447, 447i
  impure, 447
  pure, 447
"Blue bloaters," 657
Blue dot sign, in torsion of testicular appendages,
    754
"Blue toe syndrome," 774
Blunt cardiac injury. See Myocardial contusion
Blunt trauma
  abdominal, 467, **469–470**
    in pregnancy, 745–746
  bladder, 486, 487i
  and cardiac tamponade, 217
  chest, vascular injury in, 770
  eye, **618–620**
  genitourinary, 478i, 480i
  neck, **438**
    vascular injury in, 769
  nose, epistaxis in, 632
  renal, 479, 481
  spinal cord, 495
  ureteral, 484
  vascular, 767, 769
Body lice, 1023
Boehler angle, in calcaneal fractures, 544
Boerhaave syndrome, 263, 665
Bolivian hemorrhagic fever, 31t
Bone, calcium deposits in, increasing, for hypercal-
    cemia, 904–905
Bone infection. See Osteomyelitis
Bone marrow, radiation injury and, 943
Bone marrow transplantation, for multiple
    myeloma, 817
Bone marrow tumors, back pain with, 420
Bone pain, in sickle cell anemia, 809
Bone scan
  in back pain, 420
  in osteomyelitis, 839
  in tarsal injuries, 545
Borderline personality disorder, **1034**
Borrelia, 1082t–1083t
Borrelia burgdorferi infection, **863**
Botulinum antitoxin, 33, 364
Botulinum toxin, as biologic weapon, **32–33**

Botulism, **363–364**
as biologic weapon, **32–33**, 33*t*
infant, 364
symptoms and signs of, 363*t*, 363–364
weakness in, 353, **363–364**
Boutonnière deformity, **528–529, 561,** 561*i*
Bovine thrombin, 574
Bowel perforation, and abdominal pain, **273**
Box jellyfish envenomation, **957–958**
Boxer's fracture, 526–527, 565
Brachial artery injury, in humerus fractures, 519
Bradyarrhythmias, **703–706**
management of, 202, 243–244
Bradycardia, 158
in children, 1045, 1050*t*
pacemaker malfunction and, 710
sinus, **703–704,** 712, 713*i*
syncope in, 343
in urolithiasis, 761
Brain abscess, 832
and coma, **321**
delirium or confusion with, 394
in meningitis, 832
in sinusitis, 645
Brain death, criteria for, **330**
Brain tumors
and coma, **321–322**
headache with, **386**
Brainstem reflexes, in spinal cord injury, 502
Breach of duty, 61
Breast abscess, in puerperal mastitis, 748–749
Breast infection, postpartum, **748–749**
Breath sounds, in children, 1050–1051
Breathing
in abdominal trauma, 467
in basic life support, 149*i,* **150–151**
in chest trauma, 454
in head injuries, 422
in hemoptysis, 653–654
of multiply injured patient, 211
in pediatric basic life support, 164
shallow, altered mental status with, **225**
shock and, 195
Bretylium, for ventricular tachycardia, 702
British anti-lewisite (dimercaprol), for lewisite exposure, 40
Brodifacoum, poisoning/overdose of, 1010
Bromocriptine, for neuroleptic malignant syndrome, 1036–1037
Bronchial artery embolization, in hemoptysis, 654
Bronchiolitis, **835–837**
in children, **1056**
Bronchitis
acute, **667–668**
chronic, 656–661
"blue bloaters" with, 657
Bronchodilators
for asthma and COPD, 659–660
for bronchiolitis, 837, 1056
for bronchitis, 668
Bronchoscopy
in atelectasis, 667
fiberoptic, 175
for intubation in neck injury, 435
in hemoptysis, 654
in tracheobronchial injury, 463
in vascular injury to neck, 769
Broselow-Luten length-based tapes, 164
Brown recluse spider bites, 354, **954–955**
Brown-Séquard syndrome, 506
Brucella abortus, 27
Brucella canis, 27

Brucella melitensis, 27
Brucella suis, 27
Brucellosis, as biologic weapon, 24*t,* **27–28**
Brudzinski sign, 379, 383
Bruises, child abuse and, 1099, 1100*t*
Bruits
in headache patients, 383
in stroke patients, 370
in vascular trauma, 768
Brush, for wound cleansing, 580
B-type natriuretic peptide (BNP), in heart failure, 685, 686
Bubonic plague, 23*t,* 25
Buck fascia, rupture of, 490
Bucket-handle loop, in abuse-related fractures, 515
Bucket-handle tear, of menisci, 538
Buckle fracture, 513
Buddy taping, in toe fractures or dislocations, 546
Budesonide, for croup, 1052
Bulbocavernosus reflex, in spinal cord injury, 502
Bullet wounds
abdominal, 467, 468, 470
in pregnancy, 746
chest, 465–466
hand, 572
neck, 438
Bullous impetigo, 854–855
Bullous myringitis, 627*t*
Bullous pemphigoid, and exfoliative erythroderma, 1015
Bumetanide, for pulmonary edema, 227
Bunyaviridae, 31*t*
Bupivacaine
for local anesthesia, 577*t*
for rib fractures, 464
for tooth pain, 649
for zoster, 256
Buproprion, 1037
Burkholderia mallei, 29
Burkholderia pseudomallei, 29
Burkholderia spp., 24*t*
Burn center, transfer to, 923
Burns/burn injuries, **917–929**
age and, 922
associated injuries, 919–920, 922
chemical, **925–926**
chest, **928**
child abuse and, 928–929, 1099
circumferential, 922, **928**
depth of, 920–921, 921*i,* 922*t*
differential diagnosis, 1100*t*
electric, **941–942**
evaluation of, **920–923**
extremities, **928**
feathering, 940
genital, 490, 492
hand, **566–567**
and hyperkalemia, 901
life-threatening problems and, immediate management of, **917–920,** 918*i*
from lightning, **940**
linear, 940
neck, **928**
ocular, **615–617, 927**
acid, 616
alkali, 616
eyelid eversion for examination of, 616, 616*i*
thermal, 616–617
ultraviolet radiation, 617
outpatient management of, **929**
pain management for, 922
punctate, 940

severity of, **920–922,** 920*t,* 921*f,* 921*t*
site of, 921
size of, 919*i,* 920
sunburn, **927**
tar, **926–927**
thermal, 940
treatment of, **923–929**
underlying medical problems and, 922
wound care for, 922–923
Bursa aspiration, 414
Bursitis, 413, **414**
"But for" rule, 61
Butoconazole, for vaginitis, 847
Butterfly needle. *See* Scalp vein needle
"Butterfly" perineal hematoma, 490
Butyrophenones, poisoning/overdose of, 1000–1001

Ca⁺. *See* Calcium
Caffeine
for headache, 388
poisoning/overdose of, 974–975
Caisson disease, **946–947**
Caladium, toxins in, 1004*t*
Calamine lotion, for contact dermatitis, 1018
Calcaneal fractures, **544**
Calcaneofibular ligament, 540
injuries to, 543–544
Calcifications, in abdominal radiographs, 268
Calcipotriene, for psoriasis, 1022
Calcitonin, for hypercalcemia, 904–905
Calcium
deposition in bone, increasing, for hypercalcemia, 904–905
excretion of, for hypercalcemia, 904
plasma concentration, determination of, **916**
serum concentration disorders, **902–905**
Calcium channel blockers
in advanced life support, 161–162
for atrial fibrillation, 698
for atrial flutter, 699
bradycardia caused by, 704
and chest pain, 253
for multifocal atrial tachycardia, 699
for paroxysmal supraventricular tachycardia, 696–697
poisoning/overdose of, **976–977**
for preexcitation arrhythmias, 700
Calcium chloride
for calcium-channel blocker poisoning/overdose, 977
in EMS field treatment, 15
for hypocalcemia, 903
for hypokalemia, 901
Calcium gluconate
for chemical burns, 926
for ciguqtera toxin poisoning, 960
for hypocalcemia, 903
for hypokalemia, 901
Calcium pyrophosphate, in pseudogout, 409
Call outs, in team approach to cardiac arrest, 146
Caloric test
in head injuries, 422
in psychogenic coma, 347
in Wernicke encephalopathy, 398
Camphor
for contact dermatitis, 1018
toxicity, 992
Campylobacter infection
and dysentery, 307*t*
and gastroenteritis, in children, 1077
reactive arthritis in, 412

Cancer. *See specific type or organ or structure affected*
Candida albicans infection (candidiasis)
  balanitis in, 847
  in diabetes mellitus, 846–847
  foreskin, 765
  in HIV-infected patients, 863
  oral (thrush), 863
  paronychia in, 562
  vaginitis in, 846–848
Cantharellus cibarius, 1002t
Capillary ooze, 574
Capnocytophaga canimorsus infection, cellulitis in, 564–565
Capnography
  in abdominal trauma, 467
  in intubated patient, 190
Captopril
  for central venous hypervolemia, 245
  for heart failure, 686
  for hypertensive urgency, 687
Carbamate poisoning, 365, 967t
Carbamazepine, 338t
  in head injuries, 423
  and hyponatremia, 893t
  toxicity of, 338t
  for trigeminal neuralgia, 385
Carbapenem. *See* Imipenem-cilastatin
Carbogen, for central retinal artery occlusion, 605
Carbohydrate metabolism, disorders of, 867–877
  alcoholic ketoacidosis, 876–877
  diabetic ketoacidosis, 867–869
  hyperglycemic hyperosmolar nonketonic syndrome, 869–873
  hypoglycemia, 873–875
  lactic acidosis, 875–876
Carbohydrate therapy, for acute intermittent porphyria, 362
Carbon dioxide poisoning, 995t
Carbon monoxide
  poisoning, 977–979, 978t, 994, 995t
    headache in, 381
  and smoke inhalation injury, 924, 925
Carbonic anhydrase inhibitors, for pseudotumor cerebri, 386
Carbonyl chloride (phosgene), as chemical weapon, 38
Carcinoma. *See specific type or organ or structure affected*
Cardiac arrest
  in children, 163
  early prevention of, 147
  epidemiology of, 145–146
  fibrinolytic therapy for, 165–166
  lightning strike injuries and, 940
  management of, novel approaches to, 165–166
  in multiply injured patient, 211
  and respiratory distress/dyspnea, 224
  in spinal cord injury, 494
  survival, determinants of, 146
  syncope in, 342
  team approach to, 146
Cardiac arrhythmias. *See* Arrhythmias
Cardiac asthma, 226, 680
Cardiac care, in EMS field treatment, 14
Cardiac catheterization, 681
Cardiac disorders, and diarrhea and vomiting, 299
Cardiac emboli, 773
Cardiac emergencies, 675–693. *See also specific types*
  angina pectoris, 682–684
  anoxic spells in children, 692
  aortic aneurysms and dissection, 777–781
  cardiac tamponade, 689–690

cardiogenic shock, 679–680
cardiomyopathy, 690–691
coarctation of aorta, 693
congenital heart disease, 691–693
coronary syndrome, 675–684
cyanosis, 691–692
embolization, systemic or pulmonary, 681–682
heart failure, 680–681, 684–686, 692–693
hypertension and hypertensive crisis, 686–687
immediate management of, 675
mitral regurgitation, 681
myocardial infarction, 675–679
  complications of, 679–682
myocardial rupture, 681
myocarditis, 690–691
pericardial effusion, 687–690
pericarditis, 682, 687–690
pulmonary hypertension, 693
ventricular septal rupture, 681
Cardiac enzymes
  in angina, 683
  in cardiomyopathy, 691
  in myocardial contusion, 460
  in myocardial infarction, 676
Cardiac glycosides
  poisoning/overdose of, 979–980
  in poisonous plants, 1003, 1004t
Cardiac inflow obstruction, syncope in, 339t, 343
Cardiac life support. *See* Advanced life support; Basic life support
Cardiac monitoring
  in burn injuries, 919
  in calcium-channel blocker poisoning/overdose, 977
  in cardiogenic shock, 202
  in chest pain, 240
  in coma, 313
  in intubated patient, 190
  in tricyclic antidepressant poisoning/overdose, 1009
Cardiac outflow obstruction, syncope in, 339t, 340, 343–344
Cardiac pacemakers, 707–710
  bipolar, 707
  codes and settings for, 707–708, 708t, 722i
  dual-chamber, 707, 722i, 724
  failure to capture in, 709, 723i, 724
  implantable, complications of, 709
  lead complications with, 709
  malfunction of, 709–710, 723i, 724
    electrocardiogram in, 723i, 724
  oversensing by, 709, 723i, 724
  permanent, 707–710
  pocket site complications with, 709
  runaway, 709–710
  single-chamber, 707, 720–724, 722i
  types of, 707
  undersensing by, 709, 723i, 724
  unipolar, 707
  venous access complications with, 709, 710
Cardiac pacing, 705
  transcutaneous, 703, 710
Cardiac perforation, by pacemakers, 709
Cardiac rhythms, 157–158
Cardiac silhouette, in pericarditis, 688
Cardiac tamponade, 216–217, 689–690
  in aortic dissection, 779
  and cardiogenic shock, 202
  and chest pain, 243, 243t
  in chest trauma, 457–458
  classification of, 688t, 689
  clinical findings in, 457–458, 689

coexistent or antecedent findings in, 689
compensated, 688t, 690
decompensated, 688t, 689–690
general considerations in, 457, 689
imaging of, 457–458
in myocardial rupture, 681
and obstructive shock, 202
in pericarditis, 682, 687, 688
radiographic findings in, 689
and shock
  cardiogenic, 202
  obstructive, 202
symptoms and signs of, 457, 689
syncope in, 343
treatment of, 458, 689–690
Cardiac valves
  infection of (infective endocarditis), 859–861
  prosthetic, infection of, 860
Cardiogenic pulmonary edema, 226
Cardiogenic shock, 194, 197, 200–203, 459, 679–680
  arrrythmogenic, 243–244, 243t
  causes of, 193t, 201, 201t
  and chest pain, 243–244, 243t
  in children, 1047
  myocardial, 243t, 244
  in myocardial contusion, 459
  in myocardial infarction, 675, 679–680
    differential diagnosis of, 679, 680t
  nonmyocardial, 202
  and pulmonary edema, 203
Cardiomegaly
  in heart failure, 686
  in sickle cell anemia, 810
Cardiomyopathy, 690–691
  hypertrophic obstructive, syncope in, 344
  secondary, causes of, 690, 690t
Cardiopulmonary data base, 228, 230t–231t
Cardiopulmonary disease, delirium in, 1032
Cardiopulmonary examination, for gastrointestinal bleeding, 288
Cardiopulmonary resuscitation (CPR). *See also* Life support
  active compression/decompression, 165
  in cardiac arrest, 224, 342
    with spinal cord injury, 494
  in EMS field treatment, 14
  in hypothermia, 932
  in infants and children, 163–165
  "Lifestick," 165
  in lightning injuries, 941
  in near-drowning, 945–946
  in ventricular fibrillation, 703
Cardiopulmonary syncope, 342–344, 692
  causes of, 339t, 342
Cardiovascular disorders, and chest pain, 251–252
Cardiovascular emergencies, in children, 1045–1049
Cardiovascular status, esophageal varices and, 291
Cardiovascular system, radiation injury and, 943
Cardioversion. *See also* Defibrillation
  for arrhythmias, 202
  for atrial fibrillation, 698, 700
  for atrial flutter, 699
  in children, 1049
  implantable defibrillators for, 710–711
    complications of, 711
  for paroxysmal supraventricular tachycardia, 695–696
  for preexcitation arrhythmias, 700
  synchronized, 155
  for tachyarrhythmias, 244, 694
  for ventricular tachycardia, 701

Carotid artery
  blunt trauma to, 769
  dissection of, 376
  obstruction of
    and stroke, 370, 371
    surgical interventions for, 377
    and transient ischemic attacks, 376, 377
Carotid endarterectomy, 377
Carotid sinus massage
  for paroxysmal supraventricular tachycardia, 696
  for sinus tachycardia, 695
Carotid sinus syncope, 341, **345**
Carpal bone fractures, **525–526**, 526*i*
Carpal tunnel syndrome, 566
Castor bean, toxins in, 1004*t*
Cat bites, **596**
  and rabies infection, 590–593
Cataracts, formation of, corticosteroids and, 624
Catatonia, schizophrenia and, 1033
Catecholamine crisis (pheochromocytoma), **884–885**
Catharsis, for ciguqtera toxin poisoning, 960
Catheter-clad needle
  for percutaneous suprapubic cystotomy, 128–129
  for peripheral venous catheterization, **78–81**, 81*i*, 82*i*
  for thoracentesis, 112
Catheterization
  bladder/urinary
    in bladder outlet obstruction, 751–752
    in burn injuries, 920
    in gastrointestinal bleeding, 285
    in genitourinary trauma, 477–479, 490
    in hemoptysis, 654
    insertion of, **125–127**, 126*i*
    in spinal cord injury, 495, 509
    suprapubic placement in, 479
    in urethral injuries, 477–479, 488, 490
    for urine collection in females, 757
  cardiac, 681
  Coudé, 127
  external jugular vein, **83–86**, 85*i*
  femoral vein, **92–93**
  internal jugular vein, **86–89**, 87*i*, 88*i*
  peritoneal, **122–124**
  subclavian vein, **89–92**, 90*i*, 91*i*
  venous
    central, for percutaneous suprapubic cysto-
      tomy, 129
    in conscious patient with history of syncope, 337
    in EMS field treatment, **14**
    peripheral
      with catheter-clad needle, **78–81**, 81*i*, 82*i*
      with scalp vein (butterfly) needle, **81–82**, 83*i*, 84*i*
    in septic shock, 825–826
    and upper-extremity venous thrombosis, 784
    in vascular trauma, 767
Cauda equina, in spinal cord compression, 349
Cauda equina syndrome, 419
Cauliflower ear, 450
Causality, determination of, 4
Caustic agents, poisoning, **980–981**
Cauterization
  of epistaxis, 632, 632*i*, 633
  of wounds, 574
Cavernous sinus thrombosis, **606**
Cavities, dental, 649
CBC. *See* Complete blood count
CD4 cell count, in HIV/AIDS, 865

Cecum, in abdominal pain, 268
Cefaclor, for impetigo, 1019
Cefadroxil, for impetigo, 1019
Cefazolin
  for animal bites, 596
  for bursitis, 414
  for cellulitis, 855
  for mangling injuries, 572
  for peritonsillitis, 646
  prophylactic use of, 564
  for skull fractures, 425
  for suppurative tenosynovitis, 565
Cefdinir, for otitis media, 1071*t*, 1072*t*
Cefepime, for septic shock, 828*t*
Cefixime, for urinary tract infections, in children, 1076
Cefotaxime
  for brain abscess, 321
  for mastoiditis, 627*t*
  for meningitis, 834*t*
    in children, 1068*t*
  for meningococcemia, 858
  for osteomyelitis, in children, 1078*t*
  for pneumonia, 836*t*, 1060*t*
  for puerperal sepsis, 748
  for septic arthritis, 838*t*
    in children, 1078*t*
Cefotetan, for acute abdomen, 259*t*
Cefoxitin
  for acute abdomen, 259*t*
  for human bites, 565
  for infected vascular gangrene and cellulitis, 856
  for necrotizing fasciitis, 857
  for nonclostridial anaerobic celulitis, 856
  for perforated duodenum, 254
  for perforated stomach, 254
  for pneumonia, 836*t*
  for septic abortion, 736
Cefpodoxime
  for impetigo, 1019
  for otitis media, 1071*t*, 1072*t*
Cefprozil
  for impetigo, 1019
  for otitis media, 1071*t*, 1072*t*
Ceftazidime
  for glanders, 24*t*
  for melioidosis, 24*t*
  for neutropenia, 814–815
  for orbital cellulitis, 606
Ceftin. *See* Cefuroxime
Ceftriaxone
  for chancroid, 854
  for chlamydial infection, 638*t*
  for disseminated gonococcemia, 861
  for encephalitis, 314
  for epididymitis, 850
  for epiglottitis, 638*t*, 1052
  for genital abscesses, 848
  for gonorrhea, 638*t*, 848, 851
  for meningitis, 314, 834*t*
    in children, 1068*t*
  for meningococcemia, 858
  for otitis media, 1071*t*, 1072*t*
  for pelvic inflammatory disease, 846*t*
  for periorbital cellulitis, 1075
  for pharyngitis, 638*t*
  for pneumonia, 836*t*
  for pyelonephritis, 279
  for septic arthritis, 838*t*
  for syphilis, in HIV-infected patients, 853
Cefuroxime
  for acute cholecystitis, 275

  for otitis media, 1072*t*
  for pneumonia, 836*t*, 1060*t*
  for sinusitis, 643
Cefzil. *See* Cefprozil
Cell count and differential, in synovial fluid analysis, 140
Cellular immune dysfunction, 829
Cellulitis, 854–855, **1016**
  animal bites and, 564–565
  clostridial anaerobic, **856**
  facial, in sinusitis, 643–645
  hand, **564–565**
  infected vascular, **856**
  nonclostridial anaerobic, **856**
  orbital, **605–606**, 1074, 1075
  periorbital
    in children, **1074–1075**, 1074*t*
    in sinusitis, 643–645
  peritonsillar, 639*t*, **645–646**
    pharyngitis and, 1073, 1074
  preseptal, **609**
  synergistic necrotizing, **856**
  uncomplicated, 564
Central apnea, 1051
Central cord syndrome, 506
Central diabetes insipidus, **888–889**
  and hypernatremia, 896
Central nervous system (CNS)
  disorders of, and diarrhea and vomiting, 299
  infection of, and delirium, **1031**
  nerve agents and, 37
Central retinal artery occlusion, 602, **605**
Central retinal vein occlusion, 602, **614–615**
Central scotoma, 600
  in optic neuritis, 615
Central slip, 553
Central venous access, for external jugular vein
  catheterization, 83–84, 85–86
Central venous catheter
  for percutaneous suprapubic cystotomy, 129
  in septic shock, 825–826
  and upper-extremity venous thrombosis, 784
Central venous hypervolemia
  chest pain in, 240–241, 242
  hypotension or shock in, 243, 243*t*
  normal/elevated blood pressure in, 244–245
Central venous oxygen concentration, in septic
  shock, 825
Central venous pressure
  in cardiogenic shock, 201
  in resuscitation documentation, 200
  in septic shock, 825–826
Cephalexin
  for impetigo, 1019
  for infected burns, 929
  for infected sebaceous cysts, 627*t*
  for peritonsillitis, 646
  prophylactic use of, 564
  resistance to, 842–843
  for urinary tract infections, in children, 1076
Cephalic technique, of mouth-to-mask ventilation,
  151, 151*i*
Cephalosporin(s). *See also specific agent*
  for acute cholecystitis, 275
  for animal bites, 596
  for cellulitis, 855
  for COPD, 661
  for dacryocystitis, 608
  for fever, in infants, 1064
  for hepatic abscess, 276
  for human bites, 565
  for impetigo, 1019

for neutropenia, 814–815
for peritonsillitis, 646
for pneumonia, 661, 836*t*
for primary peritonitis, 281
prophylactic use of, 564
for septic arthritis, 838*t*
for suppurative tenosynovitis, 565
thrombocytopenia induced by, 792
for tooth pain, 649
for toxic shock syndrome, 862
for toxic shock-like syndrome, 862
for urinary tract infections, 842*t*
and vitamin K deficiency, 800
Cerebellum
hemorrhage in, 373–374
in stoke patients, 371
Cerebral aneurysms, in sickle cell anemia, 810
Cerebral contusion, **429**
Cerebral edema
drug therapy for, 318*i*, 319
high-altitude, **950–951**
in stroke, treatment of, 369
Cerebral hemispheres, mass lesions in, 317
Cerebral infarction. *See* Stroke
Cerebral vascular accident (CVA), and delirium,
1032
Cerebrospinal fluid (CSF)
in arsenic poisoning, 360
bloody, 132
in lumbar puncture, 132–133, 133*t*
in meningitis, 831, 831*t*
in children, 1068, 1069*t*
in meningococcemia, 858
in meningoencephalitis, 328–329
otorrhea of, following head injury, **451**
in peripheral neuropathy, 354
in seizures, 335, 341
Cerebrovascular accident. *See* Stroke
Cerebrovascular disease, syncope in, 339*t*, **345**
Cerumen impaction, **641–642**
Cervical carcinoma, **736**
Cervical collar, in EMS field treatment, 15
Cervical disk disease, and chest pain, **255**
Cervical hematoma, in neck trauma, 436
Cervical spine, unstable, and airway management,
188
Cervical spine imaging, in spinal cord injury, 495,
506–507
Cervical spine immobilization
in head injury, 421
in-line, 493, 495
in lateral position, 493
in neck injury, 435, **437**
in spinal cord injury, 493, 509
in supine position, 493
technique for moving patient in, 493
Cervical spine injury, **214**, 573. *See also* Spinal cord
injury
with head injury, 421
with neck injury, 435, 437
types of, 508*t*
Cervical spine strain (whiplash), 221, 496, **509**
Cervicitis
chlamydial, 848
gonococcal, 848, 851
mucopurulent, **848**
Cesarean delivery, perimortem, 746
C1-esterase deficiency, and angioedema, 1013
Chancre, in syphilis, 853, 864
Chancroid, **853–854**
Chauffeur's fracture, 524
Check backs, in team approach to cardiac arrest, 146

Chelating agents
for arsenic poisoning, 360–361
for heavy metal poisoning, 989*t*
iron, 988, 989*t*
lead, 989–990, 989*t*, 990*t*
mercury, 991
Chemical agents
decontamination for, **40**
in smoke inhalation, 923–924, 923*t*, 925
in systemic poisoning, 924
Chemical burns, **925–926**
ocular, 616
Chemical cautery, for hemostasis, in wound cases,
574
Chemical hemostatic agents, for hemostasis, in
wound cases, 574
Chemical injuries, vascular, 768
Chemical irritation, and conjunctivitis, 610, 611*t*
Chemical weapons, **36–41**, 36*t*
cyanide agents, **40–41**
nerve agents, **37–38**
pulmonary agents, 38
vesicants, **38–40**
Chemotherapy
extravasation of, 768
for infectious gastroenteritis, 306, 307*t*–308*t*
for multiple myeloma, 817
and neutropenia, 814
for Waldenström macroglobulinemia, 817–818
Cherry pits, toxins in, 1004*t*
Chest
circumferential burns of, **928**
flail, **215–216**, 229, 230*t*
Chest compressions, in basic life support, 151–152,
152*i*
Chest pain, **240–256**
and abdominal pain, 251
abnormal hemodynamics in, 242–245
in aortic dissection, 779
in asthma, 657
in atelectasis, 667
and back pain, 251
in cardiomyopathy, 690
in cardiovascular disorders, **251–252**
differential diagnosis of, 247*t*
by location and quality of pain, 245–251,
247*t*–250*t*
in gastrointestinal disorders, **253–254**
hypovolemia in, 242, 242*t*
initial management of, **240–242**
in interstitial pulmonary disease, 674
life-threatening problems and, immediate management of, **240–246**
in musculoskeletal disorders, 251, **254–255**
in myocardial infarction, 676, 677
in myocarditis, 690
normal hemodynamics in, **245–246**
in pleural effusion, 666
in pneumomediastinum, 665
in pneumonia, 667–668, 834–835
in pneumothorax, 655
in pulmonary disorders, **252–253**
in pulmonary embolism, 661–662
syncope with, 339, 343, 344
in tuberculosis, 669
Chest physical therapy
for atelectasis, 667
for cystic fibrosis, 673
Chest syndrome, in sickle cell anemia, 809
Chest trauma, **454–466**, 576
ABCs in, establishment of, 454
air embolism in, **464–465**

aortic injury in, **462**
asphyxia in, **465**
cardiac tamponade in, **457–458**
commotio cordis in, **465**
diaphragmatic hernia in, **460–461**
esophageal injury in, **461**
flail chest in, **458**
life-threatening problems in, immediate management of, **454–455**
massive hemothorax in, **456–457**
myocardial contusion in, **459–460**
open pneumothorax in, **456**
pain control in, 455
penetrating, **465–466**
primary survey of, immediately life-threatening
thoracic injuries identified on,
455–458
pulmonary contusion in, **458–459**
rib fractures in, **464**
secondary survey of, potentially life-threatening
injuries identified on, **458–463**
shock in, 195
sternal fracture in, **464**
tension pneumothorax in, **455–456**
thoracotomy in, emergency room, 454, **466**
tracheobronchial injury in, **462–463**
vascular injuries in, **769–771**
imaging of, 770, 770*i*, 771*t*
Chest tube (tube thoracostomy)
in abdominal trauma, 467
in hemothorax, 457
for pneumomediastinum, 252
for tension pneumothorax, 215, 225
in tension pneumothorax, 456, 656
Chest wall defects, and respiratory distress/dyspnea,
229, 230*t*
Chest wall rigidity, fentanyl and, 515
Chest wall supports, in flail chest, 458
Chest wound, 576
Chest x-rays
in abdominal pain, in children, 1081
in aortic dissection, 779, 780*t*
in aortic injury, 462, 463*i*
in asthma, 658
in atelectasis, 667
in bronchiolitis, 837
in bronchitis, 668
in cardiac tamponade, 689
in chest pain, with normal hemodynamics, 245
in chronic obstructive pulmonary disease, 658
in diaphragmatic hernia, 461, 461*i*
in diaphragmatic injuries, 470–472, 473*i*
in esophageal injury, 461
in heart failure, 685, 686
in hemothorax, 457, 457*i*
in HIV/AIDS, 865
in immunocompromised patients, 830
in interstitial pulmonary disease, 674
in penetrating chest trauma, 465
in pericarditis, 688
in pleural effusion, 666
in pneumonia, 234, 627*t*, 668, 832, 834
in pneumothorax, 455, 455*i*, 456*i*, 655
in pulmonary contusion, 459
in pulmonary edema, 685
in pulmonary embolism, 662
in thoracic aorta injury, 770, 770*i*, 771*t*
in thoracic outlet syndrome, 786
in tracheobronchial injury, 463
Cheyne-Stokes respiration, 239
CHF. *See* Congestive heart failure
Chickenpox, 1082*t*–1083*t*

Chilblains, **934**
Child, definition of, 163
Child abuse, **1097–1102**
  and burns, 928–929
  orthopedic injuries in, 515
  physical, **1097–1100**
  radial head subluxation in, 523
  reporting of, 68
  sexual, 740, 741, **1100–1102**, 1101*t*
Child neglect, and refusal to consent, 66
Children. *See also under* Pediatric
  airway management in, **186–187**
  anoxic spells in, **692**
  asthma in, 659
  atropine and, 180–181, 187
  back pain in, **419**
  bronchiolitis in, 835–837
  cardiac arrest in, 163
  cardiopulmonary resuscitation in, **163–165**
  chronic obstructive pulmonary disease in, 659
  congenital heart disease in, **691–693**
  cricothyroidotomy for, 178
  croup in, 647
  ear pain in, 626
  epiglottitis in, 237, 646–647
  fractures in, 513
  genitourinary trauma in, management of, 480*i*
  growth plate injuries in, 513, 514, 547
    classification of, 513, 513*i*
  head injuries in, special considerations in, **432**
  humerus fractures in, 519, 521
  molluscum contagiosum in, 1025
  nasal obstruction in, 633–634
  orthopedic injuries in, immobilization for, 547
  osteomyelitis in, 839
  otitis media in, 628*t*
  pneumonia in, **832–834**, 836*t*
  pulmonary hypertension in, **693**
  renal injuries in, 479
  scabies in, 1022
  scapula fractures in, 517
  shock in, 194
  sore throat in, 635
  tibial spine fractures in, 536
  tracheostomy in, 178
  tuberculosis in, 670
  ureteral injuries in, 484
  urinary tract infections in, 841–843
  viral keratoconjunctivitis in, 612
  vital signs of, 186, 186*t*
  wheezing in, differential diagnosis of, 659
Chin-lift method, in pediatric basic life support, 164
Chlamydia trachomatis infection
  cervicitis in, 848
  in children, 1101*t*
  coexistent with gonorrhea, 851
  conjunctivitis in, 610, 611*t*, 851
  culture for, 756
  pelvic inflammatory disease in, 845–846
  pelvic pain in, 728
  pharyngitis in, 638*t*, 840
  prevention of, in female rape victims, 740
  reactive arthritis in, 412
  urethritis in, 756, 844–845
  urinary tract infections in, in children, 1075
Chlorambucil, for cold agglutinin syndrome, 806
Chloramphenicol
  for botulism, 364
  for clostridial anaerobic cellulitis, 856
  for eye trauma/disorders, 622*t*
  for meningitis, 833*t*

  for meningococcemia, 858
  for plague, 26
  for Rocky Mountain spotted fever, 859
  for tularemia, 27
Chlorine gas, and conjunctivitis, 610
Chlorine poisoning, 994, 995*t*
Chlorophyllum molybdites, 1002*t*
Chlorpromazine
  poisoning/overdose of, 1000–1001
  psychiatric uses, 1036
  for psychotic confusional states, 402
Chlorpropamide, and hyponatremia, 893*t*
Choanal atresia, diagnosis and treatment of, 635*t*
Choking, foreign body airway obstruction and,
    152–153, 153*i*, 154*i*
Cholangitis
  and abdominal pain, 263
  diagnosis of, 271*t*
  suppurative, and abdominal pain, **275–276**
Cholecystitis
  in abdominal examination, 265
  abdominal pain in, 260*t*, **275**
  diagnosis of, 250*t*, 271*t*
Cholelithiasis, in sickle cell anemia, 810
Cholestasis, in sickle cell anemia, 810
Cholesteatoma, in otitis media, 642
Cholestyramine, for cardiac glycoside poisoning,
    980
Cholinergic poisoning, 967*t*
Cholinesterase inhibitors
  poisoning/overdose of, 314, **998–999**
  response in myasthenia gravis, 353
Chondritis, 627*t*
Choriocarcinoma, 742–743
Christmas disease, 795
Chromic gut sutures, 582, 585
Chronic lymphocytic leukemia (CLL), **815**
Chronic myelocytic leukemia (CML), **815–816**
Chronic obstructive lung disease, and respiratory
    distress/dyspnea, 230*t*
Chronic obstructive pulmonary disease (COPD),
    227–228, 656–661, 657*t*
  acute exacerbations, 661
  in adults, 659
  in children, 659
  clinical findings in, 657–658
  conditions associated with, 656, 657*t*
  differential diagnosis of, 659
  evaluation of, 658–659
  general considerations in, 656
  laboratory findings in, 658–659
  medical history in, 658
  mild exacerbations, 659–660
  moderate exacerbations, 660
  radiographic findings in, 658
  and respiratory distress/dyspnea, **237**
  respiratory support in, 659–660
  severe or life-threatening exacerbations, 660
  systemic corticosteroids for, 659–660
  treatment of, 659–661
Chronic obstructive pulmonary vascular disease,
    238
Chvostek test, 346
Cicuta maculata, toxins in, 1004*t*
Cicutoxin, in poisonous plants, 1004*t*
Cidofovir, for smallpox, 30
Ciguatera toxin poisoning, 363, **960**
Ciliary muscle, blunt trauma to, 618
Cimetidine
  for acute intermittent porphyria, 362
  for scrombroid poisoning, 961
Ciprofloxacin

  for anthrax, 23*t*, 25
  for chancroid, 854
  for conjunctivitis, 610
  for gonorrhea, 851
  for infectious gastroenteritis, 306
  for meningitis, 833*t*
  for otitis externa, 627*t*
  for plague, 23*t*, 26
  for pneumonia, 836*t*
  for scorpion fish envenomation, 959
  for septic arthritis, 838*t*
  for stingray wound, 957
  for suppurative cholangitis, 276
  for tularemia, 23*t*, 27
  for urinary tract infection, 842
Circulation
  in abdominal trauma, 467
  in basic life support, **151–152**, 152*i*
  in chest trauma, 454
  in hand, 551
  in head injuries, 422
  in hemoptysis, 653–654
  in multipy injured patient, 211
  in near-drowning, 945–946
  in pediatric basic life support, 164
  in poisoning victim, 964
  in septic shock, 825–826
  in shock, 195
  in spinal cord injury, 494–495
Circulatory compromise, 890
Circumcision
  elective, for phimosis, 765
  and urinary tract infection prevention, 1076
Circumferential burns, 922, **928**
Citalopram, 1037
Civil defense, and multicasualty incident/disaster
    management, 47
Civil law, 60–61
CK-MB
  in cardiomyopathy, 691
  in myocardial contusion, 460
  in myocardial infarction, 676
Clarithromycin
  for otitis media, 1072*t*
  for pharyngitis, in children, 1074
  for pneumonia, 836*t*
Clavicle fractures, **516–517**
Cleaning of wounds, 579–580
Cleansers, for skin and wounds, 580
Cleansing, of skin, 73–74
Clearance, of toxins, 969
Cleocin. *See* Clindamycin
Clindamycin
  for acute abdomen, 259*t*
  for botulism, 364
  with fluoroquinolone, for bite injuries, 564–565
  for impetigo, 1019
  for infected vascular gangrene and cellulitis, 856
  for Ludwig angina, 639*t*
  for mandibular fracture, 443
  for necrotizing fasciitis, 857
  for nonclostridial anaerobic cellulitis, 856
  for orbital cellulitis, 606
  for otitis media, 1071*t*, 1072*t*
  for pelvic inflammatory disease, 846*t*
  for periorbital cellulitis, 1075
  for peritonsillar cellulitis and abscess, 639*t*
  for pneumonia, 836*t*
  for puerperal mastitis, 749
  for synergistic necrotizing cellulitis, 856
  with TMP-SMZ, for bite injuries, 564–565
  for tooth pain, 649

for zygomaticomaxillary complex fractures, 446
Clitocybe, 1002*t*
Clobetasol propionate, for pemphigus vulgaris, 1017
Clofibrate, and hyponatremia, 893*t*
Clonidine
  bradycardia caused by, 704
  for hypertensive urgency, 687
Clopidogrel
  for chest pain with normal hemodynamics, 245
  platelet function impaired by, 794–795
  for stroke prevention, 376–377
  thrombocytopenia induced by, 793
Closed compartment syndromes, in hand trauma, **571–572**
Closed fractures, 513
  blood loss in, 511, 512*t*
Closed skull fractures, **424**
  computed tomography of, 425, 426*i*, 427*i*
Clostridial anaerobic cellulitis, **856**
Clostridial myonecrosis, **857**
Clostridium botulinum, 32, 33*t*
  and gastroenteritis, 304*t*
  weakness and paralysis caused by, 353, 362–363
Clostridium difficile
  and dysentery, 308*t*
  testing for, 302
Clostridium perfringens, and gastroenteritis, 304*t*
Clostridium perfringens infection, 856–857
Clot lysis, for arterial occlusion, 774
Clotrimazole
  for tinea, 1024
  for vaginitis, 847
Cloxacillin
  for impetigo, 1019
  for pneumonia, 836*t*
Clozapine, 1037
Clubbing, in interstitial pulmonary disease, 674
Cluster headache, 382, 383, **389–390**
CNS. *See* Central nervous system
Coagulation cascade, 790*i*
Coagulation factor(s), vitamin K-dependent, warfarin and, 800–801
Coagulation factor disorders, 789, **795–802**, 820
Coagulation factor replacement
  for disseminated intravascular coagulation, 802
  dosing regimen for, 796, 798*t*
  for hemophilia, 795–798
  inhibitors or antibodies against, 797–798
  in liver disease, 799
  plasma-derived, 796, 797*t*
  recombinant, 796, 797*t*
Coagulopathies
  in gastrointestinal bleeding, 285
  in septic shock, 826, 827
  systemic, third-trimester bleeding in, 743–744
Coarctation of aorta, 691, 692, 693, **693**
COBRA. *See* Consolidated Omnibus Reconciliation Act of 1985
Cocaine
  as anesthesia, 448, 577*t*
  and catecholamine crisis, 884
  and delirium, 1030
  delirium or confusion with, 399
  for epistaxis, 633
  for intubation, 179
  and myocardial infarction, 675
  poisoning/overdose of, 967*t*, **981–982**
  in pregnancy, third-trimester bleeding with, 744
  proarrhythmic activity of, 702
  properties of, 179*t*
  for wound care, in children, 1043

Coccyx, fractures of, 507
Codeine
  acetaminophen with, for corneal abrasion, 620
  poisoning/overdose of, 997–998
  for tooth pain, 649
Cogentin. *See* Benztropine
Cognition, in stroke patients, 371
Cognitive disorders, **1033**
Colchicine, for gouty arthritis, 409
Cold
  disorders due to, **930–936**
  extremity injury caused by, **934–936**
Cold agglutinin syndrome (CAS), 805, **806**
Cold water facial immersion, for paroxysmal supraventricular tachycardia, 696
Cold-type autoimmune hemolytic anemia, 805–807
Colic
  biliary
    abdominal pain in, 260*t*, **275**
    diagnosis of, 271*t*
  renal
    abdominal pain in, 261*t*, **278–279**
    diagnosis of, 271*t*
    rectus abdominis spasm in, 264
Coliform infection, hand, 564
Colitis. *See also* Inflammatory bowel disease
  gastrointestinal bleeding in, **295**
  ischemic
    abdominal pain in, 261*t*, **277**
    diagnosis of, 271*t*
Collateral ligaments, 533, 533*i*
  injuries of, **537**
  valgus and varus stress tests of, 533, 533*i*, 537
Colles fracture, 524
Colloids, for hypovolemic shock, 198*t*, 199
Colonic perforation, 268
Colonic polyps, and gastrointestinal bleeding, 293–295
Colonoscopy
  for angiodysplasia, 293
  for diverticulitis, 293
  for lower gastrointestinal bleeding, 289
Coma, **311–330**
  alcohol intoxication and, **327**
  associated illnesses, 964
  basilar artery thrombosis and, **323**
  brain abscess and, **321**
  brain tumor and, **321–322**
  cerebral infarction and, **322**
  cholinesterase inhibitor poisoning and, 314
  definition of, 315
  differential diagnosis of, 315*t*
  drug overdose and, **327**
  electrolyte disorders and, **328**
  embolic occlusion and, **323**
  encephalitis and, 314
  and eye movements, 316
  gamma-hydroxybutyrate and, **327**
  hepatic encephalopathy and, **327–328**
  history of, 315
  hypercapnia and, 313–314
  hyperosmolar (*See* Hyperglycemic hyperosmolar nonketotic syndrome)
  hypertensive encephalopathy and, 314
  hypertensive intracerebral hemorrhage and, **320–321**
  hyperthermia and, 314, **328**
  hypoglycemia and, 311, 313, **326–327**, 326*t*
  hypothermia and, 314, **328**
  hypoxemia and, **327**
  hypoxia and, 313–314

increased intracranial pressure and, 314
  intracerebellar hemorrhage and, **323–324**
  intracerebellar infarction and, **323–324**
  life-threatening problems and, immediate management of, **311–315**, 312*i*, 313*i*
  "locked-in" syndrome and, **324–325**
  meningitis and, 314
  meningoencephalitis and, **328–329**
  metabolic encephalopathies and, **325–329**
  myxedema, **880–881**
  narcotic overdose and, **327**
  and nasogastric intubation, 104
  neurologic examination of, 316
  opiate overdose and, 311, 313, 314
  osmolality and, **328**
  physical examination of, 315
  and pinpoint pupils, **314–315**
  poisoning and, 963–964
  pontine hemorrhage and, **323**
  postictal state and, **325**
  psychogenic, **329–330**
  and pupils, 316
  spinal cord injury and, 496
  status epilepticus and, 314
  subarachnoid hemorrhage and, **329**
  subdural hematoma and, **319–320**
  subtentorial mass lesions and, **322–325**
  supratentorial mass lesions and, **317–322**, 318*i*
  Wernicke encephalopathy and, 311, 313
Coma cocktail, 311
Combativeness, in head injuries, 423
Combitube, in EMS field treatment, 14
Comminuted fractures, 513
Commitment, involuntary, to psychiatric facility, 67
Commotio cordis, **465**
Communicable diseases. *See also* Infectious diseases
  reporting of, 68–69
Communications network
  of EMS system, 9, **16–18**
  in multicasualty incidents/disasters, 50, 54–56, 58
Compartment syndrome, **512–513**
  closed, in hand trauma, **571–572**
  in extremity trauma, 220
  in femoral shaft fractures, 533
  in forearm fractures, 524
  in hemophilia, 796
  pressure dressings and, 588
  in tibial shaft fractures, 539
Compazine. *See* Prochlorperazine
Compensated cardiac tamponade, 688*t*, 690
Compensated shock, 194
Compensatory damages, 62
Competence
  and informed consent, 65
  and refusal to consent, 66
Complete abortion, 734*t*, 735
Complete blood count (CBC)
  in abdominal pain, in children, 1081
  in asthma and COPD, 658
  in coma, 317
  in HIV/AIDS, 865
  in infants, 1063
  in stroke patients, 371
Complete heart block, **705–706**
  electrocardiogram in, 705, 720, 721*i*, 722*i*
Compression dressings, 588
Compression injuries, 575
Compressive mononeuropathies, weakness caused by, **358–359**

Compromised airway, 167–190. *See also* Airway
assessment of, 167
in children, 186–187
cricothyroidotomy for, 178
needle, **175–178**, 176*i*
extubation and, 190
foreign bodies and, 187–188
immediate management of, **167–172**, 168*i*
intubation for (*See also* Intubation)
digital, 174
drugs to assist in, **179–185**
equipment variations and, 174
fiberoptic techniques for, 174–175
patient care and, **189–190**
preparation for, 169–172
principles of, 173–174
needle cricothyroidotomy for, **175–178**, 176*i*
nonsurgical alternatives for maintenance of,
174–175
in status asthmaticus, 188
surgical intervention and, **178**
tracheostomy for, 178
in trauma patients, 188–189
Computed tomography (CT scan)
in abdominal aortic aneurysm rupture, 777
in abdominal pain, 269–270
in children, 1081
in abdominal trauma, 218–219, 468–469
in amnesia, 401
angiography with
in penetrating chest trauma, 465
in pulmonary embolism, 663
in aortic dissection, 779
in aortic injury, 462, 463*i*
in atelectasis, 667
in cardiac tamponade, 458
in cavernous sinus thrombosis, 606
in cerebrospinal fluid otorrhea, 451
in coma, 317
in delirium or confusion, 394
in diaphragmatic hernia, 461
in diffuse axonal injury, **430**, 433*i*
in distal femoral fractures, 535
in epidural hematoma, 428, 428*i*
in eye trauma, 617
in flank injuries, 476
in frontal sinus fractures, 449
in genitourinary trauma, 480, 481
in head injuries in children, 432
in head trauma, 219
in headache, 379
in hearing loss, 630
in hematuria assessment, 759
in hip fractures, 531
in HIV/AIDS, 866
in interstitial pulmonary disease, 674
in intestinal injuries, 473, 475*i*
in intracerebral hemorrhage, 373–374, 374*i*
in intracranial injury, 425–428, 506
in intracranial mass (brain tumor), 386
in mastoiditis, 629
in meningitis, 381
in multiply injured patient, 212
in nasal trauma, 440
in orbital cellulitis, 606
in orbital floor (blowout) fractures, 447, 447*i*
in osteomyelitis, 839
in otitis media, 643
in pancreatic injuries, 472
in pancreatitis, 280
in patella fractures, 534
in pelvic fractures, 530

in peroneal tendon injuries, 542
in pleural effusion, 666
in pneumothorax, 655
in pseudotumor cerebri, 386
in pulmonary contusion, 459
in pulmonary embolism, 681
in renal colic, 278
in renal injuries, 481, 484, 485*i*
in rib fractures, 464
in ruptured spleen, 278
in scalp lacerations, 424
in scapula fractures, 517
in seizures, 341
in shoulder dislocations, 519
in sinusitis, 643–645, 644*i*
in skull fractures, 424–425
closed, 425, 426*i*, 427*i*
depressed, 425, 427*i*
in sore throat, 636
in spinal cord injury, 507
in spinal infections, 420
in splenic injuries, 470, 471*i*–472*i*
in sternoclavicular joint dislocations, 516
in stroke, 369, 371, 374–375, 375, 776
in subarachnoid hemorrhage, 372*i*, 372–373,
383, 431*i*, 432*i*
in subdural hematoma, 428–429, 429*i*, 430*i*
in syncope, 340
in talar fractures, 544
in tendon rupture in knee, 539
in thoracic aorta injury, 770
in tibial plateau fractures, 535
in tibial spine fractures, 536
in traumatic aortic rupture, 218
in ureteral injuries, 481, 484
in urolithiasis, 761, 762*i*
in vascular injuries, 767, 768, 769, 770
in vertigo, 632
in zygomaticomaxillary complex fractures, 446,
446*i*
Conceptus, retained, in missed abortion, 735
Concussion, 430–431
in children, special considerations in, 432
discharge instructions in, 433–434
grading and outcome of, 431, 433*t*
hospitalization for, indications for, 433
Condom(s), for reinfection prevention, in vaginitis,
847
Conduction abnormalities, **703–706**
Conductive hearing loss, 629, 629*t*
in temporal bone fracture, **451**
testing for, 629*i*, 629–630
Condyloma lata, 853
Condylomata accuminatum, in children, 1101*t*
Confidential Morbidity Reporting, 69
Confidentiality, of medical records, 70
Confusion, **391–403**
agitated, **402**
in amnestic syndromes, 394*t*, **400–401**
assessment of, 392*i*
brain damage in, conditions associated with,
393*t*
in central anticholinergic syndrome, 399, 399*t*
definition of, 315
differential diagnosis of, 394*t*
in drug intoxication, 396, **399**
in drug withdrawal, **396–398**
electrocardiogram in, 393
evaluation of, **393–395**
examination and diagnostic tests in, 393–394
focal neurologic findings in, **394–395**
gastric contents evaluation in, 393–394

in head injuries, 430–431
in headache, 383
history of, 393
in hypertensive encephalopathy, 393
in hysteria, **402–403**
immediate measures in, 391–393
laboratory studies in, 393
life-threatening problems in, immediate management of, **391–395**, 392*i*
in meningitis, 384, **394**, 394*t*, 830
in metabolic encephalopathy, 394*t*, **395–399**
systemic disorders associated with, 396, 396*t*
neurologic examination in, 393
physical examination in, 393
postictal, **395**
in psychiatric disorders, 394*t*, **402–403**
versus organic causes, 402, 403*t*
in psychotic states, **402**
in Reye syndrome, **400**
in seizure disorders, 394*t*, **395**
special studies in, 393
in specific disorders, emergency management of,
395–403
in stroke, 394*t*, **401–402**
in trauma, **394**, 394*t*
of uncertain causes, **403**
in Wernicke encephalopathy, 393, **398–399**
Congenital heart disease, **691–693**
classification of, 691
infective endocarditis in, treatment of, 860
pathophysiology of, 691
Congestive heart failure, 226–227, **680–681**,
684–686. *See also* Heart failure
and central venous hypervolemia, 244–245
in children, **1048–1049**, 1049*t*
in infants, **692–693**
in myocardial infarction, **680–681**
Congo-Crimean hemorrhagic fever, 31*t*
Conium maculatum, toxins in, 1004*t*
Conjunctiva
blunt trauma to, 618
foreign body injuries of, **620**
Conjunctival hyperemia, in ocular burn injuries,
616, 617
Conjunctivitis, **610**, 611*t*
in allergies, 610, 611*t*
chemical irritation and, 610, 611*t*
chlamydial, 610, 611*t*, 851
differential diagnosis of, 602*t*, 611*t*
gonococcal, 851–852
in HIV-infected patients, 865
in infections, 610, 611*t*
in skin disorders, 610
in systemic disorders, 610
viral, 610, 611*t*
Consciousness
altered states of
with headache, 383
in meningitis, 384
miscellaneous rare causes of, **346–347**
loss of (*See* Loss of consciousness (LOC))
in spinal cord injury, 496
Consent, **64–69**
authority to give, 65
for blood alcohol samples, 66–67
and children, 1044–1045
implied, 64
informed, 64
intoxicated patients and, 65, 66
minors and, 65
patients in police custody and, 65
principles of, 64

psychiatric patients and, 66
  refusal to, 66
  requirements for, exceptions to, 64–65
Consolidated Omnibus Reconciliation Act of 1985
    (COBRA), 63
Constipation, and abdominal pain, 264, 1087t
Constriction band, for snake bites, 952
Constriction injuries
  hand, **566**
  penile, **491**
Consultation, 4
Contact dermatitis, **1017–1018**
Continuous positive airway pressure (CPAP)
  for asthma and COPD, 660
  for pulmonary edema, 226
Continuous positive-pressure ventilation, for acute
    high-altitude pulmonary edema, 949
Contraception
  discontinuation of, warning about, 742
  postcoital emergency, **742**
  for rape victims, 740
Contraceptive sponges, and toxic shock syndrome,
    862
Contrast venography
  in deep venous thrombosis, 782, 784
  in venous occlusion, 774–775
Contusion(s)
  arterial, 767
  bladder, 488
  cerebral, **429**
  hepatic, 473i
  myocardial, **217, 459–460**
  ocular, 618–619
  pulmonary, **216, 458–459**
  renal, 484
Convallaria majalis, toxins in, 1004t
Convergence (visual), coma and, 316
Conversion disorder, **1034–1035**
  weakness in, 355
Convulsions. *See* Seizures
COPD. *See* Chronic obstructive pulmonary disease
Copper poisoning, 995t
Copper sulfate, for chemical burns, 926
Coprinus, 1002t
Cor pulmonale, in asthma and COPD, 658
COR system, for EMS communications, 16
Cornea
  abrasions of, **620**
  acute hydrops of, **612**
  blunt trauma to, 618
  burn injuries of, 616–617
  foreign body in, **620**
    removal of, 623
  infection of, differential diagnosis of, 602t
  staining of, 623–624
Corneal edema, 604
Corneal epithelial keratitis, 612
Corneal erosion, differential diagnosis of, 602t
Corneal ulcer, 605
  bacterial, 602t, **611**
  differential diagnosis of, 602t
Coronary artery occlusion, **675–679.** *See also* My-
    ocardial infarction
  angina pectoris in, 682–684
Coronary artery stenting, 679
Coronary syndrome, acute, **675–684**
Corpus cavernosum, rupture of, 491
Corrosive agents, poisoning with, **980–981,** 981t,
    994
Corticosteroids
  for adrenal insufficiency, 858
  for aspiration, 225

for asthma, 228
for asthma and COPD, 659–660
for Bell palsy, 358
for bursitis, 414
for carbon monoxide poisoning, 979
for caustic poisoning, 981
for contact dermatitis, 1018
contraindications to, in delirium tremens, 398
for COPD, 228
for corrosive poisoning, 981
for De Quervain tenosynovitis, 566
for eye trauma, caution with, 620, 624–625
for gouty arthritis, 409
for idiopathic thrombocytopenic purpura, 1096
immunosuppression by, 825
and leukocytosis, 658
for meningitis, 384
for myxedema coma, 881
for optic neuritis, 615
for pseudotumor cerebri, 386
for pulomary fibrosis, 228
for septic shock, 205, 827
for spinal cord injury, 495, 509
for spinal cord metastases, 355
for sunburn, 927
for temporal arteritis, 387
for tendonitis, 414
for thrombotic thrombocytopenic purpura, 793
for thyroid storm, 879
for Tietze syndrome, 255
for tinea, 1024
Corticotrophin, for gouty arthritis, 409
Corynebacterium diphtheriae infection, and pharyn-
    gitis, in children, 1073
Corynebacterium hemolyticum infection, and
    pharyngitis, in children, 1073
Cosmetic appearance, wound dressings for, 589
Costochondral separation, and chest pain, **254**
Costochondritis, and chest pain, **255**
Costovertebral angle tenderness, 265
Cosyntropin, for adrenal insufficiency, 883
Coudé catheter, 127
Cough tenderness, in abdominal pain, 264
Coughing
  in asthma, 656, 657
  of blood (hemoptysis), **653–654**
  in bronchitis, 667
  in chronic obstructive pulmonary disease, 656
  in emphysema, 657–658
  in interstitial pulmonary disease, 674
  in pneumonia, 667–668, 834–835
  syncope caused by, 340, 341, 342
  in tuberculosis, 669
Coumadin, for gastrointestinal bleeding, 285
Counseling
  for genital herpes patients, 852
  for rape victims, 740, 741
  for sexual abuse victims, 1102
Cow's milk sensitivity, in children, 1089
COX-2 inhibitors
  for chronic degenerative disk disease, 417
  for lumbosacral strain, 417
  for osteoarthritis, 411
Coxiella burnetti, 24t, 28
Coxsackievirus
  and exanthems, 1082t–1083t
  and pharyngitis, in children, 1073
CPAP. *See* Continuous positive airway pressure
CPR. *See* Cardiopulmonary resuscitation
Cramps
  abdominal pain and, 262, 262i
  heat-related, **937**

Cranial dysjunction, 444i, **445**
Cranial nerve(s)
  in acute intermittent porphyria, 361
  in Bell palsy, 357–358
  in cavernous sinus thrombosis, 606
  coma and, 316
  in Guillain-Barré syndrome, 359–360
  in muscle disease, 354
  in myasthenia gravis, 353
  in neuromuscular disease, 353
  in poliomyelitis, 357
  in stroke, 371
Craniofacial dysjunction, 444i, **445**
Craniotomy, for supratentorial mass lesions, 319
Crash cart, for children, 164
Creatinine
  in coma, 316
  in diabetic ketoacidosis, 869
  in heart failure, 686
  in hyperglycemic hyperosmolar nonketonic syn-
    drome, 870
Crepitus
  in flail chest, 458
  in scapula fracture, 517
Cricoid pressure
  in basic life support, 151
  in children, 187
  positive-pressure ventilation and, 170, 172i
Cricothyroid membrane, identification of, 107,
    107i, 175, 176i
Cricothyroidotomy (cricothyrotomy), 107i,
    107–108, 175–178, 176i
  in children, 178, 187
  contraindications to, 178
  in EMS field treatment, **15**
  in laryngeal airway injury, 436
  in spinal cord injury, 494
  in vascular injury to neck, 769
Criminal law, 60–61
Critical presentation, 4
CroFab. *See* Crotalidae polyvalent immune Fab
Crohn's disease
  arthritis in, 412
  gastrointestinal bleeding in, **295**
Crotalid snakes, bites from, 951
Crotalidae polyvalent immune Fab (CroFab,
    FabAV), 952, 952t
Crotamiton, for scabies, 1022
Croup, 187, **647, 1052–1053,** 1053t
  radiographic findings in, 647, 648i
Cruciate ligaments, 533
  in hemorrhagic arthritis, 407
  injuries of, **537–538**
    avulsion, 536
    symptoms and signs of, 537, 538i
    stability of, assessment of, 537, 538i
Crush injuries, 575
  clinical findings, 220
  and hyperkalemia, 901
Cryofibrinogenemia, 567
Cryoprecipitate, **820–821**
  characteristics and doses of, 819t, 820–821
  for disseminated intravascular coagulation, 802
  for hemostatic abnormalities
    of liver disease, 799
    of renal disease, 800
  for von Willebrand disease, 799
Cryoprecipitate-poor plasma (cryosupernatant), for
    thrombotic thrombocytopenic purpura,
    793
Cryptococcus infection, in HIV-infected patients, 864
Crystal. *See* Phencyclidine

Crystalloids, for fluid resuscitation
in abdominal aortic aneurysm rupture, 777
in abdominal trauma, 468
in hemoptysis, 654
in hemorrhagic shock, 214
in hypovolemic shock, 198–199, 198*t*
in labor and delivery, 747
in multiply injured patient, 212
in septic shock, 826
in suppurative cholangitis, 276
in vascular trauma, 767
for visceral (intestinal) ischemia, 776
Crystals, in synovial fluid analysis, 140
CT scan. *See* Computed tomography
Cuboid fractures, 545
Cuffed oropharyngeal airway, and intubation
preparation, 172
Culdocentesis, in ectopic pregnancy, 196
Culture, in synovial fluid analysis, 140
Cuneiforms fracture, 545
Cutaneous anthrax, **22**, 23*t*
Cutaneous dermatophytes, **1023–1024**
Cutdown trays, prepackaged sterile
for emergency antecubital fossa venous cutdown,
77
for internal jugular vein catheterization, 86–87
for saphenous vein cutdown, 94
for subclavian vein catheterization, 90
CVA. *See* Cerebral vascular accident
Cyanide
as chemical weapon, **40–41**
poisoning, **982–984**, 994
clinical findings, 36*t*
from plants, 1003
in smoke inhalation injury, 924
Cyanoacrylate tissue adhesive, 584
Cyanocobalamin. *See* Vitamin B₁₂ₐ
Cyanogenic glycosides, in poisonous plants, 1003,
1004*t*
Cyanosis
anoxic spells in, 692
in children, 1051
in chronic bronchitis, 657
in heart disease, **691–692**
in interstitial pulmonary disease, 674
in small-vessel occlusion, 774
in venous occlusion, 774–775
Cyclizine, for vertigo, 632
Cyclobenzaprine, for tension headache, 388
Cyclones, tropical, **43**
Cyclooxygenase inhibitors, platelet function impaired by, 794–795
Cyclopentolate
for eye trauma/disorders, 622*t*
for uveitis, 613
Cyclophosphamide
for cold agglutinin syndrome, 806
and hyponatremia, 893*t*
for Waldenström macroglobulinemia, 817–818
Cyclosporine
for rheumatoid arthritis, 411
thrombocytopenia induced by, 793
Cystic fibrosis, **673**
respiratory distress/dyspnea in, 230*t*
Cystitis, 752
abdominal pain in, 1087*t*
hemorrhagic, hematuria in, 758, 759
recurrent, 842, 843
uncomplicated, **841–843**, 842*t*
Cystogram, retrograde
in bladder injuries, 473, 481, 486–488
computed tomography for, 481

Cystostomy
percutaneous suprapubic, **127–129**, 128*i*
suprapubic, for posterior urethral injuries, 490
Cytokine(s), in septic shock, 825
Cytomegalovirus infection
and exanthems, 1082*t*–1083*t*
in HIV-infected patients, 863–866
in infants, 1062
versus mononucleosis, 816
transfusion transmission of, 821–822
Cytopathic hypoxia, 826
Cytoscopy, in hematuria assessment, 759–760
Cytotoxic agents
for autoimmune hemolytic anemia, 805
for cold agglutinin syndrome, 806
and neutropenia, 814

Dacron sutures, 583
Dacryoadenitis
acute, **608–609**
viral, 609
Dacryocystitis, acute, **608**, 608*i*
Dactylitis, in sickle cell anemia, 809
Damages, negligence and, 62
Danazol, for autoimmune hemolytic anemia, 805
Dantrolene, for neuroleptic malignant syndrome,
1036
Dapsone, for brown recluse spider bites, 955
Data base, cardiopulmonary, 228, 230*t*–231*t*
Date rape drug. *See* γ-Hydroxybutyrate
Datura stramonium, toxins in, 1004*t*
DDAVP. *See* Desmopressin
DDD pacing, in cardiac pacemaker, 708, 708*t*
DDDR pacing, in cardiac pacemaker, 708, 708*t*
D-dimer assay
in deep venous thrombosis, 782
in disseminated intravascular coagulation, 802
in hemostasis assessment, 791*t*
in liver disease, 799
in pulmonary embolism, 662–663
De Quervain tenosynovitis, 566
Dead, care of, in multicasualty incidents/disasters, 51
Dead on arrival (DOA), reporting of, 69
Dead space, in wound closure, 584–585
Deadly nightshade, toxins in, 1004*t*
Death
brain, criteria for, **330**
of pediatric patients, 1045
Debridement
for frostbite, 935
for scorpion fish envenomation, 959
selective, 581
for stingray wound, 957
of wounds, 580–581, 588–589
Debriefing, after multicasualty incident/disaster, 59
Deceleration injury, and shock, 195–196
Declaration of need, of emergency department, 46
Decompensated cardiac tamponade, 688*t*, 689–690
Decompensated shock, 194
Decompression sickness, **946–947**
Decompressive hemicraniectomy, 377
Decongestants, for sinusitis, 643
Decontamination
for chemical agents, **40**
for cyanide agents, 40
for hazardous materials incidents, 54, 58–59
for lewisite, 40
for nerve agents, 38
for poisoning/overdose, 964–965
for pulmonary agents, 38
for radiation injury, 944
for sulfur mustard, 39, 40

Deep basilic vein, identification of, 77
Deep fascial space infections, hand, **564**
Deep palpation, 265
Deep reflexes, 505*t*
Deep soft tissue infections, **856–857**
Deep space bleeding, 789
Deep venous thrombosis, **782–784**, 782*t*
lower-extremity, **782–783**
and pulmonary embolism, 662, 663, 782, 783,
784
upper-extremity, **783–784**
Defensive medicine, 60
Deferoxamine, for iron poisoning, 988, 989*t*
Defibrillation, **153–156**, 155*i*. *See also* Cardioversion
automated external, 14, 155, 156*i*, 157*i*, 164
biphasic, 155, 156*i*
in EMS field treatment, **14**
implantable cardioverter, **710–711**
monophasic, 155
for polymorphic ventricular tachycardia, 702
public access, 155–156
scaling exponent of, 165
for ventricular fibrillation, 703
waveforms, 155, 156*i*
Degenerative disk disease, chronic, **417–418**
Degenerative joint disease, **410–411**
Degloving injuries, **595**
Dehydration
in children, **1046–1047**
and gastroenteritis, in children, 1077–1078
Dehydration agents, for cerebral edema, 319*t*
Delavirdine, side effects of, 865*t*
Delayed (II) (triage category), 50
Delayed hypersensitivity (type IV) reaction, *Rhus*
dermatitis and, 1018
Delirium, **391–403**, **1030–1032**
in amnestic states, 394*t*
in amnestic syndromes, **400–401**
assessment of, 392*i*
brain damage in, conditions associated with, 393*t*
in cardiopulmonary disease, **1032**
in central anticholinergic syndrome, 399, 399*t*
in central nervous system infections, 1031
in cerebral vascular accident, 1032
definition of, 315
depressants and, 1030–1031
differential diagnosis of, 394*t*
in drug intoxication, 396, **399**
in drug intoxication/withdrawal, **396–398**,
1030–1031
electrocardiogram in, 393
in electrolyte abnormalities, 1031
in endocrine disorders, **1031–1032**
evaluation of, **393–395**
examination and diagnostic tests in, 393–394
focal neurologic findings in, **394–395**
gastric contents evaluation in, 393–394
hallucinogens and, 1031
in hepatic encephalopathy, 1031
history of, 393
in hypertensive encephalopathy, 393
in hypoglycemia, 1032
immediate measures in, 391–393
in infections, **1031**
laboratory studies in, 393
life-threatening problems in, immediate management of, **391–395**, 392*i*
in meningitis, 394*t*, 830
in metabolic disorders, **1031–1032**
in metabolic encephalopathy, 394*t*, **395–399**
systemic disorders associated with, 396, 396*t*

in neurologic disorders, **1032**
neurologic examination in, 393
opioids and, 1031
physical examination in, 393
in psychiatric disorders, 394*t*, **402–403**
in Reye syndrome, **400**
in seizure disorders, 394*t*, **395**, 1032
special studies in, 393
in specific disorders, emergency management of, **395–403**
stimulants and, 1030
in stroke, 394*t*, **401–402**
in thyroid disease, 1032
in trauma, **394**, 394*t*
in Wernicke encephalopathy, 393, **398–399**, 1032
Delirium tremens, **396–398**, 1031
Delivery (birth), **746–747**
Delphinium, toxins in, 1004*t*
Deltoid ligament, 540
injuries of, 543–544
Dementia, **1030**
AIDS-related, 863–864
Demyelinating disease, optic neuritis in, 615
Dengue fever, 31*t*
Dental caries, 649
Dentin, 648, 649*i*
Department of Transportation (COT), and EMS training, 6
Depressants, and delirium, **1030–1031**
Depressed skull fractures, **425**
computed tomography of, 425, 427*i*
Depression, **1033**
syncope in, 346
tension headache in, 388
Dermabond, 584
Dermacentor andersoni, tick paralysis caused by, 362
Dermacentor variabilis, tick paralysis caused by, 362
Dermatitis
contact, **1017–1018**
Rhus, **1017–1018**
Dermatologic disorders
conjunctivitis in, 610
in HIV-infected patients, 865
in sickle cell anemia, 811
Dermatologic emergencies, **1012–1025**. *See also specific type*
angioedema, **1012–1013**
cellulitis, **1016**
contact dermatitis, **1017–1018**
cutaneous dermatophytes, **1023–1024**
erysipelas, **1016**
erythroderma, **1014–1015**
exfoliation, **1014–1015**
herpes simplex, **1020–1021**
herpes zoster, **1019–1020**
impetigo, **1018–1019**
life-threatening problems in, immediate management of, **1012–1015**
molluscum contagiosum, **1025**
pediculosis, **1022–1023**
pemphigus vulgaris, **1017**
pityriasis rosea, **1024**
psoriasis, **1021–1022**
pustular psoriasis, **1016–1017**
scabies, **1022**
staphylococcal scalded skin syndrome, **1015**
Stevens-Johnson syndrome, **1014**
tinea, **1023–1024**
toxic epidermal necrolysis, **1014**
urticaria, **1013**

Dermatologic infection, **854–857**
septic shock in, treatment of, 828*t*
Dermatomal sensation, landmarks for testing, 505*t*
Dermatophytes, cutaneous, **1023–1024**
Descemet's membrane rupture, 612
Descent
for acute high-altitude pulmonary edema, 950
for high-altitude cerebral edema, 950–951
Desmopressin
for central diabetes insipidus, 889
for hemophilia, 797
for hemostatic abnormalities of liver disease, 800
for von Willebrand disease, 799
Detergents, ionic, contraindicated for wound cleansing, 580
Developmental disorders, psychiatric, **1035**
Deviated septum, diagnosis and treatment of, 635*t*
Dexamethasone
for adrenal insufficiency, 883
for cerebral edema, 319*t*
for croup, 647, 1052
for high-altitude cerebral edema, 950
for meningitis, in children, 1069
for mountain sickness, 948, 949
for spinal cord metastases, 355
Dextran, for frostbite, 935
Dextran polymers, for absorptive dressings, 588
Dextromethorphan, poisoning/overdose of, 967*t*, 997–998
Diabetes insipidus
central, **888–889**, 896
and hypernatremia, 896
nephrogenic, 896
Diabetes mellitus
candidiasis in, 846–847
hypernatremia in, 896
necrotizing fasciitis in, 856–857
orbital cellulitis in, 606
type 2, unrecognized, **871–873**, 872*t*
Diabetic ketoacidosis, **867–869**
abdominal pain in, 259
diagnosis of, 272*t*
Diabetic retinopathy, vitreous hemorrhage in, 613
Diagnosis, 4
feasability of determining, 4
treatment response and, 4
Diagnostic peritoneal lavage (DPL), 468
in multiply injured patient, 212
in pregnant patients, 746
in visceral and hypogastric artery aneurysm, 778
Diagnostic studies, 4
Diagnostic-therapeutic concept, 4
Dialysis
for cardiac glycoside poisoning/overdose, 980
for drug elimination, 970
for hemolytic uremic syndrome, 794
for hyperphosphatemia, 906
for hyponatremia, 894
for renal disease, 800
for rewarming, 933
and septic arthritis, 837
Diamorphine, for sickle cell crisis, 808
Diamox. *See* Acetazolamide
Diaphragm
injuries of, **470–472**
radiographic findings in, 470–472, 473*i*
paralysis of, in spinal cord injury, 493–494
Diaphragmatic hernia, **460–461**
imaging of, 461, 461*i*
Diarrhea, **296–309**
and abdominal pain, 264
and acute abdominal emergencies, **297**, 297*t*

and dehydration, in children, 1046
in gastroenteritis, 306–309
bacterial, 303
in children, 1077–1078
viral, 303
history, 299–301, 301*t*
in hypotension, **296–297**, 1032
infectious causes of, **303–309**
laboratory tests for, **302–303**
life-threatening problems in, immediate management of, **296–299**
in parasitic enteritis, 303–306
physical examination, 301–302
in shock, **296–297**
in toxic exposures, **297–299**, 298*i*, 301
treatment algorithm, 298*i*
Diazepam
for acute intermittent porphyria, 362
for delirium tremens, 397–398
in EMS field treatment, 15
endotracheal administration of, 189
for hysteria, 403
for isoniazid poisoning, 996
for phencyclidine overdose, 1000
for reduction of TMJ dislocation, 652
for scorpion bites, 955
for seizures, 1008
seizures induced by, 971
for status epilepticus, 334, 336*t*
for stimulant overdose, 974
for subarachnoid hemorrhage, 329
for vertigo, 451, 632
DIC. *See* Disseminated intravascular coagulation
Dicloxacillin
for impetigo, 855
for infected burns, 929
for infected sebaceous cysts, 627*t*
for periorbital cellulitis, 1075
prophylactic use of, 564
in wound care, 590*t*, 597
Dicumarol, overdose, 1010–1011
Didanosine, side effects of, 865*t*
Dieffenbachia, toxins in, 1004*t*
Diencephalon, mass lesions in, 317, 318*i*
Diet, and diarrhea and vomiting, 301
Diet therapy, for lumbosacral strain, 418
Diethylstilbestrol, for atrophic vaginitis, 847
Dieulafoy lesion, and gastrointestinal bleeding, 290*t*
Diffuse axonal injury, **430**, 433*i*
Diffuse epigastric pain, 263
Diffuse interstitial disease, and respiratory distress/dyspnea, 230*t*, **234–235**
Diffuse peritonitis, and abdominal pain, 263
Diffuse periumbilical pain, 263
Digibind, for cardiac glycoside poisoning, 980*t*
Digit(s), small-vessel occlusion in, 774
Digital block
in fingernail removal, 558
in hand trauma, 549, 550*i*, 570–571, 578
in paronychia incision and drainage, 563
Digital flexors, 551
Digital intubation, 174
Digitalis
for heart failure in infants, 693
poisoning/overdose of, 979–980
in poisonous plants, 1003
Digitalis antibodies, for cardiac glycoside poisoning, 980, 980*t*
Digitalis purpurea, toxins in, 1004*t*
Digitoxin, poisoning/overdose of, 979–980

Digoxin
  for atrial fibrillation, 698
  for atrial flutter, 699
  for congestive heart failure, in children, 1049
  for multifocal atrial tachycardia, 699
  for paroxysmal supraventricular tachycardia, 697
  poisoning/overdose of, 979–980
  proarrhythmic activity of, 702
  toxicity of, 702
Digoxin immune Fab, for cardiac glycoside poisoning, 980, 980*t*
Dihydroergotamine, for cluster headache, 390
Dilantin. *See* Phenytoin
Dilatations, in abdominal pain, 268, 268*i*
Dilation and curettage, for postpartum hemorrhage, 748
Diltiazem
  in advanced life support, 160*t*, 162
  for atrial fibrillation, 698
  for atrial flutter, 699
  in EMS field treatment, 15
  for multifocal atrial tachycardia, 699
  for paroxysmal supraventricular tachycardia, 696–697
  poisoning/overdose of, 977
Dimenhydrinate, for vertigo, 632
Dimercaprol
  for arsenic poisoning, 361
  as chelating agent, 989*t*, 990, 991
  for lewisite exposure, 40
2,3-Dimercaptosuccinic acid (DMSA), as chelating agent, 989*t*, 990
Diphenhydramine
  for allergic reactions, 638*t*
  for anaphylactic shock, 206
  for angioedema, 1013
  for antipsychotic overdose, 1001, 1036
  for bee/wasp stings, 953
  proarrhythmic activity of, 702
  for scrombroid poisoning, 961
  for transfusion reaction prevention, 823
  for upper airway obstruction, 236, 237
  for urticaria, 1013
  for vertigo, 632
Diphenoxylate
  with atropine, for gastroenteritis, 274
  for gastroenteritis, 309
Diphtheria, sore throat in, 638*t*, 840, 841
Diphtheria-tetanus-pertussis vaccine, and autoimmune hemolytic anemia, 807–808
Diphtheritic polyneuritis, **362**
Diplopia
  in botulism, 364
  in eye injury, 440
  in orbital floor (blowout) fractures, 447
  syncope with, 339
  in zygomaticomaxillary complex fractures, 446
Dipyridamole and aspirin, for stroke prevention, 377
Direct current (DC) cardioversion
  for atrial fibrillation, 698, 700
  for atrial flutter, 699
  for paroxysmal supraventricular tachycardia, 695–696
  for preexcitation arrhythmias, 700
  for tachyarrhythmias, 694
  for ventricular tachycardia, 701
Direct laryngoscopy, 99–101, 100*i*
Direct pressure, for hemorrhagic shock, 213
Dirty bomb, 20
Disability
  in abdominal trauma, 467

  in hand trauma, 548
  in head trauma, 422
  in shock, 195
Disaster drills, 56
Disaster plans, 56
Disaster relief organizations, 56
Disaster resources, mobilization of, 56
Disasters, **42–59.** *See also specific type*
  and air medical resources, 53
  communications network and, 50, 54–56
  diffusely distributed victims, 54–56
  EMS *versus* civil defense management of, 47
  epidemiology of, 47
  hazardous materials and, 53–54
  and hospital emergency departments, **56–59**
  Incident Command System for, 47, 48*i*
  and local accessory resources, 53
  logistics of, 49–50
  and media involvement, 53
  medical management of, 47
  and mutual aid, 53
  natural, **42–45,** 43*t*
  nonnatural, **45–46**
  organization of response to, 47
  organizations and assistance, 56
  and patient distribution, 51–52
  prehospital management of, **47–56**
  and psychological support, 59
  and public safety, 52–53
  scene organization of, 49, 49*i*
  special considerations, 53–56
  and stress management, 59
  and transport, 51–52
  treatment in, 51
  and triage, 50, 57–58
Discharge instruction sheets, abandonment and, 68
Disclosure, standard of
  patient-oriented, 64
  physician-oriented, 64
Disinfectants, for skin and wound cleansing, 580
Disk disease
  and chest pain, **255**
  chronic degenerative, **417–418**
Disk herniation, 418–419
  back pain in, 415
Disk protrusion, and weakness, 351
Disk space infections, **419–420**
Dislocation(s), **513–514.** *See also specific type or structure affected*
  definition of, 513
  reduction of, 511
    procedural sedation for, 515
Disopyramide, contraindications, 1010
Disposition, 4, 5
Disseminated gonococcemia, **861**
Disseminated intravascular coagulation, 789, **801–802**
  abruptio placentae and, 744
  in meningococcemia, 858
  missed abortion and, 733
  in Rocky Mountain spotted fever, 859
  in septic shock, 205, 827
  in transfusion reactions, 822
Dissociated nystagmus, 316
Dissociative states, **1035**
Distal femur fractures, **535**
Distributive shock, 193*t*, 194, **204–207**
Diuresis, for drug elimination, 969
Diuretics
  for heart failure, 686
    in infants, 693
  for hypercalcemia, 904

  for hyponatremia, 894
  for pseudotumor cerebri, 386
Diverticula, Meckel
  in children, 1089
  and gastrointestinal bleeding, **295**
Diverticulitis
  and abdominal pain, 260*t*, **274**
  diagnosis of, 271*t*
  and gastrointestinal bleeding, **293,** 294*i*
  sigmoid, in abdominal examination, 265
Dix-Hallpike test, for vertigo and nystagmus, 630, 632
DKA. *See* Diabetic ketoacidosis
DMSA. *See* 2,3-Dimercaptosuccinic acid
DOA. *See* Dead on arrival
Dobutamine
  in advanced life support, 160*t*, 161, 162
  for cardiogenic shock, 202, 244, 679–680
  for central venous hypervolemia, 245
  for congestive heart failure, in children, 1049
  for septic shock, 826
Documentation, 4. *See also* Medical records
  of brain death diagnosis, 330
  of resuscitation efforts, 200
Dog bites, **596**
  and rabies infection, 590–593
Dog tick, paralysis caused by, 362
Donath-Landsteiner antibody, 806
DOO pacing, in cardiac pacemaker, 708*t*
Dopamine
  in advanced life support, 160*t*, 161
  for bradyarrhythmia, 243–244
  for cardiac tamponade, 689
  for cardiogenic shock, 202, 244, 679–680
  for complete heart block, 706
  for congestive heart failure, in children, 1049
  for heat stroke, 939
  for lactic acidosis, 876
  for neurogenic shock, 207
  for pulmonary embolism, 244
  for septic shock, 205, 826
  for spinal cord injury, 494–495, 509
Dopamine antagonists, for migraine, 388–389
Dopexamine, for septic shock, 827
Doppler ultrasound
  in arterial occlusion, 774
  of pulses, in vascular trauma, 768
  in testicular torsion and epididymitis, 754–755
  venous, in pulmonary embolism, 663
Doxepin, overdose of, 1008–1010
Doxycycline
  for anthrax, 23*t*, 25
  for brucellosis, 24*t*, 28
  for bullous myringitis, 627*t*
  for chlamydial infection, 610
  contraindicated in breastfeeding, 748
  for epididymitis, 850
  for gonococcal/chlamydial pharyngitis, 638*t*
  for pelvic inflammatory disease, 846*t*
  for pharyngitis, 638*t*
  for plague, 23*t*, 26
  for pneumonia, 668, 836*t*, 1060*t*
  for Q fever, 24*t*, 28
  for Rocky Mountain spotted fever, 859
  for septic abortion, 736
  for syphilis, 853
  for tularemia, 23*t*
  for urethritis, 851
  for zygomaticomaxillary complex fractures, 446
DPL. *See* Diagnostic peritoneal lavage
Drainage
  of distended bladder, 751–752

of peritonsillar abscess, 645–646, 646*i*
of wound, 585
Dressings, 585–589
absorptive, 588
for closed wounds, 588
for cosmetic appearance, 589
for debridement, 588–589
for delivery of topical antibiotics, 589
for edema control, 587–588
for elevation, 588
functions of, 585
for hand injuries, 556–557, 588
for immobilization, 587
for open wounds, 588
pressure, 588
for protection, 587
for wounds, 585–594
Droperidol, for vertigo, 632
Droplet precautions, 25*t*
Drowning. *See* Near-drowning
Drug(s). *See also specific agent*
administration of, in children, 1044
elimination of, enhancing, 969–970
in EMS field treatment, **15**
in intubation, **179–185**, 182–185
poisoning/overdose of, and coma, **327**
Drug abuse. *See also specific drugs*
infective endocarditis in, 860
intra-arterial injection of drugs in, **787**
mania in, 1034
septic arthritis in, 837
syncope in, 346
vascular injury in, 768
Drug intoxication
central anticholinergic syndrome in, 399, 399*t*
delirium or confusion in, 396, **399, 1030–1031**
head injuries in, **434**
Drug seeker, dental complaints among, 649
Drug withdrawal
clinical findings in, 397
delirium or confusion in, **396–398, 1030–1031**
sedative-hypnotic agents causing, 396*t*
seizures in, 341, 396, **397,** 398
treatment of, 397–398
Drug-adsorption type autoimmune hemolytic anemia, 807
Drug-induced immune-mediated thrombocytopenia, **792**
Drug-induced methemoglobinemia, **984–985**
Duke criteria, for infective endocarditis, 860, 860*t*
Dumb cane, toxins in, 1004*t*
DUMBELS (mnemonic), 998, 999
Duodenal disorders, and gastrointestinal bleeding, 290*t*
Duodenal ulcer
in children, 1089
perforated
and abdominal pain, 260*t*
diagnosis of, 271*t*
Duodenitis
and gastritis, 291
and gastrointestinal bleeding, 290*t*
Duodenum, perforated
and chest pain, **254**
diagnosis of, 249*t*
Duty
breach of, 61
of care, 61
to provide emergency care, **63**
Dysentery, **303–309**
Dysmenorrhea, 727*t,* **738**

Dysphagia
in botulism, 364
in sore throat, 635
Dysphonia, in botulism, 364
Dyspnea. *See also* Respiratory distress
in asthma, 657
in bronchitis, 667
in chronic bronchitis, 657
in chronic obstructive pulmonary disease, 656
in emphysema, 657
in heart failure, 686, 692
in interstitial pulmonary disease, 673–674
in pleural effusion, 666
in pneumonia, 667–668
in pulmonary aspiration syndrome, 671
in pulmonary embolism, 661–662, 681
syncope with, 339, 344
in Wernicke encephalopathy, 398
Dysuria, **756–758,** 757*t*
psychogenic, 757*t*
with urethritis, 756, 757*t,* 851
in urinary tract infections, 756–758, 757*t,* 841, 843
Dysuria-frequency syndrome, 757*t,* 758, **844–845**

EACA. *See* Epsilon-aminocaproic acid
Ear(s)
burns of, 921
disorders of, 641–643
following head trauma, **451–452**
examination of, 626
foreign body in, 627*t*
frostbite of, 642
infections of, 627*t*–628*t,* 642–643
injuries of
external, **450–451**
in facial trauma, **441**
lightning injuries of, 941
pain in, **626–629**
in children, 626
clinical findings in, 626–629
diagnosis of, 627*t*–628*t*
history of, 626
physical examination in, 626
treatment of, 627*t*–628*t,* 629
Ear canal
cerumen impaction in, **641–642**
insect in, 627*t*
Early basic life support, 147
Earthquakes, **42–43,** 44*t*
Eastern equine encephalitis (EEE), 31
Ebola virus, 31*t*
EBV infection. *See* Epstein-Barr virus infection
Ecchymosis
of eyelids (black eye), **619**
in stroke patients, 370
ECG. *See* Electrocardiogram
Echocardiogram
in cardiac tamponade, 457–458, 689
in cardiomyopathy, 691
in heart failure, 684
in hypertrophic obstructive cardiomyopathy, 344
in infective endocarditis, 860
in mitral regurgitation, 681
in myocardial contusion, 460
in myocardial rupture, 681
in pericardial effusion, 688
in pericarditis, 688
transesophageal
in aortic dissection, 779
in cardiac tamponade, 217

in infective endocarditis, 860
in thoracic aorta injury, 770
in traumatic aortic rupture, 218
in ventricular septal rupture, 681
Echovirus, and exanthems, 1082*t*–1083*t*
Ecstasy. *See* MDMA
Ecthyma, 854–855
Ectopic pregnancy, **728–733,** 743
abdominal pain in, 261*t,* **280,** 1087*t*
clinical findings in, 731
clinical presentation of, 729
diagnosis of, 271*t,* 729, 730*i*
equivocal findings of, 731–733
hemorrhagic shock in, 196
high probability of, 731
intrauterine device and, 729, 742
laboratory tests and special examinations in, 731
low probability of, 733
versus normal pregnancy, 729*i,* 731
pelvic pain in, 727*t*
ruptured, 731, 733*i*
symptoms and signs of, 731
treatment and disposition of, 731–733
ultrasound of, 729, 731, 732*i,* 733*i*
vaginal bleeding in, 726, 729
Eczema vaccinatum, smallpox vaccine and, 30
Edema
cerebral
drug therapy for, 318*i,* 319
high-altitude, **950–951**
in stroke, treatment of, 369
heat, **937**
pulmonary, **685**
acute high-altitude, **949–950**
cardiogenic, 226
in cardiogenic shock, 203
chest pain in, 243
delirium in, 1032
noncardiac, 226
respiratory distress/dyspnea in, 230*t,* **234**
severe, 226*i,* **226–227**
with wounds, control of, 587–588
Edetate calcium disodium (EDTA)
for iron poisoning, 990
for lead poisoning, 989*t*
Edrophonium, response in myasthenia gravis, 353, 366
EDTA. *See* Edetate calcium disodium
Education, 4
EEE. *See* Eastern equine encephalitis
Efavirenz, side effects of, 865*t*
Effexor. *See* Venlafaxine
EGD. *See* Esophagogastroduodenoscopy
EGT. *See* Esophageal gastric tube airway
800-MHz truncated system, for EMS communications, 16
Eikenella corrodens infection, in human bites, 565
Elapid snakes, bites from, 951
Elavil. *See* Amitriptyline
Elbow
arthrocentesis of, 136, 138, 138*i*
dislocations of, **522–523**
reduction of, 523, 523*i*
treatment of, 521*i,* 523, 523*i*
injuries of, **522–523**
nonarticular rheumatism in, 406*t*
Elderberry, toxins in, 1004*t*
Elderly
central retinal vein occlusion in, 614–615
confusion of uncertain causes in, 403
hip fractures in, 531
humerus fractures in, 519, 521

Elderly (*cont.*)
  inappropriate secretion of antidiuretic hormone in, 887
  meningitis in, 830
  multiple injuries in, 208
  myocardial contusion in, 460
  pneumonia in, 835
  tendon rupture in, 539
Electric burns, **941–942**
  hand, **567**
Electric shock, **941–942**
Electrical injuries, 922, **940–944**. *See also specific type*
Electrocardiogram (ECG)
  in abdominal pain, 267
  in adrenal insufficiency, 883
  in aortic dissection, 779, 780*t*
  in asthma and COPD, 658
  in atrial fibrillation, 697, 712, 716*i*
  in atrial flutter, 698, 712, 717*i*
  in atrial tachycardia, 695, 713*i*
  in atrioventricular block
    first-degree, 705, 720, 721*i*
    second-degree, Mobitz type I, 705, 720, 721*i*
    second-degree, Mobitz type II, 705, 720, 721*i*
    third-degree, 705, 720, 721*i*, 722*i*
  in atrioventricular junctional rhythm, 707, 719*i*, 720
  in atrioventricular nodal reentrant tachycardia, 695, 712, 713*i*–715*i*
  in atrioventricular reciprocating tachycardia, 695, 712, 715*i*
  in botulism, 364
  in burns, 919
  in cardiac tamponade, 689
  in cardiomyopathy, 690
  in catecholamine crisis, 884
  in chest pain, with normal hemodynamics, 245
  in complete heart block, 705, 720, 721*i*, 722*i*
  in acute high-altitude pulmonary edema, 949
  in delirium or confusion, 393
  in diabetic ketoacidosis, 869
  in electrical burn injuries, 567
  in EMS field treatment, **14**
  in gastrointestinal bleeding, 285
  in heart failure, 685
  in hypercalcemia, 904
  in hyperkalemia, 900–901, 900*t*
  in hypermagnesemia, 907
  in hypocalcemia, 903, 903*i*
  in hypokalemia, 898, 900*i*
  in idioventricular rhythm, 706, 717–720, 719*i*
  in multifocal atrial tachycardia, 699, 712, 717*i*
  in myocardial contusion, 459–460
  in myocardial infarction, 676, 677
  in myxedema coma, 880
  in normal sinus rhythm, 712, 712*i*
  of pacemaker activity, 720–724, 722*i*, 723*i*
    in malfunction, 723*i*, 724
  in paroxysmal supraventricular tachycardia, 695, 712, 713*i*–715*i*
  in pericarditis, 688
  in poisoning, 964, 965, 968*t*
  in polymorphic ventricular tachycardia, 702, 717, 718*i*
  in preexcitation arrhythmias, 699–700, 715*i*, 716*i*
  in premature atrial contractions, 717, 719*i*
  in premature ventricular contractions, 717, 719*i*
  in pulmonary embolism, 662
  in septic shock, 825–826
  in sinoatrial block, 720, 720*i*
  in sinus arrhythmia, 712, 713*i*
  in sinus bradycardia, 703–704, 712, 713*i*
  in sinus tachycardia, 695, 712, 712*i*
  in stroke patients, 371
  in syncope, 339, 343
  in thyroid storm, 879
  in ventricular fibrillation, 703, 717, 718*i*
  in ventricular tachycardia, 700–701, 717, 718*i*
  in Wernicke encephalopathy, 398
Electrocautery
  for epistaxis, 135
  for hemostasis, in wound cases, 574
Electrocoagulation, for angiodysplasia, 293
Electroencephalogram
  in hysteria, 403
  in psychogenic *versus* organic coma, 330
Electrolyte studies, for coma, 316
Electrolytes
  daily maintenance requirements, in children, 1046, 1046*t*
  disorders of, **890–891** (*See also* Fluid and electrolyte disorders)
    acute, weakness with, **367**
    in asthma and COPD, 658
    in coma, **328**
    in delirium, **1031**
  normal values, 891, 891*t*
  replacement of
    for central diabetes insipidus, 889
    for diabetic ketoacidosis, 870–871
    for hyperglycemic hyperosmolar nonketonic syndrome, 870–871
  serum levels of, in abdominal pain, 267
Electromyography, in postpoliomyelitis syndrome, 357
Elemental mercury poisoning, **991**
Elevated arm stress test (EAST), in thoracic outlet syndrome, 786
Elevation
  for hemostasis, 573
  of wounds, 588, 597
Elimite. *See* Permethrin
Ellis classification system, of tooth fractures, 636, 640*i*
Emancipated minors, and consent, 65, 1045
Embolectomy, for pulmonary embolism, 664
Embolic occlusion, and coma, **323**
Embolism
  air, systemic, in chest trauma, **464–465**
  arterial gas, **947–948**
  arterial occlusion by, 773
  cardiac, 773
  pulmonary, **661–664** (*See also* Pulmonary embolism)
    in myocardial infarction, **681–682**
  and stroke, 370, 370*t*, 374–377
  systemic, in myocardial infarction, **681–682**
  tumor, 773
  vascular, 773
  without infarction, 237
Embolization
  in angiodysplasia, 293
  bronchial artery, in hemoptysis, 654
  in diverticulitis, 293
  in hemobilia, 292
  septic, 238
Emergency, report of, 10
Emergency antecubital fossa venous cutdown, **76–78**, 78*i*, 79*i*
Emergency cardiac care, in EMS field treatment, **14**
Emergency care
  duty to provide, **63**
  legal aspects of, **60–72**

Emergency department
  admission orders through, 70–71
  declaration of need of, 46
  and follow-up care, 67–68
  labor and delivery in, 747
  and multicasualty incidents/disaster management, **56–59**
  thoracotomy in, 454, **466**
Emergency Medical Services (EMS) system, **6–18**
  administration of, 10
  communications network, 9, 16–18
  components of, 6–13
  dispatch of personnel from, 11, 11*i*
  field assessment, 13–14
  field treatment, 14–18
  hospital facilities of, 9–10
  layered-response system, 9, 9*t*
  and medical evaluation, 11–12
  medical supervision of, 12, 13*i*
  and multicasualty incident/disaster management, 46, 47, 52
  and multiply injured patient, 208
  operation of, 10–12
  performance evaluation of, 12–13
  professional field personnel, **6–8**
    dispatch of, 11, 11*i*
    skills and techniques of, 13–18
    special qualifications, 9
    training, 6, 7*t*–8*t*, 9
  protocols for, 16
  single-response system, 9, 9*t*
  staffing of, 9–10
  standing orders for, 16
  and transport, 12
  and treatment, 11–12
  types of systems, 9, 9*t*
  and upper airway obstruction, 224
Emergency medical technicians (EMTs), 6, **8**
  EMT-A (basic), 7*t*, **8**
  EMT-I (intermediate), 7*t*, **8**
  EMT-P (advanced), 6, **8**, 8*t*
Emergency Medical Treatment and Active Labor Act (EMTALA), 1, 61, 63, 71
Emergency medicine
  birth of, **2**, 2*t*
  definition of, **1–2**
  growth of, **2**, 2*t*
  personnel statistics for, 2, 2*t*
  principles of, **4–5**
  residency statistics for, 2, 2*t*
  scope of practice, **2–4**
Emergency physicians
  interactions with medical staff, **70–71**
  job responsibilities of, 1, **2–4**
Emergency procedures. *See specific procedures*
Emergency stabilization. *See* Stabilization
Emergency thoracotomy, **115–116**
Emergent presentation, 4
Emesis
  for ingested poisons, 965
  for iron poisoning, 988
  positive-pressure ventilation and, 170
Emphysema, 656–661
  clinical findings in, 657–658
  definition of, 656
  history of, 657
  laboratory findings in, 658
  mediastinal, arterial gas embolism and, 947, 948
  physical examination in, 657
  "pink puffers" with, 657
  subcutaneous, **664–665**
Employer, and vicarious liability, 62–63

EMS system. *See* Emergency Medical Services system

EMTALA. *See* Emergency Medical Treatment and Active Labor Act

EMTs. *See* Emergency medical technicians

EMT-Tactical courses, 9

Enalapril, for central venous hypervolemia, 245

Enalaprilat, for hypertensive emergencies, 687

Enamel, tooth, 648, 649*i*

Encephalitis
  coma in, 314
  delirium or confusion in, 394, 394*t*
  viral, **31–32**

Encephalopathy(ies)
  delirium or confusion in, 1031
  hepatic
    and coma, **327–328**
    and delirium, **1031**
  in HIV-infected patients, 864
  hypertensive
    coma in, 314
    delirium or confusion in, 393
  metabolic, **395–399**
    coma in, **325–329**
    delirium or confusion in, 394*t*, **395–399,** 396*t*
  in Reye syndrome, 400
  Wernicke, 393, **398–399,** 401
    coma in, **311, 313**
    delirium or confusion in, **1032**

Endobronchial tamponade, in hemoptysis, 654

Endocarditis, infective, **859–861**
  Duke criteria for diagnosis of, 860, 860*t*
  in HIV-infected patients, 863, 865
  pulmonary embolism in, 237
  subacute, 859

Endocrine disorders
  and delirium, **1031–1032**
  diarrhea and vomiting in, 299

Endocrine emergencies, **867–889.** *See also specific type*

Endocrine glands, radiation injury and, 944

Endometrial carcinoma, **736**

Endometriosis, **738**
  abdominal pain in, **281**
  pelvic pain in, 727*t*

Endometritis, 845
  puerperal, **748**

Endophthalmitis, 604, **606–607**

Endoscopy
  for caustic poisoning, 981
  for corrosive poisoning, 981
  for esophageal varices, 292
  for upper gastrointestinal bleeding, 288

Endotracheal intubation. *See also* Intubation
  in advanced life support, 157
  for altered mental status with shallow breathing, 225
  in asthma and COPD, 660
  in children, 164, 186, 187, 1044
  in EMS field treatment, 14
  with flexible-tipped tube, 174
  in Guillain-Barré syndrome, 360
  in head injuries, 421–422
  in hemoptysis, 654
  in massive aspiration, 225
  in myasthenia gravis, 366
  in neck injury, 769
  in pneumothorax, 655
  in poliomyelitis, 351
  in pulmonary edema, 226
  removal of, 102

in shock, in children, 1047
in spinal cord injury, 494, 508
in status epilepticus, 334–335
in tracheobronchial injury, 463
tube selection guidelines, 99, 99*t*
in weak patient, 349

Endotracheal medications, for intubated patient, 189

Enhanced 9-1-1, 9

Enophthalmos, in blowout fracture, 619–620

Enoxaparin
  for angina, 684
  for pulmonary embolism, 682

ENT emergencies, **626–652.** *See also specific types*
  cerumen impaction, **641–642**
  chronic (suppurative) otitis media, **642–643**
  croup, **647**
  ear disorders, **641–643**
  ear pain, **626–629**
  epiglottitis, **646–647**
  epistaxis, **632–633**
  frostbite, **642**
  hearing loss, **629–630**
  management of specific disorders in, **641–652**
  mouth disorders, **647–652**
  nasal obstruction, **633–634**
  oropharynx in, **645–647**
  peritonsillitis, **645–646**
  potentially harmful disorders in, immediate management of, **626–640**
  sinusitis, **643–645**
  sore throat, **634–636**
  teeth in, **636–640, 648–649**
  TMJ disorders in, **649–652**
  vertigo, **630–632**

Entamoeba histolytica infection
  and dysentery, 308*t*
  and enteritis, 306

Enteritis, parasitic, **303–306**

Enterobacter infection, and suppurative cholangitis, 276

Enterococcus infection, and suppurative cholangitis, 276

Enteroviruses
  and exanthems, 1082*t*–1083*t*
  and pharyngitis, in children, 1073

Envenomation, **951–962.** *See also specific type*

Environmental agents. *See also specific type*
  disorders due to, **930–962**

Enzyme-linked immunoassay (ELISA), for D-dimer levels
  in deep venous thrombosis, 782
  in hemostasis, 791*t*
  in pulmonary embolism, 662–663

EOA. *See* Esophageal obturator airway

Eosinophilia, in asthma and COPD, 658

Ephedrine
  in intubation, 180
  poisoning/overdose of, 974–975

Epididymitis, 752–755, **849–850**
  acute, **849–850**
  adjunctive measures in, 850
  clinical findings in, 754–755, 849–850
  gonococcal, 849–850
  orchitis with, 763
  scrotal pain with, 752–755, 753*t*
  symptoms and signs of, 849–850
  versus testicular torsion, 754–755, 763
  treatment and disposition of, 755, 850
  with urethritis, 849–850
  in urinary tract infection, 849–850

Epidural abscess, 419

Epidural anesthesia, in rib fractures, 464

Epidural compression syndrome, 415, **419**

Epidural hematoma, **428**
  coma in, **324**
  computed tomography of, 428, 428*i*

Epigastric pain
  diffuse, 263
  in myocardial infarction, 676
  in preeclampsia-eclampsia, 744

Epiglottitis, 635, **646–647,** 841
  in adults, 646–647
  in children, 187, 646–647, **1052,** 1055*i*
  diagnosis of, 638*t*
  mild, 647
  radiographic findings in, 635, 637*i*
  respiratory distress/dyspnea in, 236
  treatment of, 638*t*
  upper airway obstruction in, 224, 237

Epilepsy, **340–341.** *See also* Seizures
  in children, 1059
  reporting of, 69

Epileptic aura, 340

Epinephrine
  in advanced life support, 158, 159*t*
  for allergic reactions, 638*t*
  for anaphylactic shock, 206
  for angioedema, 1013
  for asthma, 1058
  for bradyarrhythmia, 244
  for bronchiolitis, 837, 1056
  for calcium-channel blocker poisoning, 977
  contraindications to, 574, 577–578
  for croup, 1052–1053
  in EMS field treatment, 15
  endotracheal administration of, 189
  for extubation, 190
  for hemostasis, in wound cases, 574, 577–578
  for hypotension, 1010
  and leukocytosis, 658
  with lidocaine, 576
    for drainage of peritonsillar abscess, 645
    for epistaxis, 633
    for postextraction tooth hemorrhage, 640
  nebulized racemic, for croup, 647
  in pediatric patients, 164–165
  for scorpion fish envenomation, 959
  for scrombroid poisoning, 961
  for sea urchin stings, 959
  for septic shock, 826
  for stingray wound, 956
  for upper airway obstruction, 236
  for urticaria, 1013
  for ventricular fibrillation, 703
  for wound care, in children, 1043

Epiphyseal metaphyseal fractures, child abuse and, 1099

Epistaxis, **632–633**
  cauterization for, 632*i,* 633
  in frontal sinus fractures, 449
  nasal balloon device for, 633, 634*i*
  nasal packing for, **133–136,** 134*i*
  nasal tampons for, 633, 634*i*
  in orbital floor (blowout) fractures, 447
  treatment of, 632*i,* 633, 634*i*
  in zygomaticomaxillary complex fractures, 446

Epley maneuver, for positional vertigo, 632

Eponychia, **562–563**

Epsilon-aminocaproic acid (EACA)
  for disseminated intravascular coagulation, 802
  for hemophilia, 796
  for von Willebrand disease, 799

Epstein-Barr virus (EBV) infection
  and exanthems, 1082*t*–1083*t*
  mononucleosis with, 816–817, 840
  and pharyngitis, in children, 1073
Eptifibatide, for angina, 684
Equine rabies immune globulin, 593
Equipment
  for neonatal resuscitation, 1097*t*
  for pediatric patients, 1040, 1041*t*–1042*t*
Erection, persistent (priapism), **764,** 810
Ergot derivatives
  for cluster headache, 390
  for migraine, 389
Ergotamine, for cluster headache, 390
Ergotism, **787**
Erysipelas, 854–855, **1016**
Erythema infectiosum, 1082*t*–1083*t*
Erythema multiforme, 1084*t*–1085*t*
Erythrocyte sedimentation rate
  in infective endocarditis, 860
  in mononucleosis, 816
  in stroke patients, 371
Erythroderma, **1014–1015**
Erythromycin
  for bullous myringitis, 627*t*
  for cellulitis, 1016
  for chancroid, 854
  for chlamydial infection, 610
  for diphtheria, 638*t*
  for dysuria-frequency syndrome, 845
  for erysipelas, 855, 1016
  for impetigo and ecthyma, 855
  for nasal fracture, 448
  ophthalmic ointment, 622*t*
    for conjunctivitis, 610
    for dacryocystitis, 608
  for pharyngitis, 841
    in children, 1074
  for pneumonia, 835, 836*t*, 1060*t*
  prophylactic use of, 564
    in wound care, 590*t*, 597
  for puerperal mastitis, 749
  for syphilis, 853
Erythropoietin, for multiple myeloma, 817
Escape rhythms, **703–706**
Escharotomy, for circumferential burns, 928
Escherichia coli infection
  enterohemorrhagic, and dysentery, 308*t*
  enterotoxigenic, and gastroenteritis, 304*t*
  epididymitis in, 849
  in infants, 1062
  and meningitis, 1068*t*
  in sickle cell anemia, 810
  and suppurative cholangitis, 276
  testing for, 302
  urinary tract, 841
    in children, 1075
Escherichia coli O157:H7 infection, and hemolytic
    uremic syndrome, 794
Esmolol
  in advanced life support, 160*t*, 161
  for arrhythmias, 1008
  for hypertension, in aortic dissection, 780–781
  for multifocal atrial tachycardia, 699
Esophageal detection device, and intubated patient,
    190
Esophageal disorders. *See also specific type*
  chest pain in, **253**
  gastrointestinal bleeding in, 290*t*
Esophageal foreign body, in children, **1091–1092,**
    1092*i*
Esophageal gastric tube airway, 171

Esophageal injury
  in chest trauma, **461**
  in neck trauma, 439
  pneumomediastinum with, 461, 665
Esophageal obturator airway
  complications of, 172, 172*t*
  and intubation preparation, 170–172
Esophageal spasm, diagnosis of, 249*t*
Esophageal tracheal Combitube, 171–172
Esophageal varices, gastrointestinal bleeding with,
    290*t*, **291–292**
Esophagitis
  chest pain in, 253
  in children, 1089
  diagnosis of, 249*t*
  gastritis in, 291
  gastrointestinal bleeding in, 290*t*
Esophagogastroduodenoscopy (EGD), 289–290
Esophagogram, in esophageal injury, 439
Esophagoscopy, in esophageal injury, 439, 461
Esophagus
  perforated
    chest pain in, **253**
    diagnosis of, 249*t*
  radiation injury of, 944
  traumatic injury of, **214**
Estrogen therapy
  for atrophic vaginitis, 847
  for hemostatic abnormalities in renal disease,
    800
  for idiopathic thrombocytopenic purpura, 792
ETC. *See* Esophageal tracheal Combitube
Ethambutol
  contraindications to
    in children, 670
    in pregnancy, 670
  for tuberculosis, 670
Ethanol. *See also* Alcohol
  for methanol poisoning, 985
  poisoning/overdose of, **985–986**
Ethchlorvynol, overdose, 1007
Ethinyl estradiol, for pregnancy prevention
  emergency postcoital, 742
  in female rape victims, 740
Ethmoid bone fracture, **619**
Ethylene glycol poisoning, 985, **987**
Etomidate
  adverse effects and precautions, 184
  and intubation, 184
  in reduction of fractures or dislocations, 515
Euphorbia pulcherrima, toxins in, 1004*t*
Ewart's sign, in pericardial effusion, 688
Exanthems, in children, **1080,** 1082*t*–1083*t*
Exercise
  angina in, 683
  syncope in, 340, 343
Exercise therapy
  for ankylosing spondylitis, 413
  for osteoarthritis, 411
  for tendonitis, 414
Exfoliation, **1014–1015**
Exonazol nitrate, for tinea, 1024
Expansion of trapped gas, air transport and, 18
Expectant (0) (triage category), 50
Expert witnesses, **71**
Explosions, **45**
Expressive aphasia, 401
Extensor(s)
  central wrist, 552
  extrinsic, of hand, 552–553, 553*i*
    anatomy of, 552–553, 553*i*
    testing of, 553

Extensor carpi radialis brevis, 552
Extensor carpi radialis longus, 552
Extensor carpi ulnaris, 552
Extensor digitorum communis, 553
Extensor hood mechanism, 553
Extensor pollicis brevis, 552–553
Extensor tendons of hand, 553–554
  distal, injuries of, **559–561**
  injuries of, **569**
  laceration of, **559**
  zones of injury in, 559, 560*i*
External jugular vein
  catheterization of, **83–86,** 85*i*
  identification of, 84, 84*i*
Extracorporeal blood rewarming, 933
Extraocular motility, 600
Extrapulmonary tuberculosis, 669
Extravasation, vascular injury in, 768
Extravascular hemolytic transfusion reaction, 822*t*,
    823
Extremities
  burns of, **928**
  cold injury to, **934–936**
  injuries of
    blunt, 768
    orthopedic, 512, **519–529, 532–547**
    penetrating, 768
    vascular injuries in, **767–768**
    wound care in, 576
  trauma to, **220–221**
  venous thrombosis of, **782–784**
Extrication, by EMS field personnel, **15**
Extubation, 190
Exudate, pleural, 666
Exudative retinal detachment, 607
Eye(s)
  atropine misuse in, 624
  black, **619**
  burn injuries of, **615–617,** 921, **927**
    acid, 616
    alkali, 616
    thermal, 616–617
    ultraviolet radiation, 617
  corticosteroid use in, caution with, 620, 624–625
  decontamination of, 964–965
  disorders of
    equipment and supplies required in, **621**
    errors in diagnosis of, 624
    overtreatment of, 625
    pitfalls in management of, **624–625**
    treatment of, common techniques for,
      621–625
  examination of, 600
    corneal staining for, 623–624
    eyelid eversion for, 616, 616*i*, 620, 621
    in stroke patients, 370
  herpes zoster infection in, 1020
  injuries of, 600, **615–620**
    blunt, **618–620**
    corticosteroid use in, caution with, 620
    in facial trauma, **440,** 618
    penetrating or perforating, **617–618**
  inspection of, 600
  lightning injuries of, 941
  local anesthesia for, 621, 622*t*
    dangers in use of, 624
  mechanical trauma to, **617–620**
  medications for, 621, 622*t*
    contaminated, 625
    home use of, 623
  nontraumatic conditions of, **608–615**
  pituitary apoplexy and, 886

red or painful, evaluation of, **600**, 601*t*, 601*i*
sulfur mustard exposure and, 39
Eye drops, 621
Eye emergencies, **599–625**. *See also specific types*
  acute angle-closure glaucoma, **604–605**
  acute hydrops of cornea, **612**
  acute unilateral visual loss, **600–604**, 603*i*
  atropine misuse in, 624
  bacterial corneal ulcer, **611**
  burns, **615–617**
  cavernous sinus thrombosis, **606**
  central retinal artery occlusion, **605**
  central retinal vein occlusion, **614–615**
  conjunctivitis, **610**
  corticosteroid therapy in, caution with, 620,
    624–625
  dacryoadenitis, **608–609**
  dacryocystitis, **608**
  endophthalmitis, **606–607**
  equipment and supplies for, **621**
  errors in diagnosis of, 624
  eyelid infections (preseptal cellulitis), **609**
  hordeolum (sty), **609**
  hyphema, **612–613**
  local anesthesia in, 621, 622*t*
    dangers in use of, 624
  mechanical trauma, **617–620**
  medications for, 621, 622*t*
    contaminated, 625
    home use of, 623
  nontraumatic, **608–615**
  ocular conditions requiring immediate treatment
    in, **604–608**
  ocular symptoms in, evaluation of, **600–604**
  orbital cellulitis, **605–606**
  overtreatment in, 625
  pitfalls in, **624–625**
  red or painful eye, **600**, 601*i*, 602*t*
  retinal detachment, 607
  retinal hemorrhage, **614**
  spontaneous subconjunctival hemorrhage, **610**
  toxic causes of blindness, **607–608**
  traumatic, **615–620**
  treatment of, common techniques for, **621–625**
  uveitis, **613**
  viral keratoconjunctivitis, **611–612**
  vitreous hemorrhage, **613–614**
Eye movements. *See also* Nystagmus
  in basilar artery thrombosis, 323
  in coma, 316
  in embolic occlusion, 323
  in head injuries, 422
  in psychogenic *versus* organic coma, 330
Eyeball rupture, 619
Eyebrow hair, removal contraindicated, 580
Eyelash hair, removal contraindicated, 580
Eyelids
  blunt trauma to, 618
  burn injuries of, 616–617
  ecchymosis (black eye), **619**
  eversion of, 616, 616*i*, 620, 621
  infections of, **609**
  lacerations of, **619**
  in psychogenic *versus* organic coma, 330

FabAV. *See* Crotalidae polyvalent immune Fab
Face
  abscess of, incision and drainage of, 141–142
  burns of, 921
Facet syndrome, **419**
Facial cellulitis, in sinusitis, 643–645
Facial fractures, **441–450**

Facial immersion in cold water, for paroxysmal
    supraventricular tachycardia, 696
Facial injuries, airway management in, 188
Facial lacerations
  care of, **452–453**
  closure of, 452
    timing for, 575
  delay in closing, 452
  repair technique for, 452–453
  replacement of avulsed tissue in, 452
Facial nerve
  injury to, 439–440
    in temporal bone fracture, **451**
  paralysis of, otitis media and, 1070–1071
Facial surgery, anesthesia for, 579, 579*i*
Facial trauma, **439–441**
  airway injury in, 439
  anesthesia for, 579, 579*i*
  debridement in, 581
  disposition in cases of, 441
  ear injury in, **441**
  eye injury in, **440**, 618
  mouth injuries in, **440**
  nerve injury in, 439–440
  parotid gland injury in, **440**, 440*i*
  type of injury in, 439
  vascular injury in, 439
Facial weakness, in Bell palsy, **357–358**
Factitious disorder, syncope in, 346
Factor IX
  deficiency of, 795
  replacement of, 796, 797*t*
Factor VIII
  deficiency of, 795
  replacement of, 796, 797*t*
Fainting
  emotional, 340
  heat-related, **937**
  simple, in pregnancy, 340
Fall on outstretched hand (FOOSH)
  carpal bone fractures in, 525–526
  forearm fractures in, 524
  humerus fractures in, 519
  lunate or perilunate dislocations in, 524
  radial head fractures in, 522
  scapholunate dislocations in, 525
  supracondylar fractures in, 521
False aneurysms, 768
False imprisonment, 67
False urethral passage, and urinary catheter inser-
    tion, 127
Famciclovir
  for genital herpes infection, 852
  for herpes pharyngitis, 639*t*
  for herpes simplex, 1021
  for herpes zoster, 256, 1020
Familial Mediterranean fever, diagnosis of, 272*t*
Family
  of pediatric patient, 1040
  presence during resuscitation, 146–147
Famotidine
  for allergic reactions, 638*t*
  for upper airway obstruction, 237
Fascia wounds, closure of, 584
Fasciotomy, for compartment syndrome, 512
FAST exams. *See* Focused assessment with sonogra-
    phy for trauma
Fat, suturing and closure of, 584–585
Fat pads, in elbow injuries, 522
Fatigue
  hand or arm, in thoracic outlet syndrome, 786
  in myasthenia gravis, 366

Febrile seizures, in children, 1060–1061
Febrile transfusion reactions, 822*t*, 823
Fecal cell count, for diarrhea, 302
Federal Emergency Management Agency (FEMA),
    46
Feet. *See* Foot
Felon, **563–564**, 564*i*
FEMA. *See* Federal Emergency Management
    Agency
Femoral artery aneurysm, **781**
Femoral canals, examination of, 264
Femoral fractures
  in child abuse, 1099
  distal, **535**
  spiral, in child abuse, 515
Femoral head, avascular necrosis of, 531
Femoral nerve block, 578
Femoral shaft fractures, **532–533**
Femoral vein
  catheterization of, **92–93**
  identification of, 92, 93*i*
Femoral vein phlebotomy, **92–93**
Fenoldopam
  for catecholamine crisis, 885
  for hypertensive emergencies, 687
Fentanyl
  adverse effects and precautions, 185, 515
  asthma and, 188
  for cardiogenic shock, 244
  in children, 1043
  for flail chest, 458
  and intubation, 185
  for rapid-sequence intubation, 182
  for reduction of fractures or dislocations, 515
Fetal heart rate monitoring, in trauma during preg-
    nancy, 746
Fever. *See also* Hyperthermia
  with abdominal pain, 263
  in children, **1062–1066**, 1064–1066, 1067*i*
  in delirium or confusion, 393, 394
  with diarrhea, 301–302
  with headache, 382
  in infants, **1062–1064**, 1065*i*
  in infection, in immunocompromised patient,
    829–830
  in meningitis, 379, 381, 382, 384, 830
  in otitis media, 1070
  in periorbital cellulitis, 1075
  seizure activity causing, 335, 341
  in sepsis shock, 826
  in transfusion reaction, 823
  with vomiting, 301–302
Fiberoptic bronchoscopy, 175
  for intubation in neck injury, 435
Fiberoptic intubation, 174–175
Fibrillation
  atrial, **697–698**
    in children, 1050*t*
    electrocardiogram in, 697, 712, 716*i*
    in stable patients, 698
    thromboembolic complications of, 697–698
    treatment of, 698, 700
    in unstable patients, 698
    in Wolf-Parkinson-White syndrome, 700
  ventricular, 157–158, **703**, 717, 718*i*
    in children, 164, 1050*t*
    in commotio cordis, 465
    electrocardiogram in, 703, 717, 718*i*
Fibrin degradation products, 791*t*
  in disseminated intravascular coagulation,
    802
  in liver disease, 799

Fibrinogen level, 791*t*
  in disseminated intravascular coagulation, 802
  in liver disease, 799
Fibrinogen therapy, for disseminated intravascular coagulation, 802
Fibrinolytic therapy
  for cardiac arrest, 165–166
  in EMS field treatment, 14, 15
Fibula fractures, **539–540**
Field assessment, by EMS personnel, **13–14**
Field personnel, EMS, 6, **8**
Field treatment, **14–18**
  airway control in, 14
  cardiac care in, 14
  communications in, 16–18
  extrication in, 15
  immobilization in, 15–16
  invasive procedures in, 14–15
  medications in, 15
  protocols for, 16
  splinting in, 15–16
  standing orders for, 16
"Fight bite," 527, 565
Filoviridae, 31*t*
Finger(s)
  boutonnière deformity of, **528–529, 561,** 5
    61*i*
  clawing of, in ulnar nerve injury, 570*i*
  extensor muscles of, 552–553
  flexor muscles of, 551
  injuries of, epinephrine contraindicated in, 574
  mallet, **529, 559–560,** 561*i*
  orthopedic injuries of, 526–529, 559
  splinting of, 527, 527*i,* 528*i,* 529
  swan-neck deformity of, 528–529
  trigger, 566
Finger drop, in radial nerve palsy, 358
Finger sweep, for airway obstruction, 153, 154*i*
Fingernails
  avulsion of, **558–559**
  hematoma under, **528, 558**
Fingertip amputations, **557–558**
Fingertip burns, 926
Fingertip injuries, **557–559**
Finkelstein test, in De Quervain tenosynovitis, 566
Firefighters, and multicasualty incident/disaster management, 52
Fires, **45**
First responders, 6, **7–8**
  special qualifications, 9
  training and procedures for, 7*t*
Fish, poisonous, ingestion of, **960–962**
Fistula(s)
  arteriovenous, **785**
  with vascular injuries, 768
Flail chest, **215–216, 458**
  respiratory distress/dyspnea in, **229,** 230*t*
Flank injuries, **476**
  urologic injuries in, 484
Flank pain
  in abdominal aortic aneurysm rupture, 777
  in hematuria, 758
  in pyelonephritis, 843–844
  radiating, 263
Flash burn, 617
Flaviviridae, 31*t*
Flexible-tipped endotracheal tubes, for intubation, 174
Flexion-extension imaging, of cervical spine, 507
Flexor(s)
  digital, 551

extrinsic, of hand, 551–552, 553*i*
  anatomy of, 551–552, 553*i*
  testing of, 552
  wrist, 551
Flexor carpi radialis, 551
  testing of, 552
Flexor carpi ulnaris, 551
Flexor digitorum profundus, 551–552
Flexor digitorum superficialis, 551
Flexor pollicis longus, 551
  testing of, 552
Flexor tendons of hand, injuries of, **569**
Flexor tenosynovitis, 565
  stenosing, 566
"Floaters," in vitreous hemorrhage, 613
Floods, **43–44**
Flotation tip catheter, in septic shock, 825
Flowsheet
  for diabetic ketoacidosis, 871
  for hyperglycemic hyperosmolar nonketotic syndrome, 871
Fluconazole, for tinea, 1024
Fludarabine, for cold agglutinin syndrome, 806
Fludrocortisone, for adrenal insufficiency, 883
Fluent aphasia, 394*t,* **401–402**
Fluid(s)
  daily maintenance requirements, in children, 1046, 1046*t*
  in resuscutation documentation, 200
  volume, normal values, 891, 891*t*
Fluid and electrolyte disorders, **890–916.** *See also specific disorders*
  diagnosis of, **890–891**
  of serum calcium concentration, **902–905**
  of serum magnesium concentration, **906–908**
  of serum phosphorus concentration, **905–906**
  of serum potassium concentration, **897–902**
  of serum sodium concentration, **891–897**
Fluid overload, and hyponatremia, 894
Fluid replacement/resuscitation. *See also* Volume replacement/resuscitation
  in abdominal aortic aneurysm rupture, 777
  in abdominal trauma, 467, 468, 767
  in aortic dissection, 780
  in burn injuries, 917–919, 919*t*
  in central diabetes insipidus, 889
  in chest trauma, 454, 465, 466
  in children, 1044
  in dehydration, in children, 1046
  in delirium tremens, 397
  in diabetic ketoacidosis, 870
  in disseminated intravascular coagulation, 802
  in eye trauma, 618
  in femoral shaft fractures, 533
  in gastroenteritis, in children, 1078
  in gastrointestinal bleeding, 285
  in heat-related cramps, 937
  in hemoptysis, 654
  in hemorrhagic shock, 214
  in hypercalcemia, 904
  in hyperglycemic hyperosmolar nonketotic syndrome, 870
  in hypernatremia, 896–897
  in lactic acidosis, 876
  in lightning injuries, 941
  in multiply injured patient, 212
  in myxedema coma, 881
  in neurogenic shock, 207
  in peritonsillitis, 646
  in poisoning/overdose, 964
  in pulmonary contusion, 459
  in pulmonary infections with cystic fibrosis, 673

in pyelonephritis, 844
  in rhabdomyolysis, 368
  in septic shock, 205, 826
  in sinus tachycardia, 695
  in spinal cord injury, 494, 495
  in thoracic aorta injury, 771
  in toxic shock syndrome, 862
  in toxic shock-like syndrome, 862
  in vascular trauma, 767
  in vertigo, 632
  in visceral and hypogastric artery aneurysm, 778
  in visceral (intestinal) ischemia, 776
Fluid restriction, in inappropriate secretion of antidiuretic hormone, 887
Flumazenil
  in children, 1043
  for coma, 311
  for sedative-hypnotics overdose, 1007
Fluorescein dye, for eye exam, 611, 617, 620, 621, 623–624
Fluorescent treponemal antibody-absorption test (FTA-ABS), for syphilis, 853
Fluoroquinolone(s)
  clindamycin with, for bite injuries, 564–565
  for COPD, 660, 661
  for gastrointestinal infections, in HIV-infected patients, 864–865
  for gonorrhea, 851
  for meningitis, 833*t*
  for neutropenia, 814–815
  for pneumonia, 661, 668, 836*t*
  for primary peritonitis, 281
  for prostatitis, 849
  for pyelonephritis, 279
  for Q fever, 28
  for urinary tract infections, 842*t*
  for zygomaticomaxillary complex fractures, 446
Fluoxetine, 1037
Fluvoxamine, 1037
Focal neurologic findings, in delirium or confusion, **394–395**
Focused Assessment with Sonography for Trauma (FAST), **119–121,** 120*i,* 195
  in abdominal trauma, 218–219, 468, 469, 469*i*
  in cardiac tamponade, 457
  in multiply injured patient, 212
  in penetrating chest trauma, 465
Foley catheter. *See also* Urinary catheterization
  in bladder injuries, 488
  for drainage of distended bladder, 751–752
  in genitourinary trauma, 477–479, 490
  in hemoptysis, 654
  insertion of, **125–127,** 126*i*
  selection of, 125
  in urethral injuries, 477–479, 488, 490
Folic acid therapy
  for cold agglutinin syndrome, 806
  for disseminated intravascular coagulation, 802
  for Wernicke encephalopathy, 399
Follow-up care, legal issues of, 67–68
Fomeprizole
  for ethylene glycol poisoning, 987
  for methanol poisoning, 985
Food poisoning/contamination
  botulism, 353, **363–364**
  seafood, paralytic, **363**
FOOSH. *See* Fall on outstretched hand
Foot
  abscess of, incision and drainage of, 142
  arthrocentesis of, 136, 139
  burns of, 921
  injuries of, orthopedic, 544–547

Forearm fractures, **524**
Forehead trauma, frontal sinus fractures in, 449
Foreign body
    in airway, **152–153**, 153*i*, 154*i*
        in children, 164, **1053–1055**, 1053*t*, 1055*t*
            management of, 187–188
        and respiratory distress/dyspnea, **224–225**, 236
    aspiration of, 671
    in cornea and conjunctiva, **620**
        removal of, 623
    in ear, 627*t*
    esophageal, in children, **1091–1092**, 1092*i*
    gastric, in children, **1092**
    in hand, **567–568**
    hematuria with, 759*t*, 760
    in nose, 633–634, 635*i*
    retention, in puncture wounds, 597
    small bowel, in children, **1092**
Foreskin
    dorsal slit in, 764*i*, 765
    inability to retract (phimosis), **764–765**
    retracted, constricted (paraphimosis), 764*i*, **764–765**
Fosphenytoin
    for arrhythmias, 980
    in head injuries, 423
    for prophylaxis
        in head injuries, 423
        in stroke patients, 369
        in subarachnoid hemorrhage, 373
    for status epilepticus, 335, 336*t*
        loading dose of, 334
Fournier gangrene, **764**, 856
Foxglove, toxins in, 1004*t*
Fracture(s), **513–514**. *See also specific types or structures affected*
    basilar skull, 219
    in child abuse, 1099
    closed, 513
        blood loss in, 511, 512*t*
    commonly missed, 547
    compartment syndrome in, **512–513**
    definition of, 513
    descriptive terminology in, 513, 514
    epiphyseal metaphyseal, in child abuse, 1099
    femoral, in child abuse, 1099
    open, 513
    pathologic, 513
    pelvic, genitourinary injuries in, 220
    reduction of, **511**, 512*i*
        procedural sedation for, 515
    rib
        chest pain in, 250*t*, **254**
        in child abuse, 1099
        pleuritic pain in, 238
    splinting of, 220
    types and classification of, 513–514
Francisella tularensis, 26
Frank-Starling mechanism, 684
Frazier suction device
    in drainage of peritonsillar abscess, 645
    for epistaxis, 633
Fremitus, in pleural effusion, 666
Fresh frozen plasma, **820–821**
    characteristics and doses of, 819*t*, 820
    for hemoptysis, 654
    for hemostatic abnormalities of liver disease, 799
    indications for, 820
    for thrombotic thrombocytopenic purpura, 793
Frontal sinus fractures, **449**
Frontal sinusitis, 643, 644*i*

Frostbite, **567, 642, 934–936**
    arterial injury in, 787
    auricle, 642
    clinical findings in, 642
    deep, 567
    ear, 642
    grading of injury in, 642
    hand, **567**
    nose, 642
    prevention of, 567
    superficial, 567
Fruit pits, toxins in, 1004*t*
Fugu poisoning, 961
Fugue, psychogenic, **1035**
Funduscopy, 600
Fungal infections
    orbital cellulitis in, 606
    and T-2 mycotoxins, 34–35
Fungal sepsis, 825
Furosemide
    for blood transfusion, in children, 1093
    for central venous hypervolemia, 245
    for cerebral edema, 319*t*
    for congestive heart failure, 680, 685
        in children, 1049
    in EMS field treatment, 15
    for hypercalcemia, 904
    for inappropriate secretion of antidiuretic hormone, 888
    for myocardial infarction, 677
    for pulmonary edema, 203, 227
Fusarium, 34

GA (nerve agent), 37
Gag reflex, poisoning and, 964
Galeazzi fracture, 524
Gallstone ileus, 268
Gambierdiscus toxicus, 960
Gamekeeper's thumb, 529
Gamma globulin, for idiopathic thrombocytopenic purpura, 1096
Gamma rays, 21
Gangrene
    Fournier, **764**, 856
    gas, **857**
    infected vascular, **856**
    with intra-arterial injection of drugs, 787
    venous, 774–775
Gardnerella vaginalis infection, 846–848
Gas
    toxic, **993–994**, 995*t*
    trapped, expansion of, air transport and, 18
Gas gangrene, **857**
Gas patterns, in abdominal radiographs, 267–268, 268*i*
Gas stoppage sign, 263
Gastric atony, in spinal cord injury, 495
Gastric cancer, and gastrointestinal bleeding, 290*t*
Gastric contents
    aspiration of, 671
    evaluation of, in delirium or confusion, 393–394
Gastric emptying
    for ciguqtera toxin poisoning, 960
    for ingested poisons, 965
    for paralytic shellfish poisoning, 962
Gastric erosions, and gastrointestinal bleeding, 290*t*
Gastric evacuation, nasogastric intubation for, **102–104**, 103*i*
Gastric foreign body, in children, **1092**
Gastric insufflation, basic life support and, 152
Gastric lavage
    and gastrointestinal rebleeding, 289

    for ingested poisons, 965
    nasogastric intubation for, **102–104**, 103*i*
    for poisoning/overdose, 964
Gastric ulcers
    in children, 1089
    gastrointestinal bleeding in, 290*t*
Gastritis, and gastrointestinal bleeding, **290–291**, 290*t*
Gastroenteritis. *See also* Diarrhea; Vomiting
    abdominal pain in, **274**
    bacterial, **303**
    in children, **1077–1078**
    diagnosis of, 271*t*
    management of, **306–309**
    nondysenteric, 304*t*–305*t*
    viral, **303**, 305*t*
Gastroesophageal reflux, and chest pain, 253
Gastrogaffin, in esophageal injury, 461
Gastrointestinal anthrax, **22**, 23*t*
    abdominal, 22
    oropharyngeal, 22
Gastrointestinal bleeding, **283–295**
    absence of, 286
    in children, 1085, 1090*i*, 1091*i*
    in conscious patient with history of syncope, 337
    evaluation of, 286–289
    history of, 288
    initial assessment of, 283–286
    laboratory studies for, 285
    life-threatening, immediate management of, **283–286**, 284*i*
    lower
        in children, 1089
        diagnosis of, 286
        physical examination of, 288–289
        specific disorders causing, **292–295**
    in newborn, 1089
    physical examination of, 288
    rate of, 283
    rebleeding, monitoring for, 289
    risk factors for, 283–285
    and shock, 196
    site of, 286
    stabilization procedures, 285–286
    upper
        in children, 1089
        diagnosis of, **286**, 287*i*
        physical examination of, 288
        severity of, 290*t*
        specific disorders causing, **289–292**, 290*t*
    volume of, 283
Gastrointestinal disorders
    and chest pain, **253–254**
    in children, **1080–1092**
Gastrointestinal infection, in HIV-infected patients, 864–865
Gauze packing
    for epistaxis, 633
    for wound debridement, 581
Gauze technique, for epistaxis, 135–136
GB (nerve agent), 37
GCS. *See* Glasgow Coma Scale
GD (nerve agent), 37
General anxiety disorder, syncope in, 346
Genital abscesses, female, **848**
    fluctuant, 848
    nonfluctuant, 848
Genital herpes simplex virus infection, **851–852**
    dysuria in, 757*t*
    treatment of, 852, 852*t*
Genital trauma
    external, **490–492**

Genital trauma (*cont.*)
  female, 491, **492, 737**
    in rape or sexual assault, 491, 492, 737
  male, 490–492
Genitalia, male, examination of, 264
Genitourinary emergencies, **750–765**. *See also spe-
    cific types*
  dysuria, **756–758**
  Fournier gangrene, **764**
  hematuria, atraumatic, **758–760**
  oliguria or anuria, **750–752**
  orchitis, **763–764**
  phimosis and paraphimosis, **764–765**
  priapism, **764**
  scrotal mass lesions, painless, **755–756**, 756t
  scrotal pain, **752–755**, 753t
  serious and life-threatening conditions in, imme-
      diate management of, **750–760**
  specific disorders in, emergency treatment of,
      760–765
  testicular torsion, **763**
  urolithiasis, **760–763**
Genitourinary system
  female, disorders of, **845–848**
  male, diseases of, **763–765, 849–850**
  in sickle cell anemia, 810
Genitourinary trauma, **220, 477–492**
  bladder injuries in, **486–488**
  blunt
    in children, management of, 480i
    management of, 478i
  catheterization in, 477–479
  diagnostic clues in, 477
  emergency treatment of specific injuries in,
      481–492
  genital injuries in, external, **490–492**
  immediate treatment in, 477
  intravenous pyelogram in, 480
  life-threatening injuries in, immediate manage-
      ment of, **477–481**
  in pelvic fractures, 530
  penetrating, management of, 479i
  penile rupture in, **491**
  renal injuries in, **481–484**
  skin injuries in, **492**
  special examinations and procedures in,
      477–481
  testicular injuries in, **491**
  ureteral injuries in, **484–486**
  urethral injuries in, **488–490**
Gentamicin
  for brucellosis, 28
  for cellulitis, 855
  for corneal and conjunctival foreign body in-
      juries, 620
  for eye trauma/disorders, 621, 622t
  for infected vascular gangrene and cellulitis, 856
  for infective endocarditis, 860
  for meningitis, 833t, 834t
    in children, 1068t
  for necrotizing fasciitis, 857
  for orbital floor (blowout) fractures, 620
  for osteomyelitis, in children, 1078t
  for pelvic inflammatory disease, 846t
  for perforated duodenum, 254
  for perforated stomach, 254
  for plague, 23t, 26
  for pneumonia, 836t, 1060t
  for prostatitis, 849
  for puerperal sepsis, 748
  for pyelonephritis, 279
  for septic arthritis, in children, 1078t

for synergistic necrotizing cellulitis, 856
  for tularemia, 23t, 27
  for urinary tract infections, in children, 1077
Gestational trophoblastic disease, 736–737
GF (nerve agent), 37
GHB. *See* γ-Hydroxybutyrate
GI cocktail
  for esophageal disorders, 253
  for gastritis, 291
Giardia antigen, testing for, 302
Giardia lamblia infection, gastroenteritis in, 305t
  in children, 1077
Gila monster bite, weakness with, 354
Gilanotti-Crosti syndrome, 1082t–1083t
Gingivitis, acute necrotizing ulcerative, 649, 650t
Gingko biloba, for mountain sickness, 949
Glanders, 29
Glandular tularemia, 23t, 26
Glasgow Coma Scale (GCS), 208, 210i, 422, 467,
    496
  for head trauma, 219
  for multiply injured patient, 211–212
  pediatric, 1061t
  and triage, 51
Glaucoma
  acute, differential diagnosis of, 602t
  acute angle-closure, 602, 604i, **604–605**
  central retinal vein occlusion in, 614–615
  open-angle, corticosteroids and, 624
Glomerulonephritis, hematuria in, 759, 759t, 760
Glossopharyngeal neuralgia, syncope in, 340
Glucagon
  for beta-adrenergic blocker poisoning/overdose,
      976
  for calcium-channel blocker poisoning/overdose,
      977
  for complete heart block, 706
  for hypoglycemia, 874–875
Glucocorticoids
  for anaphylactic shock, 207
  for asthma, 1058
  for brain tumor, 322
  for cerebral edema, 319t
  for croup, 1052
  deficiency of, 882
  for pemphigus vulgaris, 1017
  for septic shock, 205
  for subtentorial mass lesions, 322
  for supratentorial mass lesions, 319
  for tendonitis, 414
Glucose
  for alcoholic ketoacidosis, 877
  in coma cocktail, 311
  and delirium, 1032
  for delirium or confusion, 391–393, 393
  in EMS field treatment, 15
  for ethanol poisoning, 986
  for heat-related cramps, 937
  for hyperkalemia, in muscle disease, 355
  for hyperphosphatemia, 906
  for hypoglycemia, 326–327, 874
  for poisoning-related coma, 963–964
Glucose determination, in synovial fluid analysis,
    140
Glucose-6-phosphate dehydrogenase deficiency
    (G6PD), **812**
Glycerin
  for acute angle-closure glaucoma, 605
  for cerebral edema, 319t
Glycerol, for cerebral edema, 319t
Glycoprotein IIB/IIIA receptor antagonists
  for angina, 684

platelet function impaired by, 795
  thrombocytopenia induced by, 792
Glycopyrrolate, in children, 1044
Gold therapy, for rheumatoid arthritis, 411
Gonads, radiation injury of, 943–944
Gonococcemia, disseminated, **861**
Gonorrhea, **850–851**
  arthritis in, 404, 409–410, 838
  cervicitis in, 848, 851
  coexistent with chlamydial infection, 851
  conjunctivitis in, 851–852
  disseminated (hematogenous), **565,** 850, **861**
  dysuria in, 756, 758
  epididymitis in, 849–850
  in females, 851
  genital abscess in, 848
  in males, 851
  pelvic inflammatory disease in, 845–846
  pelvic pain in, 728
  pharyngitis in, 638t, 850
  prevention of, in female rape victims, 740
  prostatitis in, 849
  tenosynovitis in, 565
  urethritis in, 844–845, 851–852
  vaginitis in, 846
Good Samaritan laws, **63–64**
Gouty arthritis, **408–409**
Gram stain and culture
  in mucopurulent cervicitis, 848
  in septic shock, 827
  in urinary tract infections, 842
  in vaginitis, 847
Granisetron, for radiation injury, 944
Granulocyte count, in infection, in immunocom-
    promised patients, 830
Granulocytopenia, 829
Greenfield filter, for pulmonary embolism, 664
Greenstick fracture, 513
Griseofulvin, for tinea, 1024
Ground transport, 12
Growth plate injuries, 513, 514, 547
  Salter-Harris classification of, 513, 513i
Guillain-Barré syndrome
  neurogenic shock caused by, 207
  weakness caused by, **359–360**
Gunshot wounds
  abdominal, 467, 468, 470
    in pregnancy, 746
  chest, 465–466
  hand, 572
  neck, 438
  reporting of, 68
  shotgun blasts, 594–595
Gut sutures, 582
Gymnopilus, 1002t
Gynecologic cancer, **736–737**
Gynecologic disorders, abdominal pain in,
    280–281
Gynecologic emergencies, **725–749.** *See also specific
    types*
  carcinoma and other tumors, **736–737**
  contraception discontinuation in, warning
    about, **742**
  dysmenorrhea, **738**
  ectopic pregnancy, **728–733**
  endometriosis, **738**
  genital trauma, **737**
  intrauterine device problems, **741–742**
  life-threatening problems in, immediate manage-
    ment of, **725–728**
  management of specific disorders in, **728–742**
  mittelschmerz, **738**

ovarian cyst rupture, **737**
ovarian tumor torsion, **737–738**
pelvic pain, **726–728**
postcoital emergency contraception in, **742**
rape, **739–741**
septic abortion, **735–736**
spontaneous abortion, **733–735**
uterine prolapse, **738–739**
vaginal bleeding, **725–726**
vaginal disorders, **742**
vulvar disorders, **742**
Gyromitra esculenta, 1002*t*

Haemophilus ducreyi infection, 853–854
Haemophilus influenzae infection
    eyelid, 609
    meningitis in, 830, 834*t*, 1068*t*
    orbital cellulitis in, 605–606
    osteomyelitis in, 1079
    periorbital cellulitis in, 1075
    pneumonia in, 834–835
    in sickle cell anemia, 810
    sinusitis in, 643
    type B
        in children, 635, 638*t*
        epiglottitis in, 635, 638*t*
    urinary tract, in children, 1075
Haemophilus influenzae type B vaccine, 638*t*, 646,
    830
Hair loss, differential diagnosis, 1100*t*
Hair removal, from wound area, 579–580
Hair testing, in arsenic poisoning, 360
Haldol. *See* Haloperidol
Half-life, of toxin, 968
Hallucinations
    in drug withdrawal, 396–397
    in metabolic disorders, 396
    in psychosis, 402
Hallucinogens, intoxication, delirium or confusion
    in, **399, 1031**
Halogenated hydrocarbons, blindness caused by,
    607
Haloperidol
    as chemical restraint, 1028
    for mania, 1034
    for phencyclidine overdose, 1000
    poisoning/overdose of, 1000–1001
    psychiatric uses, 1036
    for psychotic confusional states, 402
    for schizophrenia, 1033
    for stimulant overdose, 974
Hamman's crunch, in pneumomediastinum,
    664–665
Hampton's Hump, in pulmonary embolism, 662
Hamstring muscles, 533
Hand
    abscess of, 562–564
        incision and drainage of, 142
    amputation of, **568–569**
    arthrocentesis of, 136, 139
    bite injuries of, 564–565, 572
    bone and joint injuries of, **524–529, 561–562**
        open or unstable, 562
        stable, 562
    burn injuries of, **566–567, 921**
    circulation in, 551
    complex injuries of, **568–572**
    constrictive problems of, minor, **566**
    dorsal, 551, 553*i*
    electrical burns of, **567**
    examination of, **551–556**
    extrinsic extensors of, 552–553, 553*i*

extrinsic flexors of, 551–552, 553*i*
    anatomy of, 551–552, 553*i*
    testing of, 552
foreign bodies embedded in, **567–568**
frostbite of, 567
function of
    active, observation of, 550
    assessment of, **551–556**
functional anatomy of, 551–556, 553*i*
high-pressure injection injuries of, **569–570**
infections of, **562–565**
innervation of, 551, 552, 553, 571*i*
intrinsic muscles of, 553–554
    anatomy of, 553–554
    testing of, 554
joints of, abbreviations for, 548
lacerations of, **557**, 559
    extensive, 557
    small, 557
mangling injuries of, **572**
nerve injuries of, 554–555, **569**
palmar, 551, 553*i*
position of function, 557, 557*i*
posture of, 550
sensory distribution in, 571*i*
skin of, 551
sling for, 557
splinting of, 527, 527*i*, 528*i*, 557, 562
terminology for, 551
thermal injuries of, **566–567**
trauma to, **524–529, 548–572**
    anesthesia in, 549–550, 550*i*, 551*i*, 552*i*,
        578, 578*i*, 579*i*
    antiseptic solutions in, 556
    bleeding in, control of, 549
    closed compartment syndromes in, **571–572**
    dressings for, 556–557, 588
    emergency evaluation and treatment of,
        548–551
    examination in, 549–551, **552–556**
    history of, 549
    instruments used in, 556
    management of specific injuries in, **557–572**
    mechanism of injury in, 549
    open wounds in, 549
    orthopedic, **524–529, 561–562**
    patient positioning for evaluation of, 549
    ring removal in, 572
    sensation in, 550–551, 555–556
    skin and wound preparation in, 556
    special emergency room problems in, **572**
    suturing in, 556
    tourniquet application in, 550
    treatment of, equipment and materials for,
        556–557
    wound inspection in, 551
    x-ray examination in, 556
    veins of, for venipuncture, 75
Hand fatigue, in thoracic outlet syndrome, 786
Hand offs, in team approach to cardiac arrest, 146
Hand surgery, anesthesia for, 578, 578*i*
"Hand trip," 787
Hand-foot syndrome, in sickle cell anemia, 809
Hand-foot-mouth syndrome, 1082*t*–1083*t*
Hanks' Balanced Salt Solution (HBSS), for avulsed
    teeth, 640
Hanks' solution, for avulsed teeth, 640
Harvesting of organs for transplantation, **72**
Hay fever, conjunctivitis in, 610
Hazardous marine life, **956–960**
Hazardous materials, and multicasualty
    incidents/disasters, 53–54

decontamination for, 58–59
    hospital management of, 58–59
    scene organization, 54, 55*i*
    training, 54–55
HBSS. *See* Hanks' Balanced Salt Solution
HCQIA. *See* Health Care Quality Improvement
    Act
Head
    abscess of, incision and drainage of, 141–142
    physical examination of
        in headache patients, 382–383
        in stroke patients, 370
Head lice, 1023
Head trauma, **219–220, 421–434**, 576
    airway management in, 188, 421–422
    breathing in, 422
    cerebral contusion in, **429**
    cerebrospinal fluid otorrhea after, **451**
    cervical spine immobilization in, 421
    in children
        child abuse and, 1099
        special considerations in, **432**
    circulation in, 422
    combativeness in, 423
    delirium or confusion in, **394**, 394*t*
    diffuse axonal injury in, **430**, 433*i*
    disability in, 422
    discharge instructions in, **433–434**
    emergency treatment of specific, **423–430**
    epidural hematoma in, **428**, 428*i*
    exposure of patient for examination, 422–423
    headache in, 379, 385
    hearing loss in, **451**
    hospitalization for, indications for, **433**
    hypertension in, **423**
    in intoxicated patients, **434**
    intracranial injury in, **425–430**
    intracranial pressure in, 422, 423
    life-threatening problems in, immediate manage-
        ment of, **421–423**
    middle and inner ear disorders following,
        451–452
    minor, **430–431**
    pain control in, 423
    reevaluation of, 434
    seizures in, 423
    skull fractures in, **424–425**, 426*i*, 427*i*
    soft tissue injuries in, **423–424**
    spinal cord injuries with, 421, 495, 496, 506
    in stroke patients, 369
    subarachnoid hemorrhage in, **429**, 431*i*, 432*i*
    subdural hematoma in, **428–429**, 429*i*, 430*i*
    vertigo in, 451, **452**
Head wound, 576
Headache, **379–390**
    acute, management of specific disorders causing,
        383–385
    associated symptoms with, 382
    in carbon monoxide poisoning, 381
    cluster, 382, **389–390**
    in delirium or confusion, 394
    diagnosis of, approach to, **381–383**
    disposition in cases of, 381
    focal neurologic abnormalities with, 379
    with head injury, 379, 382, 385
    in hemophiliacs, 795
    history of, 382
    in hypertension, 381, 382, **390**
    in intracerebral hemorrhage, 373
    intracranial mass (brain tumor) and, **386**
    life-threatening conditions caused by, immediate
        management of, **379–381**, 380*i*

Headache (*cont.*)
mass lesion, 382
in meningitis, 379–381, 382, 383, **384,** 830
in meningoencephalitis, 328
migraine (*See* Migraine)
in multiple patients from same vicinity, 381
neurologic examination in, 383
of new or recent origin, 379
pain location in, 382
pain quality in, 382
pain-sensitive structures in, 381
paracranial disease and, 381
physical examination in, 382–383
in pituitary apoplexy, 885–886
post-lumbar puncture, 132
posttraumatic, 382, **385**
postural (post-lumbar puncture), **384–385**
precipitating factors for, 382
in pseudotumor cerebri, **386**
in seizures, 379
severity of, factors influencing, 382
special signs in, 383
in stroke patients, 370, 382, **383**
subacute, management of specific disorders causing, **385–387**
in subarachnoid hemorrhage, 372, 379–381,
382, **383,** 390
syncope with, 339, 345
in temporal arteritis, 381, 382, **387**
tension, 382, **387–388**
time of onset, 382
timing of, 382
toxin exposure and, 381
in trigeminal neuralgia, 382, **385–386**
Head-tilt, in pediatric basic life support, 164
Health Care Quality Improvement Act (HCQIA),
and National Practitioner Data Bank,
71–72
HEAR network, for EMS communications, 16
Hearing loss, **629–630**
cerumen impaction and, 641
conductive, 629, 629*t*
in temporal bone fracture, **451**
testing for, 629*i,* 629–630
history of, 629
Rinne test for, 629–630, 630*i*
sensorimotor, in temporal bone fracture, **451**
sensorineural, 629
testing for, 629–630, 630*i*
sudden, causes of, 629, 629*t*
Weber test in, 629, 629*i*
Heart, examination of, in stroke patients, 370
Heart block, **704–706**
Heart disease
congenital, **691–693**
infective endocarditis in, treatment of, 860
cyanotic, **691–692**
valvular, 691
infective endocarditis in, 859–860
Heart failure, **684–686**
causes of, importance of establishing, 685
clinical findings in, 686
compensatory mechanisms in, 684
congestive, 226–227, 680–681, **684–686**
central venous hypervolemia in, 244–245
in children, **1048–1049,** 1049*t*
in infants, **692–693**
in myocardial infarction, 675, **680–681**
in infants, **692–693**
mild to moderate, **686**
severe, **685**
in spinal cord injury, 494, 495

Heart strain, right, with pulmonary embolism, 662,
664
Heat, disorders due to, **936–939**
Heat cramps, **937**
Heat edema, **937**
Heat exhaustion, **937–938**
Heat stroke, **938–939**
Heat syncope, **937**
Heavy metal poisoning, **988–991**
Heimlich maneuver, **152–153,** 153*i,* 154*i*
in pulmonary aspiration syndrome, 671
for upper airway obstruction, 224
Heinz bodies, in glucose-6-phosphate dehydrogenase deficiency, 812
Helicopter transport
for multicasualty incidents/disasters, 53
safety, 18
Helicospiral CT angiography, in pulmonary embolism, 663
Hematemesis
in children, 1085
treatment algorithm for, 1090*i*
upper gastrointestinal bleeding with, 286, 287*i*
Hematochezia, 294*i*
in children, 1085
lower gastrointestinal bleeding with, 286
treatment algorithm for, 1091*i*
upper gastrointestinal bleeding with, 286
Hematocrit
in abdominal pain, 266
in abdominal trauma, 468
in anemia, 802–803, 803*t*
in gastrointestinal bleeding, 289
in pneumonia, 668
Hematologic diseases, in children, **1093–1096**
Hematologic emergencies, **788–823.** *See also specific types*
acute leukemia, **815**
anemia, **802–813**
chronic leukemia, **815–816**
coagulation factor disorders, **795–802**
disseminated intravascular coagulation, **801–802**
drug-induced immune-mediated thrombocytopenia, **792**
glucose-6-phosphate dehydrogenase deficiency,
812
hemoglobin H disease, **811**
hemolytic anemia, **804–808**
hemolytic uremic syndrome, **792–794**
hemophilia, **795–798**
hereditary spherocytosis, **812**
idiopathic thrombocytopenic purpura, **789–792**
immune thrombocytopenia, **789–792**
leukocytosis, **815**
in liver disease, **799–800**
mononucleosis, **816–817**
multiple myeloma, **817**
neutropenia, **814–815**
platelet disorders, **789–795**
polycythemia, **813**
qualitative platelet abnormalities, **794–795**
in renal disease, **800**
sickle cell anemia, **808–811**
thalassemia, **811–812**
thrombocytopenia due to platelet sequestration,
794
thrombocytosis, **795**
thrombotic thrombocytopenic purpura,
792–794
transfusion therapy for, **818–823**
vitamin K deficiency, **800–801**
von Willebrand disease, **798–799**

Waldenström macroglobulinemia, **817–818**
warfarin complications, **800–801**
white cell disorders, **814–818**
Hematoma(s)
bilateral periorbital, 440, 449
in blunt trauma, 767
"butterfly" perineal, 490
cervical, in neck trauma, 436
ear (otohematoma), 441, **450**
epidural, **324,** 428, 428*i*
subtentorial, **324**
nasal, 635*t*
in neck trauma, 769
penile, 490, 491
in renal injury, 484, 485*i*
scalp, **424**
in scapula fracture, 517
septal, 440, 448
subdural, **428–429**
coma in, **319–320,** 320*t,* **324**
computed tomography of, 428–429, 429*i,*
430*i*
subtentorial, **324**
subungual, **528, 558**
testicular, 491
Hematopoietic tissues, radiation injury of, 943
Hematuria, **758–760**
in abdominal trauma, 468
atraumatic, **758–760**
in bladder injuries, 473
causes of, diagnostic clues to, 759*t*
dysuria associated with, 758
in genitourinary trauma, 477–479
in infective endocarditis, 860
in pyelonephritis, 843
in renal injuries, 472, 479, 481, 484
systemic conditions associated with, 758
tumor causing, 759*t,* 760
of unknown cause, 760
in ureteral injuries, 484
in urolithiasis, 758–761, 759*t*
Hemianopia, 600
Hemiataxia, in stroke patients, 371
Hemicraniectomy, decompressive, 377
Hemiparesis
ataxic, 375
in cerebellar hemorrhage, 373
in stroke patients, 371, 375
in subdural hematoma, 320
Hemiplegia, in hypertensive intracerebral hemorrhage, 320–321
Hemlock, toxins in, 1004*t*
Hemobilia, gastrointestinal bleeding in, **292**
Hemodialysis
for drug elimination, 969–970, 969*t*
for ethylene glycol poisoning, 987
for hemolytic uremic syndrome, 794
for isopropanol poisoning, 987
for lithium overdose, 997
for methanol poisoning, 987
for salicylate overdose, 1006
Hemodynamics
abnormal, and chest pain, **240–245**
normal, and chest pain, **245–246**
Hemoglobin
in abdominal trauma, 468
in anemia, 802–803, 803*t*
in gastrointestinal bleeding, 289
in pneumonia, 668
Hemoglobin H disease, **811**
Hemoglobin S (HbS), in sickle cell anemia, 808
Hemoglobinopathy, hematuria in, 759*t*

Hemolysis
  drugs precipitating, 811, 811*t*
  and hyperkalemia, 901
Hemolytic anemia
  acute, **804–808**
  alloimmune, **807**
  autoimmune, **804–807**
    cold-type, 805–807
    drug-adsorption type, 807
    drug-related, 807, **807–808**
    hereditary, 812–813
    mixed-type, 807
    warm-type, 805
  microangiopathic, 792–794
  in sickle cell anemia, 810
Hemolytic transfusion reaction
  acute, 822*t*, 822–823
  extravascular, 822*t*, 823
Hemolytic uremic syndrome, **792–794**
  in children, 1089
Hemomediastinum, in aortic dissection, 779
Hemoperfusion
  for cardiac glycoside poisoning, 980
  for drug elimination, 969*t*, 970
  for theophylline overdose, 1008
Hemoperitoneum, 484
  in pregnant patients, 746
Hemophilia, **795–798**
  bleeding manifestations in, 795, 796*t*
  factor replacement therapy for, 795–798
    dosing regimen in, 796, 798*t*
    inhibitors or antibodies against, 797–798
    plasma-derived, 796, 797*t*
    recombinant, 796, 797*t*
  type A (classic), 795
  type B (Christmas disease), 795
Hemoptysis, **653–654**
  in bronchitis, 667
  causes of, 653, 654*t*
  massive, definition of, 653
  in pneumonia, 667
  in pulmonary embolism, 662
Hemorrhage. *See also* Bleeding; Hypovolemia
  adrenal, in meningococcemia, 858
  external, in multiply injured patient, 211
  hypertensive intracerebral, **320–321**
  intracerebellar, **323–324**
  intracerebral, **373–374**
    computed tomography of, 373–374, 374*i*
    hypertensive, **320–321**
    in stroke, 370
  intracranial, thrombolytic therapy and, 677
  intraperitoneal, 124
  orbital, **619**
  pontine, 323
  postpartum, **747–748**
  retinal, 602, **614**, 614*t*
  retroperitoneal, 271*t*, **281–282**
  scalp wound, 211
  spontaneous subconjunctival, **610**
  subarachnoid (*See* Subarachnoid hemorrhage)
  subconjunctival
    spontaneous, **610**
    in viral keratoconjunctivitis, 612
  in vascular trauma, 767
  vitreous, 604, 613*t*, **613–614**
  in wound cases, control of, 573–574, 577–578
Hemorrhagic arthritis, **407**, 407*t*
  in hemophilia, 796
  in von Willebrand disease, 799
Hemorrhagic cystitis, hematuria in, 758, 759

Hemorrhagic disease, in newborn, 1089
Hemorrhagic fever, **30–31**, 31*t*
Hemorrhagic shock
  clinical findings, 213
  diagnosis of, 196, 213
  ectopic pregnancy and, 196
  in multiply injured patient, **213–214**
  treatment of, 213–214
Hemorrhagic stroke, **372–374**
Hemorrhagic telangiectasia, hereditary, gastrointestinal bleeding in, 288
Hemorrhoids, bleeding, 286, **293**
Hemostasis
  tests for, 789, 791*t*
  in wound cases, 573–574
    chemical agents for, 574
    chemical cautery for, 574
    direct, 574
    electrocautery for, 574
    elevation for, 573
    epinephrine for, 574, 577–578
    indirect, 573–574
    ligation for, 574
    pressure for, 574
    vasoconstriction for, 574
Hemostatic disorders, **789–802**
  coagulation factor, **795–802**
  in liver disease, **799–800**
  platelet, **789–795**
  in renal disease, **800**
  site of bleeding in, 789
  tests in, 789, 791*t*
Hemothorax, **456–457**, 656
  in hemorrhagic shock, 213
  imaging of, 457, 457*i*
  massive
    in aortic dissection, 779
    in chest trauma, **456–457**
  in pulmonary vascular injuries, 771
  in respiratory distress/dyspnea, **231–232**, 233*i*
Henöch-Schonlein purpura, 1084*t*–1085*t*
  in children, 1089
Heparin
  for angina, 684
  contraindications to, 682
  for deep venous thrombosis, 783
  for disseminated intravascular coagulation, 802
  for ergotism, 787
  for myocardial infarction, 678
  for pulmonary embolism, 238, 244, 664, 682
  for septic shock, 205
  thrombocytopenia induced by, 792
Hepatic abscess, abdominal pain in, 276
Hepatic encephalopathy
  coma in, **327–328**
  delirium or confusion in, **1031**
Hepatic function test, for abdominal pain, 266
Hepatic infarction, in sickle cell anemia, 809–810
Hepatitis
  abdominal pain in, **276–277**
  alcoholic, 276
  diagnosis of, 271*t*
  in hemophiliacs, 795
  with HIV infection, 865
  transmission of, via transfusions, 822*t*
  viral, 276
Hepatitis B infection
  exanthems with, 1082*t*–1083*t*
  with HIV infection, 865
  transmission of, via transfusions, 822*t*
Hepatitis B vaccine, for female rape victims, 740

Hepatitis C infection
  with HIV infection, 865
  transmission of, via transfusions, 822*t*
Hepatobiliary disorders. *See also specific type*
  abdominal pain in, **275–277**
Hepatomegaly
  in chronic myelocytic leukemia, 816
  in heart failure, in infants, 693
  in preeclampsia-eclampsia, 745
Hepatosplenomegaly, in Waldenström macroglobulinemia, 817
Herald patch, in pityriasis rosea, 1024
Hereditary angioedema, and upper airway obstruction, 237
Hereditary hemorrhagic telangiectasia, and gastrointestinal bleeding, 288
Hereditary spherocytosis, **812–813**
Hernia(s)
  diaphragmatic, **460–461**
  hiatal, diagnosis of, 249*t*
  incarcerated, scrotal pain in, 753*t*, 754
  inguinal, incarcerated, abdominal pain in, 1086*t*
Hernial rings, examination of, 264
Heroin
  delirium caused by, 1031
  poisoning/overdose of, 967*t*
Herpes simplex virus infection, **1020–1021**
  in children, 1101*t*
  genital, **851–852**
    dysuria in, 757*t*
    treatment of, 852, 852*t*
  hand, **563**
  keratitis in, corticosteroids and, 624
  ophthalmicus in, 865
  pharyngitis in, 639*t*
  primary, 1020, 1021
  recurrent, 1020–1021
  type 1, 1020
  type 2, 1020
  urinary tract, in children, 1075
Herpes zoster infection, **1019–1020**
  eyelid, 609
  ocular, 1020
Herpesvirus 6 infection, exanthems with, 1082*t*–1083*t*
Herpetic whitlow, **563**
Hexachlorophene toxicity, 580
HHNS. *See* Hyperglycemic hyperosmolar nonketonic syndrome
Hiatal hernia, diagnosis of, 249*t*
High opening pressure, and lumbar puncture, 132
High-altitude cerebral edema, **950–951**
High-altitude pulmonary edema, acute, **949–950**
High-altitude sickness, **948–951**
High-flow oxygen, and intubation preparation, 169–170
High-pressure injection injuries, **595**
  hand, **569–571**
High-stress wounds, closure of, 585, 586*i*
Highway accidents, 45
Hill-Sachs deformity, in shoulder dislocation, 519
Hip(s)
  dislocations of, **531–532**
    reduction of, 532, 532*i*
  fractures of, **531**
  injuries of, **531–532**
  nonarticular rheumatism in, 406*t*
Hirschsprung disease
  abdominal pain in, 1087*t*
  in newborns, 1084
Histamine blockers
  for allergic reactions, 638*t*

Histamine blockers (*cont.*)
  for anaphylactic shock, 207
  for upper airway obstruction, 237
Histoplasmosis, in HIV-infected patients, 864
HIV. *See* Human immunodeficiency virus; Human
      immunodeficiency virus infection
Hives. *See* Urticaria
Homans sign, in deep venous thrombosis, 782
Homatropine, for corneal abrasion, 620
Homicidal patients, **1030**
Hordeolum, acute, **609**
Hospital-acquired pneumonia, 835, 836*t*
Hospitals
  admission to, 5
    through emergency department, 70–71
  base station, for EMS systems, 9–10
  categorization of
    by areas of care, 10
    by capability, 10
  and EMS systems, 9–10
  and hazardous materials incidents, 58–59
  and multicasualty incidents/disaster manage-
      ment, 51–52, **56–59**
  and radiation incidents, 58–59
  receiving, for EMS systems, 10
  and vicarious liability, 62–63
HSV. *See* Herpes simplex virus
Human bites, **596–597**
  antibiotics for, 564, 565, 596, 597
  cellulitis with, **564–565**
  to clinician, in TMJ reduction, 652
  with metacarpal fractures, 527, 565
Human chorionic gonadotropin, in ectopic preg-
      nancy, 729–733, 730*i*
β-Human chorionic gonadotropin, in ectopic preg-
      nancy, 729–733, 730*i*
Human immunodeficiency virus (HIV) infection,
      863–866. *See also* Acquired immune
      deficiency syndrome
  clinical findings in, 863–864
  dementia in, 863–864
  disposition in cases of, 866
  drug reactions in, 866, 866*t*
  gastrointestinal presentation of, 864–865
  general considerations in, 863
  in hemophiliacs, 795
  hepatitis infection in, 865
  laboratory data in, 865–866
  and molluscum contagiosum, 1025
  neurologic presentations of, 864
  ophthalmologic presentations of, 865
  organ system-specific presentations of, 864–865
  prevention of, in female rape victims, 740
  pulmonary presentations of, 864
  renal presentations of, 865
  skin presentations of, 865
  syphilis in, 853, 864
  systemic presentations of, 865
  testing for, in female rape victims, 740
  transmission of, 863
    via transfusions, 822*t*
  treatment of, 866
  tuberculosis in, 669–670
Human papillomavirus infection, in children,
      1101*t*
Humate-P, for von Willebrand disease, 799
Humerus fractures, **519–521**
  in child abuse, 515
  pathologic, 520, 521
  supracondylar, 519, **521–522**
  treatment of, 520, 521*i*
Humoral immune dysfunction, 829

Hurricanes, **43**
Hutchinson fracture, 524
Hydatidiform mole, 736, 742–743
Hydralazine
  for hypertensive emergencies, 687
  and pericarditis, 687
  for preeclampsia-eclampsia, 745
Hydrangea, toxins in, 1004*t*
Hydrocarbons, poisoning, **992–993**, 993*t*
Hydrocele, scrotal, 755, 756*t*
Hydrocephalus, in subarachnoid hemorrhage, 373
Hydrochloric acid
  poisoning, 995*t*
  smoke inhalation injury, 924
Hydrochlorothiazide, for heart failure, 686
Hydrocodone, for tooth pain, 649
Hydrocortisone
  for adrenal insufficiency, 858, 883
  for anaphylactic shock, 207
  for balanoposthitis, 765
  for cerebral edema, 319*t*
  for pituitary apoplexy, 886
Hydrocortisone-ciprofloxacin, for otitis externa, 627*t*
Hydrocortisone-polymyxinneomycin, for otitis ex-
      terna, 627*t*
Hydrocyanic acid poisoning, 995*t*
Hydrofluoric acid, and burns, 926, 965
Hydrogen peroxide
  for aphthous stomatitis, 650*t*
  for gingivitis, 650*t*
  for pharyngitis, 638*t*
  for wound cleansing, 580
Hydrogen sulfide poisoning, 994, 995*t*
Hydrothorax, and respiratory distress/dyspnea,
      230*t*, **231–232**, 233*f*
γ-Hydroxybutyrate (GHB)
  and coma, **327**
  overdose of, 1006–1007
  withdrawal from, **397**
Hydroxyurea
  for sickle cell crisis, 809
  side effects of, 865*t*
Hyperactivity, and hyperthermia, 971
Hyperbaric oxygen therapy
  for carbon monoxide poisoning, 978
  for decompression sickness, 947
  for ergotism, 787
  for frostbite, 935
  for hydrogen sulfide poisoning, 994
Hypercalcemia, **903–905**, 904*t*
  delirium caused by, 1031
Hypercapnia
  in acute lung injury, 672
  in chronic bronchitis and emphysema, 658
  in coma, 313–314
  in delirium or confusion, 393
  in head injuries, 422
  permissive, in asthma and COPD, 660
  in pulmonary embolism, 663
Hyperemesis gravidarum, **743**
Hyperextension (whiplash) injury, 496, **509**
Hyperglycemia
  in hyponatremia, 893
  in organophosphate poisoning, 365
  in septic shock, 827
  versus stroke, 371
  without ketoacidosis, **871–873**, 872*t*
Hyperglycemic hyperosmolar nonketotic syn-
      drome, **869–873**
Hyperkalemia, 899*i*, **899–902**, 900*t*
  digitalis poisoning and, 979–980
  drug-induced, 901

  in muscle disease, 354–355
  spurious, 900*t*, 901
  true, 900*t*, 901
  weakness in, 367, 367*t*
Hyperlipidemia, in hyponatremia, 893
Hypermagnesemia, **907–908**
Hypernatremia, **895–897**
  in central diabetes insipidus, 888–889
  delirium in, 1031
  determination of, **916**
  in heat exhaustion, 938
Hyperosmolality
  in central diabetes insipidus, 888–889
  in coma, 328
Hyperosmolar coma. *See* Hyperglycemic hyperos-
      molar nonketotic syndrome
Hyperphosphatemia, **906**
  in hypocalcemia, 903
Hyperproteinemia, in hyponatremia, 893
Hyperreflexia, in preeclampsia-eclampsia, 744–745
Hypertension, **686–687**
  in aortic dissection, 196, 779–781
  central retinal vein occlusion in, 614–615
  in head injuries, 423
  headache in, 381, 382, **390**
  in heart failure, 686
  idiopathic intracranial, **386**
  management of, categories of, 687
  portal, 799
  in pregnancy, 381, 382, 744–745 (*See also*
      Preeclampsia-eclampsia)
  pulmonary
    chest pain in, **252–253**
    diagnosis of, 248*t*
    pediatric, **693**
    with pulmonary embolism, 661
    syncope in, **344**
  in spinal cord injury, 495
  stimulant overdose and, 974
Hypertensive crisis, 390, **686–687**
Hypertensive emergency, 686–687
Hypertensive encephalopathy
  coma in, 314
  delirium or confusion in, 393
Hypertensive intracerebral hemorrhage, coma in,
      320–321
Hypertensive urgency, 686–687
Hyperthermia. *See also* Fever
  coma in, 314, **328**
  in delirium or confusion, 393
  poisoning and, **971**
  postresuscitation, 162
  in status epilepticus, 335
Hyperthyroidism
  apathetic, 878
  atrial fibrillation in, 697, 698
  confusion in, 403
  delirium in, 1032
  thyroid storm in, 878–879
Hypertonic eye drops, for acute hydrops of cornea,
      612
Hypertonic saline, for hyponatremia, 894
Hypertrophic obstructive cardiomyopathy, syncope
      in, **344**
Hyperventilation
  altered states of consciousness in, **346**
  neurologic, **239**
  psychogenic, **239**, 346, 349
    and respiratory alkalosis, 912
  reflex, with pulmonary embolism, 661
Hyperviscosity, for Waldenström macroglobuline-
      mia, 817

Hypervolemia, central venous, chest pain in, 240–241, 242
Hyphema, 604, **612–613**
Hypocalcemia, **902–903**, 902*t*
  in hypomagnesemia, 907
  massive transfusion and, 821
Hypocapnia
  in asthma, 658
  in atelectasis, 667
  in pulmonary embolism, 661
Hypochondria, **1035**
Hypogastric artery aneurysm, **778**
Hypoglossal nerve injury, 437*i*, 439, 440
Hypoglycemia, **873–875**
  anoxic spells in, 692
  coma in, 311, 313, **326–327**, 326*t*
  delirium or confusion in, 391–393, 393, **1032**
  myxedema coma in, 881
  postprandial, 874
  reactive, 874
  seizures caused by, 334
  in septic shock, 827
  versus stroke, 369, 371
Hypoglycemia poisoning, 967*t*
Hypokalemia, **897–898**, 898*t*
  alkalosis in, 898
  digitalis poisoning and, 979–980
  in hypomagnesemia, 907
  in muscle disease, 354–355
  potassium depletion and, 898
  weakness caused by, **367**, 367*t*
Hypokalemic periodic paralysis, **367**
Hypomagnesemia, **906–907**, 907*t*
Hyponatremia, **891–895**, 892*i*, 893*t*
  coma in, 328
  delirium in, 1031
  determination of, **915–916**
  in fluid overload, **894**
  in heat exhaustion, 938
  in hypovolemia, **894**
  in inappropriate secretion of antidiuretic hormone, 887
  induced, for sickle cell crisis, 809
  in isovolemia, **894–895**
  in subarachnoid hemorrhage, 373
Hypoosmolality, coma in, 328
Hypophosphatemia, **905–906**, 905*t*
  respiratory alkalosis in, 912
Hypotension
  in abdominal aortic aneurysm rupture, 777–778
  beta-adrenergic blocker poisoning and, 976
  in cardiac tamponade, 457, 689
  in cardiogenic shock, 201
  chest pain in, 242–243
  in delirium or confusion, 393
  diarrhea in, **296–297**
  in head injuries, 422
  in lumbar puncture, 132
  in multipy injured patient, 211
  in myocardial infarction, 679–680
    differential diagnosis of, 679, 680*t*
  in myocardial rupture, 681
  in neurogenic shock, 207
  orthostatic, **345–346**
    patient position in, 340
    syncope in, 335–337, **345–346**
    in Wernicke encephalopathy, 398
  in pelvic fractures, 530
  poisoning and, **971**
  postresuscitation, 162
  in pulmonary agent exposure, 38
  in pulmonary embolism, 661

sepsis associated, 825–827 (*See also* Septic shock)
  in shock, 194
  in spinal cord injury, 494–495, 509
  theophylline overdose and, 1008
  tricyclic antidepressant overdose and, 1010
  in vaginal bleeding, abnormal, 725
  in visceral (intestinal) ischemia, 776
  vomiting in, **296–297**
Hypothenar intrinsics, testing of, 554
Hypothermia, **930–934**, 932*i*
  coma in, 314, **328**
  delirium or confusion in, 393
  in frostbite, 642, 935
  myxedema coma in, 881
  in near-drowning, 946
  poisoning and, **971**
  postresuscitation, 162
  protective effects of, 162–163
  in sepsis shock, 826
  underlying conditions, 931, 932–933
  and warming of blood, 214
Hypothyroidism
  delirium or confusion in, 403, 1032
  hyponatremia in, 895
  myxedema coma in, **880–881**
Hypotropia, in blowout fracture, 619–620
Hypoventilation
  in hemoptysis, 654
  in weak patient, 349
Hypovolemia. *See also* Bleeding; Hemorrhage
  in aortic dissection, 779–780
  in cardiogenic shock, 202
  chest pain in, 242, 242*t*
  in face and neck trauma, 436–437
  in hypernatremia, 896
  in hyponatremia, **894**
  in spinal cord injury, 494
  in subarachnoid hemorrhage, 373
Hypovolemic shock, 193, **197–200**
  causes of, 193*t*, 198
  nonhemorrhagic, 196
Hypoxemia
  in acute lung injury, 672
  in atelectasis, 667
  in bronchiolitis, 837
  in chronic obstructive pulmonary disease, 658
  in coma, **327**
  in delirium or confusion, 393
  in pulmonary contusion, 459
  in pulmonary embolism, 661–662, 663
Hypoxia
  air transport and, 18
  in chest trauma, 454, 455
  in chronic obstructive pulmonary disease, 656
  in coma, 313–314
  cytopathic, 826
  in flail chest, 458
  in head injury, 421–422
  in hemothorax, 456
  in pneumonia, 668
  in pulmonary contusion, 459
  in sinus tachycardia, 695
  in tension pneumothorax, 455
Hysterectomy, for septic abortion, 735
Hysteria
  confusion in, **402–403**
  versus organic disorders, 402–403, 403*t*
  weakness in, **355**
Hysterical paralysis, 497
Hysterical states, **1034–1035**
HZ. *See* Herpes zoster

IAC. *See* Interposed abdominal compression
Ibuprofen
  in children, 1044
  for dysmenorrhea, 738
  for gouty arthritis, 408
  for osteoarthritis, 410
  for otitis media, 1070
  for tooth pain, 649, 651*t*
Ibutilide, for atrial fibrillation, 698
Ice-water caloric response, in psychogenic *versus* organic coma, 330
ICS. *See* Incident Command System
Idiopathic inflammatory bowel disease. *See also* Colitis
  abdominal pain in, **274–275**
  diagnosis of, 271*t*
Idiopathic intracranial hypertension, **386**
Idiopathic thrombocytopenic purpura, **789–792**
  in children, **1094–1096**
  chronic, 789
Idioventricular rhythm, **706–707**
  accelerated, 706
  electrocardiogram in, 706, 717–720, 719*i*
Ileus, paralytic, in spinal cord injury, 495
Iliac vein injury, 772
Iliopsoas sign, 265, 265*i*
I-LMA. *See* Intubating laryngeal mask airway
Imaging studies. *See also specific types*
  in abdominal pain, in children, 1081
  in adrenal insufficiency, 883
  in central diabetes insipidus, 889
  in head trauma, 219
  in myxedema coma, 880
  in osteomyelitis, in children, 1080
  in pituitary apoplexy, 886
  sedation for, in children, 1043
  in septic arthritis, in children, 1079
  in sickle cell disease, 1094
  in traumatic aortic rupture, 218
Imidazole, for vaginitis, 847
Imipenem
  for pneumonia, 836*t*
  for suppurative cholangitis, 276
Imipenem-cilastatin
  for neutropenia, 814–815
  for otitis externa, 627*t*
  for septic abortion, 736
  for septic shock, 828*t*
Imipramine, poisoning/overdose of, 1008–1010
Immediate (I) (triage category), 50
Immersion foot/hand, **936**
Immersion syndrome, **936**
Immobilization
  cervical/vertebral spine
    in head injury, 421
    in-line, 493, 495
    in lateral position, 493
    in neck injury, 435, **437**
    in spinal cord injury, 493, 509
    for spinal trauma, 221
    in supine position, 493
    technique for moving patient in, 493
  in EMS field treatment, **15–16**
  knee
    in cruciate ligament injuries, 538
    in meniscal tears, 538
    in patella dislocation, 534
    in patella fractures, 534
    in tendon rupture, 539
  leg, in hip fractures, 531
  non-weight-bearing, in talar fractures, 544

Immobilization (*cont.*)
for orthopedic injuries in children, 547
wound, 587
Immune dysfunction, classification of, 829
Immune thrombocytopenia, **789–792**
Immunity, and reporting of child abuse, 68
Immunocompromised patients. *See also* Human immunodeficiency virus infection
infection in
isolation for, 830
suspected, evaluation of, **829–830**
septic shock in, 825
sinusitis in, 643
tuberculosis in, 669–670
type of immune dysfunction in, 829
Immunoglobulin, intravenous administration of, **821**
for autoimmune hemolytic anemia, 805
for idiopathic thrombocytopenic purpura, 792
for myasthenia gravis, 366
Immunosuppressive agents, for cold agglutinin syndrome, 806
Imodium. *See* Loperamide
Impacted fracture, 513
Impetigo, 854–855, **1018–1019**
Impetigo contagiosa, 854
Implantable cardioverter defibrillators, **710–711**
Implied consent, 64
Inappropriate secretion of antidiuretic hormone, **886–888**
Incarcerated hernia, scrotal pain in, 753*t*, 754
Incident Command System (ICS), in multicasualty incident/disaster management, 47, 48*i*
Incomplete abortion, 734*t*, 735, 742–743
pelvic pain in, 727*t*
Incontinence
in epidural compression syndrome, 419
in spinal cord injury, 495
Indanediones, poisoning/overdose of, 1010
Index finger, extensor muscles of, 553
Indinavir, side effects of, 865*t*
Indirect pressure, for hemorrhagic shock, 213
Indomethacin
for gouty arthritis, 408
and hyponatremia, 893*t*
for pericarditis, 682
for pleurisy, 252
for pleurodynia, 252
for sunburn, 927
Industrial accidents, **45**
Indwelling (Foley) urinary catheter. *See also* Urinary catheterization
insertion of, **125–127,** 126*i*
Inert gases poisoning, 994, 995*t*
Inevitable abortion, 734*t*, 735
Infant(s). *See also under* Pediatric and Newborns
apnea in, 1051
bronchiolitis in, 835–837
cardiopulmonary resuscitation in, **163–165**
congenital heart disease in, **691–693**
definition of, 163
fever in, **1062–1064**
heart failure in, **692–693**
meningitis in, 830
otitis media in, 1070
pneumonia in, **832–834,** 836*t*
scalp vein needle in, 82, 83*i*
urinary tract infection in, 841
vomiting in, 1084–1085
Infected vascular gangrene and cellulitis, **856**
Infection(s). *See also* Infectious disease emergencies; specific types or structures affected

delirium in, **1031**
diarrhea in, **303–309**
gastrointestinal bleeding in, in children, 1089
household-acquired, 1062
in immunocompromised patients, suspected, evaluation of, **829–830**
vomiting in, **303–309**
Infection control
for anthrax, 25
for botulism, 33
for brucellosis, 28
for frostbite, 935
for glanders, 29
for hemorrhagic fever, 31
for melioidosis, 29
for plague, 26
for Q fever, 28
for ricin exposure, 34
for smallpox, 30
for staphylococcal enterotoxin B, 36
for T-2 mycotoxins, 35
for tularemia, 27
for viral encephalitis, 32
Infectious disease(s), prevention of, in female rape victims, 740
Infectious disease emergencies, **824–866.** *See also* specific types
AIDS and HIV infection, **863–866**
bronchiolitis, **835–837**
cellulitis, **856**
chancroid, **853–854**
in children, **1062–1080**
clostridial myonecrosis (gas gangrene), **857**
disseminated gonococcemia, **861**
dysuria-frequency syndrome, **844–845**
epididymitis, **849–850**
female genitourinary disorders, **845–848**
genital abscess in females, **848**
genital herpes simplex virus infection, **851–852**
gonorrhea, **850–851**
in immunocompromised patients, **829–830**
infected vascular gangrene, **856**
infective endocarditis, **859–861**
life-threatening problems in, immediate management of, **825–830**
Lyme borreliosis (Lyme disease), **863**
male genitourinary disorders, **849–850**
meningitis and meningoencephalitis, **830–832**
meningococcemia, **857–858**
mucopurulent cervicitis, **848**
necrotizing fasciitis, **856–867**
nongonococcal urethritis, **851**
osteomyelitis, **838–839**
pelvic inflammatory disease, **845–846**
pharyngitis, **840–841**
pneumonia, **832–835**
prostatitis, acute bacterial, **849**
Rocky Mountain spotted fever, **858–859**
septic arthritis, **837–838**
septic shock in, **825–827**
sexually transmitted diseases, **850–854**
skin and soft tissue infections, **854–857**
specific disorders in, emergency management of, **830–857**
specific infections in, management of, **857–863**
syphilis, **852–853**
toxic shock syndrome, **861–862**
toxic shock-like syndrome, group A streptococcal infection associated with, **862**
trichomoniasis, **854**
urinary tract infections, **841–845**
vaginitis, **846–848**

Infectious mononucleosis. *See* Mononucleosis
Infectious polyneuritis. *See* Guillain-Barré syndrome
Infective endocarditis, **859–861**
Duke criteria for diagnosis of, 860, 860*t*
in HIV-infected patients, 863, 865
subacute, 859
Inflammatory arthritis, **407,** 407*t*
Inflammatory bowel disease. *See also* Colitis
abdominal pain in, 260*t*
arthritis in, 412
in children, 1089
idiopathic
abdominal pain in, **274–275**
diagnosis of, 271*t*
Influenza
abdominal pain in, 1087*t*
pharyngitis in, in children, 1073
Informed consent, 64
children and, 1044–1045
psychiatric emergencies and, 1038
Infraorbital nerve, injury of
in maxillary (Le Fort) fracture, 443–445
in orbital floor (blowout) fractures, 447
in zygomaticomaxillary complex fractures, 446
Infraorbital nerve block, 578, 579, 579*i*
Infraspinatus muscle injury, 518
Infravesical obstruction, 750
Ingested poisons. *See also* Poisoning
decontamination, 965
Inguinal canals, examination of, 264
Inguinal hernia, incarcerated, abdominal pain in, 1086*t*
Inhalants, poisoning, **993–994,** 995*t*
Inhalation anesthesia, 576
Inhalation injury, 922
Inhalational anthrax, **22,** 23*t*
Inhaled poisons. *See also* Poisoning
decontamination, 964
Injuries. *See also* Trauma
deceleration, 195–196
electrical, **940–944**
lightning, **940–941**
neck, **214–215**
pelvic, 196, 200
penetrating, 195
radiation, **943–944**
spinal cord, 196
thigh, 196, 200
Injury-scoring systems, 208
In-line cervical stabilization, 493, 495
Inner ear disorders, following head trauma, **451–452**
Inocybe, 1002*t*
Inorganic mercury poisoning, **991**
Inotropic agents
for central venous hypervolemia, 245
for septic shock, 205
Insect(s)
in ear canal, 627*t*
stings/bites, **953–956**
Insecticide poisoning, 353, 364–366, 967*t*, **998–999**
Inspection, of abdomen, 264
Inspiratory arrest, 265
Insulin
for alcoholic ketoacidosis, 877
for diabetic ketoacidosis, 871
exogenous, and hypoglycemia, 873–874
for hyperglycemia, 872–873
for hyperglycemic hyperosmolar nonketonic syndrome, 871

for hyperkalemia, 901
in muscle disease, 355
for hyperphosphatemia, 906
poisoning/overdose of, 967*t*
and hypoglycemia, 326, 326*t*
Intensive care unit (ICU), for cardiogenic shock, 203
Intercostal muscle strain, and chest pain, **254**
Intercostal muscles, paralysis of, in spinal cord injury, 493
Interictal psychosis, **395**
Internal jugular vein catheterization, **86–89**, 87*i*, 88*i*
middle (triangle) approach to, 87*i*, 87–89
posterior approach to, 88*i*, 89
International normalized ratio (INR), 791*t*
Interposed abdominal compression (IAC), 165
Interstitial pulmonary disease, **673–674**
Intestinal arthritis, **412**
Intestinal atresia, in newborns, 1084
Intestinal disorders. *See also specific type*
abdominal pain in, **272–275**
Intestinal injuries, **473–476**
computed tomography of, 473, 475*i*
Intestinal ischemia
acute, **775–776**
nonocclusive arteriolar, 775
Intestinal obstruction, 260*t*, 271*t*, **272–273**
Intestinal perforation, 268, 271*t*
Intestinal polyps, in children, 1089
Intestinal strangulation, 271*t*, **274**
Intestines, radiation injury of, 944
Intoxicated patients, and informed consent, 65, 66
Intoxication
central anticholinergic syndrome in, 399, 399*t*
delirium or confusion in, 396, **399**
head injuries in, **434**
Intra-abdominal bleeding, shock in, 195, 200
Intra-aortic balloon pump (IABP)
for cardiogenic shock, 680
for mitral regurgitation, 681
for ventricular septal rupture, 681
Intra-arterial injection of drugs, **787**
Intracerebellar hemorrhage, coma in, **323–324**
Intracerebellar infarction, coma in, **323–324**
Intracerebral hemorrhage, **373–374**
computed tomography of, 373–374, 374*i*
hypertensive, coma in, **320–321**
in stroke, 370
Intracranial hemorrhage, thrombolytic therapy and, 677
Intracranial injury, **425–428**, 573
with spinal cord injury, 495, 506
Intracranial mass, headache with, **386**
Intracranial pressure
elevated, in head injuries, 422, 423
increased, coma in, 314
Intraocular pressure
in acute angle-closure glaucoma, 604–605
in hyphema, 612–613
measurement of, 600, **623**
reduction of, 605
in retinal detachment, 607
Intraoral lacerations, **594**
Intraosseous infusion, **95–96**
in children, 1044
Intraperitoneal hemorrhage, 124
Intrathoracic neoplasm, chest pain in, **255–256**
Intrauterine devices (IUDs), **741–742**
bleeding and pain with, 741
and ectopic pregnancy, 729, 742
emergency removal of, 741

infection with, 741
lost, 741
in pelvic inflammatory disease, 846
pregnancy with IUD in place, 741–742
serious but rare problems with, 741–742
uterine perforation by, 741
Intravascular volume, decreased, 890
Intravenous access
in anaphylactic shock, 206
in burns, 917, 919*i*
in cardiogenic shock, 202
in children, 1044
in dehydration, in children, 1046
in multiply injured patient, 212
in poisoning, 963
Intravenous fluids
heated, for rewarming, 933
for hypovolemic shock, 198–199
choice of, 199
types of, 198–199, 198*t*
Intravenous immunoglobulin
for autoimmune hemolytic anemia, warm-type, 805
for idiopathic thrombocytopenic purpura, 792
Intravenous pyelogram
in genitourinary trauma, 480
in hematuria assessment, 759
one-shot
in abdominal trauma, 468, 476
in genitourinary trauma, 480
in ureteral injuries, 484–486
in urolithiasis, 761
Intravesical obstruction, 750
Intubated patient, care of, **189–190**
Intubating laryngeal mask airway (I-LMA), for airway management, 174
Intubation
in abdominal trauma, 467
in acute lung injury, 672
alternative methods of, 173, 173*t*
in anoxic spells, 692
in asthma, 188, 660, 1058
blind techniques, 173
lighted stylet for, 174–175
of children, 1044
choice of method, 173
in COPD, 660
difficult, equipment for, 169*t*
digital, 174
drugs to assist in, **179–185**
endotracheal
in advanced life support, 157
for altered mental status with shallow breathing, 225
in children, 164, 187
in EMS field treatment, 14
for massive aspiration, 225
for pulmonary edema, 226
fiberoptic, 174–175
in flail chest, 458
in Guillain-Barré syndrome, 360
in head injuries, 421–422
in head trauma, 188
in hemoptysis, 654
indications for, 169*t*
medications in, 182–185
in myasthenia gravis, 366
nasal
asthma and, 188
in children, 187
nasogastric, **102–104**, 103*i*
in comatose patients, 104

contraindicated in maxillary (Le Fort) fracture, 445
in neck injury, 436
in syncope, 337
nasotracheal, 101–102
indications for, 98
in spinal cord injury, 494
in neck injury, 435–436, 769
needle techniques, 173
orotracheal, 100*i*, 101
in head injuries, 422
indications for, 98
in maxillary (Le Fort) fracture, 445
relative contraindications for, 173*t*
in spinal cord injury, 494
in pharyngeal airway injury, 436
in pneumothorax, 655
in poliomyelitis, 351
postintubation management, 173
preparation for, 169–172
principles of, **173–174**
in pulmonary embolism, 663
rapid sequence, 180–182, 182*t*
in asthma and COPD, 660
in neck injury, 435
in spinal cord injury, 494
in respiratory effort, 167, 169*t*
retrograde, 178
in septic shock, 825
in shock, 194
in spinal cord injury, 494, 508
in status epilepticus, 334–335
in stroke, 369
surgical techniques, 173
of trachea through traumatic opening, **436**
tracheal, **98–102**
in tracheobronchial injury, 463
universal precautions and, 173
variations on, 174
in weak patient, 349
Intussusception
and abdominal pain, 1086*t*
in children, 1089
Invasive procedures, in EMS field treatment, **14–15**
Involuntary admission, **1038**
Involuntary commitment, to psychiatric facility, 67
Involuntary procedures, **1038**
Iodine, for thyroid storm, 879
Iodoquinol, for infectious gastroenteritis, 306
Ionic soaps, contraindicated for wound cleansing, 580
Ipecac
for ingested poisons, 965
for iron poisoning, 988
Ipratropium
for asthma, 660–661, 1058
for COPD, 660–661
in EMS field treatment, 15
Iridocyclitis, 605, **613**
Iris, blunt trauma to, 618
Iritis, 605, **613**
differential diagnosis of, 602*t*
in HIV-infected patients, 865
Iron
for iron-deficiency anemia, 804
in children, 1093
poisoning/overdose of, **988**
Iron-deficiency anemia, 802, **804**
in children, 1093
Irradiated packed red blood cells, 819
Irrigation, of wounds, 580
Irritant poisoning, 994, 995*t*

Irukandji jellyfish envenomation, **957–958**
Ischemia
  acute, 773–776
  acute cerebral, due to emboli, 776
  acute peripheral
    due to major arterial occlusion, 773–774
    due to small-vessel occlusion, 774
    due to venous occlusion, 774–775
  acute visceral (intestinal), **775–776**
    nonocclusive arteriolar, 775
  in arterial injury, 767
  myocardial
    angina in, 682–684
    in pulmonary embolism, 662
  in vascular trauma, minimization of, 767
  in venous injury, 767
Ischemic colitis
  abdominal pain in, 261t, **277**
  diagnosis of, 271t
Ischemic stroke, **374–377,** 776
Isolation
  for infection, in immunocompromised patients, 830
  for tuberculosis, 670
Isoniazid
  contraindicated in pregnancy, 670
  poisoning/overdose of, **994–996**
  resistance to, 670
  seizures induced by, 971
  for tuberculosis, 670
Isopropanol, poisoning/overdose of, 985, **987**
Isoproterenol
  for arrhythmias, 976
  for bradyarrhythmia, 244
  for calcium-channel blocker poisoning, 977
  for complete heart block, 706
Isovolemia, and hyponatremia, **894–895**
ITP. *See* Idiopathic thrombocytopenic purpura
Itraconazole, for tinea, 1024

Janeway lesions, in infective endocarditis, 859–860
Jarisch-Herxheimer reaction, in syphilis treatment, 853
Jaundice, neonatal
  in glucose-6-phosphate dehydrogenase deficiency, 812
  in hereditary spherocytosis, 812–813
Jaw-thrust maneuver
  in basic life support, 147, 150i
  in pediatric basic life support, 164
Jehovah's Witnesses, 66, 818
Jellyfish envenomation, **957–958**
Jequirity bean, toxins in, 1004t
Jerusalem cherry, toxins in, 1004t
Jewelry removal, in hand trauma, 572
Jimsonweed poisoning, 399, 975, 1004t
Jock itch. *See* Tinea cruris
Joint(s)
  abscesses around, incision and drainage of, 142
  examination of, in arthritis, 406
Joint aspiration, for septic arthritis, 410, 837–838
  in children, 1079
Joint Commission on the Accreditation of Health Care Organizations (JCAHO), and medical records, 70
Joint disease, degenerative, **410–411**
Joint fluid analysis, in arthritis, 407, 407t, 837–838
Jones criteria, for rheumatic fever, 411, 411t
Jones fracture, 546
Jones wrap, 544

Jugular vein catheterization
  external, **83–86,** 85i
  internal, **86–89,** 87i, 88i

Kalmia latifolia, toxins in, 1004t
Kaolin-pectin suspension, for gastroenteritis, 309
Kaopectate. *See* Kaolin-pectin suspension
Kaposi's sarcoma, 863–864
Kawasaki disease, 1082t–1083t
Kayexalate, for hyperkalemia, 901
KED. *See* Kendrick Extrication Device
Kendrick Extrication Device (KED), 15
Keratitis
  herpes simplex, corticosteroids and, 624
  in HIV-infected patients, 865
Keratoconjunctivitis, viral, **611–612**
Keratoconus, in acute hydrops of cornea, 612
Kernig sign, 379, 383
Ketamine
  asthma and, 188
  in children, 1043–1044
  for intubation, 185
  for status asthmaticus, 661
Ketoacidosis
  alcoholic, **876–877**
  diabetic, 259, 272t, **867–869**
Ketoconazole, for tinea, 1024
Ketones, in diabetic ketoacidosis, 868–869
Ketonuria, in hyperemesis gravidarum, 743
Ketorolac, for urolithiasis, 761
Kidneys. *See also under* Renal
  and calcium excretion, 904
Kienböck disease, 526
Kiesselbach area, bleeding at, 632, 632i
Klebsiella infection
  suppurative cholangitis in, 276
  urinary tract, in children, 1075
Klebsiella pneumoniae infection, 835
Kleihauer-Betke test, in trauma during pregnancy, 745
Knee
  anatomy of, 533, 533i
  arthrocentesis of, 136, 137, 137i
  dislocations of, **536–537**
    popliteal artery injury in, 536, 772
  injuries of, **533–539**
    acute, emergency department evaluation of, 533
    radiography in, rules and criteria for, 533–534
  nonarticular rheumatism in, 406t
  valgus and varus stress tests of, 533, 533i
  vasculature around, 533
Knee ligaments, 533, 533i
  injuries of, **537–538**
Knee tendons, rupture of, **539**
Knife wounds
  abdominal, 467, 470
    in pregnancy, 746
  chest, 465–466
  neck, **438,** 438i
Koebner phenomenon, and psoriasis, 1021
Korsakoff psychosis, 398, 399, 1032
KUB (kidney, urethra, and bladder) study, of urolithiasis, 761, 762i
Kussmaul's sign, in cardiac tamponade, 689

Labetalol
  for catecholamine crisis, 885
  in EMS field treatment, 15
  for hypertension, in aortic dissection, 781
  for hypertensive emergencies, 687

  for hypertensive intracerebral hemorrhage, 321
  for hypertensive urgency, 687
  for preeclampsia-eclampsia, 745
Labor and delivery, **746–747**
  emergency room, 747
    postpartum measures in, 747
  normal, 747
  premature, 746–747
Labyrinthitis, suppurative, vertigo in, 631t
Lacerations, 575
  auricle, **451**
  bladder, 488
  extensor tendon, **559**
  eyelid, **619**
  facial
    care of, **452–453**
    closure of, 452, 575
    delay in closing, 452
    repair technique for, 452–453
    replacement of avulsed tissue in, 452
  hand, **557,** 559
    extensive, 557
    small, 557
  intraoral, **594**
  lip, through-and-through, 594
  renal, 484
  scalp, **423–424,** 425
  scrotal, 492
  vaginal, 491, 492
Lachman test, of anterior cruciate ligament, 537, 538i
Lacrimal gland infection, 608–609
Lacrimal sac infection, 608
Lacrimation, with headache, 382
Lactate dehydrogenase
  in disseminated intravascular coagulation, 802
  pleural fluid levels of, 666
Lactate level, in abdominal trauma, 468
Lactating women, scabies in, 1022
Lactic acidosis, **875–876**
  seizure activity causing, 334, 341
Lacunar stroke, **375–376**
Laminectomy
  for spinal cord metastases, 355
  for spinal epidural abscess, 356
Lamivudine, side effects of, 865t
Lamotrigine, for trigeminal neuralgia, 385
Lampblack, in nail trephination, 558
Lange-Nielsen syndrome, 702
Lantana, toxins in, 1004t
Laparoscopy
  in abdominal trauma, 469
  in ectopic pregnancy, 731
  in pelvic pain, 728
Laparotomy
  in abdominal trauma
    emergency, 468
    in pregnancy, 746
  in ectopic pregnancy, 731
  in ovarian tumor torsion, 738
Laryngeal airway injury, **436**
Laryngeal anesthesia, topical, for intubation, 180
Laryngeal mask airway
  in airway management, 174
  in EMS field treatment, 14
Laryngeal mask airway-Fastrach, in EMS field treatment, 14
Laryngoscope, variations on, for intubation, 174
Laryngoscopy
  direct, 99–101, 100i
  in epiglottitis, 646–647
  for upper airway obstruction, 224

Laryngospasm, extubation and, 190
Laryngotracheobronchitis (croup), **647,**
  1052–1053
  radiographic findings in, 647, 648*i*
Lassa fever, 31*t*
Lateral collateral ligament, 540
  varus stress test of, 533, 533*i*
Lateral decubitus position, for lumbar puncture,
  129–130, 130*i*
Lateral extensor tendons (LETs), 553–554
Lateral malleolar fractures, **540**
  peroneal tendon injuries in, 542
  splinting for, 540, 540*i*
Lateral technique, of mouth-to-mask ventilation,
  151
Latex agglutination, 791*t*
Lavage, gastric. *See* Gastric lavage
Le Fort fractures, **443–445**
  classification of, 443, 444*i*
  Le Fort I, **443,** 444*i*
  Le Fort II, **443–445,** 444*i*
  Le Fort III, **445**
Lead complications, with pacemakers, 709
Lead lines, 989
Lead poisoning, **988–989,** 989*t*, 995*t*
  blindness caused by, 607
Left-to-right shunts, 691
Leg. *See also* Extremities
  burns of, **928**
  cold injury to, **934–936**
  immobilization, in hip fractures, 531
  venous occlusion in, 774–775
Legal issues, 4
  abandonment, **67–68**
  breach of duty, 61
  consent, **64–69**
  criminal *versus* civil law, 60–61
  damages, 62
  duty of care, 61
  duty to provide emergency care, **63**
  in emergency care, **60–72**
  emergency physician and medical staff interac-
    tions, **70–71**
  expert witnesses, 71
  Good Samaritan laws, **63–64**
  harvesting of organs for transplantation, **72**
  medical records, **69–70**
  National Practitioner Data Bank, **71–72**
  negligence, **61–62**
  proximate cause, 61–62
  psychiatric emergencies, 67
  reportable events, **68–69**
  res ipsa loquitur, 62
  statute of limitations, 62
  vicarious liability, **62–63**
Legionella pneumonia, 668, 835
Legionnaire disease, 835
Lens, blunt trauma to, 618
LET (lidocaine, epinephrine, and tetracaine), 576
  for wound care, in children, 1043
Lethargy
  in airway management, 970–971
  definition of, 315
  poisoning and, 964
Leukemia(s)
  acute, **815**
  chronic, **815–816**
Leukocyte-treated paced red blood cell, 819
Leukocytosis, **815**
  in asthma and COPD, 658
  in chronic myelocytic leukemia, 816
  in organophosphate poisoning, 365

seizure activity causing, 341
  in septic shock, 827
Leukopenia
  in septic shock, 827
  in Waldenström macroglobulinemia, 817
Level of consciousness, assessment of, 219
Levofloxacin
  for meningitis, 833*t*
  for neutropenia, 814–815
Lewisite, as chemical weapon, 36*t*, **40**
Liability, vicarious, **62–63**
Lice, **1022–1023**
Lidocaine, 577, 577*t*
  in advanced life support, 159*t*, 162
  for arrhythmias, 980, 1009
  for cluster headache, 390
  in EMS field treatment, 15
  endotracheal administration of, 189
  for esophageal disorders, 253
  for gastritis, 291
  for intubation, 179
  local infiltration of, 576–577
  maximum dose of, 576
  properties of, 179*t*
  for rapid-sequence intubation, 181
  safety of, 576
  for scorpion fish envenomation, 959
  for sea urchin stings, 959
  for status epilepticus, 336*t*
  for stingray wound, 956
  for Tietze syndrome, 255
  for ventricular fibrillation, 157–158, 703
  for ventricular tachycardia, 701–702
  for wound care, 576–577
    in children, 1043
Lidocaine-epinephrine, 576
  for drainage of peritonsillar abscess, 645
  for epistaxis, 633
  for postextraction tooth hemorrhage, 640
Life support
  advanced, **158–162,** 158*t*–160*t*
    adult, **156–163**
    pediatric, **164–165**
  basic, **147–156,** 148*i*
    early, 147
    pediatric, **163–164**
  termination of, **162–163**
"Lifestick" CPR, 165
Life-threatening emergency, determination of, 4
Ligament injuries, **514**
  ankle, **543–544**
  knee, **537–538**
Ligation, for hemostasis, in wound cases, 574
Light touch sensation, in spinal cord injury, 497
Lighted stylet/wand, for intubation, 174–175
Lightning injuries, **940–941**
Lily of the valley, toxins in, 1004*t*
Limb-threatening injuries
  immediate management of, **511–513**
  in knee dislocations, 536
Lindane cream
  for pediculosis, 1023
  for scabies, 1022
Lingual nerve injury, 440
Lip, through-and-through lacerations of, 594
"Lip spell," 692
Lipase, and abdominal pain, 266
Lisfranc injuries, **545–546**
Listeria infection
  in infants, 1062
  and meningitis, 1068*t*
Listeria monocytogenes infection, meningitis in, 834*t*

Lithium
  bradycardia caused by, 704
  for headache prophylaxis, 390
  poisoning/overdose of, **996–997**
  seizures induced by, 971
Livedo reticularis, 774
Liver abscess
  abdominal pain in, 276
  diagnosis of, 271*t*
Liver disease
  gastrointestinal bleeding in, 288
  hemostatic abnormalities in, **799–800**
Liver function tests, in septic shock, 827
Liver injuries, **472,** 474*i*
Liver tumor, diagnosis of, 271*t*
LMA. *See* Laryngeal mask airway
LMA-Fastrach. *See* Laryngeal mask airway-
  Fastrach
Loading officer, 51–52
Lobelia, toxins in, 1004*t*
Local accessory resources, for multicasualty inci-
  dents/disasters, 53
Local anesthesia, 576–578
  drugs used for, 577*t*
  for intubation, 179, 179*t*
  ophthalmic, 621, 622*t*
    dangers in use of, 624
  poisoning/overdose of, **981–982**
  properties of, 179*t*
  for tooth pain, 649
Local infiltration, of anesthesia, 576–578
  in hand trauma, 549, 577*i*
  method of injection, 576–577, 577*i*
Locality rule, 61
"Locked-in" syndrome, **324–325**
Logistics, of multicasualty incidents/disasters, 49,
  49*i*
Lomotil. *See* Diphenoxylate
Long QT syndrome, 702–703
Longitudinal fracture of temporal bone, **450**
Loperamide, for gastroenteritis, 309
Lorazepam
  for alcohol withdrawal, 341, 1031
  for catecholamine crisis, 885
  in EMS field treatment, 15
  for head injuries, 423
  for isoniazid poisoning, 996
  for mania, 1034
  for seizures, in children, 1062
  for status epilepticus, 334, 336*t*
  for stimulant overdose, 974
Loss of consciousness (LOC)
  in aortic stenosis, 343–344
  assessment of, 333*i*
  in cardiac arrest, 342
  episodic, 332–347
    specific disorders causing, emergency treat-
      ment of, **340–347**
  life-threatening problems in, immediate manage-
    ment of, **332–335,** 333*i*
  psychiatric causes of, **346**
  in syncope, 335–340 (*See also* Syncope)
Lost intrauterine device, 741
Lower airway disorders
  in children, **1056–1059**
  pulmonary agent exposure and, 38
Lower extremity deep venous thrombosis,
    782–783. *See also* Deep venous throm-
    bosis
Lower extremity injuries, orthopedic, **532–547**
  compartment syndrome in, 512
Lower urinary tract infections, **841–843**

Low-molecular-weight heparin (LMWH)
for angina, 684
for pulmonary embolism, 664, 682
Lown-Ganong-Levine syndrome, 699
Low-stress wounds, closure of, 585, 587*i*
Loxapine, overdose, 1009
LSD. *See* Lysergic acid diethylamide
Ludiomil. *See* Maprotiline
Ludwig angina, 639*t*, 649
Lugol's solution, for thyroid storm, 879
Lumbar puncture, **129–133,** 130*i*, 133*t*
and arterial puncture, 132
and blood in cerebrospinal fluid, 132
contraindications, 320, 321
contraindications to, 384, 831*t*, 858
in spinal cord compression, 349
and headache, 132
headache after, **384–385**
high opening pressure and, 132
in hypotension, 132
in infants, 1063–1064
in meningitis, 335, 381, 383, 384, 394, 831, 831*t*
in children, 1068, 1069*t*
in meningococcemia, 858
in obesity, 131–132
in osteoarthritis, 132
in poliomyelitis, 351, 357
previous lumbar surgery and, 132
in pseudotumor cerebri, 386
specimens, 132–133, 133*t*
in stroke patients, 371
in subarachnoid hemorrhage, 372–373, 383
in syphilis in HIV-infected patients, 853
Lumbar surgery, previous, and lumbar puncture, 132
Lumbar sympathectomy, for ergotism, 787
Lumbosacral disk, herniation of, 418–419
Lumbosacral spine imaging, in spinal cord injury, 507
Lumbosacral strain, acute, **417–418**
Lunate dislocations, **524–525,** 525*i*
Lung injury, acute, **671–673,** 672*t*
Lung parenchyma, loss of functional, respiratory distress/dyspnea in, 230*t*, **233–235**
Lung sounds, in stroke patients, 370
Luxatio erecta, 519
Lyme borreliosis (Lyme disease), **863**
Lymphocytes, radiation injury and, 943
Lymphocytosis, in mononucleosis, 816
Lymphoma(s), in HIV-infected patients, 864, 865
Lysergic acid diethylamide (LSD), and delirium, 1031

Macrocytic anemia, 803*t*
Macroglobulinemia, Waldenström, **817–818**
Macrolide(s)
for COPD, 660, 661
for pneumonia, 661, 668
Mafenide, for wounds, 589
Magnesium
in advanced life support, 159*t*, 162
for alcoholic ketoacidosis, 877
for asthma, 228, 661, 1058
for COPD, 228
deficiency, in alcohol withdrawal, 399
in EMS field treatment, 15
for hyperreflexia, in preeclampsia-eclampsia, 745
for multifocal atrial tachycardia, 699
for pulmonary fibrosis, 228
serum concentration disorders of, **906–908**
for torsades de pointes, 158, 702

Magnet application
for implantable cardioverter defibrillation malfunction, 711
for pacemaker malfunction, 710
Magnetic resonance angiography
in headache, 379
in intracerebral hemorrhage, 373
Magnetic resonance imaging
in Achilles tendon injuries, 542
in amnesia, 401
in back pain, 415
in collateral ligament injuries, 537
contraindicated
with cardiac pacemakers, 709
with implantable cardioverter defibrillators, 711
in cruciate ligament injuries, 537
in intracerebral hemorrhage, 373
in intracranial mass (brain tumor), 386
in meniscal tears, 538
in patella fractures, 534
in peroneal tendon injuries, 542
in poliomyelitis, 351
in rotator cuff injuries, 518
in spinal cord compression, 349, 351
in spinal cord injury, 507, 509
in spinal cord metastases, 355
in spinal epidural abscess, 356
in spinal infections, 420
in stroke, 369, 371, 375
in subarachnoid hemorrhage, 383
in talar fractures, 544
in tendon rupture in knee, 539
in tibial plateau fractures, 535
in tibial spine fractures, 536
in transverse myelitis, 356
in vertebral osteomyelitis, 839
in vertigo, 632
in whiplash, 509
Maisonneuve fracture, 539–540, 541, 543
Malar fracture, 445–446
Malassezia furfur, 1023
Malingering, 346, 1035
Malleolar fractures
bimalleolar and trimalleolar, 541
lateral, **540**
peroneal tendon injuries in, 542
splinting for, 540, 540*i*
medial, **540–541**
deltoid ligament rupture in, 543
posterior, **541**
Mallet finger, **529, 559–560,** 561*i*
Mallory-Weiss syndrome
abdominal pain in, 263
gastrointestinal bleeding in, 290*t*, **291**
Malpractice, 60
Malrotation, abdominal pain in, 1086*t*
Mandible
dislocation of, 652
fracture of, **441–443**
imaging of, 441–443, 442*i*
injury of, airway obstruction in, 436
Mangling injuries, hand, **572**
Manic states, **1033–1034**
Mannitol
for acute angle-closure glaucoma, 605
for carbon monoxide poisoning, 979
for cerebral edema, 319*t*
for ciguqtera toxin poisoning, 960
for eye trauma, 619
for head trauma, 220
for increased intracranial pressure, 314

for subtentorial mass lesions, 322
for supratentorial mass lesions, 319
MAOIs. *See* Monoamine oxidase inhibitors
Maprotiline, poisoning/overdose of, 1008–1010
Marburg virus, 31*t*
Marcaine. *See* Bupivacaine
Marine life, hazardous, **956–960**
Mask ventilation. *See also* Bag-mask ventilation
for high-flow oxygen, 169*t*
for tracheal intubation, 99
Mass lesion headache, 382
Mass lesions
subtentorial, **322–325**
supratentorial, **317–322,** 318*i*
Massage
carotid sinus
for paroxysmal supraventricular tachycardia, 696
for sinus tachycardia, 695
ocular, for central retinal artery occlusion, 605
Masseter spasm, in TMJ dislocation, 652
Massive aspiration, **225**
Massive transfusion, **821**
MAST trousers
for hemorrhagic shock, 213
for intrapelvic hemorrhage, 196
Mastitis, puerperal, **748–749**
Mastoiditis, 626
computed tomography in, 629
diagnosis of, 627*t*
otitis media and, 642–643, 1070, 1071
treatment of, 627*t*, 643
Maxillary fractures, **443–445**
classification of, 443, 444*i*
Le Fort I, **443,** 444*i*
Le Fort II, **443–445,** 444*i*
Le Fort III, 444*i*, 445
Maxillary sinusitis, 643, 644*i*
Maxillofacial trauma, **435–453**
airway management in, 435–436
emergency management of specific injuries in, **441–453**
life-threatening problems in, immediate management of, **435–437**
shock in, **436–437**
Maximum inspiratory force
in botulism, 364
in weak patient, 349
Mazicon. *See* Flumazenil
McMurray test, for meniscal tears, 538
MDA. *See* Methylene-dioxyamphetamine
MDMA, and delirium, 1030
Mean cellular volume (MCV), in anemia, 803–804
Measles, 1082*t*–1083*t*
Mechanical cleansing, of wounds, 580
Mechanical scrubbing, of wounds, 580
Mechanical ventilation. *See also* Ventilation
in acute lung injury, 672
in flail chest, 458
in intubated patient, 190
in pulmonary contusion, 459
in rib fractures, 464
for weak patient, 349
Meckel diverticulitis, abdominal pain in, 1086*t*
Meckel diverticulum
in children, 1089
gastrointestinal bleeding in, **295**
Meclizine
for Meniere disease, 347
for vertigo, 632
Meconium ileus, in newborns, 1084
Meconium plug syndrome, in newborns, 1084

Media involvement, in multicasualty incidents/disasters, 53, 58
Medial collateral ligament, 533, 533*i*, 540
  injuries of, 537
  valgus stress test of, 533, 533*i*
Medial malleolar fractures, **540–541**
  deltoid ligament rupture in, 543
Medial meniscal tear, 538
Median nerve, innervation of hand by, 551, 553, 554, 555, 571*i*
Median nerve block, 551*i*, 578, 579*i*
Median nerve compression, 566
Median nerve injury, 554–555
  clinical findings in, 569, 570*i*, 571*i*
  disposition in cases of, 569
  in forearm fractures, 524
  in hand trauma, 554–555, **569**
  high, 555
  low, 555
  in lunate dislocation, 525
  motor testing for, 555, 556*i*, 569, 570*i*
  sensory testing for, 555, 569, 571*i*
  in shoulder dislocation, 518–519
  treatment of, 569
Mediastinal emphysema, arterial gas embolism and, 947, 948
Mediastinum, widening of
  in aortic injury, 462, 463*i*
  in esophageal injury, 461
Medical direction
  off-line, for EMS system, 12
  on-line, for EMS system, 12
Medical evaluation, by EMS personnel, 11–12
Medical management, of multicasualty incidents/disasters, 47
Medical records
  confidentiality of, 70
  legal issues concerning, **69–70**
Medical supervision, of EMS system, 12, 13*i*
Medications. *See* Drug(s)
Medicolegal considerations. *See also* Legal issues
  with children, 1044–1045
Melena
  in children, 1085
  lower gastrointestinal bleeding in, 286
  treatment algorithm for, 1090*i*
  upper gastrointestinal bleeding in, 286
Melioidosis, 24*t*, **29**
Melphalan
  for multiple myeloma, 817
  for Waldenström macroglobulinemia, 817–818
Men
  Foley catheter insertion in, 125, 126–127
  genitalia of, examination of, 264
  radiation injury in, 943
Mendelson syndrome, 671
Meniere disease
  syncope in, 340, **347**
  vertigo in, 631*t*
Meningeal irritation, 830–831
  delirium or confusion in, **394,** 394*t*
  headache with, 379–381, 383
Meningeal signs, 328
Meningitis, **830–832**
  acute, 831–832
  acute lymphocytic, causes of, 831, 832*t*
  anthrax, **22**
  antibiotic therapy for, 381, 384, 831–832
    empiric, 831–832, 833*t*
    pathogen-specific, 834*t*
  in children, 1064, **1066–1070**
  chronic, 831

clinical findings in, 384, 830–831
and coma, 314
definition of, 830
delirium or confusion in, **394,** 394*t*, 830, 1031
disposition in cases of, 384, 832
in elderly, 830
fever in, 379, 381, 382, 384, 830
headache in, 379–381, 382, 383, **384,** 830
herpes simplex, 852
in HIV-infected patients, 863
in infants, 830
laboratory findings in, 831
lumbar puncture in, 335, 381, 383, 384, 394, 831, 831*t*
meningeal signs in, 383
  absence of, 383
with meningococcemia, 857–858
otitis media and, 642–643
purulent, 383
seizures caused by, 335, 384
septic, 831
in sickle cell anemia, 810
sinusitis and, 645
subacute, 383, 384, 831–832
supportive care in, 384, 832
symptoms and signs of, 830–831
treatment of, 384, 831–832
Meningococcemia, 1084*t*–1085*t*
  acute, **857–858**
Meningococcus, 1084*t*–1085*t*
Meningoencephalitis, **830–832**
  clinical findings in, 384, 830–831
  coma in, **328–329**
  delirium or confusion in, 394, 394*t*
  disposition in cases of, 832
  general considerations in, 830
  headache in, **384**
  symptoms and signs of, 830–831
  treatment of, 384, 831–832
Meniscectomy, 538
Menisci, 533
  tears of, **538**
Menstrual-related toxic shock syndrome, 861–862
Menstruation, painful (dysmenorrhea), 727*t*, **738**
Mental status
  altered
    lightning injuries and, 940
    shallow breathing and, **225**
    shock and, 194
  assessment of, 391
  examination of, for psychiatric emergencies, **1028–1029**
  in HIV-infected patients, 863–864, 866
Mentation, in spinal cord injury, 496, 502
Meperidine
  contraindicated in sickle cell crisis, 808
  poisoning/overdose of, 967*t*
  for sickle cell disease, in children, 1094
Mepivacaine, 576, 577*t*
Meprobamate, poisoning/overdose of, 1007
Mercury poisoning, 989*t*, **991,** 995*t*
Meropenem
  for meningitis, 833*t*
  for pneumonia, 836*t*
Mesenteric angiography, in lower gastrointestinal bleeding, 289
Mesenteric arteriography, in visceral (intestinal) ischemia, 775–776
Mesenteric thrombosis
  abdominal pain in, **277–278**
  diagnosis of, 271*t*
Mesenteric vascular occlusion, 775–776

Metabolic acidosis, **910–912**
  drugs causing, 968*t*
  and respiratory acidosis, **914**
  and respiratory alkalosis, **914**
  and respiratory distress/dyspnea, 231*t*, **238–239**
  seizure activity causing, 334
  in septic shock, 825, 826
Metabolic alkalosis, **912–913,** 913*t*
  and respiratory acidosis, **914**
  and respiratory alkalosis, **914**
Metabolic disorders, systemic, delirium or confusion in, **396,** 396*t*
Metabolic emergencies, **867–889.** *See also specific type*
  alcoholic ketoacidosis, **876–877**
  carbohydrate disorders, **867–877**
  delirium in, **1031–1032**
  diabetic ketoacidosis, **867–869**
  hyperglycemic hyperosmolar nonketotic syndrome, **869–873**
  hypoglycemia, **873–875**
  lactic acidosis, **875–876**
Metabolic encephalopathy, **395–399**
  coma in, **325–329**
  delirium or confusion in, 394*t*, **395–399**
    systemic disorders associated with, 396, 396*t*
Metabolism, of carbohydrates, disorders of, **867–877**
Metacarpal fractures, **526–527**
  human bites with, 527, 565
  splinting for, 526*i*, 527, 527*i*, 528*i*
Metacarpophalangeal joint of thumb, stress examination of, 529, 530*i*
Metal fume poisoning, 995*t*
Metallic clips, for wound closure, 582–583
Metaproterenol, for asthma and COPD, 659
Metatarsal fractures, **546**
Metered-dose inhalers (MDIs)
  for asthma and COPD, 659
  for bronchitis, 668
Metformin, for hyperglycemia, 873
Methamphetamine poisoning, 974–975
Methane poisoning, 994, 995*t*
Methanol poisoning, 985, **986–987**
  blindness caused by, 607–608
Methemoglobinemia, drug-induced, **984–985**
Methicillin, for infective endocarditis, 860
Methocarbamol
  for black widow spider bites, 954
  for tension headache, 388
Methohexital
  in children, 1043
  and intubation, 184
Methotrexate, for rheumatoid arthritis, 411
Methyl salicylate. *See* Oil of wintergreen
Methylene blue, for drug-induced methemoglobinemia, 985
Methylene-dioxyamphetamine (MDA) poisoning, 974–975
Methylergonovine, for postpartum hemorrhage, 748
Methylprednisolone
  for adrenal insufficiency, 858
  for anaphylactic shock, 207
  for asthma and COPD, 660
  for cerebral edema, 319*t*
  for idiopathic thrombocytopenic purpura, 791–792, 1096
  for spinal cord injury, 495, 509
Methylxanthines
  for asthma, 661
  poisoning/overdose of, **1007–1008**

Methyprednisolone sodium succinate, for angioedema, 1013
Methysergide, for headache prophylaxis, 390
Metoclopramide
  for dysentery, 309
  for migraine, 388–389
Metoprolol
  in advanced life support, 160*t*, 161
  for angina, 683–684
  for mitral valve prolapse, 251
  for multifocal atrial tachycardia, 699
  for myocardial infarction, 677
Metronidazole
  for acute abdomen, 259*t*
  for acute cholecystitis, 275
  for brain abscess, 321
  for hepatic abscess, 276
  for infectious gastroenteritis, 306
  for Ludwig angina, 639*t*
  for meningitis, 832
  for pelvic inflammatory disease, 846*t*
  for suppurative cholangitis, 276
  for trichomoniasis, 854
  for vaginitis, 847
Metropolitan Medical Response System, 46
Mezlocillin, for suppurative cholangitis, 276
Miconazole
  for tinea, 1024
  for vaginitis, 847
Microangiopathic hemolytic anemia, 792–793, 794
Microcytic anemia, 803*t*
Microhemagglutination-*Treponema pallidum* test (MHA-TP), 853
Micturition, syncope caused by, 340, 341, 342
Midazolam
  adverse effects and precautions, 184–185
  asthma and, 188
  in children, 1043
  contraindications, 184
  in EMS field treatment, 15
  in intubation, 184–185
  for reduction of fractures or dislocations, 515, 652
  for status epilepticus, 334, 336*t*
Midbrain, mass lesions in, 317, 318*i*
Middle ear disorders
  following head trauma, 451–452
  infections, 627*t*–628*t*, 642–643
Middle extensor tendon (MET), 553–554
  rupture of, 561
Midgut volvulus
  abdominal pain in, 1086*t*
  in newborns, 1084
Migraine, 388–389
  associated symptoms with, 382
  with aura (classic migraine), 388
  cluster variant of, 382, 383, 389–390
  pain location in, 382
  pain quality in, 382
  precipitating factors for, 382, 388
  prophylactic therapy for, 389
  severity of, factors influencing, 382
  special signs in, 383
  in stroke patients, 370
  syncope with, 345
  without aura (common migraine), 388
Miliary tuberculosis, 669
Military antishock trousers (MAST), 196, 213, 531
Military Assistance to Safety and Traffic (MAST) program, 12, 56
Military resources, for multicasualty incident/disaster management, 56

Milk
  for hypophosphatemia, 905
  for storage of avulsed teeth, 640
Milrinone, for central venous hypervolemia, 245
Mineralocorticoids, deficiency of, 882
  in hyperkalemia, 901
Minimal (III) (triage category), 50
Minimal acceptable care, 51
Minnesota tube, insertion of, 104–107, 105*i*, 106*i*
Minors
  and consent, 65
  and refusal to consent, 66
Miotics, for eye disorders, 621
Mirtazapine, 1037
Missed abortion, 733, 734*t*, 735
Missile injuries, 594–595, 767
Mistletoe, toxins in, 1004*t*
Mites, and scabies, 1022
Mithramycin, for hypercalcemia, 904
Mitral regurgitation, acute, 681
Mitral valve prolapse
  chest pain in, 251
  diagnosis of, 247*t*
  syncope in, 343
Mittelschmerz, 727*t*, 738
Mixed acid-bas disorders, 913–915
Mobitz type I atrioventricular block, 705, 720, 721*i*
Mobitz type I sinoatrial block, 704, 720, 720*i*
Mobitz type II atrioventricular block, 705, 720, 721*i*
Mobitz type II sinoatrial block, 704
Model of Clinical Practice of Emergency Medicine (ACEP), 3
Modifying factors, identification of, 4
Molar pregnancy, 736, 742–743
Molluscum contagiosum, 1025
Mollusk poisoning, 961–962
Monarthritis, 408–410
Monoamine oxidase inhibitors, 1037
  and catecholamine crisis, 884
  poisoning/overdose of, 967*t*
Monomethylhydrazine poisoning, 1001
Mononeuropathies
  compressive, 358–359
  weakness caused by, 357–359
Mononucleosis, 639*t*, 816–817
  differential diagnosis of, 816
  pharyngitis in, 840
Monophasic defibrillation, 155
Monospot test, for mononucleosis, 816
Monteggia fracture, 524
Mood disorders, 1033–1034
  assessment of, 1028
Moraxella catarrhalis infection, sinusitis in, 643
Morison pouch, 469
  in ruptured ectopic pregnancy, 731, 733*i*
Morning-after pill, 742
Morphine
  for angina, 683
  for anoxic spells, 692
  for burn injuries, 922
  for cardiogenic shock, 244
  for central venous hypervolemia, 245
  for chest pain with normal hemodynamics, 245
  for congestive heart failure, 680
    in children, 1049
  and delirium, 1031
  in EMS field treatment, 15
  for flail chest, 458
  for heart failure, 685
  and hyponatremia, 893*t*
  for mitral regurgitation, 251

for mitral stenosis, 251
  for ocular burn injuries, 616
  for perforated duodenum, 254
  for perforated stomach, 254
  for pneumomediastinum, 252
  poisoning/overdose of, 967*t*
  for pulmonary edema, 227
  for rapid-sequence intubation, 181–182
  for sickle cell crisis, 808
  for sickle cell disease, in children, 1094
Motility disorders, and chest pain, 253
Motor function
  in spinal cord injury, 496–497, 497*t*–502*t*
  in stroke patients, 371
Motor responses, coma and, 316
Motor vehicle accidents, 45
Mountain laurel, toxins in, 1004*t*
Mountain sickness, 948–951
  acute, 948–949
Mouth
  bleeding from, in hemophilia, 796
  disorders of, 647–652
  injuries of, 440
  radiation injury of, 944
Mouth-to-mask ventilation, 150*i*, 151, 151*i*
  cephalic technique, 151, 151*i*
  lateral technique, 151
  and positive-pressure ventilation, 170
Mouth-to-mouth and nose technique, in pediatric basic life support, 164
Mouth-to-mouth resuscitation, 149*i*, 150–151
MRI. *See* Magnetic resonance imaging
Mucocutaneous bleeding, in platelet disorders, 789
Mucomyst. *See* Acetylcysteine
Mucopurulent cervicitis, 848
Mucormycosis, rhinoorbitocerebral, 606
Mucous membranes, radiation injury and, 943
Mueller maneuver, in paroxysmal supraventricular tachycardia, 696
Multicasualty incidents, 42–59
  air medical resources in, 53
  classification of, 42
  communications network in, 50, 54–56
  diffusely distributed victims in, 54–56
  EMS *versus* civil defense management of, 47
  hazardous materials in, 53–54
  hospital emergency departments in, 56–59
  Incident Command System for, 47, 48*i*
  local accessory resources in, 53
  logistics of, 49–50
  media involvement in, 53
  medical management of, 47
  mutual aid in, 53
  organization of response to, 47
  organizations and assistance, 56
  patient distribution in, 51–52
  prehospital management of, 47–56
  psychological support for, 59
  public safety in, 52–53
  scene organization of, 49, 49*i*
  special considerations, 53–56
  stress management for, 59
  transport in, 51–52
  treatment in, 51
  triage in, 50, 57–58
Multifocal atrial tachycardia, 699
  electrocardiogram in, 699, 712, 717*i*
Multipartite patella, 534
Multiple myeloma, 817
  back pain in, 420
Multiply injured patient, 208–221. *See also specific injury*

hemorrhagic shock in, 213–214
initial assessment of, **210–212**
initial resuscitation of, **212–213**
intravenous access of, 212
laboratory tests for, 212
life-threatening problems in, immediate management of, **208–214**, 209*i*
neurologic examination of, 211–212
ongoing evaluation and resuscitation of, 212
preparation for, 208–210
primary survey of, 210–212
Multitasking, 4
Mumps infection
dacryoadenitis in, 609
orchitis in, 754, 763–764
scrotal pain in, 753*t*, 754
Mupirocin, for impetigo, 855, 1019
Murmurs, in vascular trauma, 768
Murphy's sign, 265
Muscle, suturing and closure of, 584–585
Muscle disease
primary acute, **367–368**
weakness in, **354–355**, 367–368
Muscle relaxants
for chronic degenerative disk disease, 417, 418
for lumbosacral strain, 417, 418
for reduction of fractures or dislocations, 515
for reduction of TMJ dislocation, 652
for tension headache, 388
for whiplash, 509
Muscle spasm
and chest pain, 255
and headache, 383
Muscle strength, in spinal cord injury, 496
Musculoskeletal disorders
and chest pain, 250*t*, 251, **254–255**
lightning injuries and, 940
Mushrooms, poisonous, **1001–1002**, 1002*t*
Mustard. *See* Sulfur mustard
Mutual aid, and multicasualty incidents/disasters, 53
Myasthenia gravis, **366**
stable, drug therapy for, 366*t*
weakness in, 353, **366**
Mycobacterium avium complex, in HIV-infected patients, 864–866
Mycobacterium tuberculosis infection, 669–670
Mycoplasma pneumoniae infection, 668, 834–835
pharyngitis in, in children, 1073
Mycotoxins, T-2, as biologic weapon, **34–35**
Mydriatic agents, 621, 622*t*
for ocular burn injuries, 616, 617
for uveitis, 613
Myelography
in spinal cord compression, 351
in spinal cord metastases, 355
in spinal epidural abscess, 356
in transverse myelitis, 356
Myelosuppressive agents, for polycythemia vera, 813
Myocardial contusion, **217, 459–460**
Myocardial enzymes
in angina, 683
in cardiomyopathy, 691
in myocardial infarction, 676
Myocardial infarction, **675–679**
abdominal pain in, 257
acute, **675–679**
diagnosis of, 247*t*
in asthma and COPD, 658
chest pain in
with hypovolemia, 242*t*
management of, 244
with normal hemodynamics, 245

clinical findings in, 676
complications of, **679–682**
congestive heart failure in, 675, **680–681**
delirium in, 1032
diagnosis of, 271*t*
differential diagnosis of, 676–677
disposition in cases of, 679
electrocardiographic findings in, 676, 677
immediate measures for, 677
laboratory findings in, 676, 677
mitral regurgitation, acute, in, **681**
myocardial rupture in, **681**
non-ST-segment-elevation, 675, 676
percutaneous coronary intervention for, 679
pericarditis in, **682**
pulmonary embolism in, **681–682**
shock in, 675, **679–680**
differential diagnosis of, 679, 680*t*
ST-segment-elevation, 675, 676
symptoms and signs of, 676
syncope in, **342**
systemic embolism in, **681–682**
thrombolytic therapy for, 677–679
treatment of, 677–679
ventricular septal rupture in, **681**
Myocardial injury, in electrical burns, 567
Myocardial ischemia
angina in, 682–684
in pulmonary embolism, 662
Myocardial reperfusion, 677–679
idioventricular rhythm in, 706–707
Myocardial rupture, **681**
Myocarditis, **690–691**
Myoclonus, in metabolic disorders, 403
Myoglobin testing
in muscle disease, 354
in myocardial infarction, 676
in rhabdomyolysis, 368
Myoglobinuria
extremity trauma and, 220
phencyclidine overdose and, 1000
Myonecrosis, clostridial, **857**
Myopathy, acute
primary, **367–368**
weakness in, **354–355**
Myringitis, 627*t*, 834
Myxedema coma, **880–881**
Myxoma, syncope with, 343

NA⁺. *See* Sodium
Nafcillin
for brain abscess, 321
for bursitis, 414
for cellulitis, 1016
for erysipelas, 1016
for impetigo, 1019
for infective endocarditis, 860
for osteomyelitis, in children, 1078*t*
for penetrating spinal cord injury, 495
for pneumonia, 836*t*
prophylactic use of, 564
for puerperal mastitis, 749
for scalded skin syndrome, 855
for septic arthritis, 838*t*
in children, 1078*t*
for staphylococcal scalded skin syndrome, 1015
Nail fold, paronychia and eponychia in, 562–563
Nailbed injury, 528, 558
Nalmefene
for opiate overdose, 998
withdrawal symptoms, 998

Naloxone
in children, 1043
in coma cocktail, 311
for delirium or confusion, 391, 393
endotracheal administration of, 189
for narcotic overdose, 327
and narcotic users, 66
for opiate overdose, 997–998
for poisoning-related coma, 964
for seizures, in children, 1062
withdrawal symptoms, 998
Naproxen
for dysmenorrhea, 738
for gouty arthritis, 408
for tooth pain, 649
Naratriptan, for migraine, 389
Narcotics/narcotic analgesics. *See also specific narcotic drugs*
for black widow spider bites, 954
for burn injuries, 922
for head injuries, 423
for musculoskeletal disorders with chest pain, 254
naloxone and, 66
for ocular burn injuries, 616
overdose of, **327**, 964
for scorpion fish envenomation, 959
for urolithiasis, 761
withdrawal symptoms of, prevention of, 998
for zoster, 256
Nasal airway
in children, 187
and intubation preparation, 170, 171*i*
Nasal balloon device, 633, 634*i*
Nasal bleeding (epistaxis), nasal packing for, **133–136**, 134*i*
Nasal fractures, **448**
reduction of, 448, 448*i*
Nasal injury, in facial trauma, **440**
Nasal intubation
in asthma, 188
in children, 187
Nasal obstruction, **633–634**, 635*t*
Nasal packing, for epistaxis, **133–136**, 134*i*
Nasal tampons, 633, 634*i*
Nasogastric intubation, **102–104**, 103*i*
in burn injuries, 920
in children, 187
in comatose patients, 104
contraindications to, in maxillary (Le Fort) fracture, 445
in gastrointestinal bleeding, 285
in neck injury, 436
in syncope, 337
Nasogastric lavage, in gastrointestinal bleeding, 286
Nasopharyngeal airway, in multiply injured patient, 210
Nasotracheal intubation, 101–102
indications for, 98
in spinal cord injury, 494
National Disaster Medical System (NDMS), 56
National Practitioner Data Bank (NPDB), **71–72**
National Registry of Emergency Medical Technicians, 6, 8
National Ski Patrol, 9
Natural disasters, **42–45**, 43*t*
Nausea. *See also* Vomiting
in abdominal pain, 263
in botulism, 364
in migraine, 382
in pregnancy, 743
Navicular fractures, 545

NDMS. *See* National Disaster Medical System
Near-drowning, **944–946**
Nebulizer therapy
  for asthma and COPD, 659–660
  for croup, 647
Nebulizers
  for asthma, 227
  for COPD, 227
  for pulomary fibrosis, 227
Neck
  abscess of, incision and drainage of, 141–142
  alignment and immobilization, in spinal cord injury, 493
  anatomic zones of, 215
  burns of, **928**
  injuries to, **214–215**
  physical examination of
    in headache patients, 383
    in spinal cord injury, 496
    in stroke patients, 370
  soft tissue x-rays of
    in croup, 647, 648*i*
    in sore throat diagnosis, 635, 637*i*
Neck pain
  in myocardial infarction, 676
  in spinal cord injury, 496, 509
Neck trauma, **435–453**, 576
  airway injury in, 436, 438–439
  airway management in, 435–436, 437
  anatomic location of, 438
  bleeding in, control of, **436–437**
  blunt, **438**, 769
  cervical spine immobilization in, 435, **437**
  diagnosis and evaluation of, **438–441**
  disposition in cases of, 439
  esophageal injury in, 439
  life-threatening problems in, immediate management of, **435–437**
  nerve injury in, 436, 437*i*, 439
  penetrating, **438**, 438*i*, 769
  shock in, **436–437**
  type of, **438**
  vascular injury in, 439, **768–769**
    zones of injury in, 769, 769*i*
  wound care in, 576
Necrolysis, toxic epidermal, **1014**
Necrotizing fasciitis, **856–857**
  of perineum, 764
Needle(s), for suturing in hand trauma, 556
Needle aspiration, of peritonsillar abscess, 645, 646*i*
Needle cricothyroidotomy, **175–178**, 176*i*
  in children, 187
Needle cricothyrotomy. *See* Transtracheal jet ventilation
Needle decompression, in abdominal trauma, 467
Needle thoracostomy
  in EMS field treatment, **15**
  for tension pneumothorax, 215, 225, 656
Needlestick injuries, in EMS field treatment, 14
Negative pressure rewarming, 933
Negligence, **61–62**
Neisseria gonorrhoeae infection. *See* also Gonorrhea
  in children, 1101*t*
  and pharyngitis, in children, 1073
  and septic arthritis, in children, 1079
  urinary tract, in children, 1075
Neisseria meningitidis infection, 834*t*, 1068*t*
Nelfinavir, side effects of, 865*t*
Neoantigen-type drug-related autoimmune hemolytic anemia, 807–808
Neomycin, for eye trauma/disorders, 622*t*

Neonate(s)
  definition of, 163
  pneumonia in, 832, 836*t*
  urinary tract infection in, 841
Neoplasms (tumors). *See also specific type*
  intrathoracic, chest pain in, **255–256**
Neostigmine, in myasthenia gravis, 353, 366, 366*t*
Nephrectomy, for renal injuries, 484
Nephrogenic diabetes insipidus, hypernatremia in, 896
Nephropathy, in HIV-infected patients, 865
Nerium oleander, toxins in, 1004*t*
Nerve(s). *See also specific nerves*
  sensory, assessment in spinal cord injury, 497–502, 503*i*, 504*i*, 505*t*
Nerve agents, as chemical weapons, 36*t*, **37–38**
Nerve block, 578
  in hand trauma, 549, 550*i*, 551*i*, 552*i*, 578, 578*i*, 579*i*
  superior laryngeal, for intubation, 180, 181*i*
  for zoster, 256
Nerve injury
  in elbow injuries, 522
  in facial trauma, 439–440
  in forearm fracture, 524
  in hand trauma, 554–555, **569**
  in humerus fractures, 519
  in lunate dislocation, 525
  in maxillary (Le Fort) fracture, 443–445
  in neck trauma, 436, 437*i*, 439
  in orbital floor (blowout) fractures, 447
  in shoulder dislocation, 518–519
  in tibial plateau fractures, 535
  in vascular trauma, prevention of, 767
  in zygomaticomaxillary complex fractures, 446
Nervous system, radiation injury and, 944
Nesiritide
  for central venous hypervolemia, 245
  for heart failure, 685
Neuralgia
  glossopharyngeal, syncope in, 340
  trigeminal, 382, **385–386**
Neurogenic shock, **207**
  causes of, 196
  differentiation from vasovagal syncope, 207
Neuroleptic malignant syndrome, **1036–1037**
Neuroleptics, as chemical restraints, 1028
Neurologic disorders
  in children, **1059–1062**
  delirium in, **1032**
  in HIV-infected patients, 864
Neurologic examination
  in abdominal trauma, 467
  in coma, **316**
  in delirium or confusion, 393
  in head injuries, 422
  in head trauma, 219
  in headache patients, 383
  in multiply injured patient, 211–212
  in spinal cord injury, **496–502**, 506
  in stroke patients, 370–371
  in vascular trauma, 768
Neurologic hyperventilation, 231*t*, **239**
Neurologic injuries, lightning injuries and, 940
Neurologic symptoms, syncope associated with, 339
Neuromuscular block, for intubated patient, 189
Neuromuscular diseases, and respiratory distress/dyspnea, 229, 230*t*
Neuromuscular junction, disease or blockage of, **363–366**
  weakness with, 353–354, **363–366**
Neuropathic bladder, 750, 751*t*

Neuropathy
  arsenical, **360–361**
  in neurogenic shock, 207
  peripheral
    weakness caused by, 354, **357–363**
    in Wernicke encephalopathy, 398
  in seafood poisoning, 363
Neurosis, pulmonary, **239**
Neurosurgical consultation, in subarachnoid hemorrhage, 373
Neutrons, 21
Neutropenia, **814–815**
Neutropenic fever, 830
Nevirapine, side effects of, 865*t*
Newborn. *See also under* Infant(s); Pediatric
  definition of, 163
  emergencies, **1096–1097**
  gastrointestinal bleeding in, 1089
  resuscitation of, 1096–1097, 1098*i*
  vomiting in, 1084
Nicotiana tabacum, toxins in, 1004*t*
Nicotine, in poisonous plants, 1003, 1004*t*
Nicotinelike toxins, in poisonous plants, 1003, 1004*t*
Nifedipine
  for acute high-altitude pulmonary edema, 950
  for high-altitude pulmonary edema, 950–951
  poisoning/overdose of, 977
Nightshade
  poisoning/overdose of, 975
  toxins in, 1004*t*
Nikolsky sign, 1014
Nimotidine, for vasospasm, 373
9-1-1 (nine-one-one), 9, 147
  enhanced, 9
NIPPV. *See* Noninvasive positive-pressure ventilation
Nitrates, for pulmonary edema, 227
Nitrites
  for cyanide poisoning, 983, 983*t*
  for hydrogen sulfide poisoning, 994
Nitrogen dioxide
  poisoning, 994, 995*t*
  and smoke inhalation injury, 924
Nitrogen poisoning, 995*t*
Nitroglycerin
  for angina, 683
  for cardiac arrest prevention, 147
  for cardiogenic shock, 244
  for central venous hypervolemia, 245
  for chest pain, 253
    with normal hemodynamics, 245
  for congestive heart failure, 680–681, 685
  in EMS field treatment, 15
  for mitral regurgitation, 251
  for mitral stenosis, 251
  for myocardial infarction, 677
  for pulmonary edema, 203
Nitroglycerin challenge, in cluster headache, 389
Nitroprusside
  for catecholamine crisis, 885
  for heart failure, 685
  for hypertension, 974
    in aortic dissection, 780–781
  for hypertensive emergencies, 687
  for preeclampsia-eclampsia, 745
Nitrous oxide, inhaled, in children, 1043
Nonabsorbable sutures, 582–583
Nonarticular rheumatism, 406, 406*t*, **413–414**
Nonclostridial anaerobic cellulitis, **856**
Nonfluent aphasia, 401
Nongonococcal (nonspecific) urethritis, **851**

Nonhemorrhagic hypovolemic shock, 196
Noninflammatory arthritis, **407,** 407*t*
Noninvasive positive-pressure ventilation (NIPPV),
  for pulmonary edema, 226
Nonionic surfactant, for wound cleansing, 580
Nonnatural disasters, **45–46**
Nonsteroidal anti-inflammatory drugs (NSAIDs)
  for ankylosing spondylitis, 413
  for bursitis, 414
  for carpal tunnel syndrome, 566
  for chronic degenerative disk disease, 417
  for flexor tenosynovitis, 566
  for gouty arthritis, 408
  for lumbosacral strain, 417
  for migraine, 388
  for musculoskeletal disorders with chest pain,
    254
  for osteoarthritis, 410–411
  for pericarditis, 682
  for peritonsillitis, 646
  platelet function impaired by, 794–795
  for pleurodynia, 665
  for pseudogout, 409
  for Reiter syndrome, 412
  for rheumatoid arthritis, 411–412
  for sickle cell crisis, 809
  for sunburn, 927
  for systemic lupus erythematosus, 413
  for tendonitis, 414
  for tension headache, 388
  for Tietze syndrome, 255
  for urolithiasis, 761
  for viral arthritis, 413
Non-ST-segment-elevation myocardial infarction,
  675, 676
Nonurgent presentation, 4
Norepinephrine
  in advanced life support, 160*t,* 161, 162
  for cardiogenic shock, 202
  for hypotension, 1010
  for neurogenic shock, 207
  for septic shock, 205, 826
Norfloxacin, for eye trauma/disorders, 622*t*
Norgestrel, for pregnancy prevention
  emergency postcoital, 742
  in female rape victims, 740
Normocytic anemia, 803*t*
Nose
  abscess of, 635*t*
  foreign body in, 633–634, 635*t*
  fractures of, **448**
    reduction of, 448, 448*i*
  frostbite of, 642
  injuries of, **440**
    epistaxis in, 632
  obstruction of, **633–634**
Nosebleed. *See* Epistaxis
Nosocomial pneumonia, 835, 836*t*
Noxious products, smoke inhalation injury, 924
NPDB. *See* National Practitioner Data Bank
N.P.O., for gastrointestinal bleeding, 285
NSAIDs. *See* Nonsteroidal anti-inflammatory drugs
α-nterferon, for cold agglutinin syndrome, 806
Nuchal rigidity
  in meningitis, 384, 830–831
  in poliomyelitis, 357
Nuclear accidents, 46
Nuclear weapons, **20–22**
Nursemaid's elbow, **523**
Nylon sutures, 583
Nystagmus
  in caloric testing, 347

dissociated, 316
Dix-Hallpike test for, 630, 632
in metabolic disorders, 396
retraction, 316
see-saw, 316
in vertigo, 630, 632
in Wernicke encephalopathy, 398

Obesity
  and chronic bronchitis, 657
  and lumbar puncture, 131–132
  and lumbosacral strain, 418
Oblique fracture, 513
Observation, 4
Obstetric emergencies, **742–749.** *See also specific*
  types
  hyperemesis gravidarum, **743**
  labor and delivery, **746–747**
  life-threatening problems in, immediate manage-
    ment of, **725–728**
  management of specific disorders in, **742–749**
  postpartum hemorrhage, **747–748**
  pregnancy, **742–743**
    discomforts of, **743**
    trauma in, **745–746**
  puerperal mastitis, **748–749**
  puerperal sepsis and endometritis, **748**
  third-trimester bleeding, **743–744**
  toxemia (preeclampsia-eclampsia), **744–745**
Obstetric patients, with multiple injuries, 208
Obstipation, and abdominal pain, 264
Obstruction, intestinal, abdominal pain in, 260*t*
Obstructive apnea, 1051
Obstructive shock, 194, 197, **203–204**
  cardiac tamponade and, 203
  causes of, 193*t*
  massive pulmonary embolism and, 203–204
Obtunded patient, poisoning and, 963–964
Obturator sign, 265, 266*i*
Occuloglandular tularemia, 24*t*
Octreotide
  for esophageal varices, 291
  for peptic ulcer disease, 290
Ocular abnormalities, in Wernicke encephalopathy,
  398
Ocular bobbing, coma and, 316
Ocular burns, **927**
Ocular conditions, requiring immediate treatment,
  604–608
Ocular massage, for central retinal artery occlusion,
  605
Ocular symptoms, important, evaluation of,
  600–604
Oculocephalic testing, 316
Oculoglandular tularemia, 26
Oculovestibular testing, 316
Odynophagia, in sore throat, 635
OEP. *See* Office of Emergency Preparedness
Office of Emergency Preparedness (OEP), 46
Off-line medical direction, for EMS system, 12
Ofloxacin
  for conjunctivitis, 610
  for eye trauma/disorders, 622*t*
  for pelvic inflammatory disease, 846*t*
Oil of wintergreen poisoning, 967*t*, 1005–1006
Olanzapine, 1037
  poisoning/overdose of, 1001
Oleander, toxicity, 1003, 1004*t*
Olecranon fractures, **522**
Oligoarthritis, 406–407, **408–411**
Oliguria, **750–752**
Omeprazole, for peptic ulcer disease, 290

Omnicef. *See* Cefdinir
Omphalotus illudens, 1002*t*
On-call physicians, 71
On-call specialty consultation, 71
Ondansetron
  for hyperemesis gravidarum, 743
  for radiation injury, 944
One-finger palpation, 264–265
One-shot intravenous pyelogram
  in abdominal trauma, 468, 476
  in genitourinary trauma, 480
On-line medical direction, for EMS system, 12
OPA. *See* Oropharyngeal airway
Opacities, in abdominal radiographs, 268
Open book fractures, 531
Open fractures, 513
Open pneumothorax, **456**
Open reduction and internal fixation (ORIF)
  of femoral shaft fractures, 533
  of hip fractures, 531
  of humerus fractures, 521
  of lunate dislocations, 525
  of pelvic fractures, 531
Open-angle glaucoma, corticosteroids and, 624
Ophthalmic medications, 621, 622*t*
  central anticholinergic syndrome caused by,
    399*t*
  contaminated, 625
  home use of, 623
Ophthalmic ointments, 621–623
Ophthalmicus, herpes, in HIV-infected patients,
  865
Ophthalmoplegia, in Wernicke encephalopathy,
  398
Opiates/opioids
  for acute intermittent porphyria, 362
  avoidance, in migraine therapy, 388
  for chronic degenerative disk disease, 417–418
  and delirium, **1031**
  for epistaxis, 633
  for gastroenteritis, 309
  for lumbosacral strain, 417–418
  for peritonsillitis, 646
  poisoning/overdose of, 967*t*, **997–998**
    coma in, 311, 313, 314
    delirium or confusion in, 393
  for sciatica, 419
  for sickle cell crisis, 808–809
  for tooth pain, 649
Optic neuritis, **615**
Oragrafin. *See* Sodium ipodate
Oral airway
  in children, 187
  and intubation preparation, 170, 171*i*
Oral contraceptives
  for female rape victims, 740
  postcoital emergency, **742**
Oral hypoglycemic agents, for hyperglycemia, 873
Oral mucosa, lacerations of, 594
Oral rehydration therapy. *See also* Fluid replace-
  ment/resuscitation
  for dehydration, in children, 1047
Orbit
  blunt trauma to, **618–620**
  examination of, in headache patients, 383
Orbital cellulitis, **605–606,** 1074, 1075
Orbital entrapment, 447
Orbital floor fractures, **447, 619–620**
  computed tomography of, 447, 447*i*
Orbital hemorrhage, **619**
Orchitis, **763–764**
  scrotal pain in, 753*t*, 754

Organ donation, 72
Organ harvesting, for transplantation, **72**
Organic causes, for psychiatric emergencies, **1030–1032**
Organic mercury poisoning, **991**
Organophosphates, poisoning, **364–366**, 967*t*, **998–999**
   clinical findings in, 365, 365*t*
   seizures induced by, 971
   weakness in, 353, **364–366**
Orientation, loss of
   in drug withdrawal, 397
   in metabolic disorders, 396
Orogastric intubation, for gastrointestinal bleeding, 285
Oropharyngeal airway
   cuffed, and intubation preparation, 172
   in multiply injured patient, 210
   in shock, 194
Oropharyngeal secretions, aspiration of, 671
Oropharyngeal tularemia, 24*t*, 26
Orotracheal intubation, 100*i*, 101. *See also* Intubation
   in head injuries, 422
   indications for, 98
   in maxillary (Le Fort) fracture, 445
   relative contraindications for, 173*t*
   in spinal cord injury, 494
ORT. *See* Oral rehydration therapy
Orthopedic emergencies, **510–547**
   common pitfalls in, **547**
   eponyms in, 514
   general principles in, **513–515**
   primary survey in, 511
   secondary survey in, 511
Orthopedic injuries, **510–547**
   to ankle joint, **540–544**
   calcaneal fracture, **544**
   in child abuse, 515
   compartment syndrome in, **512–513**
   to elbow, **522–523**
   femoral shaft fractures, **532–533**
   fibula fractures, **539–540**
   to forearm, **524**
   to hand, **524–529**, **561–562**
   to hip, **531–532**
   to knee joint, **532–539**
   life-threatening, immediate management of, **511**
   limb-threatening, immediate management of, **511–513**
   to lower extremities, **532–547**
   metatarsal fractures, **546**
   to pelvic girdle, **530–532**
   phalangeal, **546–547**
   procedural sedation for, 515
   sesamoid fractures, **547**
   to shoulder girdle, **516–519**
   to shoulder joint, **518–519**
   specific, management of, **516–547**
   splinting of, **514–515**
   subtalar dislocations, **545**
   talar fractures, **544**
   tarsal, **545**
   tarsometatarsal, **545–546**
   type I, 513
   type II, 514
   type III, 514
   type IV, 514
   type V, 514
   to upper extremities, **519–529**
   to wrist, **524–529**

Orthostatic hypotension, **345–346**
   patient position in, 340
   syncope in, 335–337, **345–346**
   in Wernicke encephalopathy, 398
Orthostatic vital signs, shock and, 194
Osgood-Schlatter disease, **535–536**
Osler nodes, in infective endocarditis, 859
Osler-Weber-Rendu disease, gastrointestinal bleeding in, 288
Osmolality
   in coma, **328**
   determination of, **915**
   in hypernatremia, 896
Osmolar gap, calculation of, 968*t*
Osteoarthritis, **410–411**
   lumbar puncture in, 132
Osteomyelitis, **838–839**
   acute, in children, 1078*t*, **1079–1080**
   in children, 1078–1080, 1078*t*
   distal phalanx, 563
   in infected vascular gangrene and cellulitis, 856
   puncture wounds and, 597
   in sickle cell anemia, 810
   in sinusitis, 643–645
   vertebral, 419, 839
Osteoporosis, humerus fractures in, 519
Otitis externa, 627*t*
   malignant, 627*t*
Otitis media
   acute, in children, **1070–1072**
   in infants, 1064, 1070
   serous or secretory, 628*t*
   suppurative (chronic), 628*t*, **642–643**
Otohematoma, 441, **450**
Otorrhea, following head injuries, **451**
Ottawa rules, for radiography
   in ankle joint injuries, 540, 543
   in knee joint injuries, 533–534
Outpatient analgesia, in children, 1044
Ova, stool testing for, 302
Ovarian carcinoma, **736**
Ovarian cyst, rupture of, **737**
   pelvic pain in, 727*t*
   vaginal bleeding in, 726
Ovarian follicle cyst, rupture of
   abdominal pain in, **281**
   diagnosis of, 271*t*
Ovarian torsion, abdominal pain in, **281**
Ovarian tumor, torsion of, **737–738**
   pelvic pain in, 727*t*
Overdose, drug. *See specific agent*
Oversensing, by cardiac pacemakers, 709, 723*i*, 724
Oxacillin
   for cellulitis, 1016
   for erysipelas, 1016
   for impetigo, 1019
   for infective endocarditis, 860
   prophylactic use of, 564
   for staphylococcal scalded skin syndrome, 1015
Oxalatelike toxins, in poisonous plants, 1004*t*
Oxalates, in poisonous plants, 1003, 1004*t*
Oxprenolol poisoning, 976
Oxygen
   in abdominal trauma, 467
   in acute high-altitude pulmonary edema, 949
   in acute lung injury, 672
   in air embolism, 465
   in altered mental status with shallow breathing, 225
   in angina, 683
   in anoxic spells, 692
   in asthma, 227, 659–660, 1058

   in atelectasis, 667
   in bronchiolitis, 837
   in burn injuries, 917
   in carbon monoxide poisoning, 978
   in cardiac tamponade, 689
   in chest pain, 240
      with normal hemodynamics, 245
   in cluster headache, 389
   in confused or delirious patient, 393
   in COPD, 227, 659–660
   in croup, 1052, 1053
   in cyanide poisoning, 983
   in dehydration, in children, 1046
   in drug-induced methemoglobinemia, 984–985
   in ergotism, 787
   in flail chest, 458
   in head injuries, 421
   in heart failure, 685
   in hemoptysis, 654
   in high-altitude cerebral edema, 950
   in inhalant poisoning, 994
   in lactic acidosis, 876
   in meningitis, in children, 1069
   in pleural effusion, 666
   in pneumomediastinum, 252
   in pneumothorax, 655
   in poliomyelitis, 351
   in pulmonary aspiration syndrome, 671
   in pulmonary contusion, 459
   in pulmonary edema, 226
   in pulmonary embolism, 682
   in pulmonary fibrosis, 227
   in pulmonary infections with cystic fibrosis, 673
   in pulmonary vascular disease, 344
   in reduction of fractures or dislocations, 515
   in septic shock, 825, 826
   in sickle cell crisis, 808
   in smoke inhalation, 917, 925
   in spinal cord injury, 493
   in traumatic asphyxia, 465
   in weak patient, 349
Oxygenation, adequacy of, and respiratory distress/dyspnea, 222–224
Oxyquinoline sulfate, for otitis media, 1070
Oxytocin, for postpartum hemorrhage, 748
Ozone. *See also* Phencyclidine
   poisoning, 995*t*

Pacemaker(s), **707–710**
   for arrhythmias, 202
   bipolar, 707
   codes and settings for, 707–708, 708, 708*t*, 722*i*
   dual-chamber, 707, 722*i*, 724
   failure to capture in, 709, 723*i*, 724
   implantable, complications of, 709
   lead complications with, 709
   malfunction of, 709–710, 723*i*, 724
      electrocardiogram in, 723*i*, 724
   oversensing by, 709, 723*i*, 724
   permanent, **707–710**
   pocket site complications with, 709
   runaway, 709–710
   single-chamber, 707, 720–724, 722*i*
   types of, 707
   undersensing by, 709, 723*i*, 724
   unipolar, 707
   venous access complications with, 709, 710
Pacemaker mediated tachycardia (PMT), 709, 710
Packed red blood cells, **818–819**
   for autoimmune hemolytic anemia, 805
   characteristics and doses of, 818, 819*t*

for hemostatic abnormalities of liver disease, 799
for hypovolemic shock, 199
for iron-deficiency anemia, 804
irradiated, 819
leukocyte-treated, 819
massive transfusion of, 821
for paroxysmal cold hemoglobinuria, 807
for thrombotic thrombocytopenic purpura, 793
washed, 819
PAD. *See* Public access defibrillation
Pain. *See also specific type or structure affected*
abdominal (*See* Abdominal pain)
chest (*See* Chest pain)
in otitis media, 1070
in pediatric patient, 1040–1044
pleuritic, 238
differential diagnosis of, **246**
referred, 1080
somatic, 1080
visceral, 1080
Pain management/relief (analgesia)
in burn injuries, 922
in chest trauma, 455
in children, 1043
in chronic degenerative disk disease, 417–418
in femoral shaft fractures, 533
in flail chest, 229, 458
in head injuries, 423
in herpes zoster infection, 1020
in lumbosacral strain, 417–418
in lunate dislocations, 525
in maxillary (Le Fort) fracture, 445
in migraine, 388
in musculoskeletal disorders with chest pain, 254
in nasal fracture, 448
outpatient, for children, 1044
in peritonsillitis, 646
in reduction of fractures or dislocations, 515
in rib fractures, 464
in scapholunate dislocations, 525
in scorpion fish envenomation, 959
in sea urchin envenomation, 959
in sickle cell crisis, 808–809
in sickle cell disease, in children, 1094
in sternal fracture, 464
in stingray envenomation, 956
in tension headache, 388
in testicular torsion, 763
in tooth pain, 649
in urolithiasis, 761
in vascular trauma, 767
in zoster infection, 256
Pain sensitivity
in hand trauma, 550–551
in spinal cord injury, 497
Pain-sensitive structures, and headache, 381
Palmar splint, 557
Palmaris longus muscle, 551
Palpation
of abdomen, 264–265
deep, 265
one-finger, 264–265
2-PAM. *See* Pralidoxime
Pamidronate, for hypercalcemia, 904
Pancreatic β cell tumor, and hypoglycemia, 874
Pancreatic injuries, **472**
Pancreatic pseudocyst, and gastrointestinal bleeding, 290*t*
Pancreatitis
acute, abdominal pain in, 261*t*, **280**
diagnosis of, 249*t*, 271*t*
lipase in, 266

Pancuronium, for intubation, 183
Panic disorder(s)
and hyperventilation, 346
and syncope, 346
Panophthalmitis, 606
Panorex imaging
in mandibular fracture, 441, 442*i*
in tooth pain, 649
Panuveitis, 613
Papilledema
as contraindication to lumbar puncture, 384
in headache, 379, 383
in pseudotumor cerebri, 386
Paracranial structures, disease in, headache with, 381
Parainfluenza virus infection
croup in, 647
pharyngitis in, in children, 1073
Paraldehyde, for status epilepticus, 336*t*
Paralysis
hypokalemia periodic, **367**
hysterical, 497
in intubated patient, 189
in neurogenic shock, 207
in shock, 196
in spinal cord injury, 496
tick, 354, **362**
Paralytic seafood poisoning, **363**
Paralytic shellfish poisoning, 305*t*, **961–962**
Paralytics, for multiply injured patient, 210
Paralyzed patients, general care of, 190
Paramedic-Critical Care training, 9
Paramedics. *See* Emergency medical technicians, ad-
vanced
Paraphimosis, **764–765**, 764*i*
Paraplegia, in shock, 196, 207
Parasites, stool testing for, 302
Parasitic enteritis, **303–306**
Parens patriae, 66
Parenteral medications
and anaphylactic shock, 206, 207
for asthma, 227
for COPD, 227
for pulmonary fibrosis, 227
Parents, and consent, 1044–1045
Parietal peritoneum, and abdominal pain, 263
Paronychia, **562–563**
incision and drainage of, 563, 563*i*
Parotid gland injury, **440**, 440*i*
Paroxetine, 1037
Paroxysmal cold hemoglobinuria (PCH), 805, **806–807**
Paroxysmal supraventricular tachycardia (PSVT), **695–697**
adenosine for, 161
AV nodal dependent or independent, 695
electrocardiogram in, 695, 712, 713*i*–715*i*
treatment of, 695–697
Particle repositioning maneuver, for positional ver-
tigo, 632
Parvovirus B19 infection, 1082*t*–1083*t*
transmission of, via transfusions, 822*t*
Pasteurella multocida infection, 564, 596
Patella dislocations, **534**
Patella fractures, **534**
Patella tendon rupture, 539
Patent ductus arteriosus, 693
Pathologic fractures, 513
of humerus, 519, 520
Patient autonomy, and refusal to consent, 66
Patient distribution, in multicasualty incidents/dis-
asters, 51–52

Patient dumping, **63**
Patient history, 4
Patient status, determination of, 4
Patient-controlled analgesia (PCA), for sickle cell
crisis, 809
Patient-oriented standard of disclosure, 64
PCP. *See* Phencyclidine
PEA. *See* Pulseless electrical activity
Peace pill. *See* Phencyclidine
Peach pits, toxins in, 1004*i*
Peak expiratory flow (PEF), in asthma, 657, 658, 1056
Pediatric. *See also* Children
Pediatric advanced life support, **164–165**
Pediatric basic life support, **163–164**
Pediatric emergencies, **1039–1102.** *See also specific
type*
abdominal pain, **1080–1081,** 1086*t*–1087*t*
acute osteomyelitis, 1078*t*, **1079–1080**
acute otitis media, **1070–1072**
anemia, **1093**
apnea, **1051–1052**
assessment of, 1039–1040, 1040*t*
asthma, **1056–1058,** 1057*i*
bleeding, **1085–1091**
bronchiolitis, **1056**
cardiac dysrhythmias, **1049,** 1050*t*
cardiovascular, **1045–1049**
child abuse, **1097–1102**
congestive heart failure, **1048–1049,** 1049*t*
dehydration, **1046–1047**
epidemiology of, 1039
equipment for, 1040, 1041*t*–1042*t*
esophageal foreign body, **1091–1092,** 1092*i*
exanthems, **1080,** 1082*t*–1083*t*
fever, **1062–1066,** 1065*i*
foreign body
in airway, 164, 187–188, **1053–1055,** 1053*t*, 1055*t*
gastrointestinal, **1092**
gastric foreign body, **1092**
gastroenteritis, **1077–1078**
gastrointestinal bleeding, 1090*i*, 1091*i*
gastrointestinal disorders, **1080–1092**
Glasgow Coma Scale for, 1061*t*
hematologic diseases, **1093–1096**
idiopathic thrombocytopenic purpura, **1094–1096**
infectious diseases, **1062–1080**
lower airway disorders, **1056–1059**
meningitis, **1066–1070**
neurologic, **1059–1062**
newborns, **1096–1097**
periorbital cellulitis, **1074–1075,** 1074*t*
pharyngitis, **1073–1074**
pneumonia, **1058–1059,** 1059*t*, 1060*t*
respiratory distress, **1050–1059**
seizures, **1059–1062**
septic arthritis, **1078–1079,** 1078*t*
shock, **1047–1048**
sickle cell disease, **1093–1094,** 1095*t*
small bowel foreign body, **1092**
upper airway obstruction, **1052–1055**
urinary tract infection, **1075–1077**
vomiting, **1081–1085,** 1088*t*
Pediatric patients
and consent, 1044–1045
death of, 1045
and drug administration, 1044
family of, 1040
and fluid administration, 1044
medicolegal considerations, 1044–1045

Pediatric patients (*cont.*)
with multiple injuries, 208
pain in, 1040–1044
sedation of, 1040–1044
vital signs, 1040, 1043*t*
Pediculosis, **1022–1023**
PEFR. *See* Peak expiratory flow
Pelvic bleeding, 728*t*
in conscious patient with history of syncope, 339
Pelvic disorders, clinical manifestations of, 728*t*
Pelvic examination
in abdominal pain, 265–266
in dysuria-frequency syndrome, 844
in rape victims, 740
Pelvic floor penetration, in female genital injuries,
491, 492
Pelvic fractures, **530–531**
bladder injuries in, 473, 481, 486
genitourinary injuries in, 220
renal injuries in, 484
stabilization of, 213
Pelvic girdle injuries, **530–532**
Pelvic inflammatory disease, **845–846**
abdominal pain in, **280**
antibiotic therapy for, 846, 846*t*
diagnostic criteria for, 846*t*
Pelvic injury
and blood loss, and hemorrhagic shock, 213
and circulation, 211
and shock, 196, 200
Pelvic pain, **726–728**, 728*t*
differential diagnosis of, 727*t*
with intrauterine device, 741
with or without bleeding, **726–728**
in pelvic inflammatory disease, 845
in pregnancy, 728, 728*t*
syncope with, 339
ultrasound in, 728, 729*i*
Pelvic peritonitis, abdominal pain in, 263
Pelvic thrombophlebitis, septic abortion and, 735
Pelvic ultrasound, in vaginal bleeding, abnormal,
726
Pelvis
examination of, in abdominal trauma, 468
stability of, evaluation of, 511, 530, 530*i*
Pemphigus vulgaris, **1017**
Penetrating trauma
abdominal, 467, **470**
in pregnancy, 745–746
and cardiac tamponade, 217
chest, **465–466**
vascular injury in, 770
eye, **617–618**
genitourinary, 479*i*
neck, **438**, 438*i*
vascular injury in, 769
renal, 479, 481
and shock, 195
vascular, 767
Penicillamine
for arsenic poisoning, 361
as chelating agent, 989*t*
for rheumatoid arthritis, 411
Penicillin(s)
for animal bites, 596
for anthrax, 25
and autoimmune hemolytic anemia, 807–808
for botulism, 364
for cellulitis, 855
for clostridial anaerobic cellulitis, 856
for diphtheria, 638*t*
for erysipelas, 855

for frostbite, 935
for hepatic abscess, 276
for impetigo, 1019
for impetigo and ecthyma, 855
for infective endocarditis, 860
for mandibular fracture, 443
for meningitis, 832, 834*t*
for meningococcemia, 858
for nonclostridial anaerobic cellulitis, 856
for open fractures, 220
for peritonsillitis, 639*t*, 646
for pharyngitis, 638*t*, 841
for pneumonia, 836*t*
prophylactic use of, 564
in wound care, 590*t*, 597
for pulmonary infections in cystic fibrosis, 673
resistance to, 851
for scalded skin syndrome, 855
for septic arthritis, 838*t*
for strep throat, 638*t*
for suppurative cholangitis, 276
for syphilis, 853
thrombocytopenia induced by, 792
for tooth pain, 649
for toxic shock syndrome, 862
for toxic shock-like syndrome, 862
for zygomaticomaxillary complex fractures, 446
Penicillin G
for bacterial pharyngitis, 638*t*
for cellulitis, 855, 1016
for erysipelas, 1016
for group B streptococcal prophylaxis, 747
and hyperkalemia, 901
for impetigo and ecthyma, 855
for mandibular fracture, 443
for meningitis, 834*t*
for meningococcemia, 858
for pharyngitis, 841
in children, 1073
for syphilis, 853
Penicillin V
for pharyngitis, 841
in children, 1073
prophylactic use of, in sickle cell anemia, 809
Penicillin VK
for animal bites, 596
for mandibular fracture, 443
Penis
foreskin of
inability to retract (phimosis), **764–765**
retracted, constricted (paraphimosis), 764*i*,
764–765
injuries of, **490–492**
constriction, **491**
epinephrine contraindicated in, 574
in pelvic fractures, 530
persistent erection of (priapism), **764**, 810
rupture of, 490, **491**
Pentobarbital
in children, 1043
for status epilepticus, 336*t*
Peptic ulcer
gastrointestinal bleeding in, **290**
perforated, abdominal pain in, **273**
Pepto-Bismol. *See* Bismuth subsalicylate
Percussion, of abdomen, 265
Percutaneous coronary intervention (PCI)
for angina, 684
for cardiogenic shock, 680
for myocardial infarction, 679, 680, 684
versus thrombolytic therapy, 679
rescue, 679

Percutaneous suprapubic cystotomy, **127–129**,
128*i*
Percutaneous transluminal angioplasty, complications of, **786**, 787*t*
Percutaneous transtracheal jet ventilation (PTTJV),
175–177, 177*t*
in children, 187
Perdnisone, for sunburn, 927
Perforated bowel, abdominal pain in, **273**
Perforated duodenal ulcer
abdominal pain in, 260*t*
diagnosis of, 249*t*
Perforated duodenum
chest pain in, **254**
diagnosis of, 271*t*
Perforated esophagus
chest pain in, **253**
diagnosis of, 249*t*
Perforated intestine, diagnosis of, 271*t*
Perforated peptic ulcer, abdominal pain in, **273**
Perforated stomach, chest pain in, **254**
Perforating injuries, to eye, **618–619**
Perianal sensation, in spinal cord injury, 497
Periapical abscess, diagnosis and treatment of, 650*t*
Pericardial disease, shock in, 197
Pericardial effusion, **687–689**
in cardiac tamponade, 457–458, 687, 688
in obstructive shock, 203
pacemakers and, 709
Pericardial friction rub, 688
Pericardiocentesis, **116–118**, 118*i*
benign, 118, 118*i*
for cardiac tamponade, 217, 243, 458, 690
for pericarditis, 689
for shock, 197
Pericarditis, **687–689**
anticoagulation contraindicated in, 682
constrictive, syncope in, 343
diagnosis of, 248*t*
immune-response, 687
in myocardial infarction, **682**
in pleurodynia, 665
Perichondritis, 627*t*
Perilunate dislocations, **524–525**
Perimortem cesarean delivery, 746
Perinephric abscess, 844
Perineum
burns of, 921
"butterfly" hematoma of, 490
necrotizing fasciitis of, 764
straddle injuries to, 490, 491*i*
Periodontal abscess, 649, 650*t*
Periodontium, 648–649
Periorbital abscess, in sinusitis, 643–645
Periorbital cellulitis
in children, **1074–1075**, 1074*t*
in sinusitis, 643–645
Peripheral aneurysms, **781**
Peripheral muscarinic stimulation, nerve agents
and, 37
Peripheral neuropathy
weakness caused by, 354, **357–363**
in Wernicke encephalopathy, 398
Peripheral nicotinic stimulation, nerve agents and,
37
Peripheral vascular disease, osteomyelitis in,
838–839
Peripheral venous access, for external jugular vein
catheterization, 83, 84–85
Peripheral venous catheterization
with catheter-clad needle, **78–81**, 81*i*, 82*i*
with scalp vein (butterfly) needle, **81–82**, 83*i*, 84*i*

Peritoneal catheter insertion, **122–124**
  operative approach, 123–124
  percutaneous approach, 123
Peritoneal dialysis
  for drug elimination, 970
  for rewarming, 933
Peritoneal fluid, and abdominal pain, 267
Peritoneal lavage, **122–124,** 124*i*, 468
  in multiply injured patient, 212
  in pregnant patients, 746
  in visceral and hypogastric artery aneurysm, 778
Peritoneum
  parietal, and abdominal pain, 263
  visceral, and abdominal pain, 263
Peritonitis
  bacterial, 259
  diagnosis of, 271*t*
  diffuse, abdominal pain in, 263
  pelvic, 845
    abdominal pain in, 263
  primary, abdominal pain in, **281**
  and rectus abdominis spasm, 264
Peritonsillar abscess, 639*t*, **645–646**
  drainage of, 645–646, 646*i*
Peritonsillar cellulitis, 639*t*, **645–646**
  pharyngitis in, 1073, 1074
Peritonsillitis, 635, 636*i*, 639*t*, **645–646**
  drainage procedure in, 645–646
Periumbilical pain, diffuse, 263
Permethrin
  for pediculosis, 1023
  for scabies, 1022
Permissive hypercapnia, in asthma and COPD, 660
Pernio, **934**
Peroneal nerve injury, in tibial plateau fractures,
  535
Peroneal nerve palsy, **359**
Peroneal tendon injuries, **542**
Personality disorders, assessment of, 1029
Personnel, mobilization of, in multicasualty inci-
  dents/disasters, 56
Petechiae
  in idiopathic thrombocytopenic purpura, 789
  in infective endocarditis, 859
  in meningococcemia, 857
  in Rocky Mountain spotted fever, 858–859
  in stroke patients, 370
Petrolatum-impregnated dressings, 587
Petroleum distillate poisoning, **992–993**, 993*t*
pH, 908–909. *See also* Acid-base disorders
  analysis of, radial artery puncture for, **96–98,**
    97*i*
  and drug elimination, 969
Phalangeal injuries, **546–547**
Phalanx fractures and dislocations, **527–528**
Phalen maneuver, in carpal tunnel syndrome, 566
Phallin, in poisonous plants, 1003
Pharmacotherapy, 4
Pharyngeal abscess, 635
Pharyngeal airway injury, **436**
Pharyngeal tracheal lumen airway (PTLA), 171
Pharyngitis, 636, **840–841**
  abdominal pain in, 1081
  anaerobic, diagnosis and treatment of, 638*t*
  bacterial, 638*t*, 840–841
    versus mononucleosis, 816
  in children, **1073–1074**
  chlamydial, 638*t*, 840
  gonococcal, 638*t*, 840, 850
  herpes, 639*t*
  streptococcal, 636, 638*t*, 816, 840–841
  viral, 840

Pharyngoconjunctival fever, 612
Pharynx, radiation injury of, 944
Phenazopyridine, for urinary tract infections, 843
  in children, 1076
Phencyclidine
  and delirium, 1031
  intoxication, 396, 399
  poisoning/overdose of, **999–1000**
Phenergan. *See* Promethazine
Phenformin, and hyponatremia, 893*t*
Phenobarbital, 338*t*
  for alcohol withdrawal seizures, 341, 398
  for head injuries, 423
  overdose, 1007
  for scorpion bites, 955
  for seizures, 974, 1008
  for status epilepticus, 336*t*
  toxicity of, 338*t*
Phenol, and burns, 926
Phenothiazine(s)
  for acute intermittent porphyria, 362
  central anticholinergic syndrome caused by,
    399*t*
  for delirium tremens, 398
  poisoning/overdose of, 971, **1000–1001**
  proarrhythmic activity of, 702
Phentolamine
  for catecholamine crisis, 884–885
  for hypertension, 974
Phenylephrine
  in advanced life support, 160*t*, 161, 162
  for calcium-channel blocker poisoning, 977
  for epistaxis, 633
  for eye trauma/disorders, 622*t*
  for intubation, 179–180
  for priapism, 764
  for septic shock, 826
Phenylpropanolamine poisoning, 974–975
Phenytoin, 338*t*
  for arrhythmias, 980, 1009–1010
  extravasation of, 768
  for head injuries, 423
  for seizures, 974
    in children, 1062
  for status epilepticus, 335, 336*t*
    loading dose of, 334
  for stroke patients, 369
  for subarachnoid hemorrhage, 373
  toxicity of, 338*t*
  for trigeminal neuralgia, 385
Phenytoin equivalents (PEs), 334
Pheochromocytoma, **884–885**
Philadelphia chromosome, 815
Philadelphia criteria, for fever in infants, 1064
Philodendron, toxins in, 1004*t*
Phimosis, **764–765**
Phlebotomy, femoral vein, **92–93**
Phlegmasia cerulea dolens, 774–775
PHN. *See* Postherpetic neuralgia
Phoradendron flavescens, toxins in, 1004*t*
Phosgene
  as chemical weapon, **38**
  clinical findings, 36*t*
  poisoning, 995*t*
Phosphate
  in diabetic ketoacidosis, 868
  for hypercalcemia, 905
Phosphorus
  and burn injuries, 926
  serum concentration disorders, **905–906**
Photophobia
  in poliomyelitis, 357

  in uveitis, 613
  in viral keratoconjunctivitis, 611–612
Phrenic nerve injury, 436, 437*i*, 439
Physical abuse, of children, **1097–1100**
Physical agents. *See also specific type*
  disorders due to, **930–962**
Physical examination, 4
Physical exertion, syncope in, 340, 343
Physician-oriented standard of disclosure, 64
Physicians, on-call, 71
Physostigmine
  for anticholinergic poisoning, 975
  contraindications, 1009
  for sedative-hypnotics overdose, 1007
Piece-of-pie sign, in lunate dislocation, 524, 525*i*
Pilocarpine
  for acute angle-closure glaucoma, 605
  for eye disorders, 605, 621
Pindolol poisoning, 976
Ping pong gaze, coma and, 316
"Pink puffers," 657
Pinpoint pupils
  in coma, **314–315,** 316
  factitious, 314–315
Piperacillin-tazobactam
  for Ludwig angina, 639*t*
  for pneumonia, 836*t*
  for septic shock, 828*t*
  for urinary tract infections, 842*t*
Piroxicam, 795
Pit vipers, bites from, 951
Pits, fruit, toxins in, 1004*t*
Pittsburgh rules, for radiography in knee joint in-
  juries, 533
Pituitary adenomas, and apoplexy, 885
Pituitary apoplexy, **885–886**
Pityriasis rosea, **1024**
Pivot shift, for testing cruciate ligaments, 537
Placenta previa, 743–744
Placental disorders, 743–744
Plague, as biologic weapon, 23*t*, **25–26**
Plain gut sutures, 582
Plain radiographs
  in abdominal trauma, 468
  in calcaneal fractures, 544
  in collateral ligament injuries, 537
  in cruciate ligament injuries, 537
  in elbow dislocations, 523
  in fibula fractures, 540
  in knee dislocations, 536
  in lateral malleolar fractures, 540
  in medial malleolar fractures, 541
  in olecranon fractures, 522
  in patella dislocations, 534
  in patella fractures, 534
  in peripheral aneurysms, 781
  in phalanx fractures and dislocations, 527
  in rotator cuff injuries, 518
  in scapula fractures, 517
  in sinusitis, 643, 644*i*
  in spinal epidural abscess, 356
  in sternoclavicular joint dislocations, 516
  in subtalar dislocations, 545
  in talar fractures, 544
  in tarsal injuries, 545
  in tarsometatarsal injuries, 546
  in thoracic outlet syndrome, 786
  in tibial shaft fractures, 539
  in tibial spine fractures, 536
  in visceral (intestinal) ischemia, 775
Plant services, multicasualty incidents/disasters and,
  58

Plants
   nontoxic, 1003*t*
   poisonous, **1003–1004,** 1004*t*
Plasma
   for gastrointestinal bleeding, 285
   for hypovolemic shock, 199
Plasma substitutes, for hypovolemic shock, 199
Plasma-derived factor replacement, 796, 797*t*
Plasma-derived products, **818–821,** 819*t*
Plasmapheresis, 817
   for cold agglutinin syndrome, 806
   for Guillain-Barré syndrome, 360
   for hemolytic uremic syndrome, 794
   in myasthenia gravis, 366
   for paroxysmal cold hemoglobinuria, 807
   for thrombotic thrombocytopenic purpura, 793
Plastic deformity, in pediatric fractures, 513
Platelet(s), function of, drugs impairing, 792*t,* 794
Platelet count, 791*t*
Platelet disorders, **789–795**
   of decreased platelet production, **789–794**
   functional or qualitative, **794–795**
     conditions associated with, 794, 794*t*
Platelet hypoplasia, 820
Platelet sequestration, thrombocytopenia due to, **794**
Platelet transfusion, **819–820**
   characteristics of products and doses in, 819*t,* 819–820
   for disseminated intravascular coagulation, 802
   for hemoptysis, 654
   for hemostatic abnormalities of renal disease, 800
   for idiopathic thrombocytopenic purpura, 792, 1096
   relative contraindications in, 820
   for von Willebrand disease, 799
Platysma muscle injury, 769
Pleural effusion, **666**
Pleural fluid lactate dehydrogenase levels, 666
Pleural fluid lactate dehydrogenase (LDH)-to-serum LDH ratio, 666
Pleural fluid protein-to-serum protein ratio, 666
Pleural fluid/blood, and respiratory distress/dyspnea, **231–232,** 233*i*
Pleural friction rub, 688
Pleurisy
   chest pain in, **252**
   diagnosis of, 248*t*
   respiratory distress/dyspnea in, 231*t,* **238**
Pleuritic pain
   differential diagnosis of, **246**
   in pleurodynia, 665
Pleurodynia, **665**
   chest pain in, **252**
Pneumastosis cystoides intestinalis, 268
Pneumatic antishock garment
   for hemorrhagic shock, 213
   for intrapelvic hemorrhage, 196
Pneumocentesis, 834
Pneumocephalus, in open skull fracture, 425, 426*i,* 427*i*
Pneumoconioses, 673–674
Pneumocystis carinii pneumonia, 234, 864, 865
Pneumomediastinum, **664–665**
   chest pain in, **252**
   diagnosis of, 248*t*
   in esophageal injury, 461, 665
Pneumonia, **667–668, 832–835**
   abdominal pain in, 1081, 1087*t*
   antibiotic therapy for, 835, 836*t*
   aspiration, 671, 835, 836*t*
   in children, **1058–1059,** 1059*t,* 1060*t,* 1064
   clinical findings in, 668

COPD in, 660, 661
   diagnosis of, 249*t*
   disposition in cases of, 668, 835
   in HIV-infected patients, 864, 865
   in immunocompromised patients, 829
   in infants and children, **832–834,** 836*t*
   in neonates, **832,** 836*t*
   nosocomial, 835, 836*t*
   in older children, **834**
   with pulmonary contusion, 459
   respiratory distress/dyspnea in, 230*t,* **234**
   right lower lobe, diagnosis of, 271*t*
   in sickle cell anemia, 810
   in teenagers and adults, **834–835,** 836*t*
   treatment of, 668, 835
Pneumonic plague, 23*t,* 25–26
Pneumonic tularemia, 24*t,* 26–27
Pneumothorax, **655–656**
   airway management in, 655–656
   arterial gas embolism in, 947, 948
   classification of, 655
   in cystic fibrosis, 673
   definition of, 655
   diagnosis of, 248*t*
   open, **456**
   pneumomediastinum in, 252, 664–665
   primary spontaneous, 655
   respiratory distress/dyspnea in, **229–231,** 230*t,* 232*i*
   secondary spontaneous, 655–656
   stable, 655
   tension, **455–456, 655–656**
     in abdominal trauma, 467
     radiographic findings in, 455, 455*i,* 456*i*
     syncope with, 343
   traumatic, **455–456, 655–656**
   unstable, 655
Pocket site complications, with pacemakers, 709
Poinsettia, toxins in, 1004*t*
Poison hemlock, toxins in, 1004*t*
Poison ivy/oak/sumac, 1018
Poisoning, **963–1011.** *See also specific agent causing*
   acceleration of elimination of poisons, **966–970**
   acetaminophen, **972–973,** 973*i*
   alcohol, **985–987**
   amphetamines, **974–975**
   anticholinergics, **975**
   anticoagulants, **1010–1011**
   antidotes for, 970, 970*t*
   antipsychotics, **1000–1001**
   arsenic, 360–361, 607, 989*t,* **990–991**
   beta-adrenergic blockers, **975–976**
   botulism, 353, **363–364**
   calcium-channel blocking agents, **976–977**
   carbamate, 365
   carbon monoxide, 381, **977–979,** 978*t*
   cardiac glycosides, **979–980**
   caustics, **980–981**
   cholinesterase inhibitors, **998–999**
   cocaine, **981–982**
   and coma, 963–964
   conditions associated with, management of, **970–972**
   corrosives, **980–981,** 981*t*
   cyanide, **982–984**
   decontamination, 964–965
   delayed severe toxicity, **972,** 972*t*
   diagnosis of, 272*t*
   drug-induced methemoglobinemia, **984–985**
   ethanol, **985–986**
   ethylene glycol, 985, **987**
   and gag reflex, 964

heavy metals, **988–991**
history, 964
hydrocarbons, **992–993,** 993*t*
and hyperthermia, **971**
and hypotension, **971**
and hypothermia, **971**
ingested, decontamination, 965
inhalants, **993–994,** 995*t*
inhaled, decontamination, 964
iron, **988**
isoniazid, **994–996**
isopropanol, 985, **987**
lead, 607, **988–989,** 989*t*
and lethargy, 964
life-threatening conditions, immediate management of, **963–964**
lithium, **996–997**
local anesthetics, **981–982**
mercury, 989*t,* **991**
methanol, 607–608, 985, **986–987**
methylxanthines, **1007–1008**
opiates, **997–998**
organophosphates, **998–999**
   clinical findings in, 365, 365*t*
   weakness caused by, 353, **364–366**
phencyclidine, **999–1000**
phenothiazines, **1000–1001**
physical examination, 965, 966*t,* 967*t*
salicylate, **1005–1006**
seafood, 363, **960–962**
and seizures, 963–964
stimulants, **974–975**
theophylline, **1007–1008**
and thermodysregulation, **971**
toxicokinetics, **966–969**
tricyclic antidepressant, **1008–1010,** 1009*i*
warfarin, **1010–1011**
Poisonous mushrooms, **1001–1002,** 1002*t*
Poisonous plants, **1003–1004,** 1003*t,* 1004*t*
Police
   in multicasualty incident/disaster management, 52–53
   patients in custody of, and informed consent, 65
Poliomyelitis, 351, **357**
Polyarthritis, 406–407, **410–413**
Polychromasia, in sickle cell anemia, 808
Polycythemia, **813–814**
   primary, **813**
   secondary, **813–814**
Polycythemia vera, **813**
Polydioxanone sutures (PDS), 582
Polydipsia, psychogenic, hyponatremia in, 895
Polyester sutures, 583
Polyethylene glycol, for burn injuries, 926
Polyglactin sutures (Vicryl), 582
Polyglycolic acid sutures (Dexon), 582
Polymorphic ventricular tachycardia, 694, **702–703**
   electrocardiogram in, 702, 717, 718*i*
Polymyxin B, for eye trauma/disorders, 621, 622*t*
Polyneuritis
   diphtheritic, **362**
   infectious (See Guillain-Barré syndrome)
Polyneuropathies, **359–363**
Polyp(s)
   colonic, **293–295**
   gastrointestinal bleeding with, 290*t,* 293–295
   intestinal, in children, 1089
   nasal, 635*t*
Polypropylene sutures, 583
Polyuria, in central diabetes insipidus, 888
Pons, mass lesions in, 318*i,* 319
Pontine hemorrhage, coma in, **323**

Popliteal artery aneurysm, **781**
Popliteal artery injury
    in knee injuries, 533, 536, 772
    in tibial plateau fractures, 535
Porcupine fish poisoning, 961
Porphyria
    acute intermittent, 361*t*, **361–362**
    diagnosis of, 271*t*
Portal hypertension, 799
Portal-hypertensive gastropathy, gastrointestinal
        bleeding in, 290*t*
Portuguese man-o-war envenomation, **957–958**
Position sense, in spinal cord injury, 497
Positional vertigo, treatment of, 632
Positive airway pressure, for asthma and COPD, 660
Positive end-expiratory pressure (PEEP)
    in acute lung injury, 672
    in pulmonary contusion, 459
Positive-pressure ventilation
    in central venous hypervolemia, 245
    in intubation preparation, 170
    in pneumothorax, 655
Postcoital emergency contraception, **742**
Postconcussion syndrome, 431
Posterior cruciate ligament, stability of, assessment
        of, 537, 538*i*
Posterior malleolar fractures, **541**
Posterior nasal packing, for epistaxis, **133–136**,
        134*i*
Postherpetic neuralgia, 1020
Postictal state, 340
    after syncope, 340
    in cardiac arrest, 342
    coma in, **325**
    confusion in, **395**
    psychosis in, **395**
    treatment during, 335
Post-lumbar puncture headache, 132
Postpartum care, in emergency department delivery,
        747
Postpartum hemorrhage, **747–748**
Postpartum infections, 748–749
Postpoliomyelitis syndrome, weakness caused by,
        357
Postprandial hypoglycemia, 874
Postresuscitation stabilization, **162**
Poststreptococcal reactive arthritis, **411**
Posttraumatic headache, 382, **385**
Postural headache, **384–385**
Postural tone, loss of, in syncope, 335
Potassium
    for alcoholic ketoacidosis, 877
    deficiency of
        in hypokalemia, 898
        in hyponatremia, 895
    in diabetic ketoacidosis, 868, 870–871
    elimination of, for hyperkalemia, 901
    for heat-related cramps, 937
    in hyperglycemic hyperosmolar nonketonic syn-
        drome, 870–871
    normal values, 897*t*
    serum levels of
        disorders of, **897–902**
        in rhabdomyolysis, 368
        and weakness, 367, 367*t*
Potassium chloride, for hypokalemia, 367
    in muscle disease, 355
Potassium chloride wet mount, for vaginitis culture,
        847
Potassium iodide
    for radiation injury, 944
    for thyroid storm, 879

Povidone-iodide, 580
PPD skin test, for tuberculosis, 670
Practolol poisoning, 976
Pralidoxime
    for drug-induced seizures, 971
    for nerve agent exposure, 37
    for organophosphate poisoning, 365, 998
Precautions
    airborne, 25*t*
    droplet, 25*t*
    standard, 25*t*
Prednisolone acetate, for uveitis, 613
Prednisone
    for asthma, 659–660, 1058
    for autoimmune hemolytic anemia, 805
    for Bell palsy, 358
    for cerebral edema, 319*t*
    for COPD, 659–660
    for gouty arthritis, 409
    for idiopathic thrombocytopenic purpura, 791
    for mononucleosis, 816
    for multiple myeloma, 817
    for pemphigus vulgaris, 1017
    for temporal arteritis, 387
    for Waldenström macroglobulinemia, 818
    for zoster, 256
Preeclampsia-eclampsia, **744–745**
    headache in, 381, 382
    mild, 745
    moderate to severe, 745
Preexcitation arrhythmias, **699–700**
    electrocardiogram in, 699–700, 715*i*, 716*i*
Preexisting medical condition, and shock, 196
Pregnancy, **742–743**
    clinical findings in, 742–743
    differential diagnosis of, 743
    discomforts of, **743**
    early symptoms and signs of, 742
    ectopic, 726, 727*t*, **728–733**, 742, 743
        abdominal pain in, 261*t*, **280**, 1087*t*
        diagnosis of, 271*t*
    epistaxis (nosebleed) in, 632
    genital herpes infection in, 852
    headache in, 381, 382
    hypertension in, 381, 382, 744–745
    with intrauterine device in place, 741–742
    laboratory tests in, 742–743
    molar, 736, 742–743
    nausea and vomiting in, 743
    normal, ultrasound of, 729*i*
    normal physiologic changes in, 745
    pelvic pain in, 728, 728*t*
    prevention of
        emergency postcoital, **742**
        in female rape victims, 740
        in sexual abuse victims, 1102
    pyelonephritis in, 843
    respiratory distress/dyspnea in, **239**
    scabies in, 1022
    syncope in, 340, 729
    third-trimester bleeding in, **743–744**
    thrombotic thrombocytopenic purpura in,
        793
    toxemia of, **744–745** (*See also* Preeclampsia-
        eclampsia)
    trauma in, **745–746**
        perimortem cesarean delivery in, 746
    tuberculosis in, 670
    vaginal bleeding in, 726
Pregnancy testing, 742–743
    in abdominal pain, 267
    in ectopic pregnancy, 731, 743

    in pelvic inflammatory disease, 845
    in pelvic pain, 728
Prehn sign, in epididymitis, 754
Prehospital care, 3
Prehospital emergency medical services. *See* Emer-
        gency Medical Services system
Premature atrial contractions, electrocardiogram in,
        717, 719*i*
Premature birth, 746–747
Premature ventricular contractions, electrocardio-
        gram in, 717, 719*i*
Prepyloric ulcers, and gastrointestinal bleeding,
        290*t*
Preseptal cellulitis, **609**
Pressors, for lactic acidosis, 876
Pressure, for hemostasis, 574
Pressure dressings, 588
Pressure garments, 588
Prevention, 4
Priapism, **764**, 810
Primary peritonitis, abdominal pain in, **281**
Prinzmetal (variant) angina, 683–684
Proarrhythmic ventricular arrhythmias, **702**
Probenecid, for pelvic inflammatory disease,
        846*t*
Procainamide
    in advanced life support, 159*t*, 162
    for atrial fibrillation, 698, 700
    contraindications, 1010
    in EMS field treatment, 15
    for paroxysmal supraventricular tachycardia, 697
    and pericarditis, 687
    for preexcitation arrhythmias, 700
    for ventricular fibrillation, 158
    for ventricular tachycardia, 702
Procaine, 577*t*
Prochlorperazine
    for dysentery, 309
    for hyperemesis gravidarum, 743
    for migraine, 388–389
    poisoning/overdose of, 1000–1001
Procidentia, 739
Proctocolitis, in HIV-infected patients, 865
Proctosigmoidoscopy, in lower gastrointestinal
        bleeding, 288
Prodrome, in vasovagal syncope, 342
Professional EMS field personnel, 6–8
Professionalism, 4
Promethazine
    for dysentery, 309
    for hyperemesis gravidarum, 743
    for vertigo, 632
Prone positioning, in acute lung injury, 672
Propane poisoning, 994, 995*t*
Proparacaine
    for corneal abrasion, 620
    for corneal and conjunctival foreign body in-
        juries, 620
    for eye trauma/disorders, 617, 620, 621, 622*t*
    for ocular burn injuries, 616
    for ocular burns, 927
    for tonometry, 623
Propoxyphene
    poisoning/overdose of, 997–998
    proarrhythmic activity of, 702
Propranolol
    for acute intermittent porphyria, 362
    for anoxic spells, 692
    for arrhythmias, 974, 1008
    contraindications to, 1009
    for hypotension, 1008
    for paroxysmal supraventricular tachycardia, 696

Propranolol (*cont.*)
poisoning/overdose of, 976
for thyroid storm, 879
Proprius tendons, 553
Propylthiouracil, for thyroid storm, 879
Prostaglandin inhibitors, for dysmenorrhea, 738
Prostate
boggy or high-riding
in abdominal trauma, 468
in genitourinary trauma, 477, 488
in urethral injuries, 488
displacement of, in urethral injuries, 488, 488*i*
examination of, in oliguria or anuria, 751
Prostatic abscess, 849
Prostatic enlargement, and urinary catheter insertion, 127
Prostatic hypertrophy, bladder outlet obstruction in, 750, 751, 751*t*
Prostatitis, 752, **849**
acute bacterial, **849**
dysuria in, 756, 757*t*
gonococcal, 849
hematuria in, 759, 759*t*
with pyelonephritis, 844
with urethritis, 849
Prosthetic cardiac valves, infection of, 860
Protective clothing, in hazardous material incidents, 53–54, 54*t*, 58
Protein, in synovial fluid analysis, 140
Protein C deficiency, warfarin and, 800
Protein S deficiency, warfarin and, 800
Proteinuria
in multiple myeloma, 817
in preeclampsia-eclampsia, 744–745
Proteus infections
suppurative cholangitis in, 276
urinary tract, in children, 1075
Prothrombin time, 791*t*
Protocols, for EMS field personnel, **16,** 17*i*
Protogonyaulax, 961
Proton-pump inhibitors
for gastritis, 291
for peptic ulcer disease, 290
Protopam. *See* Pralidoxime
Protoporphyrin IX, for acute intermittent porphyria, 362
Proximate cause, 61–62
Pruritus
in HIV-infected patients, 865
in transfusion reaction, 823
vaginal, in mucopurulent cervicitis, 848
Pseudocoarctation, 218
Pseudogout, acute, **409**
Pseudomonas aeruginosa infection
in cystic fibrosis, 673
sinusitis in, 643
Pseudomonas infections
osteomyelitis in, 1079
otitis externa in, 627*t*
in puncture wounds, 597
suppurative cholangitis in, 276
urinary tract, in children, 1075
Pseudotumor cerebri, **386**
Psilocybe, 1002*t*
Psoas shadow, 267, 267*i*
Psoriasis, **1021–1022**
and exfoliative erythroderma, 1014, 1015
pustular, **1016–1017**
Psoriasis vulgaris, 1021
Psoriatic arthritis, **412**
PSVT. *See* Paroxysmal supraventricular tachycardia

Psychiatric disorder(s)
delirium or confusion in, 394*t*, **402–403**
versus organic disorders, 402, 403*t*
syncope in, 346–347
Psychiatric emergencies, **1026–1038.** *See also specific type*
affective disorders, **1033–1034**
agitated patients, **1027–1028**
borderline personality disorder, **1034**
cognitive disorders, **1033**
delirium, **1030–1032**
dementia, **1030**
developmental disorders, **1035**
disposition, **1037–1038**
dissociative states, **1035**
functional causes for, **1032–1035**
history, 1028
homicidal patients, **1030**
hysterical states, **1034–1035**
involuntary procedures/admission, **1038**
laboratory tests, 1029
legal issues of, 67
management of, 1027*i*
mental status examination for, **1028–1029**
organic causes, **1030–1032**
organic *versus* functional cause, 1029
physical examination, 1028
psychogenic fugue, **1035**
psychopharmacotherapy, **1036–1037**
safety check, 1029–1030
schizophrenia, **1033**
screening assessment, **1028–1029**
somatoform disorders, **1034–1035**
suicidal patients, 1029–1030
violent patients, **1027–1028,** 1030
Psychiatric facility, involuntary commitment to, 67
Psychiatric patients, and consent, 66
Psychogenic coma, **329–330**
Psychogenic disorders
dysuria in, 757*t*
hyperventilation, 346, 349
syncope in, 346–347
weakness in, 348–349
Psychogenic fugue, **1035**
Psychogenic hyperventilation
respiratory alkalosis in, 912
respiratory distress/dyspnea in, 231*t*, **239**
Psychogenic polydipsia, hyponatremia in, 895
Psychological support, in multicasualty incidents/disasters, 59
Psychopharmacotherapy, **1036–1037**
Psychosis
confusion in, **402**
interictal and postictal, **395**
in Wernicke encephalopathy, 398, 399
PTLA. *See* Pharyngeal tracheal lumen airway
PTTJV. *See* Percutaneous transtracheal jet ventilation
Ptychodiscus, 961
Pubic lice, 1023
Public access defibrillation (PAD), 155–156
Public safety, in multicasualty incidents/disasters, 52–53
Puerperal mastitis, **748–749**
Puerperal sepsis, 748
Puffer fish poisoning, **961**
Pulmonary agents, as chemical weapons, **38**
Pulmonary angiography, in pulmonary embolism, 661
Pulmonary artery catheterization
in acute lung injury, 672
in intubated patients, 190

Pulmonary artery occlusion pressures, in acute lung injury, 672
Pulmonary aspiration syndrome, **671**
Pulmonary capillary wedge pressure, in acute lung injury, 672
Pulmonary collapse, **229–233,** 230*t*
Pulmonary contusion, **216,** 458–459
Pulmonary disease/disorders
chest pain in, 252–253
chronic obstructive (*See* Chronic obstructive pulmonary disease (COPD))
interstitial, 673–674
Pulmonary edema, **685**
acute high-altitude, **949–950**
cardiogenic, 226
cardiogenic shock in, 203
chest pain in, 243
delirium in, 1032
noncardiac, 226
respiratory distress/dyspnea in, 230*t*, **234**
severe, 226*i*, **226–227**
Pulmonary embolism, **661–664,** 784
acute, **661–664**
anticoagulation therapy for, 664, 682
chest pain in, 243*t*, 244
clinical findings in, 662–663, 681–682
D-dimer assay in, 662–663
deep venous thrombosis and, 662, 663, 782, 783, 784
delirium in, 1032
diagnosis of, 249*t*
diagnostic imaging of, 663
disposition in cases of, 664, 682
laboratory findings in, 662–663
management of, 244
massive, 661
syncope with, **344,** 662
in myocardial infarction, **681–682**
obstructive shock in, 197, 203–204
pleuritic pain in, 246
predisposing conditions for, 662, 662*t*
pulmonary angiography as gold standard in, 663
radiographic findings in, 662
repeated small, **238**
respiratory distress/dyspnea in, 231*t*, **237–238**
respiratory support in, 663
septic abortion and, 735
size of, 662
surgical treatment of, 664
symptoms and signs of, 662
thrombolytic therapy for, 664, 682
treatment of, 663–664, 682
ventilation-perfusion (V/Q) scans in, 661–663
Pulmonary emergencies, **653–674.** *See also specific types*
acute lung injury, **671–673**
acute respiratory distress syndrome, **671–673**
asthma, **656–661**
atelectasis, **666–667**
bronchitis, **667–668**
chronic obstructive pulmonary disease, **656–661**
cystic fibrosis, **673**
hemoptysis, **653–654**
interstitial pulmonary disease, **673–674**
life-threatening problems in, immediate management of, **653–664**
pleural effusion, **666**
pleurodynia, **666**
pneumomediastinum, **664–665**
pneumonia, **667–668**
pneumothorax, **655–656**
pulmonary aspiration syndrome, **671**

pulmonary embolism, **661–664**
specific conditions in, emergency management of, **664–674**
subcutaneous emphysema, **664–665**
tuberculosis, **669–670**
Pulmonary fibrosis, **227–228**
respiratory distress/dyspnea in, **237**
Pulmonary glanders, 29
Pulmonary hypertension
chest pain in, **252–253**
diagnosis of, 248*t*
pediatric, **693**
with pulmonary embolism, 661
syncope in, **344**
Pulmonary infections
in cystic fibrosis, 673
in HIV-infected patients, 864
septic shock in, treatment of, 828*t*
Pulmonary medications, in EMS field treatment, 15
Pulmonary melioidosis, 29
Pulmonary neurosis, **239**
Pulmonary stenosis, 691, 692, 693
syncope with, **344**
Pulmonary toilet, for intubated patient, 189
Pulmonary tuberculosis, **669–670**
emergency room goals in management of, 669
in infants, children, and adolescents, 670
latent, 670
multidrug-resistant, 669, 670
in pregnancy, 670
reporting requirements for, 670
respiratory isolation for, 670
Pulmonary vascular disease
respiratory distress/dyspnea in, 231*t*, **237–238**
syncope in, **344**
Pulmonary vascular injuries, **771**
Pulpitis, diagnosis and treatment of, 651*t*
Pulse(s)
in compartment syndrome, 512
in conscious patient with history of syncope, 335–337
in diarrhea or vomiting, 302
in vascular trauma, 768
Pulse oximetry
in abdominal trauma, 467
in acute lung injury, 672
in children, 1051
in chronic obstructive pulmonary disease, 658
in coma, 313, 317
in head injuries, 422
in hemoptysis, 654
in intubated patient, 189–190
in pleural effusion, 666
in pneumonia, 668
in pulmonary aspiration syndrome, 671
in respiratory distress assessment, 224
in septic shock, 825
in spinal cord injury, 493
Pulseless electrical activity (PEA), 158
Pulseless ventricular tachycardia, 157–158
in children, 164
Pulsus paradoxus, 689
in cardiac tamponade, 202
Pump failure, and shock, 197
Puncture wounds, 575, **597**
and osteomyelitis, in children, 1079
Punitive damages, 62
Pupillary function, assessment of, 600
Pupillary reflexes
in head injuries, 422
in stroke patients, 371

Pupils
in basilar artery thrombosis, 323
in coma, 316
in embolic occlusion, 323
in lightning injuries, 941
in multiply injured patient, 212
in narcotic overdose, 327
pinpoint
in coma, **314–315**, 316
factitious, 314–315
Purified poloxamer 188, for sickle cell crisis, 809
Purified protein derivative (PPD) skin test, for tuberculosis, 670
Purpura, in thrombocytopenia, 789
Purpura fulminans, 801
Pustular psoriasis, **1016–1017**
Pyelogram
intravenous (*See* Intravenous pyelogram)
retrograde, in ureteral injuries, 484–486
Pyelonephritis, **843–844**
abdominal pain in, 263, **279**, 1087*t*
diagnosis of, 271*t*
treatment of, 842*t*, 844
Pylephlebitis, 268
Pyloric channel ulcers, gastrointestinal bleeding in, 290*t*
Pyloric stenosis
abdominal pain in, 1086*t*
in newborns, 1084
Pyosalpinx, 845
Pyridostigmine, for myasthenia gravis, 366*t*
Pyridoxine (Vitamin B₆)
for drug-induced seizures, 971

Q fever, as biologic weapon, 24*t*, **28**
QT prolongation syndrome, 702–703
Quadriceps muscles, 533
Quadriceps tendon, 533
rupture of, 539
Quadriplegia, shock and, 196, 207
Quetiapine, 1037
Quinidine
for atrial fibrillation, 698
contraindications to, 1010
thrombocytopenia induced by, 793
Quinidinelike drugs, contraindications to, 1010
Quinsy, 645–646

Rabeprazole, for peptic ulcer disease, 290
Rabies immune globulin
equine, 593
USP, 592–593
Rabies immunization, 592*i*, 592–593, 593*i*
active, 593
passive, 592–593
Rabies infection, 590–593
management of patients at high risk for, 592–593
prophylaxis against, 592*t*, 592–593, 593*t*
risk of, 590–592, 591*i*
Raccoon eyes, 440, 449
Radial artery puncture, **96–98**, 97*i*
Radial gutter splint, 525
Radial head fractures, **522**
Radial head subluxation, **523**
Radial nerve, innervation of hand by, 552, 554
Radial nerve block, 552*i*, 578, 578*i*
Radial nerve injury, 358, 554
in forearm fractures, 524
in hand trauma, 554, **569**
in humerus fractures, 519
motor testing for, 554, 569, 570*i*

sensory testing for, 554, 555*i*, 569, 571*i*
in shoulder dislocation, 518–519
Radial nerve palsy, **358**
Radiation accidents, **45**
Radiation exposure
management of, 58–59
tolerance to, 943
Radiation injuries, **943–944**
nuclear weapons and, **20–22**
Radiation sickness, 944
Radiation therapy, for spinal cord metastases, 355
Radio communication, for EMS communications, 16
Radioactive particles, types of, 21
Radiographic studies. *See specific radiographic modalities*
Radiologic examinations
abdominal, 267–270
in diarrhea and vomiting, 302
in multiply injured patient, 212
Radionuclide scan, in testicular torsion and epididymitis, 755
Railway accidents, 45
Rales
in acute lung injury, 672
in children, 1051
in congestive heart failure, 685
in interstitial pulmonary disease, 674
in pneumonia, 667, 835
Ramsay Hunt syndrome, herpes zoster infection and, 1020
Ranitidine
for allergic reactions, 638*t*
for anaphylactic shock, 207
for scrombroid poisoning, 961
for urticaria, 1013
Rape, **739–741**
female victims of, 739–740
counseling for, 740
evaluation of, 739–740
evidence from, 739–740
follow-up for, 740
genital injuries in, 491, 492, 737
history of, 739
initial steps in care of, 739
laboratory testing in, 740
management of, 739–740
pelvic examination in, 740
physical examination of, 740
prevention of infectious diseases in, 740
prevention of pregnancy in, 740
prevention of STDs in, 740
reporting incident, 740
treatment of, 740
male victims of, 740–741
clinical findings in, 740–741
counseling for, 741
evaluation of, 740–741
evidence from, 741
history of, 741
initial steps in care of, 740
laboratory tests in, 741
management of, 740–741
physical examination in, 741
prevention of STDs in, 741
reporting of incident, 741
treatment of, 741
physician's responsibilities in, 739
Rapid plasma reagin (RPR) test, for syphilis, 853
Rapid sequence intubation (RSI)
in asthma and COPD, 660
in neck injury, 435
in spinal cord injury, 494

Rapid-sequence intubation (RSI), 180–182, 182*t*
  in asthma, 188
  in children, 187
  in multiply injured patient, 210–211
  in trauma patients, 188
Rash, smallpox and, 30
Reactivation tuberculosis, 669–670
Reactive hypoglycemia, 874
Reassessment, 4
Rebound tenderness, 265
Receiving hospitals
  duty to provide emergency care, 63
  for EMS systems, 10
Receptive aphasia, 401
Recombinant factor replacement, 796, 797*t*
Recombinant human activated protein C (RhAPC),
    for septic shock, 827
Recompression
  for arterial gas embolism, 948
  for decompression sickness, 947
Rectal examination
  in abdominal pain, 265–266
  in abdominal trauma, 468
  in back pain, 415
  in diarrhea, 302
  in gastrointestinal bleeding, 285, 288
  in genitourinary trauma, 477, 488
  in orthopedic emergencies, 511
  in pelvic fractures, 530
  in prostatitis, 849
  in urethral injuries, 488
  in vomiting, 302
Rectal infection, gonococcal, 851
Rectal ulcer, solitary, gastrointestinal bleeding in,
    295
Rectus abdominis muscle, spasm of, 264
Recurrent laryngeal nerve injury, 437*i*, 439
Red blood cell transfusion, **818–819**
  for autoimmune hemolytic anemia, 805
  characteristics of products and doses in, 818,
    819*t*
  for hemostatic abnormalities of liver disease, 799
  for iron-deficiency anemia, 804
  irradiated cells in, 819
  leukocyte-treated cells in, 819
  massive, 821
  for paroxysmal cold hemoglobinuria, 807
  for thrombotic thrombocytopenic purpura, 793
  washed cells in, 819
Red blood cell values
  in anemia, 802
  normal, 803*t*
Red cell distribution width (RDW), in anemia, 804
Red eye, evaluation of, **600**, 601*t*, 601*i*
Reduction
  of fractures and dislocations, **511**, 512*i*
    elbow, 523, 523*i*
    femoral shaft, 533
    hip, 531, 532, 532*i*
    humerus, 521
    lunate, 525
    pelvic, 531
    procedural sedation for, 515
    shoulder, 519, 521*i*
    sternoclavicular joint, 516
    TMJ, 652
  of fractures or dislocations, nasal, 448, 448*i*
Referred pain, 1080
Reflex(es)
  brainstem, in spinal cord injury, 502
  in coma, 316
  deep, 505*t*

spinal, in spinal cord injury, 502, 505*t*
  superficial, 505*t*
  visceral, 505*t*
Refusal to consent, 66
Regional anesthesia, 578
  examples of, 578
  for facial surgery, 579, 579*i*
  for hand surgery, 578, 578*i*, 579*i*
  pitfalls of, 578
Reglan. *See* Metoclopramide
Reiter syndrome, **412**
Religion, and refusal to consent, 66
Remeron. *See* Mirtazapine
Renal colic. *See also* Urolithiasis
  abdominal pain in, 261*t*, 278–279
  diagnosis of, 271*t*
  rectus abdominis spasm in, 264
Renal disease
  hemostatic abnormalities in, **800**
  hyperkalemia in, 901
  oliguria or anuria in, 750
Renal dysfunction
  in heart failure, 684, 686
  in sickle cell anemia, 810
Renal failure, in septic shock, 827
Renal function tests
  in abdominal pain, 267
  in heart failure, 686
Renal infarct
  in abdominal pain, **279**
  diagnosis of, 271*t*
Renal infections, **843–844**
Renal injuries, **481–484**
  in abdominal trauma, **472–473**
  blunt, 479, 481
  in children, 479
  classification and grading of, 481, 482*i*–483*i*
  clinical findings in, 484
  evaluation of, guidelines for, 479
  laboratory findings in, 484
  penetrating, 479, 481
  special examinations and procedures in,
    477–481
  surgical exploration in, indications for, 484
  symptoms and signs of, 484
  treatment of, 484
    guidelines for, 479
Renal insufficiency, in hypermagnesemia, 907
Renal sodium conservation, in hyponatremia, 894
Renal sodium wasting, in hyponatremia, 894
Renal stones, 762*t*
Renin, in heart failure, 684
Replantation surgery, 511, 576, 595–596
  contraindications to, 595
  hand, 568–569
Reportable events, **68–69**
Reporting, of child abuse, 68
Res ipsa loquitur, **62**
Respiratory acidosis, **909–910**, 910*t*
  acute, 910
  chronic, 910
    in chronic bronchitis and emphysema, 658
  and metabolic acidosis, **914**
  and metabolic alkalosis, **914**
Respiratory alkalosis, **912**
  acute, 912
  chronic, 912
  in hyperventilation, 346
  and metabolic acidosis, **914**
  and metabolic alkalosis, **914**
  in septic shock, 825
Respiratory arrest, in children, 1051

Respiratory distress. *See also* Dyspnea
  acute syndrome of, **671–673** (*See also* Acute res-
    piratory distress syndrome (ARDS))
  adequacy of oxygenation and, 222–224
  airway disease, **235–237**
  in asthma, 657
  in bronchiolitis, 835
  in cardiac arrest, 224
  chest wall defects, **229**
  in children, **1050–1059**
  in chronic obstructive pulmonary disease, 656
  diagnostic evaluation of, **228–229**
  in flail chest, 458
  in hemothorax, 456–457
  life-threatening problems, immediate manage-
    ment of, 222–228, 223*i*
  in loss of functional lung parenchyma, **233–235**
  in pneumothorax, 455, 655
  in pulmonary collapse, **229–233**
  in pulmonary contusion, 459
  in pulmonary vascular disease, **237–238**
  severity of, assessment of, 222
  in tracheobronchial injury, 463
Respiratory effort, patients with
  airway management in, 167
  intubation of, 167, 169*t*
Respiratory failure
  in children, 1051
  in delirium or confusion, 393
  impending, in asthma, 657
Respiratory pattern, in coma, 316
Respiratory status, in head injuries, 422
Respiratory syncytial virus (RSV) infection
  bronchiolitis in, 835, 837, 1056
  pharyngitis in, in children, 1073
Respiratory tract, radiation injury of, 944
Respondeat superior, 63
Rest, for acute high-altitude pulmonary edema, 949
Restraints
  chemical, 1028
  physical, 1028
  in psychiatric emergencies, 67
  for violent/agitated patients, 66, 1028
Resuscitation. *See also* Cardiopulmonary resuscita-
    tion; Fluid replacement/resuscitation
  in diabetic ketoacidosis, 870
  documentation of progress, 200
  family presence during, 146–147
  in frostbite, 935
  in hyperglycemic hyperosmolar nonketonic syn-
    drome, 870
  indices of, 199–200, 199*t*
  in multiply injured patient, **212–213**
  in newborn, 1096–1097, 1098*i*
  in shock, 199–200, 199*t*
  termination of, **162–163**
Reteplase (r-PA), for myocardial infarction,
    677–678
Reticulocyte count
  in anemia, 803–804
  in sickle cell anemia, 808
Retina
  abnormal, 602
  examination of, 600
  inability to visualize, 600
Retinal artery occlusion, 602, **605**
Retinal detachment, 602, **607**
  vitreous hemorrhage in, 613
Retinal hemorrhage, 602, **614**
  systemic conditions associated with, 614*t*
Retinal vein(s), boxcar appearance, in central retinal
    artery occlusion, 605

Retinal vein occlusion, 602, **614–615**
Retinitis, cytomegalovirus, 865
Retraction nystagmus, 316
Retrobulbar neuritis, 615
Retrograde angiography, complications of, **786**
Retrograde cystogram
    in bladder injuries, 473, 481, 486–488
    computed tomography for, 481
Retrograde intubation, 178
Retrograde pyelogram, in ureteral injuries, 484–486
Retrograde urethrogram
    in genitourinary trauma, 477, 480–481
    in penile rupture, 491
    in urethral injury, 477, 480–481, 488, 489*i*, 490
Retroperitoneal bleeding
    in hemorrhagic shock, 213
    in shock, 195, 200
Retroperitoneal hemorrhage
    abdominal pain in, **281–282**
    diagnosis of, 271*t*
Retroperitoneal injury, 476, 484
Retropharyngeal abscess, 635, 637*i*, 639*t*
Retrosternal discomfort, differential diagnosis,
    246
Revascularization, in stroke prevention, 377
Revised Trauma Score, 208
Rewarming
    active external methods, 933
    active internal (core) methods, 933
    for frostbite, 935
    for hypothermia, 933
Reye syndrome, **400**
Rh disease, 807
Rhabdomyolysis, **368**
    causes of, 368, 368*t*
    extremity trauma and, 220
    phencyclidine overdose and, 1000
RhAPC, for septic shock, 827
Rhegmatogenous retinal detachment, 607
Rheumatic fever
    arthritis in, **411**
    Jones criteria for, 411, 411*t*
    strep throat and, 636
Rheumatism, nonarticular, 406, 406*t*, **413–414**
Rheumatoid arthritis, **411–412**
    infection in, 837
Rhinitis
    diagnosis and treatment of, 635*t*
    epistaxis (nosebleed) in, 632
Rhinoorbitocerebral mucormycosis, 606
Rhinorrhea
    in facial trauma, 440
    in frontal sinus fractures, 449
    in headache, 382
Rhinovirus infection, pharyngitis in, in children,
    1073
Rhododendron species, toxins in, 1004*t*
Rh₀(D) immune globulin, in spontaneous abortion,
    734
Rhonchi
    in congestive heart failure, 685
    in pneumonia, 667
Rhus dermatitis, **1017–1018**
Rib, fractures of, **464**
    chest pain in, 250*t*, **254**
    in child abuse, 515, 1099
    pleuritic pain in, 238
Ribavirin
    for bronchiolitis, 837
    for hemorrhagic fever, 31
RICE treatment, for ankle sprains, 543
Richter scale, 42

Ricin
    as biologic weapon, 33*t*, **34**
    in poisonous plants, 1003, 1004*t*
Ricinus communis, toxins in, 1004*t*
Rickettsia rickettsii infection, **858–859,** 1082*t*–1083*t*
Rifampin
    for brucellosis, 24*t*, 28
    for meningococcemia prophylaxis, 858
    for tuberculosis, 670
Rift Valley fever, 31*t*
Right-to-left shunts, 691
Rigidity, nuchal
    in meningitis, 384, 830–831
    in poliomyelitis, 357
Rigors, and abdominal pain, 263
Ring finger, clawing of, in ulnar nerve injury, 570*i*
Ring removal, in hand trauma, 572
Ringworm, 1023
Rinne test, for hearing loss, 629–630, 630*i*
Risperidone, 1037
    poisoning/overdose of, 1001
Ritonavir, side effects of, 865*t*
Rizatriptan, for migraine, 389
Rocephin. *See* Ceftriaxone
Rocket fuel. *See* Phencyclidine
Rocky Mountain spotted fever, **858–859,**
    1082*t*–1083*t*
Rocuronium
    adverse effects and precautions for, 183
    in intubation, 183
Rolando fracture, 526–527
Romano-Ward syndrome, 702
Root canal pain, diagnosis and treatment of, 651*t*
Rosary bean, toxins in, 1004*t*
Roseola, 1082*t*–1083*t*
Rotation-adduction technique, for reduction of
    shoulder dislocations, 519
Rotator cuff injuries, **518**
Roth spots, in infective endocarditis, 860
RSI. *See* Rapid-sequence intubation
RSV. *See* Respiratory syncytial virus
Rubella, 1082*t*–1083*t*
    in infants, 1062
Rubeola virus, 1082*t*–1083*t*
Rule of fives, 920
Rule of nines, 920, 921*t*
Rumack-Matthew nomogram, 973, 973*i*
Runaway pacemaker, 709–710
Ruptured abdominal aortic aneurysm, shock in, 196

SA Wenckebach, 704, 720
Saccular aneurysm, and subarachnoid hemorrhage,
    372
Sacrum, fractures of, 507
Saddle anesthesia, in epidural compression syn-
    drome, 419
Safety, in psychiatric emergencies, **1029–1030**
Sag sign, in posterior cruciate ligament, 537, 538*i*
Salicylates
    poisoning/overdose of, 967*t*, **1005–1006**
        hyperthermia in, 971
        seizures induced by, 971
Saline
    nebulized, for croup, 647
    for wound irrigation and cleansing, 580
Saline wet mount, for vaginitis culture, 847
Salmonella infection
    dysentery in, 307*t*
    gastroenteritis in, in children, 1077
    reactive arthritis in, 412

Salpingitis, 845
    abdominal pain in, 261*t*, 263, **280,** 1087*t*
    diagnosis of, 271*t*
    gonococcal, 851
    pelvic pain in, 727*t*
    tubo-ovarian abscess in, 727*t*
Salt replacement, for heat-related cramps, 937
Salter-Harris classification, of growth plate injuries,
    513, 513*i*
Sambucus, toxins in, 1004*t*
Saphenous vein, identification of, 94*i*
Saphenous vein cutdown, **94–95**
Saquinavir, side effects of, 865*t*
Sarcoidosis, 673–674
Sarcoptes scabei, 1022
Sarin (nerve agent), 37
Saxitoxin poisoning, 363
Scabies, **1022**
Scalded skin syndrome, 854–855
    staphylococcal, **1015,** 1084*t*–1085*t*
Scaling exponent, of defibrillation, 165
Scalp
    examination of, in headache patients, 382–383
    hematoma of, **424**
    lacerations of, **423–424,** 425
Scalp tenderness, in headache, 383, 387, 388
Scalp vein (butterfly) needle, for peripheral venous
        catheterization, **81–82,** 83*i,* 84*i*
Scalp wound hemorrhage, 211
Scaphoid fracture, 525–526
Scapholunate dislocations, **525**
Scapula fractures, **517–518**
Scar(s), wound closure and, 585, 594
Scarlet fever, 1082*t*–1083*t*
Scene organization
    in hazardous material incidents, 54, 55*i*
    in multicasualty incidents/disasters, 49, 49*i*
Schiotz tonometer, 600
Schizophrenia, 402, **1033**
Sciatic nerve block, 578
Sciatica, **418–419**
    versus lumbosacral strain, 418
    neurologic findings in, 418, 418*t*
Scintigraphy, technetium red cell, in lower gastroin-
        testinal bleeding, 289
Sclerotherapy, in esophageal varices, 292
Scopolamine
    for eye trauma/disorders, 622*t*
    poisoning, 967*t*, 975
    for vertigo, 632
Scorpion bite, weakness with, 354
Scorpion fish sting, **958–959**
Scorpion stings, **955–956**
Scotoma, central, 600
    in optic neuritis, 615
Scrombroid poisoning, 305*t*, **960–961**
Scrotal injuries, 490, 491, 492
    pain in, 752, 753*t*
Scrotal mass lesion, painless, **755–756**
    causes of, diagnostic clues to, 756*t*
Scrotal pain, **752–755**
    acute, diagnostic clues to causes of, 753*t*
    in testicular torsion, 752–755, 753*t,* 763
Sea snake bite, 957
Sea urchin sting, **959–960**
Seafood poisoning, **960–962**
    paralytic, **363**
Seatbelt sign, in abdominal trauma, 468, 469–470
Seawater, for jellyfish stings, 958
SEB. *See* Staphylococcal enterotoxin B
Sebaceous cyst, infected, in ear, 627*t*
Second wave phenomenon, disasters and, 46

Secretions, suctioning, in spinal cord injury, 494
Security, in multicasualty incidents/disasters, 58
Sedation
    in multiply injured patient, 210
    in pediatric patient, 1040–1044
    procedural, in orthopedic emergencies, 515
    in violent/agitated patients, 1028
Sedative(s)
    for delirium tremens, 397–398
    for migraine, 388
    for pain control, in head injuries, 423
    for tension headache, 388
Sedative-hypnotics
    poisoning/overdose of, **1006–1007**
    withdrawal from
        delirium or confusion in, **396–398**
        drugs causing, 396*t*
See-saw nystagmus, 316
Seizures, **340–341**
    acidosis in, 334
    active, immediate measures for patient with,
        332–334
    acute onset, causes of, 337*t*
    in alcohol withdrawal, 341, 396, **397**, 398
    assessment of, 333*i*, 334*t*
    associated illnesses, 964
    in cardiac arrest, 342
    in children, **1059–1062**
    clinical findings in, 340–341
    in coma, 325
    delirium or confusion in, 394*t*, **395, 1032**
    deposition of cases of, 341
    drug treatment of, 336*t*, 341
    drug-induced, 971
    emergency evaluation of, 333*i*, 334*t*, 335
    general considerations in, 340
    in head injuries, 423
    headache in, 379
    in hyperthermia, 971
    in hypoglycemia, 334
    in intubated patient, 189
    in isoniazid poisoning, 994–996
    life-threatening problems in, immediate manage-
        ment of, **332–335**
    in meningitis, 335, 384
    in organophosphate poisoning, 365
    in poisoning, 963–964, 964
    in preeclampsia-eclampsia, 744–745
    reporting of, 69
    in status epilepticus, **332–335**, 340–341
    in stimulant overdose, 974
    in stroke, treatment of, 369
    in subarachnoid hemorrhage, 369, 373
    in theophylline overdose, 1008
    trauma or injury in, 341
        protection from, 335
    treatment during postictal state, 335
    in tricyclic antidepressant overdose, 1009
    underlying causes of, search for, 335
Selective serotonin reuptake inhibitors, 1037
    poisoning/overdose of, 967*t*, 1037
Selenium sulfide, for tinea, 1024
Self-harm, and restraint use, 67
Sellick maneuver
    in basic life support, 151
    positive-pressure ventilation and, 170, 172*i*
Sengstaken-Blakemore tube, insertion of, **104–107,**
        105*i*, 106*i*
Sensation
    in hand trauma, 550–551, 555–556
    in spinal cord injury, 497–502, 503*i*, 504*i*, 505*t*
Sensorcaine. See Bupivacaine

Sensorimotor hearing loss, in temporal bone frac-
        ture, **451**
Sensorineural hearing loss, 629
    testing for, 629–630, 630*i*
Sensory dysfunction, in stroke patients, 371
Sensory testing
    in hand trauma, 550–551, 555–556, 569, 571*i*
    in spinal cord injury, 497–502, 503*i*, 504*i*, 505*t*
Sepsis
    definition of, 204
    fungal, 825
    puerperal, **748**
Sepsis syndrome, defining features of, 825
Septal hematoma, 440, 448
    drainage of, 448
Septic abortion, **735–736**
    pelvic pain in, 727*t*
Septic arthritis, 407, 407*t*, **409–410, 837–838**
    antibiotic therapy for, 410, 838, 838*t*
    in children, **1078–1079**, 1078*t*
    in disseminated gonococcemia, 861
    puncture wounds and, 597
Septic embolization, 238
Septic meningitis, 831
Septic shock, 197, **204–205, 825–827**, 828*t*
    causes of, 191–193
    in children, 1047
    in meningococcemia, 858
    septic abortion and, 735
Septic thrombophlebitis, 783
Septicemic glanders, 29
Septicemic melioidosis, 29
Septicemic plague, 23*t*, 25
Septra. See Trimethoprim-sulfamethoxazole
Serotonin syndrome, 967*t*
Serratia infection, suppurative cholangitis in, 276
Sertraline, 1037
Serum amylase, and abdominal pain, 266
Serum calcium concentration disorders, **902–905**
Serum magnesium concentration disorders,
        906–908
Serum phosphorus concentration disorders,
        905–906
Serum potassium concentration disorders, **897–902**
Serum sickness, botulinum antitoxin and, 364
Serum sodium concentration disorders, **891–897**
Sesamoid fractures, **547**
Severe pulmonary edema, 226*i*, **226–227**
Severe storms, **43**
Sexual abuse, of children, 1079, **1100–1102**, 1101*t*
Sexual assault
    female genital injuries in, 491, 492, 737
    rape, **739–741**
    reporting of, 68
Sexually transmitted diseases (STDs), **850–854.** See
        also specific type
    in child abuse, 1100–1102, 1101*t*
    diarrhea and vomiting in, 301
    prevention of, in rape victims, 740, 741
Shaking, and head injuries, 1099
Shellfish poisoning, paralytic, 305*t*, **363, 961–962**
Shigella infection
    dysentery in, 307*t*
    gastroenteritis in, 303
        in children, 1077
    reactive arthritis in, 412
Shingles. See Herpes zoster
Shock, **191–207.** See also specific type
    in abdominal pain, 259
    in abdominal aortic aneurysm rupture, 777–778
    anaphylactic, 197, **206–207**
        in children, 1047

    in aortic dissection, 779–780
    in cardiac tamponade, 457
    cardiogenic (See Cardiogenic shock)
    causes of, 191–193, 193*t*, 197
        determination of, **195–197**
    in chest pain, 240, 242–243
    in chest trauma, 454, 455
    in children, **1047–1048**
    classification of, 193–194, 193*t*
    compensated, 194
    decompensated, 194
    in delirium or confusion, treatment of, 393
    diagnosis of, 191
    in diarrhea, **296–297**
    distributive, 193*t*, 194, **204–207**
    electric, **941–942**
    emergency treatment of, **197–207**
    in face or neck trauma, **436–437**
    in head injuries, 422
    in hemoptysis, 654
    hemorrhagic (See Hemorrhagic shock)
    hypovolemic (See Hypovolemic shock)
    immediate management of, **191–195**, 192*i*
    mortality rate, 191
    in multiply injured patient, 211
    in myocardial infarction, 675, **679–680**
        differential diagnosis of, 679, 680*t*
    neurogenic (See Neurogenic shock)
    obstructive (See Obstructive shock)
    in penetrating chest trauma, 466
    persistent, causes of, 200
    physical diagnosis of, 194
    in postpartum hemorrhage, 747
    in pulmonary embolism, 661, 664
    recurrent, causes of, 200
    in renal injury, 484
    resuscitation for, effectiveness of, 199–200, 199*t*
    septic (See Septic shock)
    severity of, determination of, 194
    signs of, 194
    in spinal cord injury, 494–495
    in tension pneumothorax, 455
    in trauma, **195–196,** 211
    treatment of, 194–195
    in vaginal bleeding, abnormal, 725–726
    in vascular trauma, 767, 771
    in visceral (intestinal) ischemia, 776
    in vomiting, **296–297**
    without history of trauma, approach to,
        196–197
Shotgun blast injuries, 594–595
Shoulder
    arthrocentesis of, 136, 137–138, 138*i*
    dislocations of, **518–519**
        radiographic findings in, 519, 520*i*
        reduction of, 519, 521*i*
    nonarticular rheumatism in, 406*t*
    pain in, 263
Shoulder girdle injuries, **516–519**
SIADH. See Inappropriate secretion of antidiuretic
        hormone
Sick sinus syndrome, 703, **704**
Sickle cell anemia/disease, **808–811**
    in children, 1079, **1093–1094**, 1095*t*
    crisis in, 808–811
    emergencies in, 808, 808*t*
    hematuria in, 759*t*
    osteomyelitis in, 1079
    septic arthritis in, 1079
Sickle cell gene, 808
Sickle cell trait, 808
SIDS. See Sudden infant death syndrome

Sigmoid diverticulitis, in abdominal examination, 265
Silicone ointment, for immersion syndrome, 936
Silicosis, 674
Silk sutures, 582
Silver nitrate, for cauterization
  of epistaxis, 633
  of wounds, 574
Silver nitrate-tipped sticks, for epistaxis, 135
Silver sulfadiazine (Silvadene)
  for burn injuries, 566
  for wounds, 589
Simple asphyxiants, 994, 995t
Sinequan. See Doxepin
Sinoatrial block, **704**
  first-degree, 704
  second-degree, 704
  second-degree, Mobitz type I, electrocardiogram in, 720, 720i
  second-degree, Mobitz type II, 704
  third-degree, 704
Sinus arrest, **704**
Sinus arrhythmia, electrocardiogram in, 712, 713i
Sinus bradycardia, **703–704**
  in children, 1050t
  electrocardiogram in, 703–704, 712, 713i
Sinus rhythm, electrocardiogram in, 712, 712i
Sinus tachycardia, **695**
  in children, 1050t
  electrocardiogram in, 695, 712, 712i
Sinuses
  disorders of, **643–645**
  examination of, in headache patients, 382
  transillumination of, 643
Sinusitis, **643–645**
  chronic, 643
  in immunocompromised patients, 643
  intracranial extension of, 645
  and orbital cellulitis, 606
  and periorbital cellulitis, 1074–1075
  prophylaxis against, with nasal packing for epistaxis, 633
  radiographic findings in, 643, 644i
SIRS. See Systemic inflammatory response syndrome
Sitz baths
  for epididymitis, 850
  for prostatitis, 849
6-hour limit, for wound closure, 575
Sjögren syndrome, conjunctivitis in, 610
SJS. See Stevens-Johnson syndrome
Skeletal trauma, in child abuse, 1099
Skier's thumb, 529
Skin
  cleansing of, 73
  decontamination of, 965
  examination of
    in headache patients, 382
    in stroke patients, 370
  frostbite of, 567, 642
  hand, 551
  injuries of, in genitourinary trauma, **492**
  preparation of, **73–74**
  radiation injury of, 943
  sterilization of, 73–74
  suturing and closure of, 585
Skin antimicrobials, 580
Skin cleansers, 580
Skin disinfectants, 580
Skin disorders
  conjunctivitis in, 610
  in HIV-infected patients, 865
  in sickle cell anemia, 811

Skin infection, **854–857**
  septic shock in, treatment of, 828t
Skin injuries, genital, 492
Skin lesions, in child abuse, 1100t
Skin tests, for tuberculosis, 670
Skull fractures, **424–425**
  basilar, 219, **425**, 449–450
  closed, **424**
    computed tomography of, 425, 426i, 427i
  depressed, **425**
    computed tomography of, 425, 427i
  open, **424–425**
Sleep, manic states and, 1034
Sling(s)
  for elevation of wounds, 588
  for hand injuries, 557
  for humerus fractures, 520, 521i
Slit lamp examination, 600
Small bowel foreign body, in children, **1092**
Small finger
  clawing of, in ulnar nerve injury, 570i
  extensor muscles of, 553
Smallpox, as biologic weapon, **29–30**
Small-vessel occlusion, acute peripheral ischemia due to, **774**
Smith fracture, 524
Smoke inhalation, **917–929**, 922
  evaluation of, **920–923**
  life-threatening problems and, immediate management of, **917–920**, 918i
  mechanism of injury, 923–924
  treatment of, **923–925**
Smoking
  and chronic bronchitis, 656, 657
  and chronic obstructive pulmonary disease, 656
  and emphysema, 656
Snake bites, 354, **951–952**
Sniffling position, 167, 169i
Snow blindness, 617
Soaps, ionic, contraindicated for wound cleansing, 580
Sodium
  in diabetic ketoacidosis, 868
  excessive intake of, in hypernatremia, 896
  in hyperglycemic hyperosmolar nonketonic syndrome, 869–870
  serum concentration disorders of, **891–897**
Sodium bicarbonate. See Bicarbonate
Sodium channel blockers, proarrhythmic activity of, 702
Sodium chloride, for hypovolemic shock, 198
Sodium iopanoate, for thyroid storm, 879
Sodium ipodate, for thyroid storm, 879
Sodium nitrate, for hydrogen sulfide poisoning, 994
Sodium nitrite, for cyanide poisoning, 40, 983, 983t
Sodium nitroprusside, for hypertensive intracerebral hemorrhage, 321
Sodium polystyrene sulfonate, for lithium overdose, 997
Sodium replacement, for hypernatremia, 897
Sodium thiosulfate
  for cyanide exposure, 40
  for cyanide poisoning, 983, 983t
Soft tissue infections, **854–857**
  deep, **856–857**
    septic shock in, treatment of, 828t
  superficial, **854–855**
Soft tissue injuries
  and blood loss, in hemorrhagic shock, 213
  head, **423–424**
Solanine, in poisonous plants, 1003, 1004t

Solanum nigrum, toxins in, 1004t
Solanum pseudocapsicum, toxins in, 1004t
Soman (nerve agent), 37
Somatic pain, 1080
Somatization disorder, **1035**
  and syncope, 346
Somatoform disorders, **1034–1035**
Somatostatin, for peptic ulcer disease, 290
Sore throat, **634–636, 840–841**
  airway management in, 634–635
  in children, 635
  clinical findings in, 635–636
  diagnosis of, 638t–639t
  history of, 635
  physical examination in, 635
  radiographic findings in, 635–636, 637i
  treatment of, 636, 638t–639t
Sotolol, for atrial fibrillation, 698
Spasm
  and chest pain, 253, 255
  of rectus abdominis muscle, 264
Spermatic cord block, 754
Spermatocele, 755, 756t
Spherocytosis, hereditary, **812–813**
Sphingomyelinase D, in brown recluse spider venom, **954–955**
Spider bites, 354, **953–955**
Spilled teacup sign, in lunate dislocation, 524, 525i
Spinal accessory nerve injury, 437i, 439
Spinal anesthesia, 578
  and neurogenic shock, 207
Spinal cord compression
  abscesses causing, 356
  avoidance of lumbar puncture in, 349
  axial, 508t
  cervical level, 349
  emergency imaging of, 349, 351
  emergency surgery for, 349, 351
  lesion causing, locating level of, 349
  lower or cauda equina involvement in, 349
  metastatic tumors causing, 355
  thoracic level, 349
  vertebral body involvement in, 349
  weakness caused by, 349, 351, 355, 356
Spinal cord disease, weakness in, **351, 355–356**
  differential diagnosis of, 351, 353t
Spinal cord injury, **493–509**, 573
  airway management in, 493–494, 508
  axial compression, 508t
  blood pressure in, 495
  blunt, 495
  brainstem reflexes in, 502
  cardiac arrest in, 494
  circulation in, establishing satisfactory, 494–495
  clinical findings in, 508
  complex mechanism, 508t
  complications of, treatment of, 495
  computed tomography of, 507, 509
  consultation in, 509
  cricothyrotomy in, 494
  disposition in cases of, 509
  evaluation of, **496–507**, 509
  extension-type, 508t
  flexion-rotation, 508t
  flexion-type, 508t
  gastric atony with, 495
  with head injury, 421, 495, 496, 506
  history of, 496
  hospitalization for, 507
  hypotension in, 494–495, 509
  hypovolemia in, 494
  imaging in, 506–507, 509

Spinal cord injury (*cont.*)
of cervical spine, 495, 506–507
of chest, skull, and pelvis, 506
special studies in, 507
of thoracic and lumbosacral spine, 507
immobilization in, 493, 509
intubation in, 494, 508
laboratory evaluation in, 495, 506
magnetic resonance imaging of, 507
mentation in, 496, 502
motor function in, 496–497, 497*t*–502*t*
with neck injury, 435, 437
neurologic examination in, **496–502**, 506
neurologic injury in, minimization of, 495
with or without vertebral fractures, **508–509**
paralytic ileus with, 495
penetrating, antibiotic therapy for, 495
physical examination in, general, 496
secretion suctioning in, 494
sensation in, 497–502, 503*i*, 504*i*, 505*t*
shock in, 196, 207, 494–495
specific injuries in, emergency treatment of,
507–509
spinal reflexes in, 502, 505*t*
suspected, 493
immediate management of, **493–495**
swelling in, reduction of, 495, 509
sympathetic tone in, 494–495, 509
tomography of, 507
traumatic, **221**
treatment of, 508–509
types of, 508*t*
urinary incontinence or retention in, 495
ventilation in, 493–494
whiplash (hyperextension), 496, **509**
Spinal cord lesions
complete, 505
partial, 506
Spinal cord metastases, 351, **355**
Spinal cord syndromes, **505–506**
Spinal epidural abscess, 351, **356**
Spinal infections, back pain in, **419–420**
Spinal reflexes, in spinal cord injury, 502, 505*t*
Spine
dislocation or fracture of, back pain in, 417
fractures of, in child abuse, 515
physical examination of, in spinal cord injury, 496
Spine boards, in EMS field treatment, 15
Spiral fracture, 513
in child abuse, 515
Spleen, rupture of
abdominal pain in, **278**
diagnosis of, 271*t*
Splenectomy
for autoimmune hemolytic anemia, 805
for idiopathic thrombocytopenic purpura, 791
for paroxysmal cold hemoglobinuria, 807
for thrombotic thrombocytopenic purpura, 793
Splenic artery aneurysm, 778
Splenic infarct
abdominal pain in, **278**
diagnosis of, 271*t*
in sickle cell disease, 810, 1093
Splenic injuries, **470**
computed tomography of, 470, 471*i*–472*i*
Splenic sequestration, in sickle cell anemia, 810
Splenomegaly
in chronic myelocytic leukemia, 816
in thrombocytopenia due to platelet sequestration, 794
Splints, 514–515
for ankle sprains, 543

for calcaneal fractures, 544
for carpal bone fractures, 526, 526*i*
for carpal tunnel syndrome, 566
in EMS field treatment, **15–16**
for forearm fractures, 524
for fractures, 220
for hand, 527, 527*i*, 528*i*, 557, 562
for humerus fractures, 520, 521*i*
for lateral malleolar fractures, 540, 541*i*
for lunate dislocations, 525
for mallet finger, 529
for metacarpal fractures, 526*i*, 527, 527*i*, 528*i*
for phalanx fractures and dislocations, 527
for scapholunate dislocations, 525
for teeth, 636–640
for wrist, 526, 526*i*, 527*i*, 557, 566
Spondyloarthropathies, **412–413**
Sponge, for wound cleansing, 580
Spontaneous abortion, **733–735**, 743
classification of, 734*t*
Spontaneous subconjunctival hemorrhage, **610**
Sprains, **514**
ankle, **543–544**
grading and classification of, 514
knee, **537–538**
Sputum examination
in acute lung injury, 672
in asthma and COPD, 658–659
in HIV/AIDS, 865
in pneumonia, 668, 834
in pulmonary aspiration syndrome, 671
in tuberculosis, 669
SSRIs. *See* Selective serotonin reuptake inhibitors
SSSS. *See* Staphylococcal scalded skin syndrome
Stab wounds. *See also* Penetrating trauma
abdominal, 467, 470
in pregnancy, 746
chest, 465–466
neck, **438**, 438*i*
reporting of, 68
Stabilization, 3, 4
Staffing, for EMS systems, 9–10
Stainless steel sutures, 582–583
Stains, in synovial fluid analysis, 140
Standard of care, and legal issues, 61
Standard of disclosure
patient-oriented, 64
physician-oriented, 64
Standard precautions, 25*t*
Standing orders, 6, 12, 13*i*, **16**
Staphylococcal bacteria
as biologic weapon, 33*t*, **35–36**
and toxic shock syndrome, 204, 205
Staphylococcal enterotoxin B, as biologic weapon,
33*t*, **35–36**
Staphylococcal scalded skin syndrome, 854–855,
1015, 1084*t*–1085*t*
Staphylococcus infection
impetigo in, 1018–1019
toxic shock syndrome in, 1084*t*–1085*t*
urinary tract, in children, 1075
Staphylococcus aureus infection, 35
antibiotic prophylaxis against, 564
arthritis in, 409–410, 838
breast, postpartum, 748
bursitis in, 414
in cystic fibrosis, 673
eyelid, 609
gastroenteritis in, 303, 304*t*
hand, 562, 563–564, 564
human bites and, 565
in infants, 1062

orbital cellulitis in, 605–606
osteomyelitis in, 839, 1079
paronychia and eponychia in, 562
pneumonia in, 834, 836*t*
at pocket site of cardiac pacemaker, 709
in sickle cell anemia, 810
sinusitis in, 643
soft tissue, 854–855
spinal, 419
staphylococcal scalded skin syndrome in, 1015
toxic shock syndrome in, 861–862
Staphylococcus epidermidis infection, at pocket site of
cardiac pacemaker, 709
Staples, for wound closure, 582–583, 583–584
START triage algorithm, 51*i*
Status asthmaticus, 660, 661
airway management in, 188
Status epilepticus, **332–335**, 340–341
active seizures in, immediate measures for patient with, 332–335
in children, 1059–1060, 1063*i*
coma in, 314
delirium in, 1032
diagnosis of, 333*i*
drug treatment of, 334, 335, 336*t*, 341
emergency evaluation of, 333*i*, 334*t*
versus hypoglycemia, 334
versus meningitis, 335
Statute of limitations, **62**
Stavudine, side effects of, 865*t*
STDs. *See* Sexually transmitted diseases
Steeple sign, in croup, 647, 648*i*
Stem cell transplantation, for multiple myeloma,
817
Stenosing flexor tenosynovitis, 566
Stent(s), carotid artery, 377
Stereotactic microsurgery, for arteriovenous malformations and aneurysms, 377
Stereotactic radiosurgery, for arteriovenous malformations, 377
Sterile technique, **74**
Sterilization, of skin, 73–74
Sternal fracture, **464**
Sternoclavicular joint dislocations, **516**
Steroid therapy
for adrenal insufficiency, 858
for asthma and COPD, 659–660
for autoimmune hemolytic anemia, 805, 807
for Bell palsy, 358
for bursitis, 414
for carpal tunnel syndrome, 566
contraindications to, in delirium tremens, 398
for De Quervain tenosynovitis, 566
for eye trauma, caution with, 620, 624–625
for flexor tenosynovitis, 566
for gouty arthritis, 409
for hemolytic uremic syndrome, 794
for idiopathic thrombocytopenic purpura,
791–792
and immunosuppression, 825
and leukocytosis, 658
for meningitis, 384
in children, 1069
for mononucleosis, 639*t*, 816
for multiple myeloma, 817
for optic neuritis, 615
for pemphigus vulgaris, 1017
prophylactic, for cluster headache, 390
for pseudotumor cerebri, 386
for psoriasis, 1021
for rheumatoid arthritis, 411
for sciatica, 419

for septic shock, 827
for spinal cord injury, 495, 509
for spinal cord metastases, 355
for staphylococcal enterotoxin B infection, 35–36
for temporal arteritis, 387
for tendonitis, 414
for thrombotic thrombocytopenic purpura, 793
for transverse myelitis, 356
for Waldenström macroglobulinemia, 818
Stevens-Johnson syndrome, **1014**
Stimson technique, for reduction of hip dislocation, 532
Stimulant(s)
    intoxication, delirium or confusion in, **399, 1030**
    poisoning/overdose of, **974–975**
Stingray envenomation, **956–957**
Stings
    bee, **953**
    jellyfish, **957–958**
    scorpion, **955–956**
    scorpion fish, **958–959**
    sea urchin, **959–960**
    wasp, **953**
Stitch, and chest pain, 255
    diagnosis of, 250*t*
Stomach. *See also under* Gastric
    perforated, chest pain in, **254**
    radiation injury and, 944
Stomach disorders, gastrointestinal bleeding in, 290*t*
Stomatitis, aphthous, diagnosis and treatment of, 650*t*
Stonefish sting, **958–959**
Stool
    bacterial culture of, 302
    in gastrointestinal bleeding, 289
Stool sample
    in botulism, 364
    in HIV/AIDS, 866
    in syncope, 337, 346
Storms, severe, **43**
Straddle injuries to perineum, 490, 491*i*
Strains, **514**
    lumbosacral, **417–418**
Strep throat, 636, 638*t*, 840–841
    versus mononucleosis, 816
Streptococcus infection
    acute dacryocystitis in, 608
    arthritis in, 409, **411**
    erysipelas in, 1016
    eyelid, 609
    group A, 840–841
        associated with toxic shock-like syndrome, **862**
    group B, prophylaxis, in premature birth, 747
    hand, 564
    in human bites, 565
    impetigo in, 1018–1019
    in infants, 1062
    meningitis in, 1068*t*
    orbital cellulitis in, 605–606
    osteomyelitis in, 1079
    pharyngitis in, in children, 1073
    scarlet fever in, 1082*t*–1083*t*
    soft tissue, 854–855
    throat, 636, 638*t*, 840–841
        versus mononucleosis, 816
    toxic shock syndrome in, 861–862
Streptococcus faecalis infection, urinary tract, in children, 1075
Streptococcus pneumoniae infection, 834–835
    acute dacryocystitis in, 608
    in infants, 1062
    meningitis in, 834*t*, 1068*t*
    orbital cellulitis in, 605–606
    osteomyelitis in, 1079
    periorbital cellulitis in, 1075
    in sickle cell anemia, 810
Streptococcus pyogenes infection, antibiotic prophylaxis against, 564
Streptococcus viridans infection, urinary tract, in children, 1075
Streptokinase
    for deep venous thrombosis, 783
    for massive pulmonary embolism, 203
    for myocardial infarction, 677–678
    for pulmonary embolism, 664, 682
Streptomycin
    for brucellosis, 28
    contraindicated in pregnancy, 670
    for plague, 23*t*, 26
    for tuberculosis, 670
    for tularemia, 23*t*, 27
Stress, and wound closure, 585, 586*i*
Stress fractures, 513
Stress management, in multicasualty incidents/disasters, 59
Stress ulcers, in newborn, 1089
Stretch injuries, 575
Stridor
    in children
        treatment algorithm for, 1054*t*
        in upper airway obstruction, 1052, 1053*t*
    in croup, 647
    in upper airway obstruction, 236, 1052, 1053*t*
String sign, in arterial dissection, 376
Stroke, **369–377**
    and amnesia, 401
    and aphasia, 371, 401–402
    associated symptoms in, 370
    atrial fibrillation and, 697–698
    atrial flutter and, 698–699
    versus Bell palsy, 358
    and coma, **322**
    delirium or confusion in, 394*t*, **401–402**
    embolic, 374–377
        risk factors for, 370, 370*t*
    evaluation of, **369–371**
    headache with, 370, 382, **383**
    hemorrhagic, **372–374**
    history of, 370
    imaging in, 371
    ischemic, **374–377**, 776
    laboratory tests in, 371
    lacunar, **375–376**
    life-threatening problems with, immediate management of, **369**
    lumbar puncture in, 371
    mixed sensorimotor, 375
    neurologic examination in, 370–371
    physical examination in, 370–371
    prevention of, 376–377
    pure motor, 375
    pure sensory, 375
    risk factors of, 370
    in sickle cell anemia, 810
    specific syndromes of, management of, **372–377**
    time course of deficits in, 370
    transient ischemic attacks and, 376–377
    vascular studies in, 371
    ventilation in, 369
Strongyloides stercoralis infection, and dysentery, 308*t*
Structural collapse, **45**
ST-segment-elevation, in myocardial infarction, 675, 676
Stupor, definition of, 315
Sty (acute hordeolum), **609**
Subarachnoid hemorrhage, **372–374**
    coma in, 326, **329**
    complications of, 373
    computed tomography of, 372*i*, 372–373, 383, 431*i*, 432*i*
    delirium or confusion in, 383, 394
    grading scale for, 372
    headache in, 372, 379–381, 382, **383**, 390
    neurosurgical consultation in, 373
    seizures in, 369, 373
    in sickle cell anemia, 810
    traumatic, **429**
Subclavian steal syndrome, syncope in, **345**
Subclavian vein
    catheterization of, **89–92**, 90*i*, 91*i*
    identification of, 90, 90*i*
    injury to, 772
Subconjunctival hemorrhage
    spontaneous, **610**
    in viral keratoconjunctivitis, 612
Subcutaneous emphysema, **664–665**
Subdural empyema, sinusitis and, 645
Subdural hematoma, **428–429**
    and coma, **319–320**, 320*t*, 324
    computed tomography of, 428–429, 429*i*, 430*i*
Subluxations, 513
Submental block, 578
Subscapularis muscle injury, 518
Subtalar dislocations, **545**
Subtentorial epidural hematoma, and coma, **324**
Subtentorial mass lesions. *See also specific type*
    and coma, **322–325**
Subtentorial subdural hematoma, and coma, **324**
Subungual hematoma, **528, 558**
Succimer. *See* 2,3-Dimercaptosuccinic acid
Succinylcholine
    asthma and, 188
    in intubation, 182
        in head trauma patients, 188
Sucking chest wound
    in tension pneumothorax, 215
    treatment of, 211
Suction
    in intubation preparation, 170
    for snake bites, 952
Sudden cardiac death
    in aortic stenosis, 343
    in chest trauma, **465**
    prevention of, implantable cardioverter defibrillators for, 710–711
Sudden infant death syndrome (SIDS), 163
Sugar-tong splint, 524, 541*i*, 543
Suicidal ideation, recognition of, 1029
Suicidal patients, **1029–1030**
Suicide, and wrongful death cases, 67
Sulfacetamide
    for conjunctivitis, 610
    for corneal and conjunctival foreign body injuries, 620
    for dacryocystitis, 608
    for eye trauma/disorders, 621, 622*t*
    for viral keratoconjunctivitis, 612
Sulfasalazine, for rheumatoid arthritis, 411
Sulfisoxazole, for urinary tract infections, in children, 1076
Sulfonamides, thrombocytopenia induced by, 792

Sulfonylurea
  for hyperglycemia, 873
  and hyponatremia, 893*t*
  poisoning/overdose of, 967*t*
Sulfur, for scabies, 1022
Sulfur mustard, as chemical weapon, 36*t*, 39–40
Sumatriptan
  for cluster headache, 389–390
  for migraine, 389
Sunburn, **927**
Superficial abscesses, incision and drainage of, **140–142**
Superficial reflexes, 505*t*
Superficial soft tissue infections, **854–855**
Superficial thrombophlebitis, **783**
Supergrass. *See* Phencyclidine
Superior laryngeal nerve block, for intubation, 180, 181*i*
Superior laryngeal nerve injury, 437*i*
Superwarfarins, 801
Super-warfarins, overdose, 1010
Supplies, mobilization of, in multicasualty incidents/disasters, 56
Suppurative cholangitis, abdominal pain in, 263, **275–276**
Suppurative labyrinthitis, vertigo in, 631*t*
Suppurative otitis media, 628*t*, **642–643**
Suppurative tenosynovitis, **565**
Supracondylar fractures, 519, **521–522**
Supraorbital nerve block, 579, 579*i*
Suprapubic aspiration, for urine collection in females, 758
Suprapubic catheter
  for drainage of distended bladder, 752
  placement of, 479
Suprapubic cystotomy
  percutaneous, **127–129**, 128*i*
  for posterior urethral injuries, 490
Supraspinatus muscle injury, 518
Supratentorial mass lesions. *See also specific type*
  coma in, **317–322**, 318*i*
Supraventricular arrhythmias, **695–700**
Supraventricular tachycardia, 158, 158*t*
  in children, 1050*t*
  in tricyclic antidepressant overdose, 1008–1009, 1009*i*
Supravesical obstruction, 750
Surface ambulances, 12
Surfactant, nonionic, for wound cleansing, 580
Surgical airways, **178**
  in children, 187
Surgical scars, and gastrointestinal bleeding, 288
Suture(s), 582–583
  absorbable, 582
  for facial lacerations, 452–453
  for fascia, 584
  gut, 582
  for hand injuries, 556
  for muscle and fat, 584–585
  nonabsorbable, 582–583
  removal of, 593–594
  scarring with, 585, 594
  selection of, 582
  for skin, 585
  synthetic, 582–583
  for wounds, 582–583
    deep, *versus* wound tapes, 583
    under high and low stress, 585, 586*i*, 587*i*
Suture ligation, for hemostasis, in wound cases, 574
Swan-neck deformity, of finger, 528–529, 560, 561*i*
Sweat testing, in hand trauma, 550–551, 569

Sweating, with heart failure in infants, 692
Swellfish poisoning, 961
Swelling, in spinal cord injury, reduction of, 495, 509
Swimmer's ear, 627*t*
Swimmer's view, in cervical spine imaging, 506
Sympathetic tone, in spinal cord injury, 494–495, 509
Sympathomimetics, poisoning/overdose of, 967*t*
Symphysis pubis, disruption of, in pelvic fractures, 531
Synchronized cardioversion, 155
Syncope, **335–340**
  with abdominal pain, 339
  absence or related symptoms in, 339
  in aortic stenosis, **343–344**
  arrhythmias causing, 339, 339*t*, 342, **343**
  assessment of, 333*i*
  with basilar artery insufficiency, **345**
  blood loss and, 335–339
  in cardiac arrest, 342
  in cardiac inflow obstruction, 339*t*, **343**
  in cardiac outflow obstruction, 339*t*, 340, **343–344**
  cardiopulmonary, **342–344,** 692
    causes of, 339*t*, 342
  carotid sinus, 341, **345**
  as cause of loss of consciousness, confirmation of, 335
  cerebrovascular, 339*t*, **345**
  with chest pain, 339, 343, 344
  conduction abnormalities causing, 339
  conscious patient with history of, evaluation of, **335–340**
  coughing and, 340, 341, 342
  disposition in cases of, 340
  with dyspnea, 339, 344
  evaluation of, 340
  in glossopharyngeal neuralgia, 340
  heat, **937**
  hospitalization in, risk assessment for, 340
  in hypertrophic obstructive cardiomyopathy, **344**
  in Meniere disease, 340, **347**
  micturition and, 340, 341, 342
  with migraine, **345**
  in myocardial infarction, **342**
  with neurologic symptoms, 339
  in orthostatic hypotension, 335–337, **345–346**
  pacemaker malfunction and, 710
  patient position in, 340
  with pelvic pain, 339
  in physical exertion, 340, 343
  in pregnancy, 340, 729
  psychiatric causes of, **346–347**
  with pulmonary embolism, **344,** 662
  with pulmonary hypertension, **344**
  in pulmonary stenosis, **344**
  in pulmonary vascular disease, **344**
  recovery from, 335
  situational, 341
  in subclavian steal syndrome, **345**
  vasovagal, 340, **341–342**
    common factors precipitating, 341*t*
    in urolithiasis, 761
Syndesmotic ligament, 540
Syndrome of inappropriate secretion of antidiuretic hormone, 373
Synergistic necrotizing cellulitis, **856**
Synovial fluid analysis, 139–140
  in arthritis, 407, 407*t*, 837–838
Synovitis, toxic, in children, 1079

Synthetic sutures, 582–583
  absorbable, 582
  nonabsorbable, 583
Syphilis, **852–853**
  in children, 1101*t*
  in HIV-infected patients, 853, 864
  in infants, 1062
  infectious, 853
  latent stage of, 853
  paroxysmal cold hemoglobinuria in, 806–807
  prevention of, 740
  primary stage of, 853
  reporting cases of, 853
  secondary stage of, 853
  tertiary, diagnosis of, 272*t*
  tertiary stage of, 853
Syringe irrigation, of wounds, 580
Systemic chemical poisoning, 924
Systemic coagulopathies, third-trimester bleeding in, 743–744
Systemic embolism, in myocardial infarction, **681–682**
Systemic hypothermia, **930–934**
Systemic infections, delirium in, **1031**
Systemic inflammatory response syndrome (SIRS), 191, 204, 825
Systemic lupus erythematosus, arthritis in, **413**
Systolic ejection murmur, with heart failure in infants, 692–693

T-2 mycotoxins, as biologic weapons, 33*t*, **34–35**
Tabun (nerve agent), 37
TAC, for wound care, in children, 1043
Tachyarrhythmias, **694–703**
  management of, 202, 244
  with pulse, 158
Tachycardia
  in acute intermittent porphyria, 361
  AEDs for, 14
  in asthma, 657
  atrial, 695, 712, 713*i*
  atrioventricular nodal reentrant, 695–697, 712, 713*i*–715*i*
  atrioventricular reciprocating, 695–697, 712, 715*i*
    antidromic, 699–700
    orthodromic, 699
    in Wolf-Parkinson-White syndrome, 699–700
  in cardiac tamponade, 457, 689
  in cardiogenic shock, 201
  in children, 1045, 1046, 1050*t*
  in heart failure, 684, 685, 692
  multifocal atrial, **699,** 712, 717*i*
  pacemaker mediated, 709, 710
  paroxysmal supraventricular, **695–697,** 712, 713*i*–715*i*
  in pneumothorax, 655
  polymorphic ventricular, 694, **702–703,** 717, 718*i*
  in pulmonary embolism, 661–662, 681
  pulseless ventricular, 157–158
  in shock, 194
  sinus, **695,** 712, 712*i*
  supraventricular, 158, 158*t*
    in children, 1050*t*
    in tricyclic antidepressant overdose, 1008–1009, 1009*i*
  syncope in, 343
  in urolithiasis, 761
  in vaginal bleeding, abnormal, 725
  ventricular, 158, 158*t*, **700–702,** 717, 718*i*

in children, 1050*t*
electrocardiogram in, 700–701, 717, 718*i*
polymorphic, 694, **702–703**, 717, 718*i*
pulseless, 157–158
in stable patients, 701–702
versus supraventricular tachycardia with aberrant conduction, 700–701, 701*i*
in unstable patients, 701
in Wernicke encephalopathy, 398
wide complex, 700–701, 701*i*
Tachypnea
in children, 1050
in flail chest, 458
in heart failure, 692
in hemothorax, 456
in pneumonia, 832
in pneumothorax, 455, 655
in pulmonary embolism, 661–662
Tacrolimus, thrombocytopenia induced by, 793
Talofibular ligament, 540
injuries to, 543–544
Talus, fractures of, **544**
Tamponade
balloon, for esophageal varices, 292
cardiac (*See* Cardiac tamponade)
endobronchial, in hemoptysis, 654
Tampons
nasal, for epistaxis, 633, 634*i*
vaginal, and toxic shock syndrome, 197, 205, 862
Tapes, for wound closure, 583, 584*i*, 587
Tar burns, **926–927**
Tar preparations/shampoos, for psoriasis, 1021
Tarsal bone, fractures or dislocations of, 544, **545**
Tarsometatarsal injuries, **545–546**
Taxine, in poisonous plants, 1004*t*
Taxus species, toxins in, 1004*t*
TCAs. *See* Tricyclic antidepressants
T-cell lymphoma, cutaneous, and exfoliative erythroderma, 1014
Team approach
to cardiac arrest management, 146
to trauma care, 208
Team management, 4
Tear gas, and conjunctivitis, 610
TEC. *See* Transient erythroblastopenia of childhood
Technetium red cell scintigraphy, for lower gastrointestinal bleeding, 289
TEE. *See* Transesophageal echocardiography
Teeth
anatomy of, 648–649, 649*i*
avulsion of, **450, 636–640,** 651*t*
eruption of, 651*t*
extraction of, hemorrhage after, **640**
fractures of, **450, 636,** 651*t*
Ellis classification system of, 636, 640*i*
injuries to, **450**
pain in, 649
diagnosis of, 650*t*–651*t*
as excuse for drug seekers, 649
postextraction, 650*t*
treatment of, 649, 650*t*–651*t*
subluxation of, **450, 636–640,** 651*t*
Teflon poisoning, 995*t*
Tegretol. *See* Carbamazepine
Telangiectasia, hereditary hemorrhagic, gastrointestinal bleeding in, 288
Telemetry, in EMS communications system, 18
Telepaque. *See* Sodium iopanoate
Telephone consultation, legal risks of, 68

Temperature
hypothermia and, 930
reduction of, for heat stroke, 939
Temperature sensitivity, in spinal cord injury, 497
Temporal arteries, examination of, in headache patients, 382
Temporal arteritis, **387**
headache in, 381, 382, **387**
Temporal bone, fracture of, 441, **449–450**
conductive hearing loss in, **451**
facial nerve paralysis in, **451**
longitudinal, **450**
sensorimotor hearing loss in, **451**
transverse, **450**
Temporomandibular joint
dislocation of, **652**
reduction of, 652
in headache patients, 382
pain in, **649–652**
TEN. *See* Toxic epidermal necrolysis
Ten (10)-Codes, for EMS communications, 16–18
Tendonitis, **413–414**
Tenecteplase (TNK), for myocardial infarction, 677–678, 678
Tenosynovitis
De Quervain, 566
in disseminated gonococcemia, 861
flexor, 565
stenosing, 566
gonococcal, 565
suppurative, **565**
Tension headache, 382, **387–388**
Tension pneumothorax, **215,** 229, **455–456,** 655–656
in abdominal trauma, 467
chest pain in, 243, 243*t*
radiographic findings in, 455, 455*i*, 456*i*
respiratory distress/dyspnea in, **225**
shock in, 195, 197
syncope with, 343
treatment of, 456, 656
Terbinafine, for tinea, 1024
Terbutaline
for asthma, 1058
for priapism, 764
Terconazole, for vaginitis, 847
Teres minor muscle injury, 518
Terminal extensor tendon (TET), 553–554
Terrorism. *See also* Weapons of mass destruction
acts of, **45–46**
Terry Thomas sign, in scapholunate dislocations, 525
Tertiary syphilis, diagnosis of, 272*t*
Testicular appendage, torsion of, 752–755, 763
scrotal pain in, 752–755, 753*t*
Testicular injuries, **491**
in pelvic fractures, 530
Testicular torsion, 752–755, **763**
analgesia for, 763
clinical findings in, 754–755, 763
differential diagnosis of, 763
versus epididymitis, 754–755, 763
preparation for surgery in, 763
scrotal pain in, 752–755, 753*t*
treatment and disposition of, 755, 755*i*, 763
urologic surgical consultation in, 763
Testicular tumor, 755–756, 756*t*
Tetanus immunization status, in wound cases, 575
Tetanus prophylaxis
in abdominal trauma, 470
active or passive, 590
in burn injuries, 566, 567

in eye trauma, 618
in foreign body injuries, 567, 568
in hand trauma, 557, 558
in mandibular fracture, 443
in puncture wounds, 597
recommended schedule for, 590, 590*t*
in traumatic amputation, 511
in wound care, 589–590
Tetracaine, 577*t*
for eye trauma/disorders, 616, 620, 621, 622*t*
for ocular burns, 927
for tonometry, 623
for wound care, in children, 1043
Tetracycline(s)
for animal bites, 596
for chlamydial infection, 610
contraindicated in breastfeeding, 748
for dysuria-frequency syndrome, 845
for epididymitis, 850
ophthalmic ointment, 621, 622*t*
for conjunctivitis, 610
for viral keratoconjunctivitis, 612
for puerperal sepsis, 748
for Q fever, 24*t*, 28
for Reiter syndrome, 412
resistance to, 851
for Rocky Mountain spotted fever, 859
for scorpion fish envenomation, 959
for stingray wound, 957
for tularemia, 27
Tetralogy of Fallot, 692
Tetrodotoxin poisoning, 363, **961**
Thalassemia(s), 802, **811–813**
α (alpha), 811
β (beta), 811
major, 812
minor, 812
Thenar intrinsics, testing of, 554
Theophylline
for asthma, 661
assessing serum levels of, 659
poisoning/overdose of, **1007–1008**
seizures induced by, 971
Therapeutic interventions, 4
Therapeutic privilege, doctrine of, 65
Thermal burns, 940
Thermal injuries
genital, 490, 492
hand, **566–567**
ocular, **616–617**
smoke inhalation, 923, 924
Thermodysregulation. *See also* Hyperthermia; Hypothermia
poisoning and, **971**
Thiamine
for alcoholic ketoacidosis, 877
in coma cocktail, 311
deficiency, acute, in Wernicke encephalopathy, **398–399**
for delirium or confusion, 391, 393
for delirium tremens, 397
for ethanol poisoning, 986
for hypoglycemia, 874
in alcoholic patients, 874
for Wernicke encephalopathy, 399, 401
Thiazide diuretics, for pseudotumor cerebri, 386
Thigh injury, and shock, 196, 200
Thionamides, for thyroid storm, 879
Thiopental
asthma and, 188
in intubation, 183–184
for status epilepticus, 336*t*

Thioridazine
and hyponatremia, 893*t*
psychiatric uses, 1036
Thiosulfate, for cyanide poisoning, 983, 983*t*
Third-trimester bleeding, **743–744**
Thompson test, in Achilles tendon injuries, 541–542, 542*i*
Thoracentesis, **110–112**, 111*i*
Thoracic aorta injury (TAI), **770–771**
imaging of, 770, 770*i*, 771*t*
Thoracic aortic aneurysm, **778–781**, 780*t*
Thoracic cavity lavage, for rewarming, 933
Thoracic disk disease, chest pain in, **255**
Thoracic outlet syndrome, **785–786**
Thoracic spine imaging, in spinal cord injury, 507
Thoracocentesis, for pleural effusion, 666
Thoracolumbar strain, 221
Thoracostomy
needle
in EMS field treatment, **15**
in tension pneumothorax, 215, 225, 656
in tension pneumothorax, 229–231
tube, **112–116**, 114*i*
in abdominal trauma, 467
in hemothorax, 457
in pneumomediastinum, 252
in tension pneumothorax, 215, 225, 456, 656
Thoracotomy
in cardiac tamponade, 457
contraindications to, 454
emergency, **115–116**
emergency room, 454, **466**
indications for, 454
in multiply injured patient, 211
Thorax, blood loss in
and hemorrhagic shock, 213
and shock, 200
Thorazine. *See* Chlorpromazine
Thought disorders, 1028, **1033**
Threatened abortion, 734, 734*t*
Throat, sore, **634–636, 840–841**
Throat culture, 840–841
Thrombectomy, for arterial occlusion, 774
Thrombin clotting time, 791*t*
Thrombocytopenia, **789–794**
drug-induced immune-mediated, **792**
drugs implicated in, 789, 792*t*
due to platelet sequestration, **794**
immune, **789–792**
in liver disease, 799
platelet transfusion for, 819–820
purpura in, 789
in renal disease, 800
in septic shock, 827
in Waldenström macroglobulinemia, 817
Thrombocytosis, **795**
hyperkalemia in, 901
Thrombolysis
catheter-directed
for deep venous thrombosis, 784
for venous occlusion, 775
for frostbite, 935
Thrombolytic therapy
for arterial occlusion, 774
for cardiogenic shock, 244
for central retinal artery occlusion, 605
for deep venous thrombosis, 783
for hyphema, 613
idioventricular rhythm in, 706–707
intracranial hemorrhage in, 677
for ischemic stroke, 375, 776
for massive pulmonary embolism, 203

for myocardial infarction, 677–678, 677–679
protocol for, 664
for pulmonary embolism, 238, 664, 682
for vitreous hemorrhage, 614
Thrombophlebitis
pelvic, septic abortion and, 735
septic, 783
superficial, **783**
Thrombosis
arterial occlusion by, 773
basilar artery, coma in, **323**
mesenteric
abdominal pain in, **277–278**
diagnosis of, 271*i*
Thrombotic thrombocytopenic purpura, **792–794**
Through-and-through lacerations, of lip, 594
Thrush, in HIV-infected patients, 863
Thumb
extensor muscles of, 552–553
flexor muscles of, 551
metacarpophalangeal joint of, stress examination of, 529, 530*i*
trigger, 566
Thumb sica cast, 529
Thumb sica splint, 526, 526*i*, 527, 566
Thumb web atrophy, in ulnar nerve injury, 570*i*
Thyroid disorders, **878–881**
delirium in, **1032**
Thyroid replacement, for myxedema coma, 881
Thyroid storm, **878–879**
Thyrotoxicosis, **878–879**
respiratory distress/dyspnea in, **239**
Tibial fractures, 535–536
fibula fractures with, 539
spiral, in child abuse, 515
Tibial plateau fractures, **535**
Tibial shaft fractures, **539**
Tibial spine fractures, **536**
cruciate ligament injuries in, 537
Tibial tuberosity fractures, **535–536**
Tibiocalcaneal ligament, 540
Tibiofemoral joint, dislocations of, 536–537
Tibiofibular ligaments, 540
injuries of, in posterior malleolar fractures, 541
Tibionavicular ligament, 540
Tibiotalar ligament, 540
Ticarcillin, for pulmonary infections in cystic fibrosis, 673
Ticarcillin-clavulanate
for acute abdomen, 259*t*
for human bites, 565
for Ludwig angina, 639*t*
for pneumonia, 836*t*
for septic abortion, 736
for urinary tract infections, 842*t*
Tick paralysis, 354, **362**
Ticks
and Lyme disease, 1082*t*–1083*t*
and Rocky Mountain spotted fever, 1082*t*–1083*t*
Ticlopidine
platelet function impaired by, 795
for stroke prevention, 376
Tidal waves, **44–45**
Tietze syndrome, chest pain in, 250*t*, **255**
Timolol, for acute angle-closure glaucoma, 605
Tin poisoning, 995*t*
Tincture of iodine, 580
Tinea, **1023–1024**
Tinea corporis, 1023, 1024
Tinea cruris, 1023, 1024
Tinea pedis, 1023, 1024

Tinea versicolor, 1023–1024
Tinel sign, in carpal tunnel syndrome, 566
Tinnitus, 629
Tirofiban, for angina, 684
Tissue adhesives, for wound closure, 584
Tissue necrosis, signs of, 581
Tissue plasminogen activator (t-PA)
for central retinal artery occlusion, 605
dosage and administration of, 375
for hyphema, 613
indications for, 375
for ischemic stroke, 375, 776
for massive pulmonary embolism, 203
for myocardial infarction, 677–678
versus percutaneous coronary intervention, 679
for pulmonary embolism, 664, 682
for vitreous hemorrhage, 614
TMJ dislocation, **652**
TMJ pain, **649–652**
TMP-SMZ. *See* Trimethoprim-sulfamethoxazole
Toadfish poisoning, 961
Tobacco, toxins in, 1004*t*
Tobacco use
and chronic bronchitis, 656, 657
and chronic obstructive pulmonary disease, 656
and emphysema, 656
Tobramycin
for eye trauma/disorders, 622*t*
for pulmonary infections in cystic fibrosis, 673
Tocolysis, 747
Toe(s)
buddy taping of, 546
injuries of, orthopedic, **546–547**
small-vessel occlusion in, 774
Tofranil. *See* Imipramine
Togaviridae, 31
Tolbutamide, and hyponatremia, 893*t*
Toluene diisocyanate
poisoning/overdose of, 992, 995*t*
smoke inhalation injury, 924
Tomography
computed (*See* Computed tomography)
in spinal cord injury, 507
in tarsal injuries, 545
in tibial plateau fractures, 535
Tongue, lacerations of, 594
Tongue blade test, in mandibular fracture, 441
Tongue injury, airway obstruction in, 436
Tongue-jaw lift, 153, 154*i*
in pediatric basic life support, 164
Tonometry, 600, **623**
Tono-Pen, 600
Tonsil(s), inflammation and infection of, 635, 636*i*, 645–646
Tonsillar pillars, asymmetric swelling of, 635, 636*i*
Tooth. *See* Teeth
Tooth block, 649
Toothache, **649**, 650*t*–651*t*
Topical anesthesia, 576
in children, 1043
in intubation, 99, 179, 180
Topical vasoconstrictors, in intubation, 179–180
Tornadoes, **43**
Torsades de pointes, **702–703**
electrocardiogram in, 702, 717, 718*i*
magnesium for, 158
Torus fracture, 513
Total excision of wound, 581
Touch sensation, in spinal cord injury, 497
Tourniquet, 211
in hand trauma, 550
in wound cases, 574

Toxalbumins, in poisonous plants, 1003, 1004*t*
Toxemia of pregnancy, **744–745**. *See also*
    Preeclampsia-eclampsia
Toxic epidermal necrolysis, **1014**
Toxic shock syndrome, 197, 204, 205, **861–862,**
    1084*t*–1085*t*
Toxic shock-like syndrome, group A streptococcal
    infections associated with, **862**
Toxic synovitis, in children, 1079
Toxicity, 992
    delayed severe, **972,** 972*t*
Toxicokinetics, **966–969**
Toxicology screen
    in coma, 317
    in poisoning/overdose, 966
Toxidromes, 967*t*
Toxin exposure. *See also* Poisoning
    blindness caused by, **607–608**
    headache in, 381
Toxins. *See also* Chemical weapons
    clearance of, 969
    combustible, and smoke inhalation injury,
        923–924, 923*t*
    exposure to, and diarrhea and vomiting,
        297–299, 298*i,* 301
    half-life of, 968
    radiopaque, 968*t*
    volume of distribution of, 969, 969*t*
Toxoplasmosis, in HIV-infected patients, 863, 866
t-PA. *See* Tissue plasminogen activator
Trachea, traumatic opening of, intubation through,
    436
Tracheal airway injury, **436**
Tracheal intubation, **98–102**
    in multiply injured patient, 210
Tracheobronchial injury, **462–463**
Tracheostomy, **178**
Tracheotomy, **436**
Traction retinal detachment, 607
Traction-countertraction method, for reduction of
    shoulder dislocations, 519, 521*i*
Train accidents, 45
Training
    of Emergency Medical Services personel, 6,
        7*t*–8*t,* 9
    for hazardous material incidents, 53–54
Tranexamic acid, for hemophilia, 796
Transcutaneous cardiac pacing, **142–143,** 703,
    705, 710
    for asystole, 158
Transcutaneous pacemaker, for arrhythmias, 202
Transcutaneous Pco₂ devices, 190
Transesophageal echocardiography (TEE)
    in aortic dissection, 779
    in cardiac tamponade, 217
    in infective endocarditis, 860
    in thoracic aorta injury, 770
    in traumatic aortic rupture, 218
Transfer, to burn center, 923
Transfusion reactions, 821*t,* **821–823**
    acute hemolytic, 822*t,* 822–823
    allergic, 822*t,* 823
    febrile, 822*t,* 823
    premedication against, 823
Transfusions, **818–823.** *See also specific component*
    transfusions
    albumin, **821**
    for anemia, in children, 1093
    antithrombin III, **821**
    for autoimmune hemolytic anemia, 805
    bacterial contamination in, 821–822, 822*t*
    characteristics of products and doses in, 819*t*

for chest pain with shock/hypotension, 242
for chronic myelocytic leukemia, 816
complications of, 821*t,* **821–823**
    infectious, 822*t,* 822–823
for disseminated intravascular coagulation, 802
fresh frozen plasma, **820–821**
for gastrointestinal bleeding, 285
for hemoptysis, 654
for hemorrhagic shock, 214
for hemostatic abnormalities of liver disease,
    799–800
for hemostatic abnormalities of renal disease,
    800
for hypovolemic shock, 199
for idiopathic thrombocytopenic purpura, 1096
intravenous immunoglobulin, **821**
for iron-deficiency anemia, 804
massive, **821**
for multiply injured patient, 212
packed red blood cell, **818–819**
for paroxysmal cold hemoglobinuria, 807
for penetrating chest trauma, 466
platelet, **819–820**
refusal to consent to, 66
for sickle cell anemia, 809
for splenic injuries, 470
for thrombotic thrombocytopenic purpura,
    793
typing and cross-matching for, 818
for vaginal bleeding, abnormal, 726
for vascular trauma, 767
for visceral (intestinal) ischemia, 776
Transient erythroblastopenia of childhood, 1093
Transient global amnesia, **401**
Transient ischemic attacks (TIAs), 345, 370, 374,
    376–377, 776
Transplantation, harvesting of organs for, **72**
Transport
    air, 12, **18,** 53
    by EMS personnel, 12
    ground, 12
    of hypothermic patient, 930–934
    for multicasualty incidents/disasters, 51–52, 53
Transport officer, 51–52
Transportation accidents, **45**
Transthoracic echocardiography (TTE), for cardio-
    genic shock, 201
Transtracheal jet insufflation, in vascular injury to
    neck, 769
Transtracheal jet ventilation, 107, **108–110,** 109*i,*
    110*i*
Transudate, pleural, 666
Transvaginal ultrasound, for ectopic pregnancy,
    196
Transvenous pacemaker, for arrhythmias, 202
Transverse fracture, 513
Transverse fracture of temporal bone, **450**
Transverse myelitis, weakness caused by, 351,
    355–356
Trapped gas, expansion of, air transport and, 18
Trauma. *See also specific type*
    abdominal, **218–219**
    airway management in, 188–189
    arteriography following, 215, 215*t*
    extremity, **220–221**
    and flail chest, 229
    focused assessment with sonography for,
        119–121, 120*i*
    genitourinary, **220**
    head, **219–220**
    headache after, 382, **385**
    immobilization of patient, 15

lightning injuries and, 941
major, definition of, 210*t*
and multiply injured patient, **208–214**
and orbital cellulitis, 1075
preexisting medical condition causing, 196
in pregnancy, **745–746**
seizure activity causing, 341
and shock, **195–196**
skeletal, in child abuse, 1099
spinal, **221**
and urinary catheter insertion, 127
Trauma centers, categorization of, 10
Trauma Score, 208
Traumatic aortic rupture, **217–218**
Travel, and diarrhea and vomiting, 301
Treatment response, and diagnosis, 4
Trench foot, **936**
Trench mouth, 650*t*
Trephination, fingernail, for subungual hematoma,
    528, 558
Treponema pallidum infection. *See* Syphilis
Triage
    assessment for, 50, 51*i*
    categories of, 50
    in EMS system, 9
    for multicasualty incidents/disasters, 50, 57–58
Triage tags, 50, 52*i*
Triamcinolone acetonide
    for contact dermatitis, 1018
    for sunburn, 927
Triangular bandage sling, 588
Trichomonas vaginalis infection (trichomoniasis),
    846–848, **854**
    in children, 1101*t*
Tricyclic antidepressants, 1037
    central anticholinergic syndrome caused by,
        399*t*
    poisoning/overdose of, 967*t,* 975, **1008–1010,**
        1009*f*
    proarrhythmic activity of, 702
Trifluridine, for eye trauma/disorders, 622*t*
Trigeminal nerve block, 578
Trigeminal nerve injury, 440
Trigeminal neuralgia, 382, **385–386**
Trigger finger, 566
Trigger thumb, 566
Trimethoprim, for eye trauma/disorders, 622*t*
Trimethoprim-sulfamethoxazole (TMP-SMZ)
    for brucellosis, 28
    for cellulitis, 1016
    clindamycin with
        in animal bites, 564–565
        in human bites, 565
    for epididymitis, 850
    for epiglottitis, 1052
    for erysipelas, 1016
    for gastroenteritis
        in children, 1078
        infectious, 306
    for glanders, 24*t*
    for melioidosis, 24*t*
    for otitis media, 1072*t*
    prophylactic use of, 564
    for prostatitis, 849
    for scorpion fish envenomation, 959
    for sinusitis, 643
    for stingray wound, 957
    for urinary tract infections, 842
        in children, 1076
Triptans, for migraine, 389
Tropical cyclones, **43**
Tropicamide, for uveitis, 613

Troponin
  in cardiomyopathy, 691
  in myocardial contusion, 460
  in myocardial infarction, 676
Trousseau test, 346
Tsunamis, 44–45
TTE, *See* Transthoracic echocardiography
TTJV. *See* Transtracheal jet ventilation
Tube feeding syndrome, and hypernatremia, 896
Tube thoracostomy, **112–116**, 114*i*
  in abdominal trauma, 467
  in hemothorax, 457
  in pneumomediastinum, 252
  in tension pneumothorax, 215, 225, 456, 656
Tuberculosis
  in children, 1058, 1059
  extrapulmonary, 669
  in HIV-infected patients, 863, 864, 865
  miliary, 669
  pulmonary, **669–670**
    emergency room goals in management of,
      669
    in infants, children, and adolescents, 670
    latent, 670
    multidrug-resistant, 669, 670
    in pregnancy, 670
    reporting requirements for, 670
    respiratory isolation for, 670
  reactivation, 669–670
Tubo-ovarian abscess
  abdominal pain in, 280
  in pelvic inflammatory disease, 845–846
  pelvic pain in, 727*t*
Tubular vision, 600
Tularemia
  as biologic weapon, 23*t*–24*t*, **26–27**
  occuloglandular, 24*t*
  oculoglandular, 26
  oropharyngeal, 24*t*, 26
  pneumonic, 24*t*, 26–27
  typhoidal, 24*t*, 27
  ulceroglandular, 23*t*, 26
Tumor(s). *See specific type*
Tumor emboli, 773
Twiddler syndrome, with cardiac pacemakers, 709
Tympanic bone fractures, **449–450**
Tympanic membrane rupture, in otitis media, 628*t*,
  642, 1070
Typhoidal tularemia, 24*t*, 27
Typhoons, **43**
Tyramine, in poisonous plants, 1004*t*
Tzanck test, for herpes simplex virus infection, 852

Ulcer(s)
  duodenal
    in children, 1089
    perforated, 249*t*, 260*t*
  gastric, in children, 1089
  gastrointestinal bleeding in, 290*t*
  peptic, perforated, **273**
  rectal, **295**
  stress, in newborn, 1089
Ulcerative colitis, arthritis in, 412
Ulceroglandular tularemia, 23*t*, 26
Ulnar collateral ligament, rupture of, **529**, 530*i*
Ulnar gutter splint, 527, 528*i*
Ulnar nerve, innervation of hand by, 551, 553,
  571*i*
Ulnar nerve block, 551*i*, 552*i*, 578, 579*i*
Ulnar nerve injury, 359, 555
  clinical findings in, 569, 570*i*, 571*i*
  in elbow injuries, 522

  in forearm fractures, 524
  in hand trauma, 555, **569**
  motor testing for, 555, 556*i*, 569, 570*i*
  sensory testing for, 555, 556*i*, 569, 571*i*
  in shoulder dislocation, 518–519
Ulnar nerve palsy, **359**
Ultrasonography (ultrasound)
  in abdominal aortic aneurysm rupture, 777
  in abdominal pain, 269
  in abdominal trauma, 468, 469, 469*i*
  in cardiac tamponade, 457–458
  in deep venous thrombosis, 782, 784
  Doppler
    in arterial occlusion, 774
    of pulses, in vascular trauma, 768
    in testicular torsion and epididymitis, 754–755
    venous, in pulmonary embolism, 663
  in ectopic pregnancy, 729, 731, 732*i*, 733*i*
  in genitourinary trauma, 481
  in multiply injured patient, 212
  in myocardial rupture, 681
  in ovarian tumor torsion, 738
  in pelvic inflammatory disease, 846
  in pelvic pain assessment, 728, 729*i*
  in penetrating chest trauma, 465
  in pericardial disease, 197
  in peripheral aneurysms, 781
  in pregnancy, normal, 729*i*
  in pyelonephritis, 844
  in septic abortion, 735
  in testicular injuries, 491
  in third-trimester bleeding, 744
  in thoracic outlet syndrome, 786
  transvaginal, in ectopic pregnancy, 196
  in vaginal bleeding, abnormal, 726
  in vascular injuries, 768, 769
Ultraviolet radiation, ocular burns due to, **617**
Unconscious patients, airway management in, 167
Undersensing, by cardiac pacemakers, 709, 723*i*,
  724
Unfractionated heparin (UFH)
  for angina, 684
  for pulmonary embolism, 664
United Nations Disaster Relief Office, 56
Universal precautions, for intubation, 173
Upper airway. *See also* Airway
  obstruction of, **224–225**
    in children, **1052–1055**
      differential diagnosis, 1052, 1053*t*
      treatment, 1052–1053, 1054*t*, 1055*t*
      respiratory distress/dyspnea in, 230*t*,
        236–237
    traumatic injury to, **214**
Upper extremity injuries, orthopedic, **519–529**
Upper extremity venipuncture, **74–76**, 76*i*
Upper extremity venous thrombosis, **783–784**
Upper gastrointestinal series, in upper gastrointesti-
  nal bleeding, 288
Upper respiratory system, pulmonary agent expo-
  sure and, 38
Upper urinary tract infection, **843–844**
Urea, for cerebral edema, 319*t*
Ureaplasma urealyticum infection, urinary tract, in
  children, 1075
Ureteral injuries, 476, **484–486**
  bladder outlet obstruction with, 751*t*
  special examinations and procedures in,
    477–481
Ureteral obstruction, 750
Ureteral stones, 760, 762*i*
Ureteropelvic obstruction, 750
Ureterovesical obstruction, 750

Urethral caruncle, dysuria with, 757*t*, 758
Urethral catheter, for drainage of distended bladder,
  751–752
Urethral injuries, 468, 477, **488–490**
  anterior, 490, 490*i*
  catheterization in, 477–479, 488, 490
  dysuria in, 757*t*
  imaging of, 477, 480–481, 488, 489*i*, 490, 491*i*
  in pelvic fractures, 530
  posterior, 488*i*, 488–490, 489*i*
  special examinations and procedures in, 477–481
Urethral strictures
  bladder outlet obstruction with, 750, 751*t*
  dysuria with, 757, 757*t*
  hematuria with, 759*t*, 760
Urethral syndrome, 758, 844–845
Urethritis
  chlamydial, 844–845
  dysuria with, 756, 757*t*, 844–845, 851
  epididymitis with, 849–850
  gonococcal, 844–845, 851–852
  nongonococcal (nonspecific), **851**
  prostatitis with, 849
Urethrogram, retrograde
  in genitourinary trauma, 477, 480–481
  of penile rupture, 491
  in urethral injury, 477, 480–481, 488, 489*i*, 490
Uric acid, elevated serum level of, in gouty arthritis,
  408
Urinalysis
  in abdominal pain, 266
    in children, 1081
  in abdominal trauma, 468
  in acute intermittent porphyria, 361–362
  in arsenic poisoning, 360, 361
  in coma, 317
  in cystitis, 841–842
  in diarrhea, 302
  in hematuria assessment, 759
  in infants, 1064
  in muscle disease, 354
  in poisoning/overdose, 966
  in prostatitis, 849
  in pyelonephritis, 843
  in urinary tract infection, 841–842, 842, 843
  in urinary tract infections, in children, 1076
  in urolithiasis, 761
  in vomiting, 302
Urinary anion gap, in metabolic acidosis, 911
Urinary catheterization (bladder catheterization)
  in bladder outlet obstruction, 751–752
  in burn injuries, 920
  in gastrointestinal bleeding, 285
  in genitourinary trauma, 477–479, 490
  in hemoptysis, 654
  insertion of, **125–127**, 126*i*
  in spinal cord injury, 495, 509
  suprapubic placement in, 479
  in urethral injuries, 477–479, 488, 490
  for urine collection in females, 757
Urinary disorders, abdominal pain in, **278–279**
Urinary frequency
  in dysuria-frequency syndrome, 844
  in urinary tract infections, 841, 843
Urinary incontinence, in spinal cord injury, 495
Urinary output
  decreased or absent, 750–752
  in multiply injured patient, 212
Urinary retention, 750–752
  in spinal cord injury, 495
  in uterine prolapse, 739
Urinary tract anomalies, in children, 1077

Urinary tract infections, **841–845**
acute lower (uncomplicated cystitis), **841–843**
treatment of, 842*t*, 842–843
antibiotic therapy for, 842*t*, 842–843
in children, 1064, **1075–1077**
dysuria in, 756–757, 757*t*, 758
epididymitis in, 849–850
in females, 757*t*, 758
in males, 756–757
septic shock in, treatment of, 828*t*
in sickle cell anemia, 810
upper (pyelonephritis), **843–844**
treatment of, 842*t*, 844
Urinary urgency
in dysuria-frequency syndrome, 844
in urinary tract infections, 843
Urination, painful (dysuria), **756–758**. *See also* Dysuria
Urine
blood or red blood cells in (*See* Hematuria)
collection, in females, 757–758
midstream clean-voided, 757
myoglobin in, in rhabdomyolysis, 368
protein in (*See* Proteinuria)
straining, in urolithiasis, 763
Urine collection, in children, 1076
Urine culture
in infants, 1064
in urinary tract infections, 842
Urine output
in cardiogenic shock, 202
in heat stroke, 939
in resuscutation documentation, 199–200
Urography, in pyelonephritis, 843
Urokinase
for central retinal artery occlusion, 605
for deep venous thrombosis, 783
for myocardial infarction, 678
for pulmonary embolism, 664, 682
Urolithiasis, **760–763**
abdominal pain in, 266
analgesia for, 761
hematuria in, 758–761, 759*t*
imaging of, 761, 762*i*
pyelonephritis in, 843
scrotal pain in, 753*t*, 754
Urologic injury, **477–490**
Uroshiol, hypersensitivity reaction to, 1018
Urticaria, **1013**
in transfusion reaction, 823
U-shaped splint, 524
Uterine atony, 747–748
Uterine compression, for vaginal bleeding, 726
Uterine perforation, by intrauterine device, 741
Uterine prolapse, **738–739**
Uveitis, **613**
Uvular displacement, in peritonsillitis, 635, 636*i*

Vaccine
for anthrax, 23*t*, 25
for smallpox, 29, 30
for tularemia, 27
Vaginal bleeding
abnormal, **725–726**
causes of, 726, 726*t*
in cervical cancer, 736
in ectopic pregnancy, 726, 729
in genital trauma, 737
intrauterine device and, 741
postmenopausal, 726*t*
in pregnancy, 726
premenarcheal, 726*t*

reproductive age, 726*t*
in trauma, 726
in vaginal cancer, 736
Vaginal carcinoma, **736**
Vaginal discharge
in mucopurulent cervicitis, 848
in vaginitis, 847
Vaginal injuries, 491, 492
in pelvic fractures, 530
Vaginitis, **846–848**
atrophic, 846–848
dysuria in, 757*t*
gonococcal, 846
Vagotonia, myocardial infarction with, and chest
pain with hypovolemia, 242*t*
Vagus nerve
in acute intermittent porphyria, 361
injury to, 436, 437*i*, 439
stimulation of, in paroxysmal supraventricular
tachycardia, 696
Valacyclovir
for genital herpes infection, 852
for herpes pharyngitis, 639*t*
for herpes simplex infection, 1021
for herpes zoster infection, 1020
Valgus stress test, of medial collateral ligament, 533,
533*i*, 537
Valium. *See* Diazepam
Valproic acid, 338*t*
Valsalva maneuver, in paroxysmal supraventricular
tachycardia, 696
Valvular heart disease, 691
cardiogenic shock in, 202
infective endocarditis in, 859–860
Vancomycin
for cellulitis, 855, 1016
for erysipelas, 1016
for infectious gastroenteritis, 306
for infective endocarditis, 860
for meningitis, in children, 1068*t*
for neutropenia, 814–815
for pneumonia, 836*t*
for septic arthritis, 838*t*
for septic shock, 828*t*
for toxic shock syndrome, 862
Vantin. *See* Cefpodoxime
Vapors, toxic, **993–994**, 995*t*
Varicella zoster virus
and chickenpox, 1082*t*–1083*t*
and herpes zoster, 1019–1020
Varicocele, scrotal, 755, 756*t*
Varicose veins, ruptured, **784**
Variola major, 30
Variola minor, 30
Variola virus, 29–30
Varus stress test, of lateral collateral ligament, 533,
533*i*, 537
Vascular access, in pediatric patients, 164
Vascular disorders
abdominal pain in, **277–278**
pulmonary, syncope in, **344**
Vascular emboli, 773
Vascular emergencies, **766–787**. *See also specific types*
abdominal aortic aneurysm, ruptured, **777–778**
angiography complications, **786–787**
angioplasty complications, **786–787**
arterial aneurysms, **777–781**
arteriovenous fistula, **785**
deep venous thrombosis, **782–784**
ergotism, **787**
frostbite, **787**
hypogastric artery aneurysm, **778**

intra-arterial injection of drugs, **787**
ischemic, **773–776**
not due to trauma, **773–787**
popliteal and femoral peripheral aneurysms, **781**
pulmonary embolism, **661–664, 681–682**
superficial thrombophlebitis, **783**
thoracic aortic aneurysm (aortic dissection),
778–781
thoracic outlet syndrome, **785–786**
traumatic, **766–772**
venous disease, **782–785**
venous varicosities, ruptured (varicose veins), **784**
visceral artery aneurysm, **778**
Vascular injuries, **766–772**. *See also* Vascular emergencies
in abdominal trauma, **771**
airway management in, 766
in blunt trauma, 767, 769
causes of, 767–768
chemical injuries in, 768
in chest trauma, **769–771**
imaging of, 770, 770*i*, 771*t*
control of hemorrhage in, 767
diagnostic imaging in, 768
contraindicated in unstable patient, 768
diagnostic principles in, 768
emergency management of specific, **768–772**
in extremity injuries, **767–768**
in facial trauma, 439
in frostbite, 787
general considerations in, 767–768
hospitalization for, 767
ischemia in, minimization of, 767
life-threatening injuries in, immediate management of, **766–768**
in neck trauma, 439, **768–769**
zones of injury in, 769, 769*i*
pain relief in, 767
penetrating, 767, 769
physical examination in, 768
prevention of further vascular injury in, 767
prevention of nerve injury in, 767
pulmonary, **771**
pulses in, 768
sequelae of, 768
shock in, treatment or prevention of, 767
signs of, 768
surgical consultation in, 767
traumatic, **215**
Vascular insufficiency, osteomyelitis in, 838–839
Vascular studies, in stroke patients, 371
Vascular syndromes, **785–787**
Vasoactive agents, in advanced life support, **158–161**
Vasoconstriction
for epistaxis, 135
for hemostasis, in wound cases, 574
Vasoconstrictors, for intubation, 179–180
Vasodilating agents
and cluster headache, 389
for ergotism, 787
for frostbite, 935
for visceral (intestinal) ischemia, 776
Vasoocclusive crisis, sickle cell disease and,
1093–1094
Vasopressin
in advanced life support, 159*t*, 161
for esophageal varices, 291
for septic shock, 205, 827
for ventricular fibrillation, 703
Vasopressors
extravasation of, 768
for lactic acidosis, 876

Vasopressors (*cont.*)
  for septic shock, 826
Vasospasm, in subarachnoid hemorrhage, 373
Vasovagal syncope, 340, **341–342**
  differentiation from neurogenic shock, 207
  precipitating factors, 341*t*
  in urolithiasis, 761
VAT pacing, in cardiac pacemaker, 708*t*, 722*i*
Vecuronium
  adverse effects and precautions, 183
  asthma and, 188
  in intubation, 182–183
    in head trauma patients, 188
  metabolism of, 183
  in rapid-sequence intubation, 180
VEE. *See* Venezuelan equine encephalitis
Veins, in upper extremity venipuncture, 75
Vena cava compression, in pneumothorax, 655
Vena cava injury, 772
Venereal Disease Research Laboratory (VDRL), 853
Venezuelan equine encephalitis (VEE), 31
Venezuelan hemorrhagic fever, 31*t*
Venipuncture, upper extremity, **74–76**, 76*i*
Venlafaxine, 1037
Venography
  contrast
    in deep venous thrombosis, 782, 784
    in venous occlusion, 774–775
  in thoracic outlet syndrome, 786
  in venous trauma, 772
Venomous animal injuries
  disorders due to, **951–962**
  weakness with, **353–354**
Venotomy, 77–78, 78*i*
Venous access
  with cardiac pacemakers, complications in, 709,
    710
  central, for external jugular vein catheterization,
    83–84, 85–86
  in chest pain, with normal hemodynamics, 245
  for coma, 313
  gastrointestinal bleeding and, 285
  in myxedema coma, 881
  peripheral, in external jugular vein catheteriza-
    tion, 83, 84–85
  in sickle cell disease, in children, 1094
Venous catheterization
  in conscious patient with history of syncope, 337
  in EMS field treatment, **14**
  peripheral
    with catheter-clad needle, **78–81**, 81*i*, 82*i*
    with scalp vein (butterfly) needle, **81–82**, 83*i*,
      84*i*
  in septic shock, 825–826
  and upper-extremity venous thrombosis, 784
  in vascular trauma, 767
Venous disease, **782–785**
Venous distention, with heart failure in infants, 692
Venous gangrene, 774–775
Venous injury, 767, **772**
Venous occlusion, acute peripheral ischemia due to,
  774–775
Venous pressure monitoring, in cardiogenic shock,
  679
Venous thrombosis
  and pulmonary embolism, 662, 663
  upper-extremity, **783–784**
Venous varicosities, ruptured, **784**
Ventilation. *See also* Mechanical ventilation
  in abdominal trauma, 467
  in acute high-altitude pulmonary edema, 949
  in acute lung injury, 672
  in air embolism, 465

in asthma and COPD, 660
in burn injuries, 917
in delirium or confusion, 393
in flail chest, 458
in Guillain-Barré syndrome, 360
in head injuries, 421–422
in heat stroke, 939
in hemoptysis, 654
in near-drowning, 945
in pneumothorax, 655–656
in poliomyelitis, 351
in pulmonary contusion, 459
in pulmonary embolism, 663
in rib fractures, 464
in septic shock, 825
in smoke inhalation, 917
in spinal cord injury, 493–494, 508
in status epilepticus, 334–335
in stroke, 369
in tracheobronchial injury, 463
in weak patient, 349
Ventilation-perfusion (V/Q) scan, in pulmonary
  embolism, 661–663
Ventricular arrhythmias, **700–703**
  implantable cardioverter defibrillators for, 711
  proarrhythmic, **702**
Ventricular defibrillation, AEDs for, 14
Ventricular fibrillation, 157–158, **703**
  in children, 164, 1050*t*
  in commotio cordis, 465
  electrocardiogram in, 703, 717, 718*i*
Ventricular myxoma, syncope with, 343
Ventricular preexcitation, 697, 699–700
  electrocardiogram in, 699–700, 715*i*, 716*i*
Ventricular septal defect, 693
Ventricular septal rupture, **681**
  cardiogenic shock in, 202
Ventricular tachycardia, 158, 158*t*, **700–702**
  in children, 1050*t*
  electrocardiogram in, 700–701, 717, 718*i*
  polymorphic, 694, **702–703**, 717, 718*i*
  pulseless, 157–158
  in stable patients, 701–702
  versus supraventricular tachycardia with aberrant
    conduction, 700–701, 701*i*
  in unstable patients, 701
Ventriculostomy, for hydrocephalus, after subarachnoid hemorrhage, 373
Verapamil
  for atrial fibrillation, 698
  for headache prophylaxis, 390
  for paroxysmal supraventricular tachycardia,
    696–697
  poisoning/overdose of, 977
Versed. *See* Midazolam
Vertebral artery, dissection of, 376
Vertebral body, in spinal cord compression, 349
Vertebral column injury, **493–509**. *See also* Spinal
  cord injury
Vertebral fractures
  spinal cord injury with or without, **508–509**
  without spinal cord injury, **507–508**
Vertebral osteomyelitis, 419, 839
Vertebral spine immobilization
  in head injury, 421
  in-line, 493, 495
  in lateral position, 493
  in neck injury, 435, **437**
  in spinal cord injury, 493, 509
  in supine position, 493
  technique for moving patient in, 493
Vertigo, **630–631**
  benign paroxysmal, 631*t*

central *versus* peripheral, 630, 631*t*
cerumen impaction and, 641
Dix-Hallpike test for, 630, 632
in head injuries, 451, **452**
in hearing loss, 629
history of, 630
imaging in, 632
peripheral, causes of, 630, 631*t*
positional, treatment of, 632
syncope with, 339
in temporal bone fractures, 451
treatment of, 452, 632
Vesicants
  as chemical weapons, **38–40**
  clinical findings of exposure to, 36*t*
Vesicoureteral reflux, 841
  and urinary tract infections, in children, 1076
Vestibular neuronitis, vertigo in, 631*t*
Vibration sense
  in hearing loss, 629*i*, 629–630, 630*i*
  in spinal cord injury, 497
Vibrio, and scrombroid poisoning, 960
Vibrio cholerae, and gastroenteritis, 303, 304*t*
Vibrio parahaemolyticus, and dysentery, 307*t*
Vicarious liability, **62–63**
Vincent angina, 638*t*, 840, 841
Vincristine, and hyponatremia, 893*t*
Vinegar, for jellyfish stings, 958
Violence, acts of, **45**
Violent patients, **1030**
  restraint of, 66
  S.A.F.E.S.T. approach to, 1027–1028
Viral agents, as biologic weapons, **29–32**
Viral encephalitis, **31–32**
Viral gastroenteritis, 303, 305*t*
Viral hepatitis, 276
Viral infections. *See also* specific type and structure
  affected
  arthritis in, **413**
  gastrointestinal bleeding in, in children, 1089
Virchow triad, 662
Viscera, radiation injury and, 944
Visceral artery aneurysm, **778**
Visceral disease, back pain in, 415, 417*t*
Visceral ischemia
  acute, **775–776**
  nonocclusive arteriolar, 775
Visceral pain, 1080
Visceral peritoneum, abdominal pain in, 263
Visceral reflexes, 505*t*
Viscum album, toxins in, 1004*t*
Vision
  testing of, 600
  tubular, 600
Vision loss
  in acute angle-closure glaucoma, 604–605
  acute unilateral, **600–604**, 603*i*
  in central retinal artery occlusion, 605
  in central retinal vein occlusion, 614–615
  toxic causes of, **607–608**
Visual acuity, 600
  hyphema and, 612–613
Visual field
  defects of, 600
    in migraine, 388
    in optic neuritis, 615
    in stroke patients, 371
  evaluation of, 600
Vital capacity
  in botulism, 364
  in weak patient, 349
Vital signs
  age and, 1040, 1043*t*

in back pain, 415
in children, 186, 186*t*
in conscious patient with history of syncope, 335–337
in gastrointestinal bleeding, 288
in headache, 382
in oliguria or anuria, 751
orthostatic, in shock, 194
in resuscitation documentation, 200
in seizures, 334*t*
in septic shock, 826
in stroke patients, 370
in vaginal bleeding, abnormal, 725
Vital staining, for wound debridement, 581
Vitamin A, deficiency of
conjunctivitis in, 610
hemostatic abnormalities in, 799
in liver disease, 799
Vitamin B, for Wernicke encephalopathy, 399
Vitamin B₆, for isoniazid poisoning, 996
Vitamin B₁₂ₐ, for cyanide poisoning, 983–984
Vitamin C, for Wernicke encephalopathy, 399
Vitamin K
for anticoagulant overdose, 1011
deficiency of
in liver disease, 799
warfarin and, **800–801**
for disseminated intravascular coagulation, 802
for gastrointestinal bleeding, 285
for liver disease, 799
for salicylate overdose, 1006
for warfarin complications, 800–801
Vitrectomy, for vitreous hemorrhage, 614
Vitreous, blunt trauma to, 618
Vitreous aspiration, for endophthalmitis, 607
Vitreous hemorrhage, 604, **613–614**
nontraumatic causes of, 613*t*
Volar wrist splint, 526, 526*i*, 527*i*
Volcanoes, **45**
Volkmann ischemic contracture, 521
Volume depletion, 890
Volume excess, 890
Volume expansion, for hyperphosphatemia, 906
Volume of distribution, of toxins, 969, 969*t*
Volume replacement/resuscitation. *See also* Fluid replacement/resuscitation
for apnea, in infants, 1051
for meningitis, in children, 1069
for neurogenic shock, 207
for seizures, in children, 1062
for septic shock, 205
for shock, in children, 1047
Volunteerism, and disaster relief, 56
Volvulus, diagnosis of, 271*t*
Vomiting, **296–309**
in abdominal pain, 263
in acute abdominal emergencies, **297**, 297*t*
in botulism, 364
in children, **1081–1085**, 1088*t*
in dehydration, in children, 1046
history of, 299–301, 301*t*
in hypotension, **296–297**
in infants, 1084–1085
infectious causes of, **303–309**
in intracerebral hemorrhage, 373
laboratory tests for, **302–303**
life-threatening problems, immediate management of, **296–299**
in migraine, 382
in newborn, 1084
physical examination of, 301–302
in pregnancy, 743
in shock, **296–297**

in toxic exposures, **297–299**, 298*i*, 301
treatment algorithm for, 298*i*, 300*i*
von Willebrand disease, **798–799**
classification of, 798, 798*t*
von Willebrand factor (vWF), 792–793
VOO pacing, in cardiac pacemaker, 708*t*
Vulvar abscess, **848**
Vulvar carcinoma, **736**
VVI pacing, in cardiac pacemaker, 708, 708*t*, 722*i*
VX (nerve agent), 37
VZV. *See* Varicella zoster virus

Waldenström macroglobulinemia, **817–818**
Warfarin
in atrial fibrillation, 698
complications with, 800–801
reversal of, 800, 801*t*, 820
drug interactions of, 1010, 1011*t*
poisoning/overdose of, **1010–1011**
for stroke prevention, 377
and vitamin K deficiency, **800–801**
Warm compresses, for eye trauma/disorders, 623
Warm-type autoimmune hemolytic anemia, 805
Wasp stings, **953**
Water
for chemical burns, 926
renal conservation of, in hypernatremia, 896
total bdy, variations in, 890
Water deficit (water depletion)
in heat exhaustion, 937–938
in hypernatremia, 895–897
Water hemlock, toxins in, 1004*t*
Water intake, inadequate, in hypernatremia, 896
Water restriction, in hyponatremia, 894
Waterhouse-Friderichsen syndrome, 858
Watson-Schwartz test, in acute intermittent porphyria, 361–362
Weakness, **348–369**
in acute intermittent porphyria, **361–362**
anatomic localization of, 352*t*
anterior horn cell involvement in, 351, **357**
in arsenical neuropathy, **360–361**
in botulism, 353, **363–364**
in compressive mononeuropathies, **358–359**
differential diagnosis of, 352*t*
in diphtheritic polyneuritis, 362
in electrolyte abnormalities, **367**
emergency management of specific disorders of, **355–369**
evaluation of, **351–355**
facial, in Bell palsy, **357–358**
in Guillain-Barré syndrome, **359–360**
hospitalization for, 349
in hypokalemia, **367**, 367*t*
in hysteria, **355**
life-threatening problems associated with, immediate management of, **349**, 350*i*
in mononeuropathies, **357–359**
in muscle disease (acute myopathy), **354–355**, **367–368**
in myasthenia gravis, 353, **366**
in neuromuscular disease, 353–354, **363–366**
organic *versus* psychogenic causes of, 348–349
in organophosphate poisoning, 353, **364–366**
in paralytic seafood poisoning, **363**
in peripheral neuropathy, 354, **357–363**
in poliomyelitis, 351, **357**
in polyneuropathies, **359–363**
in postpoliomyelitis syndrome, **357**
in potassium disorders, 367, 367*t*
in primary acute myopathies, **367–368**
in rhabdomyolysis, 368

spinal cord compression causing, 349, 351, 355, 356
in spinal cord disease, 351, 353*t*, **355–356**
differential diagnosis of, 351, 353*t*
with spinal cord metastases, 351, **355**
with spinal epidural abscess, 351, **356**
term, use of, 348
in tick paralysis, 354, **362**
in transverse myelitis, 351, **355–356**
with venomous animal injuries, **353–354**
ventilation in, 349
Weapons of mass destruction (WMD), 20–41
biologic weapons, **22–36**
chemical weapons, **36–41**, 36*t*
nuclear weapons, **20–22**
Weber test, in hearing loss, 629, 629*i*
WEE. *See* Western equine encephalitis
Welder's arc burn, 617
Wenckebach AV block, 705, 706
Wenckebach SA block, 704, 720
Wernicke encephalopathy, 311, 393, **398–399**, 401
coma in, 311, 313
Wernicke-Korsakoff syndrome, 396, **1032**
Wernicke's encephalopathy, delirium or confusion in, **1032**
Westermark sign, in pulmonary embolism, 662
Western equine encephalitis (WEE), 31
Whack. *See* Phencyclidine
Wheezing
in asthma, 657, 659
in children, 1051
in congestive heart failure, 680, 685
differential diagnosis of, 659
in pneumonia, 667
Whiplash injury, 496, **509**
Whirlpool therapy, for frostbite, 935
White blood cell count, in abdominal pain, 266
White cell disorders, **814–818**. *See also specific type*
acute leukemia, **815**
chronic leukemia, **815–816**
leukocytosis, **815**
mononucleosis, **816–817**
multiple myeloma, **817**
neutropenia, **814–815**
Waldenström macroglobulinemia, **817–818**
WHO. *See* World Health Organization
Whole blood transfusions. *See* Transfusions
Whole bowel irrigation, for ingested poisons, 965
Wide complex tachycardia, 700–701, 701*i*
Winter Emergency Care, 9
Winter's formula, 911
Withdrawal
from alcohol, 1031
from stimulants, 1030
WMD. *See* Weapons of mass destruction
Wolff-Parkinson-White (WPW) syndrome, 699–700
in children, 1050*t*
Women
Foley catheter insertion in, 125, 126, 126*i*
radiation injury in, 943–944
Wood tick, paralysis caused by, 362
World Health Organization (WHO), and disaster relief, 56
Wound care, **573–597**
absorption in, 588
for amputations, **595–596**
anesthesia in, 576–579
antibiotic prophylaxis in, 564, 589, 590*t*, 597
assessment in, **575–594**
for bite injuries, **596–597**
for blast injuries, **594–595**
for burn injuries, 922–923
cauterization in, 574

Wound care (*cont.*)
for children, 1043
cleaning in, 579–581
cosmetic appearance in, 589
debridement in, 580–581, 588–589
definitive, preparation for, 576
for degloving injuries, **595**
drainage in, 585
dressings for, 585–594
functions of, 585
pressure, 588
edema control in, 587–588
elevation in, 588
examination in, 575–576
extent of injury in, 575
for facial lacerations, **594**
follow-up, 593–594
hair removal in, 579–580
for hand injuries, 551, 556
hemostasis in, 573–574, 577–578
for high-pressure injection injuries, **595**
history of wound and, 575
immobilization in, 587
for intraoral lesions, **594**
irrigation in, 580, 956
life-threatening problems in, emergency management of, **573–574**
postoperative, 585–594
protection in, 587
for puncture wounds, **597**
rabies prophylaxis in, 590–593, 591*i*, 592*t*, 593*t*
for scorpion fish envenomation, 959
of specific wound types, **594–597**
for stingray wound, 956
tetanus prophylaxis in, 575, 589–590, 590*t*
topical antibiotics for, 589
total excision in, 581
Wound cleansers, 580
Wound closure, 581–585
choice of technique, 584–585
contraindications to, 581
of high-stress wounds, 585, 586*i*
of low-stress wounds, 585, 587*i*
materials for, 582–584
primary, 581–582
6-hour limit for, 575
stapling for, 582–583, 583–584
sutures for, 582–583
removal of, 593–594
taping for, 583, 587
versus deep sutures, 583
tissue adhesives for, 584
Wound contamination, 575, 581, 589
chemical hemostatic agents contraindicated in,
574
epinephrine contraindicated in, 574, 578
Wound infections, 589–593
botulism, 364
prevention of, 589, 590*t*
Wrist
abscess of, incision and drainage of, 142
anatomy of, 525*i*
arthrocentesis of, 136, 138–139
injuries of, **524–529**
nonarticular rheumatism in, 406*t*
splinting of, 526, 526*i*, 527*i*, 557, 566
Wrist block, in hand trauma, 549, 551*i*, 552*i*
Wrist drop
in radial nerve injury, 570*i*
in radial nerve palsy, 358
Wrist flexors, 551

Xanax. *See* Alprazolam
Xerosis, in HIV-infected patients, 865
X-ray studies
in abdominal pain, 267, 268*i*, 273*i*
in abdominal trauma, 468
in Achilles tendon injuries, 542
in acromioclavicular joint injuries, 517
in ankle dislocations, 543
in ankle joint injuries, criteria and rules for, 540,
543
in ankle sprains, 543
in aortic dissection, 779, 780*t*
in aortic injury, 462, 463*i*
in arsenic poisoning, 360
in asthma, 658
in atelectasis, 667
in boutonnière deformity, 528
in bronchiolitis, 837
in bronchitis, 668
in calcaneal fractures, 544
in carbon monoxide poisoning, 978
in cardiac tamponade, 689
in chronic degenerative disk disease, 417
in chronic obstructive pulmonary disease, 658
in clavicle fractures, 516
in collateral ligament injuries, 537
in cruciate ligament injuries, 537
in diaphragmatic hernia, 461, 461*i*
in diaphragmatic injuries, 470–472, 473*i*
in distal femoral fractures, 535
in elbow dislocations, 523
in elbow injuries, 522
in esophageal injury, 461
in ethmoid bone fracture, 619
in eye trauma, 617
in femoral shaft fractures, 533
in fibula fractures, 540
in hand trauma, 556
in heart failure, 685, 686
in hemothorax, 457, 457*i*
in high-altitude pulmonary edema, 949
in hip fractures, 531
in HIV/AIDS, 865
in humerus fractures, 520
in immunocompromised patients, 830
in infants, 1064
in interstitial pulmonary disease, 674
in knee dislocations, 536
in knee joint injuries, rules and criteria for,
533–534
in lateral malleolar fractures, 540
in lumbosacral strain, 417
in lunate dislocations, 525*i*
in mallet finger, 529, 559
in mandibular fracture, 441–443, 442*i*
in medial malleolar fractures, 541
in meniscal tears, 538
in multiply injured patient, 212
in near-drowning, 945
in olecranon fractures, 522
in osteomyelitis, 839
in patella dislocations, 534
in patella fractures, 534
in pelvic fractures, 530
in penetrating chest trauma, 465
in pericarditis, 688
in peripheral aneurysms, 781
in peroneal tendon injuries, 542
in phalangeal injuries, 546
in phalanx fractures and dislocations, 527
in pleural effusion, 666

in pneumonia, 627*t*, 668, 832, 834–835
in pneumothorax, 455, 455*i*, 456*i*, 655
in poisoning/overdose, 965–966, 968*t*
in pulmonary contusion, 459
in pulmonary edema, 685
in pulmonary embolism, 662
in pyelonephritis, 843–844
in radial head fractures, 522
in radial head subluxation, 523
in rheumatoid arthritis, 411
in rib fractures, 464
in rotator cuff injuries, 518
in scapholunate dislocations, 525
in scapula fractures, 517
in septic shock, 827
in sesamoid fractures, 547
in shoulder dislocations, 519, 520*i*
in sinusitis, 643, 644*i*
in sore throat, 635, 637*i*
in spinal cord injury, 506–507, 509
of cervical spine, 495, 506–507
of chest, skull, and pelvis, 506
of thoracic and lumbosacral spine, 507
in spinal cord metastases, 355
in spinal epidural abscess, 356
in spinal infections, 420
in sternoclavicular joint dislocations, 516
in subtalar dislocations, 545
in supracondylar fractures, 521
in talar fractures, 544
in tarsal injuries, 545
in tarsometatarsal injuries, 546
in tendon rupture in knee, 539
in thoracic aorta injury, 770, 770*i*, 771*t*
in thoracic outlet syndrome, 786
in tibial shaft fractures, 539
in tibial spine fractures, 536
in tracheobronchial injury, 463
in traumatic amputations, 511
in traumatic aortic rupture, 218
in vertebral fractures, 507
in visceral (intestinal) ischemia, 775
in whiplash, 509
in zygomaticomaxillary complex fractures,
446
Xylocaine. *See* Lidocaine

Yellow fever, 31*t*
Yersinia enterocolitica, 307*t*
Yersinia infection
reactive arthritis in, 412
transfusion transmission of, 822
Yersinia pestis, 25, 26
Yew, toxins in, 1004*t*
Yoke sling, 588

Zalcitabine, side effects of, 865*t*
Zebra fish sting, **958–959**
Zidovudine, side effects of, 865*t*
Zinc poisoning, 995*t*
Zirconium, cautions for use, 1018
Zithromax. *See* Azithromycin
ZMC fractures. *See* Zygomaticomaxillary complex
fractures
Zolmitriptan, for migraine, 389
Zoster infection
back pain in, **420**
chest pain in, **256**
preeruptive, abdominal pain in, 272*t*
Zygomaticomaxillary complex (ZMC) fractures,
445*i*, **445–446**, 446*i*